MAYO CLINIC CRITICAL AND NEUROCRITICAL CARE BOARD REVIEW

MAYO CLINIC SCIENTIFIC PRESS

Mayo Clinic Atlas of Regional Anesthesia and Ultrasound-Guided Nerve Blockade
Edited by James R. Hebl, MD, and Robert L. Lennon, DO

Mayo Clinic Preventive Medicine and Public Health Board Review
Edited by Prathibha Varkey, MBBS, MPH, MHPE

Mayo Clinic Infectious Diseases Board Review
Edited by Zelalem Temesgen, MD

Just Enough Physiology
By James R. Munis, MD, PhD

Mayo Clinic Cardiology: Concise Textbook, Fourth Edition
Edited by Joseph G. Murphy, MD, and Margaret A. Lloyd, MD

Mayo Clinic Electrophysiology Manual
Edited by Samuel J. Asirvatham, MD

Mayo Clinic Gastrointestinal Imaging Review, Second Edition
By C. Daniel Johnson, MD

Arrhythmias in Women: Diagnosis and Management
Edited by Yong-Mei Cha, MD, Margaret A. Lloyd, MD, and Ulrika M. Birgersdotter-Green, MD

Mayo Clinic Body MRI Case Review
By Christine U. Lee, MD, PhD, and James F. Glockner, MD, PhD

Mayo Clinic Gastroenterology and Hepatology Board Review, Fifth Edition
Edited by Stephen C. Hauser, MD

Mayo Clinic Guide to Cardiac Magnetic Resonance Imaging, Second Edition
Edited by Kiaran P. McGee, PhD, Eric E. Williamson, MD, and Matthew W. Martinez, MD

Mayo Clinic Neurology Board Review: Basic Sciences and Psychiatry for Initial Certification [vol 1] and *Clinical Neurology for Initial Certification and MOC* [vol 2]
Edited by Kelly D. Flemming, MD, and Lyell K. Jones Jr, MD

Mayo Clinic Critical Care Case Review
Edited by Rahul Kashyap, MBBS, J. Christopher Farmer, MD, and John C. O'Horo, MD

Mayo Clinic Internal Medicine Board Review, Eleventh Edition
Edited by Christopher M. Wittich, PharmD, MD

Mayo Clinic Medical Neurosciences, Sixth Edition
Edited by Eduardo E. Benarroch, MD, Jeremy K. Cutsforth-Gregory, MD, and Kelly D. Flemming, MD

Mayo Clinic Principles of Shoulder Surgery
By Joaquin Sanchez-Sotelo

Mayo Clinic Essential Neurology, Second Edition
By Andrea C. Adams, MD

Mayo Clinic Antimicrobial Handbook: Quick Guide, Third Edition
Edited by John W. Wilson, MD, and Lynn L. Estes, PharmD

MAYO CLINIC CRITICAL AND NEUROCRITICAL CARE BOARD REVIEW

EDITED BY

Eelco F. M. Wijdicks, MD, PhD
Chair, Division of Critical Care Neurology
Mayo Clinic, Rochester, Minnesota
Professor of Neurology
Mayo Clinic College of Medicine and Science

James Y. Findlay, MB, ChB
Consultant, Department of Anesthesiology and Perioperative Medicine
Mayo Clinic, Rochester, Minnesota
Associate Professor of Anesthesiology
Mayo Clinic College of Medicine and Science

William D. Freeman, MD
Consultant, Departments of Critical Care Medicine, Neurology, and Neurosurgery
Mayo Clinic, Jacksonville, Florida
Professor of Neurology and of Neurosurgery
Mayo Clinic College of Medicine and Science

Ayan Sen, MD
Chair, Department of Critical Care Medicine
Mayo Clinic Hospital, Phoenix, Arizona
Assistant Professor of Emergency Medicine and of Medicine
Mayo Clinic College of Medicine and Science

MAYO CLINIC SCIENTIFIC PRESS   OXFORD UNIVERSITY PRESS

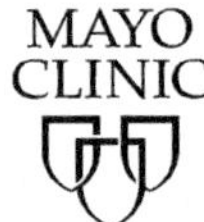

OXFORD
UNIVERSITY PRESS

Oxford University Press is a department of the University of Oxford. It furthers the University's objective of excellence in research, scholarship, and education by publishing worldwide. Oxford is a registered trade mark of Oxford University Press in the UK and certain other countries.

Published in the United States of America by Oxford University Press
198 Madison Avenue, New York, NY 10016, United States of America.

Library of Congress Cataloging-in-Publication Data
Names: Wijdicks, Eelco F. M., 1954– editor. | Findlay, James Y., editor. | Freeman, William D., editor. | Sen, Ayan.
Title: Mayo Clinic critical and neurocritical care board review / [edited by] Eelco F. M. Wijdicks, James Y. Findlay, William D. Freeman, Ayan Sen.
Other titles: Critical and neurocritical care board review
Description: New York, NY : Oxford University Press, 2019. | Includes bibliographical references and index.
Identifiers: LCCN 2019005581 | ISBN 9780190862923 (pbk.) | ISBN 9780190862930 (updf) | ISBN 9780190862947 (epub) | ISBN 9780190862954 (on-line)
Subjects: | MESH: Critical Care | Study Guide
Classification: LCC RC86.9 | NLM WX 18.2 | DDC 616.02/8076—dc23
LC record available at https://lccn.loc.gov/2019005581

9 8 7 6 5 4 3 2

Printed by LSC Communications, United States of America

Preface

Physicians have cared for patients with acute illnesses throughout history. The terminology related to these patients has changed. Sick patients became critically ill patients, and all needed intensive care. After the devastating poliomyelitis epidemics of the 1950s, a new specialty of critical care medicine emerged. Initially, respiratory care units were created for the patients affected by this severe illness, but soon they were transformed into intensive care units. Trauma units and transplant units soon followed. Specialized care for patients with acute neurologic or neurosurgical disease was established in parallel with these developments, but many of the early neuroscience intensive care units were redesigned wards. Specialized physicians and nursing staff delivered multidisciplinary care, recognizing that no one group could function well alone. Inevitably, critical care for the sickest patients was the only option to give them a fighting chance to survive.

In the United States, the Society of Critical Care Medicine brought the specialty clearly into focus in the early 1970s, and training program guidelines soon were developed in the United States and abroad. The Neurocritical Care Society was founded in 2002, and accreditation was established through the American Academy of Neurology (United Council of Neurologic Subspecialties). Most importantly, the American Board of Medical Specialties has approved creation of a neurocritical care subspecialty, and Accreditation Council for Graduate Medical Education–accredited fellowships and a new board examination are planned.

Currently, the neurocritical care board examination combines neurocritical care with general intensive care, and questions are equally divided between the 2 subjects. Accordingly, combining both areas of expertise in a single volume is appropriate.

The chapters in this book correspond with the key disorders suggested by the United Council of Neurologic Subspecialties to be studied in preparation for the examination and to assist with the critical care board examination. The book is not only detailed in basic pathophysiologic content but also describes major disorders and syndromes and their management. Because of its unprecedented complete coverage of acute neurologic disorders, it is equally useful as preparation for the critical care medicine board examination.

The success of board review books hinges on clarity of the presented information, and we focused on conciseness and readability. Readers find tables, explanatory drawings, and bullet points useful, and thus we included them throughout while keeping the text specific and informative. We edited the entire text, and we sought expert advise to fill in our gaps in knowledge or to verify our additions. All chapters were written and closely edited by Mayo Clinic faculty. The references are up-to-date and include many guidelines.

Board review books have multiple disclaimers, as does this one. Use of this book alone will not guarantee passing the examination(s), and additional texts should be consulted. The book has more than 500 multiple-choice practice questions and answers. References are included with each answer. The questions are of the type used on the board examination. Reviewing the questions may improve one's ability to take the board examination, but we all appreciate that (in essence) passing an examination is directly related to sufficient knowledge of the topics. We hope you will benefit from studying this text. It should appeal to any aspiring intensivist in training. We enjoyed selecting the material for you, and we definitely learned a few things along the way. We hope this book will help you pass the examination.

EFM WIJDICKS
JY FINDLAY
WD FREEMAN
A SEN

Table of Contents

Section VI: Procedures

Section VII: Pharmacotherapeutics

Section VIII: Ethics in the Neurointensive Care Unit

Contributors

Arnoley S. Abcejo, MD
Senior Associate Consultant, Department of Anesthesiology and Perioperative Medicine, Mayo Clinic, Rochester, Minnesota; Assistant Professor of Anesthesiology, Mayo Clinic College of Medicine and Science

Jill Adamski, MD, PhD
Chair, Division of Laboratory Medicine, Mayo Clinic Hospital, Phoenix, Arizona; Associate Professor of Laboratory Medicine and Pathology, Mayo Clinic College of Medicine and Science

Maria I. Aguilar, MD
Consultant, Department of Neurology, Mayo Clinic, Scottsdale, Arizona; Associate Professor of Neurology, Mayo Clinic College of Medicine and Science

Sikander Ailawadhi, MD
Consultant, Division of Hematology and Oncology, Mayo Clinic, Jacksonville, Florida; Associate Professor of Medicine, Mayo Clinic College of Medicine and Science

Allen J. Aksamit Jr, MD
Consultant, Department of Neurology, Mayo Clinic, Rochester, Minnesota; Professor of Neurology, Mayo Clinic College of Medicine and Science

Tariq Almerey, MD
Research Fellow in Surgery, Mayo Clinic School of Graduate Medical Education, Mayo Clinic College of Medicine and Science, Jacksonville, Florida

John L. D. Atkinson, MD
Consultant, Department of Neurologic Surgery, Mayo Clinic, Rochester, Minnesota; Professor of Neurosurgery, Mayo Clinic College of Medicine and Science

Maya A. Babu, MD
Resident in Neurosurgery, Mayo Clinic School of Graduate Medical Education, Mayo Clinic College of Medicine and Science, Rochester, Minnesota
Present address: Harvard Medical School, Boston, Massachusetts

Irina Bancos, MD
Consultant, Division of Endocrinology, Diabetes, Metabolism, & Nutrition, Mayo Clinic, Rochester, Minnesota; Assistant Professor of Medicine, Mayo Clinic College of Medicine and Science

W. Brian Beam, MD
Consultant, Department of Anesthesiology and Perioperative Medicine, Mayo Clinic, Rochester, Minnesota; Assistant Professor of Anesthesiology, Mayo Clinic College of Medicine and Science

Staci E. Beamer, MD
Senior Associate Consultant, Department of Cardiovascular and Thoracic Surgery, Mayo Clinic Hospital, Phoenix, Arizona; Assistant Professor of Surgery, Mayo Clinic College of Medicine and Science

Bernard R. Bendok, MD
Chair, Department of Neurologic Surgery, Mayo Clinic Hospital, Phoenix, Arizona; Professor of Neurosurgery, Mayo Clinic College of Medicine and Science

Joshua S. Bingham, MD
Fellow in Reconstructive Surgery, Mayo Clinic School of Graduate Medical Education and Instructor in Orthopedics, Mayo Clinic College of Medicine and Science, Scottsdale, Arizona

J. Kyle Bohman, MD
Consultant, Department of Anesthesiology and Perioperative Medicine, Mayo Clinic, Rochester, Minnesota; Assistant Professor of Anesthesiology, Mayo Clinic College of Medicine and Science

Belinda G. Bradley, APRN
Lead Nurse Practicioner, Department of Neurologic Surgery, Mayo Clinic, Jacksonville, Florida

Sherri A. Braksick, MD
Fellow in Critical Care Neurology, Mayo Clinic School of Graduate Medical Education, Mayo Clinic College of Medicine and Science, Rochester, Minnesota
Present address: University of Kansas Medical Center, Kansas City, Kansas

Jeffrey W. Britton, MD
Chair, Division of Epilepsy, Mayo Clinic, Rochester, Minnesota; Professor of Neurology, Mayo Clinic College of Medicine and Science

Benjamin L. Brown, MD
Senior Associate Consultant, Department of Neurologic Surgery, Mayo Clinic, Jacksonville, Florida; Assistant Professor of Neurosurgery, Mayo Clinic College of Medicine and Science

Robert D. Brown Jr, MD, MPH
Chair, Division of Stroke and Cerebrovascular Diseases, Mayo Clinic, Rochester, Minnesota; Professor of Neurology, Mayo Clinic College of Medicine and Science

Charles D. Burger, MD
Consultant, Division of Pulmonary, Allergy, and Sleep Medicine, Mayo Clinic, Jacksonville, Florida; Professor of Medicine, Mayo Clinic College of Medicine and Science

Hannelisa E. Callisen, PA-C
Physician Assistant, Department of Critical Care Medicine, Mayo Clinic Hospital, Phoenix, Arizona

Juan M. Canabal, MD
Senior Associate Consultant, Department of Transplantation, Mayo Clinic, Jacksonville, Florida; Assistant Professor of Medicine, Mayo Clinic College of Medicine and Science

Rodrigo Cartin-Ceba, MD
Consultant, Department of Critical Care Medicine, Mayo Clinic, Scottsdale, Arizona; Associate Professor of Medicine, Mayo Clinic College of Medicine and Science

Joseph G. Cernigliaro, MD
Chair, Division of Abdominal Imaging, Mayo Clinic, Jacksonville, Florida; Associate Professor of Radiology, Mayo Clinic College of Medicine and Science

Selby G. Chen, MD
Senior Associate Consultant, Department of Neurologic Surgery, Mayo Clinic, Jacksonville, Florida; Assistant Professor of Neurosurgery, Mayo Clinic College of Medicine and Science

Brian W. Chong, MD
Consultant, Department of Radiology, Mayo Clinic Hospital, Phoenix, Arizona; Associate Professor of Radiology, Mayo Clinic College of Medicine and Science

Michelle J. Clarke, MD
Consultant, Department of Neurologic Surgery, Mayo Clinic, Rochester, Minnesota; Professor of Neurosurgery and of Orthopedics, Mayo Clinic College of Medicine and Science

William E. Clifton III, MD
Resident in Neurologic Surgery, Mayo Clinic School of Graduate Medical Education, Mayo Clinic College of Medicine and Science, Jacksonville, Florida

Thomas B. Comfere, MD
Consultant, Department of Anesthesiology and Perioperative Medicine, Mayo Clinic, Rochester, Minnesota; Assistant Professor of Anesthesiology, Mayo Clinic College of Medicine and Science

Ryan C. Craner, MD
Consultant, Department of Anesthesiology and Perioperative Medicine, Mayo Clinic Hospital, Phoenix, Arizona; Assistant Professor of Anesthesiology, Mayo Clinic College of Medicine and Science

Amy Z. Crepeau, MD
Consultant, Department of Neurology, Mayo Clinic Hospital, Phoenix, Arizona; Assistant Professor of Neurology, Mayo Clinic College of Medicine and Science

Jonathan J. Danaraj, DO
Resident in Pulmonary and Critical Care Medicine, Mayo Clinic School of Graduate Medical Education, Mayo Clinic College of Medicine and Science, Jacksonville, Florida

Sudhir V. Datar, MBBS
Division of Critical Care Neurology, Wake Forest University Medical Center, Winston-Salem, North Carolina; Assistant Professor of Neurology and of Anesthesiology, Wake Forest School of Medicine

Bart M. Demaerschalk, MD
Consultant, Department of Neurology, Mayo Clinic Hospital, Phoenix, Arizona; Professor of Neurology, Mayo Clinic College of Medicine and Science

Onur Demirci, MD
Consultant, Department of Anesthesiology and Perioperative Medicine, Mayo Clinic, Rochester, Minnesota; Assistant Professor of Anesthesiology, Mayo Clinic College of Medicine and Science

Priya S. Dhawan, MD
Resident in Neurology, Mayo Clinic School of Graduate Medical Education, Mayo Clinic College of Medicine and Science, Rochester, Minnesota
Present address: University of British Columbia, Vancouver, British Columbia

Jose L. Diaz-Gomez, MD
Consultant, Departments of Critical Care Medicine, Anesthesiology, and Neurosurgery, Mayo Clinic, Jacksonville, Florida; Associate Professor of Anesthesiology, Mayo Clinic College of Medicine and Science
Present address: Private Practice

Dennis W. Dickson, MD
Consultant, Departments of Laboratory Medicine and Pathology and of Neuroscience, Mayo Clinic, Jacksonville, Florida; Professor of Laboratory Medicine and Pathology, Mayo Clinic College of Medicine and Science

David J. DiSantis, MD
Senior Associate Consultant, Department of Radiology, Mayo Clinic, Jacksonville, Florida; Professor of Radiology, Mayo Clinic College of Medicine and Science

Diane Donegan, MB, BCh
Research Collaborator in Endocrinology, Mayo Clinic School of Graduate Medical Education, Mayo Clinic College of Medicine and Science, Rochester, Minnesota

Oana Dumitrascu, MD
Fellow in Vascular Neurology, Mayo Clinic School of Graduate Medical Education, Mayo Clinic College of Medicine and Science, Scottsdale, Arizona

Dana Erickson, MD
Consultant, Division of Endocrinology, Diabetes, Metabolism, & Nutrition, Mayo Clinic, Rochester, Minnesota; Associate Professor of Medicine, Mayo Clinic College of Medicine and Science

Houssam Farres, MD
Consultant, Division of Vascular Surgery, Mayo Clinic, Jacksonville, Florida; Assistant Professor of Surgery, Mayo Clinic College of Medicine and Science

Anteneh M. Feyissa, MD
Senior Associate Consultant, Department of Neurology, Mayo Clinic, Jacksonville, Florida; Assistant Professor of Neurology, Mayo Clinic College of Medicine and Science

James Y. Findlay, MB, ChB
Consultant, Department of Anesthesiology and Perioperative Medicine, Mayo Clinic, Rochester, Minnesota; Associate Professor of Anesthesiology, Mayo Clinic College of Medicine and Science

Peter M. Fitzpatrick, MD
Consultant, Division of Nephrology and Hypertension, Mayo Clinic, Jacksonville, Florida; Assistant Professor of Medicine, Mayo Clinic College of Medicine and Science

Kelly D. Flemming, MD
Consultant, Department of Neurology, Mayo Clinic, Rochester, Minnesota; Associate Professor of Neurology, Mayo Clinic College of Medicine and Science

William D. Freeman, MD
Consultant, Departments of Critical Care Medicine, Neurology, and Neurosurgery, Mayo Clinic, Jacksonville, Florida; Professor of Neurology and of Neurosurgery, Mayo Clinic College of Medicine and Science

Jennifer E. Fugate, DO
Consultant, Department of Neurology, Mayo Clinic, Rochester, Minnesota; Assistant Professor of Neurology, Mayo Clinic College of Medicine and Science

Bhargavi Gali, MD
Consultant, Department of Anesthesiology and Perioperative Medicine, Mayo Clinic, Rochester, Minnesota; Assistant Professor of Anesthesiology, Mayo Clinic College of Medicine and Science

Kelly Gassie, MD
Resident in Neurologic Surgery, Mayo Clinic School of Graduate Medical Education, Mayo Clinic College of Medicine and Science, Jacksonville, Florida

Saba Ghorab, MD
Resident in Otolaryngology, Mayo Clinic School of Graduate Medical Education, Mayo Clinic College of Medicine and Science, Scottsdale, Arizona

Kevin T. Gobeske, MD, PhD
Resident in Critical Care Neurology, Mayo Clinic School of Graduate Medical Education, Mayo Clinic College of Medicine and Science, Rochester, Minnesota

Sanjeet S. Grewal, MD
Resident in Neurologic Surgery, Mayo Clinic School of Graduate Medical Education, Mayo Clinic College of Medicine and Science, Jacksonville, Florida

Pramod K. Guru, MBBS, MD
Senior Associate Consultant, Department of Critical Care Medicine, Mayo Clinic, Jacksonville, Florida; Assistant Professor of Medicine, Mayo Clinic College of Medicine and Science

Matthew R. Hall, MD
Consultant, Department of Dermatology, Mayo Clinic, Jacksonville, Florida; Assistant Professor of Dermatology, Mayo Clinic College of Medicine and Science

Mireille H. Hamdan, RDN, LD/N
Dietician, Clinical Nutrition Services, Mayo Clinic, Jacksonville, Florida; Instructor in Nutrition, Mayo Clinic College of Medicine and Science

Karen W. Hampton, MS, RRT
Respiratory Therapist, Respiratory Services, Mayo Clinic, Jacksonville, Florida

Maximiliano A. Hawkes, MD
Fellow in Critical Care Neurology, Mayo Clinic School of Graduate Medical Education and Assistant Professor of Neurology, Mayo Clinic College of Medicine and Science, Rochester, Minnesota

Walter C. Hellinger, MD
Chair, Division of Infectious Diseases, Mayo Clinic, Jacksonville, Florida; Associate Professor of Medicine, Mayo Clinic College of Medicine and Science

Denzil R. Hill, MD
Senior Associate Consultant, Department of Anesthesiology and Perioperative Medicine, Mayo Clinic, Rochester, Minnesota; Instructor in Anesthesiology, Mayo Clinic College of Medicine and Science

Sara E. Hocker, MD
Consultant, Department of Neurology, Mayo Clinic, Rochester, Minnesota; Associate Professor of Neurology, Mayo Clinic College of Medicine and Science

William W. Horn Jr, APRN
Nurse Practitioner, Department of Neurologic Surgery, Mayo Clinic, Jacksonville, Florida

Joy D. Hughes, MD
Research Fellow in General Surgery, Mayo Clinic School of Graduate Medical Education, Mayo Clinic College of Medicine and Science, Rochester, Minnesota

Gene G. Hunder, MD
Emeritus Professor of Neurology, Mayo Clinic College of Medicine and Science, Rochester, Minnesota

Cory Ingram, MD
Senior Associate Consultant, Division of Community Palliative Medicine, Mayo Clinic, Rochester, Minnesota; Assistant Professor of Family Medicine and of Palliative Medicine, Mayo Clinic College of Medicine and Science

Daniel A. Jackson, PharmD, RPh
Pharmacist, Pharmacy Services, Mayo Clinic, Jacksonville, Florida; Assistant Professor of Pharmacy, Mayo Clinic College of Medicine and Science

Jama Jahanyar, MD, PhD
Senior Associate Consultant, Department of Cardiovascular and Thoracic Surgery, Mayo Clinic Hospital, Phoenix, Arizona; Assistant Professor of Surgery, Mayo Clinic College of Medicine and Science

Norlalak Jiramethee, MD
Fellow in Critical Care Medicine, Mayo Clinic School of Graduate Medical Education, Mayo Clinic College of Medicine and Science, Jacksonville, Florida

Gretchen Johns, MD
Consultant, Department of Laboratory Medicine and Pathology, Mayo Clinic, Jacksonville, Florida; Assistant Professor of Laboratory Medicine and Pathology, Mayo Clinic College of Medicine and Science

Daniel J. Johnson, MD
Chair, Department of Surgery, Mayo Clinic Hospital, Phoenix, Arizona; Associate Professor of Surgery, Mayo Clinic College of Medicine and Science

Margaret M. Johnson, MD
Consultant, Division of Pulmonary, Allergy and Sleep Medicine, Mayo Clinic, Jacksonville, Florida; Associate Professor of Medicine, Mayo Clinic College of Medicine and Science

David T. Jones, MD
Consultant, Department of Neurology, Mayo Clinic, Rochester, Minnesota; Assistant Professor of Neurology, Mayo Clinic College of Medicine and Science

Prasuna Kamireddi, MBBS
Research Trainee, Department of Neurology, Mayo Clinic, Jacksonville, Florida

Justin C. Kao, MB, ChB
Fellow in Advanced Clinical Neurology, Mayo Clinic School of Graduate Medical Education, Mayo Clinic College of Medicine and Science, Rochester, Minnesota

Kianoush B. Kashani, MD
Consultant, Division of Nephrology and Hypertension, Mayo Clinic, Rochester, Minnesota; Professor of Medicine, Mayo Clinic College of Medicine and Science

Mira T. Keddis, MD
Consultant, Division of Nephrology, Mayo Clinic, Scottsdale, Arizona; Assistant Professor of Medicine, Mayo Clinic College of Medicine and Science

Cesar A. Keller, MD
Emeritus Professor of Medicine, Mayo Clinic College of Medicine and Science, Jacksonville, Florida

Sameer R. Keole, MD
Consultant, Department of Radiation Oncology, Mayo Clinic Hospital, Phoenix, Arizona; Assistant Professor of Radiation Oncology, Mayo Clinic College of Medicine and Science

Siva S. Ketha, MD
Research Collaborator, Mayo Clinic, Jacksonville, Florida; Assistant Professor of Medicine, Mayo Clinic College of Medicine and Science

Betty Y. S. Kim, MD, PhD
Consultant, Department of Neurologic Surgery, Mayo Clinic, Jacksonville, Florida; Associate Professor of Neurosurgery and Assistant Professor of Neuroscience, Mayo Clinic College of Medicine and Science

Theresa N. Kinard, MD
Consultant, Department of Laboratory Medicine, Mayo Clinic Hospital, Phoenix, Arizona; Assistant Professor of Laboratory Medicine and Pathology, Mayo Clinic College of Medicine and Science

Megan L. Krause, MD
Fellow in Rheumatology, Mayo Clinic School of Graduate Medical Education, Mayo Clinic College of Medicine and Science, Rochester, Minnesota

Chandan Krishna, MD
Senior Associate Consultant, Department of Neurologic Surgery, Mayo Clinic Hospital, Phoenix, Arizona; Assistant Professor of Neurosurgery, Mayo Clinic College of Medicine and Science

Fred Kusumoto, MD
Consultant, Department of Cardiovascular Diseases, Mayo Clinic, Jacksonville, Florida; Professor of Medicine, Mayo Clinic College of Medicine and Science

Minkyung Kwon, MD
Resident in Pulmonary and Critical Care Medicine, Mayo Clinic School of Graduate Medical Education, Mayo Clinic College of Medicine and Science, Jacksonville, Florida

Giuseppe Lanzino, MD
Consultant, Departments of Neurologic Surgery and Radiology, Mayo Clinic, Rochester, Minnesota; Professor of Neurosurgery, Mayo Clinic College of Medicine and Science

Biagia La Pira, MD
Research Trainee, Department of Neurologic Surgery, Mayo Clinic, Rochester, Minnesota
Present address: Private Practice, Rome, Italy

Augustine S. Lee, MD
Chair, Division of Pulmonary, Allergy and Sleep Medicine, Mayo Clinic, Jacksonville, Florida; Associate Professor of Medicine, Mayo Clinic College of Medicine and Science

Juan Carlos Leoni Moreno, MD
Consultant, Department of Transplantation, Mayo Clinic, Jacksonville, Florida; Instructor in Medicine, Mayo Clinic College of Medicine and Science

Stacy L. Libricz, PA-C, MS
Physician Assistant, Department of Critical Care Medicine, Mayo Clinic Hospital, Phoenix, Arizona; Instructor in Medicine, Mayo Clinic College of Medicine and Science

E. Paul Lindell, MD
Consultant, Department of Radiology, Mayo Clinic, Rochester, Minnesota; Assistant Professor of Radiology, Mayo Clinic College of Medicine and Science

Karthika R. Linga, MBBS
Fellow in Pulmonary and Critical Care Medicine, Mayo Clinic School of Graduate Medical Education, Mayo Clinic College of Medicine and Science, Jacksonville, Florida

Michael J. Link, MD
Consultant, Department of Neurologic Surgery, Mayo Clinic, Rochester, Minnesota; Professor of Neurosurgery, Mayo Clinic College of Medicine and Science

David G. Lott, MD
Consultant, Department of Otolaryngology-Head & Neck Surgery/Audiology, Mayo Clinic, Scottsdale, Arizona; Associate Professor of Otolaryngology, Mayo Clinic College of Medicine and Science

Amelia A. Lowell, RRT, RCP
Clinical Respiratory Care Specialist, Mayo Clinic Hospital, Phoenix, Arizona; Assistant Professor of Anesthesiology, Mayo Clinic College of Medicine and Science

Philip E. Lowman, MD
Consultant, Department of Critical Care Medicine, Mayo Clinic, Jacksonville, Florida; Instructor in Medicine, Mayo Clinic College of Medicine and Science

Patrick R. Maloney, MD
Research Collaborator, Department of Neurologic Surgery, Mayo Clinic, Rochester, Minnesota

Jennifer M. Martinez-Thompson, MD
Senior Associate Consultant, Department of Neurology, Mayo Clinic, Rochester, Minnesota; Assistant Professor of Neurology, Mayo Clinic College of Medicine and Science

Nnenna Mbabuike, MD
Fellow in Endovascular Neurosurgery, Mayo Clinic School of Graduate Medical Education, Mayo Clinic College of Medicine and Science, Jacksonville, Florida
Present address: University of Pennsylvania Medical Center, Altoona, Pennsylvania

Barbara L. McComb, MD
Emeritus Associate Professor of Radiology, Mayo Clinic College of Medicine and Science, Jacksonville, Florida

Diane C. McLaughlin, APRN
Nurse Practitioner, Department of Neurology, Mayo Clinic, Jacksonville, Florida; Instructor in Neurology, Mayo Clinic College of Medicine and Science

Margherita Milone, MD, PhD
Consultant, Department of Neurology, Mayo Clinic, Rochester, Minnesota; Professor of Neurology, Mayo Clinic College of Medicine and Science

Isabel Mira-Avendano, MD
Consultant, Division of Pulmonary, Allergy and Sleep Medicine, Mayo Clinic, Jacksonville, Florida; Assistant Professor of Medicine, Mayo Clinic College of Medicine and Science

Kevin G. Moder, MD
Consultant, Division of Rheumatology, Mayo Clinic, Rochester, Minnesota; Associate Professor of Medicine, Mayo Clinic College of Medicine and Science

Farouk Mookadam, MB, BCh
Consultant, Department of Cardiovascular Diseases, Mayo Clinic Hospital, Phoenix, Arizona; Professor of Medicine, Mayo Clinic College of Medicine and Science

January F. Moore
Special Project Associate, Division of Vascular Surgery, Mayo Clinic, Jacksonville, Florida

Monica Mordecai, MD
Consultant, Department of Anesthesiology and Perioperative Medicine, Mayo Clinic, Jacksonville, Florida; Assistant Professor of Anesthesiology, Mayo Clinic College of Medicine and Science

Pablo Moreno Franco, MD
Consultant, Department of Transplantation, Mayo Clinic, Jacksonville, Florida; Assistant Professor of Medicine, Mayo Clinic College of Medicine and Science

David S. Morris, MD
Consultant, Division of Trauma, Critical Care, & General Surgery, Mayo Clinic, Rochester, Minnesota
Present address: Intermountain Medical Center, Murray, Utah

John E. Moss, MD
Consultant, Department of Critical Care Medicine, Mayo Clinic, Jacksonville, Florida; Assistant Professor of Medicine, Mayo Clinic College of Medicine and Science

Megan S. Motosue, MD
Resident in Allergy and Immunology, Mayo Clinic School of Graduate Medical Education, Mayo Clinic College of Medicine and Science, Rochester, Minnesota

Omar Y. Mousa, MBBS
Fellow in Gastroenterology and Hepatology, Mayo Clinic School of Graduate Medical Education and Assistant Professor of Medicine, Mayo Clinic College of Medicine and Science, Jacksonville, Florida

Andrew W. Murray, MD
Consultant, Department of Anesthesiology and Perioperative Medicine, Mayo Clinic Hospital, Phoenix, Arizona; Assistant Professor of Anesthesiology, Mayo Clinic College of Medicine and Science

Santiago Naranjo-Sierra, MD
Visiting Research Fellow in Department of Critical Care Medicine, Mayo Clinic, Jacksonville, Florida
Present address: Hospital Pablo Tobon Uribe, Medellín, Colombia

Lauren K. Ng Tucker, MD
Consultant, Department of Critical Care Medicine, Mayo Clinic, Jacksonville, Florida; Assistant Professor of Medicine, Mayo Clinic College of Medicine and Science

Brandon T. Nokes, MD
Resident in Internal Medicine, Mayo Clinic School of Graduate Medical Education, Mayo Clinic College of Medicine and Science, Scottsdale, Arizona

Rahmi Oklu, MD, PhD
Chair, Division of Interventional Radiology, Mayo Clinic Hospital, Phoenix, Arizona; Professor of Radiology, Mayo Clinic College of Medicine and Science

James A. Onigkeit, MD
Consultant, Department of Anesthesiology and Perioperative Medicine, Mayo Clinic, Rochester, Minnesota; Assistant Professor of Anesthesiology, Mayo Clinic College of Medicine and Science

Yahaira Ortiz Gonzalez, MD
Resident in Cardiovascular Diseases, Mayo Clinic School of Graduate Medical Education, Mayo Clinic College of Medicine and Science, Jacksonville, Florida

Katherine M. Oshel, MD
Consultant, Division of Nephrology and Hypertension, Mayo Clinic, Jacksonville, Florida; Instructor in Medicine, Mayo Clinic College of Medicine and Science

Pragnesh P. Parikh, MD
Consultant, Department of Cardiovascular Diseases, Mayo Clinic, Jacksonville, Florida; Assistant Professor of Medicine, Mayo Clinic College of Medicine and Science

Myung S. Park, MD, MS
Consultant, Department of Surgery, Mayo Clinic, Rochester, Minnesota; Associate Professor of Surgery, Mayo Clinic College of Medicine and Science

Jeffrey J. Pasternak, MD
Chair, Division of Neuroanesthesia, Mayo Clinic, Rochester, Minnesota; Associate Professor of Anesthesiology, Mayo Clinic College of Medicine and Science

Richard K. Patch III, MD
Consultant, Department of Anesthesiology and Perioperative Medicine and Division of Critical Care Medicine, Mayo Clinic, Rochester, Minnesota; Assistant Professor of Anesthesiology and of Medicine, Mayo Clinic College of Medicine and Science

Bhavesh M. Patel, MD
Consultant, Department of Critical Care Medicine, Mayo Clinic Hospital, Phoenix, Arizona; Assistant Professor of Anesthesiology, of Medicine, and of Neurology, Mayo Clinic College of Medicine and Science

Neal M. Patel, MD
Consultant, Department of Pulmonary and Critical Care Medicine, Mayo Clinic, Jacksonville, Florida; Instructor in Medicine, Mayo Clinic College of Medicine and Science

Mark A. Pichelmann, MD
Consultant, Department of Neurologic Surgery, Mayo Clinic, Jacksonville, Florida; Assistant Professor of Neurosurgery, Mayo Clinic College of Medicine and Science

Michael R. Pichler, MD
Fellow in Cerebrovascular Neurology, Mayo Clinic School of Graduate Medical Education, Mayo Clinic College of Medicine and Science, Rochester, Minnesota

Sean J. Pittock, MD
Consultant, Department of Neurology, Mayo Clinic, Rochester, Minnesota; Professor of Neurology, Mayo Clinic College of Medicine and Science

Michael A. Pizzi, DO, PhD
Fellow in Critical Care Medicine, Mayo Clinic School of Graduate Medical Education, Mayo Clinic College of Medicine and Science, Jacksonville, Florida

Alyx B. Porter, MD
Consultant, Department of Neurology, Mayo Clinic Hospital, Phoenix, Arizona; Assistant Professor of Neurology, Mayo Clinic College of Medicine and Science

Rajiv K. Pruthi, MBBS
Consultant, Divisions of Hematology, Hematopathology, and Laboratory Genetics and Genomics, Mayo Clinic, Rochester, Minnesota; Associate Professor of Medicine, Mayo Clinic College of Medicine and Science

Juan N. Pulido, MD
Consultant, Department of Anesthesiology, Mayo Clinic, Rochester, Minnesota
Present address: Private practice, Seattle, Washington

Surakit Pungpapong, MD
Consultant, Department of Gastroenterology and Hepatology, Mayo Clinic, Jacksonville, Florida; Associate Professor of Medicine, Mayo Clinic College of Medicine and Science

Harish Ramakrishna, MD
Consultant, Department of Anesthesiology and Perioperative Medicine, Mayo Clinic Hospital, Phoenix, Arizona; Professor of Anesthesiology, Mayo Clinic College of Medicine and Science

Robert A. Ratzlaff, DO
Consultant, Departments of Critical Care Medicine and Anesthesiology and Perioperative Medicine, Mayo Clinic, Jacksonville, Florida; Assistant Professor of Anesthesiology, Mayo Clinic College of Medicine and Science

J. Ross Renew, MD
Consultant, Department of Anesthesiology and Perioperative Medicine, Mayo Clinic, Jacksonville, Florida; Assistant Professor of Anesthesiology, Mayo Clinic College of Medicine and Science

Kevin J. Renfree, MD
Consultant, Department of Orthopedic Surgery, Mayo Clinic Hospital, Phoenix, Arizona; Associate Professor of Orthopedics, Mayo Clinic College of Medicine and Science

Juan G. Ripoll Sanz, MD
Resident in Anesthesiology, Mayo Clinic School of Graduate Medical Education, Mayo Clinic College of Medicine and Science, Jacksonville, Florida

Matthew J. Ritter, MD
Consultant, Department of Anesthesiology and Perioperative Medicine, Mayo Clinic, Rochester, Minnesota; Assistant Professor of Anesthesiology, Mayo Clinic College of Medicine and Science

Mariela Rivera, MD
Consultant, Department of Surgery, Mayo Clinic, Rochester, Minnesota; Assistant Professor of Surgery, Mayo Clinic College of Medicine and Science

Christopher P. Robinson, DO, MS
Fellow in Neurocritical Care, Mayo Clinic School of Graduate Medical Education, Mayo Clinic College of Medicine and Science, Rochester, Minnesota
Present address: Department of Neurology and Neurocritical Care Division, University of Florida, Gainesville, Florida

Maisha T. Robinson, MD
Consultant, Department of Neurology, Mayo Clinic, Jacksonville, Florida; Assistant Professor of Neurology, Mayo Clinic College of Medicine and Science

Mark N. Rubin, MD
Fellow in Vascular Neurology, Mayo Clinic School of Graduate Medical Education, Mayo Clinic College of Medicine and Science, Scottsdale, Arizona
Present address: North Shore Neurological Institute, Glenview, Illinois

Carl A. Ruthman, MD
Resident in Pulmonary and Critical Care Medicine, Mayo Clinic School of Graduate Medical Education, Mayo Clinic College of Medicine and Science, Jacksonville, Florida

Arzoo Sadiqi, BS
Research Trainee, Department of Cardiovascular and Thoracic Surgery, Mayo Clinic Hospital, Phoenix, Arizona

Ankit Sakhuja, MBBS
Fellow in Critical Care Medicine, Mayo Clinic School of Graduate Medical Education, and Assistant Professor of Medicine, Mayo Clinic College of Medicine and Science, Rochester, Minnesota

Carlo Salvarani, MD
Department of Rheumatology, Azienda Ospedaliera Arcispedale Sante Maria Nuova, Reggio Emilia, Italy

Mithun Sattur, MBBS
Resident in Neurologic Surgery, Mayo Clinic School of Graduate Medical Education, Mayo Clinic College of Medicine and Science, Scottsdale, Arizona

Gregory J. Schears, MD
Consultant, Department of Anesthesiology and Perioperative Medicine, Mayo Clinic, Rochester, Minnesota; Professor of Anesthesiology, Mayo Clinic College of Medicine and Science

J. William Schleifer, MD
Fellow in Cardiovascular Diseases, Mayo Clinic School of Graduate Medical Education, Mayo Clinic College of Medicine and Science, Scottsdale, Arizona
Present address: Department of Internal Medicine, Division of Cardiology, University of Nebraska Medical Center, Omaha, Nebraska

Beth A. Schueler, PhD
Consultant, Department of Radiology, Mayo Clinic, Rochester, Minnesota; Associate Professor of Radiology and Professor of Medical Physics, Mayo Clinic College of Medicine and Science

David M. Sella, MD
Consultant, Department of Radiology, Mayo Clinic, Jacksonville, Florida; Assistant Professor of Radiology, Mayo Clinic College of Medicine and Science

Ayan Sen, MD
Chair, Department of Critical Care Medicine, Mayo Clinic Hospital, Phoenix, Arizona; Assistant Professor of Emergency Medicine and of Medicine, Mayo Clinic College of Medicine and Science

Eslam Shosha, MB, BCh
Research Fellow in Neurology, Mayo Clinic School of Graduate Medical Education, Mayo Clinic College of Medicine and Science, Rochester, Minnesota

Jason L. Siegel, MD
Senior Associate Consultant, Department of Neurology, Mayo Clinic, Jacksonville, Florida; Assistant Professor of Neurology, Mayo Clinic College of Medicine and Science

Charles R. Sims III, MD
Senior Associate Consultant, Department of Anesthesiology and Perioperative Medicine, Mayo Clinic, Rochester, Minnesota; Instructor in Anesthesiology, Mayo Clinic College of Medicine and Science

Ramachandra R. Sista, MD
Senior Associate Consultant, Division of Pulmonary Medicine, Mayo Clinic, Scottsdale, Arizona

Aurelia A. Smith, MD
Fellow in Multiple Sclerosis and Neuroimmunology, Mayo Clinic School of Graduate Medical Education, Mayo Clinic College of Medicine and Science, Rochester, Minnesota

Christina C. Smith, APRN
Nurse Practitioner, Department of Neurologic Surgery, Mayo Clinic, Jacksonville, Florida; Assistant Professor of Neurosurgery, Mayo Clinic College of Medicine and Science

David A. Sotello Aviles, MD
Fellow in Infectious Diseases, Mayo Clinic School of Graduate Medical Education, Mayo Clinic College of Medicine and Science, Jacksonville, Florida
Present address: Texas Tech University Health Sciences Center, Lubbock, Texas

Nathan P. Staff, MD, PhD
Consultant, Department of Neurology, Mayo Clinic, Rochester, Minnesota; Associate Professor of Neurology, Mayo Clinic College of Medicine and Science

John A. Stauffer, MD
Consultant, Department of Surgery, Mayo Clinic, Jacksonville, Florida; Associate Professor of Surgery, Mayo Clinic College of Medicine and Science

Glenn M. Sturchio, PhD
Consultant, Department of Radiology, Mayo Clinic, Jacksonville, Florida; Assistant Professor of Physiology, Mayo Clinic College of Medicine and Science

Matthew D. Sztajnkrycer, MD, PhD
Consultant, Department of Emergency Medicine, Mayo Clinic, Rochester, Minnesota; Professor of Emergency Medicine, Mayo Clinic College of Medicine and Science

Rabih G. Tawk, MD
Consultant, Department of Neurologic Surgery, Mayo Clinic, Jacksonville, Florida; Associate Professor of Neurosurgery, Mayo Clinic College of Medicine and Science

Jennifer A. Tracy, MD
Consultant, Department of Neurology, Mayo Clinic, Rochester, Minnesota; Assistant Professor of Neurology, Mayo Clinic College of Medicine and Science

Levan Tsamalaidze, MD
Visiting Research Fellow in Surgery, Mayo Clinic School of Graduate Medical Education, Mayo Clinic College of Medicine and Science, Jacksonville, Florida

Jamie J. Van Gompel, MD
Consultant, Department of Neurologic Surgery, Mayo Clinic, Rochester, Minnesota; Associate Professor of Neurosurgery and Otorhinolaryngology, Mayo Clinic College of Medicine and Science

Carla P. Venegas-Borsellino, MD
Senior Associate Consultant, Department of Critical Care Medicine, Mayo Clinic, Jacksonville, Florida

K. L. Venkatachalam, MD
Consultant, Department of Cardiovascular Diseases, Mayo Clinic, Jacksonville, Florida; Associate Professor of Medicine, Mayo Clinic College of Medicine and Science

Prakash Vishnu, MBBS
Senior Associate Consultant, Division of Hematology and Oncology, Mayo Clinic, Jacksonville, Florida; Assistant Professor of Medicine, Mayo Clinic College of Medicine and Science

Angela N. Vizzini, RDN, LD/N
Director, Clinical Nutrition Services, Mayo Clinic, Jacksonville, Florida; Assistant Professor of Nutrition, Mayo Clinic College of Medicine and Science

Gerald W. Volcheck, MD
Chair, Division of Allergic Diseases, Mayo Clinic, Rochester, Minnesota; Associate Professor of Medicine, Mayo Clinic College of Medicine and Science

Hani M. Wadei, MD
Senior Associate Consultant, Division of Neurology and Hypertension, Mayo Clinic, Jacksonville, Florida; Associate Professor of Medicine, Mayo Clinic College of Medicine and Science

Clarence B. Watridge, MD
Associate Consultant, Department of Neurologic Surgery, Mayo Clinic, Jacksonville, Florida; Associate Professor of Neurosurgery, Mayo Clinic College of Medicine and Science
Present address: Ponte Vedra Beach, Florida

Brian G. Weinshenker, MD
Consultant, Department of Neurology, Mayo Clinic, Rochester, Minnesota; Professor of Neurology, Mayo Clinic College of Medicine and Science

Matthew E. Welz, MS
Research Technologist for Neurosurgery, Mayo Clinic Hospital, Phoenix, Arizona

Robert E. Wharen Jr, MD
Consultant, Department of Neurologic Surgery, Mayo Clinic, Jacksonville, Florida; Professor of Neurosurgery, Mayo Clinic College of Medicine and Science

Eelco F. M. Wijdicks, MD, PhD
Chair, Division of Critical Care Neurology, Mayo Clinic, Rochester, Minnesota; Professor of Neurology, Mayo Clinic College of Medicine and Science

Nicholas D. Will, MD
Resident in Anesthesiology, Mayo Clinic School of Graduate Medical Education, Mayo Clinic College of Medicine and Science, Rochester, Minnesota

Jose C. Yataco, MD
Senior Associate Consultant, Department of Critical Care Medicine, Mayo Clinic, Jacksonville, Florida
Present address: Memphis, Tennessee

Joseph Zachariah, MD
Fellow in Critical Care Neurology, Mayo Clinic School of Graduate Medical Education, Mayo Clinic College of Medicine and Science, Rochester, Minnesota
Present address: Spectrum Hospital, Grand Rapids, Michigan

Ali A. Zaied, MD
Senior Associate Consultant, Department of Pulmonary, Critical Care, and Sleep Medicine, Mayo Clinic Health System—Northwest Wisconsin, Eau Claire, Wisconsin

Yuzana Zaw, MBBS
Fellow in Nephrology and Hypertension, Mayo Clinic School of Graduate Education, Mayo Clinic College of Medicine and Science, Scottsdale, Arizon

Section I

Fundamentals of Critical Care

Respiratory Physiology in Critical Illness

MINKYUNG KWON, MD; JOSE L. DIAZ-GOMEZ, MD

Goals

- Describe the basic lung volumes and capacities and the fundamentals of breathing mechanics.
- Describe airway resistance, lung compliance, and thoracic wall compliance as major components of pulmonary ventilation.
- Distinguish restrictive physiology from obstructive physiology.
- Describe common patterns of increased work of breathing and their associated factors.
- Describe the mechanisms of hypoxemia.

Introduction

The fundamental pillars of critical care medicine are the management of the lungs, heart, and kidneys and the provision of nutritional support. The practice of critical care medicine is often defined by abnormal respiratory physiology and requires detailed knowledge of lung mechanics, the mechanism of hypoxia, and the control of breathing. Therefore, laboratory assessment in pulmonary disorders is useful (Table 1.1; Box 1.1). Before the lungs can enable gas exchange, air must move from the upper airway down a series of branching small airways and reach the alveoli. In the walls of the alveoli, capillaries form a dense network and receive blood flowing from the pulmonary artery (from the right ventricle) before it flows to the pulmonary vein (and then to the left atrium). Between the capillary network and the alveoli lies a thin blood-gas barrier through which oxygen (O_2) and carbon dioxide (CO_2) move, chiefly by simple diffusion.

At rest, inspiration and expiration generate *tidal volume*. After the tidal volume is exhaled, further forceful expiration generates *expiratory reserve volume*. The volume of air remaining in the lung is the *residual volume*. After resting inspiration, forceful inspiration to maximal capacity generates *inspiratory reserve volume*. Volume that can be generated by maximal inspiration to maximal expiration is called *vital capacity* (Figure 1.1). Normal vital capacity is around 3 to 5 L, and normal tidal volume is approximately 500 mL. *Total minute ventilation* is the product of the tidal volume times the respiratory rate per minute.

Mechanics of Breathing

During rest, inspiration is active and expiration is passive. The most important muscle of inspiration is the diaphragm. When it contracts, the abdominal contents are forced downward and forward, and the vertical dimension of the chest cavity is increased. The external thoracic muscles make the rib margins lift and move out, increasing the transverse diameter of the thorax during forceful inspiration. At functional residual capacity, the rib cage acts as an outward force that generates negative pleural pressure. At end-expiration, the diaphragm prevents the abdominal organs from encroaching on the thoracic space and influencing the lung in the supine or prone position. During spontaneous breathing, these muscles expand the lung, creating even more negative intrapleural pressure and resulting in inspiration. During mechanical ventilation, positive pressure from the ventilator expands the chest wall, but the intrapleural pressure is positive.

Airway Resistance and Lung Compliance

Pulmonary ventilation and the work of breathing depend on the airway resistance and compliance of the lungs and the thoracic cage. *Airway resistance* is the pressure difference between the alveoli and the mouth divided by the flow rate. Most airway resistance is produced in medium-sized bronchi rather than in small bronchioles. The bronchial smooth muscles, located in medium-sized bronchi, are innervated by the autonomic nervous system. Stimulation of β-adrenergic receptors causes bronchodilation;

Table 1.1 • Useful Laboratory Values in Pulmonary Disorders

Laboratory Value	Significance in Pulmonary Disorders
Arterial blood gas	Hypoxia, hypercapnia, acidosis, alkalosis
Hemoglobin, glucose, urea nitrogen, creatinine, electrolytes, calcium, phosphorus, thyrotropin	Nonpulmonary causes of dyspnea
Plasma brain natriuretic peptide	Pulmonary edema due to heart failure
Serum bicarbonate	Chronic hypercapnia in COPD or obesity-hypoventilation syndrome
$Alpha_1$-antitrypsin	$Alpha_1$-antitrypsin deficiency, obstructive pattern
Eosinophils	Allergic asthma, parasitic infection, drug reaction, syndromes of pulmonary infiltrates with eosinophilia
Procalcitonin	Bacterial pneumonia
C-reactive protein	Pneumonia
Rheumatologic serology (ANA, RF, antisynthetase antibodies, CK, aldolase, SS-A/SS-B, Scl-70)	Interstitial lung disease
Anti-GBM antibody, ANCA	Pulmonary hemorrhage
Polycythemia	Recurrent hypoventilation or obstructive sleep apnea–associated hypoxemia

Abbreviations: ANA, antinuclear antibody; ANCA, antineutrophil cytoplasmic autoantibody; CK, creatine kinase; COPD, chronic obstructive pulmonary disease; GBM, glomerular basement membrane; RF, rheumatoid factor.

parasympathetic activity causes bronchoconstriction and increased airway resistance. Lung volume has an important effect on airway resistance: As lung volume decreases, airway resistance increases. Small airways may even close completely at low lung volumes.

Lung compliance is defined by the volume change per unit pressure change. Furthermore, it has 2 components: static and dynamic lung compliance.

Static Lung Compliance

Lung tends to collapse at any degree of pulmonary inflation, whereas the chest wall tends to recoil outward. This natural trend represents compliance of both the lung and the chest wall in static pressure-volume curves (Figure 1.2).

Lung compliance changes with various nonparenchymal conditions. Patients with obesity, ascites, or intra-abdominal hypertension have a stiffer chest wall; the lung and total respiratory system compliance curves shift down and rightward. In contrast, massive aspiration, alveolar edema, or fibrotic lung disease decreases the lung and total respiratory system compliance. In a patient with acute respiratory distress syndrome (ARDS), lung volume is further reduced and compliance is decreased. In addition, the overall volume of tissue and chest wall may be affected by illness, so that in ARDS the net effect on pleural pressure is unpredictable.

Static airway pressure of the respiratory system correlates with plateau pressure during mechanical ventilation. Moreover, the plateau pressure also represents the intra-alveolar pressure during use of an end-inspiratory hold. In passive ventilation, such as when patients are deeply sedated or paralyzed, the chest wall compliance curve tracks the pleural pressure. Thus, pressure measured with an esophageal balloon can be used to approximate these measures.

Dynamic Lung Compliance

Dynamic pressure-volume curves during inspiration and expiration exhibit a different pattern. This phenomenon, *hysteresis*, can be explained by surface tension variation at the alveolar air-fluid interface during inspiration and expiration. Pulmonary surfactant, a natural substance produced by type II epithelial cells in the lung, reduces the surface tension of the fluid layer lining the alveoli. During inspiration, alveolar surface tension increases because pulmonary surfactant spreads over a wider alveolar surface. The reverse occurs during expiration, when pulmonary surfactant condenses over a smaller alveolar surface.

Work of Breathing

Work is required to move the lung and the chest wall. The area under the dynamic pressure-volume curve of the lungs is used to estimate the work of breathing (WOB). During inspiration, the *elastic* WOB is the work needed to overcome elastic forces of the chest wall, lung parenchyma, and alveolar surface tension. In addition, *resistive* WOB is needed during inspiration to overcome tissue and airway resistance. During expiration, only resistive WOB is needed. Hence, increased WOB occurs with higher breathing rates

Box 1.1 • Interpretation of Blood Gas Data

Step 1. Determine whether the primary condition is *acidemia* (pH <7.35) or *alkalemia* (pH >7.45).

Step 2. Determine whether the disorder is *metabolic* (pH and $Paco_2$ changes are in the same direction) or *respiratory* (pH and $Paco_2$ changes are in the opposite direction).

Step 3. Determine whether compensation is adequate.

Metabolic acidosis: $Paco_2 = (1.5\ [HCO_3^-]) + 8$ (Correction ± 2)

Acute respiratory acidosis: Increase in $[HCO_3^-] = \Delta Paco_2/10$ (Correction ± 3)

Chronic respiratory acidosis: Increase in $[HCO_3^-] = 3.5\ (\Delta Paco_2/10)$

Metabolic alkalosis: Increase in $Paco_2 = 40 + 0.6\ (\Delta HCO_3^-)$

Acute respiratory alkalosis: Decrease in $[HCO_3^-] = 2\ (\Delta Paco_2/10)$

Chronic respiratory alkalosis: Decrease in $[HCO_3^-] = 5\ (\Delta Paco_2/10)$ to $7\ (\Delta Paco_2/10)$

Step 4. Calculate the anion gap (AG):

$$AG = [Na^+] - [Cl^-] + [HCO_3^-] - 12 \pm 2.$$

If the AG is elevated (>12), calculate the osmolar (OSM) gap (normal is <10):

$$\text{OSM Gap} = \text{Measured OSM} - (2\,[Na^+]) - (\text{Glucose}/18 - \text{SUN}/2.8).$$

Step 5. If an AG is present, calculate the delta-delta ratio:

$$\text{Delta} - \text{Delta Ratio} = \Delta AG / \Delta[HCO_3^-].$$

If <1, a concurrent non-AG metabolic acidosis is likely present. If >2, a concurrent metabolic alkalosis is likely present.

Abbreviations: Cl^-, chloride; Δ, change in; HCO_3^-, bicarbonate; Na^+, sodium; SUN, serum urea nitrogen.

Data from Kaufman DA. Interpretation of arterial blood gases (ABGs) [Internet]. New York: American Thoracic Society. c2017 [cited 2017 Sep 5]. Available from: http://www.thoracic.org/professionals/clinical-resources/critical-care/clinical-education/abgs.php.

and faster flow rates. With a larger tidal volume, the elastic WOB is larger. Patients with stiff lungs tend to take small rapid breaths, and patients with severe airway obstruction breathe more slowly.

Closing Capacity

Lung cannot be completely empty because of airflow-limiting segments in the small airways. Hence, expiration after development of airflow-limiting segments is effort independent. What remains in the lungs when small airways start to close is called the *closing capacity*. Patients with airway disease (eg, asthma, chronic obstructive pulmonary disease [COPD], or cystic fibrosis) are predisposed to having a higher closing capacity, leaving a large residual volume. The volume of air expired between closing capacity and residual volume is called the *closing volume*.

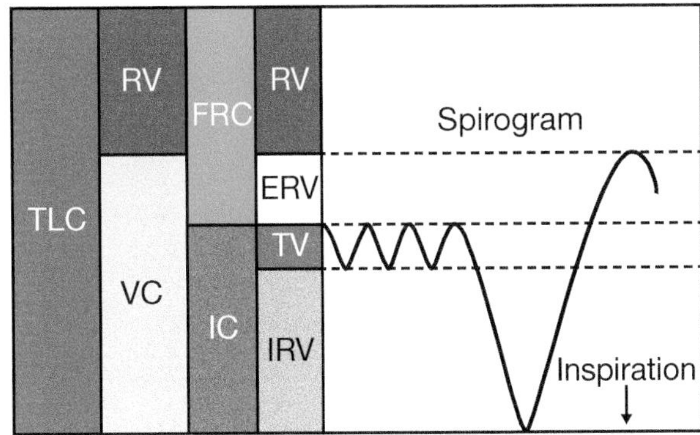

Figure 1.1. Standard Lung Volumes and Capacities. After resting inspiration, forceful inspiration to maximal capacity generates inspiratory reserve volume. The volume that can be generated by maximal inspiration to maximal expiration is the vital capacity (VC). ERV indicates expiratory reserve volume; FRC, functional residual capacity; IC, inspiratory capacity; IRV, inspiratory reserve volume; RV, residual volume; TLC, total lung capacity; TV, tidal volume.

Changes in Lung Mechanics in Acute Respiratory Failure

In patients who are critically ill with respiratory failure, 2 types of physiologic derangement occur: obstructive and restrictive.

Obstructive Physiology

In obstructive lung diseases, pulmonary compliance is normal or increased, but airway resistance is increased, especially during expiration. As mentioned above, normal expiration is passive. However, with obstructive physiology, such as in patients with asthma or COPD, extra work is needed for adequate expiration.

Restrictive Physiology

Pneumonia and ARDS are examples of diseases with restrictive physiology in which compliance of the lung, or chest wall (or both) is decreased. The static pressure-volume curve of the lungs or chest wall (or both) is shifted rightward. The transpulmonary pressure (alveolar pressure minus pleural pressure) indicates the pressure across the alveolus and therefore across the pulmonary capillary bed. Decreased compliance of the lungs requires

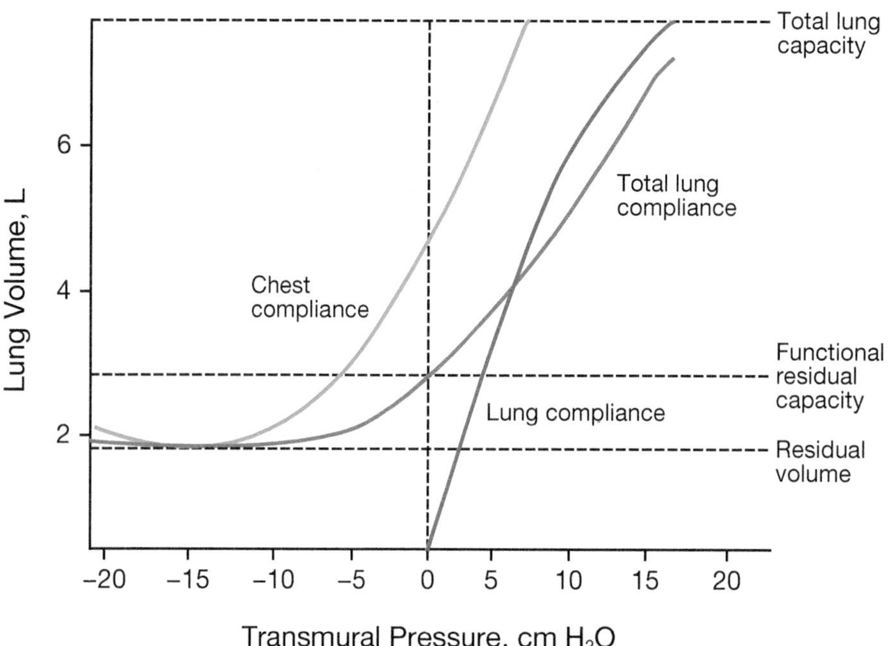

Figure 1.2. Compliance Curves. Compliance curves for lung and chest are shown along with total lung compliance. At small lung volumes, the negative transmural pressure of chest compliance indicates the chest wall's natural tendency to spring outward and expand. Lung compliance is high (ie, the slope of the curve is steep) at low lung volumes and decreases as the lung expands. Functional residual capacity is the summation of transmural pressures generated by the chest wall and lung when they are equal and opposing.

increased transpulmonary pressure for tidal inspiration. Further, the elastic WOB required for inspiration is increased and is usually compensated for by rapid shallow breathing. The intrinsic causes of restrictive physiology are interstitial lung diseases, pneumonia, and ARDS, and the extrinsic causes include respiratory muscle weakness, chest deformities, cardiomegaly, hemothorax, pneumothorax, empyema, and pleural effusion or thickening.

Respiratory Mechanics Affecting Circulation

Higher transpulmonary pressure leads to greater impedance to right ventricular outflow through the pulmonary vascular tree. A high right ventricular afterload decreases right ventricular output. Right ventricular preload depends on the degree of intrapleural pressure. With mechanical ventilation, intrapleural pressure increases during inspiration, further decreasing right ventricular preload. A stiffened chest wall increases intrapleural pressure, decreasing right ventricular preload further. Use of positive end-expiratory pressure and the prone position can also decrease right ventricular preload by increasing intrapleural pressure and stiffening the chest wall, respectively.

Neurogenic Pulmonary Edema

Acute central nervous system events such as acute head injury, seizure, tumors, and intracranial or subarachnoid hemorrhages can induce acute pulmonary edema within minutes or as late as 12 to 24 hours after the event. Besides having acute shortness of breath from pulmonary edema, patients may have fever, tachycardia, hypertension, and leukocytosis from sympathetic surge. The proposed pathophysiology is that the neuronal damage increases sympathetic tone with a catecholamine surge, which subsequently increases systemic vascular resistance and decreases left ventricular contractility, causing alveolar capillary leakage and eventually leading to a severe increase in intracranial pressure. Management is primarily supportive. α-Blockers can be used, and excessive diuresis should be avoided. The key is to treat the underlying central nervous system insult and the increased intracranial pressure.

Physiology of Hypoxia

Changes in Diffusing Capacity in Critical Illness

Gases move across the blood-gas barrier by diffusion. The O_2 diffusion reserve of the normal lung is enormous. However, in patients with alveolar hypoxia and thickening of the blood-gas barrier, O_2 diffusion is challenged.

Pulmonary Vascular Resistance

Pulmonary vascular resistance is usually small and can further decrease by recruitment and distention of capillaries. Pulmonary vascular resistance increases at high and low lung volumes. Hypoxia, serotonin, histamine, thromboxane A_2, and endothelin constrict pulmonary vasculature. Hypoxia constricts small pulmonary arteries probably by the direct effect of the low Po_2 on vascular smooth muscle. This mechanism, called *hypoxic pulmonary vasoconstriction*, directs blood flow away from poorly ventilated areas of the diseased lung in the adult.

Nitric oxide, phophodiesterase inhibitors, calcium channel blockers, and prostacyclin dilate pulmonary vasculature. Inhaled pulmonary vasodilators such as nitric oxide or inhaled phophodiesterase inhibitors reduce vascular tone locally in the well-ventilated regions, causing a shift in blood flow away from unventilated regions toward better-ventilated regions. Inhaled nitric oxide has been shown to reduce shunting and improve arterial oxygenation in patients with ARDS. Use of intravenous pulmonary vasodilators, such as prostacyclin, does not change Pao_2 much in patients with ARDS and pulmonary hypertension, probably because of the mixed effects of reduced pulmonary arterial pressure, increased cardiac output, and worsened intrapulmonary shunt.

In contrast, systemic vasodilators can produce hypoxemia. Systemic vasodilators increase cardiac output, impair hypoxic vasoconstriction in both well-ventilated and poorly ventilated pulmonary vasculature, and change intracardiac pressure or pulmonary arterial pressure, thereby altering the distribution of pulmonary blood flow. Nitroprusside, hydralazine, nitroglycerine, nifedipine, dopamine, and dobutamine can produce this effect.

Physiology of Hypoxemia

The 5 mechanisms of hypoxemia are hypoventilation, diffusion limitation, shunt, ventilation-perfusion ($\dot{V}/\dot{Q}$) mismatch, and low inspiratory O_2 pressure.

Hypoventilation

Hypoventilation always increases the alveolar Pco_2, which leads to lower alveolar Pao_2 unless additional O_2 is inspired. The treatment is to provide additional O_2.

Diffusion Limitation

Diffusion of gases is limited when the blood-gas barrier is thickened.

Shunt

This refers to blood that enters the arterial system without going through ventilated areas of the lung. Hypoxemia resulting from a shunt does not improve after adding O_2. If the shunt is caused by mixed venous blood, its size can be calculated from the shunt equation. Shunt is an important cause of hypoxemia in patients with ARDS and pneumonia.

$\dot{V}/\dot{Q}$ Mismatch

$\dot{V}/\dot{Q}$ mismatch is the most common cause of hypoxemia, especially in the perioperative period after general anesthesia. A patient with $\dot{V}/\dot{Q}$ mismatch has a problem with either ventilation (air going in and out of the lungs) or perfusion (O_2 and CO_2 diffusion at the alveoli and the pulmonary arteries). $\dot{V}/\dot{Q}$ ratios compare the amount of air reaching the alveoli to the amount of blood reaching the alveoli. The $\dot{V}/\dot{Q}$ ratio describes the gas exchange in any single lung unit. Regional differences in the $\dot{V}/\dot{Q}$ ratio in the upright lung cause regional changes in gas exchange. The normal $\dot{V}/\dot{Q}$ ratio is about 1, and decreases or increases in the ratio indicate changes in the alveolar gas and end-capillary blood composition. $\dot{V}/\dot{Q}$ mismatch impairs the uptake or elimination of all gases by the lung. Although CO_2 elimination is impaired by $\dot{V}/\dot{Q}$ mismatch, it can be corrected by increasing the ventilation to the alveoli. In contrast, hypoxemia resulting from $\dot{V}/\dot{Q}$ mismatch cannot be resolved by increased ventilation. The difference in the CO_2 and O_2 responses results from their own dissociation curve characteristics. Clinically, regions with low or high $\dot{V}/\dot{Q}$ ratios cause hypoxemia, impaired CO_2 elimination, and increased WOB in COPD patients.

Low Inspiratory O_2 Pressure

Low inspiratory O_2 pressure causes hypoxemia even with a normal alveolar-arterial difference in the partial pressure of O_2.

Changes in Dead Space in Critical Illness

Dead space is the volume (not a space) that is ventilated but does not participate in perfusion. There are 2 types of dead space: anatomical dead space and physiologic dead space. *Anatomical dead space*, normally about 150 mL, is the volume of the conducting airways. *Physiologic dead space* is the volume of gas that does not eliminate CO_2. Because physiologic dead space includes airway and alveolar dead space, it is increased in many lung diseases. Furthermore, increased $\dot{V}/\dot{Q}$ mismatch and shunt are the most likely contributors to increased dead space in ARDS.

Supplemental O_2 and CO_2 Retention in COPD Patients

High fractional supplemental O_2 may cause CO_2 retention in COPD patients because supplemental O_2 may increase the partial pressure of O_2 in the alveoli (P_{AO_2}) in lung units with a low $\dot{V}/\dot{Q}$ ratio, inhibiting regional hypoxic pulmonary vasoconstriction and increasing blood flow to these units. Consequently, blood is diverted away from better-ventilated regions, converting them to lung units with high $\dot{V}/\dot{Q}$ ratios, which increases wasted ventilation.

Supplemental O_2 may cause CO_2 retention in COPD patients through a second mechanism, the Haldane effect. In this phenomenon, increased PaO_2 decreases the binding of both hydrogen ions and CO_2 to hemoglobin, thereby increasing the amount of physically dissolved CO_2 and PCO_2. The decreased respiratory drive from low $PaCO_2$ is a less likely cause.

In clinical practice, COPD patients who receive supplemental O_2 to maintain normal PaO_2 do not retain clinically significant levels of CO_2. The use of noninvasive mechanical ventilation can alleviate CO_2 retention while providing enough O_2 in COPD patients.

Indexes of Oxygenation

Of the several indexes of oxygenation that are used, 2 are discussed here: the alveoli-arterial (A-a) gradient and the ratio of PaO_2 to the fraction of inspired O_2 (FIO_2). Both are O_2 tension–based indexes (calculated from PO_2) as opposed to a concentration-based index, such as the shunt index (calculated from the arterial O_2 content). The A-a gradient and the PaO_2/FIO_2 ratio can be affected by the following factors: a shunt, $\dot{V}/\dot{Q}$ mismatch, congenital heart disease, cardiac output, FIO_2, temperature, low PCO_2, and O_2 extraction.

A-a Gradient

The A-a gradient is the gradient between an alveolus and the arterial blood, expressed in millimeters of mercury. PAO_2 is calculated with the following simplified formula (using the sea level barometric pressure of 760 mm Hg, water vapor pressure at 37°C of 47 mm Hg, and a respiratory quotient of 0.8-0.9):

$$P_{AO_2} = (FIO_2 \times 713) - (PaCO_2 \times 1.25).$$

Subsequently, the A-a gradient is calculated as follows:

$$\text{A-a Gradient} = P_{AO_2} - PaO_2.$$

The normal value of the A-a gradient is 7 mm Hg in young patients and 14 mm Hg in elderly patients at 21% FIO_2. The A-a gradient is increased with a higher FIO_2, $\dot{V}/\dot{Q}$ mismatch, a diffusion defect, an intracardiac shunt, or an increased O_2 extraction ratio. A high $PaCO_2$ due to alveolar hypoventilation results in a normal A-a gradient, and this is the most useful situation for using the A-a gradient.

PaO_2/FIO_2 Ratio

At sea level, the PaO_2/FIO_2 ratio is normally more than 500 mm Hg; that is, PaO_2 should exceed FIO_2 by 500 times in normal lung. The PaO_2/FIO_2 ratio is used for risk stratification, such as in the Berlin definition of ARDS (eg, <100 indicates severe ARDS). The PaO_2/FIO_2 ratio, in contrast to the A-a gradient, cannot be used to distinguish hypoxemia due to alveolar hypoventilation from hypoxemia due to other causes. Like the A-a gradient, the PaO_2/FIO_2 ratio is dependent on FIO_2 and is highly dependent on the O_2 extraction ratio.

Summary

- Pulmonary ventilation depends on airway resistance and the compliance of the lungs and the thoracic cage.
- Lung compliance is defined by the volume change per unit pressure change. Massive aspiration, alveolar edema, ARDS, or fibrotic lung disease decreases lung compliance.
- A higher breathing rate is accompanied by faster flow rates and larger viscous WOB. With a larger tidal volume, the elastic work is larger.
- Restrictive physiology can occur in patients with pneumonia or ARDS. In these conditions, the compliance of the lung or chest wall (or both) is decreased.
- With obstructive physiology, airway resistance is increased, especially during expiration.
- If transmural pressure for the lungs is zero, the system is neither inflating nor deflating. For a given ventilator volume, the lateral distance between plateau pressure and the chest wall compliance curve is the transpulmonary pressure.
- The 5 mechanisms of hypoxemia are hypoventilation, diffusion limitation, shunt, $\dot{V}/\dot{Q}$ mismatch, and low inspiratory O_2 pressure.
- Dead space is the volume that is ventilated but does not participate in perfusion.

SUGGESTED READING

Adler D, Janssens J-P. The pathophysiology of respiratory failure: control of breathing, respiratory load, and muscle capacity. Respiration. 2019 Feb;97(2):93–104.

Crossley DJ, McGuire GP, Barrow PM, Houston PL. Influence of inspired oxygen concentration on deadspace, respiratory drive, and $PaCO_2$ in intubated patients with chronic obstructive pulmonary disease. Crit Care Med. 1997 Sep;25(9):1522–6.

Kaufman DA. Interpretation of arterial blood gases (ABGs) [Internet]. New York: American Thoracic Society. c2017 [cited 2017 Sep 5]. Available from: http://www.thoracic.org/professionals/clinical-resources/critical-care/clinical-education/abgs.php.

Luft UC, Mostyn EM, Loeppky JA, Venters MD. Contribution of the Haldane effect to the rise of arterial PCO_2 in hypoxic patients breathing oxygen. Crit Care Med. 1981 Jan;9(1):32–7.

Lutfi MF. The physiological basis and clinical significance of lung volume measurements. Multidiscip Respir Med. 2017 Feb 9;12:3.

Mauri T, Lazzeri M, Bellani G, Zanella A, Grasselli G. Respiratory mechanics to understand ARDS and guide mechanical ventilation. Physiol Meas. 2017 Nov;38(12):R280-H303.

Mortolla JP. How to breathe? Respiratory mechanics and breathing pattern. Respir Physiol Neurobiol. 2019 Mar;261:48–54.

Nuckton TJ, Alonso JA, Kallet RH, Daniel BM, Pittet JF, Eisner MD, et al. Pulmonary dead-space fraction as a risk factor for death in the acute respiratory distress syndrome. N Engl J Med. 2002 Apr 25;346(17):1281–6.

Ortiz-Prado E, Dunn JF, Vasconez J, Castillo D, Viscor G. Partial pressure of oxygen in the human body: a general review. Am J Blood Res. 2019 Feb;9(1):1–14.

Raoof S, Goulet K, Esan A, Hess DR, Sessler CN. Severe hypoxemic respiratory failure: part 2: nonventilatory strategies. Chest. 2010 Jun;137(6):1437–48.

Rossaint R, Falke KJ, Lopez F, Slama K, Pison U, Zapol WM. Inhaled nitric oxide for the adult respiratory distress syndrome. N Engl J Med. 1993 Feb 11;328(6):399–405.

Sassoon CS, Hassell KT, Mahutte CK. Hyperoxic-induced hypercapnia in stable chronic obstructive pulmonary disease. Am Rev Respir Dis. 1987 Apr;135(4):907–11.

Savi A, Gasparetto Maccari J, Frederico Tonietto T, Pecanha Antonio AC, Pinheiro de Oliveira R, de Mello Rieder M, et al. Influence of FIO_2 on $PaCO_2$ during noninvasive ventilation in patients with COPD. Respir Care. 2014 Mar;59(3):383–7. Epub 2013 Aug 13.

Stenqvist O, Gattinoni L, Hedenstierna G. What's new in respiratory physiology? The expanding chest wall revisited! Intensive Care Med. 2015 Jun;41(6):1110–3. Epub 2015 Feb 12.

Wandrup JH. Quantifying pulmonary oxygen transfer deficits in critically ill patients. Acta Anaesthesiol Scand Suppl. 1995;107:37–44.

West JB. Challenges in teaching the mechanics of breathing to medical and graduate students. Adv Physiol Educ. 2008 Sep;32(3):177–84.

2 Mechanical Ventilation: Basic Modes

AMELIA A. LOWELL, RRT, RCP

Goals

- Understand the basic physiology of mechanical ventilation.
- Discuss the basic modes of mechanical ventilation.
- Discuss safety and comfort measures with mechanical ventilation settings.

Introduction

The main goal of mechanical ventilation is to unload the respiratory muscles to facilitate oxygenation and ventilation. This is accomplished by providing a minute ventilation ($\dot{V}_E$) (respiratory rate × tidal volume [V_T]) that will result in adequate alveolar ventilation coupled with supplemental oxygen and a mean airway pressure that will result in adequate arterial oxygenation.

Physiology of Mechanical Breathing Assistance

The respiratory equation of motion demonstrates that the work or negative pressure that the respiratory apparatus must generate to displace volume from the atmosphere into the lungs (Pmusc) is determined by the resistance to gas flow and the compliance of the lungs.

$$\text{Pmusc} = \frac{\text{Volume}}{\text{Compliance}} + (\text{Resistance} \times \text{Flow})$$

Negative Pressure Ventilation (Normal Breathing)

When circulating hydrogen ion levels (whose major determinant is carbon dioxide) are elevated in the brain stem (medulla oblongata central chemoreceptor trigger zone), they trigger respiratory drive by means of the phrenic and intercostal nerves, resulting in contraction of the diaphragm and intercostal muscles. The diaphragm contracts downward into the abdominal cavity and, together with the activated intercostal muscles, pulls the chest wall, pleural cavity, and alveoli open. When the lungs recoil, alveolar pressure increases (compared to the pressure at the mouth), the pressure gradient is reversed, and gas flows out of the lungs.

Positive Pressure Ventilation

Positive pressure ventilation (PPV) provides ventilator support to a patient by creating a pressure gradient between the ventilator circuit and the patient's lungs. The respiratory equation of motion can be modified to include the work done by the ventilator (Pvent):

$$\text{Pmusc} + \text{Pvent} = \frac{\text{Volume}}{\text{Compliance}} + (\text{Resistance} \times \text{Flow})$$

Mechanical Ventilator Systems

The typical critical care ventilator is electrically powered and pneumatically or turbine driven. The graphical user interface allows the user to select settings and review alphanumeric and waveform data. The gas enters the machine through two 55-psig high-pressure hoses: 1 supplies oxygen and 1 supplies air. The amount of oxygen in the gas mixture is determined by the user-selected fraction of inspired oxygen (F_{IO_2}). The gas flow passes through the output control valve to the inspiratory limb and through the endotracheal tube to the patient's lungs. When the inspiratory phase is complete, the gas travels through the expiratory limb back to the ventilator.

Since the upper airway is bypassed after endotracheal intubation, the inspiratory gas must be heated and humidified before entering the lungs. Warming and humidifying are accomplished with either a heated reservoir humidifier chamber or a heat-moisture exchanger.

Operation of a Mechanical Ventilator

Five basic principles must be understood before operating a mechanical ventilator.

Flow

The output gas flow is determined by the desired volume to be delivered over the inspiratory phase.

$$\text{Flow} = \frac{\text{Volume}}{\text{Time}}$$

Volume

The volume of gas delivered is determined by the set flow rate and the inspiratory time.

$$\text{Volume} = \text{Flow} \times \text{Time}$$

Pressure

Pressure is determined by the amount of resistance the gas flow encounters as it makes its way through the ventilator circuit and airways.

$$\text{Pressure} = \text{Flow} \times \text{Resistance}$$

The 2 important pressures monitored during mechanical ventilation are the peak inspiratory pressure (PIP) and the plateau pressure (Pplat) (Figure 2.1). The PIP is measured at the end of the inspiratory phase of each breath under dynamic flow conditions and generally reflects the amount of resistance the gas encounters as it moves through the ventilator and respiratory system. The Pplat is measured during a breath hold at the end of inspiration and generally reflects the compliance of the respiratory system. It is sometimes referred to as *alveolar distending pressure*.

Resistance

Resistance is created as the gas flows through the ventilator circuit and airways. Increased airway resistance is caused by any obstruction to gas flow, which may be intraluminal (secretions and bronchoconstriction) or extraluminal (the weight of the chest wall and abdomen).

$$\text{Resistance} = \frac{\Delta\ \text{Pressure}}{\text{Flow}}$$

Compliance

Compliance is a measure of change in volume for given pressure. The amount of gas delivered is proportional to the amount of pressure it takes to move the gas through the system.

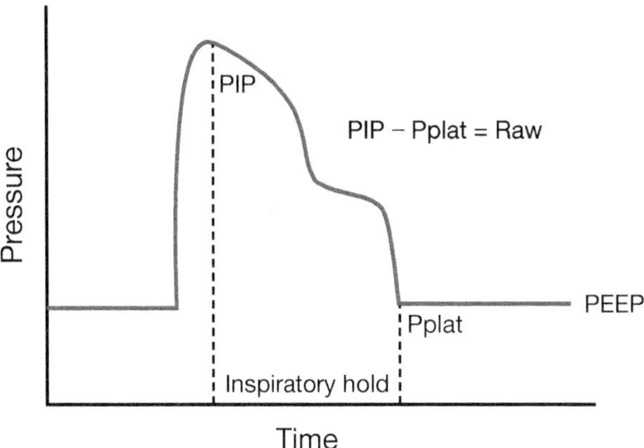

Figure 2.1. Pressures Monitored During Mechanical Ventilation. Peak inspiratory pressure (PIP) is measured at the end of the inspiratory phase. Plateau pressure (Pplat) is measured at the end of inspiration during a breath hold. Airway resistance (Raw) is the difference between PIP and Pplat. PEEP indicates positive end-expiratory pressure.

$$\text{Compliance} = \frac{\Delta\text{Volume}}{\Delta\text{Pressure}}$$

For every 1 cm H_2O of pressure applied to the system, normal lungs should receive 60 to 100 mL of gas. Lung compliance is measured in 2 ways. *Static compliance* is calculated with the Pplat (the amount of pressure in the lungs during an inspiratory hold). *Dynamic compliance* is calculated with the PIP and is not as useful clinically as the static measurement.

$$\text{Static Compliance} = \frac{V_T\ \text{Delivered (in mL)}}{\text{Pplat} - \text{PEEP}}$$

For example, if a patient has an exhaled V_T of 500 mL, a Pplat of 25 cm H_2O, and a positive end-expiratory pressure (PEEP) of 5 cm H_2O, the static compliance is 500 mL/(25 cm H_2O - 5 cm H_2O) = 25 mL/cm H_2O. Clinically this would represent poor lung compliance.

Phases of a Mechanical Breath

Initiation and Triggering

A mechanical breath is initiated by 2 methods: mechanical (timed) or patient triggered (Figure 2.2).

A mechanical (timed) breath is delivered at a set time interval. For example, if the clinician sets a respiratory rate of 10 breaths/min, a breath will be delivered by the machine every 6 seconds.

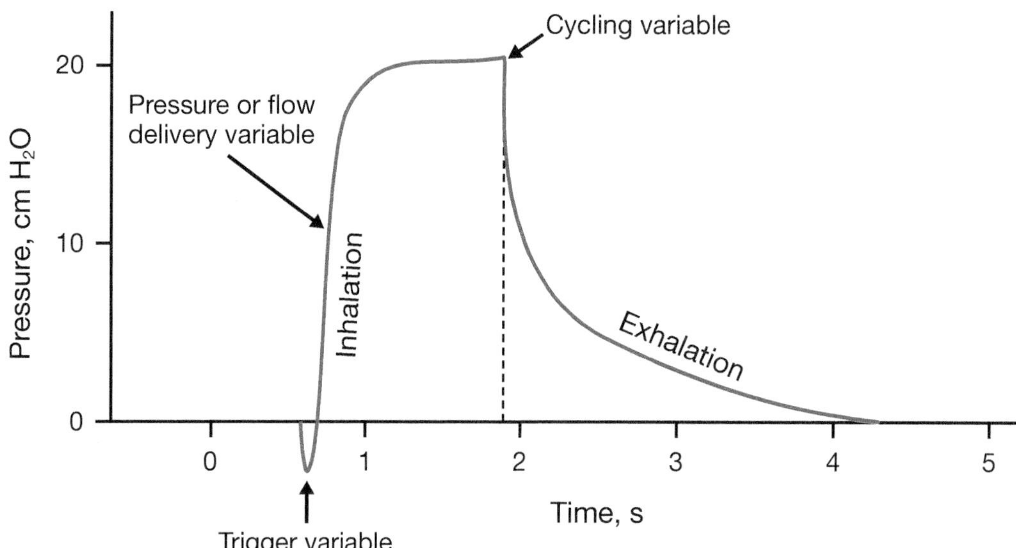

Figure 2.2. Phases of a Mechanical Breath. Pressure-time curve shows when different variables affect the inspiratory phase.

Trigger sensitivity determines the ventilator's response to a patient's inspiratory effort. When the diaphragm contracts, the ventilator measures either the decrease in pressure (*pressure trigger*) or the volume displacement (*flow trigger*) in the circuit. A patient can generally trigger a breath more easily when a flow trigger is selected.

Inspiratory Phase

When the breath is triggered, gas is released into the ventilator circuit. During this time, the circuit achieves maximum pressure and the V_T is delivered to the lungs.

Expiratory Phase

Cycling is the change from the inspiratory phase to the expiratory phase. The expiratory phase is initiated by 2 methods: One is by timing. The respiratory rate and the inspiratory time are set, and the expiratory time is a function of both. For example, if the respiratory rate is 10 breaths/min and the inspiratory time is 1 second, the expiratory phase is 5 seconds. With the second method, the inspiratory phase is stopped when the flow has decelerated to a certain percentage of peak flow. This method is used for spontaneous breaths when the inspiratory time and respiratory rate are variable instead of being set.

Ventilator Modes

Ventilator mode describes the level of support that the ventilator provides the patient (Table 2.1). It does not describe the method of breath delivery (volume controlled [VC] or pressure controlled [PC]). Although only 3 basic modes are described here, all modes of mechanical ventilation with modern ventilators allow the patient to trigger or initiate a breath. The modes vary in how the patient-triggered breaths are delivered.

Continuous Mandatory Ventilation

The commonly used term for *continuous mandatory ventilation* (CMV) mode is *assist control* (AC). The clinician selects a minimum respiratory rate, V_T, and flow rate or inspiratory pressure and inspiratory time, and the ventilator delivers a breath at that interval. An assisted breath occurs when the patient triggers the ventilator. In response to the patient's effort the machine delivers a breath with the same settings as the mechanically timed breath. In summary, the machine delivers a minimum $\dot{V}_E$, and if the patient triggers breaths above the set rate, those breaths will be assisted.

Intermittent Mandatory Ventilation

With *intermittent mandatory ventilation* (IMV), like AC mode, the ventilator delivers a minimum $\dot{V}_E$ determined by the settings (rate and volume or pressure). The critical difference between AC and IMV is how the patient-triggered breath is delivered. With AC, those breaths are mandatory by definition; with IMV, they can be both spontaneous and mandatory. With IMV, total $\dot{V}_E$ consists of a combination of controlled and spontaneous breaths.

Continuous Spontaneous Ventilation

In *continuous spontaneous ventilation* (CSV), all breaths are spontaneous. They are all patient triggered and cycled.

Table 2.1 • Ventilator Modes and Settings

Mode and Setting[a]	RR[b]	VT	Flow, L/min	Insp Time, s	PS
AC-VC	14-20	6-8 mL/kg IBW	≥60	Not set	Not set
AC-PC	14-20	Inspiratory pressure to achieve 6-8 mL/kg IBW	Not set	0.6-1.0	Not set
SIMV-VC	14-20	6-8 mL/kg IBW	≥60	Not set	Inspiratory pressure to achieve VT of 6-8 mL/kg IBW
SIMV-PC	14-20	Inspiratory pressure to achieve 6-8 mL/kg IBW	Not set	0.6-1.0	Inspiratory pressure to achieve VT of 6-8 mL/kg IBW
CSV	Not set	Not set	Not set	Not set	Inspiratory pressure to achieve VT of 6-8 mL/kg IBW

Abbreviations: AC, assist control; CSV, continuous spontaneous ventilation; IBW, ideal body weight; Insp, inspiratory; PC, pressure controlled; PS, pressure support; RR, respiratory rate; SIMV, synchronized intermittent mandatory ventilation; VC, volume controlled; VT, tidal volume.

[a] For each of these modes and settings, the fraction of inspired oxygen is 0.21 to 1.0, and the positive end-expiratory pressure is at least 5 cm H_2O.

[b] RR in breaths per minute.

The only variable that is set is the pressure support (inspiratory pressure). This mode is commonly referred to as *pressure support ventilation* (PSV).

Breath Types

Mandatory

A breath is considered mandatory when it is delivered at a timed interval. There are 2 types of mandatory breaths: 1) With VC breaths, the user selects a VT and flow rate to deliver the volume to the lungs. Volume is guaranteed and airway pressure varies depending on changes in the patient's lung mechanics (compliance and resistance). 2) With PC breaths, the user selects a driving pressure, and the VT delivered to the patient is based on the lung compliance.

Spontaneous

A spontaneous breath is both triggered and cycled by the patient. This means that the timing of breaths and the inspiration to expiration (I:E) ratio vary according to the patient's breathing pattern. Called a pressure-supported breath, the inspiratory pressure is set and the VT delivered to the patient is based on lung compliance. The breath delivery is the same as for a PC breath, but the terminology is different because it refers to a patient-triggered breath.

Summary of Mode and Breath Type

The combination of mode and breath type determines the overall ventilation strategy. If AC mode is chosen, the mandatory and patient-triggered breaths can be either VC or PC. If *synchronized IMV* (SIMV) is chosen, the mandatory breath can be VC or PC and the patient-triggered breath is spontaneous (pressure supported). In CSV mode, all breaths are spontaneous.

Determining Ventilator Settings

When choosing ventilator settings, the first step is to determine the treatment goals in terms of gas exchange, safety, and comfort for the patient (Box 2.1).

Gas Exchange

Oxygenation

Oxygen delivery and adequate tissue oxygenation are given priority in the treatment of the critically ill. However, both hypoxia and hyperoxia are related to adverse outcomes. A *U*-shaped relationship exists between Pao_2 and hospital mortality among all intensive care unit patients receiving mechanical ventilation. The lowest mortality rates have been observed among patients with a Pao_2 of 110 to 150 mm Hg; mortality increases if Pao_2 is less than 67 mm Hg or greater than 225 mm Hg. Specifically, hyperoxemia increases mortality among patients who have had cardiac arrest or traumatic brain injury. An oxygenation strategy should aim to reverse arterial hypoxemia while avoiding hyperoxemia.

Ventilation

Mechanical ventilation can facilitate improvement of alveolar ventilation and gas exchange. The goal $Paco_2$ should normalize pH. As evidence has emerged on the detrimental effects of high ventilator pressures and large tidal volumes, a strategy called *permissive hypercapnia* has become an acceptable practice for treating patients with acute respiratory distress syndrome (ARDS). The strategy requires caution if a patient has a neurologic condition because elevated $Paco_2$ levels can increase intracranial pressures, cause agitation or depressed consciousness, and decrease the seizure threshold.

For patients with intracranial hypertension, therapeutic hyperventilation to lower the $Paco_2$ to 26 to 30 mm Hg

Box 2.1 • Targets for Ventilator Settings

Safety
- Blood pressure
  - Systolic blood pressure >90 mm Hg
  - Mean arterial pressure >65 mm Hg
- Peak inspiratory pressure <35 cm H_2O
- Plateau pressure <30 cm H_2O
- Auto-PEEP—none
- Tidal volume, 6-8 mL/kg IBW

Gas exchange
- Spo_2 >88%
- Arterial blood gas analysis
  - pH 7.40
  - $Paco_2$, 35-45 mm Hg
  - Pao_2 >60 mm Hg

Comfort
- Synchrony—patient is comfortable

Abbreviations: IBW, ideal body weight; PEEP, positive end-expiratory pressure; Spo_2, oxygen saturation by pulse oximetry.

can be used as a temporizing measure when clinical herniation complicates intracranial hypertension from cerebral edema, intracranial hemorrhage, or tumor. In contrast, after traumatic brain injury, prolonged, prophylactic, induced hyperventilation with $Paco_2$ of 25 mm Hg or less is not recommended and should be avoided during the first 24 hours after injury.

Safety

Barotrauma and Volutrauma Prevention

Pulmonary barotrauma from mechanical ventilation refers to alveolar rupture due to elevated transalveolar pressure. Air leaks into extra-alveolar tissue result in various conditions, including pneumothorax, pneumomediastinum, pneumoperitoneum, and subcutaneous emphysema. The incidence of injury can be up to 50% but has been drastically reduced with the evolution of low VT (lung-protective) ventilation. Additionally, mechanical ventilation can cause trauma to the lung as in ventilator-induced lung injury or ventilator-associated lung injury. Repeated overdistention of the alveoli and cyclic atelectasis are the principal causes of alveolar injury during PPV. In the landmark Acute Respiratory Distress Syndrome Network (ARDSnet) trial, mortality decreased by 22% with use of a low VT (lung-protective) strategy. Therefore, the most effective strategies to minimize injury are to maintain a low Pplat (<30 cm H_2O) and a VT of 6 to 8 mL/kg ideal body weight (IBW) and to avoid dynamic hyperinflation.

Hemodynamic Stability

Mechanical ventilation and PPV can also have a considerable effect on hemodynamics. As positive pressure is applied to the thoracic cavity, the intrathoracic veins are compressed and the central venous and right atrial pressures are elevated. The result is a decrease in venous return to the right side of the heart and a resultant decrease in right ventricular stroke volume, preload, and pulmonary blood flow. Additionally, high impedance encountered by blood returning to the right side of the heart causes blood to pool in the abdominal visceral vasculature and the brain. The pooling of blood in the abdomen can remove blood from the general circulation and contribute to decreased left ventricular stroke volume. The resistance to cerebral drainage may also increase intracranial pressure.

In patients with decreased lung compliance (eg, ARDS), a high-PEEP open lung strategy is often used. The pressure remaining in the alveoli at the end of inspiration can compress the adjacent pulmonary vasculature and impede pulmonary blood flow. The increased intrapleural pressure can impede venous return and further reduce cardiac output.

In patients with normal cardiopulmonary systems, this effect is usually minimal and compensated for by an increased heart rate, systemic and peripheral vascular resistance, and peripheral shunting of blood. Conditions that may prevent a patient from compensating include sympathetic blockade, spinal anesthesia, spinal cord transection, and polyneuritis.

Auto-PEEP

Alveolar pressure at the end of passive expiration may exceed the set PEEP when the expiratory phase cannot be completed to the fully relaxed position of the respiratory system before the next inspiration begins. This results in unintended pressure in the lungs at the end of exhalation, which can negatively affect hemodynamics, induce pulmonary barotrauma, increase the work of breathing, cause dyspnea, cause patient-ventilator synchrony, and interfere with the effectiveness of pressure-regulated ventilation. Identifying the cause is important for determining treatment. The cause may be inappropriate timing settings (expiratory time too short) or patient physiology (obstructive disease).

Comfort

Supporting the patient's physiologic needs is not the only concern during mechanical ventilation. Ensuring patient-ventilator synchrony (PVS) should be a priority for all clinicians. Asynchrony is a cause of ineffective ventilation, impaired gas exchange, lung overdistention, increased work of breathing, and patient discomfort. The 4 categories of asynchrony are flow, trigger, cycling, and mode. All result from inappropriate matching of the ventilator settings and the patient's ventilatory demand or the presence of auto-PEEP. Classic neural injury patterns of breathing include Biot respiration, apneustic breathing, and central neurogenic hyperventilation or hypoventilation breathing, which are frequently associated with asynchrony. Generally, PC or pressure-supported breaths are more comfortable than VC, and spontaneous modes are more comfortable than AC or SIMV. Although sedation is sometimes necessary to facilitate PVS, all attempts must be made to match the ventilator output and settings to the patient's demand. Modern mechanical ventilators have been designed to address these issues by creating modes that more closely match normal physiologic breathing patterns and breath dynamics.

Ventilator Settings

Respiratory Rate

The respiratory rate is determined by the goal for $\dot{V}_E$. The clinician first calculates the V_T and then uses a rate that guarantees a minimum $\dot{V}_E$, which is 5 L/min for an adult. For example, if the V_T is 500 mL, a rate of 10 breaths/min is needed to achieve 5 L/min. The rate is then titrated to meet the goals of ventilation. The most effective way to improve ventilation (ie, decrease $Paco_2$) is to increase the respiratory rate. The limitation of this strategy is the reduction in total cycle time (TCT). For example, a rate of 20 breaths/min results in a TCT of 3 seconds. If the inspiratory time is fixed at 1 second and the rate is increased to 30 breaths/min, the resultant TCT is 2 seconds and the I:E ratio is 1:1, with a 1-second exhalation. That rate would impair ventilation and potentially induce air trapping and reduce venous return and cardiac output.

Flow

With VC breaths, the flow is set. With PC breaths, the flow is a product of the inspiratory time setting. When determining the optimum flow rate, 2 factors must be considered: the desired inspiratory time and the patient inspiratory flow demand. A flow rate that is too low or too high will cause patient-ventilator dysynchrony. A flow setting of at least 60 L/min will generally satisfy both.

Inspiratory Time and the I:E Ratio

An inspiratory time of 0.6 to 1.0 seconds generally satisfies innate neural timing with an I:E ratio of at least 1:2. With VC breaths, the inspiratory time is a product of the set volume and set flow rate (volume = flow × time). With PC breaths, the time is set by the clinician.

Tidal Volume

The currently accepted V_T is 4 to 8 mL/kg IBW. An initial V_T of 6 or 8 mL/kg IBW should be titrated down to keep Pplat less than 28 cm H_2O and driving pressure less than 15 cm H_2O.

Inspiratory Pressure

In a PC or pressure-supported breath, the delivered V_T is a result of the inspiratory driving pressure (P_I), the inspiratory time, and lung mechanics. The P_I is set to achieve the desired V_T while maintaining safe lung pressures. A reasonable strategy to determine the P_I is to start with 10 cm H_2O, observe the resultant V_T, and then titrate to achieve the desired V_T.

Oxygenation

To prevent alveolar cycling and derecruitment in acute lung injury, high levels of PEEP are necessary to counterbalance the increased lung mass resulting from edema, inflammation, and infiltrations and to maintain normal functional residual capacity. It is generally accepted that application of physiologic PEEP of 5 cm H_2O is necessary in all patients with an artificial airway because the epiglottis cannot close. When the PEEP is titrated up in response to hypoxia or atelectasis, the hemodynamics and cardiopulmonary interaction must be monitored.

The Fio_2 present in the gas mixture should be the lowest Fio_2 needed to achieve the goal oxygen saturation by pulse oximetry (Spo_2).

Summary

- Setting of the mechanical ventilator requires knowledge of flow, pressure, and volume relationships.
- Ventilator mode selection is based on the level of support required to assist $\dot{V}_E$; breath type selection is largely based on lung mechanics and patient comfort.
- Clinicians must consider the patient's physiologic needs for assistance with oxygenation and ventilation and the safety concerns of administering PPV while attempting to facilitate PVS.

SUGGESTED READING

Acute Respiratory Distress Syndrome Network, Brower RG, Matthay MA, Morris A, Schoenfeld D, Thompson BT, Wheeler A. Ventilation with lower tidal volumes as compared with traditional tidal volumes for acute lung injury and the acute respiratory distress syndrome. N Engl J Med. 2000 May 4;342(18):1301–8.

Carney N, Totten AM, O'Reilly C, Ullman JS, Hawryluk GW, Bell MJ, et al. Guidelines for the management of severe traumatic brain injury, fourth edition. Neurosurgery. 2017 Jan 1;80(1):6–15.

Curley GF, Laffey JG, Zhang H, Slutsky AS. Biotrauma and ventilator-induced lung injury: clinical implications. Chest. 2016 Nov;150(5):1109–17. Epub 2016 Jul 29.

Davis DP, Meade W, Sise MJ, Kennedy F, Simon F, Tominaga G. Both hypoxemia and extreme hyperoxemia may be detrimental in patients with severe traumatic brain injury. J Neurotrauma. 2009 Dec;26(12):2217–23.

de Vries H, Johnkman A, Shi ZH, Spoelstra-de Man A, Heunks L. Assessing breathing effort in mechanical ventilation: physiology and clinical implications. Ann Transl Med. 2018 Oct;6(19):387.

Elmer J, Scutella M, Pullalarevu R, Wang B, Vaghasia N, Trzeciak S, et al; Pittsburgh Post-Cardiac Arrest Service (PCAS). The association between hyperoxia and patient outcomes after cardiac arrest: analysis of a high-resolution database. Intensive Care Med. 2015 Jan;41(1):49–57. Epub 2014 Dec 4.

Gajic O, Dara SI, Mendez JL, Adesanya AO, Festic E, Caples SM, et al. Ventilator-associated lung injury in patients without acute lung injury at the onset of mechanical ventilation. Crit Care Med. 2004 Sep;32(9):1817–24.

Georgopoulos D, Roussos C. Control of breathing in mechanically ventilated patients. Eur Respir J. 1996 Oct;9(10):2151–60.

He HW, Liu DW. Permissive hypoxemia/conservative oxygenation strategy: Dr. Jekyll or Mr. Hyde? J Thorac Dis. 2016 May;8(5):748–50.

Hyzy RC. Diagnosis, management, and prevention of pulmonary barotrauma during invasive mechanical ventilation in adults [Internet]. UpToDate. [cited 2017 Sep 8]. Available from: https://www.uptodate.com/contents/diagnosis-management-and-prevention-of-pulmonary-barotrauma-during-invasive-mechanical-ventilation-in-adults.

Hyzy RC, Hidalgo J. Permissive hypercapnia [Internet]. UpToDate. [cited 2017 Sep 8]. Available from: https://www.uptodate.com/contents/ permissive-hypercapnia.

Kacmarek RM, Stoller JK, Heuer AJ, editors. Egan's fundamentals of respiratory care. 11th ed. St Louis (MO): Elsevier/Mosby; c2017. 1,392 p.

Luecke T, Pelosi P. Clinical review: positive end-expiratory pressure and cardiac output. Crit Care. 2005;9(6):607–21. Epub 2005 Oct 18.

Marini JJ. Dynamic hyperinflation and auto-positive end-expiratory pressure: lessons learned over 30 years. Am J Respir Crit Care Med. 2011 Oct 1;184(7):756–62.

Matthewman MC, Down J. Mechanical ventilation for the non-anaesthetist 1: physiology and mechanics. Br J Hosp med (Lond). 2018 Dec;79(12):C188–92.

Pierson DJ. Patient-ventilator interaction. Respir Care. 2011 Feb;56(2):214–28.

Sassoon CSh. Triggering of the ventilator in patient-ventilator interactions. Respir Care. 2011 Jan;56(1):39–51.

Smith ER, Amin-Hanjani S. Evaluation and management of elevated intracranial pressure in adults [Internet]. UpToDate. [cited 2017 Sep 8]. Available from: https://www.uptodate.com/contents/evaluation-and-management-of-elevated-intracranial-pressure-in-adults?source=search_result&search=cushings triad&selectedTitle=1~26#H34.

Subira C, de Haro C, Magrans R, Fernandez R, Blanch L. Respir Care. 2018 Apr;63(4):464–78. Erratum in Respir Care. 2019 Mar;64(3): e1.

3 Mechanical Ventilation: Advanced Modes

AMELIA A. LOWELL, RRT, RCP; BHAVESH M. PATEL, MD

Goals

- Describe indications for advanced mechanical ventilator modes, and describe their limitations.
- Describe advanced ventilator modes and engineering principles.
- Describe adjunctive monitoring and therapies for patients with acute respiratory disease who are undergoing mechanical ventilation.

Introduction

Chapter 2 ("Mechanical Ventilation: Basic Modes") discusses the 3 basic ventilator modes (assist control, intermittent mandatory ventilation, and continuous spontaneous ventilation), the 2 breath types (mandatory and spontaneous), and the 2 methods of breath delivery (volume controlled and pressure controlled). The present chapter focuses on advanced modes and modalities of therapy for patients receiving mechanical ventilation. The term *advanced* must be interpreted with caution because many of the newer modes of ventilation do not have substantial evidence of superiority to the basic modes of ventilation for patient outcomes. Rather, *advanced* refers to the engineering controls.

Dual-Control Ventilation

The advantage of volume-controlled breath delivery is that the operator can control the tidal volume and minute ventilation. The advantage of pressure-controlled breath delivery is that the operator can control the total airway pressure and inspiratory time, and the patient benefits from a variable flow pattern, which can be more comfortable. Dual-control ventilation combines the benefits of controlling airway pressure, delivering a target tidal volume, and using a variable flow rate.

Adaptive Pressure Control

Ventilator manufacturers use various names for breath-to-breath dual-control modes, such as the following: pressure-regulated volume control (SERVO-i ventilator; MAQUET Cardiovascular, LLC); VC+ (Puritan Bennett 840 ventilator; Medtronic); adaptive pressure ventilation (Hamilton-G5 ventilator; Hamilton Medical); and auto-flow (Dräger ventilators; Draeger, Inc). Regardless of the terminology, though, the clinician selects a target tidal volume, and the ventilator adjusts the driving pressure (within the range set by the clinician) to deliver that volume. The ventilator provides the lowest pressure needed to deliver the target tidal volume and adjusts the pressure according to measurements of lung mechanics, including dynamic compliance. If the applied pressure delivers a tidal volume that is lower than the target, the ventilator increases the pressure; if the tidal volume is higher than the target, the ventilator decreases the pressure. The main difference between ventilator designs is the algorithm by which the pressure is changed. For example, the VC+ increases or decreases the pressure by 3 cm H_2O breath to breath.

The benefit of breath-to-breath dual control is that the ventilator makes changes according to the patient's dynamic work of breathing and lung compliance. The disadvantage is that if the patient's work of breathing increases and the muscular inspiratory effort increases, the tidal volume tends to increase. In response to the increased tidal volume, which is not due to improved lung compliance, the ventilator decreases the driving pressure, which increases the work of breathing, and the cycle continues. Therefore, the clinician must closely monitor the driving pressure to determine whether the ventilator response is appropriate.

These modes have several advantages: They provide more stable gas exchange than pressure control ventilation, they provide better patient-ventilator synchrony than conventional volume control ventilation, and they probably require less human time at the bedside to ensure that the patient's ventilatory demands are met. However, there is no clear evidence that these modes improve patient outcomes.

Advanced Closed-Loop Ventilation

Achieving patient-ventilator synchrony is a constant struggle and is rarely completely achieved. Integrating the ventilator with sophisticated software to monitor and adjust to dynamic changes in the patient's lung compliance, elastance, and effort has the potential to vastly improve ventilation so that it not only facilitates gas exchange but also avoids lung injury and improves synchrony. However, there is little evidence to support the use of advanced closed-loop modes, and superiority has not been demonstrated for any mode.

Neurally Adjusted Ventilatory Assist

Neurally Adjusted Ventilatory Assist (NAVA) is a proprietary mode of ventilation on the SERVO-i ventilator that uses a nasogastric catheter to detect the electrical activity of the diaphragm and assist the patient's breathing. It can be applied to noninvasive and invasive mechanical ventilation. The proposed advantage of NAVA is that the ventilator coordinates the initiation of the breath with the patient's neuromuscular effort and thereby improves patient-ventilator synchrony. Another advantage is that breath triggering is not affected by air leaks or auto–positive end-expiratory pressure (PEEP). Two electromyographic electrodes are placed on either side of the patient's diaphragm. The signal can be used to initiate the breath or monitor the discrepancy between neuromuscular effort and ventilator output. A potential issue with using the electrical activity of the diaphragm as the main triggering mechanism is faulty nasogastric catheter placement or faulty electrode placement. The first large randomized controlled trial of NAVA in acute respiratory distress syndrome (ARDS), the NAVA in Acute Respiratory Failure (NAVIATOR) trial, is underway and will help determine the role of NAVA in ventilator management. The existing evidence suggests that NAVA can help improve patient-ventilator synchrony, decrease sedation, and improve sleep quality and patient comfort scores.

Proportional Assist Ventilation

Proportional assist ventilation software on the Puritan Bennett 840 ventilator is based on the concept of patient-driven ventilation that was first described in the early 1990s. The software couples neuroventilatory demand with ventilator output by using the respiratory equation of motion, which accounts for the compliance and elastance of the lung and the patient's effort and generates a proportional driving pressure. The operator does not preset the pressure, flow, or volume. Instead, the clinician sets the target level of assistance (percentage of support) according to the workload that a patient must overcome to breathe. For example, at 75% support, the ventilator performs 75% of the work to deliver a breath and the patient performs 25%. Work of breathing is measured in Joules per liter and reflects the change in pressure for a given volume per breath. The clinician can monitor the patient's work of breathing and adjust ventilator support according to the goals of care. It is indicated only for patients who are breathing spontaneously and have an ideal body weight greater than 25 kg. It is contraindicated if a patient has respiratory depression from either sedation or other causes and if a patient has a bronchocutaneous fistula or pleural leak.

Adaptive Support Ventilation

Adaptive Support Ventilation is a proprietary mode of ventilation (Hamilton Medical). It is a closed-loop ventilation that uses positive or negative feedback from measurements of respiratory mechanics to adjust the level of support that the patient receives. The clinician sets the percentage of minute volume (25%-350%) that the ventilator will target according to patient height and disease type, the upper pressure limit to deliver a breath, PEEP, and fraction of inspired oxygen. The ventilator adjusts the level of support depending on the patient's physiologic conditions and uses existing modes to support the patient. For example, if the patient's respiratory rate is higher than the calculated target (based on the percentage of minute volume target), the ventilator uses pressure support ventilation; if the patient is apneic, the ventilator switches to pressure control ventilation and uses synchronized intermittent mandatory ventilation when the patient's respiratory rate is lower than the target. The ventilator changes are based on the Otis equation, which states that for a given level of alveolar ventilation, there is an optimal respiratory rate for reduced work of breathing. Additionally, the percentage of minute volume, ideal body weight, and disease phenotype determine the target tidal volume to which the ventilator adjusts the driving pressure for achieving the target.

Acute Respiratory Distress Syndrome

Various new strategies to improve gas exchange and protect the lungs have emerged for managing the ventilator in patients with ARDS.

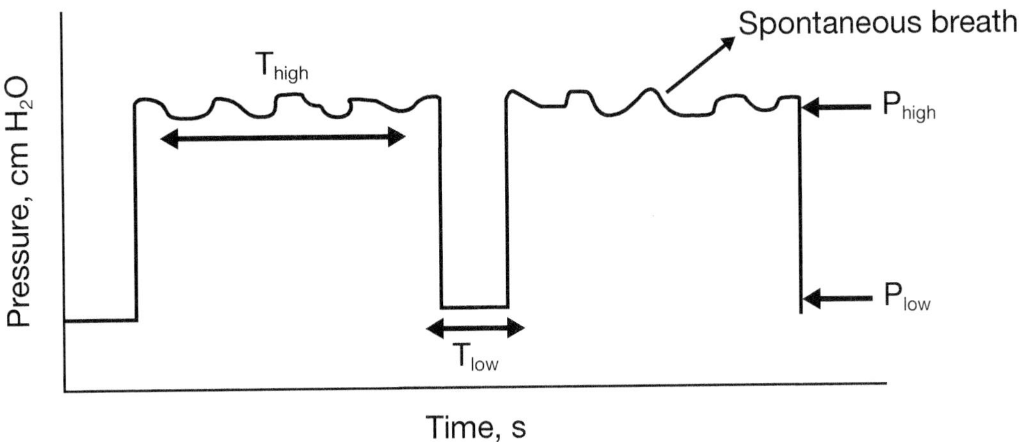

Figure 3.1. Pressure-Time Curve for Airway Pressure Release Ventilation. During the long inspiratory time (T_{high}), the driving pressure is high (P_{high}); during the short expiratory release time (T_{low}), the pressure applied is low (P_{low}). (From Daoud EG. Airway pressure release ventilation. Ann Thorac Med. 2007 Oct;2[4]:176-9; used with permission.)

Airway Pressure Release Ventilation

Airway pressure release ventilation (APRV) is an evolution of inverse-ratio ventilation that uses a long inspiratory time (T_{high}) and a short expiratory release time (T_{low}). The driving pressure during T_{high} is called P_{high}, and the pressure applied during T_{low} is called P_{low} (Figure 3.1). This is similar to setting the ventilator in pressure control mode with an applied driving pressure (pressure control setting) and an applied PEEP. The main difference is that during T_{high}, P_{low} plateaus and the patient triggers spontaneous breaths during T_{high}. Functionally, the ventilator allows the patient to breathe at a high continuous positive airway pressure for the set time and then decreases the pressure during T_{low}. The T_{low} facilitates ventilation (carbon dioxide removal) while limiting full exhalation and thus creating auto-PEEP and improving alveolar recruitment.

Clinicians and ventilator manufacturers use various settings, which are collectively called APRV. Two categories of strategies have been defined: fixed APRV and personalized APRV. Fixed APRV uses a T_{high} (<90% total cycle time) and a fixed T_{low}. In personalized APRV, the T_{low} is adjusted by analyzing the slope of the expiratory flow curve and the P_{low} is set at 0 cm H_2O (Figure 3.2). In a review of 30 years of data from using various methods of applying APRV, there was no statistically significant worse outcome when APRV was used instead of other conventional modes of mechanical ventilation. Personalized APRV has been shown to stabilize alveoli and decrease the incidence of ARDS in clinically relevant animal models and in trauma patients. The hemodynamic effects of high ventilation pressures and hypercapnia must be monitored for successful application of this mode.

Recruitment Maneuvers

A recruitment maneuver is the application of airway pressure for increasing transpulmonary pressure transiently to facilitate the opening of collapsed alveoli and improve gas exchange. Various techniques are used, but a definitive conclusion on the best method has not been reached. All maneuvers involve increasing the PEEP; some accomplish this by incrementally increasing PEEP, and others increase it quickly to reach a high PEEP (≥30 cm H_2O) and hold it for a short period. In the Alveolar Recruitment for Acute Respiratory Distress Syndrome Trial (ART), investigators found an increase in 28-day mortality when recruitment maneuvers were used instead of standard ARDS Network protocols. This finding confirmed that lung-protective ventilation is the standard of care for ARDS patients, and recruitment maneuvers should not be performed routinely.

Prone Position

In supine hospitalized patients, the dorsal pleural pressure is increased because of the weight of the heart, abdominal viscera, and ventral lungs (which is even greater with ARDS). While the dorsal alveoli are collapsed, the gravitational vascular pressure gradient improves perfusion to this region and produces a low-ventilation–high-perfusion mismatch and shunt manifesting as hypoxemia. Historically, prone positioning was reserved as a final effort to improve oxygenation but was not associated with improved mortality. In the landmark Prone Positioning in Severe ARDS (PROSEVA) trial, mortality decreased when patients were placed in a prone position soon after they were assigned to the prone group and for at least 16 consecutive hours. Current guidelines support prone positioning for more than 12 hours a day for patients with severe ARDS (Figure 3.3).

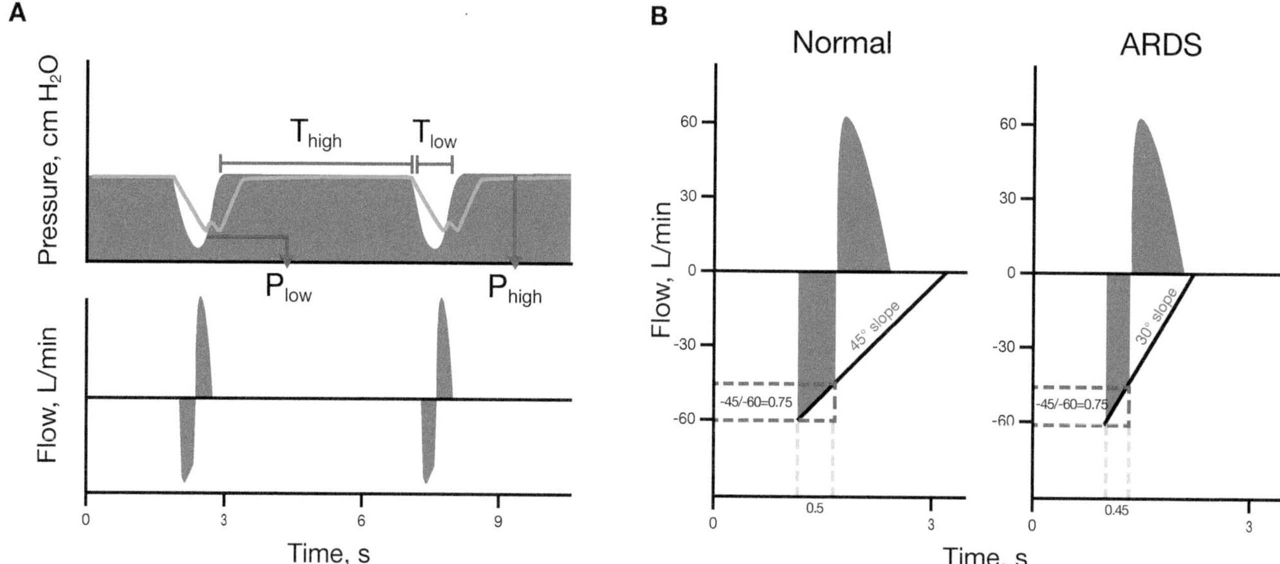

Figure 3.2. Strategies for Setting Expiratory Duration (T_{low}). A, Airway pressure release ventilation pressure-time and flow-time curves show short release phase (T_{low}), time at high pressure (T_{high}), pressure at inspiration (P_{high}), and pressure at expiration (P_{low}). With a short T_{low}, P_{low} never reaches 0 cm H_2O (measured as tracheal pressure and indicated by the green line). B, In acute respiratory distress syndrome (ARDS), the rate of lung collapse is more rapid than in normal lungs, as indicated by the steeper slope.

(From Jain SV, Kollisch-Singule M, Sadowitz B, Dombert L, Satalin J, Andrews P, et al. The 30-year evolution of airway pressure release ventilation [APRV]. Intensive Care Med Exp. 2016 Dec;4[1]:11. Epub 2016 May 20; used under Creative Common Attribution License [http://creativecommons.org/licenses/by/2.0/].)

Clinicians have been deterred from timely use of the prone position by logistic challenges, including physically turning or placing the patient on a rotating bed while maintaining the airway and vascular access devices. Patients usually have an increased amount of oral secretions and a higher risk of endotracheal tube obstruction and pressure ulcers, all of which can be managed with careful monitoring. Patients who should be excluded are those with ocular, facial, or neck trauma; spinal instability; recent sternotomy or large ventral surface burn; increased intracranial pressure (ICP); massive hemoptysis; or high risk of requiring cardiopulmonary resuscitation or defibrillation. Hemodynamic monitoring and the phlebostatic axis should be adjusted for the ventral position of the right atrium.

Extracorporeal Life Support

When conventional mechanical ventilation does not adequately facilitate gas exchange without inducing further organ injury, or if total heart failure is recognized, extracorporeal life support may be used. Extracorporeal life support facilitates gas exchange outside the body by passing blood through a membrane that can oxygenate the blood or remove carbon dioxide from the blood by using the native circulation or pump-driven blood flow. Mechanical ventilation may continue to be required to meet oxygenation and ventilation requirements. The general strategy for selecting ventilator settings during extracorporeal membrane oxygenation is to maintain global oxygen delivery while using lung-protective and right ventricular protective strategies: maintaining ultra-low tidal volumes (4 mL/kg ideal body weight), low respiratory rates (10 breaths per minute), moderate PEEP (10 cm H_2O), and relatively low plateau pressure (<25 cm H_2O). In general, challenges include selecting and locating the cannula, providing anticoagulation, being aware of drug circuit interactions, and maintaining blood protective flows while optimizing regional delivery of oxygen to organs.

Esophageal Pressure Monitoring

The best estimate of alveolar distending pressure is the plateau pressure obtained during an end-inspiratory pause. The plateau pressure provides information on static lung compliance, guides ventilator management to decrease driving pressures, and is the hallmark of risk reduction in ARDS (by maintaining plateau pressure <30 cm H_2O). However, the value of this measurement is limited because it estimates the pressure in the alveoli but does not directly measure it. A more accurate measurement of the amount of pressure required to open the lung is *transpulmonary pressure*, which can be measured indirectly with an

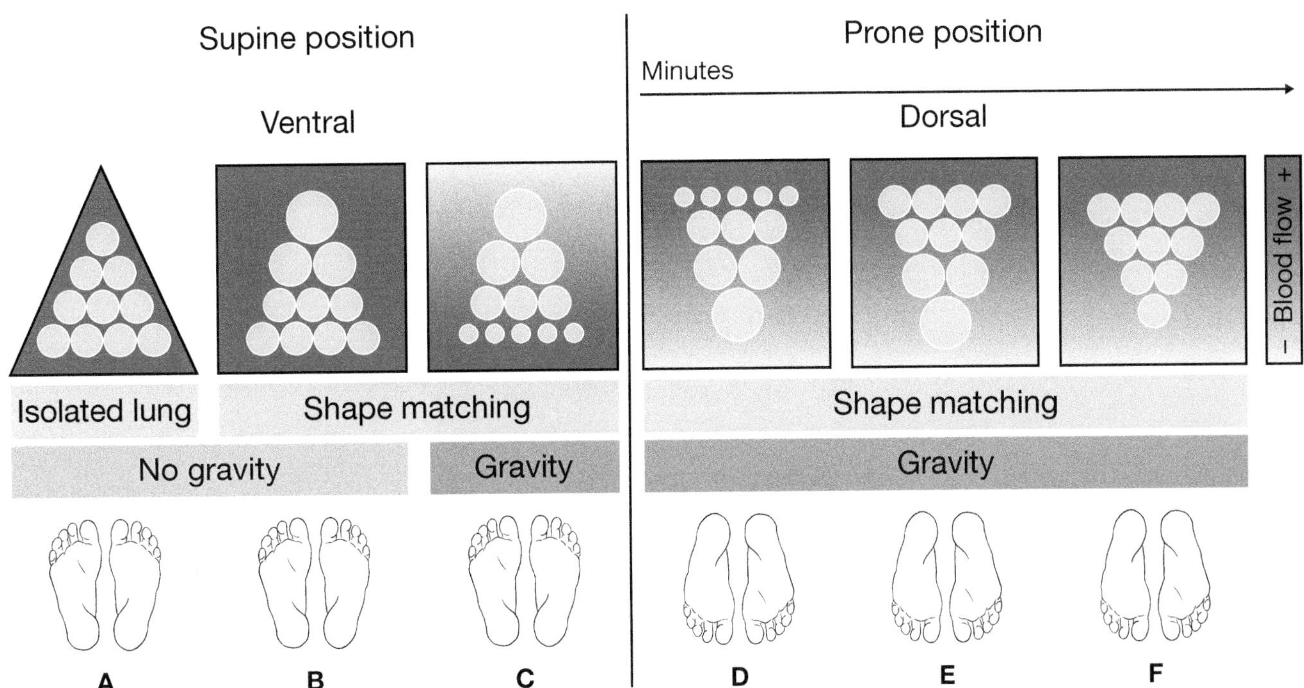

Figure 3.3. Effects of Prone Positioning on Diseased Lungs in a Patient With Acute Respiratory Distress Syndrome. A, Original shape (dorsal side is larger). B, Alveolar units are larger ventrally. C, Gravity affects ventilation and perfusion. D, Immediately after patient is placed in prone position, pulmonary blood flow in dorsal regions is unchanged. E, Dorsal regions of lungs are recruited (more than ventral derecruitment), and ventral regions are compressed (but compressive effects are dampened by shape matching). F, Oxygenation improves as transpulmonary pressure and regional inflation distribution become more homogeneous.

(From Koulouras V, Papathanakos G, Papathanasiou A, Nakos G. Efficacy of prone position in acute respiratory distress syndrome patients: a pathophysiology-based review. World J Crit Care Med. 2016 May 4;5[2]:121-36.)

esophageal catheter. Transpulmonary pressure is the difference between alveolar pressure and pleural pressure. Esophageal pressure is the surrogate for pleural pressure and can be measured continuously or during an end-inspiratory or end-expiratory hold. The esophageal pressure is the amount of pressure applied outside the lung and accounts for extrathoracic causes of increased airway pressure such as abdominal distention, obesity, and pregnancy.

$$\text{Transpulmonary Pressure} = P_{alv} - P_{es}$$

Monitoring of P_{es} allows more accurate titration of PEEP, measurement of tidal volumes and inspiratory pressures, assessment of lung recruitment ability, and management of patient-ventilator synchrony (autotriggering, ineffective triggers, and trigger delays). Evidence supports the use of P_{es} in patients with ARDS to guide PEEP titration and improve oxygenation.

High-Frequency Oscillatory Ventilation

High-frequency oscillatory ventilation differs from conventional mechanical ventilation in that it uses an oscillatory pump to deliver a fast respiratory rate measured in hertz (up to 900 breaths per minute) in an intubated patient. The purpose is to recruit alveoli and hold them open at a constant mean airway pressure with a low tidal volume (also called *amplitude*). The respiratory rate (in hertz) is set directly while the mean airway pressure is set by adjusting the flow rate and expiratory back-pressure valve. The amplitude is determined by the hertz setting and the size of the endotracheal tube. After being evaluated in adults in 6 randomized controlled trials, high-frequency oscillatory ventilation is not recommended for use in patients who have moderate or severe ARDS because the trials showed either no benefit or serious patient harm.

Nitric Oxide

Inhaled nitric oxide has been used for decades to treat persistent pulmonary hypertension in neonates, which is the only indication for its use approved by the US Food and Drug Administration. When inhaled directly, nitric oxide, a selective pulmonary vasodilator, dilates the pulmonary vasculature that it contacts by increasing the concentration of cyclic guanosine monophosphate through the action of

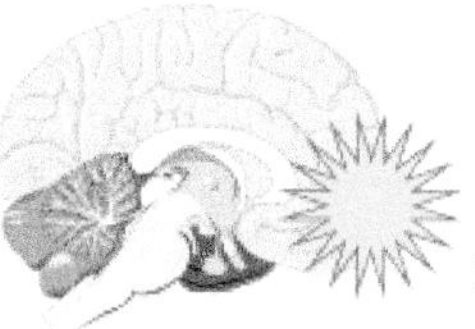

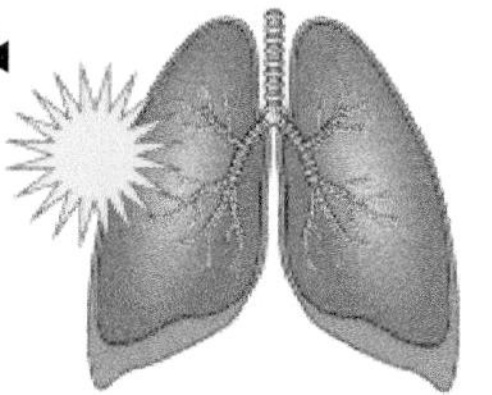

Figure 3.4. Interactions Between the Brain and Lungs in Critically Ill Patients Receiving Mechanical Ventilation. *(From Blanch L, Quintel M. Lung-brain cross talk in the critically ill. Intensive Care Med. 2017 Apr;43[4]:557-9. Epub 2016 Oct 6; used with permission.)*

guanylate cyclase. It is rapidly scavenged by hemoglobin, thereby decreasing its systemic vasodilatory effect. It is delivered through a proprietary system, the INOmax DS_{IR} (Mallinckrodt Pharmaceutical), which monitors oxygen, nitric oxide, and nitrogen dioxide levels and can be used through a mechanical ventilation circuit, high-flow nasal cannula or oxygen mask, or low-flow nasal cannula. It is used in patients who have ARDS with hypoxemic respiratory failure, in patients with right-sided heart failure (as an afterload reduction agent), in conjunction with ventricular assist device placement, and with heart or lung (or heart and lung) transplant despite lack of supporting evidence. The only well-established use in adults is for vasodilator challenges. In patients with ARDS, inhaled nitric oxide improves oxygenation and ventilation-perfusion matching, but it has not been shown to improve survival at any time point in any patient population.

Special Considerations for Patients With Neurologic Disease

Respiratory failure is the most common complication in traumatic brain injury, occurring in 20% to 25% of patients, and acute lung injury is increasingly described as a systemic complication of severe head injury that negatively affects outcomes. Massively increased sympathetic activity and the flood of inflammatory molecules have been proposed as mechanistic causes of lung injury and may render the lung more susceptible to the negative effects of mechanical ventilation (also called the double hit model). When patients with brain injury require mechanical ventilation, the clinician must balance what is good for the lungs with what is good for the brain (Figure 3.4).

Intrathoracic Pressure

The intrathoracic pressure (ITP) during positive pressure ventilation is the pressure required to deliver a tidal volume (either directly controlled as pressure control ventilation or indirectly applied as volume control ventilation) and the amount of PEEP applied to the end of exhalation. Maintenance of peak pressures less than 35 cm H_2O and plateau pressures less than 30 cm H_2O helps protect the lungs from barotrauma and volutrauma (pneumothorax, acute lung injury, and ARDS). Additionally, excess driving pressure has been linked to increased mortality among patients with ARDS. The patient with brain injury is more susceptible to lung damage because of the double hit phenomenon. Use of high PEEP is an important strategy to maintain open lungs and to improve oxygenation in respiratory failure and lung injury. The direct effect of high ITP has been shown to have a clinically insignificant effect on ICP and cerebral perfusion pressure despite the level of lung injury. However, evidence indicates that PEEP applied to lungs with normal pulmonary compliance is associated with increased ITP, decreased right atrial filling, and decreased cardiac output and mean arterial pressure (possibly from decreasing cerebral perfusion pressure). This is not necessarily true for noncompliant lungs because ITP is not transmitted to the cerebral vasculature as easily.

Patients must be monitored for the occurrence of the following mechanisms by which ITP may affect the brain: 1) PEEP increases ITP, which decreases venous return to the heart and increases jugular venous pressure, potentially increasing cerebral blood volume and ICP. 2) Decreased venous return can decrease cardiac output and mean arterial pressure, resulting in decreased cerebral perfusion pressure leading to cerebral vasodilatation and potentially increasing ICP when cerebral autoregulation is also impaired from brain injury. 3) ITP can be directly transmitted to the intracranial vasculature through the jugular vein and superior vena cava.

Partial Pressure of Arterial Carbon Dioxide

A potent mediator of cerebral vascular dilatation and relaxation, $Paco_2$ has a profound effect on cerebral blood flow and ICP. Hypercapnia causes cerebral vasodilatation and increased intracranial volume with increased ICP and decreased cerebral perfusion. Managing hypercapnia is challenging in patients with lung injury, and often permissive hypercapnia is tolerated to avoid lung overdistention and ventilator-induced lung injury. The balance between managing lung injury and brain injury can be challenging, and ICP monitoring should be instituted if feasible.

Hypocapnia directly vasoconstricts the cerebral vasculature and can decrease ICP. Hyperventilation (target $Paco_2$, 30-35 mm Hg) can be used for a short duration (15-30 minutes) as a temporizing treatment to decrease ICP after traumatic brain injury or after any condition where ICP is known to be high or suspected to be high. However, excessive hyperventilation ($Paco_2$ <30 mm Hg or long duration) is not recommended and can be harmful. Cerebral vasoconstriction decreases cerebral blood flow and can worsen secondary brain injury and brain ischemia.

Supportive Care

Suctioning

Suctioning of the endotracheal tube is an essential component of caring for a patient receiving mechanical ventilation. Some evidence suggests that suctioning can transiently but markedly increase ICP in patients with traumatic brain injury. Caution must be exercised if patients have an increased ICP (or are suspected of having an increased ICP), and the risks and benefits should be assessed before treating with suction. Additionally, patients should be well oxygenated before suctioning to avoid oxygen desaturation.

Patient Positioning

Elevating the head of the bed to 30° and maintaining a neutral head position can help decrease ICP and maintain cerebral perfusion pressure. The lateral position should be used with caution. Elevating the head of the bed is consistent with recommendations for reducing the development of ventilator-associated pneumonia.

Recommendations for positioning patients with unilateral lung disease include using the lateral position with the healthy lung down to promote ventilation-perfusion matching and improve oxygenation. Making the decision to use the lateral position in patients with unilateral lung disease and brain injury involves assessing the degree of brain injury, including ICP and cerebral perfusion pressure, and the degree of hypoxemia and weighing the risks and benefits of doing so.

As previously mentioned, prone positioning is recommended for the management of ARDS but is contraindicated for patients with increased ICP.

In the supine position, the internal jugular veins can be compressed; thus, caution should be used in patients at risk for increased ICP.

Cerebrospinal Fluid Movement

Movement of cerebrospinal fluid is influenced by respirophasic tides of cerebral venous drainage, which is largely influenced by thoracic pressure and right-sided heart compliance and function. In normal breathing, deep inhalation causes a cephalad movement of cerebrospinal fluid and a corresponding caudad movement during deep exhalation (in accordance with the Monro-Kellie doctrine). The implications of this could be applied to the introduction of high intrathoracic pressures during positive pressure ventilation and alteration of breathing patterns (such as in APRV) and could alter the natural regulation of ICP.

Summary

- Mechanical ventilation is complex, and choosing the mode involves an assessment of the patient's needs and the goals of care.
- Advanced modes couple engineering controls with sophisticated knowledge of physiology, enabling clinicians to address patient-ventilator synchrony and therapeutic treatment of lung disease.
- What truly makes a mode more advanced is the critical knowledge of how to apply it for a specific need and the ability to monitor the effect on the patient.

- Use of nonmechanical therapeutic interventions and monitoring tools that give more physiologic information should be considered.
- Understanding and recognizing the specific interactions and potential conflict between mechanical ventilation management and cerebrospinal fluid dynamics is critical in the treatment of neurocritical care patients.

SUGGESTED READING

Agency for Healthcare Research and Quality [Internet]. Daily care processes guide for reducing ventilator-associated events in mechanically ventilated patients. AHRQ Pub No. 16(17)-0018-3-EF, January 2017 [cited 2018 Jun 19]. Available from: https://www.ahrq.gov/sites/default/files/wysiwyg/professionals/quality-patient-safety/hais/tools/mvp/modules/technical/daily-care-processes-guide.pdf.

Akoumianaki E, Maggiore SM, Valenza F, Bellani G, Jubran A, Loring SH, et al; PLUG Working Group (Acute Respiratory Failure Section of the European Society of Intensive Care Medicine). The application of esophageal pressure measurement in patients with respiratory failure. Am J Respir Crit Care Med. 2014 Mar 1;189(5):520–31.

Amato MB, Meade MO, Slutsky AS, Brochard L, Costa EL, Schoenfeld DA, et al. Driving pressure and survival in the acute respiratory distress syndrome. N Engl J Med. 2015 Feb 19;372(8):747–55.

Ambrosino N, Rossi A. Proportional assist ventilation (PAV): a significant advance or a futile struggle between logic and practice? Thorax. 2002 Mar;57(3):272–6.

Boone MD, Jinadasa SP, Mueller A, Shaefi S, Kasper EM, Hanafy KA, et al. The effect of positive end-expiratory pressure on intracranial pressure and cerebral hemodynamics. Neurocrit Care. 2017 Apr;26(2):174–81.

Branson RD, Chatburn RL. Controversies in the critical care setting. Should adaptive pressure control modes be utilized for virtually all patients receiving mechanical ventilation? Respir Care. 2007 Apr;52(4):478–85.

Chatburn RL, Mireles-Cabodevila E. Closed-loop control of mechanical ventilation: description and classification of targeting schemes. Respir Care. 2011 Jan;56(1):85–102.

Dreha-Kulaczewski S, Konopka M, Joseph AA, Kollmeier J, Merboldt KD, Ludwig HC, et al. Respiration and the watershed of spinal CSF flow in humans. Sci Rep. 2018 Apr 4;8(1):5594.

Fan E, Del Sorbo L, Goligher EC, Hodgson CL, Munshi L, Walkey AJ, et al; American Thoracic Society, European Society of Intensive Care Medicine, and Society of Critical Care Medicine. An official American Thoracic Society/European Society of Intensive Care Medicine/Society of Critical Care Medicine Clinical Practice guideline: mechanical ventilation in adult patients with acute respiratory distress syndrome. Am J Respir Crit Care Med. 2017 May 1;195(9):1253–63. Erratum in: Am J Respir Crit Care Med. 2017 Jun 1;195(11):1540.

George I, Xydas S, Topkara VK, Ferdinando C, Barnwell EC, Gableman L, et al. Clinical indication for use and outcomes after inhaled nitric oxide therapy. Ann Thorac Surg. 2006 Dec;82(6):2161–9.

Guerin C, Reignier J, Richard JC, Beuret P, Gacouin A, Boulain T, et al; PROSEVA Study Group. Prone positioning in severe acute respiratory distress syndrome. N Engl J Med. 2013 Jun 6;368(23):2159–68. Epub 2013 May 20.

Haddad SH, Arabi YM. Critical care management of severe traumatic brain injury in adults. Scand J Trauma Resusc Emerg Med. 2012 Feb 3;20:12.

Hewitt NA. Lateral positioning for critically ill adult patients: a systematic review [thesis] [Internet]. Victoria (Australia): School of Nursing Faculty of Health, Deakin University. April 2013 [cited 2018 Jun 20]. Available from: https://dro.deakin.edu.au/eserv/DU:30062940/hewitt-lateralpositioning-2013A.pdf.

INOMAX (nitric oxide) for inhalation [Internet]. United Kingdom: Mallinckrodt Pharmaceuticals. c2017 [cited 2018 Jun 6]. Available from: http://inomax.com/about-inomax.

Jain SV, Kollisch-Singule M, Sadowitz B, Dombert L, Satalin J, Andrews P, et al. The 30-year evolution of airway pressure release ventilation (APRV). Intensive Care Med Exp. 2016 Dec;4(1):11. Epub 2016 May 20.

Kinoshita K. Traumatic brain injury: pathophysiology for neurocritical care. J Intensive Care. 2016 Apr 27;4:29.

Klinger JR. Inhaled nitric oxide in adults: biology and indications for use. In: Mandel J, section editor. UpToDate. Waltham (MA): UpToDate; c2018.

Koulouras V, Papathanakos G, Papathanasiou A, Nakos G. Efficacy of prone position in acute respiratory distress syndrome patients: a pathophysiology-based review. World J Crit Care Med. 2016 May 4;5(2):121–36.

Ledwith MB, Bloom S, Maloney-Wilensky E, Coyle B, Polomano RC, Le Roux PD. Effect of body position on cerebral oxygenation and physiologic parameters in patients with acute neurological conditions. J Neurosci Nurs. 2010 Oct;42(5):280–7.

Maissan IM, Dirven PJ, Haitsma IK, Hoeks SE, Gommers D, Stolker RJ. Ultrasonographic measured optic nerve sheath diameter as an accurate and quick monitor for changes in intracranial pressure. J Neurosurg. 2015 Sep;123(3):743–7. Epub 2015 May 8.

Markou N, Myrianthefs P, Malamos P, Ilieskou B, Alamanos I, Paulou E, et al. The effect of lateral positioning on gas exchange and respiratory mechanics in mechanically ventilated patients with unilateral lung disease [abstract]. Crit Care. 2002;6(Suppl 1):P23.

Mascia L, Mazzeo AT. Ventilatory management in head injury patients. Is there any conflict? Trends Anaesth Crit Care. 2011 Jun;1(3):168–74.

O'Croinin D, Ni Chonghaile M, Higgins B, Laffey JG. Bench-to-bedside review: permissive hypercapnia. Crit Care. 2005 Feb;9(1):51–9. Epub 2004 Aug 5.

Patel BM, Sen A, El-Banayosy A. Adult cardiac ECLS acute complication and comorbidity management. In: Brogan TV, Lequier L, Lorusso R, MacLaren G, Peek G, editors. Extracorporeal life support: the ELSO red book. 5th ed. Ann Arbor (MI): Extracorporeal Life Support Organization; c2017. p. 533–49.

Peripheral brain: understanding airway pressure release ventilation [Internet]. [cited 2018 Jun 18]. Available from: https://pbrainmd.wordpress.com/2015/04/17/understanding-airway-pressure-release-ventilation/.

Personalized ventilation with NAVA and Edi [Internet]. [cited 2018 Jan 24]. Available from: https://www.maquet.com/us/products/personalized-ventilation/?tab=downloads.

Proportional Assist Ventilation (PAV) Software [Internet]. Minneapolis (MN): Medtronic. [cited 2018 Aug 15]. Available from: http://www.medtronic.com/covidien/en-us/products/acute-care-ventilation/puritan-bennett-pav-plus-software.html.

Puritan Bennett 980 ventilator system: product training sample practice exercises (breathe more naturally) [Internet]. Boulder (CO): Covidien. c2013. Available from: http://www.covidien.com/imageServer.aspx/doc293914.pdf?contentID=45049&contenttype=application/pdf.

Roberts BW, Karagiannis P, Coletta M, Kilgannon JH, Chansky ME, Trzeciak S. Effects of $Paco_2$ derangements on clinical outcomes after cerebral injury: a systematic review. Resuscitation. 2015 Jun;91:32–41. Epub 2015 Mar 28.

Santos RS, Silva PL, Pelosi P, Rocco PR. Recruitment maneuvers in acute respiratory distress syndrome: the safe way is the best way. World J Crit Care Med. 2015 Nov 4;4(4):278–86.

Scholten EL, Beitler JR, Prisk GK, Malhotra A. Treatment of ARDS with prone positioning. Chest. 2017 Jan;151(1):215–24. Epub 2016 Jul 8.

Sen A, Callisen HE, Alwardt CM, Larson JS, Lowell AA, Libricz SL, et al. Adult venovenous extracorporeal membrane oxygenation for severe respiratory failure: current status and future perspectives. Ann Card Anaesth. 2016 Jan-Mar;19(1):97–111.

van der Staay M, Chatburn RL. Advanced modes of mechanical ventilation and optimal targeting schemes. Intensive Care Med Exp. 2018 Aug;6(1):30.

Writing Group for the Alveolar Recruitment for Acute Respiratory Distress Syndrome Trial (ART) Investigators, Cavalcanti AB, Suzumura EA, Laranjeira LN, Paisani DM, Damiani LP, Guimaraes HP, et al. Effect of lung recruitment and titrated positive end-expiratory pressure (PEEP) vs low peep on mortality in patients with acute respiratory distress syndrome: a randomized clinical trial. JAMA. 2017 Oct 10;318(14):1335–45.

Yamada S, Miyazaki M, Yamashita Y, Ouyang C, Yui M, Nakahashi M, et al. Influence of respiration on cerebrospinal fluid movement using magnetic resonance spin labeling. Fluids Barriers CNS. 2013 Dec 27;10(1):36.

Cardiovascular System in the Critically Ill Patient

JUAN G. RIPOLL SANZ, MD; NORLALAK JIRAMETHEE, MD;
JOSE L. DIAZ-GOMEZ, MD

Goals

- Describe the importance of vascular–cardiac pump coupling as an integrated system.
- Describe practical considerations of ventricular dysfunction.
- Explain how systemic vessels are involved in cardiac output control and fluid responsiveness.

Introduction

This chapter provides an overview of fundamental pathophysiologic concepts for the diagnosis and management of cardiovascular disorders in critically ill patients. Three major topics are presented: 1) the importance of vascular–cardiac pump coupling as an integrated system, 2) practical considerations of ventricular dysfunction, and 3) systemic vessels as a crucial factor for cardiac output (CO) control and fluid responsiveness.

Vascular–Cardiac Pump Coupling

The cardiovascular system is a closed integrated circuit. After blood is oxygenated in the lungs, the blood is pumped from the left ventricle (LV) through the high-pressure, low-volume, low-compliance, and high-resistance arterial system. Subsequently, systemic blood reaches the systemic capillary beds, where the oxygen is consumed and carbon dioxide is generated. In this closed circuit, carbon dioxide is transported to the right side of the heart through a low-pressure, low-resistance, high-volume, and high-compliance venous system.

Cardiac Cycle and Integration of Heart and Blood Vessels

After the LV systolic contraction, a stroke volume (SV) of blood is ejected into the highly resistant arterial system. A substantial portion of the SV remains stored inside the elastic arteries (the aorta and its major branches) (Figure 4.1A). The resultant net effect in the proximal arterial circulation is an increase in the pressure in inverse proportion to the capacitance of the walls of the larger arteries proximal to the resistance vessels.

$$(\text{Capacitance} = \Delta\text{Volume}/\Delta\text{Pressure})$$

At the end of systole, the ventricular systolic pressure is lower than the systemic arterial pressure, which leads to aortic valve closure as represented by the dicrotic notch in the arterial pressure waveform.

During ventricular diastole, the elastic recoil of the arterial wall ensures a continuous capillary flow. The part of the SV stored in the distended arterial bed during systole continues to run off through the peripheral vessels with a progressive decrease in arterial blood pressure (BP) until the next contraction cycle (Figure 4.1B). During this phase, the LV fills according to its diastolic volume-pressure curve while being assisted by 2 mechanisms: 1) the suction effect exerted by the lower end-diastolic pressure and volume and 2) atrial contraction.

The aforementioned interaction of the heart and blood vessels (ie, the fraction of SV stored in the major blood vessels) serves as a reliable mechanism to convert the intermittent and pulsatile nature of the cardiac motion (ie, SV) into an integrated, dynamic and continuous systemic blood flow (ie, CO). Hence, CO and systemic vascular resistance (SVR)

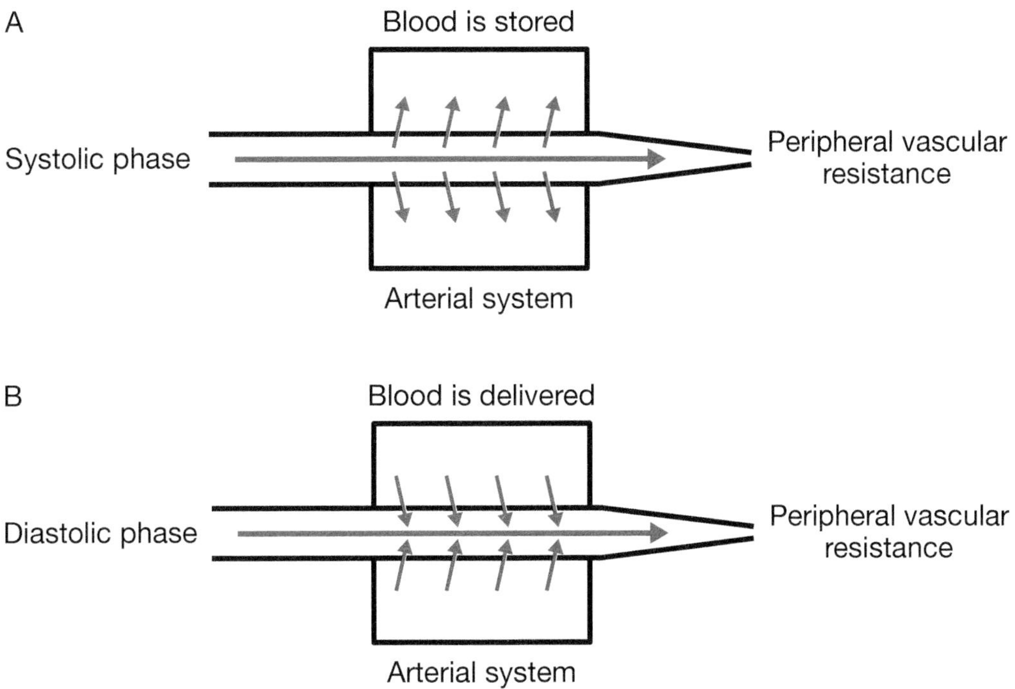

Figure 4.1. Schematic Representation of the Arterial System. A, Blood is stored in the arterial system during ventricular systole. B, Blood is delivered from the arterial system during ventricular diastole.

are the 2 main determinants of systemic BP control (BP = CO × SVR).

Practical Considerations

Performance of the cardiovascular system in critically ill patients can be characterized by interpreting surrogates for diastolic pressure, pulse pressure, and SVR such as skin temperature and capillary refill time (Boxes 4.1 and 4.2).

In healthy persons, the relation between pulse pressure and SV is not quantitative; it is determined with an unknown constant (vascular capacitance). Nevertheless, in critically ill patients, changes in vascular capacitance are usually negligible, so variation in pulse pressure is considered an early and reliable indicator of changes in SV.

Box 4.1 • Clinical Case: Cardiogenic Shock Versus Hypovolemic Shock

> A hypotensive patient has a blood pressure (BP) of 80/60 mm Hg, a heart rate of 115 beats per minute, cold skin, and increased capillary refill time (CRT). The cardiac output (CO) and pulse pressure (PP) are decreased, and the systemic vascular resistance (SVR) is increased. In this patient, the small PP (20 mm Hg) suggests a small stroke volume (and therefore a low CO). Moreover, a high SVR correlates with a preserved diastolic BP (60 mm Hg), increased CRT, and cold skin. The jugular venous pressure allows further differentiation of the type of shock (high in cardiogenic shock and low in hypovolemic shock).

Frank-Starling Curve

An increase in LV end-diastolic pressure (LVEDP) is accompanied by a curvilinear increase (a steep increase at lower filling pressures) in the ventricular performance of the heart. Therefore, at lower filling pressures, the surge in SV is more pronounced than at higher pressures (Figure 4.2).

With no changes in contractility, the volume status is modified. For example, in hypovolemia, the LV end-diastolic volume (LVEDV) is decreased, with a subsequent reduction in the SV and CO (Figure 4.2).

Changes in Contractility With Volume Unchanged

Increased contractility without a change in volume is represented by an upward and leftward shift in the Frank-Starling curve (green curve in Figure 4.2). In contrast, conditions associated with decreased myocardial contractility shift the curve down and to the right (blue curve in Figure 4.2).

Limitations of the Frank-Starling Curve in Estimating LV Function

The ventricular function analysis depicted by the Frank-Starling curve is founded on the contracting and relaxing mechanical properties of the LV. However, this analysis has its own limitations because multiple mechanisms may

Box 4.2 • Clinical Case: Septic Shock

A patient has a blood pressure (BP) of 100/30 mm Hg, a heart rate (HR) of 115 beats per minute, warm skin, and normal capillary refill time (CRT). The cardiac output (CO) and pulse pressure (PP) are increased, and the systemic vascular resistance (SVR) is decreased. The large PP (70 mm Hg) suggests a large stroke volume, which, when multiplied by the increased HR, causes a further increase in CO. Furthermore, a low SVR in the context of a high CO correlates with a low diastolic BP (30 mm Hg), warm skin, and normal CRT.

explain the same data, such as when patients have normal or increased LVEDP but decreased SV (point D in Figure 4.2):

1. Hypertrophic ventricle reducing the LVEDV
2. Reduced cardiac contractility
3. Increased LV afterload (ie, the same stroke work is required to eject a smaller SV)

Ventricular Dysfunction

Diastolic Volume-Pressure Curve: Filling Disorders

The LV transmural pressure does not exceed zero until the intraventricular volume reaches about 50 mL during diastole (unstressed volume) (point A in Figure 4.3). Subsequent addition of blood volume leads to a curvilinear increase in the cardiac pressure (point B in Figure 4.3). At this point, minor changes in LVEDV are reflected as large changes in LVEDP.

The pericardium has a major effect on the volume-pressure dynamics of the LV. It acts as a membrane loosely surrounding the heart at lower volumes and becomes stiffer as LVEDV increases (represented as a steep increase in the diastolic volume-pressure curve).

Acute myocardial ischemia or infarction directly affects ventricular relaxation and causes a leftward and upward shift of the volume-pressure curve (from point E to point F in Figure 4.3). As a consequence, a higher LVEDP is required at any given LVEDV. Indeed, for patients with acute myocardial infarction, an LVEDP pressure as high as 30 mm Hg is required to maintain adequate CO.

Occupation of the pericardial space decreases the venous return (VR) by increasing the pressure in the right atrium, thus keeping the LVEDV and CO low. Similarly, tension pneumothorax, massive pleural effusion, high abdominal pressures, and elevated levels of positive end-expiratory pressure (PEEP) increase the pressure outside the heart and thus decrease the LVEDV and SV even if LVEDP is high. Common causes of diastolic dysfunction in critically ill patients with high left atrial pressure and low LVEDV are presented in Box 4.3.

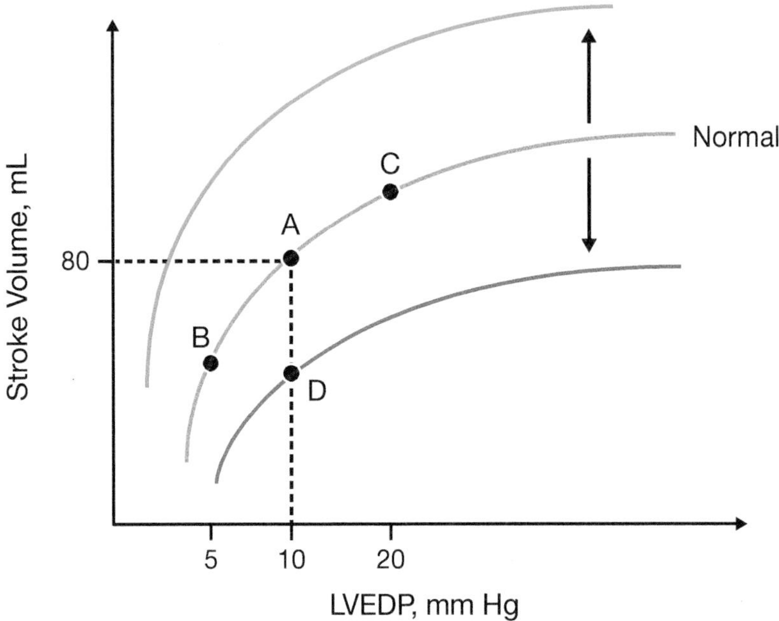

Figure 4.2. Frank-Starling Curves. Stroke volume is the measurable ventricular output in each heartbeat. The left ventricular end-diastolic pressure (LVEDP) is the preload. Myocardial contractility is represented as normal (orange), increased (green), or decreased (blue). See text for details.

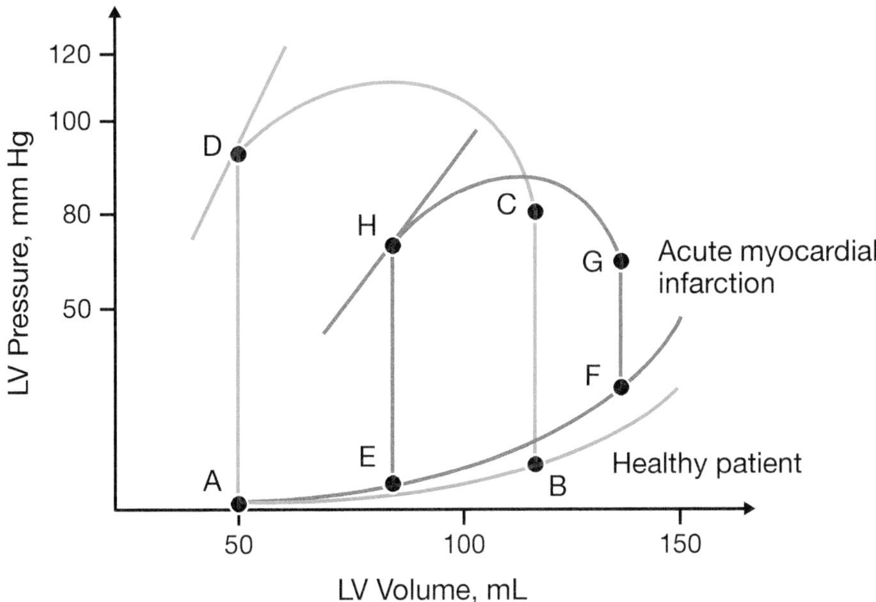

Figure 4.3. Volume-Pressure Curves. Left ventricular (LV) volume-pressure curves are shown for healthy patients (green) and patients with acute myocardial infarction (blue). See text for details.

Systolic Volume-Pressure Curve: LV Contractility

After the diastolic phase is completed, cardiac isovolumetric contraction begins (point B in Figure 4.3). Sufficient LV pressure is generated to open the aortic valve, and the systolic ejection phase begins. At an LVEDP of 10 mm Hg and an LVEDV of 120 mL, the normal heart contracts with the same volume until achieving an LVEDP of 80 mm Hg, allowing the aortic valve to open (point C in Figure 4.3). Blood is then ejected according to the pressure gradient. Finally, systolic pressure decreases from 120 mm Hg (at the beginning of the ejection phase) to 90 mm Hg, with only 50 mL of blood remaining inside the LV (point D in Figure 4.3).

Acute Ventricular Dysfunction: Myocardial Infarction and the Volume-Pressure Curve

Patients with developing acute myocardial infarction have a depressed end-systolic volume-pressure curve with an increased end-systolic volume (90 mL) at a diminished LV end-systolic pressure (75 mm Hg) (point H in Figure 4.3). The diastolic volume-pressure curve is shifted upward and leftward because of diastolic dysfunction (from point E to point F in Figure 4.3). The LVEDV is increased to 130 mL to accommodate the incoming VR and the blood volume not ejected during systole. A resultant increase in LVEDP (from 10 to 30 mm Hg) is apparent on the volume-pressure curve (point F in Figure 4.3). Despite a reflex tachycardia (heart rate 110 beats per minute), both the SV (40 mL) and the CO (4.4 mL/min) are decreased. The net effect is a decrease in blood pressure (90/70 mm Hg) despite a notable increase in SVR.

Systemic Vessels and CO Control

Although CO is the product of SV and heart rate, it is often mistakenly assumed that the heart controls CO. In fact, the systemic vessels control VR. Therefore, the heart is more precisely described as a mechanical pump with systolic and diastolic properties that regulate how VR is accommodated.

Mean systemic pressure (Pms), resistance to VR (RVR), and right atrial pressure (RAP) control VR. This conceptual model emphasizes the importance of capacitance and resistance of the systemic vessels on control of VR, especially through the baroreceptor reflexes.

Mean Systemic Pressure

Pms is the pressure measured when flow ceases within the circulatory system (at 10-15 mm Hg). This pressure is lower than the systemic arterial pressure and is similar to the RAP.

When the flow ceases, blood is drained from the arterial system (a high-pressure, low-volume system) into the venous system (a low-pressure, high-volume system), thereby accommodating the incoming blood with minor changes in pressure. When the right ventricle resumes pumping blood into the lungs, the RAP decreases with respect to the Pms; thus, a driving force suctions additional blood from the venous system into the right atrium. With

Box 4.3 • Common Causes of Diastolic Dysfunction in Critically Ill Patients With High Left Atrial Pressure and Low LVEDV

- External pressure
  - Pericardial effusion
  - Massive pleural effusion
  - PEEP
  - Tension pneumothorax
- Myocardial stiffness
  - Hypertrophic obstructive cardiomyopathy
  - Ischemic heart disease
  - Infiltrative disease
- Ventricular interdependence and right-to-left septal shift
  - Pulmonary hypertension
  - Right ventricular infarction
  - Severe acute respiratory failure
- Ventricular filling defect
  - Clot
  - Tumor
  - Vegetations
- Rhythm or valvular disease
  - Tachycardia
  - Heart block
  - Atrial fibrillation
  - Atrial flutter
  - Mitral stenosis

Abbreviations: LVEDV, left ventricular end-diastolic volume; PEEP, positive end-expiratory pressure.

subsequent heartbeats, the arterial circuit pressure increases considerably above Pms, while the venous system pressure decreases slightly below Pms. This imbalance continues until a steady state is achieved; the arterial system pressure increases sufficiently to drive the SV of each heartbeat through the arterial high-resistance system into the venous reservoir.

In general, Pms changes only slightly between no-flow and continuous-flow (steady state) states because the volume status and the compliance of the vascular system remain intact. Furthermore, it is the volume distribution from the compliant veins to the stiff arteries that is continuously modified, thus creating the driving pressure necessary to sustain a continuous flow inside the circuit.

Pms generates the driving pressure for VR to the right atrium when circulation is restarted. The 2 main mechanisms for increasing Pms while increasing VR are 1) increasing the intravascular volume and 2) decreasing the unstressed volume or compliance (or both) of the venous system. These mechanisms, controlled by baroreceptor reflexes responding to hypotension by increasing the venous tone, usually occur concurrently. The unstressed volume may also be decreased by raising the legs of supine patients or administering venoconstrictors (eg, phenylephrine). Both methods shift a portion of the unstressed volume (from large veins) into the stressed volume, thus increasing the VR and Pms. With increased cardiac contractility or reduced afterload (or both), blood is moved from the central compartment into the stressed volume, thereby increasing Pms and VR and decreasing RAP.

Venous Return

Normal Heart

In a healthy person, with each succeeding heartbeat, RAP decreases below Pms and VR increases. This sequence has been evaluated in relatively controlled conditions, keeping RAP constant while measuring VR (Figure 4.4).

As RAP decreases from 12 to 0 mm Hg (from point A to point B in Figure 4.4), VR progressively increases by the driving pressure generated through the difference between Pms and RAP:

$$\text{Driving Pressure for VR} = \text{Pms} - \text{RAP}$$

The slope of the relation between VR and Pms − RAP is the RVR:

$$\text{RVR} = \Delta(\text{Pms} - \text{RAP}) / \Delta\text{VR}$$

VR does not increase further if RAP decreases to less than zero (point B in Figure 4.4) as the flow becomes impaired when entering the thorax (the pressure in the collapsible great veins decreases below the atmospheric pressure outside them).

In the absence of right-sided heart dysfunction or pulmonary hypertension (or both), LV performance determines RAP and, consequently, VR to the right side of the heart. The corresponding interaction is depicted in Figure 4.4 (blue and red curves). The important considerations are the following: 1) When RAP decreases, CO decreases along the cardiac function curve. 2) When RAP decreases, VR increases until VR equals CO. This occurs where the VR curve and the CO curve intersect (point C in Figure 4.4).

Compensatory Mechanisms in Patients With Intact Cardiovascular Function

When CO is insufficient, the VR can be increased in different ways: 1) Pms can be increased without a change in RVR, which would be depicted as an upward shift of the VR curve (broken blue curve in Figure 4.5). This higher VR curve intersects the cardiac function curve at a higher CO (point D in Figure 4.5). 2) The contractility can be increased, or the afterload can be decreased, which would be depicted as an upward left shift in the

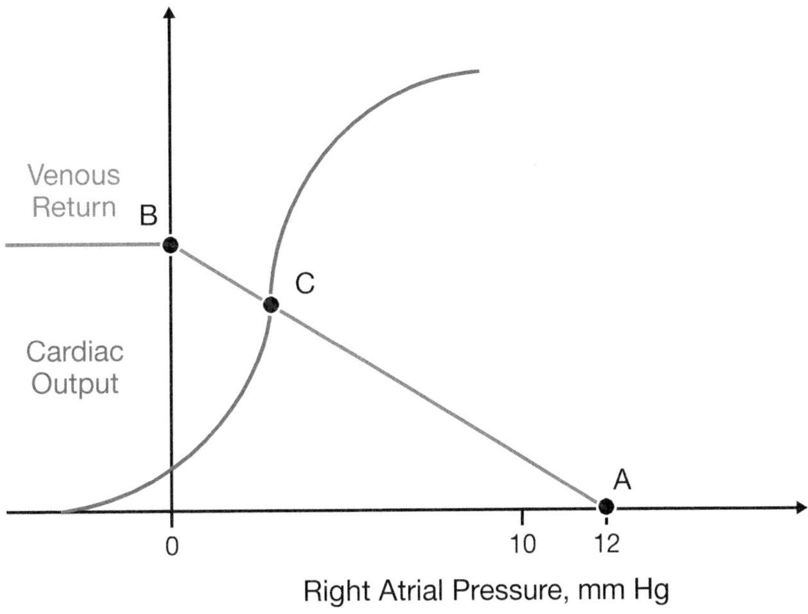

Figure 4.4. Cardiac Output Control by Systemic Vessels in a Healthy Patient. See text for details.

cardiac function curve (broken red curve in Figure 4.5). Therefore, CO increases as RAP increases, and, in this example, increased VR is associated with decreased RAP. In patients with normal cardiac function, profound decreases in RAP cause only slight increases in CO (from point C to point B in Figure 4.5). This concept illustrates why inotropic agents do not help patients with hypovolemic shock.

Pathologic States: Depressed Cardiovascular Function

In patients with depressed cardiac pumping function (broken green line in Figure 4.6), VR initially shifts down (from point A to point B in Figure 4.6) as RAP increases and Pms remains stable. However, to compensate for inadequate cardiac performance, baroreceptor reflexes are activated, resulting in fluid retention, which increases Pms until

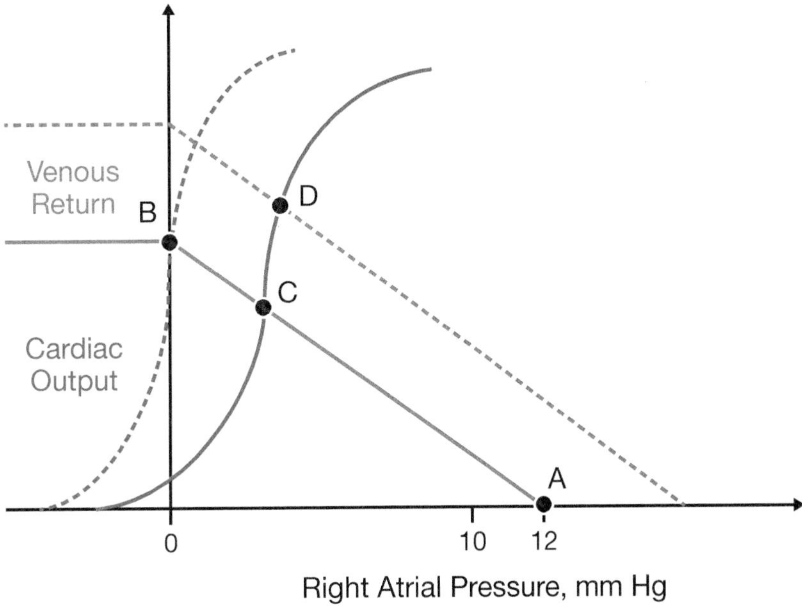

Figure 4.5. Cardiac Output Control by Systemic Vessels Through Compensatory Mechanisms. See text for details.

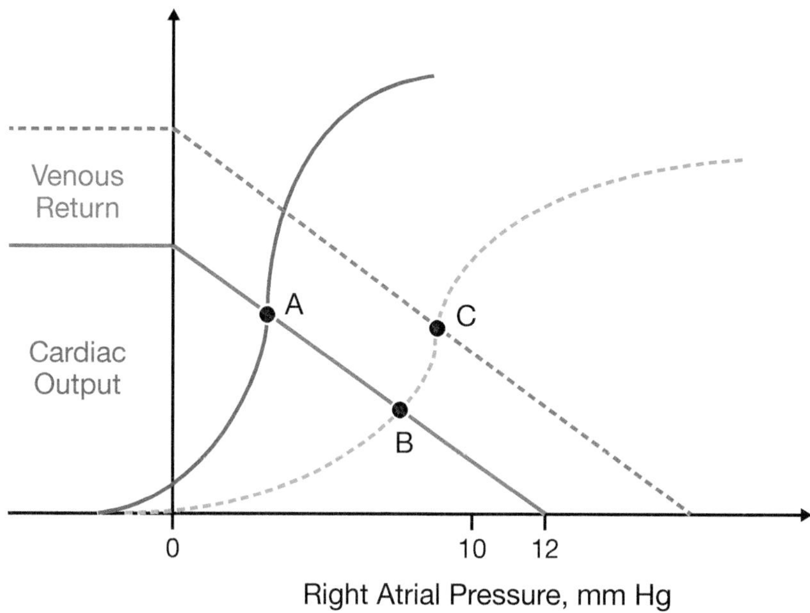

Figure 4.6. Depressed Cardiac Function. Cardiac pumping function is represented as normal (red) or depressed (green). See text for details.

CO returns to baseline (chronic congestive heart failure). Concurrently, RAP increases (from point B to point C in Figure 4.6). As a result, the patient may show signs of right heart failure, such as hepatomegaly, peripheral edema, and jugular venous distention.

Resistance to Venous Return

RVR is a relatively constant variable that changes minimally with adrenergic stimulation. A decrease in RVR (as in sepsis) is accompanied by an increase in CO. Conversely, an increase in RVR (ie, an increase in PEEP during mechanical ventilation) is associated with a decrease in CO.

Effects of Pressure Outside the Heart on CO

The pleural pressure increases under positive-pressure ventilation, thereby increasing the RAP and reducing the VR. The net effect is a decrease in VR but without modifications in cardiac function or Pms. A further increase in PEEP (ie, to 20 cm H_2O) substantially decreases the VR, so that a greater increase in Pms is required to achieve a normal state. Therefore, an increase in RVR with a subsequent decrease in VR due to PEEP is countered by increased Pms.

Effects of PEEP on CO

Patients with increased or normal circulatory volume tolerate high PEEP because their vascular reflexes, which are inactive at baseline, can be used to increase Pms with PEEP when VR is decreased. Conversely, in patients with low circulatory volume, vascular reflexes are activated at baseline and maintain VR through an increase in Pms. If these patients have not received intravascular fluids, they do not tolerate intubation and PEEP well.

Fluid Responsiveness in the Intensive Care Unit

Fluid responsiveness has generally been defined as an improvement in SV or CO by 10% to 15% after a fluid challenge. However, volume status does not equate to fluid responsiveness because it depends on cardiac function (Figure 4.7). Although 2 patients may have the same preload (ie, volume status), a fluid challenge may not result in equal increases in SV because they may not have had the same baseline cardiac function. Hence, the increase in SV is greater in patients with normal ventricular function (from point A to point B in Figure 4.7) than in patients with poor ventricular performance (from point C to point D in Figure 4.7).

Static parameters are measurements of certain hemodynamic parameters at 1 point in time. These parameters are poor predictors of fluid responsiveness. Pulmonary artery occlusion pressure (PAOP) and RAP have the same limitations for predicting fluid responsiveness: poor predictive value and low area under the receiver operating characteristic (ROC) curve. Hence, both RAP and PAOP values between responders and nonresponders overlap and therefore are not useful for predicting response to volume expansion.

In contrast to static parameters, *dynamic parameters* consider hemodynamic measurements of the heart-lung interaction during each respiratory cycle and are more

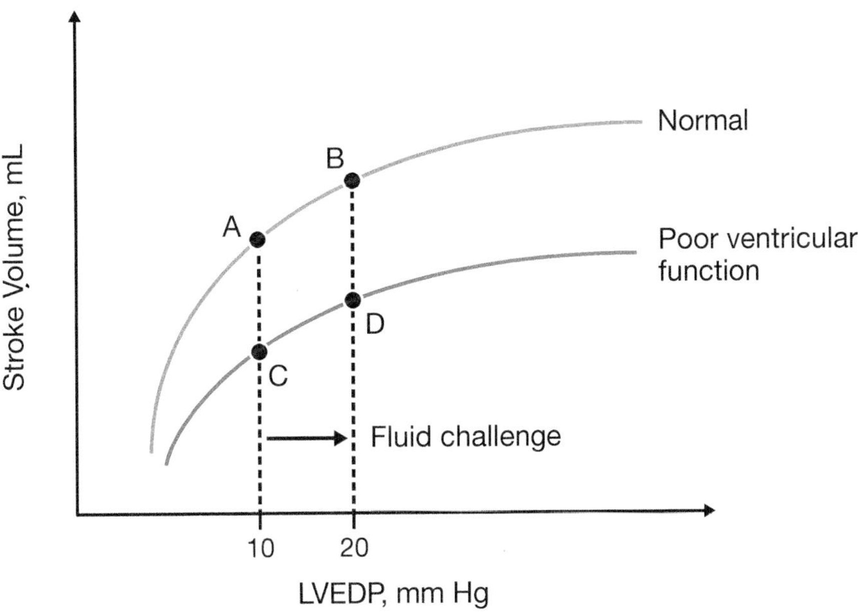

Figure 4.7. Frank-Starling Curve Variations After a Fluid Challenge. Left ventricular end-diastolic pressure (LVEDP) is the preload. Ventricular function is represented as normal (orange) or poor (blue). See text for details.

accurate predictors of fluid responsiveness. An example is *pulse pressure* (PP) *variation* (PPV).

PPV is calculated as follows:

$$\text{PPV} = \left[(\text{Maximum PP} - \text{Minimum PP})/\text{Mean PP}\right] \times 100$$

A threshold of more than 13% correlates with volume responsiveness with an area under the ROC curve of 0.98. Variation in systolic blood pressure (SBP) has also shown good correlation with fluid responsiveness but is less strongly correlated than PPV:

$$\text{SBP Variation} = [(\text{Maximum SBP} - \text{Minimum SBP}) / \text{Mean SBP}] \times 100$$

A median PPV of 12% strongly predicts fluid responsiveness among intensive care unit patients receiving mechanical ventilation (tidal volume >8 mL/kg) if they show no respiratory effort and no evidence of cardiac arrhythmia (Yang and Du, 2014; see Suggested Reading). However, to accurately predict fluid responsiveness, those conditions must be met, which precludes the use of PPV in most critically ill patients.

Among dynamic parameters for predicting fluid responsiveness in mechanically ventilated patients, maximal Doppler velocity in the LV outflow tract had the highest sensitivity for fluid responsiveness, and respirophasic variability of the superior vena cava had the highest specificity (Vignon et al, 2017; see Suggested Reading). These findings were similar for patients with septic shock, sinus rhythm, tidal volume of at least 8 mL/kg, and intra-abdominal pressure less than 12 mm Hg and for patients with hypotension and high lactate unrelated to obstructive or cardiogenic shock.

The hemodynamic measure that can reliably predict volume responsiveness in most critically ill patients is passive leg raising (PLR). PLR shifts fluid toward the central circulation, providing a reversible method of fluid challenge. If CO does not respond to PLR, giving extra fluid should not harm the patient.

Several meta-analyses have compared PLR-induced changes in PPV (mean [SD], 12% [4%]) and CO or its surrogates (Monnet et al, 2016; see Suggested Reading). Performance was superior when changes in CO or its surrogates were used in combination with PLR instead of PPV. PLR has good predictive value even in patients with spontaneous breathing effort or with cardiac arrhythmias.

Summary

- Vascular–cardiac pump coupling should be conceptualized as an integrated system mainly contributing to systemic vessel capacitance and resistance on VR.
- Performance of the cardiovascular system in critically ill patients can be characterized by interpreting surrogates for diastolic pressure, pulse pressure, and SVR such as skin temperature and capillary refill time.
- Pms, RVR, and RAP control VR. This conceptual model emphasizes the importance of capacitance and

resistance of the systemic vessels on control of VR, especially through the baroreceptor reflexes.

- Among dynamic parameters for predicting fluid responsiveness in mechanically ventilated patients, maximal Doppler velocity in the LV outflow tract had the highest sensitivity for fluid responsiveness, and respirophasic variability of the superior vena cava had the highest specificity.

SUGGESTED READING

Argulian E, Windecker S, Messerli FH. Misconceptions and facts about aortic stenosis. Am J Med. 2017 Apr;130(4):398–402. Epub 2017 Jan 18.

Cherpanath TG, Hirsch A, Geerts BF, Lagrand WK, Leeflang MM, Schultz MJ, et al. Predicting fluid responsiveness by passive leg raising: a systematic review and meta-analysis of 23 clinical trials. Crit Care Med. 2016 May;44(5):981–91.

Dalton A, Shahul S. Cardiac dysfunction in critical illness. Curr Opin Anaesthesiol. 2018 Apr;31(2):158–64.

Michard F, Boussat S, Chemla D, Anguel N, Mercat A, Lecarpentier Y, et al. Relation between respiratory changes in arterial pulse pressure and fluid responsiveness in septic patients with acute circulatory failure. Am J Respir Crit Care Med. 2000 Jul;162(1):134–8.

Michard F, Teboul JL. Predicting fluid responsiveness in ICU patients: a critical analysis of the evidence. Chest. 2002 Jun;121(6):2000–8.

Monnet X, Marik P, Teboul JL. Passive leg raising for predicting fluid responsiveness: a systematic review and meta-analysis. Intensive Care Med. 2016 Dec;42(12):1935–47. Epub 2016 Jan 29.

Monnet X, Rienzo M, Osman D, Anguel N, Richard C, Pinsky MR, et al. Passive leg raising predicts fluid responsiveness in the critically ill. Crit Care Med. 2006 May;34(5):1402–7.

Osman D, Ridel C, Ray P, Monnet X, Anguel N, Richard C, et al. Cardiac filling pressures are not appropriate to predict hemodynamic response to volume challenge. Crit Care Med. 2007 Jan;35(1):64–8.

Vignon P, Repesse X, Begot E, Leger J, Jacob C, Bouferrache K, et al. Comparison of echocardiographic indices used to predict fluid responsiveness in ventilated patients. Am J Respir Crit Care Med. 2017 Apr 15;195(8):1022–32.

Yang X, Du B. Does pulse pressure variation predict fluid responsiveness in critically ill patients? A systematic review and meta-analysis. Crit Care. 2014 Nov 27;18(6):650.

Zanger DR, Solomon AJ, Gersh BJ. Contemporary management of angina: part II: medical management of chronic stable angina. Am Fam Physician. 2000 Jan 1;61(1):129–38.

5 Renal Function in Critically Ill Patients

PRAMOD K. GURU, MBBS, MD

Goals

- Understand the basic physiology, pathogenesis, and pattern of kidney injury.
- Understand the diagnostic evaluation of kidney injury and its limitations.
- Recognize renal-specific injury commonly encountered in critically ill patients.

Introduction

Renal function serves as a window into the homeostasis of internal organs, and multiple organ system failure can occur in critically ill patients irrespective of the initial site of insult. Therefore, essential knowledge of renal pathophysiology is crucial in the diagnostic approach and management of critically ill patients. Close interaction between the kidney and other vital organs such as the heart, lungs, and brain is primarily responsible for the morbidity and mortality among critically ill patients. Pathologic renal changes can manifest in various conditions, such as acute kidney injury (AKI), chronic kidney disease, glomerulonephritis, fluid-electrolyte imbalances, and nephrotic syndrome. AKI is the most common type of abnormal renal function encountered in critically ill patients, but other less common kidney abnormalities must also be recognized for optimal care of these patients.

Overview of Renal Physiology

The kidneys help to maintain the stable body chemistries, volume and energy balance, temperature, and blood pressure that give humans the physiologic freedom to ingest different kinds of foods and fluids and to live in many environmental conditions. From a basic physiologic standpoint, the primary role of kidneys is to help form urine and balance electrolytes. However, kidneys are also responsible for many endocrine functions, such as release of renin, erythropoietin, and klotho into the systemic circulation. The 3 important aspects of renal physiology that must be understood for the care of patients are the basic mechanism of autoregulation, clearance, and the effects of diuretics.

Glomerular Function and Autoregulation

Urine formation is described by the filtration-reabsorption theory. Urine is formed by filtration of blood in the glomerulus and is then modified by reabsorption and secretion of substances in the renal tubules. The kidney filters large volumes of blood passing through the glomerular capillary system. Glomeruli are the filtering units of the kidney, and each glomerulus consists of specialized capillaries situated between 2 resistive blood vessels (afferent and efferent). The glomerular filter is formed by fenestrated endothelium, the basement membrane, and podocytes. This specialized filter is selective for both size and charge. Any damage to the components of the filtration barrier manifests clinically as a primary proteinuric disease state.

A distinct character of the glomerular circulation is autoregulation. Although the oxygen consumption of the kidneys is similar to that of other organs, the kidneys receive a large portion of the blood supply (20%-25% of the resting cardiac output). Renal blood flow autoregulation is responsible for constant glomerular plasma flow and ultrafiltration over an extended range of renal artery pressures (mean arterial pressure is about 80-120 mm Hg). The primary mediators of renal autoregulation are tubuloglomerular feedback and the myogenic response of blood vessels. Through tubuloglomerular feedback the resistive vessels are modulated by signals from the macula densa (specialized cells stimulated by the tubular fluid chloride level) in the distal renal tubules. Intrarenal shunting and efferent or afferent arteriolar vasoconstriction or dilatation are involved in the pathogenesis of kidney injury.

Tubular Functions and Urinary Concentrating Mechanisms

The primary tubular physiologic process includes reabsorption (active and passive) of the plasma ultrafiltrate, selective solute secretions to the tubular fluid (urine), and hormone production. Because of the high volume of ultrafiltrate (160-170 L daily), tubular function has high requirements for both regulation and energy. Different segments of the renal tubules contribute differentially toward the maintenance of fluids, electrolytes, and nutrient homeostasis (Table 5.1). Proximal nephron segments (proximal tubules and the loop of Henle) are mainly responsible for sodium reabsorption (about 90%), and the distal nephron (distal tubules and connecting ducts) are responsible for about only 5% to 10%. However, sodium reabsorption is highly regulated along the distal nephron, where reabsorption failure is more harmful to sodium hemostasis than when malabsorption occurs in the proximal segments.

Kidneys produce urine that is hyperosmolar to plasma, thereby allowing for excretion of solutes with minimal loss of water. Maintenance of the renal medullary osmotic gradient (increasing osmolality from the corticomedullary junction to the tip of the papillae) is essential for the urine concentrating process. Primary accumulation of sodium chloride and urea in the renal tubules, interstitium, and blood vessels of the medulla is responsible for establishment of the osmotic gradient. The critical feature for the generation of the countercurrent osmotic gradient is the transepithelial permeability of the ascending thick loop of Henle to sodium chloride and urea. Formation of ammonia in the proximal tubules is important for renal acidification and maintenance of hemostasis during an increased acid load.

Mechanisms of Action of Diuretics

In critical care patients, diuretics are main treatment agents for acute exacerbations of heart failure, hypertensive urgencies, conversion of oliguric to nonoliguric renal failure, and management of fluid overload. The 5 classes of diuretics differ in their primary sites of action and hence in their ability to inhibit sodium reabsorption (Figure 5.1): 1) *Loop diuretics* (eg, furosemide) are the most commonly used and the most potent diuretics. Their primary site of action is at the basolateral side of the thick ascending limb of the tubules, where they inhibit sodium reabsorption by acting on Na^+-K^+-$2Cl^-$ channels. 2) *Thiazide diuretics* act on Na^+-Cl^- transport channels in the distal tubule. 3) *Potassium-sparing diuretics* act in the principal cells of the collecting tubules. Amiloride and triamterene directly affect the opening of sodium channels, and spironolactone and eplerenone competitively inhibit mineralocorticoid receptors. 4) The *carbonic anhydrase inhibitor* acetazolamide acts primarily on the proximal tubules. However, the diuretic effect of acetazolamide is modest given the distal reclamation of fluids in the loop of Henle. 5) *Osmotic diuretics* (eg, mannitol) inhibit the reabsorption of sodium and water in the proximal tubule and the loop of Henle.

Abnormal Renal Function

Patterns and Pathogenesis

In general, abnormal renal function can be grouped into 10 patterns or syndromic diagnoses irrespective of the underlying pathogenic factors (Table 5.2).

The pathophysiology of abnormal kidney function leading to disease states is complex and multifactorial. Three main mechanisms are responsible for the various renal syndromes: 1) renal vascular autoregulation failure due to abnormalities of systemic mean arterial pressure; 2) direct and indirect injury (infectious, inflammatory, or toxic) to renal vessels, glomeruli, tubules, or interstitium; and 3) obstruction (intrinsic or extrinsic) of the urinary drainage system.

Kidney injury in critically ill patients is often the end result of a systemic inflammatory cascade leading to the cytokine storm initiated by the primary disease. Microcirculatory dysfunction, inflammation, and abnormal cellular metabolism are the principal mechanisms responsible for various forms of kidney injury.

Table 5.1 • Reabsorption of Substances in Segments of the Renal Tubules

	Reabsorption, %						
Renal Tubule Segment	**Sodium Chloride**	**Potassium**	**Bicarbonate**	**Water**	**Calcium**	**Magnesium**	**Phosphate**
Proximal convoluted tubule	60–70	60–70	70–90	60–70	60–70	85	10–20
Loop of Henle	15–20	15–20	15 (ascending limb)	10–15	20	10 (ascending limb)	70 (ascending limb)
Distal convoluted tubule	5–10	10	0	5	10	3	10
Collecting duct	1–2	0	0	0	5	2	0

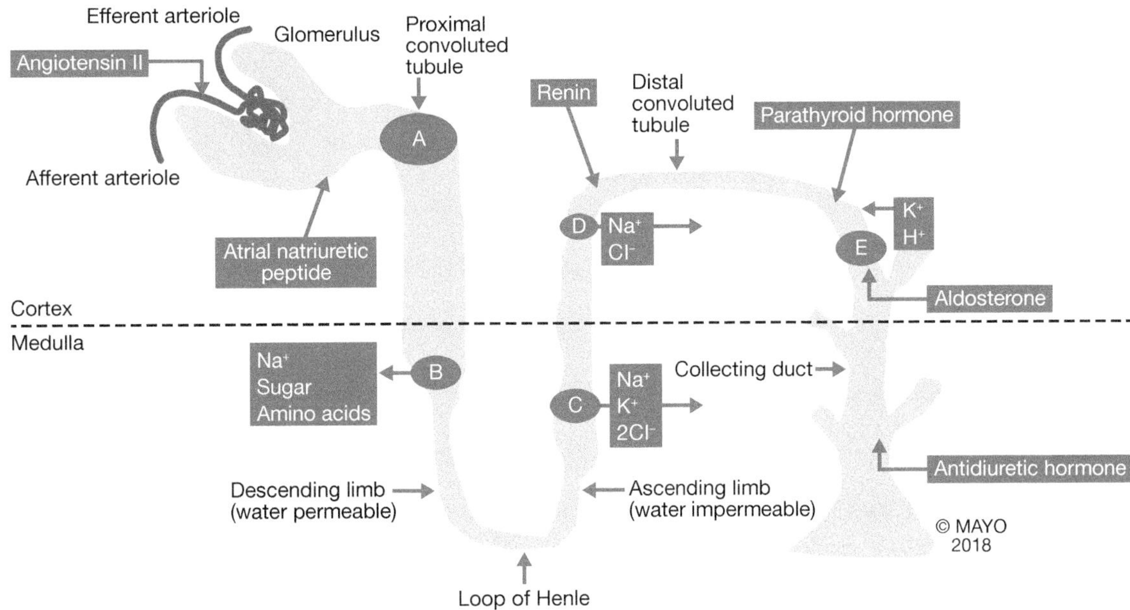

Figure 5.1. Physiologic Processes at Renal Tubule Segments. Sites of action are indicated for acetazolamide (A), osmotic diuretics (B), loop diuretics (C), thiazide diuretics (D), and potassium-sparing diuretics (E). Reabsorption of various substances in the different segments is shown in Table 5.1. Cl^- indicates chloride; H^+, hydrogen; K^+, potassium; Na^+, sodium.

Research has provided insights into the pathophysiology of kidney injury. The most relevant findings are the following: 1) The glomerular filtration rate decreases simultaneously (not sequentially) with tubular injury regardless of the site of the primary insult. 2) Persistent AKI is more severe and lasting than transient AKI (also called the prerenal state). 3) Renal tubular injury is a heterogeneous process, and all the tubules and segments are not affected simultaneously. 4) Septic AKI does not result from global ischemia but rather from localized reduction in blood flow to the renal tubules.

Clinical Manifestations

Clinically abnormal renal function follows a syndromic pattern of presentations as mentioned above. Whether the primary process is limited to the kidneys or another organ, the majority of symptoms are uniquely related to renal function. The most common abnormality in critically ill patients is decreased glomerular filtration rate leading to azotemia (increased serum levels of urea and creatinine) and abnormal urinary volumes (oliguria and anuria). Other unique clinical manifestations of renal disorders include electrolyte disturbances, abnormalities of urinary sediments (eg, casts, crystals, red blood cells, and white blood cells), polyuria, hematuria, excessive excretions of serum proteins (proteinuria), and fluid overload. Nonspecific systemic symptoms such as fever and pain are also an integral part of some renal syndromes.

Evaluation

The perfect biomarker for diagnosis of renal disease has not been identified. The standard approach to evaluation of renal function is to determine urine volume and chemistry and serum creatinine and urea levels. Recent additions to the diagnostic toolbox are serum and urine biomarkers and various imaging modalities.

Functional Markers

Traditionally the 2 most common functional markers for evaluating abnormal renal function are urine (volume and microscopy) and serum creatinine, but both are influenced by several factors, particularly in critically ill patients: 1) Serum creatinine is a late marker of kidney injury; the level increases only after more than half the renal functional mass has been lost. 2) Hemodilution in critically ill patients decreases the concentration of serum creatinine and results in inaccurate staging. 3) With severe and prolonged critical illness, serum creatinine production is low. 4) Oliguria, an appropriate response to hypovolemia, can be a sign of preserved renal function. 5) Documentation of urine output is frequently inaccurate, and oliguria is poorly validated in clinical studies.

Urine Electrolytes

Urine electrolyte studies have been among the traditional tools used in AKI management. However, studies have shown that the pattern of urine electrolyte abnormalities is no different between the prerenal state and persistent

Table 5.2 • Patterns of Abnormal Renal Function

Diagnosis	Symptoms, Signs, and Laboratory Findings
Acute kidney injury	Anuria (<100 mL daily) or oliguria (<400 mL daily) Hypertension, edema Muddy casts, hyperkalemia, elevated SUN, normal-sized kidneys
Acute nephritis	Fever, oliguria, other systemic symptoms Respiratory distress, hemoptysis, hypertension RBC casts, hematuria, mild proteinuria
Chronic kidney disease	Weakness, polyuria, nocturia, bone pain, skin changes Facial edema, hypertension Elevated urea and creatinine for ≥3 mo Bland urine sediments, isosthenuria, shrunken kidneys
Nephrotic syndrome	Facial puffiness in morning, progressive edema, and frothy urine Anasarca Proteinuria (>3.5 g/1.73 m^2/24 h) Hypoalbuminemia, lipiduria
Asymptomatic urinary abnormalities	No signs and symptoms Incidental detection of pyuria (sterile), hematuria, and mild proteinuria
Upper or lower urinary tract infections	Fever, increased urinary frequency or urgency Tender flanks and bladder Leukocyte casts Bacteriuria (>10^5 colonies/mL)
Renal tubule defects	Polyuria, nocturia, renal stones Hypovolemia Electrolyte disorders, renal calcification, large kidneys, tubular proteinuria (<1 g/24 h)
Hypertension	Headache, vision changes, weakness Systolic or diastolic hypertension, bruits Proteinuria, casts, elevated SUN or creatinine
Renal stone disorder or nephrolithiasis	Flank pain, increased urinary frequency or urgency Tender flanks Frank hematuria, pyuria, stones on imaging
Obstructive uropathy	Dysuria, slow urinary stream, sensation of fullness Prostatic enlargement, tender bladder Azotemia, oliguria, anuria

Abbreviations: RBC, red blood cell; SUN, serum urea nitrogen.

AKI in critically ill patients. Fractional excretion monitoring has no role in the evaluation of critically ill patients with AKI, and no specific indications exist for this test. Urine biochemistry is potentially useful when the baseline creatinine is unknown or very low and the creatinine level is decreasing because of hemodilution. The most important limitation of urine biochemistry is the inability to determine the adequacy of fluid resuscitation.

Injury and Stress Biomarkers

Biomarkers are proteins that are released from the injured kidney or filtered by the kidney. The 3 types are inflammatory, cell injury, and cell cycle biomarkers. Their theoretical advantages lie in their early increases in urine and serum and the relatively high sensitivity and specificity. The 2 commercially available biomarkers that can be used in the critical care setting are neutrophil gelatinase-associated lipocalin (NGAL) and insulinlike growth factor–binding protein 7 (IGFBP7) with tissue inhibitor of metalloproteinase 2 (TIMP2). Evidence suggests that both of these structural injury biomarkers aid in the early diagnosis of AKI and in ruling out AKI. The biomarkers are limited by their performance characteristics, however, and the utility of the biomarkers in short-term and long-term kidney function outcomes is yet to be determined.

Imaging

Imaging is an essential tool for evaluation of anatomical and physiologic organ abnormalities. Ultrasonography of the kidneys not only gives information about kidney size but also helps to provide information related to chronicity, obstruction, and vascular pathology. Its availability and noninvasive nature make imaging the modality of choice. Even though contrast-induced renal injury is the most feared complication of computed tomography, it has been increasingly used in the intensive care unit (ICU). Moreover, it facilitates finding the source of infection in sepsis and pyelonephritis, identifying renal malignancy, and ruling out other abdominal disease. Noncontrast computed tomography is the gold standard for diagnosis of lithiasis. The role of magnetic resonance imaging in acute critically ill patients has not been completely defined.

Renal Biopsy

Renal biopsy is another important tool, although it is less frequently performed in the critical care setting. Nevertheless, it may be necessary for identification of the exact pathology of renal dysfunction, particularly AKI, in critically ill patients to avoid future chronic kidney disease (ie, acute interstitial kidney disease and glomerulonephritis are treatable conditions). One reason that biopsy may not be used more often is the lack of correlation between disease classification and actual AKI pathology.

Management

Prevention and Early Recognition

Preventive strategies are based on identification of high-risk patients, and early recognition is important for clinical decision making and therapeutic adjustments for preventing further damage, but at least 3 barriers exist: 1) The ideal functional marker has not been identified. 2) More than 80% of patients with AKI complicating a critical illness already have AKI at ICU admission. 3) The mean arterial pressure target for prevention and the type, rate, and volume of fluid resuscitation for hypovolemic patients have not been defined.

Treatment

The goals of care are to avoid further kidney damage, to support renal function until recovery, and to prevent and treat adverse renal function abnormalities. Efforts should be made to avoid ongoing ischemia and to decrease the activity of intrarenal and extrarenal inflammatory cascades. As with any systemic disease, nutritional support and glycemic control are important for better outcomes.

Initiation of renal replacement therapy (RRT) in a patient with AKI is a daily decision-making exercise in the ICU. Dialysis is not a treatment, but it supports the deranged excretion function of the kidney. The various modalities of RRT do not appear to affect outcomes. Considerable gaps in knowledge about RRT are related to the optimal timing of initiation, selection, discontinuation, and switching among the various forms of RRT and the ideal strategy, dose, and indicators for monitoring the delivery.

Commonly Encountered Renal-Specific Abnormalities in Critically Ill Patients

Acute Kidney Injury

Critically ill ICU patients often have AKI, a grave complication of many conditions, such as shock, sepsis, trauma, burns, and drug overdose and intoxication and of various procedures, such as cardiac surgery and noncardiac surgery. General guidelines for use of pharmacologic agents and standard of care models are not available, but specific steps of care are necessary for the various types of AKI. AKI is described in more detail in Chapter 45 ("Acute Kidney Injury").

Acute Glomerulonephritis

Glomerulonephritis (GN) is inflammation of the glomerular capillary tufts. The prevalence of GN in the ICU is not known. Acute GN, also called *rapidly progressing GN*, is rare but does occur in many critically ill patients.

In patients with GN, kidney involvement is often part of a generalized vasculitis process, but vasculitis can be limited to the kidney. Renal manifestations include AKI, gross hematuria, and proteinuria. Primary glomerular disorders are heterogeneous and vary from asymptomatic proteinuria to massive proteinuria related to the nephrotic syndrome. Patients with renopulmonary syndrome have pulmonary hemorrhage and renal failure as part of the systemic vasculitis process. Rapidly progressing GN is classified according to the presence or absence of glomerular immune complexes with the use of immunofluorescent microscopy.

Most systemic vasculitis that affects the kidneys is classified as anti–glomerular basement membrane antibody GN, immune complex GN, or pauci-immune GN. Examples include systemic lupus nephritis, cryoglobulinemia, postinfectious GN, Henoch-Schönlein purpura, and antineutrophil cytoplasmic autoantibody (ANCA)-associated vasculitides (eg, microscopic or granulomatous polyangiitis and Churg-Strauss GN).

Markers of GN are red blood cell casts in the urine and dysmorphic hematuria, but diagnostic confirmation requires kidney biopsy. Acute GN is a renal emergency, and urgent treatment is mandated for all patients. Treatment options include high doses of corticosteroids, cyclophosphamide, rituximab, and plasma exchange.

Drug-Induced Renal Injury

ICU patients are frequently exposed to nephrotoxic agents, an important cause of kidney injury. The 4 drug-associated kidney diseases encountered in hospitalized patients are AKI, glomerular disorders, nephrolithiasis, and tubular dysfunction. The disease manifestations result from both dose-dependent and dose-independent mechanisms. The agents most frequently involved in drug-induced kidney injury are antibiotics, chemotherapeutic agents, and nonsteroidal anti-inflammatory drugs (NSAIDs).

In large population-based studies, nephrotoxic medications were associated with AKI in 15% to 25% of patients with AKI. Acute interstitial nephritis (AIN) is an underdiagnosed cause of AKI in critically ill patients and is responsible for AKI in 10% to 25% of patients with biopsy-proven AKI. The most common culprits of AIN in critically ill patients are medications, and less frequent causes of AIN are acute pyelonephritis, lupus nephritis, Sjögren syndrome, sarcoidosis, and malignancy. The most frequently incriminated medications are antimicrobials, proton pump inhibitors, and NSAIDs, but any medication can be associated with AIN. Idiosyncratic in nature, AIN due to drugs can occur at any stage of therapy and may not be dose dependent. Toxicity increases with the use of combination drugs, in the presence of other risk factors, and with continued use in patients with established AKI. The presence of rash, eosinophilia, and eosinophiluria is suggestive of AIN but not confirmative. Definitive diagnosis needs renal biopsy and the finding of inflammatory cell infiltrations in the interstitium.

Among the antibiotics, the nephrotoxic potential of aminoglycosides is well established. Studies have also highlighted the nephrotoxic risk of vancomycin and piperacillin-tazobactam, 2 broad-spectrum antimicrobials commonly used in the ICU. Vancomycin nephrotoxicity increases with combination nephrotoxic therapy, higher doses, higher low blood levels before the next dose, and longer duration of treatment. Two studies have shown a greater risk of AKI when vancomycin is given in combination with piperacillin-tazobactum. More studies are needed to learn the exact role of these drugs in AKI pathogenesis.

When a patient has drug-induced AIN, discontinuation of the offending agents and treatment of the underlying inflammatory disorders are the first steps. If use of the offending agent cannot be discontinued, other steps would be to limit the dose and duration of exposure, monitor the blood level, and modify other risk factors. The value of corticosteroids in drug-induced AIN has not been proved, but some advocate initiating therapy if renal function does not improve within 3 to 7 days after stopping the medication.

Kidney Injury in Malignancy

Survival of cancer patients has improved because of advances in diagnosis, targeted treatment approaches with combination chemotherapy, and stem cell transplant. These patients have unique kidney-related problems because of chemotherapy and increased longevity, and patients with malignancy may have kidney-related problems, such as AKI, glomerulonephritis, renal vein and artery thrombosis, and infiltrative disease depending on the type of malignancy and the treatment. AKI, the most common renal injury in critically ill cancer patients, is often multifactorial.

Summary

- AKI is the most commonly encountered kidney injury in ICU patients.
- Mortality among critically ill patients with kidney injury reflects complications, such as sepsis, lung injury, liver injury, cardiac dysfunction, and immunologic abnormalities, which require supportive therapy.
- No biomarkers of kidney injury are associated with improved short-term or long-term outcomes.
- Drug-induced renal injury in critically ill patients is underdiagnosed.

SUGGESTED READING

Barozzi L, Valentino M, Santoro A, Mancini E, Pavlica P. Renal ultrasonography in critically ill patients. Crit Care Med. 2007 May;35(5 Suppl):S198–205.

Burgess LD, Drew RH. Comparison of the incidence of vancomycin-induced nephrotoxicity in hospitalized patients with and without concomitant piperacillin-tazobactam. Pharmacotherapy. 2014 Jul;34(7):670–6. Epub 2014 May 22.

Calzavacca P, May CN, Bellomo R. Glomerular haemodynamics, the renal sympathetic nervous system and sepsis-induced acute kidney injury. Nephrol Dial Transplant. 2014 Dec;29(12):2178–84. Epub 2014 Mar 11.

Chmielewski J, Lewandowski RJ, Maddur H. Hepatorenal syndrome: physiology, diagnosis and management. Semin Intervent Radiol. 2018 Aug;35(3):194–7. Epub 2018 Aug 6.

Couser WG, Johnson RJ. The etiology of glomerulonephritis: roles of infection and autoimmunity. Kidney Int. 2014 Nov;86(5):905–14. Epub 2014 Mar 12.

Cupples WA. Interactions contributing to kidney blood flow autoregulation. Curr Opin Nephrol Hypertens. 2007 Jan;16(1):39–45.

Curthoys NP, Moe OW. Proximal tubule function and response to acidosis. Clin J Am Soc Nephrol. 2014 Sep 5;9(9):1627–38. Epub 2013 Aug 1.

Dantzler WH, Layton AT, Layton HE, Pannabecker TL. Urine-concentrating mechanism in the inner medulla: function of the thin limbs of the loops of Henle. Clin J Am Soc Nephrol. 2014 Oct 7;9(10):1781–9. Epub 2013 Aug 1.

Darmon M, Ostermann M, Cerda J, Dimopoulos MA, Forni L, Hoste E, et al. Diagnostic work-up and specific causes of acute kidney injury. Intensive Care Med. 2017 Jun;43(6):829–40. Epub 2017 Apr 25.

Druml W. Systemic consequences of acute kidney injury. Curr Opin Crit Care. 2014 Dec;20(6):613–9.

Ganguli A, Sawinski D, Berns JS. Kidney diseases associated with haematological cancers. Nat Rev Nephrol. 2015 Aug;11(8):478–90. Epub 2015 Jun 2.

Haraldsson B, Nystrom J, Deen WM. Properties of the glomerular barrier and mechanisms of proteinuria. Physiol Rev. 2008 Apr;88(2):451–87.
Hoenig MP, Zeidel ML. Homeostasis, the milieu interieur, and the wisdom of the nephron. Clin J Am Soc Nephrol. 2014 Jul;9(7):1272–81. Epub 2014 May 1.
Hoste EA, Bagshaw SM, Bellomo R, Cely CM, Colman R, Cruz DN, et al. Epidemiology of acute kidney injury in critically ill patients: the multinational AKI-EPI study. Intensive Care Med. 2015 Aug;41(8):1411–23. Epub 2015 Jul 11.
Kamel KS, Schreiber M, Halperin ML. Renal potassium physiology: integration of the renal response to dietary potassium depletion. Kidney Int. 2018 Jan;93(1):41–53.
Kim T, Kandiah S, Patel M, Rab S, Wong J, Xue W, et al. Risk factors for kidney injury during vancomycin and piperacillin/tazobactam administration, including increased odds of injury with combination therapy. BMC Res Notes. 2015 Oct 17;8:579.
Koyner JL, Shaw AD, Chawla LS, Hoste EA, Bihorac A, Kashani K, et al; Sapphire Investigators. Tissue inhibitor metalloproteinase-2 (TIMP-2)•IGF-binding protein-7 (IGFBP7) levels are associated with adverse long-term outcomes in patients with AKI. J Am Soc Nephrol. 2015 Jul;26(7):1747–54. Epub 2014 Dec 22.
Krishnan N, Perazella MA. Drug-induced acute interstitial nephritis: pathology, pathogenesis, and treatment. Iran J Kidney Dis. 2015 Jan;9(1):3–13.
Langenberg C, Bagshaw SM, May CN, Bellomo R. The histopathology of septic acute kidney injury: a systematic review. Crit Care. 2008;12(2):R38. Epub 2008 Mar 6.
Lin J, Denker BM. Azotemia and urinary abnormalities. In: Jameson JL, Loscalzo J, editors. Harrison's nephrology and acid-base disorders. 3rd ed. New York (NY): McGraw-Hill Education Medical; c2017.
Maciel AT, Vitorio D. Urine biochemistry assessment in critically ill patients: controversies and future perspectives. J Clin Monit Comput. 2017 Jun;31(3):539–46. Epub 2016 Apr 1.
Matejovic M, Ince C, Chawla LS, Blantz R, Molitoris BA, Rosner MH, et al; ADQI XIII Work Group. Renal hemodynamics in AKI: in search of new treatment targets. J Am Soc Nephrol. 2016 Jan;27(1):49–58. Epub 2015 Oct 28.
Mount DB. Thick ascending limb of the loop of Henle. Clin J Am Soc Nephrol. 2014 Nov 7;9(11):1974–86. Epub 2014 Oct 15.
Oppert M. Timing of renal replacement therapy in acute kidney injury. Minerva Urol Nefrol. 2016;68:72–7.
Packer RK, Desai SS, Hornbuckle K, Knepper MA. Role of countercurrent multiplication in renal ammonium handling: regulation of medullary ammonium accumulation. J Am Soc Nephrol. 1991 Jul;2(1):77–83.
Palmer LG, Schnermann J. Integrated control of Na transport along the nephron. Clin J Am Soc Nephrol. 2015 Apr 7;10(4):676–87. Epub 2014 Aug 6.
Pearce D, Soundararajan R, Trimpert C, Kashlan OB, Deen PM, Kohan DE. Collecting duct principal cell transport processes and their regulation. Clin J Am Soc Nephrol. 2015 Jan 7;10(1):135–46. Epub 2014 May 29.
Perinel S, Vincent F, Lautrette A, Dellamonica J, Mariat C, Zeni F, et al. Transient and persistent acute kidney injury and the risk of hospital mortality in critically ill patients: results of a multicenter cohort study. Crit Care Med. 2015 Aug;43(8):e269–75.
Philipponnet C, Guerin C, Canet E, Robert R, Mariat C, Dijoud F, et al. Kidney biopsy in the critically ill patient, results of a multicentre retrospective case series. Minerva Anestesiol. 2013 Jan;79(1):53–61. Epub 2012 Oct 5.
Pickkers P, Ostermann M, Joannidis M, Zarbock A, Hoste E, Bellomo R, et al. The intensive care medicine agenda on acute kidney injury. Intensive Care Med. 2017 Sep;43(9):1198–209. Epub 2017 Jan 30.
Pollak MR, Quaggin SE, Hoenig MP, Dworkin LD. The glomerulus: the sphere of influence. Clin J Am Soc Nephrol. 2014 Aug 7;9(8):1461–9. Epub 2014 May 29.
Praga M, Sevillano A, Aunon P, Gonzalez E. Changes in the aetiology, clinical presentation and management of acute interstitial nephritis, an increasingly common cause of acute kidney injury. Nephrol Dial Transplant. 2015 Sep;30(9):1472–9. Epub 2014 Oct 16.
Raghavan R, Eknoyan G. Acute interstitial nephritis: a reappraisal and update. Clin Nephrol. 2014 Sep;82(3):149–62.
Soo JY, Jansen J, Masereeuw R, Little MH. Advances in predictive in vitro models of drug-induced nephrotoxicity. Nat Rev Nephrol. 2018 Jun;14(6):378–93.
Star RA. Treatment of acute renal failure. Kidney Int. 1998 Dec;54(6):1817–31.
Stone JH, Merkel PA, Spiera R, Seo P, Langford CA, Hoffman GS, et al; RAVE-ITN Research Group. Rituximab versus cyclophosphamide for ANCA-associated vasculitis. N Engl J Med. 2010 Jul 15;363(3):221–32.
Subramanya AR, Ellison DH. Distal convoluted tubule. Clin J Am Soc Nephrol. 2014 Dec 5;9(12):2147–63. Epub 2014 May 22.
Vijayan A, Faubel S, Askenazi DJ, Cerda J, Fissell WH, Heung M, et al; American Society of Nephrology Acute Kidney Injury Advisory Group. Clinical use of the urine biomarker [TIMP-2] × [IGFBP7] for acute kidney injury risk assessment. Am J Kidney Dis. 2016 Jul;68(1):19–28. Epub 2016 Mar 4.
Vincent JL, De Backer D. Circulatory shock. N Engl J Med. 2013 Oct 31;369(18):1726–34.
Wilde B, van Paassen P, Witzke O, Tervaert JW. New pathophysiological insights and treatment of ANCA-associated vasculitis. Kidney Int. 2011 Mar;79(6):599–612. Epub 2010 Dec 8.

6 Nutrition in Critical Illness

ANGELA N. VIZZINI, RDN, LD/N; MIREILLE H. HAMDAN, RDN, LD/N

Goals

- Understand the increased nutritional risk of patients in the intensive care unit.
- Assess a patient's degree of malnutrition.
- Evaluate a patient's nutritional needs associated with a specific medical condition.
- Determine the best route of nutrition delivery.

Introduction

Nutritional care of critically ill patients prompts considerations unique to this patient population. For many years it has been postulated that the inflammation and stress response that accompany critical illness contribute to hypermetabolism and increased nutrient requirements. However, the degree of hypermetabolism is influenced by numerous factors, including severity and type of illness, recent extensive (often abdominal) surgery, and administered drugs. There is a reasonable consensus that nutrition therapy tailored to the patient's energy and protein requirements aids in recovery, maintains lean muscle mass, and decreases infectious complications. This chapter addresses nutritional issues in critically ill patients and suggests appropriate interventions and monitoring to prevent complications and facilitate recovery from critical illness.

Malnutrition and Nutritional Risk

Malnutrition and nutrient deficiencies are associated with poor wound healing, infections, respiratory dysfunction, fluid and electrolyte abnormalities, and changes in mental status. Additionally, the presence of weight loss and malnutrition may impair a response to treatment. Nutritional assessment of the critically ill patient is essential to identify nutritional deficits and then plan appropriate medical nutrition therapy, and many components of the nutritional assessment are needed to complete an accurate patient assessment. In the presence of multiple underlying diagnoses, critically ill patients may have additional difficulty adapting to severe metabolic stress because of a lack of energy stores and alterations in body composition and function. Cytokine-induced metabolic alterations, associated with shortened life expectancy, may prevent critically ill patients from regaining lean body cell mass during nutrition support.

With the risk of malnutrition in critically ill patients, early nutritional assessment should be completed within 24 to 72 hours of intensive care unit (ICU) admission to identify the intervention that may allow for the best response and recovery from critical illness. Several factors may affect the accuracy of anthropometric measurements of critically ill patients, including changes in hydration, the presence of ascites or edema, amputation, contractures and muscle wasting due to prolonged bed rest, and individual differences in body composition. Obtaining anthropometric measurements for the period before ICU admission and a detailed history before illness is often required for accurate evaluation.

Nutrition-Focused Physical Examination

The nutrition-focused physical examination, when used with other components of patient nutritional assessment, allows for a more accurate determination of the nutritional status of the critical care patient. This assessment tool can be used to help identify signs of protein-energy malnutrition and of nutritional deficiency or toxicity in rapidly proliferating tissues of the skin, hair, nails, eyes, and oral cavity (Table 6.1). Laboratory test results often do not correlate with body stores of micronutrients, and patients receiving parenteral nutrition (PN) may have misleading

Table 6.1 • Physical Symptoms Related to Deficiencies of Macronutrients and Micronutrients

Physical Symptoms	Possible Deficiency
Skin	
Delayed, poor wound healing	Protein, zinc, vitamin A, vitamin C
Xerosis	Vitamin A, essential fatty acids
Follicular hyperkeratosis	Vitamin A, vitamin C, essential fatty acids
Dermatitis, generalized	Zinc, essential fatty acids
Pellagrous dermatosis: dermatitis with hyperpigmented patches in areas exposed to sunlight	Niacin
Flaky paint dermatosis: hyperpigmented patches, usually on the back of the thighs and buttocks, that peel and reveal hypopigmented skin	Protein
Nails	
Lackluster, dull	Protein
Mottled, pale, poor blanching	Vitamin A, vitamin C
Spoon shaped, kernicterous	Iron with or without anemia
Hair	
Corkscrew hair	Copper
Depigmentation, lightening of normal hair tint	Protein, copper
Straight hair in racial groups with normally curly hair	Protein
Eyes	
Night blindness	Vitamin A
Conjunctival xerosis, abnormal dryness	Vitamin A
Pale conjunctivae (fornix area)	Iron, folate, vitamin B_{12}
Bitot spots	Vitamin A
Corneal xerosis: abnormal dryness progresses to keratomalacia	Vitamin A
Oral cavity	
Cheilosis	Vitamins B_2 and B_6, niacin
Glossitis with purple or red tongue	Vitamins B_2, B_6, and B_{12}; niacin; folate
Bleeding, spongy gums	Vitamin C
Stomatitis	Vitamin B complex, iron, vitamin C
Edematous tongue	Niacin
Dysgeusia, hypogeusia	Zinc
Other	
Ankle, sacral edema; loss of subcutaneous fat; muscle wasting; ascites	Protein-calorie malnutrition

Modified from Hammond KA. Nutrition-focused physical assessment skills for dietitians: study guide. Chicago (IL): American Dietetic Association (c2017 Dietitians in Nutrition Support); c2000; used with permission.

laboratory test results that reflect nutrient infusion rather than true nutrient status.

Determining Energy Requirements

Physiologic processes and intermediary metabolism are altered in patients who are critically ill. This alteration is caused by the stress response, which begins with a decreased metabolic rate during the shock phase and transitions to a flow phase marked by a period of regeneration and repair with an increased metabolic rate. The metabolic alterations during critical illness can accelerate glycogen and protein catabolism and lead to protein-energy malnutrition and the need for nutrition support. Depending on the type of stress, energy expenditure in critically ill patients may increase and the metabolic response may be compounded.

The resting energy expenditure (REE) in a critically ill patient is estimated to be 40% to 70% higher than in a healthy person. The gold standard is to measure REE with indirect calorimetry (IC) according to a standardized protocol. IC measures changes in the concentrations of inspired oxygen ($\dot{V}O_2$) (in milliliters per minute) and expired carbon dioxide ($\dot{V}CO_2$) (in milliliters per minute). The abbreviated Weir equation is used to calculate the total average daily REE (in kilocalories per day).

$$REE = [(3.94 \times \dot{V}O_2) + (1.11 \times \dot{V}CO_2)] \times 1.44$$

The calculated respiratory quotient (RQ) reflects substrate use and is determined by the ratio of $\dot{V}CO_2$ to $\dot{V}O_2$.

$$RQ = \dot{V}CO_2 / \dot{V}O_2$$

When the measured RQ is evaluated, the patient's history and current feeding regimen must be considered. The physiologic RQ ranges from 0.64 to 1.2. Any RQ outside this range should be evaluated further. An RQ of 0.85 indicates mixed substrate oxidation, and an RQ of 1.0 indicates complete glucose oxidation, such as immediately after a meal. An RQ less than 0.7 indicates underfeeding or prolonged fasting, with resultant ethanol and ketone oxidation. The RQ may be low with certain diseases and conditions, such as diabetes mellitus, starvation, and hypoventilation, and when technical difficulties arise during measurement. In general, an RQ greater than 1.0 indicates excess caloric intake, lipogenesis, and excess $\dot{V}_{CO_2}$. To determine an accurate RQ, the equipment must be well calibrated, and the person conducting the measurements must be experienced.

Before IC measurements are made, patients in the ICU should be awake for at least 6 to 8 hours after anesthesia, patients undergoing dialysis should have completed the procedure at least 4 hours earlier, and patients should not have received pain or sedation medications for at least 30 minutes. During measurements for resting metabolic rate (RMR), a steady state must be maintained, procedures should be avoided, and the patient should require no additional oxygen. In patients receiving continuous tube feeding, the rate and composition of infusions should remain constant for at least 12 hours before and during IC measurement. For patients receiving intermittent feedings, RMR measurements should be made 4 hours after a feeding. In addition, patients should be kept in the supine position for more accurate RMR measurement.

The American Society for Parenteral and Enteral Nutrition (ASPEN) and the Society of Critical Care Medicine (SCCM) recommend that, in the absence of IC, REE may be estimated with simple weight-based equations (Table 6.2). Published predictive equations, such as the Penn State equation, the Harris-Benedict equation, the Mifflin St Joer equation, and the Ireton-Jones equation, are no more accurate than simple weight-based equations (Box 6.1). Weight-based equations are modified for obese patients with a body mass index (BMI, calculated as weight in kilograms divided by height in meters squared) greater than 30. ASPEN and SCCM suggest using the actual body weight (ABW) for patients with a BMI of 30 to 50 and the ideal body weight (IBW) if BMI is greater than 50. IBW is calculated with the Hamwi method as follows:

Female: 100 lb for the first 5 ft and 5 lb for each additional inch
Male: 106 lb for the first 5 ft and 6 lb for each additional inch

Inadequate provision of energy causes the body to break down glycogen stores and lean muscle mass. Continued suboptimal energy intake results in an accumulated energy deficit. Energy deficits greater than 4,000 to 10,000 cal have been correlated with increased infection, organ failure, and hospital length of stay. Iatrogenic underfeeding is common in the critical care unit. Enteral regimens are frequently interrupted because of medication administration, bathing, procedures, and clogged tubes. Standardized protocols for nutrition support provide clear guidelines for optimal nutrition and may help decrease the duration of mechanical ventilation and length of stay in the ICU.

Table 6.2 • ASPEN and SCCM Weight-Based Estimations of REE

BMI	REE, kcal/kg
<30	25-30, based on ABW
30-50	11-14, based on ABW
>50	22-25, based on IBW

Abbreviations: ABW, actual body weight; ASPEN, American Society for Parenteral and Enteral Nutrition; BMI, body mass index (calculated as weight in kilograms divided by height in meters squared); IBW, ideal body weight; REE, resting energy expenditure; SCCM, Society of Critical Care Medicine.

Protein Requirements

Protein needs are increased during critical illness because of increased protein synthesis, oxidation, and breakdown. Protein breakdown is commonly exacerbated in critical care patients owing to immobilization and prolonged periods of receiving nothing by mouth or inadequate nutrition.

Box 6.1 • Energy Requirement Equations

Original Penn State equation

$$\text{RMR} = (\text{Mifflin St Joer})(0.96) + \dot{V}_E(31) + \text{Tmax}(167) - 6{,}212$$

Modified Penn State equation

$$\text{RMR} = (\text{Mifflin St Joer})(0.71) + \dot{V}_E(64) + \text{Tmax}(85) - 3{,}085$$

Mifflin St Joer value is calculated as follows:

$$\text{Men}: (10)(\text{Wt}) + (6.25)(\text{Ht}) - (5)(\text{Age}) + 5$$
$$\text{Women}: (10)(\text{Wt}) + (6.25)(\text{Ht}) - (5)(\text{Age}) - 161$$

Abbreviations: Ht, height (in centimeters); RMR, resting metabolic rate; Tmax, maximum temperature (in degrees Celsius); $\dot{V}_E$, minute ventilation (in liters per minute); Wt, weight (in kilograms).

Modified from Frankenfield DC, Coleman A, Alam S, Cooney RN. Analysis of estimation methods for resting metabolic rate in critically ill adults. JPEN J Parenter Enteral Nutr. 2009 Jan/Feb;33(1):27-36; used with permission.

Table 6.3 • Daily Protein Needs Based on BMI and Renal Function

BMI	Renal Function	Daily Protein Needs, g/kg
<30	...	Based on ABW, 1.2-2.0
<30	Receiving hemodialysis	Based on ABW, 1.5-2.0
<30	Receiving CRRT	Based on ABW, 2.0-2.5
30-40	...	Based on IBW, 2.0
≥40	...	Based on IBW, 2.5

Abbreviations: ABW, actual body weight; BMI, body mass index (calculated as weight in kilograms divided by height in meters squared); CRRT, continuous renal replacement therapy; IBW, ideal body weight.

The primary goal during critical illness is to preserve lean body mass and adequately support metabolic function. Daily protein requirements are 0.8 g/kg for a healthy person and 1.2 to 2.0 g/kg for a critically ill patient (Table 6.3). The daily protein requirement for patients receiving hemodialysis is 1.5 to 2.0 g/kg, and for patients receiving continuous renal replacement therapy, 2.0 to 2.5 g/kg because of increased loss during dialysis. Protein needs are adjusted for patients with a BMI greater than 30. When protein needs are calculated, protein loss through drains and wound output must be considered and compensated for in addition to the base protein requirements.

Nitrogen (N) balance studies can often be used to better assess the degree of catabolism and anabolism in a critical care patient. N balance (in grams per day) is determined by measuring 24-hour urine urea nitrogen (UUN) excretion, adding a factor of 3 to 5 g to allow for insensible N losses (eg, in sweat and stool) (the higher value should be used for patients with fever), and subtracting this total N output from a calculated N intake that includes all nutrition support that the patient is receiving.

$$\text{Daily N Balance (in grams)} = \text{Protein Intake (in grams)} / 6.25 - (\text{UUN} + \text{Insensible N Loss Estimate})$$

Negative N balance indicates inadequate protein intake, and positive N balance, adequate or excessive protein intake. A positive N balance is challenging to achieve during inflammation and critical illness; therefore, clinicians should aim to cover base requirements and losses. Monitoring protein requirements with 24-hour UUN measurements is not recommended for patients receiving dialysis.

Iatrogenic Underfeeding

The authors of an international, prospective study (Heyland et al, 2015; see Suggested Reading) measured the prevalence of iatrogenic underfeeding in nutritionally at-risk, critically ill patients. The study included 3,390 patients receiving mechanical ventilation in 201 patient care units. The patients received artificial nutrition for at least 96 hours. Measured variables included the time to initiate enteral nutrition and the percentage of nutrition received compared to the amount prescribed in the regimen. Nutritionally at-risk patients were defined as those receiving mechanical ventilation for more than 7 days, having a Nutrition Risk in the Critically Ill (NUTRIC) score of at least 5, and having a BMI less than 25 or a BMI of 35 or more. NUTRIC score variables include age, Acute Physiology and Chronic Health Evaluation (APACHE) II score, Sequential Organ Failure Assessment (SOFA) score, number of comorbidities, number of days from hospital admission to ICU, and, if available, interleukin 6 level. A NUTRIC score of more than 5 indicates high nutritional risk. On average, enteral nutrition was initiated 38.8 hours after admission, and 74% of patients did not receive at least 80% of the energy targets. Patients received only 61.2% of the prescribed calories and 57.6% of the prescribed protein. Results for the United States were lower, with patients receiving 51.0% of the prescribed calories and 48.1% of the prescribed protein. No significant clinical differences were found among patients grouped by BMI or NUTRIC score. The authors concluded that the majority of critically ill patients worldwide receive inadequate nutrition.

Nutrition Delivery

Enteral Nutrition

If a critically ill patient with a functioning gut requires nutrition support but cannot safely consume an oral diet, enteral nutrition (EN) is the preferred route of feeding. Feeding through an enteral route is physiologic and cost-efficient, with documented benefits. EN maintains the gut mucosal barrier, promotes efficient use of nutrients through first-pass metabolism, and supports immune function by supporting gut-associated lymphoid tissue (GALT) and mucosa-associated lymphoid tissue (MALT).

ASPEN and SCCM recommend early initiation of EN, within 24 to 48 hours of ICU admission. Early EN provides essential macronutrients and micronutrients that reduce complications associated with energy deficit. EN can be provided with a nasogastric tube or a nasoenteric tube. Nasoenteric feeding is recommended for patients at high risk for aspiration. Risk factors for aspiration include mechanical ventilation, reduced level of consciousness, inability to protect airway, and age older than 70 years. Nasoenteric tubes may be placed fluoroscopically by trained personnel. Confirmation of the tube tip location is recommended for all enteral tubes before use. Although nasogastric and nasoenteric tubes are intended for short-term use (≤4 weeks), if EN is needed for longer than 4 weeks, placement of a gastrostomy or gastrojejunostomy tube is recommended. Regardless of tube type or placement, aspiration precautions should be observed for all patients receiving EN while intubated. Precautions include elevating the head of the bed 30° to 45° and using chlorhexidine mouthwash twice daily.

Use of a standard polymeric EN formula with 1.0 to 1.5 kcal/mL is recommended for and well tolerated by most critical care patients. Although numerous disease-specific and immune-modulating enteral products are available, research does not show that patients benefit from the routine use of specialty formulas. Enteral protocols may improve the amount of calories and protein provided and decrease interruptions of EN. Such protocols provide clear guidelines pertaining to initiation rates, EN goals, water flushes, and circumstances for stopping EN. Protocols with rapid initiation and advancement should be avoided for hypotensive patients who require increasing doses of catecholamine agents. Trophic EN should be used cautiously in patients with decreasing use of vasopressors.

Tolerance of EN is assessed through physical examination and monitoring abdominal distention, stool output, and patient discomfort. Routinely checking gastric residual volume (GRV) in critically ill patients is no longer recommended by ASPEN and SCCM. An elevated GRV is not associated with aspiration or pneumonia, and interrupting EN because of an elevated GRV may lead to inadequate delivery of calories and protein. If GRV is checked, though, ASPEN and SCCM discourage withholding EN if GRV is less than 500 mL in the absence of signs of intolerance.

Parenteral Nutrition

Although EN is the preferred route of nutrition, PN can be a beneficial way to provide nutrition when a patient cannot use EN, such as when gastrointestinal tract function is inadequate or compromised. Indications for the appropriate use of PN include intestinal obstruction, distal high-output fistulas, severe gastrointestinal tract bleeding, or severe malabsorption. PN should be initiated promptly after ICU admission if a patient is malnourished or has a high nutritional risk and a nonfunctioning gastrointestinal tract. Well-nourished patients receive only limited benefits from PN administered within the first week of ICU admission. Research is inconclusive about the benefits of withholding lipids during the first week of ICU admission. The majority of lipid emulsions in the United States are soybean oil based and thought to be proinflammatory because of the ω-6 fatty acid content. Lipid emulsions containing ω-3 fatty acids have recently become available in the United States; however, only limited research supports improved clinical outcomes.

PN formulations contain dextrose, amino acids, lipids, electrolytes, vitamins, and minerals. Health care institutions should follow standardized protocols for ordering, compounding, and administering PN.

Central PN (CPN) is hyperosmolar (1,300-1,600 mOsm/L) and requires infusion into a large-diameter vein through a central line. The hypertonic solution is diluted with the rapid blood flow. The 2 methods for compounding CPN are total nutrient admixture (TNA) and 2-in-1 formulation. TNA, also commonly referred to as total parental nutrition, combines dextrose, amino acids, and lipids in 1 bag. The other method, 2-in-1 PN, also combines dextrose and amino acids in 1 bag, but lipids are administered by piggyback infusion. Both compounding methods are recognized by ASPEN and have strict guidelines for infusion times and filters. CPN is intended for patients requiring intravenous nutrition for 7 to 14 days.

Peripheral parenteral nutrition (PPN) contains similar macronutrients and micronutrients as CPN but in lower concentrations. PPN is hyperosmolar (600-900 mOsm/L) and requires a larger fluid volume; therefore, it is not desirable for patients requiring fluid restriction, and it is used infrequently in critical care patients. PPN is intended for short-term use of 5 days to 2 weeks.

CAN WE FEED Mnemonic

Many factors must be considered before a critically ill patient is given nutrition support and during administration of nutrition therapy. *CAN WE FEED* is a useful mnemonic (Box 6.2).

Complications

In critically ill patients receiving EN, diarrhea is the most frequent gastrointestinal tract–related complication that may or may not be directly associated with the formula itself. Typically, all other factors must be ruled out before diarrhea can be associated with tube feeding. The main causes for diarrhea include medications, malabsorption secondary to diagnosis or surgery, and *Clostridium difficile* infection. Antibiotic-associated diarrhea is due to disruption of intestinal flora. In addition, many medications, such as acetaminophen elixirs and furosemide, contain sorbitol, which causes diarrhea through a laxative effect.

Summary

- The inflammation and stress response that accompany critical illness contribute to hypermetabolism and increased nutrient requirements, including caloric and protein needs.
- In the presence of multiple underlying diagnoses, critically ill patients may have additional difficulty adapting to severe metabolic stress because of a lack of energy stores and alterations in body composition and function.

Box 6.2 • CAN WE FEED Mnemonic for Nutrition Support in Critically Ill Patients

C—Critical illness severity

Review comorbidities, optimize glucose control, and use appropriate critical illness scoring system.

A—Age

Age must be considered because it affects energy requirements, particularly in younger patients, who must meet continued growth requirements, and in elderly patients, among whom malnutrition is common.

N—Nutrition risk screening

Risk of RS is important in the critically ill patient.

W—Wait for resuscitation

Resuscitation takes priority over initiation of early EN or PN feeding. Evaluate potential hemodynamic instability, including serum lactate, base excess, mean arterial pressure, pressor agents, hydration status, and electrolyte levels, to assess the risk of ischemia from early enteral feeding.

E—Energy requirements

Initiate nutrition support cautiously in critically ill patients to avoid complications of RS and overfeeding. Proper protein provision may be of greater importance and can be difficult in obese patients.

F—Formula selection

Patients often can use standard EN products if use of the products is properly introduced and increased as tolerated. A small number of patients may benefit from specialty products, including elemental, semielemental, and IMD (pharmaconutrition) products.

E—Enteral access

Most patients tolerate gastric feeding, but the need for postpyloric placement should be evaluated if the patient may have gastric dysmotility.

E—Efficacy

The adequacy of intake must be evaluated repeatedly because the provision of at least 55% of caloric requirements may be required to achieve benefit from EN. Enteral protocols in the ICU have been suggested as an aid to increase the likelihood of reaching nutrition support goals.

D—Determine tolerance

A thorough physical examination is important for assessing a patient's tolerance for EN. If diarrhea occurs, the assessment should consider various causes, including medication, infectious agents, and impactions, before being attributed to the formula.

Abbreviations: EN, enteral nutrition; ICU, intensive care unit; IMD, immune-modulating diet; PN, parenteral nutrition; RS, refeeding syndrome.

Data from McClave SA, Taylor BE, Martindale RG, Warren MM, Johnson DR, Braunschweig C, et al; Society of Critical Care Medicine; American Society for Parenteral and Enteral Nutrition. Guidelines for the Provision and Assessment of Nutrition Support Therapy in the Adult Critically Ill Patient: Society of Critical Care Medicine (SCCM) and American Society for Parenteral and Enteral Nutrition (A.S.P.E.N.). JPEN J Parenter Enteral Nutr. 2016 Feb;40(2):159-211. Erratum in: JPEN J Parenter Enteral Nutr. 2016 Nov;40(8):1200 and Miller KR, Kiraly LN, Lowen CC, Martindale RG, McClave SA. "CAN WE FEED?" A mnemonic to merge nutrition and intensive care assessment of the critically ill patient. JPEN J Parenter Enteral Nutr. 2011 Sep;35(5):643-59.

- Nutritional assessment of the critically ill patient is essential to identify nutritional deficits and then plan the optimal medical nutrition therapy. Several components of nutritional assessment are needed, including a nutrition-focused physical examination, anthropometric measurements, and hydration status.
- EN therapy is the preferred route of feeding if critically ill patients cannot safely consume an oral diet, but PN can be a beneficial way to provide nutrition when a patient's gastrointestinal tract function is inadequate or compromised.
- Reevaluating and monitoring patient's tolerance of the nutrition support therapy may be detrimental to ensuring optimal delivery of nutrition.

SUGGESTED READING

Arends J, Bodoky G, Bozzetti F, Fearon K, Muscaritoli M, Selga G, et al; DGEM (German Society for Nutritional Medicine); ESPEN (European Society for Parenteral and Enteral Nutrition). ESPEN guidelines on enteral nutrition: non-surgical oncology. Clin Nutr. 2006 Apr;25(2):245–59. Epub 2006 May 12.

Ayers P, Adams S, Boullata J, Gervasio J, Holcombe B, Kraft MD, et al; American Society for Parenteral and Enteral Nutrition. A.S.P.E.N. parenteral nutrition safety consensus recommendations. JPEN J Parenter Enteral Nutr. 2014 Mar-Apr;38(3):296–333. Epub 2013 Nov 26.

Berger MM, Pichard C. Parenteral nutrition in the ICU: lessons learned over the past few years. Nutrition. 2019 Mar;59:188–94.

Cahill NE, Murch L, Jeejeebhoy K, McClave SA, Day AG, Wang M, et al. When early enteral feeding is not possible in critically ill patients: results of a multicenter observational study. JPEN J Parenter Enteral Nutr. 2011 Mar;35(2):160–8.

Casaer MP, Mesotten D, Hermans G, Wouters PJ, Schetz M, Meyfroidt G, et al. Early versus late parenteral nutrition in critically ill adults. N Engl J Med. 2011 Aug 11;365(6):506–17. Epub 2011 Jun 29.

Clark SF. Vitamins and trace elements. In: Mueller CM, editor. The A.S.P.E.N. adult nutrition support core curriculum. 2nd ed. Silver Spring (MD): American Society for Parenteral and Enteral Nutrition; c2012. p. 121–51.

Colaizzo-Anas T. Nutrient intake, digestion, absorption, and excretion. In: Mueller CM, editor. The A.S.P.E.N. adult nutrition support core curriculum. 2nd ed. Silver Spring (MD): American Society for Parenteral and Enteral Nutrition; c2012. p. 3–21.

Dvir D, Cohen J, Singer P. Computerized energy balance and complications in critically ill patients: an observational study. Clin Nutr. 2006 Feb;25(1):37–44.

Frankenfield DC, Coleman A, Alam S, Cooney RN. Analysis of estimation methods for resting metabolic rate in critically ill adults. JPEN J Parenter Enteral Nutr. 2009 Jan-Feb;33(1):27–36. Epub 2008 Nov 14.

Gerlach AT, Thomas S, Murphy CV, Stawicki PS, Whitmill ML, Pourzanjani L, et al. Does delaying early intravenous fat emulsion during parenteral nutrition reduce infections during critical illness? Surg Infect (Larchmt). 2011 Feb;12(1):43–7. Epub 2010 Dec 20.

Gottschlich M, Mattox T, DeLegge M, editors. The A.S.P.E.N. nutrition support core curriculum: a case-based approach: the adult patient. Silver Spring (MD): American Society for Parenteral and Enteral Nutrition; c2017. 851 p.

Gunst J, De Bruyn A, Van den Berghe G. Glucose control in the ICU. Curr Opin Anaesthesiol. 2019 Apr;32(2):156–62.

Haugen HA, Chan LN, Li F. Indirect calorimetry: a practical guide for clinicians. Nutr Clin Pract. 2007 Aug;22(4):377–88.

Heyland DK, Dhaliwal R, Jiang X, Day AG. Identifying critically ill patients who benefit the most from nutrition therapy: the development and initial validation of a novel risk assessment tool. Crit Care. 2011;15(6):R268. Epub 2011 Nov 15.

Heyland DK, Dhaliwal R, Wang M, Day AG. The prevalence of iatrogenic underfeeding in the nutritionally 'at-risk' critically ill patient: results of an international, multicenter, prospective study. Clin Nutr. 2015 Aug;34(4):659–66. Epub 2014 Jul 19.

Heyland DK, MacDonald S, Keefe L, Drover JW. Total parenteral nutrition in the critically ill patient: a meta-analysis. JAMA. 1998 Dec 16;280(23):2013–9.

Huhmann MB, August DA. Review of American Society for Parenteral and Enteral Nutrition (ASPEN) clinical guidelines for nutrition support in cancer patients: nutrition screening and assessment. Nutr Clin Pract. 2008 Apr-May;23(2):182–8.

Jacquelin-Ravel N, Pichard C. Clinical nutrition, body composition and oncology: a critical literature review of the synergies. Crit Rev Oncol Hematol. 2012 Oct;84(1):37–46. Epub 2012 Apr 21.

Jensen GL, Hsiao PY, Wheeler D. Nutrition screening and assessment. In: Mueller CM, editor. The A.S.P.E.N. adult nutrition support core curriculum. 2nd ed. Silver Spring (MD): American Society for Parenteral and Enteral Nutrition; c2012. p. 155–69.

Jensen GL, Mirtallo J, Compher C, Dhaliwal R, Forbes A, Grijalba RF, et al; International Consensus Guideline Committee. Adult starvation and disease-related malnutrition: a proposal for etiology-based diagnosis in the clinical practice setting from the International Consensus Guideline Committee. JPEN J Parenter Enteral Nutr. 2010 Mar-Apr;34(2):156–9.

Kuo SH, Debnam JM, Fuller GN, de Groot J. Wernicke's encephalopathy: an underrecognized and reversible cause of confusional state in cancer patients. Oncology. 2009;76(1):10–8. Epub 2008 Nov 19.

Malone A, Seres D, Lord L. Complications of enteral nutrition. In: Mueller CM, editor. The A.S.P.E.N. adult nutrition support core curriculum. 2nd ed. Silver Spring (MD): American Society for Parenteral and Enteral Nutrition; c2012. p. 218–33.

Matarese LE. Indirect calorimetry: technical aspects. J Am Diet Assoc. 1997 Oct;97(10 Suppl 2):S154–60.

McClave SA, DeMeo MT, DeLegge MH, DiSario JA, Heyland DK, Maloney JP, et al. North American Summit on Aspiration in the Critically Ill Patient: consensus statement. JPEN J Parenter Enteral Nutr. 2002 Nov-Dec;26(6 Suppl):S80–5.

McClave SA, Martindale RG, Rice TW, Heyland DK. Feeding the critically ill patient. Crit Care Med. 2014 Dec;42(12):2600–10.

McClave SA, Martindale RG, Vanek VW, McCarthy M, Roberts P, Taylor B, et al; A.S.P.E.N. Board of Directors; American College of Critical Care Medicine; Society of Critical Care Medicine. Guidelines for the Provision and Assessment of Nutrition Support Therapy in the Adult Critically Ill Patient: Society of Critical Care Medicine (SCCM) and American Society for Parenteral and Enteral Nutrition (A.S.P.E.N.). JPEN J Parenter Enteral Nutr. 2009 May-Jun;33(3):277–316.

McClave SA, Saad MA, Esterle M, Anderson M, Jotautas AE, Franklin GA, et al. Volume-based feeding in the critically ill patient. JPEN J Parenter Enteral Nutr. 2015 Aug;39(6):707–12. Epub 2014 Jun 18.

McClave SA, Taylor BE, Martindale RG, Warren MM, Johnson DR, Braunschweig C, et al; Society of Critical Care Medicine (SCCM); American Society for Parenteral and Enteral Nutrition (A.S.P.E.N.). Guidelines for the provision and assessment of nutrition support therapy in the adult critically ill patient. JPEN J Parenter Enteral Nutr. 2016 Feb;40(2):159–211. Erratum in: JPEN J Parenter Enteral Nutr. 2016 Nov;40(8):1200.

McCowen KC, Friel C, Sternberg J, Chan S, Forse RA, Burke PA, et al. Hypocaloric total parenteral nutrition: effectiveness in prevention of hyperglycemia and infectious complications: a randomized clinical trial. Crit Care Med. 2000 Nov;28(11):3606–11.

Miller KR, Kiraly LN, Lowen CC, Martindale RG, McClave SA. "CAN WE FEED?" A mnemonic to merge nutrition and intensive care assessment of the critically ill patient. JPEN J Parenter Enteral Nutr. 2011 Sep;35(5):643–59.

Miller K, Kiraly L, Martindale RG. Critical care sepsis. In: Mueller CM, editor. The A.S.P.E.N. adult nutrition support core curriculum. 2nd ed. Silver Spring (MD): American Society for Parenteral and Enteral Nutrition; c2012. p. 377–91.

Mirtallo JM, Patel M. Overview of parenteral nutrition. In: Mueller CM, editor. The A.S.P.E.N. adult nutrition support core curriculum. 2nd ed. Silver Spring (MD): American Society for Parenteral and Enteral Nutrition; c2012. p. 234–44.

Neelemaat F, van Bokhorst-de van der Schueren MA, Thijs A, Seidell JC, Weijs PJ. Resting energy expenditure in malnourished older patients at hospital admission and three months after discharge: predictive equations versus measurements. Clin Nutr. 2012 Dec;31(6):958–66. Epub 2012 Jun 1.

Pogatshnik C, Hamilton C. Nutrition-focused physical examination: skin, nails, hair, eyes, and oral cavity. Support Line. 2011 Apr;33(2):7–13.

Skipper A. Nutrition support policies, procedures, forms, and formulas. Gaithersburg (MD): Aspen; c1995. 238 p.

Suarez JI, Vizzini A, Freeman WD. The conundrum of underfeeding vs overfeeding neurocritically ill patients: is less better? Neurology. 2015 Feb 17;84(7):639–40. Epub 2015 Jan 16.

Ventura AM, Waitzberg DL. Enteral nutrition protocols for critically ill patients: are they necessary? Nutr Clin Pract. 2015 Jun;30(3):351–62. Epub 2014 Sep 23.

Villet S, Chiolero RL, Bollmann MD, Revelly JP, Cayeux M-C, Delarue J, et al. Negative impact of hypocaloric feeding and energy balance on clinical outcome in ICU patients. Clin Nutr. 2005 Aug;24(4):502–9.

Vizzini A, Aranda-Michel J. Nutritional support in head injury. Nutrition. 2011 Feb;27(2):129–32. Epub 2010 Jun 26.

White JV, Guenter P, Jensen G, Malone A, Schofield M; Academy of Nutrition and Dietetics Malnutrition Work Group; A.S.P.E.N. Malnutrition Task Force; A.S.P.E.N. Board of Directors. Consensus statement of the Academy of Nutrition and Dietetics/American Society for Parenteral and Enteral Nutrition: characteristics recommended for the identification and documentation of adult malnutrition (undernutrition). J Acad Nutr Diet. 2012 May;112(5):730–8. Epub 2012 Apr 25. Erratum in: J Acad Nutr Diet. 2012 Nov;112(11):1899.

Wong PW, Enriquez A, Barrera R. Nutritional support in critically ill patients with cancer. Crit Care Clin. 2001 Jul;17(3):743–67.

Wooley JA, Frankenfield D. Energy. In: Mueller CM, editor. The A.S.P.E.N. adult nutrition support core curriculum. 2nd ed. Silver Spring (MD): American Society for Parenteral and Enteral Nutrition; c2012. p. 22–35.

Wooley JA, Sax HC. Indirect calorimetry: applications to practice. Nutr Clin Pract. 2003 Oct;18(5):434–9.

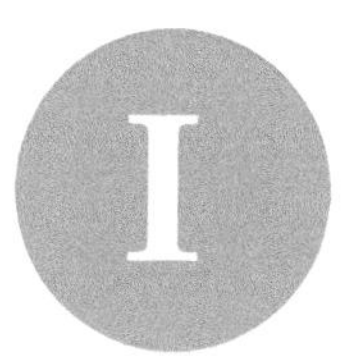

Questions and Answers

Abbreviations Used

A-a	alveoli-arterial
AKI	acute kidney injury
APRV	airway pressure release ventilation
ARDS	acute respiratory distress syndrome
BMI	body mass index
BP	blood pressure
bpm	beats per minute
CMV	continuous mandatory ventilation
CO_2	carbon dioxide
COPD	chronic obstructive pulmonary disease
CRRT	continuous renal replacement therapy
CSF	cerebrospinal fluid
ED	emergency department
FDA	US Food and Drug Administration
FEV_1	forced expiratory volume in the first second of expiration
FGF	fibroblast growth factor
FIO_2	fraction of inspired oxygen
FVC	forced vital capacity
HR	heart rate
ICU	intensive care unit
IMV	intermittent mandatory ventilation
KDIGO	Kidney Disease: Improving Global Outcomes
O_2	oxygen
PEEP	positive end-expiratory pressure
Pplat	plateau pressure
PPV	positive pressure ventilation
SpO_2	oxygen saturation by pulse oximetry
$\dot{V}E$	minute ventilation
VT	tidal volume

Questions

Multiple Choice (choose the best answer)

I.1. A 60-year-old man recovered after receiving mechanical ventilator support for months because of a severe traumatic brain injury. He was intubated for several weeks, and tracheostomy was postponed because of diffuse intravascular coagulation. He has shortness of breath. His pulmonary function test results (Table I.Q1) and a flow volume loop (Figure I.Q1) are shown.

Table I.Q1

Test	Pulmonary Function Test Results Predicted	Actual	% Predicted
FVC, L	4.35	4.73	109
FEV_1, L	3.69	2.56	69
FEV_1/FVC	0.85	0.54	...

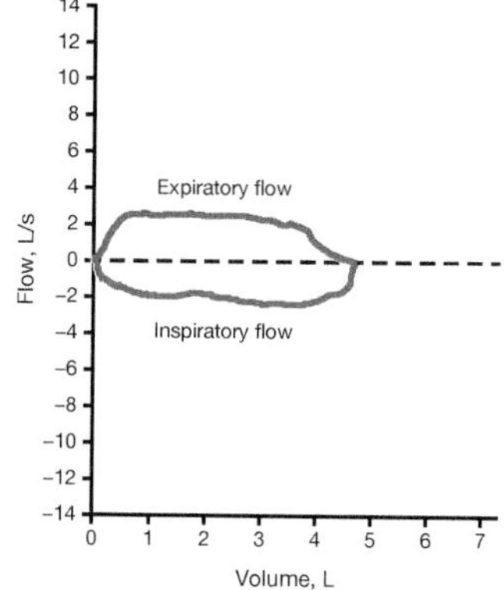

Figure I.Q1.

According to these results, which is the most likely explanation of the patient's underlying condition?

a. Unilateral mainstem bronchus obstruction
b. Variable intrathoracic upper airway obstruction
c. Variable extrathoracic upper airway obstruction
d. Fixed upper airway obstruction

I.2. A 67-year-old man presented with a middle cerebral artery infarction. In the ED, he was intubated for mechanical ventilation. Figure I.Q2 shows the initial ventilator flow-time and pressure-time waveforms.

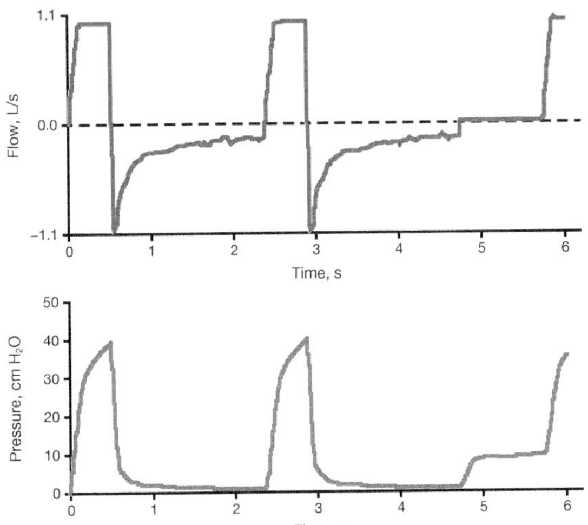

Figure I.Q2.

While he was being transported to the neurocritical care unit, however, he became progressively and profoundly hypotensive and had transient arrhythmias. The ventilator was set on volume assist-control mode, with a VT of 500 mL and a constant inspiratory flow rate of 50 L/min. The patient had a history of hypertension, atrial fibrillation, diabetes mellitus, peripheral artery disease, and COPD. What is the most appropriate first treatment?

a. Disconnect the ventilator for 30 seconds.
b. Extubate the patient and administer O_2 with a mask.
c. Place a chest tube immediately.
d. Transport the patient to the ED for chest radiography.

I.3. Which of the following will cause the end-tidal CO_2 to increase quickly?

a. Accidental extubation
b. Massive pulmonary embolism
c. Cardiopulmonary arrest
d. Mucous plugging

I.4. A 63-year-old man presented with acute respiratory failure. He was intubated and given mechanical ventilation in the ED. The initial settings for the mechanical ventilator were VT, 750 mL; respiratory rate, 10 breaths per minute; and PEEP, 5 cm H_2O. The patient was transferred to the ICU. He was deeply sedated and paralyzed, and no spontaneous breathing effort was noted. An intern decreased the VT to 500 mL and increased the respiratory rate to 15 breaths per minute. Which of the following changes would you expect to occur as a result of the intern's intervention?

a. Decreased airway resistance
b. Decreased $Paco_2$
c. Increased dead space fraction
d. Increased CO_2 production

I.5. During mechanical ventilation, what primarily influences oxygenation?

a. PEEP and Fio_2
b. Respiratory rate
c. $\dot{V}E$
d. Choices *b* and *c*

I.6. What VT range is appropriate for an adult male with an ideal body weight of 66 kg?

a. 600 to 800 mL
b. 350 to 550 mL
c. 550 to 650 mL
d. 300 to 400 mL

I.7. Lung-protective ventilation includes which of the following measures?

a. Reducing $\dot{V}E$
b. Maintaining Pplat less than 30 cm H_2O
c. Using a VT of 4 to 8 mL/kg ideal body weight
d. Choices *b* and *c*

I.8. Which mode of ventilation provides full support for all breaths (timed and patient triggered)?

a. Spontaneous
b. CMV
c. IMV
d. Noninvasive ventilation

I.9. Which of the following describes the cardiopulmonary interaction during PPV?

a. The pressure remaining in the alveoli at the end of inspiration can compress the adjacent pulmonary vasculature and impede pulmonary blood flow.
b. The intrathoracic veins are compressed, and the central venous and right atrial pressures are elevated.
c. The decrease in venous return to the right side of the heart causes increased right ventricular stroke volume, preload, and pulmonary blood flow.
d. Choices *a* and *b*

I.10. What is the benefit in selecting a dual-control adaptive pressure ventilation mode?

a. The patient must spontaneously trigger a breath.
b. The ventilator delivers a target VT while using the lowest driving pressure necessary.
c. The ventilator delivers a target VT while using the highest driving pressure necessary.
d. The patient must be comatose.

I.11. Which of the following is *not* recommended for the management of ARDS?

a. PEEP levels guided by esophageal balloon monitoring
b. APRV
c. Prone positioning
d. High-frequency oscillatory ventilation

I.12. For which patient population is the use of inhaled nitric oxide most established?

a. Patients with ARDS
b. Patients with right-sided heart failure
c. Neonates with persistent pulmonary hypertension
d. Recipients of transplanted lung

I.13. The application of high PEEP is often used for refractory hypoxemia in ARDS. Which of the following is *not* a potential consequence for patients with traumatic brain injury?

a. Improved cardiac output and cerebral perfusion pressure
b. Decreased cardiac output and cerebral perfusion pressure
c. Increased intracranial pressure
d. Decreased venous drainage from the brain to the heart

I.14. By which mechanism can hypercapnia increase intracranial pressure?

a. Prolonged elevation of $Paco_2$ produces arterial hypertension.
b. Elevated $Paco_2$ causes cerebrovascular vasodilatation.
c. Elevated $Paco_2$ decreases oxygenation of brain tissue.
d. Elevated $Paco_2$ decreases reabsorption of CSF.

I.15. A 60-year-old woman with a history of coronary artery disease and long-term use of β-blockers is transferred to the ICU from the ED with suspected abdominal sepsis due to cholangitis. While she is waiting for urgent surgical evaluation, she is in acute respiratory distress and needs emergency intubation. Immediately after she receives sedatives for tracheal intubation, refractory arterial hypotension develops (BP 70/30 mm Hg, HR stable at 70 bpm). The patient receives boluses of phenylephrine but remains hypotensive (BP 72/32 mm Hg, HR 68 bpm). Which of the following factors precipitated the arterial hypotension?

a. Increased mean systemic BP
b. Decreased isovolumetric contraction
c. Decreased systemic vascular resistance
d. Decreased HR

I.16. A 78-year-old man with a history of hypertension is admitted for an elective laparoscopic cholecystectomy. Vital signs include the following: BP 111/70 mm Hg, HR 76 bpm, respiratory rate 17 breaths per minute, and Spo_2 92% with room air. He states that he has been taking his antihypertensive medication. During the preoperative evaluation, the anesthesiologist hears a 3/6 crescendo-decrescendo systolic ejection murmur that radiates to the carotids and is immediately preceded by a systolic click. According to this patient's condition, which of the following changes would be observed in a volume-pressure curve?

a. Increased left ventricular volume and pressure due to regurgitant flow
b. Decreased left ventricular volume caused by decreased preload
c. Increased left ventricular pressure and increased end-systolic volume
d. Decreased stroke volume and decreased end-systolic volume

I.17. A 75-year-old man with a past medical history of uncontrolled hypertension and hyperlipidemia is admitted to the ED for worsening fatigue, dyspnea on exertion, and a 7-kg weight gain over the past 2 months. He is awake and alert but in moderate distress. He is using accessory respiratory muscles and says it is difficult to breathe. Vital signs include the following: BP 106/70 mm Hg, HR 106 bpm, respiratory rate 22 breaths per minute, and Spo_2 89% with room air. The patient appears uncomfortable and can speak in only short sentences. On cardiac examination, he has a regular rate and rhythm, with the apex displaced laterally to the midaxillary line in the 6th intercostal space, and a third heart sound. On lung auscultation, he has diffuse bilateral rales in the lower lung fields and his extremities have ankle edema (2+) bilaterally. How does this patient's clinical condition affect the Frank-Startling curve?

a. The curve shifts up and to the right.
b. The curve shifts down and to the left.
c. The curve shifts up and to the left.
d. The curve shifts down and to the right.

I.18. A 68-year-old man with a past medical history of uncontrolled type 2 diabetes mellitus, chronic renal insufficiency, hypertension, and hyperlipidemia is admitted to the ED with a 5-day history of productive cough with associated fevers, chills, and rigors. On examination, he is lethargic. Vital signs are HR 94 bpm, BP 80/40 mm Hg, respiratory rate 35 breaths per minute, Spo_2 89% on 3 L O_2 by nasal cannula, and temperature 39.5°C. On physical examination he has rhonchi appreciated on auscultation over the right side of his chest. Laboratory test results are as follows: white blood cell count 22×10^9/L, sodium 133 mmol/L, potassium 5.5 mmol/L, and glucose 192 mg/dL. Chest radiography shows consolidation of the right middle and lower lobe air space. Which statement is true?

a. Systolic dysfunction is at least twice as common as diastolic dysfunction in patients with septic shock.
b. Septic shock results exclusively in arterial dilatation as a result of failure of the vascular smooth muscle to vasoconstrict.
c. Diastolic dysfunction is a poor prognostic marker in patients with sepsis.
d. The adverse effects of fluid resuscitation when a patient is on the flat portion of the Frank-Starling curve is related to altered diastolic compliance at higher filling pressures.

I.19. A 65-year-old man who was admitted to the ICU with a diagnosis of septic shock and ARDS is receiving mechanical ventilator support. He appears to have increased work of breathing, and his vasopressor support has been increased for refractory shock. The intensivist wants to proceed with a fluid responsiveness test for this patient who has respiratory efforts. Which of the following would be the most reliable?

a. Inferior vena cava distensibility index
b. Inferior vena cava collapsibility index
c. Left ventricular outflow tract peak velocity variability
d. Left ventricular outflow tract area and passive leg raising

I.20. Which of the following hormones is *not* released into the systemic circulation by the kidneys?

a. Renin
b. Erythropoietin
c. Klotho
d. Antidiuretic hormone (vasopressin)

I.21. During urine acidification, which part of the renal tubular system generates most of the ammonia?

a. Proximal convoluted tubules
b. Distal convoluted tubules
c. Thick ascending loop of Henle
d. Collecting ducts

I.22. What is the main factor responsible for regulation of the glomerular filtration rate?

a. Glomerular plasma flow rate
b. Glomerular capillary hydraulic pressure
c. Tubuloglomerular feedback mechanisms
d. Myogenic response of blood vessels

I.23. Diagnosis of AKI in critically ill patients is based on an increased serum creatinine level and decreased urine output. Which of the following statements is true?

a. A small increase in creatinine (0.3 mg/dL) is associated with a poor short-term prognosis for hospitalized patients.
b. AKI classification should be done only on the basis of serum creatinine because urinary volume measurement is cumbersome.
c. Robust data are available for the use of biomarkers in the diagnosis and management of AKI.
d. AKI is not associated with in-hospital mortality.

I.24. Which of the following conditions is *not* recommended for accurately conducting indirect calorimetry?

a. The patient has been awake for at least 6 to 8 hours after anesthesia.
b. The patient is receiving nothing by mouth, and enteral nutrition is withheld for 6 hours before testing.
c. The test is conducted at least 4 hours after dialysis.
d. The test is administered at least 30 minutes after administration of pain and sedation medications.

I.25. A 65-year-old woman with subarachnoid hemorrhage is admitted to the neurocritical care unit and intubated. The team will begin enteral nutrition with a nasoenteric tube. Her BMI is 28.9. What are her protein requirements?

a. Based on actual body weight, 0.8 g/kg
b. Based on actual body weight, 1.2 to 2.0 g/kg
c. Based on ideal body weight, 2.0 g/kg
d. Based on ideal body weight, 2.5 g/kg

I.26. An 85-year-old man was transferred to the ICU with respiratory failure and was immediately intubated. He was eating well but had minimal intake in the past 24 hours. The critical care team would like to initiate enteral nutrition. What type of tube is recommended?

a. Orogastric tube
b. Nasogastric tube
c. Nasoenteric tube
d. Gastrostomy tube

I.27. On oral examination, a patient has spongy, bleeding gums. Which vitamin deficiency is most likely?

a. Vitamin A
b. Vitamin B_{12}
c. Vitamin D
d. Vitamin C

I.28. A 32-year-old man with a history of Crohn disease is admitted to the ICU with shortness of breath and recurrent small-bowel obstruction. He has lost 11.4 kg over the past 6 months and is moderately malnourished. His daily fluid limit is 1,500 mL. What form of nutrition support is recommended?

a. Peripheral parenteral nutrition
b. Central parenteral nutrition
c. Infusion of dextrose and amino acids
d. Infusion of 5% dextrose in 0.45% normal saline

Answers

I.1. Answer d.

Different patterns can appear on a flow-volume loop when patients have obstructive physiology. *Variable intrathoracic obstruction* (Figure I.A1A) is caused by lesions within the intrathoracic airways that obstruct the lumen of the airway but move in response to airway pressure changes during the respiratory cycle. An example is tracheobronchomalacia with a breakdown of the cartilaginous rings. *Variable extrathoracic obstruction* (Figure I.A1B) is caused by lesions within the extrathoracic airways that obstruct the lumen of the airway but move in response to airway pressure changes during the respiratory cycle. An example is a mobile thyroid mass compressing the trachea.

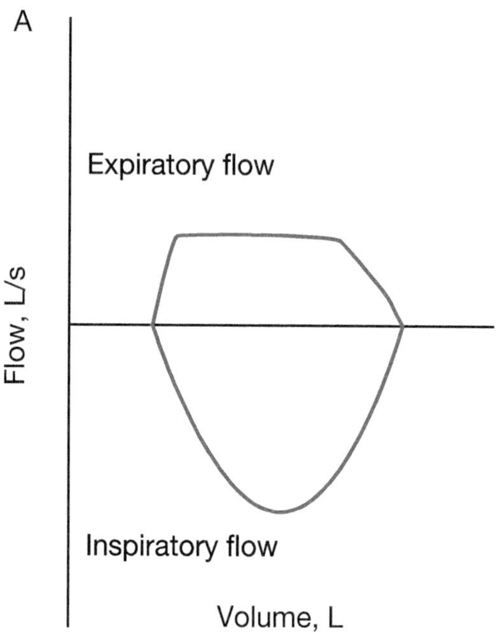

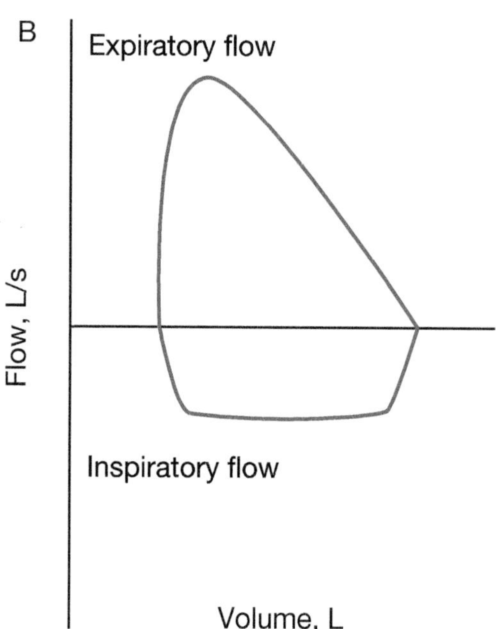

Figure I.A1.

The flow-volume loop in the question (Figure I.Q1) is the result of a fixed airway obstruction. This pattern is caused by either an intrathoracic or extrathoracic lesion that obstructs the airway lumen but does not move in response to airway pressure changes during the respiratory cycle. Examples are tracheal stenosis or bulky lymphadenopathy encasing the trachea.

Nussbaumer-Ochsner Y, Thurnheer R. Images in clinical medicine: subglottic stenosis. N Engl J Med. 2015 Jul 2;373(1):73.

I.2. Answer a.

In the patient's flow-time curve, the flow at end-expiration is not zero before the patient receives the next breath. This signifies auto-PEEP, defined as the magnitude of the end-expiratory pressure in excess of the set extrinsic PEEP. High $\dot{V}_E$ and expiratory airflow obstruction are the most important risk factors for the development of auto-PEEP. Auto-PEEP decreases venous return by mechanical compression and obstruction of the intrathoracic portion of the superior vena cava. PEEP can also decrease left ventricular afterload. Lung hyperinflation may cause bradycardia and vasodilatation through autonomic reflexes. Excessive PEEP can cause acute right ventricular failure by hyperinflation of the lungs, and shock and cardiac arrest may occur. To minimize auto-PEEP, one should minimize $\dot{V}_E$ and use small V_Ts with prolongation of the time available for exhalation. If the patient is in shock or cardiac arrest due to auto-PEEP, one should consider a brief trial of apnea or temporarily disconnect the endotracheal or tracheostomy tube from the ventilator circuit to allow complete exhalation.

Berlin D. Hemodynamic consequences of auto-PEEP. J Intensive Care Med. 2014 Mar-Apr;29(2):81–6. Epub 2012 May 15.

I.3. Answer d.

Mucous plugging can cause an increased end-tidal CO_2 if it leads to decreased V_Ts and thus decreased ventilation. All the other choices (accidental extubation, massive pulmonary embolism, and cardiopulmonary arrest) lead to decreased end-tidal CO_2 due to increased dead space ventilation (or lack of CO_2 detection with accidental extubation).

Anderson CT, Breen PH. Carbon dioxide kinetics and capnography during critical care. Crit Care. 2000;4(4):207–15. Epub 2000 Jul 12.

I.4. Answer c.

When the intern decreased the V_T, the volume of the anatomical dead space remained the same. $\dot{V}_E$ was not changed (750 mL × 10 = 500 mL × 15). Therefore, the dead space fraction of the total ventilation increased. $Paco_2$ increased because of the increased dead space fraction, while CO_2 production and airway resistance did not change.

Robertson HT. Dead space: the physiology of wasted ventilation. Eur Respir J. 2015 Jun;45(6):1704–16. Epub 2014 Nov 13. Erratum in: Eur Respir J. 2015 Oct;46(4):1226.

I.5. Answer a.

Supplemental O_2 supplies the lungs with supra-atmospheric levels of O_2, increasing the Po_2 in the alveoli. PEEP recruits collapsed alveoli and reduces alveolar collapse at the end of exhalation. $\dot{V}_E$ and respiratory rate influence ventilation and CO_2 removal.

Kacmarek RM, Stoller JK, Heuer AJ, editors. Egan's fundamentals of respiratory care. 11th ed. St Louis (MO): Elsevier/Mosby; c2017. 1,392 p.

I.6. Answer b.

The appropriate V_T range for an adult patient is 6 to 8 mL/kg ideal body weight. Therefore, the range of safe V_T delivery is 350 to 550 mL.

Kacmarek RM, Stoller JK, Heuer AJ, editors. Egan's fundamentals of respiratory care. 11th ed. St Louis (MO): Elsevier/Mosby; c2017. 1,392 p.

I.7. Answer d.

Lung-protective ventilation is widely defined as using VT of 4 to 8 mL/kg ideal body weight and maintaining a Pplat less than 30 cm H_2O. Lung-protective ventilation reduces mortality among patients with ARDS and improves outcomes for patients with ventilator-induced lung injury.

Kacmarek RM, Stoller JK, Heuer AJ, editors. Egan's fundamentals of respiratory care. 11th ed. St Louis (MO): Elsevier/Mosby; c2017. 1,392 p.

I.8. Answer b.

In CMV (commonly referred to as assist control), regardless of trigger type (timed or patient), the ventilator delivers a breath with a set VT or inspiratory pressure, inspiratory time or flow rate, PEEP, and F_{IO_2}. Each breath has the same characteristics. The patient-triggered breaths are assisted breaths, and the timed breaths are controlled breaths.

Kacmarek RM, Stoller JK, Heuer AJ, editors. Egan's fundamentals of respiratory care. 11th ed. St Louis (MO): Elsevier/Mosby; c2017. 1,392 p.

I.9. Answer d.

PPV can have a profound effect on hemodynamic parameters, including cardiac output and BP. Positive intrathoracic pressure during inspiration elevates central venous pressure and right atrial pressure, resulting in a decrease in venous return to the right side of the heart, which decreases right ventricular stroke volume, preload, and pulmonary blood flow. Additionally, PEEP can compress the pulmonary vasculature. Since HR usually does not change with PEEP, the entire decrease in cardiac output is a consequence of decreased left ventricular stroke volume. Close monitoring of hemodynamics should be coupled with mechanical ventilation, particularly when titrating PEEP to a higher level.

Kacmarek RM, Stoller JK, Heuer AJ, editors. Egan's fundamentals of respiratory care. 11th ed. St Louis (MO): Elsevier/Mosby; c2017. 1,392 p.

Luecke T, Pelosi P. Clinical review: positive end-expiratory pressure and cardiac output. Crit Care. 2005;9(6):607–21. Epub 2005 Oct 18.

I.10. Answer b.

The clinician sets the target VT and the upper and lower limits for driving pressure. The ventilator delivers the VT with the lowest pressure needed.

Puritan Bennett 980 ventilator system: product training sample practice exercises (breathe more naturally) [Internet]. Boulder (CO): Covidien. c2013. Available from: http://www.covidien.com/imageServer.aspx/ doc293914.pdf?contentID=45049&contenttype=application/pdf.

I.11. Answer d.

High-frequency oscillatory ventilation has not shown any positive effect on mortality and has harmed patients with ARDS.

Fan E, Del Sorbo L, Goligher EC, Hodgson CL, Munshi L, Walkey AJ, et al; American Thoracic Society, European Society of Intensive Care Medicine, and Society of Critical Care Medicine. An official American Thoracic Society/European Society of Intensive Care Medicine/Society of Critical Care Medicine Clinical Practice guideline: mechanical ventilation in adult patients with acute respiratory distress syndrome. Am J Respir Crit Care Med. 2017 May 1;195(9):1253–63. Erratum in: Am J Respir Crit Care Med. 2017 Jun 1;195(11):1540.

I.12. Answer c.

The FDA has approved inhaled nitric oxide for use only in neonates with persistent pulmonary hypertension. However, inhaled nitric oxide is used in patients who have other conditions, including ARDS, right-sided heart failure, and adult pulmonary hypertension, and in patients who have received a transplanted heart or lung (or both). Refractory hypoxemia has been treated successfully, but inhaled nitric oxide has not been shown to decrease mortality in any patient population.

George I, Xydas S, Topkara VK, Ferdinando C, Barnwell EC, Gableman L, et al. Clinical indication for use and outcomes after inhaled nitric oxide therapy. Ann Thorac Surg. 2006 Dec;82(6):2161–9.

INOMAX (nitric oxide) for inhalation [Internet]. United Kingdom: Mallinckrodt Pharmaceuticals. c2017 [cited 2018 Jun 6]. Available from: http://inomax.com/about-inomax.

I.13. Answer a.

PEEP has the potential to decrease cardiac output and cerebral perfusion pressure, increase intracranial pressure, and decrease venous drainage.

Boone MD, Jinadasa SP, Mueller A, Shaefi S, Kasper EM, Hanafy KA, et al. The effect of positive end-expiratory pressure on intracranial pressure and cerebral hemodynamics. Neurocrit Care. 2017 Apr;26(2):174–81.

I.14. Answer b.

Hypercapnia directly and indirectly (through alteration of CSF pH) dilates the cerebral vasculature, and hypercapnia can cause intracranial hypertension.

Roberts BW, Karagiannis P, Coletta M, Kilgannon JH, Chansky ME, Trzeciak S. Effects of $Paco_2$ derangements on clinical outcomes after cerebral injury: a systematic review. Resuscitation. 2015 Jun;91:32–41. Epub 2015 Mar 28.

I.15. Answer c.

Acute decrease in systemic vascular resistance and decreased venous return due to venodilatation are the most remarkable effects of induction of anesthesia with subsequent arterial hypotension before intubation in the ICU. At higher HRs, the relative amount of time in diastole is decreased; thus, acute myocardial ischemia can be present in patients with coronary artery disease. However, this patient's HR remained essentially the same. In addition, initiation of mechanical circulatory support and use of PEEP can worsen arterial hypotension. For this patient with suspected abdominal sepsis, the initial management should be aggressive fluid resuscitation and use of vasopressors to offset the adverse effect of sedatives. Choice *a* is incorrect because the mean systemic pressure (the pressure measured when flow ceases within the circulatory system [10-15 mm Hg]) is lower than the systemic arterial pressure and is similar to the right atrial pressure. After administration of most sedatives, venodilatation leads to lower mean systemic pressure. Choice *b* is incorrect because isovolumetric contraction remains similar if not increased because of decreased left ventricular afterload. Choice *d* is incorrect because a slight decrease in HR within the normal range would not explain the severity of arterial hypotension.

Zanger DR, Solomon AJ, Gersh BJ. Contemporary management of angina: part II: medical management of chronic stable angina. Am Fam Physician. 2000 Jan 1;61(1):129–38.

I.16. Answer c.

Aortic stenosis, the most common valvular disease worldwide, usually results from valve leaflet calcification in the sixth or seven decade of life. On auscultation, an ejection click is typically heard before a crescendo-decrescendo systolic murmur. With an increased afterload, the left ventricular pressure and end-systolic volume are increased, and the stroke volume is decreased. When the heart can no longer compensate, angina develops with heart failure or syncope (or both).

Choice *a* is incorrect because the volume-pressure curve variations are consistent with aortic regurgitation and increased regurgitant flow into the left ventricle. Choice *b* is incorrect because the volume-pressure curve variations are consistent with mitral stenosis. Choice *d* is incorrect because it is inconsistent with aortic stenosis.

Argulian E, Windecker S, Messerli FH. Misconceptions and facts about aortic stenosis. Am J Med. 2017 Apr;130(4):398–402. Epub 2017 Jan 18.

I.17. Answer d.

The patient's clinical presentation is consistent with acute decompensated congestive heart failure. Therefore, the Frank-Starling curve is shifted down and to the right. Option *c* is incorrect because it is consistent with increased cardiac contractility. Choices *a* and *b* are incorrect because they are inconsistent with congestive heart failure.

The Frank-Starling curve is affected by changes in cardiac determinants such as contractility, afterload, and preload. Modifications in preload result in changes along the same line of the Frank-Starling curve. However, changes in afterload and contractility result in a shift of the Frank-Starling curve, as follows:

An increase in contractility shifts the curve up and to the left as a result of increased cardiac output (eg, exercise).

A decrease in contractility shifts the curve down and to the right as a result of increased left ventricular end-diastolic volume and decreased cardiac output (eg, congestive heart failure).

A decrease in afterload shifts the curve up and to the left. Thus, for a given preload, the stroke volume and cardiac output are increased.

An increase in afterload shifts the curve down and to the right because of decreased stroke volume and cardiac output.

Sequeira V, van der Velden J. Historical perspective on heart function: the Frank-Starling Law. Biophys Rev. 2015 Dec;7(4):421–47. Epub 2015 Nov 19.

I.18. Answer d.

In the flat portion of the Frank-Starling curve, additional fluid administration results in increased pulmonary hydrostatic pressures and the release of atrial natriuretic peptides. The net effect is a fluid shift into the interstitial space with pulmonary and tissue edema as a result of altered O_2 delivery and extraction, distortion of the tissue architecture, disturbance of cell-to-cell interaction, limited capillary blood flow, and altered lymphatic drainage.

Choice *a* is incorrect because diastolic dysfunction is more common than systolic dysfunction among patients with septic shock. Choice *b* is incorrect because septic shock results from not only arterial vasodilatation but also from profound venous dilatation, thus resulting in an increase in the unstressed blood volume, diminished venous return, and reduced cardiac output. Choice *c* is incorrect because diastolic dysfunction is considered a good prognostic marker among patients with septic shock.

Marik P, Bellomo R. A rational approach to fluid therapy in sepsis. Br J Anaesth. 2016 Mar;116(3):339–49. Epub 2015 Oct 27.

I.19. Answer d.

Patients who are receiving mechanical ventilator support with active rather than passive breathing should be tested with passive leg raising. The other tests were validated in patients receiving passive mechanical ventilation (no respiratory efforts). This patient had increased work of breathing and ventilator dyssynchrony.

Monnet X, Rienzo M, Osman D, Anguel N, Richard C, Pinsky MR, et al. Passive leg raising predicts fluid responsiveness in the critically ill. Crit Care Med. 2006 May;34(5):1402–7.

I.20. Answer d.

Renin, an important hormone for hemostatic stability, is secreted by juxtaglomerular cells located in the walls of afferent arterioles in the renal interstitium. Erythropoietin is responsible for production of red blood cells. In adults, about 90% of erythropoietin is produced by renal interstitial fibroblasts, and 10% is contributed by extrarenal sources, primarily liver cells. Serum phosphorus regulation by the kidneys involves production of FGF 23 in osteoblasts in response to increases in serum phosphate. FGF 23 requires a cofactor to exert its action on the renal proximal tubule. Klotho is produced in the kidney and activates FGF receptor.

Vasopressin is a potent endogenous peptide influencing many biologic functions, including regulation of water balance, BP, platelet function, and thermoregulation. It is synthesized as a prohormone in the posterior hypothalamus and is stored in the posterior pituitary. Vasopressin acts on V_1, V_2, V_3, and oxytocin-type receptors. V_1 receptors are located in the vasculature, myometrium, and platelets. V_2 receptors are located along the distal tubule and collecting duct. V_3 receptors are mainly found in the pituitary gland.

Schrier RW. Vasopressin and aquaporin 2 in clinical disorders of water homeostasis. Semin Nephrol. 2008 May;28(3):289–96.

I.21. Answer a.

Ammonia excretion is the major mechanism by which the kidneys excrete acid. Of the net acid excreted or new bicarbonate generated by the kidneys, approximately one-half to two-thirds (approximately 40-50 mmol daily) is from ammonia excretion in the urine. Most of the ammonia produced is excreted from the proximal convoluted tubules into the urine rather than added to the venous blood. Synthesis and excretion of ammonia increase greatly during acid loading, in contrast to the limited increase in titratable acidity. Transport of the produced ammonia along the nephron and into the urine is a complex process.

Hamm LL, Nakhoul N, Hering-Smith KS. Acid-base homeostasis. Clin J Am Soc Nephrol. 2015 Dec 7;10(12):2232–42. Epub 2015 Nov 23.

I.22. Answer b.

The transcapillary movement of water across the glomerular capillaries is controlled by Starling forces (like in all capillary beds). Filtration results from an imbalance between the mean transcapillary hydraulic pressure gradient, which favors filtration, and the mean transcapillary oncotic pressure, which opposes filtration. The mediators of renal autoregulation are a myogenic response, which is intrinsic to the blood vessels, and a tubuloglomerular feedback mechanism by which chloride is taken up in the macula densa segment of the distal tubule. In addition, changes in the filtration fraction affect the oncotic pressure in peritubular capillaries and contribute to glomerular tubular balance.

Gong R, Dworkin LD, Brenner BM, Maddox DA. The renal circulations and glomerular ultrafiltration. In: Brenner BM, editor. Brenner & Rector's the kidney. 8th ed. Vol. 1. Philadelphia (PA): Saunders/Elsevier; c2008. p. 91–129.

I.23. Answer a.

According to the latest KDIGO guidelines, 0.3 mg/dL is the minimum serum creatinine level elevation from baseline that is associated with increased hospital mortality for AKI patients. AKI is an independent predictor of hospital mortality and is a risk factor for future chronic kidney disease. Available biomarkers are limited by their performance characteristics, and the utility of biomarkers needs to be validated for clinical outcomes.

Maciel AT, Vitorio D. Urine biochemistry assessment in critically ill patients: controversies and future perspectives. J Clin Monit Comput. 2017 Jun;31(3):539–46. Epub 2016 Apr 1.

I.24. Answer b.

In patients receiving continuous tube feeding, the rate and composition of nutrition infusion should remain constant for at least 12 hours before and during indirect calorimetry. If the patient is receiving intermittent feedings, measuring resting metabolic rate should be done 4 hours after the feeding.

Wooley JA, Frankenfield D. Energy. In: Mueller CM, editor. The A.S.P.E.N. adult nutrition support core curriculum. 2nd ed. Silver Spring (MD): American Society for Parenteral and Enteral Nutrition; c2012. p. 22–35.

Wooley JA, Sax HC. Indirect calorimetry: applications to practice. Nutr Clin Pract. 2003 Oct;18(5):434–9.

I.25. Answer b.

The daily protein requirements for a critically ill patient are 1.2 to 2.0 g/kg based on actual body weight. Protein needs would be increased if the patient were receiving hemodialysis or CRRT. Actual body weight is used for calculations when BMI is less than 30. Ideal body weight is used for calculations when BMI is 30 or more.

McClave SA, Martindale RG, Rice TW, Heyland DK. Feeding the critically ill patient. Crit Care Med. 2014 Dec;42(12):2600–10.

McClave SA, Martindale RG, Vanek VW, McCarthy M, Roberts P, Taylor B, et al; A.S.P.E.N. Board of Directors; American College of Critical Care Medicine; Society of Critical Care Medicine. Guidelines for the Provision and Assessment of Nutrition Support Therapy in the Adult Critically Ill Patient: Society of Critical Care Medicine (SCCM) and American Society for Parenteral and Enteral Nutrition (A.S.P.E.N.). JPEN J Parenter Enteral Nutr. 2009 May-Jun;33(3):277–316.

I.26. Answer c.

Nasoenteric feeding is recommended for patients at high risk for aspiration. Risk factors for aspiration include mechanical ventilation, reduced level of consciousness, inability to protect airway, and age older than 70 years. At this time, a gastrostomy tube is not recommended because the expected duration of need is less than 4 weeks.

McClave SA, Martindale RG, Rice TW, Heyland DK. Feeding the critically ill patient. Crit Care Med. 2014 Dec;42(12):2600–10.

McClave SA, Martindale RG, Vanek VW, McCarthy M, Roberts P, Taylor B, et al; A.S.P.E.N. Board of Directors; American College of Critical Care Medicine; Society of Critical Care Medicine. Guidelines for the Provision and Assessment of Nutrition Support Therapy in the Adult Critically Ill Patient: Society of Critical Care Medicine (SCCM) and American Society for Parenteral and Enteral Nutrition (A.S.P.E.N.). JPEN J Parenter Enteral Nutr. 2009 May-Jun;33(3):277–316.

I.27. Answer d.

A vitamin C deficiency could result in spongy, bleeding gums and scurvy, petechiae, and poor wound healing.

Clark SF. Vitamins and trace elements. In: Mueller CM, editor. The A.S.P.E.N. adult nutrition support core curriculum. 2nd ed. Silver Spring (MD): American Society for Parenteral and Enteral Nutrition; c2012. p. 121–51.

Pogatshnik C, Hamilton C. Nutrition-focused physical examination: skin, nails, hair, eyes, and oral cavity. Support Line. 2011 Apr;33(2):7–13.

I.28. Answer b.

Indications for the appropriate use of parenteral nutrition include intestinal obstruction, distal high-output fistulas, severe gastrointestinal tract bleeding, or severe malabsorption. Parenteral nutrition should be initiated promptly after ICU admission for malnourished or nutritionally high-risk patients with a nonfunctioning gastrointestinal tract. Peripheral parenteral nutrition is hyperosmolar at 600 to 900 mOsm/L and requires larger fluid volume; therefore, it is not desirable for patients requiring fluid restriction.

McClave SA, Martindale RG, Vanek VW, McCarthy M, Roberts P, Taylor B, et al; A.S.P.E.N. Board of Directors; American College of Critical Care Medicine; Society of Critical Care Medicine. Guidelines for the Provision and Assessment of Nutrition Support Therapy in the Adult Critically Ill Patient: Society of Critical Care Medicine (SCCM) and American Society for Parenteral and Enteral Nutrition (A.S.P.E.N.). JPEN J Parenter Enteral Nutr. 2009 May-Jun;33(3):277–316.

Mirtallo JM, Patel M. Overview of parenteral nutrition. In: Mueller CM, editor. The A.S.P.E.N. adult nutrition support core curriculum. 2nd ed. Silver Spring (MD): American Society for Parenteral and Enteral Nutrition; c2012. p. 234–44.

Section

II

Fundamentals of Neurocritical Care

7 Neurologic Examination in Neurocritical Illness

EELCO F. M. WIJDICKS, MD, PhD

Goals

- Describe the principles of localization in patients with acute brain disease.
- Describe neurologic examination of comatose patients.
- Describe lesion localization in patients with acute spinal cord disease.
- Describe clinical signs of deterioration in patients with neurocritical illness.

Introduction

Neurologic examination of critically ill neurologic patients must be the uncompromised gold standard in any evaluation. Without it or when confounded, the attending physician is prone to make errors in diagnosis, treatment, and prognosis. The localization of a disease process in a specific part of the brain (eg, the cerebrum, midbrain, pons, or medulla oblongata), spinal cord, neural plexuses, or peripheral nerves constitutes the essence of a neurologic evaluation, but neurologists resort to several neuroimaging modalities when localization is uncertain. Despite surprises delivered by magnetic resonance imaging—not infrequently used to critique the limitations of a neurologic examination—neurologic diagnosis is a deductive synthesis and is preferentially based on a full, unconfounded neurologic examination, an approach typically lacking in clinical trial–devised scales or scores.

Neurologic examination of patients admitted to intensive care units (ICUs) has unique features and follows important principles. There are major differences between outpatient practice and specialized care, and the only commonality between neurologic examinations in the neurology outpatient practice and the ICU is the use of the reflex hammer and the pin. Neurologic examination in the ICU is largely focused on cranial nerve function and motor response. The motor response can be practically divided into *spontaneous motor responses* (eg, myoclonus or focal twitches) and *evoked motor responses* (eg, decorticate and decerebrate responses). Muscle strength is evaluated for the presence or absence of symmetrical withdrawal and, if possible, shoulder abduction, elbow flexion and extension, finger spreading and closure, hip flexion, and foot elevation. Walking is often out of the question, but even if the patient is sitting, ataxia may be evident (eg, vermis hemorrhage or infarct).

The neurologic evaluation can be summarized as a series of steps: 1) interpreting key neurologic findings on examination, 2) interpreting neuroimages, 3) connecting neuroimaging findings and laboratory abnormalities to the neurologic history and critical summary of the neurologic findings, 4) examining the patient to gauge the change after treatment, and 5) predicting a clinical trajectory. The examination of the comatose patient is described below and in more detail in Chapter 14 ("Coma and Other Altered States of Consciousness").

Common Findings and Interpretation

Before specific causes are localized and identified, an initial assessment of an acutely ill patient with a neurologic condition will provide a sense of the abnormality and allow some conclusions. Common neurologic symptoms that neurologists should pursue are summarized in Table 7.1.

Lesion Localization With the Neurologic Examination

The principle of localization in acute brain injury is that a certain lesion may produce a recognizable and reproducible set of symptoms. If the brain is considered as

Table 7.1 • Common Neurologic Findings and Interpretations

Abnormality	Interpretation
Unresponsive and not awake	Coma from massive structural injury or drug effect
Unresponsive and awake	Global aphasia Nonconvulsive status epilepticus Locked-in syndrome
Fixed and dilated pupil	Expanding hemispheric mass Bihemispheric injury or brainstem injury (or both)
Retinal hemorrhage, papilledema	Aneurysmal subarachnoid hemorrhage Acute retinal artery occlusion Long-standing mass effect
Forced eye deviation	Acute hemispheric lesion Acute brainstem lesion Bihemispheric lesion (upward or downward deviation)
Nystagmus	Lesions in brainstem or cerebellum
Unable to adduct 1 eye with other eye (nystagmus with abduction)	Internuclear ophthalmoplegia with acute brainstem lesion
Anisocoria (>1 mm)	Brainstem lesion
Flaccidity of the extremities	Drug overdose Acute spinal cord injury
Spasticity of the extremities	Neuroleptic malignant syndrome Serotonin syndrome
Twitching	Focal seizures Myoclonus Asterixis clonus
Oropharyngeal weakness	Guillain-Barré syndrome Myasthenia gravis Amyotrophic lateral sclerosis (tongue atrophy, fasciculi)
Sensory deficits	Acute spinal cord injury

hemispheres and brainstem, differences become apparent. Involvement of 1 hemisphere typically produces a focal sign (ie, aphasia, alexia, agraphia, neglect, and often hemiparesis). Bilateral lesions produce a decline in consciousness and may be preceded by focal signs. Because the brainstem is a compact collection of descending fibers (long tracts) and nuclei, a lesion (even if small) can produce many neurologic findings and involve abnormalities in the cranial nerves in combination with long tract signs (hemiparesis or quadriparesis).

Many acute neurologic disorders involve a stroke, and either anterior or posterior circulation should be considered. *Acute middle cerebral artery circulation syndromes* result in face, arm, and leg motor weakness; abnormalities of sensation; a forced gaze toward the lesion; and severe multidomain aphasia (if the lesion is in the dominant hemisphere). A lesion in the opposite (nondominant) hemisphere causes hemiparesis but with apraxia, anosognosia, and loss of melodic modulation of speech.

Acute distal posterior cerebral circulation syndromes result in acute hemianopia. When the embolus is more proximal, it can involve a large territory that potentially includes the midbrain, thalamus, and a large part of the hemisphere, leading to hemispatial neglect and hemiparesis similar to an embolus in the middle cerebral artery. With bilateral posterior cerebral artery involvement, cortical blindness may occur because of involvement of both occipital lobes, such that the patient may be unaware of blindness. With bilateral proximal occlusions, the infarction of the medial temporal lobes leads to permanent amnesia.

Acute embolic occlusion of the vertebrobasilar circulation causes infarcts in the midbrain and pons. They lead mainly to major oculomotor syndromes (eg, gaze palsies, skew deviation, and third and sixth nerve palsies), hemiparesis, and ataxia.

Specific Clinical Findings

Brainstem reflexes are shown in Figure 7.1. The cranial nerves are often abnormal from structural injury, but intravenous anesthetics or neuromuscular blockers render neurologic examination impossible.

The pupils are normally round and equal in diameter, but pupillary inequality of 1 mm or less is common and of no pathologic significance. Pupils are smaller in the elderly and during sleepiness, but the normal diameter has been traditionally considered to be 2 to 7 mm. The pupil size can be small (pinpoint pupils; *miosis*), large (dilated pupils; *mydriasis*), or midway between the two. Midbrain lesions interrupt sympathetic and parasympathetic tracts, so the pupil assumes an intermediate diameter of about 5 mm. Small pupils are expected with pontine lesions because the descending sympathetic tracts are disrupted. Lateral medulla oblongata lesions also produce miosis as part of Horner syndrome. Pupillary responses remain intact even if the patient has an acute metabolic derangement or is heavily sedated, but pupillary response may be delayed and less brisk (sluggish). Opioids may cause pinpoint pupils, and the light response cannot be reliably assessed even with a pupillometer. Atropine and the condensed mist of bronchodilators can cause pupils to dilate.

Pupillometry may be more accurate than manual pupillary assessment and reduce interobserver variability, but pupils considered to be nonreactive on pupillometry may actually be slowly reacting pupils. The pupillometer does not address shape, which is important because an oval or elliptical pupil may indicate increased intracranial pressure

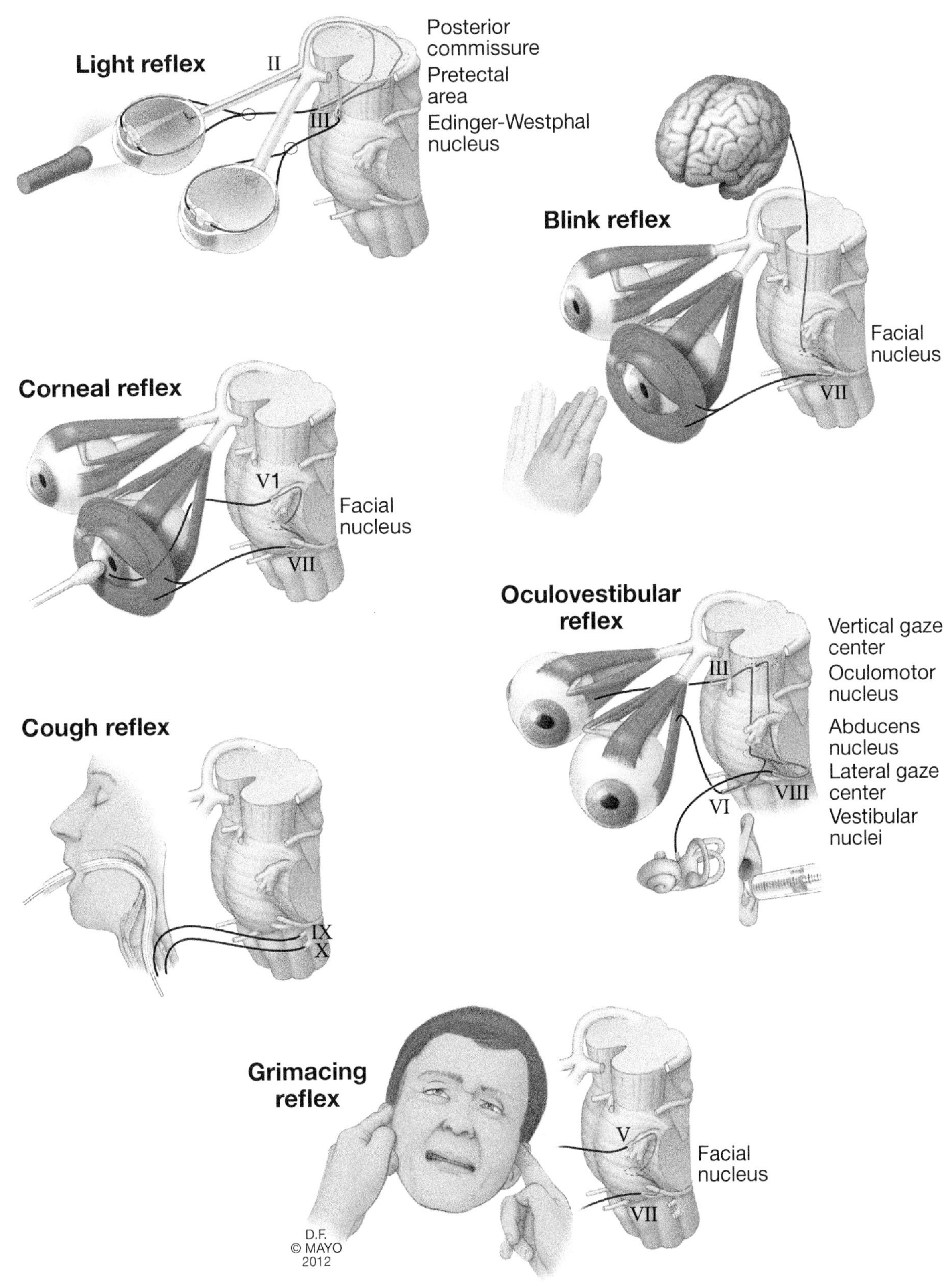

Figure 7.1. Brainstem Reflexes and Their Relations With Lesions. Roman numerals indicate cranial nerves; V1, first division of the trigeminal nerve.

(From Wijdicks EFM. Neurology of critical care. Semin Neurol. 2016;36[6]:483–91; used with permission.)

due to massive hemispheric edema, and its sudden appearance may be one of the first signs of pending change. The pupillometer has been used in many ICUs, but whether it is better than expert assessment is not clear, although it does decrease nursing staff inconsistencies.

An important test in the ICU is the blink reflex, which depends on the stimulus, such as a waving hand (stimulating the optic nerve) or loud hand clap (stimulating the acoustic nerve). An intact visual system causes a blink after a visual stimulus. This is different with the acoustic reflex, which has a reflex arc in the brainstem, and thus a blink after a loud sound excludes the cortex. (Patients in a persistent vegetative state can blink after a startling sound but not be aware of the sound.)

Eyes that do not move indicate brainstem injury or the presence of a toxin, neuromuscular junction blockers, or anesthetic drugs. Many patients with a decreased level of consciousness have spontaneous roving eye movement, and its presence is nonlocalizing.

The next part of the examination is to assess fixation or tracking. Fixation is a primitive reflex, but it differentiates coma from a minimally responsive state. To adequately address the presence of fixation, a large mirror is held in front of the patient to prove fixation and saccades. Visual tracking requires far more neuronal input and functioning of the frontal eye fields. Visual tracking in a horizontal plane requires the lateral gaze center or pontine paramedian reticular formation. These centers activate the oculomotor nucleus in the mesencephalon and the abducens nucleus in the pons.

Touching the cornea with a tissue or squirting water at the cornea elicits the corneal reflex. The corneal reflex involves the ophthalmic division of the trigeminal nerve synapsing with the facial nerve, which conveys the reflex to the orbicularis oculi, causing a blink. Another important test is the oculocephalic response elicited with rapid head movements from side to side, resulting in eyes turning in the opposite direction. As a confirmatory test (certainly if neck movements are limited or dangerous after cervical trauma) the oculovestibular reflex can be performed. The head is elevated at 30°, and approximately 50 mL of iced water is injected through a syringe. As a result, the semicircular canals are temporarily nonfunctional. When consciousness is impaired, the fast component (toward the opposite ear) is lost and the slow component gradually (within minutes) moves the eyes to the stimulated ear. The test can cause an internuclear ophthalmoplegia, with abnormal abduction of 1 eye after cold irrigation, which denotes a lesion of the medial longitudinal fasciculus.

An important part of the examination is to carefully look at forced eye deviation. Eyes usually move toward the lesion when a large structural frontotemporal parietal injury is present. Deviation away from the lesion indicates a seizure (focal initially and often generalized later). Upward gaze is expected with a more diffuse hemispheric lesion, but the pathway is not known. Deviation downward results from a thalamus or dorsal midbrain lesion. A primary brainstem lesion may cause the eyes to appear skewed.

The vagus nerve is tested with the gag reflex (which is unreliable and missing in many patients) and the cough reflex (elicited with tracheal suctioning). Typically, medulla oblongata function is poorly evaluated. In patients with catastrophic injury, the centers in the medulla provide for respiratory drive and blood pressure, and these vital signs continue the longest.

Findings in Coma

Accurate assessment of different levels of a decreased level of consciousness is difficult for many intensivists, but it should not be. Several assessments are necessary for correct interpretation of the signs of impaired consciousness, and several self-evident clinical observations must be made. More specifically, lesions in both cerebral hemispheres impair responsiveness. When 1 hemisphere is involved, consciousness is not impaired, but large territorial involvement can produce a dullness that imitates drowsiness. Only when a hemisphere pushes on the opposite hemisphere or if the ventricles become blocked does consciousness become depressed. An often poorly appreciated cause of impaired consciousness is a lesion of the thalamus (usually when the abnormality involves both structures and a number of nuclei): a thalamic tumor mass lesion compressing the opposite side or a proximal basilar artery occlusion, a thrombus in the deep cerebral veins, a pontine hemorrhage involving the thalamus, or vasculitis occluding the thalamoperforating and thalamogeniculate branches (eg, bacterial meningitis). Lower in the mesencephalon and pons, a structural lesion damages the ascending reticular activating system. This network of neurons activates the thalamus and in turn allows bilateral signal traffic from the cortex. Familiarity with these anatomical landmarks is essential in understanding coma. Moreover, if there is a discrepancy between the site of the lesion and the level of consciousness, a confounding factor (eg, sedation, intoxication, or abnormal laboratory values) may be implicated.

Neurologic examination starts with assessment of the patient's responsiveness. When the patient is comatose, the reaction to pain stimuli is one of the most important tests. A loud voice and a prod should ensure that there is no eye opening, vertical eye movement, or blinking (locked-in syndrome) before a noxious stimulus is applied (compression of the supraorbital nerve and nail beds are preferred methods).

One quick assessment is the Glasgow Coma Scale (GCS). Contrary to the intention of the originators of the GCS, users of the GCS created sum scores for the 3 components (with a total range of 3-15 points), so that GCS sum scores such

Table 7.2 • Causes of Clinical Deterioration in Common Neurocritical Illnesses

Disorder	Causes of Clinical Deterioration	Clinical Signs of Deterioration
Aneurysmal subarachnoid hemorrhage	Acute hydrocephalus Delayed cerebral ischemia Rebleeding Seizures	Decreased level of consciousness or acute coma Upward gaze palsy Pinpoint pupils New aphasia or hemiparesis
Ganglionic or lobar hemorrhage	Expanding volume Cerebral edema	Forced eye deviation Decreased level of consciousness Worsening hemiparesis Newly fixed pupil unresponsive to light and extensor posturing
Cerebellar hematoma	Compression of fourth ventricle and acute hydrocephalus Displacement of pons	New signs of Cushing syndrome Downward gaze Pinpoint pupils Worsening nystagmus Comatose
Hemispheric infarct	Hemorrhagic conversion Brain swelling	Sudden coma with extensor posturing and midposition pupils Gradually decreasing level of consciousness New-onset cerebral ptosis
Traumatic brain injury	New contusional lesions Malignant cerebral edema Extension of subdural or epidural hematoma	Newly fixed, dilated pupil New decerebrate or decorticate responses

From Wijdicks EFM. Neurology of critical care. Semin Neurol. 2016;36(6):483-91; used with permission.

as 3, 8, and 15 are now familiar. The GCS is skewed toward the motor part of the scale, which has 6 items (compared with 4 for the eye part and 5 for the verbal). Furthermore, the verbal component of the GCS is unusable for intubated patients, so most clinicians enter *T* (for *tube*) for the verbal component, but it is not clear how sum scores should be calculated when this substitution is made.

The Full Outline of Unresponsiveness (FOUR) score, a far more detailed scale, has been developed and validated and tested for accuracy with a high degree of agreement among many specialties. The FOUR score is more useful with intubated, critically ill patients because it can be used to identify different levels of coma, locked-in syndrome, uncal herniation, and brain death. However, descriptions of the separate components are best: for example, "This patient with traumatic brain injury has his eyes open but does not track a finger, has intact pupillary and corneal reflexes, localizes to pain, is intubated, and triggers the ventilator." (For more details, see Chapter 14, "Coma and Other Altered States of Consciousness.")

Examination of Patients With Clinical Deterioration

Intensivists and neurointensivists expect clinical deterioration rather than stability among patients after admission. Clinical deterioration can follow disease-specific patterns, some of which are predictable (Table 7.2).

Clinical worsening in acute brain injury is often attributed to ongoing mass effect of the primary lesion from either cerebral edema or expansion of the mass (eg, rebleeding or hemorrhage in a tumor). A classic sign, the fixed and dilated pupil, is a key warning to nursing staff and an imminent alert to physicians. A unilateral, fixed, dilated pupil (difference of 2-5 mm) is an early sign when the intracranial space is small (ie, in young patients). The explanation is stretch or compression of the third cranial nerve against the clivus rather than direct compression of the mass. Untreated, the displacement will affect both cranial nerves, but these symptoms are fully reversible. Patients who progress to brain death usually first show loss of the pontomesencephalic reflexes and then loss of medulla oblongata function, loss of vascular tone (hypotension), and apnea.

Lesions in the cerebellum may compress the pons and result in bilateral miosis and absent corneal, oculocephalic, and oculovestibular reflexes. Bradycardia with hypertensive surges may occur (Cushing reflex), and it is seen more often with posterior fossa lesions than with supratentorial lesions.

All these signs of deterioration are potentially reversible (a common misunderstanding). If the displacing mass is removed (eg, a lobar hematoma), a gradual improvement is expected, but patients may perk up quickly if the surgical delay was short and the patient was treated with osmotic diuretics. Removal of a lobar hematoma with extension into the thalamus, however, is unlikely to be beneficial when it involves such a central structure. Finally, a mass can obstruct the ventricular flow, and ventriculostomy can markedly improve the level of consciousness.

Elucidating Acute Muscle Weakness

Paraplegia or acute quadriplegia are neuroemergencies that need to be recognized and analyzed accurately. An acute neuromuscular disorder (usually Guillain-Barré syndrome and myasthenic crisis) is less common. In most surgical or trauma units, acute spinal cord injury is implicated in generalized weakness and often occurs with polytrauma.

Neurologic findings may be predictable with recognizable patterns. For example, chronic neuropathies produce distal weakness, and acute inflammatory polyneuropathies produce proximal weakness. Acute paralysis of all 4 limbs points to an acute spinal cord lesion; this is especially true when the body temperature is low, the skin is warm, and blood pressure seems unregulated. These clinical signs are hard to miss, but the circumstances often help in clinching the diagnosis (eg, trauma, anticoagulation, or aortic surgery). An acute spinal cord lesion may occur from spontaneous infarction but is exceedingly rare. Most notoriously, patients with an epidural abscess can present with sepsis and shock syndrome that may cause physicians to focus on treating the sepsis without further investigating the source in the spinal canal. Alternatively, hypotension is misinterpreted as part of dysautonomia with acute spinal shock. An astute physician who observes weakness in both legs, abnormal sensation in the buttocks area, and abnormal sphincter function should arrive at the diagnosis of spinal abscess. Magnetic resonance imaging of the spine is essential, and early surgical intervention may increase the chances of improvement.

Acute Neuromuscular Disorders

More diffuse muscle weakness with no sensory findings may point to an acute muscle, nerve, and nerve root or endplate disorder. Acute ascending weakness in a matter of days is commonly due to Guillain-Barré syndrome. Initially, patients often have distal tingling and leg weakness that later extends to the arms and bulbar muscles. Patients may need mechanical ventilation within days after onset. Along with quadriplegia, generalized areflexia is a key finding. Any patient with acute neuromuscular weakness that has progressed rapidly should undergo careful assessment of the tendon reflexes. The presence of tendon reflexes excludes several major disorders (Box 7.1).

Box 7.1 • Assessment of Tendon Reflexes for Excluding Disorders

Tendon reflexes should be carefully assessed in patients with rapidly progressing, acute neuromuscular weakness. If tendon reflexes are *present*, the following causes can be *excluded*:

- Guillain-Barré syndrome
- Neuromuscular blockade
- Botulism
- Hypermagnesemia

Another common disorder is myasthenia gravis. Patients with myasthenic crisis have excessive secretions (often after the dose of pyridostigmine bromide has been increased) that coincide with diaphragmatic weakness. Patients may be restless, reluctant to lie down, and most comfortable sitting upright. Because the patient cannot create large tidal volumes, speech is halting with a staccato delivery. Upon further examination, the patient may have weakness of the oropharyngeal muscles and may be using the accessory muscles.

Neuromuscular respiratory failure progresses as follows: 1) The diaphragm and intercostal muscles fail. 2) Accessory muscles compensate temporarily. 3) Insufficient pulmonary work leads to alveolar collapse, intrapulmonary shunting, and eventually hypoxia. Pulse oximetry may not show hypoxemia, and arterial blood gas results may be within the reference range until late in the course of respiratory failure. Nevertheless, the patient has shortness of breath and, often, a sensation of not being able to catch a full breath.

Acute Spinal Cord Injury

With the worst acute spinal cord injuries, patients have quadriplegia or paraparesis, hypotonia, loss of bladder and bowel sphincter function, loss of tendon reflexes, and an area with abrupt sensory loss to pinprick.

Several principles apply. First, complete spinal cord involvement leads to paralysis and sensation below the level of the lesion. Second, in less severely affected patients, weakness can be assessed by grading muscle strength on the British Medical Research Council Muscle Scale. Levels can be estimated by using certain key muscles such as arm abduction (C5), forearm extension (C5), forearm flexion (C5 and C6), knee extension (L3 and L4), foot and great toe dorsiflexion (L5), and plantar flexion (S1). Sensory modalities include pinprick, position, and vibration sense; light touch with a wisp of cotton; pressure touch; and temperature.

Saddle anesthesia (S3-S5) indicates a conus medullaris lesion. The sensory loss is often dissociated, with sparing of the touch sensation but loss of the pinprick sensation. Absence of dissociation suggests involvement of the cauda

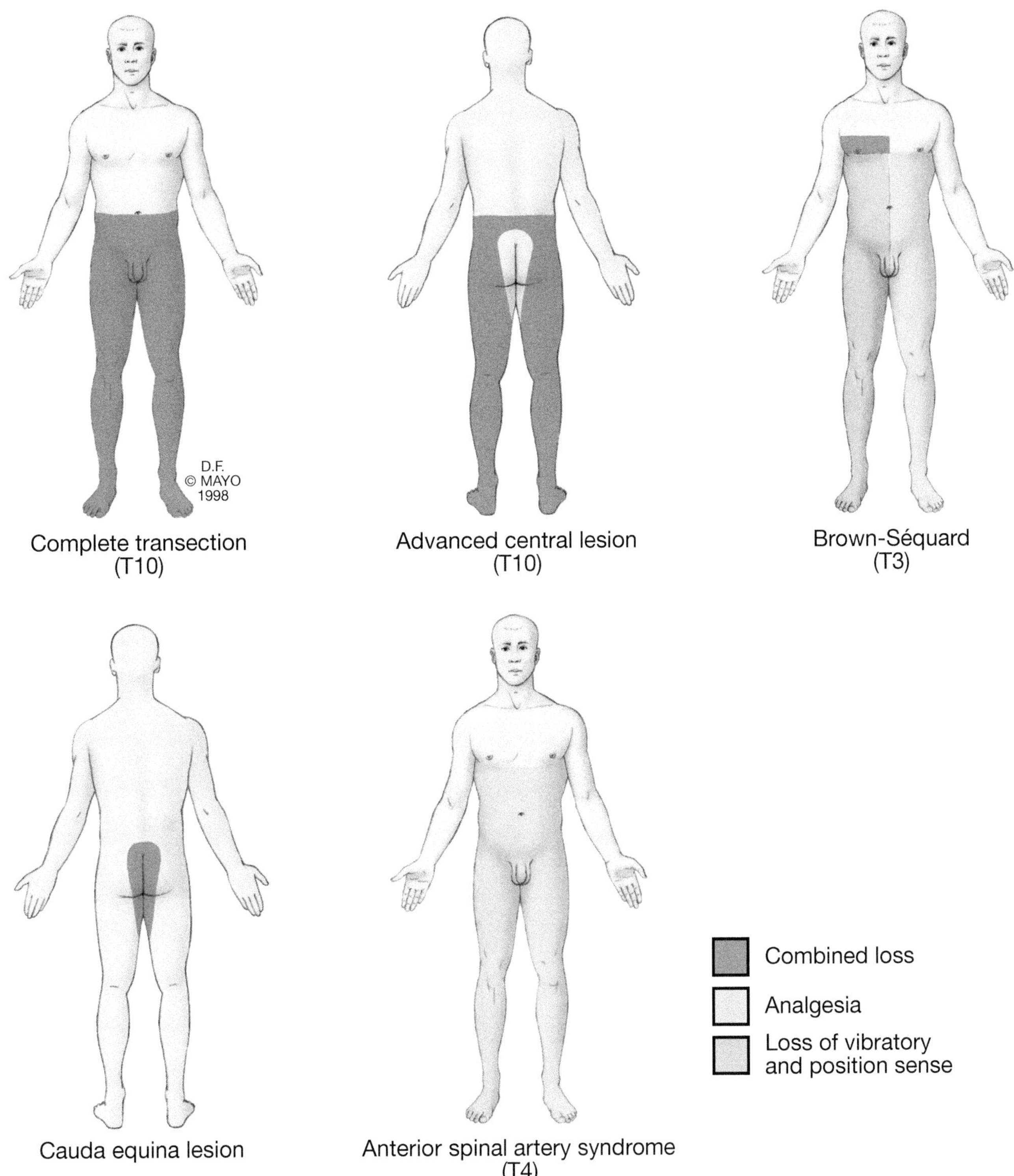

Figure 7.2. *Spinal Cord Lesions With Neurologic Findings.*

(From Wijdicks EFM. The practice of emergency and critical care neurology. New York [NY]: Oxford University Press; c2016. Chapter 36, Acute spinal cord disorders; p. 500-16; used with permission of Mayo Foundation for Medical Education and Research.)

equina in addition to the conus. Sacral sensory sparing implies a centrally located intramedullary lesion.

Important sensory landmarks are the nipples for level T4, the umbilicus for level T10, and the thumb, middle finger, and fifth digit innervated by C6, C7, and C8. The C4 and T2 dermatomes are continuous. Classic patterns of sensory loss in acute spinal cord lesions are depicted in Figure 7.2.

Summary

- Clinical expertise must be acquired and maintained because a skilled comprehensive neurologic assessment will assist in diagnosing and predicting the outcome of a neurologic disorder.
- A careful synthesis of findings from the clinical examination and neuroimaging is required to make a diagnosis.
- Eye findings (pupil size and eye movements) are key parts of the neurologic examination of the neurocritical patient.
- Specific, recognized clinical patterns help in determining clinical deterioration.

SUGGESTED READING

Berkowitz AL. Clinical neurology and neuroanatomy: a localization-based approach. New York (NY): McGraw-Hill Education; c2017. 322 p.

Caplan LR, van Gijn J, editors. Stroke syndromes. 3rd ed. Cambridge (UK): Cambridge University Press; c2012. 621 p.

O'Brien M. Aids to the examination of the peripheral nervous system. 5th ed. Edinburgh (UK): Saunders; c2010. 63 p.

Ropper AH, Samuels MA, Klein JP. Adams and Victor's principles of neurology. 10th ed. New York (NY): McGraw-Hill Education Medical; c2014. 1654 p.

Wijdicks EFM. Recognizing brain injury. Oxford (UK): Oxford University Press; c2014. 150 p. (Core principles of acute neurology series).

8 Intracranial Pressure

EELCO F. M. WIJDICKS, MD, PhD; WILLIAM D. FREEMAN, MD

Goals

- Review the intracranial compartments and the relationship between pressure and volume.
- Review the clinical consequences of increased intracranial pressure.
- Review medical and surgical treatment of increased intracranial pressure.

Introduction

One of the defining characteristics of the specialty of neurocritical care is management of increased intracranial pressure (ICP). Most injuries to the brain, however, do not result in a sustained change in ICP, at least initially. Space-occupying lesions, intracranial bleeding (epidural, subdural, or intracerebral hematoma), and large hemispheric ischemic strokes can increase the ICP and cause brain shift. The main consequence of supratentorial brain tissue shifts is brainstem injury by microvascular brain ischemia and hemorrhage due to damage to the perforating blood vessels in the brain. Crowding may also cause territorial ischemia from compression of larger arteries (eg, posterior cerebral artery from a compressing temporal uncus). If increased ICP and brainstem shift or compression are left untreated, they can cause loss of all brainstem function, clinically apparent as brainstem areflexia, apnea, and hypotension (brain death).

Increased ICP may also be evident from a computed tomographic scan (showing cerebral edema or mass effect); from specific clinical findings, such as loss of brainstem reflexes due to brain tissue shift resulting in a fixed dilated pupil; and from systemic signs such as Cushing reflex, which leads to increased systolic blood pressure, wider pulse pressure, and bradycardia.

Whether increased ICP is clinically consequential (eg, resulting in coma and associated neurologic signs) depends on the volume of the intracranial mass lesion, the rate of mass expansion, and the compensatory reserve of other intracranial compartments for accommodating the additional intracranial mass. The intracranial volumes affected first are the cerebrospinal fluid (CSF) volume, the volume of the venous sinuses, and the cerebral blood volume, which, if left unchecked, leads to reduced cerebral blood flow and critically low cerebral perfusion pressure. An important observation is that many episodes of transiently increased ICP, such as during coughing or the Valsalva maneuver, do not result in structural brain injury.

Factors Affecting ICP

The intracranial volume in adults is fixed. Therefore, when the volume of intracranial contents increases suddenly, ICP increases sharply. This intracranial pressure-volume relationship is known as the Monro-Kellie doctrine. The intracranial volume compartments include the brain parenchyma (about 1,400 g), the venous and arterial blood volumes (each 5%), CSF (10%), and brain parenchyma (80%). CSF and intracranial blood volume are each about 75 mL. The volume of intracranial contents can increase up to 10%, but the percentage depends on the volume of the brain parenchyma—a higher percentage may be tolerated in an older brain with atrophy than in a younger brain. With a rapid increase in volume of more than 10%, the pupillary light reflex changes and the Cushing reflex appears (typically after the pupils become fixed to light).

The normal ICP is 0 to 15 mm Hg, with a variable upper limit of 15 to 20 mm Hg. Nihls Lundberg observed ICP waves that correlated with poor intracranial pressure-volume states. The *A waves* (or *plateau waves*) represent sustained and severe elevations in ICP (eg, >50 mm Hg) for 5 to 20 minutes followed by a rapid decrease. Shorter and milder ICP peaks are known as *B waves* (usually up to 30-35 mm Hg for ≤5 minutes) that often occur with Cheyne-Stokes respiration. *C waves* (4-8 waves/min) are the shortest and correspond to transient oscillations of blood pressure associated with hemodynamic changes.

The pressure-volume relationship is a *J*-shaped curve when volume is plotted on the x-axis and pressure on the y-axis: When the change in volume is an increase, the change in ICP is a corresponding increase. Initially, this increase in pressure is dampened by compensatory mechanisms (exclusion of CSF and then blood) that contribute to *intracranial compliance*, but later the increase becomes rapid as those mechanisms are exhausted. Intracranial compliance is greater in elderly patients with global brain atrophy (Figure 8.1). *Intracranial elastance* is the reciprocal of intracranial compliance. The pressure-volume relationship changes after a craniectomy because the intracranial compartment is no longer closed, but cerebral blood flow does not generally influence the configuration of the pressure-volume curve until the ICP approaches the intravascular pressure.

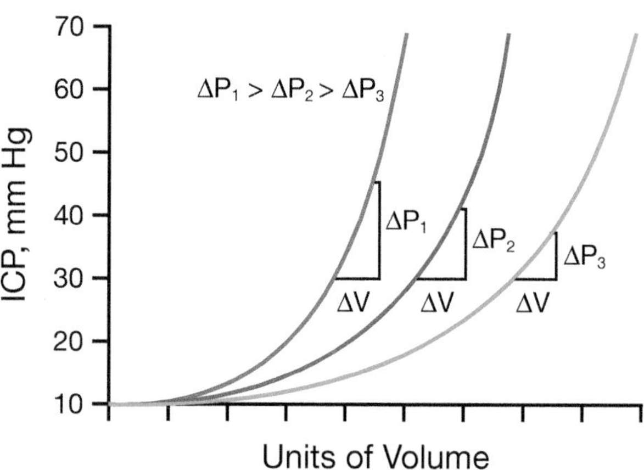

Figure 8.1. Pressure-Volume Curves. Elderly patients (green curve) tend to have more global brain atrophy and correspondingly greater intracranial compliance (represented by the more gradual ascent) than younger patients (blue curve with steep ascent). The red curve in the middle indicates the standard curve.

Consequences of ICP

Increased ICP can lead to permanent damage through several mechanisms. The main mechanism is displacement of the thalamus-brainstem complex downward, sideways, or in both directions (Figure 8.2). Eventually tissue moves through the tentorial opening and foramen magnum (Figure 8.3), but clinical signs are likely a result of the shift rather than direct compression.

There are several radiologic and pathologic descriptions of brain herniation. These designations are commonly used despite poor clinical and pathologic correlation. *Uncal herniation* refers to herniation of the parahippocampal gyrus through the tentorium. It occurs in large hemispheric masses, causing flattening of the midbrain and compression of the aqueduct. *Tonsillar herniation* is usually a consequence of an acute mass in the cerebellum. Flattening of the medulla and hemorrhagic necrosis of the tips of the cerebellar tonsils are found at autopsy.

Displacement of the brainstem may result from diffuse brain edema or from a single mass compressing the brainstem. Buckling of the brainstem usually leads to a

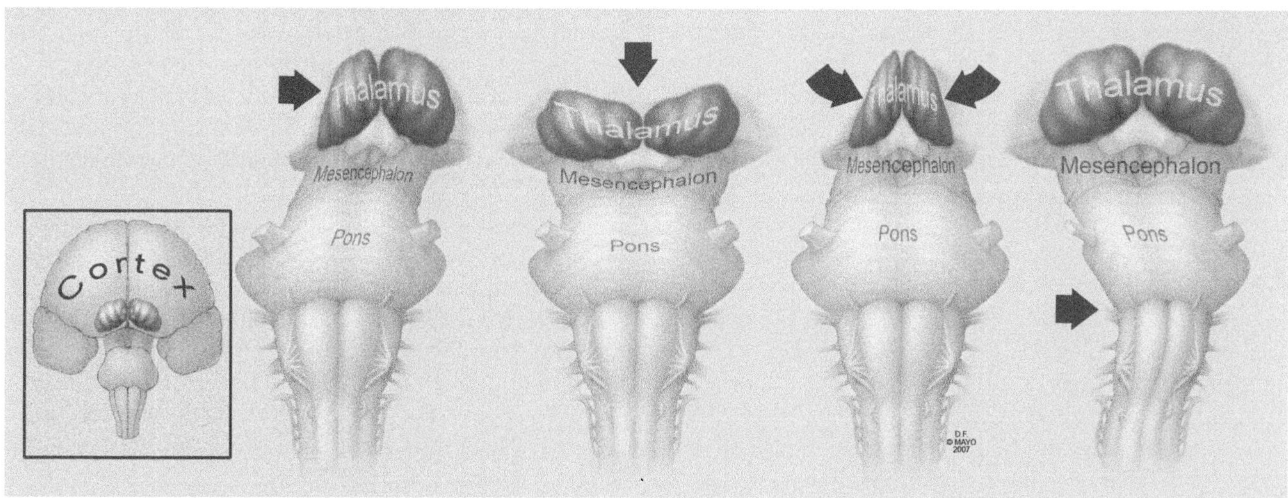

Figure 8.2. Mass Effect. Arrows indicate pressure from mass effect. The resultant types of thalamus-brainstem compression and shift are shown.

(From Wijdicks EFM. The comatose patient. 2nd ed. Oxford [UK]: Oxford University Press; c2014. Chapter 3, Neurologic examination of the comatose patient and localization principles; p. 81-110; used with permission of Mayo Foundation for Medical Education and Research.)

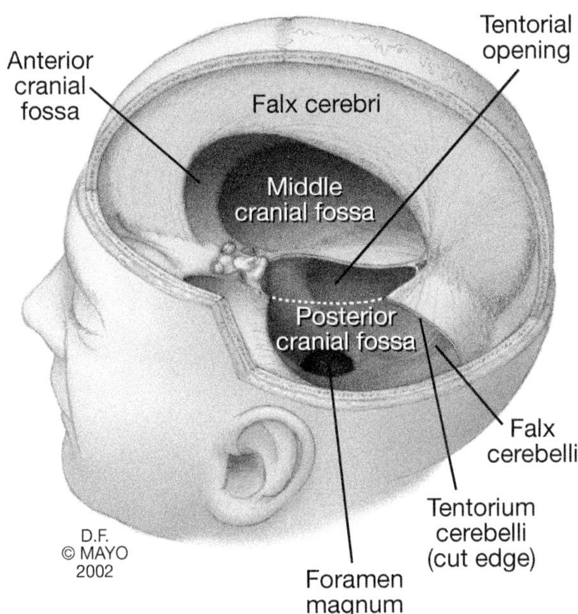

Figure 8.3. Intracranial Compartments and Openings. Brain tissue under pressure may move through the tentorial opening and foramen magnum.

(From Wijdicks EFM. The clinical practice of critical care neurology. 2nd ed. Oxford [UK]: Oxford University Press; c2003. Chapter 9, Intracranial pressure; p. 107–25; used with permission of Mayo Foundation for Medical Education and Research.)

progressive and sequential loss of function, but reflexes may be lost rapidly and completely. Damage of the pons alters the breathing drive, and breathing stops when the medulla oblongata becomes involved. Simultaneously, with involvement of the brainstem, the vagal cardiomotor centers stop providing parasympathetic activity. Unopposed sympathetic output may lead to a hypertensive response.

Eventually, ICP increases substantially and seriously reduces cerebral perfusion or causes stagnation, leading to a virtual intracranial standstill and global, profound ischemia.

Reducing ICP

Before ICP can be reduced, the cause of increased ICP must be established (Box 8.1). Increased ICP is typically caused by the introduction of a new mass, a mass effect from brain swelling, or the blockage of CSF absorption (*communicating* if arachnoid granulations are obstructed; *noncommunicating* if there is obstruction of a major ventricle or CSF pathway). Rarely, increased ICP occurs from an increase in CSF volume from a choroid plexus papilloma. Increased ICP may also be due to an increase in cerebral blood volume from vasodilatation related to hypercapnia, hypoxemia, or hyperthermia or from an obstruction to venous outflow from the intracranial cavity. Hypocapnia decreases ICP by cerebral vasoconstriction, which in turn decreases cerebral blood volume in tissue with preserved autoregulation. Thus, while brief hyperventilation can be useful for decreasing ICP in an emergency situation, prolonged hyperventilation and hypocapnia may be harmful by provoking cerebral ischemia. Hypothermia reduces brain metabolism and reduces ICP, but its long-term effect (>72 hours) has not been studied thoroughly.

Generally, the ICP threshold that prompts most providers to treat is a sustained (>5 minutes) ICP of 20 to 22 mm Hg or more, but this should be individualized according to the goal for the cerebral perfusion pressure (CPP). Most clinical studies have found that outcomes are poor if the ICP is greater than 20 mm Hg, but it is unclear whether ICP is simply a surrogate for severity of brain injury, and studies do not always report the CPP values. Current Brain Trauma Foundation guidelines recommend a CPP goal of 60 to 70 mm Hg and suggest keeping the ICP at 20 mm Hg or less. However, patients with severe traumatic brain injury may have a sustained ICP that hovers around 15 to 20 mm Hg without compromising the CPP. For those patients only, treatment should be initiated if the CPP decreases to less than 60 mm Hg.

Use of osmotic diuretics (eg, mannitol or hypertonic saline [HTS]) and brief hyperventilation should be used to reduce ICP. If the patient has a ventriculostomy, CSF drainage can be effective. If that fails, additional strategies to consider include sedation, neuromuscular paralysis, hypothermia (32°C-34°C), metabolic suppression (with high doses of propofol or barbiturates), and decompressive surgery (ie, hematoma evacuation or craniectomy).

Bedside basic ICP interventions include ensuring that the patient's head is in a neutral position (ie, not flexed or extended or turned to an extreme), the head of the bed is elevated 30° to 45°, and there is no jugular venous obstruction from an endotracheal tube or central line bandages. Patients should have adequate oxygen saturation (Spo_2) (≥95%), and $Paco_2$ should be normal or low normal (35-40 mm Hg). If transient hyperventilation is used, it should produce only mild hypocapnia ($Paco_2$ of 30-35 mm Hg), and it should be

Box 8.1 • Causes of Increased Intracranial Pressure

- Cerebral edema
- Mass lesion with shift
- Acute hydrocephalus
- Cerebral vasodilatation (hypercapnia, hypoxemia)
- Cerebral venous sinus thrombosis
- Status epilepticus
- Increased intrathoracic or intra-abdominal pressure
- Hyperthermia or febrile states

used only as a bridge to a more definitive ICP-reducing strategy because it causes global cerebral vasoconstriction.

Mannitol 20% can be given for an ICP elevation of more than 20 mm Hg or for clinical signs of herniation. The dose of mannitol ranges from 0.5 g/kg for patients with mild ICP elevations to 1.5 g/kg for patients with acute herniation that requires surgery. Mannitol can be given as a bolus or as scheduled doses depending on circumstances, but the plasma osmolality should not exceed 320 mOsm/kg to avoid increasing the risk of nephrotoxicity. Because mannitol is an osmotic diuretic, large doses can cause dehydration and electrolyte depletion.

Both mannitol and HTS are osmotically active and have equal effect when given in equivalent osmolar doses. HTS can be given through a peripheral venous access (as a 1.5% infusion), through central venous access (as a 3% infusion at 30-75 mL/h), or as boluses of higher concentrations of 7.5% (75 mL), 14.6% (24 or 48 mL), and 23.4% (15 or 30 mL). Unlike mannitol, HTS does not produce a major diuretic effect, and it is therefore a safer option in patients with renal failure or acute kidney injury. Because HTS increases circulating blood volume and acts as a volume expander, it should be used cautiously in patients with heart failure. Also, long-term use can lead to increased total body weight and blood volume (ie, anasarca). With a reflection coefficient of 1.0, HTS can pass freely between body tissue compartments. If HTS or mannitol is used, serum electrolyte and sodium levels must be monitored. In addition, if mannitol is used, the osmolar gap (OG) must be determined. The OG is the measured osmolality minus the calculated osmolality.

$$\text{Calculated Serum Osmolality} = 2 \times [\text{Sodium, in mmol/L}] + [\text{Serum Urea Nitrogen, in mg/dL}]/2.8 + [\text{Glucose, in mg/dL}]/18$$

The OG correlates well with mannitol serum concentrations. An OG less than 20 mOsm/kg indicates adequate mannitol clearance and supports safe continuation of mannitol therapy even if the measured serum osmolality is high.

The brain-plasma osmotic gradient equilibrates quickly from the buildup of intracellular osmoles, potentially rendering mannitol less effective over time. For the same reason, sudden discontinuation of osmotic agents may lead to a rapid increase in ICP.

HTS and mannitol are typically withheld if the serum sodium concentration is higher than 160 mmol/L. Enteral water can be gently administered through a nasogastric tube to reduce sodium gradually. The use of intravenous hypotonic solutions (eg, 5% dextrose in 0.45% saline or 0.45% saline) should be strictly avoided because they can worsen cerebral edema.

Targeted temperature management is critical for patients who have a brain injury and an elevated ICP because fever (core temperature >38.5°C) is associated with worse neurologic outcomes across a range of diseases, including traumatic brain injury, ischemic stroke, and subarachnoid hemorrhage. Core temperature should be measured with a Foley catheter thermistor if available; rectal or tympanic measurements are less reliable alternatives. In intubated patients, body core temperature can be measured with an esophageal temperature probe. Oral and axillary temperatures can be 0.5°C to 1°C cooler than the core temperature, and the brain temperature is often 0.25°C to 0.5°C higher than core temperature. Strict maintenance of normothermia at 37°C or fever control (<38.5°C) is advised for patients with increased ICP. Therapeutic hypothermia (32°C–34°C) can be used in patients with refractory ICP but only as a last resort. Surface cooling or intravascular cooling devices may have comparable performance. Shivering should be treated aggressively since it can raise ICP through a Valsalva-like effect and increased brain metabolism.

CPP control is affected by 2 variables: mean arterial blood pressure (MAP) and ICP. Although an increased MAP increases CPP, sustained increases in MAP and CPP can paradoxically increase ICP if cerebral autoregulation is disturbed. Also, decreases in CPP can paradoxically increase ICP by inducing compensatory venodilatation. The optimal *U*-shaped range of CPP varies from patient to patient and even for the same patient over time. Software can be used to plot MAP, ICP, and CPP and to then calculate CPP optimal values, but this multimodal monitoring (known as cerebral reactivity index) is still largely investigational.

For some agitated patients, ICP control may be achieved with adequate sedation, which can often be started with intravenous propofol (cautiously to avoid hypotension). Propofol reduces cerebral blood volume. It has a short half-life that allows neurologic assessment during interruptions in sedation, which should be done only with close ICP monitoring because sedation interruptions can provoke ICP crises in patients with exhausted intracranial compliance. Also, high-dose propofol should be used with caution, particularly in young patients, because of the risk of inducing propofol infusion syndrome, which can cause refractory shock with multiorgan failure and death. A low dose of an analgesic agent (eg, intravenous fentanyl) may be used if pain is the source of agitation. However, most patients who need sedation for increasing ICP are comatose and have less pain sensation. If a patient has received intravenous opioids, neurologic examination can be quite difficult. The use of intravenous fentanyl is indicated only if the patient is resisting use of the ventilator, if the patient has tachypnea, or if there is mechanical ventilator dyssynchrony.

If these interventions are unsuccessful, refractory ICP control methods (eg, hypothermia, barbiturates, and decompressive craniectomy) should be considered. Most clinicians no longer use barbiturates because of myocardial depression resulting in systemic hypotension with incremental use of vasopressors or inotropes, liver toxicity, risk of infection, and long elimination half-life virtually eliminating a neurologic assessment.

Summary

- The intracranial volume in adults is fixed. With a sudden increase in the volume of intracranial contents, ICP increases sharply (the Monro-Kellie doctrine).
- Control of ICP is urgent to prevent secondary brain injury or brain death.
- Mannitol is a diuretic; hypertonic saline is a volume expander.
- Refractory ICP may require surgical treatment with a craniectomy.

SUGGESTED READING

Czosnyka M, Smielewski P, Timofeev I, Lavinio A, Guazzo E, Hutchinson P, et al. Intracranial pressure: more than a number. Neurosurg Focus. 2007 May 15; 22(5):E10.

Horn P, Munch E, Vajkoczy P, Herrmann P, Quintel M, Schilling L, et al. Hypertonic saline solution for control of elevated intracranial pressure in patients with exhausted response to mannitol and barbiturates. Neurol Res. 1999 Dec;21(8):758–64.

Huang SJ, Chang L, Han YY, Lee YC, Tu YK. Efficacy and safety of hypertonic saline solutions in the treatment of severe head injury. Surg Neurol. 2006 Jun;65(6):539–46.

Johnston IH, Johnston JA, Jennett B. Intracranial-pressure changes following head injury. Lancet. 1970 Aug 29;2(7670):433–6.

Juul N, Morris GF, Marshall SB, Marshall LF; The Executive Committee of the International Selfotel Trial. Intracranial hypertension and cerebral perfusion pressure: influence on neurological deterioration and outcome in severe head injury. J Neurosurg. 2000 Jan;92(1):1–6.

Marmarou A, Maset AL, Ward JD, Choi S, Brooks D, Lutz HA, et al. Contribution of CSF and vascular factors to elevation of ICP in severely head-injured patients. J Neurosurg. 1987 Jun;66(6):883–90.

Menon DK. Cerebral protection in severe brain injury: physiological determinants of outcome and their optimisation. Br Med Bull. 1999;55(1):226–58.

Miller JD. Volume and pressure in the craniospinal axis. Clin Neurosurg. 1975;22:76–105.

Miller JD, Stanek A, Langfitt TW. Concepts of cerebral perfusion pressure and vascular compression during intracranial hypertension. Prog Brain Res. 1972;35:411–32.

Ropper AH. Hyperosmolar therapy for raised intracranial pressure. N Engl J Med. 2012 Aug 23;367(8):746–52.

9 Cerebrospinal Physiology

JOSEPH ZACHARIAH, MD

Goals

- Describe the anatomy and physiology related to the circulation of cerebrospinal fluid.
- Describe how cerebrospinal fluid changes in disease.
- Describe the dynamics of cerebrospinal fluid in disease.

Introduction

Cerebrospinal fluid (CSF) fills the subarachnoid space, spinal canal, and ventricles of the brain. CSF is enclosed within the brain by the pial layer, ependymal cells lining the ventricles, and the epithelial surface of the choroid plexus, where it is largely produced. Choroid plexus is present throughout the ventricular system with the exception of the frontal and occipital horns of the lateral ventricle and the cerebral aqueduct. The highly vascular choroid plexuses are composed of several villi lined by a monolayer of epithelial cells separated by tight junctions near the apical border facing the CSF. The ion channels, pumps, and transporters of the epithelial layer regulate the movement of ions from the uniquely fenestrated capillary arteries into the CSF. Antigen-presenting cells along the choroid plexus epithelium include epiplexus cells on the apical surface and macrophages and dendritic cells in the basal membrane on the basal surface (Figure 9.1). The epithelial cells of the choroid plexus compose the *blood-brain barrier*—more correctly called the *blood-CSF barrier*. In the blood-CSF barrier, as opposed to the blood-brain barrier, astrocytic foot processes do not cover the basement membrane of the epithelial cells.

Choroid Plexus Innervation

The vascular smooth muscle and the epithelium of the choroid plexus receive both sympathetic and parasympathetic input. The superior cervical ganglion provides the main sympathetic input to the choroid plexus. Inhibition of the sympathetic input increases the CSF volume by up to 30%; excitation decreases it by up to 30%. In the vascular bed, α-adrenergic input causes vasoconstriction and β-adrenergic input causes vasodilatation. With increased sympathetic input, CSF production decreases within the choroid plexus epithelium and blood flow decreases through the choroidal vasculature.

The choroid plexus contains the highest density of 5-hydroxytryptamine receptor 2C (5-HTR2C) in the body. With in vitro administration of 5-HTR2C, CSF production decreases, indicating its possible role in controlling the composition or production of CSF.

CSF Production

CSF is produced at a rate of 0.3 to 0.5 mL/kg hourly (about 400-600 mL daily). Typically, a total of 140 to 150 mL of CSF outlines the neuroaxis, with a turnover of 3 to 4 times daily. Choroid plexuses of the ventricles produce 70% of the CSF. Other sources of CSF production include capillary ultrafiltrate from Virchow-Robin spaces and metabolic production of water. Metabolic production of water results from the breakdown of glucose into carbon dioxide and water.

CSF production at the choroid plexus includes 1) a passive filtration of plasma in response to a pressure gradient through the fenestrated choroidal capillaries into the basement membrane and 2) an active secretory process involving the epithelial cells of the choroid plexus. Systemic blood pressure has a direct correlation to CSF production through hydrostatic pressure and passive transfer of water.

Transport Channels

Active transport of sodium (Na^+), chloride (Cl^-), and bicarbonate (HCO_3^-) into the CSF space is followed by the

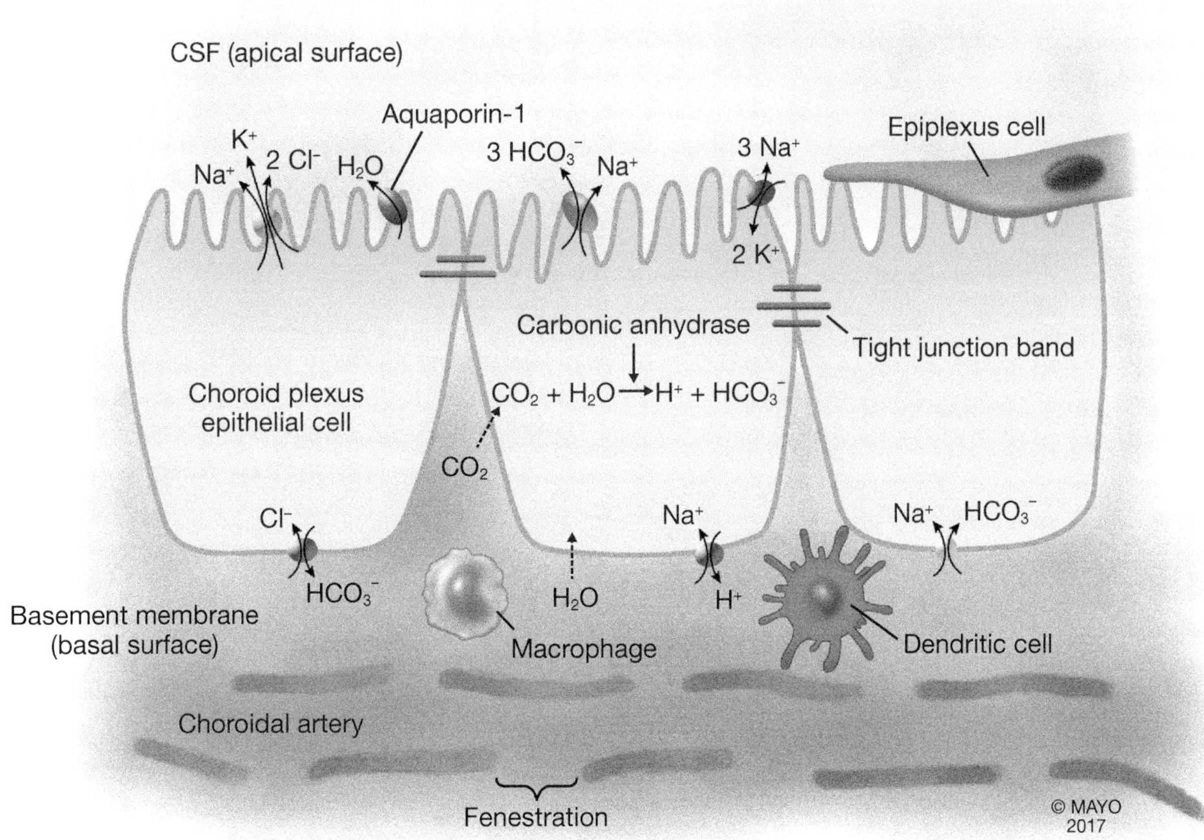

Figure 9.1. *Epithelial Cells of the Choroid Plexus Forming the Blood–Cerebrospinal Fluid (CSF) Barrier. Cl^- indicates chloride; CO_2, carbon dioxide; H^+, hydrogen ion; HCO_3^-, bicarbonate; H_2O, water; K^+, potassium; Na^+, sodium.*

osmotic introduction of water through aquaporin (AQP) channels, leading to the production of CSF. In the choroid plexus, the basal surfaces of the epithelial cells contain Na^+-coupled HCO_3^- transporters and Cl^--HCO_3^- exchangers, whereas the apical surfaces express AQP channels; potassium (K^+) channels; Na^+,K^+-adenosine triphosphatase (Na^+,K^+-ATPase); and Na^+-$2Cl^-$-K^+ cotransporters (Figure 9.1). Water transport at the basolateral membrane has not been fully elucidated but is thought to result from passive diffusion. Diffusion of water molecules is a slow process, whereas water transport through AQP channels occurs rapidly. Because of the transporters, CSF has higher concentrations of Na^+ and Cl^- and lower concentrations of other ions compared to blood. The tight junctions of the choroid plexus epithelium are leaky, allowing passive diffusion of monovalent cations. Organic anions and cations, calcium, and other trace elements also cross into the CSF.

Of the 14 AQP channels discovered, AQP1 is found in the ventricular-facing membrane of the choroid plexus epithelium. In AQP1 knockout mice, production of CSF is 20% less compared to the wild-type, suggesting that at least in mice, the majority of CSF production may be extrachoroidal.

In the choroid plexus, carbonic anhydrase catalyzes the production of HCO_3^- and hydrogen from water and carbon dioxide. Theoretically, acetazolamide decreases CSF production by inhibiting carbonic anhydrase and decreasing the levels of bicarbonate (Figure 9.1).

CSF Flow

CSF flows from the choroid plexuses in the lateral and third ventricles through the cerebral aquaduct into the fourth ventricle. From the fourth ventricle, CSF passes through the median and lateral apertures into the subarachnoid space covering the convexities of the brain and the spinal cord. Pulsatile CSF flow corresponds to the choroidal artery systolic wave and rapid respiratory waves.

Cilia found on the ependymal cells lining the ventricles direct the flow of CSF.

CSF Drainage

Most CSF is drained by absorption into the *arachnoid granulations*, which are groupings of villi that penetrate the dural layer into the venous sinuses. The arachnoid granulations drain CSF into the dural sinuses, mostly to the posterior half of the superior sagittal sinus, and eventually into the jugular system. Arachnoid villi are 1-way valves consisting of pia and an arachnoid layer. The valves open mechanically when the hydrostatic CSF pressure exceeds the hydrostatic pressure within the dural venous system.

A small component of CSF drains directly into the cerebral venules and lymphatic system. Lymphatic drainage occurs through the perineural subarachnoid spaces of the cranial nerves. Spinal arachnoid villi can also drain CSF into the spinal epidural venous plexus. Increases in intracranial pressure (ICP) directly increase CSF drainage. With marked increases in ICP, however, the ventricular ependymal layer is disrupted and a small portion of CSF infiltrates the brain parenchyma as transependymal flow.

CSF Composition

In an adult, CSF is normally acellular. A normal spinal sample may contain up to 5 white blood cells (WBCs) or red blood cells (RBCs). CSF pleocytosis with an elevated WBC count occurs in various infectious and noninfectious conditions, such as hydrocephalus, neoplasms of the blood, and subarachnoid hemorrhage. CSF pleocytosis can occur with hemorrhage into the spinal fluid at a WBC:RBC ratio ranging from 1:500 to 1:1,500.

With an increased number of RBCs, CSF is yellow or pink because of RBC degradation (*xanthochromia*). The breakdown of hemoglobin into oxyhemoglobin (pink) and bilirubin (yellow) occurs within 2 hours of RBC entry into the CSF. Thus, blood from a traumatic tap can be distinguished from blood already present in the CSF. Xanthochromia is present within 12 hours of hemorrhage in 90% of patients, persisting for up to 4 weeks. Samples analyzed hours after being obtained can be falsely reassuring because WBCs, RBCs, and malignant cells can adhere to the plastic sampling tubes. CSF can appear xanthochromic in a patient with systemic hyperbilirubinemia.

CSF protein values normally range from 23 to 38 mg/dL. The reference range may be increased in patients who are diabetic or elderly. Protein levels may be increased in hemorrhagic conditions at a ratio of 1 mg/dL per 1,000 RBCs. Infection-related protein levels may be increased for months after clearance of the infectious agent; therefore, the CSF protein level should not be used as a marker for successful treatment.

Albuminocytologic dissociation is an elevated level of CSF protein with fewer than 10 CSF WBCs. Classically, it occurs with a disruption of the blood-brain barrier, such as in inflammatory demyelinating polyneuropathies, but it has also been described in normal-pressure hydrocephalus, spinal stenosis, obesity, malignancies, and posterior reversible encephalopathy syndrome.

Glucose enters the CSF space by active transport and by simple diffusion. CSF hypoglycorrhachia, like other CSF characteristics, can be altered in infectious and noninfectious conditions. Severe hypoglycorrhachia (glucose <20 mg/dL) indicates bacterial or fungal meningitis. Viral meningitis rarely causes abnormal CSF glucose values. Unlike CSF protein, CSF glucose values normalize quickly after infections and may have utility in assessing the response to antimicrobial therapy. Normally, the ratio of CSF glucose to serum glucose is 0.6, and a ratio less than 0.4 is considered pathologic. CSF glucose values typically do not exceed 300 mg/dL even in conditions of severe systemic hyperglycemia because of the limitations of CSF glucose transport.

Like serum lactate, CSF lactate results from anaerobic metabolism in hypoxic conditions, but serum lactate elevations do not translate into increases in CSF lactate. Conditions in which CSF lactate are elevated include ischemia, head injury, subarachnoid hemorrhage, and bacterial meningitis. CSF lactate values greater than 3.5 mmol/L are considered abnormal. The main utility of CSF lactate is to differentiate bacterial meningitis from viral meningitis.

Transferrin is an iron-binding protein that facilitates the transfer of iron to cells from iron stores. The transferrin in CSF, β_2-transferrin, has increased β_2 bands on gel electrophoresis and has utility in detecting CSF rhinorrhea or otorrhea.

CSF Function

CSF allows for a route of delivery and removal of nutrients, hormones, and transmitters for the brain. The pH of CSF influences changes in respiration through actions on the medulla oblongata central chemoreceptors. The CSF volume surrounding the brain also offers a degree of mechanical support, effectively decreasing the net weight of the brain. Buoyancy is limited because CSF volume is only one-tenth of the volume of the brain parenchyma.

CSF Dynamics in Acute Neurology

Several disorders are diagnosed (or confirmed) through examination of CSF. Neoplastic meningitis may be caused by a solid tumor (carcinomatous meningitis), leukemia (leukemic meningitis), lymphoma (lymphomatous meningitis), or, rarely, primary brain tumors. Cancer cells can spread by hematogenous routes, by migration along perivascular or perineural spaces, and by direct extension of tumor. Common culprit malignancies include breast cancer, melanoma, and lung cancer. Adenocarcinoma is the most common histologic type leading to neoplastic meningitis. Patients who present with a known malignancy and multifocal neurologic deficits should be evaluated for neoplastic meningitis. Tumor deposits affecting CSF drainage may also cause hydrocephalus.

Subarachnoid hemorrhage can cause such a rapid elevation in ICP that it equals diastolic blood pressures within 1 to 2 minutes. Acute hydrocephalus, from hindrance of CSF outflow at the level of the arachnoid granulations, is proportional to the amount of blood products spilled into the subarachnoid and ventricular spaces. Patients with chronic hydrocephalus from arachnoid adhesions present 2 to 6 weeks after the ictus of hemorrhage.

The pathophysiology of idiopathic intracranial hypertension is not yet fully understood. Possible theories involve delayed CSF absorption, abnormalities in venous outflow (eg, transverse sinus thrombosis), increases in cerebral venous pressure, and an unclear association with obesity. In obese patients, increased abdominal pressure increases intrathoracic pressure and central venous pressure, which in turn decreases CSF outflow. However, this does not explain why idiopathic intracranial hypertension is a disease primarily of women and why it also occurs in patients with a normal body mass index.

Reduced CSF volume is counterbalanced by increased vascular volume, as described by the Monro-Kellie doctrine (Chapter 8, "Intracranial Pressure"). Because veins are more compliant than arteries, which have muscular walls, the extravascular volume is contained in the dural sinuses and cerebral veins. Diffuse venous engorgement is responsible for the characteristic pachymeningeal enhancement seen in magnetic resonance imaging scans of the brain. Apart from neurosurgical or chiropractic manipulation and trauma leading to a dural tear and CSF leak, CSF hypotension can also be caused by lumbar puncture or disk disease or spontaneously from a connective tissue disorder. The most common sites of dural tear are where the cervical spinal roots exit the subarachnoid space, at the cribriform plate, and at the pituitary fossa.

Reduced buoyancy and resultant sagging of the brain from decreased CSF result in traction of the cranial nerves and a holocephalic and occasionally thunderclap headache. Lying in a recumbent or supine position relieves the sagging and traction, which explains the postural nature of CSF hypotension headache. Severe CSF hypotension can cause subdural hemorrhage (from tearing of the engorged bridging veins), cortical vein thrombosis, and herniation. Cortical vein thrombosis can be caused by slow venous outflow along engorged veins.

CSF leaks can be confirmed with computed tomography or magnetic resonance myelography. If results are equivocal, a radionuclide cisternogram should help. Treatment of CSF leaks includes epidural blood patch, percutaneous fibrin glue injection, and, occasionally, surgery. Recurrence is noted in 10% of patients.

CSF examination is crucial in suspected central nervous system (CNS) infections. Mechanisms for microbial entry into the CNS have not been fully delineated, but some theories suggest that microbes may be harbored in a monocyte and then enter the CNS (Trojan horse mechanism) or that surface antigens may traverse the epithelial tissue of the blood-brain barrier.

Moreover, the prevalence of ventriculitis and nosocomial meningitis has increased with the advent of intracranial monitoring devices. Microbial catheter colonization with retrograde infection results in CNS infections. Risk factors for nosocomial infection include duration of monitoring device use, CNS sampling frequency, and whether sterile technique was used during placement of the device. Typical culprit organisms include *Staphylococcus epidermidis* (70%), *Staphylococcus aureus* (10%), and gram-negative rods (15%), such as *Klebsiella, Escherichia coli*, and *Pseudomonas*.

Diagnosis based on clinical signs may be challenging in neurocritical care patients because fevers, decreased arousal, and meningismus can be ubiquitous, and CSF laboratory markers are not reliable when taken as a singular parameter. The *cell index* is a ratio of the CSF WBC:RBC ratio to the peripheral blood WBC:RBC ratio. It is a ratio of a ratio.

$$\text{Cell Index} = \frac{(\text{WBC}/\text{RBC})_{\text{CSF}}}{(\text{WBC}/\text{RBC})_{\text{Blood}}}$$

A large increase in the cell index during surveillance testing should prompt the examiner to consider the possibility of a nosocomial infection. For this reason, some neurocritical care centers routinely draw CSF samples from ventriculostomies at various intervals. However, frequent manipulations of the closed external ventricular drain system for repeated CSF sampling carries a risk of introducing infection as well.

Antimicrobial coverage should address methicillin-resistant *S aureus* or *Pseudomonas* infections according to local infection and resistance patterns. It is not common to require CSF administration of antibiotics or to replace the offending catheter. Preventive options include use of antibiotic-impregnated catheters, silver-impregnated catheters, periprocedural antibiotic administration, or prophylactic systemic antibiotics while an intracranial monitor is used.

Summary

- CSF volume is only one-tenth of the brain parenchyma volume.

- CSF is produced through active transport of Na^+, Cl^-, and HCO_3^- into the CSF space and by the osmotic introduction of water through AQP channels.
- CSF production is approximately 400 to 600 mL daily.
- CSF flow starts in the choroid plexuses in the lateral and third ventricles.
- CSF is drained into the arachnoid granulations, which flow into the dural sinuses.

SUGGESTED READING

Bulat M, Klarica M. Recent insights into a new hydrodynamics of the cerebrospinal fluid. Brain Res Rev. 2011 Jan 1;65(2):99–112. Epub 2010 Sep 29.

Cutler RW, Page L, Galicich J, Watters GV. Formation and absorption of cerebrospinal fluid in man. Brain. 1968;91(4):707–20.

Cutler RW, Spertell RB. Cerebrospinal fluid: a selective review. Ann Neurol. 1982 Jan;11(1):1–10.

Czosnyka M, Czosnyka Z, Momjian S, Pickard JD. Cerebrospinal fluid dynamics. Physiol Meas. 2004 Oct;25(5):R51–76.

Fishman RA. Cerebrospinal fluid in diseases of the nervous system. Philadelphia (PA): Saunders; c1980. 384 p.

Lyons MK, Meyer FB. Cerebrospinal fluid physiology and the management of increased intracranial pressure. Mayo Clin Proc. 1990 May;65(5): 684–707.

10 Cerebral Circulation and Cerebral Blood Flow

ARNOLEY S. ABCEJO, MD; JEFFREY J. PASTERNAK, MD

Goals

- Describe the anatomy of the intracranial circulation.
- Describe cerebral hemodynamics and autoregulation.
- Describe the principles of measuring cerebral blood flow.

Introduction

With its high metabolic rate and lack of substrate stores, the brain is dependent on a constant supply of oxygen and glucose. If blood flow stops, alterations in brain function occur within seconds and irreversible injury can occur within a few minutes. Many patients admitted to neurosciences intensive care units have acute strokes, are eligible for endovascular procedures, and may need other measures to preserve adequate cerebral blood flow. An understanding of the blood supply, venous drainage, and factors affecting cerebral perfusion is thus pivotal to the practice of neurologic critical care. This chapter reviews the anatomical and physiologic principles governing cerebral circulation and blood flow.

Anatomy of Cerebral Circulation

The brain is supplied by 2 distinct vessel pairs: the internal carotid arteries of the anterior circulation and the vertebral arteries of the posterior circulation. The internal carotid arteries supply a larger percentage of the blood to the healthy human brain than the vertebral arteries. Anterior and posterior circulations meet at the circle of Willis, where collateral pathways help to maintain cerebral blood flow (CBF) during periods of ischemia.

Anterior Circulation

The internal carotid arteries are branches of the common carotid arteries. They enter the cranial vault through the carotid canal in the petrous portion of the temporal bone. The carotid arteries then traverse through the cavernous sinus and enter the subarachnoid space. At this point, each carotid artery gives rise to multiple branches, including the ophthalmic artery, anterior cerebral artery (ACA), anterior choroidal artery, and posterior communicating artery, before giving rise to the middle cerebral artery (MCA) (Figure 10.1). Each MCA is divided further into 4 segments, M1 through M4 (Figure 10.1). The ACAs traverse anteriorly and are connected by the anterior communicating artery that provides an avenue for collateral circulation. The ACA can be separated into up to 5 segments, A1 through A5 (Figure 10.1).

Two important smaller arteries branch off the internal carotid arteries before the MCA and ACA bifurcation: the anterior choroidal artery and the posterior communicating artery. The anterior choroidal artery supplies portions of the optic tract, medial temporal lobe, internal capsule, amygdala, caudate nucleus, inferior globus pallidus, and midbrain. The posterior communicating artery connects to the posterior cerebral artery and is the primary anastomosis between the anterior and posterior circulations of the brain.

Posterior Circulation

The vertebral arteries are branches of the subclavian artery. They travel superiorly in the neck within the transverse foramina of cervical vertebrae and enter the cranial vault through the foramen magnum. Paired vertebral arteries, traversing along the ventral surface of the medulla, each give rise to anterior spinal arteries, posterior inferior cerebellar arteries, and multiple small perforating arterioles

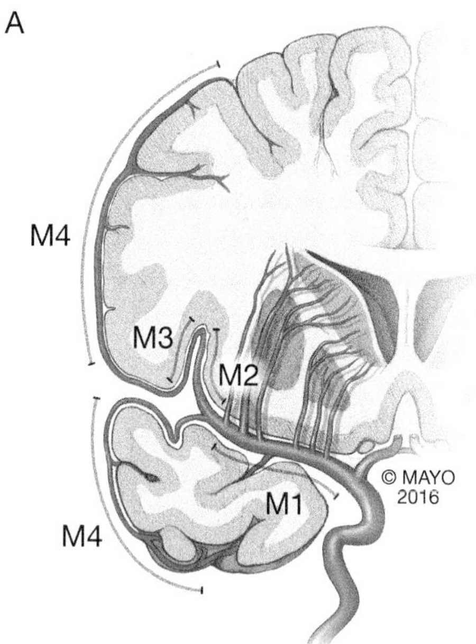
A
M4
M3
M2
M1
M4
© MAYO 2016
M1—Most proximal portion of the MCA; travels horizontally along the sphenoid
M2—Bifurcates or trifurcates around the insula
M3—Extends from the insula to the cortex
M4—Traverses and terminates along the cortex; bifurcates immediately and supplies cortical frontal, parietal, occipital, and temporal lobes

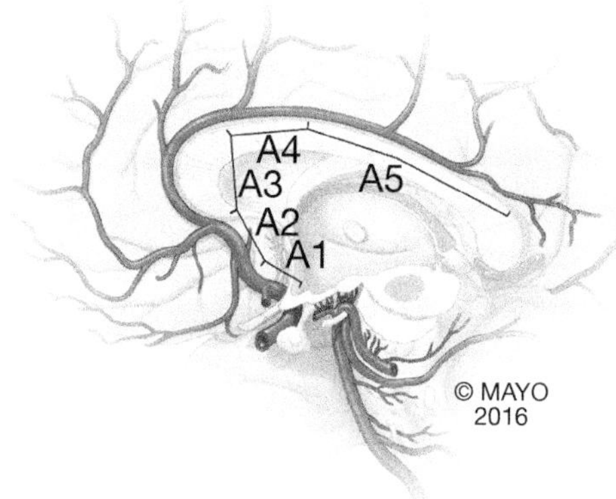
B
A4
A3
A5
A2
A1
© MAYO 2016
A1—Features the portion between the internal carotid artery and the anterior communicating artery; perforating branches from A1 help supply the caudate nucleus and internal capsule
A2—Includes the ACA until the genu of the corpus callosum
A3—Spans the genu of the corpus callosum, follows the longitudinal fissure, and ends at the rostral end of the body of the corpus callosum
A4 and A5—Follow the superior portion of the corpus callosum

Figure 10.1. Middle Cerebral Artery (MCA) and Anterior Cerebral Artery (ACA) Segmental Anatomy, Distribution, and Anatomical Correlates. A, MCA segments M1 through M4 are shown. B, ACA segments A1 through A5 are shown, although the ACA is often divided into 3 segments, where the third segment consists of A3 through A5.

that supply the medulla before joining at the pontomedullary junction and forming a single basilar artery.

The basilar artery continues along the ventral surface of the pons, giving rise to paired anterior inferior cerebellar arteries, superior cerebellar arteries, and small perforating arterioles that supply the pons.

The basilar artery terminally bifurcates into the posterior cerebral arteries (PCAs). The proximal segments of the PCAs form the posterior portion of the circle of Willis, each giving rise to posterior communicating arteries that form anastomoses with the anterior circulation. The PCA supplies most of the perfusion to the midbrain and the reticular activating system and to the medio-inferior portions of the occipital and temporal lobes.

Collateral Circulation

The circle of Willis is a hexagonal vascular ring where the anterior and posterior circulation systems meet, allowing for collateral flow between vessels on the left and right sides of the brain (Figure 10.2). The greatest benefit of collateral blood flow around the circle of Willis is observed with carotid occlusion during endarterectomy. However, the circle of Willis is not circumferentially patent in more than 50% of patients. Other potential connections for collateral circulation include the anastomoses between the middle meningeal artery and the ophthalmic artery.

Anastomoses distal to the circle of Willis can contribute to collateral circulation. Connections between the major arterial distributions—ACA, MCA, and PCA—complement CBF in vulnerable, watershed areas of the brain. These collaterals consist of small vessels. Thus, in hypoperfusion, as can occur with severe hypotension, these watershed regions can become ischemic.

Venous Drainage

Venous drainage of the brain is illustrated in Figure 10.3. Cerebral veins are small, thin-walled, valveless vessels that drain brain parenchyma. They are tributaries of larger, endothelium-lined dural venous sinuses, which are also valveless and exist between the periosteal and meningeal layers of dura mater. The dural venous sinuses then drain into the jugular veins and pterygoid venous plexus. The

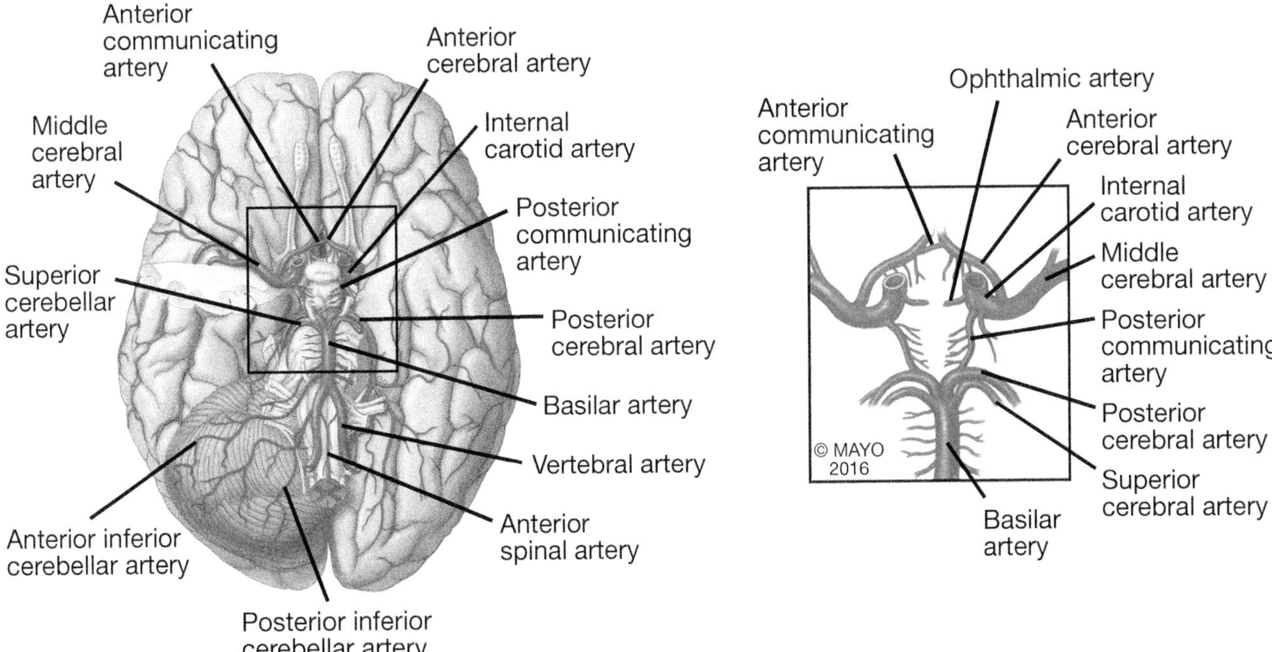

Figure 10.2. Major Arteries of the Cerebral Anterior and Cerebral Posterior Circulations.

venous system of the brain is unique in that veins do not necessarily run in parallel with the arterial circulation. Thus, occlusion of venous outflow from the brain results in injury to parenchymal regions of the brain that are different from those injured after impairment of arterial inflow.

Cerebral Hemodynamics

Global CBF in an awake adult at rest is approximately 800 mL/min or 50 mL/100 g/min. Although the brain is only a small fraction of the body's total mass (2%-3%), the brain receives 15% of total cardiac output. Cerebral metabolic rate (CMR) largely determines CBF, a phenomenon known as *flow-metabolism coupling*. For example, gray matter has a 4-fold greater CMR and CBF than white matter. Increased neuronal activity, such as with increased neuronal function or seizures, increases CBF. In contrast, decreased neuronal activity, such as with some sedative or anesthetic drugs, decreases CBF.

Under normal circumstances, mean (SD) cerebral blood volume (CBV) has been determined to be 3.77 (1.05) mL/100 g globally, with 3.93 (0.9) mL/100 g in gray matter and 2.52 (0.78) mL/100 g in white matter. A complex relationship exists between CBF and CBV: Changes in CBF and CBV can occur in parallel or in opposite directions, or 1 parameter may not change while the other does. For example, under normal circumstances with intact autoregulatory function, an increase in blood pressure leads to unchanged CBF but decreased CBV because of compensatory vasoconstriction, which is discussed further below. With impaired autoregulation, parallel changes are observed in CBF and CBV. However, in acute stroke, a decrease in CBF occurs and can cause distal vasodilatation and an increase in CBV.

Factors Affecting CBF

An important point to understand is that changes in systemic blood pressure, within reason, do not affect CBF but may affect CBV. The healthy brain can maintain a constant CBF despite changes in *cerebral perfusion pressure* (CPP), which is defined as the difference between the mean arterial pressure (MAP) and the intracranial pressure (ICP). With this autoregulation of blood flow, systemic blood pressure changes are buffered and appropriate blood delivery to the brain is maintained, usually within a CPP range of 50 to 150 mm Hg. However, the upper and lower limits of autoregulation are debatable and they likely vary among people and within the same person at different times and in different circumstances. Outside this range, CBF varies linearly with CPP. High ICP or severe systemic hypotension that compromises CPP can dangerously decrease CBF, whereas a hypertensive crisis increases CBF. Patients with chronic hypertension are more susceptible to cerebral ischemia during relative hypotension.

Autoregulation is manifested by changes in cerebral arteriolar diameter. Decreases in CPP result in vasodilatation, and increases in CPP induce vasoconstriction. Thus, within the autoregulatory range, although CBF may be

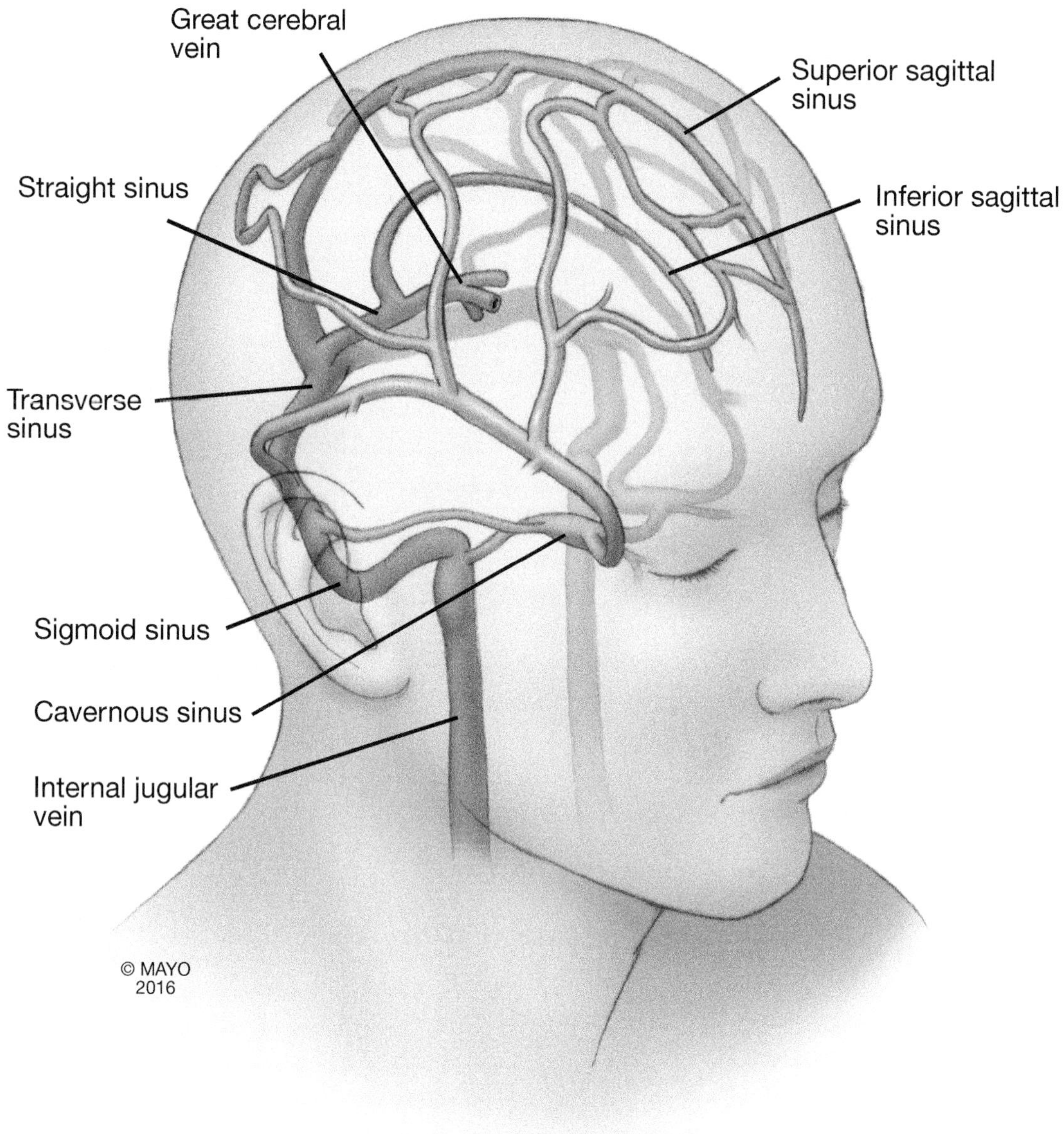

Figure 10.3. Cerebral Venous System.
(Modified from Wijdicks EFM. The practice of emergency and critical care neurology. 2nd ed. New York [NY]: Oxford University Press; c2016. p.440; used with permission of Mayo Foundation for Medical Education and Research.)

constant, CBV is not. Specifically, as CPP increases within the autoregulatory range, cerebral vasoconstriction maintains a constant CBF, but this vasoconstriction results in decreased CBV.

Control of autoregulation is complex and is dependent on several interconnected systems instead of a single mechanism. Vessel diameter is controlled by neural activity and multiple intermediary compounds, including nitric oxide, adenosine, potassium and hydrogen ions, endothelins, and prostaglandins. These mechanisms lead to myogenic changes, wherein changes in CPP, metabolism, and acid-base status promote vasomotor responses that control CBF.

Autoregulation can be impaired with brain injury, after the administration of various drugs, and with severe metabolic derangements. Cerebral autoregulatory function is not an all-or-none phenomenon—it can be intact, partially impaired, or completely impaired, leading to pressure-dependent CBF. The consequences of autoregulation failure

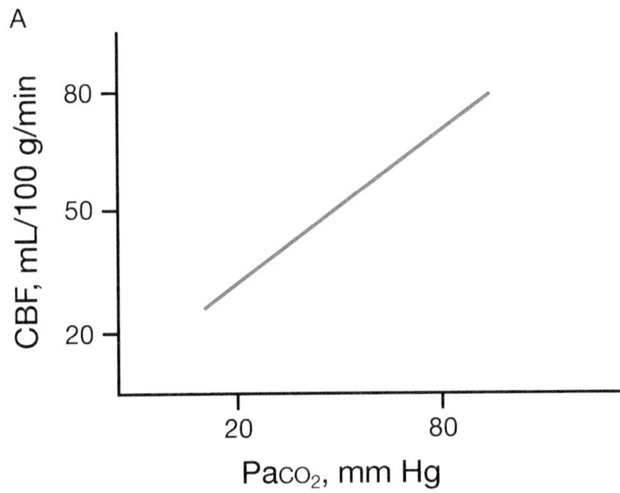

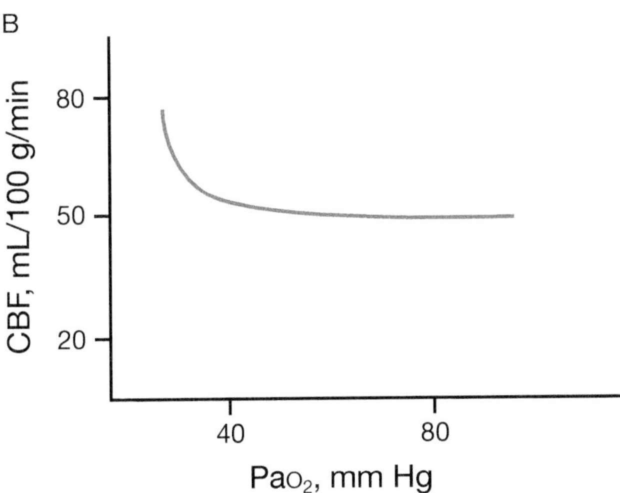

Figure 10.4. Cerebral Blood Flow (CBF) as a Function of Cerebral Perfusion Pressure. A, CBF and $Paco_2$*. B, CBF and* Pao_2*.*

depend on the disease state, with either a hypoperfusion response or a hyperperfusion response. Hypoperfusion may lead to brain ischemia at a CPP that is higher than expected. With hyperperfusion, CBF exceeds vessel capacity, manifesting as vasogenic cerebral edema or vessel rupture at a CPP that is lower than expected.

Arterial carbon dioxide tension has a profound effect on CBF because carbon dioxide is a potent cerebrovascular vasodilator. In the healthy brain, CBF is linearly dependent on carbon dioxide between a $Paco_2$ of 20 and 80 mm Hg (Figure 10.4A). Therapeutic hyperventilation can be used to treat intracranial hypertension. However, this effect is transient, lasting only 6 to 10 hours. If no ventilation changes are made, CBF approaches that associated with normocapnia despite persistent hypocapnia. This return of CBF is due to renormalization of the cerebrospinal fluid pH by alterations in the bicarbonate concentration. Thus, rapid cessation of hyperventilation can increase the CBF and the ICP.

Arterial oxygen has no direct effect on CBF until arterial oxygen tension decreases to less than 50 mm Hg, resulting in cerebral vasodilatation (Figure 10.4B).

Systemic acidosis alone does not change CBF if the blood-brain barrier is intact because hydrogen ions do not readily cross the blood-brain barrier. However, if lactic acidosis develops within the brain, such as during brain ischemia, hydrogen ions cause cerebral vasodilatation.

Brain temperature affects CMR and CBF. CMR decreases by 6% to 7% per 1°C decrease in temperature with a parallel decrease in CBF. Hyperthermia causes an increase in CMR and CBF. Severe hyperthermia (>42°C) is toxic, causing a decrease in CMR. However, in severe hyperthermia, flow-metabolism coupling is impaired and CBF continues to increase despite a decrease in CMR. This uncoupling could aggravate vascular engorgement and worsen cerebral edema.

Many drugs can augment cerebral hemodynamics. Anesthetic drugs such as propofol, barbiturates, etomidate, benzodiazepines, and opioids cause a decrease in CMR and a concomitant decrease in CBF, CBV, and ICP if ventilation is controlled. In spontaneously ventilating patients, these drugs also depress ventilation and lead to hypercapnia, which can offset the vasoconstrictive effects and cause an increase in CBF, CBV, and potentially ICP. Dexmedetomidine also decreases CMR and CBF but without a large effect on ventilation at clinically relevant doses, so it is less likely to induce hypercapnia in the spontaneously breathing patient. Ketamine seems to induce a dose-dependent increase in CBF, with frontotemporal regions of the brain appearing to be more affected than other regions of the brain, but ketamine does not appear to increase ICP, an effect that may be due to a differential effect of the drug on CBF and CBV.

Vasoactive medications can also affect cerebral hemodynamics. In hypotensive patients, catecholamines increase CBF by increasing systemic blood pressure, but when they act at adrenergic receptors on the cerebral vasculature, catecholamines can induce vasoconstriction. Cerebral vasodilators, such as nitroglycerin and nitroprusside, can increase CBV and ICP.

Measurement of CBF and Autoregulation

CBF monitoring is an evolving critical care practice, with newer modalities continuing to be developed. Jugular bulb oximetry is a traditional, indirect method for measuring the brain's use of oxygen. All else being equal, a decrease in CBF causes an increase in cerebral oxygen extraction and a decrease in jugular venous oxygen content. Doppler ultrasonography allows direct measurement of CBF velocity at the bedside and can aid in prediction of the onset and severity of vasospasm. It requires interpretation because changes in the linear velocity of blood flow (in centimeters per second) do not always correspond to similar changes in the volume flow rate of blood (in milliliters per minute). For example, distal cerebral vasoconstriction leads to a parallel decrease in CBF velocity and CBF volume flow, whereas vasospasm of major arteries can result in an increase in CBF velocity in these constricted vessels but a decrease in CBF volume flow to the parts of the brain perfused by these vessels. Computerized tomographic perfusion studies can be used to estimate CBF. Likewise, blood oxygen level dependent (BOLD) magnetic resonance imaging (MRI) is the basis for functional MRI and can highlight changes in CBF or cerebrovascular resistance. Positron emission tomography (PET) and single-photon emission computed tomography (SPECT) can also be used to estimate global and regional cerebral blood flow and metabolism.

Autoregulatory capacity can be clinically quantified by various techniques. For example, systemic blood pressure can be altered pharmacologically, and its effect on CBF velocity, as measured with transcranial Doppler sonography, can be used to judge the integrity of autoregulation because CBF velocity should not vary grossly with systemic blood pressure changes if autoregulation is intact. Changes in CBF velocity that occur in parallel with changes in systemic blood pressure indicate autoregulatory impairment.

Alternatively, a moving Pearson correlation coefficient between simultaneous values of MAP and other metrics for CBF (eg, ICP, CBF linear velocity, regional cerebral oxygen saturation, and brain tissue oxygen partial pressure) can be calculated to estimate the integrity of autoregulation. The most common is the pressure reactivity index (PRx), a moving Pearson correlation coefficient between MAP and ICP with values ranging from −1 to +1. If autoregulation is intact, an increase in MAP should induce cerebral vasoconstriction, thus decreasing ICP and PRx values, whereas autoregulatory failure would lead to parallel changes in MAP and ICP and higher PRx values.

Summary

- The carotid arteries give rise to the anterior circulation that supplies the anterior and middle cerebral arteries. The posterior circulation is derived from the vertebral arteries and supplies predominantly posterior fossa structures. This division is crucial in stroke classification.
- Normal cerebral blood flow is approximately 50 mL/100 g/min. Normal cerebral blood volume is approximately 3.77 mL/100 g. Gray matter receives more blood flow and contains a larger blood volume density than white matter.
- Flow-metabolism coupling describes the proportional increase in CBF with increases in CMR.
- Cerebral autoregulation maintains constant CBF with changes in CPP. As CPP increases, cerebral vasoconstriction occurs, decreasing CBV at the expense of maintaining CBF.
- Autoregulation can be impaired by certain drugs, in patients with brain injury, or when homeostasis is altered, leading to parallel changes in CBF in response to changes in CPP.
- CBF is linearly related to changes in $PaCO_2$ in the range of 20 to 80 mm Hg. CBF does not change in response to arterial oxygen content until hypoxia ensues, leading to increased CBF. CBF changes occur in parallel with changes in temperature. Various drugs, such as sedatives and vasoactive medications, can decrease CBF and CBV.
- Various techniques can be used to estimate regional or global changes in CBF. These include jugular bulb oximetry, transcranial Doppler sonography, and various radiologic or nuclear studies.
- Autoregulatory capacity is generally quantified by determining the relationship between CPP (or MAP) and a metric for CBF, such as ICP, CBF linear velocity, regional cerebral oxygen saturation, or brain tissue oxygen partial pressure.

SUGGESTED READING

Bulte D, Chiarelli P, Wise R, Jezzard P. Measurement of cerebral blood volume in humans using hyperoxic MRI contrast. J Magn Reson Imaging. 2007 Oct;26(4):894–9.

Czosnyka M, Miller C; Participants in the International Multidisciplinary Consensus Conference on Multimodality Monitoring. Monitoring of cerebral autoregulation. Neurocrit Care. 2014 Dec;21 Suppl 2:S95–S102.

Hatazawa J, Shimosegawa E, Toyoshima H, Ardekani BA, Suzuki A, Okudera T, et al. Cerebral blood volume in acute brain infarction: a combined study with dynamic susceptibility contrast MRI and 99mTc-HMPAO-SPECT. Stroke. 1999 Apr;30(4):800–6.

Hoffman WE, Albrecht RF, Miletich DJ. Regional cerebral blood flow changes during hypothermia. Cryobiology. 1982 Dec;19(6):640–5.

Iadecola C. The neurovascular unit coming of age: a journey through neurovascular coupling in health and disease. Neuron. 2017 Sep 27;96(1):17–42.

Krabbe-Hartkamp MJ, van der Grond J, de Leeuw FE, de Groot JC, Algra A, Hillen B, et al. Circle of Willis: morphologic variation on three-dimensional time-of-flight MR angiograms. Radiology. 1998 Apr;207(1):103–11.

Lazaridis C, Robertson CS. The role of multimodal invasive monitoring in acute traumatic brain injury. Neurosurg Clin N Am. 2016 Oct;27(4):509–17.

Madhok DY, Vitt JR, Nguyen AT. Overview of neurovascular physiology. Curr Neurol Neurosci Rep. 2018 Oct 23;18(12):99.

Memon A, McCullough LD. Cerebral circulation in men and women. Adv Exp Med Biol. 2018;1065:279–90.

Murkin JM, Kamar M, Silman Z, Balberg M, Adams SJ. Intraoperative cerebral autoregulation assessment using ultrasound-tagged near-infrared-based cerebral blood flow in comparison to transcranial Doppler cerebral flow velocity: a pilot study. J Cardiothorac Vasc Anesth. 2015 Oct;29(5):1187–93. Epub 2015 May 27.

Sanders RD, Degos V, Young WL. Cerebral perfusion under pressure: is the autoregulatory 'plateau' a level playing field for all? Anaesthesia. 2011 Nov;66(11):968–72. Epub 2011 Sep 20.

Walter EJ, Carraretto M. The neurological and cognitive consequences of hyperthermia. Crit Care. 2016 Jul 14;20(1):199.

Wang X, Ding X, Tong Y, Zong J, Zhao X, Ren H, et al. Ketamine does not increase intracranial pressure compared with opioids: meta-analysis of randomized controlled trials. J Anesth. 2014 Dec;28(6):821–7. Epub 2014 May 24.

Zeiler FA, Sader N, Gillman LM, Teitelbaum J, West M, Kazina CJ. The cerebrovascular response to ketamine: a systematic review of the animal and human literature. J Neurosurg Anesthesiol. 2016 Apr;28(2):123–40.

Consequences of Anoxia and Ischemia to the Brain

JENNIFER E. FUGATE, DO

Goals

- Describe damage to the brain from hypoxemia and ischemia.
- Describe neurologic findings associated with various prognoses.
- Describe the role of electrodiagnostic testing and neuroimaging in the assessment of anoxic-ischemic brain injury.
- Discuss pitfalls in the assessment of patients undergoing targeted temperature management.

Introduction

Cardiac arrest occurs suddenly, often without premonitory symptoms. Consciousness is lost within seconds to minutes because of insufficient cerebral blood flow in the midst of complete hemodynamic collapse. Brain cells may be salvageable if circulation is adequately restored, but time is critical because cerebral oxygen stores are lost within 20 seconds, while glucose and adenosine triphosphate stores are depleted within 5 minutes. The term *anoxia* describes the complete lack of oxygen delivery (eg, complete cessation of blood flow during cardiac arrest); *hypoxia* describes what may occur during periods of decreased oxygen delivery but with some degree of continued blood flow. Hypoxic injury is caused by severe hypoxemia (eg, asphyxia) or respiratory arrest.

Anoxic-ischemic brain injury is most commonly caused by cardiac arrest, which is frequently lethal; of the US patients with out-of-hospital cardiac arrest treated by emergency medical services, almost 90% die. Among patients who survive to hospital admission, inpatient mortality is decreasing, but a substantial number of those survivors have poor neurologic outcomes from anoxic-ischemic brain injury.

Pathophysiology

As opposed to most acute brain diseases, which are focal, anoxia induces global brain injury. The extent of damage largely reflects the duration of interrupted cerebral blood flow. Brain cells become ischemic as cerebral blood flow decreases below the levels needed to sustain brain metabolism. Although the decrease in cerebral blood flow is uniform throughout the brain, the damage to cells is not, because neuronal vulnerability varies among different regions. The brain areas most susceptible to anoxic-ischemic injury are in the hippocampus (particularly the CA1 sector), the basal ganglia (caudate nucleus and putamen), the cerebellar Purkinje cells, and the neocortex. Necrosis of the cortex is known as *laminar necrosis*. The vulnerability of these areas may be explained by the presence of excitatory neurotransmitter receptors or the high metabolic demands of neurons in these regions.

The 2 main modes of ischemic cell death are necrosis and apoptosis. Dying neurons show characteristics of both pathways. Another mechanism of neuronal and glial damage in anoxic-ischemic brain injury is "excitatory" brain injury. An efflux of the excitatory neurotransmitter glutamate increases the concentration of intracellular calcium, which causes injury by activating catabolic enzymes and endonucleases and producing free reactive oxygen species. Subsequently, proinflammatory cytokines (eg, tumor necrosis factor α and interleukins 1β and 6) are also released.

In addition to these mechanisms, the *no-reflow phenomenon* may cause further brain injury after cardiac arrest through the substantial micocirculatory perfusion deficits that exist after circulation is restored. Coagulation may occur within these reperfusion zones, with intravascular fibrin formation and microthrombosis. This concept underlies the rationale for experimental studies with recombinant tissue–type plasminogen activator in anoxic or hypoxic conditions.

One of the important questions about anoxia's effect on the brain is whether interventions can modify the degree of brain injury and, if so, whether there is an optimal time when action must be taken. Is the damage to the brain permanent and present at cardiac arrest, or are any of the detrimental processes modifiable? The concept of *neuroprotection* has garnered much research interest, but many candidates have fallen short clinically. Induced hypothermia had been considered by many to be the only beneficial neuroprotectant, but in a large randomized trial there were no differences in outcomes between patients treated with targeted normothermia (36°C) and patients treated with targeted hypothermia (33°C).

After cardiac arrest, coma often persists for days and is prolonged further by the common practice of administering sedatives and analgesics in the intensive care unit. Many comatose patients ultimately have unfavorable outcomes, but some patients do awaken, undergo rehabilitation, and resume an independent lifestyle. Neurointensivists are often responsible for the difficult task of estimating a neurologic prognosis for comatose patients early on and trying to identify which patients have a reasonable chance for recovery.

Prognostication

Estimating a neurologic prognosis for comatose patients after cardiopulmonary resuscitation (CPR) requires a multifaceted approach. Information is gathered about the details of the cardiac arrest (eg, initial cardiac rhythm, duration, and quality of CPR), serial neurologic examinations, laboratory tests, brain imaging results, and electrophysiologic studies. Certain characteristics of the cardiac arrest are associated with worse outcomes: unwitnessed arrests, longer duration of arrest, and initial cardiac rhythm of asystole or pulseless electrical activity. Other patient factors that have also been associated with worse outcomes are older age, sepsis, and malignancy.

Neurologic Examination

The neurologic examination is fundamental to the evaluation; all additional tests are ancillary and must be interpreted in the context of the clinical findings. One of the most crucial parts of the clinical assessment is to determine whether the examination is confounded by recently administered medications. If so, any decisions on prognosis must be delayed until a reliable examination can be performed that is free of the effects of recent sedatives, analgesics, or metabolic abnormalities. After a cardiac arrest, multiple organs frequently lack adequate blood flow,

Table 11.1 • Analgesics and Sedatives Commonly Used in the Intensive Care Unit

Medication	Elimination Half-life, h
Morphine	1.5-4
Fentanyl	2-5
Alfentanil	1.5-3.5
Midazolam	1-4
Lorazepam	10-20
Propofol	2

and acute kidney injury and shock liver develop. Opioids and benzodiazepines are usually administered, especially early, and elimination of these drugs from the body may take several days. Table 11.1 shows half-lives of commonly administered sedative and analgesic medications. Under normal physiologic circumstances, it takes 4 to 5 half-lives for a drug to be completely eliminated.

Traditionally, before offering a prognosis based on the neurologic examination findings of a comatose patient after CPR, clinicians have waited at least 72 hours after a cardiac arrest. However, with the widespread use of induced hypothermia or induced target temperature management—both of which often require heavy sedation—neurologic examination findings are commonly still unreliable at 72 hours, so the neurologic examination may need to be postponed even longer.

Certain clinical findings are associated with a poor outcome. Absent pupillary light reflexes, absent corneal reflexes, and a motor response that is either absent or extensor posturing are the traditional examination findings associated with a poor outcome. The most reliable of these (ie, the finding with the lowest false-positive rate) is the absence of pupillary light reflexes, most likely because it is the least affected by medications. Lingering effects of opioids and benzodiazepines may eliminate a motor response and corneal reflexes; thus, a clinician must wait to perform an accurate examination.

Another examination finding associated with a poor outcome is *myoclonic status epilepticus*, which is a spontaneous, vigorous, and continuous multifocal myoclonus that often involves the facial and axial muscles. This should be distinguished from the occasional myoclonic jerk that does not have prognostic significance. Myoclonic status epilepticus occurs early (within the first 24 hours) after cardiac arrest. An electroencephalogram (EEG) usually shows either a burst suppression pattern (Figure 11.1) or generalized periodic discharges, patterns that are also associated with unfavorable outcomes.

In most series, myoclonic status epilepticus has been invariably associated with poor outcomes (<1% of patients with myoclonic status epilepticus have good outcomes),

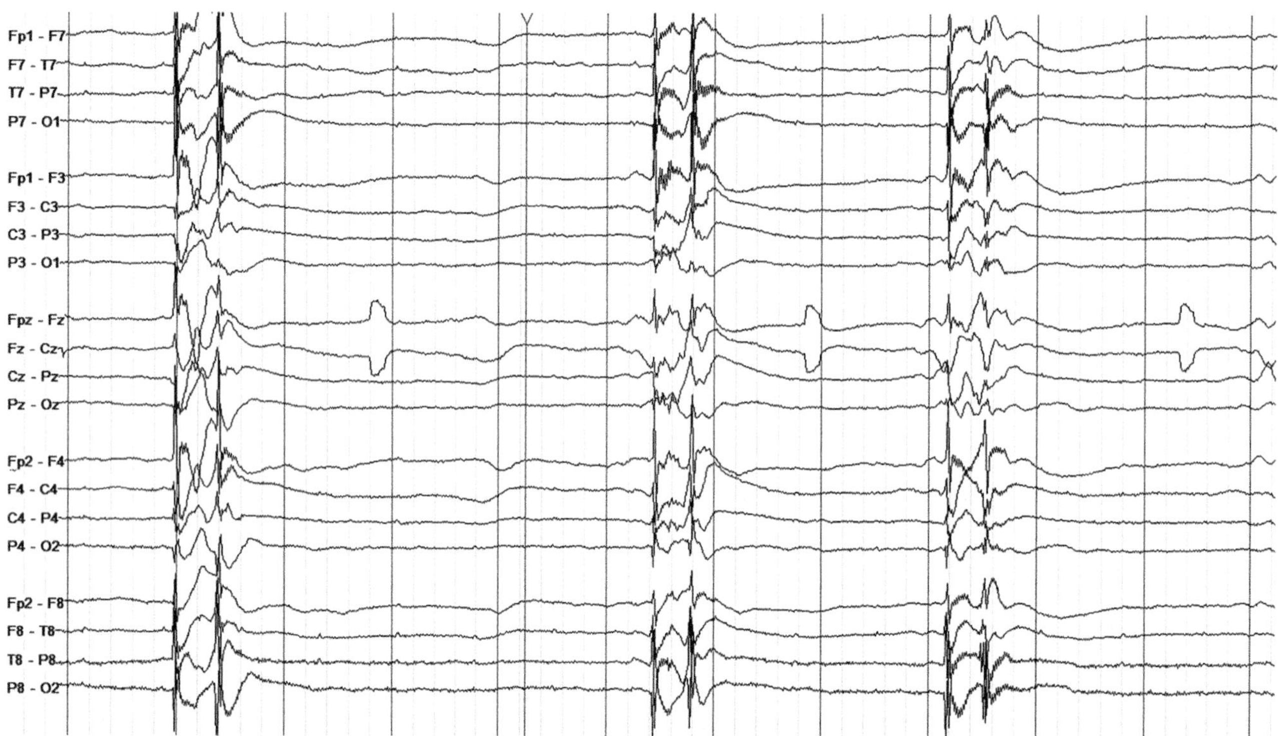

Figure 11.1. Electroencephalogram in Severe Anoxic-Ischemic Brain Injury. The bipolar montage shows a background of burst suppression with short duration bursts of polyspike activity. These bursts were sometimes clinically correlated with generalized myoclonic jerks.

but a few patients have been reported to have favorable outcomes despite having early postanoxic myoclonus. On rare occasions, the presence of myoclonic status epilepticus does not imply a poor functional outcome after cardiac arrest. Caution must be exercised in prognosticating early if patients are young, have used illicit substances, or have a primary respiratory arrest.

Electrophysiology

Somatosensory evoked potential (SSEP) testing and EEG are commonly used as ancillary tests for estimating neurologic prognosis after cardiac arrest. SSEP testing consists of stimulating both median nerves near the wrist and monitoring and averaging electrical responses at different points throughout the neuraxis. The response at the scalp (N20), the cortical response, has been well studied in prognosticating outcomes after cardiac arrest. Within 1 to 3 days after cardiac arrest, if the N20 response is absent bilaterally, the outcome is invariably poor (defined in most studies as remaining in a vegetative state or dead within 6 months). However, the study is not useful if the N20 response is present (which is the case for most patients) because the presence of the N20 response does not predict a good outcome.

Hypothermia may slow conduction velocities and alter the predictive ability of SSEP, so this test should not be performed unless the patient's temperature is normal. The use of sedative and analgesic medication does not generally alter the N20 response, but it is prudent to stop these medications before because, as emphasized above, attempts at prognostication should not be undertaken if the examination findings would still be unreliable.

EEG is used for 2 purposes when patients remain comatose after CPR. First, it is used as an adjunct in estimating neurologic prognosis. A poor neurologic prognosis is associated with several EEG patterns, including generalized suppression, suppression with periodic discharges, burst-suppression, the presense of status epilepticus, and a nonreactive background. However, prognostication should not rely on the results of 1 test alone. Even with experienced epileptologists and a standardized protocol, highly malignant EEG patterns predict outcome in about only half of patients, and any single finding generally does not predict outcome with sufficient accuracy.

The other indication for EEG in comatose patients after cardiac arrest is for seizure detection. Many centers use continuous EEG while patients are being cooled and treated with sedatives and neuromuscular blocking agents. Continuous EEG is labor and resource intensive, and not all centers have this capability. Thus, spot EEG recordings (20-30 minutes in duration) are sometimes all that can be obtained. The occurrence of electrographic seizures during cooling protocols is commonly associated with a poor prognosis. However, some patients have recovered well despite seizures, so aggressive treatment as a trial is justified for most patients. This is particularly true of seizures or status epilepticus that arises from a continuous background and during rewarming (rather than active cooling).

Serum Biomarkers

Most recent studies of biomarkers in comatose survivors of cardiac arrest have examined serum neuron-specific enolase (NSE). NSE is a gamma isomer of enolase that is located in neurons. The usefulness of this biomarker in prognostication may be more limited than electrophysiologic testing because none of the studies are automated, long laboratory turnaround times may be impractical, and standardization has not been optimal. Aside from neurons, NSE is also found in red blood cells and platelets, so hemolyzed blood specimens may show a higher level of NSE than is reflective of neuronal injury. In studies done before the routine use of cooling protocols, NSE test results predicted outcome well: An NSE level greater than 33 mcg/L 1 to 3 days after cardiac arrest was associated with a poor outcome. However, in the era of therapeutic hypothermia, several studies have shown that this cutoff is less reliable, with false-positive rates as high as 22% to 29%. Some studies have found that an NSE level as high as 80 mcg/L may be needed to reliably predict poor outcome. Others have suggested that the trend of serial NSE levels may be important, but further studies are needed. Therefore, a strict NSE threshold cannot be recommended for prognostication for patients who have had cardiac arrest and targeted temperature management until further research has been conducted and laboratory assays have been standardized.

Neuroimaging

Despite a lack of high-quality evidence, the use of neuroimaging continues to grow as an adjunct for estimating neurologic prognoses for comatose survivors of cardiac arrest. It is not uncommon that a comatose patient remains comatose but without definitive signs or tests suggesting a poor prognosis (eg, a patient may have intact brainstem reflexes, withdraw from pain, and have intact N20 responses). In those situations, imaging the brain may allow visualizing the extent of cortical damage and give insights into the severity of the anoxic injury. However, the knowledge gleaned from imaging must be tempered with the fact that no definitive validation studies exist for neuroimaging as a single modality for prognostication. Clinical context is paramount, and a multifaceted approach must be used.

If computed tomographic (CT) imaging is performed early, the findings are often normal and are usually not useful for determining the severity of anoxic-ischemic injury. In severe cases, however, after 3 to 5 days, global brain edema may be visualized. Several studies have found that the disappearance of the gray-white junction on noncontrast CT of the head has been associated with poor outcomes and failure to awaken. Those findings, though, should be interpreted cautiously because published studies on the prognostic use of CT imaging are limited mostly to retrospective case series, and the timing of CT has ranged from minutes to nearly 3 weeks after cardiac arrest.

Magnetic resonance imaging (MRI) continues to hold promise, but the current data are insufficient to systematically guide prognostication with MRI. Diffusion-weighted imaging (DWI) is particularly sensitive to ischemia, and apparent diffusion coefficient (ADC) values can provide a quantitative measure of injury. The published studies have been limited by the heterogeneity of timing for MRI and patient selection bias.

MRI parameters associated with poor outcome include widespread and persistent cortical DWI abnormalities, the combination of cortical and deep gray matter DWI and fluid-attenuated inversion recovery (FLAIR) abnormalities (Figure 11.2), and severe global ADC reduction. Still, 20% to 50% of patients with good outcomes have DWI abnormalities on MRI, and some patients have poor outcomes despite a normal MRI. Thus, decisions on continuing medical care or withdrawing life-sustaining treatments should not be made on the basis of MRI findings alone, and larger prospective studies with standardized imaging are needed. Some practical limitations that could affect the widespread use of MRI in this population include transporting patients who may be too hemodynamically unstable to move to the MRI suite and implanting temporary pacing wires and pacemakers or defibrillators.

Conclusions

A prognosis for comatose survivors of CPR is important in clinical practice. It allows discussion about the level of care, whether the patient would want another resuscitative effort, or whether medical care should be escalated. In many cases, the family will decide to withdraw support. However, all the prognosticating studies have not eliminated concern about prognostication error. Prognostication is difficult when patients have received sedative drugs, despite undergoing an examination after the drugs have been eliminated from the body, and when patients have had a cardiorespiratory arrest with drug overdose. With these patients, prudence should be exercised in making a definitive assessment.

In conclusion, anoxic-ischemic injury to the brain is damaging at ictus and often leads to prolonged coma. For many patients, a persistent unconsciousness can be expected. The continuous care of comatose patients after cardiopulmonary arrest is a major burden to the health care system, and family members should be adequately informed about the chances of recovery.

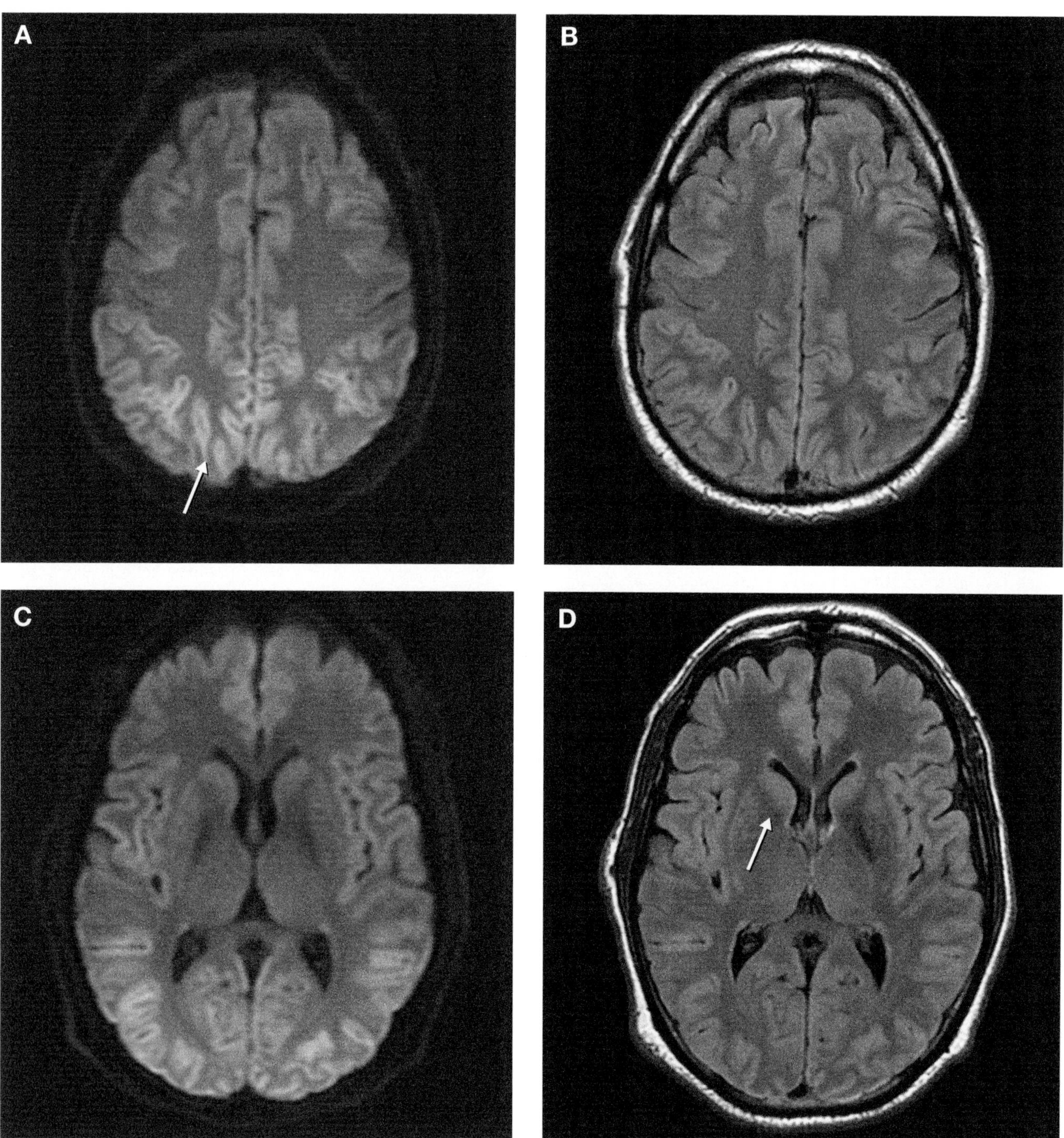

Figure 11.2. Magnetic Resonance Imaging Findings in Anoxic-Ischemic Brain Injury. A and C, Axial diffusion-weighted imaging sequences show restricted diffusion involving the majority of the neocortex, most prominent posteriorly (arrow in A). B and D, Axial fluid-attenuated inversion recovery images show a corresponding diffuse T2 signal abnormality involving the cortex and a more subtle involvement of the basal ganglia (arrow in D indicates involvement of the head of the caudate nucleus).

Summary

- Estimating a prognosis for comatose patients after cardiac arrest requires a multifaceted approach; no single test result should be used in isolation.
- Absent pupillary light reflexes are the most reliable clinical examination finding that predicts a poor outcome.
- SSEP testing is a reliable ancillary test for predicting poor outcome for comatose patients.
- NSE levels greater than 33 mcg/L may still be compatible with favorable functional outcomes for some patients treated with targeted temperature management.
- After a cardiac arrest, almost all patients should be observed for days before decisions are made about withdrawing life-sustaining therapies; if the patient underwent targeted temperature management, the observation period should be longer because drug metabolism may be delayed.

SUGGESTED READING

Bernard SA, Gray TW, Buist MD, Jones BM, Silvester W, Gutteridge G, et al. Treatment of comatose survivors of out-of-hospital cardiac arrest with induced hypothermia. N Engl J Med. 2002 Feb 21;346(8):557–63.

Bouwes A, Binnekade JM, Zandstra DF, Koelman JH, van Schaik IN, Hijdra A, et al. Somatosensory evoked potentials during mild hypothermia after cardiopulmonary resuscitation. Neurology. 2009 Nov 3;73(18):1457–61.

Geocadin RG, Wijdicks E, Armstrong MJ, Damian M, Mayer SA, Ornato JP, et al. Practice guideline summary: reducing brain injury following cardiopulmonary resuscitation: report of the Guideline Development, Dissemination, and Implementation Subcommittee of the American Academy of Neurology. Neurology. 2017 May 30;88(22):2141–9. Epub 2017 May 10.

Hypothermia After Cardiac Arrest Study Group. Mild therapeutic hypothermia to improve the neurologic outcome after cardiac arrest. N Engl J Med. 2002 Feb 21;346(8):549–56. Erratum in: N Engl J Med 2002 May 30;346(22):1756.

Kamps MJ, Horn J, Oddo M, Fugate JE, Storm C, Cronberg T, et al. Prognostication of neurologic outcome in cardiac arrest patients after mild therapeutic hypothermia: a meta-analysis of the current literature. Intensive Care Med. 2013 Oct;39(10):1671–82. Epub 2013 Jun 26.

Nielsen N, Wetterslev J, Cronberg T, Erlinge D, Gasche Y, Hassager C, et al; TTM Trial Investigators. Targeted temperature management at 33°C versus 36°C after cardiac arrest. N Engl J Med. 2013 Dec 5;369(23):2197–206. Epub 2013 Nov 17.

Scales DC, Golan E, Pinto R, Brooks SC, Chapman M, Dale CM, et al; Strategies for Post-Arrest Resuscitation Care Network. Improving appropriate neurologic prognostication after cardiac arrest: a stepped wedge cluster randomized controlled trial. Am J Respir Crit Care Med. 2016 Nov 1;194(9):1083–91.

Steffen IG, Hasper D, Ploner CJ, Schefold JC, Dietz E, Martens F, et al. Mild therapeutic hypothermia alters neuron specific enolase as an outcome predictor after resuscitation: 97 prospective hypothermia patients compared to 133 historical non-hypothermia patients. Crit Care. 2010;14(2):R69. Epub 2010 Apr 19.

Tsetsou S, Novy J, Pfeiffer C, Oddo M, Rossetti AO. Multimodal outcome prognostication after cardiac arrest and targeted temperature management: analysis at 36°C. Neurocrit Care. 2018 Feb;28(1):104–9.

Westhall E, Rossetti AO, van Rootselaar AF, Wesenberg Kjaer T, Horn J, Ullen S, et al; TTM-trial investigators. Standardized EEG interpretation accurately predicts prognosis after cardiac arrest. Neurology. 2016 Apr 19;86(16):1482–90. Epub 2016 Feb 10.

Wiberg S, Hassager C, Stammet P, Winther-Jensen M, Thomsen JH, Erlinge D, et al. Single versus serial measurements of neuron-specific enolase and prediction of poor neurological outcome in persistently unconscious patients after out-of-hospital cardiac arrest: a TTM-trial substudy. PLoS One. 2017 Jan 18;12(1):e0168894.

Wijman CA, Mlynash M, Caulfield AF, Hsia AW, Eyngorn I, Bammer R, et al. Prognostic value of brain diffusion-weighted imaging after cardiac arrest. Ann Neurol. 2009 Apr;65(4):394–402.

12 Consequences of Acute Metabolic Changes to the Brain

SHERRI A. BRAKSICK, MD; SARA E. HOCKER, MD

Goals

- Identify common metabolic derangements that affect the central nervous system.
- Review specific neurologic presentations of metabolic abnormalities.
- Review management strategies for systemic metabolic abnormalities.

Introduction

Systemic illness can have an abrupt and sometimes profound effect on the central nervous system (CNS). Organ failure and acute electrolyte disturbances may cause neurologic manifestations that are often accompanied by a decline in consciousness. Secondary injury is characterized by demyelination, cerebral edema, and anoxic-ischemic brain injury.

Hyponatremia

Acute hyponatremia (serum sodium <135 mmol/L) may result from many causes, including consequences of CNS disease. Shifts in solute and the accompanying osmotic movement can precipitate neurologic disorders such as confusion, seizure, and coma; death may be due to sudden-onset cerebral edema.

Current recommendations for the initial correction of severe hyponatremia are summarized in Box 12.1.

With overcorrection of severe hyponatremia, administer additional 5% dextrose in water (D5W) in individual doses of 6 mL/kg body weight given over 1 to 2 hours. Desmopressin (2-4 mcg daily intravenously in divided doses) can be administered. Correction should proceed with special caution in patients with alcoholic liver disease or malnutrition who are at high risk for demyelination syndromes. As the hyponatremia is being corrected, the underlying cause should be sought.

Correction of the sodium derangement is imperative for reversing acute symptoms; however, caution is required to prevent development of *osmotic demyelination syndrome* (Figure 12.1), which may result from excessively rapid correction of hyponatremia. First described in 1959 as a disorder in the pons of alcoholic patients, osmotic demyelination syndrome has since been recognized as affecting other structures within the CNS as well. Some patients recover well, but others have devastating neurologic injury.

In patients with hyperproteinemia or hyperlipidemia, laboratory testing may show a falsely low sodium level (pseudohyponatremia), which does not require specific treatment but must be recognized to prevent iatrogenic complications from erroneous therapy.

Acute Osmolar Shifts

Changes in the osmolar gradient between the extracellular and intracellular compartments can result in large fluid shifts and, in severe circumstances, cerebral edema. This has occurred in patients with diabetic ketoacidosis and hypernatremia, particularly during times of rapid solute correction. This effect may also occur in patients with nonketotic hyperosmolar states, but large studies of this condition are lacking. Other associated symptoms may be nonspecific and predominantly include altered states of consciousness.

A proposed theory to explain the mechanism for these complications involves *idiogenic osmoles*, which are

Box 12.1 • Correction of Severe, Acute, Symptomatic Hyponatremia

If patient has symptomatic, severe hyponatremia:

Step 1. Administer 150 mL hypertonic saline (3% NaCl) IV over 20 min.

Step 2. Check serum Na level 20 min after infusion.

Step 3. Repeat step 1 while waiting for test results.

Step 4. Repeat steps 1-3 twice or until serum Na level has increased by 5 mmol/L.

A. If patient has symptomatic improvement after steps 1-4:

Step A5. Stop administering hypertonic saline.

Step A6. Evaluate patient for cause of hyponatremia, and initiate cause-specific treatment.

Step A7. Do not increase serum Na level >10 mmol/L in first 24 h.

Step A8. Check serum Na level every 6-12 h until it is stable.

B. If patient has no symptomatic improvement after steps 1-4:

Step B5. Continue administering hypertonic saline (goal: increase serum Na level 1 mmol/L/h).

Step B6. Stop administering hypertonic saline if any of the following occurs:

a. Symptoms improve

b. Serum Na level increases by a total of 10 mmol/L

c. Serum Na level reaches 130 mmol/L

Step B7. Evaluate patient for cause of hyponatremia, and initiate cause-specific treatment.

Step B8. Check serum Na level every 4 h while administering hypertonic saline.

Abbreviations: IV, intravenous; Na, sodium; NaCl, sodium chloride.

Modified from Spasovski G, Vanholder R, Allolio B, Annane D, Ball S, Bichet D, et al. Clinical practice guideline on diagnosis and treatment of hyponatraemia. Intensive Care Med. 2014 Mar;40(3):320-31; used with permission.

osmotically active molecules that neurons produce when homeostasis needs to be maintained under conditions of increased extracellular osmolality. These unmeasurable molecules maintain cell volume, however, by rapidly decreasing the concentration of extracellular solutes; the osmolar shift may precipitate increased intracellular movement of fluid and subsequent edema (Figure 12.2). While this theory has not been definitively proved to be the sole explanation for this phenomenon, this understanding of hyperosmolality underlies the principle of carefully controlled correction of hyperglycemic and hypernatremic states.

Sepsis

Sepsis results in a systemic proinflammatory state as the body attempts to ward off the cause of infection. A massive release of cytokines and inflammatory mediators acts directly on the brain and affects the integrity of the blood-brain barrier. Coupled with impaired oxygen delivery to all tissues in patients with evidence of a hypoperfusion state (shock), this can result in an acute encephalopathy known as *sepsis-associated encephalopathy*.

Patients with sepsis-associated encephalopathy typically present with nonspecific symptoms, including various degrees of alteration in the level and content of consciousness. Sepsis-associated encephalopathy is an independent predictor of death among patients with sepsis. Additionally, survivors have an increased risk of later cognitive impairment.

Evaluation of the acute alterations in patients with sepsis should include evaluation for structural injury with computed tomography or magnetic resonance imaging, laboratory evaluation for metabolic abnormalities, and consideration of lumbar puncture to evaluate for CNS infection. Management centers on controlling the underlying source of infection, and patients may require both pharmacologic and nonpharmacologic interventions for associated delirium.

Acute Liver Failure

Patients who have acute hepatic dysfunction have a high risk for neurologic complications. In both acute and chronic liver disease, encephalopathy is common, and patients have various neurologic signs and symptoms (Table 12.1). The pathophysiology of hepatic encephalopathy is multifactorial and poorly understood. Prevailing theories include disruption of the blood-brain barrier and alteration of the γ-aminobutyric acid and benzodiazepine pathways.

A common treatment goal is to maintain normal ammonia levels because ammonia degradation is impaired in the diseased liver, and any degree of portocaval shunting allows for direct movement of blood from the portal circulation to the systemic circulation, effectively bypassing any possibility of ammonia breakdown. The compensatory mechanism in the brain is an increase in the size and number of Alzheimer type II cells (Figure 12.3), which are astrocytes capable of degrading ammonia. When acute and severe, this disease process may culminate in life-threatening cerebral edema. (See Chapter 41, "Acute Liver Failure," for fulminant forms and management.)

Acute Kidney Injury

Injury to the kidney causes a complex cascade of events that may precipitate neurologic worsening (Box 12.2). The most prominent acute neurologic change in acute kidney

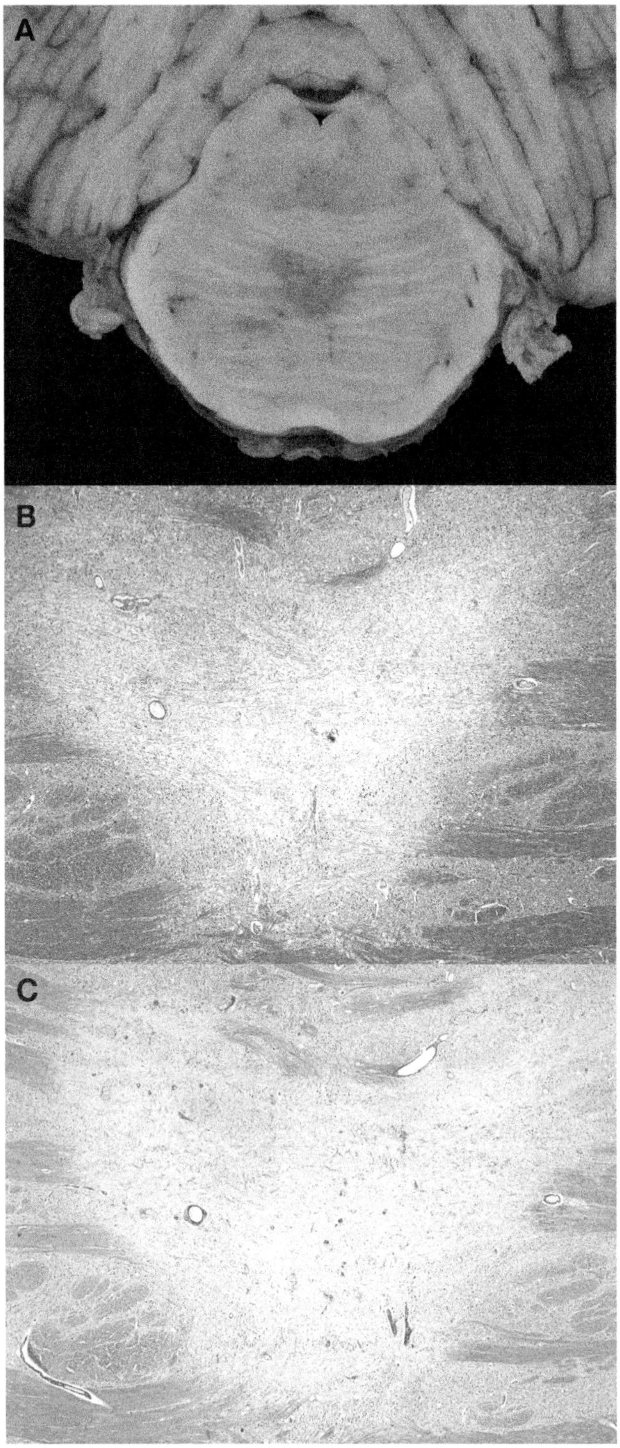

Figure 12.1. *Osmotic Demyelination Syndrome. A, Gross specimen shows a midline, triangular lesion in the basis pontis. B and C, Corresponding microscopic images show a well-circumscribed area of myelin loss with relative preservation of axons. (Courtesy of A. Raghunathan, MD, Mayo Clinic, Rochester, Minnesota; used with permission.)*

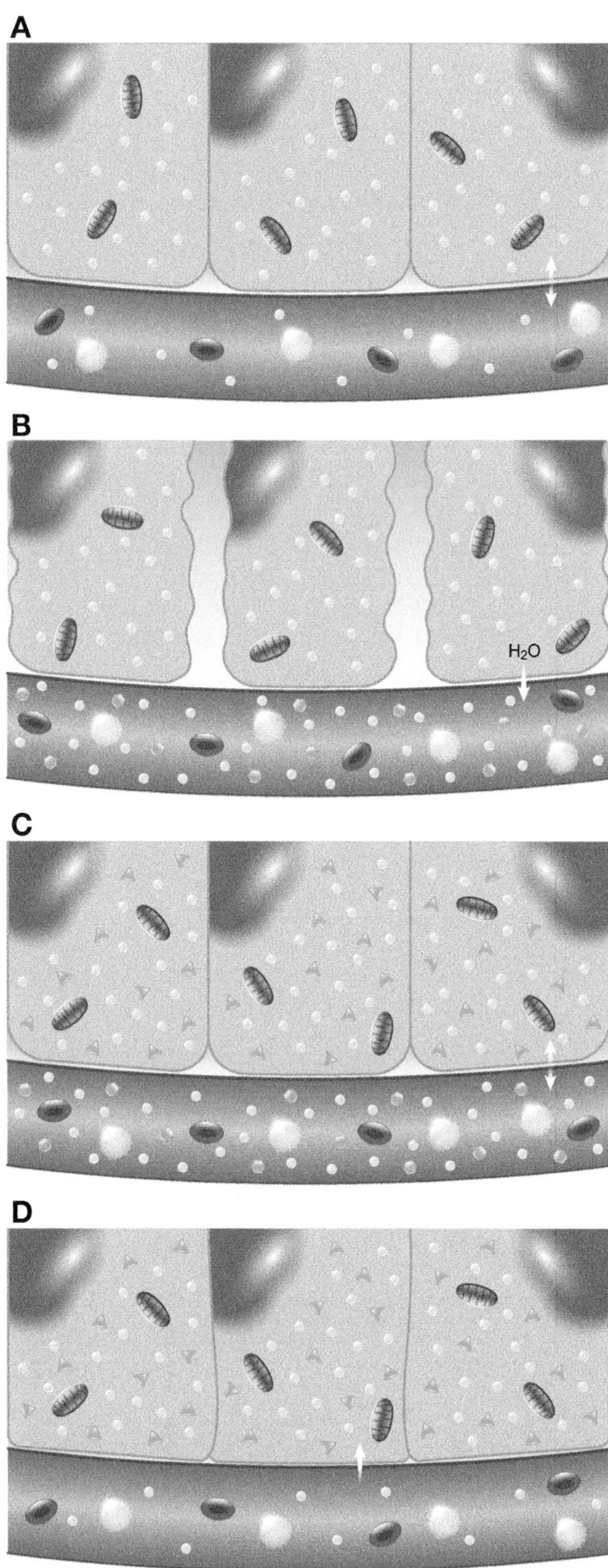

Figure 12.2. *Idiogenic Osmoles and Fluid Shifts With a Rapid Decrease in Intravascular Osmolarity. A, Normal fluid balance between cells and the extracellular environment. B, When serum osmolality increases, water (H_2O) moves out of the cells. C, Neurons produce idiogenic osmoles (green triangles). D, Rapid correction of the increased serum osmolality may lead to cellular edema.*

Table 12.1 • West Haven and FOUR Score Criteria for Grading Hepatic Encephalopathy[a]

West Haven		FOUR Score				
Grade	Features	Score	Eye Response	Motor Response	Brainstem Reflex	Respiration
0	No abnormalities detected	4	Eyelids open or manually opened; tracking or blinking on command	Thumbs up, fist, or peace sign on command	Pupillary and corneal reflexes present	Not intubated; regular breathing
1	Unawareness (mild), euphoria or anxiety, shortened attention span, impairment of calculation ability, lethargy or apathy	3	Eyelids open; not tracking	Localized response to pain	One pupil wide and fixed	Not intubated; Cheyne-Stokes breathing
2	Disorientation to time, obvious personality change, inappropriate behavior	2	Eyelids closed but open to loud voice	Flexion response to pain	Pupillary or corneal responses absent	Not intubated; irregular breathing
3	Somnolence to stupor, responsiveness to stimuli, confusion, gross disorientation, bizarre behavior	1	Eyelids closed but open to pain	Extension response to pain	Pupillary and corneal responses absent	Intubated; breathing faster than ventilator rate
4	Coma	0	Eyelids remain closed to pain	No response to pain, or generalized myoclonus status	Pupillary, corneal, and cough reflexes absent	Breathing at ventilator rate or is apneic

Abbreviation: FOUR, Full Outline of Unresponsiveness.

[a] Patients with minimal hepatic encephalopathy (West Haven grade 1) would be classified as having covert hepatic encephalopathy. Patients with West Haven grade 2 or higher encephalopathy would be classified as having overt hepatic encephalopathy. The FOUR score clinical grading scale takes into account 4 components of neurologic function. Scores range from 0 to 16, with lower scores indicating a lower level of consciousness.

Modified from Wijdicks EF. Hepatic encephalopathy. N Engl J Med. 2016 Oct 27;375(17):1660-70; used with permission.

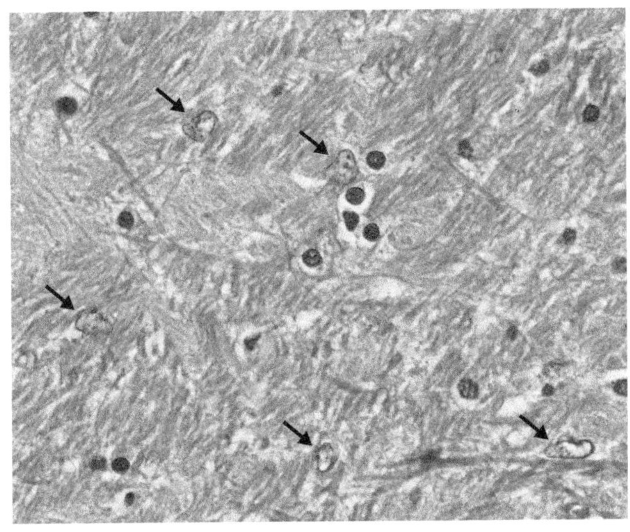

Figure 12.3. Alzheimer Type II Cells in Hepatic Encephalopathy. Characteristic of hepatic encephalopathy, Alzheimer type II astrocytes (arrows) have large nuclei with marginated chromatin and scant cytoplasm. (Courtesy of R. A. Vaubel, MD, PhD, Mayo Clinic, Rochester, Minnesota; used with permission.)

Box 12.2 • Neurologic Manifestations of Acute Kidney Injury

- Asterixis and myoclonus
- Encephalopathy to stupor
  - Increasing uremia
  - Posterior reversible encephalopathy syndrome
  - Dialysis dysequilibrium syndrome
  - Seizures (from fluid shifts during dialysis or electrolyte derangements)

injury is encephalopathy, which is often accompanied by multifocal myoclonus and asterixis. This encephalopathy is typically attributed to the accumulation of urea, other toxins, and medications that would typically be excreted by the kidney. Symptoms may include only mild confusion but can progress to coma or seizures in acute-onset, severe cases.

Many patients with acute kidney injury may also have hypertension or labile blood pressure, predisposing them to the development of *posterior reversible encephalopathy syndrome*. Common symptoms include headache, encephalopathy, cortical visual impairment, and seizures. Management includes short-term antiepileptic therapy and controlled lowering of blood pressure or discontinuation of offending agents (typically, cytotoxic medications).

In patients who require dialysis, an additional phenomenon, *dialysis dysequilibrium syndrome*, may occur. This typically affects younger patients (particularly children) and most often occurs after the initial dialysis session. It is thought to be precipitated by fluid shifts and subsequent development of cerebral edema. Symptoms can be mild, with headache and dizziness, or life-threatening, with onset of seizures or coma.

Summary

- The CNS is at risk for adverse effects relating to multiple metabolic derangements, which are more likely to occur during rapid metabolic changes than during those that develop over time.
- Hyponatremia must be carefully corrected to avoid osmotic demyelination syndrome.
- Osmolar shifts may cause accompanying large fluid shifts and provoke neurologic symptoms at onset or during correction of a hyperosmolar state.
- Patients with sepsis-associated encephalopathy are at increased risk for long-term cognitive sequelae.
- Posterior reversible encephalopathy syndrome may be associated with acute kidney injury, hypertension, labile blood pressure, or antirejection medications.

SUGGESTED READING

Adams RD, Victor M, Mancall EL. Central pontine myelinolysis: a hitherto undescribed disease occurring in alcoholic and malnourished patients. AMA Arch Neurol Psychiatry. 1959 Feb;81(2):154–72.

Angus DC, van der Poll T. Severe sepsis and septic shock. N Engl J Med. 2013 Nov 21;369(21):2063.

Arieff AI. Cerebral edema complicating nonketotic hyperosmolar coma. Miner Electrolyte Metab. 1986;12(5-6):383–9.

Arieff AI. Dialysis disequilibrium syndrome: current concepts on pathogenesis and prevention. Kidney Int. 1994 Mar;45(3):629–35.

Arieff AI, Guisado R. Effects on the central nervous system of hypernatremic and hyponatremic states. Kidney Int. 1976 Jul;10(1):104–16.

Arieff AI, Kleeman CR. Studies on mechanisms of cerebral edema in diabetic comas: effects of hyperglycemia and rapid lowering of plasma glucose in normal rabbits. J Clin Invest. 1973 Mar;52(3):571–83.

Arora SK. Hypernatremic disorders in the intensive care unit. J Intensive Care Med. 2013 Jan-Feb;28(1):37–45.

Bismuth M, Funakoshi N, Cadranel JF, Blanc P. Hepatic encephalopathy: from pathophysiology to therapeutic management. Eur J Gastroenterol Hepatol. 2011 Jan;23(1):8–22.

Burn DJ, Bates D. Neurology and the kidney. J Neurol Neurosurg Psychiatry. 1998 Dec;65(6):810–21.

Eidelman LA, Putterman D, Putterman C, Sprung CL. The spectrum of septic encephalopathy: definitions, etiologies, and mortalities. JAMA. 1996 Feb 14;275(6):470–3.

Fugate JE, Rabinstein AA. Posterior reversible encephalopathy syndrome: clinical and radiological manifestations, pathophysiology, and outstanding questions. Lancet Neurol. 2015 Sep;14(9):914–25.

Guerra C, Linde-Zwirble WT, Wunsch H. Risk factors for dementia after critical illness in elderly Medicare beneficiaries. Crit Care. 2012 Dec 17;16(6):R233.

Iwashyna TJ, Ely EW, Smith DM, Langa KM. Long-term cognitive impairment and functional disability among survivors of severe sepsis. JAMA. 2010 Oct 27;304(16):1787–94.

Kang SK, Kim W, Oh MS. Pathogenesis and treatment of hypernatremia. Nephron. 2002;92(Suppl 1):14–7.

Lawn N, Wijdicks EF, Burritt MF. Intravenous immune globulin and pseudohyponatremia. N Engl J Med. 1998 Aug 27;339(9):632.

Norenberg MD. The role of astrocytes in hepatic encephalopathy. Neurochem Pathol. 1987 Feb-Apr;6(1-2):13–33.

Singh TD, Fugate JE, Rabinstein AA. Central pontine and extrapontine myelinolysis: a systematic review. Eur J Neurol. 2014 Dec;21(12):1443–50.

Sonneville R, Verdonk F, Rauturier C, Klein IF, Wolff M, Annane D, et al. Understanding brain dysfunction in sepsis. Ann Intensive Care. 2013 May 29;3(1):15.

Spasovski G, Vanholder R, Allolio B, Annane D, Ball S, Bichet D, et al. Clinical practice guideline on diagnosis and treatment of hyponatraemia. Intensive Care Med. 2014 Mar;40(3):320–31.

Sprung CL, Peduzzi PN, Shatney CH, Schein RM, Wilson MF, Sheagren JN, et al. Impact of encephalopathy on mortality in the sepsis syndrome: the Veterans Administration Systemic Sepsis Cooperative Study Group. Crit Care Med. 1990 Aug;18(8):801–6.

Weissenborn K. Hepatic encephalopathy: definition, clinical grading and diagnostic principles. Drugs. 2019 Feb;79(Suppl 1):5–9.

Widmann CN, Heneka MT. Long-term cerebral consequences of sepsis. Lancet Neurol. 2014 Jun;13(6):630–6.

Young E, Bradley RF. Cerebral edema with irreversible coma in severe diabetic ketoacidosis. N Engl J Med. 1967 Mar 23;276(12):665–9.

13 Consequences of Acute Hypertension to the Brain

KATHERINE M. OSHEL, MD; HANI M. WADEI, MD

Goals

- Describe the role of cerebral autoregulation in maintaining cerebral blood flow in hypertension.
- Explain the effects of an acute increase in blood pressure on the brain.
- Discuss the use of antihypertensives after acute brain injury.

Introduction

Acute hypertension is a common clinical problem that accounts for almost 25% of emergency department visits in the United States. It can occur in patients who have preexisting hypertension or in patients who were previously normotensive. A large group of patients have preexisting but unidentified hypertension, but while patients with chronically elevated blood pressure (eg, systolic blood pressure of 180-200 mm Hg) may remain largely asymptomatic, a sudden increase in blood pressure has grave consequences for the heart, kidney, and brain.

One important consequence of acute hypertension to the brain is the development of posterior reversible encephalopathy syndrome (PRES), which results from changes in cerebral autoregulation and endothelial dysfunction. Other manifestations of acute hypertension to the brain, including ischemic stroke, intracranial hemorrhage, and papilledema with malignant hypertension, are discussed elsewhere in this book.

Use of intravenous antihypertensives—as a bolus or infusion—is ubiquitous for neurocritical care patients. Important characteristics of most antihypertensive drugs used to treat acute hypertension are rapid onset of action, short duration of action, and low incidence of adverse effects. However, other factors must also be considered. Costs, for example, may be prohibitive for the use of some medications, such as clevidipine, a third-generation calcium channel blocker. Caution should be exercised when sodium nitroprusside is administered, especially to patients with hepatic and renal failure.

This chapter provides an overview of cerebral autoregulation and the mechanisms of action and side effect profiles of different antihypertensive medications used to treat acute hypertension.

Cerebral Autoregulation

Cerebral autoregulation is the intrinsic capacity of the cerebral arterioles to constrict and dilate in response to changes in cerebral perfusion pressure and maintain constant cerebral blood flow (CBF). Cerebral autoregulation involves multiple mechanisms, including neurogenic stimulation, accumulation of metabolic factors (eg, adenosine and carbon dioxide), and the vasomotor activity of vascular smooth muscles either in response to variability in intravascular pressure or through the release of vasoconstrictor (eg, endothelin-1) or vasodilator (eg, nitrous oxide) substances.

Cerebral autoregulation effectively maintains constant CBF across a wide range of mean arterial pressure (MAP) (generally accepted to be 50-150 mm Hg in normotensive patients). In chronically hypertensive patients, constant CBF is maintained at higher levels of MAP than in normotensive patients, and the MAP range at which cerebral autoregulation operates is shifted higher (Figure 13.1). In hypertensive patients, however, the MAP range at which cerebral autoregulation is effective is not well defined and varies among patients. Irrespective of the operative MAP range, when MAP decreases below the cerebral autoregulation capacity, cerebral oxygen extraction from hemoglobin

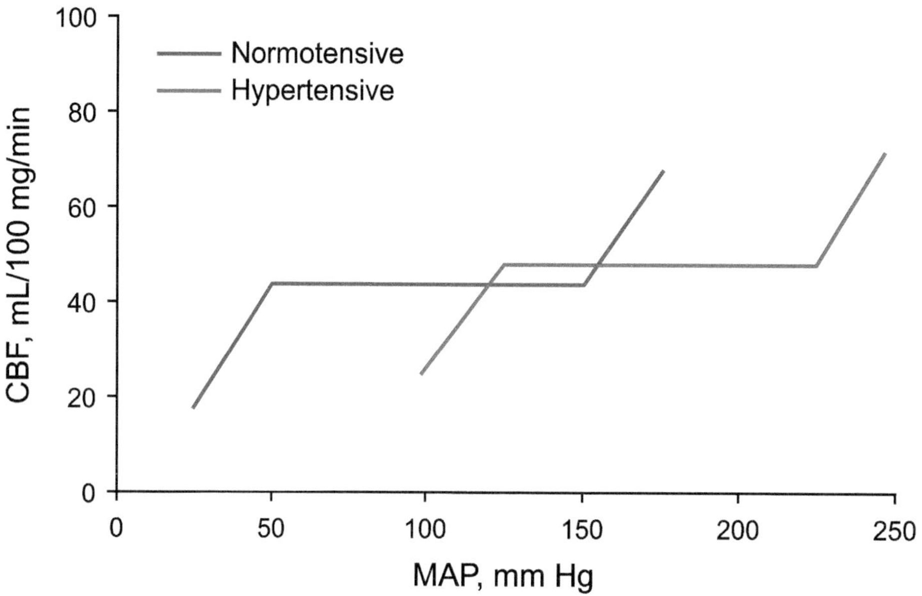

Figure 13.1. Cerebral Autoregulation. Constant cerebral blood flow (CBF) is maintained across a wide range of mean arterial pressure (MAP) whether the person is normotensive or hypertensive.

increases first before the brain becomes ischemic. When MAP increases beyond the capacity for cerebral autoregulation, CBF increases in parallel with the increase in MAP and breakthrough cerebral edema and PRES develop.

Treatment

General Measures and Target Blood Pressure Goal

Patients with neurologic complications related to an acute increase in hypertension should be managed in the intensive care unit and have continuous blood pressure monitoring. The main therapeutic goals are to decrease the blood pressure and correct the underlying precipitating cause of the acute increase in blood pressure. Early aggressive treatment increases the chances of a satisfactory outcome. The target MAP goal varies among patients and should be individualized according to age, effects of acute hypertension on the brain (eg, ischemic stroke or PRES), and underlying comorbidities. Blood pressure must be decreased promptly in patients with PRES or malignant hypertension. In patients with ischemic stroke, however, the systolic blood pressure may remain at 140 to 160 mm Hg and the diastolic blood pressure at 90 to 100 mm Hg for 24 to 48 hours after the initial event. If patients have PRES, the goal is to decrease the MAP by 20% to 25% within a few hours after initial presentation. This target is crucial because cerebral blood flow autoregulatory limits are altered in patients with long-standing hypertension (as described above), so that decreasing MAP by more than 25% of the baseline value may result in cerebral ischemia.

Blood pressure should be decreased cautiously, especially in elderly patients because if the systolic blood pressure is decreased to 110 to 140 mm Hg, the risk of acute renal failure may increase by nearly 2%. To avoid rebound hypertension, when the target blood pressure goal has been reached, oral antihypertensive medications should be administered before stopping the use of parenteral antihypertensive agents. Also, abrupt discontinuation of β-blockers and α_2-blockers should be discouraged to avoid rebound tachycardia and hypertension, respectively.

Patients with concomitant seizures should receive parenteral antiepileptic agents. Benzodiazepines, phenobarbital, and phenytoin are preferred.

Box 13.1 • *ABCDs* of Antihypertensive Drugs

A Angiotensin-converting enzyme inhibitors (benazepril, captopril, enalapril, lisinopril)

Angiotensin II receptor blockers (candesartan, losartan, valsartan)

B β-Blockers (atenolol, labetalol, metoprolol, propranolol)

C Calcium channel blockers (amlodipine, diltiazem, nifedipine, verapamil)

Central agents (clonidine, methyldopa)

D Diuretics (furosemide, hydrochlorothiazide)

Dilators (ie, vasodilators) (hydralazine, sodium nitroprusside)

Table 13.1 • Parenteral Antihypertensive Medications Used in Acute Hypertension

Drug	Route of Administration	Dosage	Onset of Action	Duration of Action	Adverse Effects and Comments
Direct-acting and dopaminergic agents					
Sodium nitroprusside	IV infusion	0.3-10 mcg/kg/min	Immediate	2-3 min	Hypotension, nausea, vomiting Risk of thiocyanate and cyanide toxicity Use lower dose in renal and hepatic insufficiency May increase intracranial pressure Shield from light Preferred agent
Nitroglycerin	IV infusion	5-100 mcg/min	1-2 min	3-5 min	Headache, nausea, vomiting No dose adjustment in hepatic and renal impairments Recommended with concomitant acute coronary event
Hydralazine	IV bolus	10-20 mg q 20 min	10-20 min	3-6 h	Hypotension, reflex tachycardia, headache, nausea, vomiting Approved for use in preeclampsia and eclampsia
Fenoldopam	IV infusion	0.03-0.1 mcg/kg/min, up to 1.6 mcg/kg/min	1-10 min	1-4 h	Angina, heart failure, hypotension, tachycardia, headache, nausea, vomiting May increase intraocular pressure; use caution with glaucoma
Centrally acting agents					
Methyldopa	IV bolus	250-500 mg q 6 h Maximum dose, 1,000 mg q 6 h	30-60 min	10-16 h	Hypotension, hepatotoxicity, and bone marrow suppression Approved for use in preeclampsia and eclampsia
α_1-Adrenergic blockers					
Phentolamine	IV bolus	5-10 mg q 5-15 min	1-2 min	3-10 min	Hypotension, tachycardia, headache, angina Recommended for perioperative management of pheochromocytoma
β-Adrenergic blockers					
Labetalol	IV bolus	20-80 mg q 5-10 min, up to 300 mg daily	5-10 min	3-6 h	Hypotension, heart block, heart failure, bronchospasm, nausea, vomiting
	IV infusion	0.5-2.0 mg/min			
Esmolol	IV bolus	500 mcg/kg/min for first 1 min	1-5 min	10 min	Hypotension, heart block, heart failure, bronchospasm
	IV infusion	50-300 mcg/kg/min			
Calcium channel blockers					
Nicardipine	IV infusion	5 mg/h, increased by 1.0-2.5 mg/h q 15 min, up to 15 mg/h	1-5 min	3-6 h	Hypotension, headache, tachycardia, nausea, vomiting
Clevidipine	IV infusion	1-2 mg/h up to 21 mg/h	1 min	<15 min	Nausea, dyslipidemia, tachycardia
ACE inhibitors					
Enalaprilat	IV bolus	0.625-2.5 mg q 6 h	5-15 min	1-6 h	Hypotension

Abbreviations: ACE, angiotensin-converting enzyme; IV, intravenous; q, every.

After initial stabilization, the cause of the acute increase in blood pressure should be sought and managed appropriately to avoid recurrent episodes. Causes include medication, lack of adherence to drug therapy, acute and chronic kidney diseases, and other secondary causes of hypertension (eg, pheochromocytoma).

Choice of Antihypertensive Agent

The *ABCD*s of antihypertensive drugs are summarized in Box 13.1. When 2 antihypertensives are used in combination, they should be from different classes (eg, labetalol and sodium nitroprusside) instead of having a similar mode of action (eg, hydralazine and sodium nitroprusside). For acute hypertension in the critical care setting, parenteral antihypertensive agents (eg, nicardipine and labetalol) are preferable because they have a rapid onset of action and can be easily titrated. Labetalol (a nonselective β-blocker and postsynaptic α_1-blocker) is a good initial choice with a low likelihood of causing hypotension; systemic vascular resistance decreases, but cardiac output does not change. Treatment with sodium nitroprusside is more complex because it is a potent vasodilator. An angiotensin-converting enzyme inhibitor, such as enalaprilat, may be useful, and hypotension is uncommon, but it is contraindicated in pregnancy and in patients with renal artery stenosis. Another useful drug is fenoldopam, a dopamine D1-like receptor agonist. Parenteral antihypertensive medications used in acute hypertension are summarized in Table 13.1.

Acute Hypertension in Pregnancy

In patients with eclampsia, magnesium sulphate and termination of nearly full-term pregnancy may be indicated. All antihypertensive agents cross the placenta to some degree, but owing to a lack of data, the efficacy of different classes of antihypertensive medications in pregnancy has not been clearly defined. Several antihypertensive agents cannot be recommended for use, and some are contraindicated in pregnancy: angiotensin-converting enzyme inhibitors, angiotensin II receptor blockers, and mineralocorticoid blockers. β-Blockers are considered acceptable, but they increase the risk of growth retardation, congenital anomalies, and maternal hepatic toxicity.

Summary

- Cerebral autoregulation maintains constant CBF across a wide range of MAP.
- Acute hypertension leads to failure of cerebral autoregulation and precipitates PRES, which is a neurologic emergency characterized by headache, seizures, mental status changes, and cerebral edema.
- If a patient has PRES, a reasonable goal is to decrease the MAP by 20% to 25% of the MAP at initial presentation.

SUGGESTED READING

Dagal A, Lam AM. Cerebral blood flow and the injured brain: how should we monitor and manipulate it? Curr Opin Anaesthesiol. 2011 Apr;24(2):131–7.

James PA, Oparil S, Carter BL, Cushman WC, Dennison-Himmelfarb C, Handler J, et al. 2014 evidence-based guideline for the management of high blood pressure in adults: report from the panel members appointed to the Eighth Joint National Committee (JNC 8). JAMA. 2014 Feb 5;311(5):507–20. Erratum in: JAMA. 2014 May 7;311(17):1809.

Magee LA, von Dadelszen P. State-of-the-art diagnosis and treatment of hypertension in pregnancy. Mayo Clin Proc. 2018 Nov;93(11):1664–77.

Olson-Chen C, Seligman NS. Hypertensive emergencies in pregnancy. Crit Care Clin. 2016 Jan;32(1):29–41. Epub 2015 Oct 6.

Papadopoulos DP, Sanidas EA, Viniou NA, Gennimata V, Chantziara V, Barbetseas I, et al. Cardiovascular hypertensive emergencies. Curr Hypertens Rep. 2015 Feb;17(2):5.

Pollack CV, Varon J, Garrison NA, Ebrahimi R, Dunbar L, Peacock WF 4th. Clevidipine, an intravenous dihydropyridine calcium channel blocker, is safe and effective for the treatment of patients with acute severe hypertension. Ann Emerg Med. 2009 Mar;53(3):329–38. Epub 2008 Jun 5.

Qureshi AI, Palesch YY, Barsan WG, Hanley DF, Hsu CY, Martin RL, et al; ATACH-2 Trial Investigators and the Neurological Emergency Treatment Trials Network. Intensive blood-pressure lowering in patients with acute cerebral hemorrhage. N Engl J Med. 2016 Sep 15;375(11):1033–43. Epub 2016 Jun 8.

14 Coma and Other Altered States of Consciousness

EELCO F. M. WIJDICKS, MD, PhD

Goals

- Explain the anatomical basis of unconsciousness and the structural causes.
- Discuss evaluation of the comatose patient.
- Discuss the reversible and irreversible causes of coma.

Introduction

The components of consciousness are classically separated into 2 major groups: level of alertness (being awake) and content of thinking (being aware). Major acute neurologic disorders affect both components. These 2 components are interrelated but sometimes dissociated. For example, a patient can be awake but not aware (eg, a patient in a vegetative state or eye-open coma) or not awake and not aware (eg, a comatose patient) (Figure 14.1). Coma is often due to an extensive structural (anoxic-ischemic) injury or to diffuse physiologic dysfunction (eg, intoxication, seizures, or acute metabolic derangement).

Anatomy of Unconsciousness

Consciousness requires functioning neurotransmitters, and the main ones are norepinephrine, dopamine, serotonin, acetylcholine, histamine, and orexin (hypocretin). Neurotransmitters are involved in pathways projecting diffusely to the cortex, but some have more specific targets. Norepinephrine and serotonin are active during waking states. The substantia nigra, ventral tegmental area, and retrorubral field all contain dopaminergic neurons. Dopamine is released during aroused waking situations, and depletion of catecholamines results in hypersomnia or slowed responsiveness.

The ascending reticular activating system (ARAS) formation areas are largely active through the neurotransmitter glutamate. The reticular formation contains neurons that use γ-aminobutyric acid, which is inhibitory. When the reticular formation is stimulated electrically, it initiates cortical activation. The ARAS also includes cholinergic neurons of the mesopontine tegmentum projecting to the thalamus and monoaminergic groups that project to the thalamus, hypothalamus, basal forebrain, and cortex.

Coma results from damage to structures such as the ARAS, thalamus, anterior cingulate cortex, and association cortex (precuneus and cuneus) (Figure 14.2). Usually transient, coma may evolve into long-term disorders of consciousness, such as persistent vegetative state, in which patients show no signs of awareness of their surroundings but have periods of wakefulness with preserved sleep-wake cycles. Coma may improve to minimally conscious state (MCS), in which patients have an inconsistent, limited awareness of self or the environment. Patients in MCS may visually fixate or track, follow simple commands, or demonstrate limited purposeful behavior, yet they cannot communicate reliably and consistently. These diagnoses require extended periods of observation and serial neurologic examinations performed with great caution. Akinetic mutism, a disorder of consciousness that is caused by lesions of the anterior cingulate gyri, shares clinical features with MCS. These patients are abulic (emotionless and neither speaking nor initiating spontaneous movements), but they maintain eye-tracking movements, facial grimacing, and blink to threat.

Other abnormalities of alertness are often labeled as encephalopathy, but the terms *metabolic encephalopathy, toxic encephalopathy*, and *delirium* are poor descriptors of acute global brain dysfunction. Often, there is no good explanation besides the more common causes, such as alcohol withdrawal, drug intoxication, drug interactions,

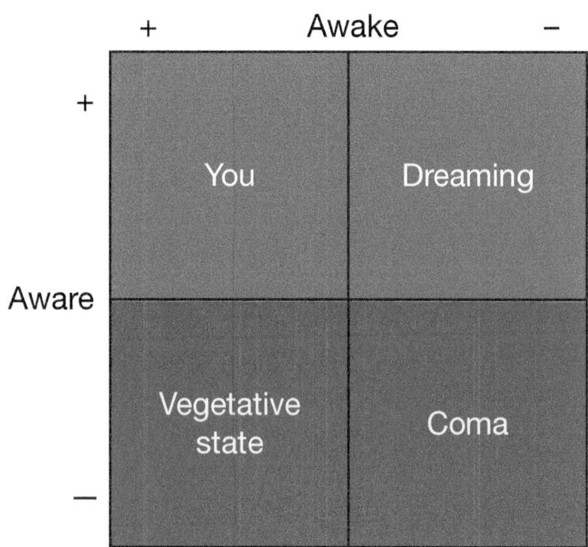

Figure 14.1. States of Consciousness Defined by Being Awake or Aware.

sepsis, or hypertensive urgency. In many patients, delirium is superimposed on a previously undiagnosed dementing illness. Delirium is common in polypharmacy, particularly when benzodiazepines and opioids are included.

Clinical Examination of the Comatose Patient

General Examination

Blood pressure, heart rate, temperature, respiratory rate, and respiratory depth suggest certain intoxications (*toxidromes*) (Table 14.1). Fever may indicate infection but also be present in neuroleptic malignant syndrome, serotonin syndrome, or drug ingestion (particularly with sympathomimetic drugs such as cocaine, amphetamines, and phencyclidine). Hypothermia may result from environmental exposure, severe hypothyroidism (myxedema coma), Wernicke encephalopathy, or structural lesions of the hypothalamus. Severe hypertension (systolic blood pressure >200 mm Hg) may lead to coma (posterior reversible encephalopathy syndrome) rather than being a result of coma.

Initial Neurologic Examination

The initial step in the assessment is to determine the depth of coma. If the patient does not respond to voice, the examiner should exclude locked-in syndrome by asking the patient to look up and blink. If the patient remains unresponsive to voice or to shaking, the examiner should apply noxious stimuli (sternal rub, pressure on the supraorbital nerve, or deep pressure on the condyles of the mandible at the temporomandibular joint).

Two commonly used coma scales are the Glasgow Coma Scale (GCS) and the Full Outline of Unresponsiveness (FOUR) score (Box 14.1). The GCS is well established and is the scale used most often for trauma patients and by emergency medical services personnel. It incorporates 3 unequally weighted responses: motor, verbal, and eye opening, with a total score ranging from 3 to 15. The FOUR score assesses 4 responses: eyelid opening and tracking, motor response, brainstem reflexes, and respiratory drive and regularity (Figure 14.3).

Comprehensive Neurologic Examination

A funduscopic examination should be routinely performed. Patients with aneurysmal subarachnoid hemorrhage or traumatic brain injury sometimes have retinal hemorrhages. Papilledema (blurring of the optic disc margins) signifies increased intracranial pressure but may not be present if the onset was hyperacute.

Pupillary size, shape, and reactivity are essential components of the neurologic examination because a change in pupillary symmetry or reactivity may herald a new or worsening intracranial disease. The autonomic system controls the pupillary light reflex by balancing sympathetic and parasympathetic inputs. The pupils should be examined with a bright light to assess the direct and consensual reflexes. Pupillary pathways are relatively resistant to metabolic influences and thus are rarely obscured, unlike other components of the examination that are more easily confounded. The size of the pupils also has localizing value. For example, hole pupils (approximately 2 mm in diameter) are characteristic of pontine lesions, midsized pupils (4-6 mm) localize to the mesencephalon with loss of both parasympathetic and sympathetic inputs, and fully dilated pupils suggest involvement of the third cranial nerve nucleus in the midbrain or peripheral nerve fibers. The spectrum of pupillary abnormalities is shown in Figure 14.4.

Forced gaze deviation can indicate destructive injury (ischemic or hemorrhagic stroke) involving the frontal eye fields ipsilaterally or an irritative focus (eg, seizure) involving the contralateral frontal lobe. In the appropriate clinical context, subtle nystagmus may be the only clue to ongoing nonconvulsive status epilepticus. Most eye movements do not localize specifically (eg, *roving eye movements*), but a rapid downward movement of the eyes with slow return to baseline (*ocular bobbing*) is characteristic of an acute pontine lesion.

Corneal reflexes are tested either by applying saline drops or by passing a cotton swab across the cornea. Coughing after deep tracheal suctioning and gag responses also should be noted.

Adventitious movements (as in myoclonus or asterixis) should be noted. In patients with an impaired level of

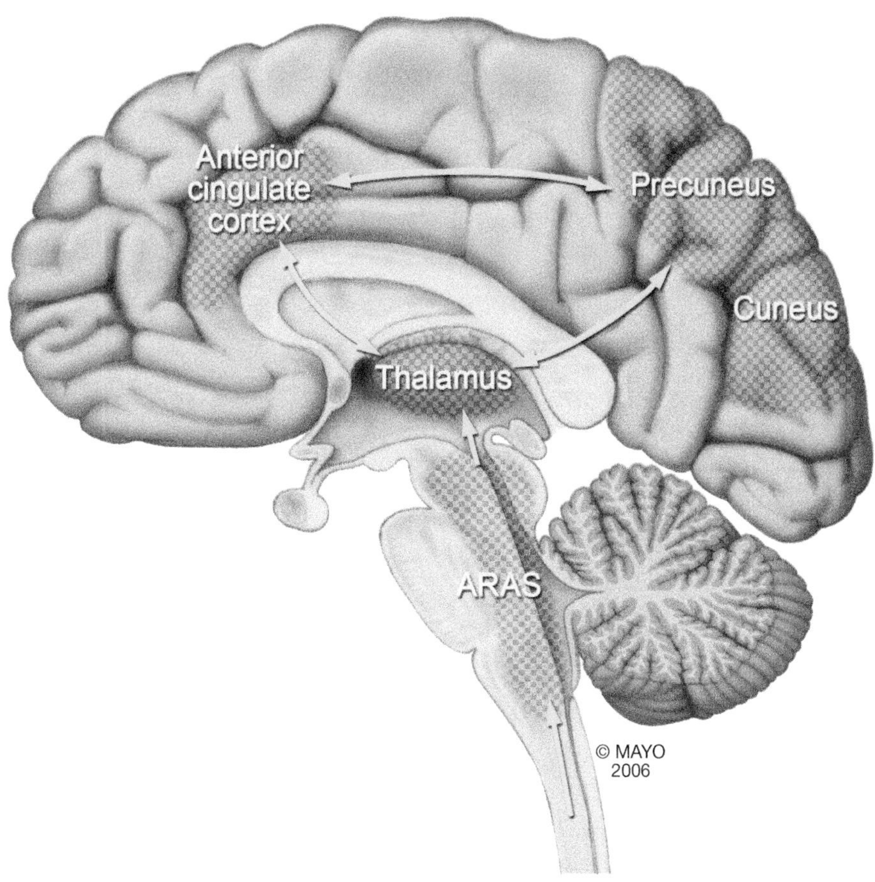

Figure 14.2. Anatomical Structures and Dorsal and Ventral Pathways Involved With the Maintenance of Consciousness. ARAS indicates ascending reticular activating system.

(From Wijdicks EFM. The comatose patient. 2nd ed. Oxford [UK]: Oxford University Press; c2014. Chapter 2, The neuroscience of the awake state; p. 60-80; used with permission of Mayo Foundation for Medical Education and Research.)

consciousness, responses range from localization to no response. A withdrawal response can be difficult to differentiate from decorticate posturing (abnormal movement with stereotyped slow flexion of the upper extremity). An abnormal extensor response is characterized by adduction and internal rotation of the upper extremity with pronation of the forearm. Decerebrate posturing indicates a more severe problem and often results from a structural lesion involving or compressing the brainstem. However, certain reversible metabolic disorders (eg, hepatic encephalopathy, hypoglycemia, or postictal states) can also produce abnormal posturing.

Localization Principles

The neurologic examination and history are integrated to localize the cause of coma. An abnormality in any of several locations within the brain and brainstem may produce a decreased level of consciousness. The ARAS, located in the dorsal upper pons and mesencephalon, is critical in the maintenance of alertness. This collection of neurons projects to the thalamus and hypothalamus, which innervate the cortex in both specific cortical regions and in a more diffuse manner. Thus, a coma can be induced by a primary brainstem lesion or, more commonly, pressure on the brainstem laterally or superiorly. Additionally, the level of consciousness can be affected by damage to both sides of the diencephalon or by bilateral or diffuse hemispheric injury. A major clinical decision is to determine whether the coma is due to a structural lesion or a widespread physiologic disturbance of neuronal function. Structural lesions that cause impaired consciousness are bihemispheric, within the brainstem parenchyma, or indicative of secondary brainstem displacement.

Table 14.1 • Toxidromes

Toxidrome	Intoxicating Substance	Clinical Features
Cholinergic	Organophosphates	Miosis Fasciculations Salivation Hypertension Tachycardia Sweating
Anticholinergic	Atropine Antihistamines Tricyclic antidepressants	Mydriasis Tremors Hypertension Tachycardia Dry skin
Sympathomimetic	Cocaine Amphetamines Theophylline	Mydriasis Tremor Hypertension Tachycardia Sweating
Serotonergic	SSRIs Lithium MAOIs	Mydriasis Myoclonus, hyperreflexia Rigidity Labile blood pressure Tachycardia
Narcotic	Opioids	Miosis Fasciculations Hypothermia Hypotension Bradycardia
Extrapyramidal	Phenothiazines Haloperidol Risperidone	Rigidity, dystonia Akathisia Mute Hypertension Tachycardia

Abbreviations: MAOI, monoamine oxidase inhibitor; SSRI, selective serotonin reuptake inhibitor.

Bihemispheric Syndromes

Possible causes of *bihemispheric syndromes* include injury to the cortex, white matter involvement in both hemispheres, and acute global physiologic dysfunction. The neurologic examination of a patient with a bihemispheric syndrome characteristically lacks features that are lateralizing or asymmetrical and shows fully preserved brainstem reflexes. Eye opening is often induced by voice or a noxious stimulus, and the full spectrum of motor responses can be observed.

Brainstem Syndromes

The 2 main types of brainstem syndromes are *intrinsic brainstem syndrome* and *brainstem displacement syndrome*. Although examination findings can be similar, the history often differentiates these 2 syndromes. Typically, the patient's eyelids remain closed to noxious stimulus.

Box 14.1 • Glasgow Coma Scale and the FOUR Score[a]

Glasgow Coma Scale

Eye response
- 4—Eyelids open spontaneously
- 3—Eyelids open to voice
- 2—Eyelids open to pain
- 1—No eyelid opening

Motor response
- 6—Obeys commands
- 5—Localizes pain
- 4—Withdraws from pain
- 3—Shows abnormal flexion to pain
- 2—Shows extension response to pain
- 1—No motor response

Verbal response
- 5—Oriented
- 4—Confused
- 3—Inappropriate words
- 2—Incomprehensible sounds
- 1—No verbal response

FOUR Score

Eye response
- 4—Eyelids open or opened; tracking or blinking to command
- 3—Eyelids open but not tracking
- 2—Eyelids closed but open to loud voice
- 1—Eyelids closed but open to pain
- 0—Eyelids remain closed to pain

Motor response
- 4—Follows commands (thumbs-up, fist, or peace sign)
- 3—Localizes pain
- 2—Flexion response to pain
- 1—Extension response to pain
- 0—No response to pain or generalized myoclonus status

Brainstem reflexes
- 4—Pupillary and corneal reflexes present
- 3—One pupil wide and fixed to light
- 2—Pupillary or corneal reflexes absent
- 1—Pupillary and corneal reflexes absent
- 0—Pupillary, corneal, and cough reflexes absent

Respiration
- 4—Not intubated; regular breathing pattern
- 3—Not intubated; Cheyne-Stokes breathing pattern
- 2—Not intubated; irregular breathing pattern
- 1—Intubated (endotracheal or tracheostomy tube); breathing faster than ventilator rate
- 0—Breathing at ventilator rate or is apneic

Abbreviation: FOUR, Full Outline of Unresponsiveness.

[a] The number before each response indicates the number of points that contribute to the total score.

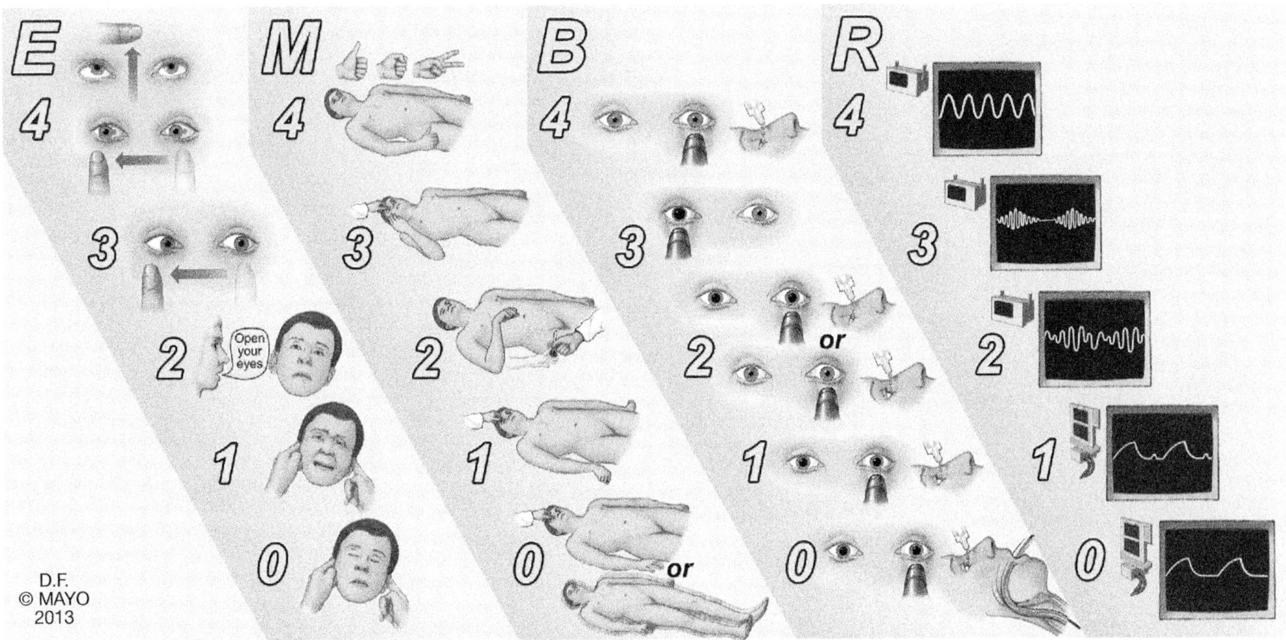

Figure 14.3. The Full Outline of Unresponsiveness (FOUR) Score. Point values (0-4) are defined in Box 14.1 for eye response (E), motor response (M), brainstem reflexes (B), and respiration (R).

(Modified from Wijdicks EFM. The practice of emergency and critical care neurology. 2nd ed. New York [NY]: Oxford University Press; c2016. Chapter 12, Comatose; p. 104-36; used with permission of Mayo Foundation for Medical Education and Research.)

Motor response may be withdrawal or extensor. Cranial nerve abnormalities are frequently observed but variable and may include skew deviation (misalignment of eyes in the vertical plane), anisocoria, and absence or asymmetry of pupillary, corneal, or oculocephalic reflexes.

Brainstem displacement can be further divided into *lateral displacement syndromes* and *central displacement syndromes*. Lateral displacement commonly compresses the thalamus and upper brainstem and causes decreased consciousness (involvement of the ARAS in the upper brainstem) with a fixed, dilated pupil unilaterally. The dilated pupil is usually ipsilateral to the mass and less commonly contralateral. Cerebellar lesions can produce lateral displacement at the pontine level with miosis and loss of corneal and oculocephalic reflexes. Distortion of the thalamus and mesencephalon in a vertical plane causes a central brainstem displacement syndrome. A characteristic at onset is fixed, midposition pupils (diameter 4-6 mm). If only the thalami are involved (sparing the mesencephalon), brainstem reflexes can be preserved (closely mimicking a bihemispheric syndrome), but a rostral-caudal progression often occurs.

Diagnostic Tests

Blood Tests

Essentially every comatose patient should undergo blood tests, including, at a minimum, levels of electrolytes (sodium, calcium, magnesium, and phosphorus), glucose, ammonia, serum urea nitrogen, bicarbonate, and hepatic transaminases; hematocrit; leukocyte count; and drug screening. A chloride level should be checked to calculate the anion gap ([sodium] - [chloride + bicarbonate]). If toxic ingestion is a reasonable possibility, specific tests should include salicylate, ethanol, and acetaminophen levels and plasma osmolality. In addition, arterial blood gas testing can be valuable to evaluate the pH and the partial pressures of oxygen and carbon dioxide. Specific blood gas abnormalities are clues to the toxin ingested (Table 14.2).

Neuroimaging

Computed Tomography

Neuroimaging supplements a thorough and careful history and neurologic examination. Noncontrast computed tomography (CT) of the head is a first-line test and should be performed for nearly all patients unless an immediately obvious cause of coma has surfaced (eg, hypoglycemia). CT is valuable to assess for acute hemorrhage, extensive subacute infarctions, and large masses (Figure 14.5). Hypodensity on CT of the head may indicate infarction, edema, or tumor; hyperdensity usually indicates acute hemorrhage, contrast agent, metals, or calcium. Air produces a very low density that appears black. CT angiography should be considered if basilar artery occlusion is suspected, particularly if the cranial nerve examination identifies abnormalities (eg, anisocoria, skew deviation,

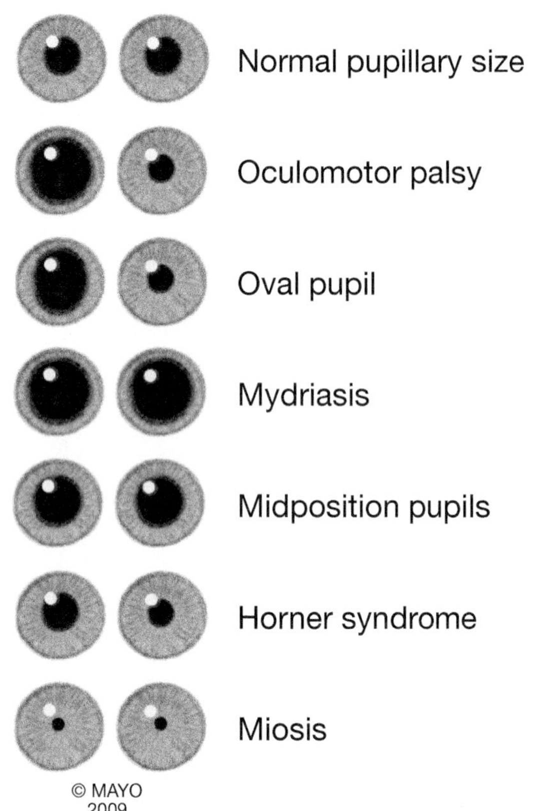

Figure 14.4. Spectrum of Pupillary Abnormalities and Causes.
(From Wijdicks EFM. The practice of emergency and critical care neurology. 2nd ed. New York [NY]: Oxford University Press; c2016. Chapter 12, Comatose; p. 104-36; used with permission of Mayo Foundation for Medical Education and Research.)

and absence or asymmetry of corneal, pupillary, or oculocephalic reflexes), if coma occurred suddenly, or if the patient has cerebrovascular risk factors. Several CT findings require prompt action (Table 14.3).

In a coma assessment, CT of the head is useful for showing other areas aside from the brain parenchyma. Bone windows highlight skull fractures after trauma; eye deviation can be a clue to hemispheric stroke; hyperdense vessels (eg, middle cerebral artery and basilar artery) may indicate the presence of acute thrombus; and the venous sinuses may appear hyperdense in venous sinus thrombosis.

Magnetic Resonance Imaging

If the cause of coma remains unknown and the patient's condition is sufficiently stabilized, magnetic resonance imaging (MRI) can provide further details. For example, MRI (particularly diffusion-weighted sequences) are useful for detecting damage from anoxic brain injury after cardiopulmonary arrest. MRI might also disclose typical lesion patterns not detectable on CT in disorders such as Wernicke encephalopathy or central pontine myelinolysis.

Table 14.2 • Blood Gas Abnormalities

Abnormality	Possible Causes
Metabolic acidosis (wide anion gap)	Methanol Ethanol Paraldehyde Isoniazid Salicylates
Metabolic alkalosis	Diuretics Nonketotic hyperglycemia Lithium
Respiratory acidosis	Barbiturates Benzodiazepines Opioids Strychnine Tetrodotoxin
Respiratory alkalosis	Salicylates Amphetamines Anticholinergics Cocaine Cyanide Paraldehyde Theophylline Carbon monoxide

Electrophysiology

A standard electroencephalogram (EEG) is an additional test in the assessment of a comatose patient. EEG is an electrophysiologic test dominated by faster frequencies (beta activity >13 Hz) in awake patients. As patients become less alert, slower frequencies predominate (theta frequency of 4-7 Hz or delta frequency <4 Hz). Characteristic EEG patterns have been associated with certain diseases, such as periodic lateralizing epileptiform discharges in herpes simplex encephalitis, generalized triphasic waves in hepatic encephalopathy, and a reactive alpha pattern in comatose patients with brainstem injury. The EEG is also helpful for patients with suspected nonconvulsive status epilepticus. The clinical presentation of these patients varies substantially, ranging from awake and confused to stuporous or comatose. Subtle clinical signs of nystagmus or eyelid twitching may be diagnostic clues, particularly if the patient is suspected of having a proclivity to seizures.

Early Actions in the Treatment of Coma

The immediate treatment of coma depends on the condition of the patient and whether vital signs are satisfactory. Improve oxygenation by delivering 40% oxygen

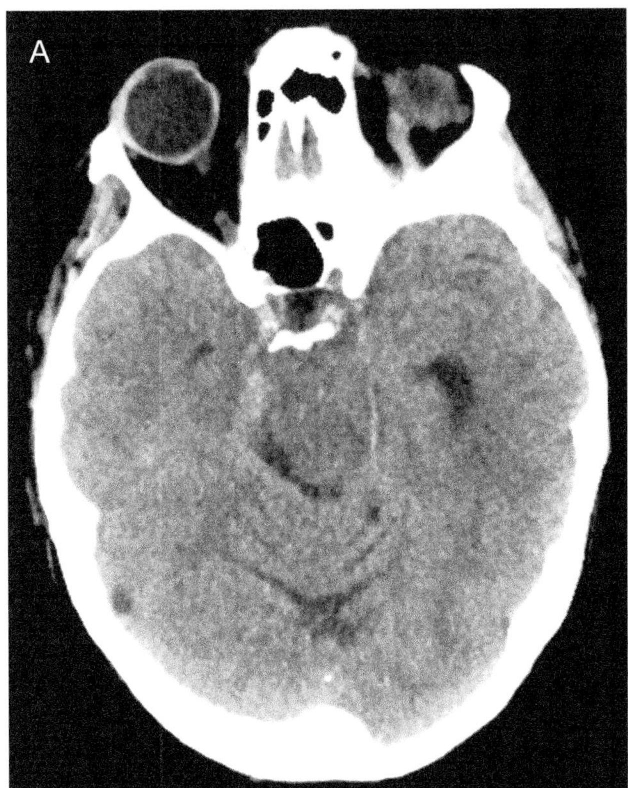

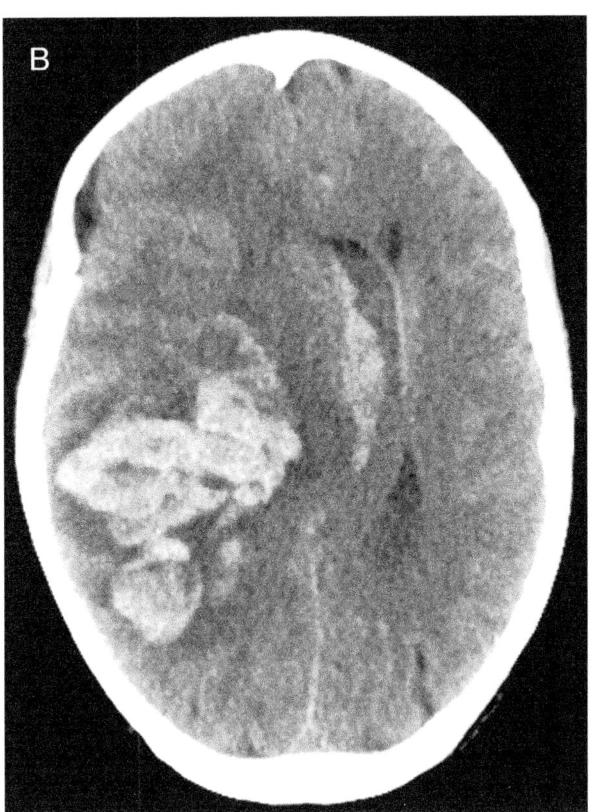

Figure 14.5. Computed Tomographic Scan With Large Cerebral Hematoma. The brainstem has shifted, with opening of the ipsilateral ambient cistern (A) and development of contralateral hydrocephalus (B).

Table 14.3 • Computed Tomographic Findings Requiring Prompt Action

Finding	Action
Hydrocephalus	Ventriculostomy to decrease the increased intracranial pressure
Mass	Consider evacuation to relieve the increased intracranial pressure
Irremovable large mass	Consider decompressive craniectomy
Suspected increased intracranial pressure	Mannitol (initial dose, 1-2 g/kg IV), often with 2 repeated doses 30-40 min apart
CNS infection	Cefotaxime (2 g every 6 h IV) *and* Vancomycin (20 mg/kg IV every 12 h) *and* Ampicillin (12 g daily in divided doses every 4 h IV) in combination with IV acyclovir (10 mg/kg every 8 h) *and* Dexamethasone (0.6 mg/kg daily IV) before administration of antibiotics and continuing for 4 d

Abbreviations: CNS, central nervous system; IV, intravenously.

with a face mask and aiming for oxygen saturation by pulse oximetry that exceeds 95%. Intubate comatose patients if they have irregular, ineffective respiratory drive and poor oxygenation or if they cannot protect their airway.

Correct hypotension by placing the patient in the Trendelenburg position and providing crystalloids (normal saline as a rapid infusion of 500-1,000 mL followed by 150 mL/h); if hypotension persists, administer vasopressors (intravenous bolus of 100 mcg phenylephrine). Correct extreme hypertension (systolic blood pressure >250 mm Hg or mean arterial pressure >130 mm Hg) with intravenous administration of labetalol (10 mg), hydralazine (10 mg), or nicardipine (10 mg/h).

To correct hypothermia, use warming blankets. To correct hyperthermia, use cooling blankets, ice packs, and ice water lavage.

If a patient has a high likelihood of hypoglycemia, give 50 mL of 50% glucose (with coadministration of 100 mg thiamine intravenously). Treat severe hyponatremia with 3% hypertonic saline and furosemide after placing a central venous catheter. Treat hypercalcemia with saline rehydration infusion followed by parenteral bisphosphonate pamidronate.

If opioid intoxication is suspected, administer naloxone intravenously (0.4-2.0 mg every 3 minutes). To reverse benzodiazepine toxicity, administer flumazenil intravenously and slowly (0.2 mg/min up to a maximum dose of 5 mg). Consider elimination of any toxin by hemodialysis or hemoperfusion.

Summary

- Physicians should distinguish between a global brain injury and an injury from mass effect, which may require neurosurgical intervention.
- CT and MRI (and less often EEG) may greatly narrow down the list of possible causes.
- If toxic ingestion is a possibility, specific tests should include salicylate, ethanol, and acetaminophen levels and plasma osmolality.
- Coma with normal CT findings may be due to seizures, central nervous system infection, or acute endocrine or electrolyte disturbances. With an embolus to the basilar artery, CT findings may be normal, but abnormal reflexes would point to the diagnosis.

SUGGESTED READING

Edlow JA, Rabinstein A, Traub SJ, Wijdicks EF. Diagnosis of reversible causes of coma. Lancet. 2014 Dec 6;384(9959):2064–76. Epub 2014 Apr 21.

Giacino JT, Ashwal S, Childs N, Cranford R, Jennett B, Katz DI, et al. The minimally conscious state: definition and diagnostic criteria. Neurology. 2002 Feb 12;58(3):349–53.

Multi-Society Task Force on PVS. Medical aspects of the persistent vegetative state (1). N Engl J Med. 1994 May 26;330(21):1499–508.

Multi-Society Task Force on PVS. Medical aspects of the persistent vegetative state (2). N Engl J Med. 1994 Jun 2;330(22):1572–9. Erratum in: N Engl J Med. 1995 Jul 13;333(2):130.

Teasdale G, Jennett B. Assessment of coma and impaired consciousness: a practical scale. Lancet. 1974 Jul 13;2(7872):81–4.

Wijdicks EF. The bare essentials: coma. Pract Neurol. 2010 Feb;10(1):51–60.

Wijdicks EFM. Who improves from coma, how do they improve, and then what? Nat Rev Neurol. 2018 Dec;14(12):694–6.

Wijdicks EF, Bamlet WR, Maramattom BV, Manno EM, McClelland RL. Validation of a new coma scale: the FOUR score. Ann Neurol. 2005 Oct;58(4):585–93.

Wijdicks EFM. The comatose patient. 2nd ed. Oxford (UK): Oxford University Press; c2014. 784 p.

15 Neuromuscular Respiratory Failure

MAXIMILIANO A. HAWKES, MD; EELCO F. M. WIJDICKS, MD, PhD

Goals

- Discuss the early clinical presentation of neuromuscular respiratory failure.
- Review the laboratory tests for patients with suspected neuromuscular respiratory failure.
- Review the management of neuromuscular respiratory failure.

Introduction

Regardless of its cause, acute neuromuscular respiratory weakness leads to alveolar hypoventilation. Additional features that complicate the clinical presentation are upper airway muscle weakness and pulmonary complications (mostly due to aspiration). Having an understanding of basic ventilatory physiology and the pathophysiologic mechanisms underlying mechanical neuromuscular respiratory failure is essential for early recognition, initial evaluation, and further etiologic investigation of neuromuscular respiratory failure.

Pulmonary Mechanics in Neuromuscular Weakness

The diaphragm is responsible for more than two-thirds of the ventilatory effort during normal breathing. Its mixed composition of slow twitch and fast twitch muscle fibers and its rich perfusion make it comparatively resistant to fatigue. Accessory inspiratory muscles are active during physiologically high rates of respiration and when pathologic conditions compromise the diaphragmatic strength or increase the workload of breathing. Unlike inspiration, expiration is a passive process mediated by elastic lung recoil, but expiratory muscles are essential for coughing and clearance of secretions.

Diaphragmatic weakness causes decreased tidal volume and alveolar hypoventilation. In the early stages of neuromuscular weakness, the minute ventilation, and thus the P_{O_2}, can be maintained within normal limits by increasing the respiratory rate. However, basal microatelectasis, mucous plugging, diminished thoracic expansion, and inefficient cough can result in oxygen desaturation early in the course of the disease because of pulmonary capillary shunting (Figure 15.1). Characteristic findings at this stage are tachypnea, contraction of accessory inspiratory muscles, normal or mildly low P_{O_2}, and normal P_{CO_2} despite the increased respiratory rate. As atelectasis worsens, pulmonary restriction and the work of breathing increase. When the compensatory action of the accessory ventilatory muscles is overwhelmed, hypercapnia and then profound hypoxia develop. If oropharyngeal muscles cannot maintain the patency of the upper airway, aspiration becomes an additional complication.

Clinical Presentation

Tachypnea, which occurs early in the course of ventilatory muscle weakness, may be accompanied by tachycardia, anxiety, discomfort, and dyspnea. In the absence of hypoxemia, dyspnea is explained by the increased firing activity of vagal fibers triggered by the increased work of breathing. Patients typically have hypophonia and interrupted speech because of frequent pauses to breathe (*staccato speech*). Forehead sweating reflects the respiratory effort. Hypoxemic patients are characteristically dyspneic and restless. When hypercapnia develops, somnolence and confusion may be additional findings.

Contraction of accessory inspiratory muscles, especially the sternocleidomastoid and scalene muscles, can be evident on inspection or palpation. This sign is known as *respiratory pulse*. Patients may also have difficulty raising their head from the bed; neck weakness, particularly in flexion, may correlate with diaphragmatic weakness. The

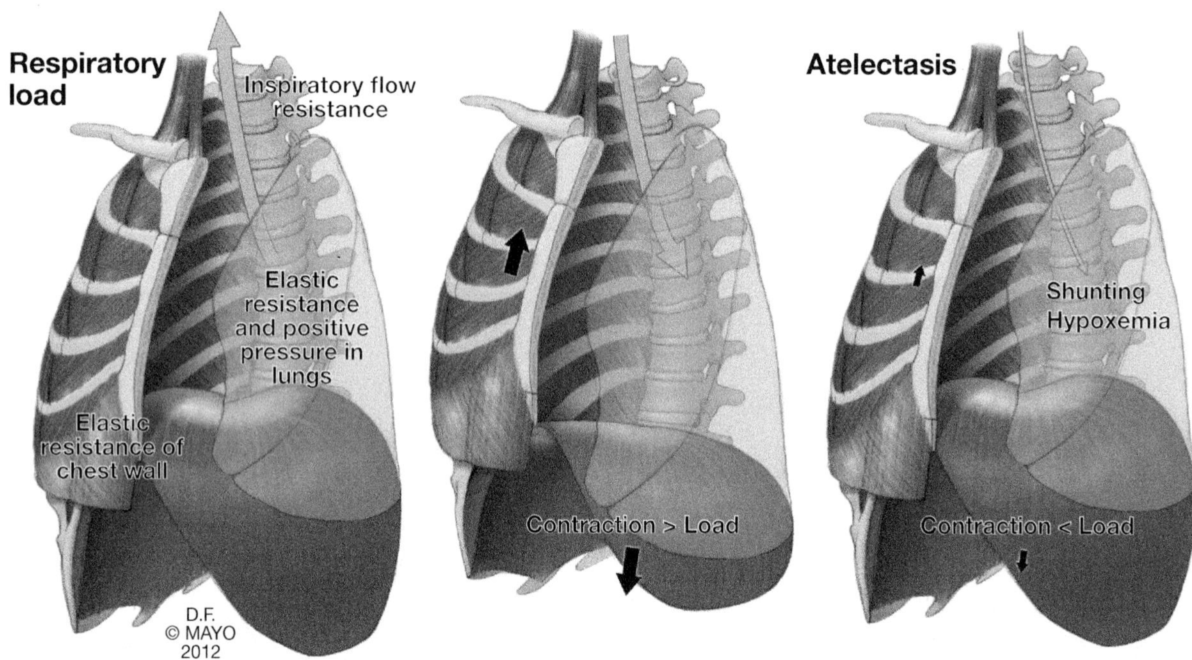

Figure 15.1. Respiratory Load and Neuromuscular Respiratory Failure. (From Wijdicks EFM. Handling difficult situations. Oxford [UK]: Oxford University Press; c2014. Chapter 8, Supporting acute respiratory muscle weakness; p. 99-114. [Core principles of acute neurology]; used with permission of Mayo Foundation for Medical Education and Research.)

hallmark of diaphragmatic weakness, *abdominal paradox*, is defined as the inward movement of the abdomen with thoracic expansion. Both abdominal paradox and dyspnea are more evident when the patient is lying supine.

Acute failure of respiratory mechanics can be recognized by 5 distress signals that begin with *D: dysphagia, dysphonia, dyssynchronous breathing*, (oxygen) *desaturation*, and *dysautonomia* (Figure 15.2). However, all 5 may not be present at the same time in every disorder.

Weakness of the oropharyngeal muscles leads to dysphonia and dysphagia. Gurgling mucus makes this element immediately recognizable, and the patient is in real danger of asphyxiation. Thoracoabdominal dyssynchrony is typical with severe respiratory muscle weakness. Normally the abdomen and chest expand and contract in synchrony. During inspiration, downward movement of the diaphragm pushes the abdominal contents down and out as the rib margins are lifted and moved out, causing both the chest and the abdomen to rise. None of this occurs if patients have mechanical respiratory failure; the movements may not be coordinated for even 2 breaths.

Evaluation of the Patient

History

Respiratory failure may be an expected complication of a previously diagnosed neuromuscular disease (eg, myasthenic crisis) or the primary manifestation of an undiagnosed entity. A detailed history will guide the neurologic examination and diagnostic workup. When patients cannot answer, collateral information should be obtained.

The onset and progression of symptoms are important. Acute onset of symptoms may increase suspicion for toxins (eg, botulism), infections (eg, West Nile virus infection), or acute neuropathies (eg, Guillain-Barré syndrome [GBS]). The faster the weakness progresses, the greater the likelihood that the patient will need mechanical ventilation. Chronic and fluctuating weakness suggests myasthenia gravis (MG). Progressive muscular weakness, dysphagia, dysarthria, and fasciculations are commonly seen in amyotrophic lateral sclerosis (ALS).

Comorbidities and recent events must be considered. For example, infectious diarrhea (from *Campylobacter jejuni*), upper airway infections, and vaccinations (in the previous 2-3 weeks) are known triggers of GBS. Concurrent infections (eg, pneumonia or urinary tract infection), some antibiotics (eg, fluoroquinolones), recent anesthesia (eg, isoflurane or ketamine), and other drugs can exacerbate MG. Ingestion of a possibly contaminated food (eg, a canned product) or the presence of a possibly infected wound should increase suspicion for botulism. Acral paresthesias and neuropathic pain are features of GBS, and dysautonomic features are characteristic in GBS and botulism. If a patient has concurrent cardiopulmonary disease with neuromuscular respiratory failure, the long-term prognosis is usually poor.

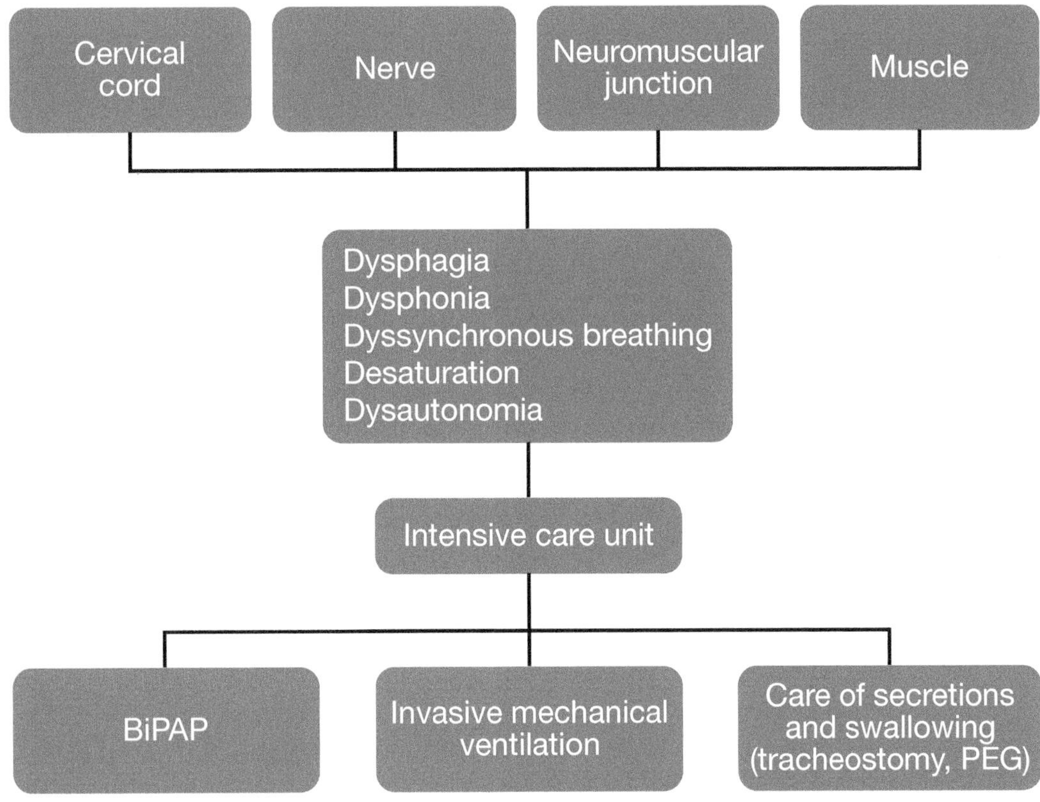

Figure 15.2. Critical Decisions in Acute Neuromuscular Respiratory Failure. Five distress signals that begin with D *are listed. BiPAP indicates bilevel positive airway pressure; PEG, percutaneous endoscopic gastrostomy.*

The site of onset, pattern of spread, and fluctuation of the weakness are useful to know: Ascending weakness is typical of GBS; weakness of ocular muscles (manifested as ptosis or diplopia) or bulbar muscles is more common in MG; weakness of axial and bulbar muscles is more common in Eaton-Lambert syndrome; fluctuations and fatigability suggest MG; and rapidly descending paralysis with prominent dysautonomic features may increase suspicion for botulism.

Physical Examination

During the physical examination, the goals are to assess for early signs of respiratory failure that require prompt intervention and to determine the most likely cause of respiratory failure. Diaphragmatic weakness can be identified by the following findings: abdominal paradox; inability to count aloud from 1 to 20 after a single maximal breath (which indicates a forced vital capacity [FVC] of <2 L); neck flexion weakness; and asymmetric thoracic expansion during breathing (which suggests a unilateral phrenic nerve lesion).

During the neurologic examination, several features should be particularly assessed: Bulbar muscle dysfunction may be apparent from drooling, nasal voice, choking, and frequent, ineffective cough. Fatigability of ocular and bulbar muscles is evaluated with the sustained upgaze test for ptosis and by observing for extraocular muscle movements after prolonged and forced eye closure. Jaw closure muscles are tested by determining whether the patient can hold a tongue depressor between molars. Fatigability can be tested by having the patient bite intermittently and seeing whether the bite holds. The presense of a sensory level suggests spinal cord injury. Distal hypoesthesia and hypopallesthesia are common features in polyneuropathies and can be features of GBS. Deep tendon reflexes are increased in some patients with motor neuron disease, abolished in patients with GBS (reflexes may be present in early GBS but absent in weak limbs), and normal in patients with myopathies and neuromuscular transmission disorders. Muscular atrophy can be evident in patients with chronic neuropathies or ALS. Central atrophy of the tongue has occurred in patients with MG and autoantibodies to muscle-specific tyrosine-kinase (MuSK) (ie, anti-MuSK MG).

Laboratory Tests

Bedside pulmonary function tests (PFTs), arterial blood gas (ABG) tests, and chest radiographs are useful to assess the initial degree of respiratory compromise and to detect early complications. Bedside PFTs also help to monitor the evolution of neuromuscular respiratory failure. Even patients without evident respiratory compromise should be closely followed with bedside PFTs because the clinical examination is not always sensitive enough to detect early respiratory compromise in patients with fluctuating or progressive neuromuscular diseases. The most valuable measures are FVC, maximal inspiratory pressure, and maximal expiratory pressure. Reference ranges and critical values are presented in Table 15.1. While critical values have been validated for GBS, reliability has not been proved for other neuromuscular diseases. Critical diaphragmatic weakness is suggested not only by absolute cutoff values but also by any decrease of 30% or more in FVC from baseline and a decrease exceeding 20% from upright to supine. These values are not firm criteria for intubation and should be interpreted within the context of the clinical examination and suspected underlying cause.

These tests are effort dependent, so the technique must be carefully explained to the patient, and proper coaching by trained respiratory therapists is essential for obtaining reliable information. If the patient has facial weakness and poor mouth sealing around the spirometer, the reliability of the test can be compromised. Other patients may have abundant oral secretions because of difficulty clearing the upper airway or because of the adverse effects of a drug (eg, myasthenia patients receiving pyridostigmine). For the measurements to be reliable, these patients must use a mask device to reduce air leakage and have secretions properly suctioned before beginning the tests. Any preexisting pulmonary conditions must be considered during interpretation of PFT results. Among patients with various causes of primary neuromuscular respiratory failure, pressures appear to have greater predictive value than FVC.

The ABG profile differs depending on the stage of the neuromuscular weakness. In the early stages of respiratory muscle weakness, for example, ABG results can be normal or show mild hypocapnia and respiratory alkalosis. If mild hypoxemia is present, basal atelectasis should be suspected. If the patient has tachypnea, normal $Paco_2$ indicates respiratory failure because the ability of the system to compensate is being overwhelmed. If hypoventilation has occurred for several days, the serum bicarbonate level may be high. Ventilatory support should be considered before a patient becomes frankly hypercapnic or hypoxemic because these are usually late findings in patients with acute neuromuscular respiratory failure.

Chest radiography is necessary to evaluate for atelectasis, pneumonia, and other forms of cardiopulmonary disease. The presence of any of these findings lowers the threshold for initiating mechanical ventilation and guides additional therapeutic efforts.

Ultrasonography is a noninvasive technique useful for assessing diaphragmatic structure and function and for guiding electromyographic needle insertion. If the diaphragm is less than 0.2 cm thick at the end of expiration, it is atrophied. Diaphragmatic thickening of less than 20% during inspiration is consistent with severe weakness. A decreased diaphragmatic excursion on deep breathing, with or without paradoxical motion on sniffing, is another indicator of diaphragmatic weakness. Side-to-side variation and velocity of contraction are additional measures for assessing diaphragmatic strength.

Table 15.1 • Pulmonary Function Tests

Pulmonary Function Test	Reference Range	Critical Value
Forced vital capacity (FVC), mL/kg	40-70	20
Maximal inspiratory pressure (MIP), cm H_2O		−30
Male	≥−100	
Female	≥−70	
Maximal expiratory pressure (MEP), cm H_2O		40
Male	>100	
Female	>40	

Modified from Wijdicks EFM. The practice of emergency and critical care neurology. 2nd ed. New York (NY): Oxford University Press; c2016. Chapter 10, Short of breath; p. 78-91; used with permission of Mayo Foundation for Medical Education and Research.

Causes of Neuromuscular Respiratory Failure

Neuromuscular respiratory failure can be caused by primary neurologic diseases, or it can be secondary to systemic diseases, toxins, drugs, or electrolyte imbalances (Box 15.1).

GBS and myasthenic crisis are the most common causes of acute primary neuromuscular respiratory failure in patients requiring admission to the intensive care unit (ICU). ALS and myopathies follow them in frequency. However, if weakness develops in a critically ill patient in the ICU, critical illness polyneuropathy or critical illness myopathy can be suspected. Given their common co-occurrence, these entities are also known as *critical illness neuromyopathy* or, more recently, *ICU-acquired weakness*. The main associated risk factors are sepsis, multiorgan failure, prolonged mechanical ventilation and ICU stay, corticosteroid administration, hyperglycemia, and renal failure. Poor nutritional status and use of neuromuscular junction blocking agents might also increase the risk. Table 15.2 lists the main clinical findings in patients with critical illness polyneuropathy or critical illness myopathy, but substantial overlap is common.

Determining a definitive diagnosis when the presumptive diagnosis is not evident is particularly challenging. Electromyography is the diagnostic test with the highest

Box 15.1 • Differential Diagnosis of Neuromuscular Respiratory Failure

Anterior horn cell disease
- Motor neuron disease
- West Nile virus infection
- Poliomyelitis
- Postpolio syndrome
- Kennedy disease

Nerve roots and peripheral nerves
- Critical illness polyneuropathy
- Guillain-Barré syndrome
- Acute onset of chronic inflammatory demyelinating polyneuropathy
- Toxins (eg, tetrodotoxin)
- Drugs (eg, chemotherapy and amiodarone)
- Vasculitis
- Paraneoplastic process
- Porphyria
- Amyloid infiltration
- Phrenic nerve injury

Neuromuscular junction
- Myasthenia gravis
- Lambert-Eaton myasthenic syndrome
- Botulism
- Organophosphate poisoning
- Tick paralysis
- Snake venom

Muscles
- Critical illness myopathy
- Inflammatory myopathies
- Metabolic myopathies (eg, hyperthyroidism, hypophosphatemia, hyperkalemia, hypokalemia, and hypernatremia)
- Toxins (eg, statins and colchicine)
- Rhabdomyolysis
- Mitochondrial myopathies
- Acid maltase deficiency

Modified from Rabinstein AA. Acute neuromuscular respiratory failure. Continuum (Minneap Minn). 2015 Oct;21(5 Neurocritical Care):1324-45; used with permission.

yield for patients without a previously known neuromuscular disease.

Ventilatory Support

The decision to intubate a patient who has neuromuscular respiratory weakness should be tailored to each patient

Table 15.2 • Characteristic Features of Critical Illness Polyneuropathy (CIP) and Critical Illness Myopathy (CIM)

Procedure	CIP	CIM
Physical examination		
Flaccid quadriparesis	Present	Present
Respiratory muscle weakness	Present	Present
Reflexes	↓↓	Normal or ↓
Sensation	↓	Normal
NCS		
CMAP amplitude	↓↓	↓
SNAP amplitude	↓	Normal
Conduction velocities	Normal or ↓	Normal
CMAP duration	Normal	↓↓
EMG	Neuropathic	Myopathic
Repetitive nerve stimulation	Normal	Normal
Direct muscle stimulation response	Normal	↓↓
Nerve or muscle biopsy	Axonal neuropathy, muscle denervation	Myosin filament loss, muscle necrosis (if severe)

Abbreviations: CMAP, compound muscle action potential; EMG, electromyography; NCS, nerve conduction study; SNAP, sensory nerve action potential; ↓, mildly reduced; ↓↓, markedly reduced.

Modified from Rabinstein AA. Acute neuromuscular respiratory failure. Continuum (Minneap Minn). 2015 Oct;21(5 Neurocritical Care):1324-45; used with permission.

and the underlying cause. Level of consciousness, ability to protect the airway, and bedside PFT results (Table 15.1) must be considered when deciding about invasive ventilation. If intubation is required, succinylcholine should be avoided because of the risk of hyperkalemia. Patients may benefit from noninvasive ventilation while the underlying cause is corrected (ie, MG exacerbation), but noninvasive ventilation often fails to benefit patients whose weakness is worsening (ie, GBS). Weaning from the ventilator can be expected if patients have acute neuromuscular respiratory failure but not a degenerative neurologic disease such as motor neuron disease.

Summary

- Neuromuscular respiratory failure is the final stage of ventilatory muscle weakness.
- Tachypnea, tachycardia, restlessness, hypophonia, halting speech, forehead sweating, use of accessory inspiratory muscles, and abdominal paradox are hallmark signs of neuromuscular respiratory failure.

- Chest radiographs, ABG tests, and bedside PFTs should complement the history and physical examination in the diagnosis of neuromuscular respiratory failure.
- ABG abnormalities are late findings; thus, initiating ventilatory support should be considered before ABG abnormalities are present.
- GBS and myasthenic crisis are the most common primary neurologic conditions causing neuromuscular respiratory failure requiring ICU admission.
- For patients with neuromuscular respiratory failure, there are no firm criteria for decisions on intubation and mechanical ventilation. ALS is another condition to consider.

SUGGESTED READING

Benditt JO. Pathophysiology of neuromuscular respiratory diseases. Clin Chest Med. 2018 Jun;39(2):297–308.

Cabrera Serrano M, Rabinstein AA. Causes and outcomes of acute neuromuscular respiratory failure. Arch Neurol. 2010 Sep;67(9):1089–94.

Cabrera Serrano M, Rabinstein AA. Usefulness of pulmonary function tests and blood gases in acute neuromuscular respiratory failure. Eur J Neurol. 2012 Mar;19(3):452–6. Epub 2011 Oct 4.

Damian MS, Wijdicks EFM. The clinical management of neuromuscular disorders in intensive care. Neuromuscul Disord. 2019 Feb;29(2):85–96.

Edmundson C, Bird SJ. Acute manifestations of neuromuscular disease. Semin Neurol. 2019 Feb;39(1):115–24.

Hutchinson D, Whyte K. Neuromuscular disease and respiratory failure. Pract Neurol. 2008 Aug;8(4): 229–37.

Kress JP, Hall JB. ICU-acquired weakness and recovery from critical illness. N Engl J Med. 2014 Apr 24;370(17):1626–35.

Lacomis D. Electrophysiology of neuromuscular disorders in critical illness. Muscle Nerve. 2013 Mar;47(3):452–63. Epub 2013 Feb 6.

Latronico N, Bolton CF. Critical illness polyneuropathy and myopathy: a major cause of muscle weakness and paralysis. Lancet Neurol. 2011 Oct;10(10):931–41.

Mehta S. Neuromuscular disease causing acute respiratory failure. Respir Care. 2006 Sep;51(9):1016–21.

Niedermeyer S, Murn M, Choi PJ. Respiratory failure in amyotrophic lateral sclerosis. Chest. 2019 Feb;155(2):401–8.

Rabinstein AA. Acute neuromuscular respiratory failure. Continuum (Minneap Minn). 2015 Oct;21(5 Neurocritical Care):1324–45.

Rabinstein AA, Wijdicks EF. Warning signs of imminent respiratory failure in neurological patients. Semin Neurol. 2003 Mar;23(1):97–104.

Sanders DB, Guptill JT. Myasthenia gravis and Lambert-Eaton myasthenic syndrome. Continuum (Minneap Minn). 2014 Oct;20(5 Peripheral Nervous System Disorders):1413–25.

Sarwal A, Walker FO, Cartwright MS. Neuromuscular ultrasound for evaluation of the diaphragm. Muscle Nerve. 2013 Mar;47(3):319–29. Epub 2013 Feb 4.

Seneviratne J, Mandrekar J, Wijdicks EF, Rabinstein AA. Noninvasive ventilation in myasthenic crisis. Arch Neurol. 2008 Jan;65(1):54–8.

Vianello A, Bevilacqua M, Arcaro G, Gallan F, Serra E. Non-invasive ventilatory approach to treatment of acute respiratory failure in neuromuscular disorders: a comparison with endotracheal intubation. Intensive Care Med. 2000 Apr;26(4):384–90.

Wijdicks EFM. The neurology of acutely failing respiratory mechanics. Ann Neurol. 2017 Apr;81(4):485–94.

Wijdicks EFM. The practice of emergency and critical care neurology. 2nd ed. New York (NY): Oxford University Press; c2016. 915 p.

Wijdicks EF, Roy TK. BiPAP in early Guillain-Barré syndrome may fail. Can J Neurol Sci. 2006 Feb;33(1):105–6.

16 Neurogenic Breathing Patterns[a]

EELCO F. M. WIJDICKS, MD, PhD

Goals

- Describe the anatomy of clinical respiratory control.
- Describe the physiology of central respiratory control.
- Describe neurogenic respiratory patterns and their importance.

Introduction

Breathing is a continuous, rhythmic, to-and-fro movement that requires a close interplay between arterial P_{CO_2}, oxygen, and respiratory centers. Certain thresholds exist for respiratory drive, and these thresholds change with acute neurologic disease. Primary structural lesions to the brainstem are most common, but decreased levels of consciousness frequently trigger episodic breathing (eg, Cheyne-Stokes respiration). Traditional teaching holds that an increase in arterial P_{CO_2} reduces cerebral spinal fluid pH and that this acidosis activates the respiratory center in the ventrolateral medulla oblongata. This chapter discusses the essentials of the respiratory pacemaker and neurologic breathing patterns.

Central Component of Breathing

Breathing originates from a pontomedullary network in the finely tuned pons. The respiratory center is a neural oscillator system that starts functioning in utero. Fetal respiratory movements of the diaphragm coincide with the start of this oscillator (the *pre-Bötzinger complex*), which is the main generator of breathing. This group of medulla oblongata neurons is the only one that, if damaged, results in complete apnea. Other main systems involved in breathing use the motor cortex and the sensory cortex. Awareness of changes in respiration and the ability to sense dyspnea involve the insula, operculum, and cingulate gyrus. The prefrontal cortex and the supramarginal gyrus integrate emotional and sensory aspects of respiration, but this function is not well understood. The functions of respiratory neurons are summarized in Table 16.1 and Figure 16.1. Most of the breathing control apparatus is in the pons and the medulla oblongata. Signals are sent to the respiratory muscles, and feedback from sensors, including central and peripheral chemoreceptors and pulmonary mechanoreceptors, relays information to the respiratory control center.

Two areas in the pons have a role in respiratory control. The *pneumotaxic center*, situated in the upper pons, induces termination of inspiration. When inspiration is shortened, the respiratory rate increases; therefore, the pneumotaxic center is responsible for regulating tidal volume and respiratory rate. An *apneustic center* has been located in the lower pons. Lesions in this area produce inspiratory gasps, possibly because the medullary respiratory neurons are uninhibited to discharge. Clinically, this occurs when moribund patients have secondary brainstem injury and breathe with inspiratory gasps before apnea.

The autonomic rhythm of breathing originates in the bilateral *ventral respiratory group*, which is ventral to the nucleus ambiguus in the medulla oblongata. The ventral respiratory group contains inspiratory and expiratory neurons, but these neurons drive both the upper airway muscles of inspiration and the spinal respiratory neurons innervating the intercostal and abdominal muscles. This explains why acute brainstem lesions not only affect respiratory rhythm but also greatly decrease the patient's ability to maintain an upper airway.

[a] Portions previously published in Wijdicks EFM. Respiration. In: Aminoff MJ, Daroff RB, editors. Encyclopedia of the neurological sciences. 2nd ed. Waltham (MA): Academic Press/Elsevier; c2014. p. 15-6. (Reference module in neuroscience and biobehavioral psychology.); used with permission.

Table 16.1 • Functions of Respiratory Neurons

Neurons	Function
Pre-Bötzinger complex	Inspiration
Bötzinger complex	Expiration
Retrotrapezoid nucleus	Chemosensation
Pontine nuclei	Regulation of respiratory cycle and control of laryngeal resistance
Rostral ventral respiratory group	Origin of relay neurons to phrenic nerve
Caudal ventral respiratory group	Shaping of expiratory drive to spinal motor neurons

Also located in the medulla oblongata (in the dorsal medial region) is the *dorsal respiratory group*, which consists of cells in the nucleus tractus solitarius. The dorsal respiratory group is responsible for inspiration and receives fibers from cranial nerves IX and X. Those nerves provide information about P_{O_2}, P_{CO_2}, and pH from peripheral chemoreceptors. The vagal nerve also relays information about pulmonary mechanics through pulmonary mechanoreceptors.

The nucleus ambiguus innervates the dilator muscles of the soft palate, pharynx, and larynx. This cluster of neurons adjusts ventilatory drive to respiratory muscle activity, but it mostly adjusts airway resistance. In acute brainstem lesions, involvement of the nucleus ambiguus contributes to mechanical dysfunction. Failure to manage secretions and maintain an open airway is thus more common than acute central apnea. Many neuronal connections controlling breathing are not known, and the brainstem center connections are modified by neuropeptides (catecholamine and cholinergic orexin-releasing [hypocretin-releasing] neurons) that are also poorly elucidated. In situations where the mechanisms are better known, pharmaceutical interventions can be considered.

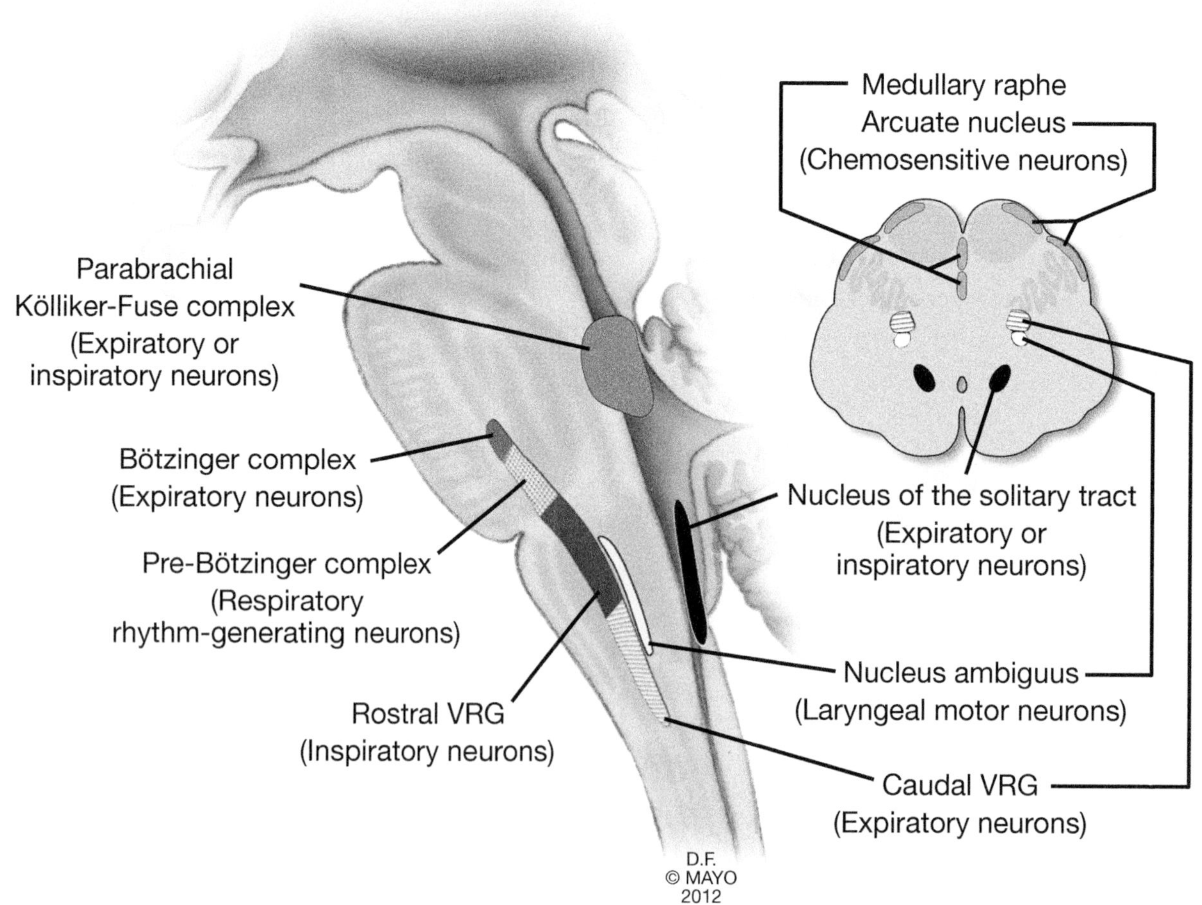

Figure 16.1. Major Respiratory Centers in the Lower Pons and the Medulla Oblongata. VRG indicates ventral respiratory group. (Modified from Wijdicks EFM. Recognizing brain injury. Oxford [UK]: Oxford University Press; c2014. Chapter 5, Neurology of breathing; p. 59-76. [Core principles of acute neurology series.]; used with permission.)

Breathing Abnormalities

Neurogenic breathing patterns are mostly abnormalities of rhythm (Table 16.2). Voluntary breathing can be affected by lesions in the pons or the basal ganglia. In affected patients, arrhythmic breathing patterns lack a cyclic pattern. *Apraxia of breathing* (often with *apraxia of swallowing*) is the inability to hold a breath and occurs in patients with acute, nondominant hemispheric lesions. Apnea may occur in neurologic lesions, such as with a large area of destruction in the lower brainstem (eg, catastrophic brain injury), but it needs to be differentiated from cervical cord lesions, which are not connected to the chest musculature.

Neurologic breathing patterns include the following: *Cluster periodic breathing* is characterized by clusters of breaths followed by apneic periods of variable duration, possibly caused by pontomedullary or diffuse cortical lesions. *Cheyne-Stokes periodic breathing* has a typical crescendo-decrescendo (spindle) breathing pattern that is common in stuporous patients, patients who are deteriorating neurologically from brain tissue displacement, and patients with congestive heart failure. Another periodic breathing pattern is *apneustic breathing*, which is an agonal breathing pattern marked by inhalation and breath-holding followed by gradual exhalation. It has been associated with tegmental lesions of the pons.

Central neurogenic hyperventilation is associated with both midbrain lesions (often lymphoma) and bihemispheric lesions. This pattern is a constant regular tachypnea with large tidal volumes that cause marked respiratory alkalosis.

Summary

- Studies on central respiratory generators have identified the primacy of the pre-Bötzinger complex.
- Central respiratory chemoreceptors that respond to hypercarbia are present in the serotonergic raphe neurons in the pons and medulla and in the retrotrapezoid nucleus.
- Despite the proximity of the nucleus ambiguus to the ventral respiratory group, the respiratory centers are relatively immune to acute injury.
- Cheyne-Stokes respiration, which is common in stuporous patients, may be the first sign of a brainstem shift.
- Central neurogenic hyperventilation is often present with midbrain lesions.

Table 16.2 • Clinically Relevant Respiratory Abnormalities

Abnormality	Site
Hypoventilation and apnea	Medulla oblongata Chemoreceptors in medullary raphe and arcuate nucleus
Sleep apnea (obstructive)	Medulla oblongata (tegmentum)
Apnea during drowsiness and sleep (Ondine curse)	Medulla oblongata (nucleus ambiguus)
Ataxic breathing	Dorsomedial area
Central neurogenic hyperventilation	Pons and midbrain
Apneustic breathing	Pons (mid or caudal)
Periodic breathing (cluster and Cheyne-Stokes)	Cortex

SUGGESTED READING

Ausborn J, Koizumi H, Barnett WH, John TT, Zhang R, Molkov YI, et al. Organization of the core respiratory network: insights from optogenetic and modeling studies. PLoS Comput Biol. 2018 Apr;14(4):e1006148.

Bolton CF, Chen R, Wijdicks EFM, Zifko UA. Neurology of breathing. Philadelphia (PA): Butterworth-Heinemann; c2004. 232 p.

Caruana-Montaldo B, Gleeson K, Zwillich CW. The control of breathing in clinical practice. Chest. 2000 Jan;117(1):205–25.

Guyenet PG, Bayliss DA. Neural control of breathing and CO_2 homeostasis. Neuron. 2015 Sep 2;87(5):946–61.

Guyenet PG, Stornetta RL, Bayliss DA. Central respiratory chemoreception. J Comp Neurol. 2010 Oct 1;518(19):3883–906.

Horn EM, Waldrop TG. Suprapontine control of respiration. Respir Physiol. 1998 Dec;114(3):201–11.

Lumb AB. Nunn's applied respiratory physiology. 7th ed. Edinburgh (UK): Churchill Livingstone/Elsevier; c2010. 556 p.

Simon RP. Respiratory manifestations of neurologic disease. Handbook Clin Neurol. 1993;19:477–501. (Series; vol. 63).

Smith JC, Abdala AP, Borgmann A, Rybak IA, Paton JF. Brainstem respiratory networks: building blocks and microcircuits. Trends Neurosci. 2013 Mar;36(3):152–62. Epub 2012 Dec 17.

Tarulli AW, Lim C, Bui JD, Saper CB, Alexander MP. Central neurogenic hyperventilation: a case report and discussion of pathophysiology. Arch Neurol. 2005 Oct;62(10):1632–4.

Wijdicks EFM. The neurology of acutely failing respiratory mechanics. Ann Neurol. 2017 Apr;81(4):485–94.

Neurogenic Cardiac Manifestations

SHERRI A. BRAKSICK, MD; EELCO F. M. WIJDICKS, MD, PhD

Goals

- Understand the spectrum of cardiac abnormalities in acute brain injury.
- Recognize clinical features of takotsubo (stress) cardiomyopathy.
- Identify known neurologic triggers of takotsubo (stress) cardiomyopathy.
- Understand treatment strategies for neurogenic cardiac abnormalities.

Introduction

Abnormalities of cardiac function and cardiac electrophysiology are not uncommon in patients with acute injury to the central nervous system, and cardiac abnormalities may be the initial signs when these patients are first evaluated. Some patients have findings that suggest an acute coronary syndrome but disappear after the intracranial pressure surge subsides.

The clinician must consider underlying neurologic disease when a patient presents with cardiac arrhythmias, new-onset pulmonary edema, hypotension, or cardiogenic shock with characteristics atypical for a primary cardiac event if the patient is in an otherwise unexplained comatose state.

Takotsubo (Stress) Cardiomyopathy

Takotsubo (stress) cardiomyopathy (TC) is considered a typically reversible phenomenon caused by a physiologic or emotional stressor. TC often results in apical hypokinesis or akinesis, although variations can occur with cardiac motion abnormalities in the midventricular segments. The Mayo Clinic criteria for diagnosis of TC are listed in Box 17.1.

Epidemiology

Of the patients with all-cause TC in a recent international TC registry, nearly 90% were women, approximately 80% were women older than 50 years (and presumably postmenopausal), and nearly 10% were reported to have an acute neurologic disorder. TC occurs in a multitude of acute neurologic conditions, including subarachnoid hemorrhage, hemorrhagic or ischemic stroke, status epilepticus, meningitis and encephalitis, myasthenia gravis, Guillain-Barré syndrome, and traumatic brain injury (Box 17.2).

Pathophysiology

The main pathophysiologic mechanism thought to be responsible for TC is a sudden catecholamine surge in response to a physical or emotional stressor. This theory has been substantiated by the finding of increased blood levels of circulating catecholamines in patients with TC but not in patients with acute coronary syndrome. The sudden increase in catecholamines acts directly on the myocardium and causes the characteristic pathologic finding of contraction band necrosis with a mononuclear infiltrate (Figure 17.1), as opposed to the neutrophilic predominance seen in acute myocardial infarction, and is thought to result from direct catecholamine toxicity on myocytes. If the sympathetic surge cannot be controlled by the afferent baroreceptors, the result is overdrive, myocardial stunning, and apical ballooning (Figure 17.2).

Clinical Presentation

Patients with TC may present with chest pain or dyspnea and with symptoms that are indistinguishable from those of acute coronary syndrome. Electrocardiography (ECG) may show diffuse ST-segment or T-wave abnormalities, and troponin levels may be elevated. With the sudden decrease in left ventricular systolic function, the initial clinical presentation may be signs of cardiac failure, arrhythmias,

Box 17.1 • Mayo Clinic Criteria for the Diagnosis of Takotsubo (Stress) Cardiomyopathy

Presence of transient akinesis, hypokinesis, or dyskinesis of the left ventricular midsegments with or without apical involvement; the regional wall motion abnormalities extend beyond a single epicardial vascular distribution

Presence of a stressful trigger (often but not always)

Presence of new electrocardiographic abnormalities (ST-segment elevation or T-wave inversion [or both]) or modest elevation of cardiac troponin

Absence of obstructive coronary disease or angiographic evidence of acute plaque rupture

Absence of pheochromocytoma and myocarditis

Modified from Prasad A, Lerman A, Rihal CS. Apical ballooning syndrome (Tako-Tsubo or stress cardiomyopathy): a mimic of acute myocardial infarction. Am Heart J. 2008 Mar;155(3):408-17. Epub 2008 Jan 31; used with permission.

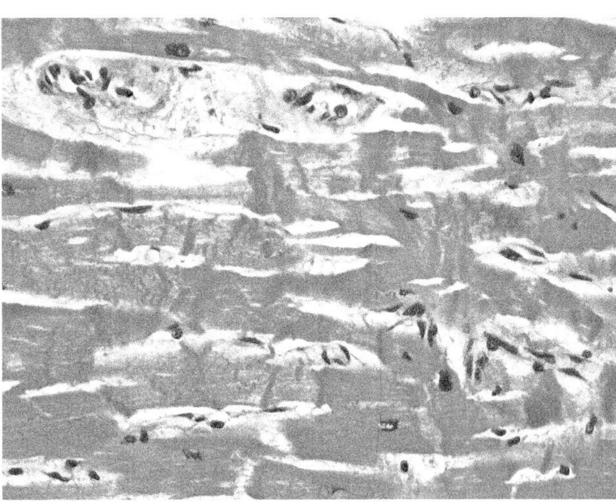

Figure 17.1. Contraction Band Necrosis in Takotsubo (Stress) Cardiomyopathy. (Hematoxylin-eosin, original magnification ×400.) (Courtesy of Melanie C. Bois, MD, Mayo Clinic, Rochester, Minnesota; used with permission.)

fulminant cardiogenic shock, syncope, or, rarely, cardiac arrest.

If an acute neurologic event results in coma and cardiac arrest, the primary neurologic abnormality may be overlooked initially while the patient is resuscitated and the patient's condition is stabilized. Emergent computed tomography of the head is warranted for a comatose patient with cardiac symptoms to evaluate for an underlying structural abnormality. If a comatose patient has unexplained symptoms (eg, hypotension or pulmonary edema) or atypical ECG changes, the patient should be evaluated for concurrent TC in addition to the primary neurologic condition.

Management

In mild cases of TC, conservative management and supportive care may be all that is required. The administration

Box 17.2 • Neurologic Conditions Associated With Takotsubo (Stress) Cardiomyopathy

Status epilepticus
Subarachnoid hemorrhage
Traumatic brain injury
Guillain-Barré syndrome
Intracerebral hemorrhage
Ischemic stroke
Meningitis and encephalitis
Myasthenia gravis
Multiple sclerosis

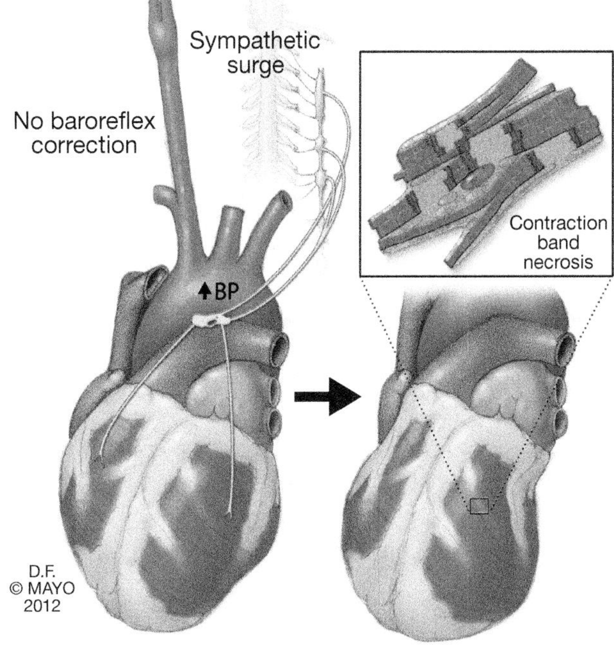

Figure 17.2. Takotsubo (Stress) Cardiomyopathy Mechanism. If the afferent baroreflex fails (left), the catecholamine surge remains uncontrolled and eventually causes apical ballooning (right). Arrow pointing up indicates increased; BP, blood pressure. (From Wijdicks EFM. Recognizing brain injury. Oxford [UK]: Oxford University Press; c2014. Chapter 7, Neurology of cardiac function; p. 91-103 [Core principles of acute neurology series]; used with permission.)

of angiotensin-converting enzyme inhibitors after TC may decrease the risk of recurrence. For patients with hypotension without pulmonary edema, judicious use of intravenous fluid boluses may be beneficial. If patients have ongoing hypotension or shock, they should be evaluated urgently for left ventricular outflow tract obstruction; management is dependent on the presence or absence of a dynamic obstruction.

For nonobstructive shock, inotropic agents (and rarely an intra-aortic balloon pump) may be required for ongoing management if normotension and end-organ perfusion cannot be maintained with vasopressors. Severe pulmonary edema may require diuretics to facilitate oxygenation. In select patients, short-term anticoagulation may also be considered to prevent or treat left ventricular thrombus formation, but if patients have an intracranial condition, these medications may be contraindicated.

Outcome

By definition, TC is a transient phenomenon. Given the variability in presentation, with some patients requiring only observation and others intensive interventions, the outcomes are dependent on the severity of the presentation and underlying comorbidity. Acute neurologic illness preceding the onset of TC is associated with an increased rate of in-hospital complications. Compared to patients without cardiogenic shock, patients with cardiogenic shock have longer hospitalization and higher mortality due to a cardiac cause. After TC, the rate of all-cause death was approximately 6% per patient-year, and the recurrence rate was about 2% per patient-year in a large registry of patients.

Other Cardiac Abnormalities in Neurologic Disease

In addition to TC, a spectrum of other cardiac abnormalities may occur with neurologic disease (Box 17.3): ECG changes, moderate troponin elevation with or without cardiac ischemia, tachyrhythmias or bradyrhythmias, atrial or ventricular arrhythmias, heart block, and, rarely, cardiac arrest.

At admission, a patient with neurologic disease may have various ECG abnormalities, symptomatic or asymptomatic, including prolongation of the corrected QT interval, T-wave abnormalities, ST-segment depression or elevation, and pathologic Q waves.

An initial troponin elevation is not uncommon in patients with neurologic disease, including subarachnoid hemorrhage, ischemic stroke, seizure and status epilepticus, and intracerebral hemorrhage, and has been independently associated with poor outcomes.

Cardiac arrest occurs uncommonly in acute neurologic disease and has been well described for patients with subarachnoid hemorrhage, who may present with cardiac arrest and coma, especially if they have high-grade hemorrhages. These patients also have an increased mortality risk and worse overall scores on the Glasgow Outcome Scale. In addition, these patients tend to present more commonly with nonshockable rhythms, but a small percentage may present with shockable ventricular arrhythmias.

Management of the cardiac abnormality depends on the severity of symptoms and whether the abnormality is sustained. Arrhythmias are the most commonly reported cardiac abnormalities in patients with neurologic disease and must be quickly recognized and addressed. Potential initial treatments for common arrhythmias are listed in Table 17.1.

Box 17.3 • Diagnostic Evaluation of Cardiac Responses to Neurologic Disease

- Cardiac enzymes—serum levels increasing moderately and then decreasing after the ictus
- Echocardiography—regional wall motion abnormality beyond a single vascular territory
- Electrocardiography—various abnormalities, including prolonged QT intervals, abnormal T waves, depressed or elevated ST segments, and pathologic Q waves
- Coronary angiography—normal coronary arteries
- Chest radiography—suggestive of pulmonary edema

Table 17.1 • Common Cardiac Arrhythmias and Initial Treatments

Arrhythmia	Initial Management
Sinus tachycardia	Administer fluid bolus Evaluate for underlying cause (eg, pain or infection)
Sinus bradycardia or atrioventricular block	If symptomatic, administer atropine and consider pacing
Atrial fibrillation	Optimize fluid status and electrolytes Control rate with β-blockade or calcium channel blockers
Multifocal atrial tachycardia	Correct electrolyte abnormalities Evaluate for other possible causes (eg, underlying primary cardiac or pulmonary disease)
Torsades de pointes	Administer magnesium sulfate
Ventricular tachycardia or ventricular fibrillation	Provide advanced cardiac life support

Summary

- Multiple cardiac abnormalities may occur in conjunction with acute neurologic disorders.
- TC is a relatively common occurrence in patients with acute catastrophic neurologic disease and recurrent seizures.
- TC has a variable presentation and should improve over time.
- TC can cause hypotension and ECG abnormalities, but it can also be detected only with echocardiography.

SUGGESTED READING

Abd TT, Hayek S, Cheng JW, Samuels OB, Wittstein IS, Lerakis S. Incidence and clinical characteristics of takotsubo cardiomyopathy post-aneurysmal subarachnoid hemorrhage. Int J Cardiol. 2014 Oct 20;176(3):1362–4. Epub 2014 Aug 6.

Akashi YJ, Goldstein DS, Barbaro G, Ueyama T. Takotsubo cardiomyopathy: a new form of acute, reversible heart failure. Circulation. 2008 Dec 16;118(25):2754–62.

Androdias G, Bernard E, Biotti D, Collongues N, Durand-Dubief F, Pique J, et al. Multiple sclerosis broke my heart. Ann Neurol. 2017 May;81(5):754–8. Epub 2017 May 9.

Brunetti ND, Santoro F, De Gennaro L, Correale M, Gaglione A, Di Biase M. Drug treatment rates with beta-blockers and ACE-inhibitors/angiotensin receptor blockers and recurrences in takotsubo cardiomyopathy: a meta-regression analysis. Int J Cardiol. 2016 Jul 1;214:340–2. Epub 2016 Apr 13.

Caretta G, Vizzardi E, Rovetta R, Evaristi L, Quinzani F, Raddino R, et al. The link between intracranial haemorrhage and cardiogenic shock: a case of Takotsubo cardiomyopathy. Acta Cardiol. 2012 Jun;67(3):363–5.

Davies KR, Gelb AW, Manninen PH, Boughner DR, Bisnaire D. Cardiac function in aneurysmal subarachnoid haemorrhage: a study of electrocardiographic and echocardiographic abnormalities. Br J Anaesth. 1991 Jul;67(1):58–63.

Diaz A, Nunez Gil IJ, Santoro F, Madias JE, Pelliccia F, Brunetti ND, et al. Takotsubo syndrome: state-of-the-art review by an expert panel—part 1. Cardiovasc Revasc Med. 2019 Jan;20(1):70–9.

Diaz A, Nunez Gil IJ, Santoro F, Madias JE, Pelliccia F, Brunetti ND, et al. Takotsubo syndrome: state-of-the-art review by an expert panel—part 2. Cardiovasc Revasc Med. 2019 Feb;20(2):153–66.

Finsterer J, Wahbi K. CNS-disease affecting the heart: brain-heart disorders. J Neurol Sci. 2014 Oct 15;345(1-2):8–14. Epub 2014 Jul 8.

Finsterer J, Wahbi K. CNS disease triggering Takotsubo stress cardiomyopathy. Int J Cardiol. 2014 Dec 15;177(2):322–9. Epub 2014 Aug 26.

Fure B, Bruun Wyller T, Thommessen B. Electrocardiographic and troponin T changes in acute ischaemic stroke. J Intern Med. 2006 Jun;259(6):592–7.

Garrett MC, Komotar RJ, Starke RM, Doshi D, Otten ML, Connolly ES. Elevated troponin levels are predictive of mortality in surgical intracerebral hemorrhage patients. Neurocrit Care. 2010 Apr;12(2):199–203. Epub 2009 Jul 21.

Hocker S, Prasad A, Rabinstein AA. Cardiac injury in refractory status epilepticus. Epilepsia. 2013 Mar;54(3):518–22. Epub 2012 Nov 13.

Komamura K, Fukui M, Iwasaku T, Hirotani S, Masuyama T. Takotsubo cardiomyopathy: pathophysiology, diagnosis and treatment. World J Cardiol. 2014 Jul 26;6(7):602–9.

Mitsuma W, Ito M, Kodama M, Takano H, Tomita M, Saito N, et al. Clinical and cardiac features of patients with subarachnoid haemorrhage presenting with out-of-hospital cardiac arrest. Resuscitation. 2011 Oct;82(10):1294–7. Epub 2011 Jul 20.

Lee VH, Oh JK, Mulvagh SL, Wijdicks EF. Mechanisms in neurogenic stress cardiomyopathy after aneurysmal subarachnoid hemorrhage. Neurocrit Care. 2006;5(3):243–9.

Oras J, Grivans C, Bartley A, Rydenhag B, Ricksten SE, Seeman-Lodding H. Elevated high-sensitive troponin T on admission is an indicator of poor long-term outcome in patients with subarachnoid haemorrhage: a prospective observational study. Crit Care. 2016 Jan 19;20:11.

Peddada K, Cruz-Flores S, Goldstein LB, Feen E, Kennedy KF, Heuring T, et al. Ischemic stroke with troponin elevation: patient characteristics, resource utilization, and in-hospital outcomes. Cerebrovasc Dis. 2016;42(3-4):213–23. Epub 2016 May 3.

Prasad A, Lerman A, Rihal CS. Apical ballooning syndrome (Tako-Tsubo or stress cardiomyopathy): a mimic of acute myocardial infarction. Am Heart J. 2008 Mar;155(3):408–17. Epub 2008 Jan 31.

Templin C, Ghadri JR, Diekmann J, Napp LC, Bataiosu DR, Jaguszewski M, et al. Clinical features and outcomes of Takotsubo (stress) cardiomyopathy. N Engl J Med. 2015 Sep 3;373(10):929–38.

Toussaint LG 3rd, Friedman JA, Wijdicks EF, Piepgras DG, Pichelmann MA, McIver JI, et al. Survival of cardiac arrest after aneurysmal subarachnoid hemorrhage. Neurosurgery. 2005 Jul;57(1):25–31.

Tsuchihashi K, Ueshima K, Uchida T, Oh-mura N, Kimura K, Owa M, et al; Angina Pectoris-Myocardial Infarction Investigations in Japan. Transient left ventricular apical ballooning without coronary artery stenosis: a novel heart syndrome mimicking acute myocardial infarction. J Am Coll Cardiol. 2001 Jul;38(1):11–8.

Wittstein IS, Thiemann DR, Lima JA, Baughman KL, Schulman SP, Gerstenblith G, et al. Neurohumoral features of myocardial stunning due to sudden emotional stress. N Engl J Med. 2005 Feb 10;352(6): 539–48.

18 Paroxysmal Sympathetic Hyperactivity

KEVIN T. GOBESKE, MD, PhD

Goals

- Understand the features of autonomic function after acute injury of the central nervous system.
- Identify components of sympathetic hyperactivity during paroxysmal events.
- Distinguish paroxysmal sympathetic hyperactivity from other illnesses in patients in the intensive care unit.
- Understand the relationship between proposed pathophysiologic mechanisms and treatment strategies.

Introduction

Paroxysmal sympathetic hyperactivity (PSH) is a form of acute dysautonomia that can occur after several types of acute (usually severe) structural brain injury. PSH typically occurs after traumatic brain injury (TBI) with diffuse axonal injury, yet it can also occur after aneurysmal subarachnoid hemorrhage, encephalitis, massive fat or air embolism, or profound anoxic-ischemic brain injury, often with each condition leading to prolonged unconsciousness. The development of PSH is associated with longer hospital stays, and it may be associated with increased mortality and worse outcomes. While the diagnostic criteria, treatment guidelines, and pathologic mechanisms underlying PSH have yet to be established, the need for early diagnosis and careful management of PSH is unmistakable.

Paroxysmal autonomic disturbances after acute brain injury have been recognized for nearly a century with various terms, including *paroxysmal autonomic storms, sympathetic storms,* and *paroxysmal autonomic instability with dystonia.* Recently, the term *PSH* has gained acceptance to ensure clarity and precision in communication and to distinguish this condition from autonomic dysreflexia due to spinal cord injury, adrenal crisis, or various toxidromes.

The diagnosis of PSH is based on clinical criteria consistent with symptoms from a potential common pathway for secondary injury progression resulting from various primary mechanisms. Although the development of PSH after a primary injury suggests that it may be a common secondary mechanism for progression of brain injury, its diagnosis is based on clinical criteria. In 2004, suggested criteria included severe brain injury (Rancho Los Amigos score ≥4); increased temperature (>38.5°C), heart rate (>130 beats per minute), and respiratory rate (>40 breaths per minute); agitation; diaphoresis; and dystonia, with at least 1 episode daily for 3 days. In 2014, a consensus paper established the conceptual definition and 11 primary criteria of PSH (Box 18.1), and a second paper tested the concordance between recorded diagnoses and the presence of at least 4 of 7 factors in patients with acute brain injury. Further validation of these criteria is necessary.

Pathogenesis

PSH involves central dysregulation of autonomic activity leading to diffuse systemic manifestations. It has been proposed that PSH may occur from "disconnection" injuries that remove the sympathoexcitatory effector pathways of the thalamus, hypothalamus, brainstem, and spinal cord from higher-order inhibitory control by diencephalic and cortical networks. An updated disconnection theory proposes that a larger imbalance in the excitatory-inhibitory ratio sensitizes inputs at excitatory autonomic centers by disrupting the tonic inhibitory drive from diffuse higher regions.

Patients with TBI accompanied by considerable hemorrhage or diffuse axonal injury may have the highest rates of PSH, and children may be more susceptible than adults. Although direct injury to the diencephalon is not necessary for PSH to develop, rates may be higher when hemorrhage, inflammation, or trauma involves the diencephalon.

Box 18.1 • Consensus Criteria for Key Features Most Consistently Identified With Paroxysmal Sympathetic Hyperactivity

- Develop after an acute brain injury
- Are paroxysmal
- Occur simultaneously
- Persist despite treatment of potential alternative diagnoses
- Sympathetic overactivity to stimuli that are normally nonpainful
- Absence of parasympathetic features during paroxysms
- Persist ≥3 consecutive days
- Persist ≥2 weeks after the injury
- Occur during ≥2 episodes daily
- Use of medications to manage sympathetic features
- Lack of alternative explanations

Clinical Features

Signs and symptoms of PSH include tachycardia, hypertension, tachypnea, hyperthermia, diaphoresis, and increased muscle tone. Pupillary dilatation, piloerection, altered gastrointestinal tract activity, and agitation may also occur. Parasympathetic features are characteristically absent. The cardinal features of PSH overlap considerably with those of other conditions affecting patients with neurologic injury in the intensive care unit (eg, sepsis, pulmonary embolism, airway obstruction, seizures, serotonin syndrome or neuroleptic malignant syndrome, withdrawal, or other toxidromes).

Unlike other diagnoses involving autonomic dysregulation, PSH is defined in relation to a preceding acute neurologic injury that is usually catastrophic. Although PSH may occur within 72 hours after injury onset, PSH typically begins within the first 2 weeks after the injury and may occur as long as 1 to 2 months afterward. PSH often persists for longer than 1 to 2 weeks after the injury, especially if diagnosis and treatment are delayed. Symptoms of PSH are episodic, with nearly complete resolution between paroxysms. The onset of clinical symptoms is paroxysmal, with co-occurrence of multiple sympathetic features, and is triggered by stimuli that normally would not yield such a response. Usually more than 2 episodes occur per day for at least 3 consecutive days.

Management

The general assumption is that better outcomes are associated with prompt recognition of paroxysmal sympathetic hyperactivity and initiation of treatment. Management of PSH can be guided by the notion that patients with PSH have abnormal sensitization to stimuli that may trigger sympathetic activity. Treatment should break the feedback cycle leading to exaggerated sympathoexcitatory responses, so management strategies logically target aggressive pain control, central sympathetic inhibition, and neuromodulation at the level of synaptic and circuit plasticity (Table 18.1).

Multidimensional management of PSH involves excluding any mimicking conditions, ensuring adequate hydration, and minimizing triggers. Pharmacologic interventions can be categorized as abortive or preventive. Intravenous

Table 18.1 • Pharmacologic Treatment of Paroxysmal Sympathetic Hyperactivity

Agent	Indication	Site of Action	Type of Medication	Main Effect
Morphine[a]	Abortive	Central	Opiate	Control paroxysms
Baclofen, benzodiazepines	Abortive, preventive	Central and peripheral	GABAergic	Mute the balance of excitation and inhibition
Dantrolene	Preventive	Peripheral	Calcium ion release blocker	Blunt feedback from spasms
Propranolol[a]	Preventive	Central	β-Antagonist sympatholytic	Blunt sympathetic activity
Clonidine, dexmedetomidine	Preventive	Central	α_2-Agonist sympatholytic	Blunt sympathetic activity
Bromocriptine	Preventive	Central	Dopamine agonist	Blunt dystonias and fever
Gabapentin[a]	Modulatory	Central	Calcium signaling, GABAergic	Limit hypersensitivity
Niaprazine	Modulatory	Central	Multiple targets	Limit hypersensitivity

Abbreviation: GABA, γ-aminobutyric acid.

[a] Preferred treatment option.

morphine is the preferred abortive agent for paroxysms of hyperalgesia and sympathetic activity. Whether opiates abort episodes of PSH by treating pain or through other central mechanisms is not known. However, an intravenous morphine bolus (2-4 mg) is so effective in improving ongoing symptoms of PSH that its failure to abate an acute episode should cause doubts about the diagnosis of PSH. Baclofen may be a useful adjunct for controlling hypertonicity.

Propranolol, a centrally acting nonselective β-blocker, is the most commonly used preventive medication for PSH. Clonidine and dexmedetomidine are central α_2-receptor agonists that can also be beneficial by reducing sympathetic outflow. Benzodiazepines may help mute the initiation of sympathetic surges when high levels of morphine are already being provided and to help manage dystonia and posturing. Gabapentin also influences γ-aminobutyric acid (GABA)-ergic activity that might similarly quell sympathetic drive, but its main effect may be sensitization through actions at the alpha-2-delta subunit of voltage-gated calcium channels (and other targets). Niaprizine, with α_2-receptor sympatholytic and other modulatory properties, has shown benefit in PSH in European studies.

Summary

- *Paroxysmal sympathetic hyperactivity* (*PSH*) is the preferred term for persistent, repeated episodes of increased sympathetic activation.
- PSH includes episodes of tachycardia, hypertension, diaphoresis, hyperthermia, tachypnea, and dystonia or posturing that is triggered by stimuli that normally would not be sufficient to produce such a response.
- PSH can arise after multiple types of severe brain injuries that can lead to impaired regulation of the cortical-diencephalic-brainstem circuits that modulate autonomic activity.
- Patients with PSH after acute brain injury have longer hospital stays and worse outcomes.
- Treatment of PSH is oral gabapentin in incremental doses; intravenous morphine is used for acute episodes.
- The goal of early recognition and treatment of PSH is to prevent it from becoming refractory and being triggered by increasingly minor stimuli.

SUGGESTED READING

Baguley IJ, Perkes IE, Fernandez-Ortega JF, Rabinstein AA, Dolce G, Hendricks HT; Consensus Working Group. Paroxysmal sympathetic hyperactivity after acquired brain injury: consensus on conceptual definition, nomenclature, and diagnostic criteria. J Neurotrauma. 2014 Sep 1;31(17):1515–20. Epub 2014 Jul 28.

Compton E. Paroxysmal sympathetic hyperactivity syndrome following traumatic brain injury. Nurs Clin N Am. 2018;53:459–67.

Fernandez-Ortega JF, Baguley IJ, Gates TA, Garcia-Caballero M, Quesada-Garcia JG, Prieto-Palomino MA. Catecholamines and paroxysmal sympathetic hyperactivity after traumatic brain injury. J Neurotrauma. 2017 Jan 1;34(1):109–14. Epub 2016 Jul 8.

Hughes JD, Rabinstein AA. Early diagnosis of paroxysmal sympathetic hyperactivity in the ICU. Neurocrit Care. 2014 Jun;20(3):454–9.

Mathew MJ, Deepika A, Shukla D, Devi BI, Ramesh VJ. Paroxysmal sympathetic hyperactivity in severe traumatic brain injury. Acta Neurochir (Wien). 2016 Nov;158(11):2047–52. Epub 2016 Aug 31.

Rabinstein AA. Paroxysmal sympathetic hyperactivity in the neurological intensive care unit. Neurol Res. 2007 Oct;29(7):680–2.

Rabinstein AA, Benarroch EE. Treatment of paroxysmal sympathetic hyperactivity. Curr Treat Options Neurol. 2008 Mar;10(2):151–7.

Takahashi C, Hinson HE, Baguley IJ. Autonomic dysfunction syndromes after acute brain injury. Handb Clin Neurol. 2015;128:539–51.

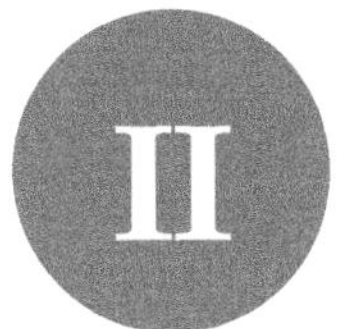

Questions and Answers

Abbreviations Used

ALS amyotrophic lateral sclerosis
ARDS acute respiratory distress syndrome
CBF cerebral blood flow
CMR cerebral metabolic rate
CSF cerebrospinal fluid
CT computed tomographic
DWI diffusion-weighted imaging
EEG electroencephalogram
GBS Guillain-Barré syndrome
HTS hypertonic saline
ICP intracranial pressure
ICU intensive care unit
IV intravenous
MAP mean arterial pressure
MRI magnetic resonance imaging
PLED periodic lateralizing epileptiform discharge
PRES posterior reversible encephalopathy syndrome
PSH paroxysmal sympathetic hyperactivity
SSEP somatosensory evoked potential
TBI traumatic brain injury

Questions

Multiple Choice (choose the best answer)

II.1. Where should you localize the lesion in a patient who has an acute traumatic spinal cord injury with paraplegia and a sensory level at the navel?
 a. T4
 b. T6
 c. T10
 d. C4

II.2. If a patient had hemianopia with alexia without agraphia, where would the lesion be located?
 a. Left occipital lobe
 b. Right occipital lobe
 c. Left temporal lobe
 d. Right temporal lobe

II.3. A patient is suddenly comatose. The examination shows anisocoria, pinpoint pupils, and extensor posturing. CT findings are normal. What is the most likely diagnosis?
 a. Intoxication with opioids
 b. Embolus to the basilar artery
 c. Brain herniation from early cerebral edema
 d. Postictal state after seizure

II.4. Which situation does *not* cause acute eye deviation to the left?
 a. Acute lesion in the left hemisphere
 b. Seizures from the right hemisphere
 c. Acute lesion in the brainstem
 d. Acute lesion in the cerebellum

II.5. Which clinical sign indicates displacement of the pons with an acute cerebellar lesion?
 a. Downward gaze
 b. Ptosis
 c. Nystagmus
 d. Bradycardia

II.6. Which of the following is used to treat refractory increased ICP?
 a. High-dose corticosteroids
 b. Prolonged hyperventilation
 c. HTS
 d. Decompressive craniotomy

II.7. Which statement correctly describes the use of osmotic diuretics to treat increased ICP?
 a. A 23% sodium chloride solution and 25% mannitol have a similar sodium content.
 b. A continuous infusion of 20% mannitol is better than a bolus.
 c. HTS is preferable to mannitol in patients with heart failure.
 d. The usual starting dose of 20% mannitol is 1 g/kg.

II.8. Which characteristic best fits with the intracranial pressure-volume curve?
 a. Initial flat segment and final steep segment with break point at 20 mm Hg
 b. Initial flat segment and final steep segment with break point at 40 mm Hg
 c. Steep for elderly patients
 d. Linear for young adult patients

II.9. What distinguishes mannitol from HTS?
 a. Potent diuretic
 b. Risk of cardiac failure
 c. Risk of infusion phlebitis
 d. Hypervolemic hypernatremia

II.10. Which disorder does *not* necessarily increase ICP?
a. Diffuse cerebral edema
b. Rapidly expanding brain tumor
c. Ongoing seizures
d. Cerebral venous thrombosis

II.11. Which innervation to the choroid plexus results in decreased production of CSF?
a. Sympathetic
b. Parasympathetic
c. Muscarinic
d. Nicotinic

II.12. What composes the blood-CSF barrier?
a. Astrocytic foot processes
b. Pial layer
c. Choroid plexus epithelial cells
d. Ependymal cells of the ventricle

II.13. A patient with a hypoglycemic encephalopathy undergoes a lumbar puncture. What is the normal ratio of CSF glucose to serum glucose?
a. 1
b. 0.8
c. 0.6
d. 0.2

II.14. What is the most common neoplastic source to metastasize to the CSF?
a. Lung cancer
b. Osteosarcoma
c. Chondrosarcoma
d. Renal cell carcinoma

II.15. After an infection, which CSF parameter takes the longest to recover to baseline?
a. Leukocyte count
b. Erythrocyte count
c. Protein
d. Glucose

II.16. Choose the correct anastomotic pair promoting successful collateral cerebral blood circulation from the internal carotid artery branch to the external carotid artery branch.
a. Ophthalmic artery—anterior communicating artery
b. Ophthalmic artery—middle meningeal artery
c. Anterior choroidal artery—anterior communicating artery
d. Anterior choroidal artery—superficial temporal artery

II.17. Which of the following statements does *not* describe the circle of Willis?
a. It is a vascular hexagonal ring where the anterior and posterior circulations meet.
b. The posterior communicating arteries are the major vessels connecting the anterior and posterior circulations.
c. The superior cerebellar artery is not a normal component of the circle of Willis.
d. The circle of Willis is wholly patent in almost all patients.

II.18. As the blood oxygen partial pressure *decreases*, what happens to CBF?
a. CBF decreases linearly.
b. CBF is unchanged for all oxygen partial pressures.
c. CBF is unchanged until hypoxia ensues.
d. CBF increases linearly.

II.19. Which of the following drugs *increases* CBF in patients receiving mechanical ventilation?
a. Ketamine
b. Propofol
c. Dexmedetomidine
d. Midazolam

II.20. Which of the following is *not* a region of the brain that is particularly susceptible to anoxic-ischemic injury?
a. Putamen
b. Neocortex
c. Supplemental motor area
d. Cerebellar Purkinje cells

II.21. How long might it take for the effects of IV fentanyl (intermittent dose) to be eliminated in a patient with normal kidney and liver function?
a. Up to 5 hours
b. Up to 10 hours
c. Up to 25 hours
d. Up to 50 hours

II.22. Which finding is the most reliable predictor of a poor outcome for a comatose patient after resuscitation?
a. Absence of pupillary light reflexes
b. Absence of corneal reflexes
c. Absence of motor response to noxious stimulation
d. Absence of facial grimace

II.23. Among patients who have been comatose after resuscitation, what percentage have good outcomes with DWI abnormalities on brain MRI?
a. 5% to 10%
b. 20% to 50%
c. 60% to 80%
d. 90% to 100%

II.24. In SSEP testing of comatose patients after cardiac arrest, the absence of which electrical response is predictive of an invariably poor neurologic outcome?
a. N13
b. P14
c. N18
d. N20

II.25. If a patient has symptomatic hyponatremia, what is the recommended correction for the serum sodium level in the first 24 hours?
a. No more than 5 mmol/L
b. No more than 8 mmol/L
c. No more than 10 mmol/L
d. No more than 12 mmol/L

II.26. Which of the following is a risk factor for the development of PRES?
a. Advanced age
b. Tacrolimus
c. Hypotension from blood loss
d. Chronic liver failure

II.27. For treating a patient with hypertension-induced PRES, which of the following is the target decrease in MAP?
a. 5% to 10%
b. 10% to 15%
c. 15% to 20%
d. 20% to 25%

II.28. A 70-year-old patient receiving long-term dialysis presents with a severe headache, confusion, and blurred vision. The CT scan shows posterior hypodensities consistent with PRES. At hospital admission, the patient's blood pressure is 250/120 mm Hg, and previous readings were nearly identical. What antihypertensive agent is preferred?
a. Nicardipine IV
b. Nitroprusside IV
c. Lisinopril orally
d. Methyldopa IV

II.29. A 64-year-old woman with a history of major depression is found unresponsive at home by a family member and brought to an emergency department. On evaluation, her vital signs are as follows: blood pressure, 92/60 mm Hg; heart rate, 124 beats per minute; respiratory rate, 12 breaths per minute; and temperature, 37°C. She is comatose. Her skin is warm and dry, her lungs are clear, and her heart rate is rapid. On neurologic examination, her eyelids open to noxious stimuli. Her pupils are symmetrical (6 mm in diameter) and have light responses. Corneal and oculocephalic reflexes are present. She withdraws all 4 extremities symmetrically to nailbed pressure. Her capillary glucose is within the reference range. According to these clinical examination findings, where is the brain dysfunction localized?

a. Pons (intrinsic brainstem)
b. Midbrain (intrinsic brainstem)
c. Both cerebral hemispheres
d. Brainstem displacement secondary to unilateral hemispheric lesion

II.30. For the patient decribed in the previous question, which medication is most likely responsible for the clinical findings?

a. Insulin
b. Oxycodone
c. Amitriptyline
d. Gabapentin

II.31. A 62-year-old man with a history of coronary artery disease, hypertension, and dyslipidemia is in the hospital recovering from an uncomplicated mitral valve repair operation. Two days postoperatively, he suddenly loses consciousness while sitting up in bed. On evaluation, his blood pressure is 217/104 mm Hg. His eyelids remain closed to noxious stimulation. His right eye is slightly higher than the left, and the right pupil is 1 mm larger than the left. Both pupils react to light. Corneal reflex is absent on the right and present on the left. He has extensor posturing of both upper extremities to pressure applied at the temporal mandibular joints. He is intubated for airway protection and hemodynamically stabilized. Emergent noncontrast CT of the head shows no abnormalities. What is the next most appropriate action?

a. Order a routine neurologic consultation.
b. Transfer the patient to the ICU for observation.
c. Administer aspirin.
d. Order an emergent CT angiogram of the head and neck.

II.32. A 52-year-old woman with an unremarkable past medical history is admitted to the hospital for "altered mental status." Her husband reports that she had some abdominal discomfort and several episodes of nausea and vomiting in the preceding days. The paramedics noted that she had a single generalized tonic-clonic seizure en route to the hospital. On examination, her temperature is 38.6°C, and her heart rate is 107 beats per minute. She is drowsy, requiring tactile stimulation to open her eyes. Brainstem reflexes are preserved, and there are no lateralizing features on motor examination. An emergent EEG shows PLEDs. Which of the following diagnoses is the most likely?

a. Herpes simplex encephalitis
b. Acute ischemic stroke
c. Metabolic encephalopathy
d. Opioid overdose

II.33. A 46-year-old woman with hypertension and a long-standing smoking history collapses at work. Paramedics are called and find the patient comatose, but she quickly starts to rouse and by the time she arrives at the hospital (within 1 hour after the witnessed collapse), she can answer questions. She is fully oriented and complains of an excruciating global headache. Her blood pressure is 146/90 mm Hg, she has a regular heart rate of 84 beats per minute, and her temperature is 36.5°C. Neurologic examination findings are nonfocal. Noncontrast CT of the head shows no acute abnormality. MRI of the brain cannot be performed until the next day. Which of the following is the most appropriate next step?

a. Treat her headache with analgesic medications, and arrange for outpatient clinical follow-up.
b. Perform a CSF examination immediately.
c. Observe for 5 hours before further testing.
d. Arrange for an EEG to be performed.

II.34. Which of the following is the most common cause of neuromuscular respiratory failure in a general ICU?

a. Critical illness polyneuropathy
b. Myasthenia gravis
c. Lambert-Eaton syndrome
d. Hypokalemia

II.35. Which of the following findings in a patient with neuromuscular weakness indicates the need for urgent intubation?

a. Dysphagia
b. Tachypnea with a normal Pco_2
c. Respiratory alkalosis
d. Dysautonomia

II.36. Which of the following is *not* a clinical sign of neuromuscular respiratory failure?

a. Tachypnea
b. Outward movement of the abdomen with deep inspiration
c. Forehead sweating
d. Use of accessory inspiratory muscles

II.37. Which of the following is *not* a major determinant in deciding whether urgent intubation is needed in patients with neuromuscular weakness and failing respiratory mechanics?

a. Clinical examination findings
b. Arterial blood gas results
c. Bedside pulmonary function test results
d. Underlying cause

II.38. In patients with neuromuscular respiratory failure, which of the following is *not* assessed with diaphragmatic ultrasonography?

a. Atrophy
b. Mobility
c. Synchrony
d. Denervation

II.39. Persistent neurogenic hyperventilation is most characteristically associated with which of the following?

a. Brainstem tumor
b. Intoxication
c. Brain herniation
d. Seizures

II.40. Which of the following does *not* characterize acute neurogenic breathing patterns caused by brainstem lesions?

a. Hyperventilation
b. Gasping or inspiratory breath-holding
c. Crescendo-decrescendo pattern
d. Stridor

II.41. Which patient has the highest risk for takotsubo cardiomyopathy?

a. A 35-year-old woman
b. A 35-year-old man
c. A 65-year-old woman
d. A 65-year-old man

II.42. What is the common pathologic finding on histologic evaluation of the myocardium in patients with takotsubo cardiomyopathy?

a. Neutrophilic infiltration
b. Contraction band necrosis
c. Cardiomyocyte autophagy
d. Apoptosis

II.43. Which of the following conditions has the highest rate of association with PSH?

a. Subarachnoid hemorrhage
b. TBI with diffuse axonal injury
c. TBI with subdural hemorrhage
d. Hemorrhagic stroke

II.44. Which of the following is the first-line therapy for severe paroxysms during PSH?

a. Propranolol
b. Gabapentin
c. Morphine
d. Lorazepam

Answers

II.1. Answer c.

Finding a sensory level is difficult and often time-consuming, but several important landmarks point to a level (eg, navel [T10], nipples [T4]).

Ropper AH, Samuels MA, Klein JP. Adams and Victor's principles of neurology. 10th ed. New York (NY): McGraw-Hill Education Medical; c2014. 1654 p.

II.2. Answer a.

This is a characteristic localization, and the lesion must be in the left occipital lobe. Alexia without agraphia is also know as pure alexia or word blindness.

Ropper AH, Samuels MA, Klein JP. Adams and Victor's principles of neurology. 10th ed. New York (NY): McGraw-Hill Education Medical; c2014. 1654 p.

II.3. Answer b.

Embolus to the basilar artery is most likely. With anisocoria and decorticate posturing, the patient has a lesion in the brainstem. These clinical findings are not seen with opioid overdose, which is a common consideration in any patient with small pupils.

Wijdicks EFM. The comatose patient. 2nd ed. Oxford (UK): Oxford University Press; c2014. 784 p.

II.4. Answer d.

Eye deviation to the left does not indicate an acute lesion in the cerebellum. With an acute lesion in the left hemisphere, the eyes move toward the lesion. With seizures, the eyes move away from the lesion.

Ropper AH, Samuels MA, Klein JP. Adams and Victor's principles of neurology. 10th ed. New York (NY): McGraw-Hill Education Medical; c2014. 1654 p.

II.5. Answer d.

Bradycardia indicates displacement of the pons with an acute cerebellar lesion. The other signs are due to primary lesions (ptosis and nystagmus) or hydrocephalus (downward gaze).

Wijdicks EFM. The comatose patient. 2nd ed. Oxford (UK): Oxford University Press; c2014. 784 p.

II.6. Answer d.

If ICP does not decrease with the usual interventions, a large bone flap must be removed, allowing brain swelling to occur without the confinement of the skull, thereby reducing ICP.

Bor-Seng-Shu E, Figueiredo EG, Amorim RL, Teixeira MJ, Valbuza JS, de Oliveira MM, et al. Decompressive craniectomy: a meta-analysis of influences on intracranial pressure and cerebral perfusion pressure in the treatment of traumatic brain injury. J Neurosurg. 2012 Sep;117(3):589–96. Epub 2012 Jul 13.

II.7. Answer d.

There are marked differences in sodium content between 23% HTS and mannitol. The best management option is to administer mannitol in a 1-g/kg dose, with a half dose for maintenance therapy and HTS if mannitol does not control ICP.

Kamel H, Navi BB, Nakagawa K, Hemphill JC 3rd, Ko NU. Hypertonic saline versus mannitol for the treatment of elevated intracranial pressure: a meta-analysis of randomized clinical trials. Crit Care Med. 2011 Mar;39(3):554–9.

II.8. Answer a.

The pressure-volume curve is determined largely by the brain tissue component. The curve is steep when there is little atrophy in younger patients. In most circumstances, ICP increases rapidly after it reaches 20 mm Hg.

Ropper AH. Hyperosmolar therapy for raised intracranial pressure. N Engl J Med. 2012 Aug 23;367(8):746–52.

II.9. Answer a.

Mannitol may have a diuresis volume 5 times greater than the volume administered. Potential concerns are hypernatremia and hypovolemia from free water loss.

Todd MM. Hyperosmolar therapy and the brain: a hundred years of hard-earned lessons. Anesthesiology. 2013 Apr;118(4):777–9.

II.10. Answer b.

Brain tumors expand and move brain tissue, but clinical signs are not a consequence of increased ICP unless massive hemorrhage is involved.

Jo JT, Schiff D. Management of neuro-oncologic emergencies. Handb Clin Neurol. 2017;141:715–41.

II.11. Answer a.

Sympathetic choroid plexus input decreases CSF production, whereas parasympathetic input increases CSF production.

Sullivan HG, Allison JD. Physiology of cerebrospinal fluid. In: Wilkins, RH, Rengahary SS, editors. Neurosurgery. Vol. 3. New York (NY): McGraw-Hill; c1985. p. 2125–35.

II.12. Answer c.

The blood-CSF barrier is made of choroid plexus epithelium that lies between choroidal arteries and the CSF.

Lyons MK, Meyer FB. Cerebrospinal fluid physiology and the management of increased intracranial pressure. Mayo Clin Proc. 1990 May;65(5):684–707.

II.13. Answer c.

The normal ratio of CSF glucose to serum glucose is 0.6.

Fishman RA. Cerebrospinal fluid in diseases of the nervous system. Philadelphia (PA): Saunders; c1980. 384 p.

II.14. Answer a.

The most common cancers to metastasize to the brain include melanoma, lung cancer, and breast cancer.

Sullivan HG, Allison JD. Physiology of cerebrospinal fluid. In: Wilkins, RH, Rengahary SS, editors. Neurosurgery. Vol. 3. New York (NY): McGraw-Hill; c1985. p. 2125–35.

II.15. Answer c.

An increased CSF protein level may persist for months and should not be used as a marker for successful antimicrobial therapy.

Fishman RA. Cerebrospinal fluid in diseases of the nervous system. Philadelphia (PA): Saunders; c1980. 384 p.

II.16. Answer b.

The ophthalmic artery is commonly known to anastomose with the middle meningeal artery. The anterior communicating and anterior choroidal arteries lie within the subarachnoid space and do not originate from the external carotid artery. The superficial temporal artery derives from the external carotid artery, but it commonly anastomoses with the supraorbital artery, which branches from the internal carotid artery.

Hayreh SS. Orbital vascular anatomy. Eye (Lond). 2006 Oct;20(10):1130–44.

II.17. Answer d.

The circle of Willis is patent in less than half of all patients. The other answers are correct.

Iqbal S. A comprehensive study of the anatomical variations of the circle of Willis in adult human brains. J Clin Diagn Res. 2013 Nov;7(11):2423–7. Epub 2013 Nov 10.

Krabbe-Hartkamp MJ, van der Grond J, de Leeuw FE, de Groot JC, Algra A, Hillen B, et al. Circle of Willis: morphologic variation on three-dimensional time-of-flight MR angiograms. Radiology. 1998 Apr;207(1):103–11.

II.18. Answer c.

During relative normoxia, changes in blood oxygen partial pressure do not affect CBF. However, during hypoxia, CBF increases in a rapid dose-dependent, nonlinear manner in response to further decreases in blood oxygen partial pressure.

Doppenberg EM, Zauner A, Bullock R, Ward JD, Fatouros PP, Young HF. Correlations between brain tissue oxygen tension, carbon dioxide tension, pH, and cerebral blood flow: a better way of monitoring the severely injured brain? Surg Neurol. 1998 Jun;49(6):650–4.

II.19. Answer a.

Propofol, dexmedetomidine, opioids, etomidate, barbiturates, and benzodiazepines decrease CBF. This decrease results from a drug-induced decrease in CMR because changes in CBF and CMR are coupled. In patients receiving mechanical ventilation, arterial carbon dioxide tension is held constant, whereas in spontaneously ventilating patients, drug-induced decreases in ventilation can cause an increase in arterial carbon dioxide tension and an increase in CBF that can offset the decrease in CBF caused by the drug. Ketamine causes an increase in CBF in humans, especially in frontotemporal regions of the brain. ICP is not greatly affected by ketamine, possibly because of differential effects on CBF and cerebral blood volume.

Wang X, Ding X, Tong Y, Zong J, Zhao X, Ren H, et al. Ketamine does not increase intracranial pressure compared with opioids: meta-analysis of randomized controlled trials. J Anesth. 2014 Dec;28(6):821–7. Epub 2014 May 24.

Zeiler FA, Sader N, Gillman LM, Teitelbaum J, West M, Kazina CJ. The cerebrovascular response to ketamine: a systematic review of the animal and human literature. J Neurosurg Anesthesiol. 2016 Apr;28(2):123–40.

II.20. Answer c.

Regions of the brain that are especially vulnerable include the basal ganglia (eg, caudate and putamen), hippocampus, neocortex, and cerebellar Purkinje cells.

Fugate JE, Wijdicks EFM. Anoxic-ischemic encephalopathy. In: Daroff RB, Jankovic J, Mazziotta JC, Pomeroy SL, editors. Bradley's neurology in clinical practice. 7th ed. Vol. 2. London (UK): Elsevier; c2016. p. 1201–8.

Maramattom BV, Wijdicks EF. Postresuscitation encephalopathy: current views, management, and prognostication. Neurologist. 2005 Jul;11(4):234–43.

II.21. Answer c.

Under normal physiologic circumstances, it takes 4 to 5 half-lives for a drug to be completely eliminated. The elimination half-life of fentanyl is 2 to 5 hours, so elimination could take up to 25 hours (5×5 hours). If the drug is given as an infusion, the half-life is prolonged because of the large volume of distribution.

Fassoulaki A, Theodoraki K, Melemeni A. Pharmacology of sedation agents and reversal agents. Digestion. 2010;82(2):80–3. Epub 2010 Apr 21.

Part V: General principles of management of critically ill neurologic patients in the neurosciences intensive care unit. In: Wijdicks EFM. The practice of emergency and critical care neurology. 2nd ed. New York (NY): Oxford University Press; c2016. p. 157–268.

II.22. Answer a.

The absence of pupillary light reflexes is the most reliable examination finding for predicting a poor outcome. Corneal reflexes and motor responses can be affected by the lingering effects of sedative and analgesic medications, so they have higher false-positive rates, especially within the first 72 hours. Facial grimace has not been systematically studied as a prognostic indicator.

Fugate JE, Wijdicks EF, Mandrekar J, Claassen DO, Manno EM, White RD, et al. Predictors of neurologic outcome in hypothermia after cardiac arrest. Ann Neurol. 2010 Dec;68(6):907–14.

Kamps MJ, Horn J, Oddo M, Fugate JE, Storm C, Cronberg T, et al. Prognostication of neurologic outcome in cardiac arrest patients after mild therapeutic hypothermia: a meta-analysis of the current literature. Intensive Care Med. 2013 Oct;39(10):1671–82. Epub 2013 Jun 26.

II.23. Answer b.

Brain MRI has not been validated by prospective studies for prognosticating for comatose patients after cardiac arrest, but it is commonly used. Several studies have shown that DWI abnormalities (of various degrees) are found in up to 20% to 50% of patients who have good outcomes. On the contrary, some patients with normal MRI scans have poor outcomes.

Choi SP, Park KN, Park HK, Kim JY, Youn CS, Ahn KJ, et al. Diffusion-weighted magnetic resonance imaging for predicting the clinical outcome of comatose survivors after cardiac arrest: a cohort study. Crit Care. 2010;14(1):R17. Epub 2010 Feb 12.

Greer D, Scripko P, Bartscher J, Sims J, Camargo E, Singhal A, et al. Clinical MRI interpretation for outcome prediction in cardiac arrest. Neurocrit Care. 2012 Oct;17(2):240–4.

II.24. Answer d.

SSEP testing with stimulation at the median nerve is one of the most reliable ancillary tests for predicting poor outcomes for comatose patients after cardiac arrest. The bilateral absence of cortical responses (N20) has been found to have a false-positive rate of 0% (95% CI, 0%-3%) for predicting poor outcomes in this population.

Greer DM. Cardiac arrest and postanoxic encephalopathy. Continuum (Minneap Minn). 2015 Oct;21(5 Neurocritical Care):1384–96.

Zandbergen EG, Hijdra A, Koelman JH, Hart AA, Vos PE, Verbeek MM, et al; PROPAC Study Group. Prediction of poor outcome within the first 3 days of postanoxic coma. Neurology. 2006 Jan 10;66(1):62–8. Erratum in: Neurology. 2006 Apr 11;66(7):1133.

II.25. Answer c.

The current recommendation states that in the first 24 hours, the serum sodium level should not be increased by more than 10 mmol/L until the sodium level reaches 130 mmol/L.

Spasovski G, Vanholder R, Allolio B, Annane D, Ball S, Bichet D, et al. Clinical practice guideline on diagnosis and treatment of hyponatraemia. Intensive Care Med. 2014 Mar;40(3):320–31.

II.26. Answer b.

Antirejection medications and immunosuppressant medications (including some chemotherapeutic agents) have been shown to increase the risk of PRES. Older adults do not have an increased risk for PRES independently, and children may be affected by this disorder. Hypertension, as opposed to hypotension, is a known risk factor. (A caveat is that sepsis with distributed shock may cause PRES.) Renal failure (often with uncontrolled hypertension) is a risk factor (liver failure is not a risk factor).

Fugate JE, Rabinstein AA. Posterior reversible encephalopathy syndrome: clinical and radiological manifestations, pathophysiology, and outstanding questions. Lancet Neurol. 2015 Sep;14(9):914–25.

Kwon S, Koo J, Lee S. Clinical spectrum of reversible posterior leukoencephalopathy syndrome. Pediatr Neurol. 2001 May;24(5):361–4.

II.27. Answer d.

Decreasing MAP by 20% to 25% of the MAP at initial presentation is a reasonable goal in managing hypertension-induced PRES.

Ruland S, Aiyagari V. Cerebral autoregulation and blood pressure lowering. Hypertension. 2007 May;49(5):977–8. Epub 2007 Mar 12.

II.28. Answer a.

Nicardipine provides more stable blood pressure control than intermittent IV boluses. Oral doses should never be used initially. Other drugs are rarely used or take too long to take effect.

Ipek E, Oktay AA, Krim SR. Hypertensive crisis: an update on clinical approach and management. Curr Opin Cardiol. 2017 Jul;32(4):397–406.

II.29. Answer c.

Both cerebral hemispheres are involved. The neurologic examination of a patient with a bihemispheric syndrome characteristically lacks lateralizing features and shows fully preserved brainstem reflexes. The preservation of brainstem reflexes argues against a condition that is primarily or secondarily causing brainstem injury.

Wijdicks EFM. The comatose patient. 2nd ed. Oxford (UK): Oxford University Press; c2014. 784 p.

II.30. Answer c.

Amitriptyline is most likely. A history of psychiatric problems or suicide attempts in a comatose patient with a bihemispheric syndrome should raise suspicion for a toxic ingestion. Hot, flushed, dry skin is typically seen with anticholinergic toxidromes, such as an overdose of tricyclic antidepressants.

Hoffman RS, Howland MA, Lewin NA, Nelson LS, Goldfrank LR, Flomenbaum NE, editors. Goldfrank's toxicologic emergencies. 10th ed. New York (NY): McGraw-Hill Education; c2015. 1882 p.

II.31. Answer d.

Emergent CT angiography of the head and neck should be ordered. If the brainstem is involved, cranial nerve abnormalities are frequently observed. These can include skew deviation (misalignment of eyes in the vertical plane), anisocoria, and absence or asymmetry of pupillary, corneal, or oculocephalic reflexes. The motor response may be withdrawal or extensor. This acutely comatose patient had cerebrovascular risk factors and was markedly hypertensive. He had abnormal findings on cranial nerve examination, extensor posturing, and normal findings on CT of the head. This is a classic presentation of a patient with basilar artery occlusion. The next step would be to confirm the clinical suspicion with noninvasive angiography of the head and neck. If an arterial occlusion is found, this patient could potentially be treated with IV thrombolysis or mechanical thrombectomy (or both).

Mak CH, Ho JW, Chan KY, Poon WS, Wong GK. Intra-arterial revascularization therapy for basilar artery occlusion: a systematic review and analysis. Neurosurg Rev. 2016 Oct;39(4):575–80. Epub 2016 Jan 25.

II.32. Answer a.

Herpes simplex encephalitis is the most likely diagnosis. PLEDs are a characteristic EEG pattern classically associated with herpes simplex encephalitis, although the pattern is not specific for this disorder. For a stuporous patient with a flulike prodrome and fever, which may indicate the presence of infection, the most likely diagnosis is herpes simplex encephalitis. IV acyclovir should be administered empirically as soon as possible (before any further diagnostic testing) because it reduces mortality and morbidity.

Rabinstein AA. Herpes virus encephalitis in adults: current knowledge and old myths. Neurol Clin. 2017 Nov;35(4):695–705. Epub 2017 Aug 10.

II.33. Answer c.

Observe for 5 hours before further testing. The clinical history suggests the possibility of acute aneurysmal subarachnoid hemorrhage. Sampling of CSF is indicated to exclude subarachnoid hemorrhage when CT of the head does not suggest a diagnosis and clinical suspicion is high. Xanthochromia, which results from erythrocyte breakdown products, is not apparent in the CSF until at least 6 hours after the onset of hemorrhage.

Carpenter CR, Hussain AM, Ward MJ, Zipfel GJ, Fowler S, Pines JM, et al. Spontaneous subarachnoid hemorrhage: a systematic review and meta-analysis describing the diagnostic accuracy of history, physical examination, imaging, and lumbar puncture with an exploration of test thresholds. Acad Emerg Med. 2016 Sep;23(9):963–1003. Epub 2016 Sep 6.

II.34. Answer b.

Myasthenia gravis is the most frequent cause of neuromuscular respiratory failure in general ICUs (with GBS and ALS close behind). In critically ill patients who have ARDS, respiratory weakness is common but rarely neurogenic. Lambert-Eaton syndrome and hypokalemia are rare disorders and are rarely associated with respiratory failure.

Cabrera Serrano M, Rabinstein AA. Causes and outcomes of acute neuromuscular respiratory failure. Arch Neurol. 2010 Sep;67(9):1089–94.

II.35. Answer b.

The expected response to tachypnea in an otherwise healthy patient is hypocapnia and respiratory alkalosis. A normal $\mathrm{Pco_2}$ in this patient may indicate failure of the compensatory mechanisms to maintain a normal minute ventilation.

Rabinstein AA. Acute neuromuscular respiratory failure. Continuum (Minneap Minn). 2015 Oct; 21(5 Neurocritical Care):1324–45.

II.36. Answer b.

Outward movement of the abdomen with deep inspiration is normal. The opposite finding, inward movement of the abdomen with deep inspiration, is called abdominal paradox and indicates critical diaphragmatic weakness.

Wijdicks EFM. The neurology of acutely failing respiratory mechanics. Ann Neurol. 2017 Apr;81(4):485–94.

II.37. Answer b.

Arterial blood gas results are typically normal until the late stages of neuromuscular respiratory failure. A thorough physical examination, bedside pulmonary function tests, and an understanding of the evolution of the underlying cause should be the mainstays in the decision to intubate a patient with neuromuscular weakness.

Rabinstein AA. Acute neuromuscular respiratory failure. Continuum (Minneap Minn). 2015 Oct; 21(5 Neurocritical Care):1324–45.

II.38. Answer d.

Diaphragmatic ultrasonography is a rapid, noninvasive test that provides a comprehensive evaluation of the structure and function of the diaphragm. It can be complemented by electromyographic examination of the diaphragm to detect evidence of denervation and distinguish between neuropathic and myopathic causes of paralysis.

Sarwal A, Walker FO, Cartwright MS. Neuromuscular ultrasound for evaluation of the diaphragm. Muscle Nerve. 2013 Mar;47(3):319–29. Epub 2013 Feb 4.

II.39. Answer a.

Central neurogenic hyperventilation is associated with both midbrain lesions (traumatic injury and, most often, lymphoma) and bihemispheric lesions.

Simon RP. Respiratory manifestations of neurologic disease. Handbook Clin Neurol. 1993;19:477–501. (Series; vol. 63).

II.40. Answer d.

Central hyperventilation, Cheyne-Stokes breathing, and terminal breathing can all be present with acute brainstem injury, but stridor is caused by mechanical airway obstruction and often occurs only in chronic conditions such as Parkinson disease.

Forsyth D, Torsney KM. Respiratory dysfunction in Parkinson's disease. J R Coll Physicians Edinb. 2017 Mar;47(1):35–9.

II.41. Answer c.

Postmenopausal women have the highest risk for all-cause takotsubo cardiomyopathy.

Bybee KA, Kara T, Prasad A, Lerman A, Barsness GW, Wright RS, et al. Systematic review: transient left ventricular apical ballooning: a syndrome that mimics ST-segment elevation myocardial infarction. Ann Intern Med. 2004 Dec 7;141(11):858–65.

Templin C, Ghadri JR, Diekmann J, Napp LC, Bataiosu DR, Jaguszewski M, et al. Clinical features and outcomes of Takotsubo (stress) cardiomyopathy. N Engl J Med. 2015 Sep 3;373(10):929–38.

II.42. Answer b.

Contraction band necrosis, with a mononuclear infiltrate, is characteristically seen in patients with takotsubo cardiomyopathy. Neutrophilic infiltrates are seen more often in acute myocardial infarction. Autophagy and apoptosis have not been described in this condition.

Akashi YJ, Goldstein DS, Barbaro G, Ueyama T. Takotsubo cardiomyopathy: a new form of acute, reversible heart failure. Circulation. 2008 Dec 16;118(25):2754–62.

Wittstein IS, Thiemann DR, Lima JA, Baughman KL, Schulman SP, Gerstenblith G, et al. Neurohumoral features of myocardial stunning due to sudden emotional stress. N Engl J Med. 2005 Feb 10;352(6):539–48.

II.43. Answer b.

TBI with severe diffuse axonal injury is often associated with extensor motor posturing. When autonomic features appear, PSH should be recognized. TBI with subdural hemorrhage may be associated with the development of seizures, which may mimic PSH. Subarachnoid hemorrhage is associated with delayed vasospasm and cerebral ischemia as a mechanism for secondary injury progression. Hemorrhagic stroke may be associated with multiple forms of secondary injury progression, and hemorrhage around the third ventricle and diencephalon may increase the rates of PSH.

Rabinstein AA, Benarroch EE. Treatment of paroxysmal sympathetic hyperactivity. Curr Treat Options Neurol. 2008 Mar;10(2):151–7.

II.44. Answer c.

Morphine is the preferred abortive therapy for paroxysms during PSH. Propranolol is a mainstay for treatment of diminishing central sympathetic activity. Lorazepam has activity to diminish the threshold for stimuli that prompt paroxysms and the symptoms of the paroxysms themselves, but the abortive action is less than with morphine. Gabapentin has multiple mechanisms to quell PSH symptoms, but it is predominantly useful in limiting the pathologic process of hypersensitization that reinforces paroxysms.

Meyfroidt G, Baguley IJ, Menon DK. Paroxysmal sympathetic hyperactivity: the storm after acute brain injury. Lancet Neurol. 2017 Sep;16(9):721–9.

Section III

Critical Care Disorders

Pulmonary Disorders

Acute Respiratory Distress Syndrome

RICHARD K. PATCH III, MD; JAMES Y. FINDLAY, MB, ChB

Goals

- Understand the underlying pathophysiology of acute respiratory distress syndrome.
- Understand how to manage acute respiratory distress syndrome.
- Be able to identify refractory hypoxemia and know the strategies for managing it.

Introduction

Acute respiratory distress syndrome (ARDS) is a clinical syndrome characterized by acute hypoxemic respiratory failure. Patients with ARDS have pulmonary damage from an acute, usually severe, diffuse inflammatory lung injury that leads to increased vascular permeability and loss of aerated tissue.

Epidemiology

Estimates of the incidence of ARDS vary widely from 1.5 to 86 cases per 100,000 annually. Incidence increases with age and varies geographically. According to a population-based study in Olmsted County, Minnesota, the incidence of ARDS decreased from 82.4 cases per 100,000 person-years in 2001 to 38.9 cases per 100,000 person-years in 2008. The decrease was attributed to improvements in the care of patients with ARDS, such as the use of lung-protective ventilation and fewer transfusions. Mortality from ARDS is estimated to range from 26% to 58%. Survivors have extensive morbidity, including neurocognitive dysfunction, physical disabilities, and psychiatric illnesses such as depression, anxiety, and posttraumatic stress disorder. Lung function may be compromised for as long as 5 years.

Pathophysiology

The main histopathologic feature of ARDS is diffuse alveolar damage with lung capillary endothelial cell injury. Classically, ARDS is divided into 2 phases, the early exudative phase and the late fibroproliferative phase.

Exudative Phase

The early exudative phase typically occurs during the first 7 days. ARDS results from cell injury to the capillary endothelium and the alveolar epithelium. Increased capillary permeability and loss of integrity in the vascular barrier allow protein-rich fluid and inflammatory mediators to accumulate inside the interstitial tissues and alveoli. Neutrophils are recruited to the lungs, and the mediators include cytokines, such as tumor necrosis factor and interleukins 1 and 6. Reactive oxygen species are also generated by activated alveolar macrophages. This cascade of events results in surfactant dysfunction, intrapulmonary shunting, and alterations in gas exchange and pulmonary mechanics. The damage to the alveolar epithelial cells impairs resorption of fluid from the alveolar space and enhances parenchymal injury and the altered gas exchange. Hyaline membranes also form in the alveolar spaces during this phase.

Fibroproliferative Phase

The late fibroproliferative phase, occurring as early as 7 to 10 days after the initial insult, is marked by ongoing injury combined with disordered repair. Increasing numbers of fibroblasts and myofibroblasts enter the alveolar walls, leading to deposition of collagens and other components of the extracellular matrix. As the process continues, lung flooding becomes less prominent and pulmonary fibrosis ensues. Clinical manifestations that parallel these events include increased dead space ventilation,

Box 19.1 • Etiology of ARDS

Pulmonary causes
- Pneumonia
- Gastric aspiration
- Inhalation injury (eg, inhaled crack cocaine)
- Near-drowning
- Lung contusion

Extrapulmonary causes
- Catastrophic acute brain injury (eg, aneurysmal subarachnoid hemorrhage)
- Sepsis
- Shock states
- Pancreatitis
- Trauma (eg, long bone fractures, fat embolism)
- Massive transfusion
- Burns
- Cardiopulmonary bypass
- Primary graft failure in lung transplant
- Drug overdose (eg, aspirin)
- Hematopoietic stem cell transplant
- Amniotic fluid embolism

Abbreviation: ARDS, acute respiratory distress syndrome.

continued abnormal gas exchange, and worsening pulmonary compliance.

Etiology

ARDS can result from various causes, which have traditionally been classified as *pulmonary* (or *direct*) and *extrapulmonary* (*indirect*) (Box 19.1). Sepsis is the most common precipitating insult, but the cause of ARDS is not always identifiable. Risk factors for ARDS developing after an insult include advanced age, alcohol use, and smoking.

Clinical Presentation

Decompensation may occur within a few hours after the inciting event or up to 72 hours after the event. Common signs and symptoms include marked respiratory distress with dyspnea, tachypnea, tachycardia, accessory muscle use, diaphoresis, and overall increased work of breathing. Arterial blood gas results indicate hypoxemia; acute respiratory alkalosis and an elevated alveolar-arterial gradient may also be present. On physical examination, the patient may be cyanotic; on auscultation, bilateral crackles may be heard. Initial chest radiography usually shows bilateral diffuse pulmonary infiltrates. Computed tomography (CT) of the chest shows asymmetric consolidation with patchy ground-glass and alveolar infiltrates throughout the lung.

Diagnosis

Since ARDS is a clinical syndrome, the diagnosis is made clinically and is not based on a single imaging finding or laboratory test result. The Berlin Definition of ARDS, published in 2012, replaced the American-European Consensus Conference definition published in 1994. Major changes to the definition included elimination of the term *acute lung injury* and removal of pulmonary capillary wedge pressure as a diagnostic criterion. In the Berlin Definition of ARDS, all the following criteria must be met:

- Respiratory symptoms must have occurred or worsened within 7 days after a precipitating event.
- Chest radiography or CT of the chest shows bilateral opacities consistent with pulmonary edema.
- Respiratory failure cannot be fully explained by cardiac failure or fluid overload, and an objective evaluation (eg, echocardiography) is required to exclude hydrostatic pulmonary edema.

A moderate to severe oxygen impairment must be present as defined by the ratio of the partial pressure of arterial oxygen ($Pa{O_2}$) to the fraction of inspired oxygen ($F{IO_2}$) (*moderate*: 100 mm Hg < $Pa{O_2}/F{IO_2}$ ≤200 mm Hg with positive end-expiratory pressure [PEEP] ≥5 cm H_2O; *severe*: $Pa{O_2}/F{IO_2}$ ≤100 mm Hg with PEEP ≥5 cm H_2O). Cardiogenic pulmonary edema can result from acute decompensated heart failure with preserved and reduced ejection fraction and from hypertensive emergencies. The patient's history, echocardiographic results, and brain natriuretic peptide levels can be useful in making the diagnosis. Other causes of hypoxemic respiratory failure that can resemble ARDS include idiopathic acute eosinophilic pneumonia and diffuse alveolar hemorrhage, but the history, bronchoscopic evaluation, and CT of the chest should provide useful diagnostic evidence (Table 19.1).

Management

The cornerstone of ARDS management is lung-protective mechanical ventilation. This involves maintaining appropriate arterial oxygenation and protecting the injured lung from further injury by limiting alveolar overdistention, trauma from repetitive opening and closing of the alveoli, and the further release of inflammatory cytokines.

Low-Tidal-Volume Ventilation

The landmark ARDS Network Lower Tidal Volume (ARMA) trial randomly assigned patients with ARDS to receive either low-tidal-volume ventilation (LTVV) (initial tidal volume [V_T] ≤6 mL/kg of ideal body weight [IBW] and plateau pressure [Pplat] ≤30 cm H_2O) or conventional ventilation

Table 19.1 • Differential Diagnosis of ARDS

Condition	Clinical Characteristics
Acute eosinophilic pneumonia	BAL with >15% eosinophils
Acute exacerbation of idiopathic pulmonary fibrosis	History and CT scan consistent with fibrosis (eg, honeycombing)
Acute interstitial pneumonia (Hamman-Rich syndrome)	Rare idiopathic form of diffuse alveolar damage with no known cause
Cardiogenic pulmonary edema	History, echocardiographic results, and BNP
Diffuse alveolar hemorrhage	Progressively bloody return on BAL with >20% hemosiderin-laden macrophages
Malignancy (leukemia or lymphoma)	History and cytology of BAL fluid

Abbreviations: ARDS, acute respiratory distress syndrome; BAL, bronchoalveolar lavage; BNP, brain natriuretic peptide; CT, computed tomography.

(initial V_T of 12 mL/kg of IBW and Pplat ≤50 cm H_2O). Use of LTVV resulted in lower 28-day mortality and hospital mortality. As a consequence of alveolar hypoventilation, hypercapnia and respiratory acidosis ensue (called *permissive hypercapnia*). The goal pH is at least 7.30, which is safe for most patients. Additional LTVV goals include Pao_2 of 55 to 80 mm Hg or oxygen saturation by pulse oximetry of 88% to 95% and Pplat of 30 cm H_2O or less.

Open-Lung Ventilation

Open-lung ventilation refers to providing LTVV with enough PEEP to maximize alveolar recruitment. The applied PEEP decreases alveolar overdistention and decreases cyclic atelectasis as more alveoli remain open throughout the respiratory cycle. Typically, PEEP and Fio_2 are titrated in concert, with incremental increases in both to achieve the aforementioned oxygenation goal. With this method, PEEP ranges from 12 to 24 mm Hg. Recruitment maneuvers include the application of high levels of positive airway pressure to open collapsed alveoli. Adverse effects include hypotension and desaturation, but these are self-limited. The Pao_2 typically increases after the maneuver, and the largest increases occur when a higher level of PEEP is used after the maneuver is completed.

Glucocorticoids

A definitive role has not been established for glucocorticoid use in patients with ARDS because the data are mixed. Trials have evaluated glucocorticoid use in both the early exudative phase and the late fibroproliferative phase. When low-dose corticosteroids were administered during the early phase, within 72 hours after presentation, patients needed mechanical ventilation for a shorter time, their intensive care unit (ICU) length of stay was shorter, and ICU mortality was lower. However, the treatment groups were small and unbalanced. Among patients who received methylprednisolone for 21 days (7-28 days after presentation), 60-day and 180-day mortality were no different.

Fluid Management

As previously stated, the cascade of events causing increased capillary permeability and noncardiogenic pulmonary edema are key aspects of ARDS. Conservative fluid management is beneficial even for patients who are not volume overloaded. Lung function improves, and the number of ventilator-free days and ICU-free days increases without worsening nonpulmonary organ failure.

Neuromuscular Blockade

Among patients with ARDS, neuromuscular blockade within 48 hours after initiating mechanical ventilation is associated with a mortality benefit. Patients treated with cisatracurium have higher 90-day survival, more ventilator-free days, and less barotrauma. ICU-acquired weakness is not increased in patients receiving paralytics. Neuromuscular blockade is thought to contribute to the elimination of ventilator asynchrony and a decrease in chest wall elastance.

Esophageal Pressure Monitoring

Esophageal balloon catheters can be used to measure esophageal pressure and thereby estimate pleural pressure, which is used to calculate transpulmonary pressure.

$$\text{Transpulmonary Pressure} = \text{Airway Pressure} - \text{Pleural Pressure}$$

With these values, a patient-specific, optimal level of PEEP can be determined. When esophageal pressure monitoring was used to assist with PEEP titration (goal transpulmonary pressure, 0-10 mm Hg) and compared with the PEEP titration algorithm outlined in the ARMA trial, patients whose PEEP was guided by esophageal monitoring had higher total levels of PEEP and better Pao_2/Fio_2 ratios but no fewer ICU-free days or ventilator-free days. As more evidence becomes available, esophageal pressure measurement may become routine.

Refractory Hypoxemia

Refractory hypoxemia does not have a standard definition, and multiple variables are used to define it. Essentially, it refers to continued hypoxemia with a Pao_2/Fio_2 ratio less than 100 mm Hg, a Pplat of at least 30 mm Hg, and an oxygenation index greater than 30 despite the patient receiving LTVV and optimal PEEP after a recruitment maneuver.

$$\text{Oxygenation Index} = (\text{F}\text{IO}_2 \times \text{Mean Airway Pressure} \times 100)/\text{Pa}\text{O}_2$$

Prone Ventilation

Prone positioning alters pulmonary mechanics by placing the more compliant ventral chest wall in contact with a firm surface, thus limiting expansion. Dorsal alveoli are recruited, and the ventral alveoli collapse. Decreased chest wall compliance does not increase Pplat during ventilation because recruitment of dorsal alveoli exceeds derecruitment of ventral alveoli, resulting in an overall increase in lung compliance. Anatomically, lung mass is greater in the dorsal regions than in the ventral regions, so that more lung is available for recruitment when the patient is prone. Blood flow in the dorsal lung and ventral lung is independent of the gravitational gradient. When a patient is in the prone position, the newly recruited dorsal alveoli continue to receive the majority of blood flow, while the newly collapsed ventral alveoli receive a minority of the blood flow. Prone positioning also decreases lung compression because the heart is dependent and, with the abdomen being unsupported, the diaphragm is displaced caudally. As a result of these physiologic effects, oxygenation is improved.

The Proning Severe ARDS Patients (PROSEVA) trial used LTVV in combination with PEEP (in accordance with the ARDS Network ARMA protocol) and prone positioning for 17 hours over 4 days. The absolute mortality risk reduction was 17%, the relative risk reduction was 50%. Contraindications to prone positioning include pregnancy, increased intracranial pressure, spinal instability, unstable fractures, active bleeding (including hemorrhagic shock or massive hemoptysis), and recent tracheal surgery or sternotomy.

Venovenous Extracorporeal Membrane Oxygenation

Extracorporeal membrane oxygenation (ECMO) is another option for treating refractory hypoxemia in patients with ARDS. In 2009, the Conventional Ventilatory Support Versus Extracorporeal Membrane Oxygenation for Severe Adult Respiratory Failure (CESAR) trial showed increased survival among patients assigned to the ECMO center compared with those assigned to conventional management. (However, some patients assigned to the ECMO center received conventional management instead of ECMO at the center.) Data related to ARDS associated with H1N1 influenza virus are mixed; some studies have shown that ECMO (compared to conventional management) benefits patients, and others have not.

Alternative Management Strategies

Alternative modes of ventilation have been used as a rescue strategy for patients with refractory hypoxemia. Examples include airway pressure release ventilation and bilevel ventilation, but neither has improved mortality. In high-frequency oscillatory ventilation (HFOV), an oscillating pump delivers a small V_T (1-4 mL/kg) at a frequency of 3 to 15 Hz. Delivering a small V_T maintains constant lung recruitment and prevents lung injury from overdistention. The 2013 Oscillation for ARDS Treated Early (OSCILLATE) trial compared patients receiving HFOV with patients receiving LTVV and high PEEP for moderate to severe ARDS. The trial was stopped early because of increased mortality in the HFOV group. In addition, the 2013 Oscillation in ARDS (OSCAR) trial compared patients receiving HFOV with patients receiving usual care. The HFOV group received more paralytics and sedative medications, and there was no mortality difference between the 2 groups at 1 month. Inhaled nitric oxide dilates the pulmonary vasculature by stimulating guanylate cyclase; the result is increased cyclic guanosine monophosphate, smooth muscle relaxation, and increased oxygenation. However, in a 2014 meta-analysis, inhaled nitric oxide had no effect on mortality, and other studies have suggested that it impairs renal function. Prostacyclin, another pulmonary vasodilator, improves oxygenation, but its efficacy in patients with ARDS is unknown: In initial small clinical trials, exogenous surfactant may have benefited ARDS patients; however, in a multicenter randomized trial, survival was not improved.

Summary

- The pathophysiologic hallmark of ARDS is diffuse alveolar damage with lung capillary endothelial cell injury.
- ARDS is divided into 2 phases, the early exudative phase and the late fibroproliferative phase.
- The Berlin Definition of ARDS is based on timing (acute respiratory symptoms of <7 days' duration); chest imaging (bilateral opacities consistent with pulmonary edema); and origin of edema (not attributed to cardiac failure or fluid overload).
- The cornerstone of management is LTVV (≤6 mL/kg of IBW) and open-lung ventilation with PEEP guided by the ARDS Network ARMA protocol.
- Prone ventilation and venovenous ECMO are good options for treating refractory hypoxemia.

SUGGESTED READING

Acute Respiratory Distress Syndrome Network, Brower RG, Matthay MA, Morris A, Schoenfeld D, Thompson BT, et al. Ventilation with lower tidal volumes as compared with traditional tidal volumes for acute lung injury and the acute respiratory distress syndrome. N Engl J Med. 2000 May 4;342(18):1301–8.

Afshari A, Brok J, Moller AM, Wetterslev J. Inhaled nitric oxide for acute respiratory distress syndrome and acute lung injury in adults and children: a systematic review with meta-analysis and trial sequential analysis. Anesth Analg. 2011 Jun;112(6):1411–21. Epub 2011 Mar 3.

Alhurani RE, Oeckler RA, Franco PM, Jenkins SM, Gajic O, Pannu SR. Refractory hypoxemia and use of rescue strategies: a U.S. National Survey of Adult Intensivists. Ann Am Thorac Soc. 2016 Jul;13(7):1105–14.

ARDS Definition Task Force, Ranieri VM, Rubenfeld GD, Thompson BT, Ferguson ND, Caldwell E, et al. Acute respiratory distress syndrome: the Berlin definition. JAMA. 2012 Jun 20;307(23):2526–33.

Bellani G, Laffey JG, Pham T, Fan E, Brochard L, Esteban A; LUNG SAFE Investigators; ESICM Trials Group. Epidemiology, patterns of care, and mortality for patients with acute respiratory distress syndrome in intensive care units in 50 countries. JAMA. 2016 Feb 23;315(8):788–800. Erratum in: JAMA. 2016 Jul 19;316(3):350.

Brower RG, Lanken PN, MacIntyre N, Matthay MA, Morris A, Ancukiewicz M, et al; National Heart, Lung, and Blood Institute ARDS Clinical Trials Network. Higher versus lower positive end-expiratory pressures in patients with the acute respiratory distress syndrome. N Engl J Med. 2004 Jul 22;351(4):327–36.

Ferguson ND, Cook DJ, Guyatt GH, Mehta S, Hand L, Austin P, et al; OSCILLATE Trial Investigators; Canadian Critical Care Trials Group. High-frequency oscillation in early acute respiratory distress syndrome. N Engl J Med. 2013 Feb 28;368(9):795–805. Epub 2013 Jan 22.

Gattinoni L, Tognoni G, Pesenti A, Taccone P, Mascheroni D, Labarta V, et al; Prone-Supine Study Group. Effect of prone positioning on the survival of patients with acute respiratory failure. N Engl J Med. 2001 Aug 23;345(8):568–73.

Guerin C, Reignier J, Richard JC, Beuret P, Gacouin A, Boulain T, et al; PROSEVA Study Group. Prone positioning in severe acute respiratory distress syndrome. N Engl J Med. 2013 Jun 6;368(23):2159–68. Epub 2013 May 20.

Li G, Malinchoc M, Cartin-Ceba R, Venkata CV, Kor DJ, Peters SG, et al. Eight-year trend of acute respiratory distress syndrome: a population-based study in Olmsted County, Minnesota. Am J Respir Crit Care Med. 2011 Jan 1;183(1):59–66. Epub 2010 Aug 6.

Madotto F, Pham T, Bellani G, Bos LD, Simonis FD, Fan E, et al. LUNG SAFE Investigators and the ESICM Trials Group. Resolved versus confirmed ARDS after 24 h: insights from the LUNG SAFE study. Intensive Care Med. 2018 May;44(5):564–77.

Matthay MA, Zemans RL. The acute respiratory distress syndrome: pathogenesis and treatment. Annu Rev Pathol. 2011;6:147–63.

National Heart, Lung, and Blood Institute Acute Respiratory Distress Syndrome (ARDS) Clinical Trials Network, Wiedemann HP, Wheeler AP, Bernard GR, Thompson BT, Hayden D, et al. Comparison of two fluid-management strategies in acute lung injury. N Engl J Med. 2006 Jun 15;354(24):2564–75. Epub 2006 May 21.

Peek GJ, Mugford M, Tiruvoipati R, Wilson A, Allen E, Thalanany MM, et al; CESAR trial collaboration. Efficacy and economic assessment of conventional ventilatory support versus extracorporeal membrane oxygenation for severe adult respiratory failure (CESAR): a multicentre randomised controlled trial. Lancet. 2009 Oct 17;374(9698):1351–63. Epub 2009 Sep 15. Erratum in: Lancet. 2009 Oct 17;374(9698):1330.

Spragg RG, Lewis JF, Walmrath HD, Johannigman J, Bellingan G, Laterre PF, et al. Effect of recombinant surfactant protein C-based surfactant on the acute respiratory distress syndrome. N Engl J Med. 2004 Aug 26;351(9):884–92.

Talmor D, Sarge T, Malhotra A, O'Donnell CR, Ritz R, Lisbon A, et al. Mechanical ventilation guided by esophageal pressure in acute lung injury. N Engl J Med. 2008 Nov 13;359(20):2095–104. Epub 2008 Nov 11.

Thompson BT, Chambers RC, Liu KD. Acute respiratory distress syndrome. N Engl J Med. 2017 Aug 10;377(6):562–72.

Young D, Lamb SE, Shah S, MacKenzie I, Tunnicliffe W, Lall R, et al; OSCAR Study Group. High-frequency oscillation for acute respiratory distress syndrome. N Engl J Med. 2013 Feb 28;368(9):806–13. Epub 2013 Jan 22.

Pulmonary Embolism: An Overview

BRANDON T. NOKES, MD; RODRIGO CARTIN-CEBA, MD

Goals

- Describe the diagnostic approach to pulmonary embolism and its classification.
- Discuss the management options for acute pulmonary embolism.
- Discuss anticoagulation for the patient with pulmonary embolism.
- Discuss the approach to recurrent pulmonary embolism.

Introduction

Venous thromboembolism (VTE) is a major public health concern with an annual incidence of 1 per 1,000 patients in the United States. VTE encompasses a spectrum of diseases including deep vein thrombosis (DVT) and pulmonary embolism (PE). DVT is a precursor to PE, and approximately 80% of patients have DVT when PE is diagnosed. The risk factors for PE are the same as those for DVT; consequently, diagnosis and management of VTE are contingent on the underlying risk factors and the extent of disease. A suspected VTE diagnosis should be pursued with risk stratification tools such as the Wells DVT and PE criteria (Table 20.1) and the Revised Geneva Score for PE (Table 20.2). This chapter reviews PE diagnosis, risk stratification, and management.

Diagnosis of PE

Patients with PE have highly variable clinical signs and symptoms, ranging from none to complete cardiopulmonary collapse. The most common signs and symptoms, however, are shortness of breath, tachypnea, tachycardia, hypoxemia, and pleuritic chest pain. With such variable presentations, though, the diagnostic algorithms for PE largely depend on clinical suspicion in conjunction with the Wells score or Revised Geneva Score for risk stratification (Tables 20.1 and 20.2). The Wells score is used more commonly in the United States and has been heavily validated. Risk stratification with the Wells score in conjunction with clinical suspicion for PE dictates the diagnostic workup: Patients with low risk for PE and a low Wells score may not need additional testing, but patients with intermediate risk should have a D-dimer test, and if those results are positive, the patients should undergo computed tomographic angiography (Figure 20.1). D-dimer levels do increase with age, so D-dimer values should be age-adjusted. Patients with a high risk for PE should undergo computed tomographic angiography directly unless they have contraindications for intravenous contrast media (eg, acute kidney failure); if they do have contraindications, they should undergo ventilation-perfusion scanning. If imaging shows dilated pulmonary vasculature or if a patient has pulmonary hypertension or right ventricular (RV) dysfunction, transthoracic echocardiography may be considered for further diagnostic evaluation.

Classification of PE

Although PE is part of the VTE spectrum, PE can be subclassified by anatomical location and, more importantly, by symptomatic severity. The broad categories of severity are massive, submassive, and other (in order of decreasing severity). *Massive PE* is characterized by hemodynamic compromise (systolic blood pressure <90 mm Hg for >15 minutes or a decrease of >40 mm Hg). *Submassive PE* is characterized by the presence of acute RV dysfunction without hemodynamic compromise. *Other PE* indicates that there is no evidence of RV strain. The RV dysfunction is typically diagnosed with echocardiography showing RV enlargement, elevated RV systolic pressure, or decreased RV systolic function or with electrocardiographic evidence of a new right bundle branch block. An

Table 20.1 • Wells Clinical Prediction Score for PE

Variable	Points
Signs and symptoms of DVT	3.0
PE is more likely than an alternative diagnosis	3.0
Heart rate >100 beats per minute	1.5
Immobilization or surgery in previous 4 wk	1.5
Previous DVT or PE	1.5
Hemoptysis	1.0
Cancer	1.0
Pretest probability of PE according to total score	
Low	<2.0
Moderate	2.0-6.0
High	>6.0
Dichotomized Wells score	
PE unlikely	≤4.0
PE likely	>4.0

Abbreviations: DVT, deep vein thrombosis; PE, pulmonary embolism.

Modified from Wells PS, Anderson DR, Rodger M, Ginsberg JS, Kearon C, Gent M, et al. Derivation of a simple clinical model to categorize patients probability of pulmonary embolism: increasing the models utility with the SimpliRED D-dimer. Thromb Haemost. 2000 Mar;83(3):416-20; used with permission.

Table 20.2 • Revised Geneva Score

Variable	Points
Age >65 y	1
Previous DVT or PE	3
Surgery (under general anesthesia) or lower limb fracture in previous month	2
Active cancer	2
Unilateral lower limb pain	3
Hemoptysis	2
Heart rate, beats per minute	
75-94	3
≥95	5
Pain on leg palpation or unilateral edema	4
Clinical probability of PE according to total score	
Low	0–3
Intermediate	4–10
High	≥11

Abbreviations: DVT, deep vein thrombosis; PE, pulmonary embolism.

From Le Gal G, Righini M, Roy PM, Sanchez O, Aujesky D, Bounameaux H, et al. Prediction of pulmonary embolism in the emergency department: the revised Geneva score. Ann Intern Med. 2006 Feb 7;144(3):165-71; used with permission.

important distinction is that this RV dysfunction is acute and is not related to chronic thromboembolic pulmonary hypertension (ie, World Health Organization group 4 pulmonary hypertension). PE can also be defined anatomically: *Central PE* occurs within the pulmonary artery, lobar arteries, or segmental arteries; *distal PE* occurs within the subsegmental arteries.

Management of PE

The mainstay of PE management is anticoagulation to prevent thrombus propagation. The body's endogenous thrombolytic mechanisms are responsible for thromboembolism clearance over time. Anticoagulation, however, prevents further thrombus formation through potentiation of antithrombin III (with heparins); inhibition of γ-carboxylation of vitamin K-dependent clotting factors (II, VII, IX, and X) (with warfarin); or inhibition of factor Xa or direct thrombin inhibition with a direct oral anticoagulant (DOAC) (Table 20.3). In the absence of an absolute contraindication, acute management should focus on optimizing the hemodynamic status, providing appropriate oxygenation, and initiating heparin infusion. However, patients with massive PE initially require either enzymatic clot lysis (with thrombolytics such as streptokinase, recombinant tissue plasminogen activator [rtPA], or tenecteplase) or mechanical removal of thromboembolism in a highly specialized medical center. The use of thrombolytics in submassive PE is controversial (Figure 20.2).

The duration of therapy is contingent on the underlying risk factors for PE (Figure 20.3). If the risk factors are transient (eg, trauma or major surgery within the past 90 days) or the patient is undergoing prolonged immobilization, the PE is considered to be *provoked* and anticoagulation is needed for only 3 months with low-molecular-weight heparin (LMWH) or DOAC. LMWH is the treatment of choice for PE if a patient is pregnant or if a patient has active malignancy. Warfarin is prescribed less frequently because its use requires cumbersome monitoring in addition to dietary and medication adjustment restrictions.

In the absence of transient risk factors, the PE is considered *unprovoked* and will require longer periods of anticoagulation, often with warfarin or DOAC. If a patient has antiphospholipid syndrome or a mechanical heart valve, lifelong use of warfarin is the treatment of choice. If PE occurred from underlying malignancy (typically hematologic malignancies or mucin-producing adenocarcinomas, such as in lung, breast, colon, gastric, and primary brain malignancies), the duration of therapy is indefinite or until the cancer is definitively treated. For patients with malignancy-related PE, LMWH has proven outcome benefits over warfarin, and DOACs have not been extensively studied. Anticoagulation provides little or no benefit to patients with tumor emboli. Patients with concurrent

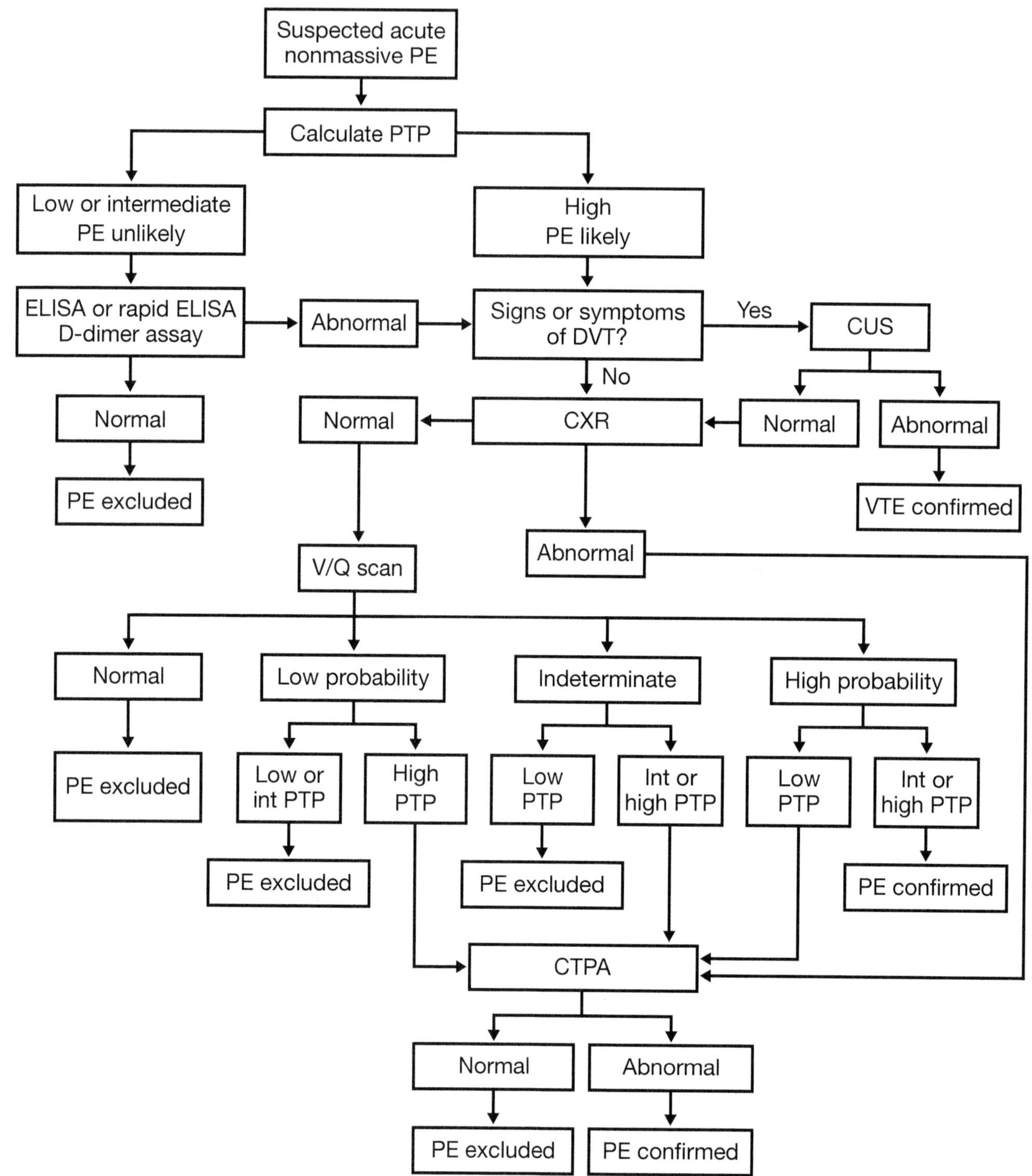

Figure 20.1. Flowchart for Diagnosis of Pulmonary Embolism (PE). CTPA indicates computed tomographic pulmonary angiography; CUS, compressive ultrasonography; CXR, chest radiography; DVT, deep vein thrombosis; ELISA, enzyme-linked immunosorbent assay; int, intermediate; PTP, pretest probability; VTE, venous thromboembolism; V/Q, ventilation-perfusion. (Data from Moores LK. Pulmonary vascular diseases. In: ACCP Pulmonary medicine board review. 26th ed. Northbrook [IL]: American College of Chest Physicians; c2009. p. 21-37.)

Table 20.3 • Anticoagulant Therapy for Pulmonary Embolism

Agent	Route of Administration	Renal Clearance, %	Half-life, h	Initial Dosage	Maintenance Dosage	Extended Therapy Dosage
Unfractionated heparin	Intravenous	30	1.5	Keep aPTT at 1.5 times upper limit of reference range	...	...
LMWH[a]	Subcutaneous	80	3-4	Weight based	Weight based	...
Fondaparinux	Subcutaneous	100	17-21	Weight based	Weight based	...
Vitamin K antagonists	Oral	Negligible	Acenocoumarol, 8-11 Warfarin, 36 Phenprocoumon, 160	Target INR, 2.0-3.0 Also give heparin for ≥5 d	Maintain INR at 2.0-3.0	Maintain INR at 2.0-3.0
Dabigatran[b]	Oral	80	14-17	Requires heparin preceding for ≥5 d	150 mg twice daily	150 mg twice daily
Rivaroxaban[c]	Oral	33	7-11	15 mg twice daily for 3 wk	20 mg once daily	20 mg once daily
Apixaban[c]	Oral	25	8-12	10 mg twice daily for 1 wk	5 mg twice daily	2.5 mg twice daily
Edoxaban[c]	Oral	35	6-11	Requires heparin preceding for ≥5 d	60 mg once daily[d]	60 mg once daily[d]
Aspirin	Oral	10	0.25	...	...	80-100 mg once daily

Abbreviations: aPTT, activated partial thromboplastin time; INR, international normalized ratio; LMWH, low-molecular-weight heparin.

[a] Recommended for patients who have active cancer or are pregnant.

[b] Contraindicated in patients with creatinine clearance less than 30 mL/min.

[c] Contraindicated in patients with creatinine clearance less than 15 mL/min.

[d] Recommended dose is 30 mg once daily for patients with creatinine clearance of 30 to 50 mL/min, patients who weigh 60 kg or less, or patients receiving certain strong P-glycoprotein inhibitors.

chronic thromboembolic disease must be evaluated for pulmonary hypertension because they may require adjunctive treatment.

If patients have unprovoked VTE, further diagnostic evaluation is required. Typically, the evaluation would include a routine history and physical examination, complete blood cell count, basic metabolic panel, liver function tests, coagulation studies, routine age-appropriate cancer screening, and a chest radiograph. Although screening for occult malignancy in patients with unprovoked VTE leads to increased early cancer detection, it does not impart a survival advantage.

Risk factors for unprovoked PE can be classified as inherited (eg, inherited hypercoagulable states) or acquired (eg, antiphospholipid syndrome). The treatment of PE due to inherited thrombophilia typically entails lifelong anticoagulation with warfarin. Lifelong anticoagulation should also be considered in patients with acquired hypercoagulable states if the recurrence risk is unacceptably high. In all other patients, therapy should be continued as long as the underlying risk factor is present (eg, malignancy, hypercoagulable state, pregnancy, or continued immobility).

Placement of an inferior vena cava filter can be considered in a limited set of circumstances. Absolute indications include the following: 1) The patient has a contraindication to anticoagulation. 2) The patient has a complication of anticoagulation. 3) Adequate anticoagulation cannot be achieved or maintained. 4) VTE recurs despite adequate anticoagulation. Relative indications include the following: 1) The patient has an iliocaval DVT or a large, free-floating

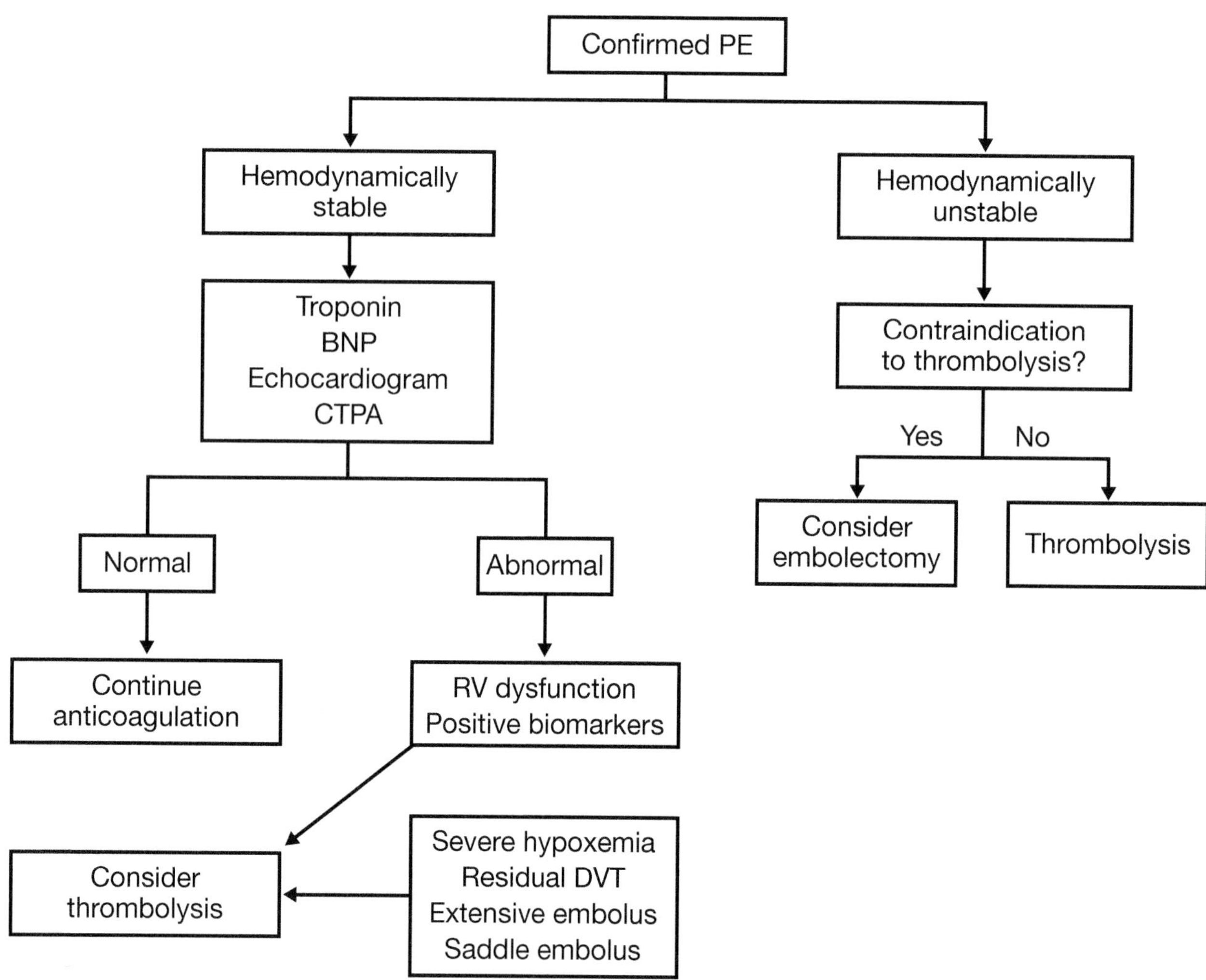

Figure 20.2. Algorithm for Thrombolysis. BNP indicates brain natriuretic peptide; CTPA, computed tomographic pulmonary angiography; DVT, deep vein thrombosis; PE, pulmonary embolism; RV, right ventricular.

proximal DVT. 2) A massive PE was treated with thrombolytics or thrombectomy. 3) Chronic PE was treated with pulmonary artery endarterectomy. 4) The patient has VTE with limited cardiorespiratory reserve. 5) The patient has not adhered to the anticoagulation regimen. 6) The patient has a high risk for complications of anticoagulation. Inferior vena cava filters are intended to be temporary, and they have decreased the PE recurrence rate, but they provide no overall mortality benefit.

As noted above, patients who have hemodynamic compromise and massive PE may benefit from administration of systemic thrombolysis (eg, streptokinase, rtPA, or tenecteplase) or from mechanical removal of thromboembolism in a highly specialized medical center. Thrombectomy may be a catheter-based procedure (ie, aspiration of the clot and balloon-guided clot removal) or, less commonly, open surgery. The decision as to which invasive approach to use is both patient-specific and contingent on local expertise. Among patients undergoing systemic thrombolysis, registries have suggested rates as high as 20% for major bleeding and 3% to 5% for intracerebral hemorrhage. In addition, if patients have not benefited from systemic thrombolysis, they may benefit from catheter-directed thrombolysis.

Specifically, ultrasound-assisted catheter-directed thrombolysis (EkoSonic Endovascular System; BTG International Ltd) may benefit patients who have persistent thrombi despite having undergone therapy with systemic thrombolysis or patients for whom systemic thrombolysis carries a large risk of bleeding. After the catheter is placed into the pulmonary artery (as an interventional radiology procedure), acoustic vibration and thrombolytic agents (in much lower doses than with systemic thrombolysis)

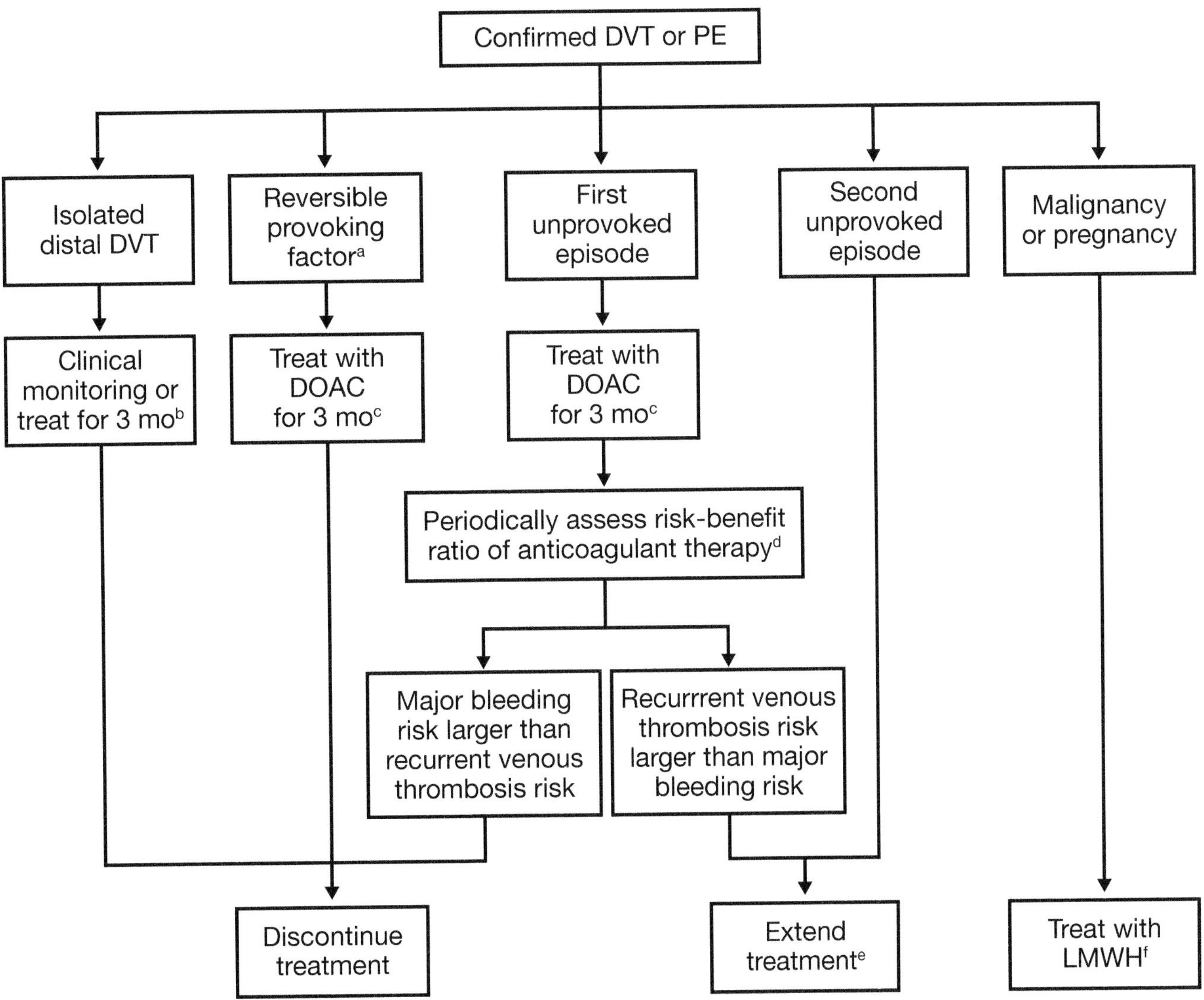

Figure 20.3. Treatment Algorithm for Pulmonary Embolism (PE). DOAC indicates direct oral anticoagulant; DVT, deep vein thrombosis; LMWH, low-molecular-weight heparin. Superscript letters indicate the following: [a] Reversible provoking factors include surgery, immobilization, and estrogen use. [b] Treatment may be preferred if patients have severe symptoms or a high risk for extension or recurrence. [c] Vitamin K antagonists are preferred if patients have a creatinine clearance of no more than 30 mL/min, if patients need to continue receiving drugs that strongly interact with DOACs (eg, strong P-glycoprotein inhibitors), or if regular monitoring is required. [d] Clinical prediction rules for recurrent venous thromboembolism and bleeding have not been prospectively validated; sex and D-dimer levels after anticoagulation therapy is stopped may be useful for assessing the risk of recurrence. [e] Treatment can be continued with the same anticoagulant given during the first 3 months; patients should be assessed periodically for bleeding risk and for reconsideration of extended treatment. [f] Patients with cancer should be treated for at least 6 months and as long as the cancer is active; a switch to vitamin K antagonists may occur post partum. (Data from Tapson VF. Treatment, prognosis, and follow-up of acute pulmonary embolism in adults [Internet]. UpToDate. [cited 2017].)

are applied directly to the thrombus for approximately 24 hours. The procedure has improved hemodynamics, RV function, and acute pulmonary hypertension. As with systemic thrombolysis, the use of ultrasound-assisted catheter-directed thrombolysis for submassive PE is controversial.

Treatment of Recurrent Thromboembolism

The risk of recurrence of PE is largely contingent on underlying risk factors for thrombus formation. Whether a patient had provoked PE or unprovoked PE, the most common risk factor for recurrence during therapy is suboptimal anticoagulation. Patient adherence to medical therapy should be assessed, and routine coagulation studies specific to the anticoagulant of choice should be performed (prothrombin time, partial thromboplastin time, and international normalized ratio, or anti–factor Xa levels). Other barriers to therapeutic anticoagulation include impaired absorption (eg, if rivaroxaban is taken without food) or a change in a patient's drug pharmacokinetics (eg, addition of a cytochrome P450 3A4 isozyme inducer to warfarin therapy or dramatic weight gain in a patient taking LMWH). If VTE has recurred despite appropriate anticoagulation, screening should be pursued for a hypercoagulable state, including tests for antithrombin mutations, protein C deficiency, protein S deficiency, factor V Leiden mutation, prothrombin G20210A mutation, and antiphospholipid syndrome. A coagulation specialist may need to be consulted for more extensive testing.

Summary

- The diagnosis of PE is largely clinical, but it can be aided with tools such as the Wells score.
- Provoked PE is treated with 3 months of anticoagulation with LMWH or DOAC therapy.
- Warfarin therapy is continued indefinitely if the cause of provoked PE is hereditary or an acquired hypercoagulable state or if the patient has a mechanical heart valve.
- The mainstay of treatment is anticoagulation; thrombolysis is indicated in massive PE, but the use of thrombolytics in submassive PE is controversial.
- Inferior vena cava filters may decrease the PE recurrence rate in certain situations, but they provide no mortality benefit.

SUGGESTED READING

Agnelli G, Buller HR, Cohen A, Curto M, Gallus AS, Johnson M, et al; AMPLIFY Investigators. Oral apixaban for the treatment of acute venous thromboembolism. N Engl J Med. 2013 Aug 29;369(9):799–808. Epub 2013 Jul 1.

Carrier M, Lazo-Langner A, Shivakumar S, Tagalakis V, Zarychanski R, Solymoss S, et al; SOME Investigators. Screening for occult cancer in unprovoked venous thromboembolism. N Engl J Med. 2015 Aug 20;373(8):697–704. Epub 2015 Jun 22.

Ceriani E, Combescure C, Le al G, Nendaz M, Perneger T, Bounameaux H, et al. Clinical prediction rules for pulmonary embolism: a systematic review and meta-analysis. J Thromb Haemost. 2010 May;8(5):957–70. Epub 2010 Feb 2.

Di Nisio M, van Es N, Buller HR. Deep vein thrombosis and pulmonary embolism. Lancet. 2016 Dec 17;388(10063):3060–73. Epub 2016 Jun 30.

Garcia MJ. Endovascular management of acute pulmonary embolism using the ultrasound-enhanced EkoSonic system. Semin Intervent Radiol. 2015 Dec;32(4):384–7.

Hoeper MM, Madani MM, Nakanishi N, Meyer B, Cebotari S, Rubin LJ. Chronic thromboembolic pulmonary hypertension. Lancet Respir Med. 2014 Jul;2(7):573–82. Epub 2014 Jun 2.

Hughes MJ, Stein PD, Matta F. Silent pulmonary embolism in patients with distal deep venous thrombosis: systematic review. Thromb Res. 2014 Dec;134(6):1182–5. Epub 2014 Oct 2.

Jaff MR, McMurtry MS, Archer SL, Cushman M, Goldenberg N, Goldhaber SZ, et al; American Heart Association Council on Cardiopulmonary, Critical Care, Perioperative and Resuscitation; American Heart Association Council on Peripheral Vascular Disease; American Heart Association Council on Arteriosclerosis, Thrombosis and Vascular Biology. Management of massive and submassive pulmonary embolism, iliofemoral deep vein thrombosis, and chronic thromboembolic pulmonary hypertension: a scientific statement from the American Heart Association. Circulation. 2011 Apr 26;123(16):1788–830. Epub 2011 Mar 21. Errata in: Circulation. 2012 Aug 14;126(7):e104. Circulation. 2012 Mar 20;125(11):e495.

Jolly M, Phillips J. Pulmonary embolism: current role of catheter treatment options and operative thrombectomy. Surg Clin North Am. 2018 Apr;98(2):279–92.

Konstantinides S, Goldhaber SZ. Pulmonary embolism: risk assessment and management. Eur Heart J. 2012 Dec;33(24):3014–22. Epub 2012 Sep 7.

Konstantinides SV. 2014 ESC guidelines on the diagnosis and management of acute pulmonary embolism. Eur Heart J. 2014 Dec 1;35(45):3145–6.

Konstantinides SV, Barco S, Lankeit M, Meyer G. Management of pulmonary embolism: an update. J Am Coll Cardiol. 2016 Mar 1;67(8):976–90.

MacCallum P, Bowles L, Keeling D. Diagnosis and management of heritable thrombophilias. BMJ. 2014 Jul 17;349:g4387.

Pasha SM, Klok FA, Snoep JD, Mos IC, Goekoop RJ, Rodger MA, et al. Safety of excluding acute pulmonary embolism based on an unlikely clinical probability by the Wells rule and normal D-dimer concentration: a meta-analysis. Thromb Res. 2010 Apr;125(4):e123–7. Epub 2009 Nov 26.

Raskob GE, Angchaisuksiri P, Blanco AN, Buller H, Gallus A, Hunt BJ, et al; ISTH Steering Committee for World Thrombosis Day. Thrombosis: a major contributor to global disease burden. Arterioscler Thromb Vasc Biol. 2014 Nov;34(11):2363–71.

Righini M, Van Es J, Den Exter PL, Roy PM, Verschuren F, Ghuysen A, et al. Age-adjusted D-dimer cutoff levels to rule out pulmonary embolism: the ADJUST-PE study. JAMA. 2014 Mar 19;311(11):1117–24. Erratum in: JAMA. 2014 Apr 23-30;311(16):1694.

Robertson L, Yeoh SE, Stansby G, Agarwal R. Effect of testing for cancer on cancer- and venous thromboembolism (VTE)-related mortality and morbidity in patients with unprovoked VTE. Cochrane Database Syst Rev. 2015 Mar 6;(3):CD010837. Update in: Cochrane Database Syst Rev. 2017 Aug 23;8:CD010837.

Schulman S, Kakkar AK, Goldhaber SZ, Schellong S, Eriksson H, Mismetti P, et al; RE-COVER II Trial Investigators. Treatment of acute venous thromboembolism with dabigatran or warfarin and pooled analysis. Circulation. 2014 Feb 18;129(7):764–72. Epub 2013 Dec 16.

Stein PD, Goodman LR, Hull RD, Dalen JE, Matta F. Diagnosis and management of isolated subsegmental pulmonary embolism: review and assessment of the options. Clin Appl Thromb Hemost. 2012 Jan-Feb;18(1):20–6. Epub 2011 Sep 23.

Tapson V. Overview of the treatment, prognosis, and follow-up of acute pulmonary embolism in adults. In: Finlay G, editor. UpToDate. Waltham (MA): UpToDate; c2016.

Vedovati MC, Germini F, Agnelli G, Becattini C. Direct oral anticoagulants in patients with VTE and cancer: a systematic review and meta-analysis. Chest. 2015 Feb;147(2):475–83.

Wells PS, Anderson DR, Rodger M, Forgie M, Kearon C, Dreyer J, et al. Evaluation of D-dimer in the diagnosis of suspected deep-vein thrombosis. N Engl J Med. 2003 Sep 25;349(13):1227–35.

Whitlock RP, Sun JC, Fremes SE, Rubens FD, Teoh KH. Antithrombotic and thrombolytic therapy for valvular disease: antithrombotic therapy and prevention of thrombosis, 9th ed: American College of Chest Physicians Evidence-Based Clinical Practice Guidelines. Chest. 2012 Feb;141(2 Suppl):e576S–e600S.

21 Asthma in the Critically Ill Patient

JONATHAN J. DANARAJ, DO; AUGUSTINE S. LEE, MD

Goals

- Recognize the signs and symptoms of severe exacerbations of asthma.
- Know the medications and interventions for critically ill patients with asthma.
- Understand specific considerations for pretreatment, induction agents, and mechanical ventilation for patients with exacerbations of asthma.

Introduction

Asthma is a common condition that affects an estimated 24 million children and adults in the United States (prevalence, 8%-10%). Globally, over 300 million people are affected and the number is expected to increase. The age distribution is bimodal, but in most patients, asthma is diagnosed before age 18 years (male to female ratio, 2:1 in children; 1:1 in adults). The World Health Organization estimates that 250,000 people die annually from asthma. In the United States, asthma mortality peaked in the mid-1990s and has since been decreasing.

Although the majority of patients have mild disease and are never admitted to the intensive care unit (ICU), patients with any severity of asthma can die of the disease. About 5% of asthmatic patients admitted to the ICU have an exacerbation requiring invasive mechanical ventilation. General prognostic factors include age, tobacco use (>20 pack-years), forced expiratory volume in 1 second (FEV_1), airflow reversibility, aspirin sensitivity, and atopy. Major risk factors for near-fatal or fatal asthma include recent history of poorly controlled asthma, prior history of mechanical ventilator support, and comorbid chronic cardiopulmonary conditions. Poor access to health care also appears to be an important risk factor because death from asthma is most common among multiracial, urban, lower-income populations.

Susceptibility to asthma is multifactorial with both genetic and environmental factors. The strongest risk factor is atopy, a sensitivity to the development of immunoglobulin E (IgE) to specific allergens. A person with atopy is 3- to 4-fold more likely to have asthma than a person without atopy. Other risk factors include birth weight, prematurity, tobacco use (including secondary exposure), and obesity.

Pathophysiology

Histologically, asthma is marked by chronic inflammation due to airway infiltration by mast cells, eosinophils, macrophages, and type 2 helper T cells with associated inflammatory cytokines such as interleukin (IL)-4, IL-5, and IL-13. Physiologically, expiratory airflow is obstructed because of excessive mucous production, mucous plugging, airway edema, smooth muscle hypertrophy, and bronchial hyperresponsiveness with resulting bronchospasm. These changes result in the cardinal signs of wheezing and shortness of breath with or without cough. When severe, these changes can lead to respiratory failure. The development of asthma likely results from various genetic factors in combination with environmental or infectious factors. The "hygiene hypothesis" attributes the increase in allergies and associated asthma in industrialized nations to immune systems altered by a decrease in "healthy" microbial exposure from living in more sanitary conditions during childhood.

Clinical Presentation

The clinical presentation of outpatients with asthma is highly variable. Some patients may be asymptomatic with flares or exacerbations triggered by exercise, aeroallergens, or infections. Others may have increasingly severe chronic

Table 21.1 • Progression of Asthma and Arterial Blood Gas Results

Blood Gas Test	Stage 1	2	3	4	5
$Paco_2$	Normal	Small decrease	Decreased	Normal	Increased
Pao_2	Normal	Normal	Small decrease	Large decrease	Large decrease

From Katsaounou PA, Sigala I, Vassilakopoulos T. Severe asthma exacerbation. In: Layon AJ, Gabrielli A, Yu M, Wood KE, editors. Civetta, Taylor, & Kirby's critical care medicine. 5th ed. Philadelphia (PA): Wolters Kluwer Health/Lippincott William & Wilkins; c2017. p. 1446-70; used with permission.

symptoms of dyspnea, wheezing, cough, or chest tightness that may interfere with rest and sleep.

Critically ill patients may be noncommunicative and thereby pose additional diagnostic challenges. In some patients, asthma may cause critical illness with respiratory failure; in others, it may complicate another primary critical illness or injury. Consideration should be given to potentially aggravating medications (eg, β-blockers or cholinergic agonists) and sensitivities to substances (eg, latex or aspirin) that are commonly used in the ICU. Examination findings may be helpful with typical expiratory-predominant wheezing (if severe, evidence of hyperinflation may be useful), but these findings are not unique to asthma. With severe exacerbations, wheezing may be paradoxically minimal or absent because of marked hyperinflation and reduced tidal volumes. Tachypnea, shallow respirations, and accessory muscle use should be evident. In the early stages, patients may have respiratory alkalosis, but respiratory acidosis and hypoxia may ensue rapidly with disease progression, fatigue, or the use of sedatives (Table 21.1). This change is important because a patient's arterial blood gas results may provide false reassurance of an inappropriate eucapnia in a patient who is tachypneic and has labored respirations.

When a patient is receiving mechanical ventilation, airflow obstruction may be indicated by elevated airway pressures, expiratory flow limitation on the flow curve, and evidence of auto–positive end-expiratory pressure (PEEP), such as incomplete exhalation before the next breath being triggered (breath stacking). If the patient has marked tachypnea with this expiratory flow limitation, achieving ventilator synchrony may be difficult, and mechanical ventilation may be complicated by hemodynamic instability due to increased intrathoracic pressure with consequently poor venous return and pneumothorax, which, if unrecognized, may be rapidly fatal in patients receiving mechanical ventilation.

Diagnosis

Pulmonary function testing can be helpful diagnostically. It is characterized by reversible airflow obstruction marked by a reduced FEV_1 to forced vital capacity ratio, with improvement after administration of a bronchodilator (increase in FEV_1 by 12% and 200 mL). If the baseline spirometry result is normal, a bronchoprovocation challenge (with methacholine, exercise, or histamine) can be administered to determine the presence of bronchial hyperresponsiveness. Typically, the diffusion capacity is preserved or increased. Although pulmonary function testing can be helpful diagnostically, it is rarely helpful in acute conditions. An adjunct diagnostic aid is the measure of exhaled nitric oxide, which correlates with eosinophil-mediated inflammation. Such testing may be helpful, but the diagnosis of asthma requires appropriate clinical context, particularly if a patient does not have established asthma and is critically ill.

For patients with known asthma, the 2007 National Asthma Education and Prevention Program Expert Panel Report 3 (EPR3) defines *severe asthma*, which requires emergency or hospital care, as the presence of dyspnea at rest that disrupts conversation and a peak expiratory flow (PEF) (or FEV_1) less than 40% of the patient's predicted value or best baseline. A subset considered to have *life-threatening asthma* is defined as patients who are too dyspneic to speak, are diaphoretic, and have a PEF (or FEV_1) less than 25% of the patient's predicted value or best baseline value. Patients in this subset should be considered for ICU admission. Other signs of imminent respiratory arrest include a decreased level of consciousness, bradycardia, pulsus paradoxus, thoracoabdominal paradox, and the absence of wheezing because of severely limited air movement.

The differential diagnosis for asthma should include pulmonary edema, chronic obstructive pulmonary disease (which may coexist with asthma), bronchiolitis from any cause (including viral infections), bronchiectasis, pneumonia, endobronchial or tracheal lesions, aspiration, excessive dynamic airway collapse, tracheomalacia, anaphylaxis, angioedema, vocal cord dysfunction, and laryngospasm. Several other asthma-related syndromes should also be considered since their management may be markedly different and affected patients may present with extrapulmonary (including neurologic) manifestations. These include allergic bronchopulmonary aspergillosis, eosinophilic granulomatosis with polyangiitis (Churg-Strauss syndrome), eosinophilic pneumonia, parasitic infections (Löffler

Table 21.2 • Differential Diagnoses for Wheezing, Dyspnea, and Cough

Wheezing	Dyspnea	Cough
Asthma	Asthma	Asthma
Bronchiectasis	Congestive heart failure	COPD
COPD	COPD	Pneumonia
Pulmonary edema	Pulmonary edema	GERD or reflux
Pulmonary embolus	Pneumonia	Malignancy
Pneumonia	Malignancy	Pneumothorax
Foreign body aspiration	Pneumothorax	Pulmonary edema
Anaphylaxis	Myocardial infarction	Anaphylaxis
Malignancy	Valvular heart disease	Tracheobronchitis
Vocal cord dysfunction	Anemia	Bronchiectasis

Abbreviations: COPD, chronic obstructive pulmonary disease; GERD, gastroesophageal reflux disease.

syndrome), and aspirin-exacerbated respiratory disease (Samter triad) (Table 21.2).

Treatment

General Considerations

The initial interventions for a patient with a severe asthma exacerbation should 1) correct any hypoxemia and 2) reverse airflow obstruction. Correction of hypoxemia may range from simply providing supplementary oxygen to administering invasive mechanical ventilator support. For most patients, a goal of 90% arterial oxygen saturation is adequate. Reversal of airflow obstruction consists primarily of providing bronchodilators and systemic corticosteroids. The EPR3 guidelines include an evidence-based algorithm for patients requiring care for asthma exacerbations (Figure 21.1). Additional considerations may include heliox, noninvasive positive-pressure ventilation (NIPPV), parenteral magnesium, and systemic β-agonists. Therapeutic value is limited or unknown for other adjunctive medications more typically used in outpatients with asthma (eg, leukotriene modifiers, anti-IgE, anti-IL5, and anti-IL13).

Bronchodilation

For acutely ill patients, bronchodilation medication should primarily be a short-acting β-agonist (eg, albuterol, levalbuterol, or pirbuterol). In the emergency department, patients may benefit from the use of a short-acting muscarinic antagonist (eg, ipratropium) for additional bronchodilator effects, although it probably does not provide additional benefit to asthmatic patients who are hospitalized or outpatients. Intravenous leukotriene-receptor antagonists can also provide bronchodilation within 10 minutes of administration, but their specific role in acute exacerbations is unclear. Aerosol bronchodilators can be administered through oral inhalers or by nebulization. Nebulization is no more effective for most asthmatic patients when oral inhalers are used with proper technique. Nebulization is recommended, however, for patients who are having a severe exacerbation, with increasing respiratory distress and worsening airflow obstruction, to ensure adequate delivery of medication. For severe exacerbations, administration can be as frequently as hourly or continuously.

Systemic β-agonists (eg, epinephrine and terbutaline) are effective bronchodilators, but they provide no proven benefit over aerosolized delivery and they may increase risk. Their use should be considered only in specific clinical contexts, such as anaphylaxis and pregnancy, or where emergency aerosol delivery is not available. The use of methylxanthines is not recommended.

Bronchodilators should be given to patients who are intubated and require mechanical ventilation. Because the ventilator circuit, endotracheal tube, and humidity may affect delivery and deposition, a pressurized metered dose inhaler (MDI) is typically used for 4 doses instead of the standard 2 doses. However, if the patient has been intubated because of a severe asthma exacerbation, repeated use of an MDI may be impractical; options include standard jet nebulization or ultrasonic nebulization. Since jet nebulization increases the flow to the ventilator circuit, ultrasonic nebulization may be preferred so that airway volumes and flows can be monitored continuously and accurately, which is particularly important for asthmatic patients, who have an increased risk for auto-PEEP and barotrauma.

Corticosteroid Therapy

Oral prednisone or methylprednisolone has excellent bioavailability and is generally recommended at 40 to 80 mg daily for most patients who require hospitalization for severe asthma exacerbation. However, parenteral glucocorticoids may be preferred for critically ill patients, especially if they have difficulties with speech or swallowing, nausea, vomiting, or a depressed level of consciousness or are receiving mechanical ventilation. Although expert opinion suggests a higher initial dosing of 60 to 80 mg every 6 to 12 hours for the first 48 hours, at least 1 randomized clinical trial has not shown an initial benefit with 100 mg compared to 500 mg when used in the emergency department. The onset of pharmacologic action is delayed by 6 to 12 hours, and immediate benefit is not expected. Preferred agents are methylprednisolone or prednisone.

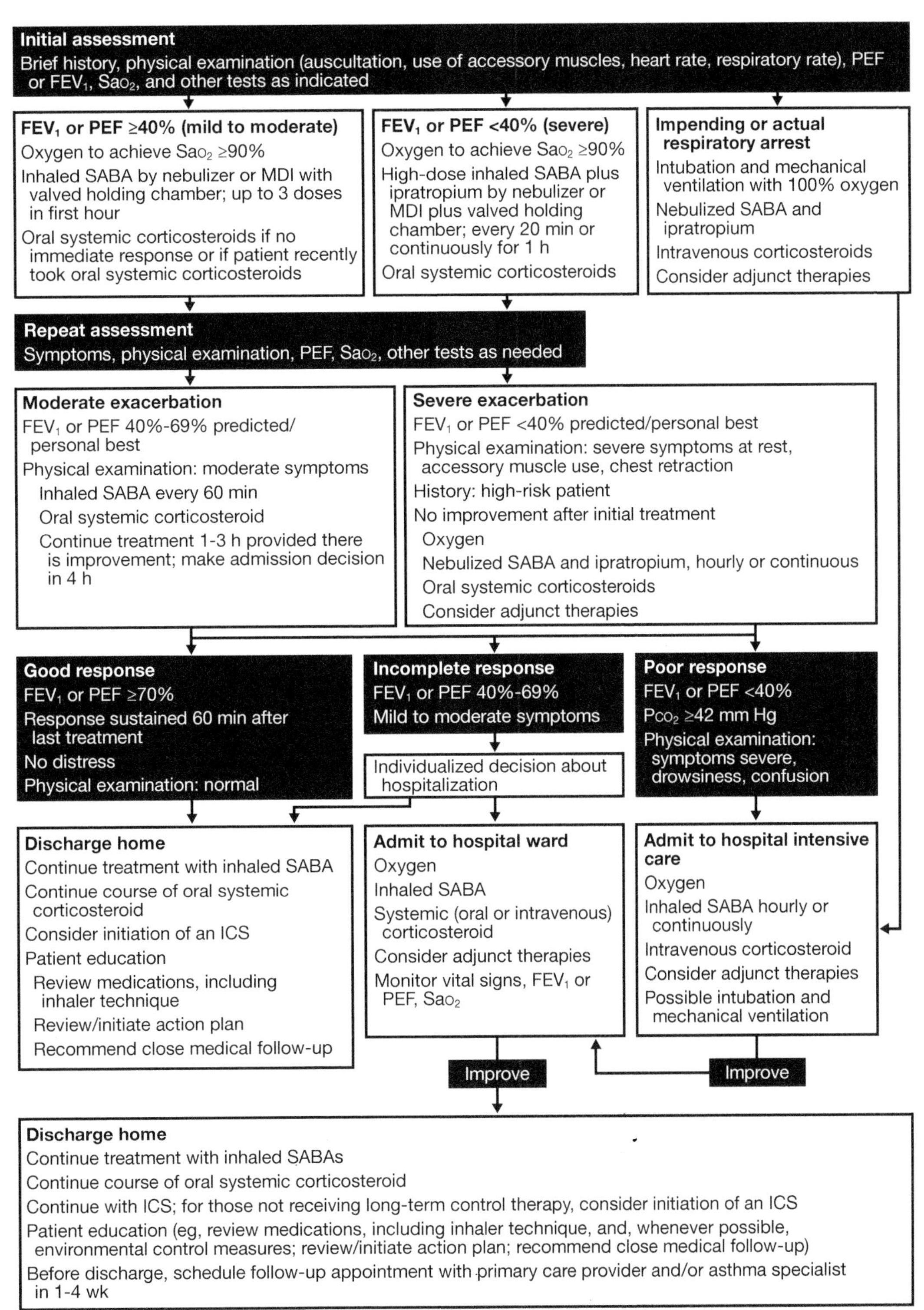

Figure 21.1. Management of Asthma Exacerbations: Emergency Department and Hospital-Based Care. FEV_1 indicates forced expiratory volume in 1 second; ICS, inhaled corticosteroid; MDI, metered dose inhaler; PEF, peak expiratory flow; SABA, short-acting β_2-agonist; SaO_2, oxygen saturation.

(From National Heart, Lung, and Blood Institute. National Asthma Education and Prevention Program: Expert Panel Report 3: Guidelines for the Diagnosis and Management of Asthma: Full Report 2007. Washington [DC]: U.S. Department of Health and Human Services; c2007. p. 373-415.)

Hydrocortisone is not recommended because it is predominantly a mineralocorticoid.

The duration of most asthma exacerbations is 10 to 14 days, and corticosteroid administration can be stopped during that time or earlier if lung function and clinical status have sustained improvement. Adverse effects of corticosteroids include hyperglycemia, hypertension, psychosis, immunosuppression, and critical illness myopathy (CIM) or critical illness polyneuropathy (CIP). Adrenal insufficiency is unlikely if corticosteroid use is limited to 2 to 3 weeks, and therapy can be stopped without tapering the dose. However, a patient's history of recent or sustained use of corticosteroids must be clarified before abrupt cessation.

Corticosteroid-induced psychosis or delirium may be particularly confusing in the neurocritical care unit, and the risk increases with the dose and duration of corticosteroid administration (typically >20 mg daily). When clinically feasible, some symptoms may be mitigated with dose reduction and with judicious use of neuroleptic agents. Neuromuscular weakness may also complicate the neurologic evaluation. Corticosteroid use, likely in combination with paralytic agents, is the primary risk factor for CIM. Clinical signs of CIM include limb flaccidity more than facial muscle weakness, slightly increased level of creatine kinase in 50% of affected patients, and possibly respiratory muscle weakness that may limit liberation from mechanical ventilator support. Patients with CIP present with similar clinical signs, but they also have sensory deficits, muscle atrophy, and reduced deep tendon reflexes. CIP has been described predominantly in the context of sepsis, but the use of corticosteroids is an additional risk factor. Electromyography may be helpful to clarify the diagnosis. Treatment is predominantly supportive: providing early physical or occupational therapy and limiting unnecessary doses or duration of corticosteroids. Blood glucose levels must also be monitored when corticosteroids are administered, even if patients are not diabetic, and patients with brain injury must receive appropriate therapy to avoid hyperglycemia. Although the development of osteonecrosis and osteoporosis may be influenced by the sustained use of corticosteroids, they are typically complications of long-term use.

Adjunctive Therapy

Adjunctive therapies to consider for the critically ill patient include parenteral magnesium and heliox. In a few studies, parenteral magnesium has decreased the need for hospitalization when used in life-threatening exacerbations. Heliox is a gas mixture of helium and oxygen (typically in a ratio of 70:30 or 60:40) that can improve laminar flow and decrease turbulent flow, thereby decreasing expiratory flow limitations, minimizing air trapping and dynamic hyperinflation, and consequently improving a patient's symptoms and work of breathing. However, clinical trials do not consistently show a clear benefit, possibly in part because of the study methods.

Mechanical Ventilation

When supplementary oxygen is inadequate, or the patient has signs of respiratory fatigue and impending respiratory arrest, endotracheal intubation and invasive mechanical ventilation may be necessary. However, the intensivist must recognize that these interventions do not correct the fundamental problem of progressive air trapping and airflow obstruction, and, if used without adequate experience, these interventions may increase the risk of hemodynamic instability and pneumothorax.

Before patients undergo rapid sequence intubation (RSI), they should receive pretreatment with corticosteroids, continuous nebulization of bronchodilators, and preoxygenation. If hemodynamic instability is expected, fluids, vasopressors, and ionotropes should be available. Epinephrine could be considered for severe hypotension and for severe bronchospasm, but its use must be weighed against its potential adverse effects if the patient is at risk for coronary ischemia, arrhythmia, or sustained tachycardias. In certain circumstances, NIPPV may be considered, although its precise role in severe exacerbations is not well defined. Pretreatment with intravenous lidocaine (1-1.5 mg/kg) 3 minutes before endotracheal intubation may also be considered for select patients to decrease bronchoconstriction and the autonomic response from laryngoscopy. It may also mitigate intracranial hypertension in a neurocritically ill patient.

Induction Agents

Induction agents recommended for asthmatic patients include propofol and ketamine; both have bronchodilator properties. Ketamine has the theoretical potential to increase intracranial pressure in patients with brain injury, but in clinical practice, when it is used in patients who have traumatic brain injury, ketamine is more likely to decrease intracranial pressure. Etomidate and benzodiazepines are acceptable alternatives, but ketamine and etomidate are probably preferred for hemodynamically unstable patients. Barbiturates (eg, thiopental) do not offer any advantages over propofol and are not commonly considered for patients in the neurocritical care unit, and, in the presence of a severe asthmatic attack, thiopental should be avoided because it may cause histamine release.

Neuromuscular Blockade

Neuromuscular blockade agents must be used for RSI, but their use should be minimized thereafter if possible because of an increased risk of CIM or CIP from concomitant corticosteroid use. Nondepolarizing agents such as rocuronium, cisatracurium, and vecuronium are preferred over succinylcholine and atracurium for minimizing histamine release that may further aggravate bronchospasm. These agents work at the presynaptic nicotinic acetycholine receptor of skeletal muscles and have little activity on smooth muscles, but they may have partial effects on muscarinic receptors that, in combination with histamine, may potentiate bronchospasm rarely or subclinically. The endotracheal tube diameter should be the largest feasible (eg, 8 mm) to facilitate ventilation and suctioning without causing additional flow limitation. After intubation, the patient and the ventilator should be carefully and continuously monitored for dyssynchrony, breath stacking or auto-PEEP, and barotrauma.

Ventilation Strategy

The optimal ventilation strategy or mode should be determined clinically at the bedside. Key concepts are to correct any hypoxia while preventing dynamic hyperinflation. To facilitate this and to improve ventilator synchrony, initial considerations may include flow triggering, decreasing the inspiration to expiration ratio (to <1:3) if possible, matching the high inspiratory flow requirements of the patient, and decreasing the respiratory rate, even at the cost of hypercapnia (ie, permissive hypercapnia), to minimize excessive breath stacking. Specifically, monitoring the patient-ventilator interaction, by using pressure-time and flow-time curves in combination with the patient's effort at the bedside, is essential to achieve synchrony and minimize complications of mechanical ventilation (Chapter 2, "Mechanical Ventilation: Basic Modes," and Chapter 3, "Mechanical Ventilation: Advanced Modes"). An exaggerated initial negative pressure deflection during inspiration along with thoracoabdominal paradox may indicate flow starvation, so the inspiratory flow should be increased to match the patient's effort. The end-expiratory and rest phases of the pressure-time and flow-time curves should also be studied to see whether there is ineffective flow (flow without additional volume), active expiration (a surge in pressure during expiration), double triggering, wasted efforts, or expiratory flow limitation (flow does not return to zero).

Sedation

Adjustments on the ventilator to match the patient's effort are often limited during extreme respiratory distress, and the breathing pattern may be injurious to the patient; thus, sedation may be necessary initially to facilitate safe and effective mechanical ventilation. Propofol may be the preferred initial choice because it has bronchodilator properties and because the expected duration of mechanical ventilator support is typically short. Rarely, isoflurane or sevoflurane might be used if an intubated patient has refractory, severe bronchospasm. Although inhaled anesthetics are typically used in the operating room, their use in the ICU as a primary sedative agent is the subject of increasing interest and study.

Dynamic Hyperinflation

If an intubated patient suddenly becomes hypotensive or has a cardiac arrest, initial considerations must include the development of tension pneumothorax and decreased cardiac preload due to excessive dynamic hyperinflation (auto-PEEP). Tension pneumothorax is an emergency. It is a clinical diagnosis, and lifesaving interventions should not be delayed until confirmatory diagnostic imaging is available. Bedside ultrasonography, which is often available at the bedside immediately, has higher sensitivity than chest radiography and with equal specificity for a pneumothorax in trauma patients evaluated by an experienced sonographer. Ventilator-aggravated hyperinflation causing shock may be partly alleviated by temporarily disconnecting the ventilator from the endotracheal tube. However, if the patient remains tachypneic and has severe bronchospasm, the dynamic hyperinflation may be intrinsic and predominantly related to a severe asthma exacerbation for which fluid challenges might help in combination with continued or adjunctive efforts at improving airflow obstruction.

Summary

- A severe asthma exacerbation can be rapidly fatal or the primary cause of critical illness, but it may also complicate the management of a neurocritically ill patient. Early recognition is important for aborting progression to frank respiratory failure and death.
- Asthma and critical illness may be aggravated by medications and interventions often used for critically ill patients, including β-antagonists, histaminergic and cholinergic agents, excessive fluids, sedatives, and various procedures.
- Intubating and managing the care of an asthmatic patient who needs mechanical ventilation require special considerations during the selection of specific pretreatment and induction agents.
- After a patient has been successfully intubated, the intensivist must balance the patient's need for oxygenation and ventilator support against complications of air trapping and barotrauma. Resolution and outcomes are usually favorable but depend on prompt recognition and timely delivery of treatment.

SUGGESTED READING

Abdelkarim H, Durie M, Bellomo R, Bergmeir C, Badawi O, El-Khawas K, et al. A comparison of characteristics and outcomes of patients admitted to the ICU with asthma in Australia and New Zealand and United States. J Asthma. 2019 Jan;31:1–7 [Epub ahead of print].

Bateman ED, Hurd SS, Barnes PJ, Bousquet J, Drazen JM, FitzGerald M, et al. Global strategy for asthma management and prevention: GINA executive summary. Eur Respir J. 2008 Jan;31(1):143–78.

Blaivas M, Lyon M, Duggal S. A prospective comparison of supine chest radiography and bedside ultrasound for the diagnosis of traumatic pneumothorax. Acad Emerg Med. 2005 Sep;12(9):844–9.

Broaddus VC, Mason RJ, Ernst JD, King TE Jr, Lazarus SC, Murray JF, et al, editors. Murray & Nadel's textbook of respiratory medicine. 6th ed. Philadelphia (PA): Elsevier/Saunders; c2016. 911 p.

Burrows B, Barbee RA, Cline MG, Knudson RJ, Lebowitz MD. Characteristics of asthma among elderly adults in a sample of the general population. Chest. 1991 Oct;100(4):935–42.

Ebina M, Takahashi T, Chiba T, Motomiya M. Cellular hypertrophy and hyperplasia of airway smooth muscles underlying bronchial asthma: a 3-D morphometric study. Am Rev Respir Dis. 1993 Sep;148(3):720–6.

Emerman CL, Cydulka RK. A randomized comparison of 100-mg vs 500-mg dose of methylprednisolone in the treatment of acute asthma. Chest. 1995 Jun;107(6):1559–63.

2011 GINA Report: Global strategy for asthma management and prevention [Internet]. c2016 Global Initiative for Asthma [cited 2016 Feb 10]. Available from: http://www.ginasthma.org/.

Kuyper LM, Pare PD, Hogg JC, Lambert RK, Ionescu D, Woods R, et al. Characterization of airway plugging in fatal asthma. Am J Med. 2003 Jul;115(1):6–11.

Li JT, O'Connell EJ. Clinical evaluation of asthma. Ann Allergy Asthma Immunol. 1996 Jan;76(1):1–13.

Li X, Wilson JW. Increased vascularity of the bronchial mucosa in mild asthma. Am J Respir Crit Care Med. 1997 Jul;156(1):229–33.

McFadden ER Jr. Acute severe asthma. Am J Respir Crit Care Med. 2003 Oct 1;168(7):740–59.

McFadden ER Jr. Pulmonary structure, physiology, and clinical correlates in asthma. In: Middleton E Jr, Reed CE, Ellis EF, Adkinson NF Jr, Yunginger JW, Busse WW, editors. Allergy: principles and practice. 4th ed. Vol. 1. St. Louis (MO): Mosby-Year Book; c1993. p. 672–93.

National Asthma Education and Prevention Program. Expert Panel Report 3 (EPR-3): Guidelines for the diagnosis and management of asthma-summary report 2007. J Allergy Clin Immunol. 2007 Nov;120(5 Suppl):S94–138. Erratum in: J Allergy Clin Immunol. 2008 Jun;121(6):1330.

Ronmark E, Lundback B, Jonsson E, Jonsson AC, Lindstrom M, Sandstrom T. Incidence of asthma in adults: report from the Obstructive Lung Disease in Northern Sweden Study. Allergy. 1997 Nov;52(11):1071–8.

Sly RM. Changing asthma mortality. Ann Allergy. 1994 Sep;73(3):259–68.

Tarlo SM, Balmes J, Balkissoon R, Beach J, Beckett W, Bernstein D, et al. Diagnosis and management of work-related asthma: American College of Chest Physicians Consensus Statement. Chest. 2008 Sep;134(3 Suppl):1S-41S. Erratum in: Chest. 2008 Oct;134(4):892.

Vignola AM, Mirabella F, Costanzo G, Di Giorgi R, Gjomarkaj M, Bellia V, et al. Airway remodeling in asthma. Chest. 2003 Mar;123(3 Suppl):417S–22S.

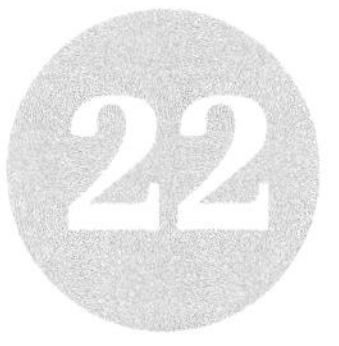

Chronic Obstructive Pulmonary Disease Exacerbation

ISABEL MIRA-AVENDANO, MD; MINKYUNG KWON, MD

Goals

- Describe exacerbation of chronic obstructive pulmonary disease.
- Discuss medical treatment of patients with exacerbation of chronic obstructive pulmonary disease.
- Describe ventilatory support for patients with exacerbation of chronic obstructive pulmonary disease.

Introduction

Patients with chronic obstructive pulmonary disease (COPD) have recurring or continuous obstruction of bronchial airflow. The disease is usually characterized by progressive chronic airway inflammation that results from smooth muscle hypertrophy, airway ciliary dysfunction, and excessive mucous production, which ultimately increases airway resistance and hyperactivity. Parenchymal destruction associated with emphysema increases lung compliance, which further decreases expiratory airflow.

During COPD exacerbation, a patient's respiratory symptoms suddenly worsen to the extent that the patient's usual therapy must be changed. In-hospital mortality is 10% to 21% for patients admitted for hypercapnic respiratory failure and requiring mechanical ventilation. COPD exacerbation can be precipitated by several factors, but the most common causes are respiratory tract infections (viral or bacterial).

Pharmacologic Therapy

Bronchodilators

Bronchodilators are the mainstay for treatment of COPD exacerbation. Inhaled short-acting β-adrenergic agonists (eg, albuterol or levalbuterol) are administered by inhaler or nebulizer every 4 to 6 hours. They can be administered in combination with inhaled short-acting anticholinergic drugs (eg, ipratropium). If patients are receiving mechanical ventilation, bronchodilators can be effectively delivered through a nebulizer or a metered dose inhaler.

Inhaled Corticosteroids

Inhaled corticosteroids decrease the severity of COPD exacerbations and modestly slow the progression of respiratory symptoms, but they have minimal or no effect on lung function and mortality. For management of COPD exacerbation, inhaled corticosteroids may be comparable to systemic corticosteroids, although the evidence is not clear.

Systemic Corticosteroids

In patients with COPD exacerbation, systemic corticosteroids can improve lung function (forced expiratory volume in 1 second [FEV_1]) and oxygenation and shorten recovery time and hospitalization duration. It is unclear whether patients who receive mechanical ventilation also receive benefit from systemic corticosteroids. Although a longer duration was previously recommended for use of oral corticosteroids, 5 to 7 days is likely sufficient. The benefit of parenteral corticosteroids over oral corticosteroids is unclear, but patients in shock (with impaired intestinal absorption) may benefit from parenteral corticosteroids.

Antibiotics

Antibiotic therapy is recommended if patients have the following 3 cardinal symptoms: increased dyspnea, increased sputum volume, and increased sputum purulence. It is also recommended if increased purulence of sputum is present in combination with 1 other cardinal symptom, or if mechanical ventilation (invasive or noninvasive) is required. The recommended duration of therapy is 5 to 7 days.

Coverage for *Pseudomonas* should be included if patients have any of the following risk factors: recent hospitalization (≥2 days during the past 90 days), frequent administration of antibiotics (≥4 courses within the past year), FEV_1 less than 50% of the predicted value, prior positive isolation, or systemic glucocorticoid use.

Mechanical Ventilation

Noninvasive Mechanical Ventilation

Noninvasive mechanical ventilation (NIMV) has a well-established role in respiratory failure associated with COPD exacerbation. It is first-line therapy for patients with acute hypercapnia or severe respiratory distress that persists despite initial use of bronchodilators and systemic corticosteroids (Box 22.1) in the absence of contraindications (Box 22.2). The use of NIMV decreases the risk of endotracheal intubation and treatment failure associated with severe exacerbations of COPD. In clinical trials, patients with more severe illness (arterial blood gases, pH <7.37 or $Paco_2$ >55 mm Hg) received the most benefit; no clear treatment effect was identified for patients with less severe illness.

Patients must be strictly monitored because mortality associated with prolonged NIMV is higher than with early invasive mechanical ventilation (IMV) when it is indicated. The best predictor of NIMV failure in acute hypercapnic respiratory failure, along with poor mental status, is severity of respiratory acidosis, both at presentation and after 1 to 2 hours of therapy.

Box 22.1 • Indications for NIMV for Patients With COPD Exacerbation

At least 1 of the following must be present:

- Respiratory acidosis ($Paco_2$ ≥6.0 kPa or 45 mm Hg *and* arterial pH ≤7.35)
- Severe dyspnea with clinical signs suggestive of respiratory muscle fatigue or increased work of breathing (or both), such as use of respiratory accessory muscles, paradoxical motion of the abdomen, or retraction of the intercostal spaces
- Persistent hypoxemia despite supplemental oxygen therapy

Abbreviations: COPD, chronic obstructive pulmonary disease; NIMV, noninvasive mechanical ventilation.

From Global Initiative for Chronic Obstructive Lung Disease (GOLD) [Internet]. Global strategy for the diagnosis, management and prevention of COPD; c2017 [cited 2017 Dec 27]. Available from: http://goldcopd.org/gold-2017-global-strategy-diagnosis-management-prevention-copd/; used with permission.

Box 22.2 • Contraindications for NIMV for Patients With COPD Exacerbation

- Respiratory or cardiac arrest
- Medical instability (hypotensive shock, myocardial infarction requiring intervention, uncontrolled ischemia or arrhythmias)
- Unable to protect airway
- Unable to fit mask
- Untreated pneumothorax
- Recent upper airway or esophageal surgery
- Excessive secretions[a]
- Uncooperative or agitated[a]

Abbreviations: COPD, chronic obstructive pulmonary disease; NIMV, noninvasive mechanical ventilation.

[a] Relative contraindications.

From Garpestad E, Brennan J, Hill NS. Noninvasive ventilation for critical care. Chest. 2007 Aug;132(2):711-20; used with permission.

Noninvasive positive-pressure ventilation (NIPPV) can be delivered with ventilatory modes preset for either volume or pressure. Pressure-preset modes (rather than volume-preset modes) have been evaluated in most randomized controlled trials of NIPPV for patients with acute respiratory failure caused by COPD. In pressure-preset modes, priority is given to reaching and maintaining a target for inspiratory pressure. This process involves decreasing the work of breathing and the spontaneous respiratory rate and increasing the expired tidal volume and the ventilator flow (to compensate for air leaks). Pressure-preset ventilation is usually administered as either *pressure-support ventilation* (PSV) or *pressure-control ventilation* (PCV). In PSV, which is used more often for patients with COPD exacerbation, each breath is triggered by the patient, and the tidal volume reflects the patient's respiratory effort and pulmonary function in combination with the preset pressure.

Mechanical Ventilator Settings

The recommendations for reducing ventilator-induced lung damage are to use low tidal volumes (6-8 mL/kg ideal body weight) and avoid plateau pressures of more than 30 mm Hg. To maintain pH at more than 7.15, permissive hypercapnia is allowed. The guiding parameter is arterial pH, not $Paco_2$, particularly in patients with chronic retention of carbon dioxide. The fraction of inspired oxygen should be set as the minimum to maintain Pao_2 above 60 mm Hg and peripheral oxygen saturation of hemoglobin above 88%; concentrations that are too high may cause oxygen toxicity, respiratory center suppression, and, most importantly, ventilation-perfusion mismatch. A high inspiratory flow rate helps most dyspneic or tachypneic patients with COPD.

Positive end-expiratory pressure (PEEP) (also called *extrinsic PEEP*) is an important consideration in ventilator setting. In auto-PEEP (also called *intrinsic PEEP*), the end-expiratory pressure exceeds the extrinsic PEEP. COPD patients, who have high airway resistance and need more time to fully empty their lungs, have an increased risk for auto-PEEP. Setting extrinsic PEEP below 75% to 85% of auto-PEEP makes triggering easier for these patients because alveolar pressure needs to be decreased below the level of extrinsic PEEP, instead of below atmospheric pressure.

High auto-PEEP can cause lung hyperinflation and result in compression and obstruction of the intrathoracic portion of the superior vena cava, so that venous return and, thus, preload are decreased. Another result of lung hyperinflation is bradycardia with vasodilation mediated through autonomic reflexes. In addition, extremely hyperinflated lungs due to auto-PEEP may cause acute right ventricular failure, shock, and cardiac arrest.

In patients with COPD, high minute ventilation further increases the risk of auto-PEEP, so minute ventilation should be kept low by using small tidal volumes and a low respiratory rate that allows enough exhalation time. If auto-PEEP has caused shock or cardiac arrest, a short trial of apnea may help the patient. To promote complete exhalation, the endotracheal or tracheostomy tube may be temporarily disconnected.

The use of higher PEEP is a concern because it may induce intracranial hypertension by transmitting intrathoracic pressure directly to the cerebral vault through a valveless spinal venous plexus. If a patient's pulmonary compliance is decreased, intrapulmonary pressure transmission is limited. Given that PEEP of less than 20 cm H_2O has no clinically significant effect on intracranial pressure, judicious use of PEEP is recommended in patients at risk for intracranial hypertension.

Insufficient data are available to support the superiority of any single mode of IMV. Pressure-targeted ventilation may cause inconsistent tidal volume, whereas volume-targeted ventilation may cause high airway pressure. Recommendations for patient care during IMV are to elevate the head of the bed, provide meticulous mouth care, give nutritional support, and manage fluids judiciously.

Complications of IMV in patients with COPD include pneumothorax and hypotension. Older patients, patients with severe comorbid disease, and patients with coexisting acute neuromuscular disease have poor outcomes. Among patients with COPD and neurologic disease, higher rates of tracheostomy have been reported for those with intracerebral hemorrhage, high hematoma volume, ganglionic location of the hematoma, or hydrocephalus.

Summary

- Respiratory tract infection is the most common cause of COPD exacerbation.
- Medical treatment of COPD exacerbation typically consists of bronchodilators, corticosteroids, and antibiotics.
- Noninvasive ventilatory support is the preferred option unless the patient has contraindications.

SUGGESTED READING

Abroug F, Ouanes I, Abroug S, Dachraoui F, Abdallah SB, Hammouda Z, et al. Systemic corticosteroids in acute exacerbation of COPD: a meta-analysis of controlled studies with emphasis on ICU patients. Ann Intensive Care. 2014 Oct 26;4:32.

Bergin SP, Rackley CR. Managing respiratory failure in obstructive lung disease. Clin Chest Med. 2016 Dec;37(4):659–67. Epub 2016 Sep 8.

Berlin D. Hemodynamic consequences of auto-PEEP. J Intensive Care Med. 2014 Mar-Apr;29(2):81–6. Epub 2012 May 15.

Bradley EH, Nallamothu BK, Stern AF, Byrd JR, Cherlin EJ, Wang Y, et al. Contemporary evidence: baseline data from the D2B Alliance. BMC Res Notes. 2008 Jun 11;1:23.

Cabrera Serrano M, Rabinstein AA. Causes and outcomes of acute neuromuscular respiratory failure. Arch Neurol. 2010 Sep;67(9):1089–94.

Celli BR, Thomas NE, Anderson JA, Ferguson GT, Jenkins CR, Jones PW, et al. Effect of pharmacotherapy on rate of decline of lung function in chronic obstructive pulmonary disease: results from the TORCH study. Am J Respir Crit Care Med. 2008 Aug 15;178(4):332–8. Epub 2008 May 29.

Crisafulli E, Barbeta E, Ielpo A, Torres A. Management of severe acute exacerbations of COPD: an updated narrative review. Multidiscip Respir Med. 2018 Oct;14(10):1057–69.

Drummond MB, Dasenbrook EC, Pitz MW, Murphy DJ, Fan E. Inhaled corticosteroids in patients with stable chronic obstructive pulmonary disease: a systematic review and meta-analysis. JAMA. 2008 Nov 26;300(20):2407–16. Erratum in: JAMA. 2009 Mar 11;301(10):1024.

Falagas ME, Avgeri SG, Matthaiou DK, Dimopoulos G, Siempos II. Short- versus long-duration antimicrobial treatment for exacerbations of chronic bronchitis: a meta-analysis. J Antimicrob Chemother. 2008 Sep;62(3):442–50. Epub 2008 May 8.

Gaude GS, Nadagouda S. Nebulized corticosteroids in the management of acute exacerbation of COPD. Lung India. 2010 Oct;27(4):230–5.

Hill NS. Where should noninvasive ventilation be delivered? Respir Care. 2009 Jan;54(1):62–70.

Huttner HB, Kohrmann M, Berger C, Georgiadis D, Schwab S. Predictive factors for tracheostomy in neurocritical care patients with spontaneous supratentorial hemorrhage. Cerebrovasc Dis. 2006;21(3):159–65. Epub 2005 Dec 23.

Keenan SP, Sinuff T, Cook DJ, Hill NS. Which patients with acute exacerbation of chronic obstructive pulmonary disease benefit from noninvasive positive-pressure ventilation? A systematic review of the literature. Ann Intern Med. 2003 Jun 3;138(11):861–70.

Lightowler JV, Wedzicha JA, Elliott MW, Ram FS. Noninvasive positive pressure ventilation to treat respiratory failure resulting from exacerbations of chronic obstructive pulmonary disease: Cochrane systematic review and meta-analysis. BMJ. 2003 Jan 25;326(7382):185.

Lindenauer PK, Stefan MS, Shieh MS, Pekow PS, Rothberg MB, Hill NS. Outcomes associated with invasive and noninvasive ventilation among patients hospitalized with exacerbations of chronic obstructive pulmonary disease. JAMA Intern Med. 2014 Dec;174(12):1982–93.

Mamary AJ, Kondapaneni S, Vance GB, Gaughan JP, Martin UJ, Criner GJ. Survival in patients receiving prolonged ventilation: factors that influence outcome. Clin Med Insights Circ Respir Pulm Med. 2011 Apr 25;5:17–26.

Peter JV, Moran JL, Phillips-Hughes J, Warn D. Noninvasive ventilation in acute respiratory failure: a meta-analysis update. Crit Care Med. 2002 Mar;30(3):555–62.

Plant PK, Owen JL, Elliott MW. Early use of non-invasive ventilation for acute exacerbations of chronic obstructive pulmonary disease on general respiratory wards: a multicentre randomised controlled trial. Lancet. 2000 Jun 3;355(9219):1931–5.

Ram FS, Picot J, Lightowler J, Wedzicha JA. Non-invasive positive pressure ventilation for treatment of respiratory failure due to exacerbations of chronic obstructive pulmonary disease. Cochrane Database Syst Rev. 2004;(3):CD004104. Update in: Cochrane Database Syst Rev. 2017 Jul 13;7:CD004104.

Ramsay M, Hart N. Current opinions on non-invasive ventilation as a treatment for chronic obstructive pulmonary disease. Curr Opin Pulm Med. 2013 Nov;19(6):626–30.

Rashid AM, Fulambarker A, Cohen ME, Patel B, Sood V. Effect of systemic corticosteroids on mechanically ventilated patients with acute exacerbation of COPD [abstract]. Chest. 2004 Oct;126(4_MeetingAbstracts):805S–6S.

Riley CM, Sciurba FC. Diagnosis and outpatient management of chronic obstructive pulmonary disease: a review. JAMA. 2019 Feb;321(8):786–97.

Souter MJ, Manno EM. Ventilatory management and extubation criteria of the neurological/neurosurgical patient. Neurohospitalist. 2013 Jan;3(1):39–45.

Vestbo J, Hurd SS, Agusti AG, Jones PW, Vogelmeier C, Anzueto A, et al. Global strategy for the diagnosis, management, and prevention of chronic obstructive pulmonary disease: GOLD executive summary. Am J Respir Crit Care Med. 2013 Feb 15;187(4):347–65. Epub 2012 Aug 9.

Vollenweider DJ, Jarrett H, Steurer-Stey CA, Garcia-Aymerich J, Puhan MA. Antibiotics for exacerbations of chronic obstructive pulmonary disease. Cochrane Database Syst Rev. 2012 Dec 12;12:CD010257.

Walters JA, Tan DJ, White CJ, Gibson PG, Wood-Baker R, Walters EH. Systemic corticosteroids for acute exacerbations of chronic obstructive pulmonary disease. Cochrane Database Syst Rev. 2014 Sep 1;(9):CD001288.

Walters JA, Tan DJ, White CJ, Wood-Baker R. Different durations of corticosteroid therapy for exacerbations of chronic obstructive pulmonary disease. Cochrane Database Syst Rev. 2014 Dec 10;(12):CD006897.

Walters JA, Wang W, Morley C, Soltani A, Wood-Baker R. Different durations of corticosteroid therapy for exacerbations of chronic obstructive pulmonary disease. Cochrane Database Syst Rev. 2011 Oct 5;(10):CD006897. Update in: Cochrane Database Syst Rev. 2014;12:CD006897.

Ward NS, Dushay KM. Clinical concise review: mechanical ventilation of patients with chronic obstructive pulmonary disease. Crit Care Med. 2008 May;36(5):1614–9.

Yang IA, Clarke MS, Sim EH, Fong KM. Inhaled corticosteroids for stable chronic obstructive pulmonary disease. Cochrane Database Syst Rev. 2012 Jul 11;(7):CD002991.

23 Pleural Diseases in Critical Care Medicine

KARTHIKA R. LINGA, MBBS; NEAL M. PATEL, MD

Goals

- Describe the etiology, clinical presentation, and management of pleural effusions and empyema.
- Elucidate the causes of pneumothorax and management in the intensive care unit.
- Discuss the usefulness of ultrasonography of the lungs for pleural effusions and pneumothorax.

Introduction

Pleural disease often affects critically ill patients and is usually related to trauma (including accidental perforation) or infection. Pneumothorax, a potentially life-threatening condition, requires early clinical recognition and sometimes urgent treatment. General intensivists often encounter pneumothorax after a procedure such as catheter placement. Neurointensivists may also encounter pneumothorax after polytrauma or recent tunneling of a ventriculoperitoneal catheter.

Pleural Effusions

Pleural effusions are identified in up to 62% of admitted patients in the medical intensive care unit (ICU) when chest radiography or ultrasonography of the lungs is used diagnostically. Effusions are broadly divided into transudates and exudates, and tests to distinguish their fluid characteristics differ in sensitivity and specificity (Table 23.1). The most commonly used criteria are the Light criteria.

Massive pleural effusion is an effusion that appears to occupy the entire hemithorax and causes marked respiratory distress, sometimes from the physiologic effects of tamponade. Common causes include traumatic hemothorax, malignancy, hepatic hydrothorax, uremic effusions, and malposition of a central venous catheter. Pleural effusions lead to compressive atelectasis with subsequent ventilation-perfusion mismatch and shunting, which can cause hypoxemia.

Supine chest radiographs do not allow for accurate evaluation of pleural effusions, and ultrasonography is increasingly preferred. The sensitivity of ultrasonography is proportional to the volume of fluid: Sensitivity is 100% with as little as 100 mL of fluid. Diagnostic or therapeutic thoracentesis is required for evaluation of almost all effusions. An exception, when observation would be sufficient, is when the diagnosis is secure, such as in heart failure. The absolute contraindications for thoracentesis are limited (patient refusal and chest wall infection), and the procedure is relatively safe in patients receiving mechanical ventilator support (the rates of pneumothorax are the same with and without ventilator support). Ultrasonographic guidance has been shown to increase procedural success rates and decrease the risk of postprocedural pneumothorax, the cost of hospitalization, and the length of stay. With ultrasonographic guidance, the risk of postprocedural pneumothorax is 2.7% and the risk of hemothorax or organ puncture is 1.2%.

Parapneumonic Effusions and Empyema

Among hospitalized patients with pneumonia, 20% to 40% have an associated effusion, and their mortality risk is 3.7 to 6.5 times higher than the risk for patients without an associated effusion. Parapneumonic effusions develop along a continuum with 3 main stages: exudative stage, fibropurulent stage, and fibroblastic stage. Ultrasonography is useful for identifying multiloculated effusions and the

Table 23.1 • Sensitivity and Specificity of Tests for Distinguishing Between Pleural Exudates and Transudates

Test	Identification of Exudate	
	Sensitivity, %	Specificity, %
Light criteria (≥1 of the following 3)	98	83
Ratio of pleural-fluid protein level to serum protein level >0.5	86	84
Ratio of pleural-fluid LDH level to serum LDH level >0.6	90	82
Pleural-fluid LDH level greater than two-thirds the upper limit of the reference range for serum LDH level	82	89
Pleural-fluid cholesterol level >60 mg/dL	54	92
Pleural-fluid cholesterol level >43 mg/dL	75	80
Ratio of pleural-fluid cholesterol level to serum cholesterol level >0.3	89	81
Serum albumin level – pleural fluid albumin level ≤1.2 g/dL	87	92

Abbreviation: LDH, lactate dehydrogenase.

From Light RW. Clinical practice: pleural effusion. N Engl J Med. 2002 Jun 20;346(25):1971-7; used with permission.

correct site. Computed tomography of the chest with contrast helps to enhance and delineate loculi.

Management considerations can begin with predicting the risk of a poor outcome for patients with parapneumonic effusions. Four categories are based on 3 variables: anatomy of the pleural space, bacteriology of the pleural fluid, and chemistry of the pleural fluid (Table 23.2). Antibiotics should be tailored for the suspected infection. Most antibiotics have good pleural space penetration, but aminoglycosides can be inactivated in an environment with low pH. Complicated parapneumonic effusions and empyemas (categories 3 and 4) should be evacuated to prevent complications. Options for evacuation include tube thoracostomy, video-assisted thoracoscopic surgery, and open decortication of lung. The First Multicenter Intrapleural Sepsis Trial (MIST1) showed similar primary outcomes for the need for open surgery with the use of small-bore, medium-bore, and large-bore tubes. On the contrary, pain, particularly that related to dissection for placement of the tubes, was markedly less with smaller tubes. Intrapleural instillation of fibrinolytic agents alone has produced various results, but studies have shown that intrapleural tissue plasminogen activator in combination with deoxyribonuclease therapy facilitated fluid drainage in patients with pleural infection, decreased the need for surgical consultation, and decreased the length of the hospital stay. Consequently, that combination is frequently used as a rescue therapy for patients who have not improved with incomplete drainage and who would otherwise be candidates for surgical débridement. Thoracoscopy is considered when

Table 23.2 • Risk Categories for Poor Outcome in Patients With Parapneumonic Effusion or Empyema

Pleural Space Anatomy		Pleural Fluid Bacteriology		Pleural Fluid Chemistry	Category	Risk of Poor Outcome	Drainage
A_0: Minimal free-flowing effusion (<10 mm on lateral decubitus)	*and*	B_x: Culture and Gram stain results unknown	*and*	C_x: pH unknown	1	Very low	No
A_1: Small to moderate free-flowing effusion (>10 mm and <0.5 of hemithorax)	*and*	B_0: Negative culture and Gram stain	*and*	C_0: pH≥7.20	2	Low	No
A_2: Large, free-flowing effusion (≥0.5 of hemithorax), loculated effusion, or effusion with thickened parietal pleura	*or*	B_1: Positive culture and Gram stain	*or*	C_1: pH<7.20	3	Moderate	Yes
		B_2: Pus			4	High	Yes

From Colice GL, Curtis A, Deslauriers J, Heffner J, Light R, Littenberg B, et al. Medical and surgical treatment of parapneumonic effusions: an evidence-based guideline. Chest. 2000 Oct;118(4):1158-71. Erratum in: Chest 2001 Jan;119(1):319; used with permission.

conservative efforts do not drain a multiloculated pleural collection or empyema.

Pneumothorax

Pneumothorax is categorized as traumatic or spontaneous. Iatrogenic causes, barotrauma, and volutrauma are the most common causes of pneumothorax in critically ill patients (Box 23.1).

Iatrogenic Pneumothorax

Central venous catheter placement, especially subclavian vein cannulation, is the most common cause of iatrogenic pneumothorax in the critical care practice, so postprocedural chest imaging is required. Furthermore, pneumothorax can occur during cardiopulmonary resuscitation maneuvers for cardiac arrest (from either barotrauma associated with bag ventilation or direct injury from rib fractures). Pneumothorax occurs in association with mechanical ventilation in patients with acute respiratory distress syndrome, chronic obstructive pulmonary disease, asthma, or intubation of the right main bronchus through direct barotrauma and volutrauma. Preventive strategies such as using low tidal volume, targeting low plateau pressures, and avoiding dynamic hyperinflation can potentially decrease the pneumothorax rate.

On chest radiography, pneumothorax is apparent in the apicolateral location in 22% of critically ill patients. An oblique view is useful for detecting occult pneumothorax. With computed tomography, pneumothorax is apparent in a larger percentage, but placement of a chest tube may not be needed for smaller pneumothoraces.

Ultrasonography shows multiple signs of pneumothorax (Figures 23.1 and 23.2). The presence of pleural sliding (negative predictive value, 99.2%-100%) in all lung regions is useful for ruling out a pneumothorax. In M-mode, the absence of pleural sliding results in a pattern that resembles a barcode (the *barcode sign*). The presence of even 1 comet-tail artifact essentially rules out the diagnosis of a pneumothorax because the ultrasound beam is being reflected in the lung interstitium. The *lung point sign* is considered a pathognomonic sign of pneumothorax (specificity, 100%). However, this sign has a much lower sensitivity (66%) and is absent with total lung collapse.

Most ICU patients tolerate poorly any degree of pneumothorax. Hence, small-bore chest tube placement should be considered. Special circumstances, such as a pneumothorax due to barotrauma even in the absence of any hemodynamic instability, should be treated with large-bore chest tubes because 30% of patients have been reported to progress into tension pneumothorax.

Box 23.1 • Causes of Pneumothorax in Critically Ill Patients

- Secondary spontaneous
  - Airway diseases
    - Status asthmaticus
    - Chronic obstructive pulmonary disease
    - Cystic fibrosis
  - Interstitial lung diseases
    - Langerhans cell histiocytosis (histiocytosis X)
    - Stage IV sarcoidosis
    - Idiopathic pulmonary fibrosis
  - Pulmonary infections
    - *Pneumocystis jiroveci*
    - Necrotizing pneumonia
    - Tuberculosis
- Barotrauma
  - Mechanical ventilation
    - Acute respiratory distress syndrome
    - Status asthmaticus
    - Chronic obstructive pulmonary disease
  - Inhalational drug use
  - Decompression injury
- Trauma
  - Rib fractures
  - Blunt chest trauma
  - Penetrating chest trauma
  - Tracheobronchial injuries
  - Esophageal rupture
- Iatrogenic
  - Central venous catheter placement
  - Thoracentesis
  - Endotracheal intubation
  - Tracheostomy
  - Nasogastric tube placement
  - Bronchoscopy with bronchoalveolar lavage or biopsies
  - Cardiopulmonary resuscitation

Tension Pneumothorax

Tension pneumothorax occurs when a 1-way valve mechanism facilitates entry of atmospheric air into the pleural

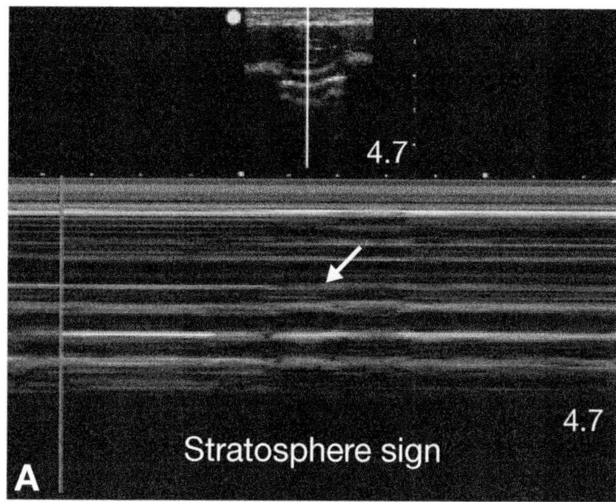

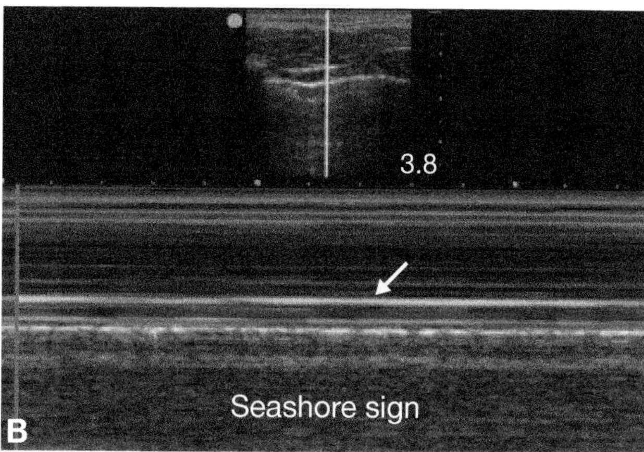

Figure 23.1. Pneumothorax on Ultrasonography. A, Stratosphere (barcode) sign (arrow) in pneumothorax. B, Seashore sign (arrow) in normal lung. (Courtesy of Michael B. Stone, MD, Portland, Oregon.)

cavity after a break in the visceral or parietal pleura. Tension pneumothorax can lead to cardiovascular collapse with pulseless electrical activity arrest. Patients receiving mechanical ventilation have a sudden increase in peak airway pressure, worsening oxygenation, and worsening lung compliance. Other signs, including prominent neck veins and contralateral shift in mediastinum, can be present. Insertion of a large-bore needle or intravenous catheter into the pleural space (at the second intercostal space and midclavicular line) is considered a valid option when a chest tube is not immediately available. Evidence of air escaping through the needle provides confirmation of the diagnosis. After this procedure, the needle is left in place until a definitive chest tube is urgently placed.

Figure 23.2. Lung Point Sign on Ultrasonography. Left, The seashore sign (white arrow) and the stratosphere sign (dotted arrow) are present as the lung intermittently contacts the chest wall. Right, B-mode shows the lung point sign (arrow) where sliding lung touches the chest wall. (From Husain LF, Hagopian L, Wayman D, Baker WE, Carmody KA. Sonographic diagnosis of pneumothorax. J Emerg Trauma Shock. 2012 Jan;5[1]:76-81; used with permission.)

Summary

- Pleural effusions are prevalent in ICU patients.
- Sampling of fluid is usually necessary to determine optimal management.
- Nonmalignant massive effusions may be due to traumatic or iatrogenic causes.
- Pneumothorax in ICU patients is typically iatrogenic and related to barotrauma or procedures; it may require chest tube placement to avoid hemodynamic and respiratory instability.
- Thoracic ultrasonography is an invaluable diagnostic tool for determining the presence or absence of a pneumothorax in critically ill patients.

SUGGESTED READING

Andrews NC, Parker EF, Shaw RR, Wilson NJ, Webb WR. Management of non tuberculous empyema: a statement of the subcommittee on surgery. Am Rev Respir Dis. 1962;85:935–6.

De Luca C, Valentino M, Rimondi MR, Branchini M, Baleni MC, Barozzi L. Use of chest sonography in acute-care radiology. J Ultrasound. 2008 Dec;11(4):125–34. Epub 2008 Nov 6.

Haynes D, Baumann MH. Management of pneumothorax. Semin Respir Crit Care Med. 2010 Dec;31(6):769–80. Epub 2011 Jan 6.

Hasley PB, Albaum MN, Li YH, Fuhrman CR, Britton CA, Marrie TJ, et al. Do pulmonary radiographic findings at presentation predict mortality in patients with community-acquired pneumonia? Arch Intern Med. 1996 Oct 28;156(19):2206–12.

Kalokairinou-Motogna M, Maratou K, Paianid I, Soldatos T, Antipa E, Tsikkini A, et al. Application of color Doppler ultrasound in the study of small pleural effusion. Med Ultrason. 2010 Mar;12(1):12–6.

Khandelwal A, Kapoor I, Goyal K, Singh S, Jena BR. Pneumothorax during percutaneous tracheostomy: a brief review of literature on attributable causes and preventable strategies. Anaesthesiol Intensive Ther. 2017;49(4):317–9. Epub 2017 Sep 27.

Lichtenstein D, Goldstein I, Mourgeon E, Cluzel P, Grenier P, Rouby JJ. Comparative diagnostic performances of auscultation, chest radiography, and lung ultrasonography in acute respiratory distress syndrome. Anesthesiology. 2004 Jan;100(1):9–15.

Lichtenstein D, Meziere G, Biderman P, Gepner A. The "lung point": an ultrasound sign specific to pneumothorax. Intensive Care Med. 2000 Oct;26(10): 1434–40.

Lichtenstein DA, Meziere G, Lascols N, Biderman P, Courret JP, Gepner A, et al. Ultrasound diagnosis of occult pneumothorax. Crit Care Med. 2005 Jun;33(6):1231–8.

Maskell NA, Davies CW, Nunn AJ, Hedley EL, Gleeson FV, Miller R, et al; First Multicenter Intrapleural Sepsis Trial (MIST1) Group. U.K. controlled trial of intrapleural streptokinase for pleural infection. N Engl J Med. 2005 Mar 3;352(9):865–74. Erratum in: N Engl J Med. 2005 May 19;352(20):2146.

Mattison LE, Coppage L, Alderman DF, Herlong JO, Sahn SA. Pleural effusions in the medical ICU: prevalence, causes, and clinical implications. Chest. 1997 Apr;111(4):1018–23.

Mercaldi CJ, Lanes SF. Ultrasound guidance decreases complications and improves the cost of care among patients undergoing thoracentesis and paracentesis. Chest. 2013 Feb 1;143(2):532–8.

Rahman NM, Maskell NA, Davies CW, Hedley EL, Nunn AJ, Gleeson FV, et al. The relationship between chest tube size and clinical outcome in pleural infection. Chest. 2010 Mar;137(3):536–43. Epub 2009 Oct 9.

Rahman NM, Maskell NA, West A, Teoh R, Arnold A, Mackinlay C, et al. Intrapleural use of tissue plasminogen activator and DNase in pleural infection. N Engl J Med. 2011 Aug 11;365(6):518–26.

Rodriguez RM, Canseco K, Baumann BM, Mower WR, Langdorf MI, Medak AJ, et al. Pneumothorax and hemothorax in the era of frequent chest computed tomography for the evaluation of adult patients with blunt trauma. Ann Emerg Med. 2019 Jan;73(1):58–65. Epub 2018 Oct 2.

Shieh L, Go M, Gessner D, Chen JH, Hopkins J, Maggio P. Improving and sustaining a reduction in iatrogenic pneumothorax through a multifaceted quality-improvement approach. J Hosp Med. 2015 Sep;10(9):599–607. Epub 2015 Jun 3.

Thommi G, Shehan JC, Robison KL, Christensen M, Backemeyer LA, McLeay MT. A double blind randomized cross over trial comparing rate of decortication and efficacy of intrapleural instillation of alteplase vs placebo in patients with empyemas and complicated parapneumonic effusions. Respir Med. 2012 May;106(5):716–23. Epub 2012 Mar 6.

Tocino IM, Miller MH, Fairfax WR. Distribution of pneumothorax in the supine and semirecumbent critically ill adult. AJR Am J Roentgenol. 1985 May;144(5):901–5.

Tulay CM, Yaldiz S, Bilge A. Oblique chest X-ray: an alternative way to detect pneumothorax. Ann Thorac Cardiovasc Surg. 2018 Jun;24(3):127–30.

24 Pulmonary Malignancy

ALI A. ZAIED, MD; MARGARET M. JOHNSON, MD

Goals

- Describe the epidemiologic characteristics of lung cancer.
- Identify complications of thoracic malignancy.
- Know how to recognize pulmonary toxicity that results from chemotherapy.

Introduction

Although the number of new lung cancer cases has decreased, most are diagnosed at an advanced stage owing to the asymptomatic nature of the disease. Furthermore, patients may need intensive care admission for paraneoplastic syndromes such as hypercalcemia, Lambert-Eaton myasthenic syndrome (LEMS), syndrome of inappropriate secretion of antidiuretic hormone (SIADH), Cushing syndrome, and superior vena cava syndrome (SVCS). Indications for intensive care unit admission can be tailored to the predicted outcome and performance status; the latest recommendations have been published as a consensus statement from several critical care organizations. Pulmonary infections must be considered in the differential diagnosis of chemotherapy-related lung toxicity.

Primary Lung Cancer

Lung cancer is the second most common cancer (excluding skin cancer) and the most common cause of cancer-related death in the United States in both sexes (approximately 160,000 deaths annually). Nearly 85% of primary lung cancers in the United States are attributable to tobacco abuse; other contributors include uranium, radon, and asbestos exposure.

Non–Small Cell Lung Cancer

Non–small cell lung cancer (NSCLC), which accounts for 75% of primary lung cancers, is subdivided by cell type (Box 24.1) and is staged according to the TNM system. Most cases are diagnosed at an advanced stage because symptoms are absent in the early stages of the disease. On the basis of a demonstrated stage shift and mortality benefit, the US Preventive Services Task Force has advocated annual screening with a low-dose computed tomographic scan of the chest for a targeted population of persons aged 55 to 79 years who are former or current smokers.

Surgical resection is recommended in the early stages of the disease if patients have adequate pulmonary reserve and overall good health. Postoperatively the predicted forced expiratory volume in 1 second should be greater than 0.80 L to allow safe resection.

Small Cell Lung Cancer

Small cell lung cancer (SCLC) accounts for 10% to 15% of primary lung cancers. It is more closely associated with tobacco exposure, including second-hand smoke exposure, than NSCLC; it has spread outside the thorax in 60% to 70% of patients at diagnosis; it is more commonly associated with paraneoplastic syndromes; and it is typically treated with radiotherapy and chemotherapy. Historically, SCLC was staged in a binary fashion (as limited or extensive), but the TNM staging system is now recommended.

Less common primary thoracic malignancies include atypical and typical carcinoid tumors, mesothelioma, pulmonary artery sarcoma, and primary pulmonary lymphoma (Chapter 51, "Hematologic and Oncologic Complications in the Intensive Care Unit").

Thoracic Metastatic Disease

Metastatic disease to the chest complicates the course of many malignancies and can involve the lung parenchyma, airways, pulmonary vasculature, mediastinal lymph nodes, and pleural space (Table 24.1).

Malignant pleural effusions are often so large that they compromise respiratory function. The most common causes

Box 24.1 • Types of Lung Cancer

Non–small cell lung cancer
- Adenocarcinoma—most common subtype; may appear as a semisolid nodule or have ground-glass opacity
- Squamous cell carcinoma—often occurs in proximal tracheobronchial tree; cavitation not uncommon
- Adenosquamous—very aggressive
- Large cell—large peripheral mass with prominent necrosis

Small cell lung cancer—strongest association with cigarette smoking

are lung cancer (most commonly adenocarcinoma), breast cancer, and lymphoma. Pleural effusions due to metastatic disease are typically exudative; often they are hemorrhagic. Diagnosis is established cytologically with the finding of malignant cells in pleural fluid. Results from a single pleural fluid sample may be negative, but repeated aspirations increase the diagnostic yield. Malignant pleural effusions portend a very poor prognosis (median survival, 6 months); thus, treatment is predicated on effective palliation of symptoms.

Treatment options include repeated needle thoracentesis, tube thoracostomy, pleurodesis (chemical or biologic), pleuroperitoneal shunt placement, and tunneled indwelling pleural catheters. Indwelling catheters allow repeated drainage and, ultimately, may cause pleurodesis. Pleurodesis is less likely to occur in patients with extensive pleural deposition, multiple pleural loculations, trapped lung, or endobronchial tumor leading to airway obstruction.

Paraneoplastic Syndromes

Hypercalcemia

Malignancy-associated hypercalcemia complicates many types of cancer (including lung cancer) and occurs by various mechanisms. Patients may have lethargy, confusion, constipation, hypovolemia, bradyarrhythmias, and electrocardiographic abnormalities. Hypovolemia results from osmotic diuresis. The cornerstones for managing malignancy-associated hypercalcemia are adequate volume resuscitation with normal saline solution (to improve glomerular filtration rate and decrease passive sodium-calcium reabsorption from the proximal tubule) and antihypercalcemic therapy. The bisphosphonates

Table 24.1 • Common Radiographic Findings in Patients With Thoracic Malignancy

Finding	Common Causes of Malignancy	Clinical Findings
Pulmonary nodule(s) (<3 cm) or mass (≥3 cm)	Single lesion: metastatic colon cancer; NSCLC Multiple nodules: metastatic cancer	Multiple nodules of various sizes suggest metastatic disease Colon cancer metastasis more commonly occurs as multiple nodules, but a single nodule or mass due to metastasis is most likely colon cancer
Mediastinal adenopathy	Lymphoma SCLC NSCLC Thyroid carcinoma Thymic carcinoma	Lymph node >1 cm in short axis on transverse CT and FDG uptake greater than mediastinal blood pool suggest malignancy, but neither is adequately sensitive or specific for confirmation
Lymphangitic pattern and pulmonary tumor emboli	Renal cell cancer Hepatocellular cancer Pancreatic cancer Lung cancer Breast cancer GI tract malignancies	Clinical presentation can mimic pulmonary embolism Poor prognosis
Endobronchial metastasis	NSCLC Melanoma Kaposi sarcoma	Potential cause of atelectasis
Pleural effusion	NSCLC Mesothelioma Breast cancer	Malignancy is common cause of large effusion (>67% of hemithorax) Exudative Bloody Can be malignant (neoplastic cells present) or paramalignant (from indirect effects of tumor on pleural space)

Abbreviations: CT, computed tomography; FDG, fludeoxyglucose F 18; GI, gastrointestinal; NSCLC, non–small cell lung cancer; SCLC, small cell lung cancer.

(pamidronate and zoledronate) are first-line therapy. Other considerations include eliminating medications associated with hypercalcemia (thiazide diuretics), increasing calcium excretion with cautious use of loop diuretics and hemodialysis, and administering glucocorticosteroids (to decrease extrarenal calcitriol production and inhibit osteoclastic resorption from bone).

Lambert-Eaton Myasthenic Syndrome

LEMS is an autoimmune disorder of the neuromuscular junction that results in decreased neuromuscular transmission. LEMS is characterized by antibodies directed against voltage-gated calcium channels (VGCCs) in the presynaptic membrane of motor nerve terminals. In approximately half the patients, LEMS is a paraneoplastic syndrome. SCLC is the most common associated malignancy; other malignant causes include prostate cancer, lymphoma, and leukemia.

Clinical features include the triad of proximal muscle weakness, autonomic dysfunction, and diminished tendon reflexes. On repetitive nerve stimulation, patients with LEMS have a low compound muscle action potential (CMAP) at rest and a further decrease in the CMAP amplitude by at least 10% at low frequency. Diagnosis is confirmed with the presence of autoantibodies against VGCCs. LEMS can be differentiated from myasthenia gravis (MG) by the pattern of progression (caudocranially in LEMS; craniocaudally in MG) and the CMAP amplitude at rest (low in LEMS; normal in MG). Evaluation for an underlying malignancy is indicated when LEMS is recognized.

First-line therapy is 3,4-diaminopyridine (DAP), which inhibits presynaptic voltage-gated potassium channels, thereby prolonging the presynaptic action potential and the VGCC opening time. If 3,4-DAP therapy is inadequate, immunosuppressive therapy is administered short-term (with plasma exchange, intravenous immunoglobulin, and rituximab) or long-term (with prednisone and azathioprine). Concomitant guideline-based management of associated malignancy is recommended.

Syndrome of Inappropriate Secretion of Antidiuretic Hormone

Hyponatremia is the most common electrolyte disturbance in cancer patients, and the most common cause of hyponatremia is SIADH, which involves paraneoplastic production of antidiuretic hormone. Other causes of hyponatremia are gastrointestinal tract fluid losses, chemotherapy, liver failure, and adrenal insufficiency. SCLC and head and neck cancers are the most common malignant causes of SIADH. Clinical manifestations, including lethargy, confusion, seizure, and coma, are related to the severity and acuity of hyponatremia. Diagnostic criteria are listed in Box 24.2.

Fluid restriction (500-1,000 mL daily) is indicated for patients with asymptomatic or mildly symptomatic hyponatremia. Other therapeutic options include demeclocycline (inhibits the effects of antidiuretic hormone in the renal tubules, thereby resulting in reversible nephrogenic diabetes insipidus) and conivaptan and tolvaptan (nonselective inhibitors of vasopressin receptors). In patients with considerable neurologic impairment from hyponatremia, 3% saline is indicated. A rate of correction of less than 8 to 10 mmol/L daily and 18 mmol/L in 48 hours is recommended to minimize the risk of osmotic demyelination.

Box 24.2 • Essential Diagnostic Criteria for SIADH

Serum osmolality <275 mOsm/kg

Urine osmolality >100 mOsm/kg

Clinically euvolemic

Urine sodium >30 mEq/L (with normal daily sodium intake)

Normal adrenal and thyroid function

No recent use of diuretics

Abbreviation: SIADH, syndrome of inappropriate secretion of antidiuretic hormone.

Cushing Syndrome

SCLC can produce ectopic adrenal corticotropin and cause Cushing syndrome, which manifests as muscle weakness, weight loss, hypertension, and hypokalemic metabolic alkalosis. The presence of Cushing syndrome is associated with a worse prognosis and may increase infectious complications.

Superior Vena Cava Syndrome

SVCS is caused by extrinsic compression of the superior vena cava by tumor, resulting in impaired venous flow. SVCS is most commonly caused by lung cancer and lymphoma. Clinical manifestations, which depend on the acuity of development and the level of obstruction, may include facial or neck swelling, arm swelling, dyspnea, cough, and dilated chest veins. Stridor (indicative of laryngeal edema) and confusion (indicative of cerebral edema) are ominous signs. In the absence of acute airway compromise or cerebral edema, expedited tissue diagnosis and staging are indicated. Therapy, which should expedite control of underlying malignancy and relieve symptoms of obstruction, may include radiotherapy, chemotherapy, and vascular stent insertion. Treatment of life-threatening manifestations, such as stridor and confusion, must take precedent over tissue confirmation of diagnosis.

Pulmonary Complications of Therapy

Pulmonary toxicity may result from many chemotherapeutic agents. No diagnostic test can confirm drug toxicity as the cause of pulmonary complications; thus, it is a diagnosis of exclusion. Drug discontinuation, with or without

Table 24.2 • Common Findings in Patients With Pulmonary Toxicity of Cancer Therapy

Finding	Therapy	Clinical Findings
Pulmonary edema	Pneumonectomy Docetaxel Doxorubicin Nivolumab	After pneumonectomy, judicious fluid management is recommended Cardiac toxicity from doxorubicin may lead to pulmonary edema; also reported to reactivate radiotherapy pneumonitis
Interstitial disease	Radiation fibrosis Bleomycin Taxanes (paclitaxel, docetaxel) Gemcitabine Fludarabine Tyrosine kinase inhibitors (erlotinib, gefitinib, osimertinib)	Administration of high F_{IO_2} potentiates bleomycin lung toxicity Gemcitabine toxicity potentiated by coadministration with taxane Fludarabine toxicity usually occurs early in course TKI-induced ILD has high mortality
Air space infiltrate	Radiotherapy Nivolumab	Radiotherapy-induced damage is most commonly confined to field of exposure but not exclusively so; usually develops 4-12 wk after radiotherapy
Bronchoconstriction	Etoposide	Infusion reaction is suggestive of anaphylaxis; likely due to vehicle
Pleural effusion	Docetaxel Nivolumab	Docetaxel is associated with capillary leakage

Abbreviations: F_{IO_2}, fraction of inspired oxygen; ILD, interstitial lung disease; TKI, tyrosine kinase inhibitor.

corticosteroid therapy, is generally indicated, but the risk-benefit ratio of drug discontinuation must be considered individually. Pulmonary infection must be excluded as the cause of symptoms or radiographic abnormalities. Table 24.2 highlights common treatment-induced pulmonary toxicity.

Thoracic radiotherapy is used in the management of lung cancer and other malignancies, including lymphoma and breast cancer. Stereotactic body radiotherapy is commonly used in early-stage NSCLC and rarely results in serious pulmonary injury. Conventional radiotherapy to the chest may result in radiation pneumonitis or fibrosis manifested as dry cough, dyspnea, and radiographic opacities. Supportive care, exclusion of alternative diagnoses, and administration of glucocorticoids are the mainstays of therapy for radiation pneumonitis. Azathioprine and cyclosporine have also been used successfully.

Summary

- NSCLC accounts for 75% of primary lung cancers, and most cases are diagnosed at an advanced stage because symptoms are absent in the early stages of the disease.
- Paraneoplastic syndromes include hypercalcemia, LEMS, SIADH, Cushing syndrome, and SVCS.
- A number of chemotherapy- and radiotherapy-related complications can affect the lungs.
- Pulmonary infection must be excluded as the cause of symptoms or radiographic abnormalities if chemotherapy-related lung toxicity is suspected.

SUGGESTED READING

Hulsbrink R, Hashemolhosseini S. Lambert-Eaton myasthenic syndrome: diagnosis, pathogenesis and therapy. Clin Neurophysiol. 2014 Dec;125(12):2328–36. Epub 2014 Jul 4.

Kieh MG, Beutel G, Boll B, Buchheidt D, Forkert R, Fuhrmann V, et al. Consensus of the German Society of Hematology and Medical Oncology (DGHO), Austrian Society of Hematology and Oncology (OeGHO), German Society for Medical Intensive Care Medicine and Emergency Medicine (DGIIN), and Austrian Society of Medical and General Intensive Care and Emergency Medicine (OGIAIN). Consensus statement of cancer patients requiring intensive care support. Ann Hematol. 2018 Jul;97(7):1271–82.

McCarty MJ, Lillis P, Vukelja SJ. Azathioprine as a steroid-sparing agent in radiation pneumonitis. Chest. 1996 May;109(5):1397–400.

McCurdy MT, Shanholtz CB. Oncologic emergencies. Crit Care Med. 2012 Jul;40(7):2212–22.

Muraoka T, Bandoh S, Fujita J, Horiike A, Ishii T, Tojo Y, et al. Corticosteroid refractory radiation pneumonitis that remarkably responded to cyclosporin A. Intern Med. 2002 Sep;41(9):730–3.

National Lung Screening Trial Research Team, Aberle DR, Adams AM, Berg CD, Black WC, Clapp JD, Fagerstrom RM, et al. Reduced lung-cancer mortality with low-dose computed tomographic screening. N Engl J Med. 2011 Aug 4;365(5):395–409. Epub 2011 Jun 29.

Rosner MH, Dalkin AC. Electrolyte disorders associated with cancer. Adv Chronic Kidney Dis. 2014 Jan;21(1):7–17.

Shepherd FA, Crowley J, Van Houtte P, Postmus PE, Carney D, Chansky K, et al; International Association for the Study of Lung Cancer International Staging Committee and Participating Institutions. The International Association for the Study of Lung Cancer lung cancer staging project: proposals regarding the clinical staging of small cell lung cancer in the forthcoming (seventh) edition of the tumor, node, metastasis classification for lung cancer. J Thorac Oncol. 2007 Dec;2(12):1067–77.

Siegel RL, Miller KD, Jemal A. Cancer statistics, 2016. CA Cancer J Clin. 2016 Jan-Feb;66(1):7–30. Epub 2016 Jan 7.

Wan JF, Bezjak A. Superior vena cava syndrome. Emerg Med Clin North Am. 2009 May;27(2):243–55.

25 Pulmonary Hypertension and Right-Sided Heart Failure in the Critically Ill

CHARLES D. BURGER, MD

Goals

- Describe the causes of pulmonary hypertension in patients in the intensive care unit.
- Discuss the diagnostic approach to pulmonary hypertension.
- Discuss the management options for pulmonary hypertension and associated right ventricular failure.

Introduction

Pulmonary hypertension (PH) was defined hemodynamically at the Fifth World Symposium on Pulmonary Hypertension (WSPH) as a mean pulmonary artery (PA) pressure (mPAP) of 25 mm Hg or more. Five diagnostic groups represent the various causes of PH. Group 1 pulmonary arterial hypertension (PAH) requires both an elevated mPAP and a pulmonary vascular resistance (PVR) of at least 3 Wood units; therefore, the left-sided heart filling pressures are not elevated (pulmonary arterial wedge pressure [PAWP] ≤15 mm Hg). Conversely, in group 2 PH, left-sided heart disease causes an elevation in PAWP. Group 3 PH is due to chronic hypoxemia typically from lung disease, group 4 PH is chronic thromboembolic PH, and group 5 PH is a miscellaneous category.

Notably, group 1 PAH is a chronic disease requiring complex PAH-specific treatments that have decreased mortality and increased quality of life. Patients with severe PH from any cause may present with right-sided heart failure (RHF) or decompensation that demands intensive care. In addition, group 1 PAH patients may be admitted to the intensive care unit (ICU) for initiation of intravenous prostanoid therapy that is titrated to a safe therapeutic level in combination with monitoring for adverse effects. Although a brief review of PAH-specific therapy is included at the end of this chapter, the primary focus of this chapter is the assessment and management of decompensated RHF due to elevated PVR and associated PH.

The importance of the physiologic interaction between the heart and lungs in critically ill patients cannot be understated. In normal circumstances, the right ventricle (RV) pumps the entire cardiac output (CO) through the low-pressure pulmonary system every minute. Conversely, pulmonary vascular disease may produce arterial narrowing, with increased PVR and resultant increases in RV afterload. Early changes include RV hypertrophy and dilatation in response to increased wall stress. The increased RV contractility generates a higher pressure upstream and overcomes the increased PVR; hence, PH develops. As the PH worsens, the RV is poorly equipped to compensate, and a vicious cycle of reduced ventricular function and increased filling pressures may ensue. Furthermore, the RV response often depends on how quickly the PVR increases. If the PVR increases suddenly, the RV may not be able to maintain adequate CO (eg, RHF and hypotension may result from a massive pulmonary embolism). If the PVR increases gradually, the RV may remodel sufficiently to maintain CO. Nonetheless, an acute exacerbation of chronic RHF may occur (eg, decompensated cor pulmonale).

Epidemiology and Etiology

The incidence of PH and RHF in critically ill patients is unknown. Specific groups, such as patients with acute respiratory distress syndrome (ARDS), provide some insight. In older studies, the prevalence of RHF was 60%, but in more recent reviews the prevalence was 10% to 25%, perhaps reflecting more effective global treatment strategies for ARDS.

Many conditions are associated with RHF; hence, the Fifth WSPH recognizes various diagnostic groups. A crucially important point is that *PH* merely denotes that the PA and associated right-sided heart pressures are elevated. PH established with echocardiography is nonspecific and does not necessarily equate to group 1 PAH without further investigation. Indeed, more common presentations include group 2 pulmonary venous hypertension (PVH) due to left-sided heart disease, which is generally systolic or diastolic left ventricular failure or valvular heart disease. Certainly, acute exacerbation of chronic decompensation may occur in any patient with group 2 or 3 PH.

Acute RHF may also occur in critically ill patients independently of conditions categorized in the Fifth WSPH diagnostic groups. For example, RV dysfunction or RHF may accompany ARDS as noted. Indeed, any acute cause of respiratory failure may produce pulmonary vascular constriction with elevated PVR and increased RV stress and associated clinical consequences. Other notable clinical scenarios include acute exacerbation of chronic left-sided heart failure or respiratory failure (eg, an acute exacerbation of chronic obstructive pulmonary disease), massive pulmonary embolism, postoperative cardiopulmonary dysfunction after major heart or lung surgery, and RV infarction. RHF may also result from high CO states such as occur in thyrotoxicosis, liver failure, congenital heart disease, and arteriovenous fistulas.

Diagnostic Approaches

The intensivist must understand the pathophysiology of PH in critically ill patients. While the explanation may be as simple as systemic volume overload with associated pulmonary edema, a more complex evaluation and intervention may be required. With an awareness of the various diagnostic groups, a clinician can secure a timely diagnosis and tailor a treatment approach. The clinical presentation is nonspecific; therefore, an increased degree of awareness and bedside echocardiography are useful to screen for PH. Symptoms include shortness of breath, fatigue, dizziness, swelling, syncope, and chest pain.

Certain presentations warrant special attention. For example, exertional syncope in a young woman may indicate the presence of group 1 PAH. Similarly, the physical examination should focus on signs of RHF: increased jugular venous distention, a blowing systolic murmur of tricuspid regurgitation, an accentuated pulmonary component of the second heart sound, abdominal distention, hepatosplenomegaly, and peripheral edema.

Echocardiography is traditionally used to screen for PAH and is quite useful in the evaluation of acute RV failure in the ICU. A complete echocardiographic study allows assessment of chamber size and function, valvular integrity, flow and Doppler studies, and right-sided pressures. More advanced echocardiographic measurements include mPAP and quantitative assessment of RV function such as fractional area change, the Tei index, and the tricuspid annulus plane systolic excursion. A less comprehensive assessment can be provided by focused bedside ultrasonography, now more widely available. Important abnormal findings include a dilated and noncollapsible inferior vena cava, an enlarged right atrium, an enlarged RV (>0.6 times the left ventricle), a *D*-shaped left ventricle, and hypokinesis of the RV. The advantages of focused echocardiography are the noninvasive nature of the test and serial assessment to evaluate response to treatment. Potential limitations include the required training, misinterpretation due to poor image quality in an ICU or limited expertise, and truncation of the evaluation in patients who should undergo right-sided heart catheterization (RHC).

The diagnostic standard is still RHC—not echocardiography. In the ICU, RHC is most commonly performed with a PA catheter (PAC). The PAC allows for direct measurement of central venous pressure, RV pressure, pulmonary arterial pressure, and oxygenation at each port and measurement of CO by thermodilution. In a wedged position, the pressure equilibrates with the left atrial pressure and is aptly named the PAWP. An accurate PAWP permits calculation of PVR and CO by the Ohm law: PVR = (mPAP – PAWP)/CO. A complete hemodynamic profile provides diagnostic and therapeutic guidance to the intensivist. Potential complications of PAH include arterial puncture, PA rupture, infection, catheter misplacement, and data misinterpretation. General use of a PAC has not changed outcomes for ICU patients; however, its use for evaluating PH is vital for proper diagnosis, prognostication, and evaluation of treatment response.

Management

Optimizing Preload

Preload is a critical component of stroke volume and therefore CO when RV function is compromised. Additionally, adequate preload is required to maintain coronary blood flow, primarily during RV diastole. Intravascular volume depletion should be avoided or treated if present. Assessment of fluid status in patients with RHF may be challenging. Despite excess total body water with peripheral edema and perhaps even ascites or pleural effusion, the intravascular volume may be inadequate to support RV preload. Bedside echocardiography and other measures (central venous pressure and PAWP) can be used initially to establish a baseline and serially to assess response to treatment. Conversely, RHF may be associated with excess fluid both intravascularly and systemically. Early recognition of fluid overload and institution of diuretics (loop diuretics or thiazide diuretics) or hemofiltration usually improves RV function and symptoms. Frequent reassessment is important to avoid fluid removal at an excessive rate.

Other factors that influence preload should also be considered. In patients receiving mechanical ventilation, excessively elevated positive inspiratory and end-expiratory pressures may impair venous return and right atrial filling. Correction of anemia may also be beneficial during resuscitation efforts (target hemoglobin ≥7 g/dL). Optimizing preload is critical for determining the overall response to treatment.

Maximizing RV Contractility

As PVR increases, the RV can compensate to only a limited extent; eventually, RV contractility decreases and systemic hypotension results. In a critically ill patient with RHF, systemic perfusion pressure must be maintained to ensure vital organ function and to preserve coronary artery flow. Reversal of the shock may require vasopressor and inotropic support. In general, norepinephrine is the recommended initial vasopressor of choice, but published evidence is weak for patients with RHF. Vasopressin can be used in conjunction with norepinephrine and, according to animal studies, may have the added advantage of PA vasodilatation. An animal model has identified vasodilator properties by way of the vasopressin V1 receptor and nitric oxide pathway.

Persistent shock due to RV systolic dysfunction warrants consideration of inotropic therapy to improve RV contractility. Dobutamine, a β_2-receptor agonist, may enhance myocardial function and decrease afterload; however, it increases myocardial oxygen demand. The usefulness of dobutamine may be limited by the induction of tachycardia and hypotension, both of which are poorly tolerated. Milrinone, a phosphodiesterase-3 inhibitor, is another option. The mechanism of action for milrinone is different from that for dobutamine, but the physiologic effect is similar, with increased cardiac contractility and pulmonary vasodilatation. Milrinone may cause less chronotropic stimulation, but its effect is limited by systemic hypotension and tachyphylaxis. Vasopressors and inotropes are summarized in Table 25.1.

More advanced treatments of RHF include extracorporeal membrane oxygenation, RV assist devices, atrial septostomy, and heart-lung or lung transplant. Appropriately selected patients may benefit from these interventions, but all except transplant are only bridging therapies. Tachyarrhythmias are poorly tolerated by the failing RV, mostly because of the loss of atrial filling. If systemic hypotension is present, electrocardioversion should be considered. Rate-controlling agents such as β-blockers and calcium channel blockers may be used in patients who have adequate blood pressure, but caution is required because of a concomitant negative inotropic effect.

Decreasing Afterload

Under normal circumstances, the pulmonary circulation requires a fraction of the systemic driving pressure because of the low PVR. Conditions or disease states that produce pulmonary venous congestion or elevated PVR increase the RV afterload and challenge the RV to compensate through increased contractile force. In addition to supporting preload and RV contractility as discussed above, strategies to decrease RV afterload should be considered. Interventions range from therapy that reverses the underlying condition that led to RHF to therapy that directly dilates the PA vasculature.

While the RV is being supported, the underlying cause should be determined and treated accordingly. The first step

Table 25.1 • Vasopressors and Inotropes Commonly Used for Pulmonary Hypertension and Right-Sided Heart Failure in the ICU

		Main Effects	
Medication	**Receptor**	**Beneficial**	**Adverse**
Norepinephrine	Strong: α_1 Moderate: β_1 and β_2	Vasoconstriction Minimal chronotropy and inotropy	Hypertension Arrhythmia Peripheral ischemia
Vasopressin	Vasopressin V1 Vasopressin V2	Vasoconstriction Water reabsorption in the collecting ducts	Arrhythmia Peripheral ischemia Cardiac ischemia
Dobutamine	β_1 β_2	Inotropy Vasodilatation	Tachycardia Arrhythmia Cardiac ischemia Hypotension
Milrinone	Phosphodiesterase-3 (inhibition)	Inotropy	Arrhythmia Hypotension Cardiac ischemia

Abbreviation: ICU, intensive care unit.

should be to provide adequate oxygenation. Hypoxia results in pulmonary vascular constriction and is exacerbated by hypercarbia and acidosis. Depending on the severity of the gas exchange derangement, treatment may range from supplemental oxygen to mechanical ventilation (including noninvasive mechanical ventilation).

The effect of mechanical ventilation on RV afterload must be monitored. Transpulmonary pressure, the main determinant of PVR, is minimal at functional residual capacity. Inadequate lung volumes lead to atelectasis, collapse of extra-alveolar vessels, and hypoxia; as a result, PVR and RV afterload increase. Conversely, overdistention leads to collapse of intra-alveolar vasculature, also increasing PVR. Excessive lung volumes may produce increased dead-space ventilation and cause undesirable hypoxemia or hypercarbia (or both).

For appropriate ventilation, the tidal volume and positive end-expiratory pressure should promote adequate gas exchange, prevent ventilator-associated lung injury, and optimize RV preload and afterload. Settings must be individualized for each patient and adjusted according to the various considerations outlined above. Although prone positioning improves oxygenation in most patients with ARDS and may also unload the RV, its effect on outcomes is debatable and the technique can be logistically challenging.

The role of pharmacologic therapy for decreasing PVR is unclear for patients with acute RHF. As noted above, reversal of the underlying cause should take precedent. The prostaglandin pathway has been studied most extensively, and agents can be delivered by mouth, inhalation, or infusion (subcutaneously or intravenously). Those agents are primarily reserved for treatment of group 1 PAH. As an example, epoprostenol is the only agent with proven mortality benefit for patients with PAH. Nonetheless, epoprostenol should not be used for other causes of PH and RHF. Indeed, systemic vasodilators may cause clinical worsening because of hypotension and worsening hypoxemia. In addition, PA vasodilators may produce or worsen pulmonary edema in patients with group 2 PVH.

Inhaled nitric oxide (iNO) has also been used to decrease PVR and improve oxygenation in various clinical settings involving RV dysfunction. The inhaled route has the theoretical advantages of avoiding both systemic hypotension and worsening ventilation-perfusion mismatch. Vasodilatation of ventilated lung segments should improve ventilation-perfusion matching and increase arterial oxygen tension. Improved CO and reduced PVR have been reported for patients with PAH, secondary causes of chronic PH, acute pulmonary embolism, ischemic RV failure, or ARDS and for patients after cardiac surgery. Although iNO improves oxygenation in approximately two-thirds of patients with ARDS, it does not decrease mortality. The short half-life of iNO offers an additional advantage in the critical care setting. The use of inhaled prostanoids (prostacyclin and analogues such as iloprost and treprostinil) is generally limited to treatment of patients with group 1 PAH. Oral agents approved for patients with group 1 PAH may present logistical challenges for administration in intubated patients. For example, because the endothelin-receptor blockers are highly teratogenic, care should be taken to prevent undue exposure to the patient and health care staff. Table 25.2 summarizes specific therapeutic interventions for the various Fifth WSPH diagnostic groups.

PAH-Specific Therapy in the ICU

Group 1 PAH therapy spans 3 targeted pathobiologic pathways. Prostaglandin I_2 (prostacyclin) binds to prostacyclin receptors, activating cyclic adenosine monophosphate and protein kinase A to produce vasodilatation and mitigate PA cellular proliferation. Endothelin-receptor antagonists block the vasoconstrictive and hyperproliferative effect on vascular smooth cells. As mentioned above, iNO is a potent vasodilator, and the effect can be enhanced by stimulating production through guanylate cyclase or inhibiting breakdown by blocking phosphodiesterase-5. Agents for PAH-specific therapy are presented in Table 25.3.

Therapy for group 1 PAH may be instituted or enhanced for ICU patients presenting with RHF and PAH if either condition is newly diagnosed. In addition, patients with known group 1 PAH may present with decompensated RHF and require additional therapy. These agents should not be used for PH not classified as group 1 PAH, with the exception of riociguat, which is approved for patients with group 4 chronic thromboembolic PE that is inoperable or persistent after pulmonary thromboendarterectomy.

Epoprostenol is commonly administered to group 1 PAH patients in RHF, and it is indicated for management of severe New York Heart Association functional class III or IV symptoms due to PAH. The drug is administered by continuous intravenous infusion. Therapy is begun in the ICU, where the dose is titrated to a therapeutic level while the patient is monitored for adverse effects and treated accordingly (eg, worsening hypoxia, headache, flushing, musculoskeletal pain, and nausea). Epoprostenol has a half-life of only a few minutes; therefore, interruptions in delivery should be avoided. In patients with compromised RV function, interruptions may produce rebound PH and an acute deterioration with hypotension and even cardiac arrest. Outpatient administration requires a permanently placed central venous catheter. As a rule, epoprostenol infusion should be prescribed only by providers experienced in the management of PAH with a protocol supported by nurses who have training and expertise in administration.

Table 25.2 • Treatment of the Primary Causes of Right Ventricular Failure in the ICU

Cause of PH	Pathophysiology	Intervention
Group 1 PAH	Pulmonary vasculature hypertrophy with increased PVR	PAH-specific therapies Endothelin receptor antagonists Nitric oxide Phosphodiesterase-5 inhibitors Stimulator of soluble guanylate cyclase Prostanoids Oxygen Diuretics
Group 2 PH (PVH)	Left-sided heart disease with increased pulmonary congestion	Diuretics Oxygen Inotropes Vasopressors
Group 3 PH (hypoxia)	Hypoxic vasoconstriction or microvasculature destruction (or both)	Oxygen or mechanical ventilation Treatment of exacerbations
Group 4 PH (CTEPH)	Unresolved PE with cellular mass adhering to the pulmonary artery intima	Pulmonary thromboendarterectomy Stimulator of soluble guanylate cyclase
ARDS	Hypoxemia and hypoxic vasoconstriction with atelectasis due to reduced lung compliance	Oxygen Ventilation Treatment of cause
Acute PE	Embolic obstruction of pulmonary artery with hypoxia and increase in dead space ventilation	Anticoagulation Thrombolytics when persistent hypotension (SBP <90 mm Hg) despite resuscitation
RV infarct	Myocardial injury or death (or both)	Acute coronary syndrome protocol Thrombolytics Intervention Percutaneous coronary intervention Coronary artery bypass graft surgery

Abbreviations: ARDS, acute respiratory distress syndrome; CTEPH, chronic thromboembolic pulmonary hypertension; ICU, intensive care unit; PAH, pulmonary arterial hypertension; PE, pulmonary embolism; PH, pulmonary hypertension; PVH, pulmonary venous hypertension; PVR, pulmonary vascular resistance; RV, right ventricular; SBP, systolic blood pressure.

Table 25.3 • Specific Therapies (and Routes of Administration) for Patients With Group 1 PAH

Mechanism of Action	Medications	Main Adverse Effects
Endothelin receptor antagonist (orally)	Bosentan Ambrisentan Macitentan	Vasodilatation: headache, flushing, edema Liver toxicity
PD5 inhibitor (orally)	Sildenafil Tadalafil	Vasodilatation: headache, flushing, nasal congestion
Stimulator of guanylate cyclase (orally)	Riociguat	Vasodilatation: headache Gastrointestinal tract symptoms: nausea, diarrhea, dyspepsia, GERD
Prostacyclin agonist	Epoprostenol (IV) Treprostinil (IV, SC, orally, inhaled) Iloprost (inhaled) Selexipag (orally)	Vasodilatation: headache, flushing Nausea Thrombocytopenia

Abbreviations: GERD, gastroesophageal reflux disease; IV, intravenously; PAH, pulmonary arterial hypertension; PD5, phosphodiesterase-5; SC, subcutaneously.

Summary

- Most PH in ICU patients is group 2 PVH or group 3 PH.
- When a patient presents with new PH, all possible causes must be considered.
- Management includes maximizing preload, increasing contractility, and reducing afterload; the goal is to achieve euvolemic fluid status.
- Maximizing RV contractility may require use of a vasopressor (norepinephrine is the recommended initial choice) and inotropic support.
- To decrease afterload by avoiding hypoxia or hypercapnia, the use of pharmacologic therapy may be considered (eg, iNO or epoprostenol).
- PAH-specific therapy may be instituted or enhanced for ICU patients presenting with RHF, but this therapy should be reserved for patients with diagnostic group 1 PAH.

SUGGESTED READING

Aduen JF, Castello R, Lozano MM, Hepler GN, Keller CA, Alvarez F, et al. An alternative echocardiographic method to estimate mean pulmonary artery pressure: diagnostic and clinical implications. J Am Soc Echocardiogr. 2009 Jul;22(7):814–9. Epub 2009 Jun 7.

Amsterdam EA, Wenger NK, Brindis RG, Casey DE Jr, Ganiats TG, Holmes DR Jr, et al; ACC/AHA Task Force Members; Society for Cardiovascular Angiography and Interventions and the Society of Thoracic Surgeons. 2014 AHA/ACC guideline for the management of patients with non-ST-elevation acute coronary syndromes: executive summary: a report of the American College of Cardiology/American Heart Association Task Force on Practice Guidelines. Circulation. 2014 Dec 23;130(25):2354–94. Epub 2014 Sep 23. Erratum in: Circulation. 2014 Dec 23;130(25):e431–2.

Burger CD, D'Albini L, Raspa S, Pruett JA. The evolution of prostacyclins in pulmonary arterial hypertension: from classical treatment to modern management. Am J Manag Care. 2016 Jan;22(1 Suppl):S3–15.

Enderby CY, Burger C. Medical treatment update on pulmonary arterial hypertension. Ther Adv Chronic Dis. 2015 Sep;6(5):264–72.

Evans DC, Doraiswamy VA, Prosciak MP, Silviera M, Seamon MJ, Rodriguez Funes V, et al. Complications associated with pulmonary artery catheters: a comprehensive clinical review. Scand J Surg. 2009;98(4):199–208.

Galie N, Humbert M, Vachiery JL, Gibbs S, Lang I, Torbicki A, et al. 2015 ESC/ERS Guidelines for the diagnosis and treatment of pulmonary hypertension: The Joint Task Force for the Diagnosis and Treatment of Pulmonary Hypertension of the European Society of Cardiology (ESC) and the European Respiratory Society (ERS): Endorsed by: Association for European Paediatric and Congenital Cardiology (AEPC), International Society for Heart and Lung Transplantation (ISHLT). Eur Heart J. 2016 Jan 1;37(1):67–119. Epub 2015 Aug 29.

Galie N, Simonneau G. The Fifth World Symposium on Pulmonary Hypertension. J Am Coll Cardiol. 2013 Dec 24;62(25 Suppl):D1–3.

Gayat E, Mebazaa A. Pulmonary hypertension in critical care. Curr Opin Crit Care. 2011 Oct;17(5):439–48.

Grinstein J, Gomberg-Maitland M. Management of pulmonary hypertension and right heart failure in the intensive care unit. Curr Hypertens Rep. 2015 May;17(5):32.

Hoeper MM, Bogaard HJ, Condliffe R, Frantz R, Khanna D, Kurzyna M, et al. Definitions and diagnosis of pulmonary hypertension. J Am Coll Cardiol. 2013 Dec 24;62(25 Suppl):D42–50.

Hoeper MM, Granton J. Intensive care unit management of patients with severe pulmonary hypertension and right heart failure. Am J Respir Crit Care Med. 2011 Nov 15;184(10):1114–24.

Kearon C, Akl EA, Ornelas J, Blaivas A, Jimenez D, Bounameaux H, et al. Antithrombotic therapy for VTE disease: CHEST Guideline and Expert Panel Report. Chest. 2016 Feb;149(2):315–52. Epub 2016 Jan 7.

Lahm T, McCaslin CA, Wozniak TC, Ghumman W, Fadl YY, Obeidat OS, et al. Medical and surgical treatment of acute right ventricular failure. J Am Coll Cardiol. 2010 Oct 26;56(18):1435–46.

Pagnamenta A, Lador F, Azzola A, Beghetti M. Modern invasive hemodynamic assessment of pulmonary hypertension. Respiration. 2018;95(3):201–11. Epub 2018 Jan 9.

Price LC, Wort SJ, Finney SJ, Marino PS, Brett SJ. Pulmonary vascular and right ventricular dysfunction in adult critical care: current and emerging options for management: a systematic literature review. Crit Care. 2010;14(5):R169. Epub 2010 Sep 21.

Circulatory and Cardiovascular Disorders

26 Anaphylaxis and Anaphylactic Shock

MEGAN S. MOTOSUE, MD; GERALD W. VOLCHECK, MD

Goals

- Describe the features of anaphylaxis and anaphylactic shock.
- Discuss the management of anaphylactic shock.

Introduction

Anaphylaxis is a serious allergic reaction that is rapid in onset and potentially fatal. Prompt recognition of the symptoms and institution of treatment are important in management. This chapter briefly discusses the background, diagnosis, and management of anaphylaxis.

Epidemiology

The lifetime prevalence of anaphylaxis is estimated to be 0.05% to 2% and appears to be increasing. Allergic reactions vary in severity, with the most severe culminating in anaphylactic shock. Common triggers include food, venom, and drugs, but up to 20% of cases have no identifiable trigger. Triggers for events vary by age. Among children and young people, food is a common trigger; among middle-aged and older people, medications and venoms are common triggers. Neuromuscular blocking agents, antibiotics, and latex are the most common causes of anesthesia-associated anaphylaxis. Risk factors for severe or fatal anaphylaxis include old age, asthma, mastocytosis, and concurrent medications, including β-blockers and angiotensin-converting enzyme inhibitors.

The pathogenesis of anaphylaxis involves immunologic mechanisms (mediated by immunoglobulin E or other substances) and nonimmunologic mechanisms. A single trigger can lead to anaphylaxis through multiple mechanisms. The end result is the activation of mast cells and basophils and the release of preformed and newly generated mediators. Histamine and tryptase are examples of mediators that act on target organs and lead to the signs and symptoms of anaphylaxis (Figure 26.1).

Clinical Features

Anaphylaxis can affect all organ systems, but the most common are the skin (flushing, itching, hives, and angioedema), the respiratory tract (cough and wheezing), and the gastrointestinal tract (abdominal pain, nausea, and vomiting). However, anaphylaxis can occur without cutaneous symptoms and without involvement of multiple organ systems. The diagnostic criteria established by the National Institute of Allergy and Infectious Disease/Food Allergy and Anaphylaxis Network (NIAID/FAAN) (Box 26.1) are 97% sensitive and 82% specific.

Symptom onset varies with the route of administration. In a series of 20 fatal anaphylactic episodes, the median times to shock, respiratory arrest, or cardiac arrest were as follows: 30 minutes for foods, 15 minutes for venom stings, and 5 minutes for iatrogenic causes (Pumphrey, 2000; see Suggested Reading).

Cardiac arrhythmias and bronchoconstriction may occur in near-fatal or fatal anaphylactic episodes. Bronchoconstriction may be so severe that patients may present with respiratory failure associated with arterial blood gas pH of 6.95 to 7.05 and P_{CO_2} greater than 90 mm Hg. The most affected organ varies from patient to patient, but in patients with asthma the organ is usually the lungs, so the patients have an increased risk of respiratory failure and death.

In anaphylactic shock, the initial hemodynamic changes are a consequence of intravascular fluid loss and vasodilatation. The loss of plasma volume in combination with a decrease in venous return leads to a transient increase in cardiac output mediated by epinephrine and norepinephrine.

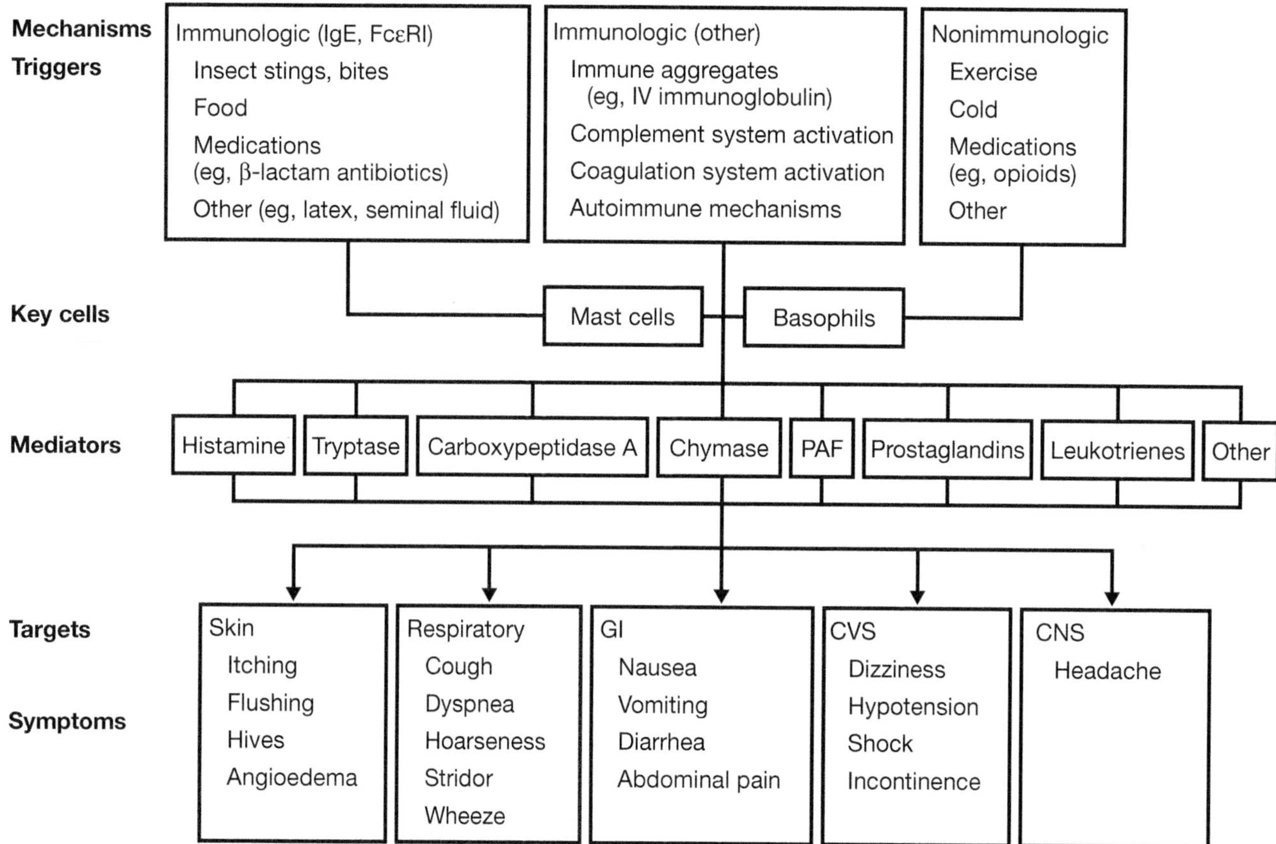

Figure 26.1. Pathogenesis of Anaphylaxis. CNS indicates central nervous system; CVS, cardiovascular system; FcεRI, receptor for Fc portion of immunoglobulin E; GI, gastrointestinal tract; Ig, immunoglobulin; IV, intravenous; PAF, platelet-activating factor.

(Modified from Simons FE. 9: Anaphylaxis. J Allergy Clin Immunol. 2008 Feb;121[2 Suppl]:S402–7; used with permission.)

This is followed by decreases in arterial pressure, right and left ventricular filling pressures, and peripheral vascular resistance. However, the subsequent loss of plasma volume and decrease in venous return ultimately lead to a decrease in cardiac output; all these factors contribute to shock. Pulmonary edema fluid associated with anaphylactic shock is characterized by a high concentration of albumin and low pulmonary artery wedge pressures, which suggest a noncardiogenic cause resulting from increased microvascular permeability.

Generally, anaphylaxis occurs in 1 of 3 clinical patterns: 1) a sudden event with rapid resolution, 2) a prolonged and protracted event that can last hours to days, 3) an event with resolution of manifestations followed by recurrence even in the absence of the initial trigger (referred to as a *biphasic reaction*). A biphasic reaction occurs in up to 20% of anaphylactic events; delayed or inadequate epinephrine dosing and response to a food allergen are common risk factors for biphasic reactions.

The laboratory marker most commonly used for supporting a diagnosis of anaphylaxis is serum tryptase. Most tryptase is found in mast cells; a small amount, in basophils. Tryptase is highly specific but lacks sensitivity. Therefore, a normal serum level of tryptase does not rule out anaphylaxis. Tryptase levels are commonly increased when anaphylaxis results from injected medications or venom. However, tryptase levels may be normal when anaphylaxis is induced by food or is not associated with hypotension. Serum tryptase levels peak at 1 to 1.5 hours after symptom onset and can remain high for up to 5 hours. Serial measurements of tryptase levels during an anaphylactic event, in addition to a baseline level, are more useful than a single measurement.

Commercial tests are also available for plasma histamine and 24-hour urine histamine metabolites. The plasma histamine level increases within the first 5 to 10 minutes of an anaphylactic event but usually returns to normal within 60 minutes after the start of the event. In contrast, 24-hour

Box 26.1 • NIAID/FAAN Clinical Criteria for Diagnosing Anaphylaxis

Anaphylaxis is highly likely when any 1 of the following 3 criteria is fulfilled:

1. Acute onset of an illness (minutes to several hours) with involvement of the skin or mucosal tissue (or both) (eg, generalized hives, pruritus or flushing, or swollen lips, tongue, or uvula) *and* at least 1 of the following:
   a. Respiratory compromise (eg, dyspnea, wheeze, bronchospasm, stridor, reduced PEF, hypoxemia)
   b. Reduced BP or associated symptoms of end-organ dysfunction (eg, hypotonia [collapse], syncope, incontinence)
2. Two or more of the following that occur rapidly after exposure to a *likely* allergen for that patient (minutes to several hours):
   a. Involvement of the skin or mucosal tissue (or both) (eg, generalized hives, pruritus or flushing, or swollen lips, tongue, or uvula)
   b. Respiratory compromise (eg, dyspnea, wheeze, bronchospasm, stridor, reduced PEF, hypoxemia)
   c. Reduced BP or associated symptoms (eg, hypotonia [collapse], syncope, incontinence)
   d. Persistent gastrointestinal tract symptoms (eg, crampy abdominal pain, vomiting)
3. Reduced BP after exposure to *known* allergen for that patient (minutes to several hours):
   a. Infants and children: low systolic BP (age specific)[a] or greater than 30% decrease in systolic BP
   b. Adults: systolic BP less than 90 mm Hg or greater than 30% decrease from that person's baseline

Abbreviations: BP, blood pressure; NIAID/FAAN, National Institute of Allergy and Infectious Disease/Food Allergy and Anaphylaxis Network; PEF, peak expiratory flow.

[a] Definition of low systolic blood pressure: aged 1 month to 1 year, less than 70 mm Hg; aged 1 to 10 years, less than the sum of 70 mm Hg plus twice the patient's age; and aged 11 to 17 years, less than 90 mm Hg.

Modified from Sampson HA, Munoz-Furlong A, Campbell RL, Adkinson NF Jr, Bock SA, Branum A, et al. Second symposium on the definition and management of anaphylaxis: summary report: Second National Institute of Allergy and Infectious Disease/Food Allergy and Anaphylaxis Network symposium. J Allergy Clin Immunol. 2006 Feb;117(2):391–7; used with permission.

urinary histamine metabolite levels can be increased for up to 24 hours and thus may be more informative. Other potential markers being examined include mediators such as carboxypeptidase A3, platelet-activating factor (PAF), and PAF hydrolase; PAF and PAF hydrolase correlate with event severity.

Treatment

As soon as anaphylaxis is suspected, the inciting trigger should be removed. The patient's airway, breathing, and cardiovascular system should be assessed. Supplemental oxygen should be given and intravenous access established. First-line treatment involves administration of intramuscular epinephrine (1 mg/mL) (0.2-0.5 mg for adults; 0.01 mg/kg for children) and volume replacement. Fluids are crucial for reversing the intravascular depletion that occurs during anaphylaxis. As soon as possible on initial presentation, patients should receive normal saline intravenously (adults, 1-2 L; children, up to 30 mL/kg).

To treat bronchospasm, inhaled short-acting β_2-agonists can be helpful. Other adjuvant therapies include histamine$_1$ and histamine$_2$ antagonists and corticosteroids, which are used for severe episodes to prevent biphasic reactions. However, there is no strong evidence supporting the role of either antihistamines or corticosteroids in the treatment of anaphylaxis. Despite a lack of established efficacy, antihistamines and corticosteroids are included in many published guidelines as second- or third-line agents.

For refractory hypotension, intravenous epinephrine should be given (2-10 mcg/min titrated according to the patient's blood pressure). Bolus doses are not recommended because they have been associated with an increased risk of overdose and adverse cardiovascular events. When patients have required additional vasopressors, dopamine and norepinephrine have been used. Additionally, glucagon can be given to patients who are unresponsive to epinephrine, such as patients who are taking β-blockers.

After the event is resolved, patients should be discharged with self-injectable epinephrine. They should also be referred to an allergy specialist for further evaluation, which may include skin testing to identify the triggering agent, and for additional management recommendations.

Summary

- Anaphylaxis is a serious allergic reaction that is rapid in onset and may cause death.
- Common triggers include food, venom, and drugs, but up to 20% of cases have no identifiable trigger.
- Anaphylactic shock is characterized by intravascular fluid loss and extensive vasodilatation leading to severe hypotension.
- Prompt recognition, epinephrine administration, and intravascular volume replacement are key elements in the first-line management of anaphylaxis.

SUGGESTED READING

Campbell RL, Bellolio MF, Knutson BD, Bellamkonda VR, Fedko MG, Nestler DM, et al. Epinephrine in anaphylaxis: higher risk of cardiovascular complications and overdose after administration of intravenous bolus epinephrine compared with intramuscular epinephrine. J Allergy Clin Immunol Pract. 2015 Jan-Feb;3(1):76–80. Epub 2014 Aug 29.

Campbell RL, Hagan JB, Manivannan V, Decker WW, Kanthala AR, Bellolio MF, et al. Evaluation of National Institute of Allergy and Infectious Diseases/Food Allergy and Anaphylaxis Network criteria for the diagnosis of anaphylaxis in emergency department patients. J Allergy Clin Immunol. 2012 Mar;129(3):748–52. Epub 2011 Nov 1.

Carlson RW, Schaeffer RC Jr, Puri VK, Brennan AP, Weil MH. Hypovolemia and permeability pulmonary edema associated with anaphylaxis. Crit Care Med. 1981 Dec;9(12):883–5.

Choo KJ, Simons FE, Sheikh A. Glucocorticoids for the treatment of anaphylaxis. Cochrane Database Syst Rev. 2012 Apr 18;(4):CD007596.

Gelincik A, Demirturk M, Yılmaz E, Ertek B, Erdogdu D, Colakoglu B, et al. Anaphylaxis in a tertiary adult allergy clinic: a retrospective review of 516 patients. Ann Allergy Asthma Immunol. 2013 Feb;110(2):96–100. Epub 2012 Dec 20.

Greenberger PA. Fatal and near-fatal anaphylaxis: factors that can worsen or contribute to fatal outcomes. Immunol Allergy Clin North Am. 2015 May;35(2):375–86. Epub 2015 Feb 27.

Lieberman P, Nicklas RA, Randolph C, Oppenheimer J, Bernstein D, Bernstein J, et al. Anaphylaxis: a practice parameter update 2015. Ann Allergy Asthma Immunol. 2015 Nov;115(5):341–84.

Lin RY, Schwartz LB, Curry A, Pesola GR, Knight RJ, Lee HS, et al. Histamine and tryptase levels in patients with acute allergic reactions: an emergency department-based study. J Allergy Clin Immunol. 2000 Jul;106(1 Pt 1):65–71.

Moss J, Fahmy NR, Sunder N, Beaven MA. Hormonal and hemodynamic profile of an anaphylactic reaction in man. Circulation. 1981 Jan;63(1):210–3.

Muraro A, Roberts G, Worm M, Bilo MB, Brockow K, Fernandez Rivas M, et al; EAACI Food Allergy and Anaphylaxis Guidelines Group. Anaphylaxis: guidelines from the European Academy of Allergy and Clinical Immunology. Allergy. 2014 Aug;69(8):1026–45. Epub 2014 Jun 9.

Pattanaik D, Yataco JC, Lieberman P. Anaphylactic and anaphylactoid reactions. In: Hall JB, Schmidt GA, Kress JP, editors. Principles of critical care. 4th ed. New York (NY): McGraw-Hill Education; c2015. p. 1269–79.

Pumphrey RS. Lessons for management of anaphylaxis from a study of fatal reactions. Clin Exp Allergy. 2000 Aug;30(8):1144–50.

Sampson HA, Munoz-Furlong A, Campbell RL, Adkinson NF Jr, Bock SA, Branum A, et al. Second symposium on the definition and management of anaphylaxis: summary report: Second National Institute of Allergy and Infectious Disease/Food Allergy and Anaphylaxis Network Symposium. J Allergy Clin Immunol. 2006 Feb;117(2):391–7.

Sheikh A, ten Broek VM, Brown SG, Simons FE. H1-antihistamines for the treatment of anaphylaxis with and without shock. Cochrane Database Syst Rev. 2007 Jan 24;(1):CD006160.

Simons FE. Anaphylaxis pathogenesis and treatment. Allergy. 2011 Jul;66 Suppl 95:31–4.

Simons FE, Ebisawa M, Sanchez-Borges M, Thong BY, Worm M, Tanno LK, et al. 2015 update of the evidence base: World Allergy Organization anaphylaxis guidelines. World Allergy Organ J. 2015 Oct 28;8(1):32.

Volcheck GW, Mertes PM. Local and general anesthetics immediate hypersensitivity reactions. Immunol Allergy Clin North Am. 2014 Aug;34(3):525–46. Epub 2014 May 27.

27 Cardiogenic Shock

ROBERT A. RATZLAFF, DO; JASON L. SIEGEL, MD

Goals

- Define *cardiogenic shock* and explain how it differs from other forms of shock.
- Review the mechanism and pathophysiology of cardiogenic shock.
- Learn how to identify and diagnose cardiogenic shock.
- Be familiar with the appropriate therapy for cardiogenic shock.

Introduction

Like all forms of shock, cardiogenic shock (CS) is a life-threatening condition of decreased blood circulation that ultimately causes systemic hypoperfusion and end-organ failure. Unlike other forms of shock, however, CS is characterized by failure of the heart itself. This chapter describes CS, including its causes and diagnosis, and provides a brief overview of management.

Definition

The diagnosis of CS is based on hemodynamic, clinical, and laboratory criteria. The hemodynamic criteria are the following:

1. Systolic blood pressure <90 mm Hg for >30 minutes.
2. Mean arterial pressure <60 mm Hg for >30 minutes.
3. High doses of 2 inotropes or vasopressors (or both) are needed to keep systolic blood pressure >90 mm Hg. Appropriate inotropes include dobutamine (>5 mcg/kg/min), epinephrine (>5 mcg/min), and milrinone (>0.0375 mcg/kg/min). Appropriate vasopressors include norepinephrine (>5 mcg/min) and vasopressin (>4 units/h).
4. Cardiac index <2.2 L/min/m^2.
5. Pulmonary capillary wedge pressure (PCWP) >18 mm Hg.

The clinical criteria are the following:

1. Pale, cool, and clammy peripheral extremities.
2. Prolonged capillary refill time.
3. Altered mental status.
4. Oliguria or anuria.
5. Pulmonary congestion.
6. Tachycardia or recurrent tachyarrhythmia.

The laboratory criteria are the following:

1. Increased serum levels of lactate (>2 mmol/L) or metabolic acidosis (pH <7.35).
2. Mixed venous saturation <55%.
3. Increasing serum levels of alanine aminotransferase and aspartate aminotransferase (>1,000 U/L).
4. Serum creatinine level >1.5 times the baseline level.

More quantitatively, the hemodynamic profile of CS is characterized by increased PCWP (preload), decreased cardiac output (pump function), increased systemic vascular resistance (afterload), and decreased mixed venous oxygen saturation (tissue perfusion) (Table 27.1), although the diagnosis can be made without the aid of these quantitative measurements. The exception is a tachyarrhythmia where the preload and afterload are decreased because of reduced filling time.

Epidemiology

The most common cause of CS is acute myocardial infarction (MI). Because patients with MI have multiple potential complications, the incidence of CS in this population is 5% to 10%. The incidence is higher among patients with

Table 27.1 • Hemodynamic Differences Between Cardiogenic Shock and Other Forms of Shock

Form of Shock	Preload (PCWP)	Afterload (SVR)	Pump Function (CO)	Tissue Perfusion (Svo_2), %
Cardiogenic	↑ >18 mm Hg	↑	↓ <2.2 L/min/m²	<55
Distributive	↔ early; ↓ late	↓	↑	>65
Hypovolemic	↔ early; ↓ late	↑	↔ early; ↓ late	>65 early; <65 late
Obstructive				
PE, PH, tension pneumothorax	↔ early; ↓ late	↑	↔ early; ↓ late	>65
Pericardial tamponade	↑	↑	↓	<65

Abbreviations: ↓, decreased; ↑, increased; ↔, normal; CO, cardiac output; PCWP, pulmonary capillary wedge pressure; PE, pulmonary embolism; PH, pulmonary hypertension; Svo_2, mixed venous oxygen saturation; SVR, systemic vascular resistance.

ST-segment elevation MI (STEMI) (7.9%) and lower among patients with non-STEMI (NSTEMI) (<3%). Patients who have CS after MI, compared with patients who do not, have a significantly higher probability of early death (65.4% vs 10.6%, $P<.001$). Even though the rate of early death is decreasing as the use of early percutaneous coronary intervention (PCI) is increasing, CS is still the leading cause of death among patients with MI.

Risk factors for CS developing after MI include older age, anterior MI, hypertension, diabetes mellitus, multivessel coronary disease, previous MI, STEMI, left bundle branch block, and female sex. Risk factors for early death include older age and history of angina or heart failure.

Pathophysiology

The 3 general mechanisms for cardiogenic shock are cardiomyopathic, arrythmogenic, and mechanical. The *cardiomyopathic* mechanism includes MI (about 80% of all CS), acute exacerbation of severe heart failure, stunned myocardium from prolonged ischemia, advanced septic shock, and myocarditis. Stress cardiomyopathy (also known as apical ballooning syndrome or takotsubo cardiomyopathy) can occur in patients with neurologic disease (eg, hemorrhagic stroke, ischemic stroke, or status epilepticus) and accounts for 4.2% of all cases of CS. The *arrythmogenic* mechanism includes tachyarrhythmia (both atrial and ventricular) and bradycardia (including Mobitz type II second-degree block and complete heart block). The *mechanical* mechanism includes severe heart valve disease (insufficiency or rupture), critical aortic stenosis, and ventricular wall defects (including septal defects and wall aneurysm).

Some disease states, such as MI, can lead to any of these mechanisms. Regardless of the underlying cause, the heart has the same underlying combination of systolic and diastolic dysfunction. The combination of systolic and diastolic heart failure causes increased metabolic demand on cardiac tissue, resulting in further cardiac damage and ultimately irreversible infarction with cessation of cardiac output. Table 27.2 summarizes how each CS mechanism decreases cardiac output and blood pressure according to the following relationships:

$$\text{Stroke volume} = \text{EDV} - \text{ESV}$$

Table 27.2 • Mechanisms for Decreased Cardiac Output in Cardiogenic Shock

Mechanism	Type of Dysfunction	Result of Dysfunction
Cardiomyopathic		
MI, heart failure, stunned myocardium, septic shock, myocarditis	Systolic Diastolic	↑ ESV; ↓ contractility ↓ EDV; ↓ myocardial relaxation
Arrythmogenic		
Tachyarrhythmia	Diastolic	↓ EDV; ↓ filling time (↓ EDV outweighs ↑ HR)
Bradyarrhythmia	Heart rate abnormality	↓ HR
Mechanical		
Aortic stenosis	Systolic	↑ ESV; ↑ afterload from stenosis
Mitral valve rupture	Systolic	↑ ESV; regurgitation of blood into LA
Ventricular wall defect	Systolic	↑ ESV; ↓ contractility

Abbreviations: ↓, decreased; ↑, increased; EDV, end-diastolic volume; ESV, end-systolic volume; HR, heart rate; LA, left atrium; MI, myocardial infarction.

(where diastolic failure decreases end-diastolic volume [EDV] and systolic failure increases end-systolic volume [ESV])

$$\text{Cardiac Output} = \text{Stroke Volume} \times \text{Heart Rate}$$

$$\text{Blood Pressure} = \text{Cardiac Output} \times \text{Resistance}$$

Although myocardial tissue can potentially benefit from a decrease in blood pressure through decreased afterload, the decrease in blood pressure ultimately decreases cardiac perfusion pressure and worsens cardiac ischemia. Diastolic dysfunction causes an increase in left ventricular end-diastolic pressure, pulmonary congestion, and hypoxemia and thereby worsens cardiac ischemia.

One compensatory mechanism of hypoperfusion is the release of catecholamines, which increase contractility but also increase myocardial oxygen demand and cause proarrhythmic and myocardiotoxic effects. Resulting increases in vasopressin and angiotensin II levels improve coronary and peripheral perfusion, although increased afterload may impair myocardial function further. The retention of excess salt and water may also worsen pulmonary edema.

Hypoperfusion also causes systemic inflammatory response syndrome, with an increase in proinflammatory cytokines (eg, interleukin 6), tumor necrosis factor α, and nitric oxide. All these substances cause peripheral vasodilatation, negating the compensatory catecholamine reflex and causing a further decrease in blood pressure.

CS is usually manifested through left ventricular (LV) failure. Right ventricular (RV) failure accounts for about only 5% of all cases of CS from MI, but the mortality rate is nearly as high when CS is related to RV failure compared with LV failure. Decreased RV output decreases pulmonary flow to the left atrium and LV, further decreasing total cardiac output. Patients with RV dysfunction have high RV end-diastolic pressures which can cause the septum to bow into the LV, impairing LV filling.

Iatrogenic CS is an important consideration in the neurocritical care unit. Increased troponin levels and stress-induced cardiomyopathy can occur after acute neurologic injury and decrease the CS threshold. β-Blockers and angiotensin-converting enzyme inhibitors are commonly used to control blood pressure in patients with acute ischemic or hemorrhagic strokes, but these drugs are associated with precipitating CS. In patients with pulmonary edema, high doses of diuretics can precipitate CS through a rapid decrease in plasma volume. In patients who already have RV failure, an overload of intravenous (IV) fluids can worsen RV failure and further decrease LV preload.

Evaluation

During evaluation of patients with CS, as with evaluation in all types of shock, rapid recognition and diagnosis are vital, and the goal is stabilization, resuscitation, and correction of the underlying problems. Often shock is initially undifferentiated, so a broad approach is appropriate.

The priorities are monitoring oxygen, securing the airway, and providing ventilation. Endotracheal intubation may be necessary, and although positive pressure ventilation may improve oxygenation, it can compromise venous return to the heart (and further decrease preload).

Hemodynamic and circulatory support involves aggressive IV fluid administration, which can be facilitated with central IV access. If a patient is in shock, IV access may require ultrasonographic guidance because the venous system may be volume depleted and easily collapsible. Arterial line access is also needed for monitoring blood pressure and for creating easy access for drawing frequent blood samples.

Invasive hemodynamic monitoring (with Swan-Ganz catheterization) may be useful for diagnosing and monitoring CS. In patients with CS, PCWP is typically greater than 15 mm Hg and the cardiac index is less than 2.2 L/min/m^2, but this procedure is not mandatory and may be deferred until after the patient's condition is stabilized.

Initial investigations should include laboratory tests for complete blood cell count, liver function tests, and serum levels of electrolytes, creatinine, urea nitrogen, lactate, brain natriuretic peptide, and troponin. Electrocardiography should be performed to identify STEMI or arrhythmias. Chest radiography should be performed to evaluate for diseases that mimic CS (eg, aortic dissection, tension pneumothorax, and pneumomediastinum) or to evaluate for complications of CS (eg, pulmonary edema).

Bedside echocardiography is recommended for diagnosis, management, and monitoring of shock; it is the best bedside tool for evaluating cardiac and hemodynamic conditions. Rapid Assessment by Cardiac Echo (RACE) is a technique that uses bedside transthoracic echocardiography with 2 modes (2-dimensional imaging and M-mode) and 5 views (parasternal long-axis, parasternal short-axis, apical 4-chamber, apical 2-chamber, and subcostal views) to answer 4 questions: 1) What is the LV function? 2) What is the RV function? 3) Is there any evidence of pericardial effusion and cardiac tamponade? 4) What is the fluid status?

Echocardiography can often replace invasive hemodynamic monitoring because the 2-dimensional Simpson multidisk method and pulsed-wave Doppler imaging across the LV output tract are accurate for cardiac output and are noninvasive. LV ejection fraction can be quantified, although visual estimates are reasonably accurate with experience. Additionally, diastolic dysfunction and valve abnormalities can also be identified, and may therefore considerably change management. When the 4 RACE questions are answered, CS can be diagnosed and managed appropriately.

Treatment

General

Patients with CS have 2 fundamental problems: decreased cardiac output and lack of oxygenated blood supply to vital organs. Therefore, delivery of supplemental oxygen (including intubation and mechanical ventilation if needed) is important for optimizing the oxygen carrying capacity of the hemoglobin, and venous access must be established. Oxygen delivery should be titrated to target a Pao_2 of more than 70 mm Hg; if patients are at risk for RV failure, a Pao_2 goal of more than 100 mm Hg may help decrease RV afterload. Volume status should also be evaluated (by echocardiography, clinical examination, or invasive monitoring tracings), and, if needed, fluid resuscitation should be given carefully. Patients with severe, refractory metabolic acidosis may benefit from treatment with sodium bicarbonate.

Hemodynamic Support

After fluid resuscitation has been initiated (with the goal of restoring euvolemia), further pharmacologic steps can be taken to achieve a mean arterial pressure that is greater than 60 to 65 mm Hg but less than 80 mm Hg. There is insufficient evidence for the use of 1 particular vasopressor or inotrope in CS. Table 27.3 describes the pertinent characteristics of various pharmacologic agents. Although vasopressors are typically first-line agents, a catecholamine response, with increased systemic vascular resistance, may already be present such that vasopressors may provide only limited benefit but worsen CS by increasing afterload.

For RV failure, inotropic therapy is indicated. Agents such as dobutamine and milrinone decrease central venous pressure and PCWP (Table 27.3) and thereby help to optimize RV end-diastolic pressure to a goal of 10 to 15 mm Hg. Inhaled nitric oxide can decrease pulmonary vascular resistance and help achieve this goal.

Antithrombotics

Aspirin and full-dose heparin infusion are indicated for all patients who have MI, regardless of whether they have CS. Use of clopidogrel is usually deferred until after PCI and stent placement, but when the decision is made to proceed with PCI, glycoprotein IIb/IIIa inhibitor therapy should be initiated. Glycoprotein IIb/IIIa inhibitors also improve outcomes among patients with NSTEMI acute coronary syndrome. In patients with CS, eptifibatide has decreased 30-day mortality, possibly by relieving microvascular obstruction.

Mechanical Support

Intra-aortic balloon pump (IABP) counterpulsation can help decrease afterload and improve diastolic coronary artery perfusion. In patients with MI who are undergoing PCI, however, IABP counterpulsation is generally not recommended because it provides no benefit for intensive care unit stay, 30-day mortality, or 1-year mortality.

LV and Biventricular Assist Devices

LV and biventricular assist devices are implanted as either a bridge to transplant or as a bridge to recovery for patients who had rapid reperfusion but with ongoing hypotension. These devices are implanted through open surgery or percutaneously through the femoral artery. Their use requires anticoagulation, which may otherwise be contraindicated because of the patient's neurologic condition (eg, intracerebral hemorrhage or large-volume ischemic stroke).

Extracorporeal Membrane Oxygenation

Extracorporeal membrane oxygenation (ECMO) machines are typically implanted in the operating room and require an experienced, multidisciplinary team to manage them postoperatively. Blood is drained from the patient through large cannulas and circulated through a mechanical pump, which oxygenates the blood and removes carbon dioxide. The 2 types of ECMO are venovenous (VV) and venoarterial (VA). In VV ECMO, blood is taken from the superior vena cava or right atrium and returned to the right atrium; VV ECMO is used to provide respiratory support for people with primary pulmonary failure. In VA ECMO, blood is taken from the right atrium and returned to the arterial system through the abdominal aorta; VA ECMO provides respiratory and hemodynamic support. VA ECMO is more appropriate than VV ECMO for CS, and several studies have shown that patients receiving VA ECMO have better hospital and long-term survival rates and better long-term functional capacity.

Complications of ECMO include lower extremity ischemia and increased afterload on the heart (because VA ECMO returns blood to the abdominal aorta against the flow of blood from the heart). Additionally, its use can lead to compartment syndrome, amputation, stroke, major bleeding, and infection.

Reperfusion

In CS due to MI, the most important treatment is early revascularization because it decreases mortality at 0.5, 1, and 6 years compared to medical therapy alone. PCI has been compared with coronary artery bypass graft (CABG) surgery in only observational studies; mortality rates appear to be similar between patients undergoing PCI and patients undergoing CABG surgery. In practice, CABG is performed in less than 5% of CS cases. No prospective randomized studies have compared multivessel PCI with PCI on only the culprit lesion. In 2017, the Culprit Lesion Only PCI Versus Multivessel PCI in Cardiogenic Shock (CULPRIT-SHOCK) trial began enrolling participants in Europe to answer this question. Fibrinolysis is indicated if PCI is not possible or is delayed.

Table 27.3 • Vasopressor and Inotropic Agents Commonly Used in Cardiogenic Shock

Agent	Mechanism of Action	Therapeutic Use	Adverse Effects	CO	SVR	MAP	HR	CVP	PCWP
Mixed activity agents									
Norepinephrine (NE)	$\alpha_1 >> \beta_1 > \beta_2$	Initial vasopressor	Bradycardia	↑ or ↓	↑↑	↑	↓	↑	↑
Dopamine	DA (15 mcg/kg/min) β_1 (6-10 mcg/kg/min) α_1 (>10 mcg/kg/min)	Second-line agent	Tachyarrythmias	↑	↑	↑	↑	↑	↑
Epinephrine	$\alpha_1 > \beta_1 > \beta_2$	Additional agent with NE First-line agent if NE is contraindicated	↑ HR Tachyarrhythmias ↑ Lactate	↑↑	↑	↑	↑↑	↑	↑
Vasopressor agents									
Phenylephrine	α_1	For use when tachyarrhythmias preclude use of other agents Can be given in bolus of 50-100 mcg	May cause ↓ stroke volume and ↓ CO	↑ or ↓	↑↑	↑	↓	↑	↑
Vasopressin	Antidiuretic hormone	Additional agent to augment efficacy	May cause ↓ CO and myocardial dysfunction (at doses >0.04 units/min) May cause myocardial ischemia in CAD	—	↑	↑	↑ or ↓	— or ↑	— or ↑
Inotropic agents									
Dobutamine	$\beta_1 > \beta_2 >> \alpha_1$	First-line choice for low CO *if* SBP is sustained at >90 mm Hg Additional agent with NE	↑ Cardiac contractility and ↑ rate May cause hypotension and tachyarrhythmias	↑↑	↓	↑	↑	—	↓
Milrinone	PDE3 inhibitor	Alternative agent for short-term ↑ CO in refractory cases	May cause peripheral vasodilatation, hypotension, ventricular arrhythmia	↑↑	↓	↓	↑	↓	↓

Abbreviations: ↓, decreased; ↑, increased; ↑↑, markedly increased; >, greater than; >>, markedly greater than; —, no effect; α_1, α_1-adrenergic receptor; β_1, β_1-adrenergic receptor; β_2, β_2-adrenergic receptor; CAD, coronary artery disease; CO, cardiac output; CVP, central venous pressure; DA, dopaminergic; HR, heart rate; MAP, mean arterial pressure; PCWP, pulmonary capillary wedge pressure; PDE3, phosphodiesterase 3 inhibitor; SBP, systolic blood pressure; SVR, systemic vascular resistance.

Dysrhythmias

Patients with CS due to dysrhythmia should be evaluated as described above. Tachyarrhythmia and bradyarrhythmia should be treated according to the American Heart Association Advanced Cardiac Life Support protocol.

Other Structural Causes

Other structural causes of CS are often identified during the initial evaluation, commonly with echocardiography. Patients with valvular dysfunction, septal defects, ventricular aneurysms, or other structural abnormalities should be referred immediately to a cardiothoracic surgeon.

Summary

- The mechanisms of cardiac dysfunction are cardiomyopathic, arrythmogenic, and mechanical.
- Bedside echocardiography is recommended for diagnosis, management decisions, and monitoring.
- Treatment should be aimed at restoring perfusion and oxygenation to vital organs and managing the underlying condition; pharmacologic therapy or mechanical techniques (or both) may be needed.

SUGGESTED READING

Aissaoui N, Puymirat E, Tabone X, Charbonnier B, Schiele F, Lefevre T, et al. Improved outcome of cardiogenic shock at the acute stage of myocardial infarction: a report from the USIK 1995, USIC 2000, and FAST-MI French nationwide registries. Eur Heart J. 2012 Oct;33(20):2535–43. Epub 2012 Aug 26.

Bagai J, Brilakis ES. Update in the management of acute coronary syndrome patients with cardiogenic shock. Curr Cardiol Rep. 2019 Mar 4;21(4):17.

Berisha S, Kastrati A, Goda A, Popa Y. Optimal value of filling pressure in the right side of the heart in acute right ventricular infarction. Br Heart J. 1990 Feb;63(2):98–102.

Cecconi M, De Backer D, Antonelli M, Beale R, Bakker J, Hofer C, et al; Task force of the European Society of Intensive Care Medicine. Consensus on circulatory shock and hemodynamic monitoring. Intensive Care Med. 2014 Dec;40(12):1795–815. Epub 2014 Nov 13.

Cheng R, Hachamovitch R, Kittleson M, Patel J, Arabia F, Moriguchi J, et al. Complications of extracorporeal membrane oxygenation for treatment of cardiogenic shock and cardiac arrest: a meta-analysis of 1,866 adult patients. Ann Thorac Surg. 2014 Feb;97(2):610–6. Epub 2013 Nov 8.

Gianni M, Dentali F, Grandi AM, Sumner G, Hiralal R, Lonn E. Apical ballooning syndrome or takotsubo cardiomyopathy: a systematic review. Eur Heart J. 2006 Jul;27(13):1523–9. Epub 2006 May 23.

Goldberg RJ, Samad NA, Yarzebski J, Gurwitz J, Bigelow C, Gore JM. Temporal trends in cardiogenic shock complicating acute myocardial infarction. N Engl J Med. 1999 Apr 15;340(15):1162–8.

Goldberg RJ, Spencer FA, Gore JM, Lessard D, Yarzebski J. Thirty-year trends (1975 to 2005) in the magnitude of, management of, and hospital death rates associated with cardiogenic shock in patients with acute myocardial infarction: a population-based perspective. Circulation. 2009 Mar 10;119(9):1211–9. Epub 2009 Feb 23.

Hasdai D, Harrington RA, Hochman JS, Califf RM, Battler A, Box JW, et al. Platelet glycoprotein IIb/IIIa blockade and outcome of cardiogenic shock complicating acute coronary syndromes without persistent ST-segment elevation. J Am Coll Cardiol. 2000 Sep;36(3):685–92.

Hochman JS, Buller CE, Sleeper LA, Boland J, Dzavik V, Sanborn TA, et al. Cardiogenic shock complicating acute myocardial infarction: etiologies, management and outcome: a report from the SHOCK Trial Registry. SHould we emergently revascularize Occluded Coronaries for cardiogenic shocK? J Am Coll Cardiol. 2000 Sep;36(3 Suppl A):1063–70.

Hochman JS, Sleeper LA, Webb JG, Sanborn TA, White HD, Talley JD, et al; SHOCK Investigators. Should We Emergently Revascularize Occluded Coronaries for Cardiogenic Shock. Early revascularization in acute myocardial infarction complicated by cardiogenic shock. N Engl J Med. 1999 Aug 26;341(9):625–34.

Hollenberg SM. Vasoactive drugs in circulatory shock. Am J Respir Crit Care Med. 2011 Apr 1;183(7):847–55. Epub 2010 Nov 19.

Jacobs AK, Leopold JA, Bates E, Mendes LA, Sleeper LA, White H, et al. Cardiogenic shock caused by right ventricular infarction: a report from the SHOCK registry. J Am Coll Cardiol. 2003 Apr 16;41(8):1273–9.

Jeger RV, Radovanovic D, Hunziker PR, Pfisterer ME, Stauffer JC, Erne P, et al; AMIS Plus Registry Investigators. Ten-year trends in the incidence and treatment of cardiogenic shock. Ann Intern Med. 2008 Nov 4;149(9):618–26.

Kolte D, Khera S, Aronow WS, Mujib M, Palaniswamy C, Sule S, et al. Trends in incidence, management, and outcomes of cardiogenic shock complicating ST-elevation myocardial infarction in the United States. J Am Heart Assoc. 2014 Jan 13;3(1):e000590.

Lindholm MG, Kober L, Boesgaard S, Torp-Pedersen C, Aldershvile J; Trandolapril Cardiac Evaluation study group. Cardiogenic shock complicating acute myocardial infarction; prognostic impact of early and late shock development. Eur Heart J. 2003 Feb;24(3):258–65.

McLean A, Huang S. Critical care ultrasound manual. Sydney (Australia): Churchill Livingstone/Elsevier; c2012. 181 p.

McLean AS. Echocardiography in shock management. Crit Care. 2016 Aug 20;20:275.

O'Gara PT, Kushner FG, Ascheim DD, Casey DE Jr, Chung MK, de Lemos JA, et al; American College of Cardiology Foundation/American Heart Association Task Force on Practice Guidelines. 2013 ACCF/AHA guideline for the management of ST-elevation myocardial infarction: a report of the American College of Cardiology Foundation/American Heart Association Task Force on Practice Guidelines. Circulation. 2013 Jan 29;127(4):e362–425. Epub 2012 Dec 17. Erratum in: Circulation. 2013 Dec 24;128(25):e481.

Overgaard CB, Dzavík V. Inotropes and vasopressors: review of physiology and clinical use in cardiovascular disease. Circulation. 2008 Sep 2;118(10):1047–56.

Platelet Glycoprotein IIb/IIIa in Unstable Angina: Receptor Suppression Using Integrilin Therapy (PURSUIT) Trial Investigators. Inhibition of platelet glycoprotein IIb/IIIa with eptifibatide in patients with acute coronary syndromes. N Engl J Med. 1998 Aug 13;339(7):436–43.

Reynolds HR, Hochman JS. Cardiogenic shock: current concepts and improving outcomes. Circulation. 2008 Feb 5;117(5):686–97.

Roffi M, Patrono C, Collet JP, Mueller C, Valgimigli M, Andreotti F, et al; Management of Acute Coronary Syndromes in Patients Presenting without Persistent ST-Segment Elevation of the European Society of Cardiology. 2015 ESC Guidelines for the management of acute coronary syndromes in patients presenting without persistent ST-segment elevation: Task Force for the Management of Acute Coronary Syndromes in Patients

Presenting without Persistent ST-Segment Elevation of the European Society of Cardiology (ESC). Eur Heart J. 2016 Jan 14;37(3):267–315. Epub 2015 Aug 29.

Sheu JJ, Tsai TH, Lee FY, Fang HY, Sun CK, Leu S, et al. Early extracorporeal membrane oxygenator-assisted primary percutaneous coronary intervention improved 30-day clinical outcomes in patients with ST-segment elevation myocardial infarction complicated with profound cardiogenic shock. Crit Care Med. 2010 Sep;38(9):1810–7.

Stephens RS, Whitman GJ. Postoperative critical care of the adult cardiac surgical patient. Part I: Routine postoperative care. Crit Care Med. 2015 Jul;43(7):1477–97.

Sylvester JT, Shimoda LA, Aaronson PI, Ward JP. Hypoxic pulmonary vasoconstriction. Physiol Rev. 2012 Jan;92(1):367–520. Erratum in: Physiol Rev. 2014 Jul;94(3):989.

Tewelde SZ, Liu SS, Winters ME. Cardiogenic shock. Cardiol Clin. 2018 Feb;36(1):53–61.

Thiele H, Ohman EM, Desch S, Eitel I, de Waha S. Management of cardiogenic shock. Eur Heart J. 2015 May 21;36(20):1223–30. Epub 2015 Mar 1.

Thiele H, Schuler G, Neumann FJ, Hausleiter J, Olbrich HG, Schwarz B, et al. Intraaortic balloon counterpulsation in acute myocardial infarction complicated by cardiogenic shock: design and rationale of the Intraaortic Balloon Pump in Cardiogenic Shock II (IABP-SHOCK II) trial. Am Heart J. 2012 Jun;163(6):938–45. Erratum in: Am Heart J. 2015 Jan;169(1):185.

Thiele H, Zeymer U, Neumann FJ, Ferenc M, Olbrich HG, Hausleiter J, et al; Intraaortic Balloon Pump in cardiogenic shock II (IABP-SHOCK II) trial investigators. Intra-aortic balloon counterpulsation in acute myocardial infarction complicated by cardiogenic shock (IABP-SHOCK II): final 12 month results of a randomised, open-label trial. Lancet. 2013 Nov 16;382(9905):1638–45. Epub 2013 Sep 3.

Unverzagt S, Buerke M, de Waha A, Haerting J, Pietzner D, Seyfarth M, et al. Intra-aortic balloon pump counterpulsation (IABP) for myocardial infarction complicated by cardiogenic shock. Cochrane Database Syst Rev. 2015 Mar 27;(3):CD007398.

28 Acute Coronary Syndrome

SIVA S. KETHA, MD; JUAN CARLOS LEONI MORENO, MD

Goals

- Describe the clinical spectrum, diagnostic approach, and contemporary management of acute coronary syndrome.
- Identify the Thrombolysis in Myocardial Infarction risk stratification in acute coronary syndrome.
- Define the indications for coronary revascularization.
- Recognize management considerations for acute coronary syndrome in specific circumstances.

Introduction

Acute coronary syndrome (ACS) encompasses all clinical manifestations caused by active myocardial ischemia and includes 3 entities: unstable angina (UA), acute non–ST-segment elevation myocardial infarction (NSTEMI), and acute ST-segment elevation myocardial infarction (STEMI). Atherosclerotic plaque rupture is the most consistent pathophysiologic event in ACS. After plaque rupture, cardiac myocytes die as a consequence of continued occlusion, thereby causing acute myocardial infarction (MI).

Prompt recognition of ACS is crucial because the greatest therapeutic effect is achieved if treatment is performed soon after presentation. Chest pain from an ACS typically starts gradually and may worsen with exertion. With *stable angina*, discomfort occurs only when activity creates an oxygen demand that outstrips the supply limitations imposed by a fixed atherosclerotic lesion. This occurs at relatively predictable points and changes slowly over time. *UA* is an abrupt change from baseline functioning, which may manifest as discomfort that begins with minimal physical activity.

Patients often describe the symptoms of ACS as discomfort rather than pain. The discomfort may feel like pressure, heaviness, tightness, fullness, or squeezing, and it often radiates to the jaw or an arm. The diagnosis of MI in patients with typical pain and possible ACS can be supported either with increased levels of cardiac biomarkers and elevation of the ST segment on electrocardiography (ECG) (as in STEMI) or with only an increased level of cardiac troponin (as in NSTEMI). In contrast, the diagnosis of UA relies mainly on the history at presentation.

Epidemiology

Each year, of the 8 million patients admitted to emergency departments for new-onset chest pain, up to 10% receive a diagnosis of ACS, and 1 million subsequent hospital admissions are registered in the United States annually. In 2013, more than 8 million people died of coronary heart disease. Mortality related to coronary heart disease has decreased since the early 2000s, especially among older patients, but mortality has remained relatively high among younger women. The decrease in mortality is due in part to a lower incidence of STEMI.

Pathogenesis

The formation of a clot within the lumen and subsequent coronary artery thrombosis is the final pathogenic mechanism in most patients with ACS. Endothelial integrity is lost because of plaque rupture or plaque erosion; further disruption leads to activation of thrombogenic contents of the plaque core and formation of thrombus in the lumen. In angiographic studies, plaque rupture has occurred more frequently in moderately occlusive lesions.

Plaque Rupture

The hallmark of acute coronary thrombosis is plaque rupture. Direct contact of blood elements with the highly thrombogenic components of the necrotic core is thought

Box 28.1 • Differential Diagnosis of NSTE-ACS

Nonischemic cardiovascular causes of chest pain
- Aortic dissection
- Expanding aortic aneurysm
- Pulmonary embolism
- Pericarditis or myopericarditis

Noncardiovascular causes of chest, back, or upper abdominal discomfort
- Pulmonary causes: pneumonia, pleuritis, or pneumothorax
- Gastrointestinal tract causes: GERD, esophageal spasm, peptic ulcer, pancreatitis, biliary disease, cholecystitis, or esophageal rupture
- Musculoskeletal causes: costochondritis or cervical radiculopathy
- Psychiatric disorders: panic attacks or anxiety
- Miscellaneous causes: sickle cell crisis or herpes zoster

Abbreviations: GERD, gastroesophageal reflux disease; NSTE-ACS, non–ST-segment elevation acute coronary syndrome.

to be directly responsible for the development of the thrombus. Plaque rupture occurs in approximately 75% of patients with acute MI; the incidence is higher in men than women.

Plaque Erosion

Plaque erosion is second to plaque rupture as a pathologic event in acute coronary thrombosis. Elevation of biomarkers (eg, myeloperoxidase) distinguishes plaque rupture from plaque erosion. Plaque erosion has been shown to be the primary lesion in sudden coronary death and acute MI in younger patients (<50 years) and in premenopausal women.

Clinical Presentation

Acute chest discomfort is the most common clinical symptom of ACS. However, acute chest discomfort can be present with several non-ACS pathologic conditions (Box 28.1). Therefore, it is essential that clinicians use a methodical assessment to establish the cause of ACS and expedite appropriate management.

Diagnostic evaluation should distinguish between the following potentially life-threatening causes of new-onset or recurrent chest pain: 1) STEMI, NSTEMI, or UA and 2) nonischemic chest pain from aortic dissection, pulmonary embolism, or esophageal rupture.

Diagnostic features of MI (STEMI or NSTEMI) include an abnormal increase in the cardiac troponin level with a typical increase or decrease in troponin levels; ECG changes suggestive of myocardial ischemia; angina or anginal equivalents; cardiac imaging showing loss of viable myocardium; or recognition of an intracoronary thrombus.

Because STEMI can be excluded by ECG, the most important distinction is between chest pain from NSTEMI and nonischemic angina (Box 28.1). Several professional organizations have created guidelines for evaluation of patients with symptoms suggestive of ACS. A reasonable approach includes an early ECG (within 10 minutes of symptom onset), physical examination, and measurement of biomarkers (eg, cardiac troponin). Serial ECGs and cardiac troponin measurement in an 8- to 23-hour observation period are recommended. Patients with non–ST-segment elevation ACS (NSTE-ACS) should receive timely delivery of specific medical therapy with a higher level of monitoring (telemetry or admission to a coronary care unit or intensive care unit).

With laboratory testing, the diagnosis of MI can often be made within 1 to 3 hours after a patient is evaluated in the emergency department. Indeed, high-sensitivity troponin assays improve only the sensitivity of the assay rather than the timeliness of the diagnosis. Cardiac troponin is not specific for the diagnosis of MI, and its interpretation relies on the clinical context and serial testing.

Complementary evaluation of patients with chest pain should include chest radiography to identify other serious causes of chest pain (eg, widened mediastinum in patients with ascending or descending aortic dissection). However, contrast computed tomography of the chest is the gold standard for confirming pulmonary embolism and aortic dissection. Transesophageal echocardiography has limitations for the identification of aortic dissection (other than proximal aortic dissection). Transthoracic echocardiographic assessment can increase suspicion for aortic dissection if a pericardial effusion or aortic regurgitation is present, and transthoracic echocardiographic evaluation is crucial for recognition of new regional wall motion abnormalities in ACS patients. Low-risk patients with chest pain can benefit from a cost-effective approach with coronary computed tomographic angiography instead of an evaluation driven by myocardial perfusion imaging.

Risk Stratification

Risk scores facilitate integration of the clinical picture, ECG, and biomarkers into a model of quantification of pretest probability. The Thrombolysis in Myocardial Infarction (TIMI) risk score was initially derived as a prognostic rule to predict 14-day outcomes for ACS patients. It includes 7 variables, with 1 variable being a composite of conventional risk factors (Box 28.2). Scores of 3 or more are associated with increased risk of death or cardiac events through day 14.

Box 28.2 • TIMI Risk Score

For the presence of each of the following 7 variables, 1 point is assigned (scores range from 0-7):

- Age 65 years or older
- Presence of 3 or more cardiac risk factors (family history of CAD, hypertension, hypercholesterolemia, diabetes mellitus, or being a current smoker)
- Known CAD
- Aspirin use within 7 days
- At least 2 episodes of angina in the preceding 24 hours
- ST-segment elevation or depression of 0.5 mm
- Elevated levels of serum cardiac biomarkers

Abbreviations: CAD, coronary artery disease; TIMI, Thrombolysis in Myocardial Infarction.

The Global Registry of Acute Coronary Events (GRACE) risk score is used to predict recurrent MI or death at 6 months after ACS. The GRACE score is well validated and includes variables from the patient's past history, physical examination, ECG, and laboratory data. Like the TIMI score, the GRACE risk score is not designed to assess whether a patient's chest pain is due to ACS.

Management

STEMI, NSTEMI, and UA are medical emergencies that require the simultaneous application of multiple therapies (Box 28.3). Patients with UA or NSTEMI should receive the same medical therapy as patients with STEMI except that they are not good candidates for thrombolysis (it provides no benefit, and it may cause harm).

Box 28.3 • Diagnostic and Management Approach to Patients With a Leading Diagnosis of Acute Coronary Syndrome

- Evaluate airway, breathing, and circulation.
- Ensure availability of cardiac monitoring and resuscitation equipment.
- Obtain comprehensive history, and perform a detailed examination.
- Interpret a 12-lead electrocardiogram.
- Provide oxygen therapy as necessary.
- Establish intravenous access, and collect blood samples for laboratory investigations (complete blood cell count and serum levels of electrolytes, creatinine, and cardiac biomarkers).
- Provide antiplatelet therapy (aspirin 162-325 mg).
- Administer coronary vasodilators (nitrates in the absence of absolute contraindications).

Coronary Revascularization

Reperfusion therapy is the most important strategy for patients with STEMI who have had symptoms for less than 12 hours. The next crucial step is to decide which reperfusion intervention would be best. Percutaneous coronary intervention (PCI) is the gold standard for revascularization if it can be performed within 90 minutes after medical evaluation. Nevertheless, patients who cannot undergo PCI in a medical facility during the first 90 minutes of emergency evaluation may be candidates for fibrinolytic therapy within 30 minutes after arrival at the hospital, especially if they do not have any contraindications.

Evidence is lacking on whether early PCI in patients presenting with NSTEMI or UA is beneficial. Patients with NSTE-ACS can receive medical management through 2 distinct pathways (an invasive strategy and an ischemia-guided strategy) (Table 28.1 and Figure 28.1). In the invasive strategy, diagnostic evaluation is pursued with coronary angiography. In contrast, the ischemia-guided strategy uses invasive evaluation only for patients who 1) have no response to conventional medical management; 2) have objective signs of myocardial ischemia (fluctuating ECG changes or abnormal results on myocardial perfusion testing) as identified on a noninvasive stress test; or 3) have a clinical profile with a high-risk stratification (eg, high TIMI or GRACE score) (Table 28.1). Regardless of which strategy is used, patients should receive optimal medical therapy (anti-ischemic and antithrombotic therapy) (Table 28.2). An early invasive strategy should not be used for patients with extensive comorbidities because risk-benefit ratio is unfavorable. Likewise, it should not be used for patients with acute chest pain who have normal levels of biomarkers and a low probability of ACS.

Medical Management

With medical management, the goal is to relieve ischemia and to reduce morbidity and mortality. Patients with compromised systemic oxygenation (oxygen saturation by pulse oximetry <90%) should receive oxygen therapy. Sublingual nitroglycerin (0.3–0.4 mg) every 5 minutes for up to 3 doses can be administered to patients with ongoing angina. Moreover, intravenous nitroglycerin is indicated for the treatment of refractory myocardial ischemia, heart failure, or concomitant hypertension.

In contrast, use of nitrates should be avoided in patients with NSTE-ACS who have recently received a phosphodiesterase inhibitor (sildenafil or vardenafil within 24 hours; tadalafil within 48 hours). Morphine sulfate can be given to patients with NSTE-ACS who have refractory angina after receiving anti-ischemic therapy.

Table 28.1 • Strategy Selection for Patients With NSTE-ACS

Strategy	Feature
Immediate invasive (within 2 h)	Refractory angina Signs or symptoms of HF or new or worsening mitral regurgitation Hemodynamic instability Recurrent angina or ischemia at rest or with low-level activities despite intensive medical therapy Sustained VT or VF
Ischemia-guided	Low-risk score (eg, TIMI, 0 or 1; GRACE <109) Low-risk female patients without diagnostic troponin levels Patient or clinician preference in the absence of high-risk features
Early invasive (within 24 h)	None of the above, but GRACE risk score is >140 Temporal change in troponin level New or presumably new ST-segment depression
Delayed invasive (within 25–72 h)	None of the above, but patient has diabetes mellitus Renal insufficiency (GFR <60 mL/min/1.73 m^2) Reduced LV systolic function (EF <40%) Early postinfarction angina PCI within 6 mo Previous CABG surgery GRACE risk score, 109-140; TIMI score ≥2

Abbreviations: CABG, coronary artery bypass graft; EF, ejection fraction; GFR, glomerular filtration rate; GRACE, Global Registry of Acute Coronary Events; HF, heart failure; LV, left ventricular; NSTE-ACS, non–ST-segment elevation acute coronary syndrome; PCI, percutaneous coronary intervention; TIMI, Thrombolysis in Myocardial Infarction; VF, ventricular fibrillation; VT, ventricular tachycardia.

Antiplatelet Agents

Antiplatelet therapy decreases the occurrence of thrombosis by affecting platelet release and aggregation. These agents include aspirin, platelet adenosine diphosphate P2Y12 receptor (P2Y12) antagonists, and glycoprotein IIb/IIIa inhibitors (GPIs). After an initial aspirin dose of 162 to 325 mg is given, aspirin 81 mg daily is used as a maintenance regimen. P2Y12 antagonists for management of ACS include clopidogrel, prasugrel, and ticagrelor (Table 28.2).

Although peri-interventional use of GPIs during PCI has been shown to effectively lower the rate of ischemic complications, their use is associated with an increased bleeding risk for patients receiving triple antiplatelet therapy. Therefore, these agents are used only selectively (for patients with a high thrombus burden) rather than routinely.

Anticoagulants

The initial management of ACS includes the use of intravenous or subcutaneous anticoagulation (unfractionated heparin [UFH], low-molecular-weight heparin, fondaparinux, or bivalirudin) and antiplatelet agents. Intravenous anticoagulation with UFH should be therapeutic for 48 hours or until the patient undergoes revascularization with PCI. An alternative regimen with enoxaparin (1 mg/kg subcutaneously every 12 hours) is recommended for the duration of hospitalization or until PCI is performed. In patients with chronic kidney disease (creatinine clearance <30 mL/min), the dosage should be reduced to 1 mg/kg once daily. Similarly, fondaparinux (2.5 mg subcutaneously daily) is used, and its administration can be continued for the duration of hospitalization or until the patient undergoes PCI. For patients having PCI while receiving fondaparinux, an anticoagulant that inhibits direct factor IIa activity (either UFH or bivalirudin) should be added because of the increased risk of catheter thrombosis. Bivalirudin at a loading dose of 0.10 mg/kg followed by 0.25 mg/kg per hour should be used only for the early invasive strategy and must be continued until the patient undergoes diagnostic angiography or PCI. Anticoagulation is not indicated for ACS at hospital discharge.

β-Blockers

β-Blocker therapy decreases myocardial oxygen consumption. Hence, use of an oral β-blocker (eg, metoprolol) is indicated within 24 hours of diagnosis of UA, NSTEMI, or STEMI except in patients with evidence of shock, signs of decompensated systolic heart failure (including pulmonary edema), or conduction system abnormalities.

Renin-Angiotensin System Inhibitors

Angiotensin-converting enzyme (ACE) inhibitor and angiotensin receptor blocker (ARB) agents decrease the risk of death after MI. If there are no contraindications, these agents should be initiated within the first 24 hours after ACS is diagnosed in patients who have signs of pulmonary congestion, congestive heart failure, extensive or anterior wall STEMI, or left ventricular ejection fraction (LVEF) less than 40%.

Aldosterone antagonist therapy (eg, spironolactone or eplerenone) is recommended for patients who have ACS 1) if they have begun receiving therapeutic doses of either an ACE inhibitor or an ARB in addition to a β-blocker and 2) if they have an LVEF less than 40% and either symptomatic congestive heart failure or diabetes mellitus. Furthermore, aldosterone antagonists improve morbidity and mortality in these selected patient populations. Their use, however, requires close monitoring for hypotension, hyperkalemia, and elevations in serum creatinine.

Statins

Statins must be initiated or continued in all patients with ACS because statins are beneficial in ACS even if patients have baseline low-density lipoprotein cholesterol levels

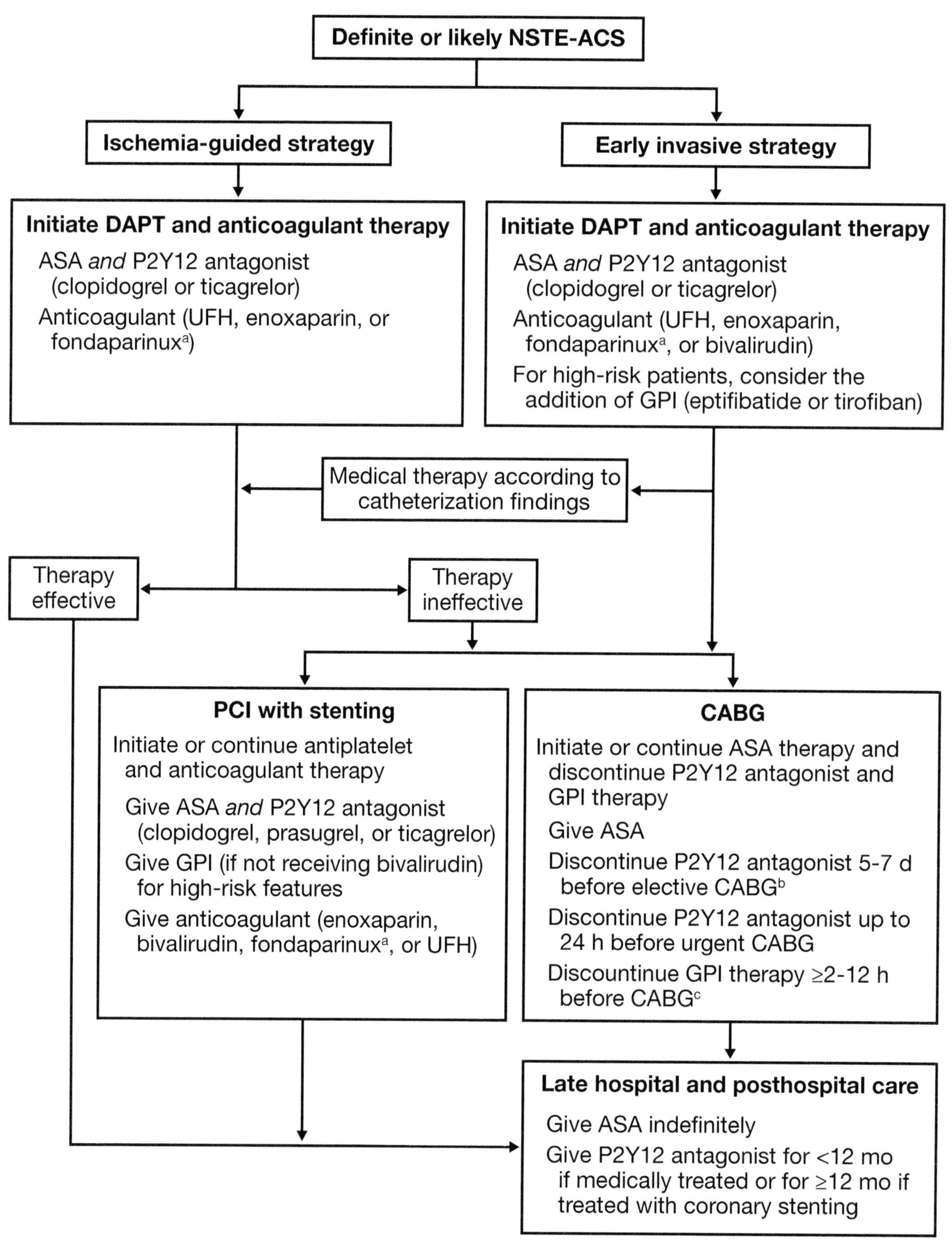

Figure 28.1. Algorithm for Management of Definite or Likely Non–ST-Segment Elevation Acute Coronary Syndrome (NSTE-ACS). Superscript a *indicates that patients who have been treated with fondaparinux who are undergoing percutaneous coronary intervention (PCI) should be given an additional anticoagulant that inhibits direct factor IIa activity because of the risk of catheter thrombosis. Superscript* b *indicates that before elective cornary artery bypass graft (CABG) surgery, clopidogrel or ticagrelor should be discontinued for 5 days and prasugrel for at least 7 days. Superscript* c *indicates that before CABG surgery, eptifibatide or tirofiban should be discontinued for at least 2 to 4 hours and abciximab for at least 12 hours. ASA indicates aspirin; DAPT, dual antiplatelet therapy; GPI, glycoprotein IIb/IIIa inhibitor; P2Y12, platelet adenosine diphosphate P2Y12 receptor; UFH, unfractionated heparin.*

Table 28.2 • Oral Antiplatelet Agents: Oral Platelet Adenosine Diphosphate P2Y12 Receptor Inhibitors

Feature	Clopidogrel	Prasugrel	Ticagrelor
Loading dose for PCI	600 mg once	60 mg	180 mg
Loading dose for medical management	300 mg once	FDA approved only for patients undergoing PCI, not medical management	180 mg
Maintenance dose	75 mg once daily	10 mg once daily (consider 5 mg if weight <60 kg)	90 mg twice daily
Onset of action	2 h with 600-mg dose 6 h with 300-mg dose	30 min	60 min
Considerations before surgical procedure	Hold for 5 d	Hold for 7 d	Hold for 5 d
Clinical considerations	Generic prescription option Genetic polymorphisms of the CYP2C19 enzyme lead to variable antiplatelet effects	Contraindicated for patients with history of stroke or TIA No net benefit for patients weighing <60 kg or for patients older than 75 years	Contraindicated for patients with daily aspirin dose >100 mg May cause dyspnea, bradyarrythmias, and ventricular pauses

Abbreviations: CYP2C19, cytochrome P450 2C19 isozyme; FDA, US Food and Drug Administration; PCI, percutaneous coronary intervention; TIA, transient ischemic attack.

of less than 70 mg/dL. For instance, high-intensity statin therapy (eg, atorvastatin >40 mg daily or rosuvastatin >20 mg daily) after an ACS event confers an absolute risk reduction of 3.9% in comparison with a lower-intensity statin regimen. Patients older than 75 years should receive a lower-intensity regimen because of limited therapeutic tolerance.

Special Circumstances

STEMI With Cardiac Arrest

Therapeutic hypothermia is indicated for STEMI patients who remain comatose immediately after out-of-hospital cardiac arrest due to ventricular fibrillation or pulseless ventricular tachycardia. Immediate angiography and PCI (when indicated) should be performed in STEMI patients after proper cardiopulmonary resuscitation.

Cocaine-Associated ACS

MI is a well-described complication among patients presenting with cocaine-induced ischemic symptoms. These patients should be treated like other ACS patients with 2 exceptions: 1) Benzodiazepines should be administered early, and 2) β-blockers should not be used in patients with acute cocaine intoxication and chest pain because of the risk of coronary artery vasospasm.

Intracoronary Stent Restenosis and Thrombosis

ACS is occasionally due to coronary stent restenosis or stent thrombosis. *Restenosis* is an insidious renarrowing of the stented segment 3 to 12 months after stent placement. Patients with restenosis may have recurrent angina or, rarely, acute MI. With drug-eluting stents, in-stent restenosis is uncommon and is usually managed with additional PCI. However, stent thrombosis is a devastating complication, and most patients present with extensive MI or sudden death. Coronary angiography is used for diagnosis, and PCI or fibrinolysis is generally indicated. The timing of stent thrombosis may provide a clue as to its cause. Despite the fact that clopidogrel resistance can be a contributory factor, the optimal medical approach for patients with clopidogrel resistance (determined with platelet function testing) is unknown. An alternative strategy would be to switch to prasugrel (10 mg daily) or ticagrelor (90 mg twice daily) in combination with aspirin. The minimum duration of dual antiplatelet therapy is 1 year; longer courses are used for patients who tolerate the therapy without having any major bleeding events.

Summary

- For patients with suspected ACS, a prompt, sequential, and evidence-based assessment is essential to determine the cause of the chest discomfort and to initiate timely, adequate therapy.
- Diagnostic evaluation should distinguish between ACS and potentially life-threatening causes of nonischemic chest pain: aortic dissection, pulmonary embolism, and esophageal rupture.
- Initial medical therapy for UA or NSTEMI is the same as for STEMI with 1 exception: Fibrinolysis provides no benefit and may cause harm.

- Patients with cocaine-associated ACS should be treated similarly to other ACS patients with 2 exceptions: Benzodiazepines should be administered early, and β-blockers should not be used because they may exacerbate coronary artery vasoconstriction.
- Most patients who have stent thrombosis, a life-threatening complication, present with cardiac arrest or massive MI. Urgent coronary angiography is essential for diagnosis, and PCI or fibrinolysis is generally indicated.

SUGGESTED READING

Amsterdam EA, Kirk JD, Bluemke DA, Diercks D, Farkouh ME, Garvey JL, et al; American Heart Association Exercise, Cardiac Rehabilitation, and Prevention Committee of the Council on Clinical Cardiology, Council on Cardiovascular Nursing, and Interdisciplinary Council on Quality of Care and Outcomes Research. Testing of low-risk patients presenting to the emergency department with chest pain: a scientific statement from the American Heart Association. Circulation. 2010 Oct 26;122(17):1756–76. Epub 2010 Jul 26. Erratum in: Circulation. 2010 Oct 26;122(17):e500–1.

Amsterdam EA, Wenger NK, Brindis RG, Casey DE Jr, Ganiats TG, Holmes DR Jr, et al. 2014 AHA/ACC Guideline for the management of patients with non-ST-elevation acute coronary syndromes: a report of the American College of Cardiology/American Heart Association Task Force on Practice Guidelines. J Am Coll Cardiol. 2014 Dec 23;64(24):e139–e228. Epub 2014 Sep 23. Erratum in: J Am Coll Cardiol. 2014 Dec 23;64(24):2713–4.

Antman EM, Cohen M, Bernink PJ, McCabe CH, Horacek T, Papuchis G, et al. The TIMI risk score for unstable angina/non-ST elevation MI: a method for prognostication and therapeutic decision making. JAMA. 2000 Aug 16;284(7):835–42.

Bandstein N, Ljung R, Johansson M, Holzmann MJ. Undetectable high-sensitivity cardiac troponin T level in the emergency department and risk of myocardial infarction. J Am Coll Cardiol. 2014 Jun 17;63(23):2569–78. Epub 2014 Mar 30.

Bernard SA, Gray TW, Buist MD, Jones BM, Silvester W, Gutteridge G, et al. Treatment of comatose survivors of out-of-hospital cardiac arrest with induced hypothermia. N Engl J Med. 2002 Feb 21;346(8):557–63.

Borger van der Burg AE, Bax JJ, Boersma E, Bootsma M, van Erven L, van der Wall EE, et al. Impact of percutaneous coronary intervention or coronary artery bypass grafting on outcome after nonfatal cardiac arrest outside the hospital. Am J Cardiol. 2003 Apr 1;91(7):785–9.

DeWood MA, Spores J, Notske R, Mouser LT, Burroughs R, Golden MS, et al. Prevalence of total coronary occlusion during the early hours of transmural myocardial infarction. N Engl J Med. 1980 Oct 16;303(16):897–902.

Eisen A, Giugliano RP, Braunwald E. Updates on acute coronary syndrome: a review. JAMA Cardiol. 2016 Sep 1;1(6):718–30.

Fox KA, Dabbous OH, Goldberg RJ, Pieper KS, Eagle KA, Van de Werf F, et al. Prediction of risk of death and myocardial infarction in the six months after presentation with acute coronary syndrome: prospective multinational observational study (GRACE). BMJ. 2006 Nov 25;333(7578):1091. Epub 2006 Oct 10.

Goldstein JA, Chinnaiyan KM, Abidov A, Achenbach S, Berman DS, Hayes SW, et al; CT-STAT Investigators. The CT-STAT (Coronary Computed Tomographic Angiography for Systematic Triage of Acute Chest Pain Patients to Treatment) trial. J Am Coll Cardiol. 2011 Sep 27;58(14):1414–22.

Gupta A, Wang Y, Spertus JA, Geda M, Lorenze N, Nkonde-Price C, et al. Trends in acute myocardial infarction in young patients and differences by sex and race, 2001 to 2010. J Am Coll Cardiol. 2014 Jul 29;64(4):337–45.

Hamm CW, Bassand JP, Agewall S, Bax J, Boersma E, Bueno H, et al; ESC Committee for Practice Guidelines. ESC Guidelines for the management of acute coronary syndromes in patients presenting without persistent ST-segment elevation: the task force for the management of acute coronary syndromes (ACS) in patients presenting without persistent ST-segment elevation of the European Society of Cardiology (ESC). Eur Heart J. 2011 Dec;32(23):2999–3054. Epub 2011 Aug 26.

Kelly AM, Klim S. Does undetectable troponin I at presentation using a contemporary sensitive assay rule out myocardial infarction? A cohort study. Emerg Med J. 2015 Oct;32(10):760–3. Epub 2014 Dec 31.

Libby P, Pasterkamp G. Requiem for the 'vulnerable plaque.' Eur Heart J. 2015 Nov 14;36(43):2984–7. Epub 2015 Jul 22.

O'Gara PT, Kushner FG, Ascheim DD, Casey DE Jr, Chung MK, de Lemos JA, et al; CF/AHA Task Force. 2013 ACCF/AHA guideline for the management of ST-elevation myocardial infarction: executive summary: a report of the American College of Cardiology Foundation/American Heart Association Task Force on Practice Guidelines. Circulation. 2013 Jan 29;127(4):529–55. Epub 2012 Dec 17.

Reichlin T, Twerenbold R, Wildi K, Rubini Gimenez M, Bergsma N, Haaf P, et al. Prospective validation of a 1-hour algorithm to rule-out and rule-in acute myocardial infarction using a high-sensitivity cardiac troponin T assay. CMAJ. 2015 May 19;187(8):E243–52. Epub 2015 Apr 13.

Roth GA, Huffman MD, Moran AE, Feigin V, Mensah GA, Naghavi M, et al. Global and regional patterns in cardiovascular mortality from 1990 to 2013. Circulation. 2015 Oct 27;132(17):1667–78.

Storrow AB, Nowak RM, Diercks DB, Singer AJ, Wu AH, Kulstad E, et al. Absolute and relative changes (delta) in troponin I for early diagnosis of myocardial infarction: results of a prospective multicenter trial. Clin Biochem. 2015 Mar;48(4-5):260–7. Epub 2014 Sep 28.

29 Cardiac Rhythm and Conduction Disturbances

YAHAIRA ORTIZ GONZALEZ, MD; FRED KUSUMOTO, MD

Goals

- Describe the arrhythmias encountered in patients in the intensive care unit.
- Discuss the classification and management of tachyarrhythmias.
- Discuss the classification and management of bradyarrhythmias.

Introduction

Patients in the intensive care unit (ICU) are exposed to several physiologic stressors that may trigger cardiac arrhythmias and lead to hemodynamic instability. Prompt recognition and initiation of appropriate therapies for arrhythmias is important because critically ill patients with arrhythmias (compared to patients without arrhythmias) have longer hospitalizations and higher mortality (30.8% vs 21.2%).

The reported incidence of symptomatic and asymptomatic arrhythmias in critically ill patients ranges from 12% to 30%. A prevalence in ICU patients of 78% has been reported; however, this included a large percentage of patients with rhythms that are not associated with hemodynamic compromise (eg, ventricular extrasystoles and first-degree atrioventricular block).

Arrhythmias are classified as tachyarrhythmias or bradyarrhythmias. The most common sustained arrhythmias are supraventricular; atrial fibrillation is the most prevalent. Among the ventricular arrhythmias, up to 50% are monomorphic ventricular tachycardias.

Risk factors that contribute to the development of arrhythmias include male sex, older age, diabetes mellitus, hypertension, congestive heart failure, coronary artery disease, and valvular heart disease. In addition, metabolic derangements, myocardial ischemia, catecholamines, inflammatory cytokines, fever, medications, and hypoxemia are also important in the development of arrhythmias. Recognition of the 5 *H*'s and the 5 *T*'s of reversible causes of cardiac arrest may assist in the diagnosis and treatment of the underlying problem (Box 29.1).

Tachyarrhythmias

Classification

An understanding of the mechanism of a tachycardia often provides insight into the best methods for managing the arrhythmia. The 3 mechanisms for tachyarrhythmias are reentry, automaticity, and triggered.

Reentry, the most common mechanism, results from 2 separate parallel conduction pathways with different conduction and recovery properties (Figure 29.1). The trigger for reentry is usually a premature beat (premature atrial contraction or premature ventricular contraction) that blocks in the "fast" pathway and conducts down the "slow" pathway. When the electrical impulse reaches the distal junction of the 2 pathways, reentry is initiated if the fast pathway has recovered and the impulse can travel retrogradely. Examples of this type of reentrant arrhythmia include supraventricular tachycardias (SVTs) such as atrioventricular (AV) nodal reentrant tachycardia (AVNRT), AV reentrant tachycardia (AVRT), atrial flutter, and most ventricular tachycardias.

Automaticity involves rapid repetitive depolarization from a cell or group of cells. Examples of this type of mechanism include ectopic atrial tachycardia, junctional tachycardia, sinus tachycardia, multifocal atrial tachycardia (MAT), and some uncommon forms of ventricular tachycardia (VT) (which are named according to the site of the automatic focus and, in MAT, where the multiple foci are involved).

Box 29.1 • Reversible Causes of Cardiac Arrest

5 *H*s
- Hypoxemia
- Hypovolemia
- Hydrogen iron (acidosis)
- Hypokalemia or hyperkalemia
- Hypothermia

5 *T*s
- Tension pneumothorax
- Tamponade, cardiac
- Toxins
- Thrombosis, pulmonary
- Thrombosis, coronary

Data from Link MS, Berkow LC, Kudenchuk PJ, Halperin HR, Hess EP, Moitra VK, et al. Part 7: Adult Advanced Cardiovascular Life Support: 2015 American Heart Association guidelines update for cardiopulmonary resuscitation and emergency cardiovascular care. Circulation. 2015 Nov 3;132(18 Suppl 2):S444-64. Erratum in: Circulation. 2015 Dec 15;132(24):e385.

Triggered tachyarrhythmias arise from spontaneous depolarizations at the terminal portion of the action potential as a result of reactivation of sodium or calcium channels (the mechanism for torsades de pointes with prolonged QT intervals) or after complete depolarization of the cell (calcium overload due to digoxin toxicity).

Clinically, tachyarrhythmias are classified first according to the QRS conduction pattern on electrocardiography (ECG) and second according to the ECG characteristics of atrial activation (Figure 29.2). If the QRS complex is narrow, the ventricles are being activated normally through the AV node and bundle of His (called an SVT). In contrast, if the QRS complex is wide, the ventricles are being activated abnormally from an SVT with aberrant conduction through the His-Purkinje system or an anomalous accessory pathway or from a VT originating in ventricular tissue. Rapid identification of VT is critical because VT is associated with rapid hemodynamic compromise and usually portends a poor prognosis. Atrial activity may be difficult to assess because of large QRS complexes due to ventricular depolarization and large T waves due to repolarization.

Narrow–QRS Complex Tachycardias

Figure 29.3 illustrates the interpretation and management of tachycardias. SVTs can be subdivided into regular and irregular. Abnormal, irregular narrow-complex tachycardias include atrial fibrillation, MAT, and atrial flutter with variable conduction.

In atrial fibrillation, the atria are activated chaotically, and low-amplitude, irregular atrial activity (fibrillatory waves) is observed rather than discrete P waves. In MAT, the atria are activated from multiple sites of abnormal automaticity within the atria with at least 3 P-wave conduction patterns, different P-P and P-R intervals, and an atrial rate faster than 100 beats per minute.

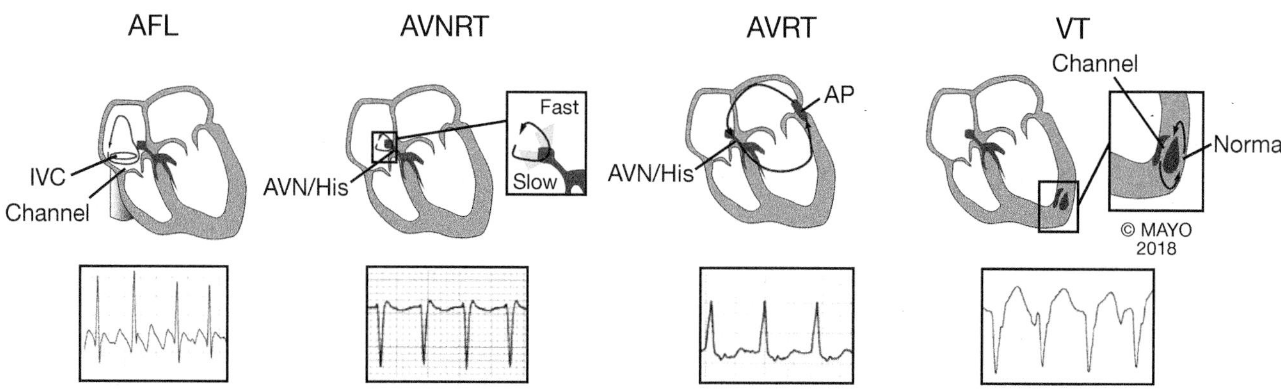

Figure 29.1. Reentry. Reentry is the most common mechanism for tachyarrhythmias in patients in the intensive care unit. Reentry mediates atrial flutter (AFL), atrioventricular (AV) nodal reentrant tachycardia (AVNRT), AV reentrant tachycardia (AVRT), and most forms of monomorphic ventricular tachycardia (VT). In reentry, 2 separate electrical pathways have different conduction properties (1 is faster; 1 is slower) and refractory periods. In AFL, the isthmus between the inferior vena cava (IVC) and the tricuspid valve forms 1 pathway, and the remainder of the right atrial tissue forms the other. In AVNRT, the 2 pathways ("fast" and "slow") are formed by separate inputs into the AV node (AVN). In AVRT, the 2 pathways are the AVN and bundle of His (AVN/His) and an accessory pathway (AP). In VT, the slowly conducting pathway is formed within a myocardial scar (generally after a myocardial infarction), and the other pathway is formed by the perimeter of normal ventricular tissue just outside the scar.

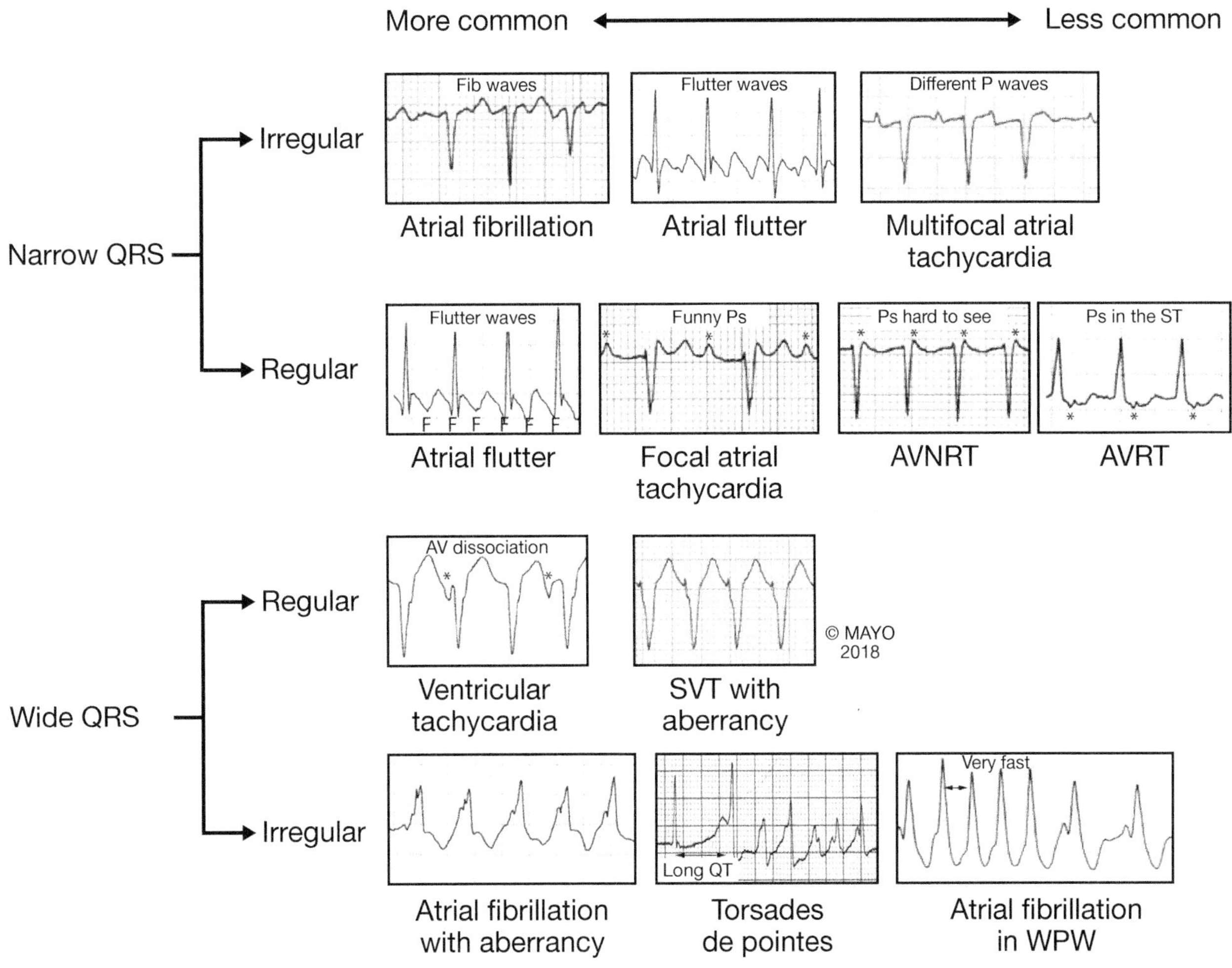

Figure 29.2. Identification of Tachyarrhythmias. Clinically, tachyarrhythmias are classified according to whether the QRS complex is narrow or wide. In a narrow–QRS complex tachycardia, the ventricles are activated normally by the His-Purkinje system; in a wide–QRS complex tachycardia, the ventricles are activated abnormally because the tachycardia is originating from ventricular tissue, the ventricles are being activated by an accessory pathway, or the His-Purkinje system is not conducting normally (aberrant conduction). Tachycardias are further categorized according to whether they are regular or irregular. The possible causes for regular wide–QRS complex tachycardias, irregular wide–QRS complex tachycardias, regular narrow–QRS complex tachycardias, and irregular narrow–QRS complex tachycardias are listed from most common to least common along with some electrocardiographic clues that can help with identification. Asterisks indicate P waves. AV indicates atrioventricular; AVNRT, atrioventricular nodal reentrant tachycardia; AVRT, atrioventricular reentrant tachycardia; Fib, fibrillary; SVT, supraventricular tachycardia; WPW, Wolff-Parkinson-White syndrome.

Atrial flutter is due to a single reentrant circuit within the atrium, and the ventricular rhythm can be regular or irregular depending on the conduction properties of the AV node. In typical atrial flutter, the ECG shows negative P waves (flutter waves) in the inferior leads II, III, and aVF because of a reentrant circuit that travels around the orifice of the tricuspid valve. Inferior-to-superior activation of the left atrium leads to the negative deflections in the inferior leads (II, III, and aVF) that have a characteristic sawtooth pattern. Less commonly, the reentrant circuit in atrial flutter does not circle around the tricuspid valve and the flutter waves may show almost any conduction pattern, depending on the general overall direction of atrial depolarization.

Regular narrow–QRS complex tachycardias include sinus tachycardia, ectopic focal atrial tachycardia, atrial flutter, AVNRT, AVRT, and automatic junctional tachycardia. The P-wave configuration and location are often helpful for distinguishing among these different possibilities (Figure

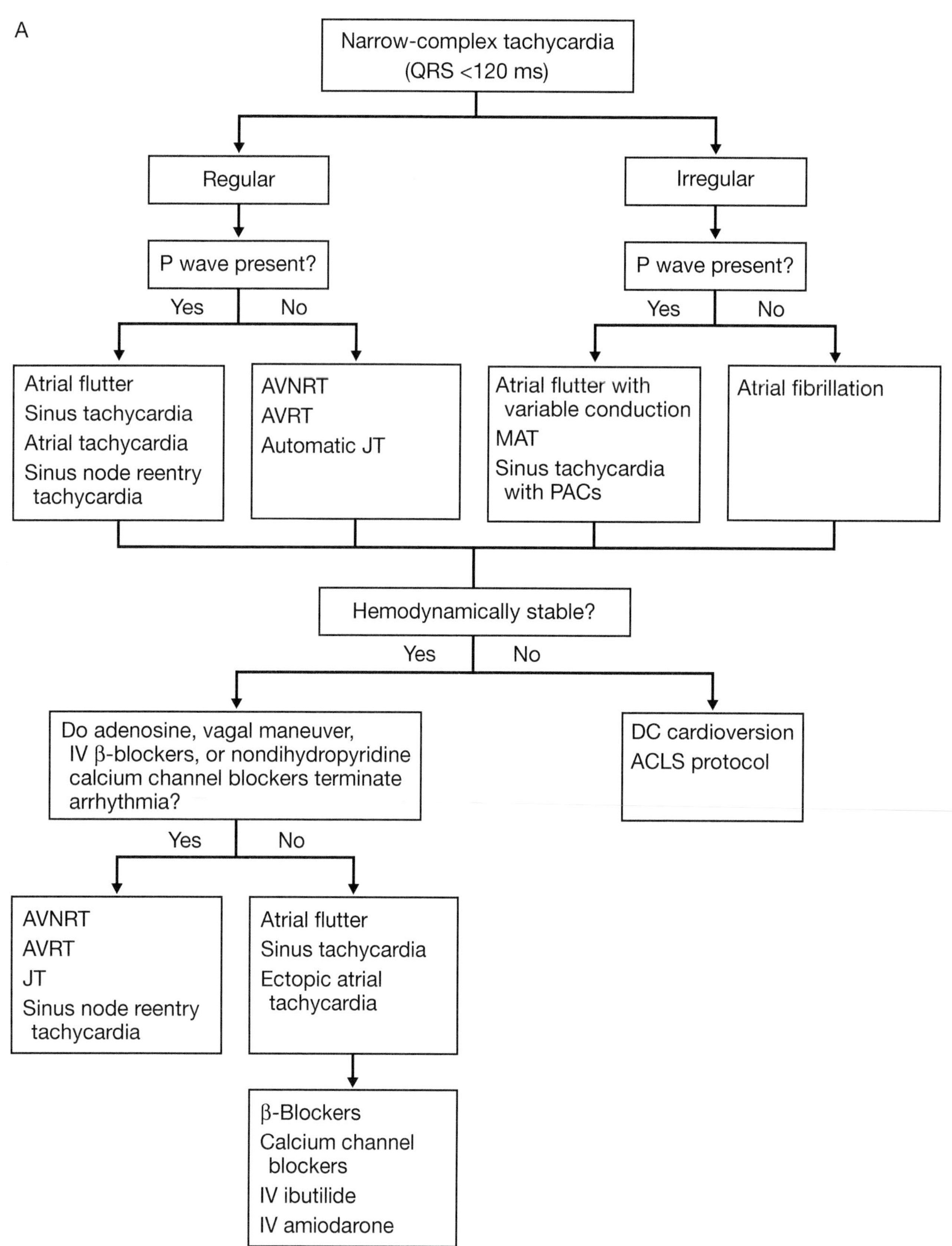

Figure 29.3. *Tachyarrhythmia Algorithm for Diagnosis and Management. A, Narrow-complex tachycardia. B, Wide-complex tachycardia. If a hemodynamically stable patient has VT and an implanted pacemaker or defibrillator, overdrive pacing may be tried. ACLS indicates Advanced Cardiac Life Support; AF, atrial fibrillation; AVNRT, atrioventricular nodal reentry tachycardia; AVRT, atrioventricular reentry tachycardia; BBB, bundle branch block; DC, direct current; IV, intravenous; JT, junctional tachycardia; MAT, multifocal atrial tachycardia; PAC, premature atrial contraction; SVT, supraventricular tachycardia; VF, ventricular fibrillation; VT, ventricular tachycardia.*

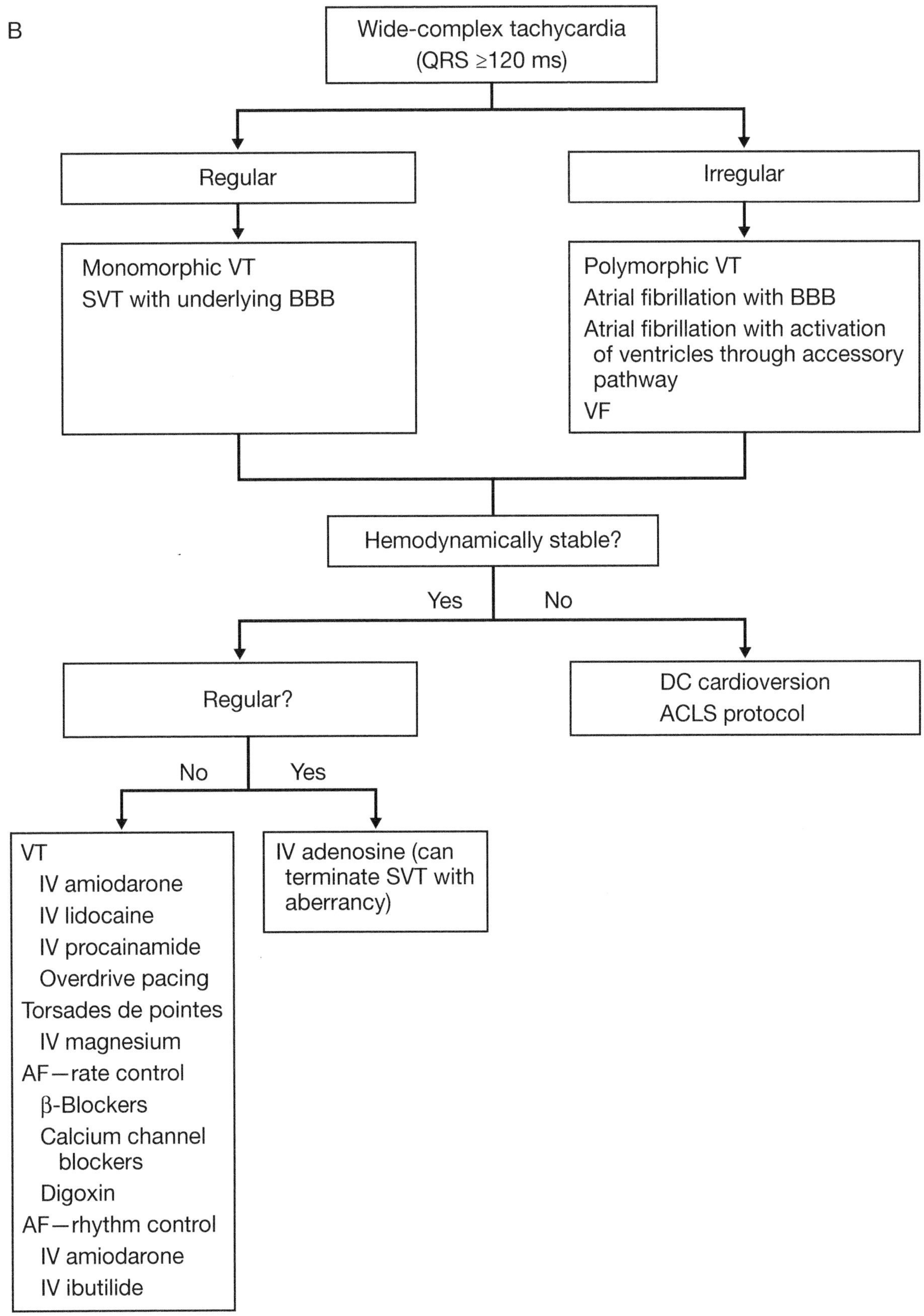

B

Wide-complex tachycardia
(QRS ≥120 ms)

Regular

Monomorphic VT
SVT with underlying BBB

Irregular

Polymorphic VT
Atrial fibrillation with BBB
Atrial fibrillation with activation of ventricles through accessory pathway
VF

Hemodynamically stable?

Yes

Regular?

No

VT
- IV amiodarone
- IV lidocaine
- IV procainamide
- Overdrive pacing

Torsades de pointes
- IV magnesium

AF—rate control
- β-Blockers
- Calcium channel blockers
- Digoxin

AF—rhythm control
- IV amiodarone
- IV ibutilide

Yes

IV adenosine (can terminate SVT with aberrancy)

No

DC cardioversion
ACLS protocol

Figure 29.3. Continued

29.2): 1) Tyically, a P wave in the usual location before the QRS complex is consistent with sinus tachycardia if the P wave has a normal configuration (negative in aVR and positive in lead II) or with ectopic focal atrial tachycardia if the P wave conduction pattern is atypical. 2) A P wave located in the ST segment is most likely observed with AVRT. 3) If the P waves cannot be identified (usually because they are obscured by the QRS complex), the arrhythmia focus may be in the region of the AV node (AVNRT or junctional tachycardia) with simultaneous activation of the atria and ventricles.

Management

Management of SVT depends on the hemodynamic stability of the patient. Rarely SVT causes hemodynamic instability, and affected patients should undergo synchronized electrical cardioversion (Figure 29.3). If patients have atrial fibrillation or atrial flutter, the risk of stroke must be considered as a result of cardioversion from atrial tissue stunning. A therapeutic and diagnostic approach for hemodynamically stable patients with regular narrow-complex SVT is the use of vagal maneuvers or adenosine. In general, intravenous adenosine terminates AV nodal–dependent pathways such as those in AVNRT, AVRT, and some focal atrial tachycardias. Adenosine can also help unmask atrial tachycardias and atrial flutter by blocking AV conduction but still allowing persistent atrial activity. If adenosine or vagal maneuvers do not terminate the tachycardia, regular and irregular SVTs are treated similarly with drugs (eg, β-blockers or nondihydropyridine calcium channel blockers) that block AV conduction and slow the ventricular rate.

For atrial flutter and atrial fibrillation, in the occasional patient where the goal of therapy is to promptly restore sinus rhythm, antiarrhythmic medications such as amiodarone and ibutilide can be considered. Ibutilide should be used cautiously, however, because it can prolong the QT interval, which may lead to polymorphic VT, especially if systolic function is decreased (left ventricular ejection fraction <30%) or if the QT interval is already prolonged.

Regardless of the type of SVT, any underlying conditions that might be contributing to the development of the arrhythmia must be treated. These conditions include hypoxia and other metabolic abnormalities, sepsis, endocrine abnormalities, and the use of medications such as exogenous catecholamines, β-agonist inhalers, or theophylline.

Wide–QRS Complex Tachycardias

When the QRS duration is 120 milliseconds or more, the arrhythmia is classified as wide QRS–complex tachycardia. Its origin can be either supraventricular (due to accompanying abnormal ventricular activation) or ventricular. VT is associated with the highest mortality in the ICU (73%). Sustained VT is defined as lasting longer than 30 seconds. In some instances, it is difficult to distinguish between VT

Box 29.2 • Some ECG Findings Suggestive of VT

AV dissociation—The ventricular rate is faster than the atrial rate. There is no relationship between the P wave and the QRS complex.

Fusion beats—A fusion beat (Figure 29.4A) results from the simultaneous firing of the ventricular foci and atrial foci that activate the ventricular conduction. A fusion beat is a hybrid between a normal QRS complex (originating in the supranodal region) and a wide QRS complex (originating from the ventricle).

Capture beats—A capture beat is a normal QRS complex that originates in the supranodal region and conducts down the bundle of His.

QRS complex width—With LBBB, the QRS duration is >160 ms; with RBBB, >140 ms.

QRS axis—The right superior axis is -90° to -180°, and the QRS complex is positive in the aVR lead.

Concordance—The QRS complex is all positive or all negative throughout the precordial leads (V_1 through V_6). A Q wave is present in the V_6 lead.

RS interval width—In precordial leads (V_1 through V_6), the RS interval is wide (>100 ms) (Figure 29.4B).

Abbreviations: AV atrioventricular; ECG, electrocardiographic; LBBB, left bundle branch block; RBBB, right bundle branch block; VT, ventricular tachycardia.

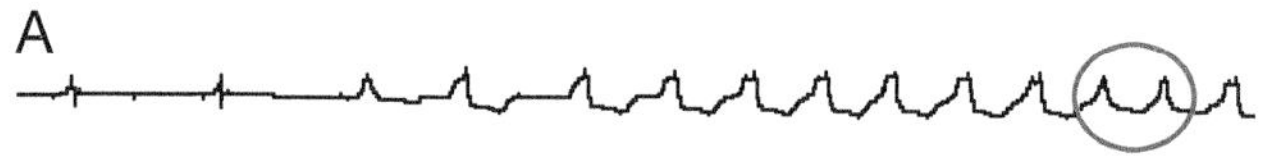

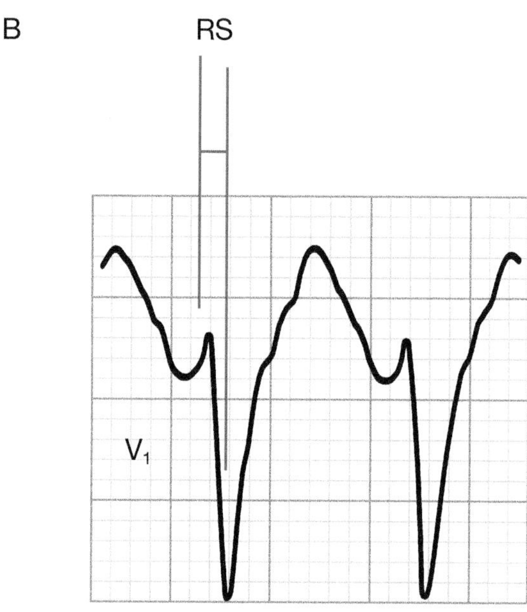

Figure 29.4. Electrocardiographic Features of Ventricular Tachycardia. A, Two fusion beats are circled. B, The RS interval is wide (>100 ms). See Box 29.2 for additional information.

and SVT with aberrant conduction. VT is more common in patients with heart disease, so a history of myocardial infarction, congestive heart failure, or recent angina has a high positive predictive value (>95%) for the diagnosis of VT. If a previous ECG is available, QRS conduction patterns that are similar during sinus rhythm and during tachycardia make SVT more likely; if the QRS complexes are different, VT is more likely. Box 29.2 and Figure 29.4 summarize ECG criteria that assist in the diagnosis of VT.

Management

The management of wide–QRS complex tachycardias depends on the hemodynamic stability of the patient (Figure 29.3). Hemodynamically unstable patients require immediate electrical cardioversion. Intravenous adenosine can be used for diagnosis and treatment of regular wide-complex arrhythmias in patients who are hemodynamically stable. Adenosine terminates AV node–dependent SVTs with aberrant ventricular conduction. In some patients with Wolff-Parkinson-White syndrome, atrial fibrillation develops with a rapid ventricular rate with conduction through either the accessory pathway or the AV His-Purkinje system. Blockade of the AV node by adenosine promotes conduction through the accessory pathway, resulting in polymorphic VT. The preferred treatment of these patients is intravenous ibutilide or procainamide.

In hemodynamically stable patients, the use of antiarrhythmics can be considered (eg, amiodarone, lidocaine, or procainamide). The use of procainamide requires caution because it may prolong the QT interval and cause hypotension; therefore, it may be a drug to avoid in the ICU. Amiodarone is the first-line medication for treatment of VT. Lidocaine may be effective in patients with underlying heart disease or ischemia. Antiarrhythmic medications are summarized in Table 29.1.

Bradyarrhythmias

Clinically significant bradyarrhythmias are uncommon in the ICU, occurring in approximately 2% to 10% of patients. *Bradycardia*, defined as a heart rate less than 60 beats per minute, can result from enhanced vagal tone, increased intracranial pressure, myocardial infarction, hypothermia, hypothyroidism, medications (eg, AV nodal blockers), intrinsic disease of the conduction system, sleep apnea, heart surgery, and electrolyte abnormalities. Sinus bradycardia may be physiologic and asymptomatic; in trained athletes, asymptomatic pauses up to 3 seconds have been observed. Bradycardia can result from sinus node dysfunction leading to sinus pauses or from AV block at the level of the AV node or at or below the bundle of His.

AV blocks are classified as first, second, or third degree. *First-degree AV block* occurs when the PR interval is longer than 200 milliseconds, but the relationship between the P wave and the QRS complex is constant. The 2 types of *second-degree AV block* are Mobitz type I and Mobitz type II. *Mobitz type I block* occurs when there is progressive prolongation of the PR interval before a nonconducted P wave. *Mobitz type II block* occurs when there is a constant PR interval before a nonconducted P wave. *Third-degree AV block* occurs when no P waves are conducted to the ventricle, resulting in no correlation between P waves and QRS complexes.

Bradycardia that results from myocardial ischemia seems to be mediated by different mechanisms, including increased vagal tone and decreased blood supply to the AV node especially when inferior wall ischemia involves the proximal right coronary artery. Bradycardia that occurs more than 24 hours after the inciting event is more likely related to myocardial edema. Advanced or complete heart block can also occur with extensive anterior myocardial ischemia or infarction. Complete heart block from myocardial ischemia is associated with increased mortality.

Postsurgical bradycardia occurs in patients who have undergone percutaneous or open heart cardiac surgery, especially if the procedure involved areas close to the AV node and if the patient had intrinsic conduction abnormalities before surgery. Pacemaker implantation has been reported as a cause of bradycardia (incidence, 2%-51%) in patients undergoing transcatheter aortic valve replacement; the most common culprit is complete heart block.

Management

Management depends on the symptoms and the extent of hemodynamic compromise. Treatment begins by identifying and addressing any reversible causes (eg, medications, electrolytes, or thyroid disease). Asymptomatic patients do not require specific treatment. If patients have ongoing symptoms, intravenous atropine is an appropriate initial therapy (0.5 mg bolus every 3-5 minutes for a maximum of 3 mg in 24 hours). If the patient has no response to atropine, or if the maximal dose has been reached, an infusion of dobutamine (2-10 mcg/kg/min) or epinephrine (2-10 mg/min) can be attempted. Temporary pacing through the transcutaneous or transvenous route may be required for patients who have no response to medications. Transcutaneous pacing is effective, but if continuous pacing for ventricular rate support is required for more than 30 minutes, placement of a temporary transvenous pacer is recommended. With sterile technique, temporary transvenous pacers are placed by way of the internal jugular vein, subclavian vein, or femoral vein with a balloon-tipped catheter that is positioned in the right ventricle.

Table 29.1 • Drugs and Their Potential Use for Tachyarrhythmias

Drug	Indications	Dosage	Adverse Effects
Metoprolol	Rate control in AF and AFL Treatment of AVNRT and AVRT	2.5-5 mg IV over 2-5 min (up to 15 mg in 15 min)	Bradycardia, AV block, hypotension, bronchospasm, fatigue, drowsiness, heart failure
Diltiazem	Rate control in AF and AFL Treatment of AVNRT and AVRT	0.25 mg/kg IV over 2 min; then 5-15 mg/h in IV drip	Hypotension, dizziness, headache, nausea, bradycardia, AV block, syncope, peripheral edema
Digoxin	Rate control in AF and AFL	0.25 mg IV every 2 h (up to 1.5 mg in 24 h)	Nausea, accelerated junctional rhythm, AV block
Esmolol	Rate control in AF and AFL	500 mcg/kg over 1 min; then 50 mcg/kg/min	Hypotension, dizziness, somnolence, headache, bronchospasm
Amiodarone	Rate control and termination and suppression of AF and AFL Treatment of VF and VT	150 mg/min over 10 min; then 1 mg/min for 6 h; then 0.5 mg/min for 18 h	Transaminitis, nausea, vomiting, constipation, anorexia, dermatologic reactions, tremor, neuropathy, abnormal gait, paresthesias, pulmonary fibrosis, hypotension, hypothyroidism, hyperthyroidism, corneal deposits, edema, flushing
Ibutilide	Termination of AF and AFL	Weight >60 kg: 1 mg over 10 min; repeat after 10 min as needed Weight <60 kg: 0.01 mg/kg	Headache, bradycardia, hypotension, palpitations, QT prolongation, torsades de pointes, heart failure, heart block, nausea
Procainamide	VT and preexcitation tachycardia	Loading dose: 15-17 mg/kg IV at 20-30 mg/min Maintenance dose: 1-4 mg/min	Hypotension, lupus, wide PR interval or QRS complex, asthenia, apraxia, depression, bone marrow suppression, nausea, myopathy, bitter taste, abdominal pain
Lidocaine	VT and VF due to ischemia	Loading dose: 1-1.5 mg/kg repeated in 5 min for a maximum of 3 mg/kg Maintenance dose: 1-4 mg/min	Dizziness, nausea, drowsiness, speech disturbance, perioral numbness, muscle twitching, psychosis, seizures, AV block, sinus arrest
Adenosine	Termination of SVT	If administered peripherally, 6-12 mg as a rapid bolus If administered centrally, 3-6 mg as a rapid bolus	Flushing, chest pain, dyspnea, headaches, light-headedness, jaw discomfort, bradycardia, bronchoconstriction, AV block, nonsustained ventricular arrhythmias
Magnesium	Torsades de pointes	2-g bolus; if arrhythmia persists, additional 2 g	Cardiovascular collapse, respiratory paralysis, hypothermia, pulmonary edema, depressed reflexes, hypotension, flushing, drowsiness, diaphoresis, hypocalcemia, hypophosphatemia, hyperkalemia, vision changes

Abbreviations: AF, atrial fibrillation; AFL, atrial flutter; AV, atrioventricular; AVNRT, atrioventricular nodal reentrant tachycardia; AVRT, atrioventricular reentrant tachycardia; IV, intravenously; SVT, supraventricular tachycardia; VF, ventricular fibrillation; VT, ventricular tachycardia.

Summary

- Arrhythmias are common in ICU patients; the most common are supraventricular, and atrial fibrillation is the most prevalent.
- Appropriate management of arrhythmias depends on the hemodynamic effects, the symptoms, and any predisposing conditions, which should be identified and corrected.
- For unstable tachyarrhythmias, electrical cardioversion is indicated.
- For unstable bradyarrhythmias, intravenous atropine is an appropriate initial therapy, but catecholamine infusions may be needed, and pacing may be required if a patient has no response to medications.

SUGGESTED READING

Annane D, Sebille V, Duboc D, Le Heuzey JY, Sadoul N, Bouvier E, et al. Incidence and prognosis of sustained arrhythmias in critically ill patients. Am J Respir Crit Care Med. 2008 Jul 1;178(1):20–5. Epub 2008 Apr 3.

Artucio H, Pereira M. Cardiac arrhythmias in critically ill patients: epidemiologic study. Crit Care Med. 1990 Dec;18(12):1383–8.

Badhwar N, Kusumoto F, Goldschlager N. Arrhythmias in the coronary care unit. J Intensive Care Med. 2012 Sep-Oct;27(5):267–89. Epub 2011 Jul 11.

Baerman JM, Morady F, DiCarlo LA Jr, de Buitleir M. Differentiation of ventricular tachycardia from supraventricular tachycardia with aberration: value of the clinical history. Ann Emerg Med. 1987 Jan;16(1):40–3.

Benjamin EJ, Levy D, Vaziri SM, D'Agostino RB, Belanger AJ, Wolf PA. Independent risk factors for atrial fibrillation in a population-based cohort: The Framingham Heart Study. JAMA. 1994 Mar 16;271(11):840–4.

Bieganowska K, Rekawek J, Szumowski L, Szymaniak E, Brzezinska-Paszke M, Miszczak-Knecht M, et al. [Morgagni-Adams-Stokes after adenosine injection in a patient with WPW syndrome: a case report]. Kardiol Pol. 2006 Dec;64(12):1453–7. Polish.

Blomstrom-Lundqvist C, Scheinman MM, Aliot EM, Alpert JS, Calkins H, Camm AJ, et al; European Society of Cardiology Committee, NASPE-Heart Rhythm Society. ACC/AHA/ESC guidelines for the management of patients with supraventricular arrhythmias: executive summary: a report of the American college of cardiology/American Heart Association task force on practice guidelines and the European Society of Cardiology committee for practice guidelines (writing committee to develop guidelines for the management of patients with supraventricular arrhythmias) developed in collaboration with NASPE-Heart Rhythm Society. J Am Coll Cardiol. 2003 Oct 15;42(8):1493–531.

Butta C, Tuttolomondo A, Di Raimondo D, Milio G, Miceli S, Attanzio MT, et al. Supraventricular tachycardias: proposal of a diagnostic algorithm for the narrow complex tachycardias. J Cardiol. 2013 Apr;61(4):247–55. Epub 2013 Mar 6.

Fleisher LA, Fleischmann KE, Auerbach AD, Barnason SA, Beckman JA, Bozkurt B, et al. 2014 ACC/AHA guideline on perioperative cardiovascular evaluation and management of patients undergoing noncardiac surgery: a report of the American College of Cardiology/American Heart Association Task Force on Practice Guidelines. Circulation. 2014 Dec 9;130(24):e278–333. Epub 2014 Aug 1.

Goldberg RJ, Zevallos JC, Yarzebski J, Alpert JS, Gore JM, Chen Z, et al. Prognosis of acute myocardial infarction complicated by complete heart block (the Worcester Heart Attack Study). Am J Cardiol. 1992 May 1;69(14):1135–41.

Goldstein JA, Lee DT, Pica MC, Dixon SR, O'Neill WW. Patterns of coronary compromise leading to bradyarrhythmias and hypotension in inferior myocardial infarction. Coron Artery Dis. 2005 Aug;16(5):265–74.

Goodman S, Shirov T, Weissman C. Supraventricular arrhythmias in intensive care unit patients: short and long-term consequences. Anesth Analg. 2007 Apr;104(4):880–6.

Griffith MJ, Linker NJ, Ward DE, Camm AJ. Adenosine in the diagnosis of broad complex tachycardia. Lancet. 1988 Mar 26;1(8587):672–5.

Harg P, Madsen S, Amlie JP. [Severe ibutilide-induced arrhythmia in patients with heart failure]. Tidsskr Nor Laegeforen. 2001 Oct 10;121(24):2834–5. Norwegian.

January CT, Wann LS, Alpert JS, Calkins H, Cigarroa JE, Cleveland JC Jr, et al; ACC/AHA Task Force Members. 2014 AHA/ACC/HRS guideline for the management of patients with atrial fibrillation: executive summary: a report of the American College of Cardiology/American Heart Association Task Force on practice guidelines and the Heart Rhythm Society. Circulation. 2014 Dec 2;130(23):2071–104. Epub 2014 Mar 28. Erratum in: Circulation. 2014 Dec 2;130(23):e270–1.

Jordaens LJ, Theuns DAMJ. Implantable cardioverter defibrillator stored ECGs: clinical management and case reports. London (UK): Springer-Verlag; c2007. 193 p.

Kafkas NV, Patsilinakos SP, Mertzanos GA, Papageorgiou KI, Chaveles JI, Dagadaki OK, et al. Conversion efficacy of intravenous ibutilide compared with intravenous amiodarone in patients with recent-onset atrial fibrillation and atrial flutter. Int J Cardiol. 2007 Jun 12;118(3):321–5. Epub 2006 Oct 17.

Kennelly C, Esaian D. Drug-induced cardiovascular adverse events in the intensive care unit. Crit Care Nurs Q. 2013 Oct-Dec;36(4):323–34.

Kobayashi Y. How to manage various arrhythmias and sudden cardiac death in the cardiovascular intensive care. J Intensive Care. 2018 Apr 11;6:23. Erratum in: J Intensive Care. 2018 May 24;6:31.

Komura S, Chinushi M, Furushima H, Hosaka Y, Izumi D, Iijima K, et al. Efficacy of procainamide and lidocaine in terminating sustained monomorphic ventricular tachycardia. Circ J. 2010 May;74(5):864–9. Epub 2010 Mar 26.

Kuipers S, Klein Klouwenberg PM, Cremer OL. Incidence, risk factors and outcomes of new-onset atrial fibrillation in patients with sepsis: a systematic review. Crit Care. 2014 Dec 15;18(6):688.

Neumar RW, Otto CW, Link MS, Kronick SL, Shuster M, Callaway CW, et al. Part 8: adult advanced cardiovascular life support: 2010 American Heart Association Guidelines for Cardiopulmonary Resuscitation and Emergency Cardiovascular Care. Circulation. 2010 Nov 2;122(18 Suppl 3):S729–67. Errata in: Circulation. 2011 Feb 15;123(6):e236. Circulation. 2013 Dec 24;128(25):e480.

Page RL, Joglar JA, Caldwell MA, Calkins H, Conti JB, Deal BJ, et al; Evidence Review Committee Chair. 2015 ACC/AHA/HRS guideline for the management of adult patients with supraventricular tachycardia: executive summary: a report of the American College of Cardiology/American Heart Association task force on clinical practice guidelines and the Heart Rhythm Society. Circulation. 2016 Apr 5;133(14):e471–505. Epub 2015 Sep 23. Erratum in: Circulation. 2016 Sep 13;134(11):e232–3.

Pedersen CT, Kay GN, Kalman J, Borggrefe M, Della-Bella P, Dickfeld T, et al; EP-Europace, UK. EHRA/HRS/APHRS expert consensus on ventricular arrhythmias. Heart Rhythm. 2014 Oct;11(10):e166–96. Epub 2014 Aug 30.

Rankin AC, Oldroyd KG, Chong E, Rae AP, Cobbe SM. Value and limitations of adenosine in the diagnosis and treatment of narrow and broad complex tachycardias. Br Heart J. 1989 Sep;62(3):195–203.

Reinelt P, Karth GD, Geppert A, Heinz G. Incidence and type of cardiac arrhythmias in critically ill patients: a

single center experience in a medical-cardiological ICU. Intensive Care Med. 2001 Sep;27(9):1466–73.
Reising S, Kusumoto F, Goldschlager N. Life-threatening arrhythmias in the intensive care unit. J Intensive Care Med. 2007 Jan-Feb;22(1):3–13.
Shine KI, Kastor JA, Yurchak PM. Multifocal atrial tachycardia: clinical and electrocardiographic features in 32 patients. N Engl J Med. 1968 Aug 15;279(7):344–9.
Siontis GC, Juni P, Pilgrim T, Stortecky S, Bullesfeld L, Meier B, et al. Predictors of permanent pacemaker implantation in patients with severe aortic stenosis undergoing TAVR: a meta-analysis. J Am Coll Cardiol. 2014 Jul 15;64(2):129–40.
Tak T, Berkseth L, Malzer R. A case of supraventricular tachycardia associated with Wolff-Parkinson-White syndrome and pregnancy. WMJ. 2012 Oct;111(5): 228–32.
Talan DA, Bauernfeind RA, Ashley WW, Kanakis C Jr, Rosen KM. Twenty-four hour continuous ECG recordings in long-distance runners. Chest. 1982 Jul;82(1):19–24.
Tracy C, Boushahri A. Managing arrhythmias in the intensive care unit. Crit Care Clin. 2014 Jul;30(3):365–90.
Valderrabano RJ, Blanco A, Santiago-Rodriguez EJ, Miranda C, Rivera-Del Rio Del Rio J, Ruiz J, et al. Risk factors and clinical outcomes of arrhythmias in the medical intensive care unit. J Intensive Care. 2016 Jan 22;4:9.

30 Hypertensive Emergencies

DENZIL R. HILL, MD; JAMES A. ONIGKEIT, MD

Goals

- Define *hypertension* and *hypertensive emergency*.
- Discuss clinical presentation and assessment of a patient with a possible hypertensive crisis.
- Discuss treatment and potential pitfalls of hypertension management.
- Review the pertinent antihypertensives and their related pharmacology.

Introduction

Hypertension is a global problem. According to the World Heart Federation, nearly 1 billion people worldwide have hypertension, and nearly two-thirds of them live in developing countries. By the year 2025, hypertension may affect more than 1.5 billion people. Uncontrolled hypertension is 1 of the main causes of premature death worldwide and the most common risk factor for heart disease, stroke, and renal diseases.

Hypertensive emergencies span a wide continuum of clinical presentations that can lead to progressive problems or, more seriously, end-organ dysfunction. In these situations, the patient's blood pressure (BP) should be decreased aggressively, generally within minutes to hours. Initially, the ability to recognize specific signs and symptoms can be difficult. Patients can present with or without a history of preexistent chronic hypertension. Historically, a diastolic BP (DBP) greater than 120 mm Hg or a systolic BP (SBP) greater than 180 mm Hg has been considered a hypertensive emergency. However, no specific thresholds exist because patients with previously normal BP can easily enter an emergency BP state after a sudden increase in their BP. Problems related to neurologic, cardiovascular, pulmonary, or renal end-organ damage are the most likely to occur and generally are the most critical to the patient's survival.

History and Physical Examination

The history and physical examination findings can be used to help determine the severity of the illness and to identify opportunities for management that will decrease the BP to a more acceptable range. The patient's hypertensive history and previous BP measurements should be identified along with any history of cardiac and renal disease. The patient should be asked about use of nonprescribed and prescribed medications and use of recreational drugs. The BP should be measured in both arms with appropriately sized cuffs.

Most patients with hypertension present with cerebral infarction (25% of patients), pulmonary edema (22%), posterior reversible encephalopathy syndrome (PRES) (16%), or congestive heart failure (12%). Patients may also present with aortic dissection, renal failure, intracranial hemorrhage, myocardial infarction, or eclampsia.

The clinical manifestations of hypertensive emergencies are generally related to end-organ damage (Box 30.1). Organ dysfunction rarely occurs with a DBP less than 120 mm Hg (except in children and some pregnant women). However, the specific DBP or SBP may be less important than the change or degree of increase. For instance, a patient with chronic hypertension may remain asymptomatic with an SBP greater than 180 mm Hg or a DBP greater than 120 mm Hg, whereas a pregnant woman may become symptomatic with a DBP greater than 95 mm Hg.

Signs and Symptoms

Patients with a hypertensive crisis can present with various symptoms and clinical signs. PRES may cause a headache with an altered level of mentation with or without findings consistent with focal neurologic deficits. Nausea and vomiting may be present, especially if intracranial pressure is increased. Papilledema is a predominant finding, but patients may also have evidence of retinopathy,

Box 30.1 • Clinical Manifestations of Hypertensive Emergencies

Eclampsia
Posterior reversible encephalopathy syndrome (PRES)
Aortic aneurysm
Acute myocardial infarction
Acute left ventricular failure
Pulmonary edema
Acute kidney injury
Hemolytic anemia

exudates, and hemorrhage on physical examination. Dyspnea on exertion and with rest can be associated with progressing pulmonary edema. The kidneys are almost always affected, and patients may present with oliguria or hematuria (or both) because of acute kidney injury.

When the cardiovascular system is affected, patients may present with angina, acute left ventricular failure, and acute myocardial infarction. In addition to these findings, the possibility of aortic dissection and its associated complications must be considered if a patient presents with acute chest pain and elevated BP. In the United States, the reported incidence of aortic dissection is 2,000 cases annually, and in Europe, 3,000 cases annually. Nearly 75% of patients with an untreated type A dissection die within 2 weeks. However, rapid and successful treatment greatly improves the 5-year survival rate. Therefore, making an accurate and timely diagnosis and applying the appropriate management techniques are essential for disease control and long-term survival. The aim of treatment is not only to lower the BP but also to decrease the velocity of left ventricular ejection, thereby halting the propagation of the dissection and decreasing the sheer stress on the aorta.

Diagnostic Evaluation and Workup

After an adequate history with an appropriate physical examination, several laboratory evaluations and diagnostic procedures should be performed to further assess the patient with a hypertensive emergency (Box 30.2). These studies are used to evaluate end-organ involvement and other potential complications that can occur with elevated BP. The kidneys are particularly susceptible to pressure fluctuations, but close attention should be given to the cardiovascular system and the strain on the heart and potential ischemia from increased work. The complete blood cell count can be helpful because some patients are at risk for hemolysis.

Treatment and Management

Most patients who present with elevated BP (ie, with a DBP about 110 mm Hg) do not show signs of end-organ damage because autoregulation maintains adequate blood flow and BP to the organ itself. These patients are in a state of *hypertensive urgency* (rather than hypertensive emergency) and generally do not require intravenous antihypertensives; instead, oral medications given in a controlled manner should gradually decrease the patient's BP over the subsequent 24 to 48 hours.

Patients who present with a true hypertensive emergency should be admitted to the intensive care unit and monitored closely (eg, with arterial line BP monitoring and telemetry) because precipitous or uncontrolled decreases in BP may be fatal. Such a decrease can occur with an upward shift from normal baseline in the autoregulation curve, most often affecting the brain, heart, and kidneys. The goal of treatment should be to decrease the mean arterial BP by 15% to 20% within 1 hour. The purpose is to stop end-organ damage quickly and safely while avoiding a more sudden decrease in BP, which has been shown to cause organ ischemia. After this primary goal has been achieved, the next goal is to adequately control the BP. Several types of medications can be used to decrease and control BP (Box 30.3).

BP Goals in Acute Brain Injury

Acute brain injury can complicate a treatment plan, especially for patients with a hypertensive crisis. Although much effort has been directed toward defining and delineating optimal BP parameters for patients with intracerebral hemorrhage, the optimal approach to management is still unknown. The data are conflicting, but they do suggest that certain pitfalls should be avoided. Specifically,

Box 30.2 • Diagnostic Evaluation of Patients With a Hypertensive Emergency

Blood tests
- Complete blood cell count
- Electrolytes
- Serum urea nitrogen and creatinine
- Cardiac enzymes (if acute coronary syndrome is a possibility)

Urinalysis
Electrocardiography
Imaging
- Chest radiography
- Computed tomography (CT) or magnetic resonance imaging of the brain
- Contrast CT of the chest or transesophageal echocardiography

Box 30.3 • Medications for Decreasing and Controlling Blood Pressure[a]

β-Blockers

Esmolol—An ultra-short-acting medication that is an ideal β-blocker for critically ill patients because of its pharmacokinetic properties.

Dose: loading dose 500 mcg/kg (infuse over 1 minute); titrate up to 300 mcg/kg/min

Onset: <1 minute

Duration: 10-30 minutes

Labetalol—Combined α_1-blocker and nonselective β-blocker (β-blockade is greater than α_1-blockade); because of its pharmacokinetics, the heart rate is maintained or slightly decreased; generally maintains cardiac output (unlike a pure β-blockade).

Dose: 10-20 mg every 10 minutes; infusion is rarely used

Onset: 2-5 minutes; peak at 5-15 minutes

Duration: 2-4 hours (variable)

Metoprolol—Selective β-blocker (β_1) that is a competitive inhibitor at the β_1-receptor site, with minimal or no interaction at the β_2-receptor site.

Dose: 5 mg every 3 minutes

Onset: 5-10 minutes

Duration: 5-8 hours

Propranolol—Nonselective β-blockade with complete block of β_1- and β_2-receptors, resulting in decreased heart rate, cardiac contractility, and blood pressure; decreases portal pressure through splanchnic vasoconstriction; not generally used for hypertensive emergency.

Dose: 1-3 mg every 2-5 minutes (maximum, 5 mg)

Onset: 5 minutes

Duration: 6-12 hours

Calcium channel blockers—Mainly impede the influx of calcium through L-type calcium channels in the vascular smooth muscle, decreasing the systemic vascular resistance through induced arteriolar dilatation.

Nicardipine—A second-generation dihydropyridine calcium channel blocker with high affinity toward vascular channels and good coronary and cerebral vasodilatory activity; it is much more water soluble than nifedipine, which makes it an excellent choice for an intravenous medication that can be titrated.

Dose: 5 mg/h initially, increasing by 2.5 mg/h every 5 minutes (maximum, 30 mg/h)

Onset: 5-10 minutes; peak at 30 minutes

Duration: 4-6 hours

Clevidipine—Another dihydropyridine calcium channel blocker similar to nicardipine; it is 99% protein bound and undergoes rapid hydrolysis (primarily by esterases in blood and extravascular tissues) to an inactive carboxylic acid metabolite and formaldehyde.

Dose: 1-2 mg/h; dose may be doubled every 2 minutes until blood pressure is near goal and then adjusted by less than double every 10-15 minutes (maximum, 32 mg/h); when dose is changed by 1-2 mg, blood pressure should change by 2-4 mm Hg

Onset: 1-2 minutes; peak at 3 minutes

Duration: 4-6 hours

Diltiazem—A nondihydropyridine calcium channel blocker that inhibits calcium from entering select voltage-sensitive areas of vascular smooth muscle and myocardium during depolarization; the result is relaxation of coronary vascular smooth muscle in conjunction with coronary vasodilatation; traditionally *not* used for control of hypertensive emergencies.

Dose: bolus 0.25 mg/kg over 2 minutes; then titrate 5-15 mg/h (maximum, 15 mg/h)

Onset: 2-7 minutes; peak at 7-10 minutes

Duration: 1-10 hours (variable)

Vasodilators

Hydralazine—A direct-acting arteriole vasodilator that should be *avoided* in hypertensive emergencies because of its variable duration of action and unpredictable effects; its antihypertensive effects are difficult to titrate.

Dose: bolus 10-20 mg every 4-6 hours (maximum, 40-mg bolus)

Onset: 5-20 minutes; peak at 30-60 minutes

Duration: up to 12 hours (duration of hypotension has been much longer in some patients)

Nitroprusside[b]—An arteriole and venous vasodilator that decreases both afterload and preload; it decreases cerebral blood flow but increases intracranial pressure, which can be detrimental in a patient with posterior reversible encephalopathy syndrome (PRES) or cerebrovascular accident.

Dose: 0.3-0.5 mcg/kg/min (bolus not recommended because onset is rapid); dose is titrated every 2-3 minutes (maximum, 10 mcg/kg/min)

Onset: 60-120 seconds; peak at 15 minutes

Duration: 1-10 minutes

Nitroglycerin—A potent venodilator that can cause arterial dilatation at high doses; blood pressure is decreased by decreasing preload and cardiac output, which can be detrimental if cerebral or renal perfusion is already compromised.

Dose: 5 mcg/min (bolus not recommended), titrated every 3-5 minutes in 5-mcg increments up to 20 mcg/min; then increase in increments of 10-20 mcg/min (maximum, 300-400 mcg/min)

Onset: 1-2 minutes; peak at 5 minutes

Duration: 5-10 minutes

[a] All doses are for intravenous administration.

[b] Cyanide is released from nitroprusside (the amount depends on the dose administered), and cyanide toxicity is a concern whenever this drug is used. Cyanide removal requires adequate liver and renal function.

in the Antihypertensive Treatment of Acute Cerebral Hemorrhage II (ATACH-2) trial and the second Intensive Blood Pressure Reduction in Acute Cerebral Hemorrhage Trial (INTERACT2), SBP less than 130 mm Hg was potentially harmful and associated with a worse outcome. An SBP goal of 135 to 165 mm Hg appears to be reasonable but is not considered the gold standard.

Defining a specific range for BP, however, addresses only a part of appropriate management. Evidence points to the risks of allowing large fluctuations in BP in patients with acute brain injury. Rapid or extreme decreases in BP should be avoided. A steady BP should be maintained because large increases or decreases tend to be associated with poorer outcomes.

Prognosis and Extended Management

Oral antihypertensives act more slowly than their intravenous counterparts, so they are not used for immediate treatment. However, their use becomes paramount after patients are discharged from the intensive care unit. Follow-up with a primary care specialist is essential for a patient's long-term survival and for management of end-organ damage that may have occurred. Depending on a patient's comorbid conditions, initial management with oral medications is usually with an angiotensin-converting enzyme inhibitor or a calcium channel blocker.

Patients' adherence to medical therapy can vary, which makes a medication such as clonidine a less popular choice because it has to be taken several times daily to be effective, and complications arise if a patient suddenly stops taking it.

Summary

- Patients who present with a hypertensive emergency may require an immediate decrease in their BP to prevent serious end-organ damage or a major cardiac event.
- Admission to the intensive care unit is warranted for BP monitoring and use of intravenous antihypertensives to control BP.
- Evaluation and diagnosis should be efficient and prompt to maximize the treatment potential and minimize the amount of time in crisis.
- The physical examination can be helpful in determining the seriousness of the hypertensive emergency and in guiding the need to focus on a particular organ system while lowering the patient's BP.
- Many antihypertensives are available, but certain indications and adverse effects should be considered.
- A titratable intravenous medication that has a short duration (eg, esmolol or nitroglycerin) is recommended if there are no outstanding contraindications. Nicardipine and clevidipine produce an adequate response with limited adverse effects. The use of hydralazine and nitroprusside should be avoided in the management of hypertensive emergency because of their potential adverse effects.

SUGGESTED READING

Abrams JH, Schulman P, White WB. Successful treatment of a monoamine oxidase inhibitor-tyramine hypertensive emergency with intravenous labetalol. N Engl J Med. 1985 Jul 4;313(1):52.

Jacobs M. Mechanism of action of hydralazine on vascular smooth muscle. Biochem Pharmacol. 1984 Sep 15;33(18):2915–9.

Katz JN, Gore JM, Amin A, Anderson FA, Dasta JF, Ferguson JJ, et al; STAT Investigators. Practice patterns, outcomes, and end-organ dysfunction for patients with acute severe hypertension: the Studying the Treatment of Acute hyperTension (STAT) registry. Am Heart J. 2009 Oct;158(4):599–606.e1.

Mayer SA, Kurtz P, Wyman A, Sung GY, Multz AS, Varon J, et al; STAT Investigators. Clinical practices, complications, and mortality in neurological patients with acute severe hypertension: the Studying the Treatment of Acute hyperTension registry. Crit Care Med. 2011 Oct;39(10):2330–6.

Rabinstein AA. Optimal blood pressure after intracerebral hemorrhage: still a moving target. Stroke. 2018 Feb;49(2):275–6. Epub 2018 Jan 4.

Rodriguez MA, Kumar SK, De Caro M. Hypertensive crisis. Cardiol Rev. 2010 Mar-Apr;18(2):102–7.

Salgado DR, Silva E, Vincent JL. Control of hypertension in the critically ill: a pathophysiological approach. Ann Intensive Care. 2013 Jun 27;3(1):17.

van den Born BH, Lip GYH, Brguljan-Hitij J, Cremer A, Segura J, Morales E, et al. ESC Council on hypertension position document on the management of hypertensive emergencies. Eur Heart J Cardiovasc Pharmacother. 2019 Jan 1;5(1):37–46. Erratum in: Eur Heart J Cardiovasc Pharmacother. 2019 Jan 1;5(1):46.

Varon J, Marik PE. Clinical review: the management of hypertensive crises. Crit Care. 2003 Oct;7(5):374–84. Epub 2003 Jul 16.

Vaughan CJ, Delanty N. Hypertensive emergencies. Lancet. 2000 Jul 29;356(9227):411–7.

Watson K, Broscious R, Devabhakthuni S, Noel ZR. Focused update on pharmacologic management of hypertensive emergencies. Curr Hypertens Rep. 2018 Jun 8;20(7):56.

31 Cardiopulmonary Resuscitation

RICHARD K. PATCH III, MD

Goals

- Describe the thoracic pump mechanism during chest compression for cardiac arrest.
- Identify the core management principles for cardiac arrest.
- Recognize the postresuscitation management measures.

Introduction

Cardiac arrest is a complex dynamic process that may occur as an end point of multiple disease states. The field of cardiopulmonary resuscitation (CPR) for cardiac arrest continues to evolve, and guidelines are updated in accordance with evidence-based evaluation of current medical literature. The American Heart Association (AHA) Guidelines for CPR and Emergency Cardiovascular Care (ECC) incorporate the most recent evidence about basic life support, advanced cardiovascular life support (ACLS), and postarrest care (https://eccguidelines.heart.org/index.php/circulation/cpr-ecc-guidelines-2/). The guidelines are the cornerstone for the management of cardiac arrest in out-of-hospital, in-hospital, and intraoperative settings. Furthermore, the implementation of comprehensive postarrest care is vital for improving patient outcomes.

Epidemiology

In 2011, out-of-hospital cardiac arrest (OHCA) occurred in 326,000 people; each year, in-hospital cardiac arrest (IHCA) occurs in 209,000 patients. Ventricular fibrillation (VF) or pulseless ventricular tachycardia (VT) accounts for 25% of OHCAs, and the other OHCAs are attributed to pulseless electrical activity (PEA) or asystole. The overall survival rate after OHCA is low (8% in North America); the estimated survival rate after IHCA is 17%. Only 10% of patients with return of spontaneous circulation (ROSC) survive to hospital discharge. Among patients with an OHCA, anoxic brain injury is the most common cause of death, and multiorgan failure is the most common cause of death among patients with an IHCA.

Physiology

Cardiac arrest is the cessation of mechanical cardiac activity and is confirmed by the lack of signs of systemic circulation. CPR provides 1) artificial circulation through chest compressions and vasoactive medications to provide blood flow to the heart and brain and 2) electrical therapy to terminate unstable tachyarrhythmias. Chest compressions provide artificial circulation by 2 mechanisms that function simultaneously: the cardiac pump and the thoracic pump.

With the cardiac pump mechanism, when the heart is compressed between the sternum and vertebral column, intraventricular gradients are generated that allow closure of the tricuspid and mitral valves with opening of the pulmonic and aortic valves so that blood is expelled into the systemic circulation. Chest decompression decreases the pressure within the ventricles, allowing the tricuspid and mitral valves to open and blood to be drawn into the ventricles.

With the thoracic pump mechanism, chest compression increases intrathoracic venous pressure compared with the extrathoracic venous pressure. Retrograde pressure and flow within the venous system is limited by venous valves, driving blood into the systemic circulation. Intracranial pressure also fluctuates during CPR.

Core Management Principles

High-quality chest compressions, the cornerstone of CPR, are associated with better survival and neurologic outcomes. Because any delay in the initiation of CPR negates those benefits, the traditional sequence of airway, breathing, and circulation (ABC) is no longer advocated. Instead, the sequence of circulation, airway, and breathing (CAB) is now the starting point in all forms of cardiac arrest.

Chest Compressions

Chest compressions for providing artificial circulation should be performed as described by the AHA—"Push hard, push fast"—with a depth of 2 inches for each compression and at least 100 compressions per minute. Between each compression, the chest must be allowed to fully recoil because any impedance will prevent the full cardiac output from reaching the systemic circulation. Compressors should rotate every 2 minutes to minimize fatigue. Mechanical devices can provide continuous chest compressions; however, data do not show that they provide any benefit over high-quality manual chest compressions. Interruptions of chest compressions (for pulse checks or placement of an endotracheal tube) need to be minimized with no more than 10-second pauses between 2-minute cycles of chest compressions.

Defibrillation

Delivery of immediate electrical shock therapy to patients with VF or pulseless VT is paramount because delays in defibrillation are associated with decreased survival. Defibrillation depolarizes the heart and prolongs the refractory period, terminating the original arrhythmia. The recommended energy delivered depends on the type of defibrillator: for a biphasic system, 120 to 200 J, and for a monophasic system, 360 J.

Airway and Ventilation

Placement of an advanced airway device is no longer considered a priority in the current ACLS guidelines. Rather, bag-valve-mask ventilation, with a 30:2 ratio of compressions to breaths delivered, is preferred because it can be performed without interrupting chest compressions. If an advanced airway device is required, it should be placed by an experienced provider, and placement should coincide with the pulse check after a 2-minutes cycle and interrupt compressions for no more than 10 seconds. When the advanced airway device is secured, 1 breath should be delivered every 6 seconds. Hyperventilation should be avoided so that increased intrathoracic pressure does not decrease venous return and subsequent cardiac output.

Physiologic Monitoring During CPR

During CPR, the end-tidal carbon dioxide ($ETCO_2$) levels should be monitored given their relationship to cardiac output and pulmonary blood flow. Levels may be less than 10 mm Hg initially, but they will increase steadily with high-quality compressions. An abrupt increase in $ETCO_2$ suggests ROSC, while a gradual decrease suggests that the compressor may be getting fatigued. $ETCO_2$ levels are also useful for prognostication: at 20 minutes of CPR, patients with $ETCO_2$ greater than 20 mm Hg have a higher chance of ROSC, while patients with $ETCO_2$ levels less than 10 mm Hg have almost no chance of ROSC. Respiratory arrest or cardiac arrest due to pulmonary embolism may confound $ETCO_2$ monitoring. High doses of epinephrine administered during an arrest will transiently decrease $ETCO_2$ because the vasoconstrictor effect increases blood pressure and decreases cardiac output. In addition, if bicarbonate is administered during resuscitation, a profound increase in $ETCO_2$ may occur and mimic ROSC.

Coronary perfusion pressure greater than 15 mm Hg during CPR is associated with ROSC. However, unless invasive monitoring is already being performed, coronary perfusion pressure is difficult to measure during CPR. Measurement of arterial relaxation or diastolic pressure, if available with invasive arterial pressure monitoring, is an alternative. Diastolic pressures greater than 20 mm Hg should be the target during high-quality chest compressions and medication administration.

Pharmacology

Pharmacologic agents are a key aspect of CPR (Table 31.1). The current guidelines have removed vasopressin from the ACLS algorithm. Epinephrine doses of 1 mg should be administered every 3 to 5 minutes. Amiodarone is the first-line antiarrhythmic agent (Table 31.2), but lidocaine is still considered an alternative. Routine use of other agents, such as calcium or bicarbonate, is not indicated unless the clinical situation warrants.

Table 31.1 • Pharmacologic Agents for CPR

Agent	Indication
Epinephrine	VF, pulseless VT, PEA, asystole
Amiodarone	VF, pulseless VT
Lidocaine	VF, pulseless VT (second-line agent)
Atropine	Symptomatic bradycardia
Sodium bicarbonate	Hyperkalemic arrest or tricyclic overdose
Calcium chloride	Hyperkalemic arrest or overdose of calcium channel blocker
Magnesium sulfate	Torsades de pointes or drug-induced QT prolongation
Fibrinolytic	Pulmonary embolism–related arrest
Intralipid or fat emulsion	Cardiac arrest due to local anesthetic toxicity

Abbreviations: CPR, cardiopulmonary resuscitation; PEA, pulseless electrical activity; VF, ventricular fibrillation; VT, ventricular tachycardia.

Table 31.2 • Arrhythmia Management

Arrhythmia	Intervention
Bradycardia Sinus bradycardia Heart block	Atropine, temporary pacing, chronotropic agents
Regular narrow-complex tachycardia Supraventricular tachycardia	Adenosine, nondihydropyridine calcium channel blocker, β-blocker
Irregular narrow-complex tachycardia Atrial fibrillation or atrial flutter Multifocal atrial tachycardia	Amiodarone, nondihydropyridine calcium channel blocker, β-blocker, cardioversion (if unstable)
Regular wide-complex tachycardia Ventricular tachycardia Supraventricular tachycardia with aberrancy	Amiodarone, procainamide, cardioversion (if unstable)
Irregular wide-complex tachycardia Atrial fibrillation with aberrancy or preexcitation	Cardioversion, amiodarone, procainamide
Irregular wide-complex tachycardia with polymorphism Torsades de pointes	Defibrillation, magnesium sulfate

Pseudo-PEA

Pseudo-PEA arrest is the presence of electrical activity with minimal myocardial contractility that cannot generate a palpable pulse. It occurs in severe shock states and is different from the electromechanical dissociation that occurs in a true PEA arrest. A waveform can be visualized with placement of an arterial line. Echocardiography showing cardiac contractility can be used to differentiate between a true PEA arrest and a pseudo-PEA arrest. The distinction is important because management with CPR depends on the absence of contractility. In addition, $ETCO_2$ is higher in intubated patients who have pseudo-PEA arrest rather than true PEA arrest.

Postresuscitation Management

Among patients with ROSC after cardiac arrest, morbidity and mortality are high and these patients require comprehensive care. Multiple issues need to be addressed simultaneously, including determining the cause of the cardiac arrest, minimizing neurologic injury, and managing cardiovascular and end-organ dysfunction. Acute coronary syndromes and cardiovascular disease are the most common causes of cardiac arrest. Other causes include pulmonary embolism, poisonings, and intracranial hemorrhage (Box 31.1).

Evaluation

Initial evaluation includes a focused history and physical examination. If patients are comatose and unable to provide a history, care providers should speak with family members, witnesses to the cardiac arrest, and emergency medical services personnel. The patient's health records from other facilities should be obtained to determine the extent and severity of preexisting medical conditions, current medications, and previous diagnostic evaluations (eg, echocardiography or other imaging). Physical examination should follow a structured approach akin to the ABC sequence. The airway should be assessed first to determine patency and type of advanced airway device. The appropriate location of an endotracheal tube should be confirmed. If a supraglottic device was used, it should be exchanged for an endotracheal tube when the patient's condition is stable. Ventilation can be assessed with ventilator waveforms, $ETCO_2$ levels, and standard auscultation. Evaluation of end-organ perfusion and circulation should include assessment of heart rate and rhythm, blood pressure, peripheral pulses, the presence of skin mottling or cold extremities, and cardiac auscultation. Comatose patients must undergo a baseline neurologic examination, and accurate assessment requires temporary avoidance of long-acting sedating medications and neuromuscular blocking agents. Prognostication tools such as the Full Outline of Unresponsiveness (FOUR) score or the Glasgow Coma Scale (GCS) should also be used.

Box 31.1 • Causes of Cardiac Arrest

Acute coronary syndrome
Acidosis
Abdominal aortic dissection or ruptured aortic aneurysm
Intracranial bleeding
Sepsis
Poisoning
Local anesthetic toxicity
Cardiac tamponade
Pulmonary embolism
Hypovolemia
Electrolyte abnormalities
Tension pneumothorax
Hypoxia
Arrhythmias

Laboratory evaluation should include arterial blood gas values, comprehensive electrolyte concentrations, complete blood cell count, coagulation profile, lactate level, and seral troponin levels. If drug ingestion is considered, serum and urine samples should be submitted for toxicology studies. Electrocardiography should be used to assist with assessing cardiac causes. Focused cardiac ultrasonography can also be performed to identify treatable causes (eg, severe hypovolemia, acute cor pulmonale, severe left ventricular dysfunction, and cardiac tamponade); however, all patients should undergo formal echocardiography after cardiac arrest. Focused lung ultrasonography should also be considered for identification of pneumothorax and large pleural effusion with tamponade physiology. Chest radiography is typically required, and other imaging studies such as computed tomography should be performed if indicated from the clinical context.

Management

Emergent percutaneous coronary intervention is indicated for patients with evidence of ST-segment elevation myocardial infarction or new left bundle branch block. In addition, patients presenting with a shockable rhythm, such as VF or pulseless VT, require urgent coronary angiography because clinically significant coronary lesions are present in 70% of patients.

Hemodynamic management is critical to maintain end-organ perfusion and to prevent episodes of hypotension that could further injure the brain and other organs. Specific goals for mean arterial pressure and systolic blood pressure have not been established. Current recommendations are from hemodynamic goals used in other critically ill populations, with a range for mean arterial pressure of 65 to 80 mm Hg. If the right ventricle is compromised, targeting a central venous pressure of 8 to 12 mm Hg may assist in ensuring adequate preload. However, the limitations of such a static measurement also need to be considered.

Maintaining urine output greater than 0.5 mL/kg per hour also assists in management. Persistent shock after cardiac arrest requires volume replacement, inotropic and vasopressor support, and possibly mechanical circulatory support such as an intra-aortic balloon pump.

The choice of a pharmacologic agent should be based on the patient's clinical condition because there is no evidence that any 1 agent is superior. Epinephrine, norepinephrine, dopamine, and dobutamine are all possible choices.

Lung-protective mechanical ventilation with tidal volumes of 6 to 8 mL/kg of ideal body weight should be used. To prevent cerebral vasoconstriction, the $Paco_2$ goal should be 35 to 40 mm Hg. In addition, avoiding hyperoxia (Pao_2 ≥300 mm Hg) is prudent because it is associated with worse outcomes. Standard principles for the care of critically ill patients should be followed. These include prevention of deep vein thrombosis and ventilator-associated pneumonia, stress ulcer prophylaxis, enteral feeding when not contraindicated, and glycemic control to maintain serum glucose values between 140 and 180 mg/dL. Hyperglycemia is associated with worse neurologic outcomes in patients with cardiac arrest.

Targeted Temperature Management and Therapeutic Hypothermia

Neurologic injury is the most common cause of morbidity and death among patients with an OHCA, and it is a common cause of death among patients with an IHCA. In initial studies, patients treated with therapeutic hypothermia (core body temperature 32°C-34°C) had better neurologic outcomes than patients not treated with temperature control. However, more recent clinical trials that used core body temperatures of 33°C to 36°C did not show any significant neurologic benefit for patients with an OHCA. In addition, survival at 6 months was no different among patients with a targeted temperature of 33°C compared with those with a target of 36°C. Furthermore, evaluation of cognitive function and quality of life at 6 months showed no difference between patients with a target of 33°C and those with a target of 36°C.

For patients with an OHCA due to a shockable rhythm (VF and pulseless VT) or a nonshockable rhythm (asystole and PEA) and for patients with an IHCA and who are comatose after ROSC, the AHA recommends targeted temperature management (TTM) of 32°C to 36°C. However, evidence continues to show that a target of 36°C confers the same neurologic benefit as 33°C but without the potential sequela of induced hypothermia. The absolute contraindications to TTM are a preexisting do-not-resuscitate order or an advance directive stating that the patient does not want aggressive care in this type of clinical situation. Relative contraindications include pregnancy, traumatic arrest, active bleeding, or a preexisting condition that precludes a meaningful recovery.

The targeted core temperature should be achieved as soon as possible and maintained for 24 hours, followed by a gradual rewarming (0.25°C-0.5°C per hour). Some patients are already mildly hypothermic at presentation; intravenous cold crystalloids can assist in initiating the process in patients who are normothermic. Intravascular or surface cooling devices should be used to maintain core temperature. Hyperthermia must be avoided, particularly after rewarming to normothermia, because it is associated with poorer outcomes for patients with cardiac arrest. Shivering increases the core body temperature and, if not controlled, can delay achieving the goal temperature. Shivering can be suppressed through sedation with propofol, dexmedetomidine, benzodiazepines, or opioids. Although intermittent administration of meperidine controls shivering in various patient populations, it may be problematic in patients with cardiac arrest because of its adverse effect profile, metabolites, and renal elimination. Neuromuscular blockade is effective but may mask seizure activity, so that continuous electroencephalographic monitoring may be required.

At core temperatures less than 35°C, platelets, clotting factors, and leukocyte function are less effective. The result is an increased risk of bleeding and infection. In addition, at hypothermic core temperatures, cardiac conduction slows, the QT interval is prolonged, and bradycardia can result. Insulin resistance may develop, resulting in hyperglycemia, and hypokalemia can occur as potassium shifts to the intracellular space. Potassium should be replaced judiciously because hyperkalemia and arrhythmias may develop as the patient is warmed and the potassium shifts back to the extracellular space. Occasionally, hypothermia can trigger a "cold diuresis" and subsequent electrolyte abnormalities. Hypothermia also prolongs the metabolism and elimination of medications.

Summary

- Anoxic brain injury is the most common cause of death among patients with OHCA.
- High-quality CPR should not be interrupted for more than 10 seconds for pulse checks or placement of an advanced airway device.
- If $ETCO_2$ levels are greater than 20 mm Hg at 20 minutes of CPR, patients have a better chance of ROSC; patients with $ETCO_2$ levels less than 10 mm Hg at 20 minutes of CPR have a minimal chance of ROSC.
- TTM between 32°C and 36°C is recommended for any unresponsive patient with an OHCA or an IHCA, regardless of the presenting rhythm.
- Hyperthermia should be avoided because it is associated with worse outcomes for patients with cardiac arrest.

SUGGESTED READING

Arrich J, Holzer M, Havel C, Mullner M, Herkner H. Hypothermia for neuroprotection in adults after cardiopulmonary resuscitation. Cochrane Database Syst Rev. 2016 Feb 15;2:CD004128.

Bernard SA, Gray TW, Buist MD, Jones BM, Silvester W, Gutteridge G, et al. Treatment of comatose survivors of out-of-hospital cardiac arrest with induced hypothermia. N Engl J Med. 2002 Feb 21;346(8):557–63.

Callaway CW, Donnino MW, Fink EL, Geocadin RG, Golan E, Kern KB, et al. Part 8: Post-cardiac arrest care: 2015 American Heart Association guidelines update for cardiopulmonary resuscitation and emergency cardiovascular care. Circulation. 2015 Nov 3;132(18 Suppl 2):S465–82. Erratum in: Circulation. 2017 Sep 5;136(10):e197.

Choi HA, Ko SB, Presciutti M, Fernandez L, Carpenter AM, Lesch C, et al. Prevention of shivering during therapeutic temperature modulation: the Columbia anti-shivering protocol. Neurocrit Care. 2011 Jun;14(3):389–94.

Cronberg T, Lilja G, Horn J, Kjaergaard J, Wise MP, Pellis T, et al; TTM Trial Investigators. Neurologic function and health-related quality of life in patients following targeted temperature management at 33°C vs 36°C after out-of-hospital cardiac arrest: a randomized clinical trial. JAMA Neurol. 2015 Jun;72(6):634–41.

Hassager C, Nagao K, Hildick-Smith D. Out-of-hospital cardiac arrest: in-hospital intervention strategies. Lancet. 2018 Mar 10;391(10124):989–98.

Heradstveit BE, Sunde K, Sunde GA, Wentzel-Larsen T, Heltne JK. Factors complicating interpretation of capnography during advanced life support in cardiac arrest: a clinical retrospective study in 575 patients. Resuscitation. 2012 Jul;83(7):813–8. Epub 2012 Feb 25.

Kleinman ME, Brennan EE, Goldberger ZD, Swor RA, Terry M, Bobrow BJ, et al. Part 5: Adult basic life support and cardiopulmonary resuscitation quality: 2015 American Heart Association guidelines update for cardiopulmonary resuscitation and emergency cardiovascular care. Circulation. 2015 Nov 3;132(18 Suppl 2):S414–35.

Link MS, Berkow LC, Kudenchuk PJ, Halperin HR, Hess EP, Moitra VK, et al. Part 7: Adult advanced cardiovascular life support: 2015 American Heart Association guidelines update for cardiopulmonary resuscitation and emergency cardiovascular care. Circulation. 2015 Nov 3;132(18 Suppl 2):S444–64. Erratum in: Circulation. 2015 Dec 15;132(24):e385.

Lurie KG, Nemergut EC, Yannopoulos D, Sweeney M. The physiology of cardiopulmonary resuscitation. Anesth Analg. 2016 Mar;122(3):767–83.

McGlinch BP, White RD. Cardiopulmonary resuscitation: basic and advanced life support. In: Miller RD, editor. Miller's anesthesia. 8th ed. Vol. 2. Philadelphia (PA): Elsevier/Saunders; c2015. p. 3182–215.

Meperidine. Micromedex Solutions [Internet]. Ann Arbor (MI): Truven Health Analytics. c2017 [cited 2016 Dec 21]. Available from: www.micromedexsolutions.com.

Mozaffarian D, Benjamin EJ, Go AS, Arnett DK, Blaha MJ, Cushman M, et al; American Heart Association Statistics Committee and Stroke Statistics Subcommittee. Heart disease and stroke statistics: 2015 update: a report from the American Heart Association. Circulation. 2015 Jan 27;131(4):e29–322. Epub 2014 Dec 17. Errata in: Circulation. 2016 Feb 23;133(8):e417. Circulation. 2015 Jun 16;131(24):e535.

Narayan SM, Wang PJ, Daubert JP. New concepts in sudden cardiac arrest to address an intractable epidemic: JACC State-of-the-Art Review. J Am Coll Cardiol. 2019 Jan 8;73(1):70–88.

Nichol G, Thomas E, Callaway CW, Hedges J, Powell JL, Aufderheide TP, et al; Resuscitation Outcomes Consortium Investigators. Regional variation in out-of-hospital cardiac arrest incidence and outcome. JAMA. 2008 Sep 24;300(12):1423–31. Erratum in: JAMA. 2008 Oct 15;300(15):1763.

Nielsen N, Wetterslev J, Cronberg T, Erlinge D, Gasche Y, Hassager C, et al; TTM Trial Investigators. Targeted temperature management at 33°C versus 36°C after cardiac arrest. N Engl J Med. 2013 Dec 5;369(23):2197–206. Epub 2013 Nov 17.

Walker AC, Johnson NJ. Critical care of the post-cardiac arrest patient. Cardiol Clin. 2018 Aug;36(3):419–28.

Wang CH, Chang WT, Huang CH, Tsai MS, Yu PH, Wang AY, et al. The effect of hyperoxia on survival following adult cardiac arrest: a systematic review and meta-analysis of observational studies. Resuscitation. 2014 Sep;85(9):1142–8. Epub 2014 Jun 2.

32 Vascular Emergencies of the Aorta

TARIQ ALMEREY, MD; JANUARY F. MOORE; HOUSSAM FARRES, MD

Goals

- Know the natural history and clinical features of abdominal aortic aneurysm and aortic dissection.
- Describe the preoperative evaluation and diagnosis of abdominal aortic aneurysm, thoracic aortic aneurysm, and aortic dissection.
- Describe the perioperative medical and surgical management of abdominal aortic aneurysm, thoracic aortic aneurysm, and aortic dissection.

Introduction

Many serious conditions require emergent vascular intervention, but the most challenging conditions that typically require admission to an intensive care unit are ruptured abdominal aortic aneurysm (AAA) and acute aortic syndrome (ie, aortic dissection, intramural hematoma, and penetrating ulcers).

Abdominal Aortic Aneurysm

AAA occurs in 6% to 13% of people older than 65 years. Unless patients with ruptured AAA receive prompt diagnosis and repair, the condition is usually fatal within a period that ranges from minutes to approximately 1 week. Even when patients receive a timely diagnosis and undergo prompt repair, mortality is as high as 50%.

The classic signs and symptoms of AAA include abdominal, back, or flank pain; circulatory instability; and a tender pulsatile mass on palpation. Patients may have episodes of dizziness or unconsciousness. Pulses in the extremities should be evaluated to establish a baseline in the event of surgical complications. Misdiagnoses of ruptured AAA include kidney stones, diverticulitis, pancreatitis, aortic dissection, and myocardial infarction.

If patients with a known history of AAA are hemodynamically unstable and present with characteristic signs and symptoms of rupture or with abdominal or pelvic pain of unknown cause, they should be referred immediately for surgical repair. If patients are hemodynamically stable, they should undergo computed tomography to confirm rupture before referral for surgical repair. If rupture is suspected in patients without known AAA, ultrasonography can be used to confirm the initial AAA diagnosis at the bedside for consideration of further treatment options.

If the patient is referred for surgery, 2 large-bore intravenous catheters should be placed, blood samples drawn for testing, the bladder catheterized, fluid infusion started, and packed red blood cells and plasma ordered. If a patient with ruptured AAA presents to an institution without appropriate surgical expertise, transferring the patient should be considered and weighed against the risk of deterioration.

For decades, open surgical repair was the mainstay therapy for ruptured AAA. However, endovascular aneurysm repair (EVAR) is rapidly becoming the preferred method of treatment, especially at institutions with an infrastructure for emergent EVAR in selected patients (who have a suitable aortic neck length, angulation, and diameter for stent graft deployment).

Open Surgical Repair

Before a patient undergoes open surgical repair, *permissive hypotension* is maintained (systolic blood pressure <80 mm Hg as long as the patient is neurologically coherent) to help in minimizing the risk of hemorrhage and free rupture. Multiple vascular agents may be administered to achieve that goal.

The preferred approach for repairing a ruptured AAA is a transperitoneal approach through a midline incision because it provides good exposure to the supraceliac aorta, the infrarenal aorta, and the iliac arteries. After the abdomen is entered, hemorrhage is controlled by compressing the aorta with direct pressure until a proximal aortic clamp is deployed. The location of the initial clamping depends on the location of the rupture and retroperitoneal hematoma. When proximal and distal control is achieved, the aneurysm sac is opened and that portion of the aorta is replaced with a tube or bifurcated graft (Dacron and polytetrafluoroethylene [PTFE] are the most commonly used materials). With the graft in place, the retroperitoneal tissue and the aneurysm sac are reapproximated over the graft to decrease the risk of aortoenteric fistula formation.

Endovascular Aortic Repair

In EVAR, after arterial access is obtained, an occlusion balloon is advanced beyond the aortic rupture area to control the bleeding. Aortography is performed to determine whether EVAR is possible. If the anatomy is suitable for EVAR, the surgeon deploys the stent graft in a manner similar to that for elective endovascular repair (Figure 32.1).

Postoperative Management

After repair, patients are treated in the intensive care unit until circulatory, respiratory, and renal functions are stable. The most common early postoperative complications are congestive heart failure, renal failure, and ischemic colitis. These patients, who often have concomitant coronary heart disease, undergo severe stress during preoperative shock and aortic clamping and declamping. Commonly, their cardiac function deteriorates and secondary hypotension requires inotropic treatment. Renal function is often impaired, and occasionally patients require dialysis. Preoperative hypotension increases creatinine and serum urea nitrogen levels in almost all patients after operation for ruptured AAA. If renal insufficiency develops with low urinary output, renal replacement therapy should be considered at an early stage. The greatest risk for developing ischemic colitis is in patients with a ruptured aneurysm and shock. The severity of ischemic colitis varies from only mucosal discharge to transmural necrosis. The risk of ischemic colitis can be determined with serial serum lactic acid levels, sigmoidoscopy, and measurement of pH at the wall of the sigmoid with a tonometer.

Thoracic Aortic Aneurysm Rupture

EVAR is the primary method for thoracic aortic aneurysm rupture repair (Figure 32.2). If the deployed stent graft covers the supra-aortic vessels for adequate sealing, a carotid-to-subclavian artery bypass is usually required. If extensive thoracic coverage (T8 to L1) is required, a spinal drain should be considered to minimize intraoperative and postoperative spinal cord ischemia. The spinal drain is placed to maintain the spinal perfusion pressure at 70 mm Hg ore more, and this can be achieved by maintaining the mean arterial pressure (MAP) at 80 mm Hg or more and the intracranial pressure (ICP) at 10 mm Hg or less. Cerebral perfusion pressure (CPP) is the difference between MAP and ICP (CPP = MAP - ICP).

Postoperatively the spinal drain is typically left in place for 48 to 72 hours (when the risk of perioperative spinal cord ischemia is highest) with the goal of maintaining ICP at 10 mm Hg or less. The cerebrospinal fluid can be drained at a rate not exceeding 30 mL/h to reach the desired ICP goal.

Aortic Dissection

Background

Acute aortic dissection is a rare, life-threatening condition. The estimated incidence is 2.6 to 3.5 per 100,000 person-years in the general population. Patients with aortic dissection present with severe chest pain and hemodynamic instability, and, if aortic dissection is not repaired, it is usually fatal. The mortality rate is 20% to 50% within the first 24 to 48 hours and 75% within 2 weeks. Death can result from any of the following: cardiac tamponade; extension of the dissection into the aortic valvular annulus, leading to aortic regurgitation; obstruction of the coronary artery, resulting in myocardial infarction; or obstruction of abdominal aortic branch vessels, resulting in organ failure.

Classification

Multiple aortic dissection classifications have been proposed, including the Stanford, DeBakey, Crawford, and DISSECT classifications. The Stanford classification simplifies management (Figure 32.3). Stanford type A dissection always involves the ascending aorta, regardless of the distal extension. Stanford type B dissection does not involve the ascending aorta. Aortic dissection is further classified as acute or chronic-acute (if symptoms began ≤14 days before presentation) or as chronic (if symptoms began >14 days before presentation).

Pathophysiology

The main event in aortic dissection is aortic intimal tear, which results in a false lumen that is created as blood passes into the aortic media through the tear (Figure 32.4). False lumen dilatation and collapse of the true lumen occur after dissection and enlarge the aortic cross-sectional area. Of the 2 types of dissection in the Stanford classification, type A is more common (60%-70% of aortic dissections) and often occurs in younger patients with connective tissue abnormalities. Type B dissection comprises approximately 25% of aortic dissections and usually affects older patients with hypertension. Anatomical variability in dissection is common, so appropriate axial imaging is critical. Multiple

A

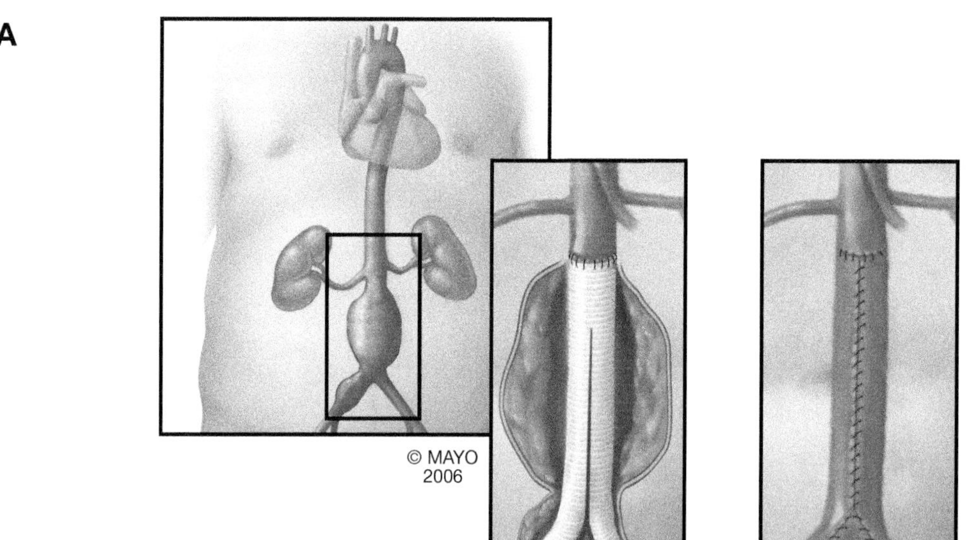

B

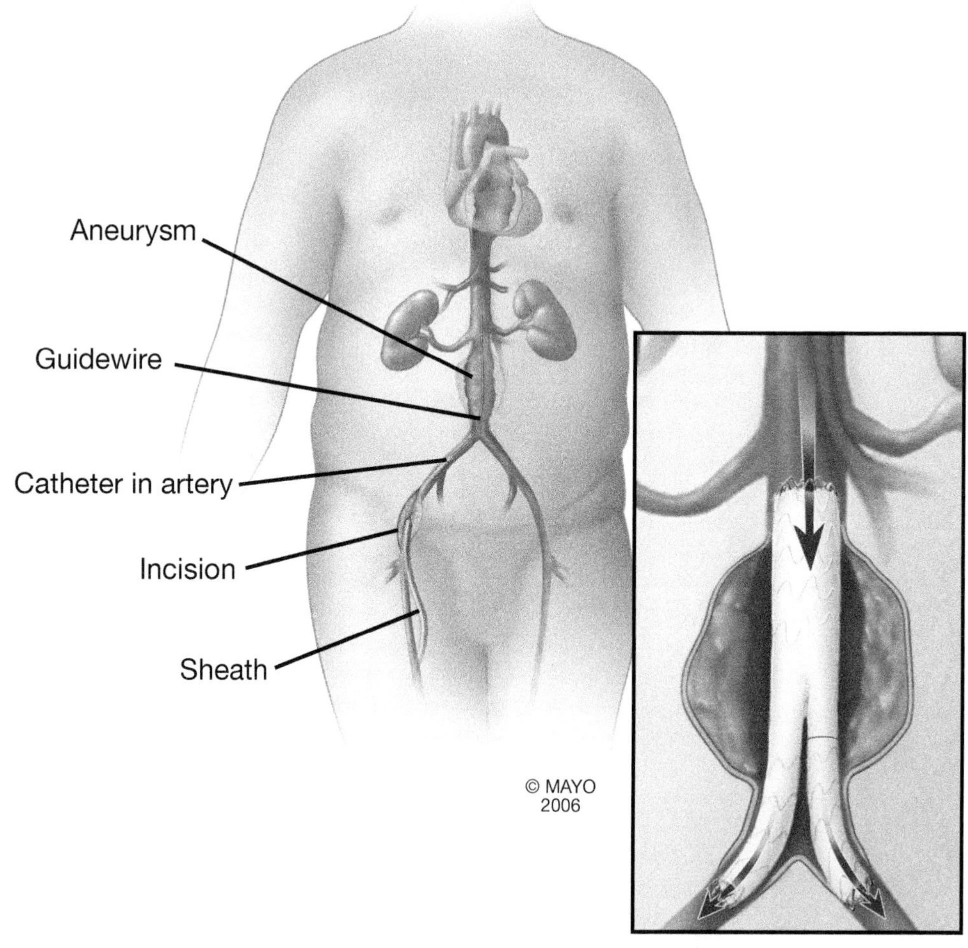

Figure 32.1. Surgical Repair of Abdominal Aortic Aneurysm. A, Open surgery. (From patient education brochure: open abdominal aortic aneurysm repair. c2006; used with permission of Mayo Foundation for Medical Education and Research.) B, Endovascular surgery. (From patient education brochure: endovascular repair of abdominal aortic aneurysms. c2008; used with permission of Mayo Foundation for Medical Education and Research.)

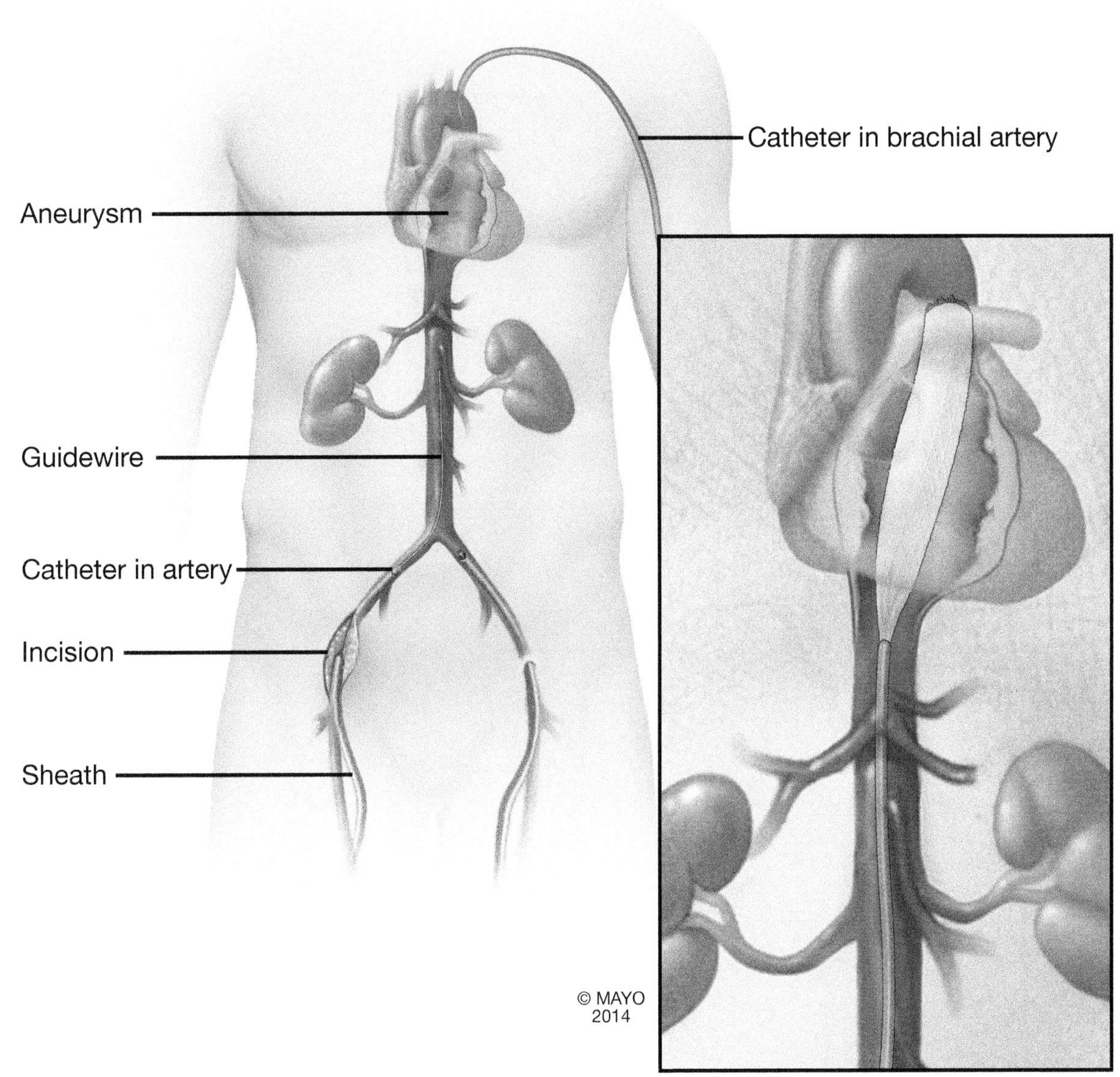

Figure 32.2. *Endovascular Repair of Thoracic Aortic Aneurysm.*
(From patient education brochure: endovascular repair of descending thoracic aortic aneurysms. c2014; used with permission of Mayo Foundation for Medical Education and Research.)

communications (*fenestrations*) may form between the true lumen and the false lumen.

Clinical Presentation

Patients with aortic dissection may pose a diagnostic dilemma. Although the dominant symptom is severe pain, which occurs in over 90% of patients, patients can have various clinical signs and symptoms depending on the extension of the dissection, including hematuria, pulse deficit, and neurologic symptoms. Accordingly, the differential diagnosis for aortic dissection is broad (Box 32.1).

Diagnostic Evaluation

Electrocardiography should be used to rule out myocardial ischemia; echocardiography should be used to rule out pericardial tamponade. Test results should be evaluated for complete blood cell count, arterial blood gases, prothrombin, creatinine, serum urea nitrogen, liver enzymes, and

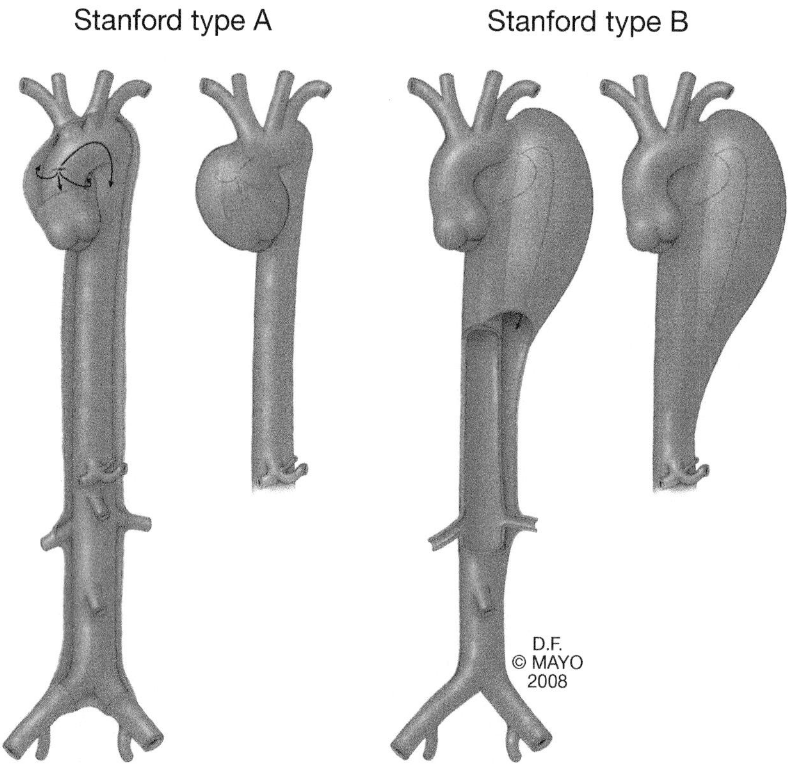

Figure 32.3. Stanford Classification of Aortic Dissection. Left, Type A involves the ascending aorta regardless of the distal extension. Right, Type B involves only the descending aorta. (Modified from Clouse WD, Hallett JW Jr, Schaff HV, Spittell PC, Rowland CM, Ilstrup DM, et al. Acute aortic dissection: population-based incidence compared with degenerative aortic aneurysm rupture. Mayo Clin Proc. 2004 Feb;79[2]:176-80; used with permission of Mayo Foundation for Medical Education and Research.)

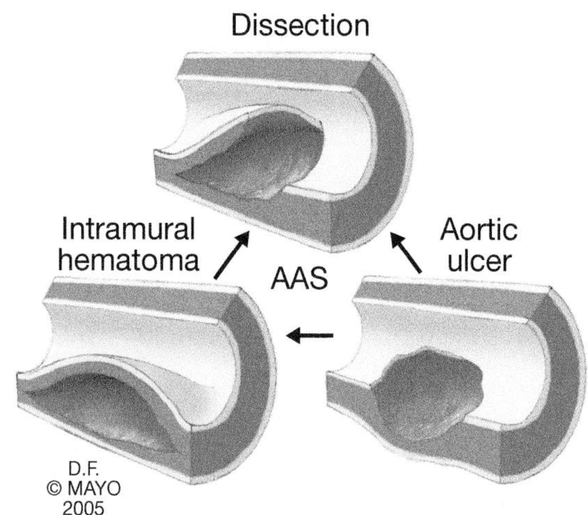

Figure 32.4. Acute Aortic Syndrome (AAS).
(From Haro LH, Krajicek M, Lobl JK. Challenges, controversies, and advances in aortic catastrophes. Emerg Med Clin North Am. 2005 Nov;23[4]:1159-77; used with permission of Mayo Foundation for Medical Education and Research.)

lactic acid. Laboratory results may indicate mild anemia, leukocytosis, hemolysis, and elevated levels of bilirubin and lactic acid. Patients may have metabolic acidosis due to malperfusion. Hematuria on urinalysis indicates kidney malperfusion.

Box 32.1 • Differential Diagnosis for Aortic Dissection

- Coronary ischemia
- Myocardial infarction
- Aortic regurgitation without dissection
- Stroke
- Pulmonary embolism
- Visceral ischemia without dissection
- Lower extremity ischemia without dissection
- Gallbladder disease
- Pericarditis
- Musculoskeletal pain
- Mediastinal tumors or cysts

Plain radiography of the chest is rarely diagnostic, but the following findings indicate the presence of aortic dissection:

- Abnormal shadow adjacent to the descending thoracic aorta.
- Deformity of the aortic knob.
- Density adjacent to the brachiocephalic trunk.
- Enlarged cardiac shadow.
- Displaced esophagus, trachea, or bronchus.
- Abnormally widened mediastinum.
- Irregular aortic contour.
- Loss of sharpness of the aortic shadow.
- Pleural effusion.

Computed tomographic angiography is accurate for diagnosing aortic dissection and provides information for classification. Magnetic resonance angiography is highly accurate and provides valuable pathoanatomical information; however, performing it is problematic if a patient is hemodynamically unstable or is receiving ventilator support. Transesophageal echocardiography is valuable, but it has limitations for visualizing the distal ascending aorta and arch. In combination with transthoracic echocardiography, however, sensitivity and specificity approach 100%.

Aortography is the gold standard for diagnosing aortic dissection. In addition, aortography can be used in combination with therapeutic endovascular management.

Management

As soon as aortic dissection is suspected, aggressive medical treatment should be started to stabilize the dissection, prevent rupture, and prevent organ ischemia. Decreasing the blood pressure is a cornerstone of treatment; however, that treatment must be balanced against the need to maintain adequate cerebral, coronary, renal, and visceral perfusion. Systolic blood pressure should be maintained at approximately 100 to 110 mm Hg and MAP at 60 to 75 mm Hg while taking into consideration urinary output and neurologic status. Multiple medications can be used to control blood pressure and heart rate; β-blockers are the first-line agents. Vasodilators such as hydralazine and sodium nitroprusside should be avoided because of the risk of reflex tachycardia and increased pulse impulse. Pain control is essential for these patients as well.

Initial treatment of acute distal aortic dissection is medical. Surgical or endovascular intervention is considered if any of the following situations occurs despite administration of maximal medical therapy:

- Aortic rupture or impending rupture.
- Rapidly expanding aortic diameter.
- Uncontrolled hypertension.
- Persistent pain despite medical therapy.
- Organ malperfusion.

Emergent surgery should be considered without a trial of medical therapy if any of the following is present:

- Type A dissection involves the intrapericardial ascending aorta and arch.
- Type B retrograde dissection involves the arch.
- A double aortic lumen involves the pericardial portion of the ascending aorta.

The most commonly considered intervention is open repair, which typically requires replacing the ascending aorta and resecting the primary tear of the intima. However, multiple endovascular techniques have emerged for covering the primary tear of the intima (typically with a covered stent graft) and for depressurizing the false lumen (through endovascular fenestration).

Aortic Intramural Hematoma and Penetrating Atherosclerotic Ulcer

Besides aortic dissection, the acute aortic syndrome includes 2 other entities: intramural hematoma and penetrating ulcer (Figure 32.4). Both are typically diagnosed and treated in a similar fashion to acute aortic dissection.

Aortic intramural hematoma is a variant of aortic dissection and is characterized by hemorrhage into the media of the aortic wall without a tear in the intimal layer. The blood within the wall quickly thromboses because of the lack of blood flow. The outer portion of the aortic wall becomes thinner, which may explain the higher risk of rupture with an intramural hematoma compared with acute dissection.

Penetrating atherosclerotic ulcers can result in aortic dissection or perforation. Noninvasive imaging shows a region of the aorta where the intima is denuded and an ulcer-like lesion projects through the aortic wall.

Summary

- If patients with a known history of AAA are hemodynamically unstable and present with characteristic signs and symptoms of rupture or with abdominal or pelvic pain of unknown cause, they should be referred immediately for surgical repair.
- Permissive hypotension before open repair of ruptured AAA is essential to minimize the risk of hemorrhage and free rupture.
- Postoperatively after AAA repair, patients must be closely monitored for common major complications such as congestive heart failure, renal failure, and ischemic colitis.
- If extensive thoracic coverage (T8 to L1) is required during endovascular repair of thoracic aortic aneurysm, a spinal drain should be considered to minimize intraoperative and postoperative spinal cord ischemia.

- The cornerstones in treatment of aortic dissection are controlling pain and decreasing blood pressure and heart rate. β-Blockers are the first-line agents. Vasodilators such as hydralazine and sodium nitroprusside should be avoided because of the risk of reflex tachycardia and increased pulse impulse.

SUGGESTED READING

Armour RH. Survivors of ruptured abdominal aortic aneurysm: the iceberg's tip. Br Med J. 1977 Oct 22;2(6094):1055–7.

Cronenwett JL, Johnston KW, editors. Rutherford's vascular surgery [online]. 8th ed. Philadelphia (PA): Saunders/Elsevier; c2014. Chapters 130-138, p. 1999.e5-2188.e4.

Golledge J. Abdominal aortic aneurysm: update on pathogenesis and medical treatments. Nat Rev Cardiol. 2019 Apr;16(4):225–42.

Lesperance K, Andersen C, Singh N, Starnes B, Martin MJ. Expanding use of emergency endovascular repair for ruptured abdominal aortic aneurysms: disparities in outcomes from a nationwide perspective. J Vasc Surg. 2008 Jun;47(6):1165–70. Epub 2008 Apr 3.

Makaloski V, Schmidli J, Wyss TR. [Ruptured abdominal aortic aneurysm]. Zentralbl Chir. 2018 Oct;143(5): 510–515. Epub 2018 Oct 24. German.

Mehta M, Byrne J, Darling RC 3rd, Paty PS, Roddy SP, Kreienberg PB, et al. Endovascular repair of ruptured infrarenal abdominal aortic aneurysm is associated with lower 30-day mortality and better 5-year survival rates than open surgical repair. J Vasc Surg. 2013 Feb;57(2):368–75. Epub 2012 Dec 21.

Mehta RH, Suzuki T, Hagan PG, Bossone E, Gilon D, Llovet A, et al. International Registry of Acute Aortic Dissection (IRAD) Investigators. Predicting death in patients with acute type A aortic dissection. Circulation. 2002 Jan 15;105(2):200–6.

Moreno DH, Cacione DG, Baptista-Silva JC. Controlled hypotension versus normotensive resuscitation strategy for people with ruptured abdominal aortic aneurysm. Cochrane Database Syst Rev. 2018 Jun 13;6:CD011664.

Nienaber CA, Eagle KA. Aortic dissection: new frontiers in diagnosis and management: Part I: from etiology to diagnostic strategies. Circulation. 2003 Aug 5;108(5):628–35.

Powell JT, Greenhalgh RM. Clinical practice: small abdominal aortic aneurysms. N Engl J Med. 2003 May 8;348(19):1895–901.

Sakalihasan N, Michel JB, Katsargyris A, Kuivaniemi H, Defraigne JO, Nchimi A, et al. Abdominal aortic aneurysms. Nat Rev Dis Primers. 2018 Oct 18;4(1):34.

Turk KA. The post-mortem incidence of abdominal aortic aneurysm. Proc R Soc Med. 1965 Nov;58(11 Part 1):869–70.

Acute Endocrine Disorders

33 Pituitary Apoplexy

SHERRI A. BRAKSICK, MD

Goals

- Identify common risk factors for pituitary apoplexy.
- Review the presenting symptoms of pituitary apoplexy.
- Review the diagnostic evaluation of suspected apoplexy.
- Understand the management strategies for pituitary apoplexy.

Introduction

Pituitary apoplexy is infarction of the pituitary gland by hemorrhage or ischemia. Although pituitary apoplexy is rare, it is a neurologic emergency and sometimes a neurosurgical and endocrine emergency that require rapid intervention to prevent severe and potentially life-threatening adrenal insufficiency, hydrocephalus, intracranial hemorrhage, or ischemic stroke.

Basic Pituitary Physiology

The pituitary gland is a complex structure that secretes multiple hormones needed to maintain homeostasis and facilitate physiologic responses to physical and environmental triggers. The anterior pituitary gland produces and releases multiple hormones in response to stimulating peptides, which originate in the hypothalamus. The products of the anterior pituitary gland are summarized in Table 33.1.

In contrast, the posterior pituitary gland secretes 2 hormones, oxytocin and vasopressin (also referred to as antidiuretic hormone), that are produced by the hypothalamus. The primary end-organ targets of oxytocin are the breasts and uterus. Vasopressin acts on vascular smooth muscle as a potent vasoconstrictor through several mechanisms and additionally at the level of the renal collecting duct, which ultimately results in water retention, decreased serum osmolality, and excretion of concentrated urine.

Risk Factors and Clinical Presentation

Pituitary apoplexy occurs more often in men and is reported most often in the sixth decade of life. Pregnancy and the postpartum period may increase the risk of apoplexy in women, but overall, apoplexy is an uncommon event. Many patients have preexisting hypertension or are receiving anticoagulants. A reported risk factor is surgery, especially cardiac surgery with its accompanying blood pressure fluctuations and anticoagulation. Other precipitating factors include bromocriptine initiation or withdrawal and estrogen therapy. Interestingly, a pituitary adenoma (either functioning or nonfunctioning) is identified in only a minority of patients who present with acute apoplexy.

The presenting symptoms of pituitary apoplexy can be nonspecific and difficult to localize. The most commonly reported symptom is classically described as severe, sudden-onset headache (ie, *thunderclap headache*). Symptoms at presentation may also include cranial nerve palsies if the hemorrhage extends into the cavernous sinus. Compression of the carotid artery in the cavernous sinus may lead to ischemia of a portion or all of the carotid territory. If the perivascular sympathetic fibers on the outer surface of the carotid artery are compressed, a partial Horner syndrome may affect the upper portion of the face. Rarely, obstructive hydrocephalus may also occur. Other common presenting symptoms and signs are listed in Box 33.1.

Table 33.1 • Hormonal Products of the Anterior Pituitary Gland

Pituitary Hormone	Systemic Product
Corticotropin	Glucocorticoids
Thyrotropin	Triiodothyronine, thyroxine
Prolactin	None
Follicle-stimulating hormone	Androgens, estrogens
Luteinizing hormone	Androgens, estrogens
Growth hormone	Insulinlike growth factor 1

Box 33.1. • Common Symptoms and Signs of Pituitary Apoplexy

- Thunderclap headache
- Diplopia
- Cranial nerve III palsy
- Cranial nerve IV palsy
- Cranial nerve VI palsy
- Photophobia
- Visual field deficit (classically bitemporal hemianopia)
- Nausea, vomiting
- Pituitary hormone deficiency
- Altered mental status
- Coma

Box 33.2. • Laboratory Evaluation of Suspected Pituitary Apoplexy

- Complete blood count
- Coagulation parameters (prothrombin time and international normalized ratio)
- Thyrotropin
- Prolactin
- Follicle-stimulating hormone
- Growth hormone
- Cortisol
- Electrolytes
- Liver function studies
- Triiodothyronine, thyroxine
- Testosterone (in men), estradiol (in women)
- Luteinizing hormone
- Insulinlike growth factor 1
- Glucose

Diagnostic Evaluation

Laboratory Evaluation

To look for evidence of hypopituitarism, the initial laboratory evaluation of a patient with suspected pituitary apoplexy should determine the levels of pituitary-derived hormones and their products (eg, insulinlike growth factor 1, thyroid hormones, cortisol). Additional laboratory studies that should be included in the initial evaluation are listed in Box 33.2.

Imaging Studies

For patients who present with a thunderclap headache or focal neurologic findings, noncontrast computed tomography (CT) should be urgently performed to evaluate more common neurologic emergencies (eg, subarachnoid hemorrhage or ischemic stroke).

Apoplexy may be difficult to identify on CT, but a large adenoma may be visible and may increase clinical suspicion for pituitary apoplexy (Figure 33.1). However, negative

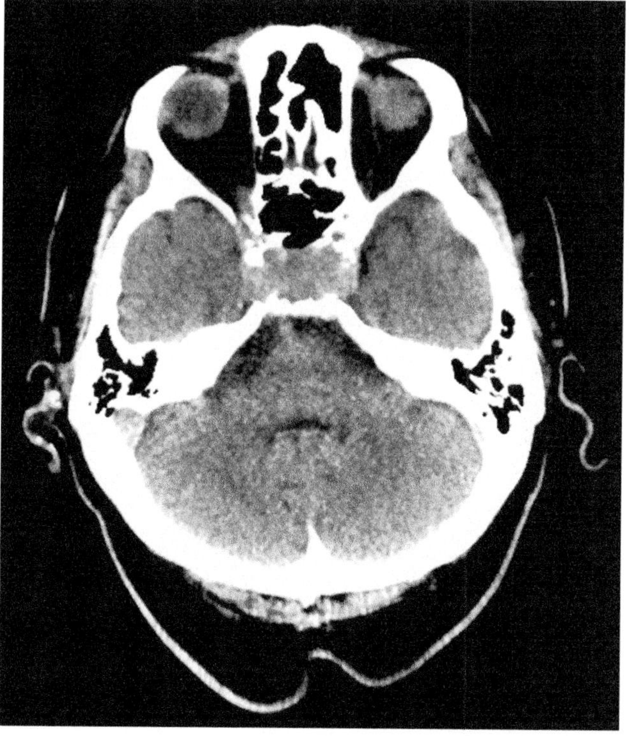

Figure 33.1. Signs of Apoplexy on Computed Tomography. Axial noncontrast computed tomographic scan of the head shows a hyperdense sellar mass. This patient presented with severe headache, bitemporal hemianopia, new right cranial nerve III palsy, and cranial nerve V1 hypoesthesia. These findings are consistent with apoplexy causing optic chiasm compression and extension into the right cavernous sinus.

findings on CT do not exclude the possibility of pituitary apoplexy.

If pituitary apoplexy is suspected clinically, but CT findings are negative, magnetic resonance imaging (MRI) should be performed. MRI is more sensitive for identifying pituitary hemorrhage and defining extension into or compression of adjacent structures (eg, cavernous sinus or optic chiasm) (Figure 33.2).

Management

Immediate management of pituitary apoplexy should focus on ensuring hemodynamic stability because of the risk of adrenal insufficiency. Stress doses of corticosteroids (eg, 50 mg hydrocortisone every 6 hours) should be administered during evaluation because adrenal insufficiency can be a life-threatening complication.

Meta-analysis indicates that some patients can be safely treated without surgery or with delayed surgery. The timing and indications for transsphenoidal resection are uncertain because no randomized controlled trials have compared conservative management with surgery, yet many clinicians advocate for urgent intervention in patients with impaired consciousness, visual field abnormalities, or progressive symptoms. Some patients, however, may need only medical management, with a primary focus on hormone replacement at the direction of an endocrinologist and electrolyte monitoring.

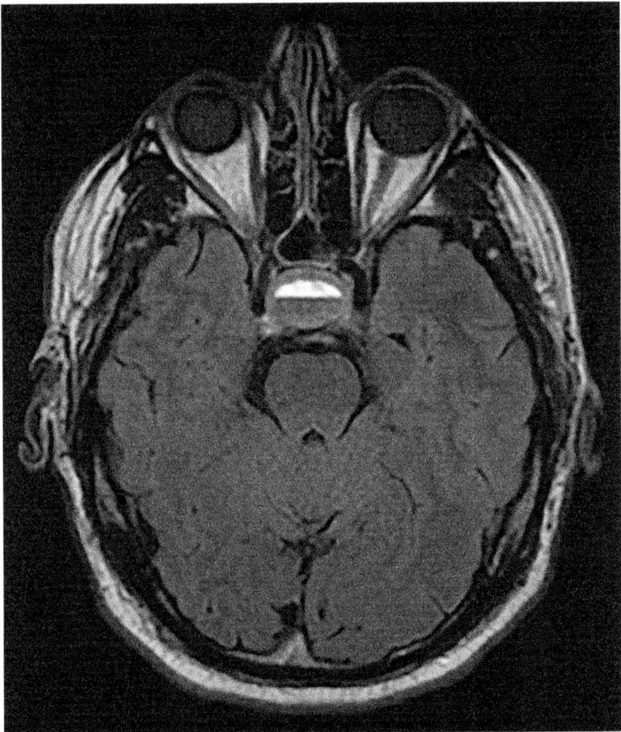

Figure 33.2. Signs of Pituitary Apoplexy on Magnetic Resonance Imaging. Axial T2-weighted fluid-attenuated inversion recovery image shows a pituitary lesion with a fluid-fluid level consistent with hemorrhage.

Outcomes

Functional outcomes are generally good for patients with pituitary apoplexy. Over time endocrine function tends to improve, but continued hormone replacement may be required. Eye movement abnormalities and visual field impairment also tend to improve but may not fully resolve. Some patients have tumor recurrence and require additional intervention, but this is uncommon.

Summary

- Pituitary apoplexy may occur with nonspecific symptoms, but thunderclap headache is often reported.
- MRI of the head is more sensitive and specific for the identification of pituitary hemorrhage and involvement of the structures adjacent to the pituitary gland.
- Acute adrenal insufficiency may be life-threatening, and steroid replacement must be started at recognition of apoplexy.
- Management includes hormone replacement and electrolyte monitoring. Surgical intervention should be considered for patients with visual field abnormalities, impaired consciousness, or progressive symptoms.

SUGGESTED READING

Amar AP, Weiss MH. Pituitary anatomy and physiology. Neurosurg Clin N Am. 2003 Jan;14(1):11–23.

Boellis A, di Napoli A, Romano A, Bozzao A. Pituitary apoplexy: an update on clinical and imaging features. Insights Imaging. 2014 Dec;5(6):753–62. Epub 2014 Oct 16.

Bujawansa S, Thondam SK, Steele C, Cuthbertson DJ, Gilkes CE, Noonan C, et al. Presentation, management and outcomes in acute pituitary apoplexy: a large single-centre experience from the United Kingdom. Clin Endocrinol (Oxf). 2014 Mar;80(3):419–24. Epub 2013 Aug 26.

de Heide LJ, van Tol KM, Doorenbos B. Pituitary apoplexy presenting during pregnancy. Neth J Med. 2004 Nov;62(10):393–6.

Dubuisson AS, Beckers A, Stevenaert A. Classical pituitary tumour apoplexy: clinical features, management and outcomes in a series of 24 patients. Clin Neurol Neurosurg. 2007 Jan;109(1):63–70. Epub 2006 Feb 20.

Giritharan S, Gnanalingham K, Kearney T. Pituitary apoplexy: bespoke patient management allows good clinical outcome. Clin Endocrinol (Oxf). 2016 Sep;85(3):415–22. Epub 2016 May 4.

Glezer A, Bronstein MD. Pituitary apoplexy: pathophysiology, diagnosis and management. Arch Endocrinol Metab. 2015 Jun;59(3):259–64.

Rajasekaran S, Vanderpump M, Baldeweg S, Drake W, Reddy N, Lanyon M, et al. UK guidelines for the management of pituitary apoplexy. Clin Endocrinol (Oxf). 2011 Jan;74(1):9–20.

Randeva HS, Schoebel J, Byrne J, Esiri M, Adams CB, Wass JA. Classical pituitary apoplexy: clinical features, management and outcome. Clin Endocrinol (Oxf). 1999 Aug;51(2):181–8.

Sahyouni R, Goshtasbi K, Choi E, Mahboubi H, Le R, Khahera AS, et al. Vision outcomes in early vs late surgical intervention of pituitary apoplexy: a meta-analysis. World Neurosurg. 2019 Mar 25. pii: S1878-8750(19)30811-3. [Epub ahead of print]

Schrupp Berg HL, Edlow JA. Post-partum pituitary apoplexy: a case report. Intern Emerg Med. 2007 Dec;2(4):311–4.

Singh TD, Valizadeh N, Meyer FB, Atkinson JL, Erickson D, Rabinstein AA. Management and outcomes of pituitary apoplexy. J Neurosurg. 2015 Jun;122(6):1450–7. Epub 2015 Apr 10.

34 Diabetes Insipidus

DANA ERICKSON, MD

Goals

- Understand the actions and regulation of antidiuretic hormone and their relationship to the development of central and nephrogenic diabetes insipidus.
- Review the evaluation of polyuria, polydipsia, and diabetes insipidus in the critical care setting.
- Understand the therapeutic approach to central diabetes insipidus.

Definitions

Diabetes insipidus (DI) results from the impaired secretion or action of antidiuretic hormone (ADH). *Central DI* occurs with partial or complete ADH deficiency; *nephrogenic DI* occurs with impaired action of ADH in the kidneys. These defects result in the production of large volumes of inappropriately dilute urine, which increases plasma osmolality and eventually stimulates thirst.

Anatomy and Physiology

ADH is a peptide hormone synthesized in the neurons of the supraoptic and paraventricular nuclei of the hypothalamus. Along with 2 additional peptides, neurophysin II and copeptin, ADH is cleaved from a preprohormone, stored in neurosecretory granules, and transported along the axonal pathway to the circulation in the posterior pituitary (ie, the neuroendocrine connection). The half-life of ADH is 15 to 30 minutes after secretion into the systemic circulation.

The main site of action is the renal system, where ADH binds to the V2 receptor in the collecting tubules and collecting duct. Receptor activation leads to the phosphorylation of aquaporin 2, which is a water channel that increases the permeability of water back into cells, thus leading to the production of more concentrated urine and a decrease in plasma osmolality. In addition, at supraphysiologic levels, ADH binds to the V1 receptors of the smooth muscle cells of blood vessels to facilitate vasoconstriction.

An increase in plasma osmolality to greater than 290 mOsm/kg (reference range, 275-295 mOsm/kg) is the main stimulus for ADH secretion from the posterior pituitary. A secondary stimulus for ADH secretion is a decrease in the effective circulating blood volume, which results in the secretion of ADH regardless of the plasma osmolality and sodium levels. The thirst mechanism is independent of ADH and mediated by osmoreceptors in the hypothalamus that detect changes in plasma osmolality; typically, plasma osmolality greater than 290 mOsm/kg stimulates thirst.

Causes

The causes of central DI are categorized as familial or acquired. The most common causes of acquired central DI are traumatic brain injury (TBI) and trauma to the pituitary or hypothalamic region caused by neurosurgical procedures performed in the anatomical areas associated with the production, transport, and storage of ADH. Moreover, brain death is another common cause of DI seen in neurocritical care units.

The exact prevalence of DI after TBI is not known but may range from 3% to 51% if the worst cases are included. The overall prevalence of permanent DI after TBI is 1% to 6%. Most cases of TBI-associated DI occur after moderate to severe head trauma, and the acute phase of DI is typically associated with cerebral edema.

Pituitary surgery or pituitary stalk injury caused by trauma can lead to 4 different patterns of DI: transient (the most common pattern), permanent, triphasic, and biphasic (Table 34.1). Factors reported to increase the risk for postoperative DI include young age, male sex, large tumor volume, and certain histologic types (eg, Rathke cleft cyst, craniopharyngioma).

Table 34.1 • Patterns of Central Diabetes Insipidus (DI) After Pituitary Surgery

Pattern	Frequency	Phase
Transient DI	Most common	. . .
Triphasic	Rare	First: decreased ADH release for 5-7 d
		Second: release of stored ADH for 2-14 d
		Third: permanent DI
Biphasic	Occasional	First: decreased ADH release for 5-7 d
		Second: release of stored ADH for 2-14 d
Permanent DI	Rare	

Abbreviation: ADH, antidiuretic hormone.

Box 34.1 • Causes of Central and Nephrogenic Diabetes Insipidus in Patients in the Intensive Care Unit

Acquired Central Diabetes Insipidus

Traumatic brain injury

Brain tumor (eg, craniopharyngioma, pituitary tumor, germinoma, meningioma, pituitary metastasis)

Infiltrative disease

- Granulomatous (eg, sarcoidosis, histiocytosis, granulomatosis with polyangiitis)
- Infectious (eg, mycobacterial infection, syphilis, meningitis, encephalitis)

Inflammatory disease (eg, hypophysitis)

Vascular disease (eg, hemorrhage, infarction [pituitary apoplexy], cerebral venous thrombosis)

Brain death

Nephrogenic Diabetes Insipidus

Acquired

- Electrolyte imbalance (eg, hypokalemia, hypercalcemia)
- Drugs (eg, lithium)

Congenital

Gestational transient central diabetes insipidus

Syndrome of inappropriate secretion of ADH (SIADH) occurs as a part of the biphasic and triphasic patterns (Table 34.1). However, SIADH can occur as an isolated entity after pituitary surgery (as a result of the uncontrolled release of ADH by degenerating neurons in the pituitary stalk). Isolated SIADH, which may occur in 2% to 37% of patients after pituitary surgery, causes accumulation of free water, decreased urine output, and concentrated urine with an inappropriately high urine osmolality in relation to plasma osmolality; these sequelae lead to hyponatremia and hypo-osmolality.

The most common causes of nephrogenic DI are acquired and result from severe electrolyte abnormalities (eg, hypokalemia or hypercalcemia) and medications (eg, lithium). Etiologic factors of DI that can occur in the critical care setting are presented in Box 34.1.

Clinical Considerations

Clinical Presentation

Patients with DI usually present with polyuria, nocturia, and polydipsia. The daily volume of urine produced varies considerably from 3 to 20 L. Neurologic signs such as decreased level of consciousness or seizures do not occur unless marked hypernatremia occurs.

If the anterior pituitary is damaged, other clinical signs of pituitary dysfunction such as adrenal insufficiency, secondary hypothyroidism, or hypogonadism can occur. Importantly, treatment of adrenal insufficiency can unmask subclinical DI because glucocorticoids suppress ADH's response to osmotic stimuli and actions in the kidney.

Diagnosis

Signs that suggest DI include polyuria, which is usually defined as dilute urine with a daily output greater than 3 L, and associated polydipsia. If water excretion surpasses water intake, elevated plasma osmolality and hypernatremia occur, which in rare situations lead to hypovolemia. In the critical care setting, clinicians must be concerned if patients have an hourly urine output greater than 200 mL for 2 to 3 consecutive hours in the absence of fluid overload or severely positive fluid balance. In these patients, polyuria can be caused by DI or osmotic diuresis due to glucose, urea, or saline. Accordingly, determination of urine osmolality, plasma osmolality, and plasma sodium levels is helpful in the initial evaluation of polyuria. In patients with DI, urine osmolality (usually <250 mOsm/kg) is lower than plasma osmolality and can be accompanied by hypernatremia if fluids are not adequately replaced or if the patient has an impaired thirst mechanism or is unconscious. If polyuria results from osmotic diuresis, urine osmolality will increase. Figure 34.1 depicts a diagnostic evaluation algorithm for polyuria.

Postoperative excretion of excessive intravenous (IV) fluids is a common cause of polyuria. In this situation, the serum sodium level is normal or low. The diagnosis of milder forms of DI is more challenging because urine osmolality can be normal or even higher than plasma osmolality

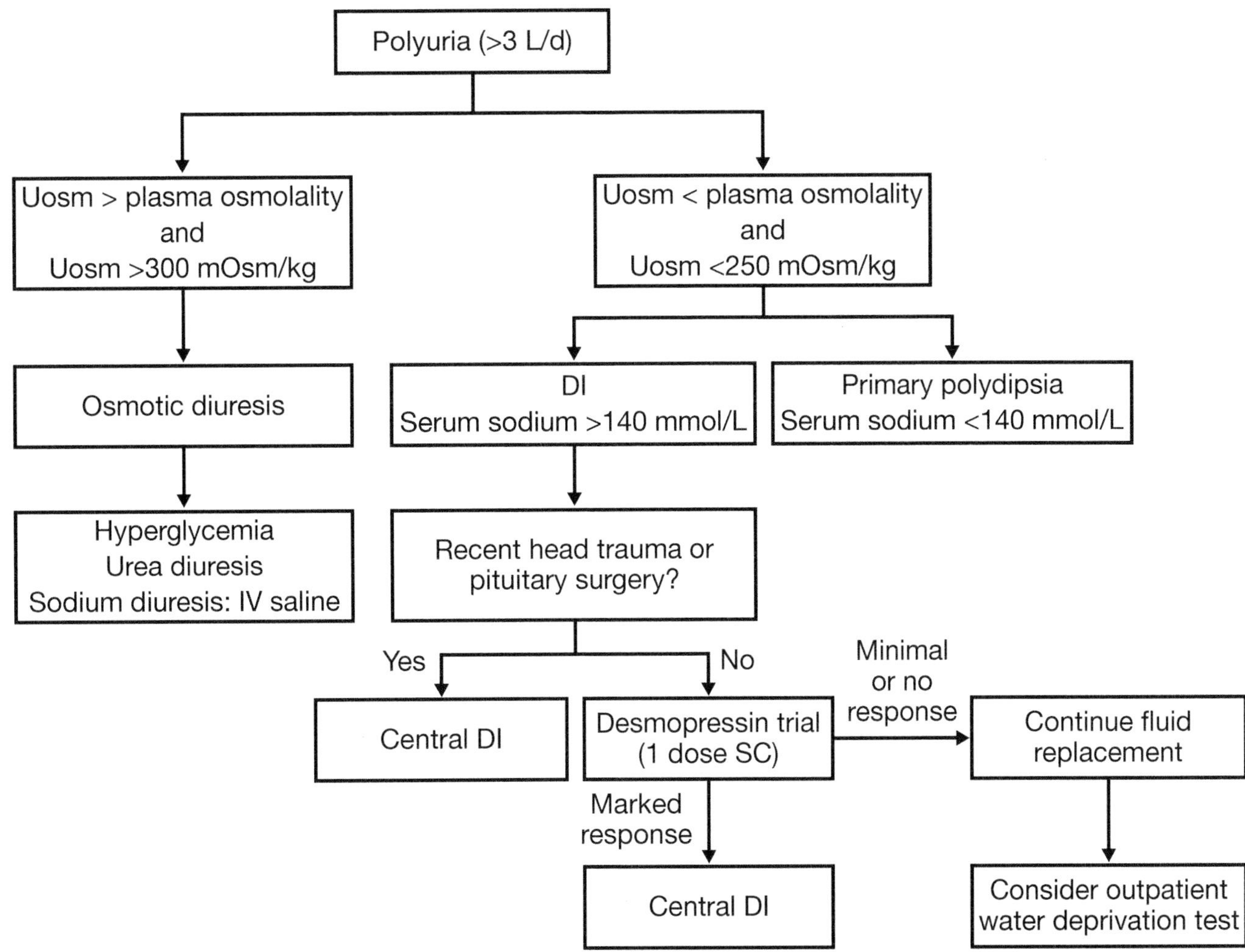

Figure 34.1. Evaluation of Polyuria and Diabetes Insipidus (DI) in the Intensive Care Unit. In the desmopressin trial, if the patient has no response to the subcutaneous (SC) dose, a higher dose may be given intravenously (IV). A marked response to the trial is defined as an increase in urine osmolality (Uosm) to more than 500 mOsm/kg and a decrease in urine volume by more than 50%. If the trial produces no response or a minimal response and the patient continues to be symptomatic, the water deprivation test may help distinguish partial central DI from nephrogenic DI.

in patients with partial central DI. Therefore, other confirmatory tests are needed such as the water deprivation test or direct plasma measurement of ADH activity and plasma copeptin, but these tests are performed in the outpatient setting.

Treatment of Central DI

The severity of central DI and the clinical circumstances of the patient (eg, neurologic status, oral intake, ability to recognize thirst) guide treatment. After central DI is diagnosed, serum sodium and osmolality should be serially monitored and the intensity of monitoring should be guided according to severity. Serum sodium might need to be measured every 4 to 6 hours depending on the degree of hypernatremia and therapeutic response. In general, sodium levels should not be decreased more than 12 mEq in 24 hours, especially in patients with hypernatremia for at least 48 hours or an unknown duration. Slowly decreasing the sodium level prevents the occurrence of brain edema, which is a rare potential complication caused by a very rapid decrease in sodium levels.

For patients with severe DI and large urine output, for patients who are intubated or unconscious, and for patients with altered thirst sensation, therapy should include fluid replacement with IV hypotonic fluids and administration of desmopressin (a vasopressin analogue).

When fluid replacement is needed, hypotonic fluids (eg, 5% dextrose in water [D5W] or half-normal saline) should be administered. Fluid intake and urinary losses should be matched milliliter for milliliter every 4 to 6 hours. If plasma

Box 34.2 • Management of Central Diabetes Insipidus

Short-term Management During Hospitalization

Replace ongoing urinary losses

- If the patient is awake with normal thirst, provide oral fluids (no more than needed to satisfy thirst)
- If the patient is lethargic or hypodipsic, administer hypotonic fluids IV (5% dextrose in water if sodium is increased; quarter- or half-normal saline if sodium is normal), and replace urinary and other fluid losses (milliliter for milliliter) every 4 to 6 hours

Correct hypernatremia

- Correct water deficit with hypotonic fluids and fluid replacement (replace half the water deficit in the first 24 hours and the remainder in the next 48 hours)[a]

Administer desmopressin

- Desmopressin is indicated if the patient cannot receive oral fluids or has impaired thirst or large urine output
- Initially administer desmopressin 0.5 to 1 mcg SC or IV every 8 to 14 hours according to urine output and osmolality[b]
- Subsequently administer desmopressin if diabetes insipidus recurs (as evidenced by decreased urine osmolality and increased urine output)
- Transition to oral or intranasal desmopressin when those routes can be used (approximately equivalent doses: 1 mcg SC or IV = 0.1 mg orally = 10 mcg intranasally)

Monitor for resolution of diabetes insipidus[c]

Long-term Management

Replace fluids

- If the patient has normal thirst, the patient may drink fluids to satisfy thirst
- If the patient is hypodipsic, prescribe fluid intake (usually 1.5-2.0 L daily)

Establish a goal weight (determined when the patient is euvolemic and normonatremic)

Measure urine output and weight daily to assess adequacy of fluid replacement

Consider whether serial plasma sodium measurements are needed

Adjust fluid intake (for 1.5-2.0 L daily) according to changes in body weight and sodium levels

Prescribe desmopressin

- Begin with 1 oral or intranasal dose at bedtime, increasing as needed to 2 to 3 doses daily
- Allow diabetes insipidus to recur between doses of desmopressin[d]

Prescribe other medications

- Less commonly, other medications with antidiuretic effects are needed (eg, carbamazepine, chlorpropamide, clofibrate, thiazide diuretics)

Abbreviations: IV, intravenously; SC, subcutaneously.

[a] Water Deficit = 0.6 × Body Weight (kg) × {[Serum Sodium (mmol/L)/140] − 1}.

[b] Patients' responses to the initial dose of desmopressin vary greatly, and the duration of action varies among patients. In addition, a higher dose has a longer duration of action.

[c] In most patients who have diabetes insipidus after pituitary surgery, and presumably in those with traumatic brain injury, diabetes insipidus is transient.

[d] Recurrence of diabetes insipidus, as indicated by increased urine output of dilute urine (with low urine osmolality), should be allowed between daily doses of desmopressin to prevent overtreatment, fluid retention, and hyponatremia.

sodium increases, the free water deficit should be calculated and replaced accordingly (Box 34.2).

Desmopressin is available in parenteral (IV or subcutaneous), oral, and intranasal preparations in North America. The parenteral route is preferable in the acute critical care setting. The initial dose can vary from 0.5 to 1 mcg (but 1 mcg is typical). The onset of action is 30 minutes, and the duration of action ranges from 6 to 14 hours depending on patient variability and the administered dose. A higher dose is associated with a longer duration of action. Subsequent doses are adjusted to the patient's response to the previous dose by reassessing urine output and osmolality. Desmopressin is administered as needed and tailored by the urine output response because DI can be transient after pituitary surgery and is sometimes followed by excessive ADH release and SIADH in patients with triphasic or biphasic

DI. Moreover, to avoid overtreatment, DI-associated polyuria should be allowed to recur before the next dose of desmopressin is administered. Recurrence is assessed by the reappearance of large urine output in conjunction with low urine osmolality. Oral or intranasal desmopressin can be administered in the outpatient setting or in the inpatient setting if desmopressin is still needed after a few days of therapy and if the nasal or oral route can be used. Box 34.2 shows treatment considerations for central DI in outpatient and inpatient settings.

The treatment of central DI is straightforward if the patient is conscious, has preserved thirst, and has free access to oral fluids because normal osmolality and serum sodium levels can be maintained by drinking fluids. Immediately after pituitary surgery, conscious patients should be encouraged to drink fluids to satisfy their thirst. Many patients do not require antidiuresis or IV fluid replacement because postoperative DI is usually mild and transient.

Summary

- Central DI results from complete or partial ADH deficiency and occurs most commonly after pituitary surgery and TBI.
- Fluid balance, urine osmolality, serum osmolality, and serum sodium levels should be initially assessed to evaluate polyuria and serially assessed if DI is confirmed.
- In most patients, DI is transient after pituitary surgery and TBI; therefore, patients with persistent DI should be reassessed periodically.
- Most nonsedated, alert patients with preserved thirst and an ample supply of water can maintain normal sodium levels. However, hypotonic fluid replacement and desmopressin are indicated for patients with central DI who are unconscious, have altered thirst, or cannot compensate for a large urine output despite oral intake.

SUGGESTED READING

Capatina C, Paluzzi A, Mitchell R, Karavitaki N. Diabetes insipidus after traumatic brain injury. J Clin Med. 2015 Jul 13;4(7):1448–62.

Fenske W, Allolio B. Clinical review: current state and future perspectives in the diagnosis of diabetes insipidus: a clinical review. J Clin Endocrinol Metab. 2012 Oct;97(10):3426–37. Epub 2012 Aug 1.

Garrahy A, Sherlock M, Thompson CJ. Management of endocrine disease: neuroendocrine surveillance and management of neurosurgical patients. Eur J Endocrinol. 2017 May;176(5):R217–33. Epub 2017 Feb 13.

Hannon MJ, Crowley RK, Behan LA, O'Sullivan EP, O'Brien MM, Sherlock M, et al. Acute glucocorticoid deficiency and diabetes insipidus are common after acute traumatic brain injury and predict mortality. J Clin Endocrinol Metab. 2013 Aug;98(8):3229–37. Epub 2013 May 20.

Hwang JJ, Hwang DY. Treatment of endocrine disorders in the neuroscience intensive care unit. Curr Treat Options Neurol. 2014 Feb;16(2):271.

Imga NN, Yildirim AE, Baser OO, Berker D. Clinical and hormonal characteristics of patients with different types of hypophysitis: a single-center experience. Arch Endocrinol Metab. 2019 Feb;63(1):47–52.

Lamas C, del Pozo C, Villabona C; Neuroendocrinology Group of the SEEN. Clinical guidelines for management of diabetes insipidus and syndrome of inappropriate antidiuretic hormone secretion after pituitary surgery. Endocrinol Nutr. 2014 Apr;61(4):e15–24. Epub 2014 Mar 1. English, Spanish.

Nemergut EC, Zuo Z, Jane JA Jr, Laws ER Jr. Predictors of diabetes insipidus after transsphenoidal surgery: a review of 881 patients. J Neurosurg. 2005 Sep;103(3):448–54.

Oiso Y, Robertson GL, Norgaard JP, Juul KV. Clinical review: treatment of neurohypophyseal diabetes insipidus. J Clin Endocrinol Metab. 2013 Oct;98(10):3958–67. Epub 2013 Jul 24.

Sav A, Rotondo F, Syro LV, Serna CA, Kovacs K. Pituitary pathology in traumatic brain injury: a review. Pituitary. 2019 Mar 29. [Epub ahead of print]

35 Panhypopituitarism

DIANE DONEGAN, MB, BCh; IRINA BANCOS, MD

Goals

- Describe the clinical presentation, diagnosis, and management of panhypopituitarism.
- Understand the pathophysiology of the hypothalamic-pituitary-adrenal axis.
- Understand the pathophysiology of the hypothalamic-pituitary-thyroid axis.
- Understand the pathophysiology of hypopituitarism and its effect on end organs.

Introduction

Hypopituitarism is defined as a deficiency in 1 or more pituitary hormones. The pituitary gland is composed of the anterior pituitary (*adenohypophysis*), which originates from an invagination of the oral ectoderm and forms the Rathke pouch, and the posterior pituitary (*neurohypophysis*), which is derived from the neural ectoderm of the diencephalon. The anterior pituitary is composed of 5 types of hormone-producing cells: 1) Somatotrophs produce growth hormone (GH); 2) gonadotrophs, follicle-stimulating hormone (FSH) and luteinizing hormone (LH); 3) thyrotrophs, thyrotropin; 4) lactotrophs, prolactin; and 5) corticotrophs, corticotropin. The posterior pituitary releases oxytocin and antidiuretic hormone (produced by the paraventricular and supraoptic neurons of the hypothalamus, respectively) through the axonal endings in the posterior lobe.

Identification of hypopituitarism is important because of its association with premature death due to respiratory and cardiovascular complications. Abrupt and severe deficiencies in corticotropin, thyrotropin, or antidiuretic hormone are potentially life-threatening complications; therefore, the use of dynamic or baseline tests to diagnose abnormal secretion of 1 or more pituitary hormones is paramount.

Etiology

The incidence of hypopituitarism is estimated to be 4 cases per 100,000 persons annually; the prevalence is estimated to be 45 cases per 100,000 persons. The risk of hypopituitarism depends on the underlying pathology, and pituitary adenoma and its treatment are the most common causes (Table 35.1). The pathophysiology of hypopituitarism also depends on the underlying etiologic factors, including vascular injury from portal vessel compression due to macroadenoma (>1 cm), pituitary hemorrhage or infarction (pituitary apoplexy), pituitary necrosis (Sheehan syndrome), trauma, radiotherapy, infiltration, genetic abnormalities, and immune activation (Table 35.1).

Presentation

Hypopituitarism may occur suddenly because of pituitary apoplexy, Sheehan syndrome, or inflammation. The resultant enlargement of the pituitary may lead to the sudden onset of severe headache, abnormal vision, or diplopia as a result of compression of adjacent structures (Chapter 33, "Pituitary Apoplexy"). In addition, nausea, vomiting, abdominal pain, and hypotension may occur if corticotropin deficiency and subsequent hypocortisolemia are present. If a patient has this constellation of symptoms, cortisol and corticotropin tests should be performed and, pending the results, a stress dose of corticosteroid should be administered immediately (Chapter 38, "Adrenal Insufficiency in Critical Care").

Patients may have more insidious presentations related to pituitary tumor, infiltrative disease, traumatic brain injury, or radiotherapy. The mass effect of a tumor may cause headache, visual changes, and oculomotor impairment; the partial or complete loss of 1 or more pituitary hormones may cause nonspecific symptoms such as fatigue,

Table 35.1 • Causes, Associated Risk Factors, and Manifestations of Hypopituitarism

Cause	Associated Risk Factors	Manifestations and Comments
Pituitary adenomas Functioning Nonfunctioning Nonpituitary tumors Craniopharyngioma Meningioma Dysgerminoma Glioma Chordoma Ependymoma Metastasis	Macroadenomas (>1 cm)	Headache, visual disturbance, and pituitary hormonal deficiency DI may occur in patients with suprasellar or stalk compression or an underlying metastatic tumor
Neurosurgery	Surgeon's experience Tumor volume, size, and infiltration	SIADH or DI may occur Assess the hypothalamic-pituitary-adrenal axis
TBI	Moderate to severe TBI, diffuse axonal injury, and skull base fracture	Signs can develop immediately or within 6 mo after injury GH, LH, and FSH deficiencies are the most common manifestations
Radiotherapy	Dose, location, and method of delivery	Most commonly affects GH; also affects LH, FSH, corticotropin, and thyrotropin
Vascular Pituitary apoplexy Sheehan syndrome Subarachnoid hemorrhage	Anticoagulation, pregnancy, severe blood loss, hypertension, and dynamic pituitary testing	Headache, vomiting, and visual impairment Failure to lactate or resume menstruation in patients with Sheehan syndrome
Infiltration Sarcoidosis Histiocytosis Hemochromatosis	Thickened pituitary stalk with or without DI with infiltration	Systemic manifestations DI with partial anterior pituitary deficiency is common
Infection	Surgery, tumor, radiotherapy, and systemic infection	Headache, visual disturbance, and pituitary hormone abnormalities Fever and leukocytosis may not occur
Immunologic Autoimmune hypophysitis	Pregnancy or postpartum period Use of CTLA-4 inhibitors or anti–PD-1 antibodies	Severe headache Corticotropin deficiency most commonly occurs
Genetic Includes mutations in the following transcription factors: HESX1, PROP1, POUF1, LHX3, LHX4, PITX1, OTX2, SOX2, and SOX3	Family history Typically occurs in infancy or adolescence	May be associated with developmental abnormalities (eg, midline structures, craniofacial defects)
Medications High doses of corticosteroids, opiates, and megestrol acetate	Dose and duration dependent Recent, sudden interruption of steroid therapy	Most commonly occurs with corticotropin deficiency and hypogonadism
Idiopathic	NA	Multiple, isolated hormonal abnormalities

Abbreviations: CTLA-4, cytotoxic T-lymphocyte–associated antigen 4; DI, diabetes insipidus; FSH, follicle-stimulating hormone; GH, growth hormone; LH, luteinizing hormone; NA, not applicable; PD-1, programmed cell death 1; SIADH, syndrome of inappropriate secretion of antidiuretic hormone; TBI, traumatic brain injury.

sleep disturbance, mental fogginess, oligomenorrhea, and reduced libido (in both sexes). An acute crisis in a patient with a chronic disease may be precipitated by a stressful event such as surgery or sepsis, which can lead to acute decompensation.

Investigation and Management

Assessment of pituitary function in critically ill patients can be hampered by altered metabolism of hormones and binding proteins, medication interactions, and associated

Table 35.2 • Evaluation and Treatment of Pituitary Hormone Deficiencies

Deficient Pituitary Hormone	Resulting Disease	Suggested Evaluation in the ICU	Criteria for Deficiency	Treatment
Corticotropin	Adrenal insufficiency	Measure cortisol and corticotropin Consider corticotropin stimulation test with 250 mcg cosyntropin	Random cortisol or peak cortisol <18 mcg/dL after corticotropin administration Corticotropin measurement differentiates pituitary deficiency and primary adrenal insufficiency	Stress dose of hydrocortisone
Thyrotropin	Hypothyroidism	Measure free thyroxine and thyrotropin	Low free thyroxine and low or normal thyrotropin Thyrotropin measurement differentiates pituitary deficiency and primary hypothyroidism	Levothyroxine 1.6 mcg/kg daily is the full replacement dose For elderly patients and patients with cardiovascular disease, start with a low dose (25 mcg) and adjust to maintain levels in the upper half of the reference range If patients have concomitant adrenal insufficiency, administer hydrocortisone before levothyroxine
GH	GH deficiency	Measure IGF-1[a]	IGF-1 less than lower limit of age-appropriate reference range	Defer GH replacement decisions until hospital discharge
Gonadotropins (LH and FSH)	Hypogonadism (testosterone or estrogen deficiency)	Measure estradiol or testosterone, and LH and FSH[a]	LH and FSH inappropriately low or normal In women, oligomenorrhea and undetectable estradiol In men, low testosterone	For premenopausal women, administer estrogen and progesterone For men, administer testosterone replacement
Prolactin	NA	Measure prolactin[a]	Less than lower limit of reference range	None

Abbreviations: FSH, follicle-stimulating hormone; GH, growth hormone; ICU, intensive care unit; IGF-1, insulinlike growth factor 1; LH, luteinizing hormone; NA, not applicable.

[a] Testing is not recommended unless the patient requires a prolonged stay.

comorbidities; therefore, results should be interpreted with caution. Identification of corticotropin or thyrotropin deficiency is essential (Table 35.2).

Hypothalamic-Pituitary-Adrenal Axis

If patients have clinical signs that are highly suggestive of adrenal insufficiency (hypotension, hyponatremia, and decreased level of consciousness), random plasma cortisol and corticotropin levels should be determined to assess function before stress doses of corticosteroids are administered. If the patient's condition is hemodynamically stable or the cortisol level is equivocal, a corticotropin stimulation test should be performed. A cortisol level of 18 mcg/dL or more effectively rules out adrenal insufficiency (Chapter 38, "Adrenal Insufficiency in Neurocritically Ill Patients").

Daily physiologic production of cortisol is estimated to be 15.5 to 19 mg; however, cortisol production increases in the presence of severe stress such as sepsis. If patients with adrenal insufficiency are ill, their daily dose of cortisol should be doubled or tripled. Intravenous corticosteroids are required in the critical care setting and preoperatively.

Hypothalamic-Pituitary-Thyroid Axis

Depending on the severity of the deficiency, the symptoms of central hypothyroidism are similar to those of primary hypothyroidism and include fatigue, constipation, cold intolerance, and decreased level of consciousness. Levels of both thyrotropin and free thyroxine should be measured to differentiate primary and secondary hypothyroidism. In secondary (central) hypothyroidism, thyrotropin is often low or inappropriately normal (ie, normal when it should not be), and free thyroxine is less than the lower limit of the reference range.

The thyroid hormone replacement dose depends on the severity of the deficiency and the presence of associated comorbidities. Cortisol reserve should be assessed and corticosteroids administered before thyroid hormone replacement because adrenal insufficiency may be precipitated by levothyroxine-induced accelerated cortisol metabolism. Replacement with a low dose of levothyroxine (25 mcg) is recommended for elderly patients and patients with cardiovascular disease; the dose should be increased as needed to maintain the free thyroxine level in the upper half of the reference range. Otherwise, higher doses (1.4-1.7 mcg/kg) may be administered to patients older than 60 years.

GH, LH, FSH, and Prolactin and Their End Organs

GH secretion is pulsatile; therefore, insulinlike growth factor 1 must be measured to assess the GH axis. In addition to estrogen and testosterone, LH and FSH can be measured to assess hypogonadism. Low levels of sex steroids in the presence of low or inappropriately low FSH and LH are consistent with hypogonadotropic (secondary) hypogonadism. Prolactin may increase from stalk compression or prolactinoma and may lead to hypogonadotropic hypogonadism; therefore, prolactin should be measured when a pituitary lesion is identified. Decisions about replacing these hormones can be postponed until hospital discharge.

In patients with chronic panhypopituitarism, levothyroxine should be continued and the corticosteroid dose adjusted. If the patient is already receiving testosterone or hormone replacement therapy and GH, these hormones may be continued in the absence of contraindications.

Summary

- Hypopituitarism may be the reason for hospital admission, it may develop as a complication, or it may be an established diagnosis.
- Identification and treatment of hypopituitarism are important, especially in adrenal or thyroid deficiency, because hypopituitarism is associated with increased morbidity and premature death.
- The most common causes of hypopituitarism are pituitary tumors and their treatment.
- Patients with hypopituitarism may present with clinical signs and symptoms that are acute or chronic.
- Appropriate laboratory testing will help identify etiologic factors, but if a patient is acutely ill, treatment (in particular, glucocorticoid replacement) should not be delayed.

SUGGESTED READING

Adams D, Kern PA. A case of pituitary abscess presenting without a source of infection or prior pituitary pathology. Endocrinol Diabetes Metab Case Rep. 2016;2016. pii: 16-0046. Epub 2016 Aug 16.

Appelman-Dijkstra NM, Malgo F, Neelis KJ, Coremans I, Biermasz NR, Pereira AM. Pituitary dysfunction in adult patients after cranial irradiation for head and nasopharyngeal tumours. Radiother Oncol. 2014 Oct;113(1):102–7. Epub 2014 Sep 15.

Bancos I, Hahner S, Tomlinson J, Arlt W. Diagnosis and management of adrenal insufficiency. Lancet Diabetes Endocrinol. 2015 Mar;3(3):216–26. Epub 2014 Aug 3.

Boonen E, Van den Berghe G. Endocrine responses to critical illness: novel insights and therapeutic implications. J Clin Endocrinol Metab. 2014 May;99(5):1569–82. Epub 2014 Feb 11.

Briet C, Salenave S, Chanson P. Pituitary apoplexy. Endocrinol Metab Clin North Am. 2015 Mar;44(1):199–209. Epub 2014 Nov 5.

Bujawansa S, Thondam SK, Steele C, Cuthbertson DJ, Gilkes CE, Noonan C, et al. Presentation, management and outcomes in acute pituitary apoplexy: a large single-centre experience from the United Kingdom. Clin Endocrinol (Oxf). 2014 Mar;80(3):419–24. Epub 2013 Aug 26.

Capatina C, Inder W, Karavitaki N, Wass JA. Management of endocrine disease: pituitary tumour apoplexy. Eur J Endocrinol. 2015 May;172(5):R179–90. Epub 2014 Dec 1.

Caturegli P. Autoimmune hypophysitis: an underestimated disease in search of its autoantigen(s). J Clin Endocrinol Metab. 2007 Jun;92(6):2038–40.

Clark PM, Gordon K. Challenges for the endocrine laboratory in critical illness. Best Pract Res Clin Endocrinol Metab. 2011 Oct;25(5):847–59.

Corsello SM, Barnabei A, Marchetti P, De Vecchis L, Salvatori R, Torino F. Endocrine side effects induced by immune checkpoint inhibitors. J Clin Endocrinol Metab. 2013 Apr;98(4):1361–75. Epub 2013 Mar 7.

Curto L, Trimarchi F. Hypopituitarism in the elderly: a narrative review on clinical management of hypothalamic-pituitary-gonadal, hypothalamic-pituitary-thyroid and hypothalamic-pituitary-adrenal axes dysfunction. J Endocrinol Invest. 2016 Oct;39(10):1115–24. Epub 2016 May 21.

Darzy KH. Radiation-induced hypopituitarism. Curr Opin Endocrinol Diabetes Obes. 2013 Aug;20(4):342–53.

Darzy KH. Radiation-induced hypopituitarism after cancer therapy: who, how and when to test. Nat Clin Pract Endocrinol Metab. 2009 Feb;5(2):88–99.

Hahner S, Loeffler M, Bleicken B, Drechsler C, Milovanovic D, Fassnacht M, et al. Epidemiology of adrenal crisis in chronic adrenal insufficiency: the need for new prevention strategies. Eur J Endocrinol. 2010 Mar;162(3):597–602. Epub 2009 Dec 2.

Higham CE, Johannsson G, Shalet SM. Hypopituitarism. Lancet. 2016 Nov 12;388(10058):2403–15. Epub 2016 Mar 31.

Jonklaas J, Bianco AC, Bauer AJ, Burman KD, Cappola AR, Celi FS, et al; American Thyroid Association Task Force on Thyroid Hormone Replacement. Guidelines for the treatment of hypothyroidism: prepared by the American Thyroid Association Task Force on Thyroid Hormone Replacement. Thyroid. 2014 Dec;24(12):1670–751.

Kelestimur F. Sheehan's syndrome. Pituitary. 2003;6(4):181–8.

Kraan GP, Dullaart RP, Pratt JJ, Wolthers BG, Drayer NM, De Bruin R. The daily cortisol production reinvestigated in healthy men: the serum and urinary cortisol production rates are not significantly different. J Clin Endocrinol Metab. 1998 Apr;83(4):1247–52.

Kurtulmus N, Mert M, Tanakol R, Yarman S. The pituitary gland in patients with Langerhans cell histiocytosis: a clinical and radiological evaluation. Endocrine. 2015 Apr;48(3):949–56. Epub 2014 Sep 11.

Littley MD, Shalet SM, Beardwell CG, Robinson EL, Sutton ML. Radiation-induced hypopituitarism is dose-dependent. Clin Endocrinol (Oxf). 1989 Sep;31(3):363–73.

Mathew V, Misgar RA, Ghosh S, Mukhopadhyay P, Roychowdhury P, Pandit K, et al. Myxedema coma: a new look into an old crisis. J Thyroid Res. 2011;2011:493462. Epub 2011 Sep 15.

McCabe MJ, Dattani MT. Genetic aspects of hypothalamic and pituitary gland development. Handb Clin Neurol. 2014;124:3–15.

Molitch ME, Clemmons DR, Malozowski S, Merriam GR, Vance ML; Endocrine Society. Evaluation and treatment of adult growth hormone deficiency: an Endocrine Society clinical practice guideline. J Clin Endocrinol Metab. 2011 Jun;96(6):1587–609.

Pappachan JM, Raskauskiene D, Kutty VR, Clayton RN. Excess mortality associated with hypopituitarism in adults: a meta-analysis of observational studies. J Clin Endocrinol Metab. 2015 Apr;100(4):1405–11. Epub 2015 Feb 6.

Pelusi C, Gasparini DI, Bianchi N, Pasquali R. Endocrine dysfunction in hereditary hemochromatosis. J Endocrinol Invest. 2016 Aug;39(8):837–47. Epub 2016 Mar 7.

Regal M, Paramo C, Sierra SM, Garcia-Mayor RV. Prevalence and incidence of hypopituitarism in an adult Caucasian population in northwestern Spain. Clin Endocrinol (Oxf). 2001 Dec;55(6):735–40.

Rupp D, Molitch M. Pituitary stalk lesions. Curr Opin Endocrinol Diabetes Obes. 2008 Aug;15(4):339–45.

Schneider HJ, Aimaretti G, Kreitschmann-Andermahr I, Stalla GK, Ghigo E. Hypopituitarism. Lancet. 2007 Apr 28;369(9571):1461–70.

Schneider HJ, Kreitschmann-Andermahr I, Ghigo E, Stalla GK, Agha A. Hypothalamopituitary dysfunction following traumatic brain injury and aneurysmal subarachnoid hemorrhage: a systematic review. JAMA. 2007 Sep 26;298(12):1429–38.

Sheehan JP, Pouratian N, Steiner L, Laws ER, Vance ML. Gamma Knife surgery for pituitary adenomas: factors related to radiological and endocrine outcomes. J Neurosurg. 2011 Feb;114(2):303–9. Epub 2010 Jun 11.

Sherlock M, Ayuk J, Tomlinson JW, Toogood AA, Aragon-Alonso A, Sheppard MC, et al. Mortality in patients with pituitary disease. Endocr Rev. 2010 Jun;31(3):301–42. Epub 2010 Jan 19.

Tanriverdi F, Schneider HJ, Aimaretti G, Masel BE, Casanueva FF, Kelestimur F. Pituitary dysfunction after traumatic brain injury: a clinical and pathophysiological approach. Endocr Rev. 2015 Jun;36(3):305–42. Epub 2015 May 7.

Tomlinson JW, Holden N, Hills RK, Wheatley K, Clayton RN, Bates AS, et al; West Midlands Prospective Hypopituitary Study Group. Association between premature mortality and hypopituitarism. Lancet. 2001 Feb 10;357(9254):425–31.

Yuen KC, Tritos NA, Samson SL, Hoffman AR, Katznelson L. American Association of Clinical Endocrinologists and American College of Endocrinology Disease State Clinical Review: update on growth hormone stimulation testing and proposed revised cut-point for the glucagon stimulation test in the diagnosis of adult growth hormone deficiency. Endocr Pract. 2016 Oct;22(10):1235–44. Epub 2016 Jul 13.

36 Thyroid Disorders in the Intensive Care Unit

JOHN E. MOSS, MD

Goals

- Describe the clinical features and management of myxedema coma.
- Elucidate the clinical presentation of patients with thyroid storm in the intensive care unit.
- Describe euthyroid sick syndrome.

Introduction

Thyroid disorders are relatively uncommon among patients in the intensive care unit (ICU) but may lead to serious morbidity and death. A working knowledge of these disorders is essential to their recognition and treatment, and an intensivist should be able to recognize and treat the 3 most common thyroid disorders in the ICU: myxedema coma, thyroid storm, and euthyroid sick syndrome.

Myxedema Coma

Myxedema coma is a severe thyroid hormone deficiency that results in an altered level of consciousness, hypothermia, and other hypothyroidism-related symptoms. Because of its high associated mortality rate, the clinical signs of myxedema coma must be immediately recognized and may include history of hypothyroidism, surgical scar on the neck, and history of hyperthyroidism treatment (including radioactive iodine administration). Myxedema coma is rare today because the widespread availability of thyrotropin assays allows early diagnosis.

Myxedema coma can be related to various nonthyroid illnesses, including heart disease and infection, and medications. Its occurrence can be isolated or associated with other autoimmune disease syndromes, and it is frequently associated with adrenal insufficiency. Patients often have low heart rate, heart failure, altered mental status, and hypothermia; they may have hyponatremia or hypoglycemia.

Objective testing for myxedema coma includes a thyroid panel and assessment of corticosteroid function to measure levels of thyrotropin, free thyroxine (T_4), and cortisol. Patients with primary hypothyroidism have a high thyrotropin level and a low T_4 level, but patients with central hypothyroidism can have low levels of both thyrotropin and T_4.

Because myxedema has been associated with mortality rates as high as 40%, treatment should not be delayed pending laboratory results. Treatment consists of thyroid hormone replacement and supportive care in addition to treatment of other associated conditions. Thyroid hormone should be administered as triiodothyronine (T_3) and T_4 because T_3 is more biologically active and T_4-to-T_3 conversion may be impaired in ill patients. A loading dose of T_4 (200-400 mcg) should be followed by a daily dose of 1.6 mcg/kg, and an initial dose of T_3 (5-20 mcg) should be followed by 2.5 to 10 mcg every 8 hours. T_3 is administered until the patient's condition is clinically stable, and then only T_4 should be administered. Because of the risk of coexisting adrenal insufficiency, patients should also be given 100 mg hydrocortisone every 8 hours until adrenal insufficiency is ruled out.

Thyroid Storm

Thyroid storm is a severe form of hyperthyroidism that requires prompt recognition and treatment because it is associated with high morbidity and mortality rates. It can be caused by severe hyperthyroidism (but the mechanism is unclear), or it can be secondary to other conditions such as nonthyroid illness, trauma, surgery, or childbirth. The symptoms of thyroid storm include tachycardia and other arrhythmias, hyperthermia, fever, agitation, anxiety, and abdominal symptoms. Patients may have other signs of thyroid disease such as exophthalmos, goiter, and tremor. If the patient's clinical signs suggest thyroid storm, blood samples should be obtained immediately for thyroid testing and the patient should be admitted to the ICU because the associated mortality rate is as high as 25%.

Laboratory findings show a low thyrotropin level and high T_4 and T_3 levels. Although total T_4 and T_3 levels are similar to those in patients with uncomplicated hyperthyroidism, free T_4 and free T_3 levels can be markedly increased. Other laboratory findings may include hyperglycemia, hypocalcemia, and abnormal results on liver function tests.

β-Blockers are often administered as the initial therapy because they help control hyperadrenergic tone; they should be administered with caution to patients with heart failure. Synthesis of new hormone is blocked with a thionamide drug such as propylthiouracil (initially 200 mg every 4 hours) or methimazole (20 mg every 4-6 hours); propylthiouracil may be preferable because it blocks T_4-to-T_3 conversion. Bile acid sequestrants are used to block enterohepatic recirculation of thyroid hormone (eg, 4 g cholestyramine 4 times daily).

Release of T_4 and T_3 from the thyroid gland is blocked by an iodine-containing solution such as strong iodine (Lugol) solution (10 drops 3 times daily) or saturated solution of potassium iodide (5 drops every 6 hours). These solutions should be administered at least 1 hour after a thionamide drug so that the iodine is not used to synthesize new hormone.

For life-threatening illness, hydrocortisone (100 mg every 9 hours) can be used to help decrease T_4-to-T_3 conversion and treat an underlying autoimmune disease.

After the patient's condition is stable, the β-blocker and steroid therapy can be stopped, but thionamide therapy should be continued and adjusted to maintain euthyroidism. Surgery may be necessary to treat Graves disease or a large toxic goiter.

Euthyroid Sick Syndrome

Thyroid function may be difficult to interpret when patients have a nonthyroid illness and variable levels of T_4, T_3, and thyrotropin. This condition, *euthyroid sick syndrome*, may be a form of acquired central hypothyroidism that protects against increased catabolism during critical illness. Measuring thyrotropin alone is inadequate for evaluating thyroid illness in these patients, and generally thyroid function tests are not performed unless thyroid disease is highly suggested. In patients with nonthyroid illness, T_4-to-T_3 conversion is impaired, and severely depressed T_4 levels during critical illness may be a marker of increased risk of death.

Thyroid hormone replacement (with T_3 or T_4) does not benefit patients who have a nonthyroid illness, and studies have shown no change in the mortality rate. Therefore, treatment is not recommended for critically ill patients with low thyroid hormone levels but no other signs of thyroid disease.

Summary

- Myxedema coma is a life-threatening hypothyroidism that is associated with various nonthyroidal illnesses.
- Myxedema coma is treated with hydrocortisone and thyroid hormone replacement.
- Thyroid storm, a severe form of hyperthyroidism, is treated with medications that block the action, release, or recirculation of thyroid hormone.
- Euthyroid sick syndrome, a common condition among patients in the ICU, should not be treated unless the patient has other signs of thyroid disease.

SUGGESTED READING

Chiha M, Samarasinghe S, Kabaker AS. Thyroid storm: an updated review. J Intensive Care Med. 2015 Mar;30(3):131–40. Epub 2013 Aug 5.

Dutta P, Bhansali A, Masoodi SR, Bhadada S, Sharma N, Rajput R. Predictors of outcome in myxoedema coma: a study from a tertiary care centre. Crit Care. 2008;12(1):R1. Epub 2008 Jan 3.

Hampton J. Thyroid gland disorder emergencies: thyroid storm and myxedema coma. AACN Adv Crit Care. 2013 Jul-Sep;24(3):325–32.

Hylander B, Rosenqvist U. Treatment of myxoedema coma: factors associated with fatal outcome. Acta Endocrinol (Copenh). 1985 Jan;108(1):65–71.

Jacobi J. Management of endocrine emergencies in the ICU. J Pharm Pract. 2019 Mar 10:897190019834771. [Epub ahead of print]

Jonklaas J, Bianco AC, Bauer AJ, Burman KD, Cappola AR, Celi FS, et al. Guidelines for the treatment of hypothyroidism: prepared by the American Thyroid Association Task Force on Thyroid Hormone Replacement. Thyroid. 2014 Dec;24(12):1670–751.

Nayak B, Burman K. Thyrotoxicosis and thyroid storm. Endocrinol Metab Clin North Am. 2006 Dec;35(4):663–86.

Wang HI, Yiang GT, Hsu CW, Wang JC, Lee CH, Chen YL. Thyroid storm in a patient with trauma: a challenging diagnosis for the emergency physician: case report and literature review. J Emerg Med. 2017 Mar;52(3):292–8. Epub 2016 Oct 11.

Glycemic Control in Neurocritically Ill Patients

CARLA P. VENEGAS-BORSELLINO, MD; MICHAEL A. PIZZI, DO, PhD; SANTIAGO NARANJO-SIERRA, MD

Goals

- Describe the importance of glycemic control in critical illness.
- Describe best practices of glycemic control.
- Describe risks of tight glycemic control.

Introduction

Hyperglycemia, hypoglycemia, and variable blood glucose levels are associated with poor outcomes in critically ill patients. This applies to both the general critical care population and the neurocritical care population. Patients with acute brain injury are sensitive to changes in glycemic levels because brain metabolism depends on a continuous, reliable supply of glucose. Hyperglycemia, which is prevalent in neurocritically ill patients, has been related to adverse outcomes after traumatic brain injury (TBI), ischemic stroke, intracranial hemorrhage, and subarachnoid hemorrhage (SAH).

Definitions and Epidemiology

Hyperglycemia

The prevalence of acute hyperglycemia in hospitalized patients ranges from 40% to 90% depending on the glycemic level cutoff used (most commonly, blood glucose >140 mg/dL or hemoglobin A_{1c} >6.5% in the absence of previous diabetes mellitus [DM]).

In critically ill patients, the diagnosis of acute hyperglycemia can be challenging because of increased capillary recruitment and poor peripheral perfusion and glucose intake. However, differentiating DM from acute hyperglycemia is important because hyperglycemia in DM patients has not been associated with worse outcomes, whereas patients with acute hyperglycemia do have higher morbidity and mortality. Acute hyperglycemia is related to a hypercatabolic state with inflammatory and neuroendocrine derangements leading to insulin resistance and gluconeogenesis.

Hypoglycemia

The lower limit of the reference range for the fasting glycemic concentration is 70 mg/dL. Hypoglycemia is considered mild if patients can self-manage it. Severe hypoglycemia requires resuscitative assistance and usually occurs when glycemic levels are less than 40 to 50 mg/dL. About 7% of patients admitted to the emergency department with altered mental status have hypoglycemia; severe hypoglycemia is more common among patients who have type 1 DM compared with type 2 DM.

In microdialysis studies, patients with acute brain injury have had profound neuroglycopenia after hypoglycemia, which contributes to metabolic distress and secondary brain injury. Undergoing intensive insulin therapy (IIT) increases a patient's risk of hypoglycemia, which can lead to coma or seizures.

Clinical Presentation

Patients with hypoglycemia or hyperglycemia usually have nonspecific signs and symptoms (eg, fatigue, weakness, and lethargy) that vary with the duration of DM, the patient's age, and accompanying metabolic changes. Hypoglycemic signs and symptoms can be divided into 3 groups: autonomic (occurring first at glycemic levels of 60-65 mg/dL); neuroglycopenic (at 45-59 mg/dL); and nonspecific (cognitive function deterioration occurring at <45 mg/dL).

Pathogenesis

Brain damage can be caused by primary and secondary injuries. Primary brain damage is irreversible and results from direct trauma, ischemia, or hemorrhage. Secondary brain damage is a consequence of the primary injury and is characterized by energy failure, oxidative stress, and production of free radicals, which lead to cerebral edema and inflammation. Hyperglycemia and hypercapnia aggravate acidosis, ischemia, and reperfusion injury, leading to cell death. An abnormal or interrupted supply of oxygen and glucose leads to catabolic deficits in brain cells with permanent tissue damage, poor neurologic outcomes, and a possible increase in in-hospital infections.

Hyperglycemia and glycemic level variability during critical illness involve multiple detrimental mechanisms, such as the production of proinflammatory cytokines and counterregulatory stress hormones. Administration of exogenous corticosteroids, parenteral nutrition, and frequent discontinuation of enteral feeding are contributing factors.

In contrast, hypoglycemia and neuroglycopenia have been associated with elevated peri-ischemic cortical depolarization and worse neurologic outcomes. Monitoring brain energy metabolism with microdialysis has shown that ischemia-induced low glucose and oxygen levels in the dialysate cause counterregulatory hyperemia and hyperglycemia and a dangerous variability in the cellular capacity for glucose uptake.

Glycemic Control in the General ICU

Management strategies for glycemic control in critically ill patients have varied. When IIT was used to maintain tight glycemic control (goal, 80-110 mg/dL) in surgical patients in the intensive care unit (ICU), ICU-related complications and mortality decreased 32% compared with traditional glucose control (goal >180 mg/dL), but the risk of hypoglycemia increased. IIT for medical patients in the ICU was beneficial if patients were in the ICU for more than 3 days, but mortality increased among patients with an ICU length of stay (LOS) less than 3 days. These differences suggest that the effects of IIT vary among types of critically ill patients.

The Normoglycemia in Intensive Care Evaluation—Survival Using Glucose Algorithm Regulation (NICE-SUGAR) trial evaluated the effect of IIT on ICU mortality. Patients receiving IIT (blood glucose goal, 81-108 mg/dL) were compared with a control group (goal <180 mg/dL). A higher percentage of patients in the IIT group had severe hypoglycemia (6.8% vs 0.5%), cardiovascular-related death (by 5.8%), absolute risk of death at 90 days (by 2.6%, with a number needed to harm of 38). The trial showed that hypoglycemia was less common and mortality was lower among patients with moderate blood glucose levels of 140 to 180 mg/dL.

A review of 36 randomized controlled trials found that very mild, mild, moderate, and tight control of blood glucose levels did not decrease short-term mortality. However, severe hypoglycemia was 5-fold more common with tight control compared with very mild or mild control. Other variables, such as cause of death, presence of DM, or type of ICU, were not significantly different between groups. After ranked analysis, the safety ranking from highest to lowest was mild control, tight control, and very mild control.

A *U*-shaped curve has been described between mean absolute glycemia and ICU mortality, with a safe margin from 126 to 162 mg/dL, and has prompted a recommendation to minimize changes in glycemic variability and avoid both hypoglycemia and hyperglycemia. Consequently, bolus administration of insulin and glucose solutions should be strictly avoided. The recommendation is to accurately monitor glycemic levels and administer insulin therapy along with adequate enteral or parenteral nutrition.

Risks Related to Hyperglycemia

Glycemic levels greater than 180 mg/dL are associated with higher mortality, longer LOS, and, most importantly, higher rates of ICU-related infections. There is evidence that the relation between mean blood glucose levels at ICU admission and mortality is represented by a *U*-shaped curve, where patients with blood glucose levels less than 120 mg/dL or greater than 162 mg/dL have increased mortality. The stress response in trauma patients triggers catabolism, which leads to protein breakdown and hyperglycemia. High glycemic concentrations have been linked to increased intracranial pressure, prolonged hospital stay, poor neurologic function, and higher mortality among patients with TBI. Prevention of hyperglycemia has decreased LOS, infection rates, pharmacy costs, laboratory testing, and imaging use.

Risks Related to Hypoglycemia

Even a sole mild hypoglycemic event (eg, blood glucose 72-81 mg/dL) can increase ICU LOS and hospital mortality, independently of the severity of disease.

Risks Related to Blood Glucose Variablity

Multiple studies have shown an association between ICU mortality and blood glucose variability with different standard deviation levels of mean absolute glycemia. In a computerized sliding-scale analysis, the hourly change in mean absolute glycemia per patient was associated with ICU death when the blood glucose level was too low or too high. This trend was apparent in the first 24 hours after surgery and has been confirmed in prospective studies.

Glycemic Control in the Neurocritical Care Unit

It is unclear whether nonphysiologic glycemic levels are markers of disease severity or contribute to secondary injury. Multiple authors have found no relationship between initial hyperglycemia and poor prognosis, but failure to achieve normoglycemia during critical illness results in a detrimental outcome. The optimal glycemic management for patients with acute brain injury requires special considerations, which may differ from those for general patient populations. For example, decreasing mortality and achieving functional recovery are essential end points.

A major concern with IIT for neurocritically ill patients is the danger of neuroglycopenia because brain glucose uptake and metabolism are esentially supply driven. Some authors have suggested that IIT can be harmful and worsen outcomes for patients with neurologic disease; other authors have reported that use of IIT may help patients avoid neurologic complications. Hence, the use of IIT in the neurocritical care unit is controversial, perhaps requiring different recommendations for specific types of acute brain injury.

The most comprehensive meta-analysis involving neurocritically ill patients compared the use of IIT with conventional glycemic control and included patients with TBI, cerebrovascular disease, encephalopathy, meningitis and encephalitis, and spinal cord injuries. In neurocritical care patients, IIT did not influence mortality and increased the risk of hypoglycemia. Although IIT resulted in fewer unfavorable neurologic outcomes, this benefit was not apparent when IIT was compared with moderate glycemic targets (110-180 mg/dL); therefore, the IIT benefits were probably derived from decreased secondary injury that resulted from keeping glycemic levels less than 180 mg/dL.

In general, a *U*-shaped curve describes the relationship between serum glycemic levels and neurologic function. Extremes at both ends of the curve (hypoglycemia and hyperglycemia) are harmful, so the optimal glucose target for neurocritical care patients is 80 to 180 mg/dL.

Stroke

Hyperglycemia is common in patients (even nondiabetic patients) who have acute ischemic stroke, especially stroke that has extensive infarcts or affects the insular cortex. Hyperglycemia can induce higher metabolic demand in the ischemia penumbra, liberating free radicals, and cause lactic acidemia, neuronal death, or deterioration of the blood-brain barrier. Hyperglycemia has been related to hemorrhagic transformation and cerebral edema in ischemic brain tissue, leading to poor neurologic functional outcomes. A glycemic level greater than 140 mg/dL and a hemoglobin A_{1c} level greater than 6.5% are independent risk factors for poor outcomes after treatment with tissue plasminogen activator, intra-arterial thrombolysis, or thrombectomy. Hemorrhagic transformation appears to be related to increased levels of matrix metalloproteinase 3, and it is best predicted with the SEDAN score, which, as part of the score, assigns 1 point for blood glucose 145 to 216 mg/dL and 2 points for blood glucose greater than 216 mg/dL. Hyperglycemia impairs recanalization, decreases tissue plasminogen activator activity, and increases coagulation through elevated thrombin-antithrombin complexes and the tissue factor pathway.

Although some studies have shown no benefit from IIT, and others have reported 30-day improvement in neurologic function as measured with the National Institutes of Health Stroke Scale score, the ideal management for this patient population remains controversial. Currently, the European Stroke Initiative and the American Heart Association/American Stroke Association guidelines recommend an optimal glucose of 140 to 180 mg/dL. An ongoing multicenter, randomized trial (Stroke Hyperglycemia Insulin Network Effort [SHINE]) is evaluating the effects of glucose control (goal, 80-130 mg/dL) on functional outcomes for patients with acute stroke.

Subarachnoid Hemorrhage

Hypoglycemia, hyperglycemia, and acute fluctuations of glycemic levels increase oxidative stress and exacerbate secondary brain injury after SAH, leading to worse functional outcome and mortality.

Hyperglycemia, linked to the development of clinical vasospasm, occurs in 70% to 90% of patients with SAH. SAH patients treated with good glycemic control have a smaller chance of poor outcome, but SAH patients treated with IIT instead of conventional glucose management show no difference in rate of clinical vasospasm, delayed ischemic neurologic deficit, or development of clinical complications.

In SAH patients, greater glycemic variability (measured with cerebral microdialysis) has been associated with symptomatic vasospasm and increased in-hospital mortality after stratification by age, the Hunt and Hess grading system, and daily score on the Glasgow Coma Scale. Although it is well documented that patients with greater blood glucose fluctuations have poorer outcomes, the best measure to evaluate the amplitude of the fluctuation is currently undefined. In comparisons of the standard deviation and mean absolute glycemia index, the absolute change in glucose per hour, and the glycemic lability index, the standard deviation and mean absolute glycemia index has been the only accurate hospital mortality predictor.

Traumatic Brain Injury

In studies of patients with TBI, IIT did not improve neurologic outcomes and IIT increased episodes of hypoglycemia. In patients with severe TBI, IIT induced an abrupt increase in cerebral metabolic crisis (as measured by microdialysis). In additional analysis, however, IIT was associated with shorter ICU stays and lower infection rates. Therefore, moderate glycemic levels (120-150 mg/dL) may be adequate to provide continuous glucose supply to the brain in this critical period.

Management

Although poor glycemic control in critical care patients carries a worse prognosis, IIT offers no mortality benefit and carries a higher risk of hypoglycemia. This effect, however, is likely not static among all subsets of ICU patients, particularly those with neurologic insults. When ICU patients were grouped into different blood glucose target levels, the range of 129 to 145 mg/dL was associated with the lowest mortality rate and least risk of hypoglycemia, indicating that this range is optimal for critically ill patients. In addition, maintaining a blood glucose level less than 180 mg/dL may improve neurologic outcomes among neurocritically ill patients.

Important variables that can affect reaching the target blood glucose level include nutritional protocols, route of nutritional support, and duration of insulin infusion, which is affected by insulin resistance over time. The duration of insulin infusion is a predictor of severe hypoglycemia, and its occurrence does not reflect illness severity. The relationship with duration of insulin infusion can possibly be explained by the induced changes in insulin sensitivity. A meta-analysis of ICU patients showed that IIT (goal, 80-110 mg/dL) may be harmful for patients receiving enteral nutrition, yet it appears to improve outcomes for patients receiving parenteral nutrition.

The current recommendation is to give insulin infusions to maintain blood glucose levels at 140 to 180 mg/dL (as in the NICE-SUGAR trial). Safe blood glucose targets and estimates of optimal insulin dose titration should include an adequate nutrition protocol, an appropriate duration of insulin infusion, and consideration of insulin sensitivity changing over time.

Glycemic control recommendations in the neurocritical care unit have changed considerably. Given their potential harm if blood glucose values are extreme or fluctuating, glycemic levels and their variability deserve committed clinical attention. Patients receiving IIT should be closely monitored and provided with appropriate enteral or parenteral nutrition to avoid iatrogenic hypoglycemia. Neurocritically ill patients require individualized therapy, with goals related to the specific type of brain injury, and any new recommendations should be supported with new technologies.

Summary

- Hyperglycemia, hypoglycemia, and high variability in blood glucose levels are associated with worse outcomes among critically ill patients.
- Ideal blood glucose control remains unknown, but studies suggest no benefit from tight control over moderate control.
- Neurocritically ill patients may benefit from therapy tailored to the specific type of brain injury.

SUGGESTED READING

Arabi YM, Tamim HM, Rishu AH. Hypoglycemia with intensive insulin therapy in critically ill patients: predisposing factors and association with mortality. Crit Care Med. 2009 Sep;37(9):2536–44.

Bilotta F, Badenes R, Lolli S, Belda FJ, Einav S, Rosa G. Insulin infusion therapy in critical care patients: regular insulin vs short-acting insulin: a prospective, crossover, randomized, multicenter blind study. J Crit Care. 2015 Apr;30(2):437.e1–6. Epub 2014 Oct 30.

Bilotta F, Rosa G. Glucose management in the neurosurgical patient: are we yet any closer? Curr Opin Anaesthesiol. 2010 Oct;23(5):539–43.

Bilotta F, Rosa G. Optimal glycemic control in neurocritical care patients. Crit Care. 2012 Oct 30;16(5):163.

Bilotta F, Spinelli A, Giovannini F, Doronzio A, Delfini R, Rosa G. The effect of intensive insulin therapy on infection rate, vasospasm, neurologic outcome, and mortality in neurointensive care unit after intracranial aneurysm clipping in patients with acute subarachnoid hemorrhage: a randomized prospective pilot trial. J Neurosurg Anesthesiol. 2007 Jul;19(3):156–60.

Bruno A, Durkalski VL, Hall CE, Juneja R, Barsan WG, Janis S, et al; SHINE investigators. The Stroke Hyperglycemia Insulin Network Effort (SHINE) trial protocol: a randomized, blinded, efficacy trial of standard vs. intensive hyperglycemia management in acute stroke. Int J Stroke. 2014 Feb;9(2):246–51. Epub 2013 Mar 19.

Chowdhury T, Kowalski S, Arabi Y, Dash HH. General intensive care for patients with traumatic brain injury: an update. Saudi J Anaesth. 2014 Apr;8(2):256–63.

Egi M, Bellomo R, Stachowski E, French CJ, Hart GK, Hegarty C, et al. Blood glucose concentration and outcome of critical illness: the impact of diabetes. Crit Care Med. 2008 Aug;36(8):2249–55.

Egi M, Bellomo R, Stachowski E, French CJ, Hart GK, Taori G, et al. The interaction of chronic and acute glycemia with mortality in critically ill patients with diabetes. Crit Care Med. 2011 Jan;39(1):105–11.

Fahy BG, Coursin DB. Critical glucose control: the devil is in the details. Mayo Clin Proc. 2008 Apr;83(4):394–7.

Gunst J, De Bruyn A, Van den Berghe G. Glucose control in the ICU. Curr Opin Anaesthesiol. 2019 Apr;32(2):156–62.

Hermanides J, Vriesendorp TM, Bosman RJ, Zandstra DF, Hoekstra JB, Devries JH. Glucose variability is associated with intensive care unit mortality. Crit Care Med. 2010 Mar;38(3):838–42.

Kramer AH, Roberts DJ, Zygun DA. Optimal glycemic control in neurocritical care patients: a systematic review and meta-analysis. Crit Care. 2012 Oct 22;16(5):R203.

Krinsley J, Schultz MJ, Spronk PE, van Braam Houckgeest F, van der Sluijs JP, Melot C, et al. Mild hypoglycemia is strongly associated with increased intensive care unit length of stay. Ann Intensive Care. 2011 Nov 24;1:49.

Krinsley JS. Glycemic variability: a strong independent predictor of mortality in critically ill patients. Crit Care Med. 2008 Nov;36(11):3008–13.

Marik PE, Preiser JC. Toward understanding tight glycemic control in the ICU: a systematic review and metaanalysis. Chest. 2010 Mar;137(3):544–51. Epub 2009 Dec 16.

NICE-SUGAR Study Investigators, Finfer S, Chittock DR, Su SY, Blair D, Foster D, Dhingra V, et al. Intensive versus conventional glucose control in critically ill patients. N Engl J Med. 2009 Mar 26;360(13):1283–97. Epub 2009 Mar 24.

Osei E, den Hertog HM, Berkhemer OA, Fransen PS, Roos YB, Beumer D, et al; MR CLEAN pretrial investigators. Increased admission and fasting glucose are associated with unfavorable short-term outcome after intra-arterial treatment of ischemic stroke in the MR CLEAN pretrial cohort. J Neurol Sci. 2016 Dec 15;371:1–5. Epub 2016 Oct 6.

Rostami E. Glucose and the injured brain-monitored in the neurointensive care unit. Front Neurol. 2014 Jun 6;5:91.

Siegelaar SE, Hermanides J, Oudemans-van Straaten HM, van der Voort PH, Bosman RJ, Zandstra DF, et al. Mean glucose during ICU admission is related to mortality by a U-shaped curve in surgical and medical patients: a retrospective cohort study. Crit Care. 2010;14(6):R224. Epub 2010 Dec 10.

Singh V, Edwards NJ. Advances in the critical care management of ischemic stroke. Stroke Res Treat. 2013;2013:510481. Epub 2013 May 16.

Smith FG, Sheehy AM, Vincent JL, Coursin DB. Critical illness-induced dysglycaemia: diabetes and beyond. Crit Care. 2010;14(6):327. Epub 2010 Nov 5.

Stoudt K, Chawla S. Don't sugar coat it: glycemic control in the intensive care unit. J Intensive Care Med. 2018 Oct 11:885066618801748. [Epub ahead of print]

Strbian D, Engelter S, Michel P, Meretoja A, Sekoranja L, Ahlhelm FJ, et al. Symptomatic intracranial hemorrhage after stroke thrombolysis: the SEDAN score. Ann Neurol. 2012 May;71(5):634–41.

Taylor BE, McClave SA, Martindale RG, Warren MM, Johnson DR, Braunschweig C, et al. Guidelines for the provision and assessment of nutrition support therapy in the adult critically ill patient: Society of Critical Care Medicine (SCCM) and American Society for Parenteral and Enteral Nutrition (A.S.P.E.N.). Crit Care Med. 2016 Feb;44(2):390–438.

Tsai SH, Lin YY, Hsu CW, Cheng CS, Chu DM. Hypoglycemia revisited in the acute care setting. Yonsei Med J. 2011 Nov;52(6):898–908.

Van den Berghe G, Schoonheydt K, Becx P, Bruyninckx F, Wouters PJ. Insulin therapy protects the central and peripheral nervous system of intensive care patients. Neurology. 2005 Apr 26;64(8):1348–53.

Van den Berghe G, Wilmer A, Hermans G, Meersseman W, Wouters PJ, Milants I, et al. Intensive insulin therapy in the medical ICU. N Engl J Med. 2006 Feb 2;354(5):449–61.

van den Berghe G, Wouters P, Weekers F, Verwaest C, Bruyninckx F, Schetz M, et al. Intensive insulin therapy in critically ill patients. N Engl J Med. 2001 Nov 8;345(19):1359–67.

Vespa P, Boonyaputthikul R, McArthur DL, Miller C, Etchepare M, Bergsneider M, et al. Intensive insulin therapy reduces microdialysis glucose values without altering glucose utilization or improving the lactate/pyruvate ratio after traumatic brain injury. Crit Care Med. 2006 Mar;34(3):850–6.

Vespa PM, McArthur D, O'Phelan K, Glenn T, Etchepare M, Kelly D, et al. Persistently low extracellular glucose correlates with poor outcome 6 months after human traumatic brain injury despite a lack of increased lactate: a microdialysis study. J Cereb Blood Flow Metab. 2003 Jul;23(7):865–77.

Viana MV, Moraes RB, Fabbrin AR, Santos MF, Gerchman F. [Assessment and treatment of hyperglycemia in critically ill patients]. Rev Bras Ter Intensiva. 2014 Jan-Mar;26(1):71–6. Portuguese.

Workgroup on Hypoglycemia, American Diabetes Association. Defining and reporting hypoglycemia in diabetes: a report from the American Diabetes Association Workgroup on Hypoglycemia. Diabetes Care. 2005 May;28(5):1245–9.

Yamada T, Shojima N, Noma H, Yamauchi T, Kadowaki T. Glycemic control, mortality, and hypoglycemia in critically ill patients: a systematic review and network meta-analysis of randomized controlled trials. Intensive Care Med. 2017 Jan;43(1):1–15. Epub 2016 Sep 16.

Zafar SN, Iqbal A, Farez MF, Kamatkar S, de Moya MA. Intensive insulin therapy in brain injury: a meta-analysis. J Neurotrauma. 2011 Jul;28(7):1307–17.

Adrenal Insufficiency in Neurocritically Ill Patients

CARLA P. VENEGAS-BORSELLINO, MD;
SANTIAGO NARANJO-SIERRA, MD

Goals

- Describe critical illness–related corticosteroid insufficiency.
- Understand common limitations in the diagnosis of critical illness–related corticosteroid insufficiency.
- Know general measures for management of critical illness–related corticosteroid insufficiency.
- Describe specific considerations for critical illness–related corticosteroid insufficiency in neurocritically ill patients.

Introduction

The hypothalamic-pituitary-adrenal (HPA) axis is a complex system that equilibrates blood levels of glucocorticoid hormones. Cortisol levels are dynamic and normally fluctuate in response to constant feedback; functional deficiency in this system results in adrenal insufficiency (AI). An elevated corticosteroid level is needed as a protective response to stress during acute illness or major surgery, but corticosteroid secretion can be altered by splanchnic and central nervous system influence, fever, acidosis, and proinflammatory cytokines. Critical illness–related corticosteroid insufficiency (CIRCI) is a relatively insufficient HPA response; often encountered in critical care patients, it can worsen outcomes.

The concept, diagnosis, and management of CIRCI are controversial. The pathophysiology is poorly understood, and cortisol levels are affected by corticotropin-releasing hormone and corticotropin stimulation, which influence tumor necrosis factor α and interleukins 1 and 6. New data suggest that CIRCI is more likely attributed to abnormal cortisol breakdown and target tissue resistance than to cortisol production, and adrenal cortex dysfunction is likely a response to high concentrations of plasma cortisol related to elevated corticotropin concentrations through feedback inhibition. This mechanism could explain why AI occurs in persistent critical disease.

In neurocritical care, disturbances in the HPA axis are a leading cause of long-term neurophysiologic sequelae after neurologic insults such as traumatic brain injury (TBI) and subarachnoid hemorrhage (SAH), so routine screening is recommended. Study results imply that HPA axis dysfunction may affect hemodynamic responses, immunomodulation, and outcomes from neurologic injuries. Both primary and secondary HPA failures may be involved.

Changes in adrenal function during persistent critical illness are poorly understood, but patients with a lower cortisol level require longer mechanical ventilator support and longer hospital and intensive care unit stays. Therefore, monitoring adrenal function in these patients is important.

Definitions

AI can be classified as absolute (primary, secondary, or tertiary AI) or relative. *Primary AI* originates in the adrenal cortex, so baseline and poststimulation concentrations of cortisol are decreased. *Secondary AI* results from impaired corticotropin secretion caused by pituitary abnormalities; the initial cortisol level is low, but it increases after stimulation (from a positive adrenal gland response). *Tertiary AI* is caused by insufficient secretion and function of arginine vasopressin or corticotropin-releasing hormone; it is commonly related to long-term glucocorticoid use, resulting in suppression of the HPA axis through negative feedback inhibition. *Relative AI* can result from CIRCI; from medications that affect cortisol production (eg, etomidate) or the

HPA axis (eg, antifungals, opioids, tricyclic antidepressants, anticoagulants, rifampin, and antiepileptics such as phenobarbital and phenytoin); or from injury due to adrenal hemorrhage or thrombosis of the adrenal vein.

The prevalence of CIRCI is unknown because there is no consensus for what constitutes an appropriate HPA-axis response in critically ill patients. Proposed diagnostic values include random cortisol levels of less than 10 mcg/dL or less than 25 mcg/dL or a corticotropin stimulation test response with a change in the serum cortisol level (delta cortisol) of less than 9 mcg/dL. An American College of Critical Care Medicine (ACCM) task force presented a consensus statement that defined *CIRCI* as AI resulting from a proinflammatory response associated with peripheral corticosteroid resistance; however, the diagnostic criteria are problematic. According to the task force, a diagnosis of CIRCI is most likely when delta cortisol is less than 9 mcg/dL after administration of 250 mcg of cosyntropin or when random total cortisol is less than 10 mcg/dL. CIRCI is less likely when serum cortisol levels surpass 34 mcg/dL.

AI may also develop during a protracted critical illness. Its diagnosis is easily missed, and there is no agreement on the appropriate frequency for testing adrenal function; however, any deteriorating clinical condition or indicators suggesting AI should prompt reevaluation for it.

Epidemiology

AI occurs in 25% of patients after TBI and in up to 40% of patients after a neurologic injury. CIRCI occurs in 55% of patients with polytrauma, and 95% of the diagnoses are made within 48 hours after the initial traumatic injury. These patients have much higher 28-day mortality (40%) than patients without CIRCI. Surprisingly, delta cortisol of less than 9 mcg/dL (but not an initially low cortisol level <10 mcg/dL) is an independent mortality risk factor.

Clinical Presentation

CIRCI with absolute AI must be considered in patients with shock and a poor response to fluid resuscitation and vasopressors. AI can coexist with or mimic sepsis, septic shock, or underlying diseases; therefore, identifying those conditions may be difficult. Clinical suspicion for AI should be increased if the patient has associated signs such as hyperpigmentation, hyponatremia, hyperkalemia, hypercalcemia, metabolic acidosis, eosinophilia, or unexplained hypoglycemia and fever.

Subarachnoid Hemorrhage

Serious dysregulation has been documented in the HPA axis after SAH. Initially cortisol levels are elevated. In the postacute period, cortisol levels approach normal concentrations, with no association between the severity of SAH and the serum level of cortisol. In the chronic phase (month to years), AI seems to be present in one-third of patients.

Traumatic Brain Injury

AI is common after severe TBI, with an incidence of 25% to 100% depending on the definition used. If patients are hemodynamically unstable, baseline and postcorticotropin cortisol levels should be measured to determine the type of AI, but controversy still surrounds cortisol cutoff values and treatment recommendations.

Spinal Cord Injury

Patients with acute or chronic spinal cord injury have a higher risk for AI. The reason is unclear, but it appears to be related to sympathetic denervation and chronic corticotropin secretion due to adrenal hypoperfusion and atrophy. The diagnosis should be considered if the patient has appropriate clinical signs and symptoms, low cortisol levels, and a positive response to replacement corticosteroid therapy.

Diagnosis

The ACCM task force recommends diagnosing CIRCI when random total cortisol levels are less than 10 mcg/dL or delta cortisol is less than 9 mcg/dL after stimulation with 250 mcg corticotropin. However, the stimulation test is not recommended for patients with septic shock or acute respiratory distress syndrome (ARDS) who may benefit from receiving glucocorticoids.

Management

If patients are receiving long-term systemic glucocorticoid therapy or are known to have primary or secondary AI, short-term stress doses of glucocorticoid replacement are recommended. Glucocorticoid replacement therapy can also be used in patients with CIRCI; mortality has decreased in up to 10% of those patients and in patients with refractory septic shock or early severe ARDS (Pao_2/fraction of inspired oxygen ≤200 within 14 days after onset). Treatment recommendations for patients with CIRCI are summarized in Box 38.1.

Neurocritical Care

For neurocritical care patients with TBI, the use of hydrocortisone to manage CIRCI seems to be associated with favorable neurologic outcomes. For patients with SAH, however, the use of steroids has caused variable outcomes, ranging from providing no benefit to being harmful: The use of fludrocortisone has been weakly associated with

Box 38.1 • Treatment of CIRCI

Hydrocortisone (50 mg every 6 hours or 10 mg/h continuous infusion [240 mg/daily] up to 7 days) is recommended for refractory septic shock after appropriate fluid resuscitation and vasopressor therapy.

Methylprednisolone (1 mg/kg daily up to 14 days) is recommended for patients with severe, early ARDS. The effectiveness of glucocorticoid therapy for ARDS has been studied, but its effect on mortality is still uncertain: It may be beneficial during the first 14 days after diagnosis but possibly harmful after that period.

The glucocorticoid dose should be decreased slowly and not terminated abruptly: After the patient is hemodynamically stable, 50 mg can be given every 6 hours; the next day, 25 mg is given every 6 hours, and the dose is tapered to the maintenance dose by days 4 to 6.

If the patient has signs of clinical deterioration (hypoxia, hypotension, or recurrent sepsis) reinitiation of the therapy may be recommended.

Use of dexamethasone is not recommended in patients with CIRCI, but it can be used temporarily if diagnostic confirmation is desired.

Abbreviations: ARDS, acute respiratory distress syndrome; CIRCI, critical illness–related corticosteroid insufficiency.

decreased cerebral ischemia and lower mortality; the use of hydrocortisone has resulted in an increased 1-month mortality rate and a higher incidence of hyperglycemia; and the use of high doses of methylprednisolone (18 mg/kg daily) has improved functional outcome (but the unusual study design excluded all patient deaths).

Postoperative Management

Patients who receive long-term corticosteroid therapy and undergo major surgery may not need stress doses of corticosteroids to improve their hemodynamic status and decrease their risk of death. Instead, administering an equivalent dose of corticosteroids intravenously may suffice. The exception is patients with Addison disease who cannot produce the extra cortisol required. For those patients, stress doses of corticosteroids improve hemodynamic parameters but not mortality, so patients should be classified according to HPA axis suppression: The HPA axis is assumed to be suppressed if a patient has taken at least 20 mg of prednisone daily for more than 3 weeks or if the patient has Cushingoid characteristics. If a patient has taken smaller doses of prednisone for shorter times, the HPA axis is probably not suppressed and specific corticosteroid coverage is not required.

Glucocorticoids in Sepsis

Various trials and heterogeneous meta-analyses, including studies that used a wide range of doses and different synthetic preparations and infusion protocols, have sought to identify beneficial effects of corticosteroid use in critical care patients. The search has been unsuccessful in general except for identifying some reduced vasopressor use and ventilator times. In 2008, the largest published study on this topic (Corticosteroid Therapy of Septic Shock [CORTICUS] trial) identified a smaller vasopressor requirement but no mortality benefit.

No conclusive benefits have been found with the use of corticosteroids in other conditions (eg, influenza, pancreatitis, liver insufficiency, cardiothoracic surgery, and other conditions in critically ill patients). Nevertheless, current data do show some benefit with systemic corticosteroid therapy for hospitalized adults who have community-acquired pneumonia, especially if they are severely ill.

Summary

- During severe illness, the HPA axis must respond to great variability, and dysfunction of the HPA axis may lead to a poor prognosis.
- Knowledge about the HPA axis in critically ill patients is incomplete; consequently, making screening and therapeutic recommendations for these patients is challenging.
- Hormonal replacement in cases of documented AI and relative critical illness AI improves mortality.

SUGGESTED READING

Annane D. Corticosteroids for severe sepsis: an evidence-based guide for physicians. Ann Intensive Care. 2011 Apr 13;1(1):7.

Annane D, Maxime V, Ibrahim F, Alvarez JC, Abe E, Boudou P. Diagnosis of adrenal insufficiency in severe sepsis and septic shock. Am J Respir Crit Care Med. 2006 Dec 15;174(12):1319–26. Epub 2006 Sep 14.

Bernard F, Outtrim J, Lynch AG, Menon DK, Matta BF. Hemodynamic steroid responsiveness is predictive of neurological outcome after traumatic brain injury. Neurocrit Care. 2006;5(3):176–9.

Bernard F, Outtrim J, Menon DK, Matta BF. Incidence of adrenal insufficiency after severe traumatic brain injury varies according to definition used: clinical implications. Br J Anaesth. 2006 Jan;96(1):72–6. Epub 2005 Nov 25.

Boonen E, Van den Berghe G. Mechanisms in endocrinology: new concepts to further unravel adrenal insufficiency during critical illness. Eur J Endocrinol. 2016 Jul;175(1):R1–9. Epub 2016 Jan 25.

Chrousos GP. Regulation and dysregulation of the hypothalamic-pituitary-adrenal axis: the corticotropin-releasing hormone perspective. Endocrinol Metab Clin North Am. 1992 Dec;21(4):833–58.

Cooper MS, Stewart PM. Corticosteroid insufficiency in acutely ill patients. N Engl J Med. 2003 Feb 20;348(8):727–34.

de Jong MF, Molenaar N, Beishuizen A, Groeneveld AB. Diminished adrenal sensitivity to endogenous and exogenous adrenocorticotropic hormone in critical illness: a prospective cohort study. Crit Care. 2015 Jan 6;19:1. Erratum in: Crit Care. 2015;19:313.

Dimopoulou I, Tsagarakis S, Kouyialis AT, Roussou P, Assithianakis G, Christoforaki M, et al. Hypothalamic-pituitary-adrenal axis dysfunction in critically ill patients with traumatic brain injury: incidence, pathophysiology, and relationship to vasopressor dependence and peripheral interleukin-6 levels. Crit Care Med. 2004 Feb;32(2):404–8.

Fernandez-Rodriguez E, Bernabeu I, Castro AI, Kelestimur F, Casanueva FF. Hypopituitarism following traumatic brain injury: determining factors for diagnosis. Front Endocrinol (Lausanne). 2011 Aug 25;2:25.

Gibbison B, Angelini GD, Lightman SL. Dynamic output and control of the hypothalamic-pituitary-adrenal axis in critical illness and major surgery. Br J Anaesth. 2013 Sep;111(3):347–60. Epub 2013 May 9.

Henley DE, Lightman SL. New insights into corticosteroid-binding globulin and glucocorticoid delivery. Neuroscience. 2011 Apr 28;180:1–8. Epub 2011 Mar 1.

Lipiner-Friedman D, Sprung CL, Laterre PF, Weiss Y, Goodman SV, Vogeser M, et al; Corticus Study Group. Adrenal function in sepsis: the retrospective Corticus cohort study. Crit Care Med. 2007 Apr;35(4):1012–8.

Marik PE, Pastores SM, Annane D, Meduri GU, Sprung CL, Arlt W, et al; American College of Critical Care Medicine. Recommendations for the diagnosis and management of corticosteroid insufficiency in critically ill adult patients: consensus statements from an international task force by the American College of Critical Care Medicine. Crit Care Med. 2008 Jun;36(6):1937–49.

Marik PE, Varon J. Requirement of perioperative stress doses of corticosteroids: a systematic review of the literature. Arch Surg. 2008 Dec;143(12):1222–6.

Meduri GU, Bridges L, Shih MC, Marik PE, Siemieniuk RA, Kocak M. Prolonged glucocorticoid treatment is associated with improved ARDS outcomes: analysis of individual patients' data from four randomized trials and trial-level meta-analysis of the updated literature. Intensive Care Med. 2016 May;42(5):829–40. Epub 2015 Oct 27.

Pastores SM, Annane D, Rochwerg B; Corticosteroid Guideline Task Force of SCCM and ESICM. Guidelines for the Diagnosis and Management of Critical Illness-Related Corticosteroid Insufficiency (CIRCI) in critically ill patients (Part II): Society of Critical Care Medicine (SCCM) and European Society of Intensive Care Medicine (ESICM) 2017. Crit Care Med. 2018 Jan;46(1):146–8.

Rhodes A, Evans LE, Alhazzani W, Levy MM, Antonelli M, Ferrer R, et al. Surviving sepsis campaign: international guidelines for management of sepsis and septic shock: 2016. Crit Care Med. 2017 Mar;45(3): 486–552.

Siemieniuk RA, Meade MO, Alonso-Coello P, Briel M, Evaniew N, Prasad M, et al. Corticosteroid therapy for patients hospitalized with community-acquired pneumonia: a systematic review and meta-analysis. Ann Intern Med. 2015 Oct 6;163(7):519–28.

Teblick A, Peeters B, Langouche L, Van den Berghe G. Adrenal function and dysfunction in critically ill patients. Nat Rev Endocrinol. 2019 Mar 8. [Epub ahead of print]

Vespa P; Participants in the International Multi-Disciplinary Consensus Conference on the Critical Care Management of Subarachnoid Hemorrhage. SAH pituitary adrenal dysfunction. Neurocrit Care. 2011 Sep;15(2):365–8.

Weant KA, Sasaki-Adams D, Dziedzic K, Ewend M. Acute relative adrenal insufficiency after aneurysmal subarachnoid hemorrhage. Neurosurgery. 2008 Oct;63(4):645–9.

Weant KA, Sasaki-Adams D, Kilpatrick M, Hadar EJ. Relative adrenal insufficiency in patients with acute spinal cord injury. Neurocrit Care. 2008;8(1):53–6.

Wu JY, Hsu SC, Ku SC, Ho CC, Yu CJ, Yang PC. Adrenal insufficiency in prolonged critical illness. Crit Care. 2008;12(3):R65. Epub 2008 May 8.

Yang Y, Liu L, Jiang D, Wang J, Ye Z, Ye J, et al. Critical illness-related corticosteroid insufficiency after multiple traumas: a multicenter, prospective cohort study. J Trauma Acute Care Surg. 2014 Jun;76(6):1390–6.

Yong SL, Marik P, Esposito M, Coulthard P. Supplemental perioperative steroids for surgical patients with adrenal insufficiency. Cochrane Database Syst Rev. 2009 Oct 7;(4):CD005367. Update in: Cochrane Database Syst Rev. 2012;12:CD005367.

Gastrointestinal Disorders

Acute Gastrointestinal Hemorrhage

PABLO MORENO FRANCO, MD; PHILIP E. LOWMAN, MD

Goals

- Discuss the initial evaluation of a patient who is suspected to have acute gastrointestinal hemorrhage.
- Understand the special circumstance of gastrointestinal hemorrhage in a neurologically injured patient.
- Explain the diagnostic approach to define anatomical location and cause of gastrointestinal hemorrhage.
- Describe available pharmacologic, nonpharmacologic, and device-based therapies for gastrointestinal hemorrhage.

Introduction

Gastrointestinal hemorrhage (GIH) is a common medical problem that is associated with considerable morbidity, mortality, and medical costs. The initial approach when GIH is suspected depends on a patient's clinical stability, which will vary depending on the amount and speed of blood loss. Therefore, if time allows, the initial evaluation should include history, physical examination, laboratory tests, and, possibly, nasogastric tube placement.

Mechanism of GIH

Pathophysiologically, GIH can start from several mechanisms, including erosions, ulcerations, vascular lesions, portal hypertension, mass lesions, brain injury, and trauma. Typically, a patient's chief complaints are 1 of 2 categories:

1. Vomiting blood (hematemesis) or black tarry stools (melena) have been associated with bleeding that occurs proximal to the ligament of Treitz, commonly referred to as upper gastrointestinal bleeding. The 3 most common causes are ulcers, esophageal varices, and Mallory-Weiss tears. The presence of fresh blood may suggest a more severe hemorrhage than if coffee-ground emesis is the presenting symptom.
2. Red or maroon blood in the stools (hematochezia) is commonly associated with lower gastrointestinal bleeding, but it can also occur in hemodynamically significant upper GIH with rapid transit. The most common causes of lower GIH include diverticulosis, infectious and ischemic colitis, and anorectal disorders such as fissures, ulcers, and hemorrhoids.

GIH in the Neurologically Injured Patient

The exact mechanism of GIH after a neurologic insult is unknown, but several hypotheses exist. Increased vagal tone due to intracranial hypertension may result in hypersecretion of gastric acid. Hypersecretion of cortisol and catecholamines, leading to vasoconstriction and mucosal damage, and ileus may also be contributing factors. Patients who have GIH after neurologic injury are at increased risk of poor functional outcomes and death. These changes in prognosis may be due to both the hemodynamic consequences of hemorrhage and the need to delay, interrupt, or discontinue use of antiplatelet and antithrombotic drugs. The incidence of GIH has been reported to be 1.5% after ischemic stroke, 2.9% after subarachnoid hemorrhage, and up to 33% in traumatic brain injury.

Primary Prevention of GIH

As noted above, patients with traumatic head injuries are at high risk for development of GIH. The high incidence of GIH lends itself to primary prevention with pharmacologic intervention. Other risk factors that predispose to the development of gastric and duodenal ulcers in critically ill patients include thrombocytopenia, coagulopathy, prolonged mechanical ventilation, and the use of corticosteroids. Pharmacologic options include histamine$_2$-receptor blockers and proton pump inhibitors, although the latter have a higher association with the development of *Clostridium difficile* infections.

Evaluation When GIH Is Suspected

Presentation

A focused history should include questions regarding chief complaints, as described above, and onset and progression of symptoms. It should also include medication exposures (timing and dosing), particularly nonsteroidal anti-inflammatory drugs, anticoagulants, antiplatelet agents, and corticosteroids. On review of systems, it is key to inquire about high-risk symptoms such as syncope, dizziness, chest pain, and diaphoresis.

Physical examination should be directed to gather further data regarding the possible source and amount of bleeding. Initial assessment of vital signs will identify hemodynamically significant bleeding, which will be accompanied by the following:

1. Tachycardia at rest *or*
2. Heart rate increasing more than 20 beats per minute or a drop in systolic blood pressure of more than 20 mm Hg when the patient is transferred from recumbent position to standing (also known as orthostatic hypotension).

A patient's general appearance, particularly in association with past medical history, may show signs of chronic conditions that predispose the patient to particular types of GIH. For example, signs of chronic liver disease (jaundice, spider angiomata, gynecomastia, loss of body hair, muscle wasting, bruising, and decreased testicular size) may suggest upper GIH, particularly from esophageal varices.

Otorhinolaryngologic examination is done to rule out possible alternative nasopharyngeal sources. A focused abdominal examination is helpful for attempting to locate the anatomical level, identifying abdominal distention, or ruling out signs of acute abdomen.

Rectal examination may show stool color changes, which could provide further clues regarding the anatomical level of the hemorrhage.

Laboratory Work-up

Complete blood count, type, and screening should be done immediately. Coagulation profiles, liver or renal function tests, and, in selected cases, thromboelastography can be obtained to assess for coagulopathy. Electrocardiography and troponins need to be considered to assess for coronary ischemia, especially in patients with concomitant chest pain or cardiovascular risk factors.

An initial increased lactate level determined in the emergency department has been associated with in-hospital mortality for patients with acute GIH. A lactate level more than 4 mmol/L has been found to confer a 6.4-fold increased odds of in-hospital mortality (94% specificity, P<.001).

Triage

Initial risk stratification is based on hemodynamic assessment, comorbidities, age, results of laboratory testing, and present history. Mortality for patients with upper GIH is usually 10% to 14%. The mean length of stay in the United States for these patients is 2.7 to 4.4 days. Hemodynamically significant GIH (hematocrit decrease >6%) has been associated with mortality rates of 20% to 39%.

Risk Assessment

Risk should be assessed before endoscopy is perfomed. There are 2 well-known validated risk assessment tools: the Rockall score and the Blatchford score. The Blatchford score has a range of 0 to 23, predicts required interventions (transfusions, endoscopy, and surgery) and death, and is based on clinical (systolic blood pressure, heart rate, melena, and syncope) and laboratory data (Table 39.1).

The Rockall score has a range of 0 to 11, serves as a predictor of rebleeding and death, and considers factors such as age, comorbidities, and shock (Table 39.2). Categories of age, shock, diagnosis, and evidence of bleeding range from 0 to 2 points, and comorbidity ranges from 0 to 3 points.

With the data obtained from risk assessment, the clinician can consider whether the patient needs to be hospitalized. A Blatchford score of 1 or less is associated with low risk of needing endoscopic intervention, and a Rockall score of 2 or less is associated with a low risk of further bleeding or death. If, for example, a patient presents with a blood urea value less than 10 mmol/L; systolic blood pressure more than 110 mm Hg (and previously normotensive); a heart rate less than 100 beats per minute; absence of melena, syncope, cardiac failure, and liver disease; and an almost normal hemoglobin level (>13 g/dL for men, >12 g/dL for women), outpatient care may be possible because of the low risk for morbidity and mortality. A Blatchford score of 7 or more is highly sensitive for predicting the need for endoscopic therapy.

Initial Management

When a patient has been evaluated, and while risk stratification is under way, the main steps to be considered include the following:

1. Initiate appropriate resuscitation. This step includes establishing adequate intravenous access, preferably with 2 large-bore intravenous catheters. Intravenous fluid resuscitation, especially if tachycardia or

Table 39.1 • Blatchford Score

Admission Risk Marker	Score Component Value
Blood urea, mmol/L	
6.5-8.0	2
>8.0-10.0	3
>10.0-25	4
>25	6
Hemoglobin, g/dL	
Men	
12.0-12.9	1
10.0-11.9	3
<10.0	6
Women	
10.0-11.9	1
<10.0	6
Systolic blood pressure, mm Hg	
100-109	1
90-99	2
<90	3
Other markers	
Pulse ≥100 beats/min	1
Presentation with melena	1
Presentation with syncope	2
Hepatic disease	2
Cardiac failure	2

From Blatchford O, Murray WR, Blatchford M. A risk score to predict need for treatment for upper-gastrointestinal haemorrhage. Lancet. 2000 Oct 14;356(9238):1318-21; used with permission.

orthostatic signs are present, can initially be done with crystalloids such as normal saline or Ringer lactate. Endotracheal intubation may be required for airway protection in cases of extensive hematemesis.

2. In select patients, consider a nasogastric tube. Expert consensus is that diagnostic nasogastric tube placement may not be necessary if early endoscopy will be done. Also, some data negate the need for a nasogastric tube. However, if one is placed, nasogastric or orogastric lavage may be helpful to clear the stomach of blood clots before endoscopy. In addition, the detection of red blood has been found to be associated with poor outcomes and the need for emergency endoscopy.
3. Consider blood product transfusions. Red blood cell transfusions should be administered in patients with a hemoglobin level of 7 g/dL or less, and the target hemoglobin level is 7 to 9 g/dL in the absence of tissue hypoperfusion, active coronary ischemia, or hemodynamically significant hemorrhage.
4. Reverse coagulopathy or anticoagulation. In anticoagulated patients, coagulopathy correction is recommended as long as endoscopy is not delayed. Reversing anticoagulation in this select patient population may enhance the outcomes of endoscopic therapy, except in patients with cirrhosis, in whom the prothrombin time and international normalized ratio do not reliably predict bleeding risk. Platelet transfusions are generally recommended for a platelet level less than 50×10^9/L, active bleeding, or recent use of antiplatelet medications.
5. Consult a gastrointestinal endoscopist. Early stratification of a patient to low-risk vs high-risk categories for rebleeding and mortality, based on both clinical and endoscopic criteria, is important for proper management. Generally, second-look endoscopies are not indicated. Also, endoscopy may need to be deferred or delayed in high-risk patients, such as those who have active acute coronary syndrome or in whom a perforated viscus is suspected.
6. Start pre-endoscopy pharmacologic therapy. Intravenous proton pump inhibitors should be used to decrease both the rebleeding and mortality risks

Table 39.2 • Rockall Score

	Score			
Variable	0	1	2	3
Age, y	<60	60-79	>80	
Shock	No shock	Pulse >100 beats/min SBP >100 mm Hg	SBP <100 mm Hg	
Comorbidity	No major		CHF, IHD, major morbidity	Renal failure, liver failure, metastatic cancer
Diagnosis	Mallory-Weiss	All other diagnoses	GI malignancy	
Evidence of bleeding	None		Blood, adherent clot, spurting vessel	

Abbreviations: CHF, congestive heart failure; GI, gastrointestinal; IHD, ischemic heart disease; SBP, systolic blood pressure.

From Rockall TA, Logan RFA, Devlin HB, Northfield TC; steering committee and members of the National Audit of Acute Upper Gastrointestinal Haemorrhage. Risk assessment after acute upper gastrointestinal haemorrhage. Gut. 1996 Mar;38(3):316-21; used with permission.

in patients with known or suspected upper GIH with high-risk stigmata who have undergone successful endoscopy therapy.

Therapies for GIH

Pharmacologic

Ulcers are the most common cause of upper GIH. Bleeding ulcers with high-risk findings on endoscopy (active bleeding, no bleeding visible vessel, adherent clots, and Forrest categories 1a or b or 2a or b) should be treated with proton pump inhibitor infusions. As an example, the recommended dose for intravenous pantoprazole is an 80 mg bolus followed by an infusion of 8 mg/h for 72 hours. There is ongoing debate regarding the need for high-cost, continuous proton pump inhibitor infusions compared with other options, such as twice-daily dosing or oral administration.

In patients with acute ulcer bleeding, neither histamine$_2$-receptor antagonists nor octreotide is routinely recommended. In the setting of suspected or known portal hypertension, the addition of octreotide as a bolus followed by infusion can lower portal venous blood flow.

Nonpharmacologic and Device-Based

Although most causes of GIH can be treated endoscopically with injection of vasoconstrictors, placement of vascular clips, and thermal therapy, surgical consultation should be considered for patients in whom endoscopic therapy fails. Increasingly available alternatives to surgical intervention

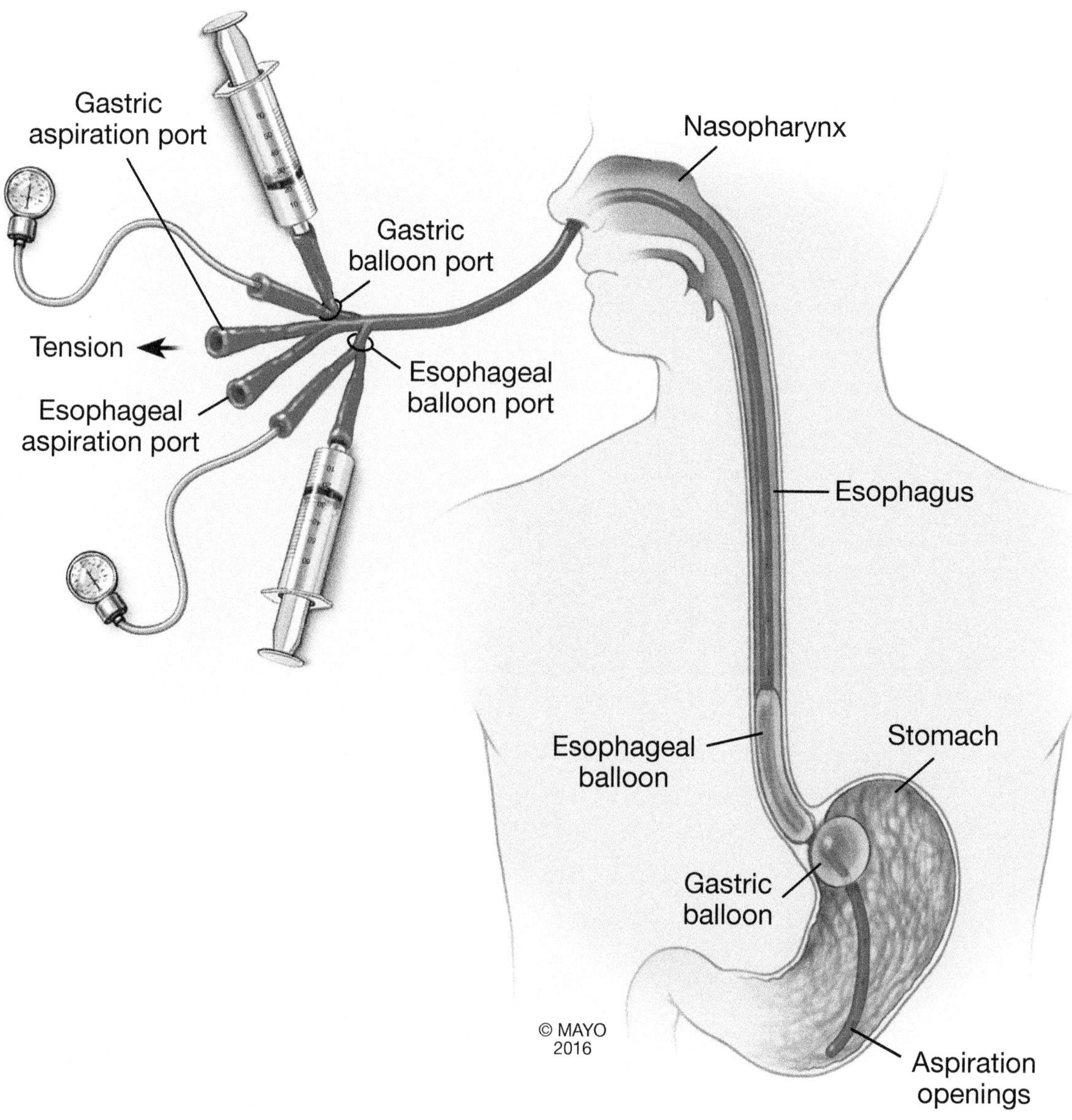

Figure 39.1. Esophageal Balloon, Minnesota Tube.

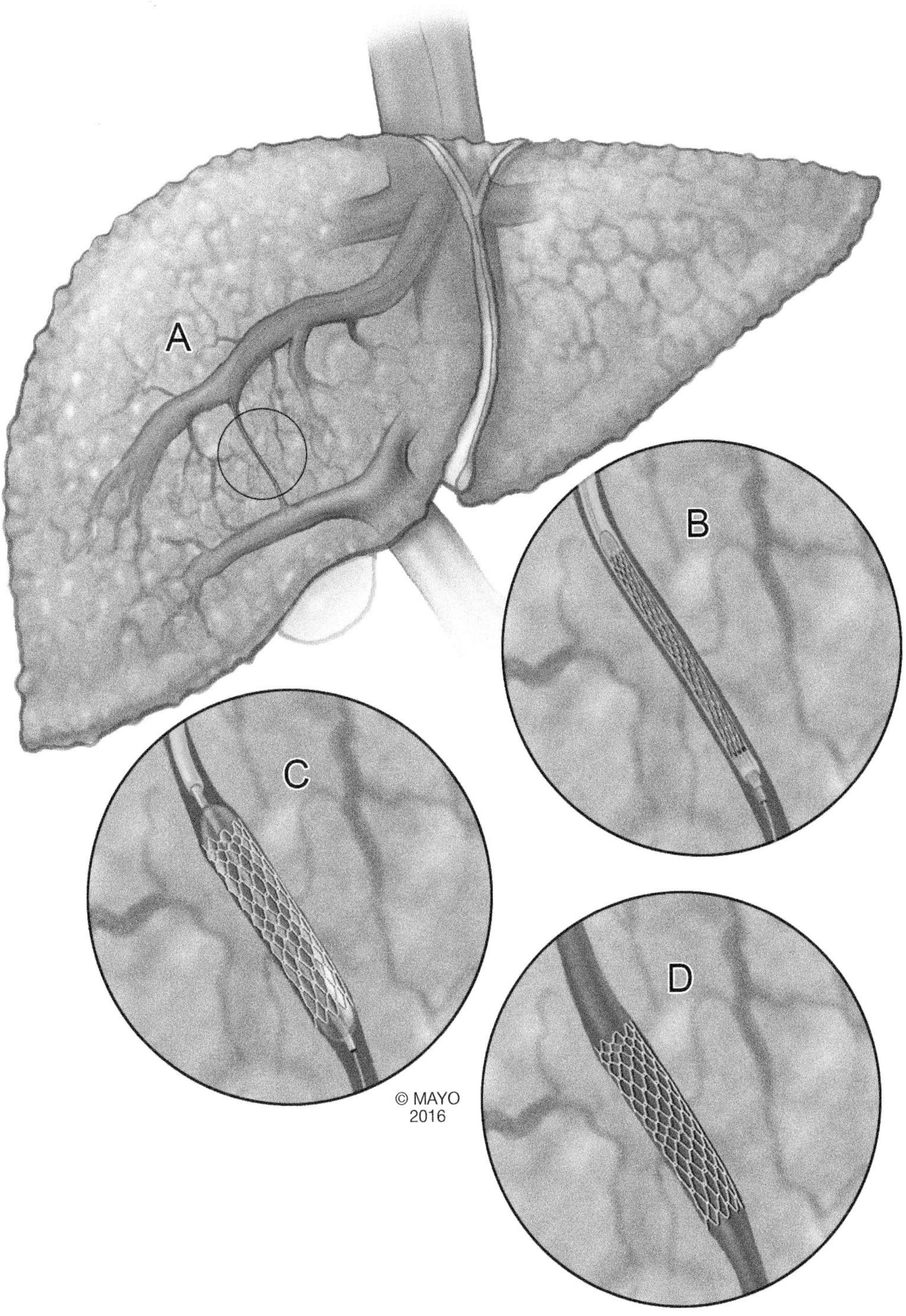

Figure 39.2. Transjugular Intrahepatic Portacaval Shunt. A, Anatomy of portal and hepatic veins, delineated to identify targets. B, Wire is advanced through the liver with a needle to connect the portal vein with one of the hepatic veins. C, Balloon is inflated to dilate the track. D, Metal stent in place. The stent keeps the track open, thus reducing portal hypertension and helping to stop variceal bleeding.

are the less invasive, catheter-based therapies performed by interventional radiologists. Catheter-based therapies use angiography for localization, and then either embolizing agents or vasoconstrictors are injected into culprit vessels to achieve hemostasis. Candidates for angiographic diagnosis and intervention include patients with massive and hemodynamically significant bleeding, those with bleeding identified on computed tomographic angiography or nuclear medicine studies, and those whose bleeding does not respond or is not amenable to endoscopic treatment.

In patients with hemodynamically significant hemorrhage, management considerations should also include massive transfusion protocol with or without the use of rapid infuser, blood warmer, and thromboelastography-guided transfusion algorithms.

Acute hemorrhage of an esophageal or gastric varix presents a challenging scenario. In such cases, airway protection followed by endoscopy with band ligation provides the safest control strategy. If this advanced endoscopic therapy is not available or it fails to provide hemostasis, then consideration should be given to placement of a balloon tamponade device (Figure 39.1) or emergency transjugular intrahepatic portacaval shunt procedure (Figure 39.2).

Summary

- Initial resuscitation for GIH includes peripheral large-bore intravenous catheters, typing and screening, and fluid resuscitation.
- Pharmocologic therapy can reduce the risk for development of stress ulcers in patients at the highest risk of bleeding.
- Laboratory work-up should include complete blood count, coagulation studies (partial thromboplastin, international normalized ratio), liver or renal profiles, electrocardiography, troponin, and lactate.
- Early clinical and endoscopic risk stratification to either low- or high-risk categories for rebleeding and mortality will dictate the required disposition and therapies.
- Initial pharmacologic therapy should include intravenous proton pump inhibitors.
- If endoscopic therapies fail, surgical consultation, catheter-based embolization, esophageal balloon placement, and transjugular intrahepatic portocaval shunting should be considered depending on the clinical scenario and available resources.

SUGGESTED READING

Barkun A, Bardou M, Marshall JK; Nonvariceal Upper GI Bleeding Consensus Conference Group. Consensus recommendations for managing patients with nonvariceal upper gastrointestinal bleeding. Ann Intern Med. 2003 Nov 18;139(10):843–57.

Barkun AN, Bardou M, Kuipers EJ, Sung J, Hunt RH, Martel M, et al; International Consensus Upper Gastrointestinal Bleeding Conference Group. International consensus recommendations on the management of patients with nonvariceal upper gastrointestinal bleeding. Ann Intern Med. 2010 Jan 19;152(2):101–13.

Blatchford O, Murray WR, Blatchford M. A risk score to predict need for treatment for upper-gastrointestinal haemorrhage. Lancet. 2000 Oct 14;356(9238):1318–21.

Bucsics T, Schoder M, Diermayr M, Feldner-Busztin M, Goeschl N, Bauer D, et al. Transjugular intrahepatic portosystemic shunts (TIPS) for the prevention of variceal re-bleeding: a two decades experience. PLoS One. 2018 Jan; 13(1):e0189414.

Liu B, Liu S, Yin A, Siddiqi J. Risks and benefits of stress ulcer prophylaxis in adult neurocritical care patients: a systematic review and meta-analysis of randomized controlled trials. Crit Care. 2015 Nov 17;19:409.

Nable JV, Graham AC. Gastrointestinal bleeding. Emerg Med Clin North Am. 2016 May;34(2):309–25. Epub 2016 Mar 16.

O'Donnell MJ, Kapral MK, Fang J, Saposnik G, Eikelboom JW, Oczkowski W, et al; Investigators of the Registry of the Canadian Stroke Network. Gastrointestinal bleeding after acute ischemic stroke. Neurology. 2008 Aug 26;71(9):650–5. Epub 2008 Aug 6.

Ramaswamy RS, Choi HW, Mouser HC, Narsinh KH, McCammack KC, Treesit T, et al. Role of interventional radiology in the management of acute gastrointestinal bleeding. World J Radiol. 2014 Apr 28;6(4):82–92.

Sachar H, Vaidya K, Laine L. Intermittent vs continuous proton pump inhibitor therapy for high-risk bleeding ulcers: a systematic review and meta-analysis. JAMA Intern Med. 2014 Nov;174(11):1755–62.

Shah A, Chisolm-Straker M, Alexander A, Rattu M, Dikdan S, Manini AF. Prognostic use of lactate to predict inpatient mortality in acute gastrointestinal hemorrhage. Am J Emerg Med. 2014 Jul;32(7):752–5. Epub 2014 Feb 17.

Strate LL. Lower GI bleeding: epidemiology and diagnosis. Gastroenterol Clin North Am. 2005 Dec;34(4):643–64.

Wang SP, Huang YH. Gastrointestinal hemorrhage after spontaneous subarachnoid hemorrhage: a single-center cohort study. Sci Rep. 2017 Oct 19;7(1):13557.

Paralytic and Obstructive Ileus

JUAN M. CANABAL, MD

Goals

- Define the 2 types of ileus: paralytic and obstructive.
- Identify common causes of ileus.
- Recognize clinical manifestations of ileus.
- Outline management of ileus and pharmacologic interventions.

Introduction

Ileus is the most common manifestation of acute gastrointestinal injury which exhibits grades of severity in the critically ill. Appropriate characterization of ileus as adynamic or mechanical in origin determines its management. This chapter discusses the most important causes, clinical and radiologic findings, and appropriate management of ileus that develops in patients in the intensive care unit.

Definitions

For many clinicians, the term *ileus* has been used interchangeably with various clinical events depending on location and cause: small bowel obstruction, paralytic (adynamic) ileus, dynamic (spastic) ileus, gallstone ileus, mechanical ileus, meconium ileus, occlusive ileus, postoperative ileus, terminal ileus, and verminous ileus. Ileus is formally defined as mechanical or adynamic obstruction of the bowel attended with severe colicky pain, vomiting, and often fever and dehydration. Unfortunately, because *ileus* is often used in vague and nonspecific ways, there can be confusion among clinicians.

A more practical and clinical definition of ileus is a temporary absence of forward peristaltic movement of the intestinal wall. With this definition, subtypes of ileus can be identified:

1. Paralytic: complete lack of peristaltic movement not due to a mechanical barrier (Tables 40.1 and 40.2).
   - Also known as adynamic ileus
   - Anatomical subdivisions (gastric, small bowel, large bowel)
2. Obstructive: a halt in peristaltic movement due to a mechanical barrier. Examples include tumor, intussusception, incarcerated hernia, retained undigested food particles, nonnutritional items such as hair or plastic, and volvulus.
3. Others
   - Postoperative ileus
   - Medically and medication-induced ileus

The incidence of ileus postoperatively has been reported to range between 3% and 30%. Inadequate definitions and lack of standardization in definitions have made it difficult to accurately report incidence, equate clinical study results of treatments, and identify potential new treatments. For example, there is confusion about the definitions of normal postoperative bowel function, early postoperative ileus, and late postoperative ileus.

Causes

Ileus has been described as a result of almost any medical situation. Functionally, the descriptions can be divided into several categories: abdominal causes, nonabdominal causes, or surgical and nonsurgical causes. Regardless of cause, the common feature is the partial or complete cessation of propulsive peristaltic movement. The underlying cause is a multifactorial combination of neurologic factors,

Table 40.1 • General Causes of Ileus (Independent of Location) and Implicated Factors

Cause	Factor
Inflammatory	Mast cells Circulating monocytes Resident macrophages Prostaglandin E_2 Nitric oxide Indirect relative intestinal ischemia or direct reduction of blood flow
Neural	Afferent pathways Glutamate at the dorsal root ganglia leads to perception and localization of pain and local autonomic response Peritoneum manipulation leads to vagus nerve stimulation, which in turn activates interleukin-1 receptors and susceptibility to early humoral changes of inflammation Efferent pathways Parasympathetic stimulation leads to acetylcholine inhibition, which increases nitric oxide production that leads to decreased vascular tone and contractility. Nitric oxide and VIP both lead to increased motility
Discontinuity of gut	Surgical resections disrupt intrinsic neural networks and the enteric nervous system
Gastrointestinal hormones and neuropeptides	VIP, motilin, and substance P cause decreased motility
Electrolyte disturbances	Hypokalemia, hypocalcemia, hypermagnesemia
Medications or iatrogenic	Mechanical Peritoneal invasion Gut integrity or resection Visceral manipulation Medication IVFs
Structural	Tumors, intussusception, meconium (children), hernia strangulation, adhesions or fibrous bands, gallstones

Abbreviations: IVFs, intravenous fluids; VIP, vasoactive intestinal peptide.

inflammatory cell factors (mast cells), opioid receptors, electrolyte imbalances, intrinsic hormone activity, and others (Table 40.1).

Clinical Findings

In general, the clinical characteristics of ileus include nausea, vomiting, abdominal distention, abdominal pain, inability to tolerate oral intake, delayed passage of stool or flatus, and fever. Any or all of those symptoms may be present. The enteric system does not act uniformly. Different parts of the intestine have different thresholds of sensitivity to changes or a noxious environment such as surgical intervention or manipulation. The resolution of nausea or the passage of flatus is not indicative of complete restoration of normal gut motility. Bowel sounds have long been used as a surrogate marker for gut activity. In reality, bowel sounds require an air-fluid interaction inside the gut (Figure 40.1). The use of nasoenteric tubes immediately postoperatively or long after surgery (days) is controversial. Some clinicians believe that the use of these tubes only eliminates the air in the air-fluid interaction in the stomach and that the stomach usually returns to function within 48 hours postoperatively.

Radiographic Findings

The radiographic test of choice is plain radiography. It can identify emergency situations such as free air (suggesting ruptured viscus); however, results can be normal even when abnormality is present. A strong clinical suspicion should not be downplayed by a normal-appearing radiograph. In a case suggestive of ileus, the appearance of air throughout the entire gut, including the rectum, likely indicates adynamic diffuse ileus (Figure 40.2). The absence of air after a section of intestine could mean that an obstruction is present. This can be small bowel or colonic. Small bowel air can be delineated in parts of the small bowel and

Table 40.2 • Common Types of Paralytic Ileus and Common Causes

Type of Paralytic Ileus	Causes
Medication-induced	Opioids and derivatives, anticholinergics, loperamide, TCAs, antiparkinsonian, phenothiazines, calcium channel blockers
Sepsis-induced	Hypotension or hypoperfusion Fluid shifts Bowel edema Circulating inflammatory mediators Any source Urinary or renal system Respiratory system Neurologic system Gastrointestinal system Viral, bacterial infection
Postoperative	Invasion of abdominal cavity Bowel manipulation Bowel resection Bowel edema or fluid shifts Electrolyte imbalances Spinal operations

Abbreviation: TCAs, tricyclic antidepressants.

obscured in others by being fluid-filled. In the colon, it can occur in any section of it: right colon, transverse colon, or left colon. Colonic pseudo-obstruction, known as Ogilvie syndrome (Figure 40.3), can be potentially life threatening if perforation ensues. After true obstruction, ischemia, or pneumatosis intestinalis is ruled out, the suggested treatment for colonic pseudo-obstruction is neostigmine.

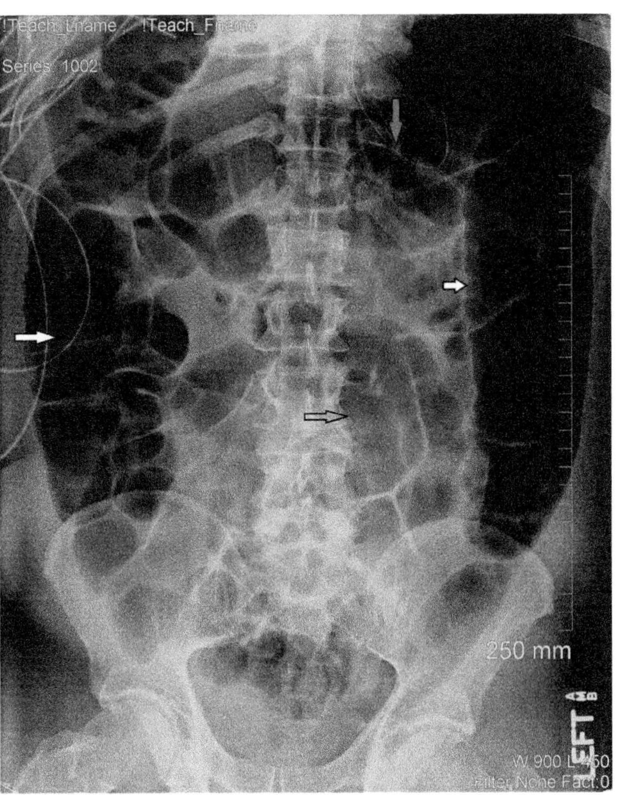

Figure 40.1. Nonobstructive Ileus. Air-fluid interface has been altered by nasogastric tube (red arrow). Air-dilated areas throughout the intestines: large intestine, ascending colon (long solid-white arrow), descending colon (short solid-white arrow), and small bowel (open arrow).

Treatment

Treatment can be implemented before, during, and after high-risk scenarios for ileus (eg, abdominal and spinal operations). The success of these interventions is difficult to assess because of lack of a standardized definition of ileus and lack of agreement on outcome metrics.

Management of ileus with nasogastric tubes can be prophylactic or therapeutic. Prophylactic use for decompression and management of ileus is not recommended. This use can actually obliterate the air-fluid interaction and delay passage of flatus. Insertion of nasogastric tubes can have its own complications, including upper airway edema, irritation, and bleeding. Use of a nasogastric tube for therapeutic purposes should be considered only at the onset of nausea with vomiting or for decompression of a clinically dilated stomach.

Careful attention to volume status is imperative. A patient with ileus can have massive redistribution of fluid

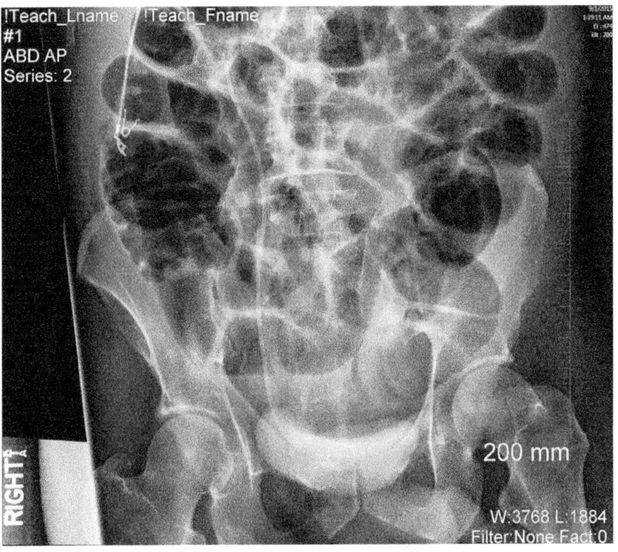

Figure 40.2. Obstructive Ileus, Distal Colon. No air noted in rectosigmoid area.

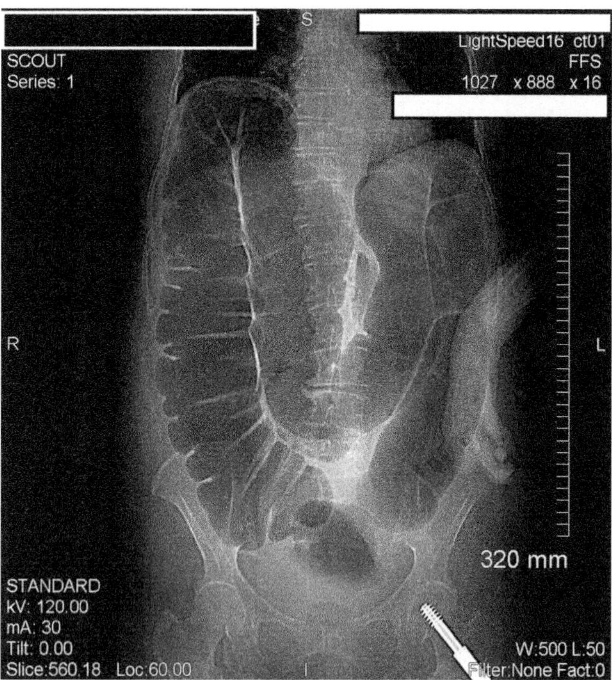

Figure 40.3. Ogilvie Syndrome.

into the interstitial space. Underresuscitation can cause electrolyte imbalance, and overresuscitation can lead to volume overload and cardiopulmonary problems, including the risk of possible anastomotic leak. Monitoring techniques for volume optimization, although available, may have risks associated with their invasiveness and may be inaccurate. Intraoperative transesophageal echocardiography, pulse index continuous cardiac output, thermodilution cardiac output techniques, and Swan-Ganz catheterization are some of the available methods that can be used for volume optimization.

Another invasive technique is mid thoracic epidural anesthesia. This effectively blocks the efferent pathways, inhibits the sympathetic nervous system and thus limits opiate use, and decreases the incidence of gastrointestinal paralysis compared with opioid-based anesthesia.

The actual operative plan or surgical technique influences the incidence of postoperative ileus. Laparoscopy decreases tissue trauma and bowel manipulation and thus decreases length of stay compared with open surgical techniques.

Nonsteroidal anti-inflammatory drugs, compared with opioids, minimizes the bowel effects and incidence of ileus. Early enteral nutrition stimulates gut motility, contributes to the formation of air-fluid interaction, and stimulates collagen formation at the anastomotic site. Chewing gum and drinking coffee also have stimulatory positive effects, but they are only temporary. Alvimopan, a μ-opioid receptor antagonist, was the first agent approved by the US Food and Drug Administration for narcotic-induced postoperative ileus. It acts on the periphery and does not cross the blood-brain barrier. Available alternatives to alvimopan are methylnaltrexone and naloxegol. They all have shown a reduction in postoperative ileus and resolution of the condition.

Agents that require randomized clinical trials are oral water-soluble radiocontrast agents such as diatrizoate meglumine and diatrizoate sodium, nicotine, magnesium sulfate, and daikenchuto. They all seem to have some questionable therapeutic benefit by either increasing colonic transit or decreasing opioid use. Daikenchuto, is a Japanese herbal combination that may act by anti-inflammatory action through nicotinic acetylcholine receptors.

Summary

- Almost any disease state, surgical and nonsurgical, can induce abnormal motility in the gastrointestinal system.
- Adjunct testing such as plain radiography or computed tomography can help define the clinical presentation.
- The most common form of ileus is postoperative ileus.
- Implementation of enhanced recovery protocols, early clinical suspicion, and early adoption of management strategies can help. These protocols include a planned surgical approach, early feeding and epidural anesthesia, limitation of opioid use and μ-receptor antagonists, use of prokinetic agents, limitation of nasogastric tube use, and early mobilization.
- The use of these protocols can improve the time to return to normal motility and thus lead to resolution of ileus.

SUGGESTED READING

Althausen PL, Gupta MC, Benson DR, Jones DA. The use of neostigmine to treat postoperative ileus in orthopedic spinal patients. J Spinal Disord. 2001 Dec;14(6):541–5.

Biondo S, Miquel J, Espin-Basany E, Sanchez JL, Golda T, Ferrer-Artola AM, et al. A double-blinded randomized clinical study on the therapeutic effect of gastrografin in prolonged postoperative ileus after elective colorectal surgery. World J Surg. 2016 Jan;40(1):206–14.

Bragg D, El-Sharkawy AM, Psaltis E, Maxwell-Armstrong CA, Lobo DN. Postoperative ileus: recent developments in pathophysiology and management. Clin Nutr. 2015 Jun;34(3):367–76. Epub 2015 Jan 31.

Coulie B, Camilleri M, Bharucha AE, Sandborn WJ, Burton D. Colonic motility in chronic ulcerative proctosigmoiditis and the effects of nicotine on colonic motility in patients and healthy subjects. Aliment Pharmacol Ther. 2001 May;15(5):653–63.

Endo M, Hori M, Ozaki H, Oikawa T, Hanawa T. Daikenchuto, a traditional Japanese herbal medicine, ameliorates postoperative ileus by anti-inflammatory action through nicotinic acetylcholine receptors. *J Gastroenterol.* 2014 Jun;49(6):1026–39. Epub 2013 Jul 12.

Flores-Funes D, Campillo-Soto A, Pellicer-Franco E, Aguayo-Albasini JL. The use of coffee, chewing-gum and gastrograffin in the management of postoperative ileus: a review of current evidence. Cir Esp. 2016 Nov;94(9):495–501. Epub 2016 Jul 22. English, Spanish.

Goldstein JL, Matuszewski KA, Delaney CP, Senagore A, Chiao EF, Shah M, et al. Inpatient economic burden of postoperative ileus associated with abdominal surgery in the United States. P & T. 2007 Feb;32(2):82–90.

Han-Geurts IJ, Hop WC, Kok NF, Lim A, Brouwer KJ, Jeekel J. Randomized clinical trial of the impact of early enteral feeding on postoperative ileus and recovery. Br J Surg. 2007 May;94(5):555–61.

Han-Geurts IJ, Hop WC, Verhoef C, Tran KT, Tilanus HW. Randomized clinical trial comparing feeding jejunostomy with nasoduodenal tube placement in patients undergoing oesophagectomy. Br J Surg. 2007 Jan;94(1):31–5.

Hiranyakas A, Bashankaev B, Seo CJ, Khaikin M, Wexner SD. Epidemiology, pathophysiology and medical management of postoperative ileus in the elderly. Drugs Aging. 2011 Feb 1;28(2):107–18.

Jorgensen H, Wetterslev J, Moiniche S, Dahl JB. Epidural local anaesthetics versus opioid-based analgesic regimens on postoperative gastrointestinal paralysis, PONV and pain after abdominal surgery. Cochrane Database Syst Rev. 2000;(4):CD001893. Update in: Cochrane Database Syst Rev. 2016;7:CD001893.

Kronberg U, Kiran RP, Soliman MS, Hammel JP, Galway U, Coffey JC, et al. A characterization of factors determining postoperative ileus after laparoscopic colectomy enables the generation of a novel predictive score. Ann Surg. 2011 Jan;253(1):78–81.

Li S, Liu Y, Peng Q, Xie L, Wang J, Qin X. Chewing gum reduces postoperative ileus following abdominal surgery: a meta-analysis of 17 randomized controlled trials. J Gastroenterol Hepatol. 2013 Jul;28(7):1122–32.

Nelson R, Tse B, Edwards S. Systematic review of prophylactic nasogastric decompression after abdominal operations. Br J Surg. 2005 Jun;92(6):673–80.

Ponec RJ, Saunders MD, Kimmey MB. Neostigmine for the treatment of acute colonic pseudo-obstruction. N Engl J Med. 1999 Jul 15;341(3):137–41.

Rahbari NN, Zimmermann JB, Schmidt T, Koch M, Weigand MA, Weitz J. Meta-analysis of standard, restrictive and supplemental fluid administration in colorectal surgery. Br J Surg. 2009 Apr;96(4):331–41.

Schwenk W, Bohm B, Haase O, Junghans T, Muller JM. Laparoscopic versus conventional colorectal resection: a prospective randomised study of postoperative ileus and early postoperative feeding. Langenbecks Arch Surg. 1998 Mar;383(1):49–55.

Shariat Moharari R, Motalebi M, Najafi A, Zamani MM, Imani F, Etezadi F, et al. Magnesium can decrease postoperative physiological ileus and postoperative pain in major non laparoscopic gastrointestinal surgeries: a randomized controlled trial. Anesth Pain Med. 2013 Dec 6;4(1):e12750.

Stengel A, Tache Y. Brain peptides and the modulation of postoperative gastric ileus. Curr Opin Pharmacol. 2014 Dec;19:31–7. Epub 2014 Jul 9.

Su'a BU, Pollock TT, Lemanu DP, MacCormick AD, Connolly AB, Hill AG. Chewing gum and postoperative ileus in adults: a systematic literature review and meta-analysis. Int J Surg. 2015 Feb;14:49–55. Epub 2015 Jan 7.

Tan EK, Cornish J, Darzi AW, Tekkis PP. Meta-analysis: alvimopan vs. placebo in the treatment of post-operative ileus. Aliment Pharmacol Ther. 2007 Jan 1;25(1):47–57. Epub 2006 Oct 17.

Vather R, O'Grady G, Bissett IP, Dinning PG. Postoperative ileus: mechanisms and future directions for research. Clin Exp Pharmacol Physiol. 2014 May;41(5):358–70.

Vather R, Trivedi S, Bissett I. Defining postoperative ileus: results of a systematic review and global survey. J Gastrointest Surg. 2013 May;17(5):962–72. Epub 2013 Feb 2.

Vlug MS, Wind J, Hollmann MW, Ubbink DT, Cense HA, Engel AF, et al; LAFA Study Group. Laparoscopy in combination with fast track multimodal management is the best perioperative strategy in patients undergoing colonic surgery: a randomized clinical trial (LAFA-study). Ann Surg. 2011 Dec;254(6):868–75.

Wattchow DA, De Fontgalland D, Bampton PA, Leach PL, McLaughlin K, Costa M. Clinical trial: the impact of cyclooxygenase inhibitors on gastrointestinal recovery after major surgery: a randomized double blind controlled trial of celecoxib or diclofenac vs. placebo. Aliment Pharmacol Ther. 2009 Nov 15;30(10):987–98. Epub 2009 Aug 20.

Acute Liver Failure

JAMES Y. FINDLAY, MB, ChB; EELCO F. M. WIJDICKS, MD, PhD

Goals

- Identify hepatic encephalopathy as a defining feature of acute liver failure.
- Describe the management of hepatic encephalopathy and cerebral edema.
- Recognize clinical conditions concomitant with acute liver failure.
- Determine candidacy for a liver transplant in patients with acute liver failure.

Introduction

Acute liver failure (ALF) is an uncommon condition in which an acute insult results in a rapid deterioration of liver function, encephalopathy, and coagulopathy in the absence of prior underlying liver disease. It is differentiated from rapid deterioration in the setting of underlying liver disease (acute on chronic liver failure) and from the gradual deterioration in liver function that can occur in chronic liver failure. The most widely used definition for ALF includes the development of encephalopathy and the presence of deranged coagulation (international normalized ratio [INR] >1.5) in a patient previously without cirrhosis and an illness of less than 26 weeks.

Epidemiology

Approximately 2,000 cases of ALF occur in the United States yearly. The most common cause of ALF in the United States and Europe is acetaminophen toxicity, deliberate or accidental. In other areas of the world, viral hepatitis is the most common, most frequently hepatitis B but also A, D, and E. Other viruses are rarely implicated. Other less common causes are mushroom poisoning, drug-induced liver injury (typically an idiosyncratic reaction), Wilson disease, acute fatty liver of pregnancy, ischemic injury (shock liver), autoimmune hepatitis, and veno-occlusive disease (Budd-Chiari syndrome). At times, no clear cause is identified. Outcomes have been improving over time; overall survival is now more than 60%.

Presentation

Initial symptoms and findings of ALF are frequently nonspecific, including nausea, malaise, and right upper quadrant pain. Jaundice is common, but it may develop later in the illness. Laboratory findings include prolonged INR, markedly increased transaminase levels, increased bilirubin level, and thrombocytopenia. Hepatic encephalopathy is a defining feature of ALF. Initial findings may be minor; with progression, increasing confusion develops, eventually superseded by coma. Hepatic encephalopathy is graded 1 to 4 (Table 41.1); increasing grade is associated with an increasing probability of cerebral edema. Initial evaluation should include a full history with emphasis on possible toxic and viral exposures, appropriate laboratory testing for diagnostic purposes and to identify the extent of liver dysfunction and associated metabolic abnormalities, and abdominal imaging, initially Doppler ultrasonography.

Management

Patients with ALF should be hospitalized and frequently monitored. Discussion with a transplant center should be initiated early so that appropriate patients can be transferred, a particular concern for those with encephalopathy and potential cerebral edema. Such patients should be considered for admission to the intensive care unit. The mainstay of management is supportive therapy, there being few specific treatments of ALF. In patients with confirmed or suspected acetaminophen toxicity, treatment with *N*-acetylcysteine should be initiated as soon as

Table 41.1 • A Comparison of West Haven and FOUR Score Criteria for Grading Hepatic Encephalopathy[a]

West Haven		FOUR Score				
Grade	**Features**	**Score**	**Eye Response**	**Motor Response**	**Brainstem Reflex**	**Respiration**
0	No abnormalities detected	4	Eyelids open or manually opened; tracking or blinking on command	Thumbs up, fist, or peace sign on command	Pupillary and corneal reflexes present	Not intubated, regular breathing
1	Unawareness (mild), euphoria or anxiety, shortened attention span, impairment of calculation ability, lethargy or apathy	3	Eyelids open but no tracking	Localized response to pain	One pupil wide and fixed	Not intubated, Cheyne-Stokes breathing
2	Disorientation to time, obvious personality change, inappropriate behavior	2	Eyelids closed but open to loud voice	Flexion response to pain	Pupillary or corneal responses absent	Not intubated, irregular breathing
3	Somnolence to stupor, responsiveness to stimuli, confusion, gross disorientation, bizarre behavior	1	Eyelids closed but open to pain	Extension response to pain	Pupillary and corneal responses absent	Breathing above ventilator rate
4	Coma	0	Eyelids remain closed to pain	No response to pain, or generalized myoclonus status	Pupillary, corneal, and cough reflexes absent	Breathing at ventilator rate or apnea

Abbreviation: FOUR, Full Outline of Unresponsiveness.

[a] Patients with minimal hepatic encephalopathy (grade 1 with the use of the West Haven criteria) would be classified as having covert hepatic encephalopathy. Patients with West Haven grade 2 or higher encephalopathy would be classified as having overt hepatic encephalopathy. The FOUR score clinical grading scale considers 4 components of neurologic function. Scores range from 0 to 16; lower scores indicate a lower level of consciousness.

From Wijdicks EFM. Hepatic encephalopathy. N Engl J Med. 2016 Oct 27;375(17):1660-70; used with permission.

possible, even if more than 48 hours from presumed ingestion. *N*-Acetylcysteine may also improve outcomes in non-acetaminophen ALF. Mushroom toxicity may respond to penicillin G administration (or silibinin, where available), nucleoside analogues can be considered for acute hepatitis B, and albumin dialysis may be used for Wilson disease to reduce the serum copper level.

Hepatic Encephalopathy and Cerebral Edema

The most serious complications of ALF are cerebral edema and intracranial hypertension (ICH). These may lead to fatal uncal herniation. The exact mechanism is not fully understood, but ammonia crosses the blood-brain barrier, where glutamine synthetase catalyzes glutamate to a non-toxic glutamine, which acts as an osmolyte and increases cerebral volume. Cerebral edema is cytotoxic, but hyperemia as a result of increased cytokines may result in extracellular edema. Concepts are depicted in Figure 41.1. The frequency of cerebral edema is related to the degree of hepatic encephalopathy, seldom occurring in grades 1 and 2, increasing to 70% or more in grade 4. Arterial ammonia concentration is also related: at less than 75 mcg/dL cerebral edema is rare, but a level of more than 200 mcg/dL is strongly associated with uncal herniation.

With progression of encephalopathy, patients should be closely monitored because deterioration may be rapid. Management of encephalopathy with either lactulose or rifaximin is of unclear benefit in ALF, unlike in chronic liver disease, but a reduction in ammonia is needed to reduce the severity of cerebral edema. Once grade 3 is reached, intubation and mechanical ventilation should be undertaken, with subsequent sedation with propofol as necessary. The patient should be nursed in a quiet environment, head elevated 30° and in a neutral position. Activities that can cause increased intracranial pressure (ICP) such as endotracheal suctioning should be minimized. Frequent neurologic evaluation for signs of ICH should be undertaken. Any seizure activity should be rapidly controlled.

ICP monitoring is controversial in ALF. The best management of increased ICP in ALF is unknown, but a goal for ICP less than 25 mm Hg is necessary. Computed tomographic scans from a patient with cerebral edema are shown in Figure 41.2. In patients with cerebral edema on computed tomography, the best option is to proceed with mannitol or a concentrated hypertonic saline bolus, maintaining the serum sodium level between 145 and 155 mmol/L. Current guidelines recommend the use of ICP monitoring in patients with high-grade encephalopathy in centers experienced with the technique. If ICP monitoring is undertaken, intraparenchymal or intraventricular placement is preferred to epidural because of better accuracy.

Maintenance of cerebral perfusion and treatment of ICP are the goals. If an ICP monitor is in place, ICP should be kept less than 20 to 25 mm Hg and cerebral perfusion pressure should be kept more than 70 mm Hg using vasopressors to augment systemic blood pressure. Hypothermia (to 33°-35°C) may also be useful for managing resistant ICP; however, it has been shown to be ineffective as a prophylactic measure. Escalation to pentobarbital treatment before transplant has major disadvantages because neurologic examination will be seriously confounded. Barbiturate infusion may be considered for severe ICH that is resistant to other therapies.

Infection

Patients with ALF are at risk for infection, both bacterial and fungal, and infection confers a considerable mortality risk. Prophylactic antimicrobial agents have not been shown to have a survival benefit, but surveillance should be regular and the threshold for initiating treatment should be low, especially in patients suspected of bloodstream infection.

Coagulopathy

An increased INR as a result of diminished clotting factor production occurs in ALF, and thrombocytopenia is common. Despite an abnormal INR, spontaneous bleeding is rare, and investigation of whole blood clotting in patients with ALF by viscoelastic testing (eg, thromboelastography) indicates normal clotting. Correction of coagulopathy in nonbleeding patients is not recommended. If bleeding occurs, or in preparation for invasive procedures, correction can be undertaken. Plasma infusion may require a large-volume infusion, which risks volume overload and may not achieve correction. The use of smaller volumes of fresh frozen plasma in combination with recombinant activated factor VII or the use of prothrombin complex concentrates can be considered as alternatives.

Kidney Failure

Acute kidney failure is a frequent accompaniment to ALF. Usual management is to maintain renal perfusion and avoid nephrotoxins as far as possible. If dialysis is required, continuous modes of replacement are preferred because they result in less hemodynamic and ICP instability than intermittent modes.

Hemodynamics

A high cardiac output, low peripheral resistance state frequently occurs in ALF. Pressors are frequently required, and hemodynamic goals should be set, keeping cerebral and systemic factors in consideration.

Metabolic Derangement

With progressing liver failure, hypoglycemia is a frequent finding. Glucose infusion should be initiated and

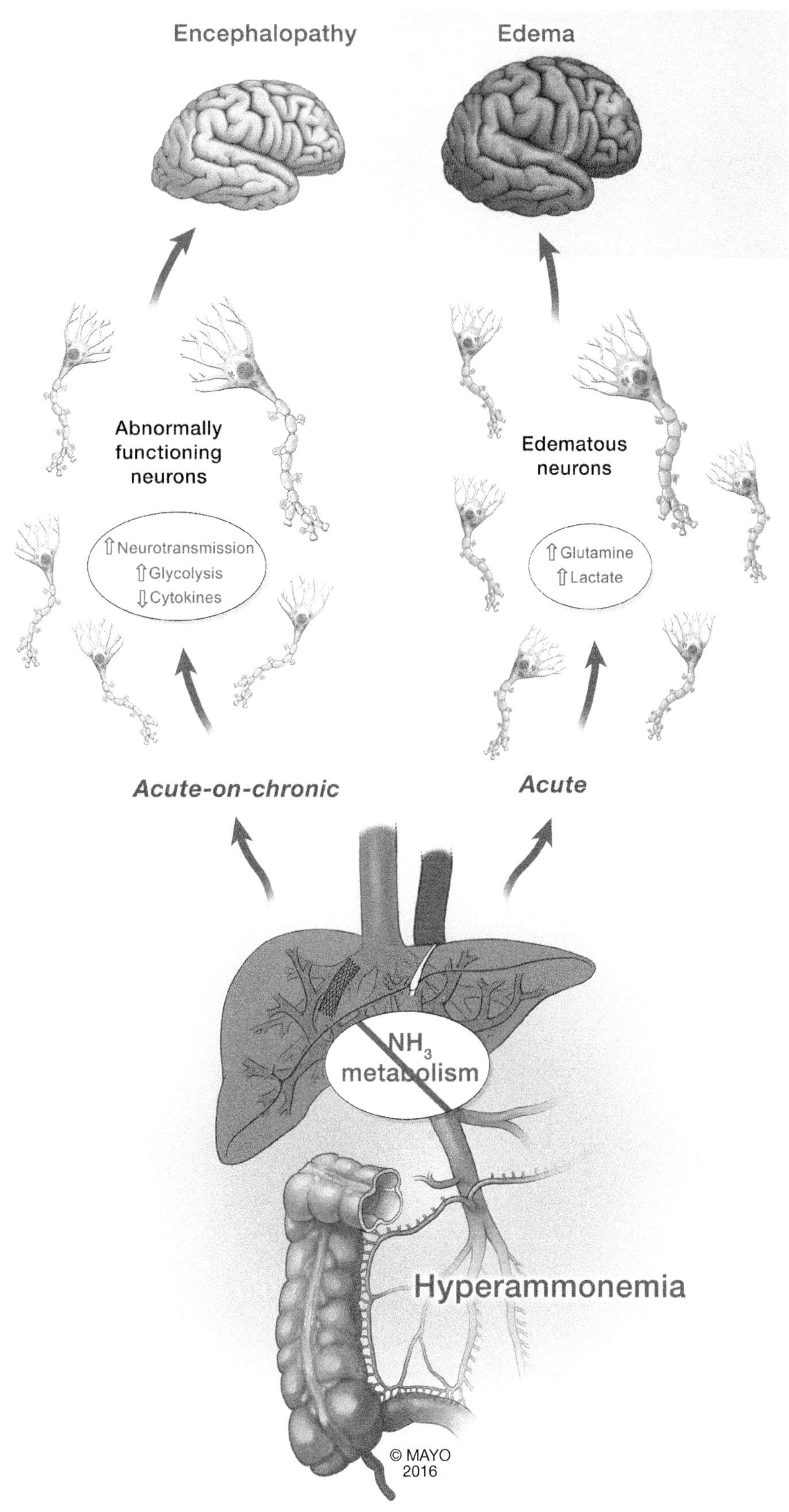

Figure 41.1. Putative Mechanism of Hepatic Encephalopathy and Brain Edema. NH_3 indicates ammonia.

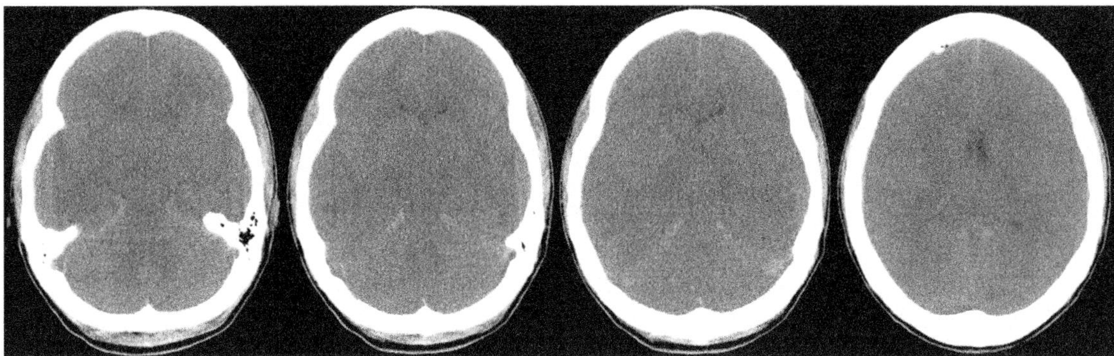

Figure 41.2. Cerebral Edema on Computed Tomography. Features include absent basal cisterns, loss of sulci, and loss of gray-white matter differentiation due to diffuse brain swelling.
(From Wijdicks EFM. Hepatic encephalopathy. N Engl J Med. 2016 Oct 27;375[17]:1660–70; used with permission.)

appropriately titrated. Phosphate, potassium, and magnesium levels should be monitored because replacement is frequently necessary.

Liver Support

Several liver support devices have been investigated, typically involving extracorporeal perfusion to replace liver function. These include hepatocyte-based systems and dialysis variants such as molecular adsorbent recirculating system. To date, none have shown conclusive benefit in clinical trials.

Decision to Transplant

Transplant is the only treatment option for patients with ALF who cannot be supported until adequate liver regeneration occurs or who sustain nonrecoverable liver injury. The determination of which patients require a liver transplant to survive ALF is an important consideration in management. Early identification of transplant candidates allows prompt listing and perhaps transplant before the development of severe multisystem failure, which can make the procedure and recovery more complex, or death. The most commonly used criteria are the King's College criteria (Box 41.1). Once these are met, listing should occur unless other contraindications are present. Patients who have had a prolonged period of ICH may have sustained irreversible brain injury and no longer be transplant candidates. Other conditions including comorbidities and psychosocial concerns may preclude proceeding to transplant.

Summary

- The most common cause of ALF in the United States is acetaminophen toxicity.
- ALF may progress rapidly, and thus patients should be closely monitored.
- Cerebral edema is the most serious complication and requires aggressive management.
- Multiple organ failure requiring high-level support is frequent.
- Liver transplant may be the only treatment; early referral to a transplant center is advised.

Box 41.1 • King's College Criteria for Transplant in Acute Liver Failure

Acetaminophen-induced ALF
- pH <7.3
- or
- Prothrombin time >100 s, creatinine >3.4 mg/dL, and grade 3 or 4 encephalopathy

Grade 4 encephalopathy

Other causes of ALF
- Prothrombin time >100 s
- or
- Any 3 of the following variables:
  - Age <10 y or >40 y
  - Duration of jaundice >7 d before onset of encephalopathy
  - Prothrombin time >50 s
  - Bilirubin >18 mg/dL
  - Cause is non-A, non-B hepatitis or idiosyncratic drug reaction

Abbreviation: ALF, acute liver failure.

Modified from O'Grady JG, Alexander GJ, Hayllar KM, Williams R. Early indicators of prognosis in fulminant hepatic failure. Gastroenterology. 1989 Aug;97(2):439-45; used with permission.

SUGGESTED READING

Bernal W, Hall C, Karvellas CJ, Auzinger G, Sizer E, Wendon J. Arterial ammonia and clinical risk factors for encephalopathy and intracranial hypertension in acute liver failure. Hepatology. 2007 Dec;46(6):1844–52.

Bernal W, Hyyrylainen A, Gera A, Audimoolam VK, McPhail MJ, Auzinger G, et al. Lessons from look-back in acute liver failure? A single centre experience of 3,300 patients. J Hepatol. 2013 Jul;59(1):74–80. Epub 2013 Feb 22.

Bernal W, Murphy N, Brown S, Whitehouse T, Bjerring PN, Hauerberg J, et al. A multicentre randomized controlled trial of moderate hypothermia to prevent intracranial hypertension in acute liver failure. J Hepatol. 2016 Aug;65(2):273–9. Epub 2016 Mar 12.

Davenport A, Will EJ, Davidson AM. Improved cardiovascular stability during continuous modes of renal replacement therapy in critically ill patients with acute hepatic and renal failure. Crit Care Med. 1993 Mar;21(3):328–38.

Fyfe B, Zaldana F, Liu C. The pathology of acute liver failure. Clin Liver Dis. 2018 May;22(2):257–68.

Lee WM. Etiologies of acute liver failure. Semin Liver Dis. 2008 May;28(2):142–52.

Lee WM, Hynan LS, Rossaro L, Fontana RJ, Stravitz RT, Larson AM, et al; Acute Liver Failure Study Group. Intravenous N-acetylcysteine improves transplant-free survival in early stage non-acetaminophen acute liver failure. Gastroenterology. 2009 Sep;137(3):856–64. Epub 2009 Jun 12. Erratum in: Gastroenterology. 2013 Sep;145(3):695.

Lee WM, Larson AM, Stravitz RT. AASLD positon paper: the management of acute liver failure: update 2011 [Internet]. American Association for the Study of Liver Diseases. c2011 [cited 2016 Nov 22]. Available from: https://www.aasld.org/sites/default/files/ guideline_documents/alfenhanced.pdf.

Lee WM, Squires RH Jr, Nyberg SL, Doo E, Hoofnagle JH. Acute liver failure: summary of a workshop. Hepatology. 2008 Apr;47(4):1401–15.

Maloney PR, Mallory GW, Atkinson JL, Wijdicks EF, Rabinstein AA, Van Gompel JJ. Intracranial pressure monitoring in acute liver failure: institutional case series. Neurocrit Care. 2016 Aug;25(1):86–93.

Montrief T, Koyfman A, Long B. Acute liver failure: a review for emergency physicians. Am J Emerge Med. 2019 Feb;37(2):329–37.

Munoz SJ. Difficult management problems in fulminant hepatic failure. Semin Liver Dis. 1993 Nov;13(4):395–413.

O'Grady JG, Alexander GJ, Hayllar KM, Williams R. Early indicators of prognosis in fulminant hepatic failure. Gastroenterology. 1989 Aug;97(2):439–45.

Squires JE, McKiernan P, Squires RH. Acute liver failure: an update. Clin Liver Dis. 2018 Nov;22(4):773–805.

Stravitz RT, Lisman T, Luketic VA, Sterling RK, Puri P, Fuchs M, et al. Minimal effects of acute liver injury/ acute liver failure on hemostasis as assessed by thromboelastography. J Hepatol. 2012 Jan;56(1):129–36. Epub 2011 May 19.

Vaquero J, Chung C, Cahill ME, Blei AT. Pathogenesis of hepatic encephalopathy in acute liver failure. Semin Liver Dis. 2003 Aug;23(3):259–69.

Wijdicks EFM. Hepatic encephalopathy. N Engl J Med. 2016 Oct 27;375(17):1660–70.

Acute Perforations of the Gastrointestinal Tract

LEVAN TSAMALAIDZE, MD; JOHN A. STAUFFER, MD

Goals

- Discuss the evolution and management of acute perforations of the gastrointestinal tract.
- Explain the algorithm of early diagnostic investigations, considering clinical features of acute abdomen in patients with neurologic conditions.
- Describe the optimal treatment of gastrointestinal tract perforations, including surgical intervention and postoperative care.
- Provide recommendations and preventive measures against acute perforations of the gastrointestinal tract in patients with neurologic conditions.

Introduction

Acute perforations of the gastrointestinal tract (GI) with subsequent release of gastric or intestinal contents into the peritoneal space have multiple causes and portend a high mortality depending on the cause. The key symptom is a sudden appearance of abdominal pain followed by signs of peritoneal irritation, severe sepsis, or shock. A proper imaging evaluation should lead to surgical intervention and aggressive supportive management.

Evolution of Acute Perforations of the GI Tract

For patients in an intensive care unit, GI hollow viscus perforation may occur under various conditions. In patients presenting emergently, acute GI perforation is a primary diagnosis. Alternatively, GI perforation may also occur and progress as a complication of critical illness. Organs that may undergo perforation include the esophagus, stomach and duodenum (ulcer perforation), gallbladder, small intestine, and colon.

GI perforation causes peritonitis, which is concomitant with the development of abdominal sepsis. The manifestations and septic complications that result are highly variable and depend on the character and location of the perforated hollow organ, the duration since the injury, the diameter of the perforation, the volume and chemical content of substance coming from the perforated organ, the abilities of neighboring tissues to resorb those contents, and the underlying comorbidities affecting a patient's immune response to the injury and functional reserve. Thus, there may be a multiplicity of different signs, symptoms, investigative findings, and clinical presentations disguised under the various diseases causing a critical condition. All of these underlying reasons make early and well-timed identification of the problem difficult. As with acute GI perforation and peritonitis, manifestations of abdominal sepsis vary with the site of perforation and contaminative agents. For example, stomach and duodenal contents provide fairly sterile, even if highly caustic, fluid compared with the high bacterial load of fecal peritonitis, a difference reflected in morbidity and mortality outcomes.

The total area of the peritoneum (visceral peritoneum) is about 50% of the total body surface. Contact of intestinal contents with peritoneum leads to increased capillary permeability and subsequent large-volume plasma exudation into the abdominal cavity, lumen of the intestine, the bowel wall, and mesentery. Within days, from 4 to 12 L of fluid may be relocated to the third space. Visceral peritoneum inflammation causes irritability and hyperkinesia for a short time, followed by bowel paralysis (paralytic ileus) and stretching. Thus, the involved colon cannot absorb fluids; instead, the quantity of intraluminal salts and water quickly increases. The resulting stretching of the hollow viscera compresses capillaries, reducing or even eliminating blood flow in the zone of inflammation, and patchy areas of ulceration lined by acute inflammatory exudates with edema and congestion are produced. Clinically, acute peritonitis is characterized by severe hypovolemia and shock. Furthermore, hypovolemia causes decreased cardiac output, compensatory vasoconstriction, and inadequate perfusion of tissues. If the condition is not resolved in a timely manner, it progresses to oliguria, metabolic acidosis, and respiratory distress. Peritonitis and subsequent septicemia can lead to septicemic shock. Local response to bacterial invasion of the perforated bowel is complex. In cases of fatal peritonitis, usually bacterial contamination takes place.

Causes

Presentation

Full-thickness injury with perforation of the GI tract is commonly caused by instrumentation or other trauma. However, methodical analysis of patients with spontaneous perforations, as a rule, exposes an etiologic factor, caused either by a full-thickness injury of the wall of the hollow organ or by a rapid and major increase of intraluminal pressure. Classic signs of acute abdomen in critically ill patients are not often expressed to the same degree as they are in healthy patients because of narcotic analgesia, medications compromising the immune system, and antibiotic use. Consequently, treatment of GI perforation is often substantially delayed because of minimal intensity of symptoms. Spontaneous esophageal perforation (Boerhaave syndrome) can be associated with intense nausea and vomiting.

Inflammation as a Pathophysiologic Factor

Inflammation can be produced by any of the following underlying etiologic factors:

- Ulceration: peptic ulcer, drugs, or chemical erosions.
- Autoimmune condition: inflammatory bowel disease or vasculitis.
- Infection: diverticulitis, *Clostridium difficile* colitis, typhoid and tuberculous perforation.
- Cardiovascular: mesenteric thrombosis and ischemia.
- Radiation: radiotherapy.
- Unknown: appendicitis.
- Lithogenesis: cholecystitis.
- Neoplastic: small bowel and colon tumors.
- Hernias and intestinal volvulus: external and internal hernias, sigmoid volvulus.
- Iatrogenic: perforation may occur as an early complication of endoscopy, such as stomach or esophageal perforation during upper GI endoscopy or damage to other intra-abdominal organs, such as the colon, during colonoscopy or endoscopic gastrostomy.
- Mechanical: obstruction or pseudoobstruction of intestine.

Clinical Approach

Primary Presentations

Symptoms associated with perforation depend on the location of the GI leakage (mediastinal, intraperitoneal, retroperitoneal and extra peritoneal). Perforation with spillage in the chest causes mediastinitis and overlap with symptoms in the peritoneal cavity that cause peritonitis. If spillage is exposed in the retroperitoneal or extraperitoneal space, the presentation is generally less dramatic and associated with more containment than free intraperitoneal perforations.

The main complaint of patients with GI perforation is persistent pain, often amplified by movement. Less commonly, esophageal perforation presents with pain in the chest or neck or with an unexplained unilateral pleural effusion.

Specific to patients in the neurocritical care unit, symptoms of GI perforation may be occult because their condition can cause a deeply comatose state or the patient may be under considerable pharmacologic sedation.

Secondary Presentations

Intestinal perforation may occur during a period of critical illness in patients with severe medical comorbidities, particularly in frail patients, those of advanced age, immunosuppressed patients, and patients with neurocritical illness. It can result in generalized abdominal infection and sepsis. In immunocompromised patients and patients undergoing antibiotic treatment for a previous source of sepsis, hospital-acquired infections may occur (approximately 50% of patients in an intensive care unit have a nosocomial infection and are at high risk for sepsis). These can include pseudomembranous colitis, which presents with diarrhea. In this case, the colon becomes colonized with *C difficile* organisms after the normal gut flora has been altered by antibiotic therapy. This condition leads to diarrhea provoked by the production of enterotoxins and cytotoxins. These pathologic processes may result in distributive shock and toxic megacolon with consequent colon perforations that are associated with high mortality in older patients and patients with neurocritical illness.

Respiratory failure, especially due to sepsis, is the main promotional factor for evolution of erosive gastritis. Erosive gastritis may be a result of compromised gastric mucosal blood flow during critical conditions. Alterations of regenerative and reparative processes caused by critical illness result in decreased production of protective factors such as prostaglandins and contribute to development of ulcerative processes in the GI tract.

Similarly, nasogastric tubes can also cause chronic irritation or pressure necrosis with perforation due to suction-related damage to the GI mucosa in patients with critical illness. This is usually identified when the aspirated gastric contents become guaiac positive or grossly bloody and requires further evaluation. Whenever possible, the nasogastric tube should be removed and upper endoscopy must be performed if signs or symptoms of ongoing upper GI bleeding are present.

Various drugs for critical illness may increase the propensity for pathologic processes to cause GI perforations. The use of nonsteroidal anti-inflammatory drugs (the most commonly implicated drugs are diclofenac and ibuprofen) and some antiplatelet medications (aspirin) have been associated with evolution of gastroduodenal erosions, colonic diverticulitis, and, rarely, jejunal ulceration. The risk of perforation increases with concurrent critical conditions. Glucocorticoids, in association with nonsteroidal anti-inflammatory drugs, are problematic because this combination suppresses the inflammatory response and subsequent recognition of a GI spillage can be delayed, as previously mentioned. Other medications, such as antibiotics, immunosuppressive drugs, iron supplementation, and cancer chemotherapy agents, also cause ulceration within the GI tract, starting as high as the esophagus and extending down the GI tract, and trigger pseudomembranous colitis, which may also cause GI perforation.

Examination

The main goal of the physical examination when GI perforation is suspected is to find signs of perforation. The following components of the examination are crucial for proper diagnosis:

- Abdominal examination: strict immobility of patient to decrease pressure on the peritoneum (sometimes referred to as "embryonic pose"), worsening pain after even lightly touching the abdomen (pain also increases during coughing or taking a breath), distended abdomen, abdominal guarding.
- Auscultation: absent bowel sounds.
- Percussion: percussion tenderness, loss of liver dullness.
- Palpation: rigid abdomen, guarding, rebound tenderness, subcutaneous emphysema.

In the later stages of GI perforation, an increasing volume of intestinal contents can be detected with a nasogastric tube. This finding may be a sign of ileus caused by peritonitis. Fever (>38.3°C) or hypothermia (<36°C), tachycardia (heart rate >90 beats per minute), weak pulse, oliguria, tachypnea (respiratory rate >20 breaths per minute, and signs of hypovolemia (turgor, decreased central venous pressure) reflect sepsis. Increasing hypotonia, cyanosis, and altered mentation point to the development of septicemia and shock.

It is important to measure intra-abdominal pressure, using a Foley catheter, if compartment syndrome caused by GI perforation and peritonitis is suspected. Normally, intra-abdominal pressure in critically ill patients is considered to be 5 to 7 mm Hg. Intra-abdominal pressure may increase as a result of many disorders or treatments, such as cirrhosis with ascites, pancreatitis, after massive resuscitation or massive transfusions, sepsis, acidosis, or respiratory failure that requires high positive end-expiratory pressure levels for treatment.

Thus, the key step in the intensive care unit is to perform vigilant investigations of the abdomen to find these complications at an early stage for elderly or obese patients, patients receiving corticosteroids or sedatives, or patients who have an unexplained presentation of developing sepsis without signs of peritoneal irritation.

Laboratory signs for surgical sepsis related to GI perforation are similar to those of other types of septic conditions (nonspecific markers: leukocytosis or leukopenia, deviation of C-reactive protein level more than 2 times above SD, coagulopathy, thrombocytopenia, hyperlactatemia, high level of plasma procalcitonin, hypoalbuminemia, azotemia). Testing of serum amylase is important in cases of acute abdomen to help determine the presence or absence of pancreatitis. It is important to exclude pancreatitis, because it will initially be a contraindication to surgical intervention. Unlike patients with pancreatitis, patients with acute abdomen from GI perforation generally have serum amylase levels less than 4 times the upper limit of normal.

Radiology

Ultrasonography

When hollow organ perforation is suspected in a patient in the intensive care unit, a focused assessment with sonography for trauma, with the patient in the Trendelenburg position, is widely used to evaluate for free fluid in the abdominal cavity. Assessment of the hepatorenal recess (Morison pouch), splenorenal space, and bladder (bladder is filled to serve as an acoustic window in the space behind the bladder) is optimal. Ultrasonography is also an emerging modality to demonstrate free air in abdomen, reaching or surpassing the sensitivity of supine chest films.

Plain Radiography

Plain upright chest radiography (without transportation of the critically ill patient from the intensive care unit), in addition to ultrasonography, is helpful for identifying GI perforation by detecting free air in the abdomen. The sensitivity for determining extraluminal air on plain radiography ranges from 50% to 75% (recent surgical or

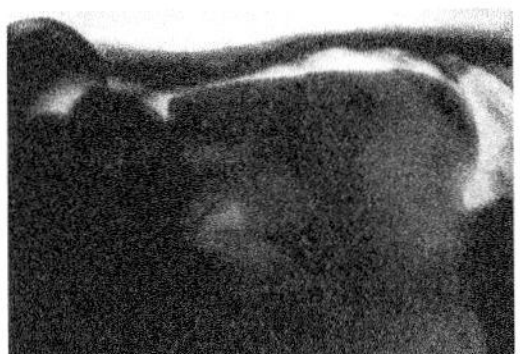

Figure 42.1. Plain Radiograph From Patient in Left Lateral Decubitus Position. Free gas is visible as a strip between the liver and the right lateral abdominal wall.

percutaneous interventions must be taken into consideration). Thus, there are several radiologic signs of pneumoperitoneum (Figure 42.1). The Rigler sign is an effect of air on both sides of the bowel wall. On a lateral image obtained with the patient in the supine position, free gas becomes visible as a strip under the front abdominal wall located in front of the liver (it has a contrasting density). If gas collects in the Morison pouch, a triangular bubble may also be seen just medial and inferior to the 11th rib. In case of the absence of free air and a high suspicion for contained perforation of the upper GI tract, esophagogastroduodenoscopy is recommended. If detection of a perforated area is difficult with endoscopy, redo radiography is recommended. If upper endoscopy is contraindicated (eg, critical condition of the patient), 200 mL of air is inserted with a nasogastric tube and radiography is repeated. If the patient's condition allows a fully upright or a left lateral decubitus position, free air can be seen on plain radiography between the liver and the right lateral abdominal wall.

If there is free air and no clinical manifestation of perforation of a hollow organ in the abdomen (in the absence of immunosuppressive therapies), the source for pneumoperitoneum could be benign (in patients on respiratory support, pneumoperitoneum can be due to continuous positive airway pressure or positive-end-expiratory pressure, endoscopy, paracentesis, peritoneal dialysis, and vaginal instrumentation), and further studies may be required.

Computed Tomography

Extraluminal air may not be demonstrable on radiographic images if the perforation is very small, self-sealed, or well contained by adjacent organs. Development of and advances in medical imaging technologies have caused computed tomography (CT) to supplant contrasted plain radiography, for the most part. This method of investigation is more informative than previous-generation imaging (Figure 42.2). Thus, for most patients, CT is the second step of imaging. Diagnosis of alimentary tract perforation is based on direct findings of extraluminal air or luminal contrast material and discontinuation of the GI wall and on indirect findings of abscess and an inflammatory mass or phlegmon related to the bowel with or without an associated enterolith or foreign body. The main disadvantage of CT is that it requires transportation of a critically ill patient with the associated risks.

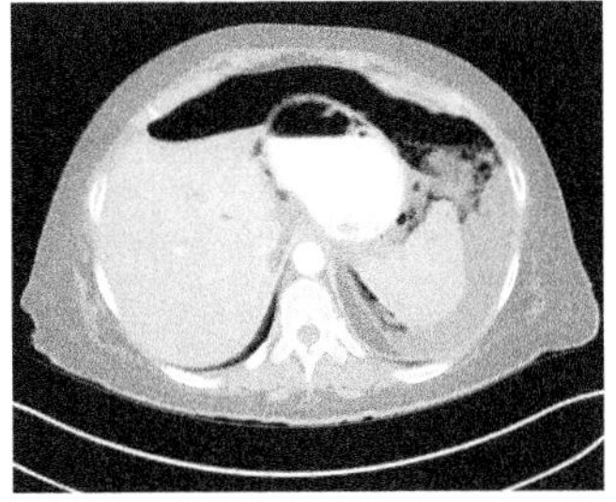

Figure 42.2. Computed Tomography Image From Patient With Gastrointestinal Perforation. Large amount of free air is seen between front abdominal wall and visceral organs.

Therefore, investigations in the intensive care unit begin with bedside ultrasonography. If no free fluid is found and clinical manifestations indicate acute abdomen, bedside radiography or CT is recommended. In a symptomatic patient, if fluid is detected without free air in the abdominal cavity, diagnostic abdominal paracentesis is indicated for identification of the character of the fluid. If GI substrate is found on paracentesis, surgery is necessary. Alternatively, if perforation is strongly suspected but not identified on imaging, laparoscopy is recommended as an invasive diagnostic method (Figure 42.3).

Treatment

Conservative

If a cervical or thoracic esophageal perforation is small, does not penetrate into the pleural cavity, and is not resulting in severe sepsis, placement of a nasogastric tube and drain in the esophagus for decompression is recommended. Also, if investigations show duodenal ulcer perforation with minimal free air and fluid in the abdomen without signs

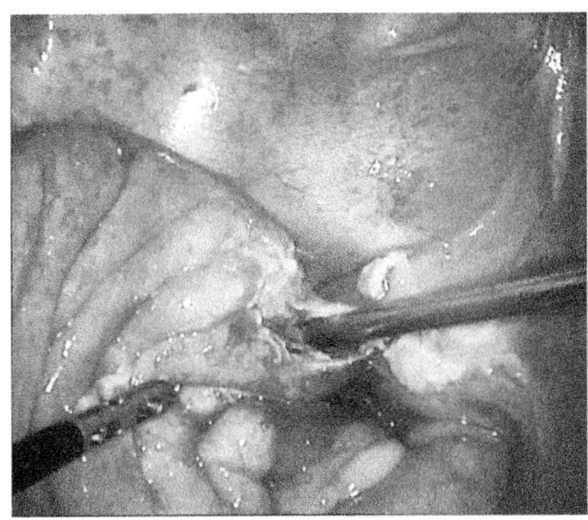

Figure 42.3. Results on Exploratory Laparoscopy in a Case of Suspected Perforation. A perforated sigmoid colon.

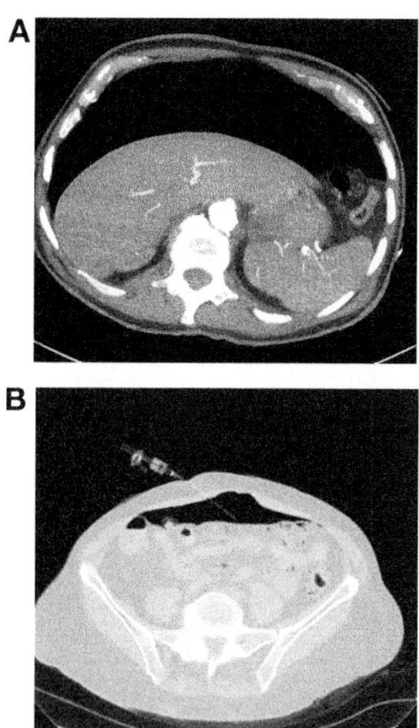

Figure 42.4. Computed Tomography in a Patient With Pneumoperitoneum. A, Extensive pneumoperitoneum. B, Guided needle decompression of pneumoperitoneum.

of generalized peritonitis, conservative treatment with a nasogastric tube and permanent suction may be attempted. However, if conservative therapy is attempted, close attention and monitoring by an experienced surgeon with serial abdominal examinations are needed. If the condition is worsening or radiologic signs show increasing volume of fluid, surgery is recommended. Intra-abdominal perforations may sometimes be walled off within an inflammatory mass (diverticular and appendix masses) and may be treated conservatively (antibiotics, anti-inflammatory agents). This approach allows for resolution of inflammation before elective surgery. Sometimes surgery may be circumvented by using radiologically guided drains for intra-abdominal collections, especially in critically ill patients, in whom surgery is associated with high mortality.

Contained GI perforation resulting in pneumoperitoneum is a rare complication of endoscopic procedures. Traditionally, GI perforation with diffuse pneumoperitoneum has been treated with surgical exploration. However, when these perforations are localized or successfully treated with endoscopic closure (with over-the-scope metallic clips or fibrin glue), operative management may not be necessary in select cases. If physical examinations show visceral peritoneal irritation resulting from pneumoperitoneum (Figure 42.4A) image-guided paracentesis is recommended (Figure 42.4B).

Surgical

An esophageal perforation of the cervical or neck region requires tissue irrigation and drainage of the contaminated spaces. Thoracic or mediastinal perforation causing clinical deterioration requires a different operative approach depending on size, site, and localization of perforation. Surgery may include repair, diversion, and exclusion, or even stenting. Large-bore chest drains may be required for pleural cavities.

Surgical treatment of intra-abdominal perforations may be accomplished with endoscopy, laparoscopy, or open surgery. If bedside endoscopy reveals acute GI perforation without considerably inflamed edges (diameter <1 cm), primary endoscopic closure of the defect may be performed by suturing or using endoscopic clips (Figure 42.5) (appropriate equipment and skills are necessary). In case of failure of endoscopic technique, laparoscopy or laparotomy is recommended. Decontamination of the abdominal cavity by suction and irrigation is followed by detection and repair of perforation. Further surgical tactics depend on the site and size of the defect in the GI tract. A small gastric or duodenal perforated ulcer may be oversewn with an omental patch. Small-bowel perforation may be treated by closing or segmental excising with primary anastomosis. Colonic perforation, as a rule, is associated with high contamination. In the majority of cases, primary anastomosis is not performed because of the risk of dehiscence. A Hartmann procedure is

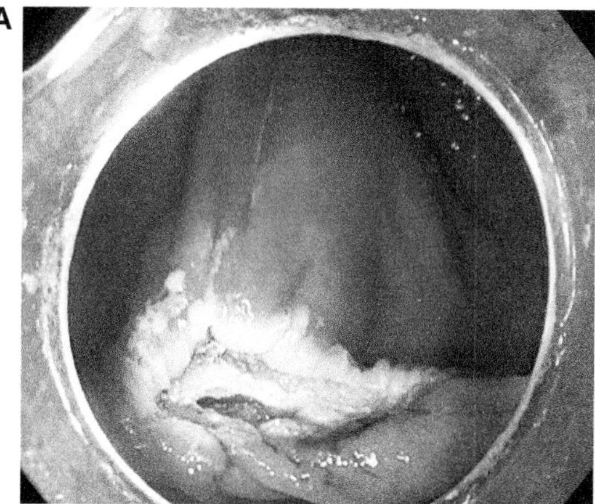

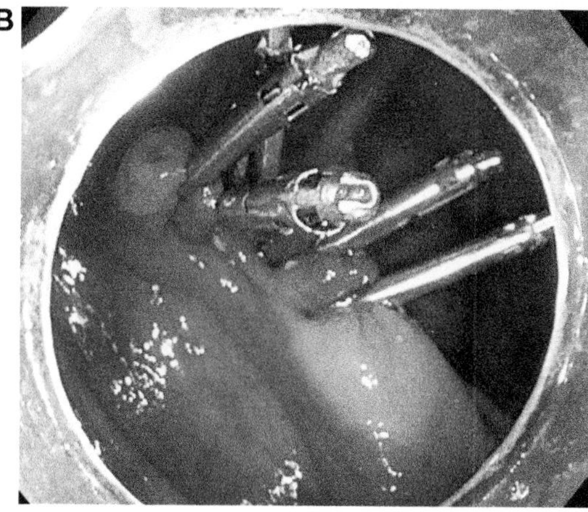

Figure 42.5. Perforated Duodenal Ulcer (A) With Primary Endoscopic Closure by Clipping (B).

recommended (proximal colon is exteriorized as a colostomy and the rectal stump is simply oversewn). Defunctioning ileostomy, with the ability to subsequently perform a simple reversion procedure, does not lessen the risk of colonic perforation but lessens the effects should it occur.

In case of severe peritonitis, laparostomy (open abdomen) may be performed in which the laparotomy wound is left open and a sterile plastic bag or vacuum dressing is sewn into the wound. It allows the abdomen to be accessed for further washout and prevents evolution of abdominal compartment syndrome. The laparostomy can be closed after peritonitis is terminated.

The surgical treatment of toxic megacolon and its complications, caused by pseudomembranous colitis, is with colectomy performed in a timely manner because of high morbidity and mortality.

Summary

- In critically ill patients, suspicion for potential perforation should be maintained because signs and symptoms may be obscured. Nausea and vomiting, progressive diarrhea, ileus, and abdominal distention should raise concerns.
- Bedside ultrasonography is the recommended initial test when perforation is suspected; CT should be the next test, depending on findings and a patient's condition.
- Measurement of intra-abdominal pressure is important if abdominal compartment syndrome is suspected.
- When perforation is suspected, imaging and laboratory studies should never substitute for the clinical judgment of an experienced surgeon.
- All patients in whom a perforation is suspected should have a surgical consultation.

SUGGESTED READING

Covarrubias DA, O'Connor OJ, McDermott S, Arellano RS. Radiologic percutaneous gastrostomy: review of potential complications and approach to managing the unexpected outcome. AJR Am J Roentgenol. 2013 Apr;200(4):921–31.

Furukawa A, Sakoda M, Yamasaki M, Kono N, Tanaka T, Nitta N, et al. Gastrointestinal tract perforation: CT diagnosis of presence, site, and cause. Abdom Imaging. 2005 Sep-Oct;30(5):524–34.

Haito-Chavez Y, Law JK, Kratt T, Arezzo A, Verra M, Morino M, et al. International multicenter experience with an over-the-scope clipping device for endoscopic management of GI defects (with video). Gastrointest Endosc. 2014 Oct;80(4):610–22. Epub 2014 Jun 5.

Jain A, Vargas HD. Advances and challenges in the management of acute colonic pseudo-obstruction (Ogilvie syndrome). Clin Colon Rectal Surg. 2012 Mar;25(1):37–45.

Malbrain ML. Abdominal pressure in the critically ill: measurement and clinical relevance. Intensive Care Med. 1999 Dec;25(12):1453–8.

Malbrain ML, Chiumello D, Pelosi P, Bihari D, Innes R, Ranieri VM, et al. Incidence and prognosis of intraabdominal hypertension in a mixed population of critically ill patients: a multiple-center epidemiological study. Crit Care Med. 2005 Feb;33(2):315–22.

Revell MA, Pugh MA, McGhee M. Gastrointestinal traumatic injuries: gastrointestinal perforation. Crit Care Nurs Clin North Am. 2018 Mar;30(1):157–66.

Rubesin SE, Levine MS. Radiologic diagnosis of gastrointestinal perforation. Radiol Clin North Am. 2003 Nov;41(6):1095–115.

Seltman AK. Surgical management of Clostridium difficile colitis. Clin Colon Rectal Surg. 2012 Dec;25(4):204–9.

Siu WT, Chau CH, Law BK, Tang CN, Ha PY, Li MK. Routine use of laparoscopic repair for perforated peptic ulcer. Br J Surg. 2004 Apr;91(4):481–4.

Squires R, Carter SN, Postier RG. Acute abdomen. In: Townsend CM, Beauchamp RD, Evers BM, Mattox KL, editors. Sabiston textbook of surgery. 20th ed. Philadelphia (PA): Elsevier; c2017. p. 1120-38.

Weaver TL, Goldberg RF, Stauffer JA, Frey ES. Needle before the knife: nonoperative management of pneumoperitoneum with image-guided aspiration after gastrointestinal perforation. Surg Laparosc Endosc Percutan Tech. 2014 Apr;24(2):e74–6. Erratum in: Surg Laparosc Endosc Percutan Tech. 2014 Jun;24(3):282.

Acute Vascular Disorders of the Intestine

OMAR Y. MOUSA, MBBS; SURAKIT PUNGPAPONG, MD

Goals

- Describe the causes and presentations of acute vascular diseases of the intestine.
- Elucidate the mechanism of intestinal injury.
- Discuss the steps to diagnosis and management of intestinal injury.

Introduction

Mesenteric ischemia is caused by insufficient blood supply to the foregut and intestines. When the blood supply does not meet the metabolic requirements of these organs, catastrophic complications may result. Death is imminent in the setting of acute mesenteric ischemia if diagnosis is delayed; associated mortality rates are as high as 60% to 80%. The severity and extent of this disease depend on the nature of the vascular obstruction and the type of occluded vessel.

The mechanism of intestinal wall injury in the setting of impaired blood flow is shown in Figure 43.1. Bacterial translocation from the intestine can eventually occur from intestinal injury.

Acute Mesenteric Ischemia

Acute mesenteric ischemia is a surgical emergency that requires prompt recognition and intervention (Figures 43.2 and 43.3). It is an uncommon cause of abdominal pain and is due to embolic occlusion in approximately 50% of cases. Other causes of acute ischemia include arterial thrombosis and complete occlusion in the setting of previous stenosis (20%-35%) or arterial dissection or inflammation (<5%). The superior mesenteric artery is classically involved. Nonocclusive mesenteric ischemia can be due to regional vasospasm and impaired perfusion (5%-15% of cases). It is related to low-flow states, hypovolemia, or heart failure or can occur after cardiac surgery and hemodialysis.

Clinical Presentation

Classically, patients present with pain out of proportion to findings on abdominal examination. However, up to a quarter of patients do not have a classic presentation. On auscultation, epigastric bruit may be found. Tenderness is present when peritonitis develops. A high level of suspicion in the appropriate clinical setting is crucial to establish the diagnosis.

Diagnosis

Obtaining a careful history and the physical examination are basic steps in establishing an early diagnosis. Any previous history of atherosclerotic vascular disease should be assessed. The acuteness of onset suggests an embolic phenomenon, mainly with a previous history of atrial fibrillation and myocardial infarction. Assessment of the acid-base status is important because the presence of leukocytosis and lactic acidosis indicates an advanced stage with full-thickness injury due to severe ischemia. Low D-dimer levels may exclude acute mesenteric ischemia.

Abdominal radiography may show ileus in the early stages and thumbprinting sign due to edematous intestinal wall or pneumatosis later on. Abdominal duplex ultrasonography has a limited role in the diagnosis. One possible reason is that emboli are usually located in the distal superior mesenteric artery, and thus the rate of false-negative results of this examination is high.

Computed tomography angiography is a highly recommended next step for the diagnosis of acute mesenteric ischemia and the exclusion of other causes. It is a rapid test and assists in evaluating the location and degree of occlusion. Its benefits outweigh its risks. Magnetic resonance angiography is a noninvasive test and is helpful in patients with kidney disease or allergy to iodinated contrast agents.

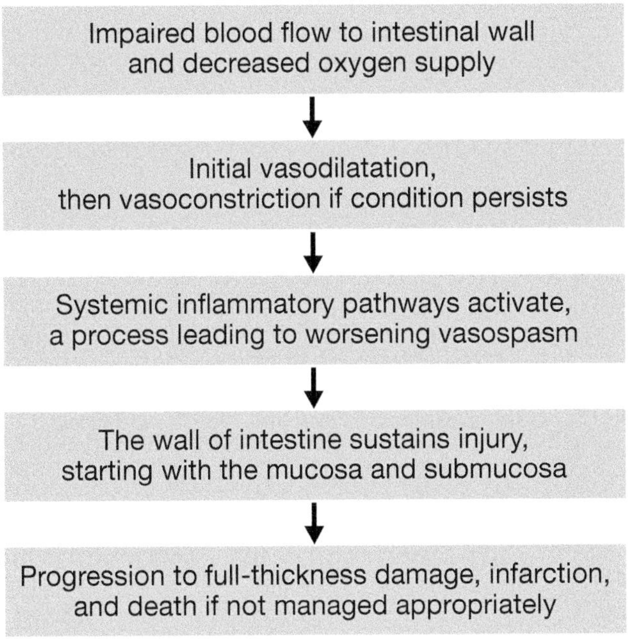

Impaired blood flow to intestinal wall and decreased oxygen supply

↓

Initial vasodilatation, then vasoconstriction if condition persists

↓

Systemic inflammatory pathways activate, a process leading to worsening vasospasm

↓

The wall of intestine sustains injury, starting with the mucosa and submucosa

↓

Progression to full-thickness damage, infarction, and death if not managed appropriately

Figure 43.1. The Mechanism of Intestinal Wall Injury.

However, evaluation is limited to the proximal parts of the superior mesenteric artery and celiac artery, and it has the potential for overestimation of the grade of stenosis.

Endoscopic evaluation is not indicated because of low sensitivity for detection of minimal ischemic changes. Advanced ischemic changes should be easily recognized with radiologic imaging, and prompt recognition allows for early surgical intervention.

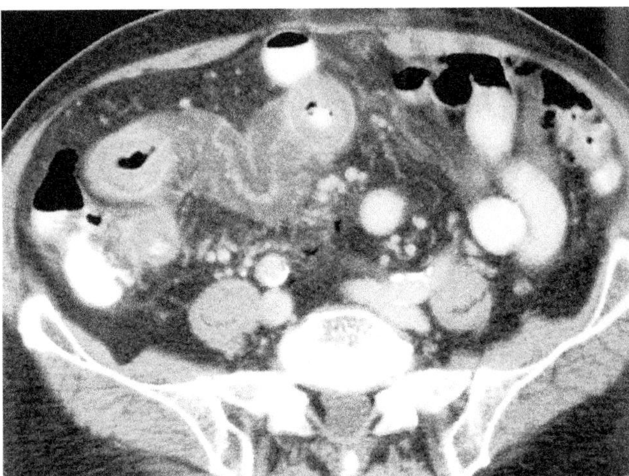

Figure 43.2. Contrast-Enhanced Computed Tomography of the Abdomen, Suggestive of Ischemic Small Bowel. *A thick-walled small bowel loop is present in the right side of the abdomen with submucosal edema.*

(From Johnson CD. Mayo Clinic gastrointestinal imaging review. 2nd ed. Oxford [UK]: Oxford University Press; c2014. Chapter 4, small bowel; p.208-322; used with permission of Mayo Foundation for Medical Education and Research.)

Management

Survival of patients with acute occlusion of the mesenteric artery depends on prompt recognition and emergency surgical intervention. Survival rates approach 50% when the diagnosis is made within 24 hours of symptom onset. Delayed recognition leads to progression of injury from ischemia to gangrene and high mortality.

Initial management should include nothing-by-mouth status, volume resuscitation, heparin treatment, and antibiotics given the risk of bacterial translocation. Emergency laparoscopy is not indicated for acute mesenteric ischemia because of its limited ability to recognize intestinal viability. Catheter angiography and revascularization are well established for management. Endovascular therapies (thrombolysis or angioplasty and stenting) are fast, safe, and associated with low mortality compared with open repairs. However, up 60% of patients who undergo endovascular therapy may have deterioration requiring exploratory laparotomy and bowel resection. Embolectomy is reserved for cases with embolism of the proximal superior mesenteric artery. Follow-up imaging after repair is crucial to detect early recurrence of the disease. Duplex ultrasonography can be performed twice a year for the first year and then annually.

Long-term management includes risk factor modification. Control of hypertension and hyperlipidemia and smoking cessation are essential measures. Antiplatelet therapies include aspirin and clopidogrel after open or endovascular repair. Total parenteral nutrition may be needed until adequate oral intake is maintained.

Mesenteric Vein Thrombosis

Mesenteric vein thrombosis can lead to mesenteric ischemia in less than 15% of cases, regardless whether of the cause is idiopathic thrombosis, thrombophilia, or trauma or due to a localized inflammatory process (eg, pancreatitis, diverticulitis, or cholangitis). Onset of symptoms is less sudden than with acute mesenteric ischemia.

Management should include systemic anticoagulation to decrease the risk of recurrence and death. Surgical intervention may include thrombectomy or thrombolysis, both of which are associated with low complication rates. Survival rates depend on the cause of thrombosis but reach up to 70% after 5 years.

Chronic Mesenteric Ischemia

Atherosclerotic disease is the cause of the majority of cases of chronic mesenteric ischemia (about 90%). It usually involves the origin of mesenteric vessels, with development

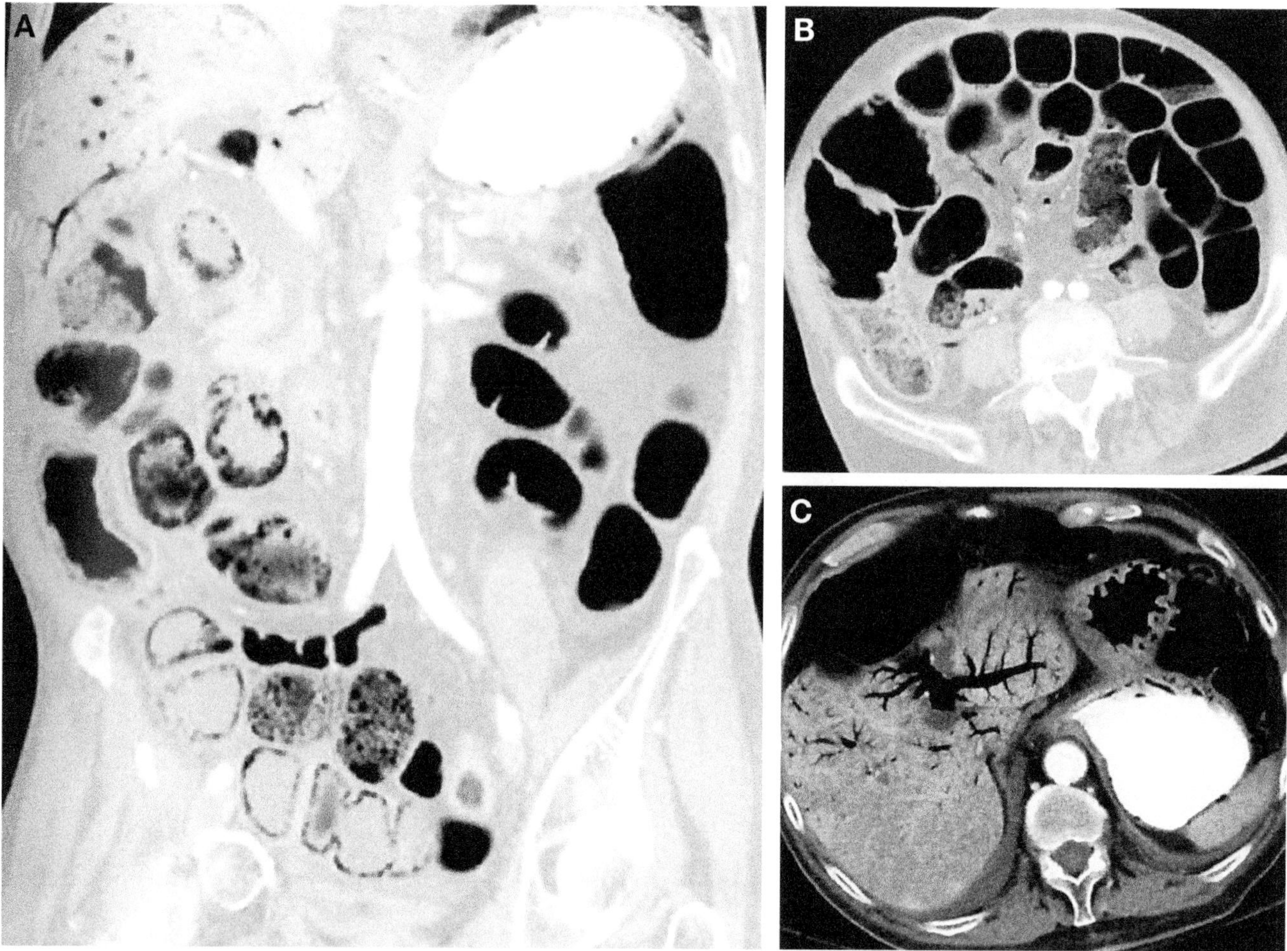

Figure 43.3. Contrast-Enhanced Computed Tomography in a Case of Mesenteric Ischemia With Secondary Pneumatosis Intestinalis and Portal Venous Gas. A, Multiple small bowel loops with pneumatosis. B, Mesenteric veins containing air. C, Portal venous gas inside the liver.

(From Johnson CD. Mayo Clinic gastrointestinal imaging review. 2nd ed. Oxford [UK]: Oxford University Press; c2014. Chapter 4, small bowel; p.208-322; used with permission of Mayo Foundation for Medical Education and Research.)

of collateral circulation over time leading to a delayed presentation until occlusion of the primary vessels.

Clinical Presentation

Abdominal pain, typically 30 to 60 minutes after meals, is the main symptom. Affected patients restrict food to avoid having pain and, therefore, lose weight. Associated symptoms include nausea, vomiting, early satiety, and changes in bowel habit.

Diagnosis

Care should be taken in patients with chronic abdominal pain who have already undergone endoscopic evaluation that had negative findings, a common scenario in chronic mesenteric ischemia. Older age, weight loss, tobacco use, and a history of atherosclerotic vascular disease should raise suspicion for this condition.

Management

Management includes elective revascularization, most commonly with endovascular repair, which has high success rates and minimal complications. Restenosis occurs in less than half of patients and requires reintervention. Stenting is superior to angioplasty alone. Open repair remains an alternative if endovascular repair alone is inadequate or in young, low-risk patients and allows vascular patency for longer duration. Enteral nutrition should be considered to improve the nutritional and immune status.

Colonic Ischemia

The mechanism of intestinal injury is similar to that of mesenteric ischemia. The duration and acuity of reduction in blood flow and the presence of collateral circulation influence the degree of injury. Damage can be reversible, and patients may be asymptomatic even though ulceration may last for several months. However, irreversible damage can develop, leading to fulminant colitis, gangrene, stricture formation, and obstruction or it may persist for a long duration and lead to chronic colitis. Risk factors for ischemic colitis include comorbidities such as cardiovascular disease, diabetes mellitus, chronic kidney disease, chronic obstructive pulmonary disease, surgical procedures that sacrifice the inferior mesenteric artery (eg, abdominal aortic aneurysm repair), and medications such as constipation-inducing agents, immunomodulators, and illicit drugs.

Clinical Presentation

The main presenting symptoms in ischemic colitis include sudden crampy, mild abdominal pain. This is associated with bright red rectal bleeding, maroon stools, or bloody diarrhea in the acute setting. These can be accompanied by an urgency to defecate. Lack of hematochezia is common in right-sided colonic ischemia, especially in patients receiving dialysis or those with sepsis and hypotension or shock.

Diagnosis

The first imaging method of choice is computed tomography of the abdomen with intravenous and oral contrast agents. This shows bowel wall thickening, edema, and thumbprinting. If imaging shows colonic pneumatosis or portomesenteric venous gas, transmural colonic infarction should be suspected. Multiphasic computed tomography angiography should be the next step if isolated right-sided colonic ischemia or acute mesenteric ischemia is suspected from the clinical presentation. Colonoscopy should be performed within the first 24 hours to confirm ischemic colitis, except when acute peritonitis, pneumatosis, or gangrene already exists.

Management

Conservative management is recommended in most patients with colonic ischemia, because the majority will have spontaneous resolution. Antibiotics are needed given the increased risk of bacterial translocation. Surgical intervention is needed in the setting of hypotension or tachycardia or if isolated right-sided colonic ischemia or pancolonic ischemia or gangrene is present.

Portal Vein Ischemia and Thrombosis

Sudden thrombosis within the portal vein (also called acute pylephlebitis) may be partial or complete. It can involve a variable part of the mesenteric veins, leading to intestinal ischemia. With complete obstruction, intestinal infarction develops, which is clinically manifested by severe abdominal pain, bloody diarrhea, ascites, metabolic acidosis, and renal or respiratory insufficiency. Prompt management with anticoagulation is highly indicated to avoid imminent complications, including intestinal perforation, peritonitis, multiorgan failure, and death. Prognosis is good in patients who have anticoagulation initiated soon after onset of the injury because it prevents intestinal infarction by keeping the superior mesenteric vein patent or recanalized. On long-term follow-up, intestinal obstruction from strictures related to prior ischemia develops in a small proportion of patients.

Summary

- Acute mesenteric ischemia is a surgical emergency that requires prompt recognition and intervention.
- Classically, patients with acute mesenteric ischemia present with pain out of proportion to findings on abdominal examination.
- Computed tomography angiography is a highly recommended next step in the diagnosis of acute mesenteric ischemia and for exclusion of other causes.
- Mesenteric vein thrombosis can lead to mesenteric ischemia in less than 15% of cases, and management should include systemic anticoagulation.
- Abdominal pain, typically 30 to 60 minutes after meals, is the main symptom in chronic mesenteric ischemia.
- The main presenting symptoms in ischemic colitis include sudden crampy abdominal pain, and bright red rectal bleeding or bloody diarrhea in the acute setting. Conservative management is recommended in most patients.
- Ischemia due to portal vein thrombosis leads to severe abdominal pain, bloody diarrhea, ascites, metabolic acidosis, and renal or respiratory insufficiency. Prompt management with anticoagulation is highly indicated.

SUGGESTED READING

Acosta S. Epidemiology of mesenteric vascular disease: clinical implications. Semin Vasc Surg. 2010 Mar;23(1):4–8.

Acosta S, Alhadad A, Svensson P, Ekberg O. Epidemiology, risk and prognostic factors in mesenteric venous thrombosis. Br J Surg. 2008 Oct;95(10):1245–51.

Beaulieu RJ, Arnaoutakis KD, Abularrage CJ, Efron DT, Schneider E, Black JH 3rd. Comparison of open and endovascular treatment of acute mesenteric ischemia. J Vasc Surg. 2014 Jan;59(1):159–64. Epub 2013 Nov 5. Erratum in: J Vasc Surg. 2014 Jul;60(1):273.

Brandt LJ, Feuerstadt P, Longstreth GF, Boley SJ; American College of Gastroenterology. ACG clinical guideline: epidemiology, risk factors, patterns of presentation, diagnosis, and management of colon ischemia (CI). Am J Gastroenterol. 2015 Jan;110(1):18–44. Epub 2014 Dec 23.

Clair DG, Beach JM. Mesenteric ischemia. N Engl J Med. 2016 Mar 10;374(10):959–68.

DeLeve LD, Valla DC, Garcia-Tsao G; American Association for the Study Liver Diseases. Vascular disorders of the liver. Hepatology. 2009 May;49(5):1729–64.

Di Minno MN, Milone F, Milone M, Iaccarino V, Venetucci P, Lupoli R, et al. Endovascular thrombolysis in acute mesenteric vein thrombosis: a 3-year follow-up with the rate of short and long-term sequaelae in 32 patients. Thromb Res. 2010 Oct;126(4):295–8. Epub 2010 Jan 25.

Kozar RA, Hu S, Hassoun HT, DeSoignie R, Moore FA. Specific intraluminal nutrients alter mucosal blood flow during gut ischemia/reperfusion. JPEN J Parenter Enteral Nutr. 2002 Jul-Aug;26(4):226–9.

Kumar S, Sarr MG, Kamath PS. thrombosis. Mesenteric venous N Engl J Med. 2001 Dec 6;345(23):1683–8.

Lim S, Halandras PM, Bechara C, Aulivola B, Crisostomo P. Contemporary management of acute mesenteric ischemia in the endovascular era. Vasc Endovascular Surg. 2019 Jan;53(1):42–50.

Oderich GS, Bower TC, Sullivan TM, Bjarnason H, Cha S, Gloviczki P. Open versus endovascular revascularization for chronic mesenteric ischemia: risk-stratified outcomes. J Vasc Surg. 2009 Jun;49(6):1472–9.e3.

Oldenburg WA, Lau LL, Rodenberg TJ, Edmonds HJ, Burger CD. Acute mesenteric ischemia: a clinical review. Arch Intern Med. 2004 May 24;164(10):1054–62.

Ryer EJ, Kalra M, Oderich GS, Duncan AA, Gloviczki P, Cha S, et al. Revascularization for acute mesenteric ischemia. J Vasc Surg. 2012 Jun;55(6):1682–9. Epub 2012 Apr 12.

Sauerland S, Agresta F, Bergamaschi R, Borzellino G, Budzynski A, Champault G, et al. Laparoscopy for abdominal emergencies: evidence-based guidelines of the European Association for Endoscopic Surgery. Surg Endosc. 2006 Jan;20(1):14–29. Epub 2005 Oct 24.

Schermerhorn ML, Giles KA, Hamdan AD, Wyers MC, Pomposelli FB. Mesenteric revascularization: management and outcomes in the United States, 1988-2006. J Vasc Surg. 2009 Aug;50(2):341–8.e1. Epub 2009 Apr 16.

Wyers MC. Acute mesenteric ischemia: diagnostic approach and surgical treatment. Semin Vasc Surg. 2010 Mar;23(1):9–20.

Abdominal Compartment Syndrome

DANIEL J. JOHNSON, MD

Goals

- Define abdominal compartment syndrome.
- Identify the systemic complications of abdominal compartment syndrome.
- Describe the diagnostic approach to and definitive management of abdominal compartment syndrome.

Introduction

In abdominal compartment syndrome (ACS), a fixed compartment (the abdomen with defined myofascial elements) is subjected to increased pressure. The result is decreased organ perfusion and subsequent dysfunction inside the abdominal cavity and the respiratory and cardiovascular systems. Given the potential for progressive organ dysfunction, identifying ACS within the context of the primary illness and instituting appropriate management can be crucial for patients in the intensive care unit.

Definitions and Description

ACS is a clinical condition brought on by a sustained increase in intra-abdominal pressure (IAP) that results in organ dysfunction. This condition occurs in patients who are otherwise critically ill and have an underlying abnormality that serves to increase IAP. A wide variety of scenarios can increase IAP, ranging from a transient increase due to a cough, sneeze, or Valsalva maneuver to a sustained, long-term increase from massive abdominal ascites. More specifically, the acute conditions that increase IAP leading to ACS in critical illness are listed in Box 44.1.

A normal IAP is rather difficult to define; however, in critical illness, it usually ranges from 5 to 7 mm Hg. Intra-abdominal hypertension (IAH) is defined as a sustained pressure more than 12 mm Hg. Although organ dysfunction does not typically occur at this level, different grades of IAH have clinical significance regarding the development and treatment of ACS (Table 44.1). Although ACS results from sustained IAH due to increased IAP, these terms are not synonymous. Organ dysfunction must be clearly demonstrated to diagnose ACS, because this implies a need to intervene. Therefore, the current definition of ACS includes a sustained IAP more than 20 mm Hg with new organ dysfunction. Primary ACS is due to intra-abdominal abnormality (eg, trauma, infection), and secondary ACS results from extra-abdominal conditions (eg, burns, massive resuscitation). A third category, called recurrent ACS, occurs after appropriate treatment has previously been rendered.

Pathophysiology

IAH can affect both abdominal and remote vital organs by restricting arterial perfusion or limiting venous drainage. Every major organ system can potentially be affected. The more notable effects are described below.

Cardiovascular

The primary cardiac changes result from diminished venous return and impaired filling of the right side of the heart caused by compression of the inferior vena cava by IAH. The reduction in forward cardiac flow can be exacerbated by hypovolemia and intra-thoracic pressure changes caused by mechanical ventilation. This manifests clinically with reduced arterial pressure and, if measured, cardiac output. Diminished tissue perfusion resulting in shock begins a dangerous cycle that needs to be reversed.

Pulmonary

Modest increases in IAP can cause elevation of the diaphragm, which is compounded in the supine patient. During mechanical ventilation, infra-diaphragmatic counterpressure affects airway and intra-thoracic pressures, interferes with ventilation, and can lead to hypercarbia,

Box 44.1 • Conditions That Predispose to Abdominal Compartment Syndrome

- Abdominal-pelvic trauma or hemorrhage
- Intra-abdominal sepsis, perforation, or anastomotic leak
- Prolonged laparotomy for any emergency or elective surgical condition with tight closure
- Severe pancreatitis, hemorrhagic pancreatitis, or pancreatic necrosis
- Massive edema (eg, burn resuscitation)
- Massive ascites (acute or due to spontaneous bacterial peritonitis)
- Abdominal wall tetany or rigidity, rigors, or status epilepticus
- Intestinal ischemia or necrosis
- Ruptured abdominal aortic or visceral aneurysm

hypoxia, and barotrauma. Appropriate ventilator strategies can ameliorate these somewhat. Massive fluid resuscitation can cause chest wall and abdominal wall edema, resulting in decreased tissue compliance and a worsening of altered pulmonary physiology. Decreasing pulmonary compliance due to these external forces may be an early sign of impending ACS.

Renal

The primary reason for the renal insufficiency that occurs with increasing IAP is compression of the renal veins. Decreased cardiac output and arterial hypoperfusion also contribute to this. Oliguria is the clinical manifestation, and this can develop with IAP as low as 15 mm Hg. Anuria and renal failure can result if measures to reverse IAH are not taken. Along with increasing airway pressures, oliguria acts as another bedside sign of potential ACS.

Table 44.1 • Grading of Intra-abdominal Hypertension

Grade	Intra-abdominal Pressure, mm Hg
1	12-15
2	16-20
3	21-25
4	>25

From Malbrain ML, Cheatham ML, Kirkpatrick A, Sugrue M, Parr M, De Waele J, et al. Results from the international conference of experts on intra-abdominal hypertension and abdominal compartment syndrome. I. Definitions. Intensive Care Med. 2006 Nov;32(11):1722-32. Epub 2006 Sep 12; used with permission.

Gastrointestinal

Unlike in the cardiovascular, pulmonary, and renal systems, early effects of increased IAP on the gut and liver are difficult to detect clinically. Hepatic and mesenteric perfusion is limited by IAH, an effect leading to progressive ischemia. The serum lactate level can be increased as a result of increased production by underperfused bowel and decreased clearance by the liver. Hypovolemia can exacerbate these findings.

Central Nervous System

Increased IAP can, through a series of mechanisms, increase central venous pressure, internal jugular vein pressure, and, ultimately, intracranial pressure. These effects can contribute to increased cerebral edema and worsening neurologic outcome in the setting of brain injury. The manifestations of these changes can be observed at the bedside when the intracranial pressure is being monitored. When some of the other signs of ACS, described above, are detected, measures to lower IAP should be initiated immediately in an effort to also control increasing intracranial pressure.

Diagnosis

Clinical suspicion for IAH should be increased when abdominal distention or abdominal wall tightness or rigidity is found on physical examination. If signs of organ dysfunction (cardiovascular, pulmonary, or renal) are present, developing ACS should be suspected and the IAP should be promptly measured. Before the development of ACS, physical signs of increased IAP may necessitate preemptive measurement of the IAP. If it is increased, serial measurements may be warranted to establish a trend and determine the need for treatment to relieve the pressure.

IAP can be measured with various means, including intraluminal or intraperitoneal catheters or transducers. Urinary bladder pressure measurement is the standard method, and this can be performed as follows: 1) empty bladder with a Foley catheter; 2) instill 25 mL of sterile saline into the bladder, and create a fluid column in the tubing; 3) clamp the tubing, and puncture the aspiration port with an 18-gauge needle connected to a pressure transducer; 4) and obtain the measurement at end-expiration with the patient calm (or even paralyzed), supine, and not bearing down or coughing. Because bladder pressures can be affected by pelvic adhesions, hematoma, or packing, interpretation of the results is not always reliable.

Sustained pressures more than 20 mm Hg warrant concern for incipient ACS, and treatment should be considered. The pressure is relative and should be correlated with the clinical condition. No standard pressure reliably predicts the diagnosis of ACS. Abdominal perfusion pressure is measured as the mean arterial pressure minus the IAP, and a value of 60 mm Hg should be targeted because this seems to correlate with improved survival.

Treatment

The management algorithm for ACS should be systematic and geared toward a sustained reduction in IAP.

Possible Measures

The following measures can be used, depending on the exact clinical scenario:

1. Volume resuscitation with fluid or blood is done to reverse shock. The ischemic consequences of increasing IAP are compounded by poor tissue perfusion.
2. Ventilator strategies should be optimized to limit tidal volume, airway pressures, and high intrathoracic pressures that may increase pressures below the diaphragm.
3. Chemical paralysis can be considered to eliminate the abdominal wall muscle contribution to IAH. Situations in which this step may be beneficial include seizures, posturing, rigors, coughing, and ventilator dyssynchrony.
4. Nasogastric or rectal tube decompression can alleviate excessive gas or fluid within the bowel lumen.
5. Paracentesis can reduce IAP when ascites is considerable.
6. Decompressive laparotomy should be considered with a sustained IAP more than 25 mm Hg and evidence of organ dysfunction. The exact threshold for intervention varies from case to case, and a level of 20 mm Hg may be appropriate in some cases.

Decompressive Laparotomy

Opening or reopening the abdomen in the setting of ACS removes abdominal wall counterpressure, allows for the evacuation of blood and clot, and permits inspection of the abdomen for necrotic or leaking bowel and any other organ abnormality. This procedure is performed in the operating room but can, if necessary, be done at the bedside. The abdomen is left open, and some type of commercially available or makeshift temporary closure device is used to cover the bowel. Negative-pressure wound therapy methods can be used. Care must be taken, however, that the increased pressure is not reproduced by the closure method. Typically, the temporary closure system is changed or reevaluated every 48 hours to determine the most optimal timing for more permanent abdominal closure. Definitive closure should be performed within 7 days to limit the risk of intestinal fistula.

Summary

- Increasing IAP can lead to IAH, defined as a pressure more than 12 mm Hg.
- ACS is defined as IAH associated with organ dysfunction.
- IAP is usually estimated by measuring the urinary bladder pressure with a Foley catheter.
- ACS can be temporized with various ancillary maneuvers; however, decompressive laparotomy should be considered with sustained pressures of 20 to 25 mm Hg and evidence of organ dysfunction.

SUGGESTED READING

Cheatham ML, White MW, Sagraves SG, Johnson JL, Block EF. Abdominal perfusion pressure: a superior parameter in the assessment of intra-abdominal hypertension. J Trauma. 2000 Oct;49(4):621–6.

Cullen DJ, Coyle JP, Teplick R, Long MC. Cardiovascular, pulmonary, and renal effects of massively increased intra-abdominal pressure in critically ill patients. Crit Care Med. 1989 Feb;17(2):118–21.

De Waele JJ, Hoste EA, Malbrain ML. Decompressive laparotomy for abdominal compartment syndrome: a critical analysis. Crit Care. 2006;10(2):R51.

Depauw PRAM, Groen RJM, Van Loon, J, Peul WC, Malbrain MLNG, De Waele JJ. The significance of intra-abdominal pressure in neurosurgery and neurological diseases: a narrative review and a conceptual proposal. Acta Neurochir (Wien). 2019 Mar. [Epub ahead of print].

Joseph DK, Dutton RP, Aarabi B, Scalea TM. Decompressive laparotomy to treat intractable intracranial hypertension after traumatic brain injury. J Trauma. 2004 Oct;57(4):687–93.

Kirkpatrick AW, Roberts DJ, De Waele J, Jaeschke R, Malbrain ML, De Keulenaer B, et al; Pediatric Guidelines Sub-Committee for the World Society of the Abdominal Compartment Syndrome. Intra-abdominal hypertension and the abdominal compartment syndrome: updated consensus definitions and clinical practice guidelines from the World Society of the Abdominal Compartment Syndrome. Intensive Care Med. 2013 Jul;39(7):1190–206. Epub 2013 May 15.

Malbrain ML, Cheatham ML, Kirkpatrick A, Sugrue M, Parr M, De Waele J, et al. Results from the international conference of experts on intra-abdominal hypertension and abdominal compartment syndrome. I. Definitions. Intensive Care Med. 2006 Nov;32(11):1722–32. Epub 2006 Sep 12.

Popescu GA, Bara T, Rad P. Abdominal compartment syndrome as a multidisciplinary challenge: a literature review. J Crit Care Med (Tarqu Mures). 2018 Oct; 4(4):114–9.

Sugrue M, Jones F, Deane SA, Bishop G, Bauman A, Hillman K. Intra-abdominal hypertension is an independent cause of postoperative renal impairment. Arch Surg. 1999 Oct;134(10):1082–5.

Renal Disorders

45 Acute Kidney Injury

ANKIT SAKHUJA, MBBS; KIANOUSH B. KASHANI, MD

Goals

- Recognize acute kidney injury in critically ill patients.
- Understand the epidemiology and outcomes of acute kidney injury.
- Discuss staging of acute kidney injury.
- Understand management options for acute kidney injury.

Introduction

Acute kidney injury (AKI) is a complex disorder that encompasses a broad spectrum of clinical presentations ranging from subclinical injury to complete loss of kidney function. AKI is fairly common in critically ill patients. Among patients who have similar conditions, those who have development of AKI have worse outcomes than those who do not. There have been significant strides in understanding the pathophysiology of AKI in recent years, but management is mostly supportive, and prevention remains critical for improving outcomes.

Definition

AKI is an acute decline in glomerular filtration rate (GFR) measured in terms of an increase in the serum creatinine value or a decrease in urine output. The definition of AKI encompasses various degrees of renal dysfunction known as the RIFLE classification (*r*isk, *i*njury, *f*ailure, *l*oss, and *e*nd-stage renal disease). The lowest stage of AKI, that is, the risk stage, was defined as an increase of 50% or more in the creatinine value, a decrease in GFR by 25% or more, or a decrease in urine output to <0.5 mL/kg per hour for 6 hours (Table 45.1).

Later studies showed that even small changes in the serum creatinine value (as low as ≥0.3 mg/dL) are associated with increased mortality. This finding was incorporated in the AKI Network definition of AKI published in 2007, for which an increase in the creatinine value of 0.3 mg/dL or more within 48 hours was also defined as AKI. The Kidney Disease Improving Global Outcomes (KDIGO) guideline merged RIFLE and AKI Network criteria (Table 45.1).

Epidemiology

Multiple studies have examined the epidemiology of AKI since the publication of RIFLE criteria in 2004; however, they are characterized by a wide range of results. The differences in the results of the studies are due to differences in populations studied, various criteria used, and timing of end points. In addition, the incidence is lower in studies that do not use urine output to detect AKI.

A study of more than 5,000 critically ill patients at a tertiary-care center found that the incidence of AKI was 67% with RIFLE criteria when both GFR and urine output were used. In-hospital mortality increased progressively with worsening RIFLE stage: 8.8% for those in the risk stage, 11.4% for those in the injury stage, and 26.3% for those in the failure stage compared with 5.5% for those without AKI. In addition, the injury and failure stages were independent predictors of in-hospital mortality (hazard ratio 1.40 [95% CI, 1.02-1.88] for injury stage and 2.70 [95% CI, 2.03-3.55] for failure stage).

In comparison, the incidence of AKI was 22% in a study of more than 300,000 patients in Veterans Affairs intensive care units according to AKI Network criteria. The study, however, did not use urine output as a criterion for AKI and thus likely underestimated its true incidence. Increasing stages of AKI were also associated with higher mortality and duration of stay (odds ratio 2.90, 6.93, and 8.93 for mortality and 7.0, 10.6, and 14.0 days for duration of stay in stages 1, 2, and 3, respectively).

In a study based on a national inpatient database, the estimated incidence of severe AKI that requires dialysis (AKI-D)

Table 45.1 • Kidney Disease Improving Global Outcomes Criteria for Diagnosis and Staging of Acute Kidney Injury

Stage	Creatinine Criteria	Urine Output Criteria
1	Increased by ≥0.3 mg/dL in 48 h OR Increased 1.5-1.9 times from baseline within 7 days	<0.5 mL/kg per hour for 6-12 h
2	Increased by 2.0-2.9 times from baseline within 7 days	<0.5 mL/kg per hour for ≥12 h
3	Increased by ≥3.0 times from baseline within 7 days OR Increased to ≥4.0 mg/dL (along with an increase of ≥0.3 mg/dL in 48 h) OR Initiation of renal replacement therapy	<0.3 mL/kg per hour for ≥24 h OR Anuria for ≥12 h

Modified from Kellum JA, Lameire N, Aspelin P, Barsoum RS, Burdmann EA, Goldstein SL, et al. Section 2: AKI definition. Kidney Int Suppl. 2012 Mar;2(1):1-138; used with permission.

in patients with severe sepsis was 6%. AKI-D was associated with an inpatient mortality of 44% (in comparison to 25% in those without) and was an independent predictor of death. This study also showed a 2% annual increase in the proportion of patients with AKI-D from 2000 through 2009, but the impact of AKI-D on mortality declined over time (for death due to AKI-D, odds ratio was 1.74 [95% CI, 1.64-1.85] in 2009 and 2.00 [95% CI, 1.84-2.18] in 2000). This decrease is likely due to improving care practices but could also be due to earlier initiation of dialysis over the years.

Hoste et al (2015; see Suggested Reading) used the KDIGO definition for identifying AKI in patients admitted to 97 intensive care units in 33 countries. They estimated AKI was present in 57.3% of 1,802 critically ill patients. Fourteen percent required dialysis for AKI. KDIGO stages 2 and 3 AKI were also associated with mortality when adjusted for other factors (odds ratio 2.94 [95% CI, 1.38-6.27] for stage 2 and 6.88 [95% CI, 3.87-12.22] for stage 3).

Etiology

The cause of AKI in intensive care units is usually multifactorial (Table 45.2). Decreased kidney perfusion, inflammatory states, kidney congestion, and obstruction have been proposed as common reasons for AKI. During hypovolemic states due to reduced blood volume caused by internal or external volume loss (eg, bleeding, diarrhea, heat shock) or decreased effective blood volume due to congestive heart failure or liver cirrhosis, kidney perfusion decreases and results in AKI. Decreased perfusion may also occur with use of nonsteroidal anti-inflammatory drugs or other nephrotoxins that cause afferent arteriolar vasoconstriction.

Alternatively, AKI could be caused by diseases of kidney parenchyma. The most common cause of AKI in intensive care units is, in fact, damage to the renal tubules, also called acute tubular necrosis. It can result from direct injury to the tubules, such as from nephrotoxic medications, or from prolonged ischemia, such as from hypotension. Allergic interstitial nephritis is another important cause of AKI in critically ill patients and can be associated even with seemingly innocuous medications such as proton pump inhibitors.

Additionally, obstruction in the urinary tract leading to a reduction in urine output and GFR can lead to AKI. Usually, bilateral obstruction is required before urine output and GFR are substantially decreased (unless there is a solitary functioning kidney). Therefore, a high index of suspicion is needed in patients who have an increased risk of obstruction. The common causes of obstructive AKI are stones, an enlarged prostate, or metastatic cancer. Retroperitoneal fibrosis is a rare condition that can also cause postrenal AKI. In a recent multicenter study of critically ill patients, slightly more than 1% of all AKI cases were due to postrenal causes.

Pathophysiology

Sepsis is a common mechanism for AKI acquired in the intensive care unit. Although AKI in patients with sepsis could be due to prolonged arterial hypotension, most cases of sepsis-associated AKI are due to an inflammatory response that affects the kidney. In a multicenter, open-label, randomized trial (SEPSISPAM), targeting a higher mean arterial pressure (80-85 mm Hg vs 65-70 mm Hg) was associated with a decreased risk of AKI and the need for dialysis in patients with a history of chronic hypertension; in patients who did not have a history of chronic hypertension, there was no difference in the incidence of AKI between the mean arterial pressure target groups.

Table 45.2 • Etiology of Acute Kidney Injury

Etiology	Mechanism	Example
Decreased effective blood volume	Ischemia-reperfusion	Dehydration Heart failure Nephrotoxins (NSAIDs, contrast agents)
Renal parenchymal disease	Glomerular	Glomerulonephritides Primary Secondary (eg, SLE, HSP)
	Interstitial	Acute and chronic interstitial nephritis Nephrotoxins (vancomycin) Infection Crystalopathies (hyperoxaluria)
	Vascular	Atheroembolic disease Vasculitides Thromboembolic disease Renal vein thrombosis
	Tubular	ATN Sepsis
Obstruction	Compressive	Retroperitoneal and pelvic cancer
	Occlusive	Prostate Nephrolithiasis

Abbreviations: ATN, acute tubular necrosis; HSP, Henoch-Schönlein purpura; NSAID, nonsteroidal anti-inflammatory drug; SLE, systemic lupus erythematosus.

Recent experimental studies have challenged the notion that most AKI in critically ill patients is due to acute tubular necrosis. In addition, septic AKI is not associated with a decrease in renal blood flow. This finding suggests that AKI in sepsis is due to the interplay of more complex mechanisms than hypovolemia and arterial hypotension. There have been recent advancements in our understanding of the pathophysiology of AKI in sepsis. Pathogenic pathways involved in the progression of sepsis are now thought to contribute to the development of septic AKI. Initial microbial infection causes a pro-inflammatory immune response involving the secretion of various cytokines (interleukin-1, tumor necrosis factor-α, interleukin-6), which ultimately progresses to a state of overwhelming inflammation, hemodynamic instability, and organ dysfunction. This is followed by a compensatory anti-inflammatory response with increased production of interleukin-10, impairment of chemotaxis and phagocytosis, and lymphocyte apoptosis. Finally, these events lead to endothelial dysfunction, thrombosis, apoptosis, and necrosis causing organ dysfunction, including AKI.

Clinical Features

Most patients with AKI are asymptomatic. Patients can present with symptoms and signs of decreased kidney function, including oliguria, anuria, edema, and hypertension. They can also present with electrolyte abnormalities, especially hyperkalemia and complications thereof. Clinical features can also depend on the underlying cause of AKI. Because of the limitations of biochemical diagnosis of AKI, its clinical identification is often delayed if clinicians rely on only the serum creatinine level for AKI detection. Using urine output as a criterion of AKI allows earlier warning about the pending clinical diagnosis of AKI.

Bleeding or other causes of hypovolemia can precipitate AKI by lowering renal blood flow. They can also present with symptoms and signs of decompensated heart–acute pulmonary edema (especially if aggressive fluid resuscitation has been implemented) or liver failure. Patients with obstructive AKI can present with oliguria or polyuria (in the case of subacute or partial obstruction such as prostate enlargement) or sudden-onset obstruction with flank pain (in those with nephrolithiasis). Defects in renal-concentrating ability due to decreased responsiveness to antidiuretic hormone can occur with partial obstruction, which can lead to polyuria as a presenting symptom.

Patients with glomerulonephritides can have various presentations from gradually to rapidly progressive kidney dysfunction. In the case of primary glomerulonephritis, the symptoms and signs can include frothy urine, hypertension, and edema. When glomerulonephritis is due to other systemic diseases (eg, systemic lupus erythematosus, Henoch-Schönlein purpura), extrarenal symptoms and signs of systemic diseases can also be noted. Patients with allergic interstitial nephritis can present with fever, rash, and eosinophilia or eosinophiluria. The triad, however, occurs in less than 10% of cases. Oliguria and hematuria can also occur in these patients.

Diagnosis

The diagnosis of AKI relies on measurement of the serum creatinine level and urine output based on KDIGO guidelines, as discussed above. However, creatinine levels are affected by age, sex, race, and muscle mass. In addition, because the production of creatinine can change in critically ill patients, diagnosing AKI can be even more challenging. Creatinine is produced by nonenzymatic cyclization of creatine, especially in skeletal muscles. Hypoperfusion leading to decreased capillary vascular perfusion can result in reduced muscle creatinine release. In addition, reduction in body mass and decreased nutritional intake while in the intensive care unit can also contribute to decreased creatinine production in critically ill patients. A careful medical history to identify the potential cause and timing of AKI onset is essential. Knowledge about potential events, such as hypovolemia, bleeding, decompensated heart or liver failure, lower urinary tract symptoms, the presence of hematuria or frothy urine, rash, and extrarenal symptoms of systemic diseases that can cause AKI, is very valuable. In addition, a meticulous review of a patient's medication list is essential to rule out drug-induced nephrotoxicity.

Reviewing the urine sediment can give invaluable information regarding the cause of AKI. Muddy-brown casts or renal tubular cells are typically found in acute tubular necrosis. Allergic interstitial nephritis and pyelonephritis are usually associated with white blood cells and white cell casts in urine. Eosinophiluria (>1% of urine white blood cells) can also occur in allergic interstitial nephritis. Glomerulonephritides are associated with dysmorphic red blood cells and red cell casts. They are, in addition, associated with proteinuria, typically more than 2 g in a 24-hour specimen.

Fractional excretion of sodium and urea can also be helpful tools for supporting the clinical diagnosis of the cause of AKI. A fractional excretion of sodium less than 1% usually suggests low renal blood flow, exposure to contrast, use of nonsteroidal anti-inflammatory drugs or angiotensin-converting enzyme inhibitors, rhabdomyolysis, and hepatorenal or cardiorenal syndrome. A fractional excretion of sodium more than 3% can indicate acute tubular necrosis, advanced chronic kidney disease, or the use of loop diuretics. Similarly, a fractional excretion of urea less than 35% is usually associated with low renal blood flow states and can be more helpful for diagnosis in the presence of diuretic use.

Renal ultrasonography with Doppler is the imaging method of choice for evaluation of patients with AKI if obstructive nephropathy or chronicity of kidney disease is under question. Increased echogenicity and small kidneys could suggest underlying chronic kidney disease. Ultrasonography also helps to exclude AKI due to obstruction, which can manifest as hydronephrosis. High-yield clinical pearls for diagnosis of AKI based on clinical scenarios are provided in Table 45.3.

Table 45.3 • Clinical Pearls for Diagnosis of AKI

Clinical Scenario	Suspected Etiology of AKI	Test Results
Bleeding, hypovolemia	Prerenal	FeNa <1%, FeUrea <35%
Sepsis, persistent hypotension	ATN	Muddy-brown casts in urine sediment
Recent antibiotics, NSAIDs, PPIs	AIN	Eosinophiluria, white cell casts in urine sediment
Recent use of indinavir, IV acyclovir	Crystal-induced nephropathy	Specific crystals seen in urine sediment
Crush injury	Rhabdomyolysis	Increased serum creatine kinase and urine myoglobin levels
Hematologic malignancy, especially with recent chemotherapy	Tumor lysis syndrome	High serum uric acid, phosphorus, and potassium levels
History of benign prostatic hypertrophy	Postrenal obstruction	Hydronephrosis on renal ultrasonography
Anemia, thrombocytopenia, AKI	TTP/HUS	Hemolysis work-up, low ADAMTS13 level
Proteinuria, hematuria	Glomerulonephritis	Dysmorphic RBCs in urine sediment, characteristic features on renal biopsy[a]

Abbreviations: ADAMTS13, *a d*isintegrin *a*nd *m*etalloprotease with *t*hrombo*s*pondin 1 repeats; AIN, allergic interstitial nephritis; AKI, acute kidney injury; ATN, acute tubular necrosis; FeNa, fractional excretion of sodium; FeUrea, fractional excretion of urea; HUS, hemolytic uremic syndrome; IV, intravenous; NSAID, nonsteroidal anti-inflammatory drug; PPI, proton pump inhibitor; RBC, red blood cell; TTP, thrombotic thrombocytopenic purpura.

[a] Search for possible causes of glomerulonephritis.

As outlined above, because of some inherent limitations, the serum creatinine level is not an optimal marker for AKI. The serum creatinine level depends on the muscle mass, fluid balance, catabolic state, or protein ingestion, and in the AKI setting it is increasingly being secreted from the proximal tubular cells. These factors can delay the diagnosis of AKI by 24 to 36 hours. Cystatin C is produced by all nucleated cells and is not affected by age, sex, race, or muscle mass, and it may be better for detecting mild GFR reductions between 60 and 90 mL/min per 1.73 m^2. The test may, however, not be as widely available as the creatinine test.

Several potential injury and stress biomarkers have also been identified for earlier diagnosis of AKI, including neutrophil gelatinase-associated lipocalin, kidney injury molecule-1, interleukin-18 and *N*-acetyl-β-D-glucosaminidase, insulin-like growth factor binding protein 7, and tissue inhibitor metalloproteinase-2. *N*-acetyl-β-D-glucosaminidase is a useful early biomarker for diagnosis of AKI; however, it is limited by its expression in systemic stress without AKI. Kidney injury molecule-1 is another promising biomarker that is expressed by proximal tubular cells in the kidney in response to ischemic or toxic injury. Urinary insulinlike growth factor binding protein-7 and tissue inhibitor metalloproteinase-2, both inducers of G_1/S cell cycle arrest, have been validated to predict the development of AKI 12 hours before a detectable increase in the creatinine level. They have also been shown to be predictors of mortality and renal recovery for AKI after cardiac surgery. A test based on these biomarkers has been approved by the US Food and Drug Administration to aid in early AKI detection in critically ill patients.

On the basis of the interactions between the functional (serum creatinine, cystatin C, and urine output) and injury biomarkers, the Acute Dialysis Quality Initiative suggested a framework for incorporation of both for the diagnosis of AKI (Figure 45.1).

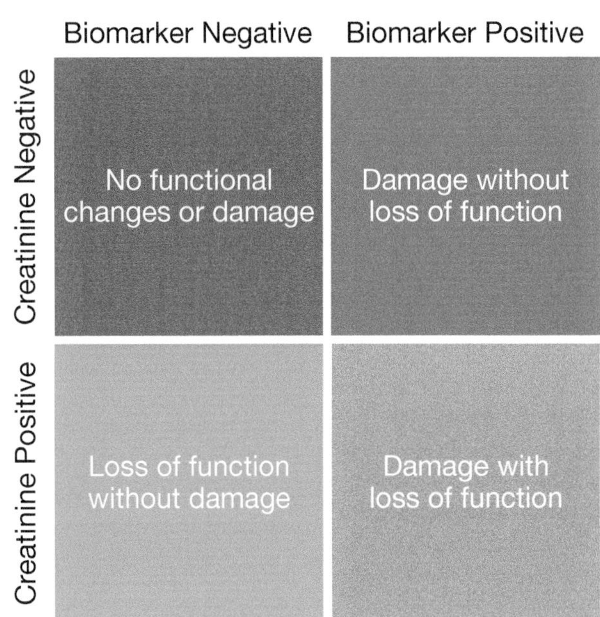

Figure 45.1. *Incorporation of Injury and Functional Markers for Diagnosis of Acute Kidney Injury.*
(Modified from Acute Dialysis Quality Initiative 10 [Internet]. c2012 [cited 2017 Nov 6]. Available from: http://www.ADQI.org; used under Creative Common Attribution License [http://creativecommons.org/licenses/by/2.0].)

Prevention and Treatment

Because the treatment of AKI is largely supportive, prevention is critical to improving outcomes. Attempts should be made to optimize hemodynamic status and avoid nephrotoxic agents (eg, iodinated contrast material, nonsteroidal anti-inflammatory drugs). Crystalloids should be the first choice for resuscitation instead of synthetic colloids, which have been associated with AKI in trials. Large human retrospective and physiologic in vitro studies indicate chloride-restricted fluids may be associated with a lower incidence of AKI than chloride-rich fluids (0.9% normal saline). However, this finding has been supported in a recent trial.

For patients at risk for contrast-induced nephropathy, especially those with an estimated GFR less than 60 mL/min per 1.73 m^2, use of low osmolar or iso-osmolar contrast agents should be considered. Intravenous volume expansion with normal saline or bicarbonate-based solutions, if clinically safe, has also been associated with a lower incidence of contrast-induced nephropathy. Because of its effect on minimizing free radical generation, *N*-acetylcysteine has been used in conjunction with isotonic saline to prevent contrast-induced nephropathy. However, this approach has been marred with conflicting results. Because of the potential for benefit and low associated toxicity and cost, oral *N*-acetylcysteine can be given at a dosage of 1,200 mg twice daily the day before and the day of the procedure.

Management of AKI is usually directed toward avoiding complications of AKI, especially hyperkalemia, metabolic acidosis, and volume overload. Diuretics can be used to manage hypervolemia, hyperkalemia, and metabolic acidosis. Renal replacement therapy in the form of either intermittent hemodialysis or continuous renal replacement therapy is needed if these complications are refractory to medical management. Other indications for renal replacement therapy are uremia (including uremic pericarditis or encephalopathy) and intoxications with dialyzable toxins. Outcomes in terms of patient survival and renal recovery are equivalent with both intermittent hemodialysis and continuous renal replacement therapy. However, continuous renal replacement therapy may be preferred in the setting of substantial volume overload or cerebral edema (because rapid changes in tissue osmolality with intermittent hemodialysis have been associated with worsening intracranial pressure), and intermittent hemodialysis may be preferable in the setting of severe hyperkalemia and toxin ingestions.

Prognosis

Development of AKI is associated with progressive decline in kidney function manifested as chronic kidney disease or end-stage renal disease. Chronic kidney disease develops in more than 50% of patients with AKI after hospital discharge. The risk of chronic kidney disease is correlated with the severity of AKI, the extent of the increase in creatinine, need for dialysis, and increasing number of AKI episodes. The high risk of chronic kidney disease persists even after recovery of kidney function. About 3% of patients with incident end-stage renal disease in the United States have acute tubular necrosis as the primary diagnosis of renal failure. Indeed, KDIGO guidelines recommend following up with a nephrologist within 3 months of an incident AKI event. Follow-up within that time frame is associated with a 24% lower hazard of death. However, only about 8% of patients are evaluated by a nephrologist within the first year after an AKI event.

Summary

- AKI is common and has grave consequences, including chronic kidney disease, end-stage renal disease, and death.
- Early detection and prevention of AKI are associated with improved outcomes. Use of both injury biomarker and functional markers is necessary for early detection of AKI.
- Management of AKI is complex, and collaboration with a nephrologist is needed. Patients with AKI should be followed by a nephrologist both short-term and long-term.

SUGGESTED READING

Asfar P, Meziani F, Hamel JF, Grelon F, Megarbane B, Anguel N, et al; SEPSISPAM Investigators. High versus low blood-pressure target in patients with septic shock. N Engl J Med. 2014 Apr 24;370(17):1583–93. Epub 2014 Mar 18.

Bagshaw SM, Adhikari NKJ, Burns KEA, Friedrich JO, Bouchard J, Lamontagne F, et al. Canadian Critical Care Trials Group. Selection and receipt of kidney replacement in critically ill older patients with AKI. Clin J Am Soc Nephrol. 2019 Apr;14(4):496–505.

Bagshaw SM, George C, Bellomo R; ANZICS Database Management Committee. A comparison of the RIFLE and AKIN criteria for acute kidney injury in critically ill patients. Nephrol Dial Transplant. 2008 May;23(5):1569–74. Epub 2008 Feb 15.

Bellomo R, Ronco C, Kellum JA, Mehta RL, Palevsky P; Acute Dialysis Quality Initiative Workgroup. Acute renal failure: definition, outcome measures, animal models, fluid therapy and information technology needs: the Second International Consensus Conference of the Acute Dialysis Quality Initiative (ADQI) Group. Crit Care. 2004 Aug;8(4):R204–12. Epub 2004 May 24.

Bhatraju PK, Zelnick LR, Katz R, Mikacenic C, Kosamo S, Hahn WO, et al. A prediction model for severe AKI in critically ill adults that incorporates clinical and biomarker data. Clin J Am Soc Nephrol. 2019 Apr;14(4):506–14.

Brenner M, Schaer GL, Mallory DL, Suffredini AF, Parrillo JE. Detection of renal blood flow abnormalities in septic and critically ill patients using a newly designed indwelling thermodilution renal vein catheter. Chest. 1990 Jul;98(1):170–9.

Bucaloiu ID, Kirchner HL, Norfolk ER, Hartle JE 2nd, Perkins RM. Increased risk of death and de novo chronic kidney disease following reversible acute kidney injury. Kidney Int. 2012 Mar;81(5):477–85. Epub 2011 Dec 7.

Chawla LS, Amdur RL, Amodeo S, Kimmel PL, Palant CE. The severity of acute kidney injury predicts progression to chronic kidney disease. Kidney Int. 2011 Jun;79(12):1361–9. Epub 2011 Mar 23.

Chertow GM, Burdick E, Honour M, Bonventre JV, Bates DW. Acute kidney injury, mortality, length of stay, and costs in hospitalized patients. J Am Soc Nephrol. 2005 Nov;16(11):3365–70. Epub 2005 Sep 21.

Doi K, Yuen PS, Eisner C, Hu X, Leelahavanichkul A, Schnermann J, et al. Reduced production of creatinine limits its use as marker of kidney injury in sepsis. J Am Soc Nephrol. 2009 Jun;20(6):1217–21. Epub 2009 Apr 23.

Harel Z, Wald R, Bargman JM, Mamdani M, Etchells E, Garg AX, et al. Nephrologist follow-up improves all-cause mortality of severe acute kidney injury survivors. Kidney Int. 2013 May;83(5):901–8. Epub 2013 Jan 16.

Herget-Rosenthal S, Bokenkamp A, Hofmann W. How to estimate GFR-serum creatinine, serum cystatin C or equations? Clin Biochem. 2007 Feb;40(3-4):153–61. Epub 2006 Nov 21.

Hoste EA, Bagshaw SM, Bellomo R, Cely CM, Colman R, Cruz DN, et al. Epidemiology of acute kidney injury in critically ill patients: the multinational AKI-EPI study. Intensive Care Med. 2015 Aug;41(8):1411–23. Epub 2015 Jul 11.

Hoste EA, Clermont G, Kersten A, Venkataraman R, Angus DC, De Bacquer D, et al. RIFLE criteria for acute kidney injury are associated with hospital mortality in critically ill patients: a cohort analysis. Crit Care. 2006;10(3):R73. Epub 2006 May 12.

Ishani A, Nelson D, Clothier B, Schult T, Nugent S, Greer N, et al. The magnitude of acute serum creatinine increase after cardiac surgery and the risk of chronic kidney disease, progression of kidney disease, and death. Arch Intern Med. 2011 Feb 14;171(3):226–33. Erratum in: Arch Intern Med. 2011 Nov 28;171(21):1919.

Jones J, Holmen J, De Graauw J, Jovanovich A, Thornton S, Chonchol M. Association of complete recovery from acute kidney injury with incident CKD stage 3 and all-cause mortality. Am J Kidney Dis. 2012 Sep;60(3):402–8. Epub 2012 Apr 27.

Kashani K, Al-Khafaji A, Ardiles T, Artigas A, Bagshaw SM, Bell M, et al. Discovery and validation of cell cycle arrest biomarkers in human acute kidney injury. Crit Care. 2013 Feb 6;17(1):R25.

Kashani K, Frazee EN, Kellum JA. Cell cycle arrest biomarkers in kidney disease. In: Patel VB, Preedy VR, editors. Biomarkers in kidney disease. Dordrecht (Netherlands): Springer Reference; c2016. p. 977-90.

Kosaka J, Lankadeva YR, May CN, Bellomo R. Histopathology of septic acute kidney injury: a systematic review of experimental data. Crit Care Med. 2016 Sep;44(9):e897–903.

Koyner JL, Shaw AD, Chawla LS, Hoste EA, Bihorac A, Kashani K, et al; Sapphire Investigators. Tissue inhibitor metalloproteinase-2 (TIMP-2)•IGF-binding protein-7 (IGFBP7) levels are associated with adverse long-term outcomes in patients with AKI. J Am Soc Nephrol. 2015 Jul;26(7):1747–54. Epub 2014 Dec 22.

Lassnigg A, Schmidlin D, Mouhieddine M, Bachmann LM, Druml W, Bauer P, et al. Minimal changes of serum creatinine predict prognosis in patients after cardiothoracic surgery: a prospective cohort study. J Am Soc Nephrol. 2004 Jun;15(6):1597–605.

Maiden MJ, Otto S, Brealey JK, Finnis ME, Chapman MJ, Kuchel TR, et al. Structure and function of the kidney in septic shock: a prospective controlled experimental study. Am J Respir Crit Care Med. 2016 Sep 15;194(6):692–700.

Meersch M, Schmidt C, Van Aken H, Martens S, Rossaint J, Singbartl K, et al. Urinary TIMP-2 and IGFBP7 as early biomarkers of acute kidney injury and renal recovery following cardiac surgery. PLoS One. 2014 Mar 27;9(3):e93460.

Murray PT, Mehta RL, Shaw A, Ronco C, Endre Z, Kellum JA, et al; ADQI 10 Workgroup. Potential use of biomarkers in acute kidney injury: report and summary of recommendations from the 10th Acute Dialysis Quality Initiative Consensus Conference. Kidney Int. 2014 Mar;85(3):513–21. Epub 2013 Oct 9.

Murugan R, Karajala-Subramanyam V, Lee M, Yende S, Kong L, Carter M, et al; Genetic and Inflammatory Markers of Sepsis (GenIMS) Investigators. Acute kidney injury in non-severe pneumonia is associated with an increased immune response and lower survival. Kidney Int. 2010 Mar;77(6):527–35. Epub 2009 Dec 23.

Myburgh JA, Finfer S, Bellomo R, Billot L, Cass A, Gattas D, et al; CHEST Investigators; Australian and New Zealand Intensive Care Society Clinical Trials Group. Hydroxyethyl starch or saline for fluid resuscitation in intensive care. N Engl J Med. 2012 Nov 15;367(20):1901–11. Epub 2012 Oct 17. Erratum in: N Engl J Med. 2016 Mar 31;374(13):1298.

Perner A, Haase N, Guttormsen AB, Tenhunen J, Klemenzson G, Aneman A, et al; 6S Trial Group; Scandinavian Critical Care Trials Group. Hydroxyethyl starch 130/0.42 versus Ringer's acetate in severe sepsis. N Engl J Med. 2012 Jul 12;367(2):124–34. Epub 2012 Jun 27. Erratum in: N Engl J Med. 2012 Aug 2;367(5):481.

Ponte B, Felipe C, Muriel A, Tenorio MT, Liano F. Long-term functional evolution after an acute kidney injury: a 10-year study. Nephrol Dial Transplant. 2008 Dec;23(12):3859–66. Epub 2008 Jul 15.

Sakhuja A, Kumar G, Gupta S, Mittal T, Taneja A, Nanchal RS. Acute kidney injury requiring dialysis in severe sepsis. Am J Respir Crit Care Med. 2015 Oct 15;192(8):951–7.

Santos WJ, Zanetta DM, Pires AC, Lobo SM, Lima EQ, Burdmann EA. Patients with ischaemic, mixed and nephrotoxic acute tubular necrosis in the intensive care unit: a homogeneous population? Crit Care. 2006;10(2):R68.

Semler MW, Self WH, Wanderer JP, Ehrenfeld JM, Wang L, Byrne DW, et al. SMART Investigators and the Pragmatic Critical Care Research Group. Balanced crystalloids versus saline in critically ill adults. N Engl J Med. 2018 Mar;378(9):829–39.

Siew ED, Peterson JF, Eden SK, Hung AM, Speroff T, Ikizler TA, et al. Outpatient nephrology referral rates after acute kidney injury. J Am Soc Nephrol. 2012 Feb;23(2):305–12. Epub 2011 Dec 8.

Thakar CV, Christianson A, Freyberg R, Almenoff P, Render ML. Incidence and outcomes of acute kidney injury in intensive care units: a Veterans Administration study. Crit Care Med. 2009 Sep;37(9):2552–8.

Thakar CV, Christianson A, Himmelfarb J, Leonard AC. Acute kidney injury episodes and chronic kidney disease risk in diabetes mellitus. Clin J Am Soc Nephrol. 2011 Nov;6(11):2567–72. Epub 2011 Sep 8.

Uchino S, Bellomo R, Goldsmith D, Bates S, Ronco C. An assessment of the RIFLE criteria for acute renal failure in hospitalized patients. Crit Care Med. 2006 Jul;34(7):1913–7.

US Renal Data System. USRDS 2011 Annual data report: atlas of chronic kidney disease and end-stage renal disease in the United States [Internet]. Bethesda (MD): National Institutes of Health, National Institute of Diabetes and Digestive and Kidney Diseases; c2011 [cited 2017 Nov 6]. Available from: https://www.usrds.org/atlas11.aspx.

Vanmassenhove J, Vanholder R, Nagler E, Van Biesen W. Urinary and serum biomarkers for the diagnosis of acute kidney injury: an in-depth review of the literature. Nephrol Dial Transplant. 2013 Feb;28(2):254–73. Epub 2012 Oct 31.

Wlodzimirow KA, Abu-Hanna A, Slabbekoorn M, Chamuleau RA, Schultz MJ, Bouman CS. A comparison of RIFLE with and without urine output criteria for acute kidney injury in critically ill patients. Crit Care. 2012 Oct 18;16(5):R200.

Young P, Bailey M, Beasley R, Henderson S, Mackle D, McArthur C, et al; SPLIT Investigators; ANZICS CTG. Effect of a buffered crystalloid solution vs saline on acute kidney injury among patients in the intensive care unit: the SPLIT Randomized Clinical Trial. JAMA. 2015 Oct 27;314(16):1701–10. Erratum in: JAMA. 2015 Dec 15;314(23):2570.

Yunos NM, Bellomo R, Hegarty C, Story D, Ho L, Bailey M. Association between a chloride-liberal vs chloride-restrictive intravenous fluid administration strategy and kidney injury in critically ill adults. JAMA. 2012 Oct 17;308(15):1566–72.

Zarjou A, Agarwal A. Sepsis and acute kidney injury. J Am Soc Nephrol. 2011 Jun;22(6):999–1006. Epub 2011 May 12.

46 Acid-Base Disorders

ONUR DEMIRCI, MD

Goals

- Describe the basics of acid-base balance.
- Introduce an approach to the evaluation of acid-base disturbances.
- Discuss the principal acid-base disorders.

Introduction

In the human body, many essential cellular processes, such as transmembrane transport and metabolic pathways, are extremely pH sensitive. Normally, systemic acid-base equilibrium is tightly controlled with an arterial pH between 7.35 and 7.45. However, because of acid production, the intracellular pH is usually slightly lower, at 7.0 to 7.2, a value closer to a neutral pH of 6.8 at 37°C. In practice, though, intracellular pH is neither measured nor directly treated. Because of the ease of measuring the pH of the blood with an arterial blood gas test, we, as clinicians, treat disturbances of acid-base hemeostasis of this extracellular compartment.

Background

The term *pH* was first used by Danish chemist Sørensen in 1909 (see Suggested Reading). It is widely believed that it stands for power of hydrogen; however, the letter *p* might have been arbitrarily assigned and derived from the 2 variables *p* and *q* from his experimental data.

pH is defined as the negative logarithm of the hydrogen ion ($[H^+]$) concentration:

$$pH = -\log([H^+])$$

At a body's normal pH of 7.4, the H^+ concentration is 40 nEq/L. Any 20% increase of H^+ concentration decreases pH by 0.1.

The major extracellular buffer in the human body is bicarbonate (HCO_3^-). First termed by Henderson in 1909 (see Suggested Reading) as *carbonic acid equilibrium* and later refined by Hasselbalch in 1916 (see Suggested Reading), this equation describes the effect of the dissociation of carbonic acid (H_2CO_3) to hydrogen ion and bicarbonate:

$$CO_2 + H_2O \rightarrow H_2CO_3 \rightarrow H^+ + HCO_3^-$$

pH can be calculated using the concentrations of carbonic acid and bicarbonate:

$$pH = pKa = \log \frac{HCO_3^-}{H_2CO_3}$$

pK_a is defined as co-logarithm of the acid dissociation constant of carbonic acid and equals 6.1.

The concentration of carbonic acid in the blood expressed as H_2CO_3 can be substituted with P_{CO_2}, which is readily obtained with a blood gas test:

$$[H_2CO_3] = k_{CO_2} \times P_{CO_2}$$

k_{CO_2} is the solubility of CO_2 in the blood, which is approximately 0.03 mmol/(L × mm Hg). Substituting pK_a and k_{CO_2} with these values finalizes the equation for the calculation of pH based on blood gas findings:

$$pH = 6.1 + \log \frac{HCO_3^-}{0.03 \times P_{CO_2}}$$

Arterial Blood Gas Measurement

An arterial blood gas test helps the clinician assess oxygenation (Pa_{O_2}), ventilation (Pa_{CO_2}), and pH. In addition

Table 46.1 • Compensatory Responses to Primary Acid-Base Disturbances and Calculation of the Adequacy of These Responses

Primary Disorder	Chronicity	Primary Change	Expected Change	Compensatory Response
Respiratory acidosis		↑ P_{CO_2}	↓ pH	↑ HCO_3^-
	Acute		↓ 0.08 per 10 mm Hg of ↑ P_{CO_2} >40 mm Hg	↑ 1 mmol/L per 10 mm Hg P_{CO_2} change
	Chronic		Reaches normal pH range	↑ 4 mmol/L per 10 mm Hg P_{CO_2} change
Respiratory alkalosis		↓ P_{CO_2}	↑ pH	↓ HCO_3^-
	Acute		↑ 0.08 per 10 mm Hg of ↓ P_{CO_2} <40 mm Hg	↓ 2 mmol/L per 10 mm Hg P_{CO_2} change
	Chronic		Reaches normal pH range	↓ 5 mmol/L per 10 mm Hg change
Metabolic acidosis	Acute or chronic	↓ HCO_3^-	$P_{CO_2} = (1.5 \times HCO_3^-) + 8\ (\pm 2)$	↓ P_{CO_2}
Metabolic alkalosis	Acute or chronic	↑ HCO_3^-	$P_{CO_2} = (0.7 \times HCO_3^-) + 21\ (\pm 2)$	↑ P_{CO_2}

Abbreviation: HCO_3^-, bicarbonate.

to these 3 directly measured values, an arterial blood gas test provides information about bicarbonate concentration (HCO_3^-) (calculated from the Henderson-Hasselbalch equation above) and base excess (calculated amount of acid that must be added to the blood sample to return the pH to 7.40 if the Pa_{CO_2} were 40 mm Hg).

Venous Blood Gas Measurement

Similarly, a venous blood gas test can be used to assess the acid-base status if an arterial sample cannot be easily obtained. Multiple studies have shown good correlation between venous and arterial blood gas results. Attention must be paid to a slightly lower pH (0.03-0.04) and slightly higher P_{CO_2} (4-6 mm Hg) for the venous blood gas results. Both bicarbonate concentration (HCO_3^-) and base excess values have shown comparable correlation between arterial and venous samples. However, hypoxemia cannot be diagnosed on the basis of the venous P_{O_2} because the arterial P_{O_2} is typically 36.9 mm Hg more than the venous P_{O_2} and has considerable variability.

Disturbances of Acid-Base Status

A decrease in blood pH to less than 7.35 is described as acidemia; inversely, an increase in pH to more than 7.45 is described as alkalemia. The underlying causes for these changes are called acidosis and alkalosis, respectively, and they can be respiratory (change in P_{CO_2}), metabolic (change in H^+), or a combination of the 2. Every primary disorder has some degree of compensatory response. These compensatory responses can be fast (increase in respiratory rate to decrease P_{CO_2}) or slow (metabolic response from the kidneys to retain bicarbonate). Their scale is different based on the chronicity of the primary disorder; however, the compensation would never be adequate to normalize the pH. These responses are summarized in Table 46.1. Figure 46.1 presents a stepwise approach to the diagnosis of the acid-base disturbances discussed below.

Respiratory Acidosis

Retention of CO_2 and associated shift of the carbonic acid equilibrium toward the buildup of hydrogen ions causes a decrease of pH to less than 7.35 from the physiologic range. Acute respiratory acidosis is commonly caused by the administration of opioids, asthma, exacerbations of chronic obstructive pulmonary disease, and diseases and processes associated with acute clouding of mental status (eg, head trauma, abrupt increase in intracranial pressure). The compensatory response from retention of bicarbonate through the kidneys is inadequate because of the abrupt onset of the primary disease. However, long-standing chronic obstructive pulmonary disease, restrictive lung disease, and neuromuscular diseases (eg, multiple sclerosis, amyotrophic lateral sclerosis, Guillain-Barré syndrome) cause chronic CO_2 retention with an almost fully compensatory response; furthermore, the pH of blood samples from patients with these disorders might be in the normal range.

Patients who have respiratory acidosis require assistance with ventilation to decrease their CO_2 levels. This can be delivered with noninvasive or invasive mechanical ventilation while the underlying cause is being treated (eg, naloxone for opioid overdose, inhaled bronchodilators for asthma and chronic obstructive pulmonary disease).

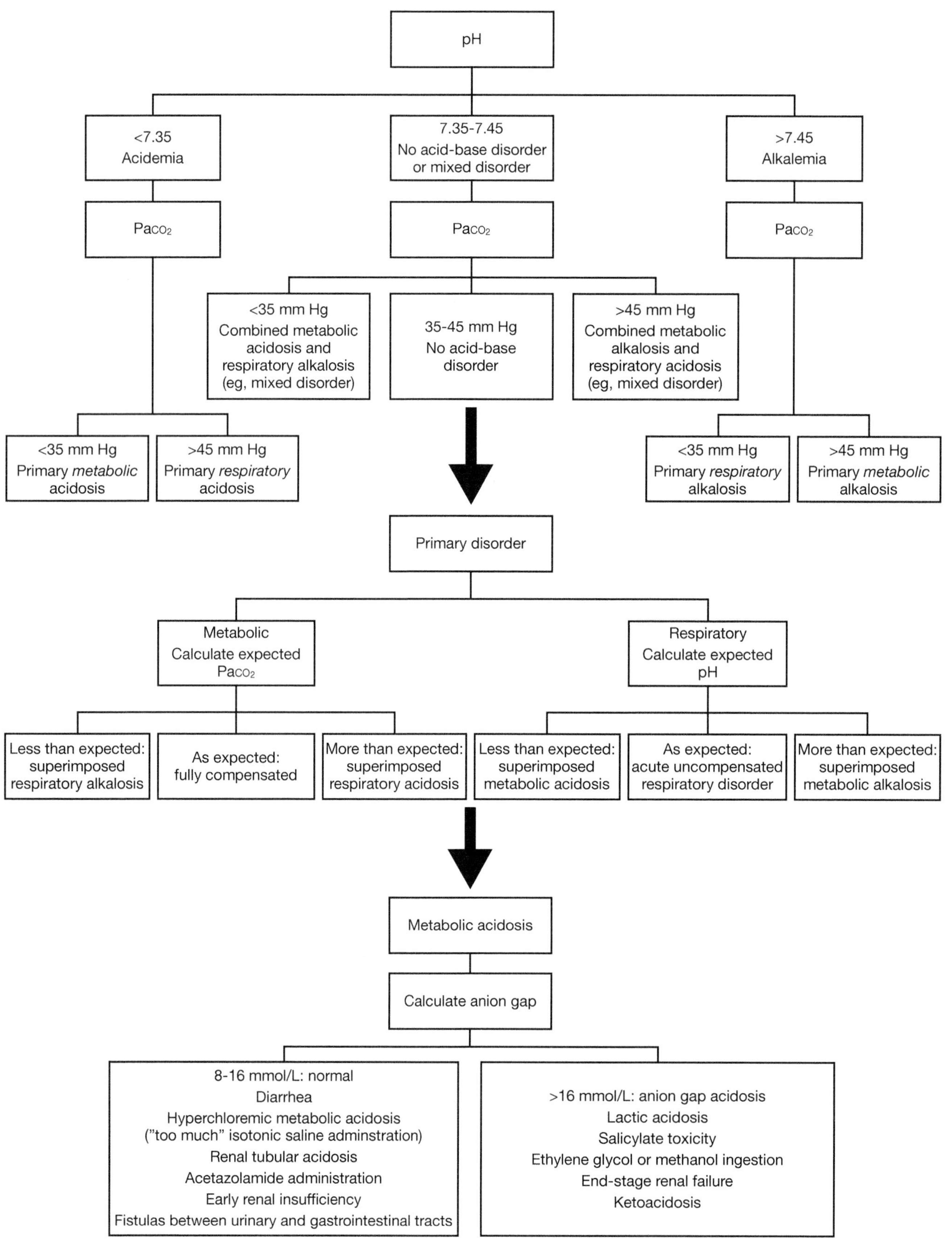

Figure 46.1. Stepwise Approach to Diagnosis of Acid-Base Disorders. Refer to Table 46.1 for the calculation of expected changes.

Respiratory Alkalosis

An increase in the minute ventilation (product of respiratory rate and tidal volume) causes hypocapnia ($Paco_2$ <40 mm Hg). Like respiratory acidosis, the chronicity of the underlying disorder influences the completeness of the compensatory response and, therefore, the degree of pH change. The most common causes of respiratory alkalosis include pregnancy, hyperventilation syndrome, pain, pulmonary embolism, early sepsis, and iatrogenic reasons in intubated patients.

Most patients with respiratory alkalosis do not require immediate intervention to normalize the $Paco_2$ unless the associated hypocalcemia results in hyperreflexia, convulsions, muscle spasm, or tetany.

Metabolic Acidosis

When the body either produces excess acids (eg, shock state with anaerobic metabolism causing lactic acid buildup) or loses bases (eg, renal tubular acidosis, diarrhea), the pH of the blood decreases to less than 7.35. The compensatory response of the body is to increase the respiratory rate and thereby cause a compensatory respiratory alkalosis to return the pH to the physiologic range. However, in cases of severe metabolic acidosis, this response can be sustained only for a certain period before the respiratory muscles fatigue and acute respiratory failure results. Also, trying to compensate for a metabolic acidosis in an intubated patient by increasing the respiratory rate above certain values causes air trapping and worsens hemodynamics.

The underlying cause of the metabolic acidosis should be initially determined by calculating the anion gap. In brief, all extracellular fluid in the human body should have an electrochemical balance; therefore, the concentration of cations and anions should be equal. The anion gap gives the clinician information about the unmeasured anions, which are usually higher than the unmeasured cations. The anion gap is calculated by subtracting the measured anions chloride (Cl^-) + HCO_3^- from the main measured cation sodium (Na^+):

$$\text{Anion gap} = Na^+ - \left(Cl^- + HCO_3^-\right)$$

Albumin makes up a large portion of the unmeasured anions. Therefore, in patients with albumin levels less than 4.5 g/dL, the anion gap should be adjusted by adding the correction factor of

$$2.5 \times (4.5 - [\text{albumin level}])$$

If the anion gap is increased from its reference range of 12 ± 4 mmol/L, the underlying cause of the acidosis is acid buildup. This is the case in lactic acidosis, salicylate toxicity, ethylene glycol or methanol ingestion, end-stage renal failure, and ketoacidosis. Inversely, in the instance of a normal anion gap, the acidosis is caused by a loss of HCO_3^-. This loss can be through the kidneys (eg, renal tubular acidosis, acetazolamide administration, early renal insufficiency) or the gastrointestinal tract (eg, diarrhea, fistulas between urinary and gastrointestinal tracts). Infusion of large amounts of isotonic saline can also cause a nonanion gap metabolic acidosis. This phenomenon is called *hyperchloremic metabolic acidosis* and is caused by chloride overload resulting in compensatory HCO_3^- excretion by the kidneys to maintain electrochemical balance.

The main objective of treatment should be correcting the underlying disease. Most acidoses, whether respiratory or metabolic, will not require base administration (sodium bicarbonate, tris-hydroxymethyl aminomethane) unless the pH decreases to less than 7.2. Also, administration of sodium bicarbonate results in CO_2 production, which will worsen the acidosis unless the patient can remove this by hyperventilating. This capability might become a problem in patients with severe underlying respiratory problems such as acute respiratory distress syndrome. In this case, tris-hydroxymethyl aminomethane might be a better choice because its acid neutralization does not produce CO_2.

Metabolic Alkalosis

An imbalance of the extracellular acid-base equilibrium due to either loss of acids or retention of HCO_3^- causes a metabolic alkalosis. The underlying causes are prolonged vomiting (HCl loss with kidneys trying to maintain electrochemical neutrality, as described above for metabolic acidosis, by retaining HCO_3^-), iatrogenic (loop or thiazide diuretics), and volume depletion (eg, contraction alkalosis). The compensatory response in this case is less pronounced than that in other acid-base disorders because metabolic alkalosis is not capable of causing substantial respiratory depression to make up for the underlying increase in pH. Neurologic sequelae of alkalosis such as depressed consciousness, generalized seizures, and muscle spasms are less pronounced in a metabolic alkalosis than in a respiratory alkalosis because the latter has markedly more influence on the central nervous system. In most cases, treatment consists of volume repletion with normal saline.

Effects of Acid-Base Status Disturbances on the Central Nervous System

Cerebral blood flow and volume are directly correlated with $Paco_2$ levels between 20 and 80 mm Hg. The increase in blood flow is a response to CO_2 crossing the blood-brain barrier (whereas it is impermeable to HCO_3^-) and dissociating to H^+. This causes a decrease in the pH of cerebrospinal fluid and results in arteriolar vasodilatation. Increased intracranial pressure can be treated with mild hyperventilation (goal $Paco_2$ of 30-35 mm Hg), which in turn decreases intracranial blood volume. However, this treatment is only temporary because the cerebrospinal fluid pH will equilibrate with the blood pH in 6 to 8 hours through active HCO_3^- transport. Hyperventilation to $Paco_2$ levels less than 30 mm Hg can predispose patients to cerebral ischemia.

Summary

- Systemic acid-base equilibrium is tightly controlled with an arterial pH between 7.35 and 7.45.
- Blood gas tests used to diagnose acid-base disorders measure pH, Pao_2, and $Paco_2$. HCO_3^- and base excess are calculated values.
- Venous blood gases correlate well with arterial blood gas pH and $Paco_2$ and HCO_3^- levels. Therefore, when an arterial blood gas value cannot be obtained, a venous sample can provide the needed information.
- A stepwise approach is needed to diagnose the underlying disorder, because many patients have mixed disturbances.
- Acidoses rarely need treatment with base administration unless the pH is 7.2 or less. Sodium bicarbonate administration might be detrimental if the patient cannot clear the resulting CO_2 load.
- Cerebral blood flow and volume are strongly influenced by $Paco_2$.

SUGGESTED READING

Berend K. Diagnostic use of base excess in acid-base disorders. N Engl J Med. 2018;378:1419–28.

Berend K, Duits AJ. The role of the clinical laboratory in diagnosing acid-base dosorders. Crit Rev Clin Lab Sci. 2019 Mar 27. [Epub ahead of print.]

Brian JE Jr. Carbon dioxide and the cerebral circulation. Anesthesiology. 1998 May;88(5):1365–86.

Byrne AL, Bennett M, Chatterji R, Symons R, Pace NL, Thomas PS. Peripheral venous and arterial blood gas analysis in adults: are they comparable? A systematic review and meta-analysis. Respirology. 2014 Feb;19(2):168–75. Epub 2014 Jan 3.

Gunnerson KJ, Kellum JA. Acid-base and electrolyte analysis in critically ill patients: are we ready for the new millennium? Curr Opin Crit Care. 2003 Dec;9(6):468–73.

Kaplan LJ, Kellum JA. Fluids, pH, ions and electrolytes. Curr Opin Crit Care. 2010 Aug;16(4):323–31.

Kelly AM, McAlpine R, Kyle E. Venous pH can safely replace arterial pH in the initial evaluation of patients in the emergency department. Emerg Med J. 2001 Sep;18(5):340–2.

Koul PA, Khan UH, Wani AA, Eachkoti R, Jan RA, Shah S, et al. Comparison and agreement between venous and arterial gas analysis in cardiopulmonary patients in Kashmir valley of the Indian subcontinent. Ann Thorac Med. 2011 Jan;6(1):33–7.

Nahas GG, Sutin KM, Fermon C, Streat S, Wiklund L, Wahlander S, et al. Guidelines for the treatment of acidaemia with THAM. Drugs. 1998 Feb;55(2):191–224. Erratum in: Drugs 1998 Apr;55(4):517.

Drug Dosing in Renal Failure

DANIEL A. JACKSON, PharmD, RPh

Goals

- Explain the equations used to estimate glomerular filtration rate in correlation with other laboratory values, signs, and symptoms when assessing the degree of renal dysfunction.
- Understand which drugs have a narrow therapeutic index and how to approach evaluation and dosing of these drugs to ensure therapeutic effects and reduced toxicity.
- Understand the fundamentals for medication dosing during continuous renal replacement therapy.

Introduction

Optimal dosing of medications can be influenced by many factors. These factors are important to consider because the therapeutic effects of drugs are frequently concentration dependent and can even result in toxicity. One factor of great importance is the pharmacokinetics of a medication. Pharmacokinetics is the way in which medications move through the body during absorption, distribution, metabolism, and excretion. This chapter focuses on the excretion of medications as it relates to renal function.

Estimating Renal Function

Renal function has been estimated with several different equations (Table 47.1). These equations are used to estimate glomerular filtration rate, a kidney function surrogate. From this estimate of kidney function, many drug manufacturers provide recommendations for modifications of drug dosing and intervals of administration. Although these recommendations are crude at best, they aim to change the drug dosing proportionally to the predicted reduction in renal function. Equations for renal function have been compared for many years, and it is not within the scope of this review to address the pros and cons for each equation. Importantly, each equation is an approximation at best and should be used in correlation with other laboratory values, signs, and symptoms when assessing the degree of renal dysfunction.

The National Kidney Foundation Kidney Disease Outcomes Quality Initiative has provided evidence-based clinical practice guidelines for all stages of chronic kidney disease. These guidelines include a table of the various stages of chronic kidney disease based on calculated glomerular filtration rate and whether dialysis is being used (Table 47.2).

Factors Affecting Dosing

As a patient's renal function decreases, renally excreted drugs accumulate. This decrease in drug clearance from the body can have minor or major impacts based on a medication's therapeutic index. The therapeutic index is defined as a comparison of the amount of drug that causes the therapeutic effect with the amount that causes toxicity. For drugs with a narrow therapeutic index, small changes in concentrations can cause toxic levels and loss of therapeutic efficacy. These medications often require therapeutic drug monitoring with drug levels, biomarkers, and clinical response to the medication. Medications with a narrow therapeutic index are listed in Table 47.3. Drugs with wide therapeutic indexes can have large changes in renal clearance with relatively low impact on the therapeutic response and low incidence of toxicity. A common class of drugs that has a wide therapeutic index is the β-lactam class of antibiotics. Although manufacturers have included dosing recommendations for decreased renal function, the incidence of toxicity is low and the therapeutic effect of the antibiotic is not altered with increased concentrations.

Another important factor to consider is the fraction of drug that is excreted unchanged by the kidneys. For drugs

Table 47.1 • Equations Used to Estimate Glomerular Filtration Rate

Name of Equation	Equation[a]
Cockcroft-Gault	CrCl = [(140 – Age) × IBW]/(SCr × 72) (× 0.85 if female)
Jelliffe	CrCl = 98 – 0.8 (Age – 20)/SCr (in mg/dL) × BSA/1.73 m^2 (× 0.9 if female)
Modification of Diet in Renal Disease	GFR (mL/min per 1.73 m^2) = 175 × $(SCr)^{-1.154}$ × $Age^{-0.203}$ × 0.742 (if female) × 1.212 (if African American)
Chronic Kidney Disease Epidemiology Collaboration	GFR = 141 × $\min(SCr/\kappa, 1)^{\alpha}$ × $\max(SCr/\kappa, 1)^{-1.209}$ × 0.993^{Age} × 1.018 (if female) × 1.159 (if African American) κ = 0.7 if female, 0.9 if male α = -0.329 if female, -0.411 if male

Abbreviations: BSA, body surface area; CrCl, creatinine clearance; GFR, glomerular filtration rate; IBW, ideal body weight; max, maximum of SCr/κ or 1; min, minimum of SCr/κ or 1; SCr, serum creatinine.
[a] Age is in years for all equations.

that have an intermediate and wide therapeutic index, this factor is used to determine whether a drug dose requires adjustment for renal dysfunction. As a drug travels through the body, it can undergo metabolism in various places, most commonly the liver. Metabolism can often convert the parent drug into active or inactive metabolites. It is important to consider the effects of active metabolites, especially in patients with renal failure, because they could lead to prolonged duration of action or toxicity. Table 47.4 lists commonly used medications with active metabolites and

Table 47.2 • National Kidney Foundation Kidney Disease Outcomes Quality Initiative Chronic Kidney Disease Stages

Stage	Description	Glomerular Filtration Rate, mL/min per 1.73 m^2
1	Slight kidney damage with normal or increased filtration	≥90
2	Mild decrease in kidney function	60-89
3	Moderate decrease in kidney function	30-59
4	Severe decrease in kidney function	15-29
5	Kidney failure	<15 or dialysis

Modified from National Kidney Foundation. K/DOQI clinical practice guidelines for bone metabolism and disease in chronic kidney disease. Am J Kidney Dis. 2003 Oct;42(4 Suppl 3):S1-201; used with permission.

Table 47.3 • Renally Cleared Drugs With a Narrow Therapeutic Index

Drug Class	Drugs	Monitoring
Aminoglycosides	Amikacin, gentamicin, and tobramycin	Drug levels
Glycopeptides	Vancomycin	Drug levels
Other	Digoxin and lithium	Drug levels

their effects in renal failure. Other medications can bypass metabolism and are excreted in their original composition. In patients with renal dysfunction, dose adjustment is important for drugs for which more than 50% of elimination occurs as excretion of the unchanged compound. This approach is also needed for medications in which the active metabolite is predominantly excreted via the kidney. Drugs that are extensively metabolized into inactive metabolites often do not require dose adjustment for renal dysfunction.

Hemodialysis can alter the dosing of medications cleared by the kidney. Patients who are dependent on hemodialysis rely on this method of extracorporeal extraction to remove toxins and medications from the bloodstream. When the dose of medications for dialysis is determined, their pharmacokinetics need to be considered. Factors of paramount consideration are how a drug is metabolized or excreted, what fraction of the drug is excreted unchanged, and the presence of active metabolites and their mode of excretion. In addition to the pharmacokinetics, whether and to what extent a medication will be removed during dialysis need to be known. Physiochemical characteristics of medications that determine the extent of removal during dialysis include molecular weight, protein binding, volume of distribution, water solubility, and plasma clearance. In addition, the type of dialysis and the dialysis membrane used can affect the degree of drug removal during dialysis. In general, drugs with low molecular weight, low protein binding, low volume of distribution, high water solubility, and a high renal clearance component of plasma clearance are more likely to be removed by dialysis.

For drugs with high removal during dialysis, dosing is often done after dialysis, if possible, or an additional dose of medication is given after each dialysis session, especially for treatment of life-threatening infections. For example, patients undergoing hemodialysis who are receiving piperacillin/tazobactam and aztreonam require the scheduled dose and an additional dose (piperacillin/tazobactam 0.75 g or aztreonam 0.25 g) after dialysis to replace the medication removed during dialysis. For renally cleared drugs that are not removed by dialysis (the fluoroquinolone antibiotics ciprofloxacin and levofloxacin), lower doses and extended intervals are used.

Table 47.4 • Commonly Used Medications With Active Metabolites and Their Effects in Renal Failure

Medication	Active Metabolite	Clinical Effects	Kinetic Effects
Diazepam	N-desmethyldiazepam	Prolonged sedation, CNS depression	Half-life prolonged up to 100 hours
Ketamine	Norketamine	Prolonged sedation, hallucinations	Prolonged half-life
Meperidine	Normeperidine	Prolonged analgesia, CNS depression, seizures	Accumulation of active metabolite, half-life prolonged up to 48 h
Midazolam	1-Hydroxy-midazolam	Prolonged sedation, CNS depression	Accumulation of active metabolite, half-life prolonged >25 h
Morphine	Morphine-6-glucuronide	Prolonged analgesia, CNS depression	Accumulation of active metabolite
Tramadol	O-desmethyltramadol	Prolonged analgesia, CNS depression	Half-life prolonged up to 17 h

Abbreviation: CNS, central nervous system.

For patients undergoing continuous renal replacement therapy (CRRT), slight dosing modifications are used. During CRRT, a patient undergoes 24-hour continuous dialysis. Removal of medications depends on characteristics similar to those in hemodialysis removal plus the type of membrane, mode of CRRT, and rate of CRRT fluid passed through the filter. The mode and membrane used are consistent, but as the fluid rates of CRRT effluent are increased, the percentage of renally cleared medications removed by the circuit increases. Dosing for renally cleared medications during high CRRT effluent rates can approach normal therapeutic doses and intervals because the CRRT is functioning like a 24-hour external kidney. Literature suggests that modern CRRT modes and higher effluent rates clear medications comparable to a creatinine clearance of 25 to 50 mL/min. Alterations in nonrenal clearance may also occur during CRRT and affect drug metabolism and elimination.

Summary

- Estimates of glomerular filtration rate can be calculated with various equations, but it is important to use an estimate in correlation with other laboratory values, signs, and symptoms when assessing the degree of renal dysfunction.
- Drugs with a narrow therapeutic index should be assessed with therapeutic drug monitoring, biomarkers, and clinical response to ensure therapeutic effects and reduced toxicity.
- Molecular weight, protein binding, volume of distribution, water solubility, and plasma clearance can affect drug removal of renally cleared medications during hemodialysis.
- Dosing for CRRT depends on dialysis mode, filter, and CRRT effluent rates.

SUGGESTED READING

Bailie GR, Mason NA. Bailie and Mason's 2016 dialysis of drugs [Internet]. Renal Pharmacy Consultants, LLC. c2013 [cited 2017 Nov 15]. Available from: http://renalpharmacyconsultants.com/.

Charhon N, Neely MN, Bourguignon L, Maire P, Jelliffe RW, Goutelle S. Comparison of four renal function estimation equations for pharmacokinetic modeling of gentamicin in geriatric patients. Antimicrob Agents Chemother. 2012 Apr;56(4):1862–9. Epub 2012 Jan 30.

Cockcroft DW, Gault MH. Prediction of creatinine clearance from serum creatinine. Nephron. 1976;16(1):31–41.

Doogue MP, Polasek TM. Drug dosing in renal disease. Clin Biochem Rev. 2011 May;32(2):69–73.

Florkowski CM, Chew-Harris JS. Methods of estimating GFR: different equations including CKD-EPI. Clin Biochem Rev. 2011 May;32(2):75–9.

Hudson JQ, Nolin TD. Pragmatic use of kidney function estimates for drug dosing: the tide is turning. Adv Chronic Kidney Dis. 2018 Jan;25(1):14–20.

Levey AS, Bosch JP, Lewis JB, Greene T, Rogers N, Roth D; Modification of Diet in Renal Disease Study Group. A more accurate method to estimate glomerular filtration rate from serum creatinine: a new prediction equation. Ann Intern Med. 1999 Mar 16;130(6): 461–70.

Levey AS, Stevens LA, Schmid CH, Zhang YL, Castro AF 3rd, Feldman HI, et al; CKD-EPI (Chronic Kidney Disease Epidemiology Collaboration). A new equation to estimate glomerular filtration rate. Ann Intern Med. 2009 May 5;150(9):604–12. Erratum in: Ann Intern Med. 2011 Sep 20;155(6):408.

Micromedex [Internet]. Truven Health Analytics. c2017 [cited 2017 Nov 15]. Available from: http://www.micromedexsolutions.com/ home/dispatch.

National Kidney Foundation Kidney Disease Outcomes Quality Initiative (NKF KDOQI) [Internet]. New York (NY): National Kidney Foundation. c2017 [cited 2017 Nov 15]. Available from: http://www.kidney.org/professionals/guidelines.

Smyth B, Jones C, Saunders J. Prescribing for patients on dialysis. Aust Prescr. 2016 Feb;39(1):21–4. Epub 2016 Feb 1.

48 Principles of Renal Replacement Therapies

PETER M. FITZPATRICK, MD

Goals

- Describe the principles of renal replacement therapy.
- Describe the types of renal replacement therapy.
- Discuss access for dialysis in the intensive care unit.
- Discuss anticoagulation for renal replacement.

Introduction

Renal replacement therapy is frequently used in the intensive care unit, primarily for the management of acute kidney injury, but it is also indicated for removal of some toxins and medications. Additionally, patients with dialysis-dependent chronic kidney failure who are admitted to the intensive care unit require their therapy to be continued. This chapter reviews the mechanisms by which renal replacement therapy operates and the types of replacement therapies that are available. Access for renal replacement and anticoagulation are also discussed.

Mechanisms of Solute Transport

All renal replacement therapies function primarily on 3 mechanisms of solute transport and removal: diffusion, ultrafiltration, adsorption. All forms of renal replacement therapy use one or more of these mechanisms.

Diffusion is the movement of molecules (solute) across a semipermeable membrane. This process is driven by concentration gradients. The movement of solutes is dependent on, for example, size and charge characteristics of the molecules and pore size and charge characteristics of the membrane. The removal of solutes by this mechanism is referred to as diffusive clearance.

Ultrafiltration is the movement of water across a semipermanent membrane. The water carries with it solutes (solvent drag) depending on the characteristics of the solute and the semipermeable membrane. This process is driven by either hydrostatic or osmotic pressure gradients. Removal of solutes by this mechanism is referred to as convective clearance.

Adsorption is a mechanism of molecules being removed from solution by adhering to the membrane or other substrate. This is referred to as adsorptive clearance.

All modern machines designed for renal replacement therapy use dialyzers (sometimes called dialysis filters) constructed of hollow fibers. The walls of these fibers constitute the semipermeable membrane mentioned above and have specific characteristics that can affect clearances. These characteristics include the type of biomaterial from which they are constructed, the pore sizes, and the thickness of the membrane.

Key factors that affect solute clearance include properties of the membrane, properties of the solute, and properties of flow on both the blood side and the dialysate side. Membrane properties include porosity, thickness, surface area, charge, and hydrophilicity. Solute properties include the molecular weight and size, charge, lipid solubility, and protein binding. The rate of blood flow through the hollow fibers and the presence or absence of unstirred blood layers can affect clearance. Likewise, dialysate flow rate, the presence or absence of unstirred layers, and the direction of dialysate flow, either countercurrent or concurrent, affect clearance. Other factors that affect clearance include treatment time, body distribution, and sequestration of solutes.

Types of Renal Replacement Therapy

Renal replacement therapies can be either intermittent or continuous. They can be provided either on a short-term basis, typically in a hospital, or on a long-term basis at a dialysis center or at home.

Hemodialysis

Hemodialysis relies primarily on diffusive clearance to remove solutes. Ultrafiltration is performed to remove a prescribed amount of fluid but does not contribute much to overall solute clearance. Hemodialysis is usually done intermittently, each treatment lasting 3 to 4 hours. The standard dialysis machine is designed to be efficient, allowing for the short treatment times. Some centers have used standard hemodialysis machines to provide extended treatments lasting 8 to 12 hours. Extended dialysis treatment times may provide more hemodynamic stability for acutely ill, hospitalized patients. Continuous renal replacement therapy machines can do continuous hemodialysis. Hemodialysis requires fluid that is called either dialysate or dialysis bath. This fluid contains sodium, chloride, potassium, bicarbonate, calcium, magnesium, and dextrose. The dialysate composition varies primarily in the potassium concentration, although different calcium levels can also be selected. The dialysis machine maintains blood flow rates of 200 to 450 mL/minute and dialysate flow rates of 500 to 800 mL/minute. These high flow rates maintain high concentration gradients between the blood and dialysate to maximize efficient solute removal. The dialysate and blood flow paths run countercurrent to enhance solute clearance efficiency. Dialysate and blood do not mix; they are always separated by the semipermeable membrane that makes up the hollow fibers.

Hemofiltration

Hemofiltration relies on convective clearance to remove solutes. There is no diffusive clearance in hemofiltration. Convective clearance is obtained by ultrafiltrating large volumes of plasma water. Hemofiltration requires large volumes of replacement fluid to avoid volume depletion from the removal of the plasma water. The patient's volume status can be adjusted by adjusting the volume of replacement fluid provided. Hemofiltration is typically a form of continuous renal replacement therapy, although it can be done intermittently. The hemofilter is also constructed of hollow fibers and looks very similar to a dialysis filter. The pore sizes tend to be larger than those of a dialysis filter to allow for high ultrafiltration rates. They also allow for removal of some larger molecule solutes. This feature can be particularly important for medications such as antibiotics and cardiac medications. The hemofiltration replacement fluid is infused into the blood line and thus it must be a sterile solution. It usually is infused proximal to the hemofilter but also can be infused distally or as a combination of proximal and distal. Blood flow rates are similar to those with hemodialysis. Flow rates of replacement fluid are based on a patient's body weight and are commonly prescribed as 25 to 35 mL/kg per hour. The replacement fluid rate equals the rate of plasma water removal. For example, a 100-kg patient would receive 3,500 mL of replacement fluid per hour and also have 3,500 mL of plasma water removed per hour. Additional fluid can be removed to correct a patient's volume status. Replacement fluid contains sodium, chloride, potassium, bicarbonate, calcium, magnesium, and dextrose. As with dialysate, the potassium and calcium concentrations may vary depending on a patient's need.

Hemodiafiltration

Hemodiafiltration combines diffusive and convective clearances. This is accomplished by adding dialysate into the hemofiltration system. The dialysate runs countercurrent to the blood flow. The replacement fluid is given just as in standard hemofiltration. Hemodiafiltration, therefore, can increase the total clearance because the diffusive and convective clearances will be additive. It does, however, increase the complexity of the machine and the cost of treatment by requiring 2 fluids.

Slow Continuous Ultrafiltration

Slow continuous ultrafiltration is designed to remove excess volume from a patient. It is typically done intermittently. Up to 1 L of fluid may be removed per hour depending on a patient's blood pressure stability. It is not useful for treating kidney failure because the solute clearances are extremely low.

Peritoneal Dialysis

Peritoneal dialysis uses the natural membrane that lines the peritoneal cavity as a dialysis filter. It also relies on diffusive clearance for solute removal and uses osmotic gradient–driven ultrafiltration for fluid removal. Peritoneal dialysis fluid contains sodium, chloride, potassium, magnesium, and calcium. It also contains acetate as a bicarbonate equivalent. The fluid uses different concentrations of dextrose to create osmotic gradient for fluid removal. The greater the dextrose concentration, the greater the fluid removal. Peritoneal dialysis fluid dwells within the abdominal cavity for a prescribed amount of time and then is drained and replaced with fresh fluid. The fluid exchange can be done either manually (continuous ambulatory peritoneal dialysis) or by a machine (continuous cycling peritoneal dialysis [automated peritoneal dialysis]).

Hemoperfusion

Solutes can be removed from the bloodstream by adsorbing onto substrates. It is most commonly used to remove toxins resulting from poisoning or drug overdoses. It can be used as a stand-alone treatment but is more commonly used along with other renal replacement therapies (but not peritoneal dialysis). The most commonly used hemoperfusion agents are activated charcoal and certain resins. These agents are usually coated and immobilized onto a membrane surface to prevent them from entering into the bloodstream. Hemoperfusion is rarely used because of possible serious complications, including thrombocytopenia, leukopenia, and increased risk of bleeding.

Access for Renal Replacement Therapy

A dual-lumen hemodialysis catheter placed in a central vein is the most commonly used access for blood-based short-term renal replacement therapy. Some temporary hemodialysis catheters include a central "nurse port" that can be used for infusions or withdrawing blood for sampling. There is some concern, however, about the increased risk for infection with a nurse port as a result of increased manipulation of the line. The tip of a dual-lumen dialysis catheter should be at the junction of the superior vena cava and right atrium or just inside the right atrium to maximize blood flow rates. A temporary dual-lumen dialysis catheter can be placed in any central vein, although the right internal jugular vein is the most desirable position. This position minimizes both the number of bends in the catheter that could limit catheter blood flow rates and the increased risk for clotting of the catheter. The left internal jugular position requires both a catheter to bend twice and a long catheter, features that increase resistance to blood flow. Subclavian catheters are discouraged because of the high risk of subclavian vein stenosis, which would limit the use of the ipsilateral arm for creating a permanent dialysis access if a patient does not regain kidney function. A femoral catheter also is discouraged because of the high risk for infection and because of the low flow present in the inferior vena cava that can compromise the efficiency of renal replacement treatment. The tip of a femoral catheter usually rests around midabdomen.

If renal replacement therapy is required for a prolonged time (>10-14 days), a tunneled dual-lumen dialysis catheter is usually recommended. This catheter exits the chest wall and is tunneled under the skin several centimeters before entering the right or left internal jugular vein. A Dacron cuff on the catheter is positioned just below the surface of the skin. The cuff and tunnel help reduce the risk for line sepsis. For long-term chronic hemodialysis, a surgically created fistula is useful to reduce the risk of sepsis and provide the most reliable access.

The most common complications of a dialysis catheter are kinking, clotting, and sepsis. Also, there is a risk of pneumothorax with insertion of the catheter.

A temporary peritoneal dialysis catheter can be used to provide short-term peritoneal dialysis, but this treatment is rarely used in the United States.

Anticoagulation for Renal Replacement Therapy

Both intermittent and continuous blood-based renal replacement therapies require extracorporeal blood flow, which can clot in the blood circuit. Peritoneal dialysis does not require anticoagulation. Several strategies can be used to prevent clotting of the extracorporeal blood lines.

No Anticoagulation

Some patients who are at a very high risk for bleeding are best not exposed to anticoagulation. Renal replacement therapy can be provided using high blood flow rates (200-300 mL/minute). The extracorporeal circuit can be flushed with 25 to 50 mL of saline every 30 minutes, but some studies have failed to show efficacy of this method.

Heparin

Heparin is typically used for intermittent hemodialysis. Patients receive a bolus of heparin (1,000-2,000 units) at the start of dialysis and then hourly infusions (500-1,000 units) until the last hour of the dialysis treatment. Because heparin has a very short half-life, most the heparin effect is gone at the end of the dialysis therapy or shortly after it is completed. For patients receiving continuous renal replacement therapy, a continuous heparin infusion is needed.

Regional Citrate Anticoagulation

For patients who cannot receive heparin or who are at increased risk for bleeding but require anticoagulation to prevent clotting of the extracorporeal circuit, regional citrate anticoagulation can be used. Citrate binds ionized calcium, which is a necessary cofactor in the coagulation cascade. Citrate is infused into the blood line before it enters the dialysis filter. Most of the citrate–calcium complexes are then removed in the filter. A calcium infusion is needed to replete the ionized calcium. Any citrate that enters into a patient's systemic bloodstream is metabolized into bicarbonate primarily by the liver. If citrate is not adequately metabolized, it can cause complications. This possibility limits the use of regional citrate anticoagulation in patients with liver failure.

Other Anticoagulants

Argatroban is a second-generation direct thrombin inhibitor. It is metabolized by the liver and has a half-life of 35 minutes. It is administered in a continuous infusion. The dose needs to be decreased in patients with liver failure. There is no antidote for the action of argatroban. Bivalirudin is another thrombin inhibitor but has a shorter half-life than argatroban. It can be used in patients with both renal and liver failure.

Summary

- Although there are several types of renal replacement therapy, they all are based on the basic principle of diffusion, ultrafiltration, and adsorption.
- The different types of renal replacement therapies have different characteristics, advantages, and disadvantages. The best therapy for a specific patient may depend on the medical condition of that patient and on the local expertise, staff, and equipment available.
- The intricacies of renal replacement therapy, such as optimal time to initiate or discontinue therapy, which type to use, dosing, solution selection, anticoagulation, and management of complications, are best managed by a nephrologist trained in delivering these therapies.

SUGGESTED READING

Bagshaw SM, Adhikari NKJ, Burns KEA, Friedrich JO, Bouchard J, Lamontagne F, et al; Canadian Critical Care Trials Group. Selection and receipt of kidney replacement in critically ill older patients with AKI. Clin J Am Soc Nephrol. 2019 Apr 5;14(4):496–505. Epub 2019 Mar 21.

Cerda J, Ronco C. Modalities of continuous renal replacement therapy: technical and clinical considerations. Semin Dial. 2009 Mar-Apr;22(2):114–22.

Joy MS, Matzke GR, Armstrong DK, Marx MA, Zarowitz BJ. A primer on continuous renal replacement therapy for critically ill patients. Ann Pharmacother. 1998 Mar;32(3):362–75.

Rachoin JS, Weisberg LS. Renal replacement therapy in the ICU. Crit Care Med. 2019 May;47(5):715–21.

Ricci Z, Romagnoli S, Ronco C. Renal replacement therapy. F1000Res. 2016 Jan 25;5. pii: F1000 Faculty Rev-103.

Yessayan L, Yee J, Frinak S, Szamosfalvi B. Continuous renal replacement therapy for the management of acid-base and electrolyte imbalances in acute kidney injury. Adv Chronic Kidney Dis. 2016 May;23(3):203–10.

49 Disorders of Water and Electrolyte Balance

YUZANA ZAW, MBBS; MIRA T. KEDDIS, MD

Goals

- Discuss the regulation of water balance.
- Describe the pathophysiology, evaluation, and treatment of hypernatremia and hyponatremia.
- Review the pathophysiology, evaluation, and treatment of cerebral salt wasting.
- Explain the common causes and treatment approach for hyperkalemia and hypokalemia.
- Review the regulation of calcium, phosphorus, and magnesium balance.

Introduction

This chapter describes the physiology of water balance; disorders of hyponatremia and hypernatremia and the approach to their evaluation, diagnosis, and treatment; and disorders of electrolyte imbalance, including those of potassium, calcium, phosphorus, and magnesium.

Water Balance

Water balance depends on both regulated and unregulated factors that determine intake of water and water losses through renal and extrarenal mechanisms. Disorders of water balance lead to hyponatremia and hypernatremia, which are disorders of serum osmolality. Hyponatremia occurs when total body water is in excess to sodium, and hypernatremia occurs when total body sodium is in excess to water. The differential diagnosis for these disorders is classically defined by a patient's volume status. Hyponatremia and hypernatremia can have determinal effects on the brain, and the rate of correction must be carefully managed. Cerebral salt wasting is characterized by hyponatremia due to renal losses of sodium in patients with intracranial disease and hypovolemic state. The low-volume state is corrected with isotonic solution. In contrast, volume replacement worsens hyponatremia in the syndrome of inappropriate antidiuretic hormone (SIADH).

Overview of Regulation of Water Balance

The 2 main compartments for total body water are intracellular fluid (ICF) and extracellular fluid (ECF). ECF includes the intravascular compartment (plasma) and the extravascular compartment (interstitial, lymph, and connective tissues). Total body water is estimated at 60% of body weight in men and 50% in women. Water balance depends on regulated and unregulated factors that affect water intake and water losses. Unregulated water intake includes water content in ingested food and beverages that are consumed in the context of taste preferences or social settings. Regulated water intake refers to the amount of water ingested in response to thirst. Water losses have regulated and unregulated components. Unregulated water losses include insensible losses from the skin and the pulmonary system through exhaled air. The degree of insensible water losses is largely influenced by activity, temperature, humidity, and dress and is estimated at 5 to 10 mL/kg of body weight. This can increase to 20 mL/kg in the setting of fever or exercise. Another determinant of unregulated water losses is the amount of solute load, which is based on body metabolism and dietary intake. An obligatory amount of water is excreted by the kidneys to eliminate that solute load. This amount of water is defined by the urine osmolality and the amount of solute load per day. A healthy person has a urine osmolality of 600 mOsm/

kg H_2O, and a typical solute load is between 900 and 1,200 mOsm per day. Therefore, the obligatory amount of water excreted in this setting can be calculated as solute load divided by urine osmolality:

$$1{,}200/600 = 2\,\text{L per day}.$$

The regulated component of water excretion is dependent on 1) the hypothalamus and posterior pituitary where arginine vasopressin (AVP) is produced and stored and 2) the renal effects of AVP. Perturbations to the regulatory and unregulatory factors that determine water balance account for disorders of water balance. Disorders of water balance manifest as hypernatremia or hyponatremia. Disorders of sodium balance manifest as hypovolemia or hypervolemia and are not physiologically under direct regulation of water balance.

The body maintains fluid osmolality within a narrow physiologic window between 285 and 290 mOsm/kg H_2O. AVP is one of the most important regulators of water balance and serum osmolality. It is produced in the hypothalamus by the supraoptic and paraventricular nuclei and released by neurophysin through calcium-dependent exocytosis. The second most important regulator of water balance is the AVP receptor, specifically the V2 receptor located in the collecting duct of the renal tubule. When serum osmolality increases, AVP binds the V2 receptor on the basolateral membrane of the renal tubule. This action activates a G-linked transmembrane protein that stimulates cyclic adenosine monophosphate and protein kinase A. Subsequently, aquaporin-2–containing vesicles are shuttled to the apical membrane (urine lumen) to increase water permeability of the tubule. Disorders of AVP and aquaporin-2, therefore, are associated with unregulated diuresis and resultant hypernatremia. Thirst is a secondary mechanism that regulates serum osmolality. Thirst is stimulated by increased serum osmolality and by low effective circulating volume. The osmotic threshold for thirst is generally higher than that for AVP and, therefore, thirst is a backup mechanism to maintain serum osmolality.

Osmoreceptors are the key mediators of AVP release in response to changes in plasma osmolality. Sodium and its anions, the most osmotically active solutes, stimulate osmoreceptors. Osmoreceptors are located in the manocellular neurons and the organum vasculosum of the lamina terminalis near the anterior hypothalamus. Each person has a set osmotic threshold, which generally ranges between 280 and 290 mOsm/kg. An increase in plasma osmolality by as little as 1 mOsm/kg H_2O will lead to an increase in AVP, which subsequently leads to an increase in urine osmolality and a decrease in urine output. Nonosmotic stimuli can also have a profound effect on AVP release. A decrease of 10% to 15% of effective circulating volume (arterial underfilling) stimulates AVP release exponentially and leads to higher AVP levels than with osmotic stimuli alone. This mechanism is the physiologic explanation for hyponatremia in patients with hepatic cirrhosis, nephrotic syndrome, and heart failure, in which low effective circulating volume stimulates AVP release. Nausea with or without vomiting can also be a nonosmotic stimulator of AVP release. Box 49.1 summarizes some of the nonosmotic regulators of AVP.

Box 49.1 • Nonosmotic Stimuli for Release of Arginine Vasopressin

- Hemodynamic stimuli
  - Hypovolemia
    - ≥15% volume loss
  - Low effective circulating volume
    - Heart failure
    - Liver cirrhosis
    - Nephrotic syndrome
  - Nausea
    - Intrinsic
    - Medication induced
- Drugs
  - Carbamazepine
  - Chlorpropamide
  - Cyclophosphamide
  - Vincristine
  - Selective serotonin reuptake inhibitors
- Hormones
  - Angiotensin II
  - Insulin

Hypernatremia Disorders

Pathophysiology of Hypernatremia

The primary disorder in hypernatremia is too little water with respect to salt and resultant high serum sodium concentration. Hypernatremia is defined as a serum sodium concentration of more than 145 mmol/L. Hypernatremia, therefore, is an increase in osmolality in the ECF compared with the ICF that drives water movement out of the cell, leading to cellular shrinkage. In the brain, this can lead to an initial decrease in brain volume. Overtime, brain cells increase uptake of inorganic and organic osmotically active ions to promote water movement back into the cell.

Hypernatremia is characterized by 2 main mechanisms: 1) sodium intake in excess to water and 2) water losses that exceed salt losses (losses of solute-free water). Sodium intake in excess to water can occur in the following situations: salt poisoning, enteral feeding without adequate free water replacement, hypertonic enemas, hypertonic sodium bicarbonate infusions, and primary hyperaldosteronism due to increased salt retention under the effect of aldosterone without a change in water reabsorption. Water losses that exceed salt losses can occur from renal and extrarenal conditions. Extrarenal conditions that lead to losses of water in excess to salt include sweating (which can be as much as 1.4 L in a 70-kg person under conditions of excessive sweating) and gastrointestinal losses from diarrhea, nasogastric suction, and enterocutaneous fistula. Osmotic diarrhea and diarrhea due to viral gastroenteritis lead to hypernatremia. However, secretory diarrhea leads to isotonic stool and does not contribute to hypernatremia.

Renal losses of solute-free water can occur with 3 main conditions. The first condition is osmotic diuresis. Nonabsorbable solutes present in the plasma and excreted by the kidney are osmotically active in the urine lumen and create a concentration gradient for water to be excreted. Examples of solutes that are osmotically active and lead to hypernatremia due to osmotic diuresis include urea (as in patients with severe renal failure), mannitol, and glucose. The second condition is central diabetes insipidus (DI), which is due to diseases that impair the production or release of AVP in the brain. The third condition is due to lack of AVP effect in the kidney, also known as nephrogenic DI. DI can be clinically detected from the following characteristics: low urine specific gravity, indicating dilute urine; high urine volume (>3.5 L/day); urine osmolality lower than serum osmolality; and high serum sodium concentrations. In DI, the kidney is unable to concentrate the urine and preserve free water. If thirst mechanisms are intact, patients can compensate by drinking more free water, resulting in polydipsia, and this generally restores the serum osmolality and serum sodium to the high normal range. However, if thirst mechanisms are impaired, then hyperosmolality and hypernatremia ensue.

Diagnosis of Hypernatremia

There are 2 crucial steps in the diagnosis of hypernatremia: 1) a detailed history, including history of head trauma and psychiatric history, and 2) adequate assessment of volume status. Once volume status is determined, hypernatremia can be categorized as hypovolemic, euvolemic, or hypervolemic (Figure 49.1). Hypovolemic hypernatremia is due to losses of water and salt, but water losses exceed salt losses. Causes can be either renal or gastrointestinal. Measurement of urine sodium concentration and urine osmolality can help differentiate renal from extrarenal causes. Extrarenal causes have low urine sodium and high urine osmolality, reflecting normal renal adaptation to low volume state (increased salt and water reabsorption). Renal causes have low urine osmolality, a suggestion that the mechanism for water reabsorption is impaired. Urine sodium may also be increased. Euvolemic hypernatremia can also result from renal and extrarenal causes. There is water loss without salt loss and, therefore, volume status is preserved. It can be due to gastrointestinal losses with inadequate water replacement caused by impaired sense of taste or thirst. Renal causes are either due to neurologic processes affecting AVP production or release or due to renal causes impairing function of AVP at the level of the kidney. If the urine osmolality is less than 300 mOsmol/kg H_2O, then central or nephrogenic DI must be considered. A urine osmolality more than 800 mOsmol/kg H_2O suggests that the cause of hypernatremia is extrarenal and that AVP and its renal effects are intact. When the urine osmolality is between 400 and 800 mOsmol/kg H_2O, a partial form of central or nephrogenic DI or an osmotic diuresis process must be considered. Hypervolemic hypernatremia is uncommon and occurs in the context of salt gain in excess to increase in total body water. This can be due to hypertonic infusions, as in sodium bicarbonate infusion, hypertonic feeding formulas, and primary hyperaldosteronism.

Water Deprivation Test

A water deprivation test is an appropriate consideration when a differentiation is needed between central and nephrogenic DI. However, it is not done in the setting of an intensive care unit.

Treatment Approach to Hypernatremia

Box 49.2 summarizes the steps in treatment approach. The options for fluid replacement depend on volume status. If a patient is hypovolemic, saline should be administered first until euvolemia is established, and then hypotonic solution or free water should be administered subsequently to correct residual hypernatremia. If the patient is euvolemic, hypernatremia should be corrected by administering free water. This can be in the form of 5% dextrose intravenously or water replacement either orally or with a nasogastric tube if thirst mechanisms are impaired. Half-normal saline (0.45%) can also be used, but higher volumes are required to correct the deficit. For patients with central DI, desmopressin therapy is required. Management of hypervolemic hypernatremia can be challenging. A combination of 5% dextrose in addition to loop diuresis can be used. If kidney failure is present in cases of hypervolemic hypernatremia, dialysis is an appropriate treatment option.

Rate of Repletion

The goal of correction is to replace the free-water deficit over 48 hours and not to correct serum sodium by more than 10 mEq per day. Overcorrection of hypernatremia increases the risk of cerebral edema. For cases of acute hypernatremia (developing in <24 hours), rapid correction (1 mEq/L per hour) is recommended. Slow correction in hypernatremia has been associated with increased mortality compared with the degree of hypernatremia. Therefore, when onset of hypernatremia is known, rapid correction

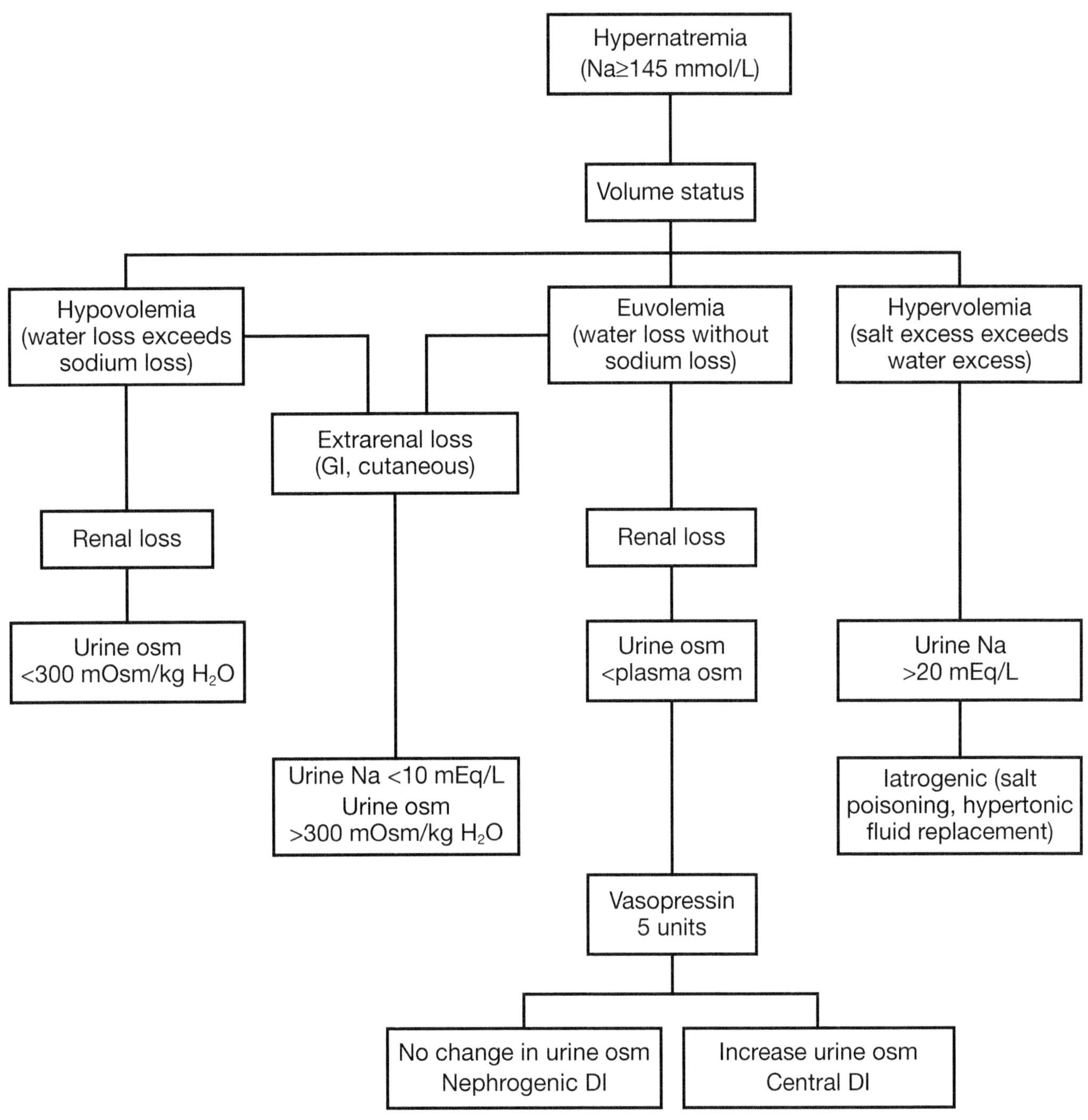

Figure 49.1. Outline for the Differential Diagnosis of Hypernatremia According to Volume Status. DI indicates diabetes insipidus; GI, gastrointestinal; Na, sodium; osm, osmolality.

can improve prognosis without increasing the risk of cerebral edema.

Hyponatremia Disorders

Pathophysiology of Hyponatremia

Hyponatremia is defined as a serum sodium level less than 135 mEq/L and is the most common electrolyte abnormality in the hospital. It is a relative excess of water in relation to sodium. Hyponatremia is a decrease in the osmolality in the ECF compared with that in the ICF. This results from impairment in the osmotic or nonosmotic regulation of AVP. The hypo-osmolar state causes water movement into ICF, leading to intracellular swelling, which may result in neuromuscular excitability, seizures, and coma, usually when the sodium level decreases acutely.

Box 49.2 • Treatment Approach to Hypernatremia

Step 1: Determine volume status
Step 2: Calculate free water deficit
Step 3: Choose a replacement fluid
Step 4: Determine rate of repletion
Step 5: Estimate ongoing "sensible" losses
Step 6: Estimate ongoing "insensible" losses
Step 7: Determine and reverse the underlying cause

Modified from Carson JM, Linas SL. 8: Hypernatremia. In: Gilbert SJ, Weiner DE, editors. National Kidney Foundation primer on kidney diseases. 7th ed. Philadelphia (PA): Elsevier; c2018. p. 77–85; used with permission.

Hyponatremia is classified by serum osmolality into 3 types. The first type, iso-osmolar hyponatremia, also known as pseudohyponatremia, is a measurement flaw in the setting of paraproteinemia and hyperlipidemia. It is characterized by normal serum osmolality and low serum sodium concentration. The second type is hypo-osmolar hyponatremia, which is the most common hyponatremic condition characterized by low serum osmolality. In the third type, hyperosmolar hyponatremia, also known as translocational hyponatremia, an osmotically active substance confined to the ECF causes fluid shift from the ICF to the ECF with resultant hyponatremia. Hyperglycemia can reduce serum sodium concentrations by 2.4 mEq/L for every 100 mg/dL increase in serum glucose.

Hypo-osmolar (serum osmolality <280 mOsm/kg H_2O), or hypotonic hyponatremia, is further classified by volume status. Hypovolemic hyponatremia occurs when salt losses exceed water losses, and this can occur in the setting of diuretics (particularly thiazides), gastrointestinal causes, third-spacing, and adrenal insufficiency. Euvolemic hyponatremia occurs when there is an excess of water without salt, and this can occur when there is excess AVP release due to medications, nausea, or pain. SIADH due to central nervous system disease, lung disease, neoplasm, and drugs presents as euvolemic hyponatremia. Other conditions that can present as euvolemic hyponatremia include hypothyroidism, glucocorticoid deficiency, and psychogenic polydipsia. Hypervolemic hyponatremia occurs when water excess exceeds salt excess, and this typically occurs in states of arterial underfilling, which include cirrhosis, heart failure, and nephrotic syndrome.

Clinical Presentation of Hyponatremia

Symptoms directly attributable to acute hyponatremia reflect neurologic dysfunction induced by cerebral edema due to a decrease in serum osmolality. Nausea and malaise are the earliest findings and may occur at serum sodium levels of less than 125 to 130 mEq/L. Headache, lethargy, obtundation, and, eventually, seizures, coma, and respiratory arrest may occur if the level decreases to less than 115 to 120 mEq/L. Patients who have chronic hyponatremia may appear to be asymptomatic despite sodium levels less than 120 mEq/L. This asymptomatic state is due to brain adaptation, which includes loss of organic osmolytes along with water loss to decrease cell swelling. Symptoms of chronic hyponatremia are more subtle and include fatigue, nausea, dizziness, gait disturbances, forgetfulness, confusion, lethargy, and muscle cramps.

Rapid correction of hyponatremia can lead to cell shrinkage, particularly damaging to the myelin-producing oligodendrocytes, which is clinically defined as osmotic demyelination syndrome (also called central pontine myelinolysis). This syndrome can result in severe and potentially irreversible neurologic symptoms. Osmotic demyelination is the most serious demyelinating disorder, typically involving the central pons but often extending into extrapontine structures. Clinical features include hyperreflexia, pseudobulbar palsy, quadriparesis, parkinsonism, locked-in syndrome, and even death. Symptoms present 1 to 7 days after overcorrection. Osmotic demyelination is potentially reversible, and one-third of patients may have full neurologic recovery. Treatment is primarily supportive. Conditions posing high risk for this complication include chronic hyponatremia with a serum sodium level of less than 110 mEq/L, alcoholism, hepatic failure, malignancy, orthotopic liver transplant, potassium depletion, and malnutrition.

Treatment Approach to Acute and Chronic Hyponatremia

The recommendations for treatment of hyponatremia rely on understanding of central nervous system adaptation to an altered serum osmolality. When the time frame of hyponatremia cannot be established with confidence, it is safest to conclude that the hypotonic state is chronic. Considering the common uncertainty and that overcorrection can lead to osmotic demyelination, current literature suggests not exceeding 6 to 8 mEq/L in any 24-hour period, regardless of clinical presentation and method of treatment, including active management and spontaneous correction. Correction by more than 10 to 12 mEq/L in 24 hours or by more than 18 mEq/L in 48 hours is commonly complicated by osmotic demyelination.

Medical emergencies such as severe symptoms mandate correction by 4 to 6 mEq/L within 4 to 6 hours. The rule of 6s can be remembered as providing 6 mEq/L of sodium in the first 6 hours. The goal should be to frontload the correction in a 24-hour period during the first 6 hours and then postpone further correction to the next day at a rate of 4 to 6 mEq/L per day.

Patients with acute symptomatic hyponatremia (<24 hours) should be treated with a 100-mL bolus of 3% saline

Box 49.3 • Formulas Used to Calculate Water Deficit and Predict Serum Na Correction

Formula 1: Relationship of serum Na to TBW

Serum Na concentration = (total body Na + K)/TBW

Formula 2: Free water deficit formula

Water deficit = TBW × ([plasma Na/140] – 1)

TBW = weight in kg × 0.6 (male) or 0.5 (female) or 0.45 (elderly)

Formula 3: Change in Na formula (Adrogue-Madias formula)

Change in Na = ([infusate Na + K] – serum Na)/(TBW +1)

Formula 4: Electrolyte free water clearance formula

Electrolyte free water clearance = urine volume × (1 – [urine Na + urine K]/serum Na)

Abbreviations: K, potassium; Na, sodium; TBW, total body water.

Data from Adrogue HJ, Madias NE. The challenge of hyponatremia. J Am Soc Nephrol. 2012 Jul;23(7):1140–8. Epub 2012 May 24.

that can be repeated with 2 additional doses every 15 minutes if there is no clinical improvement.

Treatment of chronic asymptomatic hyponatremia depends on volume status and the cause. In hypovolemic hyponatremia, isotonic saline (0.9%) increases serum sodium by approximately 1 mEq for every liter of saline. In hypervolemic hyponatremia, fluid restriction and loop diuretics remain the cornerstone. In cases of euvolemia such as SIADH, fluid restriction is recommended. Refractory cases can be treated with an antidiuretic hormone receptor antagonist, although these agents are expensive and are generally reserved for use in severe, chronic hyponatremia with a sodium value less than 120 mEq/L. These agents should not be used in patients with liver diseases because of their association with abnormal results of liver function tests. Urea has been used as an effective alternative, but unpalatability has hindered its wide application.

The rate of serum sodium correction can be calculated using the Adrogue-Madias formula (Box 49.3). Table 49.1 shows the estimated effect of infusate sodium on serum sodium concentration. When violation of the correction threshold seems likely, hypotonic saline infusate (eg, 0.45% sodium chloride, 5% dextrose in water) and desmopressin must be administered at a rate determined by the infusate formula to reverse the rapid correction.

Overview of Cerebral Salt Wasting

Cerebral salt wasting is a renal loss of sodium in patients with intracranial disease that leads to hyponatremia and

Table 49.1 • The Effect of Different Solutions on Serum Na Concentration

Solution	Infusate Na + K, mmol/L	Effect on Serum Na per 1 L, mEq/L
3% NaCl	513	↑13
0.9% NaCl	154	↑1.4
Lactated Ringer	135	↑0.8
0.45% NaCl	77	↓1.1
5% Dextrose	0	↓3.5

Abbreviations: K, potassium; Na, sodium; NaCl, sodium chloride; ↑, increase; ↓, decrease.

From Adrogue HJ, Madias NE. The challenge of hyponatremia. J Am Soc Nephrol. 2012 Jul;23(7):1140–8. Epub 2012 May 24; used with permission.

a decrease in extracellular fluid volume. Differences from SIADH are shown in Table 49.2.

Diagnostic characteristics for cerebral salt wasting include the following:

- Hypovolemic state
- Hyponatremia (serum sodium, <135 mEq/L) with low plasma osmolality
- Inappropriately increased urine osmolality (>100 mOsmol/kg H_2O and usually >300 mOsmol/kg H_2O)
- Urine sodium level >40 mEq/L
- Low serum uric acid concentration

Treatment requires volume replacement with isotonic saline and maintenance of positive salt balance. Excretion of dilute urine corrects the hyponatremia. For patients with documented cerebral salt wasting, salt tablets can be administered once they are able to take oral medications. A mineralocorticoid, such as fludrocortisone, can also be administered. Long-term therapy of cerebral salt wasting is not necessary because it tends to be transient. Resolution usually occurs within 3 to 4 weeks.

Electrolytes

Potassium Disorders

Potassium is the most abundant intracellular cation in the body; only 2% of total body potassium exists in the ECF, and only 0.4% exists in the plasma. Therefore, abnormalities in serum potassium reflect substantial change in total body potassium balance, such that for every 0.3 mmol/L decrease in potassium in the serum, the deficit in total body potassium is as much as 100 mmol. A potassium level less than 3 mmol/L is equivalent to a deficiency of almost 200 mmol. Muscles are the most abundant resource for

Table 49.2 • Characteristic Findings in CSW and SIADH

Variable	CSW	SIADH
Plasma volume	Low	High
Central venous pressure	Low	Normal or high
Pulmonary capillary wedge pressure	Low	High
Dehydration	Yes	No
Hematocrit value	High	Normal
Albumin value	Increased	Normal
BNP value	High	Normal
Plasma ADH value	Normal	High
BUN:creatinine ratio	High	Low to normal
Urine output	Increased	Decreased
Fractional excretion of phosphate	High	Low
Urine osmolality	Low	High
Urine Na value	Very high	High
Treatment	Fluid administration	Fluid restriction
Response to normal saline	Dilute urine	Lower serum Na

Abbreviations: ADH, antidiuretic hormone; BNP, brain natriuretic peptide; BUN, blood urea nitrogen; CSW, cerebral salt wasting; Na, sodium; SIADH, syndrome of inappropriate secretion of antidiuretic hormone.

potassium, storing more than 2,000 mmol/L, followed by the liver, storing up to 250 mmol/L. The ECF has 4 mmol/L of potassium.

Potassium balance is dependent on several factors, including diet, gastrointestinal system, cellular shifting, and renal excretion. It is rare for diet alone to contribute to disorders of potassium balance, except for cases of starvation or severe eating disorders that can present with hypokalemia. In normal homeostasis, only 5% of potassium is excreted in the feces. However, gastrointestinal potassium losses can increase to as much as 70 mmol/L in the colon under the effect of aldosterone. Fecal losses are largely dependent on stool volume.

Cellular shifting is regulated by factors that impact the sodium-potassium adenosine triphosphatase pump. The sodium-potassium adenosine triphosphatase pump is upregulated by β_2-adrenoceptor agonist and α-adrenoceptor antagonist and insulin, a process that can result in hypokalemia. The pump is downregulated by hyperglycemia, β_2-adrenoceptor antagonists, and α-adrenoceptor agonists, a process resulting in hyperkalemia.

Table 49.3 • Medications That Can Impair Potassium Excretion

Mechanism	Medication
Decreased aldosterone levels	Angiotensin receptor blockers, ACE inhibitors, heparin, ketoconazole, nonsteroidal anti-inflammatory medications, calcineurin inhibitors
Collecting tubule	
eNaC blockade	Trimethoprim, pentamidine, amiloride, triamterene
Na-K ATPase blockade	Cyclosporine, tacrolimus

Abbreviations: ACE, angiotensin-converting enzyme; eNaC, epithelial sodium channel; Na-K ATPase, sodium-potassium adenosine triphosphatase.

Renal handling is the most powerful regulator of potassium excretion in the body. Of ingested potassium, 95% is excreted by the kidney. Four factors determine renal excretion: aldosterone and its effects on the epithelial sodium channel (Table 49.3), urine flow rate, delivery of sodium to the distal tubule, and plasma potassium concentration.

Pseudohyperkalemia and Hyperkalemia Disorders

Pseudohyperkalemia can occur from phlebotomy or specimen handling methods such as use of a tourniquet, fist clenching, or trauma. The serum potassium value tends to be higher than that of plasma by 0.1 to 0.5 mEq/L. Both thrombocytosis and leukocytosis can cause pseudohyperkalemia. A whole blood sample would be required to assess for this effect.

Hyperkalemia is defined as a serum potassium level more than 5.3 mEq/L. Hyperkalemia disorders can be characterized by 2 main mechanisms: internal potassium shifting and impaired renal excretion of potassium. Factors that promote shifting of potassium outside the cell include hyperglycemia and insulin deficiency, organic metabolic acidosis, tissue catabolism (rhabdomyolysis), nonselective β-blockers such as propranolol and labetalol, and exercise. Impaired renal excretion of potassium can be due to decreased aldosterone secretion from the adrenal gland, aldosterone resistance at the renal tubule, and renal failure caused by decreased potassium filtration.

Hyperkalemia is typically clinically silent; severe cases present with muscle weakness and a pattern of ascending paralysis. Electrocardiographic changes are the most common abnormalities; 39% of patients have these changes when the potassium level increases to more than 7.0 mEq/L. When the potassium level exceeds 6.0 mEq/L in the presence of electrocardiographic changes, treatment is warranted.

The 3 approaches to treatment are stabilization of the myocardium with calcium (Table 49.4), internal potassium

Table 49.4 • Treatment Options for Hyperkalemia

Treatment	Dose	Onset of Action
Calcium gluconate (chloride, if in central vein)	1 g IV	3-5 min, effect up to 1 h
Insulin and D5W	20 U IV with 50 mL of 50% D5W	10 min, peak 1 h, effect for 6 h
$NaHCO_3$	50 mEq IV	Avoid mixing with Ca, risk of precipitation
Albuterol>	10-20 mg in 4 mL Saline nebulized	30 min, up to 90-120 min

Abbreviations: Ca, calcium; D5W, dextrose 5% in water; IV, intravenously; $NaHCO_3$, sodium bicarbonate.

shifting, and potassium removal. Potassium removal can be mediated by the gastrointestinal system by using sodium polystyrene (effect delayed for at least 2 hours with peak effect between 4-6 hours). The use of sodium polystyrene should be avoided for patients at risk for colonic necrosis, such as patients with recent abdominal surgery, bowel injury, or intestinal dysfunction. Potassium removal by prompting excretion with loop diuretics should be the first choice in patients who are not in severe renal failure. For patients in renal failure, dialysis is the best treatment approach.

Hypokalemia Disorders

Hypokalemia is defined as a serum potassium level less than 3.5 mEq/L. The 3 main mechanisms for potassium losses include cellular shifting, gastrointestinal losses, and renal losses. Cellular uptake is enhanced by alkalemia, insulin, and β_2-adrenergic agonists. Gastrointestinal causes are typically due to diarrhea and can occur in patients with celiac disease and villous adenoma. Renal losses of potassium can be due to excess aldosterone or increased distal delivery of sodium in the setting of diuretic therapy. Assessment of the urine potassium to urine creatinine ratio can help differentiate renal from gastrointestinal causes of hypokalemia. A urine potassium to urine creatinine ratio less than 1.5 is consistent with diarrhea, whereas a ratio more than 1.5 is consistent with renal losses. The general treatment approach to potassium replacement is to replace 10 mEq of potassium for every 0.1 mEq decrease in serum level. Intravenous replacement should not exceed a rate of 20 mEq/hour.

Other Mineral Disorders

Calcium Regulation

Calcium has an important role in bone mineralization, muscular contraction, blood coagulation, nerve pulse transmission, and enzymatic activity. Calcium is more abundant intracellularly. The extracellular component exists as protein bound (45%) and diffusible (55%). Calcium homeostasis is regulated by 3 organs: kidneys, intestine, and skeleton. There are several key factors in the regulation of calcium, including parathyroid hormone, activated vitamin D, plasma calcium levels, effective circulating volume, and acid-base balance.

Activated vitamin D or calcitriol is the most important hormone for regulating calcium absorption in the gut. Parathyroid hormone is the most important regulator of renal calcium reabsorption. Calcitriol has a synergistic effect with parathyroid hormone. Volume expansion leads to renal losses of calcium, whereas volume contraction leads to hypercalcemia. Alkalosis is associated with hypercalcemia, whereas acidemia can be associated with hypocalcemia. Loop diuretics cause hypocalcemia, and thiazide diuretics cause hypercalcemia.

Phosphorus Regulation

Phosphorus is found most abundantly in bones and is an essential component of soft tissues and cell structures. Up to 90% of plasma phosphate is free, and about 10% is protein bound. Only 1% of phosphorus is in the ECF. Phosphorus is regulated by parathyroid hormone, phosphorus intake, calcitriol, pH balance, and fibroblast growth factor-23. Factors that lead to increased phosphorus excretion by the kidney include acidemia, fibroblast growth factor-23, and parathyroid hormone. Calcitriol upregulates phosphorus absorption in the gut and in the kidney.

Magnesium Regulation

Magnesium is distributed almost evenly in the bones and in the intracellular compartment and is most abundant in cardiac and skeletal muscles. It is the second most abundant cation intracellularly after potassium and has an important role in nerve conduction, muscle contraction, and potassium and calcium balance. Normal magnesium level ranges between 1.8 and 2.2 mg/dL. Magnesium is primarily regulated by the kidneys. Claudin-16 is a tight junction protein that enables paracellular absorption of magnesium in the kidney. Genetic mutations of claudin-16 can lead to severe renal wasting of magnesium. Factors that increase magnesium absorption include parathyroid hormone, hypomagnesemia, and volume contraction. Factors that decrease magnesium absorption include hypercalcemia and hypermagnesemia, loop and thiazide diuretics, mannitol, aminoglycosides, antineoplastic medications including cisplastin, proton pump inhibitors (through inhibition of magnesium absorption in the gut), and gastrointestinal losses from diarrhea.

The causes, clinical syndromes, and management of disorders of calcium, phosphate, and magnesium are presented in Table 49.5.

Table 49.5 • Mineral Disorders: Causes and Treatment

	Disorder					
Characteristics	**Hypocalcemia**	**Hypercalcemia**	**Hypophosphatemia**	**Hyperphosphatemia**	**Hypomagnesemia**	**Hypermagnesemia**
Definitions	Ca <8.7 mg/dL	Ca >10.4 mg/dL	Phos <2.5 mg/dL	Phos >4.5 mg/dL	Mg <1.8 mEq/L	Mg >2.2 mg/dL
Causes	1. Hypoparathyroidism 2. Low magnesium 3. Vitamin D deficiency 4. Pancreatitis 5. Hungry bone syndrome 6. Respiratory alkalosis 7. Tumor lysis 8. Rhabdomyolysis 9. Loop diuretics	1. Primary hyperparathyroidism 2. Milk-alkali syndrome 3. Lithium, thiazides, vitamins A and D intoxication 4. Immobilization 5. Granulomatous diseases 6. Hypercalcemia of malignancy	1. Starvation 2. Vitamin D deficiency 3. Alcoholism 4. High PTH 5. Fanconi syndrome 6. Diuresis 7. Respiratory alkalosis 8. Calcium or aluminum antacids	1. Renal failure 2. Vitamin D intoxication 3. Acidemia 4. Tumor lysis 5. Rhabdomyolysis 6. Phosphate enema 7. Hypoparathyroidism	1. GI losses such as with NGT suction, vomiting, diarrhea, intestinal bypass, short bowel, laxative abuse, villous adenoma, enteric fistula 2. Chronic alcoholism 3. Protein calorie malnutrition 4. Medications: PPI, amphotericin, cyclosporine, cisplatin, foscarnet, aminoglycosides, pentamidine 5. Diuresis	1. Rare 2. Excessive use of Mg-containing laxatives, enemas, antacids 3. Renal failure 4. Rhabdomyolysis
Clinical presentation	1. Positive Trousseau and Chvostek signs 2. Paresthesias 3. Seizures 4. Depression 5. Muscle spasm	1. Altered mental status 2. Depression 3. Fatigue 4. Muscle weakness 5. Constipation, nausea, vomiting 6. Polyuria, polydipsia	1. Muscle weakness 2. Confusion	Asymptomatic	1. Tremor 2. Seizures 3. Nystagmus	1. Lethargy 2. Hypotension 3. Nausea, vomiting 4. Ileus 5. Urinary retention
Complication	1. Prolonged QT 2. Hypotension 3. Arrythmia	1. Nephrolithiasis 2. Arrhythmia	1. Rhabdomyolysis 2. Hemolysis 3. Encephalopathy 4. Respiratory failure 5. Impaired bone mineralization	Vascular and metastatic calcifications	1. Arrhythmia 2. Hypertension 3. Insulin resistance 4. Osteoporosis	1. Paralysis 2. Bradycardia 3. Respiratory depression 4. Coma
Evaluation	Blood gas, Mg, PTH, phosphorus	PTH, PTHrP, vitamin D, 1,25-vitamin D, skeletal survey	24-hour urine phosphorus	Potassium, PTH, phosphorus, vitamin D, calcium	24-hour urine Mg. High urine Mg consistent with renal Mg wasting	Mg, Ca, phosphorus
Treatment	1. Calcium gluconate or chloride IV 2. Calcium carbonate or citrate 3. Correct low Mg	1. Volume expansion 2. Loop diuretics to prevent volume overload 3. Bisphosphonates 4. Calcitonin 5. Steroids	1. Sodium phosphate IV 2. Potassium phosphate or sodium phosphate oral preparations 3. Dairy products	1. Phosphate binders such as calcium acetate with meals, sevelamer, lanthanum 2. Dialysis	1. 1-2 g $MgSO_4$ IV 2. Mg oxide, Mg citrate, Mg chloride oral replacement 3. Amiloride and triamterene can decrease renal Mg wasting	1. Volume expansion 2. Loop diuretics 3. Dialysis

Abbreviations: Ca, calcium; GI, gastrointestinal; IV, intravenously; Mg, magnesium; $MgSO_4$, magnesium sulfate; NGT, nasogastric tube; Phos, phosphorus; PPI, proton pump inhibitor; PTH, parathyroid hormone; PTHrP, parathyroid hormone-related peptide.

Summary

- Water balance is determined by vasopressin and its renal effects and is influenced by osmotic and nonosmotic variables.
- Hypernatremia can be caused by 2 main mechanisms: sodium intake in excess to water (hypertonic fluids or feeding) or water losses that exceed salt losses (renal or gastrointestinal).
- Correction of hypernatremia depends on the volume status and determination of free water deficit.
- Treatment of asymptomatic hyponatremia depends on determining the underlying volume status and cause.
- Overly rapid correction of hyponatremia can lead to osmotic demyelination syndrome.
- Acute symptomatic hyponatremia can be treated with a 100-mL bolus of 3% saline; chronic symptomatic hyponatremia requires correction of serum sodium by 6 mEq in the first 6 hours.
- Hyperkalemia treatment includes cardiac stabilization with calcium in patients with abnormal electrocardiographic changes, internal cellular shifting of potassium, and potassium excretion with diuretics or dialysis.
- Disorders of parathyroid hormone and vitamin D cause most disorders of calcium balance.

SUGGESTED READING

Adrogue HJ, Madias NE. Hyponatremia. N Engl J Med. 2000 May 25;342(21):1581–9.

Adrogue HJ, Madias NE. The challenge of hyponatremia. J Am Soc Nephrol. 2012 Jul;23(7):1140–8. Epub 2012 May 24.

Anderson RJ, Chung HM, Kluge R, Schrier RW. Hyponatremia: a prospective analysis of its epidemiology and the pathogenetic role of vasopressin. Ann Intern Med. 1985 Feb;102(2):164–8.

Ashraf N, Locksley R, Arieff AI. Thiazide-induced hyponatremia associated with death or neurologic damage in outpatients. Am J Med. 1981 Jun;70(6):1163–8.

Chung HM, Kluge R, Schrier RW, Anderson RJ. Clinical assessment of extracellular fluid volume in hyponatremia. Am J Med. 1987 Nov;83(5):905–8.

Clayton JA, Le Jeune IR, Hall IP. Severe hyponatraemia in medical in-patients: aetiology, assessment and outcome. QJM. 2006 Aug;99(8):505–11. Epub 2006 Jul 22.

Danziger J, Zeidel ML. Osmotic homeostasis. Clin J Am Soc Nephrol. 2015 May 7;10(5):852–62. Epub 2014 Jul 30. Erratum in: Clin J Am Soc Nephrol. 2015 Sep 4;10(9):1703.

Edelman IS, Leibman J, O'Meara MP, Birkenfeld LW. Interrelations between serum sodium concentration, serum osmolarity and total exchangeable sodium, total exchangeable potassium and total body water. J Clin Invest. 1958 Sep;37(9):1236–56.

Ellison DH, Berl T. Clinical practice: the syndrome of inappropriate antidiuresis. N Engl J Med. 2007 May 17;356(20):2064–72.

Fenske WK, Christ-Crain M, Horning A, Simet J, Szinnai G, Fassnacht M, et al. A copeptin-based classification of the osmoregulatory defects in the syndrome of inappropriate antidiuresis. J Am Soc Nephrol. 2014 Oct;25(10):2376–83. Epub 2014 Apr 10.

Harrois A, Anstey JR. Diabetes insipidus and syndrome of inappropriate antidiuretic hormone in critically ill patients. Crit Care Clin. 2019 Apr;35(2):187–200. Epub 2019 Jan 28.

Muhsin SA, Mount DB. Diagnosis and treatment of hypernatremia. Best Pract Res Clin Endocrinol Metab. 2016 Mar;30(2):189–203. Epub 2016 Mar 4.

Pham PC, Pham PM, Pham PT. Vasopressin excess and hyponatremia. Am J Kidney Dis. 2006 May;47(5):727–37.

Rose BD, Post TW. Clinical physiology of acid-base and electrolyte disorders. 5th ed. New York (NY): McGraw-Hill; c2001. 992 p.

Spasovski G, Vanholder R, Allolio B, Annane D, Ball S, Bichet D, et al; Hyponatraemia Guideline Development Group. Clinical practice guideline on diagnosis and treatment of hyponatraemia. Nephrol Dial Transplant. 2014 Apr;29 Suppl 2:i1–i39. Epub 2014 Feb 25. Erratum in: Nephrol Dial Transplant. 2014 Jun;40(6):924.

Sterns RH. Disorders of plasma sodium: causes, consequences, and correction. N Engl J Med. 2015 Jan 1;372(1):55–65.

Sterns RH, Hix JK, Silver SM. Management of hyponatremia in the ICU. Chest. 2013 Aug;144(2):672–9.

Sterns RH, Silver SM. Complications and management of hyponatremia. Curr Opin Nephrol Hypertens. 2016 Mar;25(2):114–9.

Hematologic and Inflammatory Disorders

Anemia and Blood Transfusion

JOY D. HUGHES, MD; MARIELA RIVERA, MD; MYUNG S. PARK, MD, MS

Goals

- Discuss causes of acute anemia in the intensive care unit.
- Discuss the diagnosis and management of anemia in patients requiring neurocritical care.
- Review transfusion strategies for patients with anemia.

Introduction

Critically ill patients commonly present with anemia, defined as a hemoglobin level less than 13.0 g/dL in men and less than 11.6 g/dL in women or as clinical signs of bleeding, including tachycardia and low urine output with active hemorrhage. Anemia is common, occurring in up to a third of critically ill patients, and is associated with high morbidity and mortality rates, particularly in patients with central nervous system injuries and disease. The causes of anemia can vary from chronic conditions such as kidney disease or malnutrition to acute conditions such as bleeding or consumptive coagulopathy. For proper management, patients must be assessed for hemorrhagic shock, which would necessitate a resuscitative treatment strategy initially. If a patient is anemic but hemodynamically stable, a thorough work-up for the underlying cause of the anemia must be performed in addition to treatment of the symptoms of the critical illness. In a neurocritical care unit, special consideration should be given to maintaining adequate perfusion for recovery of central nervous system deficits and prevention of further neurologic insult.

The Patient With Anemia

Anemia in Symptomatic Patients

In a neurocritical care unit, patients presenting with anemia should be evaluated for a source of hemorrhage; an unrecognized source may result in shock. The definition of shock is inadequate perfusion of the tissues resulting in end-organ damage. Hemorrhagic shock falls into the broader category of hypovolemic shock with reduction in diastolic filling pressures and volume. The causes of hemorrhagic shock include trauma, surgical blood loss, yet undiagnosed medical conditions, spontaneous hematoma, and iatrogenic causes such as cerebral angiogram–associated retroperitoneal hemorrhage. Hemorrhagic shock is a clinical diagnosis. Classically, a patient in hemorrhagic shock has sluggish capillary refill with cool, mottled extremities, worsening tachycardia, low blood pressure (systolic blood pressure <90 mm Hg), and oliguria. Marked hypotension results in a decline in consciousness. The 4 classes of hemorrhagic shock are defined in Table 50.1. A careful history of the patient should include any medical conditions associated with coagulopathy or medications that are associated with bleeding such as aspirin, warfarin, heparin, or platelet inhibitors.

Management of hemorrhagic shock is focused on both control of the bleeding source and volume resuscitation with blood products. If there is visible hemorrhage, manual pressure is applied over the affected area until definitive surgical management. If a bleeding source is suspected within the chest, abdomen, or pelvis, radiologic imaging, such as computed tomography with an intravenous contrast agent, is used to identify areas of bleeding. If indicated, an

Table 50.1 • Classification of Hemorrhagic Shock

	Class			
Factor	**1**	**2**	**3**	**4**
Blood loss	<750 mL	750-1,500 mL	1,500-2,000 mL	>2,000 mL
Heart rate, bpm	<100	100-120	120-140	>140
Systolic blood pressure	Normal	Normal	Decreased	Decreased
Pulse pressure	Normal	Decreased	Decreased	Decreased
Respiratory rate, breaths/min	Normal	20-30	30-40	>40
Urine output, mL/h	>30	20-30	5-15	Oliguria
Mental status	Normal or slightly anxious	Anxious	Confused	Lethargic

Abbreviation: bpm, beats per minute.

Modified from Cinat ME, Hoyt DB. Hemorrhagic shock. In: Gabrielli A, Layon AJ, Yu M, editors. Civetta, Taylor, & Kirby's critical care. 4th ed. Philadelphia (PA): Wolters Kluwer Health/Lippincott Williams & Wilkins; c2009. p. 893–923; used with permission.

interventional radiologist should be consulted for bleeding control. Transferring a patient to a radiology suite should be considered only for patients who are stable; if available, hybrid operating rooms, which have combined interventional radiologic and operative capabilities, should be used for unstable patients. Patients with ongoing bleeding may require massive transfusion (discussed below in Management of Anemia). Crystalloid resuscitation is minimized to avoid hemodilution, which worsens coagulopathy. The use of hemoglobin levels to gauge the adequacy of resuscitation is inaccurate because of the time needed for equilibration of the hemoglobin concentration.

Anemia in Stable Patients

Critically ill patients requiring neurocritical care may have concurrent medical conditions causing anemia with or without coagulopathy. In fact, the majority of patients presenting to an intensive care unit with hemoglobin levels in the normal range will become anemic during hospitalization. Management of anemia in critically ill patients has evolved to a goal of minimizing a patient's exposure to unnecessary blood products; this management strategy is largely due to the Transfusion Requirements in Critical Care trial published in 1999. The trial concluded that maintenance of hemoglobin concentrations between 7.0 and 9.0 g/dL resulted in improved outcomes compared with maintenance at higher concentrations. A threshold hemoglobin value of 7 to 8 g/dL for most patients was supported by a 2016 Cochrane systematic review and meta-analysis of 31 randomized clinical trials that included patients from a range of specialties (eg, surgery, critical care). Historically, neurointensivists have interpreted these outcomes with caution because of the belief that patients with neurologic injuries may benefit from high transfusion thresholds. A randomized trial comparing a transfusion threshold of 7 to 10 g/dL found no improvement in neurologic outcomes and a higher incidence of thromboembolic events for the high-threshold transfusion group. The ideal threshold for transfusion in patients with acute neurologic injury remains elusive.

Patient Assessment

The diagnostic evaluation of a critically ill patient with anemia is broad. Evaluation may begin with whether red blood cells are being lost (hemorrhage), destroyed prematurely, or underproduced. Peripheral blood smears may show dysmorphia of red blood cells due to hereditary disorders or malnutrition and findings of either microcytic or macrocytic anemias. These findings are associated with different chronic medical conditions, which are beyond the scope of this chapter.

In patients with an acute drop in hemoglobin level, intensivists should investigate for a source of hemorrhage. If no external blood loss is obvious, the patient should be evaluated for gastrointestinal hemorrhage (see Chapter 39, "Acute Gastrointestinal Hemorrhage"). A nasogastric tube may elucidate whether there is an upper gastrointestinal bleed. In patients with acute increases of intracranial pressure or any catastrophic brain injury, a stress ulcer should be suspected as a possible cause of an upper gastrointestinal bleed. A stress ulcer (also called a Cushing ulcer, named after Harvey Cushing) may form at the distal esophagus, stomach, or duodenum as a result of increased gastric acid secretion; the cause of this acid hypersecretion is believed to be vagus nerve overstimulation. If there is sanguineous effluent from the nasogastric tube, upper endoscopy is indicated for confirmation of the bleeding source and management of the bleeding. Further work-up after nasogastric tube placement includes a rectal examination to evaluate for a potential lower gastrointestinal bleed. If no other source of bleeding is identified and the hemoglobin level continues to decrease, colonoscopy is indicated.

In the absence of suspected hemorrhage, the differential diagnosis for anemia includes 2 broad categories: failure of red blood cell production (bone marrow) and destruction of red blood cells (intravascular and extravascular hemolysis). Initial laboratory evaluation of anemia should include a complete blood count, including mean corpuscular volume; a reticulocyte count; and a peripheral blood smear. Nucleated red blood cells correlate with septicemia, profound hypoxia, massive hemorrhage, and a high mortality rate. Renal failure, malnutrition, and chronic illness may all effect red blood cell production. Sepsis may correlate with decreased red blood cell count, thrombocytopenia, or leukopenia. Decreased iron intake is a common cause of anemia, but low dietary intake of many other nutrients and minerals can be implicated in chronic anemia. Particular attention should be paid to monitoring phosphate levels, because severe hypophosphatemia may be associated with hemolytic anemia. Certain infections, such as malaria infection ith *Plasmodium* organisms, may manifest as anemia with central nervous system symptoms of seizure or obtundation. Treatment focuses on both addressing the underlying problem and transfusing blood products if hemoglobin levels are below the accepted threshold (usually 7-8 g/dL).

Coagulopathy

Anemia in the setting of critical illness may be associated with coagulopathy. The cause of coagulopathy may be consumption of coagulation factors (eg, in disseminated intravascular coagulation), hypothermia, iatrogenic from medications, acidosis, or myriad other causes. It is crucial to identify and treat microvascular bleeding, which occurs due to coagulopathy. Historically, bleeding time, prothrombin time, and partial thromboplastin time were the laboratory markers used to establish intrinsic versus extrinsic pathways of coagulopathy; thromboelastography is a whole blood viscoelastic assay that can be used to diagnose coagulopathy and guide appropriate colloid resuscitation.

Management of abnormal factors generally includes transfusion of fresh frozen plasma or prothrombin factor concentrate for increased prothrombin time and fresh frozen plasma for increased activated partial thromboplastin time. Thromboelastography measures several factors (Figure 50.1):

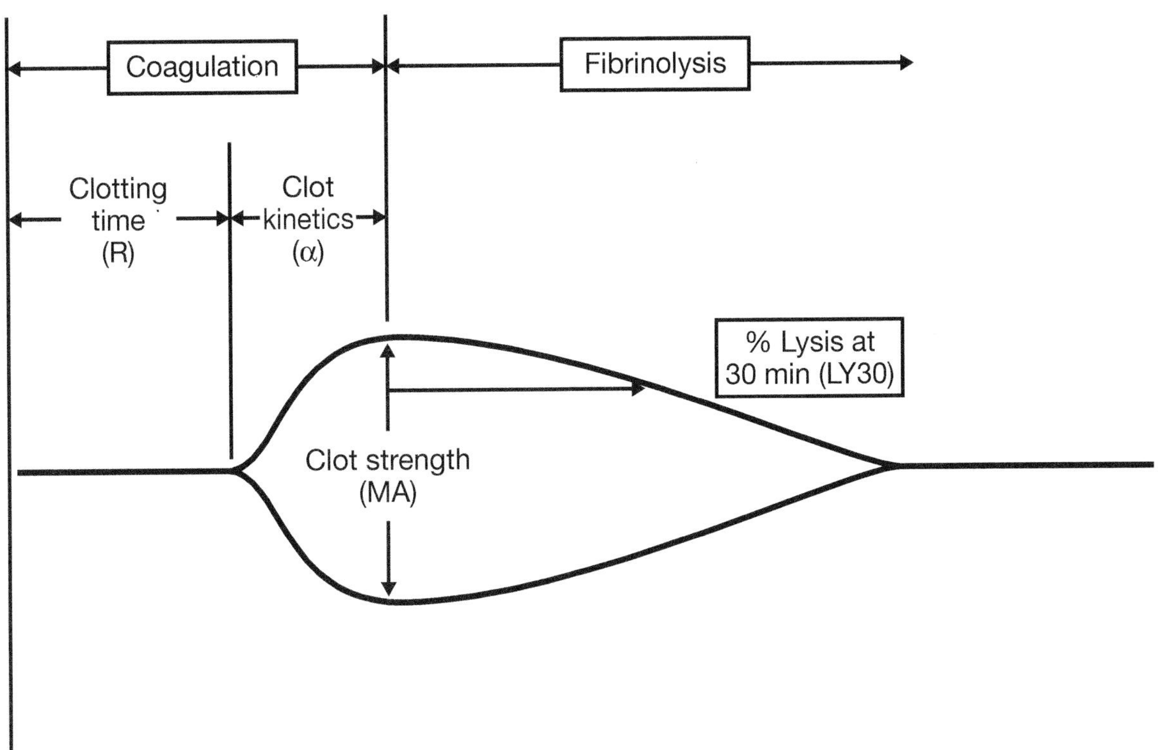

Figure 50.1. Thromboelastogram. MA indicates maximum amplitude.

1. Time to clot formation (R value)
2. Kinetics of clot development (α angle)
3. Maximum strength of the clot
4. The percentage of clot lysis 30 minutes after reaching maximum amplitude (LY30)

These factors are affected by distinguishable traits of the clotting cascade. Normal R time indicates that adequate clotting factors are present. The α angle is largely affected by fibrinogen, but depletion of coagulation factors can lead to decreasing values. Platelet count and function determine the maximum amplitude. The LY30 is determined by fibrinolysis. Selection of type of blood product transfusion can be guided by these measurements. Fresh frozen plasma is used for treatment of increased R time. Platelets are transfused for a low maximum amplitude. Transfusion of cryoprecipitate and fresh frozen plasma (400 mg fibrinogen in 200-250 mL) should be considered for a low α angle. Thromboelastography is not useful for guiding packed red blood cell transfusions.

Management of Anemia

After thorough evaluation of the causes of anemia in a critically ill patient, the intensivist must determine whether transfusion of red blood cells is appropriate. In patients without cardiovascular instability and no suspicion of hemorrhage, transfusion guidelines based on hemoglobin level could direct therapy. Studies in patients with ischemic cardiac disease support a transfusion to a hemoglobin threshold of less than 10 g/dL. This guideline has been applied to patients with neurologic injury also, whereas patients without neurologic injury are generally managed with a transfusion threshold of less than 7 g/dL. If transfusion of red blood cells is planned, blood typing, screening, and crossmatching should be performed to minimize the risks of transfusion-related complications. When 1 unit of packed red blood cells is administered, the expected increase in hemoglobin is 1.0 to 1.5 g/dL. According to available data, patients should be assessed clinically when transfusion is considered. If the patient is stable, transfusion may not be needed even when the hemoglobin level is 7 to 8 g/dL.

Patients with symptomatic anemia should be evaluated for shock, and blood products should be administered to normalize vital signs. Transfusion should not be delayed for laboratory evaluation, because there is a period during which the hemoglobin concentration has not equilibrated with total body water, and hemoglobin concentration may appear normal despite massive blood loss. In particular, for patients with neurologic injuries, periods of hypotension should be minimized. If large-volume resuscitation is anticipated and consistent neurologic examinations cannot be obtained at the bedside, an intracranial pressure monitoring device should be considered to gauge the effect of resuscitation on intracranial pressure.

If multiple units of blood products are necessary, most institutions have a massive transfusion protocol that follows a transfusion ratio of packed red blood cells to platelets to fresh frozen plasma of 1:1:1. The formulaic approach of the massive transfusion protocol then needs to be tempered to avoid unnecessary resuscitation. Thus, we recommend that thromboelastography be used to guide the need for ongoing blood transfusions. The massive transfusion protocol is associated with improved outcomes and better use of blood products. Hypothermia, which impedes thrombin generation and platelet activation, should be avoided, and blood warmers should be used early in the resuscitation.

Transfusion Complications

Risks of blood transfusion include infection, transfusion reaction, and volume overload. The most common transfusion-related pathogens are hepatitis C, cytomegalovirus, and (rarely) bacteria. Transfusion-related acute lung injury manifests as acute lung injury within 6 hours of blood product transfusion. Patients may also have anaphylaxis to blood transfusion. Transfusion-associated circulatory overload is a risk for patients with congestive heart failure and manifests as pulmonary edema. The volume of the transfusion correlates with the risk. If patients have an ABO incompatibility reaction, hemolysis may also develop.

Pharmacologic Adjuncts

In cases of life-threatening coagulopathy, treatment with antifibrinolytics, such as tranexamic acid or ε-aminocaproic acid, might be attempted. However, these medications should be used with caution, because they have been shown in multiple trials to increase the risk of cerebral infarction and deep vein thrombosis. In the Clinical Randomisation of an Antifibrinolytic in Significant Haemorrhage 2 (CRASH-2) trial of patients with trauma, the overall mortality rate was lower in the tranexamic acid group (14.5%) than in the placebo group (16%) (relative risk, 0.91; 95% CI, 0.85-0.97), as was death from hemorrhage (4.9% vs 5.7%; relative risk, 0.85; 95% CI, 0.76-0.96), but the relative risk of mortality increased if tranexamic acid was given more than 3 hours after traumatic injury. Thus, use of antifibrinolytics warrants close monitoring for thrombotic complications, and timing of their use, especially in patients with traumatic injuries, should be assessed on a case-by-case basis.

Summary

- Anemia is common among patients in neurocritical care units.
- The causes of anemia vary widely, and expeditious evaluation and management are required to stabilize patients and prevent increased morbidity.
- Adjunctive investigative measures rely heavily on laboratory evaluation to determine underlying conditions such as coagulopathy and to correct these derangements.
- A conservative transfusion strategy is increasingly supported by peer-reviewed evidence for improved outcomes.
- A threshold hemoglobin value of 7 to 8 g/dL, achieved with a restrictive transfusion approach, can be used as a guide in most patients.
- For hemodynamically stable patients, a transfusion rate of 1 unit of red blood cells at a time is advised.
- Symptomatic patients whose hemoglobin level is less than 10 g/dL should have transfusion to improve hemodynamic instability and symptoms of myocardial ischemia.
- For patients with ischemic cardiac disease the transfusion threshold is less than 8 g/dL, and for patients with symptoms or ongoing ischemia the target hemoglobin level is 10 g/dL or more.
- Patients requiring massive transfusion should be evaluated clinically for shock, and blood products should be administered to normalize vital signs. Transfusion should not be delayed for laboratory evaluation.
- A blood warmer should be used whenever multiple units are transfused. Hypothermia should be either avoided or minimized.

SUGGESTED READING

Bhalla PK, Zhou T, Levine JM. How should aneurysmal subarachnoid hemorrhage be managed? In: Deutschman CS, Neligan PJ, editors. Evidence-based practice of critical care. 2nd ed. Philadelphia (PA): Elsevier; c2016. p. 450–60.

Carson JL, Guyatt G, Heddle NM, Grossman BJ, Cohn CS, Fung MK, et al. Clinical Practice Guidelines From the AABB: red blood cell transfusion thresholds and storage. JAMA. 2016 Nov 15;316(19):2025–35.

Carson JL, Kleinman S. Indications and hemoglobin thresholds for red blood cell transfusion in the adult. In: Tirnauer JS, editor. UpToDate. Waltham (MA): UpToDate; c2016.

Carson JL, Stanworth SJ, Roubinian N, Fergusson DA, Triulzi D, Doree C, et al. Transfusion thresholds and other strategies for guiding allogeneic red blood cell transfusion. Cochrane Database Syst Rev. 2016 Oct 12;10:CD002042.

Chestnut RM. Intracranial pressure. In: Le Roux PD, Levine JM, Kofke WA, editors. Monitoring in neurocritical care. Philadelphia (PA): Elsevier/Saunders; c2013. p. 338–47.e4.

CRASH-2 trial collaborators, Shakur H, Roberts I, Bautista R, Caballero J, Coats T, Dewan Y, et al. Effects of tranexamic acid on death, vascular occlusive events, and blood transfusion in trauma patients with significant haemorrhage (CRASH-2): a randomised, placebo-controlled trial. Lancet. 2010 Jul 3;376(9734):23–32. Epub 2010 Jun 14.

Docherty AB, Turgeon AF, Walsh TS. Best practice in critical care: anaemia in acute and critical illness. Transfus Med. 2018 Apr;28(2):181–9. Epub 2018 Jan 25.

Gabrielli A, Layon AJ, Yu M, editors. Civetta, Taylor, & Kirby's critical care. 4th ed. Philadelphia (PA): Wolters Kluwer Health/Lippincott Williams & Wilkins; c2009. 2765 p.

Greer SE, Rhynhart KK, Gupta R, Corwin HL. New developments in massive transfusion in trauma. Curr Opin Anaesthesiol. 2010 Apr;23(2):246–50.

Hebert PC, Wells G, Blajchman MA, Marshall J, Martin C, Pagliarello G, et al; Transfusion Requirements in Critical Care Investigators, Canadian Critical Care Trials Group. A multicenter, randomized, controlled clinical trial of transfusion requirements in critical care. N Engl J Med. 1999 Feb 11;340(6):409–17. Erratum in: N Engl J Med 1999 Apr 1;340(13):1056.

Hess JR. Massive blood transfusion. In: Tirnauer JS, editor. UpToDate. Waltham (MA): UpToDate; c2016.

Holcomb JB, Tilley BC, Baraniuk S, Fox EE, Wade CE, Podbielski JM, et al; PROPPR Study Group. Transfusion of plasma, platelets, and red blood cells in a 1:1:1 vs a 1:1:2 ratio and mortality in patients with severe trauma: the PROPPR randomized clinical trial. JAMA. 2015 Feb 3;313(5):471–82.

Kang YG, Martin DJ, Marquez J, Lewis JH, Bontempo FA, Shaw BW Jr, et al. Intraoperative changes in blood coagulation and thrombelastographic monitoring in liver transplantation. Anesth Analg. 1985 Sep;64(9):888–96.

Kumar MA. Hematology and coagulation. In: Le Roux PD, Levine JM, Kofke WA, editors. Monitoring in neurocritical care. Philadelphia (PA): Elsevier/Saunders; c2013. p. 131–47.e6.

Robertson CS, Hannay HJ, Yamal JM, Gopinath S, Goodman JC, Tilley BC; Epo Severe TBI Trial Investigators, Baldwin A, Rivera Lara L, Saucedo-Crespo H, Ahmed

O, Sadasivan S, Ponce L, et al. Effect of erythropoietin and transfusion threshold on neurological recovery after traumatic brain injury: a randomized clinical trial. JAMA. 2014 Jul 2;312(1):36–47.

Schrier SL. Approach to the adult patient with anemia. In: Tirnauer JS, editor. UpToDate. Waltham (MA): UpToDate; c2016.

Shah A, Fisher SA, Wong H, Roy NB, McKechnie S, Doree C, et al. Safety and efficacy of iron therapy on reducing red blood cell transfusion requirements and treating anaemia in critically ill adults: a systematic review with meta-analysis and trial sequential analysis. J Crit Care. 2019 Feb;49:162–71. Epub 2018 Nov 10.

Stinger HK, Spinella PC, Perkins JG, Grathwohl KW, Salinas J, Martini WZ, et al. The ratio of fibrinogen to red cells transfused affects survival in casualties receiving massive transfusions at an army combat support hospital. J Trauma. 2008 Feb;64(2 Suppl):S79–85.

Hematologic and Oncologic Complications in the Intensive Care Unit

CARL A. RUTHMAN, MD; JOSE C. YATACO, MD

Goals

- Describe the presentation and management of common cancer-related problems that occur in patients in intensive care units.
- Discuss complications of chemotherapeutic and biological agents.
- Discuss the common complications of bone marrow transplant.

Introduction

Up to 15% of all patients admitted to the intensive care unit (ICU) have some type of cancer. As the aging population and also immunosuppressed organ-transplant recipients continue to increase, this percentage is expected to increase.

Patients with cancer can present to the ICU with the complications and conditions of the general population, but a few are particular to their type of cancer or treatment. Some of the most common of cancer-related ICU complications are reviewed in this chapter, particularly those that need complex and urgent management.

Endocrine Complications

Tumor Lysis Syndrome

This syndrome occurs when many neoplastic cells are rapidly killed, a process causing the release of intracellular contents into the systemic circulation. It includes the constellation of hyperuricemia, hyperkalemia, hyperphosphatemia, hypocalcemia, and acute renal failure. It typically occurs in the setting of initial chemotherapy for acute leukemias and high-grade non-Hodgkin lymphoma. However, it has also occurred in association with some solid tumors such as hepatoblastoma and stage IV neuroblastoma and in patients receiving immunotherapy such as interleukin-2 (IL-2), sunitinib, imatinib, and rituximab. The critical observation period starts a few hours after chemotherapy and continues up to 5 to 7 days after treatment.

The principles of therapy for tumor lysis syndrome are identification of high-risk patients (high-grade hematologic malignancy, baseline lactate dehydrogenase level >150 U/L, and uric acid level more than 10 mg/dL), active chemistry monitoring, and early supportive therapy.

Treatment includes intravenous hydration with crystalloids, allopurinol orally or rasburicase intravenously, alkalinization of urine, calcium replacement, exchange resins for hyperkalemia, and phosphate binders for hyperphosphatemia. Hemodialysis may be required for patients unresponsive to medical treatment or with established acute renal failure.

Hypercalcemia

This is the most common metabolic abnormality that occurs in patients with cancer. Cardiovascular and renal dysfunctions are the most serious end-organ effects of hypercalcemia. The symptoms are nonspecific and include nausea, anorexia, lethargy, and confusion. The final path for all cases of cancer-related hypercalcemia is osteoclast-enhanced bone resorption mediated through receptor activator of nuclear factor-κB ligand. Parathyroid hormone is usually suppressed, and the osteoclastic activation and proliferation are mediated by factors produced by the tumor, such as parathyroid hormone–related protein, activated vitamin D, and multiple cytokines (eg, interleukin-1, tumor necrosis factor, granulocyte-macrophage colony-stimulating factor, prostaglandin E_2, platelet-derived growth factor).

The first therapeutic intervention should be vigorous intravenous hydration with normal saline to replete the intravascular volume, increase renal perfusion, and favor calciuresis. Further renal excretion of calcium can be increased with furosemide diuresis. These important initial steps should be followed by definitive treatment. Calcitonin subcutaneously and saline will quickly lower calcium levels, usually in the first 12 to 24 hours. The bisphosphonates zoledronic acid intravenously and pamidronate intravenously have been effective for the long-term treatment of hypercalcemia, and their effects can occur in 48 hours from the initial dose. Denosumab (a receptor activator of nuclear factor-κB ligand inhibitor) is now available and is an option for patients with hypercalcemia refractory to zoledronic acid.

Cardiac, Pulmonary, and Gastrointestinal Complications

Cardiac

Cardiac dysfunction can be a direct consequence of tumor invasion in the mediastinum or an effect from therapy, including chemotherapy, immunotherapy, and radiation.

Superior vena cava syndrome is a known complication caused by obstruction of blood flow through the superior vena cava. Lymphomas and lung carcinomas are the most common causes of this condition. Symptoms include facial and upper extremity edema, development of collateral circulation, life-threatening respiratory failure, and increased intracranial pressure. Initiation of specific chemotherapy is paramount for lymphomas or small cell lung cancers, for which biopsy confirmation is absolutely necessary. Radiation therapy in high-grade fractions can be used for tumors unresponsive to chemotherapy, achieving symptomatic response in most cases. Other treatments include thrombolysis and endovascular stents.

Different chemotherapy and new biological agents can cause considerate cardiac toxicity, either early or months after drug administration. Chemotherapy-induced cardiac dysfunction can be classified in two types. Type I dysfunction, such as the one caused by doxorubicin, is dose related and cumulative, and the underlying cardiac damage is mostly permanent and irreversible. Type I cardiac dysfunction has a higher risk of recurrent dysfunction with progression to heart failure and death when patients are rechallenged with the same agent. Type II myocardial dysfunction is a new type of dysfunction that has been described in association with new biological agents, such as trastuzumab. Patients with type II dysfunction have a high likelihood of full recovery in a relatively short time. Type II dysfunction is not dose related, and it is relatively safe to rechallenge patients with the same agent.

The risk of development of cardiac toxicity is higher in older patients and in those with preexisting cardiac disease or ventricular dysfunction. Doxorubicin and other anthracycline agents are among the most common drugs responsible for development of congestive heart failure. Low-dose boluses or continuous infusions seem to reduce the frequency of clinically significant cardiac dysfunction. Cyclophosphamide, commonly used for treatment of lymphomas and for stem cell transplant–conditioning regimens, is associated with sporadic development of congestive heart failure, sometimes acute and severe, especially at high doses. A new agent, trastuzumab, an anti-HER2 antibody, used commonly for the treatment of breast carcinoma, is known to cause congestive heart failure in 3% to 4% of patients. The treatment of cardiac toxicity induced by cancer drugs includes diuretics, angiotensin-converting enzyme inhibitors, digoxin, and β-blockers. Radiation therapy delivered to the mediastinum for the treatment of Hodgkin disease, lung malignancies, and breast cancer can result in cardiac complications such as pericarditis, myocardial fibrosis, and accelerated coronary disease. These complications typically take several years to present.

Pulmonary

The development of symptomatic pulmonary infiltrates in patients with cancer is common. The causes vary from infectious to noninfectious and include direct tumor invasion, leukostasis, hemorrhage, and radiation- and chemotherapy-induced pneumonitis.

The chemotherapy drugs most likely to cause pneumonitis are bleomycin and mitomycin, but many others can also cause pulmonary toxicity: nitrosureas, gemcitabine, taxanes, and vinca alkaloids. Everolimus, an inhibitor of the mTOR (mammalian target of rapamycin) pathway, used in treatment of renal cancer, and erlotinib, an inhibitor of the phosphorylation of epidermal growth factor receptor, used in treatment of lung cancer, can also cause severe and irreversible pneumonitis. New therapeutic biological agents targeted against vascular endothelial growth factor (eg, bevacizumab) have shown improved outcomes in lung cancer. Unfortunately, they have been associated with life-threatening hemoptysis, especially in patients with squamous cell cancer. Aggressive supportive treatment is recommended for these cases, given the potential benefits of this new therapy.

Gastrointestinal

Neutropenic enterocolitis (typhlitis) often occurs a week after chemotherapy for leukemia. Common agents include doxorubicin, vinka alkaloids, and cytosine arabinoside. Patients present with abdominal pain, fever, bloody stools, and diarrhea. The cause is multifactorial, including chemotherapy-induced colonic mucosal wall damage, thrombocytopenia-related bleed, and colonic colonization by pathogenic bacteria. Computed tomography may show bowel wall thickening, colonic pneumatosis, and pneumoperitoneum. Bowel rest and broad-spectrum antibiotics may be successful, but surgery is sometimes required for bowel perforation, uncontrolled sepsis, or life-threatening bleed.

Ipilimumab, a recombinant monoclonal antibody (which binds cytotoxic T-lymphocyte–associated antigen 4) used in the treatment of melanoma, can cause colitis in up to 40% of patients. Biopsies have shown neutrophilic and lymphocytic infiltrates in colonic crypts, supporting the hypothesis that ipilimumab can cause tissue injury by breaking self-tolerance. Active monitoring for early symptoms (4-6 stools per day) is important. Discontinuation of therapy could be sufficient for mild cases, but more severe symptoms require steroid treatment with a slow taper when symptoms resolve. Emergency surgery is indicated for severe cases with bowel perforation.

Ileus, from decreased bowel motility, is common with different chemotherapy drugs: paclitaxel, vincristine, and cytosine arabinoside are common culprits. Treatment is mostly supportive with bowel rest and decompression.

Hematologic Complications

Hyperleukocytosis

Most commonly occurring in acute myeloid leukemia, hyperleukocytosis (HL) is a white blood cell count more than 100×10^9/L in the setting of leukemia. The most devastating complication of HL is leukostasis. Leukostasis is a clinicopathologic syndrome caused by the increased viscosity and metabolic activity of blood in the setting of HL and is defined pathologically by the presence of white blood cell plugs within arterioles. This causes global tissue hypoperfusion with myriad signs and symptoms thereof and is associated with a poor prognosis. Disseminated intravascular coagulation and tumor lysis syndrome are additional known complications of HL.

Treatment for HL is aimed at reducing the leukemic burden and preventing complications. In patients with newly diagnosed acute myeloid leukemia who are candidates, cytarabine-based chemotherapy is generally offered. Administration of rasburicase or allopurinol, along with adequate hydration, can help reduce the risk of tumor lysis syndrome. Pretreatment with hydroxyurea has been described but has not been shown to be beneficial. Leukapheresis is reserved for cases of HL complicated by leukostasis.

Disseminated Intravascular Coagulation

Disseminated intravascular coagulation can result from various systemic insults, including solid tumors and hematologic malignancies, most commonly acute promyelocytic leukemia or mucinous tumors. This topic is covered in more detail in Chapter 53, "Disseminated Intravascular Coagulation: Clinical Diagnosis and Management."

Biological Therapy Complications

In the past few years, several biologically active compounds have been approved for patient use, including interleukins, colony-stimulating factors, monoclonal antibodies, anti-CD20, T-cell–directed antibodies, and antibody-radioisotope conjugates. The adverse effects and toxicities of these new therapies are just now being described. Synthetic IL-2 and T-cell–directed antibodies (eg, ipilimumab) are the biological agents most likely to induce toxicities that will require management in the ICU.

Recombinant IL-2, or aldesleukin, is used for treatment of melanoma and renal cell carcinoma. Capillary leak is the main mechanism by which IL-2 can cause end-organ toxicity. Increased levels of nitric oxide and adhesion of activated lymphocytes to vascular endothelium have been shown to cause vascular leaks in animal models. The primary clinically relevant manifestations of IL-2 administration are systemic hypotension, renal dysfunction, and cardiovascular disturbances.

Systemic hypotension is an expected adverse effect of IL-2 as a result of the widespread capillary leak and systemic vasodilatation. Anticipation of hypotension with gradual discontined use of all antihypertensive drugs is recommended before administration of IL-2. If hypotension persists or is severe, supportive management with administration of colloids or α-agonists such as phenylephrine is recommended.

IL-2–triggered renal dysfunction is mediated predominantly by systemic vasodilatation and capillary leak resulting in "pre-renal" physiology. Urine output should be maintained at a rate of 1 to 1.5 mL/kg per hour with administration of intravenously administered fluids, with the understanding that excessive volume administration exacerbates the peripheral edema associated with IL-2 therapy. If acidosis or oliguria becomes severe, low-dose dopamine (2-5 μg/kg per minute) can be given. If this is ineffective, the IL-2 therapy can be discontinued until renal function has recovered rather than increasing the dopamine dose, which is associated with an increased risk of tachyarrhythmias.

Cardiovascular complications are the most severe consequences of IL-2 therapy. In fact, aldesleukin has a black box warning encouraging cardiovascular stress testing before administration of the drug. Reflex sinus tachycardia due to systemic vasodilatation is an expected adverse effect of IL-2. However, other tachyarrhythmias, including supraventricular tachycardia, atrial fibrillation or flutter, and ventricular tachycardia, have been described. If an arrhythmia occurs, decisions regarding whether to discontinue use of the drug should be based on the severity of the complication in relation to the expected clinical benefit of continuing

IL-2 therapy. Myocarditis has also been described in up to 5% of all patients treated with IL-2. This is generally mild and manifests with a mild global decrease in left ventricular function, but it further underscores the importance of pretreatment cardiopulmonary testing.

Allergic and Anaphylactic Reactions to Monoclonal Antibodies

The number of clinically available monoclonal antibodies is expected to top 70 by the year 2020. Allergic reactions to them occur in 10% to 15% of patients.

When assessing a patient with a reaction to monoclonal antibody therapy, the first step is to delineate between so-called standard infusion reactions and anaphylaxis. Diagnosis and treatment of anaphylaxis is discussed in detail in Chapter 27, "Cardiogenic Shock." The antineoplastic monoclonal antibody agents most commonly implicated in causing both standard infusion reactions and anaphylaxis are rituximab, cetuximab, and trastuzumab.

Symptoms of standard infusion reactions include myalgias, fever, nausea, bronchorrhea, flushing, urticaria, rashes, headache, tachycardia, dyspnea, abdominal pain, and rhinitis. Management of standard infusion reactions depends on the severity of symptoms. Mild cases generally respond to temporary interruption of infusion and symptomatic management with acetaminophen and antihistamines. When symptoms resolve, the infusion can be resumed at half the initial rate. More severe cases require cessation of the infusion with consideration of desensitization before any additional doses. Pretreatment with acetaminophen and antihistamines can attenuate the severity of standard infusion reactions. Severe cases causing upper airway edema with or without bronchospasm must be monitored in the ICU for fiberoptic examination or potential intubation.

Anaphylactic reactions with circulatory collapse are rare and not necessarily predicted with test doses of the antibody. They are associated with a high mortality rate despite ICU support.

Bone Marrow Transplant Complications

Hematopoietic stem cell transplant (HSCT) is a potentially curative procedure used in the treatment of various hematologic cancers. The procedure generally involves myeloablative chemotherapy with or without adjuvant radiation, followed by infusion of either donor (allogenic) or patient-derived (autologous) hematopoietic stem cells with the goal of reconstituting healthy marrow (engraftment). In the period between myeloablation and engraftment, profound transfusion-dependent pancytopenia is present with associated complications, including bleeding, infections, and pulmonary edema. During and after engraftment, however, additional morbidity can occur. A few of the common complications of HSCT are discussed here. A timeframe of noninfectious complications are shown in Table 51.1.

Acute and Chronic Graft-Versus-Host Disease

Graft-versus-host disease (GVHD) is a condition specific to allogenic HSCT wherein donor-derived leukocytes mount an immune response to recipient cells or tissue. Generally, GVHD is designated as acute in the first 100 days after HSCT and chronic after 100 days.

Acute GVHD classically involves the skin, gastrointestinal tract, or liver. The dermatologic manifestations range from mild maculopapular rash to severe widespread bullous disease mimicking Stevens-Johnson syndrome. Likewise, the gastrointestinal manifestations range in severity from mild abdominal discomfort to severe hemorrhagic diarrhea. Liver function test abnormalities mimic cholestasis with an out-of-proportion increase in alkaline phosphatase caused by immune-mediated injury to bile ducts. Diagnosis is usually clinical, but in uncertain cases a biopsy may be necessary. Glucocorticoids (methylprednisolone at 2 mg/kg) constitute the cornerstone of management for acute GVHD; intravenous immunoglobulin has shown to be effective and is used in very severe or refractory cases.

Chronic GVHD may target skin; liver; all mucosal surfaces, including aerodigestive, gut and genitourinary, eyes; fascia; and joints. The manifestations within these organ systems are diverse, and, because of the implications associated with treatment, biopsy is generally recommended to confirm a diagnosis. Management is corticosteroid based with the addition of adjuvant mTOR inhibitor or cyclosporine in refractory cases.

Engraftment Syndrome

Engraftment syndrome may occur after either autologous or allogenic HSCT and is thought to be caused by the relative flood of pro-inflammatory mediators that are released around the time bone marrow reconstitutes. The usual clinical and laboratory manifestations include noncardiogenic pulmonary edema, fevers, rash, diarrhea, eosinophilia, thrombocytopenia, liver function test abnormalities, and acute kidney injury. Symptoms are usually self-limited and generally responsive to a short course of methylprednisolone. Pulmonary edema in engraftment syndrome is notoriously nonresponsive to loop diuretics; thus, if considerable respiratory distress is present, noninvasive positive-pressure ventilation or, if necessary, intubation should be pursued.

Diffuse Alveolar Hemorrhage

Diffuse alveolar hemorrhage is a dreaded complication of HSCT with high associated morbidity and mortality. Classic cases present within the first 2 weeks after HSCT, and the peri-engraftment period seems to be associated with the highest risk. Clinical features include hypoxemia and

Table 51.1 • Timeframe of Common Noninfectious Pulmonary Complications of Hematopoietic Stem Cell Transplant

	Days		
Complication	**0-30**	**>30-100**	**>100**
Recipient immune defects	Neutropenia, invasive devices, mucositis	Impaired cellular immunity (iatrogenic)	Impaired cellular immunity (iatrogenic) Impaired humoral immunity
Noninfectious pulmonary	Acute GVHD Engraftment syndrome CHF Veno-occlusive disease Diffuse alveolar hemorrhage	Acute GVHD Diffuse alveolar hemorrhage Veno-occlusive disease Idiopathic pneumonia syndrome Cryptogenic organizing pneumonia	Posttransplant lymphoproliferative disorder Bronchiolitis obliterans Cryptogenic organizing pneumonia

Abbreviations: CHF, congestive heart failure; GVHD, graft-versus-host disease.

diffuse multifocal pulmonary infiltrates. The diagnosis of diffuse alveolar hemorrhage is established with bronchoscopy, wherein sequential bronchoalveolar lavage aliquots will be progressively bloodier. Early recognition and management with corticosteroids have been shown to attenuate mortality risk; however, the need for aggressive supportive care measures should be anticipated because of the grim overall prognosis associated with this complication.

Idiopathic Pneumonia Syndrome

Idiopathic pneumonia syndrome is a complication of HSCT that occurs after engraftment and usually within the first 4 months. It is a diagnosis of exclusion that requires the presence of alveolar infiltrates, evidence of impaired gas exchange, and exclusion of infections, cardiovascular disease, and renal dysfunction as explanations for the infiltrates. The importance of an exhaustive search for infections within bronchoalveolar lavage specimens before establishing a diagnosis cannot be overemphasized. Medical therapy for idiopathic pneumonia syndrome generally yields disappointing results. High-dose glucocorticoids are used, and clinical trials into the use of tumor necrosis factor-α inhibitors are under way.

Veno-occlusive Disease

Pulmonary veno-occlusive disease is a relatively rare, late complication of HSCT. Clinically, it manifests with signs or symptoms of pulmonary hypertension, including pulmonary vascular congestion, increased pulmonary artery diameter on chest computed tomography, pleural effusions, decreased diffusing capacity of the lungs for carbon monoxide on pulmonary function tests, or echocardiographic evidence of right ventricular strain. In the absence of left heart disease or another explanation for increased pulmonary artery pressures, a diagnosis of pulmonary veno-occlusive disease should be considered. Lung biopsy will confirm the diagnosis. Prognosis is poor. One small case series has shown a modest response to treatment with corticosteroids.

Summary

- The mere presence of solid cancer is not an independent predictor of an adverse outcome after an ICU admission.
- Hypercalcemia is the most common metabolic abnormality in oncologic patients. Hydration remains the first therapeutic intervention in all cases.
- Chemotherapy can be initiated in the ICU for urgent indications such as superior vena cava syndrome and hyperleukocytosis with leukostasis.
- The survival rate of patients in the ICU who have most types of hematologic malignancies has improved tremendously.
- The overall prognosis for recipients of allogenic bone marrow transplants who are admitted to the ICU remains poor.
- Patients with HSCT can have a particular set of complications that usually follow a particular timeline, which is very helpful in the diagnostic work-up (Table 51.1).

SUGGESTED READING

Chi AK, Soubani AO, White AC, Miller KB. An update on pulmonary complications of hematopoietic stem cell transplantation. Chest. 2013 Dec;144(6):1913–22.

Daver N, Kantarjian H, Marcucci G, Pierce S, Brandt M, Dinardo C, et al. Clinical characteristics and outcomes in patients with acute promyelocytic leukaemia and hyperleucocytosis. Br J Haematol. 2015 Mar;168(5):646–53. Epub 2014 Oct 14.

Davis EJ, Salem JE, Young A, Green JR, Ferrell PB, Ancell KK, et al. Hematologic complications of immune checkpoint inhibitors. Oncologist. 2019 Feb 28. pii: theoncologist.2018–0574. [Epub ahead of print]

Dubbs SB. Rapid fire: tumor lysis syndrome. Emerg Med Clin North Am. 2018 Aug;36(3):517–25.

Ewer MS, Vooletich MT, Durand JB, Woods ML, Davis JR, Valero V, et al. Reversibility of trastuzumab-related cardiotoxicity: new insights based on clinical course and response to medical treatment. J Clin Oncol. 2005 Nov 1;23(31):7820–6.

Hande KR, Garrow GC. Acute tumor lysis syndrome in patients with high-grade non-Hodgkin's lymphoma. Am J Med. 1993 Feb;94(2):133–9.

Hu JR, Florido R, Lipson EJ, Naidoo J, Ardehali R, Tocchetti CG, et al. Cardiovascular toxicities associated with immune checkpoint inhibitors. Cardiovasc Res. 2019 Apr 15;115(5):854–68.

Jasek AM, Day HJ. Acute spontaneous tumor lysis syndrome. Am J Hematol. 1994 Oct;47(2):129–31.

Lucena CM, Torres A, Rovira M, Marcos MA, de la Bellacasa JP, Sanchez M, et al. Pulmonary complications in hematopoietic SCT: a prospective study. Bone Marrow Transplant. 2014 Oct;49(10):1293–9. Epub 2014 Jul 21.

Merrill SP, Reynolds P, Kalra A, Biehl J, Vandivier RW, Mueller SW. Early administration of infliximab for severe ipilimumab-related diarrhea in a critically ill patient. Ann Pharmacother. 2014 Jun;48(6):806–10. Epub 2014 Mar 20.

Naidoo J, Page DB, Li BT, Connell LC, Schindler K, Lacouture ME, et al. Toxicities of the anti-PD-1 and anti-PD-L1 immune checkpoint antibodies. Ann Oncol. 2015 Dec;26(12):2375–91. Epub 2015 Sep 14.

Porcu P, Cripe LD, Ng EW, Bhatia S, Danielson CM, Orazi A, et al. Hyperleukocytic leukemias and leukostasis: a review of pathophysiology, clinical presentation and management. Leuk Lymphoma. 2000 Sep;39(1-2):1–18.

Sawaya H, Sebag IA, Plana JC, Januzzi JL, Ky B, Cohen V, et al. Early detection and prediction of cardiotoxicity in chemotherapy-treated patients. Am J Cardiol. 2011 May 1;107(9):1375–80. Epub 2011 Mar 2.

Spitzer TR. Engraftment syndrome: double-edged sword of hematopoietic cell transplants. Bone Marrow Transplant. 2015 Apr;50(4):469–75. Epub 2015 Jan 12.

Williams KJ, Grauer DW, Henry DW, Rockey ML. Corticosteroids for the management of immune-related adverse events in patients receiving checkpoint inhibitors. J Oncol Pharm Pract. 2019 Apr;25(3):544–50. Epub 2017 Dec 9.

52 Thrombocytopenia and Thrombocytopathy

GRETCHEN JOHNS, MD

Goals

- Describe causes of thrombocytopenia.
- Elucidate clinical features of, diagnostic approaches to, and management of thrombocytopenia due to platelet destruction.
- Catalog drugs associated with thrombocytopenia and its management.

Introduction

Platelet disorders are quantitative or qualitative, or both. Either markedly increased or decreased numbers of platelets can cause harmful sequelae. Platelet disorders can be divided into acquired or hereditary; acquired disorders are much more common than congenital disorders. Platelet disorders can be due to increased platelet destruction or decreased platelet production (Box 52.1). Pseudothrombocytopenia, dilutional effects, or possible splenic sequestration should be considered when the platelet count is low for the first time. The recent addition of a drug, commonly used in intensive care units, is also an important consideration for patients with newly acquired thrombocytopenia.

Platelets are produced in the bone marrow, released into the peripheral blood circulation, and removed by the reticuloendothelial system after 7 to 10 days. Platelets have no nucleus, have alpha and dense granules, and are smaller than red blood cells (2-4 μm vs 6-8 μm). Occasional larger platelets are present that are younger and more active in clotting than the smaller, older platelets. Giant platelets (as large as or larger than red blood cells) are normally not present. The mean platelet volume can be helpful to assess the size (volume) of the platelets. Normal platelet counts are fairly stable throughout life and are 150 to 400 × 10^9/L. Bleeding risk increases at lower platelet counts; platelet counts more than 50 × 10^9/L generally do not require treatment. Patients who are going to have surgery or procedures may require a platelet transfusion to reach a platelet count of 50 × 10^9/L before proceeding.

Bleeding due to platelet disorders tends to be mucocutaneous bleeding (oral and nasal cavities; gastrointestinal and genitourinary tracts; skin, such as petechiae, purpura, ecchymoses, excessive bleeding following minor cuts) or immediate bleeding with invasive procedures. In contrast, bleeding related to clotting factor deficiencies tends to involve deep tissue bleeding (joints and muscles) or delayed bleeding after invasive procedures.

Evaluation for a possible platelet disorder includes a detailed family and personal history of abnormal bleeding or clotting in response to hemostatic challenges, a complete blood count with peripheral blood smear review, and a physical examination. Additional testing is added according to the symptoms and history. In the intensive care unit, rapid-onset thrombocytopenia can be associated with heparin use, and the platelet decrease can be precipitous. Thrombocytopenia associated with critical illness or drug induced results in a slow decline.

Pseudothrombocytopenia

The term *pseudothrombocytopenia* is generally reserved for platelets clumping in the presence of the anticoagulant EDTA. The platelet clumps can easily be seen on the peripheral blood smear. When the calcium is bound by the EDTA, antibodies from the patient cause the platelets to agglutinate. The phenomenon is artifactual, and the platelets are normal in number and function in vivo. Platelet satellitism is a similar in vitro phenomenon in which the platelets adhere to the neutrophils in the EDTA-anticoagulated

Box 52.1 • Causes of Thrombocytopenia

Pseudothrombocytopenia (EDTA-related artifact, clot)
Dilutional (massive transfusion, pregnancy, contamination)
Increased platelet destruction
- Immune
  - Autoimmune ([idiopathic] autoimmune thrombocytopenic purpura, thrombotic thrombocytopenic purpura, posttransfusion purpura)
  - Idiopathic
  - Secondary (drug-induced thrombocytopenia, connective tissue diseases)
- Nonimmune
  - Consumptive (disseminated intravascular coagulation)
  - Sepsis

Decreased platelet production
- Bone marrow failure
  - Primary (aplastic anemia)
  - Secondary (metastatic malignancies, hematologic malignancies, causes of necrosis or fibrosis)
- Nutritional deficiency (vitamin B_{12}, folate)
- Infections (HIV, hepatitis, cytomegalovirus)
- Drug-induced (chemotherapy)

From Pruthi RK. Hemostatic disorders. In: Wittich CM, editor. Mayo Clinic internal medicine board review. 11th ed. New York (NY): Oxford University Press; c2016. p. 415-25. (Mayo Clinic Scientific Press series); used with permission of Mayo Foundation for Medical Education and Research.

blood. Recollecting the blood in a sodium citrate anticoagulant tube usually results in an accurate platelet count without the clumping or satellitism.

Once pseudothrombocytopenia is eliminated, investigation of the cause of the low platelet count generally begins by trying to rule out the most serious causes of thrombocytopenia, such as heparin-induced thrombocytopenia (HIT), thrombotic thrombocytopenic purpura (TTP), and the HELLP syndrome of pregnancy (*h*emolysis, *e*levated *l*iver enzymes, and *l*ow *p*latelet count).

Acquired Thrombocytopenia Due to Increased Platelet Destruction

Idiopathic Thrombocytopenic Purpura

Idiopathic (also called autoimmune) thrombocytopenic purpura (ITP) is caused by autoimmune destruction of a patient's own platelets due to antibodies directed against glycoproteins on the platelet surface. Most commonly, only platelets are affected, and the red blood cells and white blood cells are normal in number. In children, the onset is acute with mucosal bleeding, petechiae, and purpura. It frequently follows an upper respiratory tract infection or other viral infection. The large majority of children have a spontaneous resolution within 4 to 6 weeks. In adults, ITP may be found when a minor injury results in a large bruise or hematoma out of proportion to the injury. A patient may have had a low platelet count for some time without realizing it. It is more common in women than men. ITP in adults is less likely to be associated with a recent viral infection or to resolve spontaneously. Splenomegaly is uncommon, and another diagnosis should be considered if it is present.

ITP is a diagnosis of exclusion (Table 52.1). Examination of the peripheral blood smear shows large platelets (increased mean platelet volume), indicative of increased turnover. Some hematology analyzers can calculate the percentage of immature platelets that are present, which will also be increased. The platelet count is often less than 50×10^9/L. Platelet counts of less than 10×10^9/L put the patient at risk for spontaneous bleeding, including cerebral or subarachnoid hemorrhage.

Treatment is according to the American Society of Hematology guidelines, as follows:

1. No treatment is routinely required for patients with no bleeding or mild bleeding regardless of the platelet count.
2. For patients with platelet counts of less than 30×10^9/L, consider treatment with prednisone 1 mg/kg for up to 1 month. About 70% of patients respond, and the chance of a long-term remission is 40%. For severe bleeding, treat with 1 g/kg intravenous immunoglobulin, 1 dose, repeated as necessary.

Splenectomy is used to treat corticosteroid-refractory ITP and is thought to decrease antibody production and platelet destruction. The remission rate is about 75%, and about 60% of patients remain in long-term remission. Vaccines for pneumococcus, meningococcus, and *Haemophilus influenzae* organisms should be administered 2 weeks before splenectomy. Howell-Jolly bodies (nuclear remnants) are present on peripheral blood smears after splenectomy, unless an accessory spleen is present. Patients with an accessory spleen will need to have it removed as well.

Other options include pulsed dexamethasone, azathioprine, cyclophosphamide, colchicine, cyclosporine, rituximab, vincristine, vinblastine, anti-Rh (D) immunoglobulin, danazol, immunoadsorption apheresis with staphylococcal protein A columns, and thrombopoietin receptor agonists (eltrombopag and romiplostim). Prophylactic platelet transfusions are not contraindicated in patients with ITP, but they are generally not needed because patients with ITP have young, large, thrombogenic platelets and clotting occurs even at fairly low platelet counts.

Table 52.1 • Comparison of 3 Types of Thrombocytopenia

	Type		
Factor	**ITP**	**TTP**	**HIT**
Cause of thrombocytopenia	Autoantibodies to glycoproteins on platelet surface	Most commonly autoantibodies to ADAMTS13	Autoantibodies to platelet factor 4–heparin complex
Risk factors	More frequent in women than men Children: recent viral illness	Autoimmune diseases, pregnancy, pancreatitis, cancer, bone marrow transplant, infections, surgery, medications Often no known risk factor	Unfractionated heparin more often than LMWH Women more than men Patients with major surgery or trauma more likely than medical or obstetric patients
Characteristics or complications	Splenomegaly uncommon Usually an isolated platelet abnormality Young, larger platelets result in less bleeding at low platelet counts	Microangiopathic hemolytic anemia (increased LDH, low hemoglobin, schistocytes) Two-thirds of patients have neurologic abnormalities One-tenth as common as ITP	Thrombosis (HITT) (arterial or venous) Skin necrosis at heparin injection site Anaphylactoid reaction DIC Adrenal hemorrhage and shock
Treatment	Glucocorticoids, rituximab, splenectomy	Therapeutic plasma exchange Treatment of underlying cause, if known	Stop use of heparin and LMWH, and start use of a nonheparin anticoagulant Transition carefully to warfarin
Platelet nadir and timing	10×10^9/L or less Acute onset in children; insidious onset and more likely to be chronic in adults	20×10^9/L or less, but variable Acute onset, but some patients have multiple relapses	Fall of 50% or more of baseline platelet count Nadir usually $>20 \times 10^9$/L Nadir may exceed the lower end of the reference range in patients with a high baseline platelet count Occurs 4-15 days after first exposure to heparin or 1-2 days with heparin exposure in the last 30-100 days
Prophylactic platelet transfusions	Not usually required, but no contraindication	Contraindicated because of increased risk of arterial thrombosis and death (in actively bleeding patients, platelet transfusion should be carefully monitored for thromboembolic events)	Contraindicated because of increased risk for arterial thrombosis and death (in actively bleeding patients, platelet transfusion should be carefully monitored for thromboembolic events)

Abbreviations: ADAMTS13, *a disintegrin and metalloprotease with a thrombospondin type 1 motif, member 13*; DIC, disseminated intravascular coagulation; HIT, heparin-induced thrombocytopenia; HITT, heparin-induced thrombocytopenia with thrombosis; ITP, idiopathic (autoimmune) thrombocytopenia; LDH, lactate dehydrogenase; LMWH, low-molecular-weight heparin; TTP, thrombotic thrombocytopenic purpura.

Thrombotic Thrombocytopenic Purpura

TTP is not a disorder of platelets but a severe deficiency of or antibody against the von Willebrand factor–cleaving metalloprotease ADAMTS13 (*a disintegrin and metalloprotease with a thrombospondin type 1 motif, member 13*). This metalloprotease cleaves the ultralarge multimers of von Willebrand factor as they exit their storage sites in platelets and endothelial cells. Because the ultralarge von Willebrand factor multimers are highly thrombogenic, the inability to cleave them results in systemic microvascular thrombi containing large numbers of platelets. The current diagnostic criteria for TTP requires only 2 elements: microangiopathic hemolytic anemia and thrombocytopenia without another clinically apparent cause. Two-thirds of patients have neurologic abnormalities, but this criterion is no longer required for diagnosis.

TTP is most commonly diagnosed in middle-aged black women with systemic lupus erythematosus or other autoimmune diseases. Additional risk factors include the third trimester of pregnancy, pancreatitis, cancer, bone marrow transplant, congenital mutations, infections (including HIV), surgery, and medications (quinine, mitomycin C, gemcitabine, cyclosporine, vascular endothelial growth factor inhibitors, ticlopidine, and, less commonly, clopidogrel), but many cases have no obvious precipitating factor(s). Laboratory features include an increased lactate dehydrogenase level related to hemolysis, low platelet count, and schistocytes on the peripheral blood smear.

The waxing and waning of the neurologic deficits, which may include seizures or nonconvulsive status epilepticus, have been tentatively explained by intermittent ischemia caused by microthrombi, but reversible brain lesions and a posterior reversible encephalopathy syndrome have also been reported.

Treatment with therapeutic plasma exchange using plasma blood products that contain ADAMTS13 (not albumin) has greatly reduced mortality from more than 90% in the 1960s to approximately 20% currently. Glucocorticoid therapy may be used in conjunction with therapeutic plasma exchange. For patients with relapses, a standard regimen of rituximab may be tried. Patients with nonclassic forms of TTP may be less responsive to treatment. Prophylactic platelet transfusion is contraindicated in patients with TTP to avoid increasing the risk of arterial thrombosis and death. However, in actively bleeding patients, platelet transfusions may be given with careful monitoring for thromboembolic complications.

Heparin-Induced Thrombocytopenia

HIT is an immune-mediated adverse drug reaction caused by an immunoglobulin G antibody that recognizes the complex of platelet factor 4 bound to heparin. It occurs in 1% to 8% of patients administered unfractionated heparin and in a lower percentage of patients given low-molecular-weight heparin. The latter cannot be substituted for heparin in patients who experience HIT after administration of unfractionated heparin because of some cross-reactivity. HIT can develop at any dose, including with line flushes or low-dose prophylaxis for patients with reduced mobility. Nonimmune heparin-associated thrombocytopenia is a separate entity in which patients have a decrease in platelet count during heparin administration but it is not associated with the HIT antibodies. Heparin-associated thrombocytopenia is considered clinically insignificant and does not require treatment.

HIT is clinically significant and is suspected when the platelet count decreases 50% or more between days 5 to 14 after heparin exposure. In patients who have previously had heparin exposure, the count may decrease in less time, as soon as 24 hours after their subsequent heparin exposure. The thrombosis may be either venous (deep vein thrombosis, pulmonary embolism, adrenal vein thrombosis, cerebral vein thrombosis, mesenteric vein thrombosis) or arterial (occlusion of large limb arteries, stroke, myocardial infarction, mesenteric artery thrombosis). Other complications include skin necrosis at the site of heparin injection, anaphylactoid reaction within 30 minutes of intravenous or subcutaneous administration of heparin, decompensated disseminated intravascular coagulation, adrenal hemorrhagic necrosis, and shock.

HIT is a clinical diagnosis, and scoring systems are available, including the 4 Ts scoring system. Zero to 2 points are assigned for responses to each of 4 categories in this system; a score of 4 or 5 points indicates an intermediate probability of HIT, and a score of 6 to 8 points indicates a high probability. If the probability is intermediate or high, use of heparin should be discontinued and an alternative nonheparin anticoagulant should be used.

The 4 Ts scoring system is as follows:

- Thrombocytopenia: percentage of decrease of platelet count and level of platelet nadir.
- Timing of decrease of platelet count: 4-15 days with no previous exposure or <4 days with heparin exposure in the past 30-100 days.
- Thrombosis or other sequelae: new thrombosis versus recurrent, progressive, suspected, or no thrombosis.
- Other causes of thrombocytopenia: no other cause, possible cause, or other known cause.

Laboratory testing includes 2 categories: immunologic (antigen) assays, which often are enzyme-linked immunosorbent assays, and functional (activation) assays. The enzyme-linked immunosorbent assays are more readily available and are sensitive but not as specific. The functional assays, such as the serotonin release assay and the heparin-induced platelet activation assay, are sensitive and specific but have limited availability.

Treatment involves the use of nonheparin anticoagulants after the use of heparin is stopped, which should be done before the laboratory test results are known in patients who have an intermediate or high clinical probability because of the high risk of thrombosis. Argatroban, bivalirudin, or fondaparinux can be used with dose adjustments for liver or renal dysfunction, as needed. Currently, few or no studies support using the new direct oral anticoagulants, which are not approved for this use by the US Food and Drug Administration but have potential to be used in these patients. Prophylactic platelet transfusion is contraindicated in patients with HIT to avoid increasing the risk of arterial thrombosis and death. However, in actively bleeding patients, platelet transfusions may be given with careful monitoring for thromboembolic complications. Patients with HIT are at risk for skin necrosis and limb gangrene during initiation of warfarin therapy. Warfarin use should not be started until the platelet count is at the lower end of the normal reference range, and there should be about a 5-day overlap (until the target international normalized ratio is reached) with the nonheparin anticoagulant. Low doses of warfarin should be used initially. Unfractionated heparin may be given again in the future if a patient's immunologic assay result returns to negative and the platelet count is once again in the normal reference range.

Drug-Induced Thrombocytopenia

Drug-induced thrombocytopenia is often misdiagnosed and mistreated as ITP. Documenting a drug as the cause of the thrombocytopenia requires that several criteria be met, including recovery of the platelet count when use of the drug is stopped and decrease of the platelet count when use of the drug is restarted. Drug-induced thrombocytopenia can be divided into 2 types: 1) those that decrease platelet production and 2) those that increase platelet destruction, often through immune mechanisms. Reactions may occur in all patients using a particular medication or may be idiosyncratic, affecting only isolated patients.

Selective inhibition of megakaryocytes is common with chronic use of large quantities of alcohol, high doses of estrogens, histone deacetylase inhibitors, linezolid, imatinib mesylate, anagrelide, and interferons. Chemotherapeutic agents often suppress all myeloid lines, but severe thrombocytopenia may be a limitation for continuing therapy. Drug-induced aplastic anemia usually is idiosyncratic; implicated drugs include anticonvulsants, nonsteroidal anti-inflammatory drugs, and sulfonamides.

Drug-induced platelet destruction can occur through nonimmune or immune mechanisms. Nonimmune platelet destruction can occur with granulocyte-macrophage colony-stimulating factor, tumor necrosis factor α with interferon gamma, porcine factor VIII, desmopressin in type IIB or platelet-type von Willebrand disease, protamine sulfate, and amrinone. Drugs can cause platelet destruction through several different immune mechanisms, such as a hapten-dependent antibody, immune complex formation, or autoantibody formation. HIT is one of the most concerning types because of the thrombotic complications. Other drugs that cause platelet destruction through immune mechanisms include penicillin, cephalosporins, amphotericin B, vancomycin, other antibiotics, nonsteroidal anti-inflammatory drugs, valproic acid, carbamazepine, other anticonvulsants, quinine, gold salts, L-dopa, procainamide, eptifibatide, tirofiban, and abciximab (Table 52.2).

Reactions due to preformed antibodies, such as the murine antibodies that react with abciximab, can cause platelet counts to decrease in minutes. Other drug reactions require the formation of antibodies, and thus the decrease in the platelet count may occur up to 14 days after initiating medication use. With the exception of gold salts, platelet counts recover within 4 to 14 days after discontinuing use of the drug. Platelet counts may take much longer to recover after stopping use of gold salts. Low platelet counts due to viral infections generally take longer to reach normal values again (weeks to months).

Table 52.2 • Drugs Strongly Associated With Antibody-Mediated Thrombocytopenia

Drug Classification	Specific Drugs
Analgesics and nonsteroidal anti-inflammatory	Acetaminophen, ibuprofen, naproxen
Antiarrhythmic	Quinidine
Anticonvulsant	Carbamazepine, phenytoin, valproic acid
Antimicrobial	Ampicillin, ethambutol, piperacillin, quinine, rifampin, sulfisoxasole, trimethoprim-sulfamethoxazole, vancomycin
Antineoplastic	Irinotecan, oxaliplatin
Antipsychotic	Haloperidol
Glycoprotein IIb/III inhibitors	Abciximab, eptifibatide, tirofiban
Histamine$_2$ blockers	Ranitidine
HMG CoA inhibitors	Simvastatin

Abbreviation: HMG CoA, 3-hydroxy-3-methylglutaryl coenzyme A.

Thrombocytopenia Due to Decreased Platelet Production

Decreased bone marrow production of platelets can occur from bone marrow–infiltrating malignancy (primary or metastatic), infections (HIV, *Helicobacter pylori*, Epstein-Barr virus, rickettsial infections, ehrlichiosis, leptospirosis, sepsis, cytomegalovirus, fungal infections), or bone marrow–failure states (myelodysplastic syndrome, aplastic anemia). Nutritional deficiencies (vitamin B_{12} or folate), autoimmune diseases, medications, radiation, antiphospholipid antibody syndrome, and causes of bone marrow necrosis or fibrosis can result in thrombocytopenia. Treatment of the underlying disorder and management of the thrombocytopenia through minimum blood draws and platelet transfusions are both required.

Congenital Platelet Disorders

Congenital platelet disorders are relatively rare; patients have a personal and family history of abnormal mucocutaneous and immediate postoperative bleeding. Platelet function testing is used to identify some congenital bleeding disorders; others require electron microscopy, flow cytometry, or genetic testing for diagnosis. Family members may also want to be tested if they have a history of increased bleeding. With severe congenital disorders, platelet transfusion may be necessary for prophylaxis. Mild to moderate disorders may need platelet transfusions with hemorrhage or on standby for major invasive procedures.

Thrombocytopenia in Pregnancy

In a little more than 5% of women, mild thrombocytopenia develops during an uncomplicated pregnancy, called gestational thrombocytopenia. This is benign and does not require treatment; the thrombocytopenia resolves after delivery. One-fourth of women with preeclampsia have mild thrombocytopenia. HELLP syndrome is a severe form of hypertensive disease in pregnancy and requires delivery of the baby. Other causes of low platelet counts in pregnancy include ITP, disseminated intravascular coagulation, TTP, acute fatty liver of pregnancy, infections (bacterial, viral such as HIV and hepatitis), antiphospholipid antibodies, medications (quinine, heparin), and nutritional deficiency.

Summary

- Exclude pseudothrombocytopenia or dilution in patients with first-time thrombocytopenia.
- Most thrombocytopenias are acquired and result from increased platelet destruction or decreased platelet production.
- Causes of thrombocytopenia due to increased platelet destruction include ITP (autoimmune), TTP, HIT, and drug-induced thrombocytopenia. Specific diagnostic and management steps exist for these conditions.
- Thrombocytopenia can also be due to decreased platelet production or congenital platelet disorders.
- Thrombocytopenia in pregnancy can be life-threatening and associated with the HELLP syndrome.

SUGGESTED READING

American Society of Hematology. 2011 Clinical Practice Guideline on the Evaluation and Management of Immune Thrombocytopenia (ITP). Washington (DC): American Society of Hematology; c2011.

Burrus TM, Wijdicks EF, Rabinstein AA. Brain lesions are most often reversible in acute thrombotic thrombocytopenic purpura. Neurology. 2009 Jul 7;73(1):66–70.

Cuker A, Crowther MA. 2013 Clinical Practice Guideline on the Evaluation and Management of Adults with Suspected Heparin-Induced Thrombocytopenia (HIT). Washington (DC): American Society of Hematology; c2013.

East JM, Cserti-Gazdewich CM, Granton JT. Heparin-induced thrombocytopenia in the critically ill patient. Chest. 2017 Dec 16. pii: S0012-3692(17)33223-3. [Epub ahead of print]

Goodnight SH, Hathaway WE, editors. Disorders of hemostasis and thrombosis: a clinical guide. 2nd ed. New York (NY): McGraw-Hill Medical Pub. Division; c2001. p. 76–126.

Kappler S, Ronan-Bentle S, Graham A. Thrombotic microangiopathies (TTP, HUS, HELLP). Hematol Oncol Clin North Am. 2017 Dec;31(6):1081–1103.

Kitchens CS, Kessler CM, Konkle BA, editors. Consultative hemostasis and thrombosis [electronic resource]. 3rd ed. Philadelphia (PA): Elsevier/Saunders; c2013. p. 103–49.

Marder VJ, Aird WC, Bennett JS, Schulman S, White GC II, editors. Hemostasis and thrombosis: basic principles and clinical practice. 6th ed. Philadelphia (PA): Wolters Kluwer Health/Lippincott Williams & Wilkins; c2013. p. 751–828.

Michelson AD, editor. Platelets. 3rd ed. London (UK): Elsevier/AP; c2013. p. 813–1017.

Mitta A, Curtis BR, Reese JA, George JN. Drug-induced thrombocytopenia: 2019 Update of clinical and laboratory data. Am J Hematol. 2019 Mar;94(3):E76–8. Epub 2018 Dec 27.

53 Disseminated Intravascular Coagulation: Clinical Diagnosis and Management

PRAKASH VISHNU, MBBS; SIKANDER AILAWADHI, MD

Goals

- Describe the pathophysiologic basis of disseminated intravascular coagulation.
- Identify the underlying conditions that lead to disseminated intravascular coagulation.
- Delineate supportive management of disseminated intravascular coagulation.

Introduction

Disseminated intravascular coagulation (DIC) is a phenomenon with the potential for causing thrombosis and bleeding. DIC, typically occurring in patients with critical illness, can manifest as an acute, life-threatening emergency or as a chronic, subclinical process depending on the influence of morbidity from the underlying cause. The presence of DIC increases the risk of mortality by twofold in patients with trauma and severe sepsis and is an independent predictor of mortality. The pathogenesis of DIC is not only related to abnormal coagulation activation and platelet consumption but also involves multiple mechanisms of the inflammatory system and innate immunity.

Epidemiology

The incidence of DIC may be underestimated because many cases are mild, subclinical, or transient. It reportedly occurs in about 1% of patients hospitalized in tertiary-care medical centers. The occurrence of DIC also largely varies according to the underlying medical condition that causes it and ensues at a greater rate in patients with sepsis (83%), trauma (31%), and cancer (7%). Among patients with bacterial sepsis, the likelihood of DIC is related to the severity of the systemic inflammatory response. DIC can occur in a considerable number of patients with cancers, such as acute promyelocytic leukemia, pancreatic cancer, and other solid tumors such as ovarian, gastric, prostate, and breast. Some of the risk factors for development of DIC in patients with cancer include older age (>60 years), male sex, and advanced stage of cancer. Among patients with obstetric complications, the incidence of DIC ranges from 66% in patients with amniotic fluid embolism to 20% in patients with hemolysis, elevated liver function results, and low platelet level (HELLP syndrome). In general, DIC resolves if the underlying condition is self-limiting or can be aptly managed as the status of hemostasis normalizes.

Causes

DIC does not occur in isolation but is due to several underlying conditions (Tables 53.1 and 53.2) that are responsible for its initiation and propagation, generally by 1 of the following 2 pathways: 1) a systemic inflammatory response, which leads to instigation of the cytokine system and a consequent activation of coagulation (eg, major trauma or sepsis) and 2) exposure or release of procoagulant factor into the bloodstream (eg, obstetric cases, cancer, or crush injury).

The common causes of DIC include the following:

1. Sepsis due to bacterial, fungal, viral, or parasitic infections.
2. Trauma, particularly to the central nervous system.
3. Malignancy, especially acute promyelocytic leukemia, mucin-producing tumors (eg, pancreatic, gastric, ovarian), and brain tumors.
4. Obstetric complications such as acute fatty liver of pregnancy, HELLP syndrome, preeclampsia, and retained dead fetus.

Table 53.1 • Causes of Acute DIC

Category	Cause
Traumatic	Motor vehicle accidents, head injury Burns Snake envenomation
Obstetric	Abruptio placentae Acute peripartum hemorrhage Amniotic fluid embolism Acute fatty liver of pregnancy Preeclampsia, eclampsia, HELLP syndrome Retained dead fetus
Infectious	Bacterial (eg, sepsis due to gram-positive and gram-negative bacterial infection, rickettsia) Viral (eg, CMV, HIV, VZV) Fungal (eg, *Histoplasma*) Parasitic (eg, malaria)
Transfusion	Hemolytic reactions Massive transfusion
Neoplastic	Acute myeloid leukemia Metastatic mucin-producing adenocarcinoma
Other	Prosthetic devices Peritoneovenous shunts Ventricular assist devices Heat stroke, hyperthermia Hemorrhagic skin necrosis (purpura fulminans) Catastrophic antiphospholipid syndrome

Abbreviations: CMV, cytomegalovirus; DIC, disseminated intravascular coagulation; HELLP, hemolysis, elevated liver enzymes, and low platelet count; VZV, varicella-zoster virus.

Data from Levi M, Toh CH, Thachil J, Watson HG; British Committee for Standards in Haematology. Guidelines for the diagnosis and management of disseminated intravascular coagulation. Br J Haematol. 2009 Apr;145(1):24-33. Epub 2009 Feb 12.

Table 53.2 • Causes of Chronic DIC

Category	Cause
Obstetric	Retained products of conception Retained dead fetus syndrome
Cardiovascular	Raynaud disease Myocardial infarction Aortic aneurysm
Neoplastic	Solid tumors
Hematologic	Myeloproliferative syndromes
Inflammatory	Rheumatoid arthritis Sarcoidosis Crohn disease, ulcerative colitis
Localized DIC	Renal allograft rejection Giant hemangioma (Kasabach-Merritt syndrome)

Abbreviation: DIC, disseminated intravascular coagulation.

Data from Levi M, Toh CH, Thachil J, Watson HG; British Committee for Standards in Haematology. Guidelines for the diagnosis and management of disseminated intravascular coagulation. Br J Haematol. 2009 Apr;145(1):24-33. Epub 2009 Feb 12.

5. Intravascular hemolysis, often due to acute hemolytic transfusion reaction in the setting of ABO-incompatible transfusion or to hemolysis such as in severe malaria.

Other causes of DIC are less frequent but can be considered if none of the above conditions are evident or in certain clinical situations such as the following:

1. Heat stroke
2. Crush injuries
3. Amphetamine overdose
4. Insertion of a peritoneovenous shunt
5. Fat embolism
6. Vascular aberrations (eg, aortic aneurysm, kaposiform hemangioendothelioma)
7. Hereditary protein C deficiency
8. Acute solid-organ transplant rejection
9. Catastrophic antiphospholipid antibody syndrome

Pathogenesis

Normal hemostasis by means of intravascular coagulation and fibrinolysis confirms formation of a blood clot at the location of injury to the vasculature, followed by clearance of the clot to allow tissue repair. Multiple feedbacks are built into this system to prevent a generalized activation of coagulation and limit the clot to the site of injury. However, in DIC, these processes of coagulation and fibrinolysis become abnormally activated within the vasculature, a result leading to ongoing coagulation and fibrinolysis.

A typical sequence of events and pathways in DIC is as shown in Figure 53.1 and is initiated by exposure of blood to a procoagulant such as tissue factor (TF), from which it is generally protected. Sources and components of these procoagulants depend on the underlying condition. Some bacterial products, such as lipopolysaccharides, can trigger coagulation. In meningococcal sepsis, microparticles containing TF are found in circulation. Traumatic injury to the vascular endothelium and tissues can release TF, procoagulant enzymes, or phospholipids. A proteolytic enzyme produced by some mucinous tumors and placenta acts as a "cancer procoagulant" that can activate factor X. In severe intravascular hemolysis such as acute hemolytic transfusion reaction, coagulation is activated by a combination of processes including TF release, generation of cytokines such as tumor necrosis factor and interleukin-1, and reduced nitric oxide function. In patients with inherited or acquired protein C deficiency, an imbalance between thrombin generation and fibrinolysis may be responsible for overwhelming normal mechanisms that protect against inappropriate coagulation. Neutrophils can also contribute to the development of neutrophil extracellular traps, which have procoagulant properties.

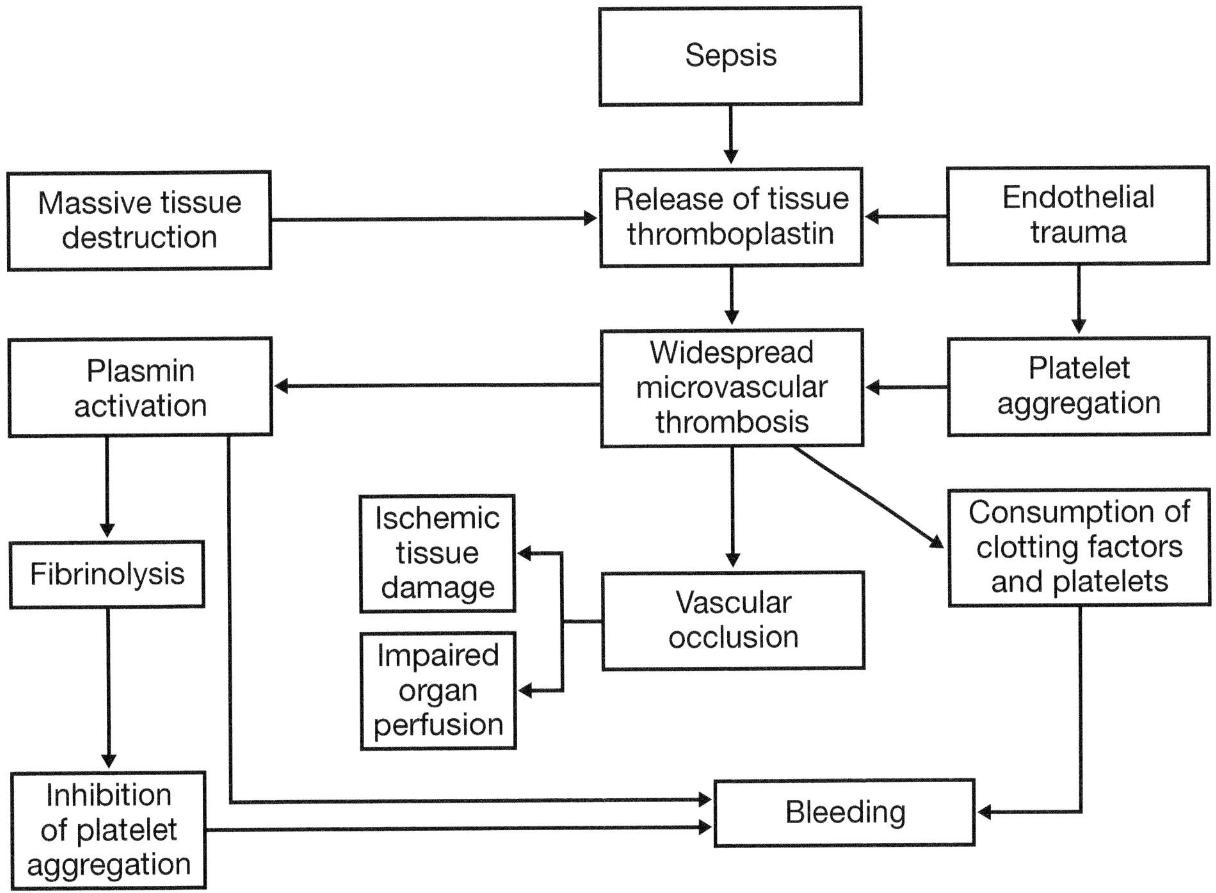

Figure 53.1. Pathophysiologic Pathways in Disseminated Intravascular Coagulation.

Further, the thrombus produced by activation of the coagulation cascade leads to consumption of endogenous coagulation factors, creating a "consumption coagulopathy," and of anticoagulant factors such as protein C, protein S, and antithrombin (AT), and also platelets. Fibrinolysis is activated by the generation of fibrin degradation products (FDPs) at the locations of thrombus formation. When present in substantial quantifies, FDPs can hinder fibrin clot formation and also platelet aggregation. With thrombus formation or bleeding, tissue or organ damage can ensue from reduced perfusion. Other vascular causes that could contribute to the pathogenesis of DIC are endothelial damage, which can result in the release of procoagulant substances and the loss of endothelial antithrombotic properties; reduced local blood flow, which slows diffusion of procoagulant and anticoagulant factors away from the site; and reduced organ perfusion, which may delay hepatic clearance of coagulation by-products. Levels of nitric oxide may be reduced, an effect causing increased vascular tone and enhanced platelet aggregation and activation.

Clinical Manifestations

Clinical findings consistent with acute DIC include bleeding, especially oozing from sites of trauma, catheters, or drains; thrombocytopenia; prolonged in vitro coagulation times (activated partial thromboplastin time [aPTT] and prolonged prothrombin time [PT]); increased D-dimer level but low level of plasma fibrinogen; increased thrombin time; and reduced levels of procoagulant factors such as factors II, V, VII, and X and natural anticoagulants such as protein C, protein S, and AT. Peripheral blood smear may show microangiopathic changes. The bleeding in acute DIC can be life-threatening if it involves the gastrointestinal tract, lungs, or central nervous system.

Chronic (compensated) DIC, usually occurring in patients with advanced malignant tumors, particularly ovarian, gastric, pancreatic, and brain tumors, manifests when blood is intermittently or continuously exposed to smaller quantities of TF or other procoagulant substances. Coagulation factors and platelets are consumed, but production can compensate, and the liver is able to clear the

FDPs. In vitro coagulation times may be normal, and thrombocytopenia may be mild or absent. Thrombosis generally predominates over bleeding, although many patients are asymptomatic with laboratory-only evidence of increased thrombin generation and fibrinolysis. Although none of the clinical findings are highly specific to chronic DIC, a combination of the following findings may be consistent with chronic DIC: venous or arterial thromboembolism, especially without another clear precipitating factor; mild or no thrombocytopenia; normal or mildly prolonged PT and aPTT; normal or even slightly increased plasma fibrinogen level; increased plasma D-dimer level, and microangiopathic changes on peripheral blood smear. Thromboembolic manifestations of DIC include venous thromboembolism and arterial thrombosis with tissue or organ ischemia. Also, patients with chronic DIC in the setting of a malignant tumor can also have development of nonbacterial thrombotic endocarditis (marantic endocarditis, Libman-Sacks endocarditis, verrucous endocarditis) and superficial migratory thrombophlebitis (Trousseau syndrome).

Unlike some of the other thrombotic microangiopathies (TMAs), such as complement-mediated hemolytic uremic syndrome and thrombotic thrombocytopenic purpura, which are characterized by platelet-rich microthrombi without substantial fibrin clot formation or consumption coagulopathy, DIC is associated with microvascular thrombi that contain fibrin and platelets. Thus, other TMAs generally present with thrombocytopenia and normal results of coagulation studies. However, both DIC and TMAs can cause microangiopathic hemolytic anemia and show schistocytes on peripheral blood smear. Schistocytes in DIC are formed as red blood cells pass through fibrin strands and microthrombi and become mechanically sheared.

Organ dysfunction occurs more often with acute DIC than with chronic DIC and can be due to various mechanisms, including vascular thrombosis, hemorrhage, and hypoperfusion. Jaundice from hepatic dysfunction is common in DIC. Preexisting liver failure can exacerbate DIC by impairing hepatic production or clearance of clotting factors. Pulmonary hemorrhage with hemoptysis and dyspnea can result from injury to the pulmonary vascular endothelium. This may be particularly concerning in patients with acute respiratory distress syndrome because of their underlying condition. Several neurologic abnormalities including delirium, coma, and transient focal neurologic symptoms can occur in patients with DIC.

Purpura fulminans, a rare, life-threatening condition with extensive tissue thrombosis and hemorrhagic skin necrosis, can occur with DIC. Many patients with this condition have inherited protein C deficiency (homozygous or compound heterozygous deficiency). Presentation in early infancy is common, but older patients are also occasionally affected. Purpura fulminans can also manifest in the setting of severe acquired protein C deficiency and also in severe meningococcal infections.

Table 53.3 • ISTH Scoring System for Diagnosis of DIC

Underlying Clinical Condition Predisposing to DIC	Essential
Platelet count, $\times 10^9$/L	50-100: 1 point <50: 2 points
Fibrin-related marker (eg, D-dimer, FDP)	Moderate increase: 2 points Marked increase: 3 points
Fibrinogen, g/L	<1: 1 point
Prothrombin time	Prolonged by 3-6 seconds: 1 point Prolonged by >6 seconds: 2 points
DIC diagnosis	≥5 points

Abbreviations: DIC, disseminated intravascular coagulation; FDP, fibrin degradation product; ISTH, International Society on Thrombosis and Haemostasis.

Data from Taylor FB Jr, Toh CH, Hoots WK, Wada H, Levi M; Scientific Subcommittee on Disseminated Intravascular Coagulation (DIC) of the International Society on Thrombosis and Haemostasis (ISTH). Towards definition, clinical and laboratory criteria, and a scoring system for disseminated intravascular coagulation. Thromb Haemost. 2001 Nov;86(5):1327-30.

Diagnostic Evaluation

No laboratory test can accurately confirm or eliminate the diagnosis of DIC. The findings of thrombocytopenia, low fibrinogen level, and increased D-dimer level are sensitive, but not specific, for DIC. It is a clinical diagnosis based on the findings of fibrinolysis or coagulopathy in an appropriate setting. The Scientific Subcommittee on DIC of the International Society on Thrombosis and Haemostasis developed a 5-step diagnostic algorithm to calculate a DIC score (Table 53.3). The presence of an underlying illness that is known to be associated with DIC is essential for diagnosis of acute or overt DIC. A score of 5 or more is compatible with DIC, but a score of less than 5 may be suggestive but not affirmative of chronic or nonovert DIC. For patients with findings suggestive of DIC who do not have an obvious underlying cause, the underlying condition causing coagulopathy and other plausible causes of bleeding, thrombosis, and laboratory abnormalities should be evaluated.

In patients suspected to have DIC, the laboratory assessment should include a complete blood count, review of the peripheral blood smear, and screening tests of coagulation (ie, PT, aPTT, fibrinogen, and D-dimer). The frequency of these tests may depend on the severity of DIC. Once- or twice-daily testing may be appropriate in an acutely ill patient with active bleeding or thrombosis, whereas less frequent testing would be reasonable in a patient with only laboratory abnormalities. It is imperative to note that several conditions other than DIC, such as venous thromboembolism, recent surgery, or trauma, could be associated with increased D-dimer and FDP levels. In critically ill patients, a prolonged PT cannot be routinely attributed to DIC, because they may not have received adequate nutrition and would have received several antibiotics causing vitamin K deficiency, factors affecting vitamin K-dependent hemostasis. Also, because FDPs are metabolized in the liver and eliminated by the kidneys, hepatic and renal impairment can influence the levels. Thus, determining the FDP level must not be considered as a stand-alone test in DIC, but it can be a useful indicator when the D-dimer level is increased concomitantly with a decrease in the platelet count and abnormal coagulation times. Natural anticoagulants such as AT and protein C are frequently reduced in DIC, and such decreases may have prognostic significance.

The differential diagnosis of DIC includes other disorders associated with bleeding and hypercoagulability and other causes of microangiopathic hemolytic anemia and thrombocytopenia. Some conditions, such as liver failure, can be either a cause of DIC or a consequence of DIC. In such cases, the diagnosis of the other condition does not reject the possibility of DIC. Akin to DIC, severe liver disease is associated with reductions in both procoagulant and anticoagulant factors and thrombocytopenia, and patients can have bleeding or thrombosis. Thrombocytopenia in severe liver disease is often caused by a combination of hypersplenism and thrombopoietin deficiency because the liver is the primary site of thrombopoietin synthesis. Checking the plasma factor VIII level can be considered. Because factor VIII is not produced by hepatocytes, its level is often low in DIC and high in severe liver disease. Patients with TMAs present with microangiopathic hemolytic anemia and thrombocytopenia due to platelet consumption in microvascular thrombi. They may be acutely ill and thrombocytopenic and have schistocytes on the peripheral blood smear, as in DIC, but they have a normal coagulation profile because the microvascular thrombi in these conditions are primarily platelet-rich and fibrin-poor thrombi and are not associated with consumption coagulopathy. Occasionally, TMA that leads to organ ischemia can in turn trigger DIC.

Heparin-induced thrombocytopenia, which is due to the production of autoantibodies to platelet factor epitope incited by heparin binding to platelets after exposure to heparin, mostly manifests as thrombocytopenia and occasionally with thrombosis and rarely bleeding. Unlike DIC, patients with heparin-induced thrombocytopenia typically have recent heparin exposure and a positive serologic result for heparin-platelet factor epitope antibodies (heparin-induced thrombocytopenia antibodies). Also, patients with heparin-induced thrombocytopenia do not have global coagulation abnormalities, except for abnormalities caused by their anticoagulant or an increased D-dimer level associated with thromboembolism.

Treatment

DIC typically develops as a consequence of other disorders, and thus the basis of its treatment is management of the underlying disease. Treating DIC is usually not very effective if the provoking process cannot be stopped. In general, systemic therapies such as prohemostatic or anticoagulant agents are not used prophylactically to prevent bleeding or thrombosis. However, patients are closely monitored for bleeding and thrombotic complications, and these complications should be treated promptly if they occur. Furthermore, ancillary measures and supportive care (eg, hemodynamic and ventilatory support) should be initiated for a good clinical outcome. The ancillary measures can be categorized as blood product transfusion support and treatments that modify thrombin generation. Given its ubiquity, modulating thrombin generation can target procoagulant and profibrinolytic activities in DIC.

Transfusion Support

In patients with DIC, blood product transfusion includes platelets, fibrinogen replacement in the form of cryoprecipitate or fibrinogen concentrates, and fresh frozen plasma. Platelet transfusion should be considered when the patient has bleeding and the platelet count is less than 50×10^9/L. A lower threshold of 20 to 30×10^9/L can be used in patients without bleeding. The threshold for platelet transfusion depends on the clinical situation and the severity of thrombocytopenia. Fresh frozen plasma is usually given if there is bleeding and the PT or aPTT is prolonged (more than 1.5 times the upper limit of normal range). The preferred dose is 15 to 20 mL/kg, but a higher dose may be needed in patients with severe bleeding. Notably, prolongation of the PT or aPTT in DIC may also be related to interference by FDPs. Certain coagulation factors such as factor V are absent in prothrombin complex concentrates. Thus, prothrombin complex concentrate is used only if fresh frozen plasma is contraindicated because of volume overload. Cryoprecipitate should be considered in patients with bleeding and a fibrinogen level less than 100 mg/dL. Fibrinogen concentrates might offer more consistent fibrinogen replacement, but such products are not currently approved for management of DIC.

Modulating Thrombin Generation

Despite sparse evidence that heparin administration reverses organ dysfunction associated with DIC, it has been used historically as a treatment option. In recent years, low-molecular-weight heparin has been used more often in lieu of unfractionated heparin because of its reliable pharmacokinetics and lower bleeding risks. A Japanese study involving 125 patients with DIC showed the substantial improvements of reduced bleeding symptoms and organ failure and higher safety with dalteparin compared with unfractionated heparin. In patients who are deemed to be at high risk of bleeding, unfractionated heparin may still be considered because of its shorter half-life and quick reversibility of its effect.

In DIC, AT, a natural anticoagulant, is depleted early in the course of excessive thrombin generation. A low AT level is known to be an indicator of poor clinical outcome in patients with sepsis and also an independent prognosticator of mortality in DIC. A randomized study of 51 patients with DIC and shock found that administration of AT considerably shortened the duration of DIC compared with heparin alone. Similarly, a post hoc exploration of a much larger clinical trial (KyberSept) in which 229 patients with DIC received high-dose AT without concomitant heparin found a considerable decrease in 28-day mortality compared with placebo. AT treatment for DIC is not yet approved worldwide, although a tailored dosing of AT has been approved in Japan.

The efficacy of activated protein C (drotrecogin alfa) in severe sepsis was shown in a randomized controlled trial (Protein C Worldwide Evaluation in Severe Sepsis, PROWESS). Mortality was reduced (24.7%) in the activated protein C cohort compared with that in the placebo cohort (30.8%), and patients with DIC had the highest benefit. Conversely, a conflicting report of its efficacy in patients with septic shock prompted another study, PROWESS-SHOCK, which did not show any difference in 28-day all-cause mortality in the group receiving activated protein C (26.4%) compared with that in the placebo group (24.2%), even in those with severe protein C deficiency. The results led to withdrawal of activated protein C from the market.

Patients with purpura fulminans seem to benefit from the administration of protein C concentrate, according to the data from a small series of 12 patients with purpura fulminans. Despite a predicted mortality rate of 60% to 80%, none of the patients who received protein C concentrate infusion (administered as a continuous infusion to maintain the plasma concentration between 0.8 and 1.2 IU/mL) died.

Soluble thrombomodulin is being evaluated in clinical trials. Its anticoagulant property is dependent on the amount of thrombin generated and, thus, theoretically has less bleeding risk than other anticoagulants such as activated protein C. In a multicenter, randomized controlled clinical trial comparing the effects of recombinant soluble thermomodulin to those of heparin in patients with DIC due to infection and cancer, the resolution rate of DIC was 66.1% with soluble thermomodulin and 49.9% with heparin. Patients with infection-related DIC treated with soluble thermomodulin also had a substantially decreased mortality rate (28.0% vs 34.6%) and also favorable changes in hematologic markers and bleeding-related events. More recently, a trial of 65 patients with DIC due to sepsis who required ventilator management had considerably lower 28-day mortality with recombinant soluble thermomodulin than the control group (25% vs 47%) and a quick reduction in the Sequential Organ Failure Assessment score on day 1, a suggestion of an organ-protective effect of soluble thermomodulin in the setting of sepsis.

Modulating Profibrinolytic Activity

Hyperfibrinolysis, a common phenomenon in DIC, is a natural reactionary process to deal with the uncontrolled thrombin generation. Thus, inhibiting excessive fibrinolysis with antifibrinolytic agents such as ε-aminocaproic acid, tranexamic acid, or aprotinin may be harmful for patients with DIC. In the acute coagulopathy of trauma, wherein hyperfibrinolysis is extensive, antifibrinolytic agents are beneficial only for patients with persistent bleeding after adequate replacement of fresh frozen plasma. In this situation, administration of tranexamic acid (loading dose of 1 g given over 10 minutes followed by an 8-hour infusion of 1 g) substantially decreased the risk of hemorrhage-related death in patients with trauma while not increasing the vascular occlusive events. Another clinical context in which tranexamic acid has been beneficial is massive postpartum hemorrhage, in which fibrinolysis is a major pathophysiologic factor in causing coagulopathy.

Summary

- DIC is a maladaptive responsiveness of coagulation and hemostatic systems with simultaneous hemorrhagic and microvascular thrombotic events. With an important cross-talk among inflammatory pathways, coagulation cascade, and innate immune processes, treatment for DIC is likely to require multimodality approaches.
- DIC is a clinical and laboratory diagnosis, based on findings of coagulopathy or fibrinolysis in the appropriate setting. No single laboratory test can accurately confirm or eliminate the diagnosis.
- The management strategy, in addition to addressing the underlying cause, should be individualized, dependent on the clinical scenario of thrombosis or hemorrhage.

SUGGESTED READING

Arepally GM. Heparin-induced thrombocytopenia. Blood. 2017 May 25;129(21):2864–72. Epub 2017 Apr 17.

Bernard GR, Vincent JL, Laterre PF, LaRosa SP, Dhainaut JF, Lopez-Rodriguez A, et al; Recombinant human protein C Worldwide Evaluation in Severe Sepsis (PROWESS) study group: efficacy and safety of recombinant human activated protein C for severe sepsis. N Engl J Med. 2001 Mar 8;344(10):699–709.

Capon SM, Goldfinger D. Acute hemolytic transfusion reaction, a paradigm of the systemic inflammatory response: new insights into pathophysiology and treatment. Transfusion. 1995 Jun;35(6):513–20. Erratum in: Transfusion 1995 Sep;35(9):794.

Chang JC. Disseminated intravascular coagulation: is it fact or fancy? Blood Coagul Fibrinolysis. 2018 Apr;29(3):330–7.

Choi Q, Hong KH, Kim JE, Kim HK. Changes in plasma levels of natural anticoagulants in disseminated intravascular coagulation: high prognostic value of antithrombin and protein C in patients with underlying sepsis or severe infection. Ann Lab Med. 2014 Mar;34(2):85–91. Epub 2014 Feb 13.

CRASH-2 trial collaborators, Shakur H, Roberts I, Bautista R, Caballero J, Coats T, Dewan Y, et al. Effects of tranexamic acid on death, vascular occlusive events, and blood transfusion in trauma patients with significant haemorrhage (CRASH-2): a randomised, placebo-controlled trial. Lancet. 2010 Jul 3;376(9734):23–32. Epub 2010 Jun 14.

Delabranche X, Stiel L, Severac F, Galoisy AC, Mauvieux L, Zobairi F, et al. Evidence of netosis in septic shock-induced disseminated intravascular coagulation. Shock. 2017 Mar;47(3):313–7.

Drolz A, Horvatits T, Roedl K, Rutter K, Staufer K, Kneidinger N, et al. Coagulation parameters and major bleeding in critically ill patients with cirrhosis. Hepatology. 2016 Aug;64(2):556–68. Epub 2016 Jun 9.

Ducloy-Bouthors AS, Jude B, Duhamel A, Broisin F, Huissoud C, Keita-Meyer H, et al; EXADELI Study Group, Susen S. High-dose tranexamic acid reduces blood loss in postpartum haemorrhage. Crit Care. 2011;15(2):R117. Epub 2011 Apr 15.

Fourrier F, Chopin C, Goudemand J, Hendrycx S, Caron C, Rime A, et al. Septic shock, multiple organ failure, and disseminated intravascular coagulation. Compared patterns of antithrombin III, protein C, and protein S deficiencies. Chest. 1992 Mar;101(3):816–23.

Gando S, Nanzaki S, Kemmotsu O. Disseminated intravascular coagulation and sustained systemic inflammatory response syndrome predict organ dysfunctions after trauma: application of clinical decision analysis. Ann Surg. 1999 Jan;229(1):121–7.

Gando S, Wada H, Thachil J; Scientific and Standardization Committee on DIC of the International Society on Thrombosis and Haemostasis (ISTH). Differentiating disseminated intravascular coagulation (DIC) with the fibrinolytic phenotype from coagulopathy of trauma and acute coagulopathy of trauma-shock (COT/ACOTS). J Thromb Haemost. 2013 May;11(5):826–35.

Kienast J, Juers M, Wiedermann CJ, Hoffmann JN, Ostermann H, Strauss R, et al; KyberSept investigators. Treatment effects of high-dose antithrombin without concomitant heparin in patients with severe sepsis with or without disseminated intravascular coagulation. J Thromb Haemost. 2006 Jan;4(1):90–7.

Kitchens CS. Thrombocytopenia and thrombosis in disseminated intravascular coagulation (DIC). Hematology Am Soc Hematol Educ Program. 2009 Jan;2009(1):240–6.

Kujovich JL. Coagulopathy in liver disease: a balancing act. Hematology Am Soc Hematol Educ Program. 2015;2015:243–9.

Kyowa Hakko Kirin Company. Approval for ACOALAN in Japan. c2015 [cited 2018 Sep 10]. Available from: http://www.kyowa-kirin.com/news_releases/2015/e20150703_01.html.

Levi M, Ten Cate H. Disseminated intravascular coagulation. N Engl J Med. 1999 Aug 19;341(8):586–92.

Levi M, Toh CH, Thachil J, Watson HG; British Committee for Standards in Haematology. Guidelines for the diagnosis and management of disseminated intravascular coagulation. Br J Haematol. 2009 Apr;145(1):24–33. Epub 2009 Feb 12.

Matsuda T. Clinical aspects of DIC: disseminated intravascular coagulation. Pol J Pharmacol. 1996 Jan-Feb;48(1):73–5.

Ranieri VM, Thompson BT, Barie PS, Dhainaut JF, Douglas IS, Finfer S, et al; PROWESS-SHOCK Study Group. Drotrecogin alfa (activated) in adults with septic shock. N Engl J Med. 2012 May 31;366(22):2055–64. Epub 2012 May 22.

Saha M, McDaniel JK, Zheng XL. Thrombotic thrombocytopenic purpura: pathogenesis, diagnosis and potential novel therapeutics. J Thromb Haemost. 2017 Oct;15(10):1889–1900. Epub 2017 Jul 27.

Saito H, Maruyama I, Shimazaki S, Yamamoto Y, Aikawa N, Ohno R, et al. Efficacy and safety of recombinant human soluble thrombomodulin (ART-123) in disseminated intravascular coagulation: results of a phase III, randomized, double-blind clinical trial. J Thromb Haemost. 2007 Jan;5(1):31–41. Epub 2006 Oct 13.

Sakuragawa N, Hasegawa H, Maki M, Nakagawa M, Nakashima M. Clinical evaluation of low-molecular-weight heparin (FR-860) on disseminated intravascular coagulation (DIC): a multicenter co-operative double-blind trial in comparison with heparin. Thromb Res. 1993 Dec 15;72(6):475–500.

Sallah S, Wan JY, Nguyen NP, Hanrahan LR, Sigounas G. Disseminated intravascular coagulation in solid tumors: clinical and pathologic study. Thromb Haemost. 2001 Sep;86(3):828–33.

Sibai BM, Ramadan MK, Usta I, Salama M, Mercer BM, Friedman SA. Maternal morbidity and mortality in 442 pregnancies with hemolysis, elevated liver enzymes, and low platelets (HELLP syndrome). Am J Obstet Gynecol. 1993 Oct;169(4):1000–6.

Smith OP, White B, Vaughan D, Rafferty M, Claffey L, Lyons B, et al. Use of protein-C concentrate, heparin, and haemodiafiltration in meningococcus-induced purpura fulminans. Lancet. 1997 Nov 29;350(9091):1590–3.

Squizzato A, Hunt BJ, Kinasewitz GT, Wada H, Ten Cate H, Thachil J, et al. Supportive management strategies for disseminated intravascular coagulation: an international consensus. Thromb Haemost. 2016 May 2;115(5):896–904. Epub 2015 Dec 17.

Taylor FB Jr, Toh CH, Hoots WK, Wada H, Levi M; Scientific Subcommittee on Disseminated Intravascular Coagulation (DIC) of the International Society on Thrombosis and Haemostasis (ISTH). Towards definition, clinical and laboratory criteria, and a scoring system for disseminated intravascular coagulation. Thromb Haemost. 2001 Nov;86(5):1327–30.

Toh CH, Alhamdi Y. Current consideration and management of disseminated intravascular coagulation. Hematology Am Soc Hematol Educ Program. 2013;2013:286–91.

Umemura Y, Yamakawa K, Hayakawa M, Hamasaki T, Fujimi S; Japan Septic Disseminated Intravascular Coagulation (J-Septic DIC) study group. Screening itself for disseminated intravascular coagulation may reduce mortality in sepsis: a nationwide multicenter registry in Japan. Thromb Res. 2018 Jan;161:60–6. Epub 2017 Nov 26.

Wada H, Thachil J, Di Nisio M, Mathew P, Kurosawa S, Gando S, et al; The Scientific Standardization Committee on DIC of the International Society on

Thrombosis Haemostasis. Guidance for diagnosis and treatment of DIC from harmonization of the recommendations from three guidelines. J Thromb Haemost. 2013 Feb 4. [Epub ahead of print]

Yamakawa K, Fujimi S, Mohri T, Matsuda H, Nakamori Y, Hirose T, et al. Treatment effects of recombinant human soluble thrombomodulin in patients with severe sepsis: a historical control study. Crit Care. 2011;15(3):R123. Epub 2011 May 11.

Yatabe T, Inoue S, Sakamoto S, Sumi Y, Nishida O, Hayashida K, et al. The anticoagulant treatment for sepsis induced disseminated intravascular coagulation; network meta-analysis. Thromb Res. 2018 Nov;171:136–42. Epub 2018 Oct 6.

Diagnosis and Management of Acquired Bleeding Disorders[a]

RAJIV K. PRUTHI, MBBS

Goals

- Review the pathophysiology of coagulation.
- Know the clinical presentation and differential diagnosis of acquired bleeding disorders.
- Recall the appropriate laboratory evaluation of acquired bleeding disorders.
- Formulate an optimal management plan for acquired bleeding disorders.
- Understand the pathophysiology, clinical presentation, and evaluation of acquired coagulopathy.

Introduction

The hemostatic response to vascular injury consists of vascular constriction, platelet activation resulting in platelet adhesion (mediated by von Willebrand factor [VWF]), and platelet aggregation resulting in an initial platelet plug formation at the site of vascular injury. This platelet plug is stabilized by formation of fibrin, which results from activation of the procoagulant coagulation factors. Congenital or acquired abnormalities of the procoagulant factors result in a bleeding and thrombotic tendency of variable severity. Acquired abnormalities of the procoagulant system are typically associated underlying systemic disorders; however, they may also be idiopathic. Recognition, laboratory diagnosis, and principles of management of acquired coagulopathy are reviewed in this chapter.

Pathophysiology, Clinical Presentation, and Evaluation of Acquired Coagulopathy

Acquired perturbations of the coagulation system predispose patients to hemorrhage and characteristically present with adulthood onset of bleeding symptoms and lack of a family history of a bleeding disorder. The acquired coagulopathy may come to light because of incidental findings on routine laboratory testing or presentation with acute or subacute (spontaneous or trauma- or surgery-induced) hemorrhage. It is typically associated with medications, underlying autoimmune disorders, or a malignant condition. Knowing a patient's comorbid illnesses may facilitate diagnosis of the bleeding disorder.

Initial evaluation consists of obtaining a detailed history (including personal and family history of bleeding), physical examination, and assessment of all prescription and, particularly, nonprescription (herbal) medicaments. Spontaneous onset of bleeding portends a severe bleeding disorder, whereas bleeding provoked by surgery or trauma suggests a mild or moderate disorder. Initial laboratory testing typically consists of routine tests (discussed below and in Table 54.1), and more specialized testing is used as needed. Results, when interpreted within the context of a patient's clinical presentation, generally provide sufficient information for immediate management while results of additional, more specialized tests are pending. However, while these results are awaited, a differential diagnosis of acquired bleeding disorder should be considered.

[a] Portions previously published in Pruthi RK. Hemostatic disorders. In: Wittich CM, editor. Mayo Clinic internal medicine board review. 11th ed. New York (NY): Oxford University Press; c2016. p. 415-25. (Mayo Clinic Scientific Press series); used with permission of Mayo Foundation for Medical Education and Research.

Table 54.1 • Underlying Disorders and Associated Findings on Coagulation Test Results

Condition	CBC (Platelet Count)	PT	aPTT	Fibrinogen	D-Dimer	VWF Levels
Artifact of high hematocrit	High hemoglobin/ hematocrit	Prolonged[a]	Prolonged[a]	No effect	No effect	Normal
Anticoagulant contamination[b]	No effect	Prolonged[c]	Prolonged[d]	No effect	No effect	Normal
Acquired von Willebrand syndrome	No effect	No effect	May prolong[a]	No effect	No direct effect[b]	Reduced
Autoimmune factor VIII inhibitors	No effect	No effect	Prolonged[c]	No effect	No direct effect[b]	Normal
Autoimmune factor V inhibitors	No effect	Prolonged[c]	Prolonged[c]	No effect	No direct effect[b]	Normal
Liver disease	Thrombocytopenia	Prolonged[a]	Prolonged[a]	Decreased	Increased	Increased
DIC	Thrombocytopenia	Prolonged[a]	Prolonged[a]	Decreased	Increased	Increased

Abbreviations: aPTT, activated partial thromboplastin time; CBC, complete blood count; DIC, disseminated intravascular coagulation and fibrinolysis; PT, prothrombin time; VWF, von Willebrand factor.

[a] Corrects on mixing study with normal pooled plasma.

[b] Heparin or direct thrombin inhibitor; may be increased as a result of hemorrhage.

[c] With direct thrombin inhibitors.

[d] Inhibited on mixing study.

Common Differential Diagnosis of Acquired Bleeding Disorders

Acquired bleeding disorders can be broadly categorized into those that primarily affect platelets or coagulation factors (including von Willebrand factor) and those that affect multiple components. Platelet disorders were discussed in Chapter 52 ("Thrombocytopenia and Thrombocytopathy"). Acquired abnormalities of 1 or more coagulation factors can be broadly categorized into coagulation factor deficiencies or inhibitors. Diagnosis requires specialized assays.

Overview and Interpretation of Laboratory Assays

A complete blood count (CBC) with white blood cell differential count provides information on platelet count and the presence or absence of circulating leukemic blasts. It is important to exclude pseudothrombocytopenia, an in vitro phenomenon due to EDTA-mediated platelet clumping for which a peripheral blood smear or repeat CBC in citrate anticoagulant will help differentiate from true thrombocytopenia. Prolonged prothrombin time (PT) or activated partial thromboplastin time (aPTT) may be artifactual (high hematocrit, diluted sample), contaminated with anticoagulant (eg, heparin-coated central venous or arterial catheters), or due to coagulation factor deficiency or the presence of an inhibitor (Figure 54.1).

Once artifact or contamination has been excluded, the next step is to perform mixing studies with normal pooled plasma. Correction of the clotting time into reference range suggests a coagulation factor deficiency (congenital or acquired), whereas shortening but not complete correction into the reference range suggests the presence of an inhibitor. Three broad types of inhibitors should be considered: medications (eg, heparins and direct thrombin and factor Xa inhibitors); specific coagulation factor inhibitors (eg, factor VIII or factor V inhibitors), which are risks for bleeding; or nonspecific inhibitors (eg, lupus anticoagulants), which pose a risk for thrombosis. Follow-up specialized coagulation factor assays or inhibitor testing typically leads to diagnosis of the underlying cause of the prolonged PT and aPTT. Typical findings in various coagulopathies are listed in Table 54.1.

It is very important to consider bleeding disorders that do not prolong the PT or aPTT. These disorders include platelet function defects, mild von Willebrand disease, factor XIII abnormalities, and deficiencies of components of the fibrinolytic proteins such as α_2-antiplasmin and plasminogen activator-1 inhibitor.

Acquired Bleeding Disorders

Acquired von Willebrand Syndrome

Pathophysiology and Clinical Presentation

Acquired von Willebrand syndrome (AVWS) is associated with various diseases that, through multiple mechanisms, lead to a variable reduction of VWF (Box 54.1). Deficiency or dysfunction of VWF leads to the inability of platelets to form a hemostatic platelet plug at sites of vascular injury.

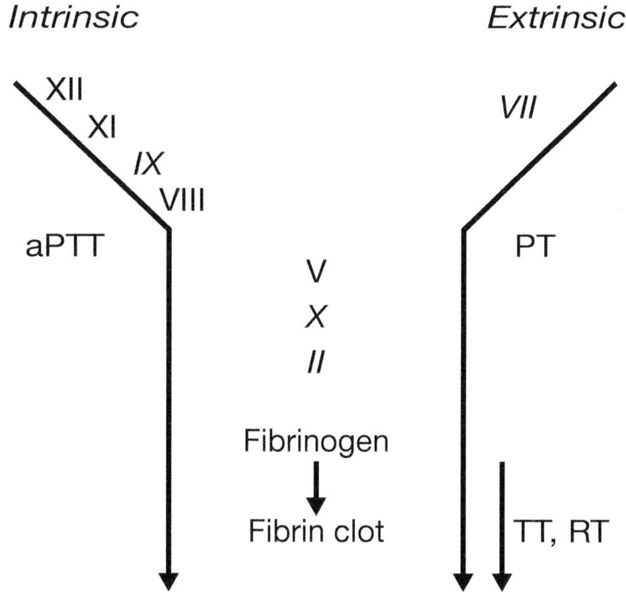

Figure 54.1. Simplified Coagulation Cascade Showing Coagulation Factors in the Intrinsic, Extrinsic, and Final Common Pathways. aPTT indicates activated partial thromboplastin time; PT, prothrombin time; RT, reptilase time; TT, thrombin time. Factors in italics are vitamin K–dependent coagulation factors.

Box 54.1 • Disorders Associated With Acquired von Willebrand Syndrome

- Malignancy
  - Monoclonal protein–associated disorders[a]
  - Lymphoproliferative disorders[b]
  - Myeloproliferative disorders[c]
  - Wilms tumor
- Autoimmune diseases
  - Systemic lupus erythematosus
  - Autoimmune thyroiditis
- Cardiovascular disorders
  - Ventricular assist device
  - Aortic stenosis
  - Hypertrophic cardiomyopathy
- Drugs
  - Valproic acid
  - Ciprofloxacin
  - Griseofulvin
  - Hydroxyethyl starch
- Other disorders
  - Inflammatory bowel disease
  - Hypothyroidism

[a] Including monoclonal gammopathy of undetermined significance, multiple myeloma, Waldenström macroglobulinemia, and systemic amyloidosis.

[b] Including non-Hodgkin lymphoma and chronic lymphocytic leukemia.

[c] Including essential thrombocythemia, polycythemia vera, and primary myelofibrosis.

Laboratory Diagnosis

Results of routine laboratory testing are listed in Table 54.1. VWF is a carrier protein for factor VIII, and thus it may result in low factor VIII and prolongation of the aPTT (Figure 54.1). However, the majority of patients with von Willebrand disease (congenital or acquired) have a normal aPTT, and thus a normal test result does not exclude the diagnosis. For suspected AVWS, assays for VWF antigen, VWF activity (eg, ristocetin cofactor activity), and factor VIII should be performed.

Management

Options for management of hemorrhage include desmopressin and VWF concentrate. In addition, potential underlying or associated disorders should be investigated. The response to desmopressin is typically short-lived. In fact, desmopressin is ineffective for severe deficiency of VWF, for which VWF concentrate should be used. If VWF concentrate is not available, cryoprecipitate, which contains VWF, may be used. Repeated dosing is typically needed and should be based on postinfusion VWF levels; the half-life of the infused concentrate may be very short, a characteristic feature of AVWS associated with monoclonal protein disorders. For AVWS associated with immunoglobulin G monoclonal proteins, administration of intravenous gamma globulin infusions typically increases endogenous VWF levels, and repeated infusions (generally every 3-4 weeks) may obviate VWF concentrate administration. Immunoglobulin M monoclonal protein–associated AVWS seldom responds to intravenous gamma globulin infusions.

Acquired (Autoimmune) Hemophilia

Pathophysiology and Clinical Presentation

Neutralizing autoantibodies against factor VIII cause the most commonly recognized acquired bleeding disorder due to coagulation factor inhibitors: acquired hemophilia. The autoantibodies occur spontaneously and, unlike in AVWS, are typically idiopathic, but occasionally they are associated with an underlying disorder (Box 54.2). Presentation is typically with mucocutaneous or potentially life- or limb-threatening soft tissue hemorrhage.

Laboratory Diagnosis

Results of laboratory tests are listed in Table 54.1. A mixing study of the prolonged aPTT will be inhibited (the clotting time fails to normalize), and reflexive coagulation factor (Figure 54.1) assays will show a markedly reduced factor VIII. Specialized assays to confirm and quantitate the factor VIII inhibitor are required.

Management

Up to 34% of patients may not require hemostatic therapy given their asymptomatic presentation or minor, non–life-threatening bleeding symptoms. When treatment is indicated, options for management of hemorrhage vary with inhibitor titer and institutional availability. For low titer (less than 5 Bethesda units), high doses of plasma-derived or recombinant factor VIII concentrates may be used (pending availability of alternative agents). However, this treatment typically results in an anamnestic increase in inhibitor titer, thus reducing hemostatic efficacy. The majority of patients eventually require bypassing agents.

Other agents, which may be available only at specialized centers, include bypassing agents such as activated prothrombin complex concentrates and recombinant factor VIIa. Plasma-derived porcine factor VIII has been used successfully; however, it is not currently available. Recombinant porcine factor VIII has been shown to be very effective. A limitation of bypassing agents (activated prothrombin complex concentrates and recombinant factor VIIa) is the lack of generally available coagulation assays to monitor effectiveness. However, the efficacy of recombinant porcine factor VIII concentrate can be monitored with use of factor VIII activity assays.

Measures to eliminate the inhibitor should be instituted once the diagnosis has been confirmed. The general approach is glucocorticoid as first-line therapy, as either a single agent or with a steroid-sparing agent (eg, cytotoxic chemotherapy such as cyclophosphamide or anti-CD20 antibody [rituximab]), for high-titer antibodies. With this approach, approximately 70% of patients achieve remission from the inhibitor at a median of 57 days.

Box 54.2 • Disorders Associated With Autoantibodies Against Factor VIII

- Associated disorder
- None (idiopathic)
- Malignancy
  - Solid-organ tumors
  - Lymphoproliferative disorders
- Autoimmune diseases
  - Systemic lupus erythematosus
  - Rheumatoid arthritis
  - Polymyalgia rheumatic
- Other disorders
  - Dermatologic conditions (eg, pemphigoid)
  - Pregnancy

Autoimmune Factor V Antibodies

Pathophysiology and Clinical Presentation

After factor VIII inhibitors, autoantibodies against factor V are likely the next most common cause of antibody-mediated acquired bleeding disorders. The antibodies are most commonly immunoglobulin G antibodies directed against functional epitopes on factor V. The majority of cases occur in association with antibiotic use, malignant conditions, or other autoimmune disorders (Box 54.3). The majority of patients present with mucocutaneous hemorrhage (gastrointestinal, genitourinary, and airway tracts).

Laboratory Diagnosis

Results of screening coagulation tests are listed in Table 54.1. Given that factor V is within the final common pathway (Figure 54.1), both PT and aPTT are prolonged and inhibited on a mixing study with normal pooled plasma. Additional coagulation factor assays typically lead to the diagnosis of factor V deficiency, and specialized tests are required to determine the titer.

Management

In the asymptomatic patient, expectant management with close observation is reasonable because spontaneous

Box 54.3 • Disorders Associated With Autoantibodies Against Factor V

- Associated disorder
- Idiopathic
- Surgery (cardiovascular, abdominal, and neurologic)
- Exposure to bovine protein (fibrin glue)
- Exposure to β-lactam antibiotics
- Malignancy
- Autoimmune disease

resolution of the inhibitor is common. For the symptomatic patient, as with management of autoimmune factor VIII inhibitors, there are 2 goals of therapy: 1) achievement and maintenance of hemostasis and 2) elimination of the inhibitor. Patients in whom the disorder is related to antibiotics seem to have the best prognosis: spontaneous resolution of the inhibitor with discontinuation of use of the offending antibiotic. Patients who have inhibitors occurring in association with autoimmune disorders or malignant conditions seem to have a worse prognosis. Options for maintaining hemostasis include fresh frozen plasma. However, the infused factor V present in fresh frozen plasma generally gets neutralized. Infusion of platelet concentrates results in achievement of hemostasis in up to 70% of patients. Intravenous immunoglobulin has been used.

Additional options include off-label use of activated prothrombin complex concentrates or recombinant factor VIIa. Immunosuppressive regimens including glucocorticoids alone or in association with alkylating agents (typically cyclophosphamide) result in suppression of the antibody in close to 60% of cases; anti-CD20 monoclonal antibody (rituximab) provides another alternative.

Liver Disease

Pathophysiology and Clinical Presentation

In advanced liver disease, there is a balanced reduction in procoagulant (except VWF and factor VIII, which are increased to variable degrees), anticoagulant, and fibrinolytic proteins with thrombocytopenia, the thrombocytopenia being due to splenomegaly and sequestration and decreased production of thrombopoietin. In aggregate, in stable liver disease, as measured by specialized thrombin-generation assays, hemostasis is balanced and the patient is not at substantially increased risk of either bleeding or thrombosis unless there is a triggering event (eg, infection, renal disease). Progressive liver disease leads to an imbalance in the hemostatic proteins, which tips the balance toward thrombosis or bleeding. The dogma that patients with severe liver disease are at high risk for bleeding may be due to their increased risk of variceal hemorrhage (an anatomical defect) and to findings of thrombocytopenia and prolonged PT and aPTT, which measure only the procoagulant component of the coagulation proteins. Patients with liver failure are also at risk for thromboses such as portal vein thrombosis.

Laboratory Diagnosis

The CBC shows mild to moderate thrombocytopenia. Screening coagulation tests (PT, aPTT) have prolonged results because of deficiencies in the procoagulant proteins. The thrombin time is generally prolonged if fibrinogen levels are substantially reduced. If measured, anticoagulant proteins (eg, protein C, antithrombin) are reduced to a variable extent. Although not assayed routinely, the fibrinolytic proteins (α_2-antiplasmin and plasminogen) are also reduced.

Distinguishing between severe liver disease and disseminated intravascular coagulation and fibrinolysis (DIC) is complex. However, in severe liver disease, VWF and factor VIII are markedly increased, whereas the factor VIII may be reduced in DIC.

Management

The majority of patients with advanced liver disease do not experience major hemorrhage, except perhaps for those with large varices, for which endoscopic therapy may be required. Indiscriminate infusion of fresh frozen plasma in an attempt to correct laboratory abnormalities should be avoided. Given that patients with advanced liver disease may be in more of a prothrombotic state, use of activated prothrombin complex concentrates and recombinant factor VIIa for management of hemorrhage should be avoided. Replenishment of the deficient coagulation factors with fresh frozen plasma and cryoprecipitate (more concentrated form for fibrinogen and factor XIII) may be indicated until the liver recovers or is replaced by a transplanted liver.

Disseminated Intravascular Coagulation

Pathophysiology and Clinical Presentation

DIC is a clinicopathologic syndrome associated with one or more underlying disorders (Box 54.4) that, through perturbation in proinflammatory cytokines, coagulation factors, and anticoagulant and fibrinolytic systems, result in microvascular thrombosis, consumption of clotting factors, and thrombocytopenia, which in turn predispose patients to hemorrhage.

Bleeding manifestations include bleeding from surgical wounds and venipuncture sites, whereas thrombotic manifestations include macrovascular thrombosis such as venous thromboembolism and acute arterial occlusions (stroke and myocardial infarction) or microvascular thrombosis including necrotic skin lesions, renal infarction, and acute kidney injury.

Laboratory Diagnosis

No single laboratory test is diagnostic of DIC. Because DIC is a clinicopathologic syndrome, the laboratory data need to be interpreted within the context of the clinical scenario (Box 54.4). Routine tests of coagulation typically identify thrombocytopenia, prolonged PT and aPTT (due to consumption of coagulation factors), and low levels of fibrinogen due to consumption. In addition, breakdown products of fibrin and fibrinogen (fibrin degradation products and D-dimers) provide evidence of ongoing fibrinolysis. An assay for the presence of soluble fibrin monomer complexes, which occur as a result of thrombin action on fibrinogen, is

Box 54.4 • Clinical Conditions Associated With Disseminated Intravascular Coagulation

Acute
- Sepsis, bacterial infections
- Trauma
- Obstetric complication (eg, abruptio placentae, amniotic fluid embolism)
- Snakebite (eg, viper and rattlesnake)
- Acute hemolytic transfusion reactions (eg, ABO-incompatible blood)

Chronic
- Malignancy
  - Hematologic (eg, acute leukemia)
  - Solid-organ (eg, pancreatic, gastric, prostate)
- Vascular malformations (eg, aortic aneurysm, congenital vascular malformations)
- Obstetric complication (eg, retained dead fetus)
- Advanced liver disease

a sensitive test for diagnosis of DIC. Other possible findings are consumption of the anticoagulants and a reduction in the fibrinolytic components (eg, α_2-antiplasmin, plasminogen activator inhibitor, and plasminogen). The complexity of diagnosing DIC has led to development of scoring systems to aid in the diagnosis (Box 54.5).

Box 54.5. • International Society on Thrombosis and Haemostasis Diagnostic Scoring System for Disseminated Intravascular Coagulation[a]

Platelet count, 10^9/L
- >100 = 0
- <100 = 1
- <50 = 2

Increased fibrin marker (eg, D-dimer, fibrin degradation products)
- No increase = 0
- Moderate increase = 2
- Strong increase = 3

Prothrombin time prolongation, seconds
- <3 = 0
- >3 but <6 = 1
- >6 = 2

Fibrinogen level, mg/dL
- >100 = 0
- <100 = 1

Calculate score
- ≥5 = compatible with overt DIC; repeat score daily
- <5 = suggestive for non-overt DIC; repeat score next 1-2 days

Abbreviation: DIC, disseminated intravascular coagulation.

[a] System is to be used with patient's identifiable underlying disorder known to be associated with overt disseminated intravascular coagulation.

Modified from Toh CH, Hoots WK; SSC on Disseminated Intravascular Coagulation of the ISTH. The scoring system of the Scientific and Standardisation Committee on Disseminated Intravascular Coagulation of the International Society on Thrombosis and Haemostasis: a 5-year overview. J Thromb Haemost. 2007 Mar;5(3):604-6. Epub 2006 Nov 10; used with permission.

Management

Approach to management varies with clinical presentation (eg, acute versus chronic) and whether the patient is experiencing hemorrhage. If underlying disease is not already apparent, identifying and treating it are important while managing the clinical manifestations of the coagulopathy. Judicious blood component replacement therapy is critical and should be avoided to treat solely laboratory abnormalities.

Transfusion of platelet concentrates should be avoided in thrombocytopenic patients with platelet counts more than 50×10^9/L who are not experiencing hemorrhage. This threshold may even be lowered, to 20×10^9/L, in patients at low risk of hemorrhage. For patients experiencing hemorrhage and those with platelet counts less than 20×10^9/L, therapeutic and prophylactic transfusions, respectively, should be considered. Infusion is with 1 unit of platelet concentrate at a time; additional infusions are based on clinical and laboratory assessment. Cryoprecipitate infusion is indicated for consumptive hypofibrinogenemia; the typical threshold is 100 mg/dL. Posttransfusion measurement of fibrinogen is important.

There are no clear PT or aPTT cutoffs for fresh frozen plasma infusion. Asymptomatic prolongation up to twice the upper reference range may be tolerated in the nonbleeding patient. However, in the actively bleeding patient, the goal of fresh frozen plasma infusions should be to control hemorrhage as opposed to correcting abnormally prolonged PT or aPTT. The role of prophylactic fresh frozen plasma infusion is unclear. At the other end of the spectrum, for patients presenting with low-grade compensated DIC with mild coagulopathy and no bleeding, withholding transfusion support pending a search for and management of the underlying disease is reasonable.

In addition to blood component support, adjunctive therapies may be indicated depending on the underlying disorders. Although unfractionated heparin inhibits thrombin and interrupts the cycle of consumptive coagulopathy, it is also associated with hemorrhage, including intracranial hemorrhage. Thus, in patients with acute DIC, heparin usually has a limited role, if any (except with acute DIC associated with promyelocytic leukemia), but it may have a role in chronic DIC, as found with solid tumors, the retained dead fetus syndrome, aortic aneurysm, and giant hemangiomas. Antithrombin concentrate has not been clearly shown to improve mortality among patients with DIC, and fibrinolysis inhibitors, such as ε-aminocaproic acid or tranexamic acid, are generally contraindicated in DIC.

Summary

- Adult onset of bleeding in a patient with no previous personal history of spontaneous or trauma- or surgery-induced hemorrhage or a family history of hemorrhage strongly suggests development of an acquired bleeding disorder.
- Laboratory abnormalities noted on initial testing (Table 54.1) are not generally diagnostic of any particular coagulopathy. Thus, clinical correlation with the patient's underlying comorbidities and specialized testing are important in pursuing the diagnosis.
- An existing comorbidity such as a malignant condition or other autoimmune disorders and performance of coagulation assays generally lead to the diagnosis of the underlying coagulopathy.
- Results of special coagulation testing generally confirm the underlying diagnosis and thus direct optimal management of bleeding.
- Management options for achieving and maintaining hemostasis vary with the underlying coagulopathy and should be judiciously applied.

SUGGESTED READING

Bar-Natan M, Hymes KB. Management of intraoperative coagulopathy. Neurosurg Clin N Am. 2018 Oct;29(4):557–65.

Bobba RK, Garg P, Arya M, Freter CE. Postoperative bleeding in an elderly patient from acquired factor V inhibitor: rapid response to immunosuppressive therapy. Am J Med Sci. 2011 Mar;341(3):253–6.

Collins PW, Hirsch S, Baglin TP, Dolan G, Hanley J, Makris M, et al; UK Haemophilia Centre Doctors' Organisation. Acquired hemophilia A in the United Kingdom: a 2-year national surveillance study by the United Kingdom Haemophilia Centre Doctors' Organisation. Blood. 2007 Mar 1;109(5):1870–7. Epub 2006 Oct 17.

Di Nisio M, Baudo F, Cosmi B, D'Angelo A, De Gasperi A, Malato A, et al; Italian Society for Thrombosis and Haemostasis. Diagnosis and treatment of disseminated intravascular coagulation: guidelines of the Italian Society for Haemostasis and Thrombosis (SISET). Thromb Res. 2012 May;129(5):e177–84. Epub 2011 Sep 17.

Federici AB, Stabile F, Castaman G, Canciani MT, Mannucci PM. Treatment of acquired von Willebrand syndrome in patients with monoclonal gammopathy of uncertain significance: comparison of three different therapeutic approaches. Blood. 1998 Oct 15;92(8):2707–11.

Franchini M, Lippi G. Acquired factor V inhibitors: a systematic review. J Thromb Thrombolysis. 2011 May;31(4):449–57.

Franchini M, Mannucci PM. Von Willebrand disease-associated angiodysplasia: a few answers, still many questions. Br J Haematol. 2013 Apr;161(2):177–82. Epub 2013 Feb 23.

Hay CR, Negrier C, Ludlam CA. The treatment of bleeding in acquired haemophilia with recombinant factor VIIa: a multicentre study. Thromb Haemost. 1997 Dec;78(6):1463–7.

Kamal AH, Tefferi A, Pruthi RK. How to interpret and pursue an abnormal prothrombin time, activated partial thromboplastin time, and bleeding time in adults. Mayo Clin Proc. 2007 Jul;82(7):864–73.

Kitchens CS. Prolonged activated partial thromboplastin time of unknown etiology: a prospective study of 100 consecutive cases referred for consultation. Am J Hematol. 1988 Jan;27(1):38–45.

Kruse-Jarres R, St-Louis J, Greist A, Shapiro A, Smith H, Chowdary P, et al. Efficacy and safety of OBI-1, an antihaemophilic factor VIII (recombinant), porcine sequence, in subjects with acquired haemophilia A. Haemophilia. 2015 Mar;21(2):162–70. Epub 2015 Jan 27.

Laursen MA, Larsen JB, Hvas AM. Platelet function in disseminated intravascular coagulation: a systematic review. Platelets. 2018 May;29(3):238–48. Epub 2018 Mar 8.

Lebrun A, Leroy-Matheron C, Arlet JB, Bartolucci P, Michel M. Successful treatment with rituximab in a patient with an acquired factor V inhibitor. Am J Hematol. 2008 Feb;83(2):163–4.

Levi M, Ten Cate H. Disseminated intravascular coagulation. N Engl J Med. 1999 Aug 19;341(8):586–92.

Levi M, Toh CH, Thachil J, Watson HG. Guidelines for the diagnosis and management of disseminated intravascular coagulation. British Committee for Standards in Haematology. Br J Haematol. 2009 Apr;145(1):24–33. Epub 2009 Feb 12.

Lian EC, Tzakis AG, Andrews D. Response of factor V inhibitor to rituximab in a patient who received liver transplantation for primary biliary cirrhosis. Am J Hematol. 2004 Dec;77(4):363–5.

Ma ES, Liang RH, Chu KM, Lau GK. Complete response of acquired FV inhibitor to rituximab. Int J Hematol. 2015 Apr;101(4):421–2. Epub 2015 Jan 24.

Morrison AE, Ludlam CA, Kessler C. Use of porcine factor VIII in the treatment of patients with acquired hemophilia. Blood. 1993 Mar 15;81(6):1513–20.

Perdekamp MT, Rubenstein DA, Jesty J, Hultin MB. Platelet factor V supports hemostasis in a patient with an acquired factor V inhibitor, as shown by prothrombinase and tenase assays. Blood Coagul Fibrinolysis. 2006 Oct;17(7):593–7.

Rios R, Sangro B, Herrero I, Quiroga J, Prieto J. The role of thrombopoietin in the thrombocytopenia of patients with liver cirrhosis. Am J Gastroenterol. 2005 Jun;100(6):1311–6.

Sallah S. Treatment of acquired haemophilia with factor eight inhibitor bypassing activity. Haemophilia. 2004 Mar;10(2):169–73.

Taylor FB Jr, Toh CH, Hoots WK, Wada H, Levi M; Scientific Subcommittee on Disseminated Intravascular Coagulation (DIC) of the International Society on Thrombosis and Haemostasis (ISTH). Towards definition, clinical and laboratory criteria, and a scoring system for disseminated intravascular coagulation. Thromb Haemost. 2001 Nov;86(5):1327–30.

Tefferi A, Hanson CA, Inwards DJ. How to interpret and pursue an abnormal complete blood cell count in adults. Mayo Clin Proc. 2005 Jul;80(7):923–36.

Thachil J. The elusive diagnosis of disseminated intravascular coagulation: does a diagnosis of DIC exist anymore? Semin Thromb Hemost. 2019 Feb;45(1):100–7. Epub 2019 Jan 11.

Tripodi A, Mannucci PM. The coagulopathy of chronic liver disease. N Engl J Med. 2011 Jul 14;365(2):147–56.

Tripodi A, Salerno F, Chantarangkul V, Clerici M, Cazzaniga M, Primignani M, et al. Evidence of normal thrombin generation in cirrhosis despite abnormal conventional coagulation tests. Hepatology. 2005 Mar;41(3):553–8.

Wada H, Asakura H, Okamoto K, Iba T, Uchiyama T, Kawasugi K, et al; Japanese Society of Thrombosis Hemostasis/DIC Subcommittee. Expert consensus for the treatment of disseminated intravascular coagulation in Japan. Thromb Res. 2010 Jan;125(1):6–11. Epub 2009 Sep 25.

Yamada Y, Miyakawa Y, Sawano M, Okano Y. Successful treatment of severe lung hemorrhage caused by acquired factor V inhibitor with rituximab. Intern Med. 2014;53(10):1083–5.

Anticoagulation Monitoring and Reversal

THERESA N. KINARD, MD

Goals

- Understand the mechanism of action for unfractionated heparin, warfarin, and direct thrombin inhibitors and direct Xa inhibitors.
- Recognize appropriate laboratory tests for monitoring anticoagulation therapy in patients with complex, critical conditions.
- Describe the limitations of laboratory tests for monitoring anticoagulation therapy.
- Discuss therapeutic options for anticoagulation reversal.

Introduction

The balance of natural procoagulant and anticoagulant activity within the body is delicate, and a minor disruption may lead to bleeding or clotting complications. Anticoagulation in critical illness is often necessary for a host of reasons, either prophylactic or therapeutic.

This chapter reviews common anticoagulation management issues in the critically ill patient, such as optimal laboratory monitoring of anticoagulation therapy and urgent reversal options, focusing on the most common anticoagulants used in current practice.

Mechanisms of Action

Coagulation proteins are present in plasma as zymogens (inactivated) and, when cleaved, the proteins are activated, a state designated with the suffix *a*. The contact activation pathway begins with activation of factor XI and subsequent downstream activation of additional coagulation proteins to ultimately generate thrombin (factor [F]IIa). Thrombin cleaves fibrinogen to form fibrin monomers, which become crosslinked to form the structural support for a clot. The tissue factor pathway is a complementary mechanism to initiate coagulation at the site of damaged vessels. Damaged tissue releases tissue factor, which promotes formation of activated factor VII (FVIIa). FVIIa converges with the contact activation pathway at the formation of factor Xa (FXa), meeting at the common pathway to generate thrombin. Reduction of functional factor levels and inhibition of thrombin and thrombin generation are effective mechanisms for anticoagulation therapy.

Unfractionated Heparin

Unfractionated heparin (UFH) therapy is a preferred approach in intensive care units because of its relatively short half-life, the ability to quickly reverse its effects, and its nonrenal elimination. It is administered intravenously or by subcutaneous injection for the treatment or prevention of thrombotic diseases. Proper weight-based administration of UFH has been shown to effectively reduce morbidity and mortality associated with thromboembolic processes. It is also a common medication for extracorporeal anticoagulation during procedures such as apheresis, hemodialysis, and extracorporeal membrane oxygenation and during invasive surgical interventions that use cardiopulmonary bypass.

Heparin is a negatively charged, sulfated polysaccharide, in which UFH is a mixture of large and small heparin fractions. It is an indirect inhibitor of multiple procoagulant enzymes, and its primary anticoagulation effect is mediated by antithrombin (AT). AT is a naturally occurring anticoagulant protein found in blood whose anticoagulant effect is magnified many-fold when interacting with heparin. Interestingly, only one-third of heparin molecules contain the high-affinity pentasaccharide required for anticoagulant activity, and thus heparin responses are heterogeneous.

Although heparin targets multiple factors in the contact activation pathway and tissue factor pathway, FXa and FIIa are the most responsive to inhibition. Binding of FXa or heparin to antithrombin causes a conformational change at the AT's reactive center that accelerates its interaction with FXa. Heparin's high-negative charge surrounding large-molecular-weight heparins results in binding to positively charged proteins and surfaces. The nonselective binding to cells and proteins reduces the anticoagulant response and pharmacokinetics.

Therapeutic monitoring of the anticoagulation activity of UFH includes measurement 6 hours after a bolus and 6 hours after each rate change. At least 6 hours is required to achieve steady-state kinetics. Therefore, monitoring heparin therapy more frequently than 6 hours results in non–steady-state analysis and can lead to erroneous dosing adjustments.

Laboratory monitoring is generally performed on the basis of the activated partial thromboplastin time (aPTT) or the chromogenic anti-Xa assay. The aPTT continues to be the principal basis on which most laboratories monitor intravenous UFH therapy. The aPTT offers many advantages. The test is quick, inexpensive, and widely available. However, it is a clot-based test and does not directly measure heparin. Numerous aPTT reagents exist, and each has a variable response to heparin therapy and can be influenced by patient-dependent physiologic factors. Pre-analytic and analytic factors may result in erroneous prolongation or blunting of the aPTT and subsequent under- or over-anticoagulation, respectively.

Clinical conditions, especially common conditions that occur in critically ill patients, can alter the aPTT but do not correlate with bleeding or protection from thrombosis. A common situation is concurrent administration of anticoagulation, usually a vitamin K antagonist, or the presence of antiphospholipid antibodies. Factor deficiencies, for example, as a result of liver disease or consumptive coagulopathy in disseminated intravascular coagulopathy, also result in a poor reflection of heparin anticoagulation. All of these clinical situations produce an increased baseline aPTT and can potentially result in under-anticoagulation with heparin. Acute-phase reactants factors VIII and fibrinogen are the most important confounders and may be dramatically increased and shorten the baseline aPTT. At the same time, acutely ill patients are also known to have AT deficiency. These conditions can result in potential over-anticoagulation when monitoring heparin therapy according to the aPTT.

A 1972 prospective study of patients with venous thromboembolism treated with heparin found that the risk for recurrent thromboembolic disease is associated with failure to obtain an aPTT ratio of approximately 1.5 to 2.5 times the control value, and this became the standard for the therapeutic range, which corresponded to a heparin level of 0.3 to 0.7 IU/mL by the anti-Xa assay. Additional studies found that anti-Xa levels more than 0.74 to 0.88 IU/mL were associated with more bleeding complications, a finding supporting the avoidance of exceeding an Xa level of more than 0.7 to 0.8 IU/mL to minimize bleeding risk. In the 1990s, the American College of Chest Physicians and the College of American Pathologists recommended that specific therapeutic goal ranges of aPTT for individual institutions should be determined according to a corresponding heparin level of 0.3 to 0.7 IU/mL by the anti-Xa assay. Alternatively, UFH can be monitored directly with the anti-Xa assay, which is becoming widely available in hospital laboratories.

The anti-Xa assay is affected by hemolysis, icterus, and hypertriglyceridemia, which affect the instrument's ability to measure and discriminate the chromogenic reaction. Therefore, affected patients should have their heparin monitored with aPTT and not the anti-Xa assay. Furthermore, anti-Xa reagents that do not supplement with AT may underestimate heparin concentrations in the presence of a substantial AT deficiency. Conversely, a suspicion or diagnosis of AT deficiency may be missed if AT is supplemented in the reagent.

An advantage of anticoagulating with UFH is its relatively short half-life, which allows quick or brief anticoagulant interruption for bleeding or invasive procedures. A major portion of UFH is cleared by a rapid, dose-dependent mechanism.

For rapid reversal, protamine sulfate should be administered. Protamine neutralizes heparin by binding to it and preventing its interaction with AT, and the protamine-heparin complex is rapidly cleared by the reticuloendothelial system. Protamine, 1 mg, neutralizes 80 to 100 IU of heparin within 15 minutes of heparin administration. This guideline is based on the initial or total dose of heparin without taking its elimination into account. Intravenous protamine has a half-life of 7 minutes. When UFH is given as an intravenous infusion, only the UFH administered in the preceding 2 to 2.5 hours should be considered for dosing protamine. Relative protamine overdose can result in increased anticoagulation and decreased platelet function. Ideally, the protamine dose should be based on plasma levels of heparin. Adverse effects of protamine include hypotension (most common) and a clinical range of hypersensitivity reactions, which can be avoided by slow infusions. Plasma infusion is ineffective for reversing the effect of heparin, and it is a source of AT, which increases the anticoagulation effect of UFH. Plasma should not be used for reversing the effect of UFH.

Warfarin

Vitamin K antagonists (VKAs) have been prescribed to patients for the past 60 years as prophylaxis for and treatment of venous and arterial thromboembolism. VKAs are effective for 1) prevention of thromboembolism; 2) prophylaxis against systemic emboli in patients with prosthetic heart valves or atrial fibrillation or who have had myocardial infarction; and 3) reducing the risk of recurrent myocardial infarction and strokes. However, clinical management of the therapy is complicated by the narrow therapeutic range, variability in individual dose response and laboratory monitoring, and bleeding adverse events.

Vitamin K is essential for the posttranslational modification of specific proteins produced by the liver: factors II, VII, IX, and X and proteins C and S. γ-Glutamyl carboxylase is a vitamin K-dependent enzyme that renders these factors functional and allows the factors to participate in the formation of coagulation complexes for generation of thrombin. Vitamin K is fat soluble, and any condition that inhibits or prevents absorption, particularly absorption of fats, affects the production of functional vitamin K-dependent factors (VKDFs).

Although VKAs affect both procoagulant and anticoagulant VKDFs, procoagulant inhibition is more dominant. The biologic effects of warfarin are not apparent until the functional VKDFs are reduced to less than 30%. Because of the varied half-lives of the VKDFs, VKAs are generally bridged with a UFH therapy to prevent the transient increased risk of thrombosis from rapid reduction of protein C (half-life, 3 hours). It takes 3 to 5 days after initiation of warfarin to achieve this effect. The elimination half-life of warfarin is approximately 40 hours (range, 36-42 hours).

Warfarin therapy is monitored according to the international normalized ratio (INR), which is a calculated value based on the prothrombin time. The therapeutic range for patients receiving VKAs depends on the indication for treatment.

The individual dose response to VKAs is highly variable, and the intensity of anticoagulation is an important determinant of the bleeding risk in patients receiving VKAs. Patients with INRs more than 6 are at greater risk for development of any type of major bleeding, and the risk of intracranial hemorrhage increases when the INR is more than 4. Fluctuation in the INR is an indicator of poor management of warfarin therapy and increases bleeding risk. These hemorrhagic complications require an effective and rapid antidote for reversal of the effect of VKA.

Before the availability of prothrombin complex concentrates (PCC), the standard of care for reversing the VKA effect and bleeding was plasma transfusion. However, plasma requires ABO blood typing, a long preparation time, a large volume, and slow infusion rate. Additionally, transfusion of plasma also has the potential for adverse events, including allergic reactions, transfusion-related acute lung injury, transfusion-associated circulatory overload, and a risk of infectious disease transmission. Currently, several published guidelines recommend withholding warfarin and administering vitamin K and PCC for reversal of the VKA effect if they are available.

PCCs are available as activated or nonactivated. Nonactivated PCCs can be classified as 4-factor PCC (4F-PCC) or 3-factor PCC (3F-PCC). 3F-PCCs contain very low concentrations of factor VII and probably no protein C or S. The 4F-PCCs contain all VKDFs, including protein C and S. 4F-PCC is approved by the US Food and Drug Administration for the urgent reversal of VKA effect in patients with acute major bleeding and reversal for an urgent procedure. Supplemental vitamin K should also be given to sustain the hemostatic effects beyond 6 hours.

The recommended dosage is based on a patient's weight in kilograms and pretreatment INR. In clinical trials, 4F-PCC was able to reduce the INR to 1.3 or less at 30 minutes in 62% of patients, but it was reduced in only 9.6% of patients who received plasma. The 4F-PCC effect was superior to plasma for INR reduction and non-inferior for hemostatic efficacy in patients with major bleeding due to VKA.

4F-PCC is contraindicated in patients with a known severe reaction to 4F-PCC or any of the components and in patients with disseminated intravascular coagulation. Although patients with a history of heparin-induced thrombocytopenia are potentially at risk for recurrence because of heparin in the 4F-PCC, there have been no reports of heparin-induced thrombocytopenia type 2 in postmarket surveillance studies.

Clinical studies examining the use of 4F-PCC have found that thrombotic complications are rare. The reduced risk of thromboembolic events with 4F-PCC may be attributed to lack of activated factors and the presence of natural anticoagulants protein C and protein S. These traits allow balance of procoagulants and anticoagulants, which may prevent excessive thrombin generation.

Direct Oral Anticoagulants

Direct oral anticoagulants (DOACs) have gained preference over warfarin since being introduced in 2010. Unlike warfarin, which indirectly reduces the level of functional VKDFs, DOACs can directly inhibit critical enzymes in the coagulation cascade. Unlike UFH, which indirectly inhibits free FXa or FIIa, DOACs can specifically target both free and clot-bound FXa or FIIa, a feature that makes them more effective anticoagulants than warfarin. Clinical trials have shown that DOACs are as effective as warfarin but are associated with an overall reduced incidence of intracranial hemorrhage.

Patients and medication prescribers are favoring DOACs because of their efficacy, ease of use, and favorable safety profile. Although the number of visits for treatment of atrial fibrillation and venous thromboembolism have steadily increased in past years, between 2009 and 2014 visits related to warfarin treatment declined, and visits related to DOAC treatment have increased to more than 1 million per quarter. In 2014, rivaroxaban became the most commonly prescribed DOAC for atrial fibrillation, followed by apixaban and dabigatran. In 36% of visits for venous thromboembolism, treatment was with DOACs.

Currently, DOACs have 2 categories of mechanism. Dabigatran etexilate is the only oral direct thrombin inhibitor approved by the US Food and Drug Administration. It is an orally inactive prodrug that, when hydrolyzed to its active metabolite, dabigatran, reversibly inhibits the active site of FIIa and prevents the cleavage of fibrinogen to fibrin. Dabigatran is predominantly eliminated by the kidneys; thus, periodic assessment of renal function is necessary, and use of the drug should be discontinued with acute renal failure.

Rivaroxaban, apixaban, and edoxaban are direct FXa inhibitors, hence the suffix -xaban. FXa is a critical factor at the convergence of the contact factor (extrinsic) pathway and tissue factor (intrinsic) pathway, and its inhibition is sufficient for the prevention and treatment of thrombosis. Creatinine clearance is also important to consider when determining whether a direct Xa inhibitor is the optimal anticoagulant for the patient and at which precise dose.

DOACs quickly reach maximal concentrations between 1 to 4 hours after ingestion, have predictable pharmacodynamics and pharmacokinetics, and have relatively short half-lives from 5 to 17 hours in healthy persons. Therapeutic drug monitoring and dose adjustments, with the exception of concomitant renal dysfunction, are not necessary. In addition, specific laboratory tests for monitoring DOAC are not widely available.

Dabigatran prolongs aPTT, ecarin clotting time, and thrombin time, but the degree of prolongation does not necessarily correlate with the degree of anticoagulation. A laboratory-validated dilute thrombin time may be used for monitoring of dabigatran therapy. A normal thrombin time most likely excludes therapeutic anticoagulation with dabigatran, and a normal aPTT likely rules out excessive anticoagulation with dabigatran. Direct factor X inhibitors have variable effects on routine laboratory tests. A normal prothrombin time may rule out excess drug levels of rivaroxaban and edoxan but not apixaban. Anti-Xa assays specifically calibrated to each direct FXa inhibitor may also be used to evaluate the level of therapeutic anticoagulation, but these tests are not widely available.

The risk of gastrointestinal bleeding with DOACs is increased compared with that of warfarin, but the risks of intracranial hemorrhage and life-threatening bleeding are less.

Before idarucizumab was approved by the US Food and Drug Administration, no reversal options were available for any DOAC, and limited data existed to recommend administration of factor concentrates for life-threatening or uncontrolled bleeding. Because of the short half-lives of these medications, if the last administration of a DOAC was more than 24 hours prior, approximately 2 half-lives would have passed (excluding concomitant renal failure), and specific reversal may not be indicated. Some patients may be supported with transfusion resuscitation in the event of bleeding.

When bleeding is life-threatening or uncontrolled, or when an urgent invasive procedure is needed within recent administration of dabigatran, administration of 5 g of idarucizumab should be considered. It is a humanized monoclonal antibody fragment and binds to dabigatran and its metabolite with higher affinity than the binding affinity of dabigatran to FIIa. Coagulation tests results may re-increase 12 to 24 hours after idarucizumab administration, but additional doses of this reversal agent should be limited to situations with persistent clinical bleeding. The short half-life of dabigatran facilitates rapid restoration of normal hemostasis, a result that obviates an antidote in the majority of patients.

Andexanet alfa is a recombinant modified human FXa decoy protein that has been shown to reverse the direct and indirect inhibition of FXa. In a recent study of patients with acute major bleeding (mostly intracranial or gastrointestinal) who received factor Xa inhibitor, treatment with andexanet alfa markedly reduced anti–factor Xa activity, and 82% of patients had excellent or good hemostatic efficacy at 12 hours.

Summary

- Familiarity with available coagulation testing assays in one's laboratory is important. Knowledge of available testing and alternative testing methods provides opportunities to optimize management of anticoagulation therapy.
- The anti-Xa assay measures heparin concentration and is a more reliable method to monitor heparin therapy than the PTT. This assay has become automated, and turnaround times for results are similar to those of performing the traditional aPTT.
- 4F-PCC, approved by the US Food and Drug Administration, is indicated for reversal of the effect of warfarin for major bleeding or urgent surgical intervention. Vitamin K should also be administered to sustain coagulation effects. Minor bleeding or procedures that may be delayed can be managed by holding warfarin administration and administering vitamin K.
- Idarucizumab should be administered for reversal of the effect of dabigatran. Andexanet alfa is a potent reversal agent for direct Xa inhibitors.

SUGGESTED READING

Adcock DM, Gosselin R. Direct oral anticoagulants (DOACs) in the laboratory: 2015 review. Thromb Res. 2015 Jul;136(1):7–12. Epub 2015 May 8.

Ageno W, Gallus AS, Wittkowsky A, Crowther M, Hylek EM, Palareti G. Oral anticoagulant therapy: antithrombotic therapy and prevention of thrombosis, 9th ed: American College of Chest Physicians

Evidence-Based Clinical Practice Guidelines. Chest. 2012 Feb;141(2 Suppl):e44S–e88S.

Ansell J, Hirsh J, Hylek E, Jacobson A, Crowther M, Palareti G. Pharmacology and management of the vitamin K antagonists: American College of Chest Physicians Evidence-Based Clinical Practice Guidelines (8th Edition). Chest. 2008 Jun;133(6 Suppl):160S–98S.

Avecilla ST, Ferrell C, Chandler WL, Reyes M. Plasma-diluted thrombin time to measure dabigatran concentrations during dabigatran etexilate therapy. Am J Clin Pathol. 2012 Apr;137(4):572–4.

Barnes GD, Lucas E, Alexander GC, Goldberger ZD. National trends in ambulatory oral anticoagulant use. Am J Med. 2015 Dec;128(12):1300–5.e2. Epub 2015 Jul 2.

Basu D, Gallus A, Hirsh J, Cade J. A prospective study of the value of monitoring heparin treatment with the activated partial thromboplastin time. N Engl J Med. 1972 Aug 17;287(7):324–7.

Bates SM, Weitz JI. Coagulation assays. Circulation. 2005 Jul 26;112(4):e53–60.

Bechtel BF, Nunez TC, Lyon JA, Cotton BA, Barrett TW. Treatments for reversing warfarin anticoagulation in patients with acute intracranial hemorrhage: a structured literature review. Int J Emerg Med. 2011 Jul 8;4(1):40.

Breckenridge A, Orme M. Kinetics of warfarin absorption in man. Clin Pharmacol Ther. 1973 Nov-Dec;14(6):955–61.

Connolly SJ, Crowther M, Eikelboom JW, Gibson CM, Curnutte JT, Lawrence JH, et al; ANNEXA-4 Investigators. Full study report of andexanet alfa for bleeding associated with factor Xa inhibitors. N Engl J Med. 2019 Apr 4;380(14):1326–35. Epub 2019 Feb 7.

Connolly SJ, Ezekowitz MD, Yusuf S, Eikelboom J, Oldgren J, Parekh A, et al; RE-LY Steering Committee and Investigators. Dabigatran versus warfarin in patients with atrial fibrillation. N Engl J Med. 2009 Sep 17;361(12):1139–51. Epub 2009 Aug 30. Erratum in: N Engl J Med. 2010 Nov 4;363(19):1877.

Connolly SJ, Milling TJ Jr, Eikelboom JW, Gibson CM, Curnutte JT, Gold A, et al; ANNEXA-4 Investigators. Andexanet alfa for acute major bleeding associated with factor Xa inhibitors. N Engl J Med. 2016 Sep 22;375(12):1131–41. Epub 2016 Aug 30.

Cuker A, Burnett A, Triller D, Crowther M, Ansell J, Van Cott EM, et al. Reversal of direct oral anticoagulants: guidance from the anticoagulation forum. Am J Hematol. 2019 Mar 27. [Epub ahead of print]

Cuker A, Siegal D. Monitoring and reversal of direct oral anticoagulants. Hematology Am Soc Hematol Educ Program. 2015;2015:117–24.

Eliquis [package insert]. Princeton (NJ): Bristol-Myers Squibb Company; c2017. [cited 2017 Jan 3]. Available from: http://packageinserts.bms.com/pi/pi_eliquis.pdf.

Fihn SD, McDonell M, Martin D, Henikoff J, Vermes D, Kent D, et al; Warfarin Optimized Outpatient Follow-up Study Group. Risk factors for complications of chronic anticoagulation: a multicenter study. Ann Intern Med. 1993 Apr 1;118(7):511–20.

Garcia DA, Baglin TP, Weitz JI, Samama MM. Parenteral anticoagulants: antithrombotic therapy and prevention of thrombosis, 9th ed: American College of Chest Physicians Evidence-Based Clinical Practice Guidelines. Chest. 2012 Feb;141(2 Suppl):e24S–e43S. Errata in: Chest. 2012 May;141(5):1369. Chest. 2013 Aug;144(2):721.

Giugliano RP, Ruff CT, Braunwald E, Murphy SA, Wiviott SD, Halperin JL, et al; ENGAGE AF-TIMI 48 Investigators. Edoxaban versus warfarin in patients with atrial fibrillation. N Engl J Med. 2013 Nov 28;369(22):2093–104. Epub 2013 Nov 19.

Granger CB, Alexander JH, McMurray JJ, Lopes RD, Hylek EM, Hanna M, et al; ARISTOTLE Committees and Investigators. Apixaban versus warfarin in patients with atrial fibrillation. N Engl J Med. 2011 Sep 15;365(11):981–92. Epub 2011 Aug 27.

Hanke AA, Joch C, Gorlinger K. Long-term safety and efficacy of a pasteurized nanofiltrated prothrombin complex concentrate (Beriplex P/N): a pharmacovigilance study. Br J Anaesth. 2013 May;110(5):764–72. Epub 2013 Jan 18.

Hankey GJ, Eikelboom JW. Dabigatran etexilate: a new oral thrombin inhibitor. Circulation. 2011 Apr 5;123(13):1436–50.

Hewick DS, McEwen J. Plasma half-lives, plasma metabolites and anticoagulant efficacies of the enantiomers of warfarin in man. J Pharm Pharmacol. 1973 Jun;25(6):458–65.

Hignite C, Uetrecht J, Tschanz C, Azarnoff D. Kinetics of R and S warfarin enantiomers. Clin Pharmacol Ther. 1980 Jul;28(1):99–105.

Hirsh J, Anand SS, Halperin JL, Fuster V; American Heart Association. Guide to anticoagulant therapy: heparin: a statement for healthcare professionals from the American Heart Association. Circulation. 2001 Jun 19;103(24):2994–3018.

Holbrook A, Schulman S, Witt DM, Vandvik PO, Fish J, Kovacs MJ, et al. Evidence-based management of anticoagulant therapy: antithrombotic therapy and prevention of thrombosis, 9th ed: American College of Chest Physicians Evidence-Based Clinical Practice Guidelines. Chest. 2012 Feb;141(2 Suppl):e152S–e84S.

Hylek EM, Chang YC, Skates SJ, Hughes RA, Singer DE. Prospective study of the outcomes of ambulatory patients with excessive warfarin anticoagulation. Arch Intern Med. 2000 Jun 12;160(11):1612–7.

Hylek EM, Singer DE. Risk factors for intracranial hemorrhage in outpatients taking warfarin. Ann Intern Med. 1994 Jun 1;120(11):897–902.

Jobes DR, Aitken GL, Shaffer GW. Increased accuracy and precision of heparin and protamine dosing reduces blood loss and transfusion in patients undergoing primary cardiac operations. J Thorac Cardiovasc Surg. 1995 Jul;110(1):36–45.

Keeling D, Baglin T, Tait C, Watson H, Perry D, Baglin C, et al; British Committee for Standards in Haematology. Guidelines on oral anticoagulation with warfarin: fourth edition. Br J Haematol. 2011 Aug;154(3):311–24. Epub 2011 Jun 14.

Kumar S, Haigh JR, Tate G, Boothby M, Joanes DN, Davies JA, et al. Effect of warfarin on plasma concentrations of vitamin K dependent coagulation factors in patients with stable control and monitored compliance. Br J Haematol. 1990 Jan;74(1):82–5.

Ni Ainle F, Preston RJ, Jenkins PV, Nel HJ, Johnson JA, Smith OP, et al. Protamine sulfate down-regulates thrombin generation by inhibiting factor V activation. Blood. 2009 Aug 20;114(8):1658–65. Epub 2009 Jun 16.

O'Reilly RA. Studies on the optical enantiomorphs of warfarin in man. Clin Pharmacol Ther. 1974 Aug;16(2):348–54.

Patel MR, Mahaffey KW, Garg J, Pan G, Singer DE, Hacke W, et al; ROCKET AF Investigators. Rivaroxaban versus warfarin in nonvalvular atrial fibrillation. N Engl J Med. 2011 Sep 8;365(10):883–91. Epub 2011 Aug 10.

Paul B, Oxley A, Brigham K, Cox T, Hamilton PJ. Factor II, VII, IX and X concentrations in patients receiving long term warfarin. J Clin Pathol. 1987 Jan;40(1):94–8.

Pradaxa [package insert]. Ridgefield (CT): Boehringer Ingelheim Pharmaceuticals, Inc; c2017. [cited 2017 Jan 3]. Available from: http://docs.boehringer-ingelheim.com/Prescribing%20Information/PIs/Pradaxa/Pradaxa.pdf.

Samama MM, Guinet C. Laboratory assessment of new anticoagulants. Clin Chem Lab Med. 2011 May;49(5):761–72. Epub 2011 Feb 3.

Saraf K, Morris PD, Garg P, Sheridan P, Storey R. Non-vitamin K antagonist oral anticoagulants (NOACs): clinical evidence and therapeutic considerations. Postgrad Med J. 2014 Sep;90(1067):520–8. Epub 2014 Aug 1. Erratum in: Postgrad Med J. 2014 Oct;90(1068):575.

Sarode R, Milling TJ Jr, Refaai MA, Mangione A, Schneider A, Durn BL, et al. Efficacy and safety of a 4-factor prothrombin complex concentrate in patients on vitamin K antagonists presenting with major bleeding: a randomized, plasma-controlled, phase IIIb study. Circulation. 2013 Sep 10;128(11):1234–43. Epub 2013 Aug 9.

Savaysa [package insert]. Parsippany (NJ): Daiichi Sankyo, Co, LTD; c2015. [cited 2017 Jan 3]. Available from: http://www.accessdata.fda.gov/drugsatfda_docs/label/2015/206316lbl.pdf.

Smith M, Wakam G, Wakefield T, Obi A. New trends in anticoagulation therapy. Surg Clin North Am. 2018 Apr;98(2):219–38. Epub 2018 Feb 3.

Sorensen B, Spahn DR, Innerhofer P, Spannagl M, Rossaint R. Clinical review: prothrombin complex concentrates: evaluation of safety and thrombogenicity. Crit Care. 2011;15(1):201. Epub 2011 Jan 12. Erratum in: Crit Care. 2011;15(2):409.

Tornkvist M, Smith JG, Labaf A. Current evidence of oral anticoagulant reversal: a systematic review. Thromb Res. 2018 Feb;162:22–31. Epub 2017 Dec 6.

Vandiver JW, Vondracek TG. Antifactor Xa levels versus activated partial thromboplastin time for monitoring unfractionated heparin. Pharmacotherapy. 2012 Jun;32(6):546–58. Epub 2012 Apr 24.

Vang ML, Hvas AM, Ravn HB. Urgent reversal of vitamin K antagonist therapy. Acta Anaesthesiol Scand. 2011 May;55(5):507–16. Epub 2011 Mar 21. Erratum in: Acta Anaesthesiol Scand. 2011 Jul;55(6):766.

Wittkowsky AK. Warfarin. In: Murphy JE, editor. Clinical pharmacokinetics. 5th ed. Bethesda (MD): American Society of Health-System Pharmacists; c2012. p. 351–72.

Wittkowsky AK. Why warfarin and heparin need to overlap when treating acute venous thromboembolism. Dis Mon. 2005 Feb-Mar;51(2–3):112–5.

Xarelto [package insert]. Titusville (NJ): Janssen Pharmaceuticals, Inc; c2011. [cited 2017 Jan 3]. Available from: https://www.xareltohcp.com/shared/product/xarelto/prescribing-information.pdf.

Yang L, Stanworth S, Hopewell S, Doree C, Murphy M. Is fresh-frozen plasma clinically effective? An update of a systematic review of randomized controlled trials. Transfusion. 2012 Aug;52(8):1673–86. Epub 2012 Jan 18.

Yeh CH, Fredenburgh JC, Weitz JI. Oral direct factor Xa inhibitors. Circ Res. 2012 Sep 28;111(8):1069–78.

Therapeutic Plasma Exchange for Acute Hematologic Disorders

JILL ADAMSKI, MD, PhD

Goals

- Describe technical considerations associated with therapeutic plasma exchange.
- Review the indications for therapeutic plasma exchange.
- Elucidate the grade of evidence for therapeutic plasma exchange in different disorders.

Introduction

Therapeutic plasma exchange (TPE) is a process by which whole blood is removed from a patient and separated into 3 components: red blood cells, white blood cells (buffy coat), and plasma. After separation, the plasma is discarded, and the other blood components are returned to the patient along with exogenous fluid to replace the removed plasma. The replacement fluid is typically 5% albumin or donor plasma, and the choice of replacement fluid depends on the indication for TPE or clinical status of the patient. Numerous apheresis instruments have been approved by the US Food and Drug Administration to perform TPE with either centrifugal- or membrane-filtration–based cell-plasma separation. TPE is an important tool to remove pathogenic substances (eg, antibodies) from plasma, and this technique is considered first-line therapy for numerous conditions that affect patients in the critical care unit. This chapter describes the role of TPE in management of hematologic disorders, some of which have neurologic manifestations. Neurologic indications for TPE are addressed in Chapter 93, "Myasthenia Gravis"; Chapter 94, "Guillain-Barré Syndrome"; and Chapter 104, "Autoimmune Encephalitis."

Technical Considerations

Vascular Access

TPE requires blood flow rates ranging from 50 to 200 mL/min, depending on the type of instrument being used. Centrifugal-based instruments use lower flow rates than membrane-filtration–based instruments. Peripheral access may be achieved in some patients with large-bore needles. For peripheral access to be successful, the patient must have sufficiently large peripheral veins and the ability to consciously participate in the procedure by fist clenching to augment blood flow and lying still to prevent infiltration. Double-lumen apheresis or dialysis central venous catheters are often used in the critical care unit because of the nature of the patient population. Temporary central venous catheters may be used for acute cases or when relatively few procedures are indicated. If a patient requires TPE for more than 1 week, a tunneled central venous catheter should be considered.

Access for TPE also may be achieved in tandem with that for other extracorporeal procedures (eg, extracorporeal membrane oxygenation, continuous renal replacement therapy).

Anticoagulation

Like other extracorporeal devices, apheresis instruments require anticoagulation to prevent clotting in the apheresis circuit. Citrate, in the form of anticoagulant citrate dextrose solution A, is commonly used for a centrifugal-based instrument. Citrate mediates anticoagulation by binding ionized calcium, which is required for clot formation. Patients may experience symptoms of hypocalcemia if the citrate infusion rate exceeds their ability to metabolize the anticoagulant. Heparin tends to be reserved for membrane-filtration–based instruments with faster blood flows.

Replacement Fluid

Patient plasma is exchanged with a replacement fluid during TPE to maintain intravascular volume. When possible, 5% albumin is used as the replacement fluid because it has a very low risk of adverse reactions and transmission of infectious diseases. The disadvantages of using albumin are that this fluid does not replace clotting factors and other plasma proteins that are removed during the procedure, and albumin is substantially more expensive than other replacement fluids.

Donor plasma (fresh frozen plasma) is used when plasma proteins must be replaced during the exchange. Typically, plasma is used in patients with underlying coagulopathies or immediately before or after invasive surgical procedures to prevent dilutional coagulopathy and increased risk of bleeding. Plasma may also be used to replace important plasma proteins that are missing in certain disease states, such as ADAMTS13 (*a* *d*isintegrin *a*nd *m*etalloprotease with *t*hrombo*s*pondin-type motifs) enzyme in the setting of thrombotic thrombocytopenic purpura. Plasma replacement is associated with higher risks of adverse events during the procedure: allergic reactions, anaphylaxis, transfusion-related acute lung injury, hypocalcemia, and transfusion-transmitted infections.

Number and Frequency of TPE Procedures

The duration and timing of TPE procedures are determined by the intravascular and extravascular distribution of the protein that is targeted for removal. When one plasma volume is exchanged, approximately 63% of intravascular plasma proteins are removed. The removal of plasma proteins is nonlinear because of continuous mixing of replacement fluid with plasma in the intravascular space, and exchanging more than 1 to 1.5 plasma volumes has minimal effect on the amount of targeted substance removal.

If the targeted component is primarily found in the intravascular space (eg, immunoglobulin M antibodies), then daily TPE may be considered. If the targeted component is distributed equally between the intravascular and extravascular spaces (eg, immunoglobulin G antibodies), then the interval between procedures needs to allow for reequilibration from the extravascular space into the intravascular compartment. Reequilibration of immunoglobulin G typically occurs within 48 hours. Approximately 70% to 85% of total body immunoglobulin G can be removed with 5 to 7 one plasma volume exchanges over a 2-week period when done in combination with immunosuppression.

Table 56.1 • American Society for Apheresis Categories of Indications

Category	Definition
I	Apheresis, alone or in conjuction with other therapies, is considered a first-line intervention for these indications
II	Apheresis, alone or in conjuction with other therapies, is considered a second-line intervention for these indications
III	Role of apheresis therapy has not been established for these indications. Decisions should be made on case-by-case basis
IV	Apheresis therapy is ineffective or harmful. Institutional review board approval should be sought if apheresis is performed for these indications

From Adamski J. Thrombotic microangiopathy and indications for therapeutic plasma exchange. Hematology Am Soc Hematol Educ Program. 2014 Dec 5;2014(1):444–9. Epub 2014 Nov 18; used with permission.

Hematologic Indications for TPE

The American Society for Apheresis regularly publishes evidence-based guidelines to direct the use of TPE and other apheresis therapy. Each indication is assigned a category, I to IV (Table 56.1), and a strength of recommendation based on the Grading of Recommendations Assessment, Development and Evaluation system. Hematologic indications categorized for TPE by the Society are listed in Table 56.2. Key points for some of these indications are described below.

Thrombotic Thrombocytopenic Purpura

Thrombotic thrombocytopenic purpura is a hematologic emergency and a first-line indication for TPE. If the disease is untreated, the mortality rate is more than 80%. Neurologic involvement at presentation and later has been reported in many patients with thrombotic thrombocytopenic purpura, and TPE is warranted and associated with improvement of brain lesions. This condition is caused by an autoantibody directed against the von Willebrand factor cleaving enzyme ADAMTS13, which is characterized by microangiopathic hemolytic anemia, thrombocytopenia, and end-organ damage due to microvascular thrombi. TPE is performed daily until the platelet count normalizes. Relapses are common, thus patients must be monitored closely in the days after cessation of TPE. Plasma is used as a replacement to provide exogenous ADAMTS13 enzyme and to prevent coagulopathy due to daily exchanges.

Table 56.2 • Hematologic Indications for Therapeutic Plasma Exchange

Category	Indication
I	Hyperviscosity in monoclonal gammopathies
	Thrombotic microangiopathy
	Factor H autoantibodies in aHUS
	Drug-associated, limited to ticlopidine
	Thrombotic thrombocytopenic purpura
II	Cold agglutinin disease, severe presentation
	Catastrophic antiphospholipid syndrome
	Cryoglobulinemia
	Myeloma cast nephropathy
III	Autoimmune hemolytic anemia, severe warm
	Coagulation factor inhibitors, autoimmune
	HELLP syndrome, antepartumk
	Hemophagocytic syndrome
	Henoch-Schönlein syndrome
	Heparin-induced thrombocytopenia
	Immune thrombocytopenia, refractory
	Thrombotic microangiopathy
	Complement factor mutations, aHUS
	Associated with hematopoietic stem cell transplant
	Shiga toxin–induced HUS with severe neurologic symptoms
	Drug: clopidogrel, calcineurin inhibitors
IV	Thrombotic microangiopathy
	Shiga toxin–induced HUS in absense of severe neurologic symptoms
	Drug: gemcitabine, quinine

Abbreviations: aHUS, atypical hemolytic uremic syndrome; HELLP, *h*emolysis, *e*levated *l*iver enzymes, *l*ow *p*latelet count; HUS, hemolytic uremic syndrome.

Cold Agglutinin Disease

Cold agglutinin disease is caused by immunoglobulin M autoantibodies that bind to and fix complement on red blood cells at temperatures less than normal body temperature, 37°C. Severe hemolytic anemia may occur in mildly hypothermic patients, and they should be kept warm during acute exacerbations. TPE replacement fluid is typically prewarmed 5% albumin and, when possible, the instrument should be equilibrated to 37°C in the patient's warmed room to prevent agglutination within the extracorporeal circuit.

Heparin-Induced Thrombocytopenia

Patients with acute or subacute heparin-induced thrombocytopenia who require cardiopulmonary bypass during surgery can undergo TPE preoperatively. Immediate, albeit temporary, removal of the heparin-induced thrombocytopenia antibody allows for heparin to be used to anticoagulate the cardiopulmonary bypass circuit as an alternative to using a direct thrombin inhibitor. In the absence of heparin-induced thrombocytopenia antibodies, TPE is not necessary, and cardiopulmonary bypass with heparin used for anticoagulation is usually well tolerated. TPE may also be used to treat acute heparin-induced thrombocytopenia and new or progressing thrombosis.

Summary

- TPE is a procedure that facilitates removal of pathogenic substances from plasma.
- Several technical aspects must be considered before TPE, including how to achieve vascular access, anticoagulation of the instrument, and replacement fluid type.
- Many hematologic conditions can be treated with TPE.

SUGGESTED READING

Barcellini W. Current treatment strategies in autoimmune hemolytic disorders. Expert Rev Hematol. 2015 Oct;8(5):681–91. Epub 2015 Jul 31.

Burrus TM, Wijdicks EF, Rabinstein AA. Brain lesions are most often reversible in acute thrombotic thrombocytopenic purpura. Neurology. 2009 Jul 7;73(1):66–70.

Coppo P; French Reference Center for Thrombotic Microangiopathies. Treatment of autoimmune thrombotic thrombocytopenic purpura in the more severe forms. Transfus Apher Sci. 2017 Feb;56(1):52–6. Epub 2016 Dec 30.

Jaeschke R, Guyatt GH, Dellinger P, Schunemann H, Levy MM, Kunz R, et al; GRADE Working Group. Use of GRADE grid to reach decisions on clinical practice guidelines when consensus is elusive. BMJ. 2008 Jul 31;337:a744.

Kaplan AA. Therapeutic plasma exchange: a technical and operational review. J Clin Apher. 2013 Feb;28(1):3–10.

Kes P, Janssens ME, Basic-Jukic N, Kljak M. A randomized crossover study comparing membrane and centrifugal therapeutic plasma exchange procedures. Transfusion. 2016 Dec;56(12):3065–72. Epub 2016 Oct 5.

Linkins LA, Dans AL, Moores LK, Bona R, Davidson BL, Schulman S, et al. Treatment and prevention of heparin-induced thrombocytopenia: Antithrombotic Therapy and Prevention of Thrombosis, 9th ed: American College of Chest Physicians Evidence-Based Clinical Practice Guidelines. Chest. 2012 Feb;141(2 Suppl):e495S–e530S. Erratum in: Chest. 2015 Dec;148(6):1529.

Pham HP, Schwartz J. New apheresis indications in hematological disorders. Curr Opin Hematol. 2016 Nov;23(6):581–7.

Roman PE, DeVore AD, Welsby IJ. Techniques and applications of perioperative therapeutic plasma exchange. Curr Opin Anaesthesiol. 2014 Feb;27(1):57–64.

Sanford KW, Balogun RA. Therapeutic apheresis in critically ill patients. J Clin Apher. 2011;26(5):249–51. Epub 2011 Aug 10.

Schwartz J, Padmanabhan A, Aqui N, Balogun RA, Connelly-Smith L, Delaney M, et al. Guidelines on the use of therapeutic apheresis in clinical practice-evidence-based approach from the Writing Committee of the American Society for Apheresis: The seventh special issue. J Clin Apher. 2016 Jun;31(3):149–62.

Warkentin TE, Sheppard JA, Chu FV, Kapoor A, Crowther MA, Gangji A. Plasma exchange to remove HIT antibodies: dissociation between enzyme-immunoassay and platelet activation test reactivities. Blood. 2015 Jan 1;125(1):195–8. Epub 2014 Nov 18.

Welsby IJ, Um J, Milano CA, Ortel TL, Arepally G. Plasmapheresis and heparin reexposure as a management strategy for cardiac surgical patients with heparin-induced thrombocytopenia. Anesth Analg. 2010 Jan 1;110(1):30–5. Epub 2009 Nov 21.

Williams ME, Balogun RA. Principles of separation: indications and therapeutic targets for plasma exchange. Clin J Am Soc Nephrol. 2014 Jan;9(1):181–90. Epub 2013 Oct 31.

Zanatta E, Cozzi M, Marson P, Cozzi F. The role of plasma exchange in the management of autoimmune disorders. Br J Haematol. 2019 Mar 28. [Epub ahead of print]

Rheumatologic and Autoimmune Emergencies

MEGAN L. KRAUSE, MD; KEVIN G. MODER, MD

Goals

- Discuss the evaluation and management of acute arthritis.
- Describe the presentation and management of other rheumatologic emergencies.

Introduction

Rheumatologic emergencies are overall very rare. However, when they do occur, they must be recognized quickly to prevent severe morbidity and mortality. Examples are acute arthritis, catastrophic antiphospholipid antibody syndrome, giant cell arteritis, and transverse myelitis.

Acute Arthritis

Presentation

In the setting of acute arthritis, patients can present with pain, erythema, swelling, reduced range of motion of any joint, and fever.

Evaluation

Acute arthritis can be infectious or crystalline (gout or pseudogout). Aspiration is the initial step in evaluation. Ultrasound guidance can be helpful for aspiration, particularly of small joints. If sufficient fluid is aspirated, then studies should include Gram stain, bacterial culture, cell count, and crystal analysis. If limited fluid is obtained, then culture should be the priority. Crystals can be evaluated from a single drop of fluid with a polarizing microscope.

When there is concern for septic arthritis because of an erythematous or swollen joint, a source for infection should be sought with tests including blood cultures. Septic arthritis is often the result of hematogenous spread. Inflammatory markers, such as erythrocyte sedimentation rate and C-reactive protein, will usually be increased in both septic arthritis and acute crystalline arthritis. The uric acid value can be determined, but the value may be normal during an acute gout flare.

Treatment

Orthopedic surgery is necessary when there is concern for septic arthritis. Treatment of septic arthritis includes a combination of antibiotics and washout procedures in the operating room as opposed to repeated aspiration. While culture results are awaited, empiric treatment with antibiotics should be started. However, preferably, aspiration is done before antibiotic therapy is initiated.

The finding of crystals can be consistent with crystalline arthritis, either gout (uric acid crystals, needle shaped) or pseudogout (calcium pyrophosphate crystals, rhomboid shaped). However, the presence of crystals does not rule out infection; both conditions can occur in the same joint concurrently.

Catastrophic Antiphospholipid Antibody Syndrome

Presentation

Catastrophic antiphospholipid antibody syndrome occurs in a minority of patients with antiphospholipid antibody syndrome and presents with multiple organ failure. Typically, it is defined as 3 affected organs within 1 week as a result of thrombosis. The symptoms are variable and are dependent on the organ affected but can include respiratory failure as the result of diffuse alveolar hemorrhage or pulmonary embolism.

Catastrophic antiphospholipid antibody syndrome can be the first presentation of antiphospholipid antibody syndrome, but more commonly it occurs in the setting of a known diagnosis of antiphospholipid antibody syndrome. Inciting events for catastrophic antiphospholipid antibody syndrome can include interruption of anticoagulation, malignancy, infection, and trauma. Antiphospholipid antibody syndrome can occur in isolation but can also occur in association with systemic lupus erythematosus.

Evaluation

Evaluation requires exclusion of other causes of multiorgan failure. Complete blood counts and coagulation studies are needed for evaluation. Organ-specific assessments may include laboratory tests and imaging. If a patient does not have known antiphospholipid antibody syndrome, then testing for lupus anticoagulant, anticardiolipin immunoglobulin (Ig) M and IgG, and anti–β_2-glycoprotein 1 IgM and IgG is warranted.

Treatment

Catastrophic antiphospholipid antibody syndrome is associated with a high mortality rate. Multiple interventions are often attempted in parallel because of the severity of the disease. If there is no evidence of active bleeding, then anticoagulation should be used. High-dose corticosteroids are recommended. In addition, intravenous Ig and plasma exchange are options for therapy, but they should not be done concurrently because of the removal of intravenous Ig with plasma exchange. Sometimes immunosuppressants such as cyclophosphamide and rituximab are considered, but they do not have an immediate onset of action.

Emergency Giant Cell Arteritis

Presentation

Giant cell arteritis is a form of large-vessel vasculitis that affects elderly persons. The classic cranial symptoms include vision loss (due to disrupted blood flow to the posterior ciliary artery) or diplopia, headache, scalp tenderness, and jaw claudication. Symptoms of polymyalgia rheumatica, such as aching about the shoulder and hip girdle, are common. The aorta and its branches can also be involved, the symptoms of which are arm claudication and disparate upper-extremity blood pressures. Constitutional symptoms (fever, weight loss, fatigue) can also occur.

Evaluation

A full physical examination, with careful attention to the vascular examination, should be performed. This should include palpation of the temporal arteries with attention for abnormal appearance and tenderness, evaluation for bruits of the subclavian and carotid arteries, and evaluation of radial, femoral, and pedal pulses. Blood pressures should be obtained in both arms to evaluate for asymmetry. Laboratory evaluation should include inflammatory markers, erythrocyte sedimentation rate, and C-reactive protein, which are almost always increased. Temporal artery biopsy can confirm the diagnosis. If the result on the first side is negative, the additional yield from bilateral biopsy is 15%. Results of temporal artery biopsy may remain positive for weeks to months after treatment. Imaging of the aorta and its branches to look for other areas of involvement is done in selected patients, especially those with disparate blood pressures or arm claudication.

Treatment

Treatment includes high-dose corticosteroids. If visual symptoms are present, often methylprednisone, 1,000 mg intravenously is given for 3 days. Otherwise, oral prednisone, 40 to 60 mg daily, is the usual initial treatment. If giant cell arteritis is strongly suspected, then corticosteroid therapy should be initiated while results of temporal artery biopsy are awaited.

Transverse Myelitis Due to a Rheumatologic Cause

Presentation

Transverse myelitis can be associated with many rheumatologic conditions, including systemic lupus erythematosus, Sjögren syndrome, and antiphospholipid antibody syndrome. Clinical symptoms can be diverse and include bilateral motor deficits, sensory symptoms typically with a sensory level, and bowel or bladder symptoms. Symptoms develop rapidly over the course of days to weeks.

Evaluation

Magnetic resonance imaging of the entire spine (to evaluate for myelopathy, with gadolinium consistent with inflammation) and brain (to evaluate for other abnormalities to provide etiologic clues) is indicated in cases of suspected transverse myelitis. Analysis of cerebrospinal fluid (to evaluate for evidence of inflammation, including increased white blood cell count, oligoclonal bands, and increased protein level) is also indicated. Multiple sclerosis and neuromyelitis optica should be included in the differential diagnosis. Serologic testing for underlying rheumatic disease includes antinuclear antibody, SS-A, SS-B, Smith, ribonucleoprotein, complement (C3, C4), lupus anticoagulant, and anticardiolipin IgM and IgG.

Treatment

High-dose corticosteroids and plasma exchange are often used to treat transverse myelitis. In the setting of an associated rheumatologic condition, additional immunosuppression such as cyclophosphamide is given.

Summary

- Rheumatologic emergencies are rare but require prompt identification and management.
- Acute arthritis may be infective or crystalline. In infective cases, orthopedic surgery should be part of management. The presence of crystals does not exclude an infective cause.
- Other rheumatologic emergencies include catastrophic antiphospholipid antibody syndrome, giant cell arteritis, and transverse myelitis.

SUGGESTED READING

Bertolaccini ML, Amengual O, Andreoli L, Atsumi T, Chighizola CB, Forastiero R, et al. 14th International Congress on Antiphospholipid Antibodies Task Force: report on antiphospholipid syndrome laboratory diagnostics and trends. Autoimmun Rev. 2014 Sep;13(9):917–30. Epub 2014 May 10.

Cervera R, Rodriguez-Pinto, Espinosa G. The diagnosis and clinical management of the catastrophic antiphospholipid syndrome: a comprehensive review. J Autoimmun. 2018 Aug;92:1–11. Epub 2018 May 18.

Chighizola CB, Raimondo MG, Meroni PL. Management of thrombotic antiphospholipid syndrome. Semin Thromb Hemost. 2018 Jul;44(5):419–26. Epub 2017 Mar 9.

Dejaco C, Brouwer E, Mason JC, Buttgereit F, Matteson EL, Dasgupta B. Giant cell arteritis and polymyalgia rheumatica: current challenges and opportunities. Nat Rev Rheumatol. 2017 Oct;13(10):578–92. Epub 2017 Sep 14.

Graf J. Central nervous system manifestations of antiphospholipid syndrome. Rheum Dis Clin North Am. 2017 Nov;43(4):547–60.

Pradeep S, Smith JH. Giant cell arteritis: practical pearls and updates. Curr Pain Headache Rep. 2018 Jan 17;22(1):2.

Samson M, Corbera-Bellalta M, Audia S, Planas-Rigol E, Martin L, Cid MC, et al. Recent advances in our understanding of giant cell arteritis pathogenesis. Autoimmun Rev. 2017 Aug;16(8):833–44. Epub 2017 May 28.

Schreiber K, Sciascia S, de Groot PG, Devreese K, Jacobsen S, Ruiz-Irastorza G, et al. Antiphospholipid syndrome. Nat Rev Dis Primers. 2018 Jan 11;4:17103. Erratum in: Nat Rev Dis Primers. 2018 Jan 25;4:18005.

Sepsis and Other Infectious Diseases

Infectious Diseases Complicating Critical Care

DAVID A. SOTELLO AVILES, MD; WALTER C. HELLINGER, MD

Goals

- Describe the evaluation of new-onset fever or suspected sepsis in the intensive care unit.
- Recognize a reasonable empiric antibiotic management for each nosocomial infection in the intensive care unit.
- Identify the most relevant strategies for prevention of nosocomial infections in the intensive care unit.

Introduction

Infection is a common complication in the intensive care unit (ICU). Furthermore, infection more than doubles the mortality rate in the ICU. Antibiotic resistance in *Staphylococcus aureus, Enterococcus*, Enterobacteriaceae, and fungal infection is among the most challenging issues in the ICU. In addition, critical illness affects antibiotic pharmacokinetics. Thus, implementation of strategies to prevent infection is of utmost importance to improve patient outcome.

Epidemiology

Patients admitted to ICUs are at increased risk for nosocomial infections due to 1) complications of their acute disease; 2) immune impairment related to acute and, for some, chronic illness; and 3) insertion of therapeutic and diagnostic devices that breach anatomical barriers between internal and, in some cases, sterile compartments and the external environment. The incidence of nosocomial infection in ICUs is 2 to 5 times higher than that in other medical inpatient services. The risk of death related to nosocomial infections acquired in ICUs can be up to 50% if they are associated with septic shock.

The most common nosocomial infections in patients in ICUs are central line–associated bloodstream infections, catheter-associated urinary tract infections, and ventilator-associated pneumonias. The frequencies of these infections vary somewhat among different types of ICUs because of differences in the populations of patients served and the types of care delivered. The incidence of catheter-associated urinary tract infections has been higher in neurology ICUs and in neurosurgical ICUs than in other ICUs, and the incidence of ventilator-associated pneumonia has been highest in neurosurgical ICUs. Infections associated with external cerebral spinal fluid collection systems are largely confined to neurology ICUs, neurosurgical ICUs, and general ICUs that serve patients with critical neurologic illness. The incidences of health care–associated infections have been changing since the introductions of new preventive measures.

The pathogens responsible for these infections have been gram-negative bacilli (50%) including Enterobacteriaceae and *Pseudomonas*, gram-positive cocci (35%) including coagulase-negative staphylococci, methicillin-resistant *Staphylococcus aureus*, enterococci, and yeast (15%), primarily *Candida* species. The prevalence of antimicrobial resistance in these pathogens is increasing.

Diagnosis

The development of nosocomial infection in ICUs is usually, although not always, associated with the development of fever (temperature ≥38°C or ≥100.4°F). Infection may also be associated with hypothermia, hemodynamic instability, organ system dysfunction, leukopenia, or leukocytosis without fever. The new consensus definitions for sepsis and septic shock capture the many ways that nosocomial infection complicated by organ system dysfunction may present.

The incidence of fever in patients in ICUs ranges from 8% to 37%. In up to 50% of cases of new fever the cause is noninfectious. Fever may be a consequence of aseptic processes such as surgery-related tissue injury and aseptic cytokine release, deep venous thrombosis, pulmonary embolism, drugs, malignant hyperthermia, neuroleptic malignant syndrome, serotonin syndrome, acute allograft rejection, or withdrawal syndromes. In neurology and neurosurgical ICUs, another noninfectious cause to consider is central fever resulting from resetting of the hypothalamic thermostat from traumatic brain injury or intracranial hemorrhage.

The evaluation of new-onset fever or suspected sepsis in ICUs should be a systematic process that considers all the possible causes without substantial delay of initiation of empiric treatment. A thorough history and physical examination are essential. Important to evaluate in all patients are the reason for admission, recent hospitalizations, comorbidities, immunosuppressive conditions or treatments, recent surgical procedures, medical and surgical interventions during the current hospitalization, transfusions of blood products, presence of invasive support devices (vascular or urinary catheters, endotracheal and thoracostomy tubes, ventricular drains), recent antibiotic exposure, pathogen colonization, and history of recurrent infection syndromes or infectious pathogens. Symptoms, complaints, or problems that have appeared since hospitalization should be determined.

During the physical examination, attention needs to be paid to hemodynamic stability, need (if any) for ongoing fluid resuscitation or vasopressors to maintain blood pressure, recent changes in respiratory rate or oxygen requirements, changes in respiratory secretions, new heart murmurs, appearance of erythema or purulence at the skin exit sites of vascular catheters and other drains, new or asymmetric swelling in the extremities, new sites of tenderness to palpation, changes in the skin, appearance of surgical wounds, and changes in results of the neurologic examination.

Laboratory results that generally should be reviewed include complete blood counts, chemistry panels inclusive of liver function tests, chest radiographs, and, in the setting of acute respiratory infection or suspected sepsis, procalcitonin (see below). Additional radiographic studies may be indicated for evaluation of recent abdominal surgical procedures (eg, computed tomography of the abdomen or pelvis), new swelling or discharge from surgical wounds (eg, computed tomography or ultrasonography), or changes of consciousness (eg, computed tomography of the head).

On the basis of the history, physical examination, and initial laboratory results, a differential diagnosis of the likely cause of fever will need to be developed. Specimens to collect for culture should be directed by the suspected site(s) of infection. In general, at least 2 blood specimens should be collected for culture. If there is no specific evidence to raise concern for infection associated with an indwelling percutaneous vascular device (eg, erythema or purulence at the exit site), 2 blood specimens collected by peripheral venipuncture are recommended; indiscriminate collection of blood from vascular catheters will increase the rate of false-positive blood culture results and unnecessary antibiotic administration and catheter removal. If, in the absence of hemodynamic instability or tunnel or exit site inflammation, central venous catheter infection is suspected, 2 blood specimens can be collected at the same time, 1 by peripheral venipuncture and 1 from the catheter. Growth of the same pathogen in both specimens with earlier growth in the catheter specimen (differential time to positivity ≥2 hours) is consistent with catheter infection. If evidence of vascular catheter infection is identified, or if, in the presence of hemodynamic instability or tunnel or exit site inflammation, central venous catheter infection is suspected, the catheter should be removed immediately and the tip of the catheter should be sent for culture.

The American Thoracic Society and the Infectious Diseases Society of America have defined hospital- or ventilator-associated pneumonia as a new lung infiltrate on chest radiography plus clinical evidence (eg, fever, purulent sputum, leukocytosis) that the infiltrate is of infectious origin. When pneumonia is suspected, lower respiratory tract secretions need to be collected for Gram stain and bacterial and fungal culture. In the nonintubated patient, bronchoscopic evaluation may be necessary if an adequate sputum specimen cannot be collected. In the intubated patient, the most recent guidelines of the American Thoracic Society and the Infectious Diseases Society of America are to obtain a lower respiratory tract specimen for Gram stain and culture noninvasively (ie, by endotracheal aspiration).

Obtaining urine specimens for urinalysis and culture from patients with indwelling bladder catheters should be limited to those with signs or symptoms of urinary tract infection (eg, unexplained suprapubic or flank pain, bladder spasm), kidney transplant recipients, patients with granulocytopenia, patients who have had urologic surgery, and patients with urinary tract obstruction. If a catheter has been in place for more than 14 days, it should be replaced and a specimen should be collected from the newly placed catheter. For patients with new fever in an ICU who do not have symptoms of urinary tract infection or who are not in the aforementioned groups, evaluating urine from bladder catheters is not recommended because the results of cultures are likely to indicate asymptomatic bacteriuria or funguria, for which treatment would not be advised.

Stool specimens should be submitted for testing for *Clostridium difficile* infection if the stools are unformed and 3 or more have been passed in the preceding 24 hours without other causes for diarrhea such as laxatives, gastrointestinal hemorrhage, and recent initiation of enteric nutrition. Current available methods for *C difficile* testing are highly sensitive, and therefore repeat testing is not recommended if a test result is negative. Because toxigenic *C difficile* colonization may persist after treatment, submitting stool for a test of cure after diarrhea has resolved is also not recommended.

Meningitis or parameningeal cranial and spinal infections may complicate craniotomy, internal cerebrospinal fluid shunts, external ventricular drains, external lumbar cerebrospinal fluid drains, epidural injections, lumbar

Table 58.1 • Empiric Antibiotic Management for Nosocomial Infections in the Intensive Care Unit

Infectious Syndrome	Treatment Recommendation	Duration of Therapy
Catheter-associated urinary tract infection	Urinary catheter removal if possible Exchange catheter if in place >14 days and still required Empiric antipseudomonal cephalosporin, antipseudomonal β-lactam/β-lactamase inhibitor, or carbapenem De-escalate to narrowest spectrum of effective therapy based on results of cultures	7 days if signs and symptoms subside rapidly, otherwise 10-14 days
Central line–associated bloodstream infection	Remove catheter whenever possible; this is critical if associated with septic thrombosis, metastatic infection, or septic shock Empiric vancomycin (or daptomycin) for MRSA (when methicillin resistance in *Staphylococcus aureus* is unknown or exceeds 10%–15%) and an empiric 4th-generation cephalosporin, antipseudomonal penicillin-β-lactamase inhibitor, or carbapenem for multidrug-resistant gram-negative bacilli Consider empiric antifungal (*Candida* spp) therapy with an echinocandin in settings of septic shock, total parenteral nutrition, neutropenia, and femoral vein catheterization De-escalate to narrowest spectrum of effective therapy based on culture results	Treatment duration varies from 7-42 days depending on the pathogen and the presence or absence of metastatic infection
Ventilator-associated pneumonia	Empiric vancomycin (or linezolid) for MRSA (when methicillin resistance in *Staphylococcus aureus* is unknown or exceeds 10%-15%) and an empiric 4th-generation cephalosporin, antipseudomonal penicillin-β-lactamase inhibitor, or carbapenem for multidrug-resistant gram-negative bacilli De-escalate to narrowest spectrum of effective therapy based on culture results	7 days
Clostridium difficile infection	Avoid unnecessary use of antibiotics Metronidazole is usually recommended as first-line drug for mild-moderate disease and first recurrence For severe disease (WBC >15×10^9/L or serum Cr >1.5-fold over premorbid level), oral vancomycin is preferred For severe disease complicated by ileus, concomitant administration of vancomycin rectally and metronidazole intravenously may be necessary For severe disease complicated by invasive colitis, broad-spectrum antibiotic therapy (eg, antipseudomonal penicillin + β-lactamase inhibitor or antipseudomonal cephalosporin + metronidazole) is indicated Early surgical evaluation for severe disease should be considered	10-14 days Longer therapy may be required for refractory or recurrent cases
External ventricular device infection	Remove the device Vancomycin plus ceftazidime, cefepime, or meropenem Intraventricular antibiotic (eg, vancomycin, aminoglycoside) administrations is not FDA approved and indications are not clearly defined. Consultation with infectious disease and pharmacy staff should be considered before pursuing	Treatment duration determined by susceptibilities of pathogens to administered antimicrobials, management of foreign bodies at sites of infection, and clinical course

Abbreviations: Cr, creatinine; FDA, US Food and Drug Administration; MRSA, methicillin-resistant *Staphylococcus aureus*; WBC, white blood cell count.

punctures, and trauma. These infections may present with fever, local pain, headache, meningismus, inflammation of surgical wounds or device exit sites, or deteriorations in levels of consciousness or of cognitive function. Imaging; cerebrospinal fluid sampling for cell counts, protein level, glucose level, Gram stain, and bacterial and fungal cultures; surgical exploration with Gram stain; or bacterial and fungal culture of deep wound specimens may be indicated depending on the site of concern.

Pleural space or intra-abdominal infection may complicate ongoing pneumonia, chest tube insertions, gastric tube insertions, recent thoracic or abdominal surgery, bloodstream infection, or underlying organ system disease or dysfunction (eg, colonic diverticulitis). Computed tomography can identify rim-enhancing fluid collections, which may be amenable to diagnostic percutaneous aspiration, Gram stain and culture, and therapeutic drainage.

Management

After the suspected site of infection has been established and appropriate specimens for cultures have been collected, empiric antibiotic treatment should be initiated in the moderately or severely ill patient. Table 58.1 lists empiric antibiotic treatment regimens based on the suspected infection syndrome. Modifications of these suggestions should be directed by facility and, preferably, ICU-specific antibiogram and may be indicated for known colonization with multiple antibiotic-resistant pathogens. Removal of infected devices, drainage of abscesses, or

Table 58.2 • Strategies for Prevention of Nosocomial Infections in the Intensive Care Unit

Infectious Syndrome	Recommended Prevention
Catheter-associated urinary tract infection	Insert urinary catheters Only when indicated: selected surgical procedures, hourly assessment of urine output, management of retention or obstruction, assisting care of adjacent wounds Aseptically, using sterile technique Consider alternatives (eg, condom catheters, intermittent catheterizations, suprapubic catheterization) Maintain unobstructed urine flow in a closed system Remove catheters when no longer needed
Central line–associated bloodstream infection	Bathe patients >2 years old with chlorhexidine preparation daily Avoid femoral vein for central venous access in obese adults, as possible Prepare insertion site with an alcoholic chlorhexidine antiseptic Insert central line using maximum sterile barrier precautions: Mask, cap, sterile gown and gloves, large sterile drape Disinfect hubs, needleless connectors, injection ports with alcoholic chlorhexidine preparation or 70% alcohol or povidone-iodine before access Change dressing and perform site care with chlorhexidine-based antiseptic every 5-7 days for transparent dressings, every 2 days for gauze dressings, and whenever dressing is soiled, loose, or damp Remove central line when no longer needed for patient care
Ventilator-associated pneumonia	Avoid intubation when possible Minimize sedation Maintain and improve physical conditioning Minimize pooling of secretions above the endotracheal tube cuff Elevate the head of the bed Change ventilator circuits only if visibly soiled or malfunctioning Optimize and minimize use of antibiotics across hospital through stewardship
Clostridium difficile infection	Place patients with suspected or confirmed *C difficile* infection in single rooms on contact precautions Gloves and gowns donned and doffed at room entry and exit Meticulous hand hygiene before and after donning and doffing gloves and gowns Soap and water preferred in outbreak settings Dedicate equipment to care of patient as possible; clean and disinfect all other equipment with sporicidal agent at room entry and exit Use Environmental Protection Agency–approved, hospital-grade sporicidal disinfectant (eg, sodium hypochlorite) for environmental cleaning of rooms of patients with *C difficile* infection
External ventricular devices	Insert the device using sterile technique One dose of antibiotics before device insertion is recommended as prophylaxis Antimicrobial impregnated devices are recommended to decrease the risk of infection Cerebrospinal fluid sampling is recommended only when clinically indicated; this should not be done routinely. Routine change of catheters is not recommended

débridement of surgical wounds is essential for adequate therapy. When infected devices cannot be removed (eg, cranioplasties, external ventricular drains), options for optimal management may best be identified through cross-disciplinary reviews with surgeons and infectious diseases subspecialists.

During the 24 to 72 hours after initiation of an empiric antibiotic regimen, results of cultures and other laboratory studies and the patient's clinical course must be assessed to determine whether this additional information supports diagnosis of the infectious syndrome suspected at initiation of antibiotic treatment. If it does, the empiric regimen generally should be narrowed to treat the pathogens recovered in culture, and the duration of the therapeutic regimen needs to be determined. Serum procalcitonin levels may be useful for determination of duration of antibiotic treatment, especially in the setting of lower respiratory tract infection and sepsis. However, other clinical scenarios need further investigation. Recommended durations of antibiotic treatment of common infection syndromes are provided in Table 58.1. If the clinical course and culture and laboratory findings do not support an infection syndrome, the antibiotic treatment should be stopped and other additional diagnostic evaluation should be pursued as clinically indicated.

Prevention

Prevention of nosocomial infection in the ICU is critically important. Strategies for reducing the risk of the predominant nosocomial infections in the ICU are described in Table 58.2.

Summary

- Fever does not necessarily indicate an infectious process; noninfectious causes of fever should always be comprehensively considered.
- The evaluation of a patient with fever in an ICU can be challenging. A thorough history and physical examination are required. Further evaluation tests and procedures should be done based on clinical and epidemiologic considerations.
- Prompt empiric antibiotic administration is beneficial for patients with sepsis. Broad-spectrum empiric antibiotic regimens should be narrowed to therapeutic regimens within 48 to 72 hours of initiation when results of cultures become available.
- Most nosocomial infections can be prevented by methodic implementation of preventive strategies.

SUGGESTED READING

Angus DC, Linde-Zwirble WT, Lidicker J, Clermont G, Carcillo J, Pinsky MR. Epidemiology of severe sepsis in the United States: analysis of incidence, outcome, and associated costs of care. Crit Care Med. 2001 Jul;29(7):1303–10.

Barlam TF, Cosgrove SE, Abbo LM, MacDougall C, Schuetz AN, Septimus EJ, et al. Implementing an antibiotic stewardship program: guidelines by the Infectious Diseases Society of America and the Society for Healthcare Epidemiology of America. Clin Infect Dis. 2016 May 15;62(10):e51–77. Epub 2016 Apr 13.

Baron EJ, Weinstein MP, Dunne WM Jr, Yagupsky P, Welch DF, Wilson DM. Blood cultures IV. Washington (DC): ASM Press; c2005. (Cumitech: cumulative techniques and procedures in clinical microbiology series).

Chenoweth CE, Gould CV, Saint S. Diagnosis, management, and prevention of catheter-associated urinary tract infections. Infect Dis Clin North Am. 2014 Mar;28(1):105–19. Epub 2013 Dec 8.

Cohen SH, Gerding DN, Johnson S, Kelly CP, Loo VG, McDonald LC, et al; Society for Healthcare Epidemiology of America; Infectious Diseases Society of America. Clinical practice guidelines for *Clostridium difficile* infection in adults: 2010 update by the Society for Healthcare Epidemiology of America (SHEA) and the Infectious Diseases Society of America (IDSA). Infect Control Hosp Epidemiol. 2010 May;31(5):431–55.

Drugs for bacterial infections. Treat Guidel Med Lett. 2010 Jun;8(94):43–52.

Dubberke ER, Carling P, Carrico R, Donskey CJ, Loo VG, McDonald LC, et al. Strategies to prevent *Clostridium difficile* infections in acute care hospitals: 2014 update. Infect Control Hosp Epidemiol. 2014 Jun;35(6):628–45.

Dudeck MA, Edwards JR, Allen-Bridson K, Gross C, Malpiedi PJ, Peterson KD, et al. National Healthcare Safety Network Report, data summary for 2013, device-associated module. Am J Infect Control. 2015 Mar 1;43(3):206–21. Epub 2015 Jan 6.

Dudeck MA, Horan TC, Peterson KD, Allen-Bridson K, Morrell C, Pollock DA, et al. National Healthcare Safety Network (NHSN) Report, data summary for 2010, device-associated module. Am J Infect Control. 2011 Dec;39(10):798–816.

Fried HI, Nathan BR, Rowe AS, Zabramski JM, Andaluz N, Bhimraj A, et al. The insertion and management of external ventricular drains: an evidence-based consensus statement: a statement for healthcare professionals from the Neurocritical Care Society. Neurocrit Care. 2016 Feb;24(1):61–81.

Hooton TM, Bradley SF, Cardenas DD, Colgan R, Geerlings SE, Rice JC, et al; Infectious Diseases Society of America. Diagnosis, prevention, and treatment of catheter-associated urinary tract infection in adults: 2009 International Clinical Practice Guidelines from the Infectious Diseases Society of America. Clin Infect Dis. 2010 Mar 1;50(5):625–63.

Kalil AC, Metersky ML, Klompas M, Muscedere J, Sweeney DA, Palmer LB, et al. Management of adults with hospital-acquired and ventilator-associated pneumonia: 2016 Clinical Practice Guidelines by the Infectious Diseases Society of America and the American Thoracic Society. Clin Infect Dis. 2016 Sep 1;63(5):e61–e111. Epub 2016 Jul 14.

Klompas M, Branson R, Eichenwald EC, Greene LR, Howell MD, Lee G, et al; Society for Healthcare Epidemiology of America (SHEA). Strategies to prevent ventilator-associated pneumonia in acute care hospitals: 2014 update. Infect Control Hosp Epidemiol. 2014 Aug;35(8):915–36.

Laws C, Jallo JI. Fever and infection in the neurosurgical intensive care unit. JHN J. 2010;5(2):23–7.

Leone M, Bouadma L, Bouhemad B, Brissaud O, Dauger S, Gibot S, et al. Hospital-acquired pneumonia in ICU. Anaesth Crit Care Pain Med. 2018 Feb;37(1):83–98. Epub 2017 Nov 15.

Lo E, Nicolle LE, Coffin SE, Gould C, Maragakis LL, Meddings J, et al. Strategies to prevent catheter-associated urinary tract infections in acute care hospitals: 2014 update. Infect Control Hosp Epidemiol. 2014 May;35(5):464–79.

Maki DG, Tsigrelis C. Nosocomial infection in the intensive care unit. In: Parrillo JE, Dellinger RP, editors. Critical care medicine: principles of diagnosis and management in the adult. 4th ed. Philadelphia (PA): Elsevier/Saunders; c2014. p. 825–69.

Marschall J, Mermel LA, Fakih M, Hadaway L, Kallen A, O'Grady NP, et al; Society for Healthcare Epidemiology of America. Strategies to prevent central line-associated bloodstream infections in acute care hospitals: 2014 update. Infect Control Hosp Epidemiol. 2014 Jul;35(7):753–71.

Martin GS, Mannino DM, Eaton S, Moss M. The epidemiology of sepsis in the United States from 1979 through 2000. N Engl J Med. 2003 Apr 17;348(16):1546–54.

Mermel LA, Allon M, Bouza E, Craven DE, Flynn P, O'Grady NP, et al. Clinical practice guidelines for the diagnosis and management of intravascular catheter-related infection: 2009 update by the Infectious Diseases Society of America. Clin Infect Dis. 2009 Jul 1;49(1):1–45. Errata in: Clin Infect Dis. 2010 Apr 1;50(7):1079. Clin Infect Dis. 2010 Feb 1;50(3):457.

Mitchell JD, Grocott HP, Phillips-Bute B, Mathew JP, Newman MF, Bar-Yosef S. Cytokine secretion after cardiac surgery and its relationship to postoperative fever. Cytokine. 2007 Apr;38(1):37–42. Epub 2007 Jun 14.

Mitharwal SM, Yaddanapudi S, Bhardwaj N, Gautam V, Biswal M, Yaddanapudi L. Intensive care unit-acquired infections in a tertiary care hospital: an epidemiologic survey and influence on patient outcomes. Am J Infect Control. 2016 Jul 1;44(7):e113–7. Epub 2016 Mar 2.

O'Grady NP, Barie PS, Bartlett JG, Bleck T, Carroll K, Kalil AC, et al; American College of Critical Care Medicine; Infectious Diseases Society of America. Guidelines for evaluation of new fever in critically ill adult patients: 2008 update from the American College of Critical Care Medicine and the Infectious Diseases Society of America. Crit Care Med. 2008 Apr;36(4):1330–49. Erratum in: Crit Care Med. 2008 Jun;36(6):1992.

Raad I, Hanna HA, Alakech B, Chatzinikolaou I, Johnson MM, Tarrand J. Differential time to positivity: a useful method for diagnosing catheter-related bloodstream infections. Ann Intern Med. 2004 Jan 6;140(1):18–25.

Rhee C. Using procalcitonin to guide antibiotic therapy. Open Forum Infect Dis. 2016 Dec 7;4(1):ofw249.

Richards MJ, Edwards JR, Culver DH, Gaynes RP. Nosocomial infections in combined medical-surgical intensive care units in the United States. Infect Control Hosp Epidemiol. 2000 Aug;21(8):510–5.

Singer M, Deutschman CS, Seymour CW, Shankar-Hari M, Annane D, Bauer M, et al. The Third International Consensus Definitions for Sepsis and Septic Shock (Sepsis-3). JAMA. 2016 Feb 23;315(8):801–10.

van de Beek D, Drake JM, Tunkel AR. Nosocomial bacterial meningitis. N Engl J Med. 2010 Jan 14;362(2):146–54.

Vazquez-Guillamet C, Kollef MH. Treatment of Gram-positive infections in critically ill patients. BMC Infect Dis. 2014 Nov 28;14:92.

Weiner LM, Fridkin SK, Aponte-Torres Z, Avery L, Coffin N, Dudeck MA, et al. Vital signs: preventing antibiotic-resistant infections in hospitals: United States, 2014. MMWR Morb Mortal Wkly Rep. 2016 Mar 11;65(9):235–41.

Weinstein MP. Blood culture contamination: persisting problems and partial progress. J Clin Microbiol. 2003 Jun;41(6):2275–8.

Young PJ, Saxena M. Fever management in intensive care patients with infections. Crit Care. 2014 Mar 18;18(2):206.

59 Antibiotics in the Intensive Care Unit

DAVID A. SOTELLO AVILES, MD; WALTER C. HELLINGER, MD

Goals

- Provide a background of different antibiotics and their mechanisms of action.
- Elucidate antibiotic activity against different organisms.
- Describe antibiotic resistance and stewardship.

Introduction

Antimicrobial therapy is a critical component in the management of many infections. Antimicrobial therapy should not be initiated before a susceptible pathogen is suspected or confirmed or before appropriate diagnostic specimens, including those for cultures, are collected. The limited and adjunctive role of antibiotics in the management of many infections that require source control (eg, removal of infected devices, drainage of abscesses) or mitigation of predisposing anatomical or physiologic conditions (eg, recurrent respiratory aspiration, obstruction of the urine collection system) needs to be respected. Recognizing indications for antibiotic administration and appropriately selecting agents based on clinical and microbiologic findings are required. Distinguishing between empiric prescribing, when infection syndromes and pathogens are suspected, and therapeutic prescribing, when infection syndromes are confirmed and pathogens identified, is critically important.

Working knowledge of drug dosing, adjustment of dosing for renal or hepatic insufficiency, drug-drug interactions, and antibiotic allergies or intolerances is required, and ready access to and liberal use of reference guides help ensure good patient care. The ultimate goal of prescribing is to choose the safest, narrowest, shortest, and least expensive regimen. The first step that must be taken on the path to rational use of antibiotics is to understand the drugs themselves and their spectrum of activities, pharmacology, toxicity, and potential therapeutic roles.

This chapter reviews the pharmacologic characteristics and clinical applications of the antibiotic agents most frequently used in the intensive care unit. The spectrums of activity of the most commonly used antibiotics in critical care units are summarized in Table 59.1.

Antibiotics

β-Lactam Antibiotics

These agents inhibit synthesis of the bacterial peptidoglycan cell wall by attachment to, and inactivation of, bacterial penicillin-binding proteins, the peptidases that extend and cross-link cell wall peptides. This class of antibiotics encompasses several families, including penicillins, cephalosporins, carbapenems and monobactams, which share a common core structure, the β-lactam ring, but differ in their spectrums of activity, pharmacology, and therapeutic applications.

Penicillins

Penicillin is the naturally occurring parent compound, produced by the mold *Penicillium*. It is active against many gram-positive cocci, gram-positive bacilli, anaerobes, and spirochetes. Resistance to penicillin and to all of its derivatives discussed below is mediated through 1) production of a β-lactamase, which hydrolyzes its β-lactam ring; 2) alterations in the outer cell membranes of gram-negative bacteria that prevent penicillin from reaching peptidases at the peptidoglycan cell wall; or 3) alteration in conformation of peptidases that prevents penicillin and other β-lactam antibiotic binding and thereby results in intrinsic β-lactam antibiotic resistance, as observed in methicillin-resistant staphylococci and penicillin-resistant pneumococci.

Penicillinase-resistant, antistaphylococcal penicillins (eg, nafcillin, oxacillin) are not inactivated by the β-lactamase (penicillinase) that is produced by 80% of strains of

Table 59.1 • Summarized Antibiotic Spectrum of Agents Most Commonly Used in the ICU

	Coverage									
Group	**GP**	**GN**	***Pseudomonas aeruginosa***	**Anaerobes**	**MSSA**	**MRSA**	***Listeria* spp**	**GN ESBL**	**GN CRE**	**Other**
Antistaphylococcal penicillins	+++	+	–	–	+++	–	–	–	–	
Aminopenicillins	++	++	–	+	–	–	+++	–	–	Enterococci (not VRE)
Carboxypenicillins/ ureidopenicillins	+++	+++	+++	+	–	–	++	–	–	
Ureidopenicillin + β-lactamase inhibitor	+++	+++	+++	+++	++	–	++	+	–	
Cephalosporins										
First-generation	+++	+	–	+	+++	–	–	–	–	
Second-generation	+++	++	–	+	++	–	–	–	–	
Third-generation	++	+++	–	+	++	–	–	–	–	*Borrelia* spp, *Neisseria gonorrhoeae*
Fourth-generation	++	+++	+++	+	++	–	–	–	–	
Ceftaroline	+++	+++	–	+	+++	+++	–	–	–	
Carbapenems	+++	+++	+++	+++	+++	–	++	+++	–	Enterococci (not including ertapenem)
Vancomycin	+++	–	–	–	++	+++	–	–	–	Enterococci, *Clostridium difficile* (oral)
Daptomycin	+++	–	–	–	+++	+++	–	–	–	Enterococci
Linezolid	+++	–	–	–	+++	+++	+	–	–	
Quinolones	++	+++	++	–	+	–	++	+/–	+/–	*Chlamydia* spp, *Mycoplasma* spp, *Legionella* spp, *Salmonella* spp, *Brucella* spp
Macrolides	++	+	–	–	++	–	–	–	–	*Chlamydia* spp, *Mycoplasma* spp, *Legionella* spp, *Rickettsiae* spp, *Corynebacterium diphtheriae*, *Bordetella pertussis*
Tetracyclines	+++	++	–	–	++	++	–	+/–	+/–	*Mycoplasma* spp, *Chlamydia* spp, *Coxiella burnetii*, *Rickettsia* spp, *Anaplasma*, *Borrelia* spp
Tigecycline (glycylcycline)	+++	+++	–	–	++	+++	–	++	++	Same as tetracyclines
Clindamycin	+++	–	–	++	++	++	–	–	–	
Metronidazole	–	–	–	+++	–	–	–	–	–	*C difficile*, many protozoal microorganisms
Trimethoprim-sulfamethoxazole	++	++	–	–	++	++	++	+	+	*Pneumocystis jiroveci*, *Nocardia* spp, *Stenotrophomonas* spp, *Burkholderia* spp, *Toxoplasma gondii*
Aminoglycosides	+	+++	++	–	–	+	++	+	+	Synergy for enterococci, streptococci, *Staphylococcus aureus*

Abbreviations: CRE, carbapenem-resistant Enterobacteriaceae; ESBL, extended-spectrum β-lactamases; GN, gram-negative; GP, gram-positive; ICU, intensive care unit; MRSA, methicillin-resistant *Staphylococcus aureus*; MSSA, methicillin-susceptible *Staphylococcus aureus*; VRE, vancomycin-resistant enterococci; plus and minus symbols indicate degree of effectiveness.

Staphylococcus aureus and most health care–related coagulase-negative staphylococci.

Aminopenicillins (eg, ampicillin, amoxicillin), by virtue of their greater lipid solubility compared with penicillin, are able to cross the outer cell membrane of gram-negative bacteria and are thereby active against many non–β-lactamase-producing strains of common gram-negative pathogens, such as *Escherichia coli, Proteus*, and *Salmonella*. The aminopenicillins, unlike the antistaphylococcal penicillins discussed above, share penicillin's excellent activity against streptococci, including enterococci.

The extended-spectrum penicillins (carboxypenicillins and ureidopenicillins), like the aminopenicillins, retain the base spectrum of activity of penicillin while extending it to provide activity against gram-negative bacteria that are not susceptible to the aminopenicillins. They are active against *Pseudomonas aeruginosa* organisms.

In general, penicillins are minimally metabolized. They are cleared primarily by the renal system and are cleared quickly. The serum half-life of penicillins is less than 60 minutes; optimally, they must be administered every 4 to 6 hours. The antistaphylococcal penicillins, the aminopenicillins, and the ureidopenicillins are excreted in the bile; biliary excretion of the antistaphylococcal penicillins is such that they can be administered without dose adjustment to patients in renal failure receiving dialysis with unimpaired hepatic function. With the exception of the antistaphylococcal penicillins, dose reduction is generally required in the setting of renal dysfunction.

One of the more common adverse effects of the penicillins is hypersensitivity reactions, including rash, anaphylactic shock, and interstitial nephritis. Hepatobiliary toxicity (hepatocellular enzyme increase) may occur during administration of antistaphylococcal penicillins. The penicillins have poor central nervous system (CNS) penetration, which is improved in the setting of meningeal inflammation.

Cephalosporins

Cephalosporins are grouped by the generations in which they were released, chronologically. The generations do differ in their spectrum of activity and pharmacology. The first- and second-generation cephalosporins are more active against gram-positive bacteria, and the third- and fourth-generations are more active against gram-negative bacteria. Some third-generation cephalosporins (eg, ceftazidime) and the fourth-generation cephalosporins (eg, cefipime) are active against *P aeruginosa*. Neither the cephalosporins nor the penicillins are active against *Legionella* spp, *Mycoplasma* spp, *Chlamydia* spp, or *Rickettsia* spp. With the single exception of ceftaroline (see below), the cephalosporins are not active against enterococci. The mechanisms of bacterial resistance, excretion, and adverse reactions are similar to those of penicillins. The serum half-lives of the third- and fourth-generation agents, particularly ceftriaxone, are, in general, longer than those of the first- and second-generation agents. All agents are principally eliminated by renal excretion and must be adjusted for renal insufficiency except for ceftriaxone, which is so efficiently excreted in the bile that it can be given, like the antistaphylococcal penicillins, without dose adjustment to patients in renal failure receiving dialysis with unimpaired hepatic function. All of the third-generation cephalosporins, except cefoperazone, and the only fourth-generation agent, cefepime, can penetrate the blood-brain barrier and achieve CNS concentrations suitable for treatment of susceptible pathogens.

Recently released fifth-generation cephalosporins are, unlike all other β-lactam antibiotics, active against methicillin-resistant staphylococci and penicillin-resistant pneumococci. Agents in this class include ceftaroline and ceftobiprole (not available in the United States). Neither agent is active against *P aeruginosa*.

Carbapenems

This family of β-lactam antibiotics includes agents with the broadest spectrum of activity of all antimicrobials approved for systemic administration to humans. Imipenem, the first carbapenem to be released, is active against streptococci, enterococci, methicillin-susceptible *S aureus*, most anaerobes, and most gram-negative bacteria (including *Pseudomonas*). Subsequently released meropenem and doripenem have spectrums of activity and pharmacology similar to those of imipenem without imipenem's epileptogenicity and infusion-related emesis. Imipenem, meropenem, and doripenem must be administered every 6 to 8 hours to patients with normal renal function. The most recently released ertapenem can be administered once every 24 hours because of its longer serum half-life. Ertapenem, however, lacks activity against enterococci and *Pseudomonas* and *Acinetobacter* organisms. Because of their very broad spectrum, these agents can be used to treat various infections, including polymicrobial infections, and meropenem has been shown to be safe and effective in a wide range of bacterial CNS infections. Given their exceptional activity against common nosocomial aerobic gram-negative bacterial pathogens, however, many institutions have elected to discourage frequent use of these agents when other less broadly active agents can be used together or in combination so as to prevent the appearance and spread of carbapenem resistance.

Monobactams

Aztreonam is the single member of this family. Its spectrum of activity is limited to aerobic gram-negative pathogens, including *P aeruginosa*. Aztreonam has the unusual property of infrequently producing cross-reactive hypersensitivity in patients who are allergic to penicillins or cephalosporins, the exception being ceftazidime, from which aztreonam was created by removal of its 6-member dihydrothiazine ring.

β-Lactam–β-Lactamase Inhibitor Combinations

β-Lactamase inhibitors are relatively small compounds that serve as suicide inhibitors of β-lactamases produced by staphylococci, anaerobes, and aerobic gram-negative bacilli. When combined with β-lactam antibiotics, these inhibitors extend the spectrum of the co-administered agents to second-line antistaphylococcal activity, first-line antianaerobic activity, and broader aerobic gram-negative activity. Examples of these agents include clavulanate, sulbactam, and tazobactam, which have been combined with aminopenicillins (amoxicillin-clavulanate, ampicillin-sulbactam), ureidopenicillins (ticarcillin-clavulanate, piperacillin-tazobactam), and cephalosporins (ceftazidime-tazobactam). The spectrum of activity and pharmacology of the β-lactam antibiotics remain unchanged when administered with the β-lactamase inhibitor.

Two recently released β-lactam–β-lactamase inhibitor combinations, ceftazidime-avibactam and ceftolozane-tazobactam, provide reliable activity against an array of extended spectrum β-lactamases that are responsible for conferring broad resistance of common gram-negative bacterial pathogens (eg, *E coli, Klebsiella pneumoniae*) to most penicillins and cephalosporins. Ceftazidime-avibactam is also active against many carbapenem-resistant Enterobacteriaceae, although not metallo-β-lactamase– (eg, New Delhi metallo-β-lactamase-1) producing strains.

Quinolones

The quinolone antibiotics block bacterial DNA gyrase and topoisomerase IV, which are responsible for bacterial DNA synthesis and postreplication DNA modification. Most are fluorinated derivatives of nalidixic acid, which was released in the 1960s. The first fluoroquinolone antibiotics to be released (eg, norfloxacin, ciprofloxacin, ofloxacin) were active against *S aureus* and aerobic gram-negative bacilli and cocci, including, with respect to ciprofloxacin, *P aeruginosa*. A subsequent generation of fluoroquinolones (eg, levofloxacin, moxifloxacin, gemifloxacin), also known as respiratory quinolones, have reliable activity against penicillin-resistant *Streptococcus pneumoniae*. Levofloxacin is distinguished in this later generation by activity against many aerobic gram-negative bacteria, including *Pseudomonas* organisms. The fluoroquinolones are active in vivo against a wide array of intracellular pathogens, including *Mycoplasma, Chlamydia, Legionella, Salmonella*, and *Brucella*. They are also active against *Mycobacterium tuberculosis* and *Bacillus anthracis*.

Quinolones are efficiently absorbed from the gastrointestinal tract, more than 95% for many compounds, a feature that facilitates administration and reduces cost of therapy. They achieve excellent penetration of the genitourinary tract, lungs, prostate, bones, and joints. They can be used to treat respiratory, gastrointestinal, genitourinary, and musculoskeletal infections. Most may be administered once or twice daily and require dose adjustment for renal impairment. Toxicities include tendinopathy (more common in older patients); impairment of bone development in immature animals, which has restricted their use in the pediatric population; neuropathy; and prolongation of the QT interval. Bacterial resistance to fluoroquinolones, especially in health care–associated infection, has increased because of their widespread use. As for all other antibiotics, susceptibility to these agents must be examined in pathogens for which they are prescribed.

Glycopeptides

These antibiotics, of which vancomycin is the best known, are frequently used to treat infections of patients in the intensive care unit. Most importantly, they are active against methicillin-resistant staphylococci, both coagulase-positive (ie, *S aureus*) and coagulase-negative. In addition, they are active against *Bacillus* spp, *Corynebacterium* spp, *Actinomyces* spp, *Clostridium* spp, and many *Enterococcus* spp. They are not active against gram-negative bacteria or mycobacteria. Because of their negligible absorption after oral administration, their use is restricted to parenteral administration, with the exception of intraluminal therapy of *Clostridium difficile* infection. Their bactericidal mechanism of action is through inhibition of the cell wall synthesis by binding to the D-alanyl-D-alanine terminus of peptide cell wall precursors. Resistance is most common among *Enterococcus* spp (especially *E faecium*) and is rare, fortunately, in *S aureus*.

Vancomycin is inferior to antistaphylococcal penicillins for treatment of methicillin-susceptible *S aureus*. Vancomycin can pass the blood-brain barrier to a limited degree, achieving therapeutic concentrations in the cerebrospinal fluid, most reliably so in the setting of meningeal inflammation. It is excreted without metabolism renally. A not infrequent toxicity is infusion-related red man syndrome that follows histamine release from direct, nonallergic vancomycin-mediated mast cell destabilization. It can usually be mitigated or avoided by slowing the rate of infusion. Nephrotoxicity was a common complication of originally released vancomycin formulations in the 1960s. Although less common now, nephrotoxicity still occurs, and its risk is reduced by monitoring serum levels to avoid excessive increases. Ototoxicity has also been reported with supratherapeutic levels.

Newer Agents Active Against Gram-Positive Bacterial Pathogens

Daptomycin is a lipopeptide that disrupts the bacterial cell membrane function in a calcium-dependent mechanism, which in turn results in depolarization, loss of membrane potential, and cell death. Its spectrum of activity is very similar to that of vancomycin. Muscular toxicity is the most common adverse effect. It is inactivated by pulmonary surfactant and, therefore, cannot be used for treatment of pneumonia. Bacterial resistance may appear during treatment, particularly in settings of high inocula or foreign body–associated infection. Therefore, appropriate dosing, sometimes in combination with other agents, and appropriate source control of infection (ie, débridement of devitalized tissues, removal of infected foreign bodies) are indicated.

Linezolid is an oxazolidinone that has excellent coverage against gram-positive organisms, including *Staphylococci* spp and *Enterococci* spp. It inhibits protein synthesis by binding to the 50S ribosomal subunit. It achieves excellent absorption after oral administration and is commonly used for treatment of infections caused by *S aureus* (including methicillin-resistant *S aureus*), *E faecium* (vancomycin-resistant), and other streptococcal infections. Major adverse effects include myelosuppression, usually appearing after 14 or more days of administration, and, because of its nonspecific inhibition of monoamine oxidase, interaction with commonly used drugs such as selective serotonin reuptake inhibitors to provoke the serotonin syndrome.

Other Antibiotic Agents Used in the Intensive Care Unit

The macrolides are useful for treatment of gram-positive infections such as *Streptococci* spp and for treatment of *Moraxella catarrhalis*, nontuberculous mycobacteria, and intracellular organisms including *Chlamydia, Mycoplasma, Legionella*, and *Rickettsiae* spp. They are agents of choice when treating *Corynebacterium diphtheriae*, and *Bordetella pertussis*. Some have substantial gastrointestinal adverse effects and can prolong the QT interval.

Tetracyclines are active against a broad range of intracellular pathogens, including *Mycoplasma, Chlamydia, Legionella, Coxiella burnetti, Rickettsia* spp, and *Anaplasma phagocytophilum*, and spirochetes, including *Borrelia* spp (eg, *B burgdorferi*, the agent of Lyme disease), *Treponema pallidum*, and *Listeria*. Members including doxycycline and minocycline have near 100% oral bioavailability and readily cross the blood-brain barrier, reaching therapeutic cerebrospinal fluid concentrations. Dosage adjustment is generally not required for renal dysfunction, but caution is advised during administration in the setting of hepatic dysfunction. Common important adverse effects include gastrointestinal upset, esophageal ulceration, and photosensitizing rash. Tigecycline is a glycylcycline derivative of minocycline that has broad antimicrobial activity including methicillin-resistant *S aureus, Acinetobacter baumannii*, and some multiple–drug-resistant aerobic gram-negative pathogens, excluding *P aeruginosa*. The therapeutic niche of tigecycline remains to be determined.

Clindamycin is active against many gram-positive pathogens, including *Streptococcus* spp and *S aureus*, and has broad activity against anaerobic pathogens, including *Bacteroides fragilis*. Its administration may be more strongly associated with a risk of *C difficile* colitis than many other antibiotics. Metronidazole is a nitroimidazole active against many anaerobic protozoal and bacterial microorganisms. It has excellent oral bioavailability and tissue distribution, including the CNS. It is commonly used for CNS infections when anaerobic coverage is required and for treatment of mild to moderate *C difficile* infections. Trimethoprim-sulfamethoxazole is active against many strains of methicillin-resistant *S aureus, Streptococcus* spp, and other aerobic gram-positive and gram-negative pathogens, including multiple–drug-resistant pathogens such as *Burkholderia* spp and *Stenotrophomonas*. It is also a first-line agent in the treatment of *Pneumocystis jiroveci, Toxoplasma gondii*, and many *Nocardia* spp.

Aminoglycosides exert their antimicrobial effect by inhibiting bacterial protein synthesis. They are active against aerobic gram-negative bacteria and some mycobacteria. In combination with agents that interfere with bacterial cell wall synthesis or repair, they can synergistically inhibit some bacterial pathogens, including strains of *Enterococcus* spp, *Streptococcus* spp, *S aureus*, and *Pseudomonas*. They are not used as monotherapy when equally active agents in less toxic classes of antibiotics are available. They are not absorbed after oral administration. Their distribution after parenteral administration is primarily the extracellular fluid space, except for the CNS because they do not efficiently cross the blood-brain barrier. Their most important toxicities are nephrotoxicity, ototoxicity, and vestibular toxicity, which can be prevented or mitigated by appropriate dosing, laboratory monitoring of renal function and serum drug concentrations, and clinical monitoring of hearing, tinnitus, and vertigo. These toxicities can occur even with optimal therapeutic monitoring. If identified early, many reverse after immediate discontinuation of aminoglycoside use.

Summary

- Antibiotics are routinely used in intensive care units; a comprehensive understanding of their pharmacodynamic and pharmacokinetic properties is essential for their rational use and avoidance of potential adverse effects or interactions with other drugs.
- A strong knowledge of the different spectra of activity of the different antibiotic groups is crucial for adequate therapy.
- Empiric and therapeutic selection of antimicrobials must be made in light of possible antibiotic resistance of potential pathogens, both to ensure optimal clinical outcomes and to prevent unnecessary selective pressure that will promote the appearance and further spread of antibiotic resistance.

SUGGESTED READING

Ali M, Naureen H, Tariq MH, Farrukh MJ, Usman A, Khattak S, et al. Rational use of antibiotics in an intensive care unit: a retrospective study of the impact on clinical outcomes and mortality rate. Infect Drug Resist. 2019 Feb 26;12:493–9.

Baddour LM, Wilson WR, Bayer AS, Fowler VG Jr, Tleyjeh IM, Rybak MJ, et al; American Heart Association Committee on Rheumatic Fever, Endocarditis, and Kawasaki Disease of the Council on Cardiovascular Disease in the Young, Council on Clinical Cardiology, Council on Cardiovascular Surgery and Anesthesia, and Stroke Council. Infective endocarditis in adults: diagnosis, antimicrobial therapy, and management of complications: a scientific statement for healthcare professionals from the American Heart Association. Circulation. 2015 Oct 13;132(15):1435–1486. Epub 2015 Sep 15. Errata in: Circulation. 2015 Oct 27;132(17):e215. Circulation. 2016 Aug 23;134(8):e113.

Campion M, Scully G. Antibiotic use in the intensive care unit: optimization and de-escalation. J Intensive Care Med. 2018 Dec;33(12):647–55. Epub 2018 Mar 13.

Craig WA, Andes DR. Cephalosporins. In: Bennett JE, Dolin R, Blaser MJ, editors. Mandell, Douglas, and Bennett's principles and practice of infectious diseases. 8th ed. Vol. 1. Philadelphia (PA): Elsevier/Saunders; c2015. p. 278–292.

Doi Y, Chambers HF. Penicillins and β-lactamase inhibitors. In: Bennett JE, Dolin R, Blaser MJ, editors. Mandell, Douglas, and Bennett's principles and practice of infectious diseases. 8th ed. Vol. 1. Philadelphia (PA): Elsevier/Saunders; c2015. p. 263–277.

Hooper DC, Strahilevitz J. Quinolones. In: Bennett JE, Dolin R, Blaser MJ, editors. Mandell, Douglas, and Bennett's principles and practice of infectious diseases. 8th ed. Vol. 1. Philadelphia (PA): Elsevier/Saunders; c2015. p. 419–439.

Leggett JE. Aminoglycosides. In: Bennett JE, Dolin R, Blaser MJ, editors. Mandell, Douglas, and Bennett's principles and practice of infectious diseases. 8th ed. Vol. 1. Philadelphia (PA): Elsevier/Saunders; c2015. p. 310–321.

Leone M, Bouadma L, Bouhemad B, Brissaud O, Dauger S, Gibot S, et al. Hospital-acquired pneumonia in ICU. Anaesth Crit Care Pain Med. 2018 Feb;37(1):83–98. Epub 2017 Nov 15.

MacDougall C, Chambers HF. Protein synthesis inhibitors and miscellaneous antibacterial agents. In: Brunton LL, editor. Goodman & Gilman's: the pharmacological basis of therapeutics. 12th ed. New York (NY): McGraw-Hill Medical; c2011. p. 1521–1547.

Marston HD, Dixon DM, Knisely JM, Palmore TN, Fauci AS. Antimicrobial resistance. JAMA. 2016 Sep 20;316(11):1193–1204.

Moffa M, Brook I. Tetracyclines, glycylcyclines, and chloramphenicol. In: Bennett JE, Dolin R, Blaser MJ, editors. Mandell, Douglas, and Bennett's principles and practice of infectious diseases. 8th ed. Vol. 1. Philadelphia (PA): Elsevier/Saunders; c2015. p. 322–338.

Murray BE, Arias CA, Nannini EC. Glycopeptides (vancomycin and teicoplanin), streptogramins (quinupristin-dalfopristin), lipopeptides (daptomycin), and lipoglycopeptides (telavancin). In: Bennett JE, Dolin R, Blaser MJ, editors. Mandell, Douglas, and Bennett's principles and practice of infectious diseases. 8th ed. Vol. 1. Philadelphia (PA): Elsevier/Saunders; c2015. p. 377–s400.

Nagel JL, Aronoff DM. Metronidazole. In: Bennett JE, Dolin R, Blaser MJ, editors. Mandell, Douglas, and Bennett's principles and practice of infectious diseases. 8th ed. Vol. 1. Philadelphia (PA): Elsevier/Saunders; c2015. p. 350–357.

Pappas PG, Kauffman CA, Andes DR, Clancy CJ, Marr KA, Ostrosky-Zeichner L, et al. Clinical Practice Guideline for the Management of Candidiasis: 2016 update by the Infectious Diseases Society of America. Clin Infect Dis. 2016 Feb 15;62(4):e1-50. Epub 2015 Dec 16.

Petri WA Jr. Penicillins, cephalosporins, and other β-lactam antibiotics. In: Brunton LL, editor. Goodman & Gilman's: the pharmacological basis of therapeutics. 12th ed. New York (NY): McGraw-Hill Medical; c2011. p. 1477–1503.

Petri WA Jr. Sulfonamides, trimethoprim-sulfamethoxazole, quinolones, and agents for urinary tract infections. In: Brunton LL, editor. Goodman & Gilman's: the pharmacological basis of therapeutics. 12th ed. New York (NY): McGraw-Hill Medical; c2011. p. 1463–1476.

Sivapalasingam S, Steigbigel NH. Macrolides, clindamycin, and ketolides. In: Bennett JE, Dolin R, Blaser MJ, editors. Mandell, Douglas, and Bennett's principles and practice of infectious diseases. 8th ed. Vol. 1. Philadelphia (PA): Elsevier/Saunders; c2015. p. 358–376.

Timsit JF, Bassetti M, Cremer O, Daikos G, de Waele J, Kallil A, et al. Rationalizing antimicrobial therapy in the ICU: a narrative review. Intensive Care Med. 2019 Feb;45(2):172–89. Epub 2019 Jan 18.

Zinner SH, Mayer KH. Sulfonamides and trimethoprim. In: Bennett JE, Dolin R, Blaser MJ, editors. Mandell, Douglas, and Bennett's principles and practice of infectious diseases. 8th ed. Vol. 1. Philadelphia (PA): Elsevier/Saunders; c2015. p. 410–418.

Sepsis and Septic Shock

CHARLES R. SIMS III, MD; THOMAS B. COMFERE, MD

Goals

- Define the evolving classifications of sepsis.
- Review epidemiologic factors, predisposing conditions, and clinical manifestations of a critically ill patient with sepsis.
- Summarize evidence-based protocols for evaluation and management of sepsis.
- Review common neurologic complications associated with sepsis.

Introduction

Sepsis is the most common cause of admission to the intensive care unit (ICU). Although its incidence has increased during the past decade, its short-term mortality has decreased. Furthermore, organ dysfunction caused by dysregulated host immune response to infection resulting in systemic hypoperfusion and end-organ dysfunction is associated with long-term outcomes including frequent morbidity (secondary infections, hospital readmission, decreased quality of life) and mortality in the ICU.

Definitions and Epidemiology

Sepsis is a syndrome defined as life-threatening organ dysfunction caused by a dysregulated host response to infection. Sepsis is one of the most common reasons for admission to an ICU and is associated with extensive use of resources and high mortality. Its underlying pathobiologic details remain poorly defined, and no standard test for diagnosis exists.

Previous concepts used to identify sepsis relied on criteria defining a systemic inflammatory response syndrome (SIRS) paired with an identifiable source of infection. Progression to severe sepsis and septic shock involved clinical signs of end-organ perfusion. The lack of specificity of these criteria, especially the inability to differentiate simple infection from evolving organ failure, prompted a revision of definitions and the elimination of the terms *SIRS* and *severe sepsis*.

The current definition of sepsis uses the Sequential Organ-Failure Assessment (SOFA) score, and progression to septic shock is defined as circulatory, cellular, and metabolic disruptions that are profound enough to increase mortality. The SOFA score (Table 60.1) indicates actual organ dysfunction, as opposed to SIRS criteria, which tend to indicate an inflammatory response that has the potential to progress to organ dysfunction.

A SOFA score of 2 or more reflects an overall mortality risk of approximately 10% in a general hospital population with suspected infection, which is higher than the mortality associated with ST-elevation myocardial infarction (8.1%). Recent studies have shown divergent mortality for a given SOFA score based on patient location and admission source.

The quick SOFA score (qSOFA) is an abbreviated score of alteration in mental status, systolic blood pressure of 100 mm Hg or less, or respiratory rate of 22 or more breaths per minute, assigning 1 point for each. It is used as a bedside prompt to identify patients who might have sepsis. Patients with 2 or more points at the onset of infection have an increased mortality.

The SOFA score has shown improved diagnostic accuracy over SIRS criteria and qSOFA in patients with suspected infection admitted to the ICU. The performance of SOFA and qSOFA in the neurology ICU remains less well characterized. Confounders in this setting include the high rate of central fever (considered to be around 50%) and frequent nonsepsis-related mental status, respiratory, and

Table 60.1 • The Sequential Organ-Failure Assessment (SOFA) Score

Organ System Factor	SOFA Score 0	1	2	3	4
Respiration					
Pao_2/Fio_2, mm Hg	≥400	<400	<300	<200 with respiratory support	<100 with respiratory support
Coagulation					
Platelets, $\times 10^9$/L	≥150	<150	<100	<50	<20
Liver					
Bilirubin, mg/dL	<1.2	1.2-1.9	2.0-5.9	6.0-11.9	≥12
Cardiovascular					
Hypertension	MAP ≥70 mm Hg	MAP <70 mm Hg	Dopamine <5 mcg/kg per min or dobutamine (any dose)	Dopamine 5.1-15 mcg/kg per min or epinephrine ≤0.1 mcg/kg per min or norepinephrine ≤0.1 mcg/kg per min	Dopamine >15 mcg/kg per min or epinephrine >0.1 mcg/kg per min or norepinephrine >0.1 mcg/kg per min
Central nervous system					
Glasgow Coma Scale score	15	13-14	10-12	6-9	<6
Renal					
Creatinine, mg/dL	<1.2	1.2-1.9	2.0-3.4	3.5-4.9	>5.0
Urine output, mL/d	NA	NA	NA	<500	<200

Abbreviations: MAP, mean arterial pressure; NA, not applicable; Pao_2/Fio_2, ratio of the partial pressure of arterial oxygen and fraction of inspired oxygen.

From Vincent JL, Moreno R, Takala J, Willatts S, De Mendonca A, Bruining H, et al; on behalf of the Working Group on Sepsis-Related Problems of the European Society of Intensive Care Medicine. The SOFA (Sepsis-related Organ Failure Assessment) score to describe organ dysfunction/failure. Intensive Care Med. 1996 Jul;22(7):707-10; used with permission.

hemodynamic changes. Central fever can be differentiated from infectious fever by a history of prior blood transfusion; the absence of infiltrates on chest radiography; underlying diagnosis of subarachnoid hemorrhage, intraventricular hemorrhage, or tumor; negative results of blood cultures; and onset of fever within 72 hours of admission.

Lactate levels and lactate clearance are sensitive, albeit nonspecific, stand-alone indicators of cellular or metabolic stress rather than shock. Lactate levels can be increased because of tissue hypoperfusion but also because of endogenous and exogenous catecholamines and decreased hepatic clearance. Current guidelines suggest use of lactate levels to identify early shock that is manifesting with hypotension and use of lactate clearance to evaluate the success of resuscitation.

Globally, the incidence of sepsis has increased because of improved clinical recognition, aging populations with more comorbidities, and, in some countries, reimbursement-favorable coding. In-hospital mortality has decreased regardless of severity, geography, or facility as a result of this increased recognition and early intervention. Demographic risk factors for sepsis include male sex, being African-American, being elderly, having cancer or immunosuppression, and having polymorphisms of certain genes (*TLR1* and *TLR4, SVEP1, FER*). Modifiable risks include alcoholism, smoking, vitamin D deficiency, and inadequate vaccinations.

Pathophysiology: Immunologic, Cellular, and Molecular Disruption Mechanisms

The defining characteristic of sepsis is severe disruption of the normal host immune-mediated response to infection. The molecular sequence of events is a dynamic process that is triggered by an inciting pathogen and results in a complex condition, which is briefly reviewed below.

Cells have the ability to recognize pathogen-associated molecular patterns that occur when components of bacterial, fungal, or viral pathogens interact with cellular receptors (Toll-like and C-type lectin) or cytosol receptors (nucleotide-binding oligomerization domain–like or retinoic acid-inducible gene 1). These same patterns can present as a result of cellular damage (damage-associated molecular patterns). Recognition of these patterns signals the innate immune system to begin transcription of interferons and proinflammatory cytokines such as tumor necrosis factor α and interleukins. Some of these molecules can assemble into inflammasomes responsible for immune cell maturation and initiation of the caspase-mediated programmed cell death cascade, termed *pyroptosis*, in attempts to stop pathogen spread.

The goal of proinflammatory cytokines is early damage control to prevent the spread of minor or local infections. In a severe infection, the response may exceed its own regulation and result in the overproduction of reactive oxygen species. This process induces the excessive formation of nitric oxide, impairs mitochondrial function, and prevents formation of adenosine triphosphate with subsequent disruption of cellular operations, all of which can result in widespread systemic injury. Complement activation and disruption of endothelial molecular interaction can lead to increased vascular permeability. The extreme end of this spectrum leads to immune-mediated thrombosis that results in disseminated intravascular coagulation and further organ damage.

The terminal events in septic shock and multiorgan system failure occur with metabolic disturbances and global catabolism. Mitochondrial damage from both reactive oxygen species and antibiotics decreases adenosine triphosphate production. Without energy, cells enter a state of hibernation that reduces tissue oxygen tension and exacerbates organ damage. Cells with specialized function are especially vulnerable.

Resolution of proinflammatory processes is a coordinated cellular effort termed *efferocytosis* that relies on separate molecular signals. Anti-inflammatory pathways, mediated by leukocyte production of interleukin-10 and transforming growth factor-β, antagonize cytokines and interleukin activity. Damage-associated and pathogen-associated molecular patterns that are activated undergo autophagy by vesicles that target and degrade the pathogen-bound complex and damaged cellular components. Reduction in reactive oxygen species, repair of endothelial permeability, and clearance of cytotoxic cells occur through bioactive lipoxins, resolvins, protectins, maresins, regulator T cells, and myeloid-derived suppressor cells in a coordinated effort to restore immune homeostasis.

Organ-Specific Damage: Organ Systems and Immune Progression

The common key principle to multiorgan system disruption in sepsis is the propagation of a proinflammatory cytokine cascade. This leads to increased vascular permeability with alterations in microcirculation, cellular congestion, and impaired oxygen use. These disruptions result in tissue hypoxia, anaerobic glycolysis, and lactatemia.

The cardiovascular response to sepsis is one of high cardiac output and low systemic vascular resistance. Capillary permeability in alveoli creates ventilation-perfusion mismatches and reduced lung compliance that can lead to acute respiratory distress syndrome and progressive arterial hypoxemia. Gut epithelium disruption increases bacterial translocation, autodigestion with vasoconstriction, and edema that decreases nutrient absorption and can lead to ischemia. Systemic inflammation is perpetuated by disruptions in hepatobiliary clearance, transport, and processing functions. Immune-mediated microvascular dysfunction of renal epithelial cells leads to tubular necrosis, tubular congestion, and a rapidly progressive acute kidney injury.

The central nervous system is important for mitigating early injury in that vagal nuclei inhibit cytokine production by innate immune cells throughout the body. Clinical findings of encephalopathy, or delirium, result from infiltration of inflammatory cytokines through the blood-brain barrier, leading to progressive edema, oxidative stress, and neurotransmitter dysfunction. These effects can lead to potentially long-lasting neurocognitive deficits independently associated with mortality, especially in ventilated patients. Disruptions in perfusion, coagulopathy, and clearance can lead to further ischemic and hemorrhagic insult.

Clinical Tools and Initial Evaluation

Controversy surrounds nearly every aspect of sepsis management, and additional large randomized clinical trials are needed. The clinical aspects of intervention and management that are frequently used are the recommendations summarized by the Surviving Sepsis Campaign, most recently updated in 2018. The bundles have been criticized for the lack of any prospective evidence.

The major tenets of sepsis management are prompt recognition of sepsis and, if it is present, source control, initiation of antimicrobial therapy, and restoration of tissue perfusion and oxygenation.

Source Control

The primary therapy for sepsis includes identification and eradication of the septic focus. All other treatments are merely supportive.

The most common sites of infection in order of prevalence are the lungs, abdomen, bloodstream, kidney, and genitourinary tract. In hospitalized patients, central and arterial lines and surgical sites are frequent foci of infection. The majority of isolates are a combination of gram-positive cocci (*Staphylococcus*, *Streptococcus*, and *Enterococcus* spp), gram-negative rods (*Escherichia coli* and *Pseudomonas* spp), and fungus (*Candida* spp, *Aspergillus* spp). Drug-resistant organisms with increasing prevalence include methicillin-resistant *Staphylococcus aureus*, gram-negative rods with extended-spectrum β-lactamases, vancomycin-resistant *Enterococcus*, and carbapenem- or fluoroquinolone-resistant *Pseudomonas* and *Acinetobacter*. Resistance patterns show geographic preference. Sepsis due to fungal infections, candidemia, hematologic cancers, cirrhosis, and required mechanical ventilator or renal replacement therapy has been associated with increased mortality in ICUs. Patients with cirrhosis alone have a higher incidence of infection than those without cirrhosis, specifically with methicillin-resistant *S aureus*, and a higher hospital mortality. In children, according to data from the Sepsis PRevalence, OUtcomes, and Therapies (SPROUT) study, the most common sites of infection are the lungs, bloodstream, abdomen, central nervous system, and genitourinary tract. In one-third to one-half of all patients who have the clinical picture of sepsis, blood culture results remain negative. The exact cause of this phenomenon remains unclear, but possible explanations are inadequate cultures, administration of antibiotics before obtaining culture specimens, viral infections, trauma, or pancreatitis.

Initiation of Antimicrobial Therapy

Timing of Antimicrobial Therapy

Observational studies have shown that delay of appropriate antimicrobial therapy after presentation of initial hypotension can increase mortality by 8% per hour during the first 6 hours. Thus, time to administration of appropriate antimicrobial therapy is one of the strongest predictors of outcome in sepsis. Guidelines of the Surviving Sepsis Campaign recommend initiation of antimicrobial therapy within 1 hour both in patients with sepsis and in patients with septic shock.

Choice of Antimicrobials

Inadequate antibiotic coverage has been shown to be relatively common (up to 32% of cases) and associated with a high mortality (34% vs 18%).

When there is no obvious pathogen in a patient presenting with sepsis, broad empiric therapy should be initiated. Our initial approach includes vancomycin, because methicillin-resistant *S aureus* cannot be ruled out even in community dwellers without recent hospitalization, combined with either a fourth-generation cephalosporin (cefepime) or β-lactam or β-lactamase inhibitor (eg, piperacillin-tazobactam). If there is known resistance to those combinations, antipseudomonal carbapenems (imipenem, meropenem) can be used.

Antimicrobial therapy can be de-escalated when culture results confirm a specific infection. If no positive culture result confirms a specific infection but the patient responds to empiric therapy, de-escalation of antimicrobial coverage can be considered in select cases.

Fluid Resuscitation

Enthusiasm for increasing oxygen delivery has waned because prospective trials have shown no difference in anaerobic metabolism thresholds in patients with sepsis compared with patients without sepsis, and neither high mixed venous oxygen nor supranormal cardiac output targets have influenced survival. Standard therapy targets a mean arterial pressure goal of 65 to 90 mm Hg and a urine output of more than 0.5 mL/kg per hour with use of a combination of crystalloids, colloids, and vasopressors. Early goal-directed therapy, a phrase coined by Rivers and colleagues in 2001 in a single-center randomized clinical trial involves a treatment bundle consisting of standard therapy, a central venous pressure goal of 8 to 12 mm Hg, red blood cell transfusions, and inotropes. With this approach, the absolute reduction in mortality was 16%. Subsequent multicenter randomized clinical trials (Protocolized Care for Early Septic Shock [ProCESS], Protocolised Management in Sepsis [ProMISe], Australasian Resuscitation in Sepsis Evaluation [ARISE]) were not able to show that early goal-directed therapy itself improves outcomes but rather prompted the creation and organization of system processes that improved early recognition and treatment (Nguyen et al, 2016; see Suggested Reading).

Isotonic crystalloid solutions are the fluid of choice for resuscitation of patients with sepsis and septic shock. To date, there is no consensus on the superiority of balanced crystalloid solution such as lactated Ringer solution and PlasmaLyte (Baxter) over normal saline (NaCl 0.9%). Use of normal saline has been shown to result in hyperchloremic metabolic acidosis and, in some retrospective analyses, a higher rate of renal injury. No prospective studies have shown increased renal injury in patients receiving normal saline compared with balanced salt solutions. One caveat in a neurology ICU population is the relative hypotonicity of lactated Ringer solution (273 mOsm/L) compared with normal saline (308 mOsm/L) and possible resultant effects on formation of cerebral edema.

Hydroxyethyl starch solutions are the only fluid with level 1 evidence against use and contain a US Food and Drug Administration boxed restriction citing concerns of increased mortality, severe renal failure, and bleeding.

Albumin 5% is isotonic and may be preferred in early sepsis, and some evidence suggests a mortality benefit in patients with nontraumatic sepsis.

In patients at risk for increased intracranial pressure, such as many of those in the neurology ICU, albumin 5% should likely be avoided because of its tendency to increase intracranial pressure when the blood-brain barrier is disrupted. The likely mechanism of this increase is migration of hypertonic molecules into the interstitial fluid with subsequent worsening of edema and exacerbation of organ dysfunction.

The optimal amount of fluid for resuscitation and its type remain a matter of controversy. A positive fluid balance is an independent risk factor for death without clear evidence of causality. Under-resuscitation equally worsens outcomes. Currently, expert opinion remains that the decrease in mortality in patients with septic shock supports the benefit of an early and balanced fluid resuscitation to maintain standard therapy targets that must evolve to serve the physiologic needs of the patient. The recommended initial fluid resuscitation goal is 30 mL/kg over 3 hours.

Our approach to fluid resuscitation uses lactated Ringer solution as the main fluid if no contraindications to its relative hypotonicity exist. A patient's fluid responsiveness to a bolus administration of fluid is observed and, if blood pressure or perfusion is improved, fluid administration is repeated. The fluid challenge serves as one component of a multifaceted evaluation that also includes an array of hemodynamic monitoring and assessment, including central venous pressure, pulse pressure variation, or inferior vena cava diameter and collapsibility by bedside ultrasonography. Measurement of serial serum lactate levels, with an aim of rapid normalization, continues to guide resuscitation targets.

Vasopressor Therapy

Recent evidence comparing mean arterial pressure goals failed to establish an optimal target, and there was no difference in survival between a blood pressure goal of 60 to 65 mm Hg and 80 to 85 mm Hg, although higher incidences of atrial fibrillation were reported with a pressure goal of 80 to 85 mm Hg. In patients in neurology ICUs, blood pressure goals are often dictated by the need to maintain cerebral perfusion pressure. Given the absence of a clear harm signal with a low or a high blood pressure management approach in sepsis, the cerebral perfusion pressure goal can reasonably be used as the main determinant of the goal blood pressure. To achieve this, vasopressors are used.

A 2011 systematic review of 23 randomized trials found no convincing evidence of vasopressor superiority in patients with shock. The one exception is dopamine, with which a 2012 meta-analysis reported a higher mortality compared with norepinephrine (Vasu et al, 2012; see Suggested Reading). Phenylephrine is often avoided because of lack of efficacy in septic shock and because it is a pure α-agonist without inotropic effects. In our practice, we tend to use phenylephrine in select patients with sepsis if it is thought that norepinephrine will unduly increase heart rate, such as in cases of atrial fibrillation with rapid ventricular response and underlying ischemic heart disease. The addition of vasopressin to norepinephrine lowers norepinephrine requirements without a change in morbidity or mortality. The recent Vasopressin vs Norepinephrine as Initial Therapy in Septic Shock (VANISH, Gordon et al, 2016; see Suggested Reading) and the Vasopressin Versus Norepinephrine for the Management of Shock After Cardiac Surgery (VaNCS) (see Suggested Reading) studies suggest improved renal function and a lower rate of atrial fibrillation if vasopressin is used as the first-line vasopressor.

The most recent Surviving Sepsis Campaign guidelines recommend norepinephrine as first-line therapy, followed by epinephrine or vasopressin as second- and third-line agents, respectively.

Additional Supportive Therapies

In the ProCESS, ProMISe, and ARISE trials, survival was not improved with early goal-directed therapy strategies using red cell transfusions to increase oxygen delivery. The Transfusion Requirements in Septic Shock (TRISS) study (see Suggested Reading) found no difference in 90-day mortality or rate of ischemic events with transfusion thresholds of 7 mg/dL or 9 mg/dL.

Implementation of hospital protocols guided by the ICU Liberation Bundles helps reduce unnecessary sedation, which improves rehabilitation potential, allows early mobilization, and improves delirium. Short-acting sedatives such as propofol and, most recently, dexmedetomidine have been shown to decrease delirium and shorten time to liberation from mechanical ventilation. In the neurology ICU, propofol is the most commonly used sedative to facilitate mechanical ventilation because of its rapid titratability.

Low tidal ventilation lung protection strategies have shown a marked survival benefit not only in patients with acute respiratory distress syndrome but also in patients with sepsis at risk for development of acute respiratory distress syndrome. Analyses of the impact of implementing protocols to prevent acute respiratory distress syndrome in patients in ICUs have found an absolute reduction in hospital mortality of 8.9%.

Renal Replacement Therapy

Continuous and intermittent renal replacement therapy have shown similar outcomes in most trials. Continuous renal replacement therapy is usually associated with less hemodynamic instability and less need to adjust vasopressors.

Blood Glucose Management

Blood glucose management should follow a protocol and aim for a blood glucose level less than 180 mg/dL but avoid hypoglycemia. More aggressive blood glucose management goals have historically been advocated after single-center trials showed a benefit, but they were subsequently abandoned when multicenter trials showed a lack of benefit and increased risk of hypoglycemia, which is particularly deleterious in a neurology ICU population.

Corticosteroids

The use of corticosteroids in sepsis has been studied extensively. High-dose corticosteroids have consistently been shown to increase mortality, likely due to immunosuppression and subsequent risk for secondary infections, but low-dose corticosteroids can be useful in shock refractory to vasopressors. Although corticosteroids reduce vasopressor requirements, even low doses can increase infectious risk and should be used with caution and for the shortest duration possible.

Nutrition

Patients with septic shock should receive enteral nutrition within 24 to 48 hours of the diagnosis of sepsis and after the resuscitation is complete and the patient is hemodynamically stable. Nutritional guidelines suggest the provision of trophic feeding (defined as 10-20 kcal/h or up to 500 kcal/day) for the initial phase of sepsis and increasing the intake as tolerated after 24 to 48 hours to more than 80% of the target energy goal during the first week. We suggest delivery of 1.2 to 2 g protein/kg per day.

The use of parenteral nutrition is discouraged because of multiple trials showing worse outcomes in patients receiving parenteral nutrition within 1 week of the onset of critical illness, regardless of their prior nutritional state. Immune-modulating formulas have been extensively studied but have not shown consistent benefit.

Sepsis-Specific Non-antimicrobial Drugs

In past decades, multiple attempts have been made to treat sepsis with disease-modifying drugs that mainly aim to modify the inflammatory cascade. Drug classes studied included, among others, high- and low-dose corticosteroids, tumor necrosis factor-α inhibitors, and activated protein C. Although these sepsis-specific therapies were promising in the laboratory setting, all failed to show a consistent benefit in randomized clinical trials.

Neurologic Complications of Sepsis

Neuropathy and myopathy associated with critical illness are discussed in Chapter 97, "Myopathy and Neuropathy Acquired in the Intensive Care Unit."

Sepsis-associated encephalopathy (SAE) is global brain dysfunction due to altered brain perfusion and inflammation, the presentation of which ranges from delirium to coma. It is an early marker of sepsis. The overall mechanisms involved in SAE have not been fully defined but include neuronal loss or loss of function with resultant changes in cholinergic signaling due to microcirculatory dysfunction and inflammation.

SAE is a diagnosis of exclusion. The differential diagnosis includes, among others, primary brain abnormality such as encephalitis, meningitis, or other central nervous system disorders; electrolyte abnormalities; hepatic dysfunction; renal failure; and drug effects. The presence of mental status changes in sepsis increases mortality substantially. Although severe degrees of the SAE spectrum might have an increased mortality, there is no exact way to quantify this impact.

No specific treatment of SAE addresses the underlying pathophysiologic mechanism of microcirculatory changes and inflammation. The current focus of intervention is on avoiding the known additive deleterious effect of sedatives, especially benzodiazepines. Dexmedetomidine, used as a sedative to facilitate mechanical ventilation, has been shown to reduce the incidence of delirium compared with lorazepam. Sedation with low-dose propofol also seems to be superior to benzodiazepines.

Summary

- Sepsis is a dynamic syndrome that affects every organ system in the body.
- Prompt recognition of sepsis and shock, source control, antimicrobial therapy, and restoration of organ perfusion improve outcomes.
- SOFA and qSOFA scores indicate actual organ dysfunction more accurately than SIRS criteria.
- Implementation of a clinical protocol to support organ systems and associated complications during sepsis may improve survival.
- SAE is a spectrum of neurocognitive dysfunction caused by sepsis that has considerable impact on mortality.

SUGGESTED READING

Gordon AC, Mason AJ, Thirunavukkarasu N, Perkins GD, Cecconi M, Cepkova M, et al; VANISH Investigators. Effect of early vasopressin vs norepinephrine on kidney failure in patients with septic shock: the VANISH Randomized Clinical Trial. JAMA. 2016 Aug 2;316(5):509–18.

Hajjar LA, Vincent JL, Barbosa Gomes Galas FR, Rhodes A, Landoni G, Osawa EA, et al. Vasopressin versus norepinephrine in patients with vasoplegic shock after cardiac surgery: the VANCS Randomized Controlled Trial. Anesthesiology. 2017 Jan;126(1):85–93.

Holst LB, Haase N, Wetterslev J, Wernerman J, Guttormsen AB, Karlsson S, et al; TRISS Trial Group; Scandinavian Critical Care Trials Group. Lower versus higher hemoglobin threshold for transfusion in septic shock. N Engl J Med. 2014 Oct 9;371(15):1381–91. Epub 2014 Oct 1.

Levy MM, Evans LE, Rhodes A. The surviving sepsis campaign bundle: 2018 update. Intensive Care Med. 2018 Jun;44(6):925–8. Epub 2018 Apr 19.

Levy MM, Rhodes A, Evans LE; Steering and Executive Committee of the Surviving Sepsis Campaign.

COUNTERPOINT: Should the surviving sepsis campaign guidelines be retired? No. Chest. 2019 Jan;155(1):14–7.
Levy MM, Rhodes A, Evans LE; Steering and Executive Committee of the Surviving Sepsis Campaign. Rebuttal from Drs Levy, Rhodes, and Evans. Chest. 2019 Jan;155(1):19–20.
Marik PE, Farkas JD, Spiegel R, Weingart S; collaborating authors. POINT: Should the surviving sepsis campaign guidelines be retired? Yes. Chest. 2019 Jan;155(1):12–4.
Marik PE, Farkas JD, Spiegel R, Weingart S; collaborating authors. Rebuttal from Drs Marik, Farkas, Spiegel et al. Chest. 2019 Jan;155(1):17–8.
Mukherjee V, Evans L. Implementation of the surviving sepsis campaign guidelines. Curr Opin Crit Care. 2017 Oct;23(5):412–6.
Napolitano LM. Sepsis 2018: definitions and guideline changes. Surg Infect (Larchmt). 2018 Feb/Mar;19(2):117–25.
Nguyen HB, Jaehne AK, Jayaprakash N, Semler MW, Hegab S, Yataco AC, et al. Early goal-directed therapy in severe sepsis and septic shock: insights and comparisons to ProCESS, ProMISe, and ARISE. Crit Care. 2016 Jul 1;20(1):160.
Rhodes A, Evans LE, Alhazzani W, Levy MM, Antonelli M, Ferrer R, et al. Surviving sepsis campaign: international guidelines for management of sepsis and septic shock: 2016. Crit Care Med. 2017 Mar;45(3):486–552.
Rivers E, Nguyen B, Havstad S, Ressler J, Muzzin A, Knoblich B, et al; Early Goal-Directed Therapy Collaborative Group. Early goal-directed therapy in the treatment of severe sepsis and septic shock. N Engl J Med. 2001 Nov 8;345(19):1368–77.
Vasu TS, Cavallazzi R, Hirani A, Kaplan G, Leiby B, Marik PE. Norepinephrine or dopamine for septic shock: systematic review of randomized clinical trials. J Intensive Care Med. 2012 May-Jun;27(3):172–8. Epub 2011 Mar 24.

Dermatologic Concerns

Dermatologic Emergencies in the Intensive Care Unit

MATTHEW R. HALL, MD

Goals

- Discuss drug hypersensitivity syndromes.
- Describe the clinical presentation of common dermatologic emergencies in the intensive care unit.
- Discuss the diagnosis and management of dermatologic emergencies.

Introduction

Rashes are relatively common in hospitalized patients, but only rarely are they life threatening. Emergent skin conditions in these patients are usually sequelae of medication reactions (drug eruptions) or complications from sepsis. Drug eruptions are the most common cause of rashes that occur while a patient is hospitalized. The prototypic drug rash is morbilliform (maculopapular) in appearance and consists of coalescing, erythematous macules and papules. Most drug eruptions are benign and resolve if the offending medication is discontinued. However, the drug hypersensitivity syndrome, Stevens-Johnson syndrome (SJS), and toxic epidermal necrolysis (TEN) are urgent conditions that require prompt diagnosis and management. Purpura fulminans can develop in patients with sepsis and disseminated intravascular coagulation.

Drug Hypersensitivity Syndrome

Drug hypersensitivity syndrome, also known as drug reaction with eosinophilia and systemic symptoms (DRESS), can be a life-threatening medication reaction due to internal organ involvement. The most common causes of DRESS include aromatic anticonvulsants (eg, phenytoin, carbamazepine, and phenobarbital) and sulfonamides. DRESS typically begins within 2 months after patients initiate therapy with the medication, most commonly within the first 2 to 6 weeks. Patients with DRESS may first have a fever and pruritus; a diffuse morbilliform eruption then occurs, often with facial edema.

DRESS can be associated with multiorgan manifestations involving the lymphatic system (lymphadenopathy), hematopoietic system (leukocytosis with eosinophilia), liver (elevated liver enzymes), kidneys, lungs, heart (myocarditis), nervous system (encephalitis), gastrointestinal tract (gastroenteritis), or endocrine system (thyroiditis and pancreatitis). DRESS-induced myocarditis can be fatal, and liver involvement can lead to fulminant hepatitis. The liver is the most commonly affected visceral organ.

If DRESS is suspected, the use of all potentially causative medications should be discontinued. Patients should be treated with systemic corticosteroids at an initial daily dose of at least 1 mg/kg of prednisone or its equivalent, which should be tapered gradually over 3 to 6 months to avoid relapses. Despite supportive care, patients with DRESS have a 10% risk of death, usually due to hepatic necrosis.

The validity of assessment tools for predicting adverse dermatologic reactions is questionable. Guidelines from a National Institutes of Health working group were published in 2017.

SJS and TEN

SJS and TEN are life-threatening, blistering, hypersensitivity reactions of the skin and mucous membranes, most commonly the result of medications. SJS and TEN are commonly considered to be various degrees of severity of the same pathologic process. These conditions are differentiated by the percentage of body surface area (BSA) involved. SJS is characterized by involvement of less than 10% BSA; SJS/TEN overlap syndrome, 10% to 30%; and TEN, more than 30%.

Patients with SJS have purpuric macules or atypical targetoid patches with blisters and erosions. Patients with TEN have dusky purpuric patches with epidermal sloughing, leading to an eroded, denuded base. SJS and TEN are also characterized by erosions of mucous membranes of the mouth, eyes, and genitalia. The areas of cutaneous involvement are often tender, and the Nikolsky sign can be elicited when tangential lateral pressure induces sloughing of the epidermis from the dermis. Patients also often have fever and malaise. Systemic involvement can occur from sloughing of epithelial linings of the conjunctivae, gastrointestinal tract, trachea, bronchi, and kidneys.

Most cases of SJS/TEN result from drug reactions. The majority are caused by antibiotics (sulfonamides, aminopenicillins, cephalosporins, and quinolones); anticonvulsants (lamotrigine, carbamazepine, phenytoin, and phenobarbital); nevirapine; sulfasalazine; allopurinol; and oxicam nonsteroidal anti-inflammatory drugs. SJS/TEN usually occurs within 6 to 14 days after administration of the causative medication.

This drug reaction is thought to lead to activation of cytotoxic $CD8^+$ T cells, which cause epithelial cell apoptosis induced by the T-cell Fas ligand binding to its receptor on the target cell. SJS and TEN can be fatal, commonly from sepsis, gastrointestinal tract hemorrhage, pulmonary embolism, pulmonary edema, or myocardial infarction. The mortality rate for patients with SJS ranges from 1% to 5%; for patients with TEN, 25% to 30%. The severity-of-illness score for toxic epidermal necrolysis (SCORTEN) was developed to assess severity and predict mortality (Box 61.1).

Box 61.1 • Severity-of-Illness Score for Toxic Epidermal Necrolysis (SCORTEN)

The following criteria are each worth 1 point:

- Age >40 y
- Heart rate >120 beats per minute
- Comorbid malignancy
- Epidermal detachment involving >10% body surface area on day 1
- Serum urea nitrogen >28 mg/dL
- Serum glucose >252 mg/dL
- Serum bicarbonate <20 mmol/L

The total score is used to predict the mortality rate as follows:

Total score (mortality rate, %)

- 0 or 1 (3)
- 2 (12)
- 3 (36)
- 4 (58)
- ≥5 (90)

Modified from Bastuji-Garin S, Fouchard N, Bertocchi M, Roujeau JC, Revuz J, Wolkenstein P. SCORTEN: a severity-of-illness score for toxic epidermal necrolysis. J Invest Dermatol. 2000 Aug;115(2):149-53; used with permission.

Patients who survive SJS and TEN may have chronic sequelae involving the eyes (dry eye syndrome, photophobia, corneal scarring, decreased visual acuity, or blindness); mouth (xerostomia or periodontal disease); genitourinary system (dyspareunia, adhesions, or phimosis); or lungs (bronchitis, bronchiectasis, or organizing pneumonia).

Treatment of SJS and TEN involves stopping all potential causative medications and providing supportive care in an intensive care unit or preferably a burn unit, if available. Burn units can deliver optimum wound care and supportive care for patients with extensive cutaneous necrosis. Early consultation with an ophthalmologist can help prevent ocular damage. The patient's fluid and electrolyte status should be monitored closely for imbalances, and prompt initiation of antibiotics with wound cultures should be performed if signs of infection develop. There is no convincing evidence for initiation of systemic anti-inflammatory therapy, but some studies have shown survival benefit from initiation of intravenous immunoglobulin, which may inhibit Fas-mediated apoptosis of keratinocytes.

Purpura Fulminans

If disseminated intravascular coagulation develops in patients with sepsis, the skin may have widespread, symmetric, necrotic, and gangrenous purpuric patches. This clinical cutaneous presentation is termed *purpura fulminans*. Prompt recognition of this condition is crucial because mortality is high and, among survivors, morbidity is serious. Severe infection (most often meningococcemia) and underlying malignancy are the most common causes of this condition. Because purpura fulminans can be a sign of meningococcemia, prompt initiation of antibiotics and supportive care can be lifesaving. Widespread gangrene may necessitate amputation, so multidisciplinary care involving wound care and vascular surgery is important.

Summary

- SJS, TEN, and the drug hypersensitivity syndrome are urgent conditions that require prompt diagnosis and management.
- Purpura fulminans can develop in patients with sepsis and disseminated intravascular coagulation.
- DRESS can be a life-threatening medication reaction due to internal organ involvement; patients should receive corticosteroid therapy.
- SJS and TEN are life-threatening, blistering, hypersensitivity reactions of the skin and mucous membranes, most commonly the result of medications.
- Treatment of SJS and TEN involves stopping all potential causative medications and providing supportive care in an intensive care unit or preferably a burn unit, if available.

SUGGESTED READING

Bastuji-Garin S, Fouchard N, Bertocchi M, Roujeau JC, Revuz J, Wolkenstein P. SCORTEN: a severity-of-illness score for toxic epidermal necrolysis. J Invest Dermatol. 2000 Aug;115(2):149–53.

Bastuji-Garin S, Rzany B, Stern RS, Shear NH, Naldi L, Roujeau JC. Clinical classification of cases of toxic epidermal necrolysis, Stevens-Johnson syndrome, and erythema multiforme. Arch Dermatol. 1993 Jan;129(1):92–6.

Chiou CC, Yang LC, Hung SI, Chang YC, Kuo TT, Ho HC, et al. Clinicopathological features and prognosis of drug rash with eosinophilia and systemic symptoms: a study of 30 cases in Taiwan. J Eur Acad Dermatol Venereol. 2008 Sep;22(9):1044–9. Epub 2008 Jul 4.

Goldman JL, Chung WH, Lee BR, Chen CB, Lu CW, Hoetzenecker W, et al. Adverse drug reaction causality assessment tools for drug-induced Stevens-Johnson syndrome and toxic epidermal necrolysis: room for improvement. Eur J Clin Pharmacol. 2019 Mar 27. [Epub ahead of print]

Harr T, French LE. Toxic epidermal necrolysis and Stevens-Johnson syndrome. Orphanet J Rare Dis. 2010 Dec 16;5:39.

Mockenhaupt M, Viboud C, Dunant A, Naldi L, Halevy S, Bouwes Bavinck JN, et al; The EuroSCAR-study. Stevens-Johnson syndrome and toxic epidermal necrolysis: assessment of medication risks with emphasis on recently marketed drugs. J Invest Dermatol. 2008 Jan;128(1):35–44. Epub 2007 Sep 6.

Newell BD, Moinfar M, Mancini AJ, Nopper AJ. Retrospective analysis of 32 pediatric patients with anticonvulsant hypersensitivity syndrome (ACHSS). Pediatr Dermatol. 2009 Sep-Oct;26(5):536–46.

Tas S, Simonart T. Drug rash with eosinophilia and systemic symptoms (DRESS syndrome). Acta Clin Belg. 1999 Aug;54(4):197–200.

Tas S, Simonart T. Management of drug rash with eosinophilia and systemic symptoms (DRESS syndrome): an update. Dermatology. 2003;206(4): 353–6.

Trauma and Burns

Initial Approach to the Management of Multisystem Trauma

DAVID S. MORRIS, MD

Goals

- Review the epidemiology of trauma and the most common causes of early death.
- Describe the airway, breathing, circulation, disability, and exposure (ABCDE) approach to the initial evaluation and management of patients with multisystem trauma.
- Discuss lifesaving interventions and surgical damage control.

Introduction

Nearly 200,000 people die of injury-related causes in the United States each year, and injury is the leading cause of death for all patients aged 1 to 44 years. Approximately 30 million people sustain nonfatal injuries each year, which results in about 29 million emergency department visits and 3 million hospital admissions. The total estimated cost of injury, including the costs for medical care and lost productivity, is $671 billion annually.

Most deaths from traumatic injury occur at 3 specific times after the injury. The first is immediately after a severe injury, such as decapitation, dismemberment, rapid blood loss, or massive direct trauma to the brain or heart. These injuries are so severe that survival is usually not possible even if medical care is immediately available. The second time when deaths often occur is in the minutes to hours after injury, when death may be due to airway loss, head injury, or hemorrhage. This period is the "golden hour" of trauma care, and all trauma resuscitation is aimed at identifying patients in this category and treating the potentially reversible causes. The third period of frequent deaths is days to weeks after an injury, when patients die of complications from the injury, such as ventilator-associated pneumonia, wound infections, and other causes familiar to most clinicians in the intensive care unit (ICU).

Management of severely injured patients, typically defined as having an Injury Severity Score greater than 15 (Box 62.1 and Table 62.1), is best managed in a level I or level II trauma center. Hospitals without trauma centers may provide essential lifesaving care and stabilization before the patient is transferred. In addition, those hospitals may admit patients who are injured as a consequence of other medical issues (eg, a driver who has a motor vehicle accident during a seizure). For these patients, care of the primary process must be integrated into the care of the resulting injuries. Thus, any physician who provides care for critically ill patients should have a basic familiarity with the fundamentals of trauma care.

Initial management of a severely injured patient can be challenging because of the acuity and severity of the injury and because so many unknowns exist at presentation. Clinicians must make serious and often nonreversible decisions about treatment even though they have limited information about the patient. The stakes are high and so is the stress on the team and the hospital's resources.

This chapter focuses on the initial approach to patients with multisystem trauma. The key principles in an ideal resuscitation are described with the airway, breathing, circulation, disability, and exposure (ABCDE) approach outlined in the Advanced Trauma Life Support course. Potential pitfalls are discussed.

Evaluation

Preparation Before the Patient Arrives

When possible, the team that will be caring for the patient should be assembled and briefed before the patient's arrival. This briefing allows the team leader to outline a

Box 62.1 • Abbreviated Injury Score (AIS)

The AIS classifies injuries in the following 9 body regions:

- Head
- Face
- Neck
- Thorax
- Abdomen
- Spine
- Upper extremity
- Lower extremity
- External

For each of the 9 body regions, the severity of the injury is scored from 1 to 6 according to expert consensus definitions for levels of severity for each body region injury:

- Minor—1
- Moderate—2
- Serious—3
- Severe—4
- Critical—5
- Unsurvivable—6

Data from Civil ID, Schwab CW. The Abbreviated Injury Scale, 1985 revision: a condensed chart for clinical use. J Trauma. 1988 Jan;28(1):87-90.

Table 62.1 • Calculation of the Injury Severity Score (ISS) From the Abbreviated Injury Score (AIS)[a]

Body Region	Description	AIS
Head, neck, cervical spine	Loss of consciousness	2
Face	Corneal abrasion	1
Chest, thoracic spine	Flail chest	4
Abdomen, lumbar spine	Major liver laceration	4
Extremities, pelvis	Femoral fracture	3
External	Superficial abrasion	1

[a] The ISS is the sum of the square of each of the 3 highest AIS body region scores. In this example, ISS = $4^2 + 4^2 + 3^2 = 16 + 16 + 9 = 41$. By convention, the maximum ISS is 75. If any single AIS is 6, the patient is automatically given an ISS of 75, regardless of other body region involvement.

Data from Civil ID, Schwab CW. The Abbreviated Injury Scale, 1985 revision: a condensed chart for clinical use. J Trauma. 1988 Jan;28(1):87-90.

plan of care and gather equipment or supplies. At a minimum, the resuscitation space should have the capacity for definitive airway management (including a surgical airway if needed), pleural space decompression with needle thoracostomy or chest tubes, intravenous (IV) access, IV fluids and blood product administration, and spinal immobilization. An adequate number of care providers should be assembled to help with the evaluation and procedures required. Assistance may be needed from providers in various specialties, including emergency medicine, anesthesia, and surgical specialties (trauma, orthopedics, and neurosurgery). Proper preparation can mean the difference between success and failure in situations when minutes matter.

Primary Survey

In the trauma primary survey, the conditions that may pose an immediate threat to the patient's life are quickly identified through the ABCDE sequence, which should be followed in a stepwise fashion. For example, airway patency and adequacy are confirmed before breathing is assessed. Breathing issues, such as a pneumothorax, are addressed before circulation is assessed, and so on. If a larger team is present to assess a trauma patient, multiple steps in the sequence may be addressed simultaneously. For example, the *airway* may be assessed by the airway provider while the assisting provider places a chest tube (addressing *breathing*) and blood products are administered by the bedside nurse (addressing *circulation*). The team leader must direct the team members efficiently so that resuscitation proceeds appropriately.

The use of a systematic approach is critical to success, and failure to follow a defined sequence often results in poor outcomes for the injured patient if the team misses injuries or does not recognize impending decompensation. A team can easily focus on 1 aspect of a patient's injury (eg, a broken bone protruding through the skin) and lose sight of other problems, which may be subtle but immediately life threatening. In military parlance, this is called "losing situational awareness," and similar situations have been described during cockpit emergencies for flight crews. The most important function of the team leader is to maintain situational awareness and keep the team oriented to the ABCDE sequence.

The importance of the ABCDE sequence must be emphasized as the recommended process for trauma patients. The American Heart Association has changed the recommended sequence for cardiac resuscitation from airway, breathing, and circulation (ABC) to circulation, airway, and breathing (CAB) to reflect the importance of early, effective chest compressions. Injured patients, however, require resuscitation from different causes, namely hemorrhagic shock and severe head injury. For these reasons, the resuscitation sequence for injured patients is still ABCDE. Cardiopulmonary resuscitation for patients with cardiac arrest due to traumatic causes is not beneficial and may prevent or delay potentially lifesaving interventions, such as decompression of a tension pneumothorax with a chest tube or needle.

At the conclusion of the primary survey, the team should have identified all immediately life-threatening problems and taken steps to address them. Excluding the time spent performing interventions, an efficient primary survey should take no more than 1 or 2 minutes. At the end of the primary survey, the team should have an overall sense of the patient's clinical stability. The most common causes of illness are severe head injury and hemorrhage, and all further investigations should be aimed at determining the sequence of surgical interventions required. A hypotensive patient should be taken to the operating room as quickly as possible for surgical control of hemorrhage. For patients who are not hypotensive and in whom hemorrhage is not suspected, a secondary survey is performed in the resuscitation area to identify all injuries (as discussed below).

Adjuncts to the Primary Survey

Several interventions and diagnostic studies are considered adjuncts to the primary survey. These adjuncts are used to quickly identify sources of massive blood loss. A person can lose life-threatening amounts of blood into 5 locations: the pleural space, the peritoneal cavity, the retroperitoneal space, the muscular compartments of the thighs, and the external environment. Some adjuncts to the primary survey are used for cavitary triage: chest radiography to look for massive hemothorax; ultrasonography of the peritoneal cavity (ie, focused assessment with sonography in trauma [FAST]); and pelvic radiography to assess for fracture, which is commonly associated with retroperitoneal hemorrhage. Other adjuncts to the primary survey include laboratory assessments, nasogastric tube and urinary catheter placement, electrocardiography, and splinting of fractures. In certain circumstances, these adjuncts may be omitted because of the patient's clinical status or because of concern about a specific injury. For example, a nasogastric tube should not be placed if a basilar skull fracture is present or suspected. Similarly, blood at the urethral meatus may indicate an anterior pelvic fracture and disruption of the urethra; a urinary catheter should not be placed blindly. As soon as the source of hemorrhage is identified, the patient should be rapidly transferred to the operating room for appropriate surgical treatment.

Secondary Survey

After the primary survey, if a patient is hemodynamically stable or responds to volume restoration and then becomes hemodynamically stable, a secondary survey is performed. The goal of the secondary survey is to identify all injuries that may be present and to help plan imaging studies and the patient's destination after the resuscitation area (ie, ICU, computed tomographic [CT] scanner, interventional radiology suite, or general care floor). The secondary survey consists of a complete physical examination, including the back (if not examined as part of the exposure component in the ABCDE sequence of the primary survey). Other information obtained at this time, if possible, includes the patient's past medical history, allergies, and relevant social and family history. If lacerations or puncture wounds are present, a tetanus immunization should be given if the patient's vaccination status is not current or is unknown.

Imaging Studies

For several reasons clinicians should have a relatively low threshold for obtaining axial imaging to evaluate adult patients with polytrauma: The patient may be unresponsive, may have a decreased mental status, or may be unable to participate in the evaluation because of distracting injuries. In busy trauma centers, a CT scan may be the quickest way to determine which patients can be safely discharged from the emergency department and which should be admitted. In addition, because many injury situations involve complex medicolegal issues, the CT scan may help provide documentation of injuries. Despite these reasons, however, clinicians should still exercise good clinical judgment about the cost-benefit ratio for imaging studies because the exposure to ionizing radiation is a real, albeit small, risk over a patient's lifetime. For this reason, pediatric patients (who potentially have many more years at risk) should undergo CT only when a high suspicion of injury exists, typically when physical examination findings or the mechanism of injury warrants such suspicion. National consensus recommendations are available from the American College of Radiology, but local practice guidelines should be followed whenever available.

Therapy

Lifesaving Interventions

As mentioned above, several key interventions may be required during the primary survey. These include definitive airway control, decompression of pneumothorax or hemothorax with chest tubes, hemorrhage control and restoration of circulatory volume, and splinting or stabilizing fractures when possible. The patient should not leave the trauma bay before the need for these interventions has been evaluated and any necessary procedures have been performed. In addition, if a patient's status suddenly decompensates, the team should repeat the primary survey to determine the source of the problem.

Surgical Phase of Resuscitation and Damage Control

Patients who are hypotensive should be moved from the resuscitation area directly to the operating room for definitive surgical hemostasis and control of life-threatening injuries. For many years, lengthy, complex, surgical repair of injuries resulted in intraoperative coagulopathy, worsening acidosis, and protracted hypothermia. This *lethal triad* resulted in a mortality rate higher than what would be expected from the injury severity.

In recent years, the concept of *damage control surgery* has gained popularity in the trauma community as a way to avoid subjecting the patient to physiologic exhaustion in the operating room. First described in 1983, the concept of abbreviated surgical treatment became the standard of care during the 1990s after being championed by trauma surgeons in busy urban trauma centers who were treating a high number of patients who had penetrating trauma. Damage control surgery focuses on only controlling compelling hemorrhage and contamination (eg, gastrointestinal tract spillage or urine leakage) without definitive surgical reconstruction or closure of the abdomen or chest during the initial operation. Techniques used to avoid lengthy procedures include vascular shunting rather than time-consuming definitive vascular repair, intestinal resection without immediate reanastomosis, external fixation of fractures, and liberal use of temporary abdominal closure.

Along with damage control surgery, the concept of *damage control resuscitation* has been developed for patients with the lethal triad. Also known as *permissive hypotension*, the concept of damage control resuscitation is based on a lower systolic blood pressure goal (typically around 90 mm Hg for adult patients) during resuscitation until definitive hemorrhage control has been achieved. Injured patients who are bleeding have been shown to have worse outcomes when higher systolic blood pressures (ie, >90 mm Hg) are used as resuscitation targets. Injured patients have also been shown to benefit from resuscitation with blood products given in a balanced 1:1:1 ratio of erythrocytes to plasma to platelets. Damage control resuscitation should begin in the resuscitation area (or in the prehospital setting, if possible) and continue through and beyond the operative phase of care.

ICU Phase and Ongoing Resuscitation

ICU care for a patient with multisystem trauma should focus on reversing the lethal triad of acidosis, hypothermia, and coagulopathy. Typically during the ICU phase of resuscitation, definitive surgical control of bleeding is accomplished and traditional end points of resuscitation are targeted for vital signs, thromboelastography, prothrombin time or international normalized ratio, partial thromboplastin time, serum lactate level, base excess, pH, and tissue oxygenation. The end points are best achieved through ongoing resuscitation with a balanced-ratio blood product and a target of euvolemia. Aggressive use of crystalloid solutions in supraphysiologic volumes is discouraged because of the risk of pulmonary edema, acute respiratory distress syndrome, intra-abdominal hypertension, and abdominal compartment syndrome. Large volumes of crystalloid also may lead to dilution of clotting factors and prolonged coagulopathy. The patient should be rewarmed using ambient heating techniques, and all IV fluids and blood products should be infused through a warmer. If definitive hemorrhage and contamination control has been achieved, physiologic stabilization typically occurs in 12 to 36 hours. If the above end points are not normalized, the ICU team should suspect ongoing hemorrhage or an untreated source of sepsis, and operative reexploration should be performed.

When the patient has been adequately resuscitated, the identified injuries can be definitively repaired. The role of the ICU clinician is to help coordinate the care of the patient with the multiple surgical teams that are frequently involved. The ICU clinician is in the best position to determine whether the patient's condition is stable enough to endure the planned procedure on the scheduled day. For example, the condition of a patient who has only recently been adequately resuscitated may be stable enough for cleaning a wound but not for a 12-hour spine stabilization surgery. Or a patient with persistently elevated intracranial pressure may not be able to lie flat in the operating room, so procedures that require level supine positioning should be postponed. Priority should be given to reconstruction of vascular injuries and gastrointestinal tract reanastomosis or stoma creation whenever possible because these injuries have a shorter window for definitive repair. The temptation to try to accomplish too much in a single trip to the operating room must be controlled.

Many multisystem trauma patients require multiple operations and lengthy ICU stays. These operative procedures may lead to "ICU inertia," a tendency to leave a patient intubated longer than necessary or to hold nutrition unnecessarily for future operations. The caloric requirements for severely injured patients can be much higher than for the average ICU patient, and enteral nutrition should be used early whenever possible. With intestinal continuity, an open abdomen is not a contraindication to enteral nutrition. If a patient has a cuffed airway protection device (an endotracheal tube or tracheostomy tube), tube feedings do not need to be withheld the night before nonaerodigestive procedures. In general, patients with multisystem trauma should be extubated as soon as they meet the criteria, regardless of their intubation needs for future operative procedures. A patient who arrives in the operating room without an endotracheal tube is more likely to leave the operating room without one.

Management Summary

A systematic evaluation and treatment strategy should be followed for all patients with multisystem trauma. In the initial phases, emphasis should be on identifying and treating injuries that pose an immediate threat to the patient's life. Patients in unstable condition belong in the operating room or in the interventional radiology suite. If patients are in stable condition, a comprehensive history should be obtained and a complete physical examination performed if possible. Resuscitation should be guided by restoration of euvolemia and reversal of coagulopathy with blood products given in a balanced ratio and minimal use of crystalloid solution. Definitive hemorrhage control should not be delayed.

Summary

- Follow the Advanced Trauma Life Support ABCDE systematic strategy.
- Do not delay lifesaving interventions.
- Minimize crystalloid use.
- Restore euvolemia and reverse coagulopathy with balanced-ratio blood product resuscitation.
- Achieve definitive hemorrhage control as soon as possible.
- Resuscitate in the ICU after damage control surgery.

SUGGESTED READING

American College of Surgeons, Committee on Trauma. Advanced trauma life support: student course manual. 9th ed. Chicago (IL): American College of Surgeons; c2012. 366 p.

Baker SP, O'Neill B, Haddon W Jr, Long WB. The injury severity score: a method for describing patients with multiple injuries and evaluating emergency care. J Trauma. 1974 Mar;14(3):187–96.

Borgman MA, Spinella PC, Perkins JG, Grathwohl KW, Repine T, Beekley AC, et al. The ratio of blood products transfused affects mortality in patients receiving massive transfusions at a combat support hospital. J Trauma. 2007 Oct;63(4):805–13.

Civil ID, Schwab CW. The Abbreviated Injury Scale, 1985 revision: a condensed chart for clinical use. J Trauma. 1988 Jan;28(1):87–90.

Duchesne JC, McSwain NE Jr, Cotton BA, Hunt JP, Dellavolpe J, Lafaro K, et al. Damage control resuscitation: the new face of damage control. J Trauma. 2010 Oct;69(4):976–90.

Fatal injury data [Internet]. Atlanta (GA): Centers for Disease Control and Prevention. [cited 2017 Nov 27]. Available from: http://www.cdc.gov/injury/wisqars/fatal.html.

Holcomb JB, Wade CE, Michalek JE, Chisholm GB, Zarzabal LA, Schreiber MA, et al. Increased plasma and platelet to red blood cell ratios improves outcome in 466 massively transfused civilian trauma patients. Ann Surg. 2008 Sep;248(3):447–58. Erratum in: Ann Surg. 2011 Feb;253(2):392.

Kovacs G, Sowers N. Airway management in trauma. Emerg Med Clin North Am. 2018 Feb;36(1):61–84.

Parent BA, Mandell SP, Maier RV, Minei J, Sperry J, Moore EE, et al. Safety of minimizing preoperative starvation in critically ill and intubated trauma patients. J Trauma Acute Care Surg. 2016 Jun;80(6):957–63.

Peev MP, Yeh DD, Quraishi SA, Osler P, Chang Y, Gillis E, et al. Causes and consequences of interrupted enteral nutrition: a prospective observational study in critically ill surgical patients. JPEN J Parenter Enteral Nutr. 2015 Jan;39(1):21–7. Epub 2014 Apr 7.

Rotondo MF, Schwab CW, McGonigal MD, Phillips GR 3rd, Fruchterman TM, Kauder DR, et al. 'Damage control': an approach for improved survival in exsanguinating penetrating abdominal injury. J Trauma. 1993 Sep;35(3):375–82.

Shand S, Curtis K, Dinh M, Burns B. What is the impact of prehospital blood product administration for patients with catastrophic haemorrhage: an integrative review. Injury. 2019 Feb;50(2):226–34. Epub 2018 Dec 12.

Stone HH, Strom PR, Mullins RJ. Management of the major coagulopathy with onset during laparotomy. Ann Surg. 1983 May;197(5):532–5.

Travers AH, Rea TD, Bobrow BJ, Edelson DP, Berg RA, Sayre MR, et al. Part 4: CPR overview: 2010 American Heart Association guidelines for cardiopulmonary resuscitation and emergency cardiovascular care. Circulation. 2010 Nov 2;122(18 Suppl 3):S676–84.

63 Chest and Abdominal Trauma

JOY D. HUGHES, MD; DAVID S. MORRIS, MD

Goals

- Discuss the basics of thoracic and abdominal injuries that are most commonly encountered in neurocritical care.
- Review the resuscitation strategies for patients with hemorrhagic shock and concurrent neurologic injuries.

Introduction

Injuries to the chest or abdomen frequently affect management of traumatic brain injury (TBI). Neurocritical care clinicians must be familiar with management principles for these injuries. This chapter reviews common injuries to the torso, with particular attention to problems affecting neurologic management, but it cannot provide an exhaustive list of injuries and management principles for this broad topic. Close interaction with clinicians familiar with the management of nonneurologic traumatic injury is recommended. Guidelines have been published.

Thoracic Injuries

Chest Wall Trauma

Rib fractures are common after blunt trauma, and the number and severity of fractures may be underestimated from chest radiography. *Flail chest,* defined as 2 or more fractures in 2 or more adjacent ribs, can disturb respiratory mechanics and may necessitate prolonged mechanical ventilation. Additionally, underlying pulmonary contusion may profoundly impair gas exchange. Higher positive end-expiratory pressure (PEEP) may be required to maintain adequate oxygenation; however, if higher PEEP is contraindicated because of elevated intracranial pressure (ICP) or lack of ICP monitoring, alternative strategies for oxygenation may be necessary. These strategies may include preferential increases in the fraction of inspired oxygen over PEEP, inhaled vasodilators, reversed-ratio ventilation, and a lower threshold for chemical paralysis. High-frequency oscillatory ventilation (HFOV) and independent lung ventilation strategies have been used with some success. The use of mannitol or hypertonic saline may be indicated to decrease ICP if cerebral perfusion pressure can be maintained. Supporting evidence for these strategies is scant, and consequences of these methods (ie, hypercapnia during HFOV) need to be considered and weighed against the benefits of higher oxygenation. ICP should always be carefully evaluated during trials of these various strategies.

Even without a true flail chest injury, simple rib fractures may impair respiratory function. Most patients with rib fractures can be treated nonoperatively with aggressive analgesia, supplemental oxygen, and aggressive pulmonary hygiene. For patients with multiple rib fractures and flail chest, operative fixation has been effective in decreasing ventilator time, hospital length of stay, and incidence of pneumonia.

Pneumothorax and Hemothorax

Up to 20% of trauma patients present with pneumothorax or hemothorax. For a large or symptomatic pneumothorax, management includes tube thoracostomy and supplemental oxygen. A large hemothorax may impair expansion of the lung; initial management with tube thoracostomy is usually sufficient, but a persistent or massive hemothorax (>1 L) may require operative intervention.

Mediastinal Injuries

Trauma to the anterior chest wall (common in motor vehicle accidents because of impact with the seatbelt, airbag, or steering wheel) can also cause injury to mediastinal structures. Pericardial tamponade may be recognized with the classic presentation of the Beck triad: muffled heart tones, jugular venous distention, and hypotension. In the absence of tamponade, blunt myocardial injury may cause hemodynamic compromise, although most commonly the initial presenting sign is sinus tachycardia. Electrocardiography should be used to rule out conduction abnormalities, and patients should be observed with telemetric monitoring. If electrocardiographic abnormalities are present, or if the clinician has concerns about labile arterial blood pressure and cardiac function, echocardiography should be used to help guide treatment. Blunt injury can also result in aortic dissection, which should be suspected with any high-energy trauma to the anterior chest wall. Computed tomographic (CT) angiography is the diagnostic modality of choice, and prompt consultation with vascular and cardiothoracic surgical specialists is indicated if aortic dissection is identified.

Abdominal Injuries

Abdominal injuries are common in the multitrauma patient and may necessitate laparotomy. In recent years, nonoperative management has been used more frequently for solid organ injuries; however, these injuries may result in delayed hemorrhage. Hollow viscous injuries are notoriously difficult to identify on CT imaging, and failure to identify them may lead to delayed sepsis. Among patients who do require laparotomy, damage control techniques—such as temporary abdominal closure—are frequently used as well, which may complicate management of polytrauma patients with TBI.

Liver and Spleen

Injuries to the solid organs are a large portion of injuries causing hemorrhagic shock in patients with torso trauma. The liver and spleen are the most commonly injured intra-abdominal organs, and these injuries are commonly managed conservatively or with intravascular embolization. When patients have concomitant TBI, trauma surgeons may have a lower threshold for choosing operative management (ie, splenectomy with lower grade injuries) to decrease the likelihood of delayed hemorrhage and resulting hypotension. Maintenance of systolic blood pressure greater than 90 mm Hg and cerebral perfusion pressure at 60 mm Hg are the goals of resuscitation for hemorrhage in patients with TBI. Permissive hypotension is contraindicated for patients with severe TBI because this strategy places patients at high risk for worse neurologic outcomes. Patients who have had splenic embolization are at risk for delayed bleeding because of the dual blood supply of the spleen. Close observation is key to management.

Patients who undergo splenectomy or embolization should receive immunization against encapsulated organisms: *Haemophilus influenzae* type B, *Streptococcus pneumoniae*, and *Neisseria meningitidis*. The optimal timing of immunization is at least 14 days after splenectomy. Overwhelming sepsis after splenectomy is a rare but severe complication. The use of prophylactic antibiotics to prevent sepsis is controversial.

Open Abdomen and Abdominal Compartment Syndrome

Patients with abdominal injuries and patients receiving high-volume resuscitation for other injuries are at risk for *abdominal compartment syndrome*, characterized by ventilation impairment, decreased cardiac output, abdominal wall distention, and, subsequently, increased intrathoracic pressures. Bladder pressures greater than 25 mm Hg (ideally measured while the patient is paralyzed) may aid diagnosis. As mentioned above, increased intra-abdominal pressure transmits to the thoracic cavity and in turn can increase ICP. The combination of low cardiac output and high ICP can be catastrophic for patients with injury to the central nervous system. Therefore, maintaining a high degree of awareness, providing judicious fluid resuscitation, and seeking prompt consultation with a trauma surgeon are paramount to managing abdominal compartment syndrome. Decompressive laparotomy with temporary abdominal closure (ie, *open abdomen*) is the definitive treatment for abdominal compartment syndrome and may be carried out in the intensive care unit if a patient's condition is too unstable for transport to the operating room.

Pelvic Fractures

Pelvic fractures may cause considerable blood loss in patients after blunt trauma and are often associated with TBI (in up to 50% of patients). Pelvic fractures rarely occur in isolation, and because they are significantly correlated with aortic injury, the mediastinum must be carefully evaluated with radiography and CT of the chest. Patients with pelvic fractures may also have injury to the bladder, pelvic vasculature, or rectum. As usual with multitrauma patients, hemorrhage control is a high priority because even transient episodes of hypotension may worsen neurologic outcomes. Patients with open-book pelvic fractures are treated initially with a pelvic binder. An orthopedic surgeon should be consulted for definitive management.

Summary

- Chest injuries are common in trauma patients.
- Mediastinal injury can result in life-threatening conditions.
- Injury to any organ in the abdomen is a potential source of bleeding and thus hemorrhagic shock, which may develop in a delayed fashion.
- When treating trauma patients, the neurointensivist should have suspicion that injury is a source of ventilatory or hemodynamic instability and be prepared to seek prompt surgical consultation for evaluation and management.

SUGGESTED READING

American College of Surgeons, Committee on Trauma. Abdominal and pelvic trauma. In: Advanced trauma life support: student course manual. 9th ed. Chicago (IL): American College of Surgeons; c2012. p. 122–45.

American College of Surgeons, Committee on Trauma. Thoracic trauma. In: Advanced trauma life support: student course manual. 9th ed. Chicago (IL): American College of Surgeons; c2012. p. 94–118.

Coccolini F, Roberts D, Ansaloni L, Ivatury R, Gamberini E, Kluger Y, et al. The open abdomen in trauma and non-trauma patients: WSES guidelines. World J Emerg Surg. 2018 Feb 2;13:7.

de Campos JRM, White TW. Chest wall stabilization in trauma patients: why, when, and how? J Thorac Dis. 2018 Apr;10(Suppl 8):S951–62.

Furak J, Athanassiadi K. Diaphragm and transdiaphragmatic injuries. J Thorac Dis. 2019 Feb;11(Suppl 2):S152–7.

Kourouche S, Buckley T, Munroe B, Curtis K. Development of a blunt chest injury care bundle: an integrative review. Injury. 2018 Jun;49(6):1008–23. Epub 2018 Apr 7.

Mattox KL, Moore EE, Feliciano DV, editors. Trauma. 7th ed. New York (NY): McGraw-Hill Medical; c2013. 1224 p.

Molnar TF. Thoracic damage control surgery. J Thorac Dis. 2019 Feb;11(Suppl 2):S158–66.

Ramin S, Charbit J, Jaber S, Capdevila X. Acute respiratory distress syndrome after chest trauma: epidemiology, specific physiopathology and ventilation strategies. Anaesth Crit Care Pain Med. 2018 Oct 17. pii: S2352-5568(18)30303-5. [Epub ahead of print]

Rendeki S, Molnar TF. Pulmonary contusion. J Thorac Dis. 2019 Feb;11(Suppl 2):S141–51.

Schuurmans J, Goslings JC, Schepers T. Operative management versus non-operative management of rib fractures in flail chest injuries: a systematic review. Eur J Trauma Emerg Surg. 2017 Apr;43(2):163–8. Epub 2016 Aug 29.

Schellenberg M, Inaba K. Critical decisions in the management of thoracic trauma. Emerg Med Clin North Am. 2018 Feb;36(1):135–47.

Simon B, Ebert J, Bokhari F, Capella J, Emhoff T, Hayward T 3rd, et al; Eastern Association for the Surgery of Trauma. Management of pulmonary contusion and flail chest: an Eastern Association for the Surgery of Trauma practice management guideline. J Trauma Acute Care Surg. 2012 Nov;73(5 Suppl 4):S351–61.

Tieu B, Schipper P, Sukumar M, Mayberry JC. Pertinent surgical anatomy of the thorax and mediastinum. In: Asensio JA, Trunkey DD, editors. Current therapy of trauma and surgical critical care. 2nd ed. Philadelphia (PA): Elsevier; c2016. p. 205–28.

Verma N, White CS, Mohammed TL. Blunt cardiothoracic trauma: common injuries and diagnosis. Semin Roentgenol. 2018 Apr;53(2):171–7. Epub 2018 Feb 6.

64 Skeletal Trauma

JOSHUA S. BINGHAM, MD; KEVIN J. RENFREE, MD

Goals

- Review the basic evaluation and management of skeletal trauma.
- Describe the critical complications of skeletal trauma.
- Discuss the management steps for complications of skeletal trauma.

Introduction

In critically ill patients with polytrauma, a surge in the inflammatory response can lead to further injury and multisystem organ failure if not treated appropriately. During this acute inflammatory period, only life-threatening injuries should be treated. This chapter discusses the appropriate workup and management of skeletal trauma in critically ill patients.

Radiographic Evaluation

The initial radiographic workup for all trauma patients should include an anteroposterior view of the chest, an anteroposterior view of the pelvis, and a lateral view of the cervical spine. Computed tomography of the cervical spine, abdomen, and pelvis may also need to be performed during the initial workup to rule out life-threatening injuries.

Inadequate imaging is the most common cause of a delayed diagnosis of skeletal injuries. Complete radiographic evaluation of an extremity must include the joint above the fracture and the joint below the fracture. Without a complete radiographic evaluation of femoral shaft fractures, 3% to 10% of ipsilateral femoral neck fractures may be missed.

Damage Control Orthopedics

During the acute inflammatory window (2-5 days after injury), the risk of acute respiratory distress syndrome is increased. Only life-threatening injuries should be treated in this period. Temporary stabilization should be performed and definitive management delayed until after adequate resuscitation. Although helpful, vital signs alone are not sufficient indicators of adequate resuscitation (Table 64.1). A serum lactate level less than 2.5 mmol/L is the most sensitive indicator of adequate resuscitation.

Parameters for staging definitive treatment are based on the severity of injuries. If patients have an Injury Severity Score (ISS) greater than 20 with a thoracic injury or an ISS greater than 40 without a thoracic injury, multiple long-bone fractures, or severe pelvic abdominal trauma, they should undergo temporary stabilization and staged definitive management. Examples of temporary stabilization include splinting, skeletal traction, and external fixation.

Principles of Reduction and Immobilization

Closed reduction and stabilization of long-bone fractures prevents further soft tissue and neurovascular injuries. A neurovascular examination should be performed before and after any reduction. After reduction, the joint above the injury and the joint below the injury should be immobilized in a functional position (eg, intrinsic plus position for the hand) (Figure 64.1). Splints often require a 3-point mold to maintain reduction, but they must allow for swelling.

Common methods of immobilization include splints, traction (skin and skeletal), external fixation, and pelvic binders. Circumferential immobilization (ie, a cast) should

Table 64.1 • Indicators of Adequate Resuscitation

Component	Finding
Heart rate, beats per minute	<100
Mean arterial pressure, mm Hg	>60
Urine output, mL/kg/h	0.5-1.0
Base deficit	−2 to +2
Serum lactate, mmol/L	<2.5

be avoided for acute injuries because it does not allow for swelling. Skeletal traction and external fixation are often the temporary immobilization methods of choice for length-unstable, lower extremity, long-bone fractures in polytrauma patients.

Pelvic ring injuries are associated with a high mortality rate (15%-25%); hemorrhage from venous plexus injuries is the leading cause of death. Pelvic binders can decrease the intrapelvic volume, thereby decreasing hemorrhage (Figure 64.2). The appropriate position for binder application is over the greater trochanters (not the iliac crests).

Open Fractures

A high degree of awareness is required for open fractures whenever a soft tissue injury is overlying a fracture because the infection rate is high without early treatment. Open fractures are classified according to the Gustilo-Anderson classification (Table 64.2). Type I fractures are generally clean, low-energy wounds; types II and III have more contamination and soft tissue injuries.

Initial management of open fractures should include intravenous antibiotics and tetanus prophylaxis. Early initiation of antibiotics is the most important factor in minimizing infection. The type and duration of antibiotic therapy is determined according to the type of open fracture (Table 64.3). Antibiotic therapy should be continued for 24 to 48 hours after definitive soft tissue coverage.

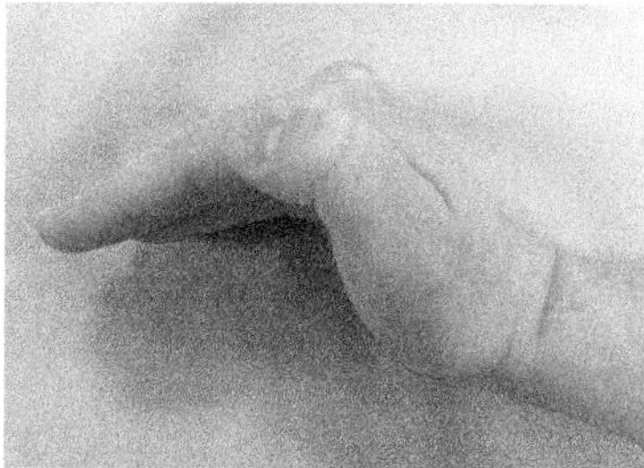

Figure 64.1. Hand in the Intrinsic Plus Position.

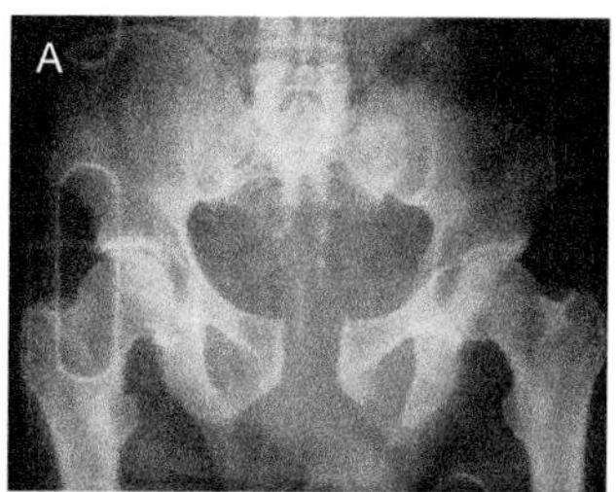

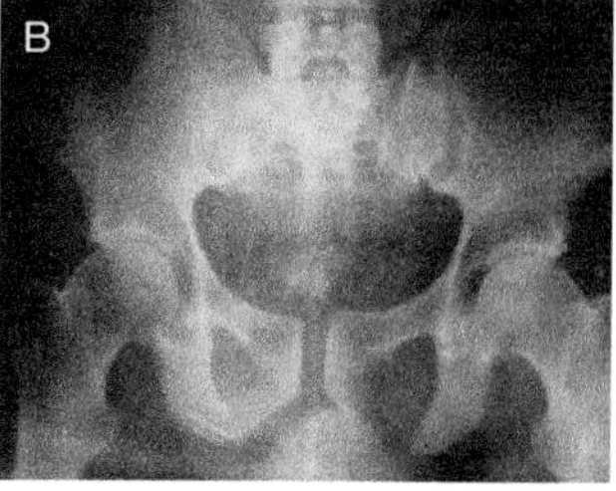

Figure 64.2. Pelvic Ring Injury. A, Without pelvic binder. B, With pelvic binder.

In addition to early antibiotic treatment, operative irrigation and débridement should be performed within 12 hours after the injury. Subsequent débridement every 24 to 48 hours may be required because of the severity of the injury and level of contamination. If definitive soft tissue coverage is delayed for more than 7 days, the risk of infection increases.

Compartment Syndrome

Compartment syndrome occurs when a sudden increase in interstitial pressure from local injury leads to inadequate perfusion and irreversible muscle and nerve damage. Common causes of compartment syndrome include fractures, vascular injuries, crush injuries, compressive dressings, and burns. Clinical signs and symptoms of compartment syndrome are pain, pallor, paralysis, paresthesia, and pulselessness, but they may be late findings. Disproportionate pain with passive motion is the most sensitive and specific clinical finding.

Pressure monitoring may be useful in the obtunded patient when a clinical examination is inadequate. All muscle groups within each compartment should be tested. The needle should be perpendicular to the floor and within 5 cm of the injury site. Compartment pressure greater than 30 mm Hg or within 30 mm Hg of the diastolic pressure is diagnostic. Compartment syndrome is a surgical emergency that requires complete decompression of all involved fascial compartments by fasciotomy.

Table 64.2 • Gustilo-Anderson Classification for Open Fractures

	Gustilo Type				
Criterion	**I**	**II**	**IIIA**	**IIIB**	**IIIC**
Amount of energy dissipated	Low	Moderate	High	High	High
Degree of contamination	Clean	Moderate	Extensive	Extensive	Extensive
Wound size, cm	<1	1-10	>10	>10	>10
Extent of soft tissue injury	Local	Local	Local	Requires flap coverage	Typically requires flap coverage
Extent of neurovascular injury	None	None	None	None	Requires repair

Fat Emboli Syndrome

Fat emboli syndrome (FES) results from an inflammatory response to embolized fat globules in the bloodstream after long-bone fracture or intramedullary reaming. FES occurs in 3% to 4% of patients who have an isolated long-bone fracture and in 10% to 15% of patients with polytrauma; the mortality rate is up to 15%.

FES usually occurs within 24 hours after the initial event and is diagnosed when 1 major criterion and 4 minor criteria are met. The *major criteria* are depression, hypoxemia (Pao_2<60 mm Hg), pulmonary edema, and petechial rash. The *minor criteria* are tachycardia, retinal emboli, fat in sputum or urine, pyrexia, thrombocytopenia, and decreased hematocrit.

Treatment is mainly supportive and includes mechanical ventilation with high positive end-expiratory pressure. Early temporary stabilization of the fracture (within 24 hours) is the most important factor in preventing FES.

Summary

- The most common cause of a delayed diagnosis of skeletal trauma is inadequate imaging.
- Performing temporary stabilization and staging definitive management until after adequate resuscitation minimizes the risk of secondary complications such as acute respiratory distress syndrome.
- Closed reduction and immobilization of fractures limits further neurovascular and soft tissue injuries.
- Early antibiotic therapy for open fractures is the most important factor in decreasing the risk of infection.
- Disproportionate pain with passive motion is the most sensitive and specific clinical finding in a patient with compartment syndrome.
- Treatment of FES is mainly supportive and includes mechanical ventilation with high positive end-expiratory pressure.

Table 64.3 • IV Antibiotic Therapy for Open Fractures

	Likely Organism			IV Antibiotic			Duration of Antibiotics	
Gustilo Type	**G+**	**G–**	**An**	**Ceph**	**Amino**	**Pen**	**24 h**	**24-48 h**
I	Y			Y			Y	
II	Y			Y				Y
IIIA	Y	Y		Y	Y			Y
IIIB	Y	Y		Y	Y			Y
IIIC	Y	Y		Y	Y			Y
III—Bowel contamination or farm injury	Y	Y	Y	Y	Y	Y		Y

Abbreviations: Amino, aminoglycoside; An, anaerobe; Ceph, first-generation cephalosporin; G–, gram-negative rod; G+, gram-positive cocci; IV, intravenous; Pen, penicillin; Y, yes.

SUGGESTED READING

Anderson PA, Muchow RD, Munoz A, Tontz WL, Resnick DK. Clearance of the asymptomatic cervical spine: a meta-analysis. J Orthop Trauma. 2010 Feb;24(2):100–6.

Caba-Doussoux P, Leon-Baltasar JL, Garcia-Fuentes C, Resines-Erasun C. Damage control orthopaedics in severe polytrauma with femur fracture. Injury. 2012 Dec;43 Suppl 2:S42–6.

D'Alleyrand JC, O'Toole RV. The evolution of damage control orthopedics: current evidence and practical applications of early appropriate care. Orthop Clin North Am. 2013 Oct;44(4):499–507. Epub 2013 Aug 21.

Frink M, Hildebrand F, Krettek C, Brand J, Hankemeier S. Compartment syndrome of the lower leg and foot. Clin Orthop Relat Res. 2010 Apr;468(4):940–50. Epub 2009 May 27.

Gustilo RB, Anderson JT. Prevention of infection in the treatment of one thousand and twenty-five open fractures of long bones: retrospective and prospective analyses. J Bone Joint Surg Am. 1976 Jun;58(4):453–8.

Hauser CJ, Adams CA Jr, Eachempati SR; Council of the Surgical Infection Society. Surgical Infection Society guideline: prophylactic antibiotic use in open fractures: an evidence-based guideline. Surg Infect (Larchmt). 2006 Aug;7(4):379–405.

Kim PH, Leopold SS. In brief: Gustilo-Anderson classification. [corrected]. Clin Orthop Relat Res. 2012 Nov;470(11):3270–4. Epub 2012 May 9. Erratum in: Clin Orthop Relat Res. 2012 Dec;470(12):3624.

Krieg JC, Mohr M, Ellis TJ, Simpson TS, Madey SM, Bottlang M. Emergent stabilization of pelvic ring injuries by controlled circumferential compression: a clinical trial. J Trauma. 2005 Sep;59(3):659–64.

Levy D. The fat embolism syndrome: a review. Clin Orthop Relat Res. 1990 Dec;(261):281–6.

Michaleff ZA, Maher CG, Verhagen AP, Rebbeck T, Lin CW. Accuracy of the Canadian C-spine rule and NEXUS to screen for clinically important cervical spine injury in patients following blunt trauma: a systematic review. CMAJ. 2012 Nov 6;184(16):E867–76. Epub 2012 Oct 9.

Mutschler M, Nienaber U, Brockamp T, Wafaisade A, Fabian T, Paffrath T, et al; TraumaRegister DGU. Renaissance of base deficit for the initial assessment of trauma patients: a base deficit-based classification for hypovolemic shock developed on data from 16,305 patients derived from the TraumaRegister DGU®. Crit Care. 2013 Mar 6;17(2):R42.

Odom SR, Howell MD, Silva GS, Nielsen VM, Gupta A, Shapiro NI, et al. Lactate clearance as a predictor of mortality in trauma patients. J Trauma Acute Care Surg. 2013 Apr;74(4):999–1004. Erratum in: J Trauma Acute Care Surg. 2014 Mar;76(3):902.

Pape HC, Giannoudis PV, Krettek C, Trentz O. Timing of fixation of major fractures in blunt polytrauma: role of conventional indicators in clinical decision making. J Orthop Trauma. 2005 Sep;19(8):551–62.

Porter JM, Ivatury RR. In search of the optimal end points of resuscitation in trauma patients: a review. J Trauma. 1998 May;44(5):908–14.

Rothberg DL, Makarewich CA. Fat embolism and fat embolism syndrome. J Am Acad Orthop Surg. 2019 Apr 15;27(8):e346–55.

Shaikh N. Emergency management of fat embolism syndrome. J Emerg Trauma Shock. 2009 Jan;2(1):29–33.

Turen CH, Dube MA, LeCroy MC. Approach to the polytraumatized patient with musculoskeletal injuries. J Am Acad Orthop Surg. 1999 May-Jun;7(3):154–65.

Whitesides TE, Heckman MM. Acute compartment syndrome: update on diagnosis and treatment. J Am Acad Orthop Surg. 1996 Jul;4(4):209–18.

Zalavras CG, Patzakis MJ. Open fractures: evaluation and management. J Am Acad Orthop Surg. 2003 May-Jun;11(3):212–9.

65 Burns and Electrical Injuries

BRANDON T. NOKES, MD; AYAN SEN, MD

Goals

- Know how to classify burns according to the American Burn Association criteria.
- Understand management of burns and fluid resuscitation of patients with burn injuries.
- Describe electrical burn injuries.

Introduction

Burn injuries may cause morbidity and death, and patients may have widely variable presentations and outcomes. This chapter focuses on the critical care aspects of burn injury and management issues of burn and electrical injuries.

Classification of Burns

Burns are classified according to the amount of total body surface area (TBSA) affected, the depth of burn, and the type of exposure associated with the burn. More specifically, burns can be chemical, electrical, or thermal. Burn severity is determined by the depth of involvement (Table 65.1): First-degree burns affect only the epidermis; second-degree burns include the epidermis and some dermis; third-degree burns extend into the subcutaneous tissue; and fourth-degree burns include underlying structures, such as muscles, bones, tendons, and nerves. Burns are also classified according to the extent of TBSA involved. The 2 commonly used methods of assessing TBSA in adults are the Lund-Browder classification (Figure 65.1) and the *rule of nines* (9% for each arm, 18% for each leg, 18% for the front of the torso, 18% for the back of the torso, 9% for the head, and 1% for the perineum). When the burn is irregular or patchy, the *palm method* may be useful: The palm of the patient's hand, excluding the fingers, is approximately 0.5% of the TBSA, and the entire palmar surface, including the fingers, is 1% in children and adults.

Management of Burns

Early Steps

Early management of burns typically occurs in the field or in the emergency department. As with other trauma, the first step in management is the primary survey (airway, breathing, circulation, and disability). Assessing for a patent airway is of the utmost importance because burns are characterized by capillary leak with marked tissue edema. Edema involving the airway, through thermal injury or associated inhalational injury, may result in morbidity. If patients cannot protect their airway or if respiratory compromise is a possibility, endotracheal intubation may be necessary. In addition to increasing the risk for direct and indirect airway compromise, burn injuries can predispose patients to metabolic acidosis resulting from traumatic cell lysis, thereby increasing the work of breathing. Carbon monoxide poisoning with fire-associated burn injuries may lead to concurrent impairment of oxygen delivery.

Circulatory collapse is an important consideration in the management of burn injuries. Capillary leak can lead to extensive interstitial edema and, in turn, a shock state. Because cardiac dysrhythmia is another consideration, especially with electrical burn injuries, blood pressure should be rapidly assessed with a peripheral cuff, an arterial line should be established for hemodynamic monitoring, and telemetric monitoring should be used early for arrhythmia assessment. Early intravenous access should be established with 2 large-bore intravenous catheters.

Disability assessment is especially important in the context of automobile-related and electrical burn injuries. A cervical collar, if applicable, is typically placed in the field. Disability assessment should be targeted toward trauma, such as facial fractures, which may hinder the

Table 65.1 • Burn Classification

Depth	Appearance	Sensation	Healing Time
Superficial burn	Dry, red Blanches with pressure	Painful	3-6 d
Superficial partial-thickness burn	Blisters Moist, red, weeping Blanches with pressure	Painful to temperature and air	7-21 d
Deep partial-thickness burn	Blisters (easily unroofed) Wet or waxy dry Variable color (patchy to cheesy white to red) Does not blanch with pressure	Perceptive of pressure only	>21 d Usually requires surgical treatment
Full-thickness burn	Waxy white to leathery gray to charred and black Dry and inelastic No blanching with pressure	Deep pressure only	Rarely heals without surgical treatment
Fourth-degree burn	Extends into fascia or muscle	Deep pressure	Never heals without surgical treatment

From Rice PL Jr, Orgill DP. Classification of burn injury. In: Post TW, editor. UpToDate. Waltham (MA): UpToDate; c2018 [cited 2018 Sep 7]; used with permission as modified from data in Mertens DM, Jenkins ME, Warden GD. Outpatient burn management. Nurs Clin North Am. 1997 Jun;32(2):343-64; Peate WF. Outpatient management of burns. Am Fam Physician. 1992 Mar;45(3):1321-30; and Clayton MC, Solem LD. No ice, no butter: advice on management of burns for primary care physicians. Postgrad Med. 1995 May;97(5):151-5.

assessment of the patient's airway, breathing, and circulation during resuscitation. After disability is assessed, the secondary survey can proceed. Simultaneously, fluid resuscitation should be initiated, and burns should be cooled to prevent further thermal injury. A patient with second- or third-degree burns is highly likely to have other forms of intracranial, thoracoabdominal, or musculoskeletal trauma. Full primary and secondary surveys should be repeated, and imaging should be performed as needed to rule out missed injuries. Criteria for transfer to a burn center should be considered (Box 65.1).

Fluid Resuscitation

Although the importance of early fluid resuscitation in burn management is undisputed, the appropriate fluid resuscitation formula is still debated. Since the 1970s, the *Parkland formula* has been widely used: In the first 24 hours, crystalloid (typically, lactated Ringer solution) is given at a dose of 4 mL/kg for each 1% of TBSA burned, with half the amount given in the first 8 hours. Criticisms of this approach are that it may lead to inappropriate fluid administration, most commonly overadministration, and cause complications such as abdominal compartment syndrome. As a result, some advocate for lower initial volumes according to the *modified Brooke formula*: Crystalloid is given at a dose of 2 mL/kg for each 1% of TBSA burned. In the second 24 hours of resuscitation, a recommended colloid dose is 0.3 to 0.5 mL/kg for each 1% of TBSA burned, although the role of colloids is controversial. The US Army Institute of Surgical Research has implemented the *rule of tens*, where the initial fluid rate is calculated as the percentage of burned TBSA multiplied by 10, with another 100 mL/h added for every 10 kg of body weight if the patient weighs more than 80 kg. This formula has not been widely validated, but it eliminates the need for cumbersome calculation.

Regardless of the initial approach to fluid resuscitation, ongoing and frequent evaluation of the patient is necessary to determine whether the resuscitation goals are being met, with therapy modified as indicated (Figure 65.2). In addition to the traditional markers of volume status (heart rate, blood pressure, and urine output), more advanced markers have been investigated, particularly indexes from noninvasive cardiac monitoring, but they lack validation or widespread acceptance. Vasopressors may be used, but the best vasopressor for burn-related shock has not been determined.

Other Considerations

If patients have extensive, severe burns, the chance of survival may be low, and palliation may be appropriate. No index of survival is perfect; however, if the *Baux score* (sum

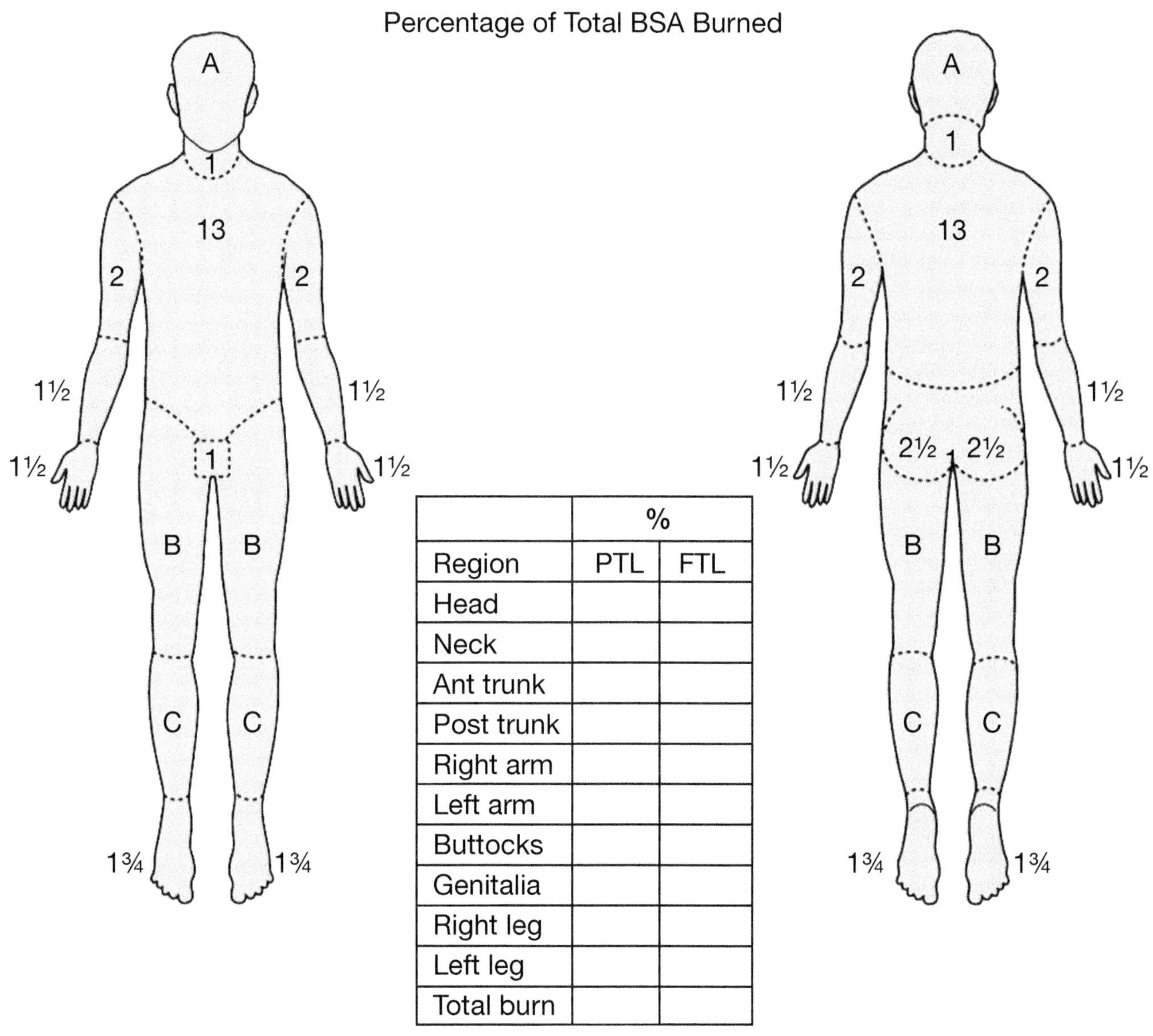

	%	
Region	PTL	FTL
Head		
Neck		
Ant trunk		
Post trunk		
Right arm		
Left arm		
Buttocks		
Genitalia		
Right leg		
Left leg		
Total burn		

Relative Percentage of BSA Affected by Growth According to Age

Area	**0 y**	**1 y**	**5 y**	**10 y**	**15 y**	**Adult**
A = ½ of head	9½	8½	6½	5½	4½	3½
B = ½ of 1 thigh	2¾	3¼	4	4½	4½	4¾
C = ½ of 1 lower leg	2½	2½	2¾	3	3¼	3½

Figure 65.1. Lund-Browder Classification. The numbers with the human figures are percentages assigned to burned areas. Erythematous areas are excluded. Ant indicates anterior; BSA, body surface area; FTL, full-thickness loss; Post, posterior; PTL, partial-thickness loss.

(Modified from Hettiaratchy S, Papini R. Initial management of a major burn: II—assessment and resuscitation. BMJ. 2004 Jul 10;329[7457]:101–3; used with permission.)

Box 65.1 • Burn Injury Criteria for Transfer to a Burn Center

1. Partial-thickness burns on more than 10% of the total body surface area
2. Burns that involve the face, hands, feet, genitalia, perineum, or major joints
3. Third-degree burns regardless of patient's age
4. Electrical burns, including lightning injury
5. Chemical burns
6. Inhalational injury
7. Burn injury in patients with preexisting medical disorders that could complicate management, prolong recovery, or cause death
8. Any patient with burns and concomitant trauma (eg, fractures) in which the burn injury poses the greater risk of morbidity or mortality
   a. If the trauma poses the greater immediate risk, the patient may be initially stabilized in a trauma center before being transferred to a burn unit
   b. Physician judgment is necessary, and decisions should be made in concert with the regional medical control plan and triage protocols
9. Burned children in hospitals that do not have qualified personnel or equipment for the care of children
10. Burn injury in patients who require special social, emotional, and rehabilitative intervention

Data from American College of Surgeons. Committee on Trauma. Resources for optimal care of the injured patient: 2006. Chicago (IL): American College of Surgeons; c2006.

of the patient's age and the percentage of TBSA burned) is greater than 150, the injury will most likely be fatal.

After initial resuscitative measures have been instituted, other aspects of management should be considered: 1) Pain management, which can be challenging, should be initiated early. Opiates are typically the mainstay, but the addition of ketamine or dexmedetomidine can be useful both for procedures and for further analgesia. 2) Enteral nutrition should be initiated early (unless the patient has gastric ileus with mesenteric edema). 3) Early surgical consultation for consideration of débridement and skin grafting is particularly important with circumferential burns where eschar may compromise the patient's limbs or airway (neck involvement) or interfere with mechanical ventilation (chest involvement). 4) Physical and occupational therapy should be started early. 5) Infection is a large risk. Burned areas should be inspected frequently and dressings changed. Topical antimicrobial use is common. The need for empirical antibiotics is unclear, and their use is guided largely by individual clinical practice.

Electrical Injury

Electrical injuries, which account for 3% of burn injuries, include thermal injuries, dysrhythmias and central nervous system injury. Triage and management for burns from electrical injuries are similar to those for other burns, with special consideration for cardiac arrhythmia. Any arrhythmias that arise should be treated like arrhythmias after myocardial infarction. Patients who have ectopic beats after electrical burn injury should be admitted to a telemetry unit for observation.

Summary

- Burn management is a multidisciplinary practice that starts with assessment of the patient's airway, breathing, and circulation and classification of the burn.
- The optimal fluid resuscitation protocol has not been established, although the Parkland formula is widely used.
- The response to resuscitation should be carefully monitored and adjustments made as indicated.
- Early management should include wound cooling, local dressing, pain management, and enteral nutrition.
- Early surgical consultation for débridement and skin grafting is important.

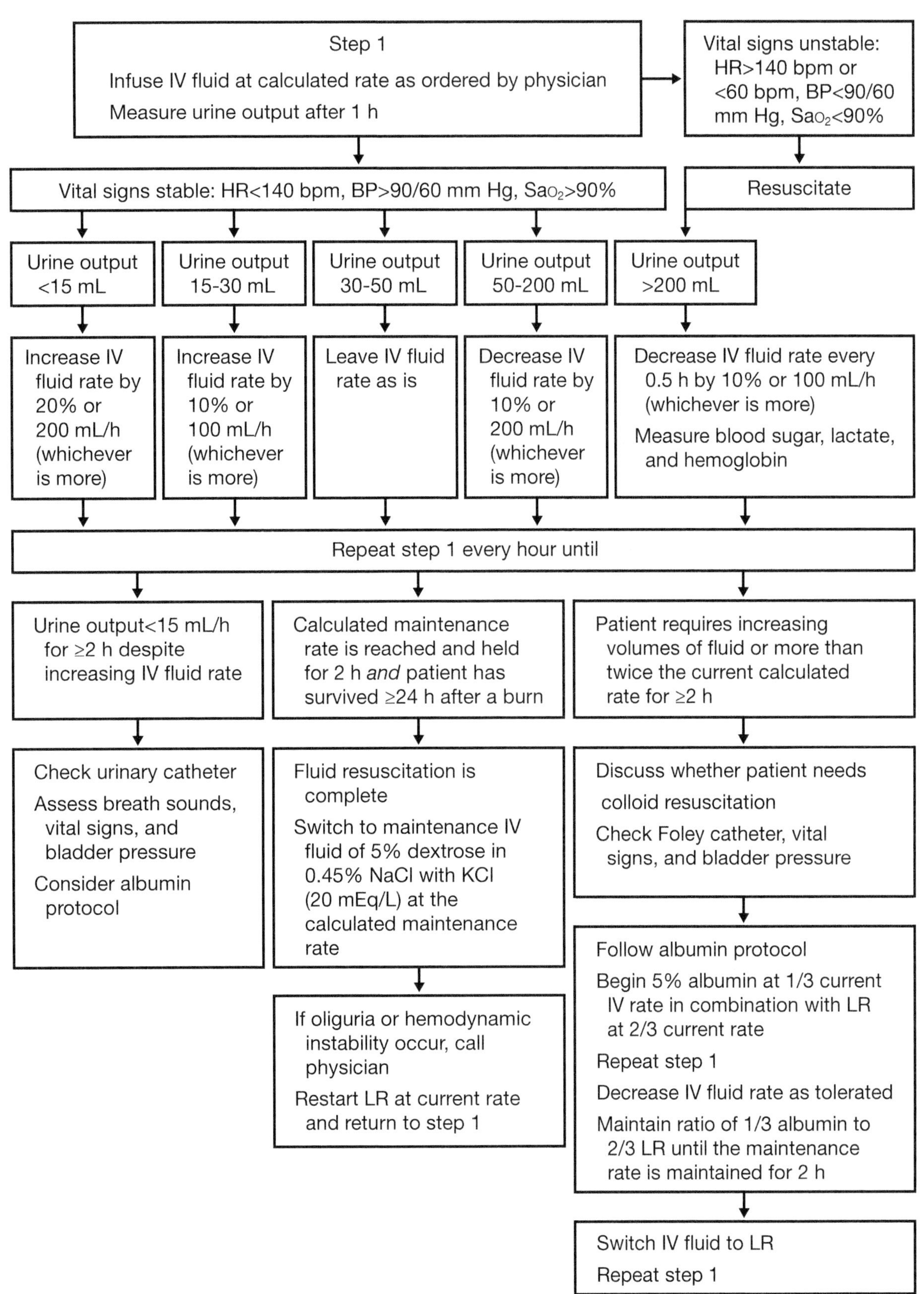

Figure 65.2. Fluid Resuscitation Protocol for Use in Patient Care Units. The initial infusion rate is calculated with the Parkland formula. BP indicates blood pressure; bpm, beats per minute; HR, heart rate; IV, intravenous; LR, lactated Ringer solution; Sa_{O_2}, arterial oxygen saturation.

(Modified from Saffle JI. The phenomenon of "fluid creep" in acute burn resuscitation. J Burn Care Res. 2007 May-Jun;28[3]:382-95; used with permission.)

SUGGESTED READING

Allison K, Porter K. Consensus on the prehospital approach to burns patient management. Emerg Med J. 2004 Jan;21(1):112–4.

Alvarado R, Chung KK, Cancio LC, Wolf SE. Burn resuscitation. Burns. 2009 Feb;35(1):4–14. Epub 2008 Jun 9.

Kearns RD, Rich PB, Cairns CB, Holmes JH, Cairns BA. Electrical injury and burn care: a review of best practices. EMS World. 2014 Sep;43(9):34–40, 55.

Palmieri TL. Infection prevention: unique aspects of burn units. Surg Infect (Larchmt). 2019 Feb/Mar;20(2):111–4. Epub 2019 Jan 24.

Pham TN, Cancio LC, Gibran NS; American Burn Association. American Burn Association practice guidelines burn shock resuscitation. J Burn Care Res. 2008 Jan-Feb;29(1):257–66.

Smolle C, Cambiaso-Daniel J, Forbes AA, Wurzer P, Hundeshagen G, Branski LK, et al. Recent trends in burn epidemiology worldwide: a systematic review. Burns. 2017 Mar;43(2):249–57. Epub 2016 Sep 3.

Tricklebank S. Modern trends in fluid therapy for burns. Burns. 2009 Sep;35(6):757–67. Epub 2009 May 30.

Cardiothoracic Critical Care

Cardiothoracic Surgery and Postoperative Intensive Care

JUAN G. RIPOLL SANZ, MD; ROBERT A. RATZLAFF, DO

Goals

- Describe the basic principles and common indications for cardiopulmonary bypass.
- Review the most common cardiothoracic surgical procedures and their indications.
- Describe general and specific complications after cardiothoracic surgical procedures.

Introduction

Cardiothoracic surgical (CTS) critical care responsibilities have progressively shifted away from surgeons and toward intensivists in the past several decades. CTS patients present unique challenges, and optimal patient care in the intensive care unit is a main factor for the prevention of deaths after any type of open heart surgery.

Cardiopulmonary Bypass

Principles

Cardiopulmonary bypass (CPB) is a surgical technique that allows transient replacement of cardiovascular and pulmonary function during CTS procedures. The CPB circuit has 5 main functions: 1) preservation of a bloodless surgical field; 2) blood-gas exchange; 3) thermoregulation for organ protection (systemic cooling and rewarming); 4) preservation of vital organ perfusion; and 5) protection and support of the heart and lungs.

Typically, deoxygenated blood is gravity drained into a venous reservoir by cannulation of large systemic veins. The amount of blood drainage is almost exclusively dependent on the column height between the patient and the pump, the central venous pressure, and the resistance to flow inside the venous circuit. From the venous reservoir, the blood is pumped to an oxygenator (also known as a gas exchanger) and heat exchanger. After rapidly passing through an arterial filter, the blood is returned to the systemic circulation through an arterial cannula. The standard CPB circuits also include blood-gas monitors; roller pumps (useful for cardioplegia delivery, suction, and venting); safety mechanisms (eg, bubble detectors); real-time monitors (eg, flow and pressure); and blood filters (Figure 66.1).

Indications

CPB is used to provide cardiac and respiratory support during surgical procedures involving the heart or great vessels (Box 66.1). The most common indication is coronary artery bypass graft (CABG) surgery. Although CPB is used in around 80% of CABG procedures performed in the United States, nearly 20% are performed with the patient's own heart and lungs to ensure perfusion of vital organs (called *off-pump CABG [OPCABG] surgery*).

Physiologic Sequelae

CTS under CPB provokes systemic inflammatory response syndrome (SIRS). The development of SIRS during CPB is caused mainly by the interaction of blood products within the artificial surface, surgical-induced trauma, a massive release of free radicals after ischemia-reperfusion injury, and increased production of proinflammatory cytokines. Clinically, postoperative complications from SIRS vary from cardiopulmonary damage to multiorgan failure.

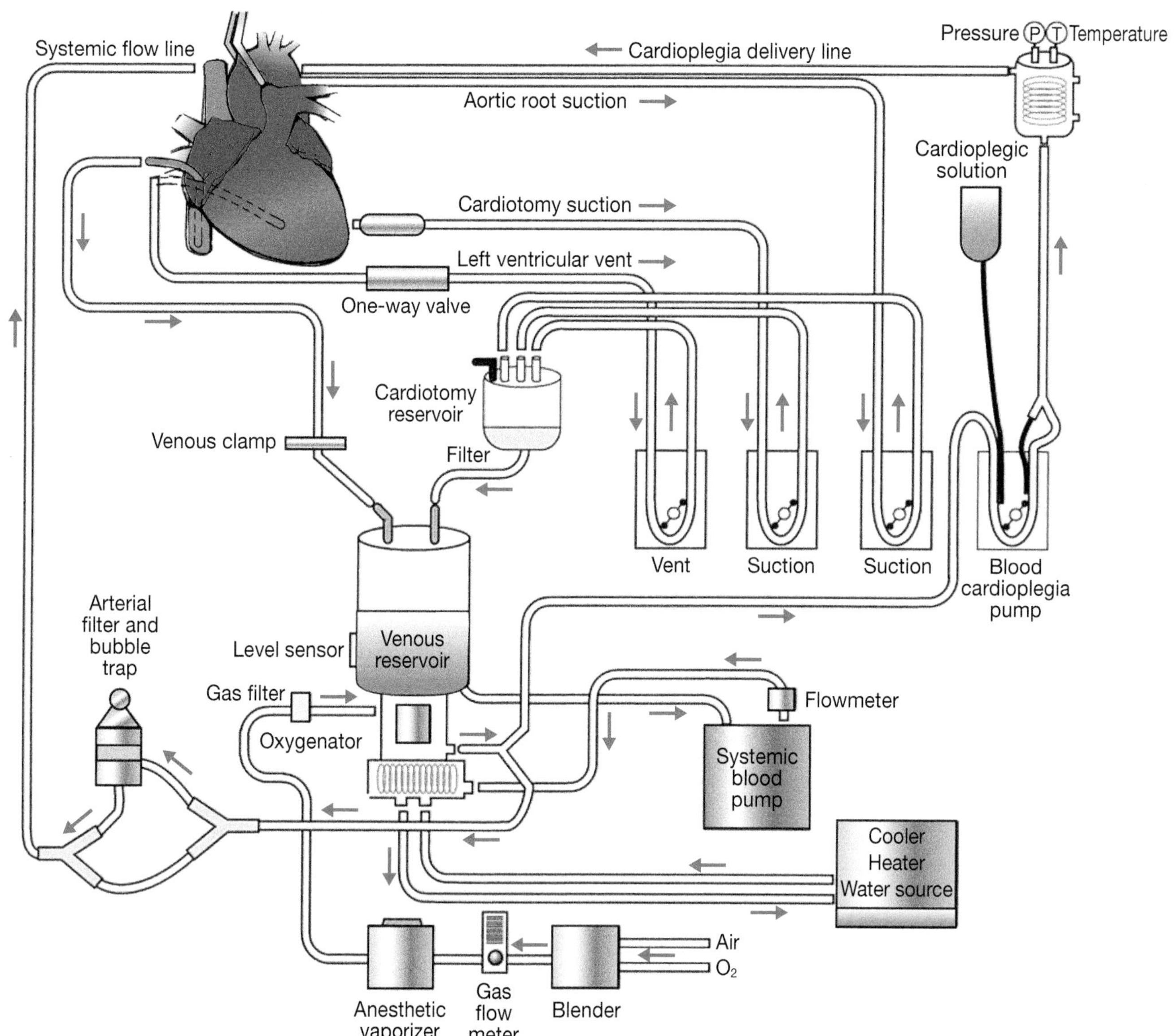

Figure 66.1. Cardiopulmonary Bypass Circuit. The main components are the oxygenator, the systemic blood pump, and the venous reservoir. O_2 indicates oxygen.

(From Bassin L, Bell D. Temporary extracorporeal bypass modalities during aortic surgery. Best Pract Res Clin Anaesthesiol. 2016 Sep;30[3]:341-57. Epub 2016 Aug 17; used with permission.)

Box 66.1 • Common Indications for Cardiopulmonary Bypass

- Coronary artery bypass graft surgery
- Heart valve replacement or repair
- Surgical repair of aneurysm (eg, aortic aneurysm or intracranial aneurysm)
- Repair of atrioventricular or ventricular septal defects
- Transplants (heart, lung, or combined heart-lung)
- Pulmonary thromboendarterectomy and thrombectomy
- Repair of congenital heart defects (eg, tetralogy of Fallot)

Common CTS Procedures

CABG Surgery

In CABG surgery, a partial or complete atherosclerotic occlusion of the coronary arteries is bypassed with the use of autologous arteries or veins. Typically, CABG surgery is performed through a median sternotomy, which offers optimal exposure of the heart. The procedure is considered relatively safe; major complications occur in about 0.4% of patients. To allow for proper manipulation during surgery, the heart is arrested by occluding the ascending aorta and then perfusing the heart with a cold, high-potassium cardioplegic solution. The CPB machine supports the systemic circulation during the cardiac arrest (1-2 hours).

Autologous grafts used for bypass include the left internal thoracic artery (or the left internal mammary artery [LIMA]) and the great saphenous vein. Although infrequently used, left internal thoracic artery grafts to bypass the left anterior descending (LAD) coronary artery result in better clinical outcomes and longer patency than great saphenous vein grafts. Similarly, grafts from other arteries have better patency than the great saphenous vein (eg, gastroepiploic artery, radial artery, and right internal thoracic artery), but they are not routinely used mainly because of technical limitations.

The duration of a CABG procedure is usually 3 to 5 hours, depending on the expertise of the surgeon and other factors. The average in-hospital stay after an uncomplicated procedure is 5 to 7 days, and full recovery is expected 6 to 12 weeks after the surgical intervention.

Valvular Heart Disease and Surgical Valve Repair

Valvular heart disease is among the most common causes of heart failure. In the United States, nearly 4.0 million to 5.5 million adults have valvular heart disease and about 20,000 patients die of valvular heart disease annually (incidence, 7 per 100,000 patients). The most common causes are presented in Box 66.2.

Although the aortic and mitral valves are the most frequently compromised, the pulmonic and tricuspid valves can be affected. All the heart valves are amenable to surgical repair or replacement, and the specific procedure depends on the location and lesion characteristics of the affected valve. However, the most common cardiac surgical procedures in adults are designed to mitigate stenoses or regurgitant lesions of the aortic or mitral valve and secondary regurgitation of the tricuspid valve. The most common valve lesion requiring surgery is aortic stenosis.

Box 66.2 • Causes of Valvular Heart Disease

- Congenital abnormalities and connective tissue diseases
  - Connective tissue disorders (eg, Marfan syndrome)
  - Congenital valve disease (eg, bicuspid aortic valve disease)
  - Environmentally determined (eg, rubella causing pulmonary stenosis)
- Immunologic and inflammatory diseases (eg, rheumatic fever, syphilis, ankylosing spondylitis, AIDS, and systemic lupus erythematosus)
- Myocardial diseases (eg, ischemic, nonischemic, and hypertrophic cardiomyopathy)
- Neoplasia (eg, myxoma, fibroelastoma, and carcinoid)
- Degenerative processes (related to aging, with possible genetic and environmental predisposing factors)
- Iatrogenic valve diseases (eg, after valve repair surgery)
- Drugs and other agents (eg, radiation and trauma)
- Infiltrative causes (eg, hypereosinophilic syndrome and mucopolysaccharidoses)
- Idiopathic

Thoracic Surgery

Pneumonectomy

The first multistage pneumonectomy was performed in 1895 in a patient with tuberculous empyema. However, it was not until 1933 that a 1-stage pneumonectomy was successfully accomplished in a patient with lung carcinoma.

Single pneumonectomy is the total removal of the diseased lung. *Extrapleural pneumonectomy* is a more invasive procedure that involves the resection of not only the compromised lung but also the mediastinal lymph nodes, the visceral and parietal pleura, the pericardium, and the ipsilateral hemidiaphragm.

Although pneumonectomy conveys a substantial risk of cardiovascular and pulmonary complications, the procedure has been commonly indicated for patients with large thymomas and malignant lung tumors such as mesotheliomas. In general, this approach is frequently accompanied by chemotherapy and radiotherapy to increase survival. The overall 30-day mortality after pneumonectomy ranges from 5% to 13% and correlates inversely with the institutional surgical case volume.

Lobectomy

Lobectomy is the resection of a single lung lobe. Because it preserves pulmonary function, lobectomy is considered a paramount technique for patients with a diagnosis of early-stage non–small cell lung cancer.

Pulmonary Wedge Resection

Pulmonary wedge resection is a nonanatomical wedge resection of the lung for diagnostic or therapeutic purposes. The area of the lung designated for excision must be mobile, and resections that include a draining vein or a branch of a pulmonary artery will require proximal vascular control to prevent further bleeding. If the lesion is small or difficult to visualize on the lung surface, instruments or a finger can be inserted into the chest cavity to palpate the lung and localize the lesion. Landmarks can also be used to estimate the location of the lesion. However, some interpolation is required because radiologic imaging is usually performed with the lung inflated, while the surgical procedure is performed on the deflated lung. Nodules that are difficult to find can be localized by various methods, including computed tomographically guided methods, radionuclide imaging, navigational bronchoscopy, and real-time imaging. As with open thoracotomy, surgical staplers offer fast and reliable hemostasis of the edge of resected lung and minimize air leakage.

Video-Assisted Thoracoscopic Surgery

Video-assisted thoracoscopic surgery (VATS) is a minimally invasive surgical intervention that does not require a formal thoracotomy incision. It provides adequate visualization of the surgical field despite reduced access to the thorax, thus allowing the procedure to be performed in patients who are severely compromised or who have limited pulmonary reserve. The overall mortality is estimated to be 0% to 2%, which is more favorable than the mortality with conventional thoracotomy.

Initially, VATS was used exclusively for diagnostic and therapeutic interventions involving the lungs, mediastinum, and pleura, but now VATS is used for all structures in the chest. The heart, spinal column, esophagus, great vessels, diaphragm, and nerves are all easily accessible with VATS (Box 66.3). Compared with conventional thoracotomy, VATS results in a shorter operating time, an earlier return to normal activity, and less postoperative morbidity.

Box 66.3 • Indications for Video-Assisted Thoracoscopic Surgery

- Lung
  - Wedge resection
  - Segmentectomy
  - Lobectomy
  - Closure of bronchopleural fistula
  - Lung tumor resection or staging
- Pleura
  - Decortication
  - Adhesiolysis
  - Pleurodesis
- Intrathoracic cavity (diagnosis and treatment)
  - Pleural effusions
  - Foreign body
  - Intrathoracic lesions (eg, cyst or tumor)
- Mediastinum
  - Mediastinal tumor resection or staging
  - Cyst removal
  - Thymectomy
- Heart and vessels
  - Minimally invasive valvular surgical interventions
  - Coronary artery surgical procedures
  - Pericardectomy
- Nerves and spine
  - Diskectomy
  - Spinal deformity assessment and correction
  - Sympathectomy
  - Spinal abscess drainage
- Esophagus and diaphragm
  - Esophageal tumor resection or staging
  - Complete or partial esophageal resection
  - Diaphragm biopsy or repair

Minimally Invasive CTS Procedures

Minimally invasive cardiothoracic surgery (MICS) has gained more popularity among cardiothoracic surgeons. Interest in MICS was initially low because of concerns related to increased risk of perioperative complications resulting from a prolonged surgical time and a smaller surgical field for complex procedures. Nevertheless, with recent innovations in transthoracic echocardiography, robotic technology, development of novel surgical instruments, and improved perfusion techniques, minimally invasive cardiothoracic approaches have advanced. The most common MICS procedures are minimally invasive direct CABG (MIDCABG) surgery and transcatheter aortic valve replacement (TAVR).

MIDCABG Surgery

In MIDCABG surgery, a small anterolateral thoracotomy is made and a single-vessel (usually the LIMA) off-pump bypass is used to overcome the area of atherosclerotic obstruction in the LAD coronary artery. It is the preferred approach for treating isolated disease of the LAD and is gaining more popularity for multivessel revascularization in Europe and the United States.

Various series have shown promising results for MIDCABG surgery; compared with standard CABG surgery, MIDCABG surgery involves a shorter postoperative in-hospital length of stay, earlier return to full activity, decreased use of resources, excellent graft patency, and fewer perioperative transfusion requirements.

The first MIDCABG procedures were performed through anterolateral thoracotomies and without CPB (ie, OPCABG). The benefits of OPCABG are controversial, but the outcome of an OPCABG procedure compared with an on-pump MIDCABG procedure depends more on the expertise of the surgeon and the institutional protocol than on the technique itself. Despite the controversy, there is agreement that the selection of the appropriate surgical technique must be individualized among patients undergoing myocardial revascularization.

Transcatheter Aortic Valve Replacement

Aortic stenosis is the most prevalent valvular heart disease in the Western world. The disease process has a prolonged latent asymptomatic phase, but after symptoms occur, patients have a poor prognosis, with 5-year survival rates varying from 10% to 50%. Aortic valve replacement (AVR) by sternotomy extends and enhances the quality of life, even in selected elderly patients. Nevertheless, many patients do not undergo an AVR because of the perceived or real increased risks associated with the surgical procedure. TAVR is an alternative to AVR by sternotomy for elderly patients or patients with multiple comorbidities that put them at high surgical risk. During TAVR, a prosthetic heart valve is implanted within the damaged native aortic valve (or sometimes within a previously repaired aortic valve) without the requirement for open-heart surgery and CPB. Since the first TAVR in 2002, more than 60,000 procedures have been performed worldwide. Multiple randomized clinical trials have validated the efficacy and safety of TAVR; it is a good alternative for patients who have high surgical risk and symptomatic degenerative aortic stenosis.

Postoperative CTS Complications

In general, CTS patients tend to have similar postoperative problems (Table 66.1), but certain postoperative problems are characteristic of specific procedures (Table 66.2).

The clinical approach to a CTS patient in the intensive care unit varies according to the procedure and the patient. Often, however, such as after a first-time or primary CABG or a first-time single valve repair, patients arrive intubated and may be receiving low-dose inotropic support or vasopressor therapy. Within 12 to 24 hours, they are warmed, resuscitated, extubated, and weaned from the chemical support. This approach is commonly referred to as *fast-tracking*. Patients who may be candidates for fast-tracking (eg, because they have few or clinically insignificant comorbidities) are often identified preoperatively by the cardiothoracic surgical, anesthesia, and intensive care unit teams. During the perioperative period, fast-tracking requires a multidisciplinary approach. Although primary or first-time heart surgery can be uneventful, the potential for problems exists. The risk of complications is higher for patients who have subsequent CABG or valve surgery, so they may not be suitable candidates for fast-tracking.

After a CTS procedure, multiple complications can arise, including poor perfusion, bleeding, arrhythmias, and cardiovascular instability. Poor perfusion can be characterized by high or increasing serum lactic acid levels or low mixed venous oxygen saturation (or both). Low mixed venous oxygen saturation may be a marker of additional underlying problems such as low circulating blood volume (from bleeding or hypovolemia); hypotension (due to hypovolemia, bleeding, or vasoplegia); and low cardiac output (eg, bradyarrhythmias, atrial fibrillation, and conduction abnormalities). Another common complication of CTS interventions is bleeding, which is defined as chest tube output of more than 200 mL/h or more than 1,500 mL in 8 hours. Generally, chest tube output that is increasing or not decreasing usually prompts reoperation or reexploration by the surgical team. Administering appropriate fluid volume, warming the patient to 37°C, increasing positive-end expiratory pressure, and evaluating results from specific laboratory tests (eg, thromboelastography, coagulation tests, and activated clotting time) are initial steps that may precede the decision to surgically explore the chest.

If the patient's condition has not stabilized after appropriate diagnostic steps and interventions, functional cardiothoracic abnormalities must be considered (eg, left ventricular failure, right ventricular failure, and valvular dysfunction.). Echocardiography (transthoracic or transesophageal) is the gold standard for assessing the cardiovascular system (Table 66.2). Additional postoperative CTS complications can be assessed with point-of-care ultrasonography, chest radiography, pulmonary artery catheter tracings and trends, and electrocardiography.

Table 66.1 • General Postoperative Complications of Cardiothoracic Surgery

Complication	Clues to Aid Diagnosis	Intervention
Poor perfusion	High or increasing lactate (>2 mmol/L) Low blood pressure Low mixed venous oxygen saturation	Fluid resuscitation Blood transfusion Inotropes, vasopressors Pacing (atrial, atrioventricular, ventricular)
Bleeding	Chest tube output >200 mL/h or >1,500 mL in 8 h	Warming patient Fluid resuscitation Blood transfusion Laboratory tests (coagulation tests, thromboelastography, activated clotting time) Chest reexploration (typically a last resort) Increasing positive end-expiratory pressure
Arrhythmias	Electrocardiography, echocardiography	Replenishing electrolytes

Table 66.2 • Organ-Specific Postoperative Complications of Cardiothoracic Surgery

Complication	Clues to Aid Diagnosis	Intervention
Cardiovascular		
LV failure	ECHO	See Chapter 113[a]
RV failure	ECHO	See Chapter 113[a]
Myocardial ischemia	ECHO	See Chapter 113[a]
Valvular dysfunction	ECHO	See Chapter 113[a]
Vasoplegia	ECHO; PA catheter	Vasopressors; intotropes; methylene blue
Pericardial effusion	ECHO; PA catheter	IVF; vasopressors
Cardiac tamponade	ECHO; PA catheter	Immediate pericardiocentesis
Atrial fibrillation	ECG	Amiodarone; β-blockers
Ventricular arrhythmias	ECG	Cardioversion
Bradyarrhythmias	ECG	Atrial pacing; inotropes
Atrioventricular conduction block	ECG	Permanent pacemaker
Pulmonary		
Malposition of ETT	Clinical examination; US; CXR	Reposition with or without bronchoscopy
Pneumothorax	Clinical examination; US; CXR	Chest tube/pigtail catheter
Hemothorax	Clinical examination; US; CXR	Chest tube/pigtail catheter
Respiratory failure	Clinical examination; US; CXR	NIPPV; mechanical ventilation; diuresis
Pleural effusion	Clinical examination; US; CXR	Chest tube/pigtail catheter; thoracentesis; diuresis; ambulation
Neurologic		
Stroke	Clinical examination; CT; CT angiography; MRI	Consider CTA/CTP to evaluate for endovascular clot retrieval
Limb ischemia	Clinical examination; CT angiography; MRI	If descending aortic surgery, consider placement of lumbar drain (if not already present) Increase SCPP similar to cerebral perfusion pressure (SCPP = MAP – ICP)

Abbreviations: BP, blood pressure; CT, computed tomography; CTA, computed tomographic angiography; CTP, computed tomographic perfusion; CXR, chest radiography; ECG, electrocardiography; ECHO, echocardiography; ETT, endotracheal tube; ICP, intracranial pressure; IVF, intravenous fluids; LV, left ventricular; MAP, mean arterial pressure; mPAP, mean pulmonary arterial pressure; MRI, magnetic resonance imaging; NIPPV, noninvasive positive-pressure ventilation; PA, pulmonary artery; RV, right ventricular; SCPP, spinal cord perfusion pressure; US, ultrasonography.

[a] Chapter 113, "Transesophageal Echocardiography."

Summary

- The main functions of CPB are preservation of a bloodless surgical field, blood-gas exchange, thermoregulation for organ protection (systemic cooling and rewarming), preservation of vital organ perfusion, and protection and support of the heart and lungs.
- CPB is used to provide cardiac and respiratory support during surgical procedures involving the heart or great vessels.
- Over the past decade, recent innovations in transthoracic echocardiography, robotic technology, development of novel surgical instruments, and improved perfusion techniques have led to an increase in the popularity of MICS procedures (eg, MIDCABG surgery and TAVR).
- Postoperative complications of CTS procedures commonly result from poor perfusion, arrhythmias, and bleeding.
- Specific postoperative complications of CTS procedures are mainly related to cardiovascular, pulmonary, and neurologic dysfunction.

SUGGESTED READING

Adams DH, Popma JJ, Reardon MJ, Yakubov SJ, Coselli JS, Deeb GM, et al; U.S. CoreValve Clinical Investigators. Transcatheter aortic-valve replacement with a self-expanding prosthesis. N Engl J Med. 2014 May 8;370(19):1790–8. Epub 2014 Mar 29.

Ailawadi G, Zacour RK. Cardiopulmonary bypass/extracorporeal membrane oxygenation/left heart bypass: indications, techniques, and complications. Surg Clin North Am. 2009 Aug;89(4):781–96.

Alexander JH, Smith PK. Coronary-artery bypass grafting. N Engl J Med. 2016 May 19;374(20):1954–64.

Awais O, Reidy MR, Mehta K, Bianco V, Gooding WE, Schuchert MJ, et al. Electromagnetic navigation bronchoscopy-guided dye marking for thoracoscopic resection of pulmonary nodules. Ann Thorac Surg. 2016 Jul;102(1):223–9. Epub 2016 May 5.

Barry AE, Chaney MA, London MJ. Anesthetic management during cardiopulmonary bypass: a systematic review. Anesth Analg. 2015 Apr;120(4):749–69.

Carabello BA, Paulus WJ. Aortic stenosis. Lancet. 2009 Mar 14;373(9667):956–66. Epub 2009 Feb 21.

Desai ND, Cohen EA, Naylor CD, Fremes SE; Radial Artery Patency Study Investigators. A randomized comparison of radial-artery and saphenous-vein coronary bypass grafts. N Engl J Med. 2004 Nov 25;351(22):2302–9.

ElBardissi AW, Aranki SF, Sheng S, O'Brien SM, Greenberg CC, Gammie JS. Trends in isolated coronary artery bypass grafting: an analysis of the Society of Thoracic Surgeons adult cardiac surgery database. J Thorac Cardiovasc Surg. 2012 Feb;143(2):273–81.

Ginsberg RJ, Rubinstein LV; Lung Cancer Study Group. Randomized trial of lobectomy versus limited resection for T1 N0 non-small cell lung cancer. Ann Thorac Surg. 1995 Sep;60(3):615–22.

Hillis LD, Smith PK, Anderson JL, Bittl JA, Bridges CR, Byrne JG, et al; American College of Cardiology Foundation; American Heart Association Task Force on Practice Guidelines; American Association for Thoracic Surgery; Society of Cardiovascular Anesthesiologists; Society of Thoracic Surgeons. 2011 ACCF/AHA guideline for coronary artery bypass graft surgery: a report of the American College of Cardiology Foundation/American Heart Association Task Force on Practice Guidelines: developed in collaboration with the American Association for Thoracic Surgery, Society of Cardiovascular Anesthesiologists, and Society of Thoracic Surgeons. J Am Coll Cardiol. 2011 Dec 6;58(24):e123–210. Epub 2011 Nov 7.

Holmes DR Jr, Brennan JM, Rumsfeld JS, Dai D, O'Brien SM, Vemulapalli S, et al; STS/ACC TVT Registry. Clinical outcomes at 1 year following transcatheter aortic valve replacement. JAMA. 2015 Mar 10;313(10):1019–28.

Iribarne A, Easterwood R, Chan EY, Yang J, Soni L, Russo MJ, et al. The golden age of minimally invasive cardiothoracic surgery: current and future perspectives. Future Cardiol. 2011 May;7(3):333–46.

James TW, Faber LP. Indications for pneumonectomy: pneumonectomy for malignant disease. Chest Surg Clin N Am. 1999 May;9(2):291–309.

Kofidis T, Emmert MY, Paeschke HG, Emmert LS, Zhang R, Haverich A. Long-term follow-up after minimal invasive direct coronary artery bypass grafting procedure: a multi-factorial retrospective analysis at 1000 patient-years. Interact Cardiovasc Thorac Surg. 2009 Dec;9(6):990–4. Epub 2009 Sep 4.

Leon MB, Smith CR, Mack M, Miller DC, Moses JW, Svensson LG, et al; PARTNER Trial Investigators. Transcatheter aortic-valve implantation for aortic stenosis in patients who cannot undergo surgery. N Engl J Med. 2010 Oct 21;363(17):1597–607. Epub 2010 Sep 22.

Mark JB. Multimodal detection of perioperative myocardial ischemia. Tex Heart Inst J. 2005;32(4):461–6.

Mason AC, Krasna MJ, White CS. The role of radiologic imaging in diagnosing complications of video-assisted thoracoscopic surgery. Chest. 1998 Mar;113(3):820–5.

Mozaffarian D, Benjamin EJ, Go AS, Arnett DK, Blaha MJ, Cushman M, et al; American Heart Association Statistics Committee; Stroke Statistics Subcommittee. Heart Disease and Stroke Statistics—2016 Update: A Report From the American Heart Association. Circulation. 2016 Jan 26;133(4):e38–360. Epub 2015 Dec 16. Erratum in: Circulation. 2016 Apr 12;133(15):e599.

Murphy GJ, Angelini GD. Side effects of cardiopulmonary bypass: what is the reality? J Card Surg. 2004 Nov-Dec;19(6):481–8.

Paul S, Altorki NK, Sheng S, Lee PC, Harpole DH, Onaitis MW, et al. Thoracoscopic lobectomy is associated with lower morbidity than open lobectomy: a propensity-matched analysis from the STS database. J Thorac Cardiovasc Surg. 2010 Feb;139(2):366–78.

Perkins JG, Cap AP, Weiss BM, Reid TJ, Bolan CD. Massive transfusion and nonsurgical hemostatic agents. Crit Care Med. 2008 Jul;36(7 Suppl):S325–39. Erratum in: Crit Care Med. 2008 Sep;36(9):2718.

Predina JD, Kunkala M, Aliperti LA, Singhal AK, Singhal S. Sleeve lobectomy: current indications and future directions. Ann Thorac Cardiovasc Surg. 2010 Oct;16(5):310–8.

Ramnath N, Demmy TL, Antun A, Natarajan N, Nwogu CE, Loewen GM, et al. Pneumonectomy for bronchogenic carcinoma: analysis of factors predicting survival. Ann Thorac Surg. 2007 May;83(5):1831–6.

Rosamond W, Flegal K, Friday G, Furie K, Go A, Greenlund K, et al; American Heart Association Statistics Committee and Stroke Statistics Subcommittee. Heart disease and stroke statistics—2007 update: a report from the American Heart Association Statistics Committee and Stroke Statistics Subcommittee. Circulation. 2007 Feb 6;115(5):e69–171. Epub 2006 Dec 28. Errata in: Circulation. 2007 Feb 6;115(5):e172. Circulation. 2010 Jul 6; 122(1):e9.

Sarkar K, Sarkar M, Ussia GP. Current status of transcatheter aortic valve replacement. Med Clin North Am. 2015 Jul;99(4):805–33.

Sellke FW, Chu LM, Cohn WE. Current state of surgical myocardial revascularization. Circ J. 2010 Jun;74(6):1031–7. Epub 2010 May 8.

Sellke FW, DiMaio JM, Caplan LR, Ferguson TB, Gardner TJ, Hiratzka LF, et al; American Heart Association. Comparing on-pump and off-pump coronary artery bypass grafting: numerous studies but few conclusions: a scientific statement from the American Heart Association council on cardiovascular surgery and anesthesia in collaboration with the interdisciplinary working group on quality of care and outcomes research. Circulation. 2005 May 31;111(21): 2858–64.

Singh M, Sporn ZA, Schaff HV, Pellikka PA. ACC/AHA Versus ESC guidelines on prosthetic heart valve management: JACC guideline comparison. J Am Coll Cardiol. 2019 Apr 9;73(13):1707–18.

Sivarajan M, Amory DW, Everett GB, Buffington C. Blood pressure, not cardiac output, determines blood loss during induced hypotension. Anesth Analg. 1980 Mar;59(3):203–6.

Suma H, Tanabe H, Takahashi A, Horii T, Isomura T, Hirose H, et al. Twenty years experience with the gastroepiploic artery graft for CABG. Circulation. 2007 Sep 11;116(11 Suppl):I188–91.

Tapson VF. Acute pulmonary embolism. N Engl J Med. 2008 Mar 6;358(10):1037–52.

Yim AP. VATS major pulmonary resection revisited: controversies, techniques, and results. Ann Thorac Surg. 2002 Aug;74(2):615–23.

67 Mechanical Circulatory Assist Devices

AYAN SEN, MD; BHAVESH M. PATEL, MD

Goals

- Describe the common mechanical circulatory assist devices.
- Review clinical presentations of patients with left ventricular assist devices.
- Review complications, including neurologic complications, of left ventricular assist devices.

Introduction

Mechanical circulatory assist devices (MCADs) are used in patients with decompensated heart failure refractory to medical therapy. The devices are used as a bridge to transplant, as a bridge to recovery for reversible conditions, as a bridge to decision while a patient's eligibility for transplant is determined, and as destination therapy to support left-sided heart function when a patient is not eligible for transplant. MCADs restore tissue circulation by increasing blood flow and, thereby, improving organ function.

Types of Devices

MCADs can be paracorporeal or extracorporeal (ie, placed outside the body) or intracorporeal (ie, implanted inside the body above or below the diaphragm). Left ventricular assist devices (LVADs) support left ventricular (LV) function, right ventricular assist devices support right ventricular (RV) function, and biventricular assist devices support both the RV and the LV. A total artificial heart is pulsatile and consists of 2 ventricles and 4 valves that pump blood throughout the body and replace the function of the native heart.

The first LVADs were pulsatile or displacement (pusher-plate) pumps that simulated the native heart. However, owing to complications, continuous-flow LVADs have become prevalent. They produce 2 types of blood flow: centrifugal or axial. Device-related terminology and abnormalities are summarized in Table 67.1.

Postoperative Management of LVADs

Postoperative hemodynamic optimization of LVADs requires invasive monitoring through a pulmonary artery catheter (PAC) and noninvasive monitoring with echocardiography. Fluids and inotropes are typically used to maintain mean arterial pressure (MAP) at 60 to 80 mm Hg and central venous pressure (CVP) and pulmonary capillary wedge pressure at less than 15 mm Hg. Cardiac output measurements with the PAC may not correlate with the LVAD flows. A common target is a pump index corresponding to a cardiac index of more than 2 L/min/m^2. A high MAP (>90 mm Hg) increases the risk of hemorrhagic stroke because the patients will need anticoagulation by the second or third day.

Hypotension can be due to many causes, including hypovolemia, hemorrhage, pump failure, native heart dysfunction (either LV or RV), or postoperative vasoplegia (Figure 67.1). Vasoplegia requires norepinephrine or vasopressin (or both). Hypovolemia should be treated judiciously with small boluses and frequent hemodynamic assessment. Cardiac tamponade should be ruled out when hypotension occurs with low LVAD flows and high filling pressures. Urgent bedside echocardiography or transesophageal echocardiography may be necessary. Pneumothorax rarely occurs because the pleural space is rarely breached during surgery, but the possibility should be assessed with chest radiography or bedside ultrasonography for a comprehensive workup.

Arrhythmias are not uncommon after LVAD surgery and are treated with antiarrhythmics, such as amiodarone and digoxin. Lidocaine may be beneficial in ventricular tachyarrhythmias. Cardioversion may be needed if the loss of atrial

Table 67.1 • LVAD Abnormalities

Abnormality	Cause	Intervention
High power	Pump thrombus	Anticoagulation therapy, pump exchange
Low power	Device problem	Check batteries, power source
High pulsatility index	Recovery of LV function Lead damage	Wean from LVAD support Check LVAD and driveline
Low pulsatility index	Worsening native ventricular function Hypovolemia Excess pump speed	Increase pump speed, inotropic therapy Administer fluid therapy Lower pump speed
High flow rate	Vasodilation (SALAD [sepsis, anaphylaxis, liver dysfunction, adrenal insufficiency, drugs])	Identify and treat causes of sepsis; administer vasopressors for low mean arterial pressure
Low flow rate	Hypovolemia, bleeding, RV failure, tamponade, hypertensive emergency Arrhythmias	Administer intravenous fluids, blood Assess and treat Assess and treat
Suction events	All causes of low flow Excessive LV unloading	Administer fluid therapy Lower pump speed

Abbreviations: LV, left ventricular; LVAD, left ventricular assist device; RV, right ventricular.

Modified from Feldman D, Pamboukian SV, Teuteberg JJ, Birks E, Lietz K, Moore SA, et al; International Society for Heart and Lung Transplantation. The 2013 International Society for Heart and Lung Transplantation guidelines for mechanical circulatory support: executive summary. J Heart Lung Transplant. 2013 Feb;32(2):157–87; used with permission.

kick in patients with atrial fibrillation, atrial flutter, or ventricular rhythms leads to reduced LVAD flows and hypotension. Most patients require an automatic implantable cardioverter-defibrillator (AICD) for this reason, and AICD shocks or overdrive antitachycardia pacing can occur during episodes of ventricular arrhythmias. An uncontrollable ventricular arrhythmia can be an indication for temporary extracorporeal membrane oxygenation because it can lead to RV failure, which is not supported by the LVAD.

Aortic valve degeneration could be another cause of low cardiac output and hypotension. When used for extended periods, continuous-flow LVADs can lead to aortic valve degeneration and aortic regurgitation, which are usually diagnosed with echocardiography.

LVADs have several types of alarms (battery alarms, advisory alarms, and hazard alarms) that can indicate mechanical issues. When a device fails, emergency and critical care providers should consult the instruction booklet and contact the LVAD coordinator. When device failure occurs in patients with long-term LVADs, the LVAD coordinator and coordinating center should be contacted urgently.

Clinical Presentations

Device Thrombosis

LVAD pump thrombosis, which can impede blood flow, occurs in approximately 8% of patients with implanted, continuous-flow LVADs. Pathophysiologic causes include blood-device surface interactions, shear stress of blood flow from altered blood-flow dynamics (especially in continuous-flow LVADs), cannula malposition, acquired von Willebrand factor deficiency, and heparin-induced thrombocytopenia.

Typically, patients present in cardiogenic shock with a scratching, grating, rough sound on auscultation. As blood flow decreases, more power may be necessary to drive the impeller; this change can be diagnostic. Increased levels of plasma free hemoglobin (>40 mg/dL) or lactate dehydrogenase can be suggestive of a pump thrombus. Diagnosis can be confirmed with serial estimation of LV end-diastolic diameter with increasing LVAD speeds (in a ramp study). Treatment options include additional anticoagulation, thrombolytic therapy, or use of an LVAD pump exchange.

Gastrointestinal Tract Bleeding

Gastrointestinal tract (GI) bleeding is common in patients with an LVAD (reported incidence, 22%-40%). Altered blood flow patterns with a continuous-flow device (as in Heyde syndrome) lead to formation of arteriovenous malformations, which are prone to bleeding. Patients with acquired von Willebrand factor deficiency have an increased risk for GI bleeding. Gastric antral vascular ectasia is a rare cause.

Management consists of stopping and reversing anticoagulation and performing upper and lower GI endoscopy to identify and treat the source of bleeding. A capsule study or push enteroscopy may be needed if the source of the bleeding cannot be identified on endoscopy. Octreotide has been used as a somatostatin analogue to decrease splanchnic arterial blood flow to treat GI bleeding. If other therapy fails,

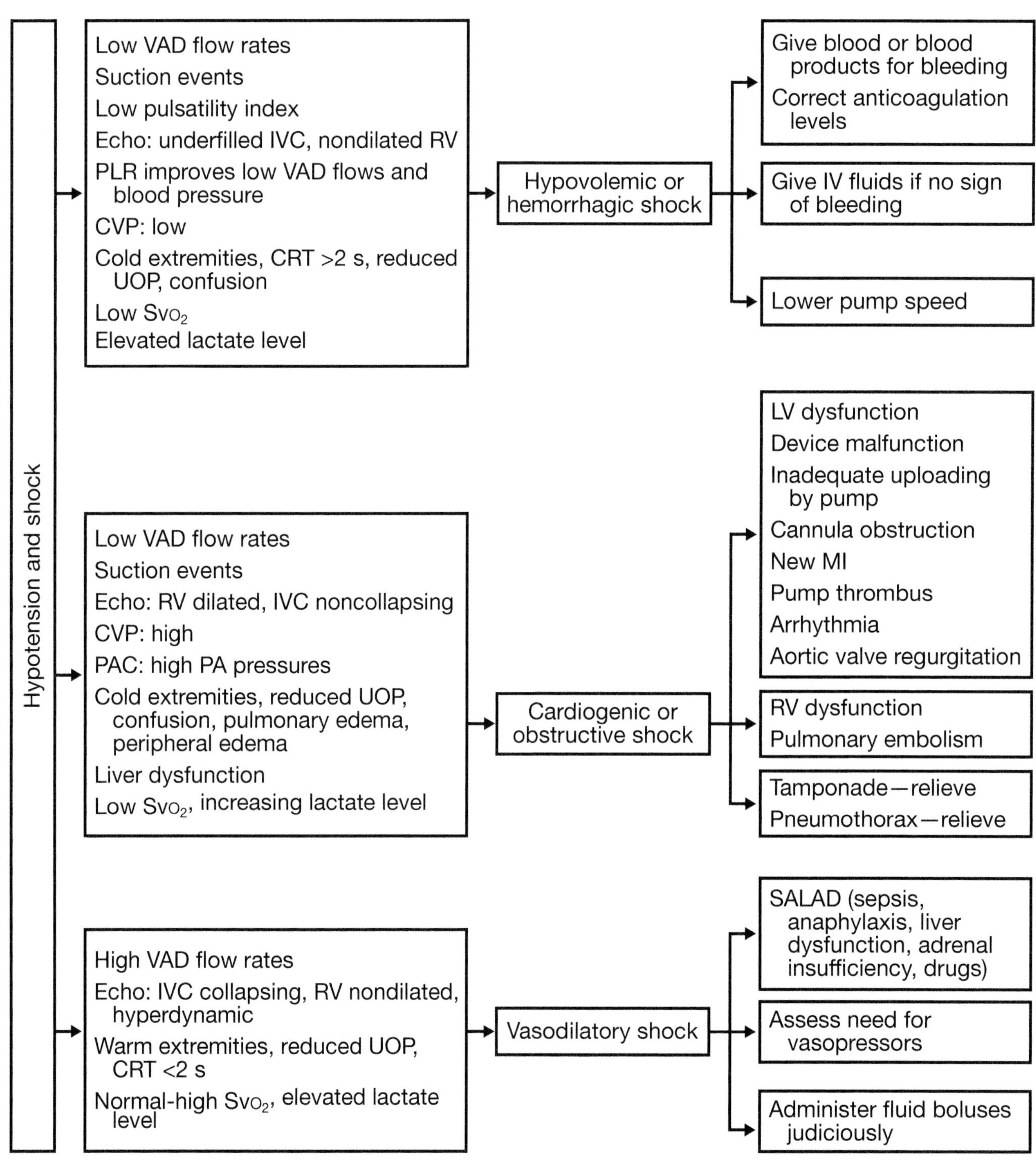

Figure 67.1. Causes and Treatment of Hypotension and Shock in Patients With a Left Ventricular Assist Device. CRT indicates capillary refill time; CVP, central venous pressure; Echo, echocardiography; IV, intravenous; IVC, inferior vena cava; LV, left ventricular; MI, myocardial infarction; PA, pulmonary artery; PAC, pulmonary artery catheter; PLR, passive leg raising; RV, right ventricular; Svo_2, mixed venous oxygen saturation; UOP, urinary output; VAD, ventricular assist device.

(Modified from Sen A, Larson JS, Kashani KB, Libricz SL, Patel BM, Guru PK, et al. Mechanical circulatory assist devices: a primer for critical care and emergency physicians. Crit Care. 2016 Jun 25;20[1]:153. Open access article distributed under the Creative Commons Attribution License [https://creativecommons.org/licenses/by/4.0/legalcode].)

angiography and embolization may be needed. Resumption of anticoagulation is vital for avoiding pump thrombosis, but the timing of initiation depends on the patient's clinical status.

Acute Kidney Injury

The incidence of acute kidney injury (AKI) after LVAD implantation has been reported to range from 7% to 56%. Usually cardiorenal syndrome improves after LVAD placement. AKI that develops postoperatively is usually due to hemodynamic issues, prolonged cardiopulmonary bypass time, or hemolysis. Patients with AKI that is refractory to hemodynamic optimization need renal replacement therapy.

Infection

Among patients with LVADs, the reported long-term infection rates are 30% to 50%. Patients with sepsis present with hypotension and vasoplegic syndrome. Fluid administration should be judicious and determined according to the patient's clinical hemodynamic status, echocardiographic findings, and results of invasive monitoring (eg, CVP and PAC). Management of sepsis should include use of blood cultures, antibiotics, and lactate clearance.

Infections specific to LVADs involve the pump pocket, cannula, or driveline and may require ultrasonography or computed tomography (CT) for diagnosis. LVAD-related infections include endocarditis, pericarditis, pneumonia, mediastinitis, central line infections, and urinary tract infections.

Infections typically involve *Staphylococcus, Enterococcus, Pseudomonas, Enterobacter*, or *Candida*. Driveline infections should be treated with oral or intravenous antibiotics according to the severity of the infection. Management of pump pocket infections includes drainage and débridement of the device pocket and empirical use of broad-spectrum antibiotics. In some patients, long-term suppressive antibiotic therapy may be indicated. In refractory infections and bacteremia, device removal and urgent transplant may be needed if the LVAD was used as a bridge to recovery.

Neurologic Complications

When patients with an LVAD present with acute encephalopathy, they should have a comprehensive workup that includes ruling out metabolic, infectious, and drug-related systemic causes. Neurologic issues, such as, acute stroke and seizure, should be investigated. A hemolysis panel (including lactate dehydrogenase, haptoglobin, and plasma free hemoglobin) is necessary to rule out embolic causes of stroke.

These patients have a high risk for ischemic and hemorrhagic stroke. Predisposing factors include a need for anticoagulation, acquired von Willebrand factor deficiency, infections, and device thrombosis causing an embolic event. Right-sided strokes are more common because of the anatomical alignment of the outflow cannula of the LVAD directing emboli to the right brachiocephalic trunk (58% of ischemic strokes occur in the right hemisphere, 28% in the left, and 6.5% in both hemispheres; 6.5% are vertebrobasilar in origin). CT and CT angiography should be performed for all patients who present with signs concerning for acute stroke. Although systemic thrombolytic therapy is indicated, it should be used only with the consensus of all key stakeholders. Endovascular strategies have been used for proximal large-vessel occlusions. If a patient has hemorrhagic stroke, anticoagulation should be stopped. The use of prothrombotic agents for reversal should be based on the clinical symptoms, size and location of the hemorrhage, and the risk of a pump thrombus. If a patient has been taking warfarin, therapy should include prothrombin complex concentrate, fresh frozen plasma, or vitamin K. If a patient has been receiving antiplatelet agents, desmopressin and a platelet transfusion can be used. Therapy for postthrombolytic bleeding includes cryoprecipitate and antifibrinolytic agents, such as ε-aminocaproic acid or tranexamic acid.

Summary

- LVADs are used in patients with decompensated heart failure refractory to medical therapy and can serve as a bridge to transplant.
- Patients with LVADs have a high risk for right-sided ischemic and hemorrhagic stroke.
- Among patients with LVADs, long-term infection rates are 30% to 50%.

SUGGESTED READING

Allen SJ, Sidebotham D. Postoperative care and complications after ventricular assist device implantation. Best Pract Res Clin Anaesthesiol. 2012 Jun;26(2):231–46.

Cowger JA, Grafton G. Candidate selection for durable mechanical circulatory support. Cardiol Clin. 2018 Nov;36(4):487–94.

Crowther MA, Cook DJ, Albert M, Williamson D, Meade M, Granton J, et al; Canadian Critical Care Trials Group. The 4Ts scoring system for heparin-induced thrombocytopenia in medical-surgical intensive care unit patients. J Crit Care. 2010 Jun;25(2):287–93. Epub 2010 Feb 10.

DeVore AD, Patel PA, Patel CB. Medical management of patients with a left ventricular assist device for the non-left ventricular assist device specialist. JACC Heart Fail. 2017 Sep;5(9):621–31. Epub 2017 Aug 16.

EMS guide January 2014: mechanical circulatory support organization [Internet]. Thoratec Corporation. ©2014 [cited 2018 Nov 26]. Available from: https://www.mass.gov/files/documents/2017/10/31/Field%20Guides%20Master%20Document.pdf.

Gopinathannair R, Cornwell WK, Dukes JW, Ellis CR, Hickey KT, Joglar JA, et al; American Heart Association Electrocardiography and Arrhythmias Committee; Heart Failure and Transplantation Committee of the Council on Clinical Cardiology; and Council on

Cardiovascular and Stroke Nursing. Device Therapy and arrhythmia management in left ventricular assist device recipients: a scientific statement from the American Heart Association. Circulation. 2019 Apr 4:CIR0000000000000673. [Epub ahead of print]

Gordon RJ, Weinberg AD, Pagani FD, Slaughter MS, Pappas PS, Naka Y, et al; Ventricular Assist Device Infection Study Group. Prospective, multicenter study of ventricular assist device infections. Circulation. 2013 Feb 12;127(6):691–702. Epub 2013 Jan 11.

Gurbel PA, Shah P, Desai S, Tantry US. Antithrombotic strategies and device thrombosis. Cardiol Clin. 2018 Nov;36(4):541–50. Epub 2018 Sep 15.

Kadakkal A, Najjar SS. Neurologic events in continuous-flow left ventricular assist devices. Cardiol Clin. 2018 Nov;36(4):531–9.

Kanwar MK, Bailey S, Murali S. Challenges and future directions in left ventricular assist device therapy. Crit Care Clin. 2018 Jul;34(3):479–92.

Kato TS, Ota T, Schulze PC, Farr M, Jorde U, Takayama H, et al. Asymmetric pattern of cerebrovascular lesions in patients after left ventricular assist device implantation. Stroke. 2012 Mar;43(3):872–4. Epub 2011 Dec 29.

Kirklin JK, Naftel DC, Kormos RL, Pagani FD, Myers SL, Stevenson LW, et al. Interagency Registry for Mechanically Assisted Circulatory Support (INTERMACS) analysis of pump thrombosis in the HeartMate II left ventricular assist device. J Heart Lung Transplant. 2014 Jan;33(1):12–22. Epub 2013 Nov 27. Erratum in: J Heart Lung Transplant. 2015 Oct;34(10):1356.

Mohite PN, Popov AF, Zych B, Dhar D, Capoccia M, Simon AR. Organ donation following brain stem death after ventricular assist device implantation. Asian Cardiovasc Thorac Ann. 2014 Mar;22(3):345–6. Epub 2013 Aug 14.

Nakahara S, Chien C, Gelow J, Dalouk K, Henrikson CA, Mudd J, et al. Ventricular arrhythmias after left ventricular assist device. Circ Arrhythm Electrophysiol. 2013 Jun;6(3):648–54.

Nienaber J, Wilhelm MP, Sohail MR. Current concepts in the diagnosis and management of left ventricular assist device infections. Expert Rev Anti Infect Ther. 2013 Feb;11(2):201–10.

Oswald H, Schultz-Wildelau C, Gardiwal A, Lusebrink U, Konig T, Meyer A, et al. Implantable defibrillator therapy for ventricular tachyarrhythmia in left ventricular assist device patients. Eur J Heart Fail. 2010 Jun;12(6):593–9. Epub 2010 Apr 20.

Patel AM, Adeseun GA, Ahmed I, Mitter N, Rame JE, Rudnick MR. Renal failure in patients with left ventricular assist devices. Clin J Am Soc Nephrol. 2013 Mar;8(3):484–96. Epub 2012 Oct 11.

Sen A, Larson JS, Kashani KB, Libricz SL, Patel BM, Guru PK, et al. Mechanical circulatory assist devices: a primer for critical care and emergency physicians. Crit Care. 2016 Jun 25;20(1):153.

Slaughter MS, Pagani FD, Rogers JG, Miller LW, Sun B, Russell SD, et al; HeartMate II Clinical Investigators. Clinical management of continuous-flow left ventricular assist devices in advanced heart failure. J Heart Lung Transplant. 2010 Apr;29(4 Suppl):S1–39. Epub 2010 Feb 24.

Timms D. A review of clinical ventricular assist devices. Med Eng Phys. 2011 Nov;33(9):1041–7. Epub 2011 Jun 12.

Extracorporeal Membrane Oxygenation

J. KYLE BOHMAN, MD; GREGORY J. SCHEARS, MD

Goals

- Understand the basic physiology of extracorporeal membrane oxygenation.
- Compare the risks of venovenous and venoarterial extracorporeal membrane oxygenation.
- Discuss the basic management principles in extracorporeal membrane oxygenation.

Introduction

Extracorporeal membrane oxygenation (ECMO) is a general term describing an extracorporeal circuit with a pump and a gas exchange membrane that can be used for cardiac support or respiratory support (or both) depending on its configuration. The 2 basic configurations of ECMO are venoarterial (VA) and venovenous (VV). VA ECMO removes blood from the venous circulation and pumps it through the oxygenator and back into the patient's arterial circulation (Figure 68.1). VV ECMO removes blood from the venous circulation and pumps it through the oxygenator and back into the patient's venous circulation. Thus, VV ECMO does not afford any direct cardiac support but functions only to oxygenate and decarboxylate the blood. In contrast, VA ECMO can support or temporarily replace the patient's cardiac and respiratory functions. Common indications for VA ECMO include postcardiotomy (if it is difficult to separate the patient from cardiopulmonary bypass during cardiac surgery), malignant ventricular arrhythmias, cardiogenic shock, and extracorporeal cardiopulmonary resuscitation (which is the use of ECMO during cardiopulmonary resuscitation for cardiac arrest).

Neurophysiologic Implications

Depending on the ECMO configuration and blood flow settings and on the patient's cardiac function, systemic blood flow during ECMO can be pulsatile or nonpulsatile. Nonpulsatile flow has been shown to interfere with normal cerebral autoregulation. A disruption of autoregulation coupled with systemic anticoagulation is thought to increase the risk of hemorrhagic strokes. After long-term exposure to nonpulsatile flow, such as with left ventricular assist devices, cerebral autoregulation may normalize over time.

Abnormal cerebral autoregulation can also be caused by the events preceding the use of ECMO. Even with pulsatile systemic blood flow, cerebral autoregulation may still be disrupted. For example, cardiac arrest, severe hypoxia, and severe hypercarbia have been shown to transiently disrupt cerebral autoregulation. This defect in autoregulation may persist after restoration of normal blood flow and normalization of arterial blood gases (ABGs). Patients receiving VV ECMO (with normal cardiac function and normal pulsatility) have also been found to have abnormal cerebral autoregulation.

Anticoagulation Management

The reaction between the ECMO circuit surface and the patient's blood can trigger clot formation within the ECMO circuit, and areas of blood stagnation in the patient's body or the ECMO circuit may precipitate clot formation. These clots within the patient or the circuit can break free and cause embolization in the patient. Because of this risk of clot formation, anticoagulation is nearly ubiquitous during ECMO. Generally, anticoagulation is more intense during

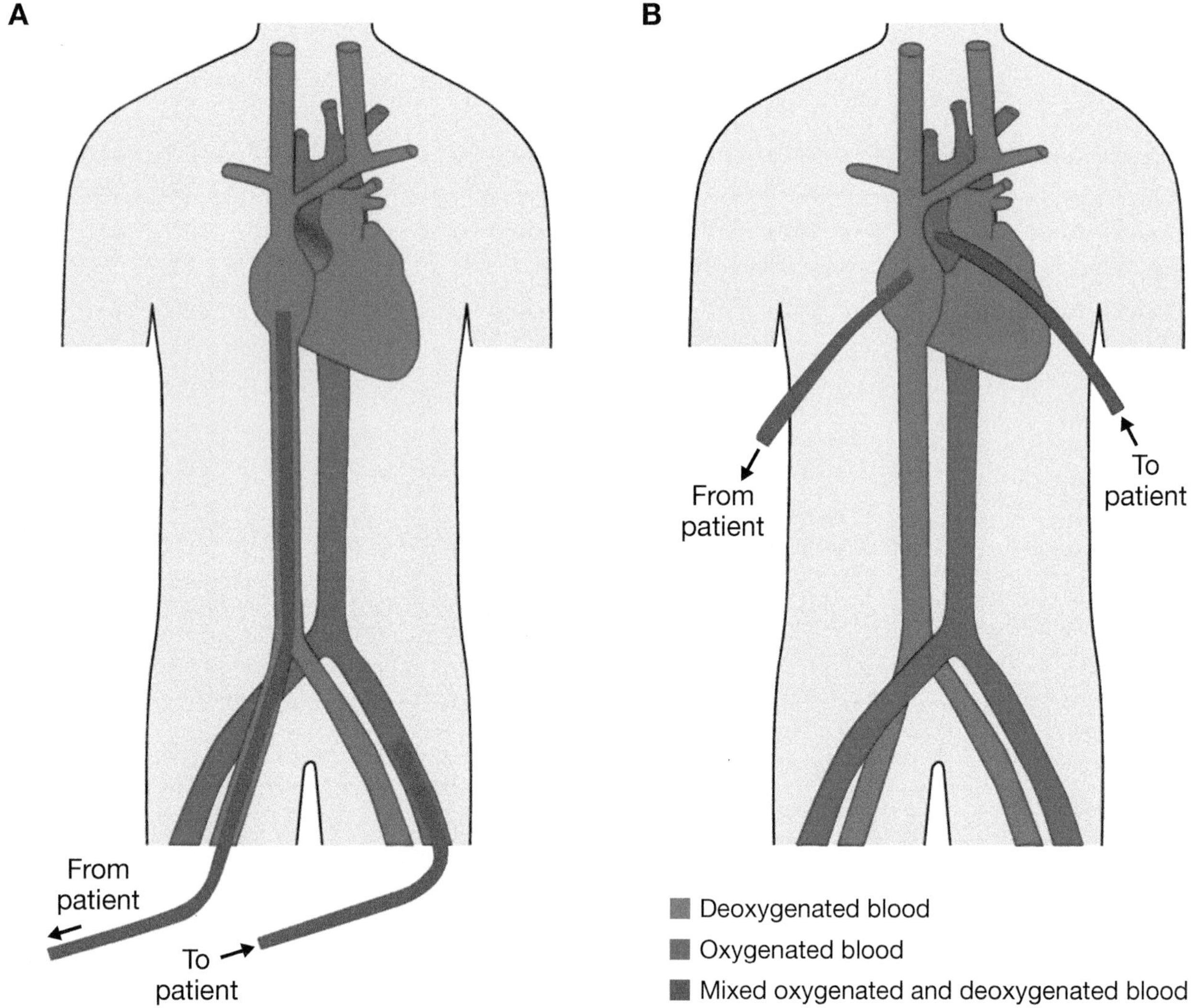

Figure 68.1. *Venoarterial (VA) Extracorporeal Membrane Oxygenation (ECMO). A, During peripheral VA ECMO, blood is drained from near the inferior vena cava–right atrium junction through a femoral venous cannula and then ejected into the common iliac artery through a femoral arterial cannula. B, During central VA ECMO, blood is drained directly from the right atrium and ejected directly into the proximal aorta.*

(From Chung M, Shiloh AL, Carlese A. Monitoring of the adult patient on venoarterial extracorporeal membrane oxygenation. ScientificWorldJournal. 2014;2014:393258; open access article distributed under the Creative Commons Attribution License [https://creativecommons.org/licenses/by/3.0/legalcode].)

VA ECMO because any emboli ejected from the ECMO circuit enter the patient's arterial circulation. In contrast, unless there is a right-to-left shunt (eg, a patent foramen ovale), emboli ejected from the ECMO circuit during VV ECMO are collected in the patient's pulmonary vascular bed and are generally of much less clinical consequence than systemic arterial emboli.

Fully understanding the clinical coagulation status of a patient receiving ECMO is often challenging even with all the available coagulation tests, including activated partial thromboplastin time (aPTT), prothrombin time, platelet counts, thromboelastography, factor Xa level, and activated clotting time. Complications may vary considerably among patients who have identical laboratory values: Some patients may have more bleeding complications, some may have more clots in their ECMO circuits, and some may have both bleeding and clotting complications. At many institutions, a target for aPTT is 40 to 60 seconds during VV ECMO and 60 to 80 seconds during VA ECMO; either heparin or bivalirudin is administered to achieve these aPTT values.

Neurologic Complications

Neurologic injuries are common in patients treated with ECMO; the reported incidence ranges from 10% to 50%. A retrospective clinicopathologic study reported that the incidence of neurologic injuries was 50% among patients treated with ECMO. These neurologic injuries are often attributed to the events prompting initiation of ECMO (eg, cardiac arrest) or to the ECMO circuit and its associated systemic anticoagulation.

Central Nervous System Complications

Ischemic Stroke

Central embolic strokes likely account for the majority of ischemic strokes during ECMO. During VA ECMO (or VV ECMO in a patient with a patent foramen ovale), small clots may develop on the arterial side of the ECMO circuit and cause embolization in the patient's arterial vasculature. Systemic anticoagulation minimizes but usually does not eliminate clot formation within the ECMO circuit. If a large clot is identified in the arterial side of the ECMO circuit, ECMO teams often temporarily stop ECMO blood flows to remove the clot from the circuit. Despite these precautions, ischemic strokes occur in 3.6% to 4.1% of all adults treated with ECMO. The incidence of stroke is similar but possibly slightly higher (5.4%) in patients who receive VA ECMO after cardiotomy (after cardiopulmonary bypass for cardiac surgery).

Intracranial Hemorrhage

Intracranial hemorrhage during ECMO is often attributed to systemic anticoagulation in patients with impaired cerebral autoregulation. Alternatively, some intracranial hemorrhages result from hemorrhagic conversion of acute ischemic strokes. The reported incidence of intracranial hemorrhage during ECMO is 3.6% to 4.7%.

Diffuse Anoxic Brain Injury

Diffuse anoxic brain injury is most often related to cardiac or respiratory arrest that occurred before initiation of ECMO. However, another important cause of diffuse anoxic brain injury is proximal aortic hypoxemia (often referred to as *harlequin syndrome* or *mixing cloud*). Harlequin syndrome is specific to VA ECMO (particularly peripheral VA ECMO) and is caused by poorly oxygenated blood being ejected from the left ventricle and perfusing the proximal aortic branches. During VA ECMO, if pulmonary function is impaired, any blood that flows through the native heart and lungs will be hypoxemic when it is ejected from the left ventricle (Figure 68.2). The extent of proximal aortic hypoxemia depends on the severity of lung dysfunction and on the amount of blood flowing through the native

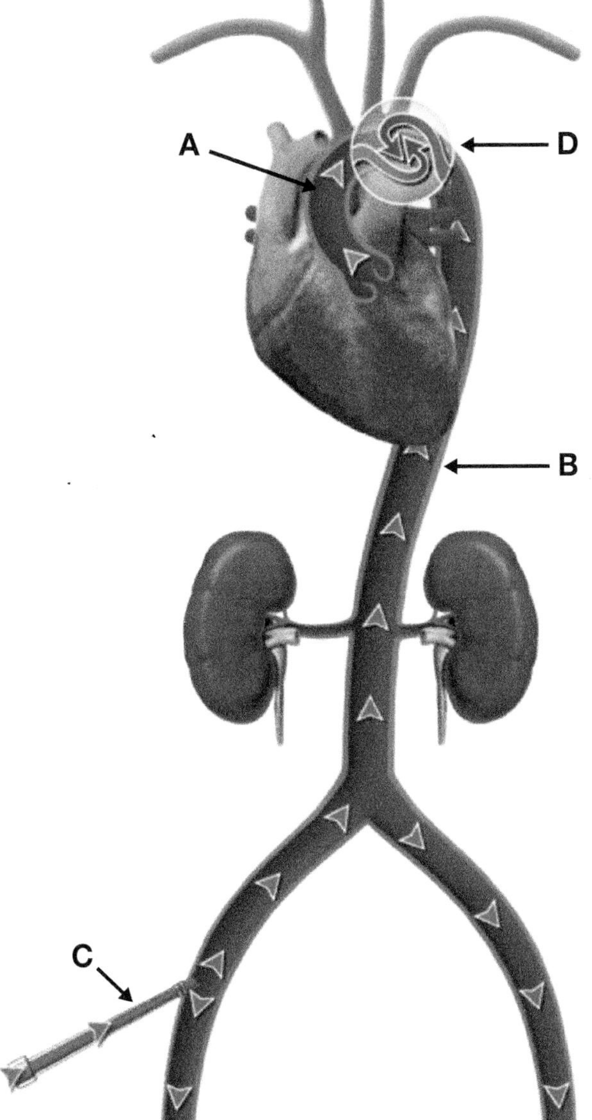

Figure 68.2. *Proximal Aortic Hypoxemia in Venoarterial (VA) Extracorporeal Membrane Oxygenation (ECMO). Blood ejecting from the heart (A) competes with the retrograde flow of blood (B) pumped from the femoral artery peripheral VA ECMO cannula (C) and creates a mixing cloud in the aorta (D). The location of the mixing cloud in the aorta depends on the relative blood flow from the heart and from the ECMO cannula. The degree of oxygenation of the blood ejecting from the heart is primarily dependent on the patient's native lung function.*

(From Alwardt CM, Patel BM, Lowell A, Dobberpuhl J, Riley JB, DeValeria PA. Regional perfusion during venoarterial extracorporeal membrane oxygenation: a case report and educational modules on the concept of dual circulations. J Extra Corpor Technol. 2013 Sep;45(3):187–94; used with permission.)

heart and not through the ECMO circuit. VA ECMO with central cannulation (ie, with the outflow cannula in the proximal aorta) greatly decreases but does not eliminate the risk of harlequin syndrome. During VA ECMO, oxygen saturation and ABGs should be measured in the right upper extremity (the most proximal aortic arch branch) to detect and prevent harlequin syndrome.

Cognitive Impairment

Long-term cognitive deficits are fairly common in ECMO survivors. When 28 adult patients were examined an average of 5 years after ECMO, 41% had impaired neuropsychological performance. These neuropsychological deficits were associated with neuroradiologic lesions (cerebral infarcts, microemboli, and intracranial hemorrhage), which were evident in 52% of the 28 patients. The neuroradiologic findings were far more common in patients who received VA ECMO than in patients who received VV ECMO (75% vs 17%), but not all microhemorrhages have prognostic importance.

Peripheral Nervous System Complications

Limb Ischemia and Compartment Syndrome

Limb ischemia during ECMO is usually caused by retrograde peripheral cannulation of the femoral artery for VA ECMO with occlusion of antegrade flow through the superficial femoral artery. To prevent limb ischemia, a common practice is to routinely place an antegrade reperfusion catheter in the superficial femoral artery distal to the femoral ECMO cannulation site. Another cause of distal limb ischemia is embolism of a clot from the ECMO circuit. Lower extremity ischemia has been reported to develop in 16.9% to 19.9% of VA ECMO patients.

Compartment syndrome typically results from swelling due to lower extremity hypoperfusion and ischemia. The reported incidence of compartment syndrome during VA ECMO is 9.2% to 10.3%. While compartment syndrome is developing, an awake patient experiences pain and paresthesias in the affected limb. In sedated patients, the first signs of compartment syndrome are pallor and a loss of pulses or arterial Doppler flows in the affected limb.

Critical Illness Polyneuropathy and Myopathy

Critical illness polyneuropathy (CIP) and critical illness myopathy (CIM) are other causes of peripheral neurologic deficits during ECMO. CIP and CIM are not specific to ECMO, but they are not infrequent during the course of ECMO because patients receiving ECMO may have severe illness and require prolonged sedation. Additionally, acute motor axonal neuropathy has been associated with H1N1 influenza virus, and historically some patients with this strain of influenza have required ECMO for severe acute respiratory distress syndrome.

Neurologic Testing

Magnetic Resonance Imaging

All ECMO circuits are not compatible with magnetic resonance imaging (MRI). The ECMO operating console contains many metallic components, and even many modern ECMO cannulae contain wire reinforcement, thus making them incompatible with MRI.

Computed Tomography

Patients can undergo computed tomography during ECMO treatment, but the risks and benefits must be weighed: The procedure involves transporting a critically ill patient and risking disruption of flow or accidental decannulation while transporting the patient and moving the patient into the scanner. An adequate number of knowledgeable persons must be present to safely care for the patient and manage all the lines.

Sedation

During ECMO, sedation and analgesia may be needed to decrease oxygen consumption, to decrease the risk of dislodging the cannula with excessive movement, and to decrease the risk of reduced venous return (ie, "suckdown") during a patient's Valsalva maneuver (from straining or agitation). Furthermore, ECMO appears to have a considerable effect on drug pharmacokinetics. Lipophilic drugs are sequestered in the ECMO cannula and oxygenator membrane, which can alter the sedative and analgesic effects and the rate of clearance during ECMO. Drug pharmacokinetics are also affected by the increased volume of distribution resulting from the blood volume within the ECMO circuit. The magnitude of many of the effects of ECMO on drug pharmacokinetics is still being elucidated.

Brain Death Examination

A full brain death apnea test can be performed while a patient is receiving ECMO. Because the ECMO circuit removes carbon dioxide, modified apnea tests have been proposed for patients receiving VA ECMO. The prerequisites for the standard apnea test apply (normothermia, no residual sedation, normoxia, and normocarbia).

In 1 proposed modified apnea test, a sample is drawn for baseline ABG analysis, the patient receives continuous positive airway pressure through the endotracheal tube with either the ventilator (with no pressure support ventilation) or an anesthesia bag, and the ECMO sweep flow is decreased to the lowest setting to maintain oxygen saturations greater than 90%. After the patient is observed for respiratory efforts for 8 minutes, another sample is drawn for ABG analysis.

A much more controlled method is to blend carbon dioxide into the ECMO system. Titration of carbon dioxide is controlled and predictable, and an 8% volume ratio enables the maintenance of the same ECMO sweep gas flow.

The primary modification of the modified apnea examinations is the reduction of ECMO sweep gas flow to a minimal level (to prevent normalization of carbon dioxide by the ECMO circuit) without ceasing ECMO sweep gas flow (otherwise hypercarbic and hypoxic blood would be delivered directly into the arterial circulation). In a patient with severe lung dysfunction, hypercarbia may still develop during an apnea test even if the patient has an adequate respiratory effort (and intact medullary function).

Ancillary Testing for Brain Injury

Plasma biomarkers of brain injury have been investigated in patients receiving ECMO but not as extensively as in patients not treated with ECMO. After the use of ECMO for refractory cardiac arrest, neuron-specific enolase (NSE) serum levels are correlated with poor neurologic outcomes. In adults, an NSE serum level greater than 100 mcg/L within 24 hours after initiation of ECMO is predictive of poor neurologic outcomes and death. Similarly, a peak NSE serum level greater than 80 mcg/L within 4 days after initiation of ECMO has a high specificity (100%) but only modest sensitivity (63%) for a poor neurologic outcome. An important caveat relevant to ECMO is that hemolysis can falsely elevate NSE levels.

Summary

- ECMO cannulation configuration greatly affects the frequency and type of neurologic injuries.
- ECMO can disrupt normal cerebral autoregulation.
- Blood stagnation and contact with the foreign materials in the ECMO circuit cause clot formation.
- Neurologic complications develop in 10% to 50% of patients treated with ECMO.
- The events preceding the use of ECMO heavily influence the risk of neurologic injuries.
- ECMO circuits are not MRI compatible.
- The ECMO circuit can considerably affect drug pharmacokinetics.
- Traditional brain death apnea testing requires modification while a patient is receiving ECMO.

SUGGESTED READING

Alwardt CM, Patel BM, Lowell A, Dobberpuhl J, Riley JB, DeValeria PA. Regional perfusion during venoarterial extracorporeal membrane oxygenation: a case report and educational modules on the concept of dual circulations. J Extra Corpor Technol. 2013 Sep;45(3):187–94.

Cheng R, Hachamovitch R, Kittleson M, Patel J, Arabia F, Moriguchi J, et al. Complications of extracorporeal membrane oxygenation for treatment of cardiogenic shock and cardiac arrest: a meta-analysis of 1,866 adult patients. Ann Thorac Surg. 2014 Feb;97(2):610–6. Epub 2013 Nov 8.

Chung M, Shiloh AL, Carlese A. Monitoring of the adult patient on venoarterial extracorporeal membrane oxygenation. ScientificWorldJournal. 2014;2014:393258. Epub 2014 Apr 3.

Cornwell WK 3rd, Tarumi T, Aengevaeren VL, Ayers C, Divanji P, Fu Q, et al. Effect of pulsatile and nonpulsatile flow on cerebral perfusion in patients with left ventricular assist devices. J Heart Lung Transplant. 2014 Dec;33(12):1295–303. Epub 2014 Aug 28.

Eleuteri K, Koerner MM, Horstmanshof D, El Banayosy A. Temporary Circulatory support and extracorporeal membrane oxygenation. Cardiol Clin. 2018 Nov;36(4):473–85.

Floerchinger B, Philipp A, Foltan M, Keyser A, Camboni D, Lubnow M, et al. Neuron-specific enolase serum levels predict severe neuronal injury after extracorporeal life support in resuscitation. Eur J Cardiothorac Surg. 2014 Mar;45(3):496–501. Epub 2013 Jul 21.

Hoeper MM, Tudorache I, Kuhn C, Marsch G, Hartung D, Wiesner O, et al. Extracorporeal membrane oxygenation watershed. Circulation. 2014 Sep 2;130(10):864–5.

Hoskote SS, Fugate JE, Wijdicks EF. Performance of an apnea test for brain death determination in a patient receiving venoarterial extracorporeal membrane oxygenation. J Cardiothorac Vasc Anesth. 2014 Aug;28(4):1027–9.

Hund E. Neurological complications of sepsis: critical illness polyneuropathy and myopathy. J Neurol. 2001 Nov;248(11):929–34.

Kutlesa M, Santini M, Krajinovic V, Raffanelli D, Barsic B. Acute motor axonal neuropathy associated with pandemic H1N1 influenza A infection. Neurocrit Care. 2010 Aug;13(1):98–100.

Mateen FJ, Muralidharan R, Shinohara RT, Parisi JE, Schears GJ, et al. Neurological injury in adults treated with extracorporeal membrane oxygenation. Arch Neurol. 2011 Dec;68(12):1543–9. Epub 2011 Aug 8.

Muralidharan R, Mateen FJ, Shinohara RT, Schears GJ, Wijdicks EF. The challenges with brain death determination in adult patients on extracorporeal membrane oxygenation. Neurocrit Care. 2011 Jun;14(3):423–6.

Nasr DM, Rabinstein AA. Neurologic complications of extracorporeal membrane oxygenation. J Clin Neurol. 2015 Oct;11(4):383–9. Epub 2015 Aug 21.

Ono M, Joshi B, Brady K, Easley RB, Kibler K, Conte J, et al. Cerebral blood flow autoregulation is preserved after continuous-flow left ventricular assist device implantation. J Cardiothorac Vasc Anesth. 2012 Dec;26(6):1022–8.

Ramont L, Thoannes H, Volondat A, Chastang F, Millet MC, Maquart FX. Effects of hemolysis and storage condition on neuron-specific enolase (NSE) in cerebrospinal fluid and serum: implications in clinical practice. Clin Chem Lab Med. 2005;43(11):1215–7.

Rastan AJ, Dege A, Mohr M, Doll N, Falk V, Walther T, et al. Early and late outcomes of 517 consecutive adult patients treated with extracorporeal membrane oxygenation for refractory postcardiotomy cardiogenic shock. J Thorac Cardiovasc Surg. 2010 Feb;139(2):302–11.

Reisinger J, Hollinger K, Lang W, Steiner C, Winter T, Zeindlhofer E, et al. Prediction of neurological outcome after cardiopulmonary resuscitation by serial determination of serum neuron-specific enolase. Eur Heart J. 2007 Jan;28(1):52–8. Epub 2006 Oct 23.

Risnes I, Wagner K, Nome T, Sundet K, Jensen J, Hynas IA, et al. Cerebral outcome in adult patients treated with extracorporeal membrane oxygenation. Ann Thorac Surg. 2006 Apr;81(4):1401–6.

Shekar K, Fraser JF, Smith MT, Roberts JA. Pharmacokinetic changes in patients receiving extracorporeal membrane oxygenation. J Crit Care. 2012 Dec;27(6):741.e9–18. Epub 2012 Apr 18.

Shekar K, Roberts JA, Mullany DV, Corley A, Fisquet S, Bull TN, et al. Increased sedation requirements in patients receiving extracorporeal membrane oxygenation for respiratory and cardiorespiratory failure. Anaesth Intensive Care. 2012 Jul;40(4):648–55.

Short BL. The effect of extracorporeal life support on the brain: a focus on ECMO. Semin Perinatol. 2005 Feb;29(1):45–50.

Sidebotham D, McGeorge A, McGuinness S, Edwards M, Willcox T, Beca J. Extracorporeal membrane oxygenation for treating severe cardiac and respiratory failure in adults: part 2-technical considerations. J Cardiothorac Vasc Anesth. 2010 Feb;24(1):164–72. Epub 2009 Oct 28.

Tweed A, Cote J, Lou H, Gregory G, Wade J. Impairment of cerebral blood flow autoregulation in the newborn lamb by hypoxia. Pediatr Res. 1986 Jun;20(6):516–9.

Walker LK, Short BL, Gleason CA, Jones MD Jr, Traystman RJ. Cerebrovascular response to carbon dioxide in lambs receiving extracorporeal membrane oxygenation. Crit Care Med. 1994 Feb;22(2):291–8.

Walker LK, Short BL, Traystman RJ. Impairment of cerebral autoregulation during venovenous extracorporeal membrane oxygenation in the newborn lamb. Crit Care Med. 1996 Dec;24(12):2001–6.

Wijdicks EFM. Critical synopsis and key questions in brain death determination. Intensive Care Med. 2019 Mar;45(3):306–9. Epub 2019 Feb 6.

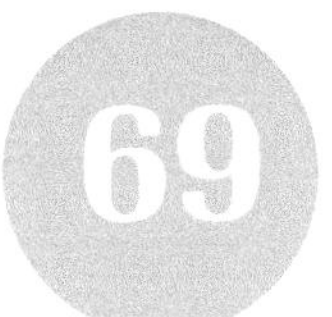

Cardiac Pacing in the Intensive Care Unit

J. WILLIAM SCHLEIFER, MD; FAROUK MOOKADAM, MB, BCh; HARISH RAMAKRISHNA, MD

Goals

- Describe the most relevant radiographic features for identification of an unknown cardiac implantable electronic device.
- Identify conditions requiring implantation and extraction of a cardiac implantable electronic device.
- Know how to recognize pacing malfunction.

Introduction

Patients with pacemakers and implantable cardioverter-defibrillators (ICDs) are commonly encountered in the intensive care unit (ICU). Knowledge of device function and indications for device implantation and extraction are required for safe perioperative and critical care management.

Identification of an Unknown Device

The term *cardiac implantable electronic device* (CIED) includes all types of pacemakers and ICDs. All are radiopaque, and important information for identifying the nature of the device can be obtained from the chest radiograph (Figure 69.1). *Permanent pacemakers* have small-profile pulse generators connected to transvenous leads that terminate in 1 or more of the following locations: right atrium, right ventricle, and coronary sinus (Figure 69.1A). *ICDs* have a larger pulse generator connected to a lead with at least 1 defibrillation coil, potentially in addition to other pacing leads (Figure 69.1B). *Subcutaneous ICDs* have a pulse generator connected to a lead with defibrillation coils that lie entirely in the subcutaneous tissue with no intracardiac pacing function (Figure 69.1C and 1D). *Leadless pacemakers* are fixed to the endocardium and pace only the ventricle (Figure 69.1E and 1F). Device programming information can be obtained from device interrogation with manufacturer-specific programmers.

The type of lead is also identifiable from the chest radiograph (Figure 69.2). *Passive fixation* leads maintain their position with tines that rest on the endocardium, or, as with temporary leads, they may not have any stabilizing structures (Figure 69.2A). *Active fixation* leads have a screw that is advanced into the myocardium to maintain position (Figure 69.2B). Active fixation leads can also be used for temporary pacing if maximum lead stability is required. The fixation screw must be fully retracted before a temporary active fixation lead is removed to prevent damage to the myocardium.

Device Malfunction

Pacemakers pace at the lower programmed rate unless they are triggered to pace faster or are inhibited by sensed electrical activity. Therefore, device troubleshooting involves answering the following questions:

- Is the device behaving according to its programmed settings?
- Are the programmed settings appropriate to the clinical situation?
- Is the device sensing appropriately?
- Is the device capturing when it attempts to pace?

Device troubleshooting requires device interrogation. However, sensing and capturing abnormalities can frequently be inferred from the electrocardiogram (ECG). A rate that is slower than the programmed lower rate limit, with no pacing spikes, probably indicates an *oversensing problem* (ie, the device is inappropriately inhibited by sensed electrical signals). Pacing spikes inappropriately interposed within a normal rhythm that is faster than the lower rate limit probably indicate an *undersensing problem.* Pacing spikes that do not produce a P wave or a QRS complex and do not occur during a myocardial refractory period indicate a *failure to capture.*

Responses to Magnets

A magnet placed on a pacemaker will cause it to pace at a manufacturer-specific rate that is not inhibited by sensed events. A magnet placed on a defibrillator will inhibit tachycardia treatment (ie, antitachycardia pacing and shocks) but not the pacing rate. If a patient is receiving inappropriate shocks, the immediate treatment is to place a magnet over the device.

Pacing Programmed Settings

Device programming is indicated with a code (eg, VVIR 60-120 beats per minute). The first letter indicates the chamber paced (*A*, atrium; *V*, ventricle; or *D*, dual). The second

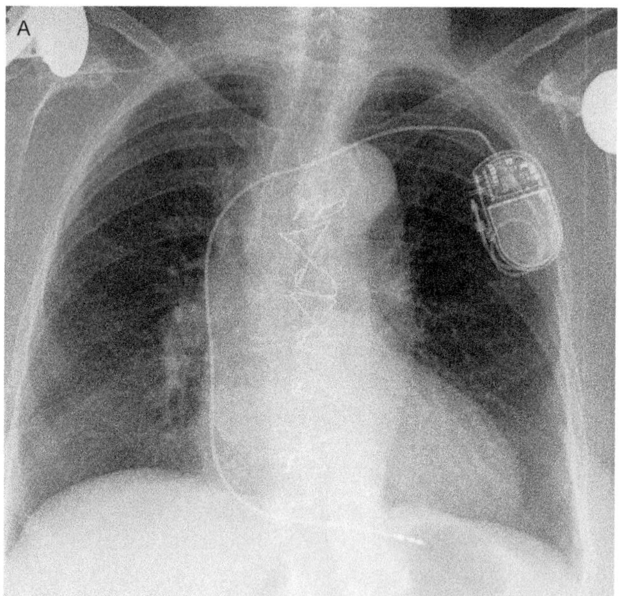

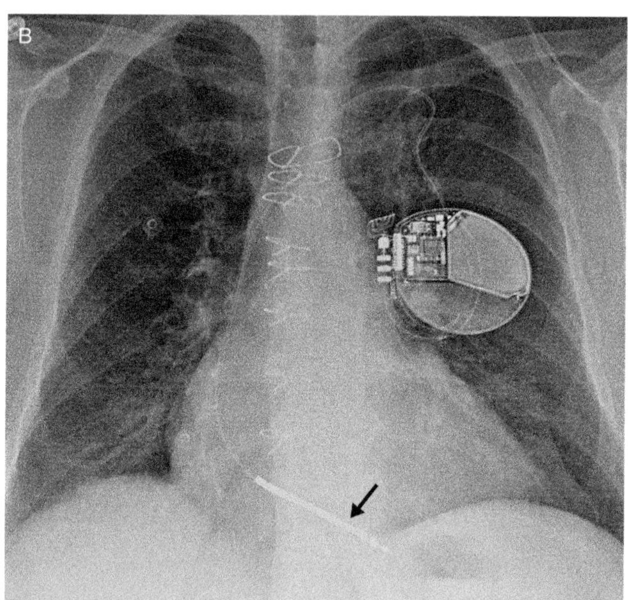

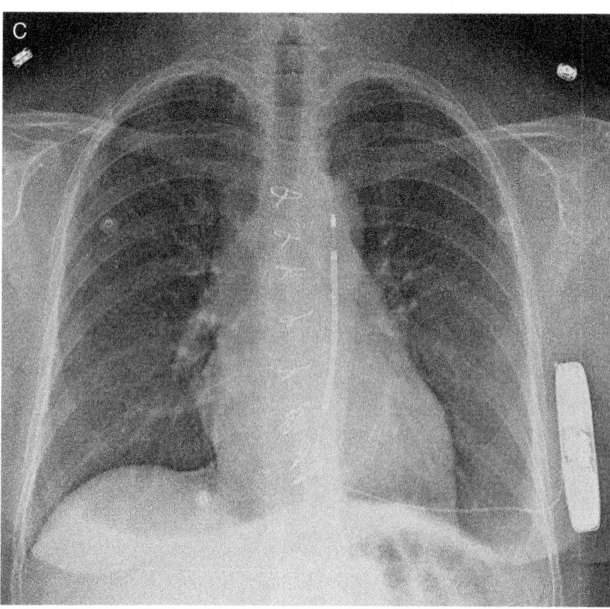

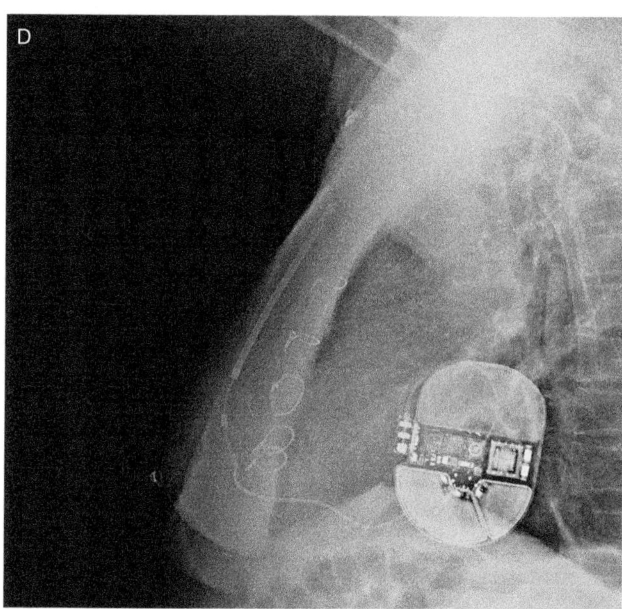

Figure 69.1. Radiographs of Various Cardiac Implantable Electronic Devices for Pacing and Defibrillation. A, Single-chamber pacemaker. B, Single-chamber implantable cardioverter-defibrillator (ICD) with defibrillation coil (arrow). C and D, Subcutaneous ICD. E and F, Leadless pacemaker (arrows).

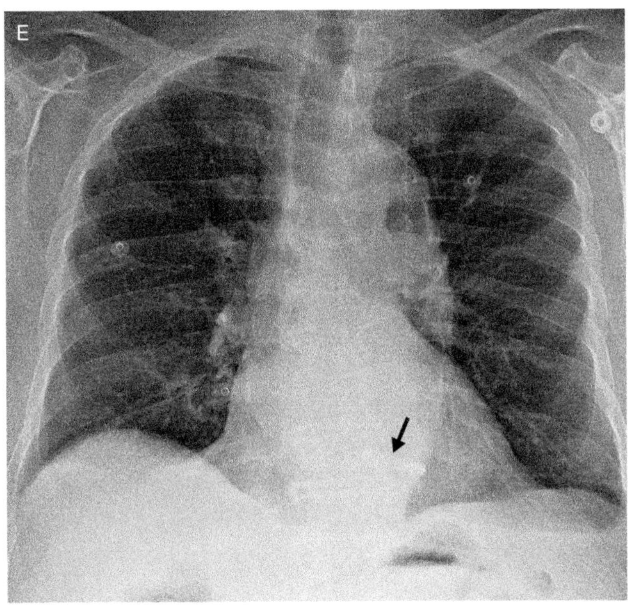

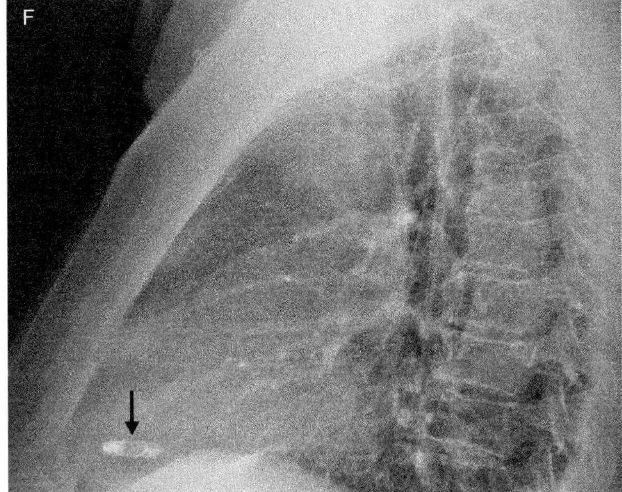

Figure 69.1 Continued

letter indicates the chamber sensed (*A*, atrium; *V*, ventricle; or *D*, dual). The third letter indicates how the device responds to a sensed event. In single-chamber devices, *I* indicates that the device is inhibited (ie, it will not pace) if it senses electrical activity. In dual-chamber devices, D indicates that in response to electrical activity sensed by the atrial lead, atrial pacing is inhibited and ventricular pacing is triggered at a predetermined atrioventricular (AV) delay. In the example above, the fourth letter, *R*, indicates that the rate response is on; if the rate response is off, the code has only 3 letters. The 2 mechanisms of rate response are accelerometer and minute ventilation. With the *accelerometer rate response*, physical movement of the device increases the heart rate. This can occur in the ICU in a supine patient if the device is mechanically moved (eg, during chest physiotherapy). With the *minute ventilation rate response*, if the device senses changes in thoracic

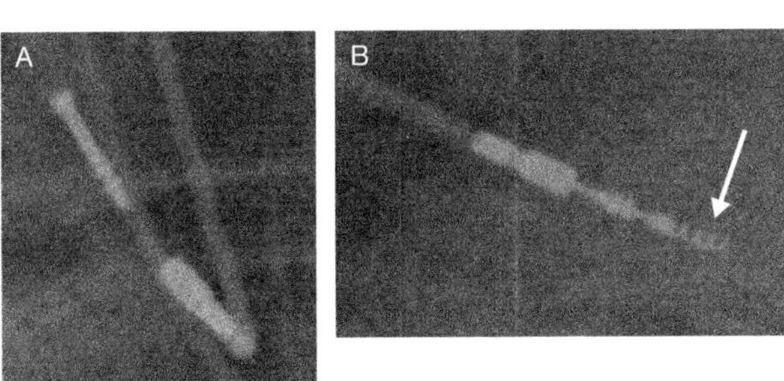

Figure 69.2. Radiographs of Types of Leads. A, Passive fixation leads do not have a deployable screw. B, Active fixation leads have a deployable screw (arrow).

impedance that correlate with changes in minute ventilation, the device increases the heart rate. As a result, unexpected increases in pacing rates may occur in patients with pulmonary disease.

A range of rates is given in which the pacemaker will pace, with rate increases based on a tracked atrial rate or a rate response sensor. The device will pace slower than the programmed rate or fail to pace because of oversensing, special settings, or battery life. *Oversensing* occurs when other electrical activity inhibits pacing. This electrical activity may be from T waves, electrical activity in other cardiac chambers, or extracardiac electrical activity (eg, electrocautery, transcutaneous electrical nerve stimulation, magnetic resonance imaging, or welding). *Special settings* include sleep modes and hysteresis modes in which the device temporarily slows down to detect native electrical activity. A third reason is that the battery may be at the end of its life.

The device will pace at or near the upper rate limit when it is tracking sinus tachycardia or atrial tachycardia; during pacemaker-mediated tachycardia (ventricular pacing travels retrograde up the AV node, stimulates the atrium, and is sensed by the atrial lead, which paces the ventricle, etc); or when it is sensing the rate response (eg, movement of accelerometer or increased minute ventilation).

Defibrillator Programmed Settings

All transvenous ICDs have pacing settings as described above in addition to defibrillation settings. ICDs are usually programmed to provide pace termination (ie, antitachycardia pacing) and then shocks to terminate tachycardia depending on the rate. At slower rates of tachycardia, supraventricular tachycardia discriminators can be enabled, and additional bursts of antitachycardia pacing can be used. At very fast rates, a single burst of antitachycardia pacing may be used before shocks begin; supraventricular tachycardia discriminators are not applied in the fastest tachycardia zone.

Shocks are intended to treat life-threatening ventricular arrhythmias. Shocks administered in any other situation are considered *inappropriate*. Inappropriate shocks can result from *oversensing*, in which other electrical activity, whether intracardiac or extracardiac, is interpreted as QRS complexes making the rate faster. This electrical activity may be external noise (eg, from electrocautery) or internal noise (eg, from lead fracture). Inappropriate shocks can also result from *supraventricular tachycardias*, including sinus tachycardias that are incorrectly considered ventricular tachycardia or are in the fastest rate of the treatment zone.

Shocks may be inappropriately withheld for ventricular tachycardia and ventricular fibrillation. The most likely causes of shocks being withheld inappropriately are ventricular tachycardia that is slower than the programmed detection zone; incorrect application of supraventricular tachycardia discriminators indicating that the rhythm is supraventricular rather than ventricular tachycardia; undersensing of fine ventricular fibrillation, so that the device senses a rate that is slower than it actually is; and a battery at the end of its life.

Circumstances Requiring Pacing

The many indications for pacing can be categorized into 4 groups:

1. Symptomatic bradycardia, including sinus bradycardia, chronotropic incompetence (ie, the heart rate does not increase appropriately with physiologic demand), sinus pauses and arrest, any AV block that causes symptoms, and hypotension and physiologically inappropriate bradycardia.
2. High-grade conduction system disease (symptomatic or asymptomatic), including Mobitz type II block, 2:1 AV block, third-degree AV block, alternating bundle branch block, any AV block in a patient with myotonic dystrophy or muscular dystrophy, a regular and slow escape rhythm in atrial fibrillation, and a sinus pause >3 seconds or a ventricular pause >5 seconds in atrial fibrillation.
3. Pacing to prevent pause-dependent ventricular arrhythmias, particularly those associated with a prolonged QT interval (as in torsades de pointes).
4. Overdrive pacing to terminate reentry arrhythmias, including atrial flutter and ventricular tachycardia.

Each of these situations can occur in ICU patients, and the nature of the situation dictates whether the pacemaker should be permanent or temporary. Transcutaneous pacing can be used in emergency situations, but it contracts the intercostal muscles and causes considerable discomfort, so patients should be heavily sedated. Because the esophagus is near the left atrium, a pacing lead can be advanced down the esophagus if only atrial pacing is needed. Temporary transvenous pacing can be performed with either a passive or an active fixation lead through any access site; however, if fluoroscopy is not immediately available, the easiest access sites for temporary pacing are the right internal jugular and the left subclavian veins. When lead stability is required, an active fixation lead (with a screw) should be placed under fluoroscopy. In emergency situations, a passive fixation lead, in particular, a balloon-tipped lead, is useful, but patients should be maintained on strict bed rest for as long as pacing is required.

Temporary pacing is useful for situations that are reversible, including complete AV block due to Lyme disease; drug overdose (eg, digoxin, β-blockers, or calcium channel blockers); and AV block immediately after cardiac surgery. Permanent pacing should be considered for any situation that is irreversible or that has resolved but may recur without warning (eg, a prolonged sinus pause with no identifiable cause).

Frequently, temporary pacers are used for cardiac procedures and certain conditions that place patients at high risk for AV block or sinus node dysfunction. For these temporary pacers, epicardial wires may be placed while the patient is in the operating room, or endocardial wires may be placed percutaneously. Appropriate situations include cardiac surgery (eg, coronary artery bypass grafting, maze procedure, valve replacement or repair, myectomy, and heart transplant); acute myocardial infarction, particularly of the right coronary artery; complex interventions (eg, rotation atherectomy or alcohol septal ablation); and transcatheter aortic valve implantation.

Temporary damage to the conduction system should resolve; after several days, either the temporary pacemaker should be removed or a permanent pacemaker should be implanted. The exception is the self-expanding transcatheter aortic valves that may cause further delayed damage to the conduction system; pacemakers may be required despite partial conduction recovery, but formal guidelines for this situation have not been established.

Several complications may occur during pacemaker or ICD implantation, including pneumothorax, cardiac perforation and tamponade, bleeding and pocket hematoma, and infection, particularly device pocket infection and wound dehiscence.

Circumstances Requiring Device Extraction

Persistent bacteremia in patients with CIEDs may be related to device infection, and in many patients, the only way to clear this infection is to extract the device. Risk factors for serious complications with device extraction include duration of lead implantation (longer durations increase the risk); bulky leads (especially defibrillation leads with coils in the superior vena cava); and vascular disease, renal dysfunction, and vascular calcification. Because of the risks associated with lead extraction, the procedure should be coordinated with a multidisciplinary team, including cardiac surgery, electrophysiology, echocardiography, cardiac anesthesiology, and critical care clinicians.

In a patient with infection, the entire device must be extracted for a cure. The infection may be in the CIED pocket, the lead may have a vegetation, or the patient may have persistent bacteremia with an organism likely to cause device infection, such as gram-positive cocci. If the patient is device dependent, implantation of a temporary pacemaker is required, with extended hospitalization for treatment with intravenous antibiotics. Device reimplantation can occur when the infection has cleared.

Sometimes complete extraction of the lead is not required. These indications include lead malfunction (insulation or wire fracture), lead dislodgement, venous occlusion, and tricuspid valve impingement causing severe tricuspid regurgitation.

Several complications may occur during device extraction, including cardiac avulsion, perforation, and tamponade; laceration of the great veins, causing catastrophic bleeding; and damage to the tricuspid valve.

End-of-Life Management of Pacemakers and Defibrillators

Discontinuing any medical intervention, including pacing and defibrillator therapies, at the request of the patient is generally considered ethical. Defibrillator shocks are associated with considerable discomfort and distress, so it is reasonable to turn off defibrillator therapies when patients with terminal illness make the request. Turning off pacing in a pacemaker-dependent patient is likely to cause immediate hemodynamic effects from profound bradycardia or asystole; additionally, the burdens of pacing are minimal. In end-of-life situations, if a pacemaker-dependent patient requests that the device be turned off, the request should prompt discussion of several topics: the difference between defibrillator and pacing functions, the effect of turning off pacing functions, and how pacing does not cause additional discomfort or prolong the dying process.

Summary

- The chest radiograph provides important information for identifying the nature of the CIED.
- Device troubleshooting requires device interrogation. However, sensing and capturing abnormalities can be frequently inferred from the ECG.
- Temporary pacing is useful for situations that are reversible, including complete AV block due to Lyme disease; drug overdose (eg, digoxin, β-blockers, or calcium channel blockers); and AV block immediately after cardiac surgery.

SUGGESTED READING

Cingolani E, Goldhaber JI, Marban E. Next-generation pacemakers: from small devices to biological pacemakers. Nat Rev Cardiol. 2018 Mar;15(3):139–50. Epub 2017 Nov 16.

Drew BJ, Ackerman MJ, Funk M, Gibler WB, Kligfield P, Menon V, et al; American Heart Association Acute Cardiac Care Committee of the Council on Clinical Cardiology, the Council on Cardiovascular Nursing, and the American College of Cardiology Foundation. Prevention of torsade de pointes in hospital settings: a scientific statement from the American Heart Association and the American College of Cardiology Foundation. Circulation. 2010 Mar 2;121(8):1047–60. Epub 2010 Feb 8. Erratum in: Circulation. 2010 Aug 24;122(8):e440.

Epstein AE, DiMarco JP, Ellenbogen KA, Estes NA 3rd, Freedman RA, Gettes LS, et al; American College of Cardiology Foundation; American Heart Association Task Force on Practice Guidelines; Heart Rhythm Society. 2012 ACCF/AHA/HRS focused update incorporated into the ACCF/AHA/HRS 2008 guidelines for device-based therapy of cardiac rhythm abnormalities: a report of the American College of Cardiology Foundation/American Heart Association Task Force on Practice Guidelines and the Heart Rhythm Society. Circulation. 2013 Jan 22;127(3):e283–352. Epub 2012 Dec 19.

Lampert R, Hayes DL, Annas GJ, Farley MA, Goldstein NE, Hamilton RM, et al; American College of Cardiology; American Geriatrics Society; American Academy of Hospice and Palliative Medicine; American Heart Association; European Heart Rhythm Association; Hospice and Palliative Nurses Association. HRS Expert Consensus Statement on the Management of Cardiovascular Implantable Electronic Devices (CIEDs) in patients nearing end of life or requesting withdrawal of therapy. Heart Rhythm. 2010 Jul;7(7):1008–26. Epub 2010 May 14.

Wilkoff BL, Love CJ, Byrd CL, Bongiorni MG, Carrillo RG, Crossley GH 3rd, et al; Heart Rhythm Society; American Heart Association. Transvenous lead extraction: Heart Rhythm Society expert consensus on facilities, training, indications, and patient management: this document was endorsed by the American Heart Association (AHA). Heart Rhythm. 2009 Jul;6(7):1085–104. Epub 2009 May 22.

Transplant Critical Care

Clinical Management of Heart Transplant Recipients

ARZOO SADIQI, BS; JAMA JAHANYAR, MD, PhD

Goals

- Appreciate the key aspects in the evolution of heart transplant.
- Understand the basic principles involved in the clinical management of heart transplant recipients.

Introduction

The challenges of managing heart transplant recipients postoperatively relate to right ventricular failure, immunosuppression, and the unique physiology of the donor heart. Clinical management of heart transplant recipients requires a multidisciplinary team approach with a coordinated effort between intensivists, cardiac surgeons, heart transplant cardiologists, and infectious disease specialists.

Historical Perspective

The foundation for the surgical treatment of heart failure was laid by Norman Shumway, MD, PhD, and Richard R. Lower, MD, when they introduced the biatrial anastomotic technique for orthotopic heart transplant in the 1960s at Stanford Hospital (Stanford, California). This technique was later modified to the bicaval technique, with a lower incidence of sinus node dysfunction and tricuspid regurgitation.

Although the first successful orthotopic heart transplant was performed in 1967, another decade passed before transplant was truly considered to be a treatment option. Early attempts were compromised by rejection and failure due to inadequate immunosuppression. After the introduction of cyclosporine, a calcineurin inhibitor, in the 1970s and with the development of more potent immunosuppressants, the prognosis improved. Today the goal with cardiac transplant is to provide high quality of life and long-term survival for patients with end-stage heart disease.

The International Society for Heart & Lung Transplantation reports over 118,000 adult and pediatric heart transplants worldwide, with a median survival of 10.5 years for adult patients and 15.6 years for pediatric patients. These patients are now increasingly common at most major academic medical centers in the world.

General Approach to Management

The goals for clinical management of heart transplant recipients should be 1) maintenance of graft function; 2) recovery or maintenance of organ subsystem function; 3) establishment of immunologic tolerance toward the allograft; 4) prevention and treatment of early infectious complications; 5) prevention of right-sided heart failure; and 6) promotion of a psychological and educational milieu for long-term rehabilitation and compliance.

The function of the donor heart is unique because it reflects factors derived from both the donor and the recipient. The donor heart can sustain injuries from donor trauma (myocardial contusion) or brain death that occurs from inadequate cardioprotection during procurement, implantation, or reperfusion. Some degree of donor heart dysfunction occurs in 30% to 50% of transplanted hearts, but less than 2% of patients die of early graft failure. Most forms of early graft dysfunction are reversible with normal donor heart function if the heart is properly supported during the recovery period.

Long-standing left-sided heart failure in the recipient leads to secondary pulmonary hypertension, which adversely affects the donor heart posttransplant. Patients with severe pulmonary hypertension (transpulmonary gradient >15 mm Hg) should therefore receive a left ventricular assist device (LVAD) as a bridge to transplant to alleviate the pulmonary hypertension over time, to restore and improve end-organ perfusion and function, and to prevent right-sided heart failure or end-organ failure posttransplant. In the past, patients with severe pulmonary hypertension would have been treated with a heterotopic heart transplant instead.

The cardiectomy of the native heart on cardiopulmonary bypass leaves a surgical situs that requires the anastomosis of 4 or 5 structures. In the bicaval technique, the 5 structures are the left atrium, inferior vena cava, main pulmonary artery, aorta, and superior vena cava. In the biatrial technique, the 4 structures are the left atrium, right atrium, main pulmonary artery, and aorta. The result, however, is denervation of the heart, which is a unique feature of the transplanted heart that affects the intrinsic heart rate of around 100 beats per minute and how the heart responds to medications postoperatively.

Medical Therapy

Generally when the heart transplant recipient leaves the operating room, inotropes and pulmonary vasodilators (epoprostenol or nitric oxide) have been administered with the aim of preventing posttransplant right-sided heart failure. Doses of these drugs should be carefully tapered over time with particular attention paid toward right-sided heart filling pressures, mixed venous oxygen saturation, and carbon monoxide. Hence, use of a pulmonary artery catheter in the early postoperative period helps guide treatment.

Commonly used inotropic agents and vasopressors include dopamine, dobutamine, milrinone, norepinephrine, epinephrine, and vasopressin. Agents such as atropine and digoxin are rendered ineffective because of the cardiac denervation, and hence they are not used after cardiac transplant. For chronotropic activity, isoproterenol is the drug of choice in heart transplant recipients. However, it is rarely used now because temporary atrial and ventricular pacing wires are usually available to help achieve the desired heart rate in patients with an escape rhythm due to temporary sinus node dysfunction or atrioventricular block. Most instances of escape rhythm resolve over time, however, and the percentage of patients receiving a permanent pacemaker after heart transplant (which was 20%-30% in the past) is now exceedingly low because of refinements in surgical technique, improved cardioprotection, and overall shorter durations of ischemia.

Patients who have had previous surgical procedures, in particular for an LVAD, and preoperative warfarin treatment have an increased risk of a bleeding diathesis and are treated with vitamin K preoperatively. After completion of cardiopulmonary bypass and heparin reversal, the surgeon will evaluate the extent of the patient's bleeding and determine whether additional blood products, factor VII, or anti-inhibitor coagulant complex is needed. If the patient is bleeding in the intensive care unit, aggressive rewarming and additional administration of blood products may be required. The transplant surgeon should be involved in this decision. Rarely, patients must be returned to the operating room to stop ongoing bleeding.

Immunosuppressants, such as cyclosporine and tacrolimus, are nephrotoxic, and the dosage must be adjusted according to serum creatinine and serum urea nitrogen levels. Many centers use induction treatment with antithymocyte globulin (for calcineurin-inhibitor–sparing therapy), which can aid in decreasing the overall dosage of nephrotoxic immunosuppressants in the early postoperative period. Perioperative high doses of intravenous corticosteroids are also commonly given after heart transplant according to protocol. Another commonly used drug is mycophenolate mofetil, which has widely replaced azathioprine. Heart transplant recipients typically continue to receive a triple immunosuppressive regimen of tacrolimus, mycophenolate mofetil, and corticosteroids in the early posttransplant period. At our center, prophylactic antibiotics are administered until the chest tubes are removed.

Ventricular Dysfunction

If left ventricular dysfunction occurs in the allograft postoperatively, the patient must receive temporary mechanical support with an intra-aortic balloon pump or possibly venoarterial extracorporeal membrane oxygenation (VA-ECMO) as a bridge to myocardial recovery. Postoperative vasoplegia is often encountered; it is temporary and often related to either preoperative angiotensin-converting enzyme inhibitor therapy for heart failure or temporary systemic inflammatory response from cardiopulmonary bypass. The drugs of choice are vasopressin, norepinephrine, and phenylephrine. We prefer to use vasopressin in this situation because it preferably increases systemic vascular resistance and spares pulmonary vascular resistance.

As mentioned above, right ventricular dysfunction is commonly encountered after heart transplant because vascular resistance is increased. Patients known to have high pulmonary resistance must be recognized and this must be considered during donor heart selection. The donor heart is allocated according to compatibility factors, such as ABO blood type, preformed allogenic antibodies, and patient's height and weight; in patients with increased pulmonary pressures, the heart must not be undersized, and the sex is an important factor also. The rescue strategy for a patient with profound right ventricular dysfunction and cardiogenic shock is mainly support with VA-ECMO until ventricular function recovers.

Summary

- The goals for clinical management of heart transplant recipients should be 1) maintenance of graft function; 2) recovery or maintenance of organ subsystem function; 3) establishment of immunologic tolerance toward the allograft; 4) prevention and treatment of early infectious complications; 5) prevention of right-sided heart failure; and 6) promotion of a psychological and educational milieu for long-term rehabilitation and compliance.
- Right ventricular dysfunction and postoperative vasoplegia are often encountered after heart transplant.

SUGGESTED READING

Bhatia SJ, Kirshenbaum JM, Shemin RJ, Cohn LH, Collins JJ, Di Sesa VJ, et al. Time course of resolution of pulmonary hypertension and right ventricular remodeling after orthotopic cardiac transplantation. Circulation. 1987 Oct;76(4):819–26.

Costanzo MR, Dipchand A, Starling R, Anderson A, Chan M, Desai S, et al; International Society of Heart and Lung Transplantation Guidelines. The International Society of Heart and Lung Transplantation Guidelines for the care of heart transplant recipients. J Heart Lung Transplant. 2010 Aug;29(8):914–56.

Kirklin JK, Naftel DC, Kirklin JW, Blackstone EH, White-Williams C, Bourge RC. Pulmonary vascular resistance and the risk of heart transplantation. J Heart Transplant. 1988 Sep-Oct;7(5):331–6.

Kirklin JK, Young JB, McGiffin DC. Heart transplantation. New York (NY): Churchill Livingstone; c2002. 883 p.

Critical Care of Heart-Lung and Lung Transplant Recipients

RAMACHANDRA R. SISTA, MD

Goals

- Understand the complex, multidisciplinary approach to the posttransplant care of heart-lung and lung recipients.
- Understand the unique posttransplant management principles and guidelines for the care of heart-lung and lung recipients.
- Know how to identify and manage the unique complications that can occur in heart-lung and lung recipients in the early posttransplant phase.

Introduction

Lung transplant is a complex procedure that has been a successful therapy for various end-stage lung diseases since the 1980s. Combined heart-lung transplant, however, is performed much less frequently than in the past (only 69 were reported to the International Society for Heart & Lung Transplantation [ISHLT] registry in 2014, and 27 of those were in North America). In contrast, about 3,917 lung transplants were performed in adults worldwide in 2014, and 2,327 were performed in adults in the United States in 2016. Survival rates after lung transplant have been stable over the past several years (90% survival at 3 months, 80% at 1 year, 60% at 3 years, and 45% at 5 years). The types of transplant procedures available and the general indications for lung transplant are listed in Boxes 71.1 and 71.2.

The posttransplant clinical course and management strategies for lung recipients have a considerable degree of overlap in the immediate, short-term, and long-term periods. In heart-lung recipients, postoperative bleeding and the need for a follow-up operation are not uncommon.

Guidelines for Clinical Management

Sedation, Analgesia, and Delirium

Optimal use of opiate analgesics in combination with sedatives should be provided as infusions titrated according to the patient's comfort level (eg, fentanyl, propofol, and dexmedetomidine). Rarely, epidural analgesia is required. Delirium is fairly common, but for successful outcomes, it must be identified and treated to decrease the number of days that a ventilator is required and to decrease the number of days in the intensive care unit (ICU). After extubation, when the patient can resume oral intake, analgesia is provided orally with intermittent intravenous (IV) analgesia for breakthrough pain.

Ventilator Management

Standard modes of ventilation and weaning techniques are satisfactory after single-lung transplant (SLT) or bilateral lung transplant (BLT) except in rare circumstances. After SLT for chronic obstructive pulmonary disease or emphysema (obstructive airway disease), positive end-expiratory pressure (PEEP) is kept low to prevent hyperinflation of the more compliant, native lung. Dynamic hyperinflation of the native lung can cause severe mediastinal shift with compression of the lung allograft, leading to severe hypoxemia from ventilation-perfusion mismatch and to hypotension from intrinsic PEEP.

Box 71.1 • Types of Lung Transplant Procedures

Single-lung transplant (SLT)
Bilateral lung transplant (BLT)
Bilateral sequential single-lung transplant (BSSLT)
Transplant of lobes from living related donors
Heart-lung transplant

At many centers, bronchoscopy is routinely performed before extubation to reexamine anastomotic sites. If they do not have complications, SLT recipients are extubated 8 to 24 hours after transplant. Patients with pulmonary hypertension are predisposed to reperfusion injury, and after BLT or heart-lung transplant, patients may have more severe reperfusion injury and often require mechanical ventilation for a longer period.

After extubation, pulmonary clearance measures are mandatory. These include the use of incentive spirometry and a mucus clearance device. The use of daily bronchoscopy is a common practice to facilitate clearance of secretions that accumulate because of impaired mucociliary function due to lung denervation.

Box 71.2 • Indications for Lung Transplant

Group A
- COPD, emphysema with or without alpha$_1$-antitrypsin deficiency
- Non–cystic fibrosis bronchiectasis, including primary ciliary dyskinesia
- Lymphangioleiomyomatosis (LAM)
- Sarcoidosis with mPAP ≤30 mm Hg

Group B
- Idiopathic pulmonary arterial hypertension (primary pulmonary hypertension)
- Eisenmenger syndrome
- Other pulmonary vascular diseases: pulmonary venoocclusive disease, pulmonary capillary hemangiomatosis, chronic thromboembolic pulmonary hypertension

Group C
- Cystic fibrosis–related bronchiectasis
- Immune deficiency syndromes

Group D
- Idiopathic pulmonary fibrosis/usual interstitial pneumonitis (IPF/UIP)
- All other restrictive lung diseases, including hemosiderosis
- Eosinophilic granulomatosis
- Sarcoidosis with mPAP >30 mm Hg
- Scleroderma, CREST syndrome
- Bronchoalveolar carcinoma (BAC)
- Retransplant (bronchiolitis obliterans syndrome [BOS] or chronic rejection after lung transplant; primary graft failure after lung transplant)

Abbreviations: COPD, chronic obstructive pulmonary disease; CREST, calcinosis cutis, Raynaud phenomenon, esophageal dysfunction, sclerodactyly, and telangiectasia; mPAP, mean pulmonary arterial pressure.

From McCurry KR, Shearon TH, Edwards LB, Chan KM, Sweet SC, Valapour M, et al. Lung transplantation in the United States, 1998-2007. Am J Transplant. 2009 Apr;9(4 Pt 2):942-58; used with permission.

Hemodynamic Management

Lung and heart-lung transplant recipients should not be treated the same as patients who have had routine cardiopulmonary bypass. A newly transplanted lung allograft has some degree of pulmonary edema because of increased vascular permeability and disruption of lymphatic vessels, so fluid restriction is paramount for protecting the pulmonary allograft. The lungs of heart-lung transplant recipients seem to be less prone to reperfusion injury than those of SLT or BLT recipients.

Central venous pressure greater than 7 mm Hg has been associated with higher mortality rates in the ICU and hospital. Pulmonary capillary wedge pressure should be kept as low as possible while maintaining adequate urine output, optimal values for cellular oxygen delivery indexes, and appropriate systemic blood pressure. To achieve this balance, vasoactive, inotropic, and diuretic drugs are often necessary in the first 24 to 48 hours (α-agonists are usually less preferred). In addition, inotropic agents are routinely used after heart-lung transplant and after lung transplant if recipients have right ventricular dysfunction. The optimal fluid (crystalloid or colloid) for volume replacement after lung transplant is unknown and controversial, but colloids are favored if the resuscitative goal is to achieve a hemodynamic end point.

Immunosuppression

At most centers, a dual strategy is used for immunosuppression: initial induction and a lifelong maintenance regimen. Induction is achieved with several agents, such as monoclonal (murine) antilymphocytic antibody (muromonab-CD3) and polyclonal rabbit antithymocyte globulin; rarely, systemic inflammatory response syndrome and anaphylaxis occur with these agents. Interleukin 2 receptor antagonists (eg, basiliximab) are also used. After heart-lung and lung transplant, a maintenance regimen is implemented indefinitely with 3 classes of immunosuppressive agents: corticosteroids (eg, IV methylprednisolone or prednisone); calcineurin inhibitors (eg, cyclosporine or tacrolimus); and cell cycle inhibitors or antimetabolites (eg, mycophenolate mofetil or azathioprine) (Table 71.1 and Figure 71.1).

In a patient with intravascular depletion, calcineurin inhibitors can cause renal impairment, so they should be

Table 71.1 • Agents Used for Immunosuppression After Heart-Lung and Lung Transplant

Agent	Class	Dose and Schedule	Goal Level	Dosage Adjustment Guidelines
Methylprednisolone sodium succinate	Corticosteroid	One 500-mg dose IV before perfusion of the allograft; then 125 mg IV every 8 h for 3 doses (first dose upon arrival in ICU)	NA	NA
Prednisone	Corticosteroid	1 mg/kg orally in 2 divided doses (every 12 h) daily, beginning the day after completion of IV methylprednisolone therapy	NA	NA
Basiliximab (for induction; transplant center dependent)	Interleukin 2 inhibitor (anti-CD25 monoclonal antibody)	1 mg/kg IV, beginning in operating room (along with methylprednisolone sodium succinate) and continuing on day 7 and every other week for 3 additional doses (total of 5 doses)	NA	NA
Mycophenolate mofetil (MMF)	Purine synthesis and cell cycle inhibitor	On postoperative day 0, start 500 mg IV every 12 h, and switch to oral administration when patient can tolerate oral medication; increase to a goal of 1,000 mg every 12 h over the next 3-7 d as patient can tolerate it	NA	Hold if WBC count $<5.0\times10^9$/L Decrease or hold if patient has diarrhea or other gastrointestinal tract intolerance
Azathioprine	Purine synthesis and cell cycle inhibitor	Start if patient cannot tolerate MMF at 2 mg/kg orally or 1 mg/kg IV daily	NA	Hold if WBC count $<5.0\times10^9$/L
Tacrolimus	Calcineurin inhibitor	On postoperative day 1, start 0.5-1 mg orally every 12 h (delay the starting dose if creatinine level is increasing)	12-15 ng/mL	If <12 ng/mL, increase by 0.5 mg If >15 ng/mL, decrease by 0.5 mg
Cyclosporine	Calcineurin inhibitor	On postoperative day 1, start 2.5-5 mg/kg orally every 12 h (delay the starting dose if creatinine level is increasing)	350-400 ng/mL	If <350 ng/mL, increase by 25 mg If >400 ng/mL, decrease by 25 mg

Abbreviations: ICU, intensive care unit; IV, intravenously; NA, not applicable; WBC, white blood cell.

Data from Knoop C, Haverich A, Fischer S. Immunosuppressive therapy after human lung transplantation. Eur Respir J. 2004 Jan;23(1):159-71.

withheld or administered at a lower dose until the serum creatinine level decreases and urine output increases. Because calcineurin inhibitors are metabolized by the cytochrome P450 3A4 isozyme (CYP3A4), if they are administered with medications that induce or inhibit CYP3A4, the blood levels of the calcineurin inhibitors will be affected and will require daily monitoring.

Antimicrobial Prophylaxis

Posttransplant immunosuppressive therapies necessitate routine use of prophylaxis against opportunistic infections for an indefinite period. The most important opportunistic infections are caused by cytomegalovirus (CMV), *Pneumocystis jiroveci* (formerly *Pneumocystis carinii*), and other fungi.

Cytomegalovirus

CMV is the most important pathogen after solid organ transplant. Primary infection is most severe in a CMV-negative recipient who receives lungs from a CMV-positive donor (ie, a mismatch). Routine prophylaxis against CMV disease is started with IV ganciclovir postoperatively upon arrival in the ICU; oral valganciclovir is then used during the first year. If the donor and recipient are CMV negative, IV acyclovir alone is sufficient; the oral form is then used indefinitely. In addition to receiving pharmacoprophylaxis, the patient should undergo CMV surveillance with quantitative polymerase chain reaction testing of the blood every week initially and then every month indefinitely.

Pneumocystis jiroveci

Trimethoprim-sulfamethoxazole (co-trimoxazole) is used daily (single-strength preparation) or 3 times weekly (double-strength preparation). If patients have sulfa allergy or intolerance, pentamidine (300 mg) may be inhaled with a nebulizer monthly; atovaquone (100 mg orally twice daily) is another alternative.

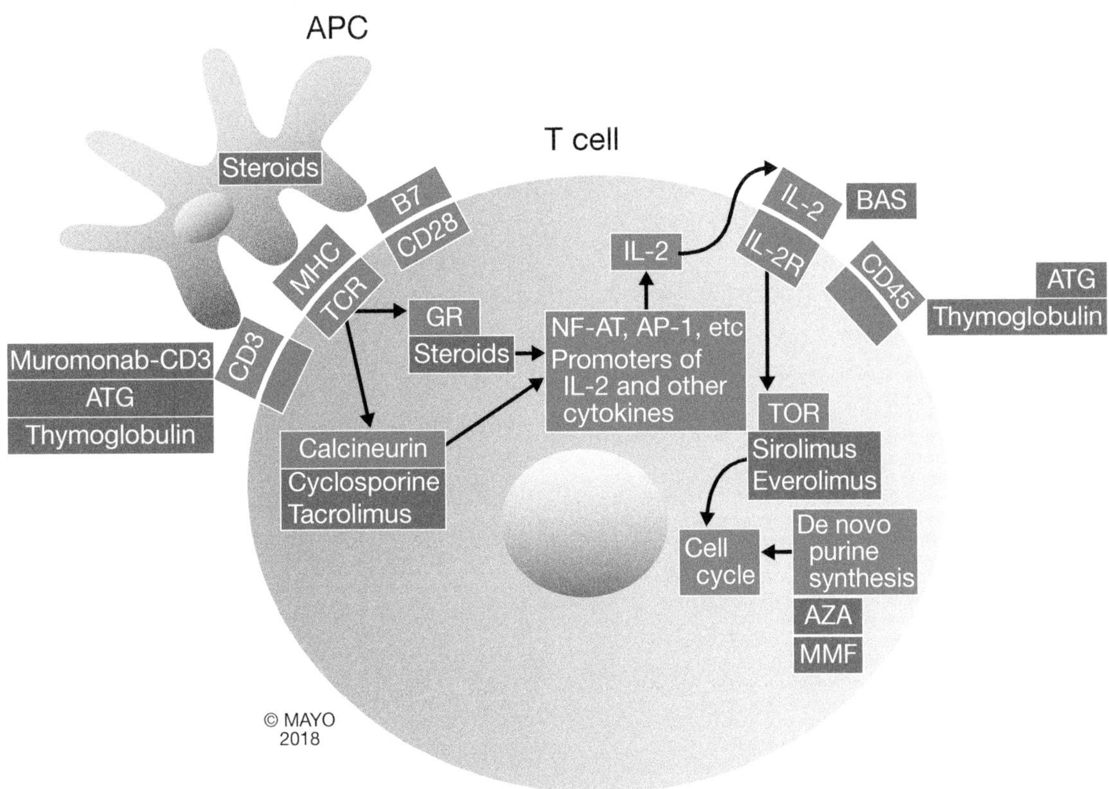

Figure 71.1. Immunologic Mechanisms in Acute Rejection and Targets for Immunosuppressive Agents. Donor antigens are recognized by a recipient antigen-presenting cell (APC) (indirect allorecognition). Alloantigens carried by an APC are recognized by a T-cell receptor (TCR)-CD3 complex on the surface of the T cell. When accompanied by costimulatory signals such as those from CD28 and its ligand B7, the T-cell is activated, resulting in activation of calcineurin. Calcineurin dephosphorylates nuclear factor of activated T cells (NF-AT), allowing it to enter the nucleus and bind to promoters of interleukin (IL)-2 and other cytokines. IL-2 activates an IL-2 cell surface receptor (IL-2R) and stimulates clonal expansion of T cells (helper T cells). IL-2, along with other cytokines produced by helper T cells, stimulates expansion of other immune system cells. Activation of IL-2R stimulates the target of rapamycin (TOR) pathway, which regulates translation of messenger RNAs to proteins that regulate the cell cycle. Sites of action of specific drugs (in red) show the multiple sites of action of these drugs and underscore the rationale for combination therapy. ATG indicates equine antithymocyte globulin; AP-1, activator protein 1; AZA, azathioprine; BAS, basiliximab; GR, glucocorticoid receptor; MHC, major histocompatability complex; MMF, mycophenolate mofetil.

Fungal Infections

Fungal infections after lung transplant are associated with relatively high morbidity and mortality. They are more common in the first 2 to 3 months after transplant. The risk may be higher with more intense immunosuppression related to treating rejection soon after transplant. *Aspergillus* infection in the lung allograft can be asymptomatic and invasive. At several centers, nebulized, inhaled amphotericin B is routinely used as a precaution until the patient is discharged. Oral itraconazole or fluconazole has been suggested for lifelong prophylaxis against fungal infections in areas where coccidioidomycosis is endemic.

Complications

Lung Ischemia-Reperfusion Injury and Primary Graft Dysfunction

Lung ischemia-reperfusion injury (LIRI), or *reimplantation response*, is a form of acute lung injury. Characterized by progressively worsening gas exchange, lung compliance, and pulmonary infiltrates on chest radiography within 72 hours after transplant, LIRI is similar to noncardiogenic pulmonary edema that is typical of acute respiratory distress syndrome (Figure 71.2). To some degree, all transplanted lungs have LIRI; when LIRI has these clinical manifestations, the term *primary graft dysfunction* is

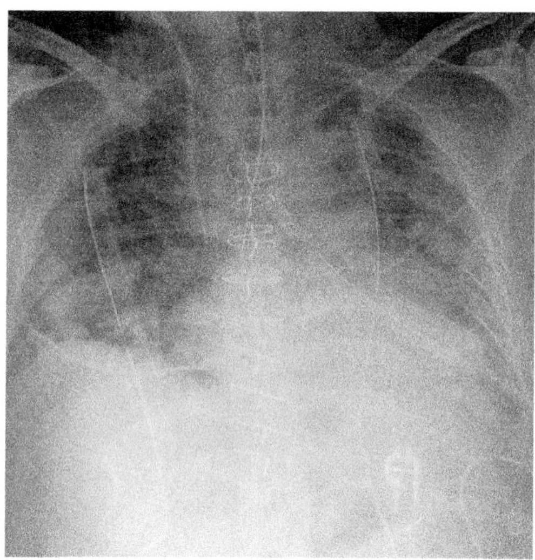

Figure 71.2. Chest Radiograph 24 Hours After Bilateral Lung Transplant. The patient had lung ischemia-reperfusion injury. In addition to the radiographic evidence of diffuse bilateral infiltrates, clinical findings included severe hypoxemia and worsening lung compliance as in acute respiratory distress syndrome.

often used. LIRI is an important cause of morbidity and mortality within 30 days after lung transplant (occurring in 11%-25% of recipients) and is attributed to donor lung abnormalities such as aspiration, contusion, inadequate lung perfusion, and lymphatic disruption.

Treatment is largely supportive, with lung-protective ventilation and a higher level of PEEP. Diuretics and vasoactive agents are preferentially used to optimize hemodynamic parameters with volume restriction. Inhaled nitric oxide, with its potent, selective, pulmonary vasodilator and anti-inflammatory effects, may improve hemodynamic parameters and ventilation-perfusion matching and assist in short-term resuscitation, although no long-term survival data exist to support its benefit. In patients with severe cases, extracorporeal membrane oxygenation (ECMO) has been used with some success as a short-term bridge to recovery, but long-term survival has been lower among patients receiving ECMO than among those who did not receive ECMO.

Acute Rejection

Acute rejection is a short-term and long-term threat to allograft survival and function. *Hyperacute rejection* is a rare antibody-mediated process that occurs within minutes to hours after transplant and is caused by preformed recipient antibodies against donor lung allograft vascular endothelium. Acute rejection is less common in the first 2 weeks after transplant, but it may occur in up to 40% of patients in the first month after transplant.

Patients may be asymptomatic, or they may have nonspecific symptoms such as fatigue, malaise, cough, fever, chest tightness, and dyspnea, which can also occur with an infectious process. Patients with severe cases may be hypoxic at rest or with exertion. Radiographic studies may not be useful. Bronchoscopically guided transbronchial lung biopsy is the gold standard for diagnosis of acute lung rejection.

Treatment of acute rejection includes high doses of corticosteroids (methylprednisolone 10 mg/kg IV daily for 3 consecutive days). If the patient has little or no improvement (ie, *steroid-resistant rejection*), other therapeutic agents should be considered (eg, rabbit antithymocyte globulin or muromonab-CD3). Plasmapheresis has been used as adjunctive therapy. An infectious process must be ruled out before immunosuppression is intensified.

Airway Complications

Airway complications may lead to morbidity and death. Bronchial dehiscence, a serious early airway complication, contributes to early graft failure and high mortality from acute mediastinitis. More commonly, stenosis and bronchomalacia are often late sequelae of ischemic injury that can be relieved with periodic balloon dilatation and stent placement as indicated.

Vascular Complications

Vascular complications may occur immediately after surgery and, if undiagnosed, are associated with high mortality in the early posttransplant phase. Pulmonary artery stenosis and pulmonary venous obstruction cause graft dysfunction in the early posttransplant phase and mimic primary graft dysfunction. Although patients with pulmonary artery stenosis may have a chest that appears clear on radiography, the radiologic findings in pulmonary venous obstruction can resemble those in reperfusion injury. Pulmonary venous obstruction can be identified with pulmonary angiography, however, and reperfusion injury can be identified with transesophageal echocardiography. Pulmonary venous thrombosis is another potentially life-threatening complication that can occur soon after lung transplant. Early reoperation is usually required with cardiopulmonary bypass for venous complications. In high-risk patients, vascular dilation or stent insertion can be a therapeutic option for pulmonary artery stenosis.

Cardiac Dysrhythmias

Atrial flutter occurs frequently in BLT recipients. The likely proposed mechanism is circus electrical movement around left atrial cuff suture lines. At some centers, digoxin is administered prophylactically. Amiodarone and diltiazem can be used for short-term treatment of atrial dysrhythmias. β-Blockers should be used with caution, particularly in patients with right ventricular dysfunction.

Pleural Complications

After bilateral sequential SLT, chest tubes are removed sequentially. Both pleural spaces are communicating after a double-lung transplant, and a single chest tube is often adequate to drain them. Small air leaks are common immediately after lung transplant and usually resolve within 2 weeks without the need for surgical intervention. Airway dehiscence must be ruled out with early bronchoscopy and inspection of the bronchial anastomosis for persistent air leak.

Pleural effusion is common in the first month after transplant and indicates poor pleural drainage (with a low serum albumin level and interrupted peribronchial lymphatic vessels). Rarely, pleural effusion occurs in association with acute rejection and infections. Usually, the pleural effusion is serosanguineous and exudative (neutrophil rich); it often decreases with diuretics and concomitant colloid administration. Persistent pleural effusion requires thoracentesis and bronchoscopy to rule out empyema and rejection. Other causes include postoperative hemothorax or chylothorax (triglyceride rich) from injury to the thoracic duct. Pleural fluid analysis is useful for making an early diagnosis.

Neurologic Complications

Although routine, meticulous, intraoperative phrenic nerve preservation is usually pursued, phrenic nerve injury leading to diaphragmatic paralysis occurs in 3% to 9% of patients after lung transplant; it is more common after heart-lung transplant. Diaphragmatic dysfunction increases hospital length of stay but without serious long-term negative outcomes.

Gastrointestinal Tract Complications

Gastroparesis, which may occur after heart-lung and lung transplant, responds to promotility agents (eg, metoclopramide and erythromycin) and frequent small meals. Gastroesophageal reflux disease (GERD) occurs frequently and responds well to histamine$_2$ blockers, proton pump inhibitors, and antireflux measures, but GERD may lead to microaspiration or silent aspiration episodes and trigger acute lung rejection with decreased lung function. If these episodes are identified early, they may be treated with laparoscopic fundoplication.

Diarrhea is frequently an adverse effect of mycophenolate mofetil. If diarrhea does not resolve, azathioprine can be substituted for mycophenolate mofetil. Colonic perforation has occurred in patients with CMV colitis or non-CMV colitis. Because corticosteroid use can mask symptoms that normally accompany acute abdomen, the physician must maintain a high degree of awareness.

Nosocomial Infections

Infections occurring immediately after transplant are related to the surgical procedure and ventilator dependence. The use of all vascular lines and tubes should be discontinued as soon as possible. In the first month after transplant, the most common infections are bacterial (eg, nosocomial bacterial pneumonia, empyema, catheter-related infections, wound infections, and urinary tract infections). Common nosocomial organisms include *Staphylococcus aureus* and enteric gram-negative bacilli (*Pseudomonas, Proteus, Klebsiella*, and *Escherichia coli*). Rarely, *Legionella* has been reported. Denervation of the lung allograft impairs the cough reflex and mucociliary clearance. In addition, complications at the anastomotic site may enhance colonization and result in bronchial anastomotic dehiscence, leading to mediastinitis, which can be fatal. Latent infection or colonization that occurred before transplant may reactivate during immunosuppressive therapy (eg, tuberculosis or aspergillosis).

Summary

- Several unique and specific, postoperative complications may occur soon after heart-lung and lung transplant.
- Optimal early posttransplant outcomes require a dedicated, multidisciplinary team approach that involves cardiothoracic surgery, lung transplant, ICU, and ancillary staff members.
- An awareness of potential problems and early intervention lead to improved short-term and long-term outcomes for critically ill transplant recipients.

SUGGESTED READING

Alsaeed M, Husain S. Infections in heart and lung transplant recipients. Crit Care Clin. 2019 Jan;35(1):75–93. Epub 2018 Oct 25.

Arcasoy SM. Medical complications and management of lung transplant recipients. Respir Care Clin N Am. 2004 Dec;10(4):505–29.

Christie JD, Carby M, Bag R, Corris P, Hertz M, Weill D; ISHLT Working Group on Primary Lung Graft Dysfunction. Report of the ISHLT Working Group on Primary Lung Graft Dysfunction part II: definition: a consensus statement of the International Society for Heart and Lung Transplantation. J Heart Lung Transplant. 2005 Oct;24(10):1454–9. Epub 2005 Jun 4.

Bermudez CA, Adusumilli PS, McCurry KR, Zaldonis D, Crespo MM, Pilewski JM, et al. Extracorporeal membrane oxygenation for primary graft dysfunction after lung transplantation: long-term survival. Ann Thorac Surg. 2009 Mar;87(3):854–60.

International Society for Heart & Lung Transplantation [Internet]. Addison (TX): International Society for Heart & Lung Transplantation. [cited 2017 Dec 18]. Available from: https://www.ishlt.org/registries/slides.asp?slides=heartLungRegistry.

Knoop C, Haverich A, Fischer S. Immunosuppressive therapy after human lung transplantation. Eur Respir J. 2004 Jan;23(1):159–71.

Le Pavec J, Hascoet S, Fadel E. Heart-lung transplantation: current indications, prognosis and specific considerations. J Thorac Dis. 2018 Oct;10(10):5946–52.

Mattner F, Fischer S, Weissbrodt H, Chaberny IF, Sohr D, Gottlieb J, et al. Post-operative nosocomial infections after lung and heart transplantation. J Heart Lung Transplant. 2007 Mar;26(3):241–9.

McCurry KR, Shearon TH, Edwards LB, Chan KM, Sweet SC, Valapour M, et al. Lung transplantation in the United States, 1998-2007. Am J Transplant. 2009 Apr;9(4 Pt 2):942–58.

Meyers BF, de la Morena M, Sweet SC, Trulock EP, Guthrie TJ, Mendeloff EN, et al. Primary graft dysfunction and other selected complications of lung transplantation: a single-center experience of 983 patients. J Thorac Cardiovasc Surg. 2005 Jun;129(6):1421–9.

Organ procurement and transplantation network [Internet]. Washington (DC): U.S. Department of Health & Human Services. [cited 2017 Dec 18]. Available from: https://optn.transplant.hrsa.gov/.

Patterson GA, Cooper JD, Goldman B, Weisel RD, Pearson FG, Waters PF, et al. Technique of successful clinical double-lung transplantation. Ann Thorac Surg. 1988 Jun;45(6):626–33.

Reitz BA, Wallwork JL, Hunt SA, Pennock JL, Billingham ME, Oyer PE, et al. Heart-lung transplantation: successful therapy for patients with pulmonary vascular disease. N Engl J Med. 1982 Mar 11;306(10):557–64.

Remund KF, Best M, Egan JJ. Infections relevant to lung transplantation. Proc Am Thorac Soc. 2009 Jan 15;6(1):94–100.

Starnes VA, Bowdish ME, Woo MS, Barbers RG, Schenkel FA, Horn MV, et al. A decade of living lobar lung transplantation: recipient outcomes. J Thorac Cardiovasc Surg. 2004 Jan;127(1):114–22.

Weill D, Benden C, Corris PA, Dark JH, Davis RD, Keshavjee S, et al. A consensus document for the selection of lung transplant candidates: 2014: an update from the Pulmonary Transplantation Council of the International Society for Heart and Lung Transplantation. J Heart Lung Transplant. 2015 Jan;34(1):1–15. Epub 2014 Jun 26.

Zamora MR. Cytomegalovirus and lung transplantation. Am J Transplant. 2004 Aug;4(8):1219–26.

72 Clinical Management of Liver Transplant Recipients

BHARGAVI GALI, MD

Goals

- Understand the basics of liver transplant surgery, including anesthetic management.
- Review the immediate posttransplant complications that may occur.
- Know what should be included in the immediate posttransplant assessment.

Introduction

Improvements in surgical, anesthetic, and critical care management since the 1990s have led to better outcomes for liver transplant (LT) recipients. Estimated 1-year survival after LT increased from 64% in 1989 to 89% in 2014. Of all transplants performed in the United States, 23% are LTs, and more than 7,000 LTs were performed in 2015. In most medical centers, LT recipients are initially cared for in an intensive care unit (ICU). With changes in the intraoperative surgical and anesthetic management, the typical time and resources required for immediate postoperative care have decreased, allowing for rapid recovery protocols to be instituted in some centers for patients without clinical complications.

The surgical procedure is divided into preanhepatic, anhepatic, and neohepatic stages. The *preanhepatic stage* includes incision, dissection, and mobilization of the liver and ends when the liver is isolated from the circulation. The *anhepatic stage* begins when the liver is isolated from the circulation and ends with reperfusion (between the anhepatic and neohepatic phases), when the transplanted liver is placed into the recipient's circulation. The *neohepatic phase* is from reperfusion to the end of the surgical procedure.

Anesthetic management includes invasive arterial blood pressure monitoring and central venous access for monitoring. Some centers use pulmonary artery catheters for all LTs, and others use central venous pressure and another method for cardiac index or stroke volume assessment. Large-bore venous access is required for rapid transfusion of blood products and fluids; often a rapid-infusion device is available in preparation for possible massive blood loss. Transesophageal echocardiography is now more commonly used to assess volume status and wall motion abnormalities and to monitor for thrombi or air emboli.

Postoperative Management

In most centers, LT recipients are transferred to the ICU for clinical management (Box 72.1). Many centers have rapid recovery pathways for patients without clinical complications. Patients who have acute liver failure, hepatopulmonary syndrome, portopulmonary hypertension, or a need for ICU care before LT may have prolonged postoperative courses.

Cardiovascular

Patients may be hemodynamically unstable in the immediate posttransplant period. The most frequent cause is vasodilatation, which can result from the preexisting low-resistance and high-output state of end-stage liver disease and from reperfusion of the liver. Patients may require vasopressors (eg, norepinephrine or vasopressin), and volume resuscitation may be necessary along with careful observation for ongoing bleeding. The target for mean arterial pressure is 65 to 70 mm Hg. Hypertension may result from hypervolemia, pain, hypothermia, or immunosuppressants (eg, cyclosporine or tacrolimus). Typically, patients

Box 72.1. • Initial Assessment of Liver Transplant Recipients in the Intensive Care Unit

- Laboratory test results
  - Complete blood cell count
  - Coagulation profile (may include thromboelastography)
  - Serum levels of electrolytes
  - Liver function tests
  - Arterial blood gas analysis
  - Serum level of lactate
  - Doppler ultrasonography of the right upper quadrant of the abdomen (within 6-12 h)
- Hemodynamic status
  - Assess the need for 1) ongoing volume resuscitation (often with albumin) or 2) titration of vasoactive medications.
- Respiratory status
  - Assess the need for 1) high minute ventilation if the patient has ongoing metabolic acidosis or 2) oxygenation if the patient has hepatopulmonary syndrome, acute liver failure, or high transfusion requirements.
- Active bleeding
  - Monitor 1) serial laboratory studies, including conventional coagulation studies (prothrombin time, activated partial thromboplastin time, fibrinogen, and platelet count) in addition to viscoelastic studies (eg, thromboelastography); 2) abdominal girth assessments; and 3) drain output.
- Allograft function
  - Determine whether 1) coagulopathy has been corrected, 2) metabolic acidosis has resolved, and 3) blood flow is satisfactory (with ultrasonography).

are treated if their systolic blood pressure is greater than 160 mm Hg or if their diastolic blood pressure is greater than 100 mm Hg. Dysrhythmias can result from electrolyte abnormalities, hypoxemia, hypercapnia, anemia, hypothermia, or myocardial ischemia. Acute left ventricular dysfunction (possibly related to hypothermia, volume overload, or acid-base abnormalities) can lead to pulmonary edema and possibly posttransplant cardiomyopathy.

Pulmonary

In uncomplicated LT, patients may be able to be weaned from ventilatory support within several hours. However, patients with preexisting pulmonary problems, including hepatopulmonary syndrome, portopulmonary hypertension, and pleural effusions, may require a longer period of postoperative intubation. The right hemidiaphragm may be paralyzed if the right phrenic nerve was injured intraoperatively during suprahepatic caval clamping. Acute respiratory distress syndrome can result from multiple causes, including severe reperfusion injury, transfusion-related acute lung injury, sepsis, or surgical events.

Hematologic

Bleeding in the immediate postoperative period may be related to coagulopathy, thrombocytopenia, surgical causes, hypothermia, and hypocalcemia. Correction of coagulopathy is typically based on evidence of clinical bleeding because standard algorithms do not exist for transfusion of fresh frozen plasma, cryoprecipitate, or platelets. The need for transfusion is often determined from the results of conventional coagulation tests (prothrombin time, activated partial thromboplastin time, fibrinogen, and platelet count) and viscoelastic tests (eg, thromboelastography or thromboelastometry). When a patient has ongoing bleeding, transfusion may be indicated if thromboelastographic findings include a prolonged reaction time (consider fresh frozen plasma), a narrow alpha angle (consider cryoprecipitate), or a narrow maximum amplitude (consider platelets). Viscoelastic methods are also useful for assessment of hypercoagulability. Conventional coagulation tests may be used in combination with viscoelastic studies to guide transfusion. The risk of bleeding is weighed against the risk of hepatic artery thrombosis and portal vein thrombosis. Approximately 10% of patients require surgical reexploration for bleeding.

Renal

Renal dysfunction may be preexisting in patients undergoing LT. Worsening or new-onset renal injury can result from hypotension, cardiac dysfunction, hypovolemia, nephrotoxic medications, or acute tubular necrosis. Renal replacement therapy is needed in 8% to 17% of LT patients. Electrolyte abnormalities may occur postoperatively; hyperkalemia commonly results from transfusions, organ preservation solutions, preexisting renal dysfunction, and metabolic acidosis.

Metabolic

Hypocalcemia may develop after transfusion of packed red blood cells because calcium may be chelated by the citrate in the preservative solution. Patients undergoing living donor LT or split LT require phosphate supplementation for regeneration of liver parenchyma. The lactate level is often abnormally high initially because the liver converts lactate to pyruvate. A persistently high lactate level may indicate poor graft function.

Glycemic

Hyperglycemia commonly occurs and can be related to administration of corticosteroids, catecholamine infusions, surgical stress, sepsis, or calcineurin inhibitors (cyclosporine or tacrolimus). Glucose levels above 200 mg/dL may affect graft function, and insulin infusion is often used to manage hyperglycemia. Hypoglycemia may indicate hepatic dysfunction or a nonfunctioning graft.

Neurologic

Neurologic complications may affect 15% to 30% of patients after LT. Seizures, which occur in 1% to 8% of patients after LT, are often related to toxicity from a calcineurin inhibitor (cyclosporine or tacrolimus). Encephalopathy is another common complication in approximately 12% of patients after LT. Many patients who had pretransplant encephalopathy may have prolonged awakening after LT, but prolonged awakening can also indicate poor initial graft function. Cerebrovascular events, including ischemic and embolic events and intracranial bleeding, occur in 2% to 6% of LT patients. Central pontine myelinolysis caused by rapid fluctuations in serum sodium and osmolality now occurs in less than 1% of LT patients.

Infectious

Infections are an important complication in LT recipients, although the incidence has decreased. Patients with liver failure have impaired immunity, and immunosuppression postoperatively further increases the risk of infection. Postoperative antibiotic prophylaxis is aimed at causes of surgical site infections and at respiratory or abdominal pathogens. Gram-positive bacteria (enterococci and staphylococci) are more common than previously thought, although respiratory infections may also be caused by gram-negative bacteria or fungi. Risk factors for early infections include portal vein thrombosis, recipient age older than 45 years, bile leak, severe hyperglycemia, preoperative hyponatremia, and ICU stay exceeding 9 days.

Surgical

After LT, 8% to 15% of patients may have vascular complications, including thrombosis of the hepatic artery or portal vein, stenosis, or dissection. Vascular complications may be detected with Doppler ultrasonography of the hepatic vessels and may require urgent reexploration. Biliary complications are most common in patients who undergo living donor LT or split LT (incidence, 23%); initial management is often endoscopic.

Graft Function

Determination of initial graft function is typically based on routine laboratory assessment and ultrasonographic imaging. Metabolic acidosis and coagulopathy improve rapidly with optimal initial graft function but may be delayed if the organ is from an expanded criteria donor. Intraoperative ischemic injury or prolonged preservation of the organ before transplant may also affect initial graft function. Primary nonfunction of the graft is rare but is indicated by continued acidosis, coagulopathy, hypoglycemia, and systemic inflammatory response syndrome; it requires urgent retransplant. Hyperacute rejection is rare, but it is characterized by rapid deterioration in graft function on days 1 to 10 after transplant. Acute cellular rejection is most likely to occur 5 to 7 days after transplant, usually after the patient has left the ICU.

Summary

- After LT, a multidisciplinary approach to intensive care management is necessary to optimize outcomes.
- The ICU team, surgeons, and hepatologists must remain in close communication to address many potential problems, including hemodynamic instability, respiratory management and weaning, coagulation and bleeding, maintenance of renal function, and optimization of graft success.
- Early identification of medical and surgical problems decreases morbidity in the immediate posttransplant period.

SUGGESTED READING

Aduen JF, Hellinger WC, Kramer DJ, Stapelfeldt WH, Bonatti H, Crook JE, et al. Spectrum of pneumonia in the current era of liver transplantation and its effect on survival. Mayo Clin Proc. 2005 Oct;80(10):1303–6.

Barri YM, Sanchez EQ, Jennings LW, Melton LB, Hays S, Levy MF, et al. Acute kidney injury following liver transplantation: definition and outcome. Liver Transpl. 2009 May;15(5):475–83.

Braun N, Dette S, Viebahn R. Impairment of renal function following liver transplantation. Transplant Proc. 2003 Jun;35(4):1458–60.

Cabezuelo JB, Ramirez P, Rios A, Acosta F, Torres D, Sansano T, et al. Risk factors of acute renal failure after liver transplantation. Kidney Int. 2006 Mar;69(6):1073–80.

De Pietri L, Mocchegiani F, Leuzzi C, Montalti R, Vivarelli M, Agnoletti V. Transoesophageal echocardiography during liver transplantation. World J Hepatol. 2015 Oct 18;7(23):2432–48.

Feltracco P, Barbieri S, Galligioni H, Michieletto E, Carollo C, Ori C. Intensive care management of liver transplanted patients. World J Hepatol. 2011 Mar 27;3(3):61–71.

Gupta A, Cottam S, Wendon J. Liver transplantation. In: Bersten AD, Soni N, editors. Oh's intensive care manual. 7th ed. Oxford (UK): Butterworth-Heinemann/ Elsevier; c2014. p.1040–52.

Hall TH, Dhir A. Anesthesia for liver transplantation. Semin Cardiothorac Vasc Anesth. 2013 Sep;17(3):180–94. Epub 2013 Mar 12.

Hannaman MJ, Hevesi ZG. Anesthesia care for liver transplantation. Transplant Rev (Orlando). 2011 Jan;25(1):36–43.

Hartmann M, Szalai C, Saner FH. Hemostasis in liver transplantation: pathophysiology, monitoring, and treatment. World J Gastroenterol. 2016 Jan 28;22(4):1541–50.

Keegan MT, Kramer DJ. Perioperative care of the liver transplant patient. Crit Care Clin. 2016 Jul;32(3):453–73.

Kim SI. Bacterial infection after liver transplantation. World J Gastroenterol. 2014 May 28;20(20):6211–20.

Kramer DJ, Siegal EM, Frogge SJ, Chadha MS. Perioperative management of the liver transplant recipient. Crit Care Clin. 2019 Jan;35(1):95–105.

Krenn CG, De Wolf AM. Current approach to intraoperative monitoring in liver transplantation. Curr Opin Organ Transplant. 2008 Jun;13(3):285–90.

Liang TB, Bai XL, Li DL, Li JJ, Zheng SS. Early postoperative hemorrhage requiring urgent surgical reintervention after orthotopic liver transplantation. Transplant Proc. 2007 Jun;39(5):1549–53.

Lui JK, Spaho L, Holzwanger E, Bui R, Daly JS, Bozorgzadeh A, et al. Intensive care of pulmonary complications following liver transplantation. J Intensive Care Med. 2018 Nov;33(11):595–608. Epub 2018 Mar 18.

Mandell MS, Campsen J, Zimmerman M, Biancofiore G, Tsou MY. The clinical value of early extubation. Curr Opin Organ Transplant. 2009 Jun;14(3):297–302.

Navasa M, Feu F, Garcia-Pagan JC, Jimenez W, Llach J, Rimola A, et al. Hemodynamic and humoral changes after liver transplantation in patients with cirrhosis. Hepatology. 1993 Mar;17(3):355–60.

Nemes B, Gaman G, Doros A. Biliary complications after liver transplantation. Expert Rev Gastroenterol Hepatol. 2015 Apr;9(4):447–66. Epub 2014 Oct 21.

Niemann CU, Kramer DJ. Transplant critical care: standards for intensive care of the patient with liver failure before and after transplantation. Liver Transpl. 2011 May;17(5):485–7.

Ozier Y, Klinck JR. Anesthetic management of hepatic transplantation. Curr Opin Anaesthesiol. 2008 Jun;21(3):391–400.

Perez-Saborido B, Pacheco-Sanchez D, Barrera-Rebollo A, Asensio-Diaz E, Pinto-Fuentes P, Sarmentero-Prieto JC, et al. Incidence, management, and results of vascular complications after liver transplantation. Transplant Proc. 2011 Apr;43(3):749–50.

Ramalingam VS, Ansari S, Fisher M. Respiratory complication in liver disease. Crit Care Clin. 2016 Jul;32(3):357–69.

Ramsay M. Justification for routine intensive care after liver transplantation. Liver Transpl. 2013 Nov;19 Suppl 2:S1–5.

Randall HB, Klintmalm GB. Postoperative intensive care unit management: adult liver transplant recipients. In: Busuttil RW, Klintmalm GB, editors. Transplantation of the liver. 2nd ed. Philadelphia (PA): Elsevier/Saunders; c2005. p. 833–51.

Sampathkumar P, Lerman A, Kim BY, Narr BJ, Poterucha JJ, Torsher LC, et al. Post-liver transplantation myocardial dysfunction. Liver Transpl Surg. 1998 Sep;4(5):399–403.

Saner F, Gu Y, Minouchehr S, Ilker K, Fruhauf NR, Paul A, et al. Neurological complications after cadaveric and living donor liver transplantation. J Neurol. 2006 May;253(5):612–7. Epub 2006 Mar 6.

Shah SA, Levy GA, Adcock LD, Gallagher G, Grant DR. Adult-to-adult living donor liver transplantation. Can J Gastroenterol. 2006 May;20(5):339–43.

Wallia A, Parikh ND, Molitch ME, Mahler E, Tian L, Huang JJ, et al. Posttransplant hyperglycemia is associated with increased risk of liver allograft rejection. Transplantation. 2010 Jan 27;89(2):222–6.

Weiss N, Thabut D. Neurological complications occurring after liver transplantation: role of risk factors, hepatic encephalopathy, and acute (on chronic) brain injury. Liver Transpl. 2019 Mar;25(3):469–87.

Zivkovic SA. Neurologic complications after liver transplantation. World J Hepatol. 2013 Aug 27;5(8):409–16.

73 Clinical Management of Kidney Transplant Recipients

JAMES A. ONIGKEIT, MD

Goals

- Describe intraoperative challenges with kidney transplant.
- Review postoperative complications in kidney transplant recipients.
- Elucidate posttransplant immunosuppression.

Introduction

Kidney transplant is common. More than 19,000 kidney transplants were performed in the United States in 2017. About two-thirds were deceased donor transplants, and about one-third were living donor transplants.

Intraoperative Management

The clinical management of a kidney transplant recipient begins in the operating room. The surgical procedure usually involves placement of the allograft in an extraperitoneal, heterotopic position in the right or left iliac fossa.

Three main anastomoses are required: arterial, venous, and ureteral. First, the vascular anastomoses are created. The donor renal artery is anastomosed to the external or internal iliac artery, and the donor renal vein is anastomosed to the external iliac vein. The last anastomosis involves the donor ureter, which is anastomosed to the recipient bladder or, if the native kidney is removed, to the native ureter.

The surgical field is observed for hemostasis, and the kidney is observed for signs of adequate perfusion (appropriate color, texture, and urine production). Levels of electrolytes, especially magnesium, calcium, and potassium, are monitored. The patient's volume status is continually assessed and maintained to be euvolemic to slightly hypervolemic.

Posttransplant Complications

Posttransplant complications can be divided into 2 categories: surgical and medical. Although these categories overlap, surgical complications typically occur earlier than medical complications owing to their mechanical source.

Surgical Complications

Thrombosis of the renal artery or vein is the most concerning immediate surgical complication associated with graft loss. It has several causes, including hypotension, torsion, kinking, hypercoagulable state, donors with multiple renal arteries, technical anastomotic errors, disparity in vessel size during anastomosis, extension of existing thrombus, extrinsic compression from hematoma or lymphocele, and accelerated rejection. Diagnosis is typically made with Doppler ultrasonography showing diminished or absent blood flow.

Renal artery stenosis is the most common vascular complication and usually occurs months to years after transplant. It is more common with living donor transplants owing to the end-to-end anastomoses of the donor arteries. Clinical signs include refractory hypertension and graft dysfunction. The best diagnostic test is arteriography, but Doppler ultrasonography can be used to avoid the use of a contrast agent. Treatment includes angioplasty, stenting, and surgical correction.

Leakage from the urinary tract typically results from technical factors or devascularization. Clinical signs include fever, pain, swelling over the graft, decreased urine output, and urine leakage from the incision. Diagnosis can involve checking the creatinine level of the leaking fluid or performing an isotope scan or cystography. Small leaks typically resolve on their own, but larger leaks may require surgical correction.

Lymphoceles occur from inadequate ligation of the lymphatics overlying the iliac vessels. This leakage of lymph can lead to compression and subsequent graft dysfunction. Patients may have unilateral lower limb swelling on the affected side. Diagnosis is made with ultrasonography, and treatment involves aspiration and catheter drainage. Sclerosants can be instilled to obliterate the cavity, but they increase the risk of chemical peritonitis. Alternatively, the lymphocele can be surgically drained into the peritoneal cavity.

Medical Complications

The intensivist needs to be aware of potential posttransplant medical complications. These include graft failure, infection, fever, electrolyte imbalances, neurologic disorders, hematologic disorders, and posttransplant diabetes mellitus.

Graft Failure

Acute graft failure can occur anytime from many causes. It is characterized by the same signs as acute kidney injury, with an increased creatinine level and low urine output, and the workup should follow the same approach as for acute kidney injury. Ultrasonography is often helpful, particularly to rule out surgical complications. Efforts should be made to optimize prerenal factors, postrenal factors, and intravascular volume. Graft failure necessitating dialysis within the first postoperative week is characteristic of delayed graft function. This distinction is important because the diagnosis has been associated with increased allograft immunogenicity, increased risk of rejection, and decreased long-term survival.

Infection

Infections are the leading cause of morbidity and death, particularly in the early posttransplant period, and more than 80% of recipients have at least 1 episode of infection in the first year. Kidney transplant patients are at risk for opportunistic infections, but among all types of transplant recipients, they have the lowest incidence of pulmonary complications.

Fever

Although fever can be infectious, noninfectious causes must also be considered. Noninfectious causes include pulmonary atelectasis, severe acute rejection, administration of antilymphocyte antibodies (eg, antithymocyte globulin [rabbit]), and posttransplant lymphoma.

Electrolyte Imbalances

Electrolytes must be monitored because abnormalities can occur from graft dysfunction and from immunosuppressive therapy. Calcineurin inhibitors (eg, cyclosporine and tacrolimus) can cause marked electrolyte abnormalities. They cause decreased potassium excretion in urine, leading to hyperkalemia. Hypophosphatemia, hypomagnesemia, and hypocalcemia result from increased urinary excretion.

Neurologic Disorders

Immunosupression itself can lead to neurologic and psychiatric symptoms. Immunosupression is lifelong, and current regimens include cyclosporine or tacrolimus, mycophenolate mofetil or azathioprine, and corticosteroids. Tacrolimus and cyclosporine can cause tremors, insomnia, and paresthesias. Corticosteroids, particularly prednisone in doses larger than 40 mg daily, are associated with psychosis.

Posterior reversible encephalopathy syndrome (PRES) is related to immunosuppression. Although no specific diagnostic criteria have been identified, common features include visual disturbance, seizures, altered mentation, and headaches that are unresponsive to analgesia. Diagnosis involves neuroimaging, which typically shows subcortical edema without infarction in a distribution not confined to a single vascular territory. PRES is usually reversible with a decrease in dosage or discontinuation of the offending agent.

Immunosuppression can also lead to inappropriate proliferation of B cells, termed posttransplant lymphoproliferative disorder. This disorder can lead to lymphoma and, if the central nervous system is involved, various neurologic presentations. For this reason, headache in a transplant recipient must be considered potentially life-threatening. Diagnosis is typically made with imaging or lumbar puncture.

Hematologic Disorders

Hematologic disorders are common in kidney transplant recipients. The prevalence of anemia after transplant exceeds 20% at 1 year and 30% at 3 years. The development of hemolytic uremic syndrome has been associated with the use of calcineurin inhibitors, acute rejection, and cytomegalovirus infection.

Corticosteroids can lead to leukocytosis because of demargination of leukocytes adherent to the vascular endothelium. Band cells are characteristically absent in corticosteroid-associated leukocytosis. Thus, the presence of band cells should prompt a search for infection.

Posttransplant erythrocytosis occurs in approximately 10% to 20% of renal transplant recipients during the first posttransplant year. It persists in approximately half the affected patients.

Diabetes Mellitus

When diabetes mellitus develops in posttransplant patients, the disorder is associated with increased graft failure and mortality. The annual incidence is high (5%-20%).

Summary

- Three main anastomoses are required in kidney transplant: arterial, venous, and ureteral.
- Posttransplant complications can be divided into 2 categories: surgical and medical.
- Thrombosis of the renal artery or vein is the most concerning immediate complication that can lead to graft loss.
- Other complications include graft failure, infection, fever, electrolyte imbalances, neurologic disorders, hematologic disorders, and posttransplant diabetes mellitus.

SUGGESTED READING

Bechstein WO. Neurotoxicity of calcineurin inhibitors: impact and clinical management. Transpl Int. 2000;13(5):313–26.

Buttigieg J, Agius-Anastasi A, Sharma A, Halawa A. Early urological complications after kidney transplantation: an overview. World J Transplant. 2018 Sep 10;8(5):142–9.

Dahdaleh S, Malhotra P. Treatment of central nervous system complications of renal dialysis and transplantation. Curr Treat Options Neurol. 2019 Mar 11;21(3):13.

De Gasperi A, Feltracco P, Ceravola E, Mazza E. Pulmonary complications in patients receiving a solid-organ transplant. Curr Opin Crit Care. 2014 Aug;20(4):411–9.

DiMartini A, Crone C, Fireman M, Dew MA. Psychiatric aspects of organ transplantation in critical care. Crit Care Clin. 2008 Oct;24(4):949–81.

Einollahi B, Nemati E, Rostami Z, Teimoori M, Ghadian AR. Electrolytes disturbance and cyclosporine blood levels among kidney transplant recipients. Int J Organ Transplant Med. 2012;3(4):166–75.

Gonwa T, Johnson C, Ahsan N, Alfrey EJ, Halloran P, Stegall M, et al. Randomized trial of tacrolimus + mycophenolate mofetil or azathioprine versus cyclosporine + mycophenolate mofetil after cadaveric kidney transplantation: results at three years. Transplantation. 2003 Jun 27;75(12):2048–53.

Himmelfarb J, Sayegh MH, editors. Chronic kidney disease, dialysis, and transplantation: companion to Brenner & Rector's the kidney. 3rd ed. Philadelphia (PA): Saunders/Elsevier; c2010. 737 p.

Hinchey J, Chaves C, Appignani B, Breen J, Pao L, Wang A, et al. A reversible posterior leukoencephalopathy syndrome. N Engl J Med. 1996 Feb 22;334(8):494–500.

Karuthu S, Blumberg EA. Common infections in kidney transplant recipients. Clin J Am Soc Nephrol. 2012 Dec;7(12):2058–70. Epub 2012 Sep 13.

Kasiske BL, Snyder JJ, Gilbertson D, Matas AJ. Diabetes mellitus after kidney transplantation in the United States. Am J Transplant. 2003 Feb;3(2):178–85.

Lee CH, Kim GH. Electrolyte and acid-base disturbances induced by clacineurin inhibitors. Electrolyte Blood Press. 2007 Dec;5(2):126–30. Epub 2007 Dec 31.

Loren AW, Porter DL, Stadtmauer EA, Tsai DE. Post-transplant lymphoproliferative disorder: a review. Bone Marrow Transplant. 2003 Feb;31(3):145–55.

Mix TC, Kazmi W, Khan S, Ruthazer R, Rohrer R, Pereira BJ, et al. Anemia: a continuing problem following kidney transplantation. Am J Transplant. 2003 Nov;3(11):1426–33.

Nakagawa M, Terashima T, D'yachkova Y, Bondy GP, Hogg JC, van Eeden SF. Glucocorticoid-induced granulocytosis: contribution of marrow release and demargination of intravascular granulocytes. Circulation. 1998 Nov 24;98(21):2307–13.

Nassi L, Gaidano G. II. Challenges in the management of post-transplant lymphoproliferative disorder. Hematol Oncol. 2015 Jun;33 Suppl 1:96–9.

Perico N, Cattaneo D, Sayegh MH, Remuzzi G. Delayed graft function in kidney transplantation. Lancet. 2004 Nov 13–19;364(9447):1814–27.

Rodgers SK, Sereni CP, Horrow MM. Ultrasonographic evaluation of the renal transplant. Radiol Clin North Am. 2014 Nov;52(6):1307–24. Epub 2014 Sep 4.

Rubin RH. Infectious disease complications of renal transplantation. Kidney Int. 1993 Jul;44(1):221–36.

Tapiawala SN, Tinckam KJ, Cardella CJ, Schiff J, Cattran DC, Cole EH, et al. Delayed graft function and the risk for death with a functioning graft. J Am Soc Nephrol. 2010 Jan;21(1):153–61. Epub 2009 Oct 29.

Transplant trends [Internet]. Richmond (VA): United Network for Organ Sharing. c2018 [cited 2018 May 18]. Available from: https://unos.org/data/transplant-trends/#transplants_by_organ_type+year+2017.

Wu WK, Famure O, Li Y, Kim SJ. Delayed graft function and the risk of acute rejection in the modern era of kidney transplantation. Kidney Int. 2015 Oct;88(4):851–8. Epub 2015 Jun 24.

74 Small Intestinal Transplant

AYAN SEN, MD

Goals

- Review indications for small bowel transplant.
- Know the critical care issues associated with small bowel transplant.
- Understand the neurologic complications associated with small bowel transplant.

Introduction

Intestinal transplant (ITx) is becoming a valid option for patients with intestinal failure who are receiving long-term parenteral nutrition and have associated complications. Multivisceral transplant was first reported by Starzl et al in 1989 (see Suggested Reading). Since then the number of intestinal transplants performed in the United States has increased dramatically (from 5 in 1990 to 146 in 2016). Furthermore, 1-year graft and patient survival rates are similar to those for solid abdominal organ transplants (up to 80%).

Indications

Short gut syndrome and functional bowel problems are the most common clinical conditions leading to intestinal failure and subsequent eligibility for ITx. Less common, recently identified indications include complicated abdominal vascular disorder and specific low-grade neoplastic tumors (eg, mesenteric desmoids and neuroendocrine pancreatic tumors). Nonetheless, a timely referral for transplant is crucial before the patient has complications related to total parenteral nutrition (TPN) (eg, liver failure). Simultaneous liver transplant is indicated if the patient has advanced liver disease and cholestasis. The American Society of Transplantation and the Centers for Medicare and Medicaid Services recommend intestinal transplant under the following conditions:

- Failure of long-term home TPN with 1 or more of the following complications: impending or overt liver failure; thrombosis of 2 or more central veins; 2 or more episodes of sepsis per year, particularly if they require in-hospital care; shock and fungemia; and recurrent episodes of dehydration.
- Relatively high risk of death.
- Severe short gut syndrome (residual small bowel <10 cm in infants and <20 cm in adults).
- Frequent hospital admissions, long-term opioid dependency, or pseudo-obstruction.
- Unwillingness to accept long-term home TPN.

Contraindications

Contraindications for intestinal transplant include the following: cardiopulmonary insufficiency, history or presence of systemic aggressive or incurable malignancy, coexistent severe systemic autoimmune disease, diagnosis of AIDS, and life-threatening intra-abdominal or severe systemic infections.

Technique

The majority of donors are hemodynamically stable after brain death and have no intestinal pathology. The organs are harvested and usually preserved in University of Wisconsin solution, although histidine-tryptophan-ketoglutarate solution has also been used. Cold ischemia time is minimumized by coordinating the timing of the donor and recipient operations. The intestinal anastomosis is constructed in side-to-side fashion to overcome any size discrepancy between the graft and the recipient intestine.

After a feeding jejunostomy or gastrostomy is performed, the distal end of the graft is left as an end ileostomy or a loop ileostomy. Usually the arterial inflow is from the recipient infrarenal aorta and the venous outflow is from the portal vein. If mesenteric venous return is compromised, such as in mesenteric thrombosis, the venous outflow is created through the inferior vena cava (for systemic drainage).

Closure of the abdominal wall can be difficult because of adhesions associated with previous surgical operations, chronic infections, and an abdominal wall with a tendency to contract. Thus, abdominal closure under these circumstances may require temporary mesh or Gore-Tex grafts or rotation flaps.

Postoperative Management

Hemodynamic optimization is important postoperatively, and invasive monitoring with a central venous catheter or pulmonary artery catheter is typical. However, vascular access may be challenging because of the use of long-term parenteral nutrition through a peripherally inserted central catheter and the high incidence of venous thrombosis. In these situations, transesophageal echocardiography may be required. Avoiding high doses of vasopressors may be beneficial for graft survival.

Hyperventilation should be avoided in patients receiving cyclosporine or tacrolimus because of the lower seizure threshold with hypocapnia. Hypoalbuminemia predisposes patients to ascites and pleural effusions. Ascites, intestinal edema, or pleural effusions may affect respiratory mechanics in the perioperative period. Hence, spontaneous breathing is considered beneficial because it promotes venous drainage and intestinal or intestinal-liver graft perfusion. Ambulation, mobilization, and aggressive physical and respiratory therapy are advised. Tracheal extubation within 3 to 4 hours can be achieved safely if postoperative recovery is unremarkable (absence of shock, acute respiratory failure, electrolyte imbalance, and encephalopathy). Postoperative analgesia is more effective with neuraxial opioids and local anesthetics. Otherwise, intravenous patient-controlled analgesia and a subsequent regimen of oral opioids for the first 94 hours should suffice for appropriate pain relief.

Patients with a protein C, protein S, or antithrombin III deficiency as an indication for transplant have a higher risk for perioperative thrombotic events. Electrolyte imbalance may result from diarrhea and dehydration. After ITx, patients may have severe secretory diarrhea that must be distinguished from rejection or new infection. Unexplained severe metabolic acidosis should raise concern for an acute complication of the graft (eg, a major artery thrombosis). In the early posttransplant period, patients may have renal dysfunction and a decreased glomerular filtration rate as a result of hypovolemia, antibiotic therapy, or immunosuppression. Red blood cell transfusion should be considered if the hematocrit is 28% to 30%. Overtransfusion of blood products may predispose to graft arterial thrombosis, which is highly lethal. Thromboelastography facilitates coagulation monitoring, although conventional coagulation tests can also provide valuable information and guide management. Prophylaxis against infection consists of trimethoprim-sulfamethoxazole for *Pneumocystis jiroveci* infection, nystatin swish and swallow or a clotrimazole troche 4 times daily for fungi, and prophylaxis for cytomegalovirus.

Adequate nutritional support can preserve the trophism of the transplanted intestine. Therefore, a main objective of postoperative care is to provide enteral nutrition as soon as signs of intestinal function are apparent without evidence of anastomotic complications. Nevertheless, TPN should be continued if the daily nutritional support goal is not achieved.

Complications

Technical

Various technical complications can occur, including bleeding, thrombosis, and anastomotic leaks in 10% to 15% of patients, although much higher rates have been reported. Common infectious causes that result in high mortality include intra-abdominal sepsis, catheter-related bloodstream infections, and bacterial translocation from the graft. In addition to broad antibiotic coverage, treatment may include removal of the implicated catheter, treatment against cytomegalovirus infection, and gut decontamination (when bacterial translocation is suspected). Patients are given a mixture of polymyxin, amphotericin B, and gentamicin orally every 6 hours.

Posttransplant lymphoproliferative disease (associated with Epstein-Barr virus) develops in up to 30% of ITx recipients. Treatment involves a substantial decrease in the immunosuppression regimen and initiation of antiviral therapy and chemotherapy with a regimen such as cyclophosphamide, doxorubicin, vincristine, and prednisone (CHOP) or rituximab in combination with CHOP.

The incidence of graft-vs-host disease (GVHD) after ITx is approximately 7% to 9% because of the high reservoir of lymphocytes in Peyer patches, lamina propria, and mesenteric lymph nodes. GVHD most often involves the skin, liver, lungs, bone marrow, and gastrointestinal tract. Patients usually present with a skin rash, mouth or tongue lesions, diarrhea, gastrointestinal tract ulcerations, liver dysfunction, and bone marrow suppression.

Most current antirejection protocols include induction immunosuppression with antilymphocyte agents (eg, thymoglobulin) given perioperatively in conjunction with a short course of glucocorticoids and calcineurin inhibitors as maintenance therapy. The incidence of acute cellular rejection has decreased with improved immunosuppression protocols. Six-month mortality from severe rejection is approximately 25% to 45%. Patients with acute rejection may have increased stoma output, fever, abdominal pain, distention, and ileus. Acute rejection also predisposes to sepsis from bacterial translocation and fungal infections.

Diagnosis is made from pathologic specimens obtained during endoscopy. In the early postoperative period, serial endoscopy is performed through the stoma, and intestinal biopsy specimens are commonly used for graft surveillance because most rejections occur within the first month posttransplant. Zoom endoscopy (up to 100-fold magnification) has been described (sensitivity, 45%; specificity, 98%). After the first month, endoscopy is performed less frequently. The mainstay of treatment of mild rejection typically involves corticosteroids and intensification of the baseline immunosuppressive regimen. Attempts have been made to decrease the rejection rates with radiotherapy of donor grafts (ex vivo), infusion of the donor bone marrow, or leukocyte depletion before transplant. However, radiotherapy can lead to radiation-induced small bowel injury.

Neurologic

Neurologic complications are common after ITx and are associated with considerable morbidity. Extensive loss of intestinal mucosa decreases the absorptive surface for nutrients, electrolytes, and vitamins, leading to deficiencies and associated neurologic signs and symptoms (Table 74.1). TPN can also be associated with neurologic symptoms and signs, such as metabolic encephalopathy due to metabolic and electrolyte abnormalities, sepsis, and poor glucose control:

- The rate of neurologic complications after ITx is higher (85%) than after other solid organ transplants. The high prevalence has been attributed to metabolic disturbances in the pretransplant and posttransplant periods and to aggressive immunosuppression necessitated by the increased immunogenicity of the intestine.
- Headaches occur in about 50% of patients. The high incidence is attributed to high doses of tacrolimus. In addition, rebound headaches occur from opiate withdrawal.
- Encephalopathy occurs in 43% of patients from multifactorial causes. These causes are not specific to ITx.
- Seizures occur in 17% of patients. Usually they are associated with metabolic disturbances or structural brain lesions.
- Central nervous system infection occurs in about 7% of patients. This percentage is much higher than for patients with liver or heart transplants. Immunosuppressive regimens can increase translocation of bacteria across intestinal barriers and permit dissemination to the brain. Infections with *Aspergillus, Toxoplasma, Cryptococcus, Echinococcus, Strongyloides*, and *Acanthamoeba* have been reported after ITx.
- Tacrolimus may lead to neurotoxicity. ITx recipients require higher immunosuppressive doses of tacrolimus to prevent rejection, but the use of higher doses may lead to neurotoxicity.
- Ischemic strokes may occur in patients with hypercoagulable disorders, which may have led to bowel ischemia and short gut syndrome. Many of these patients require lifelong anticoagulation to prevent ischemic strokes.

The diagnostic workup of ITx recipients with neurologic complications should include a description of any pretransplant neurologic dysfunction, the type of transplant (small intestine only or both liver and intestine), time course of the symptoms, type and intensity of immunosuppression, identification of risk factors for opportunistic infections, and consideration of the neurologic complications being a manifestation of graft dysfunction. Laboratory testing should include bloodwork (metabolic panel, blood cell count, and electrolytes). Cultures of fluids and tissues as indicated and comprehensive cerebrospinal fluid analysis are critical. Computed tomography, magnetic resonance imaging, electroencephalography, and electromyography should be done as needed to determine the cause of the neurologic deficits.

Therapy should be directed toward the cause of the neurologic complications. Neurologic injuries may necessitate changes in the dosage or type of immunosuppressive therapy. Mycophenolate mofetil or sirolimus should replace tacrolimus to lessen the neurologic toxicity.

Table 74.1 • Neurologic Signs and Symptoms From Deficiencies of Vitamins and Nutrients

Deficient Substance	Signs and Symptoms
Vitamin B_{12}	Subacute degeneration of the spinal cord (paresthesias of the extremities and spastic weakness and incoordination of the limbs) Dementia (may be reversible)
Folate	Peripheral neuropathy and encephalopathy
Biotin	Peripheral neuropathy and seizures
Pantothenic acid	Peripheral neuropathy and generalized motor weakness
Thiamine	Wernicke encephalopathy and peripheral neuropathy
Vitamin A	Impaired nocturnal vision
Vitamin E	Spinocerebellar degenerative disorder with weakness, ataxia, loss of proprioception, dysphagia, dysarthria, ophthalmoplegia, and dementia
Vitamin D	Proximal myopathy
Magnesium and calcium	Tetany, encephalopathy, and seizures

Summary

- ITx is becoming a valid option for patients with intestinal failure due to severe short gut syndrome who are receiving long-term parenteral nutrition and have associated complications.
- Various technical complications can occur, including bleeding, thrombosis, and anastomotic leaks in 10% to 15% of patients, while intra-abdominal sepsis, catheter-related bloodstream infections, and bacterial translocation from the graft lead to high morbidity and mortality.
- Six-month mortality from severe acute rejection is approximately 25% to 45%.
- Most current antirejection protocols include induction immunosuppression with antilymphocyte agents (eg, thymoglobulin) given perioperatively in conjunction with a short course of glucocorticoids and calcineurin inhibitors as maintenance therapy.
- Posttransplant lymphoproliferative disease (associated with Epstein-Barr virus) develops in up to 30% of ITx recipients and requires chemotherapy.
- Neurologic complications are common after ITx and can be due to extensive loss of intestinal mucosa, which decreases the absorptive surface for nutrients, electrolytes, and vitamins, leading to deficiencies and associated neurologic signs and symptoms.

SUGGESTED READING

Abu-Elmagd K, Reyes J, Bond G, Mazariegos G, Wu T, Murase N, et al. Clinical intestinal transplantation: a decade of experience at a single center. Ann Surg. 2001 Sep;234(3):404–16.

Abu-Elmagd KM. Intestinal transplantation for short bowel syndrome and gastrointestinal failure: current consensus, rewarding outcomes, and practical guidelines. Gastroenterology. 2006 Feb;130(2 Suppl 1):S132–7.

Berden JH, Hoitsma AJ, Merx JL, Keyser A. Severe central-nervous-system toxicity associated with cyclosporin. Lancet. 1985 Jan 26;1(8422):219–20.

Buchman AL, Scolapio J, Fryer J. AGA technical review on short bowel syndrome and intestinal transplantation. Gastroenterology. 2003 Apr;124(4):1111–34.

Cai J, Wu G, Qing A, Everly M, Cheng E, Terasaki P. Organ Procurement and Transplantation Network/Scientific Registry of Transplant Recipients 2014 Data Report: intestine. Clin Transpl. 2014:33–47.

Furukawa H, Reyes J, Abu-Elmagd K, Mieles L, Hutson W, Kocoshis S, et al. Intestinal transplantation at the University of Pittsburgh: six-year experience. Transplant Proc. 1997 Feb-Mar;29(1–2):688–9.

Jacewicz M, Marino CR. Neurologic complications of pancreas and small bowel transplantation. Handb Clin Neurol. 2014;121:1277–93.

Kato T, Gaynor JJ, Nishida S, Mittal N, Selvaggi G, Levi D, et al. Zoom endoscopic monitoring of small bowel allograft rejection. Surg Endosc. 2006 May;20(5):773–82. Epub 2006 Mar 16.

Kato T, Gaynor JJ, Selvaggi G, Mittal N, Thompson J, McLaughlin GE, et al. Intestinal transplantation in children: a summary of clinical outcomes and prognostic factors in 108 patients from a single center. J Gastrointest Surg. 2005 Jan;9(1):75–89.

Kaufman SS, Atkinson JB, Bianchi A, Goulet OJ, Grant D, Langnas AN, et al; American Society of Transplantation. Indications for pediatric intestinal transplantation: a position paper of the American Society of Transplantation. Pediatr Transplant. 2001 Apr;5(2):80–7.

Kesseli S, Sudan D. Small bowel transplantation. Surg Clin North Am. 2019 Feb;99(1):103–16.

Khan FA, Tzakis AG. Intestinal and multivisceral transplantation. In: Ginns LC, Cosimi AB, Morris PJ, editors. Transplantation. Malden (MA): Blackwell Science; c1999. p. 422–37.

Khan FA, Selvaggi G. Overview of intestinal and multivisceral transplantation. In: Robson KM, editor. UpToDate. Waltham (MA): UpToDate; c2016.

Kostopanagiotou G, Sidiropoulou T, Pyrsopoulos N, Pretto EA Jr, Pandazi A, Matsota P, et al. Anesthetic and perioperative management of intestinal and multivisceral allograft recipient in nontransplant surgery. Transpl Int. 2008 May;21(5):415–27. Epub 2008 Jan 14.

Lauro A, Altimari A, Di Simone M, Dazzi A, Cescon M, Zanfi C, et al. Acute cellular rejection monitoring after intestinal transplant: utility of serologic markers and zoom videoendoscopy as support of conventional biopsy and clinical findings. Transplant Proc. 2008 Jun;40(5):1575–6.

Lewis MB, Howdle PD. Neurologic complications of liver transplantation in adults. Neurology. 2003 Nov 11;61(9):1174–8.

Masetti M, Cautero N, Lauro A, Di Benedetto F, Begliomini B, Siniscalchi A, et al. Three-year experience in clinical intestinal transplantation. Transplant Proc. 2004 Mar;36(2):309–11.

Mazariegos GV, Abu-Elmagd K, Jaffe R, Bond G, Sindhi R, Martin L, et al. Graft versus host disease in intestinal transplantation. Am J Transplant. 2004 Sep;4(9):1459–65.

Organ Procurement and Transplantation Network [Internet]. National data. Richmond (VA): United Network for Organ Sharing; c2018 [cited 2018 Sep 17]. Available from: https://optn.transplant.hrsa.gov/data/view-data-reports/national-data/.

Patchell RA. Neurological complications of organ transplantation. Ann Neurol. 1994 Nov;36(5):688–703.

Pustavoitau A, Bhardwaj A, Stevens R. Neurological complications of transplantation. J Intensive Care Med. 2011 Jul-Aug;26(4):209–22.

Reyes J, Mazariegos GV, Bond GM, Green M, Dvorchik I, Kosmach-Park B, et al. Pediatric intestinal transplantation: historical notes, principles and controversies. Pediatr Transplant. 2002 Jun;6(3):193–207.

Starzl TE, Rowe MI, Todo S, Jaffe R, Tzakis A, Hoffman AL, et al. Transplantation of multiple abdominal viscera. JAMA. 1989 Mar 10;261(10):1449–57.

Sudan D. The current state of intestine transplantation: indications, techniques, outcomes and challenges. Am J Transplant. 2014 Sep;14(9):1976–84. Epub 2014 Aug 6.

Varkey J, Simren M, Jalanko H, Oltean M, Saalman R, Gudjonsdottir A, et al. Fifteen years' experience of intestinal and multivisceral transplantation in the Nordic countries. Scand J Gastroenterol. 2015 Mar;50(3):278–90. Epub 2015 Jan 16.

Wu G, Selvaggi G, Nishida S, Moon J, Island E, Ruiz P, et al. Graft-versus-host disease after intestinal and multivisceral transplantation. Transplantation. 2011 Jan 27;91(2):219–24.

Zivkovic SA, Eidelman BH, Bond G, Costa G, Abu-Elmagd KM. The clinical spectrum of neurologic disorders after intestinal and multivisceral transplantation. Clin Transplant. 2010 Mar-Apr;24(2):164–8. Epub 2009 Aug 24.

Toxicity and Toxins

75 Serotonin Syndrome

KEVIN T. GOBESKE, MD, PhD; EELCO F. M. WIJDICKS, MD, PhD

Goals

- Understand the clinicopathologic framework of serotonin toxicity and its underlying mechanisms.
- Identify the clinical features of serotonin syndrome that facilitate early diagnosis and treatment.
- Distinguish the characteristics of serotonin syndrome from those of other pathologic conditions in critically ill patients.
- Understand the principles of clinical management of serotonin syndrome.

Introduction

Serotonin syndrome affects the central nervous system, the autonomic nervous system, and the neuromuscular system and can have acute and potentially life-threatening manifestations. By definition, serotonin syndrome is associated with changes in serotonin exposure and thus might be described more accurately as *serotonergic excess* or *serotonin toxicity*. The central nervous system effects of serotonin involve regulation of attention, arousal, mood, learning, appetite, and temperature. Peripheral nervous system activity includes vasoconstriction, gastrointestinal tract motility, spinal–motor action pattern generation, and muscle contraction threshold gating. Systemic actions of serotonin include bronchoconstriction, bone metabolism, and platelet aggregation. Serotonergic toxicity thus includes the constellation of encephalopathy, agitation, diaphoresis, vital sign changes, hyperreflexia, abnormal movements, vomiting, and diarrhea.

Serotonin syndrome is a clinical diagnosis that requires the presence of a serotonergic agent (Box 75.1) along with a cluster of symptoms, and the syndrome typically occurs after a change in serotonin exposure or in the processing of established doses during injury. Serotonin syndrome is becoming increasingly common as the number and use of serotonergic drugs increase. Nevertheless, serotonin toxicity is often underdiagnosed and undertreated. Most undetected cases are mild and self-resolving and may be misattributed to adverse effects of new medications. Yet even severe cases in patients who are already critically ill can be easily missed or mistaken; the consequences of an inaccurate diagnosis are compounded further in intensive care unit patients who already have other neurologic dysfunction. Since serotonin syndrome is purely a clinical diagnosis, rapid semiologic pattern recognition and evaluation of recent medication exposure is essential. Early consideration of serotonin syndrome may limit additional exposure and prevent serious complications.

Pathogenesis

Serotonin, also called 5-hydroxytryptamine (5-HT), is an indolamine neurotransmitter in the monoamine superfamily. Serotonin is the endogenous ligand for the 5-HT receptor family. With the exception of 5-HT$_3$, the 5-HT receptor family consists of G protein–coupled receptors linked to adenylyl cyclase or phospholipase C–signaling cascades. The 2 major subfamilies of 5-HT receptors and numerous other receptor subtypes are each implicated in different processes. The wide-ranging physiologic actions of these pathways mirror the breadth of symptoms that occur in serotonin toxicity. Furthermore, most physiologic and pharmacologic triggers for serotonin signaling also involve changes in the activity of other monoamine neurotransmitters. Indeed, few medications or neural circuits are purely serotonergic at a particular presynaptic or postsynaptic receptor pathway.

The concept that serotonin toxicity is also expressed as a syndromic combination of mechanisms at the cellular level may be challenged by a series of laboratory studies. Specific manipulations at different receptor types have shown that

Box 75.1 • Serotonergic Agents

Serotonin precursors or agonists

Tryptophan, 5-HTP, SAMe, DHE, triptans, LSD, 5-MeO-DIPT, lithium, mirtazapine, buspirone

Decreased serotonin reuptake

Serotonin reuptake inhibitors: fluoxetine, paroxetine, fluvoxamine, sertraline, citalopram, escitalopram, trazodone, nefazodone, vilazodone

Serotonin-norepinephrine reuptake inhibitors: duloxetine, venlafaxine, desvenlafaxine, milnacipran, atomoxetine, sibutramine

Tricyclic antidepressants: amitriptyline, nortriptyline, clomipramine, imipramine, desipramine, doxepin

Antiemetics: ondansetron, granisetron, metoclopramide

Others: dextromethorphan, cyclobenzaprine, chlorpheniramine, St John's wort, yohimbine

Decreased serotonin breakdown

Monoamine oxidase inhibitors: selegiline, rasagiline, phenelzine, tranylcypromine, isocarboxazid, moclobemide

Antibiotics: linezolid, tedizolid, cycloserine

Others: methylene blue, procarbazine, Syrian rue, nutmeg, ginseng

Opiates with mixed serotonin agonism

Tramadol, tapentadol, meperidine, fentanyl, pentazocine, buprenorphine, dextropropoxyphene

Stimulants with serotonergic activity

Drugs of abuse: amphetamines, MDMA, MDA, cocaine

Anorectics: phentermine, fenfluramine, dexfenfluramine, sibutramine, amfepramone

Other agonists

Antipsychotics: risperidone, olanzapine, clozapine

Antiepileptics: valproate, carbamazepine

Peripheral inhibitors of metabolism

Fluconazole, erythromycin, ciprofloxacin, ritonavir

Abbreviations: DHE, dihydroergotamine; 5-HTP, hydroxytryptophan; 5-MeO-DIPT, 5-methoxy-N,N-diisopropyltryptamine; LSD, lysergic acid diethylamide; MDA, methylenedioxyamphetamine; MDMA, 3,4-methylenedioxymethamphetamine; SAMe, *S*-adenosyl-L-methionine.

5-HT_{1A} and 5-HT_2 (or 5-HT_{2A}) receptor activity may be the primary driver for observed pathologic features. In studies of animal models, specific 5-HT_{1A} agonists have been suggested to influence hyperactivity and abnormal movements. Specific 5-HT_2 and 5-HT_{2A} agonists induce hyperthermia and axial muscle contractions; however, these may be blocked by the coadministration of 5-HT_{1A} selective antagonists applied at equal concentrations. Since 5-HT_{1A} receptors have high binding affinity, they may be nearly fully occupied at standard doses of serotonergic medications. Yet when serotonin concentrations are high, occupation of 5-HT_2 receptors becomes more important. However, cross-talk and reciprocal modulation occur between 5-HT_{1A} and 5-HT_{2A} receptor pathways, and 5-HT_{2A} activation potentiates many 5-HT_{1A}-mediated behaviors. Importantly, severe hyperthermia appears to be prevented by 5-HT_{2A} antagonists even in the presence of high serotonin concentrations. Patients with the C/C genetic variant of 5-HT_2 receptors have a 3-fold higher rate of discontinuation of paroxetine from adverse effects. Figure 75.1 is a simplified illustration of how uptake receptors are blocked.

Clinical Presentation

Although it may have protean manifestations, serotonin syndrome is classically described as the triad of neuromuscular excitability, altered mental status, and autonomic dysregulation (including gastrointestinal tract hypermotility) (Table 75.1). Of these features, diaphoresis, myoclonus, and increased gastrointestinal tract activity are among the most common and, along with the timing of onset, can best help to distinguish serotonin excess from other toxidromes (Table 75.2). Conceptually, serotonin syndrome covers a spectrum from the mild adverse effects of selective serotonin reuptake inhibitors to the consequences of severe autonomic instability and muscle hyperactivity. Neuromuscular dysfunction such as agitation, hyperactivity, and tremor are nonspecific findings; hyperreflexia or induced myoclonus that is more pronounced in the legs than in the arms suggests serotonin excess; and spontaneous myoclonus, rigidity, or tonic-isometric contractions increase the concern for severe disease. Similarly, cognitive dysfunction includes nonspecific findings such as neurocognitive slowing, confusion, anxiety, and delirium; more specific clinical manifestations of serotonin toxicity include hallucinations in combination with stupor that does not wax and wane; and coma is possible in the most severe cases. Nonspecific autonomic findings include tachycardia, nausea, and mild fever with diaphoresis; notable gastrointestinal tract hypermotility, diaphoresis, and pupillary changes suggest serotonin activity; and severe hyperthermia, tachycardia, and labile blood pressure increase the concern for severe disease.

The diagnosis of serotonin syndrome is made from the clinical history and examination findings; no laboratory or ancillary testing has proved reliable. Clinical decision rules have been codified for the diagnosis of serotonin syndrome (Box 75.2). These criteria are based on the presence of a serotonergic agent and certain combinations of symptoms, which have 84% sensitivity and 97% specificity when compared with the formal diagnosis by a medical toxicologist.

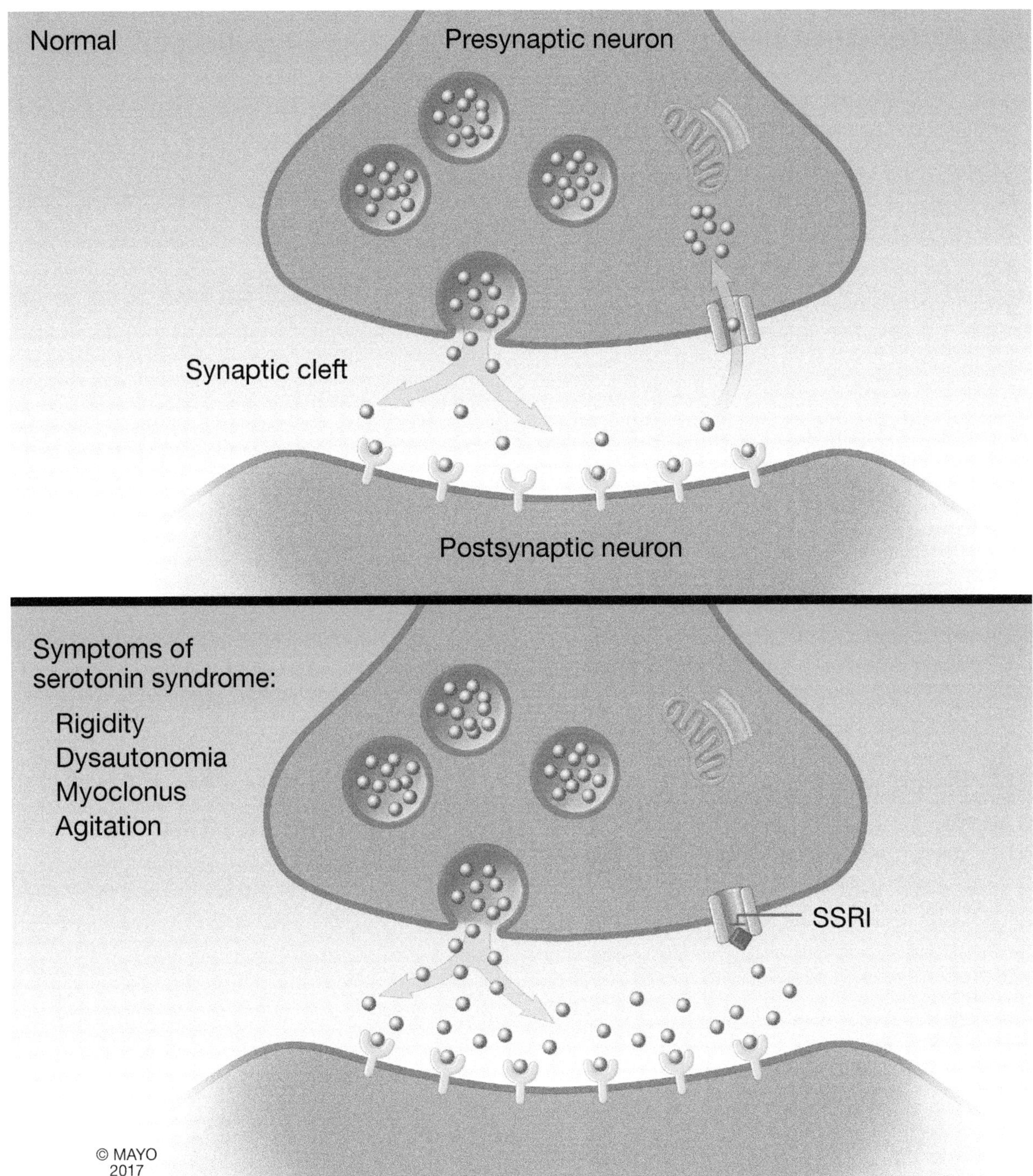

Figure 75.1. Serotonin Syndrome. Blocking of uptake receptors by selective serotonin reuptake inhibitors (SSRIs) results in increased serotonin levels and clinical symptoms.

If features of serotonin syndrome can be distinguished from those of other causes of altered mental status, fever, and vital sign abnormalities in critically ill patients, clinicians may avert progression to even more severe disease. Furthermore, since the medication history of these patients is often complicated or unknown, astute observance of clinical signs and symptoms may drive the search for potentially serotonergic drug combinations. If serotonergic excess is identified, the use of inciting agents can be stopped, and if severe features of serotonergic excess are recognized, potentially lifesaving interventions can be instituted.

Table 75.1 • Clinical Manifestations of Serotonin Syndrome

	Type of Dysfunction		
Severity	**Autonomic**	**Neuromuscular**	**Cognitive**
Severe	Labile blood pressure Hyperthermia (>40°C) Tachycardia (>140 bpm)	Severe clonus or rigidity Respiratory failure Rhabdomyolysis	Delirium Stupor Coma
Moderate	Hypertension Hyperthermia (37°C-40°C) Tachycardia (100-140 bpm) Nausea, vomiting, diarrhea	Moderate hyperreflexia Provoked or spontaneous clonus Spontaneous myoclonus Opsoclonus	Agitation Confusion
Mild	Diaphoresis Pupillary dilatation Tachycardia (80-100 bpm)	Mild hyperreflexia Mild myoclonus Mild tremor	Listlessness Anxiety Insomnia

Abbreviation: bpm, beats per minute.

Clinical Management

The 3 pillars in the management of serotonin syndrome in acute care settings are 1) rapid cessation of the use of all serotonergic agents, 2) supportive care targeted at restoration of homeostasis of vital functions, and 3) surveillance and management of complications due to severe disease.

Laboratory tests are used for the management of serotonin syndrome rather than for diagnosis or prognostication. Initial studies should assess electrolyte abnormalities associated with muscle and membrane instability, including calcium, magnesium, and phosphorous, along with a basic blood chemistry panel. Myocyte instability and breakdown can be monitored with serial measurements of levels of serum potassium, creatine kinase, aldolase, and urine myoglobin. Potential development of rhabdomyolysis can be tracked with levels of creatinine and creatine kinase while the patient receives robust hydration and diuresis. Hepatic and hematologic complications of moderate to severe serotonin syndrome can be screened for with levels of transaminases, bilirubin, and fibrinogen and coagulation studies.

Even if a patient has mild to moderate disease, intravenous fluids should be provided to ensure volume repletion. Benzodiazepines can be useful for sedation and can help improve tachycardia and hypertension. Since blood pressure and heart rate can be labile, great care must be taken to avoid rapid overcorrection. In particular, when hypertension cannot be quelled with sedation, only short-acting antihypertensives should be used so as not to cause or prolong dangerous hypotension. Often hyperthermia can be prevented by calming neuromuscular hyperexcitability with benzodiazepines, yet when fevers develop they should be

Table 75.2 • Comparison of Serotonin Toxicity and Related Toxidromes

Feature	Serotonin Toxicity	Dopamine Deficiency (NMS)	Anticholinergic Toxicity
Onset	12-48 h	Days to weeks	Hours
Duration	12-24 h	Days to weeks	Hours to days
Distinct features	Myoclonus Increased GI motility Hyperreflexia (more pronounced in legs than in arms)	Extrapyramidal signs Bradyreflexia Lead pipe rigidity	Dry skin Urinary retention Decreased bowel sounds
Overlapping features		Hyperthermia Increased tone Diaphoresis Autonomic instability Altered mental state	Hyperthermia Pupillary dilatation Muscle jerks (occasionally) Tachycardia, hypertension Altered mental state

Abbreviations: GI, gastrointestinal tract; NMS, neuroleptic malignant syndrome.

Box 75.2 • Criteria for the Diagnosis of Serotonin Syndrome

The diagnosis of serotonin syndrome requires that a patient meet both of the following criteria:

1. Patient has taken a serotonergic agent
2. Patient has 1 of the following:
   - Spontaneous clonus
   - Inducible clonus *and* either agitation or diaphoresis
   - Ocular clonus *and* either agitation or diaphoresis
   - Tremor *and* hyperreflexia
   - Hypertonia *and* hyperthermia *and* ocular clonus

Modified from Boyer EW, Shannon M. The serotonin syndrome. N Engl J Med. 2005 Mar 17;352(11):1112-20. Errata in: N Engl J Med. 2007 Jun 7;356(23):2437. N Engl J Med. 2009 Oct 22;361(17):1714; used with permission.

managed rigorously. Typical antipyretics such as acetaminophen are less effective in serotonin-induced hyperthermia, in which the fever is generated by myocyte hyperactivity rather than central hypothalamic regulation. Contact, evaporative, and environmental cooling are the mainstays of management for mild or moderate fevers. Persistent fever, especially when accompanied by tachycardia, rigidity, myoclonus, or rhabdomyolysis, may prompt treatment with cyproheptadine, which is usually initiated as a loading dose with a lower maintenance dose every 2 to 4 hours until the fever improves. Patients with a fever of 40°C to 41°C may require treatment with paralysis, intubation, and more aggressive sedation.

Summary

- Serotonin syndrome is a clinical toxidrome due to excess serotonergic activity on the central nervous system and neuromuscular system.
- Features of serotonergic excess may be obscured in patients who also have neurologic injuries and a complicated critical illness.
- Serotonin toxicity exists along a broad spectrum from mild to life-threatening.
- Symptoms of serotonin toxicity gradually start to resolve within 1 to 3 days after stopping therapy with the offending agents; however, consequences of severe or unrecognized toxicity may be more profound and persistent.
- Management of serotonin syndrome is focused on identifying the syndrome, stopping the use of serotonergic drugs, providing supportive care, and quieting neuromuscular excitation with benzodiazepines and often with cyproheptadine.

SUGGESTED READING

Baldo BA. Opioid analgesic drugs and serotonin toxicity (syndrome): mechanisms, animal models, and links to clinical effects. Arch Toxicol. 2018 Aug;92(8):2457–73. Epub 2018 Jun 18.

Boyer EW, Shannon M. The serotonin syndrome. N Engl J Med. 2005 Mar 17;352(11):1112–20. Errata in: N Engl J Med. 2007 Jun 7;356(23):2437. N Engl J Med. 2009 Oct 22;361(17):1714.

Brunton LL, editor. Goodman & Gilman's the pharmacological basis of therapeutics. 12th ed. New York (NY): McGraw-Hill Medical; c2011. 2,084 p.

Haberzettl R, Bert B, Fink H, Fox MA. Animal models of the serotonin syndrome: a systematic review. Behav Brain Res. 2013 Nov 1;256:328–45. Epub 2013 Sep 1.

Iqbal MM, Basil MJ, Kaplan J, Iqbal MT. Overview of serotonin syndrome. Ann Clin Psychiatry. 2012 Nov;24(4):310–8.

Isbister GK, Buckley NA. The pathophysiology of serotonin toxicity in animals and humans: implications for diagnosis and treatment. Clin Neuropharmacol. 2005 Sep-Oct;28(5):205–14.

Klaassen CD, editor. Casarett and Doull's toxicology: the basic science of poisons. 8th ed. New York (NY): McGraw-Hill Education/Medical; c2013. 1,454 p.

Pedavally S, Fugate JE, Rabinstein AA. Serotonin syndrome in the intensive care unit: clinical presentations and precipitating medications. Neurocrit Care. 2014 Aug;21(1):108–13.

Rajan S, Kaas B, Moukheiber E. Movement disorders emergencies. Semin Neurol. 2019 Feb;39(1):125–36. Epub 2019 Feb 11.

Tormoehlen LM, Rusyniak DE. Neuroleptic malignant syndrome and serotonin syndrome. Handb Clin Neurol. 2018;157:663–75.

Wang RZ, Vashistha V, Kaur S, Houchens NW. Serotonin syndrome: preventing, recognizing, and treating it. Cleve Clin J Med. 2016 Nov;83(11):810–7.

76 Neuroleptic Malignant Syndrome and Hyperthermia

J. ROSS RENEW, MD; MONICA MORDECAI, MD

Goals

- Discuss the risk factors for neuroleptic malignant syndrome.
- Recognize the diagnostic criteria that are the hallmark features of neuroleptic malignant syndrome.
- Understand the therapy and supportive care for patients with neuroleptic malignant syndrome.

Introduction

Neuroleptic malignant syndrome (NMS) is an uncommon, potentially fatal reaction to antipsychotic medications. Most cases occur in men between the ages of 20 and 50 because they have the highest proportion of antipsychotic consumption. The prevalence of NMS has been reported as 0.07% to 2.2%, but the published diagnostic criteria for NMS varied widely until the *Diagnostic and Statistical Manual of Mental Disorders* (Fifth Edition) (*DSM-5*) addressed the issue in 2013.

NMS is characterized by a constellation of clinical symptoms and laboratory abnormalities, including hyperthermia, muscle rigidity, and increased serum creatine kinase (CK) levels. Patients may also present with tremor, altered mental status, autonomic dysfunction, and leukocytosis (Box 76.1). The symptoms and clinical signs develop over 1 to 3 days, and patients present with a history of exposure to a neuroleptic agent, although metoclopramide and tricyclic antidepressants have also been implicated because of their antidopaminergic properties.

Pathogenesis of NMS

The pathogenesis of NMS is unclear, although various mechanisms have been proposed. The central dopaminergic theory arose from the finding that injecting dopamine directly into the hypothalamus decreased core temperatures in mammals. Conversely, the blockade of dopamine receptors by neuroleptics may increase core temperature because it disrupts central thermoregulation. Furthermore, the overlap between NMS and malignant hyperthermia (MH) has led to the proposal that NMS patients have similar skeletal muscle defects. Indeed, dantrolene sodium has been used successfully to treat both conditions, and in vitro studies have found similar responses to contractility testing; however, further efforts have not confirmed that NMS patients are susceptible to MH. NMS patients may have a genetic predisposition due to a defect in the sarcolemma, but neuroleptics have also been shown to have direct toxic effects on skeletal muscle. Regardless of the mechanism, NMS carries a mortality of 11%, and acute kidney injury is the strongest predictor of NMS-related death.

Risk Factors for NMS

Although NMS is often described as an idiosyncratic reaction, several risk factors have been described: taking high doses of neuroleptics, taking multiple neuroleptics, instituting large changes in dosing (either increases or abrupt cessation), and using intravenous or intramuscular routes. Dehydration, exposure to high ambient temperature, and serious medical comorbidities have also been implicated, and the existence of genetic susceptibility supports a channelopathy mechanism.

Diagnosis of NMS

When a clinician suspects NMS, a broad evaluation is often necessary to exclude other conditions such as central

Box 76.1 • *DSM-5* Criteria for Neuroleptic Malignant Syndrome

- Temperature
  - Oral temperature >38°C on ≥2 occasions
- Physical examination
  - Rigidity
  - Altered mental status
  - Diaphoresis
  - Urinary incontinence
  - Pallor
- Laboratory testing
  - CK >4× upper limit of reference range
- Hemodynamics
  - HR >25% above baseline
  - SBP or DBP ≥25% above baseline
  - SBP fluctuations ≥25 mm Hg above baseline
  - DBP fluctuations ≥20 mm Hg above baseline
  - RR >50% above baseline

Abbreviations: CK, creatine kinase; DBP, diastolic blood pressure; *DSM-5, Diagnostic and Statistical Manual of Mental Disorders* (Fifth Edition); HR, heart rate; RR, respiratory rate; SBP, systolic blood pressure.

anticholinergic syndrome, MH, infection (including tetanus), and various drug reactions (Box 76.2). In addition to a thorough history and physical examination, appropriate studies may include CK concentrations, white blood cell count, blood cultures, kidney and liver profiles, electroencephalography, urinalysis, thyroid testing, lumbar puncture, and computed tomography. Arterial blood gas analysis typically indicates metabolic acidosis.

Box 76.2. • Differential Diagnosis for Neuroleptic Malignant Syndrome

- Drug reaction
  - Acute lethal catatonia
  - Malignant hyperthermia
  - Lithium toxicity
  - MAOI reaction
  - Neuroleptic-induced heat stroke
  - Central anticholinergic syndrome
  - Serotonin syndrome
- Infection
  - Tetanus
  - Sepsis
- Tumor
  - Cerebral tumor

Abbreviation: MAOI, monoamine oxidase inhibitor.

Treatment of NMS

Treatment of NMS is largely supportive. After use of the offending agent is stopped, neuroleptic levels decrease slowly; neuroleptics are not removed with hemodialysis. The value of other pharmacologic interventions has been debated, and insufficient data are available to definitively establish their efficacy. Nonetheless, bromocriptine mesylate, dantrolene sodium, and benzodiazepines have been used alone or in combination as adjunct therapy to supportive measures in the treatment of NMS. Bromocriptine mesylate is a dopamine agonist that can reverse the centrally mediated effects of hyperthermia, muscle rigidity, and autonomic instability. Dantrolene sodium has also been used, either as a sole treatment or in combination with bromocriptine. The utility of dantrolene supports the notion that NMS and MH overlap pathophysiologically.

Atypical NMS

Atypical NMS has been described when 1 or more of the usual NMS diagnostic criteria are absent. Not all the diagnostic criteria need to be present for the diagnosis. The varied nature of presentation can lead to difficulty with both diagnosis and treatment. One case of atypical NMS was reported after metoclopramide and haloperidol were administered. The patient did not have muscle rigidity but did meet other diagnostic criteria. After treatment with bromocriptine and supportive care, the patient had a good response.

Other Causes of Hyperthermia

As mentioned above, NMS overlaps with other potentially fatal conditions. Patients with MH also present with elevated temperature, rigidity, and increased CK level, but MH occurs after exposure to a triggering anesthetic such as volatile gases or succinylcholine, whereas NMS patients have been exposed to neuroleptic medications. Furthermore, patients with various reactions to other medications can have presentations similar to those of patients with NMS. Central anticholinergic syndrome from atropine poisoning can result in hyperthermia and altered mental status. However, resolution of these and other anticholinergic symptoms after administration of physostigmine helps to differentiate central anticholinergic syndrome from NMS. Monoamine oxidase inhibitor (MAOI) overdose or the use of MAOIs with narcotics or tricyclic antidepressants can lead to an exaggerated sympathetic response that includes delirium and hyperthermia.

Classic heat stroke occurs when the body's thermoregulatory mechanisms are overwhelmed from metabolic and environmental sources. Patients receiving neuroleptic agents are predisposed to hyperthermia because these medications have anticholinergic properties that block sweating and subsequent heat dissipation. This neuroleptic-induced heat stroke can be distinguished from NMS because the patient does not have extrapyramidal symptoms and has been exposed to high ambient temperatures.

Infectious causes of fever and altered mental status must also be addressed because a delay in therapy can have serious consequences. Patients with central nervous system infections such as meningitis generally have abnormal lumbar puncture results and neurologic focality on physical examination.

Serotonin syndrome (SS) involves a constellation of symptoms that overlap with NMS symptoms. However, the 2 conditions are distinguished by muscle rigidity (more frequent and more pronounced in NMS) and myoclonus with hyperreflexia (seen in SS). Patients with either NMS or SS can present with altered mental status, autonomic dysfunction, and increased CK levels.

Indeed, the many causes of hyperthermia necessitate broad initial evaluations. The combination of exposure to neuroleptics, muscle rigidity, hyperthermia, and increased CK levels is suggestive of NMS. The importance of the clinical history and physical examination must be emphasized when working with such diagnostic challenges.

Summary

- The diagnosis of NMS is one of exclusion and typically includes a constellation of symptoms, including hyperthermia, muscle rigidity, altered mental status, increased CK level, autonomic dysfunction, and leukocytosis.
- Patients with NMS or atypical NMS have varied presentations, so both conditions need to be considered when at least 1 of the typical NMS diagnostic criteria is absent.
- Treatment options are largely supportive, but pharmacologic agents to consider include bromocriptine mesylate, dantrolene sodium, and benzodiazepines.

SUGGESTED READING

Adnet P, Lestavel P, Krivosic-Horber R. Neuroleptic malignant syndrome. Br J Anaesth. 2000 Jul;85(1):129–35.

American Psychiatric Association. Diagnostic and statistical manual of mental disorders. 5th ed. Arlington (VA): American Psychiatric Association; c2013. 947 p.

Boss MJ, Diaz-Gomez JL, Koch C. The great masquerader: atypical neuroleptic malignant syndrome after cardiac surgery. J Cardiothorac Vasc Anesth. 2014 Feb;28(1):121–3. Epub 2012 Aug 31.

Denborough MA, Collins SP, Hopkinson KC. Rhabdomyolysis and malignant hyperpyrexia. Br Med J (Clin Res Ed). 1984 Jun 23;288(6434):1878.

Friedman LS, Weinrauch LA, D'Elia JA. Metoclopramide-induced neuroleptic malignant syndrome. Arch Intern Med. 1987 Aug;147(8):1495–7.

Gelenberg AJ, Bellinghausen B, Wojcik JD, Falk WE, Sachs GS. A prospective survey of neuroleptic malignant syndrome in a short-term psychiatric hospital. Am J Psychiatry. 1988 Apr;145(4):517–8.

Hermesh H, Aizenberg D, Lapidot M, Munitz H. Risk of malignant hyperthermia among patients with neuroleptic malignant syndrome and their families. Am J Psychiatry. 1988 Nov;145(11):1431–4.

Keck PE Jr, Pope HG Jr, Cohen BM, McElroy SL, Nierenberg AA. Risk factors for neuroleptic malignant syndrome: a case-control study. Arch Gen Psychiatry. 1989 Oct;46(10):914–8.

Keck PE Jr, Sebastianelli J, Pope HG Jr, McElroy SL. Frequency and presentation of neuroleptic malignant syndrome in a state psychiatric hospital. J Clin Psychiatry. 1989 Sep;50(9):352–5.

Madakasira S. Amoxapine-induced neuroleptic malignant syndrome. DICP. 1989 Jan;23(1):50–1.

Nisijima K. Serotonin syndrome overlapping with neuroleptic malignant syndrome: a case report and approaches for differentially diagnosing the two syndromes. Asian J Psychiatr. 2015 Dec;18:100–1. Epub 2015 Oct 14.

Shalev A, Hermesh H, Munitz H. Mortality from neuroleptic malignant syndrome. J Clin Psychiatry. 1989 Jan;50(1):18–25.

Tse L, Barr AM, Scarapicchia V, Vila-Rodriguez F. Neuroleptic malignant syndrome: a review from a clinically oriented perspective. Curr Neuropharmacol. 2015;13(3):395–406.

van Rensburg R, Decloedt EH. An approach to the pharmacotherapy of neuroleptic malignant syndrome. Psychopharmacol Bull. 2019 Feb 15;49(1):84–91.

Clinical Toxicology: Selected Drugs of Abuse and Chemical and Biological Warfare Agents

MATTHEW D. SZTAJNKRYCER, MD, PhD

Goals

- Describe the clinical presentation of patients who are using selected drugs of abuse.
- Review the clinical management of critically ill patients intoxicated with opioids, stimulants, hallucinogens, or dissociative agents.
- Discuss the clinical management of patients exposed to nerve agents and the risk of secondary contamination.
- Distinguish between the clinical presentations of patients who have anthrax, smallpox, or pneumonic plague.

Selected Drugs of Abuse

Introduction

Approximately 10% of the US population 12 years or older uses illicit drugs. Although illicit drug use is typically considered a disease of the young, substance misuse is also a serious risk for older persons.

Marijuana and Synthetic Cannabinoids

The most commonly used illicit drug is marijuana, which is derived from the dried flowers and leaves of *Cannabis sativa, Cannabis indica,* and *Cannabis ruderalis.* The active ingredient is Δ^9-tetrahydrocannabinol (THC). Sensemilla, derived from the seedless tops of female plants, has the highest THC concentration. Hashish oil is extracted from *Cannabis* with a nonpolar solvent.

Marijuana exerts its effects through the cannabinoid receptors CB1 and CB2. The immediate results of marijuana use are variable psychologic effects, increased heart rate, decreased systemic vascular resistance, decreased airway resistance, and conjunctival injection. Toxic effects include exaggerated physiologic and psychologic effects, decreased coordination, and decreased psychomotor activity. In children, marijuana ingestion is associated with central nervous system (CNS) depression and respiratory depression. After use of marijuana was legalized in Colorado, health authorities reported an increased prevalence of burns (attributed to THC extraction with butane), cyclic vomiting syndrome, and health care visits due to edible product ingestions.

Synthetic cannabinoids (SC) were developed initially as nonopioid analgesics and subsequently as research tools. In 2012, as part of the Synthetic Drug Abuse Prevention Act, 26 SCs were classified as Schedule I agents by the US Drug Enforcement Administration. In contrast to marijuana use, SC use is associated with a serious potential for toxicity, including severe psychomotor agitation, seizures, acute kidney injury, acute stroke, and acute coronary syndrome. At least 25 deaths have been attributed to SCs, especially to newer-generation agents such as ADB-PINACA and ADB-CHMINACA. No specific antidote exists and management is supportive.

Opioids

Classically, the term *opiate* referred to a drug derived from opium, including codeine, morphine, and heroin, and *opioid* referred to naturally occurring or synthetic drugs with opiatelike properties. Although the term *opioid* is used for both groups, this distinction is important in the interpretation of drug screens based on enzyme-linked

Table 77.1 • Typical ELISA-Based Testing and Detection Times for 7 Drugs of Abuse

Drug	Analyte	Detection Time
Amphetamine	Amphetamine	≤24 h
Barbiturates	Secobarbital	18-29 h
Benzodiazepines	Oxazepam	5-6 h
Cannabis	Δ^9-THC	1 d to 3 wk
Cocaine	Benzoylecgonine	2-3 d
Opiates	Morphine	1-3 d
Phencyclidine	Phencyclidine	≤3 d

Abbreviations: ELISA, enzyme-linked immunosorbent assay; THC, tetrahydrocannabinol.

immunosorbent assays (Table 77.1), many of which detect opiates but inconsistently detect opioids.

An opioid abuse epidemic is occurring in the United States. Heroin deaths increased 6-fold from 2001 through 2014, with 10,574 deaths recorded in 2014. Deaths from prescription opioids have quadrupled since 1999, accounting for more than 165,000 deaths from 1999 through 2014. Clinically, opioids cause analgesia, but toxic effects include respiratory depression, CNS depression, and miosis; this triad is commonly referred to as the *opioid toxidrome* (Box 77.1). Acute lung injury may occur, although the cause is unclear. Often associated with naloxone administration (see below), acute lung injury more likely results from opioid-associated hypoventilation and central sympathetic effects and is simply unmasked when spontaneous ventilation returns after naloxone administration. Prolongation of the corrected QT interval and torsades de pointes have been reported, especially after methadone administration, and QRS prolongation, which occurs with tricyclic antidepressant toxicity, may occur after propoxyphene use. Seizures typically occur from hypoxia, although they commonly occur with meperidine, propoxyphene, and tramadol toxicity. Novel synthetic opioids, such as U-47700 and the nonpharmaceutical fentanyls acetylfentanyl and furanylfentanyl, are an increasing concern because their use has resulted in fatal clusters.

Few specific antidotal therapies exist for acute poisoning or for immediately altering the clinical management of the critically ill patient. The exception is naloxone. Administration of naloxone to the unresponsive opioid-intoxicated patient may mitigate the need for airway management. Titration of naloxone is recommended for treatment of an unresponsive patient who is otherwise clinically stable and has a history of long-term opioid use. An initial dose of 0.04 mg is therapeutic without unnecessarily inducing acute opioid withdrawal. If a patient has an inadequate response, the dose may be increased to 10 mg. A continuous infusion of two-thirds the response dose per hour can be initiated to maintain this level of arousal. Certain agents may require naloxone doses that are higher than expected.

Box 77.1 • Selected Chemical Toxidromes

Opioid—heroin, fentanyl
- Respiratory depression
- Central nervous system depression
- Miosis

Sympathomimetic—cocaine, methamphetamine, ethanol withdrawal
- Hypertension
- Tachycardia
- Hyperpyrexia
- Mydriasis
- Delirium or anxiety
- Diaphoresis

Anticholinergic (antimuscarinic)—jimsonweed, belladonna, diphenhydramine[a]
- "Red as a beet" (flushed skin)
- "Dry as a stone" (dry mucous membranes, dry skin)
- "Blind as a bat" (mydriasis)
- "Mad as a hatter" (delirium)
- "Hot as hell" (hyperthermia)

Cholinergic (muscarinic)—organophosphate pesticides, nerve agents
- SLUDGEM mnemonic
  - Salivation
  - Lacrimation
  - Urination
  - Defecation
  - Gastric emptying
  - Miosis
- DUMBELS mnemonic
  - Defecation
  - Urination
  - Miosis
  - Bradycardia
  - Bronchorrhea
  - Emptying (gastric)
  - Lacrimation
  - Salivation

[a] Diphenhydramine, an antihistamine, has potent anticholinergic effects rather than purely antimuscarinic effects.

Stimulants

Stimulants, a broad category of psychoactive substances used for increased alertness and euphoria, include cocaine, methamphetamine, and cathinone derivatives. Cocaine (benzoylmethylecgonine) is a water-soluble alkaloid derived from the plant *Erythroxylon coca*. The crystalline freebase of cocaine, commonly referred to as *crack*, can be smoked because it is heat stable. Coingestion of ethanol results in the production of cocaethylene (benzoylethylecgonine), an active metabolite with a longer duration of action and increased toxicity. Cocaine blocks the reuptake of multiple biogenic amines, including serotonin, dopamine, epinephrine, and norepinephrine.

Methamphetamine is a phenethylamine structurally related to norepinephrine. *Ice* refers to a high-purity, clear crystalline form that is typically smoked. Methamphetamine causes effects by the release of catecholamines (especially dopamine, norepinephrine, and serotonin) from presynaptic nerve terminals, resulting in a hyperadrenergic state.

Synthetic cathinones are derived from khat (*Catha edulis*), a flowering plant native to the Horn of Africa and the Arabian Peninsula. Methylenedioxypyrovalerone (MDPV) (also called bath salts) and α-pyrrolidinopentiophenone (α-PVP) (also called gravel or flakka) are common synthetic cathinones that cause both norepinephrine-dopamine reuptake inhibition and serotonergic effects.

Patients with acute stimulant toxicity present with a sympathomimetic toxidrome (Box 77.1). The presence of diaphoresis may help to distinguish a sympathomimetic toxidrome from an anticholinergic toxidrome. Acute cardiovascular toxicity includes cardiac and noncardiac chest pain, dysrhythmias, vasospasm, and aortic dissection. Cocaine activates the coagulation cascade and impairs clot lysis. Abdominal pain may be due to vasospasm and ischemia. Rhabdomyolysis occurs secondary to psychomotor agitation, as does hyperthermia (Figure 77.1), which may cause multiorgan dysfunction. MDPV toxicity is associated with serotonin syndrome, and unusual compartment syndromes, including the paraspinal musculature, have been reported.

Seizures are common after use of cocaine, especially crack. Other problems described with sympathomimetic use include subarachnoid, intraparenchymal, and intraventricular cerebral hemorrhage; vasospastic and thrombotic infarctions; and transient ischemic attacks. Psychosis is more prominent after methamphetamine use than after cocaine use. Use of synthetic cathinones is associated with a prolonged psychosis, including self-mutilating behaviors, suicidal and homicidal ideation, and episodes of cannibalism. After MDPV use, one-fourth of patients presenting to an emergency department require admission to an intensive care unit for agitation.

Management of acute stimulant toxicity is supportive. Benzodiazepines are considered first-line agents for psychomotor agitation and may be at least as effective as

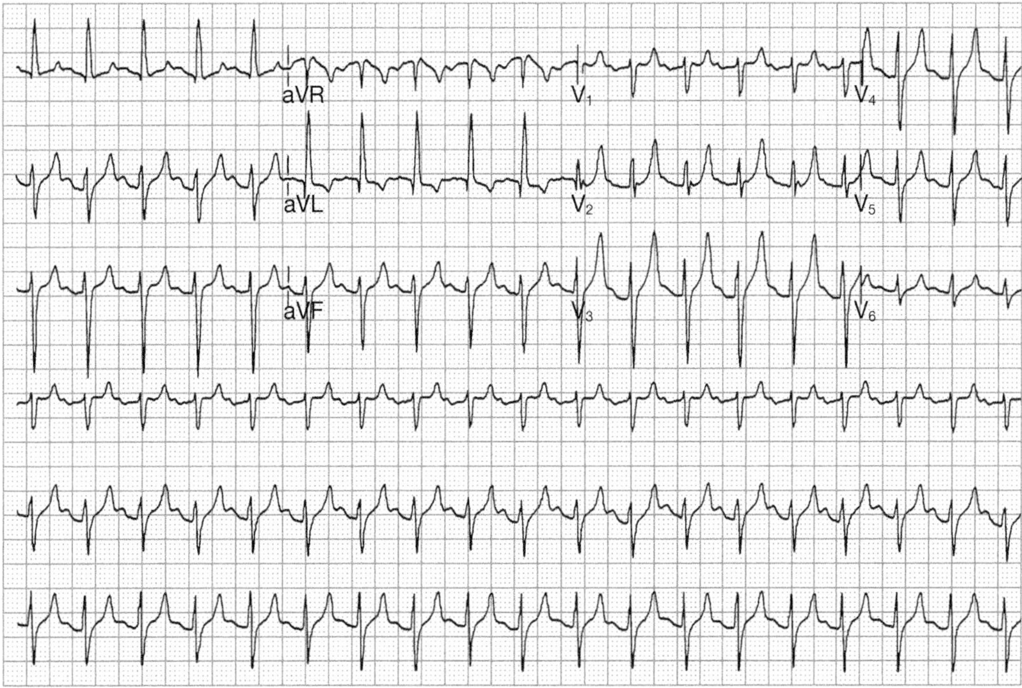

Figure 77.1. Acute Cocaine Toxicity. Electrocardiogram shows tachycardia (heart rate, 143 beats per minute) and QRS widening (126 milliseconds) that are probably the result of cocaine-induced sodium channel blockade. Peaked T waves reflect hyperkalemia (potassium, 6.7 mmol/L) due to psychomotor agitation and rhabdomyolysis.

nitroglycerin for cocaine-associated chest pain. The use of β-adrenergic blocking agents for cocaine toxicity is controversial. Paradoxical hypertension and increased coronary vasospasm have been reported and are thought to result from the loss of β_2-mediated vasodilatation and unopposed α_1-mediated vasoconstriction. The use of β-adrenergic blocking agents should be avoided in patients with suspected cocaine toxicity. Although thrombolytics appear to be safe to use in patients with cocaine-associated myocardial infarction, the value of thrombolytics in acute ischemic stroke is uncertain.

Hallucinogens and Dissociatives

Hallucinogens alter perception of reality without clouding the sensorium. They include phenethylamines, lysergides, and tryptamines. Mood-modifying phenethylamines, such as 3,4-methylenedioxymethamphetamine (MDMA) (also called ecstasy), 2,5-dimethoxy-4-bromophenethylamine (2C-B), and 25I-NBOMe (also called N-Bomb), have more pronounced serotonergic effects than typical phenethylamines. Lysergic acid diethylamide (LSD) is a lysergide. Psilocybin, found in hallucinogenic mushrooms, is a tryptamine.

Dissociative agents produce a sensation of detachment from the environment, typically through antagonism of the *N*-methyl-D-aspartate (NMDA) receptor (eg, phencyclidine and ketamine) or agonism of the opioid κ receptor (eg, ibogaine and *Salvia divinorum*). NMDA-receptor antagonist dissociatives can produce general anesthesia; hallucinogenic effects occur at subdissociative doses.

When hallucinogens are used, acute physiologic effects precede or coincide with the development of psychoactive perceptual changes. The physiologic effects are sympathomimetic and include hyperthermia, tachycardia, hypertension, and diaphoresis. In addition to life-threatening sympathomimetic toxicity, other conditions that may occur are serotonin syndrome, coagulopathy, seizures, and vasoconstriction. Bruxism is common with MDMA use. Profound hyponatremia and subsequent cerebral edema, which is more common in women, may be secondary to serotonin-mediated syndrome of inappropriate secretion of antidiuretic hormone.

NMDA-antagonizing dissociative agents are associated with less pronounced sympathomimetic toxicity. Although rare, respiratory depression has occurred with rapid administration of ketamine. Psychomotor abnormalities are frequently the inciting factor for medical presentation. Neurologic findings include rotatory and vertical nystagmus, ataxia, and altered gait.

Treatment of excessive psychomotor agitation is supportive and involves sedation, temperature management, and prevention of rhabdomyolysis. Because they affect thermoregulation and have proarrhythmogenic and proepileptogenic properties, antipsychotic agents are not considered appropriate first-line agents for drug-induced psychomotor agitation. Use of antipsychotics to manage hallucinogen-induced agitation is associated with hallucinogen-persisting perception disorder.

Internal Concealment of Drugs of Abuse

Concealment with premeditated intent to smuggle large quantities of a substance, typically cocaine or heroin, is termed *body packing*. Packages may cause clinical signs and symptoms resulting from mechanical bowel obstruction. Microperforation may cause severe toxicity, including ischemic bowel if cocaine or other sympathomimetic agents are involved. Sudden cardiovascular collapse has been reported, and intravaginal concealment has resulted in uterine ischemia. Asymptomatic patients should undergo imaging, with either plain radiography or computed tomography, and gastrointestinal tract decontamination with whole-bowel irrigation. Pregnant women have been used for internal concealment to discourage the use of radiographic imaging.

Body stuffing is typically the unplanned ingestion of contraband while being arrested. Occasionally the agent may be concealed in the vagina or rectum. Because the substances are packaged for street sales, they may be poorly wrapped or unwrapped, and multiple agents may be involved. Patients typically become symptomatic within 6 hours, although the packaging may delay the effects.

Chemical and Biological Warfare Agents

Introduction

Chemical and biological agents have been used in warfare for millennia. Chemical weapons are regulated under the 1993 Chemical Weapons Convention. Classic chemical weapons include nerve agents, vesicants, blood agents (cellular asphyxiants [eg, cyanide]), choking agents (pulmonary toxicity [eg, phosgene and chlorine]), and incapacitating agents (nonlethal [eg, 3-quinuclidinyl benzilate]) (Figure 77.2A). However, many other substances, including toxic industrial chemicals, may cause mass casualties (Figure 77.2B). The Centers for Disease Control and Prevention (CDC) classifies biological warfare agents into Category A, B, or C. Category A agents are of greatest concern.

Vesicants

Also known as *blister agents*, vesicants include sulfur mustard derivatives (also called H, HS, and HD) and the arsenical lewisite (also called L). Although cellular toxicity occurs rapidly after exposure to mustard agents, clinical effects may be delayed several hours. In contrast, lewisite exposure causes immediate symptoms. Vesicants

A

The Box

Nerve agents

Botulism

Vesicants

Cyanide

Plague

Viral hemorrhagic fever

Anthrax

Smallpox

Incapacitants

Pulmonary agents

Tularemia

B

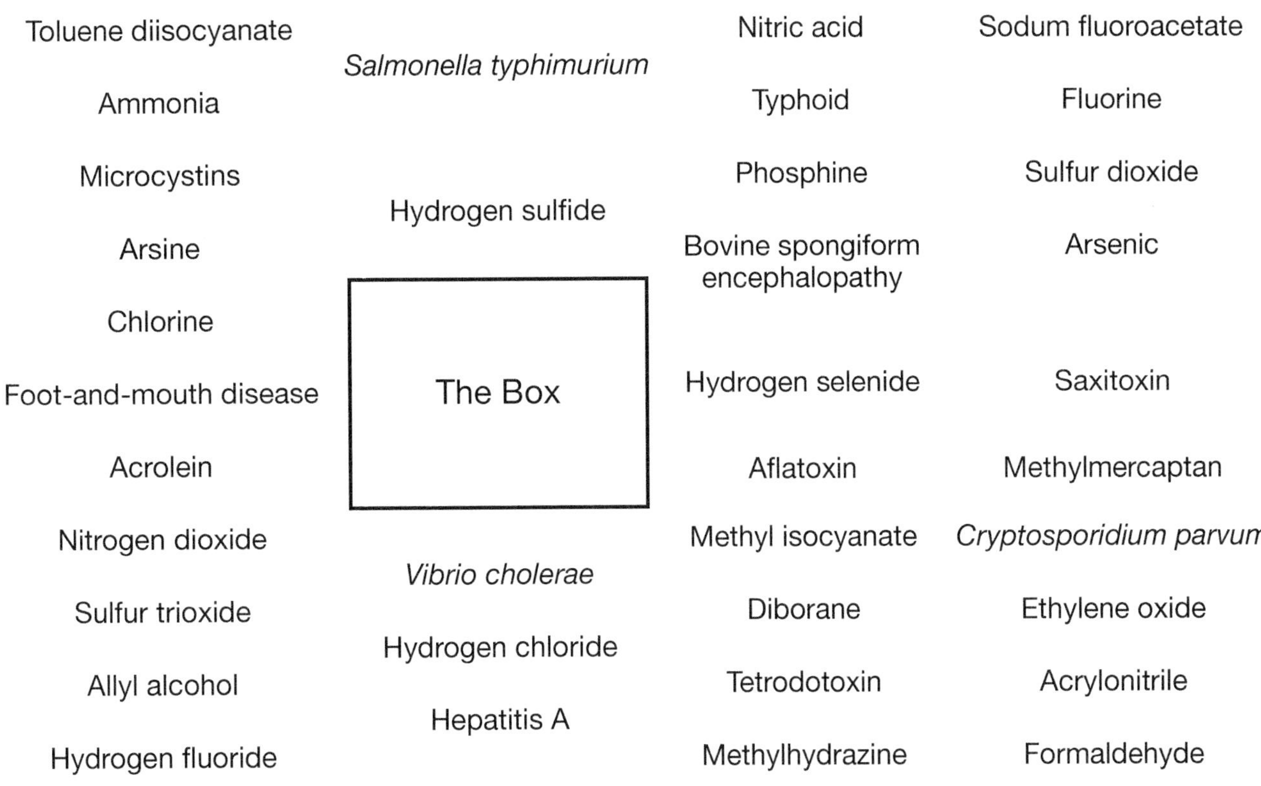

Figure 77.2. Chemical and Biological Agents: Thinking Outside the Box. A, Category 1 chemical agents and Category A biological agents and diseases are of high concern. B, Many other more common substances, however, may cause mass casualties or fatalities.

primarily exert toxic effects on the skin, eyes, and lungs; lewisite causes additional systemic toxicity from arsenic compounds.

Blistering occurs with exposure to 10 mcg liquid mustard agent; the median lethal dose (LD_{50}) is 100 mg/kg, which is equivalent to involvement of 20% of the total body surface area. A patient presenting with burns covering 50% of the total body surface area would have received a dose equivalent to an LD_{50} of about 2.5 and, in a mass casualty event, would typically be deemed *expectant* (ie, not expected to survive).

Management is primarily supportive, focusing on infection prevention and aggressive pulmonary hygiene. Systemic toxicity due to lewisite can be treated with British antilewisite (BAL). Skin decontamination within 1 to 2 minutes is the only effective means of mitigating subsequent tissue injury. Vesicant injuries are often described as being analogous to thermal burns, and fluid resuscitation is managed according to burn replacement formulas; however, patients with vesicant injuries lose less fluid than patients with thermal burns, so the use of burn formulas for fluid therapy results in overresuscitation and clinical decompensation.

Nerve Agents

Of the classic chemical agents, the most toxic include tabun (GA), sarin (GB), soman (GD), and VX. Nerve agents cause toxicity by inhibiting the enzyme acetylcholinesterase (AChE), resulting in acetylcholine accumulation and continued stimulation of the target organ. Initially reversible, AChE inhibition eventually becomes permanent through a process called *aging*. The aging period is relatively long, but exposure to GD is unique in that aging may occur in less than 2 minutes.

Nerve agents affect organs that have cholinergic receptors, resulting in muscarinic, nicotinic, and CNS toxicity. Patients with muscarinic toxicity present with a cholinergic toxidrome (Box 77.1). Skeletal muscle nicotinic effects include fasciculations, weakness, and flaccid paralysis; ganglionic effects include tachycardia and hypertension. CNS toxicity causes seizures and coma.

Initial management of nerve agent casualties should focus on decontamination and staff protection. Volatile nerve agents have the potential to off-gas and secondarily contaminate health care providers. Specific antidotal therapy for nerve agent toxicity includes atropine and oximes. Atropine, which is effective against muscarinic symptoms, is titrated with the goal of decreasing pulmonary secretions and ventilatory resistance rather than heart rate or pupillary size. Doses of 10 to 20 mg may be required in the first few hours. Oximes, such as pralidoxime chloride (2-PAM), restore AChE activity before aging begins; the effects are most noticeable in organs with nicotinic receptors. In the prehospital or mass casualty setting, intramuscular autoinjectors containing both atropine and oximes can be rapidly administered. In the hospital, oximes are best administered by intravenous infusion. The neuromuscular blocking agents succinylcholine and mivacurium should be used with caution because of nerve agent–induced plasma cholinesterase inhibition.

Category A Biological Warfare Agents

The CDC classifies 6 biological agents and diseases in category A: anthrax (*Bacillus anthracis*), plague (*Yersinia pestis*), tularemia (*Francisella tularensis*), variola major and variola minor (smallpox viruses), viral hemorrhagic fevers (eg, filoviruses and arenaviruses), and botulism (*Clostridium botulinum* toxin). After a biological warfare attack, the disease pattern is expected to differ from a naturally occurring epidemic. Attack indicators include a compressed infection curve, a high attack rate (lower attack rates among persons working indoors), predominantly respiratory signs and symptoms in affected persons, and increased numbers of sick or dead animals.

The name *anthrax* (from the Greek word for *coal*) reflects the black necrotic eschar that forms with cutaneous anthrax. The binary toxins, edema toxin and lethal toxin, each contain protective antigen and are responsible for causing anthrax-related morbidity and death. Of the 3 clinical syndromes that occur (cutaneous anthrax, gastrointestinal anthrax, and inhalational anthrax), inhalational anthrax causes the greatest concern in biological warfare events. After an incubation period of 1 to 6 days, influenzalike illness (ILI) develops; in the next 24 to 36 hours, rapid decompensation, septic shock, and death occur. Hemorrhagic meningitis develops in 50% of patients. The hallmark findings on chest radiography are a widened mediastinum (due to lymphadenopathy) and a lack of infiltrates.

Patients with plague characteristically have bubonic, primary septicemic, or pneumonic plague. After an incubation period of 2 to 3 days, patients with pneumonic plague have a productive cough with bloody sputum, and shock and frequently disseminated intravascular coagulation develop; chest radiography shows evidence of bronchopneumonia.

Smallpox lesions are similar to those of varicella, especially in the early stages of the disease. After an incubation period of 16 days, ILI symptoms develop; several days later, a centrifugal rash develops on the face and extremities. The rash becomes pustular over the next week, gradually extending centrally, although the lesions remain more abundant on the face and extremities, which may help to distinguish smallpox from varicella. In contrast to varicella, smallpox lesions are synchronous in development. Pustules develop into scabs, which subsequently separate from the body, heralding the loss of infectivity.

Pneumonic plague, smallpox, and the viral hemorrhagic fevers all pose a secondary transmission hazard. Owing to delays in presentation, decontamination is not typically required. Management predominantly involves supportive care and rapid antibiotic administration, although biological warfare stocks may have been genetically modified for antibiotic resistance. Vaccines exist for anthrax and smallpox, and research on a vaccine for Ebola virus disease is in progress. A monoclonal antibody against the *B anthracis* protective antigen, raxibacumab, has been approved by the US Food and Drug Administration under the Animal Rule.

Summary

- Approximately 10% of the US population 12 years or older uses illicit drugs.
- Knowledge of clinical toxidromes may permit rapid recognition of general classes of toxins but not identification of specific agents.
- Antidotal therapy for drugs of abuse is limited, with the exception of naloxone for opioid toxicity.
- The primary focus in caring for a critically ill, intoxicated patient is to provide supportive care with airway management and maintenance of hemodynamic stability.
- Deliberate chemical releases, especially those involving classic chemical warfare agents, pose a secondary contamination risk to emergency medical responders and other health care providers.

SUGGESTED READING

Adalja AA, Toner E, Inglesby TV. Clinical management of potential bioterrorism-related conditions. N Engl J Med. 2015 Mar 5;372(10):954–62.

Baumann BM, Perrone J, Hornig SE, Shofer FS, Hollander JE. Randomized, double-blind, placebo-controlled trial of diazepam, nitroglycerin, or both for treatment of patients with potential cocaine-associated acute coronary syndromes. Acad Emerg Med. 2000 Aug;7(8):878–85.

Borek HA, Holstege CP. Hyperthermia and multiorgan failure after abuse of "bath salts" containing 3,4-methylenedioxypyrovalerone. Ann Emerg Med. 2012 Jul;60(1):103–5. Epub 2012 Mar 3.

Boyer EW. Management of opioid analgesic overdose. N Engl J Med. 2012 Jul 12;367(2):146–55.

Breman JG, Henderson DA. Diagnosis and management of smallpox. N Engl J Med. 2002 Apr 25;346(17):1300–8. Epub 2002 Mar 28.

Center for Behavioral Health Statistics and Quality. Behavioral health trends in the United States: results from the 2014 National Survey on Drug Use and Health [Internet]. Washington (DC): Substance Abuse and Mental Health Services Administration. (HHS Publication No. SMA 15–4927, NSDUH Series H-50). Available from: https://www.samhsa.gov/data/sites/default/files/NSDUH-FRR1-2014/NSDUH-FRR1-2014.pdf.

Center for Substance Abuse Treatment. Substance abuse among older adults [Internet]. Treatment Improvement Protocol (TIP) Series, No. 26. HHS Publication No. (SMA) 12-3918. Rockville (MD): Substance Abuse and Mental Health Services Administration, 1998. Available from: http://integratedrecovery.org/wp-content/uploads/2010/08/TIP26-SA.and_.Older_.Adults.pdf.

Centers for Disease Control and Prevention. Prescription opioid overdose data [Internet]. Atlanta (GA): CDC [cited 2016 Sep 29]. Available from: http://www.cdc.gov/drugoverdose/data/overdose.html.

Cordero DR, Medina C, Helfgott A. Cocaine body packing in pregnancy. Ann Emerg Med. 2006 Sep;48(3):323–5. Epub 2006 May 2.

Costanzi S, Machado JH, Mitchell M. Nerve agents: what they are, how they work, how to counter them. ACS Chem Neurosci. 2018 May 16;9(5):873–85. Epub 2018 Apr 25.

Derlet RW, Heischober B. Methamphetamine: stimulant of the 1990s? West J Med. 1990 Dec;153(6):625–8.

Dixon TC, Meselson M, Guillemin J, Hanna PC. Anthrax. N Engl J Med. 1999 Sep 9;341(11):815–26.

Duberstein JL, Kaufman DM. A clinical study of an epidemic of heroin intoxication and heroin-induced pulmonary edema. Am J Med. 1971 Dec;51(6):704–14.

Farah R, Farah R. Ecstasy (3,4-methylenedioxymethamphetamine)-induced inappropriate antidiuretic hormone secretion. Pediatr Emerg Care. 2008 Sep;24(9):615–7.

Farooq MU, Bhatt A, Patel M. Neurotoxic and cardiotoxic effects of cocaine and ethanol. J Med Toxicol. 2009 Sep;5(3):134–8.

Gold LH, Geyer MA, Koob GF. Neurochemical mechanisms involved in behavioral effects of amphetamines and related designer drugs. NIDA Res Monogr. 1989;94:101–26.

Goldfrank L, Weisman RS, Errick JK, Lo MW. A dosing nomogram for continuous infusion intravenous naloxone. Ann Emerg Med. 1986 May;15(5):566–70.

Green SM, Clark R, Hostetler MA, Cohen M, Carlson D, Rothrock SG. Inadvertent ketamine overdose in children: clinical manifestations and outcome. Ann Emerg Med. 1999 Oct;34(4 Pt 1):492–7.

Hine CH, Wright JA, Allison DJ, Stephens BG, Pasi A. Analysis of fatalities from acute narcotism in a major urban area. J Forensic Sci. 1982 Apr;27(2):372–84.

Hoffman RS, Hollander JE. Thrombolytic therapy and cocaine-induced myocardial infarction. Am J Emerg Med. 1996 Nov;14(7):693–5.

Holland RW 3rd, Marx JA, Earnest MP, Ranniger S. Grand mal seizures temporally related to cocaine use: clinical and diagnostic features. Ann Emerg Med. 1992 Jul;21(7):772–6.

Klock JC, Boerner U, Becker CE. Coma, hyperthermia, and bleeding associated with massive LSD overdose, a report of eight cases. Clin Toxicol. 1975;8(2):191–203.

Kugelmass AD, Oda A, Monahan K, Cabral C, Ware JA. Activation of human platelets by cocaine. Circulation. 1993 Sep;88(3):876–83.

Leikin JB, Krantz AJ, Zell-Kanter M, Barkin RL, Hryhorczuk DO. Clinical features and management of intoxication due to hallucinogenic drugs. Med Toxicol Adverse Drug Exp. 1989 Sep-Oct;4(5):324–50.

Levine M, Levitan R, Skolnik A. Compartment syndrome after "bath salts" use: a case series. Ann Emerg Med. 2013 Apr;61(4):480–3. Epub 2013 Jan 12.

Lozier MJ, Boyd M, Stanley C, Ogilvie L, King E, Martin C, et al. Acetyl fentanyl, a novel fentanyl analog, causes

14 overdose deaths in Rhode Island, March-May 2013. J Med Toxicol. 2015 Jun;11(2):208–17.

Macnab A, Anderson E, Susak L. Ingestion of cannabis: a cause of coma in children. Pediatr Emerg Care. 1989 Dec;5(4):238–9.

Martin JA, Campbell A, Killip T, Kotz M, Krantz MJ, Kreek MJ, et al; Substance Abuse and Mental Health Services Administration. QT interval screening in methadone maintenance treatment: report of a SAMHSA expert panel. J Addict Dis. 2011 Oct;30(4):283–306. Erratum in: J Addict Dis. 2012 Jan;31(1):91.

Martin-Schild S, Albright KC, Misra V, Philip M, Barreto AD, Hallevi H, et al. Intravenous tissue plasminogen activator in patients with cocaine-associated acute ischemic stroke. Stroke. 2009 Nov;40(11):3635–7. Epub 2009 Sep 10.

McCord J, Jneid H, Hollander JE, de Lemos JA, Cercek B, Hsue P, et al; American Heart Association Acute Cardiac Care Committee of the Council on Clinical Cardiology. Management of cocaine-associated chest pain and myocardial infarction: a scientific statement from the American Heart Association Acute Cardiac Care Committee of the Council on Clinical Cardiology. Circulation. 2008 Apr 8;117(14):1897–907. Epub 2008 Mar 17.

Migone TS, Subramanian GM, Zhong J, Healey LM, Corey A, Devalaraja M, et al. Raxibacumab for the treatment of inhalational anthrax. N Engl J Med. 2009 Jul 9;361(2):135–44.

Monte AA, Bronstein AC, Cao DJ, Heard KJ, Hoppe JA, Hoyte CO, et al. An outbreak of exposure to a novel synthetic cannabinoid. N Engl J Med. 2014 Jan 23;370(4):389–90.

Monte AA, Zane RD, Heard KJ. The implications of marijuana legalization in Colorado. JAMA. 2015 Jan 20;313(3):241–2.

Moritz ML, Kalantar-Zadeh K, Ayus JC. Ecstacy-associated hyponatremia: why are women at risk? Nephrol Dial Transplant. 2013 Sep;28(9):2206–9. Epub 2013 Jun 26.

Mugele J, Nanagas KA, Tormoehlen LM. Serotonin syndrome associated with MDPV use: a case report. Ann Emerg Med. 2012 Jul;60(1):100-2. Epub 2012 Jan 10.

National Institute on Drug Abuse. National survey of drug use and health [Internet]. Bethesda (MD): National Institute on Drug Abuse: Advancing Addiction Science [cited 2016 Sep 29]. Available from: https://www.drugabuse.gov/national-survey-drug-use-health.

Nozaki H, Hori S, Shinozawa Y, Fujishima S, Takuma K, Sagoh M, et al. Secondary exposure of medical staff to sarin vapor in the emergency room. Intensive Care Med. 1995 Dec;21(12):1032-5.

Okumura T, Suzuki K, Fukuda A, Kohama A, Takasu N, Ishimatsu S, et al. The Tokyo subway sarin attack: disaster management, Part 1: community emergency response. Acad Emerg Med. 1998 Jun;5(6):613-7.

Richardt A, Hulseweh B, Niemeyer B, Sabath F, editors. CBRN protection: managing the threat of chemical, biological, radioactive and nuclear weapons. Weinheim (Germany): Wiley-VCH Verlag GmbH; c2013. 514 p.

Schwartz MD, Trecki J, Edison LA, Steck AR, Arnold JK, Gerona RR. A common source outbreak of severe delirium associated with exposure to the novel synthetic cannabinoid ADB-PINACA. J Emerg Med. 2015 May;48(5):573-80. Epub 2015 Feb 26.

Sener EB, Ustun E, Kocamanoglu S, Tur A. Prolonged apnea following succinylcholine administration in undiagnosed acute organophosphate poisoning. Acta Anaesthesiol Scand. 2002 Sep;46(8):1046-8.

Sidell FR, Urbanetti JS, Smith WJ, Hurst CG. Vesicants. In: Sidell FR, Takafuji ET, Franz DR, editors. Medical aspects of chemical and biological warfare. Washington (DC): Borden Institute, Walter Reed Army Medical Center; Falls Church (VA): Office of the Surgeon General, United States Army, c1997. (Textbook of military medicine. Part I: warfare, weaponry, and the casualty; vol. 3).

Sidney S. Cardiovascular consequences of marijuana use. J Clin Pharmacol. 2002 Nov;42(11 Suppl):64S-70S.

Tashkin DP. Airway effects of marijuana, cocaine, and other inhaled illicit agents. Curr Opin Pulm Med. 2001 Mar;7(2):43-61.

Tomassoni AJ, French RN, Walter FG. Toxic industrial chemicals and chemical weapons: exposure, identification, and management by syndrome. Emerg Med Clin North Am. 2015 Feb;33(1):13-36. Epub 2014 Nov 15.

Traub SJ, Hoffman RS, Nelson LS. Body packing: the internal concealment of illicit drugs. N Engl J Med. 2003 Dec 25;349(26):2519-26.

Waldhoer M, Bartlett SE, Whistler JL. Opioid receptors. Annu Rev Biochem. 2004;73:953-90.

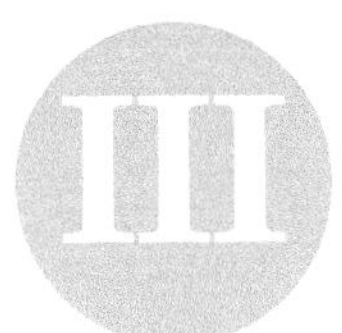

Questions and Answers

Abbreviations Used

4F-PCC 4-factor prothrombin complex concentrate
5-HT 5-hydroxytryptamine
ABC airway, breathing, and circulation
ABCDE airway, breathing, circulation, disability, and exposure
ABG arterial blood gas
ACCM American College of Critical Care Medicine
ACLS advanced cardiovascular life support
ACS acute coronary syndrome
ADAMTS13 a disintegrin and metalloprotease with a thrombospondin type 1 motif, member 13
AI adrenal insufficiency
AIN allergic interstitial nephritis
AKI acute kidney injury
AMPLE allergies, medications, past illness, last meal, events
ANC absolute neutrophil count
aPTT activated partial thromboplastin time
α-PVP α-pyrrolidinopentiophenone
ARDS acute respiratory distress syndrome
AT antithrombin
ATN acute tubular necrosis
AV atrioventricular
BNP brain natriuretic peptide
BP blood pressure
bpm beats per minute
CABG coronary artery bypass graft
CIRCI critical illness–related corticosteroid insufficiency
CK creatine kinase
CKD chronic kidney disease
CK-MB creatine kinase MB
Cl^- chloride
CNS central nervous system
COPD chronic obstructive pulmonary disease
CORTICUS Corticosteroid Therapy of Septic Shock
CPB cardiopulmonary bypass
CPR cardiopulmonary resuscitation
CT computed tomography
CVP central venous pressure
D5W 5% dextrose in water
DI diabetes insipidus
DIC disseminated intravascular coagulation
DNase deoxyribonuclease
DOAC direct oral anticoagulant
DVT deep vein thrombosis
ECG electrocardiography
ECMO extracorporeal membrane oxygenation
ED emergency department
$ETCO_2$ end-tidal carbon dioxide
FAST focused assessment with sonography in trauma
FDPs fibrin degradation products
FeNa fractional excretion of sodium
FIO_2 fraction of inspired oxygen
GCS Glasgow Coma Scale
HbA_{1c} hemoglobin A_{1c}
HCO_3^- bicarbonate
HELLP hemolysis, elevated liver enzymes, low platelet count
HIT heparin-induced thrombocytopenia
HPA hypothalamic-pituitary-adrenal
HR heart rate
ICD implantable cardioverter-defibrillator
ICU intensive care unit
IGF-1 insulinlike growth factor 1
IIT intensive insulin therapy
INR international normalized ratio
ITP idiopathic thrombocytopenic purpura
IV intravenous
IVC inferior vena cava
LMWH low-molecular-weight heparin

LVAD	left ventricular assist device
MAP	mean arterial pressure
MCA	middle cerebral artery
MDMA	3,4-methylenedioxymethamphetamine
MI	myocardial infarction
MIST1	First Multicenter Intrapleural Sepsis Trial
MRI	magnetic resonance imaging
MRSA	methicillin-resistant *Staphyloccocus aureus*
MSSA	methicillin-susceptible *Staphylococcus aureus*
NA	not applicable
Na$^+$	sodium
NETs	neutrophil extracellular traps
NICE-SUGAR	Normoglycemia in Intensive Care Evaluation—Survival Using Glucose Algorithm Regulation
NMS	neuroleptic malignant syndrome
NSE	neuron-specific enolase
NSTEMI	non–ST-segment elevation myocardial infarction
NYHA	New York Heart Association
OHCA	out-of-hospital cardiac arrest
PAH	pulmonary arterial hypertension
PCP	phencyclidine hydrochloride
PE	pulmonary embolism
PEEP	positive end-expiratory pressure
PFO	patent foramen ovale
PH	pulmonary hypertension
PRES	posterior reversible encephalopathy syndrome
PT	prothrombin time
ROSC	return of spontaneous circulation
SIADH	syndrome of inappropriate secretion of antidiuretic hormone
SNRI	serotonin-norepinephrine reuptake inhibitors
SOFA	Sequential Organ-Failure Assessment
Spo_2	oxygen saturation by pulse oximetry
SSRI	selective serotonin reuptake inhibitor
SUN	serum urea nitrogen
TBSA	total body surface area
TCA	tricyclic antidepressant
TF	tissue factor
tPA	tissue plasminogen activator
TPE	therapeutic plasma exchange
TPN	total parenteral nutrition
TTM	targeted temperature management
TTP	thrombotic thrombocytopenic purpura
UFH	unfractionated heparin
VA ECMO	venoarterial extracorporeal membrane oxygenation
VA	venoarterial
VKA	vitamin K antagonist
VV	venovenous
WBC	white blood cell

Questions

Multiple Choice (choose the best answer)

Pulmonary Disorders

III.1. Which of the following is *not* involved in the pathophysiology of ARDS?
- a. Reactive oxygen species
- b. Surfactant dysfunction
- c. Tumor necrosis factor
- d. Eosinophils

III.2. Which of the following is appropriate for management of refractory hypoxemia?
- a. Inhaled nitric oxide
- b. Prone ventilation
- c. Airway pressure release ventilation
- d. High-frequency oscillatory ventilation

III.3. Which of the following is *not* a known cause of ARDS?
- a. Pancreatitis
- b. Aspiration
- c. Intracranial hemorrhage
- d. Sepsis

III.4. Which of the following is *not* a physiologic alteration in ARDS?
- a. Decreased lung compliance
- b. Ventilation-perfusion mismatch
- c. Intrapulmonary shunt
- d. Decreased dead space ventilation

III.5. Which of the following has *no* benefit in the management of ARDS?
- a. Neuromuscular blockade
- b. Glucocorticoids
- c. Conservative fluid management
- d. Surfactant

III.6. A 52-year-old man with no relevant medical history comes to the ED reporting dyspnea and chest pain. On physical examination he has tachycardia (HR 117 bpm) and low oxygen saturation in room air (89%). A chest radiograph is normal, and an ECG showed only sinus tachycardia with no ischemic changes. He has a previous history of CKD and allergy to intravenous contrast media. What should you obtain next?
- a. Ventilation-perfusion scan
- b. CT angiogram
- c. Lower extremity ultrasonogram
- d. Serum D-dimer level

III.7. If the patient described in the previous question has acute kidney failure with CKD and an elevated D-dimer level, what is the most appropriate next diagnostic test for identifying PE?
- a. Ventilation-perfusion scanning
- b. Lower extremity ultrasonography
- c. CT angiography
- d. No further testing is needed; begin anticoagulation for PE.

III.8. If a ventilation-perfusion scan is indeterminate, CT pulmonary angiography is often pursued with caution. If a segmental PE is found for which the patient is symptomatic, for how long should the patient undergo anticoagulation treatment?
- a. 6 months
- b. 12 months
- c. Indefinitely
- d. More information is needed.

III.9. A 49-year-old healthy man presents to the ED with shortness of breath and chest pain. His Wells score is 5. CT angiography shows a large saddle PE. While he is in the CT scanner, he becomes hemodynamically unstable and his systolic BP decreases to 60 mm Hg. What is the most appropriate therapy for this PE?
- a. Intravenous heparin drip
- b. Systemic thrombolysis with tPA

c. Ultrasound-assisted catheter-directed thrombolysis
d. Immediate placement of an IVC filter

III.10. A 73-year-old man had a provoked PE after prolonged immobilization during a recent flight overseas. He presents for follow-up 3 months after beginning treatment with LMWH. He reports right calf pain and concedes that he stopped LMWH therapy 1 month ago because he was beginning to feel better. He is worried, however, because he has been reading online and now thinks that he might need an IVC filter. On physical examination he has a positive Homans sign. What should you tell him?
a. He will probably need an IVC soon because a DVT has developed.
b. He should switch to a DOAC for 6 months because it would have better efficacy with concurrent PE and DVT.
c. He has not been receiving anticoagulation therapy long enough to conclude that anticoagulation has failed, but he should undergo compression ultrasonography to assess for DVT.
d. He should receive LMWH for 1 year.

III.11. A 22-year-old college student presents to the ED with dyspnea, wheezing, and chest tightness. He has a history of asthma and reports adhering to a regimen of twice-daily use of a corticosteroid inhaler (he does not recall its name). His housemate, who provides the history because the patient is dyspneic, acquired a cat 1 week ago, which is when the patient increased his use of albuterol (18 puffs in the past 24 hours). He could not sleep the past night. On examination, he is mildly hypertensive (BP 150/85 mm Hg) and tachycardic (HR 105 bpm and regular). He appears to be in mild respiratory distress, drowsy but verbally arousable, oriented, and behaving appropriately. Breathing is labored, with visible use of accessory muscles and a respiratory rate of 30 breaths per minute. He does not have pulsus paradoxus or thoracoabdominal paradox. Auscultation is notable for quiet, shallow respirations, with minimal expiratory wheezing. A medical student ordered a chest radiograph, which shows clear but hyperinflated lungs, and a room air ABG analysis. The medical student recommends a corticosteroid pack, albuterol nebulization, a dose of lorazepam, and ceftriaxone with discharge instructions to follow-up with his asthma physician in 2 days. You disagree with the medical student. Which of the following ABG results could represent impending respiratory failure?
a. pH 7.38, $Paco_2$ 43 mm Hg, Pao_2 74 mm Hg
b. pH 7.48, $Paco_2$ 30 mm Hg, Pao_2 95 mm Hg
c. pH 7.48, $Paco_2$ 30 mm Hg, Pao_2 60 mm Hg
d. pH 7.49, $Paco_2$ 32 mm Hg, Pao_2 62 mm Hg

III.12. The college student described in the preceding question became progressively more obtunded, bradycardic, and hypoxic and was urgently intubated. Endotracheal intubation was performed by the ED physician without apparent complications, and the patient was administered IV methylprednisolone and continuous albuterol nebulization. He was transferred to the ICU. The critical care fellow, who received a call about the patient's progressive hypotension 30 minutes after intubation, finds that the patient is breathing faster than the set ventilator rate of 12 breaths per minute. The flow-time ventilator waveform is shown in Figure III.Q12.

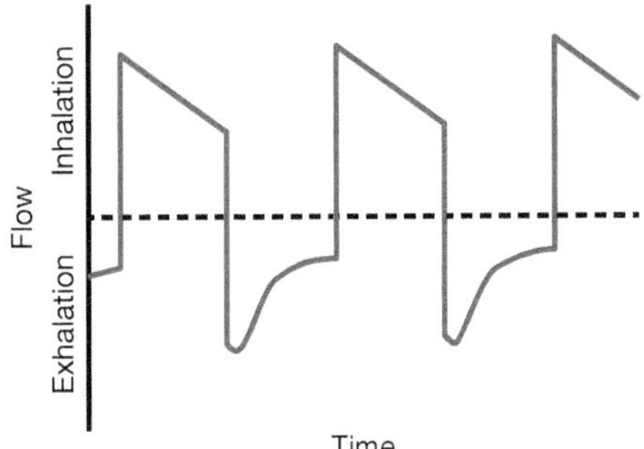

Figure III.Q12.

Which of the following interventions is *least* likely to be required to correct the patient's hypotension?
a. Needle decompression of the chest
b. Disconnecting the endotracheal tube from the ventilator
c. Reducing the inspiration to expiration ratio from 1:1 to 1:3
d. The medical student was right. The patient has septic shock from a cat scratch and requires vasopressors and antibiotics immediately.

III.13. Which of the following statements correctly describes pharmacologic management of COPD in a patient in the neurocritical care unit?
a. For severe but not life-threatening COPD exacerbation, the frequency of short-acting bronchodilators should be increased.
b. Use of an inhaled corticosteroid in combination with an inhaled long-acting β-agonist is superior to use of an inhaled corticosteroid alone in patients who have COPD and are in stable condition.
c. Acute exacerbation of COPD must be treated with a systemic corticosteroid for 10 to 14 days.
d. Systemic corticosteroid therapy greatly benefits patients who are receiving mechanical ventilation during an acute exacerbation of COPD.

III.14. A 67-year-old man presented with MCA infarction. His initial GCS score was 2, and he was intubated and administered mechanical ventilation in the ED. Figure III.Q14 shows his initial ventilator flows and pressure waveforms before he was transported to the neurocritical care unit, where he became progressively and profoundly hypotensive and had arrhythmias.

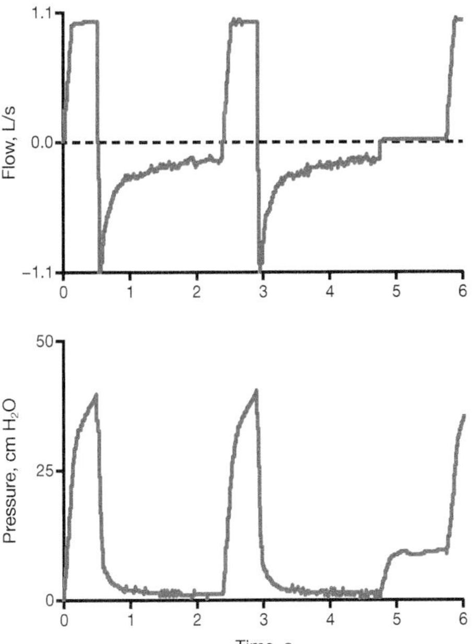

Figure III.Q14.

He was receiving volume assist-control mode ventilation with a tidal volume of 500 mL and a constant inspiratory flow rate of 50 L/min. He has a history of hypertension, atrial fibrillation, diabetes mellitus, peripheral artery disease, and COPD. What is the most appropriate first management step?
a. Disconnect the ventilator for 30 seconds.
b. Extubate the patient and change to an oxygen mask for ventilation.
c. Start chest compressions.
d. Return the patient to the ED for an urgent chest radiograph.

III.15. A 54-year-old man was admitted to the ICU with myasthenic crisis. At admission, the patient had right basilar infiltrates suggestive of aspiration pneumonia. On hospitalization day 5, bedside ultrasonography showed evidence of a moderately large multiloculated pleural effusion (500-750 mL). Diagnostic and therapeutic thoracentesis was performed, and 100 mL of straw-colored fluid was removed. Results of fluid analysis were pH 7.15, lactate dehydrogenase 350 U/L, protein 5 mg/dL, cholesterol 75 mg/dL, and WBC count notable for 10 cells/mcL with predominant neutrophilia. Given concern for an infectious process in the pleural space, a small-bore (10F) pigtail catheter was inserted into the pleural space. Over the next 48 hours, approximately 75 mL of fluid drained from the chest tube. Bedside ultrasonography allowed confirmation of the persistence of a moderately sized, multiloculated pleural effusion. What course of action should be recommended?

a. Broad-spectrum antibiotics
b. Antibiotics and replacing the chest tube with a larger 16F pigtail catheter
c. Antibiotics and instilling tPA through the pigtail catheter
d. Antibiotics and instilling tPA and DNase

III.16. A 65-year-old woman was admitted to the ICU with embolic cerebrovascular accident. The hospital course was complicated by aspiration, and subsequent ARDS. You are called to the patient's bedside to evaluate a high peak pressure alarm. The ventilator settings for volume control are respiratory rate 16 breaths per minute, tidal volume 400 mL, PEEP 7 cm H_2O, and F_{IO_2} 80%. Peak pressure is 45 mm Hg, and plateau pressure is 40 mm Hg. Concerned about a pneumothorax, you perform a limited thoracic ultrasonographic examination to assess for the presence of a pneumothorax. Two-dimensional and M-mode images are shown in Figure III.Q16.

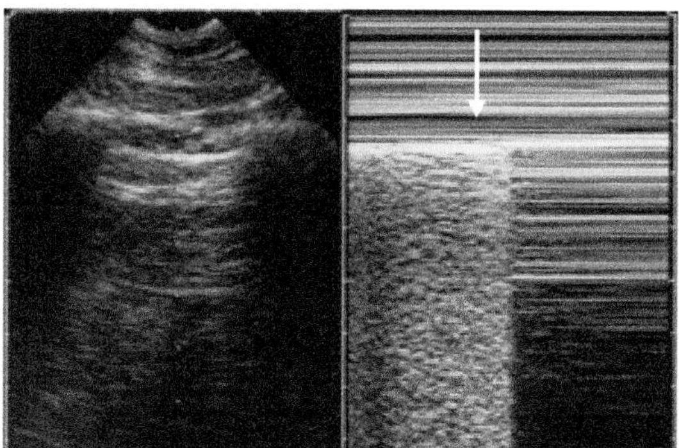

Figure III.Q16.

What is the name of this finding, which has been reported to be 100% specific for the presence of pneumothorax?

a. Seashore sign
b. Stratosphere sign
c. Lung sliding sign
d. Lung point sign

III.17. A 70-year-old man with a 55–pack-year smoking history presents with lethargy and confusion. The chest radiograph is shown in Figure III.Q17.

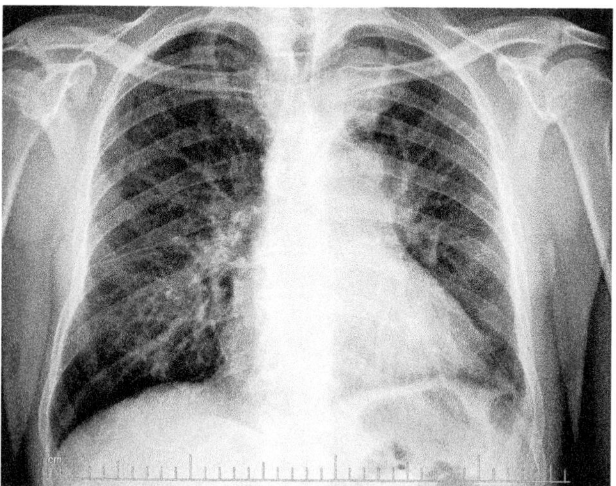

Figure III.Q17.

Laboratory analysis is notable for the following: hemoglobin 11.0 g/dL, platelet count 550×10^9/L, potassium 4.0 mmol/L, Na^+ 124 mmol/L, calcium 8.2 mg/dL, and creatinine 0.9 mg/dL. No previous laboratory test results are available. Which of the following is true?

a. Cytology of lymph node aspirate most likely will show squamous cell carcinoma.
b. Urgent administration of 3% saline solution is indicated.
c. Serum osmolality would be expected to be less than 275 mOsm/kg.
d. Urine Na^+ would be expected to be less than 30 meq/L.

III.18. A 76-year-old man who recently received a diagnosis of small cell lung cancer presents with neck fullness, progressive dyspnea, and hypoxemia. A representative CT image is shown in Figure III.Q18.

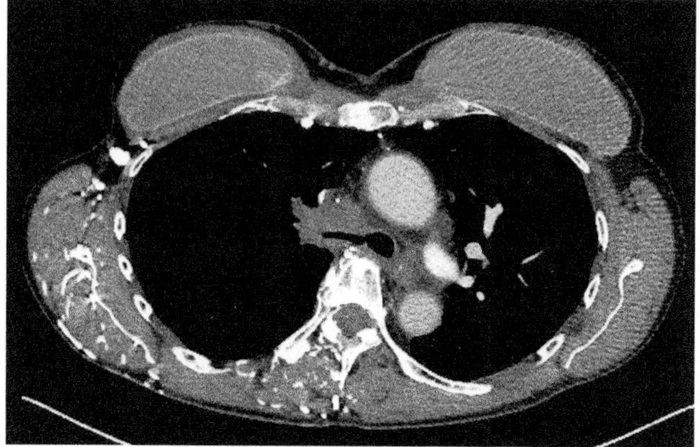

Figure III.Q18.

After initial supportive care has been provided, what should be the next step in management?

a. Administration of a high dose of corticosteroids (methylprednisolone 60 mg IV every 6 hours)
b. Urgent radiotherapy
c. Administration of cisplatin and etoposide
d. Stent placement in the superior vena cava

III.19. What is the best screening test for PH?
a. Right-sided heart catheterization
b. ECG
c. Echocardiography
d. Pulmonary function tests

III.20. An ICU patient presents with submassive PE with the following clinical findings: systemic BP 110/60 mm Hg, HR 96 bpm, Spo_2 92% with 5 L/min supplemental oxygen by open mask, normal first heart sound, accentuated second heart sound, and no evidence of peripheral edema. In addition, bedside echocardiography shows a dilated right ventricle but an IVC of normal size with partial collapse on inspiration. What is the recommended fluid management for this patient?
a. Begin aggressive fluid resuscitation.
b. Maintain euvolemia.
c. Begin aggressive diuresis.
d. Begin noninvasive mechanical ventilation.

III.21. A patient presents to the ICU with a 10-day history of fevers, chills, and cough. He had exposure to sick contacts. On admission he is hypoxic with a room air Spo_2 of 83%. He is intubated in the ED, administered volume assist-control mode ventilation (tidal volume 6 mL/kg, rate 10 breaths per minute, PEEP 10 cm H_2O, and Fio_2 60%), and transferred to the ICU, where ABG analysis shows pH 7.32, $Paco_2$ 45 mm Hg, and Pao_2 50 mm Hg. Mean systemic BP is 65 mm Hg; HR, 92 bpm. As determined with urinary catheterization, urine output is adequate. Bedside echocardiography shows a dilated right ventricle with decreased systolic function. The IVC has a diameter of 2.5 cm with minimal change during the respiratory cycle. What is the best next step?
a. Place a pulmonary artery catheter (ie, a Swan-Ganz catheter).
b. Begin fluid resuscitation.
c. Maximize Fio_2 and PEEP to increase oxygenation.
d. Administer inhaled nitric oxide.

III.22. A 43-year-old woman with scleroderma and group 1 PAH is admitted to the ICU after presenting with dyspnea at rest and recent exertional syncope. What therapy should be initiated?
a. IV epoprostenol
b. Inhaled nitric oxide
c. Oral bosentan
d. Oral sildenafil

III.23. Which of the following patients most likely has group 1 PAH?
a. A 68-year-old man with chronic congestive heart failure and a left ventricular ejection fraction of 35%
b. A 45-year-old woman who presents with dyspnea on exertion and a history of taking prescription weight loss medication for 1 year
c. A 78-year-old woman with chronic hypoxemia from severe COPD
d. A 40-year-old morbidly obese man who has mild dyspnea with exertion, excessive daytime sleepiness, and loud snoring

Cardiovascular Disorders

III.24. Which of the following is true for serum tryptase levels in anaphylaxis?
a. The tryptase level will be elevated for only 30 to 60 minutes after the onset of the event.
b. Tryptase is found primarily in basophils, and a small amount is in mast cells.
c. A normal tryptase level rules out anaphylaxis.
d. Serial measurements of tryptase levels during an anaphylactic event, in addition to a baseline level, are more useful than a single measurement.

III.25. Which statement best describes the hemodynamics of anaphylactic shock?
a. Anaphylactic shock is characterized by increased venous return and cardiac output.
b. Anaphylactic shock is characterized by intravascular fluid loss and extensive vasodilatation.
c. Pulmonary edema fluid in patients with anaphylactic shock is associated with low albumin concentrations and high pulmonary artery wedge pressures.
d. Anaphylactic shock is characterized by increases in arterial pressure, right and left ventricular filling pressures, and peripheral vascular resistance.

III.26. What is the most common cause of cardiogenic shock?
a. Acute mitral regurgitation
b. Acute MI
c. Atrial fibrillation with rapid ventricular response
d. Aortic stenosis

III.27. Which of the following does *not* support the diagnosis of cardiogenic shock?
a. Systolic BP less than 90 mm Hg for 30 minutes while receiving norepinephrine 15 mcg/min and vasopressin 4 units/h
b. Serum lactate level of 1.9 mmol/L
c. Alert to person but not to place and time
d. Pulmonary capillary wedge pressure greater than 18 mm Hg

III.28. What diagnostic tool is the most sensitive and specific for establishing the diagnosis of cardiogenic shock?
a. Serial ECGs
b. Serial transthoracic echocardiographic studies
c. Pulmonary artery catheterization with cardiac indices
d. Serial troponin measurements

III.29. What is the first-line medication for a patient who has cardiogenic shock with a low cardiac output but a sustained systolic BP greater than 90 mm Hg?
a. Epinephrine
b. Norepinephrine
c. Dobutamine
d. Vasopressin

III.30. For patients with cardiogenic shock and concomitant perioperative right ventricular failure or ischemia, which of the following is *not* a treatment goal?
a. Pco_2 less than 45 mm Hg
b. Pao_2 greater than 80 mm Hg
c. HR less than 55 bpm
d. Inhaled nitric oxide at 20 ppm

III.31. A 55-year-old woman presented to the ED with acute chest pain. The ECG showed a 2-mm ST-segment elevation in leads II, III, and aVF that was consistent with an acute MI. The patient received a drug-eluting stent in her proximal right coronary artery. She felt well afterward but told you that she had normal results on a stress test 1 month ago and was perplexed that she had a cardiac event. You explain that the stress test can detect severe obstructions but not milder, nonobstructive plaques that can rupture. What pathogenic mechanism did this patient most likely have?
a. Low systemic myeloperoxidase levels
b. Thick fibrous cap
c. Enlarged lipid-filled plaque core
d. Normal levels of inflammatory markers

III.32. A 55-year-old woman with a history of hypertension comes to the ED with acute-onset chest pain. She describes an acute onset of knife-like chest pain that radiates to her back in the interscapular area, and she has bilateral leg weakness. She is diaphoretic. Her BP is 170/100 mm Hg, her pulse is 104 bpm, and her respiratory rate is 18 breaths per minute. Her lungs are clear. On cardiac examination, she has a fourth heart sound with no murmurs. Her ECG shows ST-segment elevation in leads II, III, and aVF. What is the appropriate next step?
a. Two-dimensional echocardiography
b. Chest radiography
c. CT angiography of the chest
d. Cardiac enzyme levels

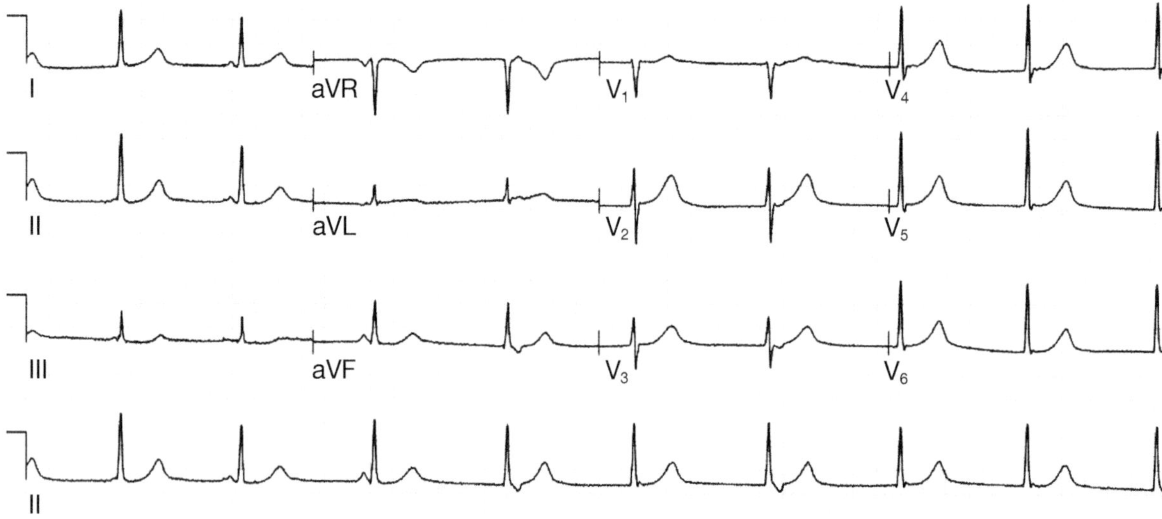

Figure III.Q36.

III.33. A 55-year-old man presented to the ED with a 1-hour history of substernal chest pressure radiating to the jaw and left arm at rest. He has no relevant medical history, but he does not visit any physician regularly. His resting ECG is normal. What biomarker would you use to diagnose an ACS in this patient?

a. Troponin I at 0, 3, and 6 hours
b. CK and CK-MB at 0, 3, and 6 hours
c. High-sensitivity troponin at 0 hours
d. BNP at 0 hours

III.34. A 60-year-old woman with a history of diabetes mellitus, cerebrovascular accident, and hypertension is admitted in stable condition with an NSTEMI. Coronary angiography showed a 90% stenosis of the mid left anterior descending coronary artery. You are asked to start her antiplatelet therapy. Which of these regimens is optimal after the coronary lesion is treated with a drug-eluting stent?

a. Aspirin 325 mg daily and ticagrelor 90 mg twice daily
b. Aspirin 81 mg daily and ticagrelor 90 mg twice daily
c. Aspirin 325 mg daily, ticagrelor 90 mg twice daily, and warfarin 5 mg every night
d. Aspirin 81 mg daily and ticagrelor 180 mg twice daily

III.35. A 66-year-old man presented to the ED with new constant precordial chest pressure for the past 3 hours. When he is given oxygen supplementation and nitroglycerin sublingually, his pain is relieved. He does not take any medications at home. ECG shows a 1- to 2-mm ST-segment depression in the lateral leads (V_4 through V_6). What medication should he receive before he is transferred to the cardiac catheterization laboratory?

a. Aspirin 81 mg and prasugrel 60 mg
b. Aspirin 325 mg and clopidogrel 600 mg
c. Clopidogrel 300 mg
d. Ticagrelor 180 mg

III.36. A 67-year-old man is in the ICU after uneventful surgery for an abdominal aortic aneurysm. He has a history of hypertension and a previous coronary artery angioplasty. He is currently taking metoprolol 50 mg twice daily and lisinopril 20 mg once daily. Preoperative echocardiography showed an ejection fraction of 50% with mild mitral regurgitation. The ECG is shown in Figure III.Q36.

The patient is asymptomatic. What should be the next step?

a. Stop the metoprolol therapy.
b. Prepare the patient for transcutaneous pacing.

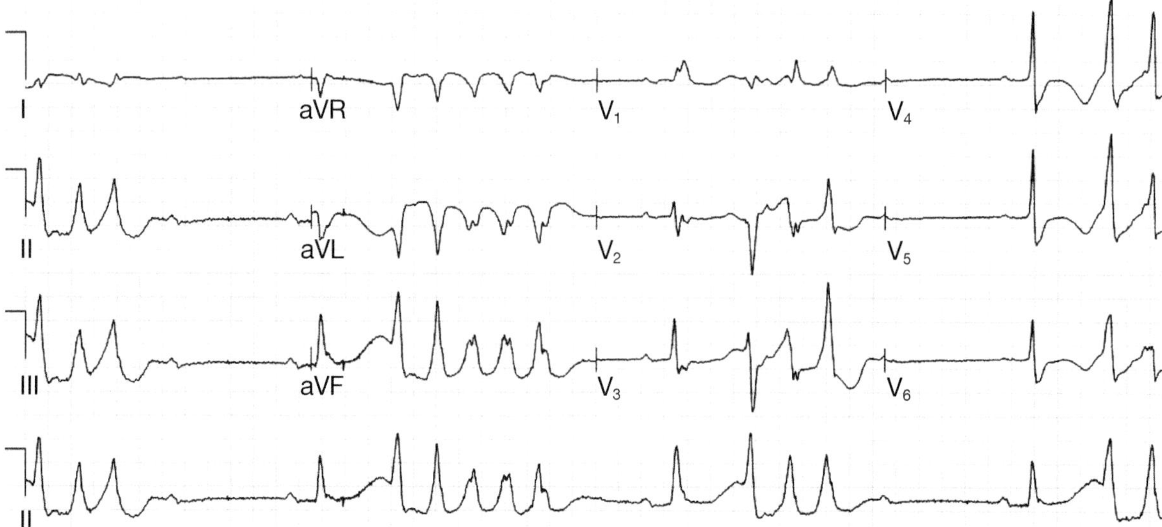

Figure III.Q37.

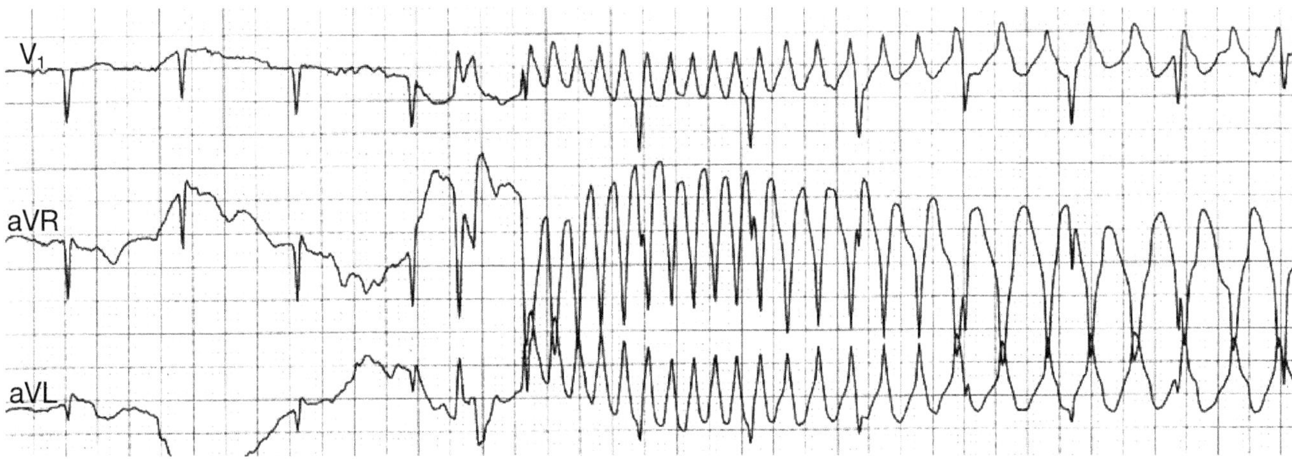

Figure III.Q38.

c. Begin a dobutamine infusion at 5 mcg/kg/min.
d. Observe the patient.

III.37. A 72-year-old man is admitted because he has an intracranial hemorrhage. The ECG is shown in Figure III.Q37.

What should be the next step?

a. Administer amiodarone 150 mg IV.
b. Administer lidocaine 75 mg IV.
c. Initiate transcutaneous pacing at a rate of 80 bpm.
d. Administer calcium gluconate 10 mg IV.

III.38. The ECG in Figure III.Q38 was received by telemetry.

What should be the next step?

a. Initiate transcutaneous pacing at 80 bpm.
b. Administer atropine 0.5 mg IV.
c. Administer amiodarone 150 mg IV.
d. Observe the patient.

III.39. An 87-year-old woman is admitted to the ICU with "failure to thrive." She has a long history of atrial fibrillation and is treated with digoxin 0.25 mcg/daily and warfarin. Her systolic BP is 90 mm Hg. Her lungs are clear. On cardiovascular examination, she has a II/VI systolic murmur. Her ECG is shown in Figure III.Q39.

What should be the next step?

a. Initiate transcutaneous pacing.
b. Stop the digoxin therapy.
c. Administer amiodarone 200 mg twice daily.
d. Observe the patient.

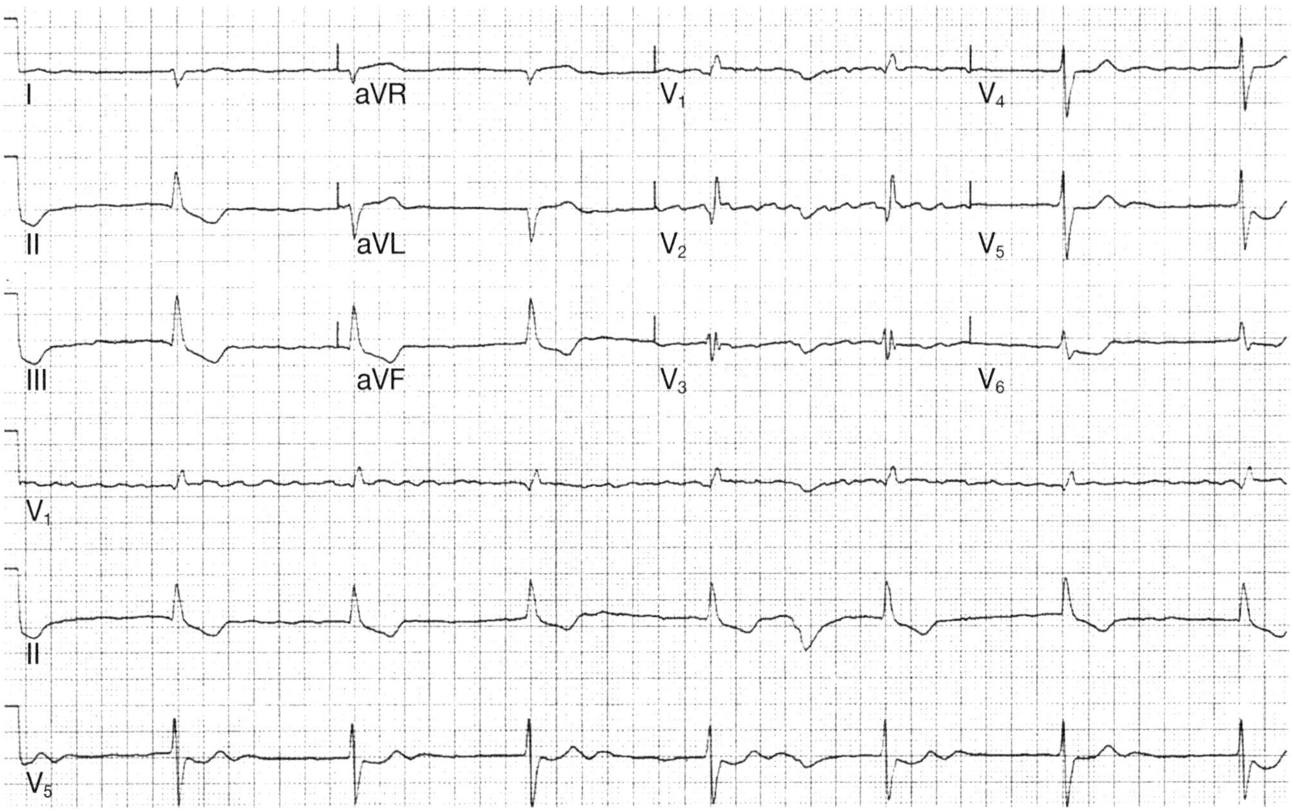

Figure III.Q39.

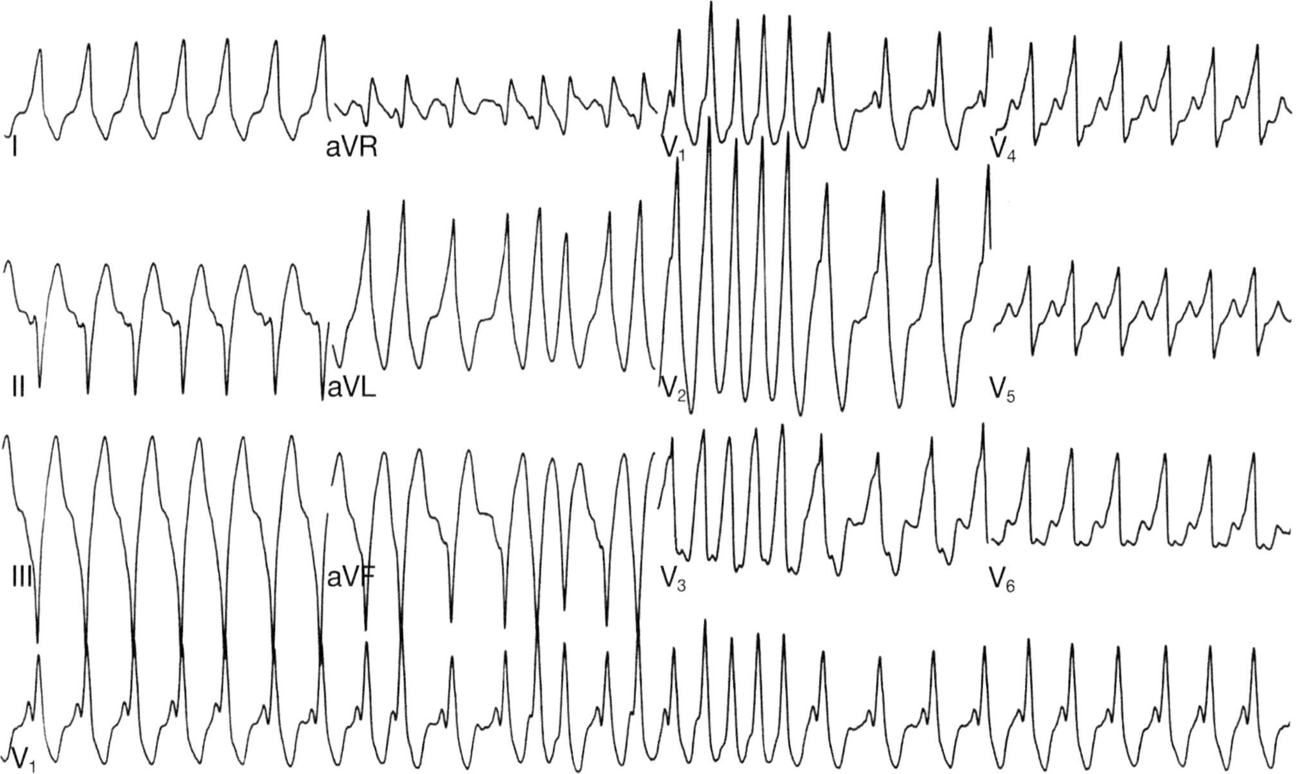

Figure III.Q40.

III.40. A 29-year-old man is recovering from an emergent appendectomy. A rapid HR suddenly develops. He has no history of other medical problems. His family history is unremarkable, but his grandfather died in his 30s from an unknown cause. The patient is uncomfortable but not short of breath. His BP is 95/60 mm Hg, and his physical examination findings are unremarkable other than a rapid HR. His ECG is shown in Figure III.Q40.

What should be the next step?

a. Immediately begin synchronized cardioversion at 150 J.
b. Administer adenosine 6 mg IV.
c. Administer amiodarone 150 mg IV.
d. Administer procainamide 1 g IV.

III.41. Which of the following distinguishes hypertensive emergency from hypertensive urgency?

a. History of drug abuse (ie, cocaine)
b. Greater elevations in mean arterial BP
c. Diastolic BP greater than 120 mm Hg
d. Evidence of end-organ damage

III.42. A 57-year-old man presents with symptoms of dyspnea on exertion associated with progressive pulmonary edema after a motor vehicle accident. He has bruising on his thorax and complains of chest pain. Later he receives a diagnosis of hypertensive crisis and is transferred to the ICU. What must be ruled out before completing a workup for hypertensive emergency?

a. Pulmonary contusions
b. Sternal fractures and rib fractures
c. Aortic dissection
d. Acute left ventricular aneurysm with partial rupture

III.43. For which of the following patients would TTM be *inappropriate*?

a. A 67-year-old woman who had an anterior ST-segment elevation MI subsequently had a pulseless ventricular tachycardia cardiac arrest during catheterization and is now unresponsive.
b. A 23-year-old man had a cardiac arrest after a motor vehicle accident and has active intra-abdominal bleeding that requires emergent surgical intervention.
c. A 25-year-old woman had an in-hospital cardiac arrest attributed to pulseless electrical activity due to PE. Thrombolytics were administered, and she remains unresponsive.
d. A 74-year-old man had a witnessed OHCA due to ventricular fibrillation. After resuscitation for 35 minutes, return of spontaneous circulation was achieved.

III.44. Which of the following would *not* alter the $ETCO_2$ value during CPR?

a. Administration of epinephrine during cardiac arrest
b. Cardiac arrest due to PE
c. Administration of amiodarone
d. Administration of HCO_3^- during cardiac arrest

III.45. A 75-year-old woman is undergoing TTM at 36°C after having a witnessed ventricular fibrillation cardiac arrest at the local shopping mall. She has AKI, her creatinine is 3.4 mg/dL, and her urine output is minimal. She is shivering, and the medical team is having difficulty maintaining her core body temperature at 36°C. Which of the following is *not* an appropriate method for controlling her shivering?

a. Neuromuscular blockade
b. Intermittent administration of meperidine IV
c. Increasing the dose of a propofol infusion as hemodynamically tolerated
d. Adding a fentanyl infusion to a midazolam infusion for sedation

III.46. A 45-year-old woman had an OHCA due to ventricular fibrillation. She is undergoing TTM at 36°C. Which of the following is *not* appropriate in this patient's management?

a. Allowing blood glucose values to fluctuate above 200 mg/dL
b. Titrating vasopressors or inotropes for a mean arterial pressure greater than 70 mm Hg

c. Providing lung-protective mechanical ventilation
d. Administering a crystalloid bolus to increase the CVP of 4 mm Hg

III.47. A 62-year-old man was admitted to the medical cardiac ICU for unstable angina and then had a ventricular fibrillation arrest. He received 2 rounds of high-quality CPR with appropriate ACLS medications, and ROSC was achieved with bradycardia as the post-ROSC rhythm. The patient did not respond to an initial 0.5-mg dose of atropine nor to a second 0.5-mg dose 3 minutes later. Now he is hemodynamically unstable (HR, 35 bpm; BP, 65/30 mm Hg). Which of the following is the *least* appropriate next step?
a. Epinephrine infusion
b. Dopamine infusion
c. Transcutaneous pacing
d. A third 0.5-mg dose of atropine in 3 minutes

III.48. A 59-year-old man presents with acute chest pain. CT angiography shows a type B aortic dissection. His BP is 150/70 mm Hg with an MAP of 98 mm Hg. Urine output is normal. The patient has no other symptoms. What is your best course for managing his BP?
a. Decrease the systolic BP to 100 to 110 mm Hg, and keep the MAP at 60 to 75 mm Hg.
b. Decrease the systolic BP to 100 to 110 mm Hg, and keep the MAP at less than 60 mm Hg.
c. Increase the systolic BP to 160 mm Hg to improve perfusion, and maintain the MAP at 60 to 75 mm Hg.
d. Maintain the MAP at 70 mm Hg or more, independently of the systolic BP.

III.49. A 48-year-old man presents with acute, severe chest pain radiating to his back. ECG and troponin levels are normal. Chest radiography shows a density adjacent to the brachiocephalic trunk. CT angiography shows a type A aortic dissection involving the intrapericardial ascending aorta and arch. The patient's BP is 110/65 mm Hg; the MAP is 80 mm Hg. What is the best course of action?
a. Perform transesophageal echocardiography to confirm the dissection.
b. Order magnetic resonance angiography for better visualization.
c. Provide medical management.
d. Proceed with emergent surgical repair.

Acute Endocrine Disorders

III.50. A patient presents to the ED with sudden-onset headache and double vision. On examination the patient has cranial nerve VI palsy on the right side and paresthesia along the distribution of the first division of cranial nerve V on the right side. The patient also has bitemporal hemianopia. What should be the next diagnostic step?
a. Evaluate laboratory markers of endocrine function.
b. Perform ECG.
c. Perform lumbar puncture.
d. Perform MRI of the head.

III.51. Which of the following is a reported risk factor for pituitary apoplexy in many patients?
a. Pregnancy
b. Female sex
c. Hypertension
d. Recent infection

III.52. A 38-year-old man is admitted to the ICU after transsphenoidal resection of a sellar mass performed earlier that morning. At 8 hours after surgery, his urine output was increased (200 mL/h for 3 consecutive hours) and his electrolyte levels were abnormal. The sellar mass was diagnosed 2 months earlier when he presented with concerns about his vision. At that time, he was given a diagnosis of DI and secondary adrenal insufficiency, and the radiographic appearance of the mass was suggestive of craniopharyngioma. At home, his medications included oral desmopressin 0.1 mg twice daily and hydrocortisone at a physiologic replacement dose. Five days before admission he was prescribed high-dose prednisone for asthma exacerbation. On the day of surgery, he took his morning dose of desmopressin preoperatively and received stress doses of dexamethasone in the operating room. In the ICU, the patient is extubated but somnolent. His BP is 120/60 mm Hg, and his HR is 110 bpm. The route of administration for desmopressin was changed from oral to subcutaneous with the same twice-daily schedule he had followed at home, and he was given D5W (200 mL/h) because he had a high urine output. Laboratory test results are shown in Table III.Q52.

Table III.Q52 •

Component	Result
Na^+, mmol/L	148
Potassium, mmol/L	4.5
Calcium, mg/dL	10
Glucose, mg/dL	400
Creatinine, mg/dL	1.5
SUN, mg/dL	18
Plasma osmolality, mOsm/kg	299
Urine osmolality, mOsm/kg	380

What is the best next step in the management of this patient's polyuria?
a. Immediately administer 1 mcg IV desmopressin.
b. Increase the rate of D5W to 400 mL/h.
c. Start IV insulin and change the fluids to normal saline.
d. Immediately administer 0.1 mg oral desmopressin.

III.53. You receive a call in the middle of the night from an ICU nurse about a patient with a large urine output. The patient is a 65-year-old woman with a nonfunctioning pituitary macroadenoma that was diagnosed 3 weeks ago. Earlier in the day, the patient underwent an uncomplicated transsphenoidal resection of a pituitary tumor. Preoperatively she had no evidence of pituitary dysfunction, but she has had increased urine output (300 mL/h) for the past 4 hours. On examination the patient is extubated, conscious, and thirsty. She has been drinking water for the past 3 hours and is uncomfortable because of frequent urination. The patient's BP is 130/80 mm Hg; her HR is 90 bpm. The findings from the cardiopulmonary examination are normal. The patient received 3 L of 0.9% normal saline in the operating room. Laboratory results are as follows: Na^+ 147 mmol/L, glucose 120 mg/dL, plasma osmolality 305 mOsm/kg, and urine osmolality 130 mOsm/kg. What is the best next step in the management of this patient's polyuria?
a. Immediately administer 10 mcg intranasal desmopressin.
b. Start D5W at 300 mL/h.
c. No other management is required for now.
d. Immediately administer 1 mcg IV desmopressin.

III.54. A 70-year-old man with a history of obstructive sleep apnea, bilateral carpal tunnel syndrome, hypertension, type 2 diabetes mellitus, and atrial fibrillation (he is receiving warfarin) is admitted to the ICU with a sudden and severe headache, blurred vision, and a decreased level of consciousness.

The patient is hypotensive on admission. His BP is 80/65 mm Hg despite having received 2 L of normal saline in the ED. He is given pressure support. On neurologic examination, the only deficit is left cranial nerve III palsy. He has several skin tags and large hands and feet; his hands feel soft like bread dough. Laboratory results are as follows: Na^+ 133 mmol/L, potassium 5 mmol/L, creatinine 1.2 ng/mL, and INR 1.5. CT of the head does not show subarachnoid hemorrhage or intracerebral bleeding, but a pituitary tumor with a possible fluid-fluid level is apparent. MRI is being arranged. In the meantime, which is the most appropriate next step?

a. Immediately determine the IGF-1 level.
b. Immediately determine random cortisol and corticotropin levels, and then administer IV corticosteroids.
c. Request an urgent neurosurgical consultation.
d. Measure the HbA_{1c} level to determine whether the patient's cranial nerve III palsy is related to type 2 diabetes mellitus.

III.55. A 45-year-old man with a history of panhypopituitarism due to severe traumatic brain injury after a motor vehicle accident 10 years ago is admitted to the ICU with shortness of breath, cough, and fever. He is febrile (body temperature 38.5°C) and hypotensive. Chest radiography indicates left lower lobe consolidation consistent with pneumonia. Blood samples are obtained for cultures. He is given IV antibiotics and fluids.

His family provided a list of his prescription medications and said that he had received his medications that morning. He receives 15 mg hydrocortisone in the morning, 10 mg hydrocortisone in the midafternoon, 150 mcg levothyroxine daily, and 200 mg intramuscular testosterone cypionate every 2 weeks (his latest injection was administered 1 week ago). Table III.Q55 shows the results of the blood tests performed when he arrived in the ICU at 10 am.

Table III.Q55 •

Component	Result (Reference Range)
WBC count, $\times10^9$/L	18
Creatinine, mg/dL	1.5
Na^+, mmol/L	133
Potassium, mmol/L	5
Thyrotropin, mIU/mL	0.1 (0.3-4.2)
Random cortisol, mcg/dL	15
Total testosterone, ng/dL	400 (240-950)
IGF-1, ng/mL	68 (69-266)

In addition to administering IV antibiotics and fluids, what should be done next?

a. Administer a stress dose of corticosteroid and decrease the levothyroxine dose.
b. Administer a stress dose of corticosteroid and measure the free thyroxine level.
c. Do not administer a corticosteroid because the random cortisol level indicates recovery of the hypothalamic-pituitary-adrenal axis.
d. Continue the patient's current regimen of hormone replacement therapy.

III.56. A 26-year-old woman was found unresponsive at home. In the ED, she is accompanied by her husband who says that she had been getting ready for bed because she felt tired. Peripheral blood glucose testing by the paramedics showed hypoglycemia (glucose 30 mg/dL). When she was treated with dextrose, she became more responsive. On arrival in the ED, she was hypoglycemic (glucose 45 mg/dL) and hypotensive (BP 80/60 mm Hg). Her HR was 98 bpm; her body temperature was 36.5°C. A 10% dextrose drip was required to maintain an adequate glucose level.

Her husband states that the patient has been nauseated, tired, and dizzy since she gave birth to their 2-month-old infant. They had attributed these symptoms to sleepless nights. In addition, he states that the delivery was difficult, and she required several blood transfusions because of bleeding. She has not been able to breastfeed. She has not been taking any new medications except iron supplements. She does not have diabetes mellitus, and she has no relevant past medical history. Laboratory test results are shown in Table III.Q56.

Table III.Q56 •

Component	Result
WBC count, $\times10^9$/L	8
Hemoglobin, g/dL	11
Platelet count, $\times10^9$/L	200
Na^+, mmol/L	130
Potassium, mmol/L	5.1
Creatinine, mg/dL	1.2
Glucose, mg/dL	45
Random cortisol, mcg/dL	2
Corticotropin, pg/mL	18
Thyrotropin, mIU/mL	0.15
Free thyroxine, ng/dL	0.6

What is the best next step in treating this patient?

a. Administer a stress dose of corticosteroid and order 8 am cortisol and corticotropin tests to determine whether she has primary or secondary adrenal insufficiency.
b. Administer levothyroxine and then a stress dose of corticosteroid as soon as possible.
c. Perform a corticotropin stimulation test and then administer a stress dose of corticosteroid.
d. Administer a stress dose of corticosteroid and then levothyroxine.

III.57. Which of the following is *not* a sign or symptom of myxedema coma?

a. Hyponatremia
b. Hyperthermia
c. Hypoglycemia
d. Hypoventilation

III.58. If a patient with thyroid storm is given an iodine-containing solution to block new hormone synthesis, the solution should be given at least 1 hour after which type of medication?

a. β-Blocker
b. Thionamide agent (eg, propylthiouracil or methimazole)
c. Bile acid sequestrant
d. Glucocorticoid

III.59. A 74-year-old obese (weight, 95.5 kg) man who has no other previous medical history is admitted to the neurocritical care unit after receiving a diagnosis of ischemic stroke 12 hours earlier, which is associated with slurred speech and right hemiparesis. On admission, his glucose level is 313 mg/dL and HbA_{1c} is 8.1%. The patient's father had a history of type 2 diabetes mellitus controlled with insulin. The patient does not smoke or drink alcohol. According to his clinical situation, which of the following is true?

a. Regardless whether this man has "stress hyperglycemia" or unrecognized diabetes mellitus, an insulin drip should be started immediately for glycemic control.
b. To improve clinical outcomes in a neurocritically ill patient, tight glycemic control should be performed to keep glucose levels as low as possible.

c. In-hospital glucose levels have no effect on morbidity and mortality for patients who have had stroke, bypass surgery, or MI.
d. Bolus administration of insulin and glucose solutions should be used for glycemic control.

III.60. Hyperglycemia, hypoglycemia, and glycemic variability carry a worse neurologic prognosis for neurocritically ill patients, especially after stroke, intracranial bleeding, subarachnoid hemorrhage, and traumatic brain injury. The injured brain is sensitive to changes in the glycemic level because brain metabolism depends on a permanent, reliable supply of glucose. Which blood glucose level should be maintained for critically ill patients?
a. 80-110 mg/dL
b. 110-140 mg/dL
c. 140-180 mg/dL
d. 180-200 mg/dL

III.61. A 76-year-old man with a previous medical history of hypertension, type 2 diabetes mellitus, and early-stage Alzheimer dementia has a recent urinary outflow obstruction requiring long-term use of an indwelling urinary catheter. In the past 5 days, his interaction with his family has decreased, his oral intake has been poor, and he seems more confused than usual. His primary care physician diagnosed a urinary tract infection. His initial outpatient oral antibiotic therapy did not seem to help, his delirium worsened, and he is dehydrated and has nonoliguric AKI, so he has been admitted to the hospital in the neurocritical care unit. On admission, he has lethargy, systemic inflammatory response syndrome, hypotension, and dry mucous membranes, and his urine appeared purulent. The rest of the physical examination was unremarkable. Laboratory test results included the following: WBC count 14.5×10^9/L, blood glucose on admission 238 mg/dL, creatinine 2.5 mg/dL, SUN 48 mg/dL, and lactic acid 3.4 mmol/L. In the hospital, what should his initial treatment include?
a. Trimethoprim-sulfamethoxazole 2 tablets orally every 6 hours
b. Hydrocortisone 50 mg IV every 6 hours
c. Fludrocortisone 0.1 mg orally once
d. IV fluids and IV antibiotics

III.62. Controversy over glycemic control includes the blood glucose level that should prompt IV insulin control, the appropriate degree of control, the safety of various blood glucose levels, and the appropriate monitoring interval. For optimal management of glycemic control in the ICU, which of the following is *not* a safe recommendation?
a. Provide IIT with appropriate nutritional support and frequent glucose monitoring.
b. Maintain blood glucose levels at less than 180 mg/dL.
c. Minimize glycemic variability.
d. Maintain blood glucose levels at less than 90 mg/dL.

III.63. The diagnostic criteria for CIRCI are controversial. Which of the following is consistent with the latest recommendations of the ACCM?
a. Delta serum cortisol less than 9 mcg/dL after a corticotropin stimulation test (250 mcg of cosyntropin)
b. Hypereosinophilia
c. Hyponatremia with hypokalemia
d. Hypotension

III.64. Which of the following may be caused by IV etomidate?
a. Hypoglycemia due to insulin release
b. Hyperglycemia due to insulin suppression
c. Increased glucagon release
d. AI

III.65. A 41-year-old woman is admitted after a motor vehicle accident complicated with polytrauma, hip fracture requiring surgical repair, and stupor from closed head trauma with no abnormal findings on CT of the head. She has a past medical history of rheumatoid arthritis diagnosed 5 years ago. She is admitted to the neurocritical care unit for close neurologic monitoring of her brain concussion. Her clinical course 48 hours after admission has evolved with hypotension despite generous normal saline infusions and vasopressor therapy, moderate body temperature, appropriate tachycardia, and no evidence of blood loss. Other data include a normal hemoglobin level, moderate eosinophilia, no ECG changes, low blood glucose, normal levels of cardiac enzymes, and mild hyponatremia. What should urgent treatment include?
a. 100 mcg levothyroxine IV
b. 25 mcg liothyronine orally
c. 6 mg dexamethasone IV
d. 3% saline infusion to replace the sodium deficit

Gastrointestinal Disorders

III.66. A 63-year-old man is admitted to the hospital after a home fire that caused him smoke-inhalation injury and second-degree skin burns to 30% of his body. He is later transferred to an ICU with respiratory failure due to pneumonia complicated by severe ARDS and hypotension. Low tidal volume ventilation and neuromuscular blockade are instituted. Central venous access is obtained for the provision of fluids, norepinephrine, and empiric antibiotics for septic shock. Laboratory results are notable for the following: hemoglobin, 13.3 g/dL; platelet count, 120×10^9/L; lactate, 1.9 mmol/L; and INR 1.9.

The patient's past medical history is significant for osteoarthritis treated with acetaminophen and basal cell carcinoma of the skin treated with excision and electrocautery. He takes enteric-coated aspirin 81 milligrams daily for primary prevention of cardiovascular disease.

Which of the following is *not* a risk factor for stress-related gastric mucosal damage (stress ulcers)?
a. Mechanical ventilation for less than 48 hours
b. Severe burn
c. Platelet count of 120×10^9/L
d. INR more than 1.5

III.67. A 45-year-old woman with alcoholic cirrhosis presents after 2 episodes of hematemesis. She has known portal hypertension complicated by ascites, mild hepatic encephalopathy, and grade 3 esophageal varices that were last banded 4 months ago. Home medications include milk thistle, lactulose, and tramadol. She requires therapeutic paracentesis every 4 to 6 weeks.

At presentation, the patient's BP is 132/94 mm Hg, HR is 94 bpm, and Spo_2 is 97% while the patient is breathing room air. Physical examination is remarkable for asterixis, lethargy, a distended abdomen with fluid wave, and palmar erythema. Laboratory results are notable for the following: hemoglobin, 11.5 g/dL; INR, 1.9; creatinine, 1.6 mg/dL; albumin, 3.2 g/dL; and total bilirubin, 2.8 mg/dL. Which of the following interventions is *least* appropriate for the management of this patient?
a. Ceftriaxone 1 g IV every 24 hours
b. Octreotide 50 mcg bolus followed by 50 mcg/hour infusion
c. Pantoprazole 80 mg IV followed by 8 mg/hour infusion
d. Transfusion of red blood cells

III.68. The patient described in the previous question undergoes upper endoscopy with findings of bleeding esophageal varices. Endoscopic ligation therapy and sclerotherapy are attempted but are unsuccessful in achieving hemostasis. Which of the following interventions is *least* appropriate?
a. Administration of recombinant factor VIIa
b. Placement of esophageal tamponade balloon
c. Endotracheal intubation
d. Transjugular intrahepatic portosystemic shunt

III.69. A 78-year-old man presents with a 5-day history of black tarry stool, light-headedness with standing, and worsening fatigue. He denies abdominal pain, chest pain, syncope, and use of any new medications. His past medical history is significant for diet-controlled type 2 diabetes mellitus and dyslipidemia. He takes rosuvastatin 20 mg daily and aspirin 81 mg daily.

At presentation, vital signs are as follows: HR, 114 bpm; BP, 98/60 mm Hg; and Spo_2, 97% while breathing 2 L of oxygen through nasal cannula. Results of abdominal examination are normal, and rectal examination shows no abnormalities other than melena. A nasogastric tube placed while in the ED yields a nonbloody aspirate. ECG shows sinus tachycardia without signs of ischemia. Results of laboratory studies are as follows: hemoglobin, 6.9 g/dL; creatinine, 1.5 mg/dL (baseline 0.9 mg/dL); and INR, 0.9. Which of the following is the most appropriate next step in management?

a. CT with oral and IV contrast agent
b. Mesenteric angiography
c. Resuscitation with IV fluids and blood products
d. Esophagogastroduodenoscopy

III.70. A 65-year-old woman is hospitalized with DVT of the right lower extremity that developed after a cross-country flight. She denies any prior cardiac history and does not take antiplatelet or nonsteroidal anti-inflammatory agents. A heparin infusion is started with a goal aPTT 60 to 90 seconds. She receives warfarin 5 mg on the evening of admission. The following day, you are called emergently to the patient's room because she is hypotensive and unresponsive. On examination, she has pallor, bradypnea, and no response to voice. HR is 140 bpm, and BP is 60/38 mm Hg. While the patient is being positioned for intubation, more than 1,000 mL of bright red blood is noted, consistent with massive hematochezia.

Immediate laboratory results are remarkable for the following: hemoglobin, 4.6 g/dL; INR, 1.0; platelet count, 95×10^9/L; creatinine 0.9 mg/dL; and aPTT, 116 seconds.

In addition to discontinuing the use of heparin and resuscitating with IV fluids and red blood cells, which of the following therapies is indicated in this patient?

a. 3- or 4-Factor prothrombin complex concentrate
b. Protamine sulfate
c. Idarucizumab
d. Platelet pheresis pack transfusion

III.71. A 65-year-old man with a history of nonalcoholic cirrhosis was admitted to the ICU for sepsis with fever, hypotension, AKI, and hyperlactatemia (lactate level, 4.2 mmol/L). You effectively resuscitated the patient with 30 mL/kg of crystalloid, cultured the blood, and administered broad-spectrum antibiotics. Bedside limited and focused echocardiography after resuscitation showed that the IVC was not collapsible and that moderate right-sided pleural effusion and ascites were present. You aspirated the ascites, and analysis results were leukocytes 850 mcL and neutrophils 90%. At 4 hours after admission, the lactate level is 2 mmol/L. BP is maintained with vasopressin and norepinephrine infusions.

On the third day, increasing abdominal distention, nausea, and pain developed. Examination shows silent abdomen. Fentanyl, 50 mcg every hour, is ordered because the patient's abdominal pain level is 8 of 10. You decide to use ultrasonography to look for ascites and decompressed abdomen only to find only trace ascites. Amylase and lipase levels are normal. What is your next step?

a. Place a nasogastric tube and order methylnaltrexone, 12 mg subcutaneously every other day.
b. Order CT of the abdomen and pelvis.
c. Order plain anteroposterior abdominal radiography.
d. Order anteroposterior and lateral abdominal radiography.

III.72. The patient described in the previous question still seems to have occasional flatus. The abdominal pain worsens as time passes. Results of abdominal radiography are shown in Figure III.Q72.

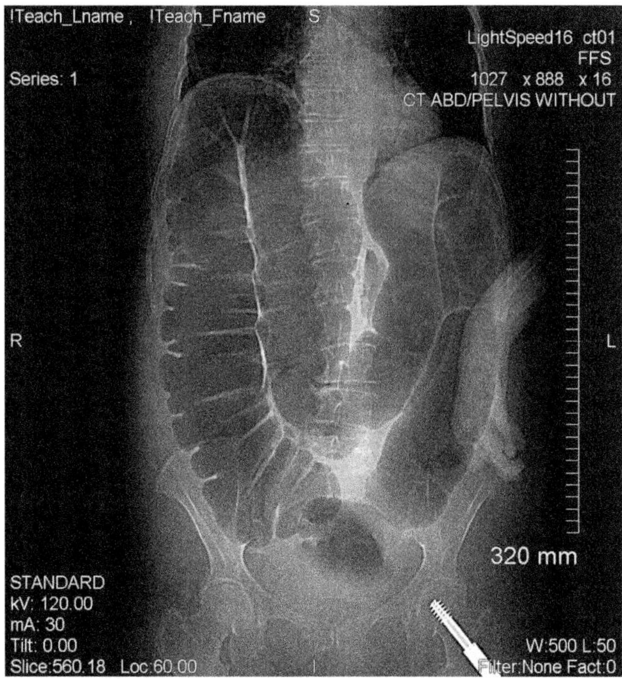

Figure III.Q72.

CT of the abdomen and pelvis shows no clear obstruction, and there is no evidence of pneumatosis intestinalis or ischemic changes. You start conservative treatment for 24 to 48 hours with methylnaltrexone, erythromycin IV, and laxative suppositories. What is your next step?

a. Call the gastrointestinal team to do a decompression colonoscopy.
b. Administer neostigmine, 2 mg IV.
c. Insert a rectal tube.
d. Order serial enemas.

III.73. In patients with acute liver failure, which of the following complications does *not* occur commonly?

a. Acute kidney failure
b. Variceal bleeding
c. Cerebral edema
d. Hypotension

III.74. A 19-year-old woman with acute liver failure due to acetaminophen poisoning is transferred from an outside hospital. On arrival, she is drowsy but rouses to stimulation and has garbled, unintelligible speech. What is your initial management?

a. Urgent CT of the head
b. Close monitoring with frequent neurologic assessment
c. Initiate *N*-acetylcysteine therapy.
d. Endotracheal intubation and mechanical ventilation

III.75. A 76-year-old man with severe cerebrovascular disease requiring antibiotics, nonsteroidal anti-inflammatory drugs, and antiplatelet medications also has respiratory failure necessitating mechanical ventilation. Unrecognized sepsis develops, and an abdominal source is suspected. Which of the following is an objective sign of perforation of hollow viscus?

a. Absent bowel sounds
b. Percussion tenderness
c. Loss of liver dullness
d. Distended abdomen

III.76. In the patient described in the previous question, abdominal distention develops and he has high nasogastric tube residuals from enteral feeding. On plain abdominal radiography, no free air is identified. At this point, which of the following statements is accurate?
a. Perforation has been excluded, and another source of sepsis should be sought.
b. Perforation is still a possibility, and further imaging should be pursued.
c. Abdominal radiography is of no value for identifying gastrointestinal spillage.
d. Surgical service should be contacted, and the patient should be readied for urgent laparotomy.

III.77. In the patient described in the 2 previous questions, concern is raised for the development of an abdominal compartment syndrome. What is the appropriate next test?
a. Abdominal ultrasonography
b. Plain abdominal radiography
c. Abdominal CT
d. Measurement of intra-abdominal pressure with a Foley catheter

III.78. The manifestations and septic complications caused by perforation depend on which of the following?
a. Location of the perforated hollow organ
b. Duration since the injury
c. The volume and chemical content of substance coming from the perforated organ
d. All of the above

III.79. Which of the following treatments has been successful for gastrointestinal perforations?
a. Conservative management with nasogastric tube aspiration
b. Percutaneous needle aspiration
c. Endoscopy
d. All of the above

III.80. A 76-year-old woman has a known history of an incidentally found 6.9-cm aortic aneurysm. She underwent elective open repair of her aneurysm without complications. Intraoperatively, the aneurysm was found to be infrarenal, and the surgeon did not reimplant any vessels. On postoperative day 1, severe abdominal pain and bloody diarrhea developed. Which of the following is true regarding her probable condition?
a. Occlusion of the mesenteric vessels is responsible for producing ischemia in most cases.
b. The most common clinical presentation includes lower abdominal pain and bleeding.
c. It most commonly involves the cecum and rectum.
d. The best next step for diagnosis is abdominal radiography.

III.81. A 74-year-old man with end-stage renal disease is receiving hemodialysis triweekly. In the previous year, he had a left MCA stroke, and 2 weeks ago he had an acute MI. He was brought to the ED after waking up with severe abdominal pain. The ED physician noticed mild epigastric discomfort, but otherwise the results of physical examination were unremarkable. IV administered fentanyl was provided for pain control. Which of the following accurately describes acute occlusion of the superior mesenteric artery?
a. Acute occlusion of the superior mesenteric artery usually results in complete foregut infarction.
b. Emboli most commonly arise from aortic atheromatous plaques.
c. The ascending colon and descending colon are generally spared as a result of sparing of the middle colic artery.
d. Sudden complete occlusion is most often caused by embolism rather than by thrombosis.

III.82. The cardiovascular changes in patients who have ACS are due to which of the following?
a. Decreased filling of the right side of the heart by direct pressure of the diaphragm on the right side of the heart
b. Decreased filling of the left side of the heart by increased intrathoracic pressure
c. Direct pressure on the abdominal aorta leading to increased afterload
d. Direct pressure on the IVC leading to decreased filling of the right side of the heart

III.83. Decompressive laparotomy should be strongly considered in patients with which of the following findings?
a. A tight abdomen on physical examination
b. Sustained intra-abdominal pressure more than 25 mm Hg and evidence of organ dysfunction
c. Sustained intra-abdominal pressure more than 20 mm Hg
d. Failure of all other measures to control abdominal pressure

Renal Disorders

III.84. A 57-year-old male patient is admitted to the hospital with pneumonia. He requires 3 L of oxygen by nasal cannula. After appropriate cultures, he is given nafcillin and levofloxacin, in addition to chest physiotherapy. He is also given subcutaneous heparin as prophylaxis for DVT and pantoprazole for stress ulcer prevention. By day 3 of hospitalization, he is improving from a respiratory standpoint, but he is noted to have a generalized erythematous rash and a temperature of 38.3°C. His creatinine level is increased from 0.8 mg/dL on admission to 1.5 mg/dL. Which one of the following findings is most likely in this case?
a. Muddy-brown casts in urine sediment
b. Hyaline casts in urine sediment
c. White cell casts in urine sediment and eosinophiluria
d. Granular casts in urine sediment

III.85. A 67-year-old woman is admitted to the ICU with gram-negative bacteremia and sepsis. She is receiving appropriate antibiotics; however, she needs norepinephrine and vasopressin for persistent hypotension. She is intubated and is receiving 40% Fio_2 with PEEP 5 cm H_2O, tidal volume 350 mL, and respiratory rate 18 breaths per minute. During the past 24 hours, her urine output has decreased to only 400 mL, and her serum creatinine level has increased to 3.5 mg/dL from the baseline of 0.7 mg/dL. Her urine sediment shows muddy-brown casts consistent with ATN. Her serum potassium level is 3.8 mEq/L, and serum HCO_3^- level is 20 mmol/L. Which one of the following statements is true?
a. Intermittent hemodialysis should be started immediately.
b. Continuous renal replacement therapy should be started immediately.
c. She does not currently have any indication for dialysis.
d. Give high-dose loop diuretics to increase urine output because they will decrease her chance of dying.

III.86. A 54-year-old woman is admitted to the ICU with atrial fibrillation and rapid ventricular rate. Rate control is achieved with β-blockers, and anticoagulation with heparin drip is started. Her course is complicated by intracranial hemorrhage. She is intubated for airway protection. Her further course is notable for the increase in creatinine level from 0.6 mg/dL to 4 mg/dL, decrease in urine output to

200 mL during the past 24 hours, and hyperkalemia with serum potassium level of 6.2 mEq/L despite her receiving insulin/dextrose and Na^+ polystyrene sulfonate. Which one of the following is the best response?

a. Intermittent hemodialysis should be started.
b. Continuous renal replacement therapy should be started.
c. She does not currently have any indication for dialysis.
d. Give high-dose loop diuretics to increase urine output.

III.87. A 65-year-old woman with a past medical history remarkable for diabetes mellitus, coronary artery disease, and hypertension is admitted to the ICU for severe sepsis due to hospital-acquired pneumonia and AKI. Which one of the following indicates that ATN is the most likely cause of AKI?

a. 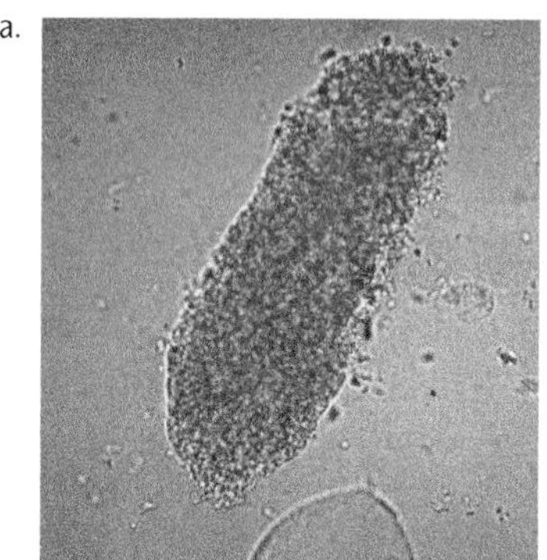

b. 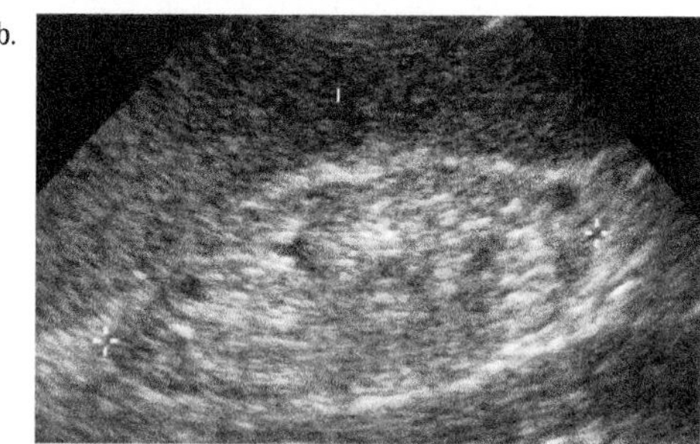

c. 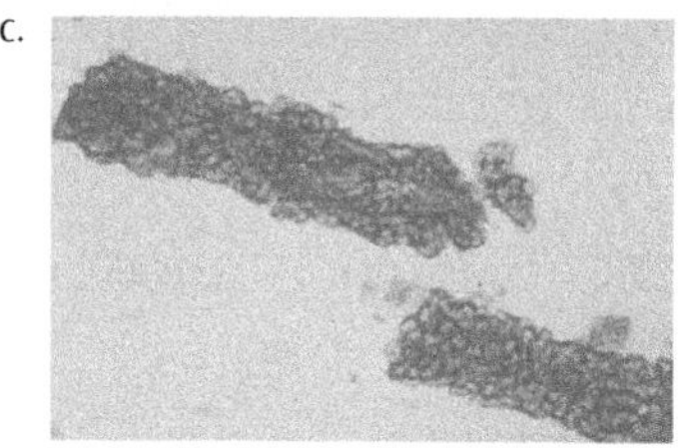

d. Plasma values: Na^+ 140 mEq/L and creatinine 4.2 mg/dL; urine values: Na^+ 10 mEq/L and creatinine 42 mg/dL

III.88. Which one of the following graphs represents the temporal trends of the incidence of AKI among hospitalized patients?

a. 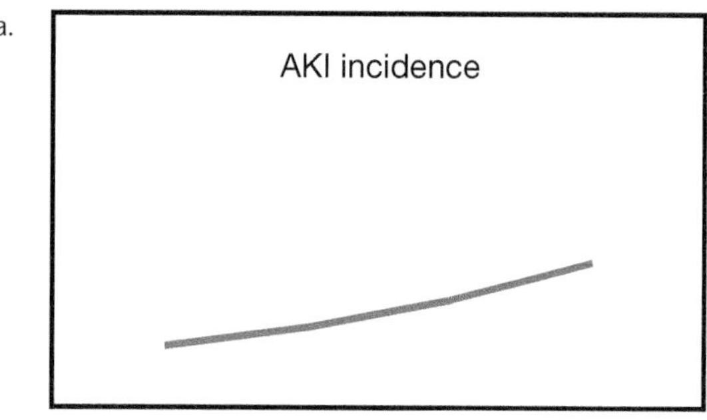

b. 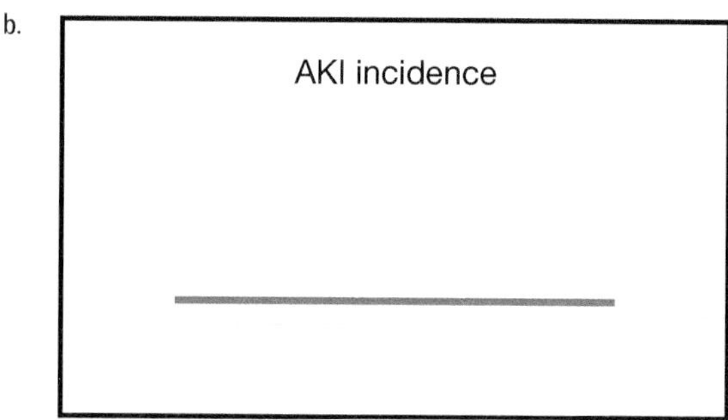

c. 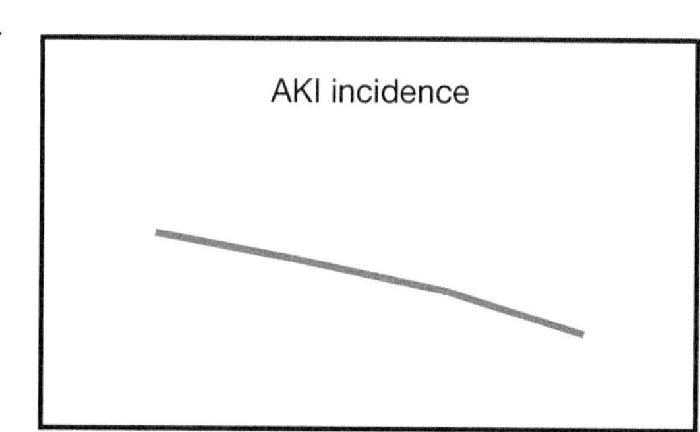

d. 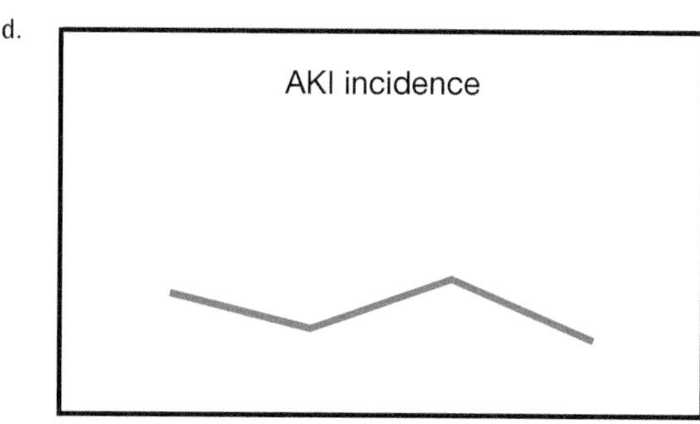

III.89. An 80-year-old woman with severe peripheral vascular disease is admitted to the ICU with severe obtundation. She has slow and shallow respirations. An ABG test has been ordered; however, after multiple attempts, a sample could not be obtained. If a venous sample were to be obtained, which of the following values would not show a good correlation with an arterial sample?

a. pH
b. PO_2
c. PCO_2
d. HCO_3^-

III.90. A patient has the ABG results shown in Table III.Q90.

Table III.Q90 •

Component	Result
pH	7.25
$PaCO_2$, mm Hg	25
PaO_2, mm Hg	85
HCO_3^-, mmol/L	10
Base excess, mmol/L	14
Na^+, mmol/L	135
Cl^-, mmol/L	100

Which of the following diagnoses is unlikely?
a. Renal tubular acidosis
b. Lactic acidosis
c. Salicylate toxicity
d. Methanol ingestion

III.91. Which of the following is *not* a characteristic of a medication that will be removed by hemodialysis?
a. Low lipid solubility
b. Small molecular size
c. High nonrenal plasma clearance
d. Low protein binding

III.92. In patients with renal dysfunction, which of the following antibiotics requires therapeutic drug monitoring and adjustment because of its narrow therapeutic index?
a. Gentamicin
b. Meropenem
c. Ceftriaxone
d. Levofloxacin

III.93. Which of the following does *not* contribute to solute clearance during renal replacement therapy?
a. Convection
b. Amalgamation
c. Adsorption
d. Diffusion

III.94. Which statement is true about hemodiafiltration?
a. It is better than hemodialysis.
b. It is less expensive to perform than hemodialysis.
c. It combines diffusive and convective clearances.
d. It eliminates the need for dialysis fluids.

III.95. Which of the following is the preferred catheter access site for short-term dialysis?
a. Femoral vein
b. Left subclavian vein
c. Left internal jugular vein
d. Right internal jugular vein

III.96. A 21-year-old woman was brought by her friend to the ED because of seizures. The patient has a history of depression managed with citalopram. She had been at a graduation party where recreational drugs were used. On presentation, she is confused and diaphoretic. Her temperature is 38.6°C, BP 139/98 mm Hg, and HR 105 bpm. No focal deficits are found on neurologic examination. Laboratory results are as follows: Na^+, 119 mEq/L; Cl^-, 89 mEq/L; HCO_3^-, 23 mEq/L; and creatinine, 0.8 mg/dL. Serum osmolality is 260 mOsm/kg H_2O, urine osmolality 500 mOsm/kg H_2O, and urine Na^+ 45 mEq/L. Which of the following is the most likely cause of hyponatremia in this patient?
a. Alcohol
b. Hypovolemia
c. MDMA (ecstasy)
d. Psychogenic polydipsia

III.97. A 44-year-old man with history of bipolar disorder who is receiving lithium therapy was brought to the ED because of a 3-day history of irritability, weakness, and lethargy. He had had a diarrheal illness for 2 weeks before presentation. On examination, his weight is 60 kg, BP 88/60 mm Hg, and HR 120 bpm. His neurologic examination is notable for his being alert and oriented to person only. Laboratory results are as follows: Na^+, 158 mEq/L; Cl^-, 120 mEq/L; HCO_3^-, 19 mEq/L; and creatinine 1.2 mg/dL.

Which of the following is the most appropriate treatment?
a. 0.9% normal saline until euvolemic state is achieved
b. D5W with the goal of lowering the serum Na^+ level by 10 mEq in the first 24 hours
c. 0.45% saline
d. Encourage free water intake.

III.98. A 51-year-old man with a history of hepatitis C complicated by hepatic cirrhosis was admitted for severe hyponatremia. Two weeks before admission, nausea and abdominal discomfort developed after he ate a hamburger. Since then his appetite has decreased, and oral intake is minimal. A week before presentation, slow progressive weakness, confusion, and blurry vision developed. Medications include spironolactone, midodrine, lactulose, and ranitidine. On examination, his weight is 60 kg, BP 90/56 mm Hg, and HR 96 bpm. His neurologic examination is notable for slurred speech. He does not have edema. Laboratory results are as follows: Na^+, 114 mEq/L; Cl^-, 84 mEq/L; HCO_3^-, 23 mEq/L; potassium, 5.3 mmol/L, and creatinine 0.9 mg/dL. Serum osmolality is 258 mOsm/kg, urine osmolality 409 mOsm/kg H_2O, and urine Na^+ 25 mEq/L.
What is the best treatment approach for this patient?
a. 1 L of fluid restriction, discontinue use of spironolactone, and 1 L of 3% saline during first 6 hours
b. 1 L of fluid restriction, discontinue use of spironolactone, and give loop diuretic
c. 1 L of normal saline and discontinue use of spironolactone
d. 1 L of fluid restriction, discontinue use of spironolactone, and 300 mL of 3% saline during first 6 hours

III.99. A 44-year-old man was admitted to the hospital for severe headache and found to have a subarachnoid hemorrhage. Three days later, hyponatremia develops. Which of the following laboratory findings distinguishes cerebral salt wasting from SIADH?
a. Hematocrit level
b. Urine osmolality
c. Urine Na^+ level
d. Uric acid level

III.100. A 40-year-old man with a history of alcohol abuse is brought to the ED for seizure-like activity. On examination, his BP is 90/56 mm Hg, and HR is 118 bpm. He appears disheveled and smells of alcohol. His neurologic examination is notable for postictal state. Laboratory results are as follows: Na^+, 109 mEq/L; Cl^-, 84 mEq/L; HCO_3^-, 28 mEq/L; potassium, 2.6 mmol/L; and creatinine, 0.9 mg/dL. Serum osmolality is 240 mOsm/kg, and urine osmolality is 150 mOsm/kg H_2O. He is admitted to the ICU and receives the following therapeutic interventions: 80 mEq of potassium Cl−, 500 mL of 3% normal saline, and thiamine and glucose therapy. At 24 hours later, mental status improved, and his serum Na+ level corrected to 120 mEq/L and potassium to 3.4 mmol/L. Later that evening he became obtunded and respiratory distress requiring emergency intubation developed.

Which of the following is the most appropriate treatment at this time?
a. Resume therapy with 3% saline for a correction rate of 6 mEq/L/day.
b. Replace potassium with potassium Cl^- in half-normal saline.
c. Administer desmopressin and D5W.
d. Administer half-normal saline at 100 mL/hour.

Hematologic and Inflammatory Disorders

III.101. A patient is recovering from lumbar disk laminectomy; on postoperative day 2, he complains of crushing chest pain. His vital signs are within normal limits. Results of laboratory evaluation are as follows: hemoglobin, 7.5 g/dL; troponin, 0.3 ng/L on admission with an increase to 0.4 ng/dL after 3 hours. In addition to management of ACS, what is the appropriate treatment?
a. Transfusion to attain a hemoglobin level of 10 g/dL
b. Administration of 2 L of crystalloid

c. Transfusion to attain the patient's baseline hemoglobin level (13 g/dL on admission)
d. Transfusion to attain a hemoglobin level of 8 g/dL

III.102. A 45-year-old man has a recent diagnosis of high-grade non-Hodgkin lymphoma and completed his first round of chemotherapy 48 hours ago. His renal function was normal, lactic acid level was 4 mg/dL, and lactate dehydrogenase level was 180 U/L before initiation of therapy. He presented to the ED with generalized weakness, nausea, and palpitations. On physical examination, his HR is 120 bpm, BP is 100/60 mm Hg, respiratory rate is 28 breaths per minute, and Spo_2 is 96% while breathing room air. His mucosa and skin seem dry, mentation is normal, and results of cardiovascular and pulmonary examinations are normal. He has profound muscle weakness and depressed tendon reflexes. Laboratory test results are shown in Table III.Q102.

Table III.Q102.

Component	Result
Hemoglobin, g/dL	10
WBCs, × 10^9/L	4
Platelets, × 10^9/L	70
Na^+, mmol/L	139
Potassium, mmol/L	7.9
HCO_3^-, mmol/L	15
Phosphorus, mg/dL	9
Creatinine, mg/dL	3.5
Lactic acid, mg/dL	4
Uric acid, mg/dL	19

Electrocardiography shows diffuse peaked T waves, prolonged PR interval, and widening of the QRS complex. Chest radiography results are normal. What is the first action to take in the management of this patient?
a. IV hydration and correction of acidosis
b. IV administration of calcium gluconate, insulin, and 50% dextrose
c. IV administered fluids and electrolytes replacement
d. Renal replacement therapy

III.103. Which statement is *not* correct about cardiac complications after chemotherapy?
a. They are more likely to occur in young patients with previous left ventricular dysfunction.
b. Type I cardiotoxicity is usually dose related and more likely to be permanent.
c. Type II cardiotoxicity is not dose related and more likely to be reversible.
d. Trastuzumab causes congestive heart failure (type II cardiotoxicity) in 3% to 4% of patients.

III.104. A 53-year-old man with no significant past medical history is directly admitted to the ICU from the ED. His main initial symptom was progressive abdominal pain for several days. When evaluated, the patient is disoriented, lethargic, and complaining of shortness of breath, chest pain, and abdominal pain. On examination, he is in clear distress. Vital signs are as follows: HR 124 bpm; BP, 164/94 mm Hg; respirations, 41 breaths per minute; temperature, 39.2°C; and oxygen saturation, 84% while breathing 10 L/min supplemental oxygen. Crackles are heard bilaterally in all lung fields. His abdomen is nondistended and soft but diffusely tender with rebound tenderness. Several digits are cool. Initial laboratory results are shown in Table III.Q104.

Table III.Q104.

Component	Result
Hemoglobin, mg/dL	7.3
WBCs, × 10^9/L	134 (60% myeloblasts)
Platelets, × 10^9/L	40
Na^+, mmol/L	133
Potassium, mmol/L	6.7
Cl^-, mmol/L	102
Creatinine, mg/dL	4.5
HCO_3^-, mmol/L	10
Lactate, mmol/L	12.3
Troponin T, ng/dL	0.42
ABG	
pH	7.19
Pco_2, mm Hg	27
Pao_2, mm Hg	62

Chest radiography shows diffuse bilateral pulmonary infiltrates and small bilateral pleural effusions. ECG shows mild ST-segment depressions in leads aVL, V_1, and V_2. Which of the following is indicated to treat the most likely underlying cause of the patient's signs and symptoms?
a. Initiate IV heparin infusion and consult a cardiologist for management of non–ST-segment elevation MI.
b. Urgent plasma exchange transfusion
c. Urgent cytotoxic chemotherapy with concurrent leukapheresis
d. Broad-spectrum antibiotics after obtaining a bronchoalveolar lavage specimen for atypical pneumonia

III.105. A 57-year-old woman who received an unrelated-donor allogenic hematopoietic stem cell transplant 23 days ago for myelofibrosis due to polycythemia vera is admitted to the ICU in respiratory distress. On arrival, the patient is disoriented to time and place, intermittently combative, and unable to provide any meaningful history information. According to the admitting physician, the patient was alert and oriented until this morning. On review of her chart, from day 0 to day 20, the ANC was 0.0 cells/mcL. On day 21 the ANC was 0.2 cells/mcL, yesterday it was 3.2 cells/mcL, and today it is 9.2 cells/mcL. The patient has been having periodic fevers throughout her hospital stay. Since her admission, 4 sets of blood cultures have been negative for bacteria. She received empiric treatment with cefepime and vancomycin. On examination, her vitals are as follows: HR, 102 bpm; BP, 110/74 mm Hg; respirations, 29 breaths per minute; temperature, 38.4°C; and Spo_2, 89% while breathing 2 L oxygen by nasal cannula. Bilateral crackles are heard in all lung fields, greater at the bases bilaterally. No murmurs or rubs are appreciated, and rhythm is regular. The abdomen is soft and nontender. Erythroderma is noted diffusely. Laboratory test results (obtained today) are shown in Table III.Q105.

Table III.Q105. •

Component	Result
Hemoglobin, mg/dL	8.1
WBCs, $\times 10^9$/L	9.2
Platelets, $\times 10^9$/L	23
Na^+, mmol/L	142
Potassium, mmol/L	4.1
Cl^-, mmol/L	99
Creatinine, mg/dL	2.4
HCO_3^-, mmol/L	22
Lactate, mmol/L	1.6
Aspartate aminotransferase, U/L	220
Alanine aminotransferase, U/L	206
Alkaline phosphatase, U/L	40
ABG	
pH	7.48
Pco_2, mm Hg	30
Pao_2, mm Hg	57

Chest radiography shows diffuse pulmonary congestion with B lines. ECG results are within normal limits. What is the most likely diagnosis?

a. Acute graft-vs-host disease
b. Engraftment syndrome
c. Chronic graft-vs-host disease
d. Pneumocystis pneumonia

III.106. Which one of the following is correct concerning a patient who may have HIT?

a. Wait for the laboratory test results before deciding whether to stop the use of heparin.
b. Warfarin administration may be started while the platelet count is still low but is increasing.
c. Line flushes of heparin are safe to use because of the low amount of heparin involved.
d. A clinical probability scoring system assessment should be performed first.

III.107. Which of the following is an unlikely presentation for a patient with ITP?

a. A 65-year-old man with a low platelet count who has hepatosplenomegaly, night sweats, bone pain, lymphadenopathy, and weight loss
b. A 6-year-old child who had recent upper respiratory tract infection and now has petechiae
c. A 50-year-old woman who was in a minor car accident and has massive bruising.
d. A 59-year-old man with bruising and purpura who is negative for HIV, hepatitis C, alcohol use, and DIC and has not changed any medications recently.

III.108. A 37-year-old woman with systemic lupus erythematosus is admitted with confusion, anemia, and a platelet count of 18×10^9/L. Which of the following answers is the most reasonable approach in caring for this patient?

a. Order next-generation sequencing for congenital platelet disorders.
b. Consider splenectomy.
c. Test for congenital TTP by ordering genetic mutational testing.
d. Promptly initiate therapeutic plasma exchange with plasma blood products.

III.109. Which of the following is correct concerning drug-induced thrombocytopenia?

a. Over-the-counter nutritional supplements and herbal remedies do not cause platelet dysfunction or thrombocytopenia.
b. Drug-induced thrombocytopenia usually resolves quickly (7-14 days) after stopping use of the medication.
c. The number of cases of drug-induced thrombocytopenia is accurately reported.
d. Chronic ingestion of large quantities of alcohol does not affect megakaryocytopoiesis.

III.110. Which of the following statements is true concerning congenital platelet disorders?

a. Congenital platelet disorders are the most common causes of thrombocytopenia.
b. Patients with congenital platelet disorders characteristically bleed into their muscles and joints and have delayed bleeding after surgery.
c. Platelet transfusions may be required for hemorrhage or may need to be available on standby for procedures.
d. Congenital platelet disorders respond well to the same drugs used for ITP and to splenectomy.

III.111. Which of the following statements is true about DIC?

a. It is a systemic process with bleeding and risk of thrombosis.
b. It is an inherited condition.
c. It is transmissible and spreads from one person to another.
d. It occurs independently and is not associated with any other illness.

III.112. DIC does not occur in isolation and is due to several underlying conditions that are responsible for its initiation and propagation. Although the majority of patients manifest with acute DIC, which of the following is most likely to cause chronic DIC?

a. Motor vehicle accidents with head injury
b. Bacterial sepsis
c. Myeloproliferative disorders
d. HELLP syndrome

III.113. Which of the following statements accurately describes the pathogenic process of abnormal activation of coagulation and fibrinolysis within the vasculature in DIC?

a. DIC is initiated by exposure of blood to prekallikrein.
b. In acute hemolytic transfusion reaction, DIC is caused by increased nitric oxide function and lack of cytokines such as interleukin-1 and tumor necrosis factor.
c. Neutrophils protect against activation of clotting cascade by formation of NETs, which have anticoagulant properties.
d. Cell-free DNA induces platelet aggregation and proteolytic degradation of anticoagulants such as tissue factor pathway inhibitor.

III.114. Which of the following sets of laboratory findings typically is found in DIC?

a. Increased fibrinogen, increased antithrombin, reduced platelets
b. Increased FDPs, decreased PT or aPTT, reduced platelets, increased antithrombin
c. Increased FDP, prolonged PT or aPTT, reduced platelets, increased antithrombin
d. Increased FDP, prolonged PT or aPTT, reduced platelets, decreased antithrombin

III.115. Which of the following statements is true about ancillary treatment of DIC?

a. Platelet transfusion is considered if the patient has bleeding and the platelet count is less than 50×10^9/L, whereas a lower threshold of 20 to 30×10^9/L may be used in patients without bleeding.

b. Although a low plasma AT level is known to be a prognosticator of poor clinical outcome in patients with sepsis and an independent marker of mortality in DIC, therapeutic infusion of AT in DIC is not yet medically approved.
c. Excess fibrinolysis is typical of DIC. However, preventing excessive fibrinolysis with antifibrinolytic agents such as tranexamic acid can be harmful in DIC.
d. All of the above.

III.116. In a patient who has a prolonged PT or aPTT, which of the following is the next most appropriate step in evaluation?
a. Coagulation factor assays
b. Mixing studies with normal pooled plasma
c. von Willebrand factor assays
d. Platelet aggregation studies

III.117. A 70-year-old man with a history of monoclonal gammopathy of undetermined significance of 10 years' duration complains that he has noted increased bruising with minimal trauma for the past 6 months. He has no coexisting chronic illnesses and is currently taking atorvastatin. Apart from scattered bruises on his arms and legs, results of his physical examination are normal. Results of the following laboratory studies are normal: complete blood count, PT, aPTT, and fibrinogen. Which of the following acquired bleeding disorders may best explain his clinical presentation?
a. Factor VIII inhibitor
b. Factor V inhibitor
c. DIC
d. Acquired von Willebrand syndrome

III.118. A 62-year-old man is admitted to the critical care unit with extremity bruising, hematomas, and gastrointestinal hemorrhage. He has a long-standing history of systemic lupus erythematosus, which has been managed with hydroxychloroquine. With the exception of extensive cutaneous bruises, the results of physical examination are normal. Results of laboratory studies are listed in Table III.Q118.

Table III.Q118. •

Component	Result
Complete blood count	Normal
Fibrinogen	Normal
aPTT, s	72 (normal, 25–37)
1:1 Mixing study with normal pooled plasma, s	58
D-Dimer	Markedly increased

Which of the following acquired coagulopathies does this patient most likely have?
a. Factor VIII inhibitor
b. Factor V inhibitor
c. DIC and fibrinolysis
d. Acquired von Willebrand syndrome

III.119. A 78-year-old woman with a history of atrial fibrillation who is receiving warfarin was admitted to the ED after she was found unconscious at her home. Her family suspects that she had fallen down the stairs. Point-of-care testing in the ED found the following: hemoglobin level, 13.4 g/dL; platelet count, 243 × 10^9/L; and INR, 4.4. CT of the head showed an acute subdural hematoma and substantial midline shift. On neurosurgical consultation, urgent decompression was recommended. The patient weighs 90 kg and has a body mass index of 38. Besides holding warfarin administration, what is the best option for reversing the effect of warfarin?
a. Immediately determine ABO-Rh type and transfuse 10 to 15 mL/kg of fresh frozen plasma.
b. Administer 10 mg of vitamin K IV, check the INR every 6 hours, and delay surgery until the INR is normal.
c. Administer 5 to 10 mg of vitamin K IV and 3,150 IU of 4F-PCC now and take the patient to surgery immediately.
d. Administer 10 mg of vitamin K subcutaneously and 3,150 IU of 4F-PCC now and take the patient to surgery immediately.

III.120. A 28-year-old woman with a history of thrombophilia due to antiphospholipid antibodies receives maintenance therapy with warfarin and has an INR goal of 2.0 to 3.0. She is admitted for acute right-sided weakness and is found to have multiple acute ischemic infarcts. She admits that she has not been compliant with her anticoagulation therapy. Results of laboratory studies are listed in Table III.Q120.

Table III.Q120. •

Component	Reference Range	Patient's Baseline Value at Admission
PT, s	11.0-14.2	13.8
aPTT, s	25.0-35.0	52.0
aPTT UFH therapeutic range, s	62.0-95.0	NA
INR	NA	1.3

IV UFH therapy is started. What is the UFH therapeutic anticoagulation goal for this patient?
a. 1.5 to 2.5 times the patient's baseline aPTT
b. aPTT of 62 to 95 seconds
c. aPTT of 96 to 126 seconds
d. Plasma UFH concentration of 0.3 to 0.7 U/mL by anti-Xa assay

III.121. An 87-year-old man with a history of prostate cancer is examined in the ED for shortness of breath. During his evaluation, a PE is found. UFH infusion is initiated, and therapeutic anticoagulation is achieved within 24 hours at 18 U/kg per hour. The patient weighs 70 kg and received maintenance therapy with heparin at a rate of 1,260 units/h until he started complaining of abdominal pain on day 3 of admission. Urgent CT showed an acute, large retroperitoneal hematoma. He had become hemodynamically unstable, and the heparin therapy was discontinued. What is the most appropriate next step?
a. Administer 12 mg of protamine sulfate IV to neutralize the UFH.
b. Administer 30 mg of protamine sulfate IV to neutralize the UFH.
c. Administer 1 unit of plasma to neutralize the UFH.
d. Administer 700 mL of plasma to neutralize the UFH.

III.122. A 76-year-old man in whom a DVT was diagnosed 4 months ago is receiving oral therapy with daily dabigatran. The patient now presents to the ED after he fell in the shower, hit his head, and had subsequent loss of consciousness. The patient is drowsy, and CT of the head shows a large subdural hematoma with substantial midline shift. According to family, the patient took dabigatran 14 hours ago. He takes no other prescription medication and has not taken any over-the-counter medications in the past 14 days. The patient's laboratory values are shown in Table III.Q122.

Table III.Q122. •

Component	Reference Range	Patient's Baseline Value at Admission
WBC count, × 10^9/L	3.5-10.5	10.3
Hemoglobin, g/dL	12-15	14.5
Hematocrit, %	35-45	44
Platelet count, × 10^9/L	150-350	277
PT, s	11.0-14.2	20
aPTT, s	25.0-35.0	41.0
Fibrinogen, mg/dL	200-375	412
INR	NA	1.5

What is the next best management plan to prepare him for immediate surgery?

a. The patient's surgery must be delayed by 24 to 48 hours after his last dose of dabigatran.
b. Administer 10 to 15 mL/kg of fresh frozen plasma, then take the patient immediately to surgery.
c. Dialyze the patient now and take him to surgery.
d. Administer a total of 5 g of idarucizumab before taking the patient to surgery.

III.123. A 67-year-old man with a history of recurrent DVT who is receiving life-long anticoagulation presents to the ED complaining of extreme fatigue. He had been feeling tired for the past 2 weeks. He reports having dark tarry stools for approximately 3 weeks. He is currently receiving 20 mg of rivaroxaban daily to reduce the risk of recurrent DVT; he last took the medication 30 hours ago. On examination, he is hypotensive, tachycardic, and markedly pale. Your laboratory does not offer rivaroxaban level testing with an anti-Xa assay, but the ED physician ordered it anyway. Results of liver and renal function tests on admission are normal, but the admission laboratory values of other tests were remarkable for the values shown in Table III.Q123.

Table III.Q123. •

Component	Reference Range	Patient's Baseline Value at Admission
WBC count, × 10^9/L	3.5-10.5	12.5
Hemoglobin, g/dL	12-15	5.6
Hematocrit, %	35-45	16
Platelet count, × 10^9/L	150-350	117
PT, s	11.0-14.2	18
aPTT, s	25.0-35.0	32
Fibrinogen, mg/dL	200-375	389
Therapeutic UFH Xa level, U/mL	0.3-0.7	2.3
INR	NA	1.4

Other than herbal and vitamin supplements, the patient denies taking other over-the-counter medications. You provide transfusion support with 3 units of packed red blood cells. The patient becomes hemodynamically stabilized, and gastrointestinal bleeding is suspected to have slowed or stopped. In addition to the therapies initiated, you should consider which of the following?

a. Administration of prothrombin complex concentrate to counter the effects of residual rivaroxaban, as evidenced by the increased anti-Xa level
b. Administration of recombinant activated factor VII to counter the effects of rivaroxaban, as evidenced by the increased anti-Xa level
c. Recheck the PT and INR and, if increased above the normal reference range, administer prothrombin complex concentrate.
d. Monitor the patient's vital signs and hematologic factors frequently, and provide transfusion support as necessary. No reversal therapies are needed at this time.

III.124. A 27-year-old obtunded woman is admitted to the critical care unit while undergoing TPE for TTP. Which of the following statements is correct?

a. Vascular access should be achieved with peripheral veins if they are palpable in the antecubital fossa.
b. Because of profound thrombocytopenia, all anticoagulation should be held, including anticoagulation for the apheresis instrument.
c. Albumin should be used as replacement fluid to minimize adverse reactions in this critically ill patient.
d. Plasma should be used as replacement fluid to provide exogenous enzymes and clotting factors.

III.125. A 52-year-old man with dilated cardiomyopathy and a remote history of HIT is hospitalized while waiting for a heart transplant. He is currently receiving prophylactic anticoagulation with argatroban. Which of the following statements is correct?

a. Laboratory tests show no evidence of HIT antibodies; it is not necessary to perform TPE if heparin is used to anticoagulate the CPB circuit during transplant.
b. Laboratory tests show no evidence of HIT antibodies; however, TPE should still be performed before transplant if heparin is used to anticoagulate the CPB circuit.
c. Laboratory tests show no evidence of HIT antibodies; it is not necessary to perform TPE before transplant because heparin is absolutely contraindicated for CPB in patients with a history of HIT.
d. Laboratory tests are positive for HIT antibodies; it is not necessary to perform TPE if heparin is used to anticoagulate the CPB circuit during transplant.

III.126. An 82-year-old man is admitted to the neurologic critical care unit after a stroke complicated by aspiration pneumonia. His past medical history includes hypertension, hyperlipidemia, diabetes mellitus, and gout. Outpatient medications include metoprolol, furosemide, simvastatin, metformin, and allopurinol. On the third day of admission, an erythematous, warm right knee and associated effusion are noted. Laboratory results are WBC count, 18×10^9/L; creatinine, 2.3 mg/dL; erythrocyte sedimentation rate, 60 mm in 1 hour, C-reactive protein, 90 mg/L; and uric acid, 9 mg/dL. On polarized microscopy of aspirated fluid, negatively birefringent crystals consistent with monosodium urate crystals are found. What is the next best step?

a. Initiate indomethacin therapy.
b. Obtain blood cultures and start empiric antibiotic therapy.
c. Inject corticosteroids intra-articularly.
d. Initiate colchicine therapy.

III.127. An 84-year-old woman is admitted after transient monocular vision loss. In the past few weeks, she has had considerable anorexia, weight loss, and low-grade fever. She has also had fatigue in the setting of disrupted sleep from the discomfort of placing her head on her pillow. Initial evaluation includes CT, which does not show any acute abnormalities. On examination, she has a difficult time getting from the chair to the bed because of pain. No murmurs are noted, and no carotid bruits are appreciated. She does have tenderness to palpation over the temporal region bilaterally. Results of laboratory evaluation are hemoglobin, 10.4 mg/dL; WBCs, 12×10^9/L; platelets, 485, erythrocyte sedimentation rate, 85 mm in 1 hour, C-reactive protein, 120 mg/L; and creatinine, 0.8 mg/dL. What is the next best step?

a. Start methylprednisolone therapy now, 1,000 mg IV, and order temporal artery biopsy.
b. Order temporal artery biopsy and, after it is completed, start methylprednisolone therapy 1,000 mg IV.
c. Start prednisone therapy, 15 mg daily, and order temporal artery biopsy.
d. Order temporal artery biopsy and, after it is completed, start prednisone therapy, 15 mg daily.

Sepsis and Other Infectious Diseases

III.128. Which of the following recommendations regarding the diagnosis and management of *Clostridium difficile* infections is *not* correct?

a. Use of all unnecessary antibiotics should be discontinued.
b. Vancomycin is the drug of choice of severe *C difficile* infections.
c. Stool specimens should be collected only if the patient has had passage of 3 or more unformed stools.
d. Test of cure is recommended at the completion of treatment.

III.129. Which one of the following statements is correct regarding diagnosis, management, and prevention of catheter-related urinary tract infections?

a. Routine urine specimens for cultures should be drawn from all patients with indwelling urinary catheters at 72 hours of placement.
b. The presence of pyuria is useful for differentiating asymptomatic bacteriuria from catheter-related urinary tract infection.
c. Urine specimens for cultures should not be obtained for evaluation of fever in a patient in ICU in the absence of symptoms of urinary tract infection (eg, suprapubic pain or bladder spasms, flank pain) unless the patient is a kidney transplant recipient, is granulocytopenic, has recently undergone urologic surgery, or has an obstructed renal collection system.
d. Treatment of asymptomatic bacteriuria is recommended in all patients admitted to an ICU.

III.130. Which of the following options to prevent central line–associated bloodstream infection is correct?

a. All central lines should be routinely cultured.
b. Patients should receive prophylactic vancomycin before all central line insertions.
c. Central venous lines should be rotated periodically.
d. Daily chlorhexidine baths have shown benefit for preventing central line–associated bloodstream infection.

III.131. A 65-year-old man with a past medical history of metastatic malignant melanoma was admitted to the ICU 3 days ago for status epilepticus. His seizure activity has resolved for the past 2 days, although he is not ready to be extubated. A right femoral catheter was placed during admission; today you notice considerable erythema and some purulence at the access site of the catheter and new-onset fever and hypotension. You decide to remove the catheter and start empiric IV vancomycin. After 24 hours, the patient is still febrile and has worsening leukocytosis and persistent hypotension requiring vasopressors. What would be your next action?

a. Perform brain MRI with and without contrast agent.
b. Add cefepime to the current antibiotic treatment.
c. Continue current treatment with IV vancomycin.
d. Add cefepime and caspofungin to the current antibiotic treatment.

III.132. A 65-year-old man was admitted 20 days ago for management of Guillain-Barré syndrome. He received treatment with levofloxacin 4 to 5 weeks ago for an upper respiratory tract infection. His neurologic status has recovered satisfactorily. Today he is transferred to the neurology ICU because of encephalopathy associated with fever, hypotension, and profuse watery diarrhea. His BP has not improved after multiple IV fluid boluses. His WBC is 27.5×10^9/L, and a *Clostridium difficile* toxin assay is reported as having positive results. What would you do next?

a. Start oral vancomycin therapy.
b. Start IV metronidazole therapy.
c. Perform rapid surgical evaluation.
d. Choices *a, b,* and *c,* are correct.

III.133. A patient admitted to the ICU has development of fever, and blood cultures are positive for *Enterococcus faecalis*. Which of the following antibiotics is never effective against *E faecalis*?

a. Daptomycin
b. Linezolid
c. Ceftriaxone
d. Ampicillin

III.134. A patient is admitted for a decompressive procedure for an epidural abscess. Intraoperative cultures are positive against MSSA. The patient has no allergies to any medication. Which of the following antibiotics is the preferred choice?

a. Nafcillin
b. Ceftriaxone
c. Vancomycin
d. Linezolid

III.135. Which of the following agents does *not* have activity against *Pseudomonas aeruginosa*?

a. Levofloxacin
b. Aztreonam
c. Ceftolozane-tazobactam
d. Cefotaxime

III.136. A patient was admitted to the ICU for new- onset seizures that, after extensive workup, were found to be due to a brain abscess caused by *Candida albicans* (pansusceptible). Which of the following is *not* an adequate option in the management of this infection?

a. Fluconazole
b. Caspofungin
c. Voriconazole
d. Amphotericin B

III.137. A 24-year-old man with a past medical history of systemic lupus erythematosus has been receiving high-dose prednisone for the past few weeks for lupus nephritis. He was admitted to the neurology ICU after new-onset seizures. Brain MRI shows a frontal abscess. Blood cultures are positive for *Pseudomonas aeruginosa*, resistant to all β-lactam antibiotics except to carbapenems. The microorganism is also resistant to ciprofloxacin and aminoglycosides. What antibiotic do you administer?

a. Imipenem- cilastin
b. Meropenem
c. Ertapenem
d. Cefepime

III.138. An 84-year-old African-American man presents to the ED complaining of severe abdominal pain. He has a history of coronary artery disease, COPD, diabetes mellitus, and long-standing CKD. He has been a smoker for 30 years. Initial findings are as follows: temperature, 35.4°C; BP, 70/40 mm Hg; respirations, 30 per minute; arterial Spo_2, 92% breathing 2L of oxygen through a nasal cannula (oxygen he brought from home). On examination, he is not responsive to questioning, and his extremities are cool and slightly mottled. CT shows a colonic abscess. What is your diagnosis?

a. Systemic inflammatory response
b. Sepsis
c. Septic shock
d. Multi-organ dysfunction syndrome

III.139. Which of the following is *not* part of the SOFA score?
a. Ratio of Pao_2/Fio_2
b. Bilirubin level
c. Platelet level
d. INR

III.140. For the patient described in Question III.138, what therapeutic intervention will most benefit his morbidity and mortality after cardiopulmonary stabilization?
a. Broad-spectrum antibiotics
b. CT-guided drainage
c. Early renal replacement therapy
d. Lung-protective mechanical ventilation strategies

III.141. ARDS develops in the patient described in Question III.138 and he has to be intubated for refractory hypoxemia. What medication is *not* preferred for maintenance sedation?
a. Ketamine
b. Propofol
c. Fentanyl
d. Midazolam

Dermatologic Concerns

III.142. Which of the following is *not* a common cause of drug hypersensitivity syndrome?
a. Doxycycline
b. Trimethoprim-sulfamethoxazole
c. Phenytoin
d. Carbamazepine

III.143. Which of the following is *not* a prognostic factor for determining the risk of death from toxic epidermal necrolysis?
a. Preexisting malignancy
b. HR greater than 120 bpm
c. SUN greater than 28 mg/dL
d. Aspartate aminotransferase greater than 98 units/L

Trauma and Burns

III.144. A 34-year-old man is brought comatose to the ED after a motor vehicle accident in which his vehicle sustained considerable damage. His BP is 60/40 mm Hg, and his pulse is 130 bpm. He is gasping for breaths. His abdomen is distended, and both ankles have actively bleeding open fractures. If simultaneous interventions are not possible, which of the following interventions should be performed *first*?
a. Place tourniquets on both lower extremities.
b. Start resuscitation with a balanced-ratio blood product.
c. Obtain a chest radiograph to look for pneumothorax.
d. Establish a definitive airway.

III.145. Which of the following is considered an adjunct to the primary survey?
a. Nasogastric tube placement
b. Airway examination
c. AMPLE history
d. Tetanus toxoid administration

III.146. A patient has been admitted comatose to the neurocritical care unit for management of a severe head injury after a fall from 30 feet. He is intubated. He has left rib fractures, a low-grade splenic laceration, and left femoral and acetabular fractures. Two hours after ICU admission, his BP suddenly decreases to 60/40 mm Hg and his HR is 110 bpm. Which of the following is the appropriate initial response by the ICU clinician?
a. Repeat the primary survey (assess the patient for ABC).
b. Page a general surgeon for the splenic laceration.
c. Perform a needle decompression of the pleural spaces bilaterally.
d. Order angiography for embolization of retroperitoneal hemorrhage.

III.147. A 49-year-old man is brought to the ED by paramedics after a head-on motor vehicle collision in which he was a restrained driver. His HR is 130 bpm, BP 95/55 mm Hg, and Spo_2 90%. He opens his eyes in response to pain, is mumbling incomprehensibly, and withdraws with painful stimuli. He has bruising over his sternum. The cardiac monitor shows frequent ectopic beats. He undergoes CT of the head, spine, chest, abdomen, and pelvis. What is the most appropriate next additional test to order?
a. Formal echocardiography
b. Troponin levels
c. ECG (12-lead)
d. Abdominal aortography

III.148. A 19-year-old woman is admitted to the ICU after undergoing selective angioembolization of the spleen for a grade III splenic laceration. Her GCS score is 5T with minimal sedation. Initially, she is hemodynamically stable. On day 2, her HR progressively increases to 140 to 150 bpm, and her BP is 85/45 mm Hg. You suspect delayed splenic bleeding. After initiation of resuscitation, what should be the next step in management?
a. General angioembolization of the spleen
b. Permissive hypotension to prevent further hemorrhage
c. Tranexamic acid, massive transfusion protocol, and blood products directed with thromboelastography.
d. Emergent splenectomy

III.149. A 38-year-old woman is involved in a pedestrian-automobile accident. On initial trauma evaluation, she has an open fracture of the left femoral shaft, a closed fracture of the right femur, an open fracture of the right tibial shaft, and a closed fracture of the right humeral shaft. Her systolic BP is 100 mm Hg; her HR is 123 bpm. Her initial hematocrit is 34.3%, and serum lactate is 4.8 mmol/L. What is the most appropriate next step in treatment?
a. Irrigation and débridement of the open fractures; intramedullary nailing of both femoral fractures and the tibial fracture; and splinting of the humeral shaft fracture
b. Irrigation and débridement of the open fractures; intramedullary nailing of both femoral fractures and the tibial fracture; and open reduction and internal fixation of the humeral shaft fracture
c. Irrigation and débridement of the open fractures; external fixation of both femoral fractures and the tibial fracture; and splinting of the humeral shaft fracture
d. Irrigation and débridement of the open fractures; splinting of both femoral fractures, the tibial fracture, and the humeral shaft fracture

III.150. A 16-year-old adolescent girl sustained a closed fracture of the proximal tibia after a fall at a trampoline park. The fracture is reduced and placed in a long-leg splint in the ED, and the patient is admitted for definitive fixation. Throughout the night, she requires increasing doses of narcotics for uncontrolled pain. What is the earliest and most sensitive sign of impending compartment syndrome?
a. Decreased sensation in the foot
b. Decreased pulses in the foot
c. Pain out of proportion for the injury
d. Inability to move the toes of the affected extremity

III.151. A 25-year-old man is brought to the ED after the fire department rescued him from a house fire. His clothing is charred, and exposed skin, including the skin on his face, shows signs of burn injury. He is drowsy but rousable, and he moans with movement. What is the first step in management?

a. Initiate local cooling of the burn.
b. Obtain IV access with a large-bore catheter and start immediate fluid resuscitation according to the Parkland formula.
c. Assess the airway.
d. Administer IV analgesia.

III.152. According to the Parkland formula for fluid resuscitation in burn management, in the first 24 hours, fluid is given at a dose of 4 mL/kg for each 1% of TBSA burned. What is an important concern with this approach?

a. It may lead to overadministration of fluid.
b. The formula underestimates the circulating volume in a burn patient.
c. It does not offer guidance beyond the first 24 hours.
d. Colloid is not included in the recommendation.

Cardiothoracic Critical Care

III.153. A 67-year-old man with a past medical history of hypothyroidism, type 2 diabetes mellitus, hypertension, coronary artery disease, and atrial fibrillation had 4-vessel CABG surgery the previous day. He now reports having retrosternal chest pain that is nonreproducible. His BP is 85/43 mm Hg, and his HR is 95 bpm with frequent premature ventricular contractions on the ECG. His respiratory rate is 18 breaths per minute (mildly labored), and his Spo_2 is 93% with oxygen delivered by nasal cannula at 5 L/min. He says that his chest pain is similar to what he felt before the surgical procedure. You suspect that he may be having an ischemic event possibly related to a failed bypass graft. Which of the following is the most specific and sensitive test to help diagnose his ischemia?

a. Serum lactate level greater than 2.0 mmol/L
b. Serial ECG
c. Transthoracic echocardiography
d. Serial troponin levels

III.154. A 32-year-old man with a past medical history of congenital bicuspid aortic valve stenosis (treated with aortic valve replacement at the age of 22), obstructive sleep apnea, and type 1 diabetes mellitus had a reoperation with sternotomy and mechanical aortic valve replacement today. His BP is 79/55 mm Hg, and his HR is 112 bpm (sinus rhythm). The patient is intubated and receiving mechanical ventilation with the following settings: pressure control ventilation with pressure support of 15 mm Hg; PEEP, 5 cm H_2O; ventilator rate, 12 breaths per minute; minute ventilation, 12.4 L/min; Fio_2, 0.50; and Spo_2, 98%. In the first hour after the surgical procedure, his chest tube output was 300 mL; in the second hour, 325 mL; and in the third hour, 350 mL. The obvious concern is bleeding. Which of the following is *not* an acceptable management strategy?

a. Aim for a fibrinogen level greater than 150 mg/dL.
b. Maintain a systolic BP greater than 110 mm Hg.
c. Aim for a pH between 7.35 and 7.42.
d. Maintain a hemoglobin level greater than 8 g/dL.

III.155. A 90-year-old man with a past medical history of hypothyroidism, coronary artery disease, and hypertension is referred to a cardiologist for a 3-month history of progressive dyspnea on exertion and an episode of syncope while walking to the house of his daughter about a month ago. On admission to the office, his BP is 136/65 mm Hg, his HR is 82 bpm, and his respiratory rate is 18 breaths per minute. After multiple diagnostic tests, transthoracic echocardiography showed that the patient has aortic stenosis. Which of the following is *most* important in deciding whether to replace the aortic valve in this patient?

a. Mean transvalvular gradient
b. Systolic pulmonary artery pressure
c. Ejection fraction
d. Left ventricular end-diastolic pressure

III.156. A 65-year-old man with a past medical history of hypertension and type 2 diabetes mellitus is admitted to the hospital for elective CABG surgery. Five days after undergoing an uneventful procedure, he had acute dyspnea and chest pain accompanied by oxyhemoglobin desaturation. According to your clinical suspicion, which of the following ABG values is most likely present in this patient?

a. pH 7.5, Pao_2 60, $Paco_2$ 30, HCO_3^- 22 mmol/L
b. pH 7.3, Pao_2 60, $Paco_2$ 30, HCO_3^- 20 mmol/L
c. pH 7.5, Pao_2 60, $Paco_2$ 50, HCO_3^- 28 mmol/L
d. pH 7.3, Pao_2 60, $Paco_2$ 50, HCO_3^- 24 mmol/L

III.157. A 45-year-old man with a past medical history of a previously repaired bicuspid aortic valve, CKD, type 2 diabetes mellitus, and hypertension is in the ICU after a reoperation for aortic valve replacement. Owing to the complexity of the repair, the cardiac bypass time was 360 minutes, and the patient received 6 units of packed red blood cells and 4 packs of fresh frozen plasma. His BP is 79/55 mm Hg; his HR is 122 bpm (sinus rhythm). He is intubated and receiving mechanical ventilation as follows: pressure controlled ventilation with a pressure support of 15 cm H_2O; PEEP, 10 cm H_2O; ventilator rate, 12 breaths per minute; minute ventilation, 12.4 L/min; Fio_2, 0.50; and Spo_2, 98%. Despite increasing doses of epinephrine and vasopressin, his BP does not increase. The pulmonary artery catheter reading is 45/25 mm Hg; mean pulmonary artery pressure, 32 mm Hg; and CVP, 25 mm Hg. In the first hour after he arrived from the operating room, his chest tube output was 50 mL; in the second hour, 25 mL; and in the third hour, 25 mL. Pericardial tamponade is the main concern. Which of the following is *not* a key diagnostic consideration or management strategy?

a. Early diastolic collapse of the right ventricular free wall
b. Late diastolic compression or collapse of the right atrium
c. Transfusing packed red blood cells to maintain a hemoglobin level of more than 8 mg/dL
d. Giving a 500-mL bolus of lactated Ringer solution

III.158. Which of the following causes low LVAD flows?

a. Adrenal insufficiency
b. Sepsis
c. Anaphylaxis
d. Saddle PE

III.159. If a patient with a destination LVAD has intracranial hemorrhage, is receiving warfarin, and needs reversal of coagulopathy, which agent should be used first?

a. Platelets
b. Tranexamic acid
c. 4F-PCC
d. Idarucizumab

III.160. A 34-year-old man in the ICU is receiving VV ECMO for severe influenza-associated ARDS. New-onset left arm weakness prompts a consultation with a neurologist, and a CT scan of the head shows acute ischemic changes in the right MCA territory. A baseline transthoracic echocardiogram for an incidental murmur was obtained when the patient was 32 years old. It showed trivial tricuspid regurgitation and a small PFO with a left-to-right shunt. His ECMO therapy was complicated by clot formation in the ECMO tubing that required an increase in heparin anticoagulation, from an initial aPTT range of 40 to 60 seconds up to the latest aPTT range of 60 to 80 seconds. What is the most likely cause of his ischemic stroke?

a. Intracardiac thrombus formation due to blood stagnation in the left atrium
b. An embolic event during cannulation of the aorta for ECMO
c. Spontaneous dissection of the MCA
d. Embolism of a clot from the ECMO circuit across the PFO

III.161. During cardiac arrest due to arrhythmia, a 68-year-old man is treated with VA ECMO. The ECMO team orders serial NSE levels to aid prognostication. Which of the following is true about serum NSE levels during ECMO?

a. There is no evidence to support the validity of NSE levels during ECMO.
b. Serum NSE levels greater than 100 mcg/L within 24 hours after initiation of ECMO are predictive of poor neurologic outcomes and death.
c. Serum NSE levels greater than 80 mcg/L during ECMO have excellent sensitivity but only modest specificity for poor neurologic outcomes.
d. Hemolysis has no effect on serum NSE levels.

III.162. A 60-year-old woman presents with an ST-segment elevation MI that results in ventricular fibrillation arrest in the coronary catheterization laboratory. After 2 minutes of CPR, she regains a pulse and awakens enough to follow commands symmetrically with all 4 extremities. Owing to her high inotropic requirements and worsening hypoxemia from severe pulmonary edema, the cardiologist proceeds with peripheral cannulation for VA ECMO (through the femoral vein and femoral artery). The patient is anesthetized during the femoral cannulation. While the patient receives peripheral VA ECMO, the pulse oximetry readings in her right hand are lower than expected (68%). A sample for ABG analysis is drawn from the left radial arterial line and shows pH 7.39, $Paco_2$ 40 mm Hg, and PaO_2 347 mm Hg. Since cannulation, ECMO blood flows have been 5 L/min (cardiac index >2.2 L/min/m^2), and mean arterial BPs have been 65 to 80 mm Hg. Sedation is held for 48 hours, but the patient does not awaken. Findings from CT of the head are consistent with diffuse anoxic brain injury. What is the most likely cause of the patient's diffuse anoxic brain injury?

a. Proximal aortic hypoxemia (harlequin syndrome)
b. The initial ventricular fibrillation arrest
c. ECMO oxygenator membrane failure
d. ECMO pump failure

III.163. Which of the following is true about cerebral autoregulation?

a. Cerebral autoregulation is normal immediately after initiation of nonpulsatile blood flow, such as with VA ECMO.
b. Even after restoration of normal pulsatile blood flow and normalization of ABGs, cerebral autoregulation may be impaired for hours after cardiac arrest.
c. Cerebral autoregulation does not normalize after long-term exposure to nonpulsatile blood flow, such as with LVADs.
d. Systemic anticoagulation but not impaired cerebral autoregulation is thought to predispose ECMO patients to hemorrhagic stroke.

III.164. A 58-year-old man treated with peripheral VA ECMO (through right femoral vein and right femoral artery cannulations) was weaned from sedation and extubated, while ECMO was continued. He reports numbness in his right leg and foot. On examination, he has no motor strength in his right foot and ankle (dorsiflexion and plantarflexion). The right leg distal to the knee is cool and cyanotic, with no palpable distal pulses. His other extremities have normal sensation, normal motor strength, and normal signs of distal perfusion. What is the most likely cause of the patient's right leg and foot numbness?

a. Compartment syndrome
b. Critical illness polyneuropathy
c. Compression of the femoral nerve near the cannulation site
d. Acute intermittent porphyria

III.165. An 86-year-old woman presents to the ED with light-headedness, nausea, and chest discomfort that is worse with inspiration. She underwent pacemaker implantation 3 days ago. Her BP is 92/54 mm Hg, but the systolic BP decreases to 78 mm Hg with inspiration. Her ECG shows atrial and ventricular pacing and capture. What should be the next step in the clinical management of this patient?

a. Perform coronary angiography.
b. Increase the pacing output.
c. Reposition the pacing lead.
d. Perform urgent echocardiography and pericardiocentesis.

III.166. A 52-year-old woman with a history of renal transplant is undergoing therapy for community-acquired pneumonia and is urgently transferred to the ICU after resuscitation for in-hospital ventricular fibrillation arrest. She was rapidly resuscitated and has recovered consciousness. She has no history of coronary artery disease, and a coronary angiogram performed 2 months ago showed no clinically significant coronary artery disease. The ECG strip recorded while she was resting in the ICU is shown in Figure III.Q166.

A 12-lead ECG shows sinus bradycardia with frequent premature ventricular contractions and a corrected QT interval of 640 ms. In addition to reviewing her current medication regimen and electrolyte levels, what should be the next step in the clinical management of this patient?

a. Administer IV insulin and glucose.
b. Request a consultation for ICD implantation.
c. Initiate sotalol therapy.
d. Insert a temporary pacing wire.

III.167. A 68-year-old man is hospitalized with recurrent bacteremia and septic shock after completing a 2-week course of nafcillin therapy for MSSA bacteremia. He has a history of complete heart block and a dual-chamber pacemaker, but otherwise he has no history of heart disease. Follow-up blood cultures again grow MSSA. After hemodynamic stabilization, a transesophageal echocardiogram shows no vegetations on the valves or on the device wires, and the ejection fraction is 70% and hyperdynamic. A CT scan is negative for abscesses, and no other source of infection is identified. What should be the next step in the clinical management of this patient?

a. Extraction of the entire pacing system, with placement of a temporary pacemaker
b. Extraction of the pacing pulse generator only
c. Treatment with vancomycin for 2 weeks
d. A longer course of nafcillin and a follow-up transesophageal echocardiogram in 2 weeks

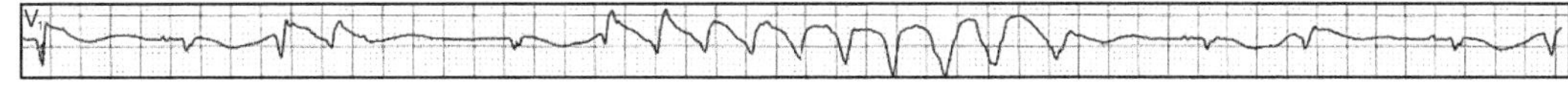

Figure III.Q166.

III.168. A 64-year-old man presents with a history of 5 defibrillator shocks within the past hour. He was awake and conscious and has felt well otherwise over the course of the day. An ECG shows normal sinus rhythm (HR 92 bpm). What should be the next step in the clinical management of this patient?
a. Administer a bolus of amiodarone.
b. Perform chest radiography to evaluate defibrillator lead integrity.
c. Interrogate the device.
d. Place a magnet over the device.

III.169. An 82-year-old man with ischemic cardiomyopathy, an ejection fraction of 25%, and previous ventricular arrhythmias with a biventricular ICD implanted 5 years ago, is admitted to the hospital with community-acquired pneumonia, shock, and multiorgan failure. He previously underwent atrioventricular node ablation because of a history of atrial fibrillation; he is pacemaker dependent. He is encephalopathic, and the adult named in his medical power of attorney indicates a desire to pursue comfort care and requests having the ICD turned off. Which of the following is most correct in describing inactivation of the device in this situation?
a. Both defibrillation and pacing functions can be inactivated without changing the patient's clinical status.
b. Inactivating pacing and defibrillation functions is comparable to physician-assisted suicide.
c. Pacing and defibrillation are medical interventions that can be ethically withdrawn; however, the adult named in the medical power of attorney must understand that asystole may result from discontinuing pacing in a pacemaker-dependent patient.
d. Placing a magnet over the device would inhibit both pacing and defibrillation functions.

Transplant Critical Care

III.170. Which statement correctly describes high CVP and low cardiac output in a heart transplant recipient?
a. They are normal and expected as the heart adjusts to the new host and the blunted neurohormonal response due to the inadvertent cardiac denervation.
b. They should be treated with nitrates and preload reduction.
c. They should be treated with IV fluids and improved preload to help the donor heart overcome the low cardiac output.
d. They are alarming signs of right-sided heart failure due to the recipient's preexisting PH.

III.171. Which of the following should *not* be used to treat heart transplant recipients who have bradycardia postoperatively?
a. Isoproterenol
b. Atropine
c. Atrial pacing
d. Atrial and ventricular pacing

III.172. A 59-year-old man had double lung transplant for severe PH. On postoperative day 1, reintubation was required (after initial, successful extubation) for worsening lung infiltrates and hypoxemia. Chest radiography shows bilateral diffuse infiltrates. Which of the following is the likely cause?
a. Pulmonary contusion
b. Severe acute rejection
c. Primary graft dysfunction
d. Cytomegalovirus pneumonia from immunosuppression

III.173. A 43-year-old man is successfully extubated and is recovering in the ICU after combined heart-lung transplant. On postoperative day 3, he has atrial fibrillation with a rapid ventricular response that is successfully converted with an IV diltiazem infusion. AKI develops after 3 days (creatinine increased to 1.9 mg/dL). The serum level of tacrolimus rapidly increased to 19.3 ng/mL from 8.5 ng/mL the day before. What caused the AKI and sudden increase in the tacrolimus level?
a. Rhabdomyolysis with decreased drug clearance
b. Drug-to-drug interaction
c. AKI from atrial fibrillation
d. Obstructive uropathy

III.174. Which of the following may indicate poor graft function in the early period after liver transplant?
a. Low albumin level
b. Fever
c. High lactate level
d. Increased creatinine level

III.175. Which of the following is *least* likely to lead to a prolonged stay in the ICU after liver transplant?
a. Renal dysfunction
b. Acute liver failure
c. Pleural effusion
d. Portopulmonary hypertension

III.176. A 35-year-old man who had diabetic nephropathy received a transplanted kidney from a donor after cardiac death. Postoperatively, the patient had adequate urine output, but on postoperative day 7, he had severe flank pain, hematuria, decreased urine output, and signs of hyperkalemia (potassium, 6.1 mmol/L) with peaked T waves on ECG. What is the best next diagnostic step?
a. CT scan of the abdomen and pelvis
b. Doppler ultrasonography of the transplanted kidney
c. MRI of the abdomen and pelvis
d. Urinalysis

III.177. A 61-year-old woman received a transplanted kidney 3 months ago. She presented to the ED with acute onset of altered mental status and seizures. She was intubated for airway protection. Which of the following would *not* be included in the differential diagnosis of her acute encephalopathy?
a. Drug (tacrolimus) toxicity
b. Sepsis
c. PRES
d. Subarachnoid hemorrhage

III.178. Which of the following is *not* an indication for small bowel transplant?
a. Short gut syndrome
b. Failure of home TPN
c. Adenocarcinoma of the small intestine with liver metastasis
d. Recurrent intestinal pseudo-obstruction

III.179. Which of the following is *not* a cause of higher rates of neurologic complications in patients who have received a small intestinal transplant?
a. Greater immunosuppressive needs
b. Vitamin deficiencies
c. Anesthetic agents used intraoperatively
d. Metabolic disturbances related to TPN

Toxicity and Toxins

III.180. Which set of features may help to distinguish serotonin syndrome from other toxidromes?
a. Onset within hours, confusion, dry mucous membranes, decreased bowel peristalsis, urinary retention, tachycardia, hyperthermia
b. Onset within the first day, agitation, hallucinations, abnormal eye movements, hypertension, dilated pupils, potentially dangerous response to long-acting β-blockers

c. Onset within 12 to 48 hours, increased gastrointestinal tract motility, hyperreflexia with increased tone in the legs more than the arms, myoclonus
d. Onset within 1 to 10 days, bradyreflexia or variable reflexes, lead pipe rigidity, extrapyramidal signs, autonomic instability, hyperthermia

III.181. Which of the following scenarios would *not* raise concern for relative serotonin excess leading to serotonin syndrome?
a. A man receiving a stable dose of fluoxetine sustains a severe cerebral anoxic injury after cardiac arrest and then is treated with fentanyl.
b. A young woman who takes amitriptyline and frovatriptan for migraines and nutritional supplements for memory begins treatment with linezolid for MRSA pneumonia.
c. A young man with a history of amphetamine abuse recently began taking topiramate for seizures, melatonin for sleep, and clonazepam for anxiety and now, on the eighth day after hospital admission, begins treatment with gabapentin and levofloxacin.
d. An elderly woman who takes valproate for seizures, trazodone for sleep, and tramadol for pain begins treatment with fluconazole and erythromycin for mixed infections and then receives metoclopramide and ondansetron for nausea.

III.182. Which of the following is *not* a typical diagnostic feature of NMS?
a. Altered mental consciousness
b. Muscle rigidity
c. Hypothermia
d. Increased CK level

III.183. Which of the following carries the highest risk of NMS for a patient?
a. Use of anxiolytics
b. Use of SSRIs
c. Hypothermia
d. Genetic predisposition from a defect in the sarcolemma

III.184. Which of the following statements about drugs of abuse is correct?
a. Approximately 5% of the US population 12 years or older uses illicit drugs.
b. The most commonly used illicit drug is marijuana.
c. US deaths from prescription opioids have decreased since 1999.
d. Synthetic cannabinoids are safer than marijuana.

III.185. A 24-year-old man presents to the ED with miosis, respiratory depression, and CNS depression. On the basis of the clinical toxidrome, 0.04 mg naloxone is administered without clinical effect. A second dose of 0.4 mg naloxone is administered, again without effect. CT of the head shows a preserved gray matter–white matter interface and no evidence of infarction or bleeding. With which of the following agents is the patient most likely intoxicated?
a. Acetylfentanyl
b. Cocaine
c. Heroin
d. Marijuana

III.186. A 19-year-old woman is admitted to the ICU intubated and unresponsive. She is tachycardic and moderately hypertensive with dilated pupils. Before she arrived in the ED, she had a generalized tonic-clonic seizure at an electronic dance festival. In the ED, laboratory test results were unremarkable except for Na^+ (108 mmol/L); head CT showed cerebral edema. Which of the following agents is most likely responsible for this presentation?
a. Furanylfentanyl
b. Ketamine
c. MDMA
d. α-PVP

III.187. You are called to the ED to assist in the care of several critically ill patients who have had an unknown exposure. While caring for a patient in extremis, you notice that your eyes hurt and your nose is running. Others in the room complain of eye pain and difficulty breathing. Looking about, you notice that the medical provider next to you has miosis, lacrimation, and rhinorrhea. Local news reports state that a terrorist organization is claiming responsibility for these events. Which of the following agents most likely caused these findings?
a. Cyanide
b. Lewisite
c. Phosgene
d. Sarin

III.188. A patient is admitted to the ICU with acute respiratory failure and severe sepsis during a recognized biological warfare event. A chest radiograph shows multilobar pneumonia and a normal mediastinum. No pustular lesions exist. Bloody diarrhea and body fluids are absent. Which disease or biological agent caused these findings?
a. Anthrax (*Bacillus anthracis*)
b. Plague (*Yersinia pestis*)
c. Smallpox (variola virus)
d. Ebola virus disease

Answers

Pulmonary Disorders

III.1. Answer d.

Eosinophils are not involved in the pathophysiology of ARDS. They are involved in acute eosinophilic pneumonia, which resembles ARDS. Reactive oxygen species, surfactant dysfunction, and tumor necrosis factor all contribute to the development of ARDS.

Matthay MA, Zemans RL. The acute respiratory distress syndrome: pathogenesis and treatment. Annu Rev Pathol. 2011;6:147–63.

III.2. Answer b.

Prone ventilation is associated with reduced mortality. Inhaled nitric oxide has no benefit and may increase the risk of renal failure. Airway pressure release ventilation has not improved mortality compared with conventional low-tidal-volume ventilation, and high-frequency oscillatory ventilation appears to increase mortality.

Afshari A, Brok J, Moller AM, Wetterslev J. Inhaled nitric oxide for acute respiratory distress syndrome and acute lung injury in adults and children: a systematic review with meta-analysis and trial sequential analysis. Anesth Analg. 2011 Jun;112(6):1411–21. Epub 2011 Mar 3.

Guerin C, Reignier J, Richard JC, Beuret P, Gacouin A, Boulain T, et al; PROSEVA Study Group. Prone positioning in severe acute respiratory distress syndrome. N Engl J Med. 2013 Jun 6;368(23):2159–68. Epub 2013 May 20.

Young D, Lamb SE, Shah S, MacKenzie I, Tunnicliffe W, Lall R, et al; OSCAR Study Group. High-frequency oscillation for acute respiratory distress syndrome. N Engl J Med. 2013 Feb 28;368(9):806–13. Epub 2013 Jan 22.

III.3. Answer c.

Intracranial hemorrhage may be associated with neurogenic pulmonary edema or aspiration, but by itself it does not cause ARDS. Aspiration, pancreatitis, and sepsis are all known causes.

Thompson BT, Chambers RC, Liu KD. Acute respiratory distress syndrome. N Engl J Med. 2017 Aug 10;377(6):562–72.

III.4. Answer d.

ARDS is associated with increased—not decreased—dead space ventilation. Lung compliance is decreased, and both intrapulmonary shunt and ventilation-perfusion mismatch are present in patients with ARDS.

Matthay MA, Zemans RL. The acute respiratory distress syndrome: pathogenesis and treatment. Annu Rev Pathol. 2011;6:147–63.

III.5. Answer d.

Neuromuscular blockade, glucocorticoids, and conservative fluid management have all shown some benefit to patients with ARDS. Surfactant administration has no benefit.

Spragg RG, Lewis JF, Walmrath HD, Johannigman J, Bellingan G, Laterre PF, et al. Effect of recombinant surfactant protein C-based surfactant on the acute respiratory distress syndrome. N Engl J Med. 2004 Aug 26;351(9):884–92.

III.6. Answer d.

According to the Wells score, this patient has a low risk for PE because the only criterion he meets is tachycardia (1.5 points). He does not have any known PE risk factors, and several conditions could be contributing to his symptoms. If patients are unlikely to have PE (Wells score ≤4), a D-dimer test is the first step in PE evaluation. Assessing for fibrinogen breakdown products (D-dimer) is a rapid, widely available, and highly sensitive test that enables patients with negative test results to forego expensive and potentially dangerous imaging. However, D-dimer test results can be positive in several nonspecific inflammatory conditions. This fact should be considered before the test is performed because a positive result requires follow-up imaging as part of a PE evaluation.

Pasha SM, Klok FA, Snoep JD, Mos IC, Goekoop RJ, Rodger MA, et al. Safety of excluding acute pulmonary embolism based on an unlikely clinical probability by the Wells rule and normal D-dimer concentration: a meta-analysis. Thromb Res. 2010 Apr;125(4):e123–7. Epub 2009 Nov 26.

Wells PS, Anderson DR, Rodger M, Forgie M, Kearon C, Dreyer J, et al. Evaluation of D-dimer in the diagnosis of suspected deep-vein thrombosis. N Engl J Med. 2003 Sep 25;349(13):1227–35.

III.7. Answer a.

Patients who have an allergy to contrast media or acute kidney failure and have sufficient indications for imaging for PE should undergo ventilation-perfusion scanning instead of CT angiography. Ventilation-perfusion scanning has a high negative predictive value and should also be considered for young or pregnant women with normal chest radiographs.

Konstantinides S, Goldhaber SZ. Pulmonary embolism: risk assessment and management. Eur Heart J. 2012 Dec;33(24):3014–22. Epub 2012 Sep 7.

Konstantinides SV. 2014 ESC Guidelines on the diagnosis and management of acute pulmonary embolism. Eur Heart J. 2014 Dec 1;35(45):3145–6.

III.8. Answer d.

The duration of anticoagulation depends on whether the PE was provoked or unprovoked and on the likelihood of recurrence. Provoked PE in a patient with transient risk factors (eg, prolonged immobility or recent surgery) can be treated for 3 to 6 months with either LMWH or a DOAC with no difference in benefit between the 2 treatment durations. Patients with unprovoked PE should undergo further diagnostic evaluation. Patients with an underlying malignancy should receive LMWH until the malignancy has been definitively treated. Patients with a hypercoagulable state should receive lifelong anticoagulation with warfarin.

Di Nisio M, van Es N, Buller HR. Deep vein thrombosis and pulmonary embolism. Lancet. 2016 Dec 17;388(10063):3060–73. Epub 2016 Jun 30.

Konstantinides SV, Barco S, Lankeit M, Meyer G. Management of pulmonary embolism: an update. J Am Coll Cardiol. 2016 Mar 1;67(8):976–90.

III.9. Answer b.

Massive PE is characterized by hemodynamic compromise, and it is the only PE subtype for which systemic thrombolysis is absolutely indicated. Ultrasound-assisted catheter-directed thrombolysis can be considered if the clot burden or hemodynamic compromise persists after systemic thrombolysis. Surgical thrombectomy can also be considered in massive PE.

Garcia MJ. Endovascular management of acute pulmonary embolism using the ultrasound-enhanced EkoSonic system. Semin Intervent Radiol. 2015 Dec;32(4):384–7.

Jaff MR, McMurtry MS, Archer SL, Cushman M, Goldenberg N, Goldhaber SZ, et al; American Heart Association Council on Cardiopulmonary, Critical Care, Perioperative and Resuscitation; American Heart Association Council on Peripheral Vascular Disease; American Heart Association Council on Arteriosclerosis, Thrombosis and Vascular Biology. Management of massive and submassive pulmonary embolism, iliofemoral deep vein thrombosis, and chronic thromboembolic pulmonary hypertension: a scientific statement from the American Heart Association. Circulation. 2011 Apr 26;123(16):1788–830. Epub 2011 Mar 21. Errata in: Circulation. 2012 Aug 14;126(7):e104. Circulation. 2012 Mar 20;125(11):e495.

III.10. Answer c.

The absolute indications for an IVC filter include contraindication to anticoagulation, complication of anticoagulation, failure to achieve adequate anticoagulation despite appropriate dosing, and recurrence of venous thromboembolism despite appropriate treatment. This patient has not completed his treatment course, so there is insufficient evidence that anticoagulation has failed. He likely has a DVT due to nonadherence with his prescribed regimen, and he should be evaluated further with compression ultrasonography. He does not have an absolute indication for an IVC filter at this time.

Konstantinides S, Goldhaber SZ. Pulmonary embolism: risk assessment and management. Eur Heart J. 2012 Dec;33(24):3014–22. Epub 2012 Sep 7.

Konstantinides SV, Barco S, Lankeit M, Meyer G. Management of pulmonary embolism: an update. J Am Coll Cardiol. 2016 Mar 1;67(8):976–90.

III.11. Answer a.

An otherwise healthy, young patient with a respiratory rate of 30 breaths per minute should have a clear respiratory alkalosis as in choices *b, c,* and *d*. However, the pseudonormal Paco_2 and pH in choice *a* is inappropriate for the degree of tachypnea and may represent impending respiratory failure. A Paco_2 of 60 mm Hg, although not normal for this patient, is adequate. Benzodiazepine in this situation is contraindicated because suppressing the patient's respiratory drive would precipitate acute respiratory acidosis and failure. Antibiotics have no empirical use in a patient with asthma exacerbations and neither does a routine chest radiograph. Other clues to the severe asthma exacerbation and possibly impending respiratory failure include the patient's drowsiness, inability to provide his own history because of dyspnea and tachypnea, and the late-stage diminishment of wheezing and tidal respirations due to severe dynamic hyperinflation.

McFadden ER Jr, Lyons HA. Arterial-blood gas tension in asthma. N Engl J Med. 1968 May 9;278(19):1027–32.

Rodriguez-Roisin R. Acute severe asthma: pathophysiology and pathobiology of gas exchange abnormalities. Eur Respir J. 1997 Jun;10(6):1359–71.

Trawick DR, Holm C, Wirth J. Influence of gender on rates of hospitalization, hospital course, and hypercapnea in high-risk patients admitted for asthma: a 10-year retrospective study at Yale-New Haven Hospital. Chest. 2001 Jan;119(1):115–9.

III.12. Answer d.

The medical student in choice *d* remains incorrect, and vasopressors and antibiotics are least likely to correct the patient's hypotension. The ventilator waveform shows an inspiration to expiration ratio of 1:1, with incomplete exhalation before delivery of the next mechanical breath. This will lead to progressive air trapping and hyperinflation, putting the patient at risk for barotrauma, including tension pneumothorax and hypotension due to reduced venous return (preload). Thus, needle decompression, if tension pneumothorax is clinically evident, can be lifesaving. Hyperinflation leading to poor venous return can be partially alleviated through decompressing the chest by disconnecting the ventilator. Similarly, changes to minimize air trapping and dynamic hyperinflation on the ventilator may help to reduce the recurrence of hypotension; these changes include allowing a longer expiratory time and reducing the respiratory drive of the patient with sedatives to the extent of allowing hypercapnia if necessary.

Dhand R. Ventilator graphics and respiratory mechanics in the patient with obstructive lung disease. Respir Care. 2005 Feb;50(2):246–61.

Leatherman J. Mechanical ventilation for severe asthma. Chest. 2015 Jun;147(6):1671–80.

Oddo M, Feihl F, Schaller MD, Perret C. Management of mechanical ventilation in acute severe asthma: practical aspects. Intensive Care Med. 2006 Apr;32(4):501–10. Epub 2006 Jan 27.

III.13. Answer b.

The general rules for pharmacologic management of COPD also apply to patients in a neurocritical care unit who have comorbid COPD. Pharmacologic therapy for COPD is used to reduce symptoms, reduce frequency and severity of exacerbations, and improve the patient's health status and exercise tolerance. Long-acting formulations for β_2-agonists and anticholinergics are preferred over short-acting formulations. Long-term treatment with inhaled corticosteroids in combination with long-acting bronchodilators is recommended for patients at high risk for COPD exacerbation, which is a worsening of symptoms to the extent that medication must be changed. Short-acting inhaled β_2-agonists with or without short-acting anticholinergics are used to treat an exacerbation. Systemic corticosteroids and antibiotics can shorten recovery time, improving lung function and arterial hypoxemia, and shorten the length of hospital stay. There is no clear evidence that parenteral corticosteroid treatment provides benefit over oral treatment. Five days of oral corticosteroid therapy is probably sufficient for treatment of adults who have acute exacerbations of COPD (previously, longer courses of 10-14 days were used). It is unclear whether systemic corticosteroid therapy benefits patients who are receiving mechanical ventilation during an acute exacerbation of COPD.

Rashid AM, Fulambarker A, Cohen ME, Patel B, Sood V. Effect of systemic corticosteroids on mechanically ventilated patients with acute exacerbation of COPD [abstract]. Chest. 2004 Oct;126(4_MeetingAbstracts):805S–6S.

Vestbo J, Hurd SS, Agusti AG, Jones PW, Vogelmeier C, Anzueto A, et al. Global strategy for the diagnosis, management, and prevention of chronic obstructive pulmonary disease: GOLD executive summary. Am J Respir Crit Care Med. 2013 Feb 15;187(4):347–65. Epub 2012 Aug 9.

Walters JA, Tan DJ, White CJ, Wood-Baker R. Different durations of corticosteroid therapy for exacerbations of chronic obstructive pulmonary disease. Cochrane Database Syst Rev. 2014 Dec 10;(12):CD006897.

III.14. Answer a.

In the flow-time curve, flow at end-expiration is not zero before the patient receives the next breath. This signifies auto-PEEP, in which the end-expiratory pressure exceeds the extrinsic PEEP. Risk factors for auto-PEEP include high minute ventilation and expiratory airflow obstruction. Auto-PEEP causes lung hyperinflation, which compresses and obstructs the intrathoracic portion of the superior vena cava. Auto-PEEP can also decrease left ventricular afterload. Lung hyperinflation may cause bradycardia and vasodilation mediated through autonomic reflexes. Hyperinflation can also cause acute right ventricular failure, shock, and cardiac arrest. To minimize auto-PEEP, one should minimize minute ventilation and use small tidal volumes with prolongation of the time available for exhalation. If auto-PEEP has caused shock or cardiac arrest, a brief trial of apnea may help. To promote complete exhalation, the endotracheal or tracheostomy tube may be temporarily disconnected.

Berlin D. Hemodynamic consequences of auto-PEEP. J Intensive Care Med. 2014 Mar-Apr;29(2):81–6. Epub 2012 May 15.

III.15. Answer d.

The patient's pleural effusion is consistent with a parapneumonic effusion. Laboratory and imaging findings suggest that the patient is at high risk for complications, so drainage is recommended. A trial (MIST1) showed that there was no difference with the use of small-bore, medium-bore, and large-bore tubes for primary outcomes of mortality or need for open surgery. On the contrary, pain related to dissection for placement of the tubes, was markedly less with the smaller tubes. Intrapleural instillation of fibrinolytic agents alone has produced various results, but studies have shown that intrapleural tPA in combination with DNase therapy improved fluid drainage in patients with pleural infection and decreased the frequency of surgical referral and the duration of the hospital stay.

Maskell NA, Davies CW, Nunn AJ, Hedley EL, Gleeson FV, Miller R, et al; First Multicenter Intrapleural Sepsis Trial (MIST1) Group. U.K. controlled trial of intrapleural streptokinase for pleural infection. N Engl J Med. 2005 Mar 3;352(9):865–74. Erratum in: N Engl J Med. 2005 May 19;352(20):2146.

Rahman NM, Maskell NA, West A, Teoh R, Arnold A, Mackinlay C, et al. Intrapleural use of tissue plasminogen activator and DNase in pleural infection. N Engl J Med. 2011 Aug 11;365(6):518–26.

III.16. Answer d.

The lung point sign (arrow) involves visualizing the point where the visceral pleura (lung) begins to separate from the parietal pleural (chest wall) at the margin of a pneumothorax. The lung point sign is 100% specific for pneumothorax and defines its border. Although the specificity is high, the sensitivity of the lung point sign is relatively low (66%). The sign is not seen in cases of total lung collapse.

Lung sliding is a normal finding that represents a pleural line (parietal and visceral layers of the pleura) that slides back and forth during the respiratory cycle. Its presence suggests the absence of pneumothorax. With M-mode imaging, in the presence of a pneumothorax (thus in the absence of pleural sliding), horizontal lines are visualized throughout in a laminar pattern. The appearance resembles a barcode and is thus named the stratsophere sign. In a patient without a pneumothorax, a homogenous granular pattern is seen below the pleural line (seashore sign).

De Luca C, Valentino M, Rimondi MR, Branchini M, Baleni MC, Barozzi L. Use of chest sonography in acute-care radiology. J Ultrasound. 2008 Dec;11(4):125–34. Epub 2008 Nov 6.

Lichtenstein D, Meziere G, Biderman P, Gepner A. The "lung point": an ultrasound sign specific to pneumothorax. Intensive Care Med. 2000 Oct;26(10):1434–40.

III.17. Answer c.

The patient's clinical presentation and laboratory test results are consistent with SIADH. The chest radiograph showed left lung nodular opacity. Small cell lung cancer is the most common malignant cause of SIADH. Diagnostic criteria include serum osmolality less than 275 mOsm/kg, urine osmolality greater than 100 mOsm/kg, and urine Na^+ greater than 30 mEq/L (Box 24.2 lists other criteria). Mildly symptomatic hyponatremia is treated with fluid restriction.

Rosner MH, Dalkin AC. Electrolyte disorders associated with cancer. Adv Chronic Kidney Dis. 2014 Jan;21(1):7–17.

III.18. Answer b.

The clinical and radiologic findings are consistent with superior vena cava syndrome. Initial management includes supportive measures and urgent radiotherapy to acutely relieve the obstruction. The delayed therapeutic effect of other options (chemotherapy and stent insertion) preclude their use in an urgent setting.

Wan JF, Bezjak A. Superior vena cava syndrome. Emerg Med Clin North Am. 2009 May;27(2):243–55.

III.19. Answer c.

Echocardiography is the test of choice to screen for PH because it is noninvasive and widely available. The pulmonary arterial systolic pressure, often reported as right ventricular systolic pressure, is calculated from the peak tricuspid regurgitant velocity and right atrial pressure according to an assessment of the IVC. Echocardiography is also useful for evaluating the size and function of the right side of the heart and for examining for any left-sided heart or valvular abnormalities.

Right-sided heart catheterization (also known as pulmonary artery catheterization or Swan-Ganz catheterization) offers direct measurement of hemodynamic pressures and is the confirmatory test to diagnose PH. Nonetheless, it is invasive, and correct interpretation of the results can be challenging for clinicians. Typically, after screening echocardiography has been used to identify elevated right-sided heart pressures, right-sided heart catheterization is the next step. It is the only test that can reliably diagnose left-to-right shunting and left-sided heart disease as potential causes of the PH. ECG is most useful in the diagnosis of arrhythmias and acute coronary syndromes. Evidence of acute or chronic PH may include right-axis deviation, right bundle branch block, right ventricular hypertrophy or strain, or the so-called pulmonary pattern (S1Q3T3 pattern), which is most often seen with acute right ventricular strain, perhaps with massive PE. Pulmonary function test results are useful for outpatient evaluation of PH to ensure that pulmonary disease (eg, severe COPD) is not the cause. Subtle patterns may indicate early pulmonary vasculature disease, such as an isolated diffusion abnormality. The test, however, is complex and requires full patient cooperation and equipment that is not mobile, so complete testing with diffusing capacity is rarely performed in the ICU.

Aduen JF, Castello R, Lozano MM, Hepler GN, Keller CA, Alvarez F, et al. An alternative echocardiographic method to estimate mean pulmonary artery pressure: diagnostic and clinical implications. J Am Soc Echocardiogr. 2009 Jul;22(7):814–9. Epub 2009 Jun 7.

Galie N, Simonneau G. The Fifth World Symposium on Pulmonary Hypertension. J Am Coll Cardiol. 2013 Dec 24;62(25 Suppl):D1–3.

Gayat E, Mebazaa A. Pulmonary hypertension in critical care. Curr Opin Crit Care. 2011 Oct;17(5):439–48.

III.20. Answer b.

Accurate assessment of this patient's fluid status is challenging. Since the cause of the right ventricular strain is acute, volume overload is unlikely. The systemic BP, HR, and IVC assessment suggest euvolemia. The current adequate volume status should be maintained because preload is a critical component of stroke volume and therefore cardiac output when right ventricular function is compromised. Intravascular volume depletion is to be avoided or treated if present. Bedside echocardiography can be used to establish a baseline and to serially assess the response to treatment.

Aggressive fluid resuscitation is not indicated when a patient is hemodynamically stable, and it may lead to fluid overload and worsening gas exchange. Aggressive diuresis with intravascular volume depletion should be avoided because low preload will compromise stroke volume and therefore cardiac output. The echocardiographic assessment of the IVC does not suggest volume overload.

Galie N, Simonneau G. The Fifth World Symposium on Pulmonary Hypertension. J Am Coll Cardiol. 2013 Dec 24;62(25 Suppl):D1–3.

Price LC, Wort SJ, Finney SJ, Marino PS, Brett SJ. Pulmonary vascular and right ventricular dysfunction in adult critical care: current and emerging options for management: a systematic literature review. Crit Care. 2010;14(5):R169. Epub 2010 Sep 21.

III.21. Answer c.

Hypoxia produces pulmonary vascular constriction and is exacerbated by hypercarbia and acidosis. Depending on the severity of the gas exchange derangement, treatment ranges from supplemental oxygen to mechanical ventilation (including noninvasive mechanical ventilation). Use of the ARDS Network protocol with high PEEP may increase oxygenation. In addition, the ventilator rate may be increased to address the hypercarbia.

Hemodynamic parameters obtained with a pulmonary artery catheter are used to confirm a diagnosis of PAH; however, the clinical presentation of this patient is consistent with hypoxic respiratory failure, most likely ARDS with a respiratory infection. Pulmonary artery catheterization is invasive, and its routine use has not been shown to change mortality for patients in the ICU. Maximizing fluid status and aiming for euvolemia is important, but the clinical presentation does not suggest hypovolemia (as shown by the adequate perfusion pressure and dilated IVC); therefore, fluid resuscitation would not be the first step. Although inhaled nitric oxide improves oxygenation in patients with ARDS, survival is not improved.

Brower RG, Lanken PN, MacIntyre N, Matthay MA, Morris A, Ancukiewicz M, et al; National Heart, Lung, and Blood Institute ARDS Clinical Trials Network. Higher versus lower positive end-expiratory pressures in patients with the acute respiratory distress syndrome. N Engl J Med. 2004 Jul 22;351(4):327–36.

Murdoch SD, Cohen AT, Bellamy MC. Pulmonary artery catheterization and mortality in critically ill patients. Br J Anaesth. 2000 Oct;85(4):611–5.

Price LC, Wort SJ, Finney SJ, Marino PS, Brett SJ. Pulmonary vascular and right ventricular dysfunction in adult critical care: current and emerging options for management: a systematic literature review. Crit Care. 2010;14(5):R169. Epub 2010 Sep 21.

III.22. Answer a.

Epoprostenol is indicated for management of severe NYHA functional class III or IV symptoms due to PAH. The patient presented with NYHA functional class IV heart failure. Epoprostenol is administered by continuous IV infusion. Initiation of therapy is often performed in the ICU, particularly if the patient presents with NYHA functional class IV heart failure. Generally, a pulmonary artery catheter is used to confirm the diagnosis and monitor dose titration to a therapeutic level. Adverse effects such as headache and gastrointestinal tract dysfunction (eg, nausea and vomiting or diarrhea) must be anticipated and treated. The dose may also be limited by systemic hypotension because epoprostenol is a potent vasodilator of both pulmonary and systemic arteries.

Inhaled nitric oxide is often used to test acute vasoresponsiveness, but it can also be used in patients with acute decompensated PAH and right ventricular failure. Challenges with long-term delivery, short half-life, and expense, however, preclude its long-term use. Bosentan is an endothelin-1 receptor antagonist, approved for use in patients with group 1 PAH; however, published guidelines recommend prompt initiation of infusion prostanoid for NYHA functional class IV symptoms. Bosentan (and ambrisentan and macitentan) are generally reserved for patients in NYHA functional class II or III or for patients requiring combination therapy. Administration in an ICU can be challenging, because the general recommendation is to avoid crushing these medications if they are given through a feeding tube. Sildenafil is a phosphodiesterase-5 inhibitor that relaxes vascular smooth muscle and decreases pulmonary vascular resistance. Published guidelines recommend prompt initiation of infusion prostanoid for NYHA functional class IV symptoms. Sildenafil (and tadalafil) are generally reserved for patients who are in NYHA functional class II or III or who require combination therapy.

Badesch DB, Tapson VF, McGoon MD, Brundage BH, Rubin LJ, Wigley FM, et al. Continuous intravenous epoprostenol for pulmonary hypertension due to the scleroderma spectrum of disease. A randomized, controlled trial. Ann Intern Med. 2000 Mar 21;132(6):425–34.

Burger CD, D'Albini L, Raspa S, Pruett JA. The evolution of prostacyclins in pulmonary arterial hypertension: from classical treatment to modern management. Am J Manag Care. 2016 Jan;22(1 Suppl):S3–15.

Enderby CY, Burger C. Medical treatment update on pulmonary arterial hypertension. Ther Adv Chronic Dis. 2015 Sep;6(5):264–72.

Galie N, Humbert M, Vachiery JL, Gibbs S, Lang I, Torbicki A, et al. 2015 ESC/ERS Guidelines for the diagnosis and treatment of pulmonary hypertension: The Joint Task Force for the Diagnosis and Treatment of Pulmonary Hypertension of the European Society of Cardiology (ESC) and the European Respiratory Society (ERS): Endorsed by: Association for European Paediatric and Congenital Cardiology (AEPC), International Society for Heart and Lung Transplantation (ISHLT). Eur Heart J. 2016 Jan 1;37(1):67–119. Epub 2015 Aug 29.

III.23. Answer b.

Risk factors for group 1 PAH include certain weight loss medications (anorexigens), particularly fenfluramines. The 68-year-old man with chronic congestive heart failure and a left ventricular ejection fraction of 35% most likely has group 2 pulmonary venous hypertension. The 78-year-old woman with chronic hypoxemia from severe COPD most likely has diagnostic group 3 PH owing to hypoxemia from severe COPD. The 40-year-old morbidly obese man who has mild dyspnea with exertion, excessive daytime sleepiness, and loud snoring most likely has diagnostic group 3 PH related to obstructive sleep apnea.

Galie N, Humbert M, Vachiery JL, Gibbs S, Lang I, Torbicki A, et al. 2015 ESC/ERS Guidelines for the diagnosis and treatment of pulmonary hypertension: The Joint Task Force for the Diagnosis and Treatment of Pulmonary Hypertension of the European Society of Cardiology (ESC) and the European Respiratory Society (ERS): Endorsed by: Association for European Paediatric and Congenital Cardiology (AEPC), International Society for Heart and Lung Transplantation (ISHLT). Eur Heart J. 2016 Jan 1;37(1):67–119. Epub 2015 Aug 29.

Galie N, Simonneau G. The Fifth World Symposium on Pulmonary Hypertension. J Am Coll Cardiol. 2013 Dec 24;62(25 Suppl):D1–3.

Hoeper MM, Bogaard HJ, Condliffe R, Frantz R, Khanna D, Kurzyna M, et al. Definitions and diagnosis of pulmonary hypertension. J Am Coll Cardiol. 2013 Dec 24;62(25 Suppl):D42–50.

Cardiovascular Disorders

III.24. Answer d.

Choice *a* is incorrect because, unlike plasma histamine (which usually returns to a normal level in <60 minutes), tryptase levels can remain high much longer and be elevated for up to 5 hours. The recommended time frame for measuring tryptase is thus much longer (up to 3 hours after symptom onset) compared with that for plasma histamine (up to 1 hour after symptom onset). Tryptase is released during an anaphylactic event primarily by mast cells, with a small amount from basophils, so choice *b* is incorrect. Choice *c* is incorrect because an elevated serum tryptase level can support a diagnosis of anaphylaxis, but a normal tryptase level does not rule out anaphylaxis. In fact, while elevated tryptase levels commonly occur in anaphylaxis secondary to injected medications and venom, tryptase levels may be normal in food-induced anaphylaxis and in anaphylaxis not associated with hypotension. Published guidelines have emphasized that obtaining a baseline tryptase level along with serial tryptase levels during an anaphylactic event is more useful than obtaining a single measurement, so choice *d* is the correct answer.

Lieberman P, Nicklas RA, Randolph C, Oppenheimer J, Bernstein D, Bernstein J, et al. Anaphylaxis: a practice parameter update 2015. Ann Allergy Asthma Immunol. 2015 Nov;115(5):341–84.

Simons FE, Ebisawa M, Sanchez-Borges M, Thong BY, Worm M, Tanno LK, et al. 2015 update of the evidence base: World Allergy Organization anaphylaxis guidelines. World Allergy Organ J. 2015 Oct 28;8(1):32.

III.25. Answer b.

Intravascular fluid loss and vasodilatation lead to hypotension, the hallmark of anaphylactic shock. Choices *a*, *c*, and *d* are incorrect because venous return and cardiac output are decreased; the pulmonary edema fluid is characterized by a high concentration of albumin and low pulmonary wedge pressures; and patients have overall decreases in arterial pressure, right and left ventricular filling pressures, and peripheral vascular resistance.

Carlson RW, Schaeffer RC Jr, Puri VK, Brennan AP, Weil MH. Hypovolemia and permeability pulmonary edema associated with anaphylaxis. Crit Care Med. 1981 Dec;9(12):883–5.

Pattanaik D, Yataco JC, Lieberman P. Anaphylactic and anaphylactoid reactions. In: Hall JB, Schmidt GA, Kress JP, editors. Principles of critical care. 4th ed. New York (NY): McGraw-Hill Education; c2015. p. 1269–79.

III.26. Answer b.

The most common cause of cardiogenic shock is acute MI, typically from an ST-segment elevation MI. Acute mitral regurgitation causing papillary muscle dysfunction, atrial fibrillation with rapid ventricular response, and critical aortic stenosis can all contribute to the lack of blood pumped by the heart, leading to cardiogenic shock. However, they are not the most common causes.

Hochman JS, Buller CE, Sleeper LA, Boland J, Dzavik V, Sanborn TA, et al. Cardiogenic shock complicating acute myocardial infarction: etiologies, management and outcome: a report from the SHOCK Trial Registry. SHould we emergently revascularize Occluded Coronaries for cardiogenic shocK? J Am Coll Cardiol. 2000 Sep;36(3 Suppl A):1063–70.

Lindholm MG, Kober L, Boesgaard S, Torp-Pedersen C, Aldershvile J; Trandolapril Cardiac Evaluation study group. Cardiogenic shock complicating acute myocardial infarction; prognostic impact of early and late shock development. Eur Heart J. 2003 Feb;24(3):258–65.

III.27. Answer b.

Traditionally, a serum lactic acid level greater than 2.0 mmol/L is considered to indicate hypoperfusion. All the other criteria listed are either hemodynamic signs or clinical signs that support the diagnosis of cardiogenic shock.

Reynolds HR, Hochman JS. Cardiogenic shock: current concepts and improving outcomes. Circulation. 2008 Feb 5;117(5):686–97.

Thiele H, Ohman EM, Desch S, Eitel I, de Waha S. Management of cardiogenic shock. Eur Heart J. 2015 May 21;36(20):1223–30. Epub 2015 Mar 1.

III.28. Answer b.

Early echocardiography is of utmost importance to rule out mechanical causes of cardiogenic shock, such as rupture of the ventricular septum, free wall, or papillary muscles. Echocardiography is also useful for differentiating the type of shock and whether it was caused by a combination of 2 or more factors.

Cecconi M, De Backer D, Antonelli M, Beale R, Bakker J, Hofer C, et al; Task force of the European Society of Intensive Care Medicine. Consensus on circulatory shock and hemodynamic monitoring. Intensive Care Med. 2014 Dec;40(12):1795–815. Epub 2014 Nov 13.

McLean AS. Echocardiography in shock management. Crit Care. 2016 Aug 20;20:275.

III.29. Answer c.

All the medications listed have utility in the treatment of cardiogenic shock, but for patients with low cardiac output and a sustained systolic BP greater than 90 mm Hg, dobutamine is the recommended first-line medication. In patients with a low cardiac output and a low systolic BP (<90 mm Hg), norepinephrine is the drug of choice. Epinephrine can be used as well, typically in addition to norepinephrine. Vasopressin can be used to augment either norepinephrine or epinephrine, but caution is advised if patients have coronary artery disease because vasopressin may cause myocardial ischemia.

Overgaard CB, Dzavik V. Inotropes and vasopressors: review of physiology and clinical use in cardiovascular disease. Circulation. 2008 Sep 2;118(10):1047–56.

Thiele H, Ohman EM, Desch S, Eitel I, de Waha S. Management of cardiogenic shock. Eur Heart J. 2015 May 21;36(20):1223–30. Epub 2015 Mar 1.

III.30. Answer c.

Patients with cardiogenic shock and concomitant right ventricular failure (or ischemia) are susceptible to the adverse effects of bradyarrhythmias. Therefore, biventricular output is HR dependent, and bradycardia, even in the absence of AV dyssynchrony, may be deleterious in patients with right ventricular ischemia. Hypoxic pulmonary vasoconstriction can occur in response to decreases in oxygen tension in the alveoli, pulmonary arterial blood, or bronchial arterial blood and is enhanced by hypoxemia, hypercarbia, or acidemia. Inhaled nitric oxide can be used in the management of perioperative right ventricular dysfunction.

Berisha S, Kastrati A, Goda A, Popa Y. Optimal value of filling pressure in the right side of the heart in acute right ventricular infarction. Br Heart J. 1990 Feb;63(2):98–102.

Stephens RS, Whitman GJ. Postoperative critical care of the adult cardiac surgical patient. Part I: Routine postoperative care. Crit Care Med. 2015 Jul;43(7):1477–97.

Sylvester JT, Shimoda LA, Aaronson PI, Ward JP. Hypoxic pulmonary vasoconstriction. Physiol Rev. 2012 Jan;92(1):367–520. Erratum in: Physiol Rev. 2014 Jul;94(3):989.

III.31. Answer c.

Plaques that tend to rupture are usually composed of a core filled with lipids and are associated with increased levels of inflammatory markers and a thin fibrous cap. Coronary obstructions larger than 70% can be detected with a well-performed stress test; however, lesions that are nonobstructive (ie, not limiting blood flow) can be missed during a stress test but still can be vulnerable to rupture.

Nair A, Kuban BD, Tuzcu EM, Schoenhagen P, Nissen SE, Vince DG. Coronary plaque classification with intravascular ultrasound radiofrequency data analysis. Circulation. 2002 Oct 22;106(17):2200–6.

Pasterkamp G, den Ruijter HM, Libby P. Temporal shifts in clinical presentation and underlying mechanisms of atherosclerotic disease. Nat Rev Cardiol. 2017 Jan;14(1):21–9. Epub 2016 Oct 20.

III.32. Answer c.

The patient's symptoms are classic for acute aortic dissection, which if extended to the base of the aortic root can compromise the right coronary ostium and flow to the right coronary artery, thus explaining the ECG findings. Emergent chest CT and a cardiothoracic consultation are indicated. Transesophageal echocardiography of the aorta could be used, but 2-dimensional echocardiography would not be useful for assessing the ascending or descending dissecting aorta. Chest radiography would show a widened mediastinum but would not be sensitive or specific for an aortic dissection. Measurement of cardiac enzyme levels would not be helpful in this situation and would only delay care.

Hiratzka LF, Bakris GL, Beckman JA, Bersin RM, Carr VF, Casey DE Jr, et al; American College of Cardiology Foundation/American Heart Association Task Force on Practice Guidelines; American Association for Thoracic Surgery; American College of Radiology; American Stroke Association; Society of Cardiovascular Anesthesiologists; Society for Cardiovascular Angiography and Interventions; Society of Interventional Radiology; Society of Thoracic Surgeons; Society for Vascular Medicine. 2010 ACCF/AHA/AATS/ACR/ASA/SCA/SCAI/SIR/STS/SVM Guidelines for the diagnosis and management of patients with thoracic aortic disease: a report of the American College of Cardiology Foundation/American Heart Association Task Force on Practice Guidelines, American Association for Thoracic Surgery, American College of Radiology, American Stroke Association, Society of Cardiovascular Anesthesiologists, Society for Cardiovascular Angiography and Interventions, Society of Interventional Radiology, Society of Thoracic Surgeons,and Society for Vascular Medicine. J Am Coll Cardiol. 2010 Apr 6;55(14):e27–e129. Erratum in: J Am Coll Cardiol. 2013 Sep 10;62(11):1039–40.

International Registry of Acute Aortic Dissections (IRAD). Aortic dissection: information for patients from the International Registry of Acute Aortic Dissection [Internet]. Ann Arbor (MI): University of Michigan Health System [cited 2018 Sep 17]. Available from: http://www.iradonline.org/irad.html.

III.33. Answer a.

Diagnosis of ACS can be made from the sensitive measurements of cardiac troponin alone within 1 to 3 hours of a patient's arrival in the ED. CK and CK-MB are not sensitive or specific enough for a diagnosis of myocardial injury; although they were used in the past, their use has been replaced by the use of troponins. High-sensitivity troponin can be elevated at 0 hours, but subsequent serial measurements are required to exclude ACS. BNP is a biomarker for heart failure.

Kelly AM, Klim S. Does undetectable troponin I at presentation using a contemporary sensitive assay rule out myocardial infarction? A cohort study. Emerg Med J. 2015 Oct;32(10):760–3. Epub 2014 Dec 31.

Storrow AB, Nowak RM, Diercks DB, Singer AJ, Wu AH, Kulstad E, et al. Absolute and relative changes (delta) in troponin I for early diagnosis of myocardial infarction: results of a prospective multicenter trial. Clin Biochem. 2015 Mar;48(4-5):260–7. Epub 2014 Sep 28.

III.34. Answer b.

A low dose of aspirin (81-100 mg daily) should be given in combination with ticagrelor 90 mg twice daily. Triple therapy that includes warfarin has not been studied for ACS and can increase the bleeding risk.

Amsterdam EA, Wenger NK, Brindis RG, Casey DE Jr, Ganiats TG, Holmes DR Jr, et al. 2014 AHA/ACC Guideline for the management of patients with non-ST-elevation acute coronary syndromes: a report of the American College of Cardiology/American Heart Association Task Force on Practice Guidelines. J Am Coll Cardiol. 2014 Dec 23;64(24):e139–e228. Epub 2014 Sep 23. Erratum in: J Am Coll Cardiol. 2014 Dec 23;64(24):2713–4.

Eisen A, Giugliano RP, Braunwald E. Updates on acute coronary syndrome: a review. JAMA Cardiol. 2016 Sep 1;1(6):718–30.

III.35. Answer b.

This patient has an NSTEMI. Antiplatelet therapy should be part of the initial management plan before the patient undergoes coronary angiography. Platelet adenosine diphosphate receptor antagonists (eg, prasugrel, clopidogrel, and ticagrelor) are given in conjunction with aspirin and not as monotherapy. The loading dose for aspirin is 325 mg. Prasugrel is usually given if a patient is undergoing revascularization during an NSTEMI, although the guidelines recommend that it not be given unless there is evidence of anatomical obstruction.

Amsterdam EA, Wenger NK, Brindis RG, Casey DE Jr, Ganiats TG, Holmes DR Jr, et al. 2014 AHA/ACC Guideline for the management of patients with non-ST-elevation acute coronary syndromes: a report of the American College of Cardiology/American Heart Association Task Force on Practice Guidelines. J Am Coll Cardiol. 2014 Dec 23;64(24):e139–e228. Epub 2014 Sep 23. Erratum in: J Am Coll Cardiol. 2014 Dec 23;64(24):2713–4.

Eisen A, Giugliano RP, Braunwald E. Updates on acute coronary syndrome: a review. JAMA Cardiol. 2016 Sep 1;1(6):718–30.

III.36. Answer d.

The ECG shows isorhythmic dissociation. The AV junctional rate is faster than the sinus node rate. P waves due to sinus node depolarization are positive in lead II, and P waves from the AV junction are negative in lead II. The second QRS complex is earlier because the sinus node P wave is conducting normally to the ventricles. The patient is asymptomatic, so no specific treatment is required. Stopping the metoprolol therapy is unnecessary and may be deleterious if a patient has had an MI.

Kusumoto F. ECG interpretation: from pathophysiology to clinical application. New York (NY): Springer; c2009. 298 p.

Kusumoto F, Bernath P. ECG interpretation for everyone: an on-the-spot guide. Chichester (UK): Wiley-Blackwell; c2012.

III.37. Answer c.

The patient has torsades de pointes, a special form of ventricular tachycardia associated with QT-interval prolongation (notice the QT intervals of the 3 normal beats). Amiodarone would likely exacerbate the arrhythmia by further prolonging the QT interval. Lidocaine is generally most effective for ischemia. In this patient, the ventricular arrhythmia appears to be associated with a slow ventricular rate due to AV block. Transcutaneous pacing would be the most likely maneuver to quickly and reliably increase the ventricular rate. Bradycardia due to increased vagal tone and

QT-interval prolongation are not uncommon in patients with intracranial bleeding. IV magnesium or an IV β-agonist would also be reasonable choices.

Kusumoto F. ECG interpretation: from pathophysiology to clinical application. New York (NY): Springer; c2009. 298 p.

Kusumoto F, Bernath P. ECG interpretation for everyone: an on-the-spot guide. Chichester (UK): Wiley-Blackwell; c2012.

III.38. Answer d.

The apparent episode of ventricular tachycardia is due to artifact. Regular QRS complexes occur at the beginning of the strip and during the "ventricular tachycardia."

Kusumoto F. ECG interpretation: from pathophysiology to clinical application. New York (NY): Springer; c2009. 298 p.

Kusumoto F, Bernath P. ECG interpretation for everyone: an on-the-spot guide. Chichester (UK): Wiley-Blackwell; c2012.

III.39. Answer b.

The patient has atrial fibrillation (no discrete P waves can be seen), but her ventricular rhythm is regular. This apparent paradox is due to the presence of complete heart block most likely due to digoxin toxicity. Amiodarone would worsen it. Although transcutaneous pacing might increase the ventricular rate, the patient does not have acute symptoms that would mandate either of these options.

Kusumoto F. ECG interpretation: from pathophysiology to clinical application. New York (NY): Springer; c2009. 298 p.

Kusumoto F, Bernath P. ECG interpretation for everyone: an on-the-spot guide. Chichester (UK): Wiley-Blackwell; c2012.

III.40. Answer d.

This patient has an irregular, rapid, wide-complex rhythm. This triad is very suggestive of atrial fibrillation with rapid activation of the ventricles through an accessory pathway that connects the atria and the ventricles. Normally in atrial fibrillation, the ventricular rate is limited by the decremental conduction properties of the AV node. Incomplete formation of the mitral and tricuspid annuli in utero results in a small strand of tissue other than the AV node that "connects" the atria to the ventricles. This was originally described in the early 1900s and is often called the Wolff-Parkinson-White syndrome. When a patient has an accessory pathway, rapid conduction to the ventricles can lead to rapid ventricular rates (with an abnormal, wide QRS complex since the His-Purkinje system is not used); it may lead to sudden cardiac death. Treatment is directed at blocking conduction through the accessory pathway because blocking activation of the AV node can lead to even faster heart rates. Of the medications listed in the answer choices, only procainamide has this effect. Cardioversion can be used in patients with clinically significant hemodynamic compromise.

Kusumoto F. ECG interpretation: from pathophysiology to clinical application. New York (NY): Springer; c2009. 298 p.

Kusumoto F, Bernath P. ECG interpretation for everyone: an on-the-spot guide. Chichester (UK): Wiley-Blackwell; c2012.

III.41. Answer d.

Both hypertensive urgency and hypertensive emergency are characterized by large increases in BP. However, patients who present with a hypertensive emergency also present with end-organ damage, whereas those who present with hypertensive urgency do not. The organs most often affected by elevated BP are the kidneys, brain, and heart. Drugs such as cocaine are more likely associated with hypertensive emergency, but their use is not a distinguishing feature.

Henny-Fullin K, Buess D, Handschin A, Leuppi J, Dieterle T. [Hypertensive urgency and emergency]. Ther Umsch. 2015 Jun;72(6):405–11. German.

Katz JN, Gore JM, Amin A, Anderson FA, Dasta JF, Ferguson JJ, et al; STAT Investigators. Practice patterns, outcomes, and end-organ dysfunction for patients with acute severe hypertension: the Studying the Treatment of Acute hyperTension (STAT) registry. Am Heart J. 2009 Oct;158(4):599–606.e1.

III.42. Answer c.

Aortic dissection must be ruled out in a patient who presents in a hypertensive crisis and has chest pain. Echocardiography, along with checking troponin levels and serial ECGs, should be performed to help evaluate for left ventricular failure and acute MI. A patient with an aneurysm could present with similar clinical signs and symptoms but would usually present with hypotension rather than hypertension. Fractures and lung involvement are certainly possible after a motor vehicle accident, but evaluation for those conditions would be secondary to an evaluation for a possible dissection.

Hiratzka LF, Bakris GL, Beckman JA, Bersin RM, Carr VF, Casey DE Jr, et al; American College of Cardiology Foundation/American Heart Association Task Force on Practice Guidelines; American Association for Thoracic Surgery; American College of Radiology; American Stroke Association; Society of Cardiovascular Anesthesiologists; Society for Cardiovascular Angiography and Interventions; Society of Interventional Radiology; Society of Thoracic Surgeons; Society for Vascular Medicine. 2010 ACCF/AHA/AATS/ACR/ASA/SCA/SCAI/ SIR/STS/SVM guidelines for the diagnosis and management of patients with thoracic aortic disease: a report of the American College of Cardiology Foundation/American Heart Association Task Force on Practice Guidelines, American Association for Thoracic Surgery, American College of Radiology, American Stroke Association, Society of Cardiovascular Anesthesiologists, Society for Cardiovascular Angiography and Interventions, Society of Interventional Radiology, Society of Thoracic Surgeons, and Society for Vascular Medicine. Circulation. 2010 Apr 6;121(13):e266–369. Epub 2010 Mar 16. Erratum in: Circulation. 2010 Jul 27;122(4):e410.

Li JZ, Eagle KA, Vaishnava P. Hypertensive and acute aortic syndromes. Cardiol Clin. 2013 Nov;31(4):493–501. Epub 2013 Sep 20.

III.43. Answer b.

Both traumatic cardiac arrest and active bleeding are relative contraindications for TTM. The duration of resuscitation does not preclude use of TTM, and both pulseless ventricular tachycardia and in-hospital cardiac arrest resulting from PE are indications for TTM.

Callaway CW, Donnino MW, Fink EL, Geocadin RG, Golan E, Kern KB, et al. Part 8: Post-cardiac arrest care: 2015 American Heart Association guidelines update for cardiopulmonary resuscitation and emergency cardiovascular care. Circulation. 2015 Nov 3;132(18 Suppl 2):S465–82. Erratum in: Circulation. 2017 Sep 5;136(10):e197.

III.44. Answer c.

The administration of epinephrine may transiently decrease $ETCO_2$ because of the vasoconstrictor effect. Massive PE may alter the $ETCO_2$ because of the vascular obstruction and dead space ventilation. Bicarbonate administration transiently increases $ETCO_2$. Amiodarone administration has no effect on $ETCO_2$.

Heradstveit BE, Sunde K, Sunde GA, Wentzel-Larsen T, Heltne JK. Factors complicating interpretation of capnography during advanced life support in cardiac arrest: a clinical retrospective study in 575 patients. Resuscitation. 2012 Jul;83(7):813–8. Epub 2012 Feb 25.

III.45. Answer b.

Meperidine may be appropriate, but patients with cardiac arrest are at risk for anoxic brain injury, and meperidine lowers the seizure threshold. In addition, this patient has AKI, and meperidine is partially eliminated by the kidney; the meperidine metabolite, normeperidine, can promote seizure activity.

Choi HA, Ko SB, Presciutti M, Fernandez L, Carpenter AM, Lesch C, et al. Prevention of shivering during therapeutic temperature modulation: the Columbia anti-shivering protocol. Neurocrit Care. 2011 Jun;14(3):389–94.

Meperidine. Micromedex Solutions [Internet]. Ann Arbor (MI): Truven Health Analytics. c2017 [cited 2016 Dec 21]. Available from: www.micromedexsolutions.com.

III.46. Answer a.

Hyperglycemia is associated with worse neurologic outcomes among patients with cardiac arrest. Serum glucose values should be maintained at 140 to 180 mg/dL. The other choices are all appropriate management options.

Callaway CW, Donnino MW, Fink EL, Geocadin RG, Golan E, Kern KB, et al. Part 8: Post-cardiac arrest care: 2015 American Heart Association guidelines update for cardiopulmonary resuscitation and emergency cardiovascular care. Circulation. 2015 Nov 3;132(18 Suppl 2):S465–82. Erratum in: Circulation. 2017 Sep 5;136(10):e197.

III.47. Answer d.

Current ACLS guidelines for the management of symptomatic, unstable bradycardia include administering atropine at 0.5 mg every 3 to 5 minutes up to a total of 3 mg. However, the patient is in postarrest shock and has not responded to a total of 1 mg of atropine. Waiting an additional 3 minutes to give another dose of atropine could precipitate further deterioration in his condition. Epinephrine and dopamine infusions and pacing, either transcutanesouly or transvenously, are all appropriate.

Link MS, Berkow LC, Kudenchuk PJ, Halperin HR, Hess EP, Moitra VK, et al. Part 7: adult advanced cardiovascular life support: 2015 American Heart Association guidelines update for cardiopulmonary resuscitation and emergency cardiovascular care. Circulation. 2015 Nov 3;132(18 Suppl 2):S444–64. Erratum in: Circulation. 2015 Dec 15;132(24):e385.

III.48. Answer a.

It is necessary to maintain a balance between decreasing the systolic BP (to reduce the force on the aortic wall) and maintaining adequate perfusion to end organs (MAP 60-75 mm Hg).

Nienaber CA, Rousseau H, Eggebrecht H, Kische S, Fattori R, Rehders TC, et al; INSTEAD Trial. Randomized comparison of strategies for type B aortic dissection: the INvestigation of STEnt Grafts in Aortic Dissection (INSTEAD) trial. Circulation. 2009 Dec 22;120(25):2519–28. Epub 2009 Dec 7.

Scott AJ, Bicknell CD. Contemporary management of acute type B dissection. Eur J Vasc Endovasc Surg. 2016 Mar;51(3):452–9. Epub 2015 Dec 9.

III.49. Answer d.

Type A aortic dissection that involves the intrapericardial ascending aorta and arch is a surgical emergency. This type of dissection carries a high risk of rupture and extension of the dissection to the coronary arteries and aortic valve resulting in myocardial ischemia or infarction, severe aortic regurgitation, or pericardial tamponade.

Mehta RH, Suzuki T, Hagan PG, Bossone E, Gilon D, Llovet A, et al; International Registry of Acute Aortic Dissection (IRAD) Investigators. Predicting death in patients with acute type A aortic dissection. Circulation. 2002 Jan 15;105(2):200–6.

Nienaber CA, Eagle KA. Aortic dissection: new frontiers in diagnosis and management: Part I: from etiology to diagnostic strategies. Circulation. 2003 Aug 5;108(5):628–35.

Acute Endocrine Disorders

III.50. Answer d.

This patient is presenting with symptoms of pituitary apoplexy. Urgent imaging is necessary, and MRI is the preferred choice. CT of the head is fast and readily available but less sensitive and specific than MRI for identifying pituitary hemorrhage and involvement of nearby structures. However, MRI is more time-consuming and cannot always be performed. CT should be performed if the patient's condition is unstable, the patient's diagnosis is unclear, or MRI is unavailable.

Glezer A, Bronstein MD. Pituitary apoplexy: pathophysiology, diagnosis and management. Arch Endocrinol Metab. 2015 Jun;59(3):259–64.

Rajasekaran S, Vanderpump M, Baldeweg S, Drake W, Reddy N, Lanyon M, et al. UK guidelines for the management of pituitary apoplexy. Clin Endocrinol (Oxf). 2011 Jan;74(1):9–20.

III.51. Answer c.

Although pregnancy is a reported risk factor, apoplexy is rare in pregnant women. Overall, men are more often affected than women. Additional reported risk factors include hypertension, use of antithrombotic medications, initiation or withdrawal of hormonally active substances (eg, bromocriptine), and surgery (in particular, cardiac surgery).

Glezer A, Bronstein MD. Pituitary apoplexy: pathophysiology, diagnosis and management. Arch Endocrinol Metab. 2015 Jun;59(3):259–64.

Rajasekaran S, Vanderpump M, Baldeweg S, Drake W, Reddy N, Lanyon M, et al. UK guidelines for the management of pituitary apoplexy. Clin Endocrinol (Oxf). 2011 Jan;74(1):9–20.

III.52. Answer c.

Disturbances in water and Na^+ balance occur in as many as 75% of patients after transsphenoidal surgery for sellar or parasellar masses. Moreover, hypernatremia is common in patients in the ICU and is frequently caused by excessive renal water loss.

This case shows the differential diagnosis of polyuria with hypernatremia in the neurocritical care setting. In this patient, central DI occurred before surgery, thereby raising the possibility of postoperative polyuria secondary to worsening DI. However, it is important to consider other common causes of polyuria and hypernatremia after transsphenoidal surgery such as osmotic diuresis induced by saline, urea, or elevated glucose. Determination of serum and urine osmolality helps distinguish DI and osmotic diuresis. In patients with DI, urine osmolality is lower than serum osmolality and usually less than 250 mOsm/kg. In contrast, in patients with osmotic diuresis, urine is relatively concentrated and urine osmolality is greater than 300 mOsm/kg. Therefore, this case is an example of polyuria caused by osmotic diuresis because the urine was concentrated (urine osmolality 380 mOsm/kg). The increased urine osmolality was higher than the serum osmolality, which is typical of osmotic diuresis, and caused by marked hyperglycemia and subsequent glucosuria. Correcting hyperglycemia by administering insulin and changing the IV fluids from D5W to normal saline should correct glucosuria and polyuria.

Administering extra doses of desmopressin is not appropriate because, despite the history of DI, the patient's urine is not diluted and polyuria is not caused by antidiuretic hormone deficiency. Moreover, increasing the rate of D5W administration from 200 to

400 mL/h would only worsen hyperglycemia, which could further exacerbate polyuria.

Kristof RA, Rother M, Neuloh G, Klingmuller D. Incidence, clinical manifestations, and course of water and electrolyte metabolism disturbances following transsphenoidal pituitary adenoma surgery: a prospective observational study. J Neurosurg. 2009 Sep;111(3):555–62.

Lindner G, Funk GC. Hypernatremia in critically ill patients. J Crit Care. 2013 Apr;28(2):216.e11–20. Epub 2012 Jul 2.

III.53. Answer d.

This patient has DI (she has polyuria, dilute urine with low urine osmolality, and mild hypernatremia). The cause is most likely central and is a complication of transsphenoidal surgery.

The treatment of central DI depends on the mental status of the patient, the patient's ability to perceive thirst, and the severity of DI as estimated from the urine output. This patient is awake with an intact thirst, and she is partially compensating by drinking water. Desmopressin administration would help to confirm the diagnosis of central DI and help with management. In patients with central DI, desmopressin reduces urine output, increases urine osmolality, and improves hypernatremia; therefore, 1 dose of parenteral desmopressin (IV or subcutaneous) is indicated. Moreover, the patient has a large urine output with frequent urination, which causes discomfort; therefore, continued observation with no other management is incorrect.

To avoid overtreatment, which can lead to water intoxication and hyponatremia, subsequent doses of desmopressin should be administered only after reassessing the clinical situation, Na^+ levels, urine output, and urine osmolality.

Desmopressin is available in 3 preparations (intranasal, oral, and parenteral), but in the acute hospital setting, parenteral administration is preferable given the more reliable bioavailability of the drug. Moreover, the intranasal route should not be used immediately after transsphenoidal surgery because the absorption of desmopressin could be affected.

Fluid replacement is essential in the management of DI. IV hypotonic fluids are indicated for central DI if the sedated patient cannot receive oral fluids, thirst is impaired, or DI is severe enough to cause large urine output with concomitant marked hypernatremia. Consequently, to avoid overtreatment of conscious patients with an intact thirst, such as the patient presented here, oral fluid intake is preferable to IV fluids.

Kim RJ, Malattia C, Allen M, Moshang T Jr, Maghnie M. Vasopressin and desmopressin in central diabetes insipidus: adverse effects and clinical considerations. Pediatr Endocrinol Rev. 2004 Nov;2 Suppl 1:115–23.

Lamas C, del Pozo C, Villabona C; Neuroendocrinology Group of the SEEN. Clinical guidelines for management of diabetes insipidus and syndrome of inappropriate antidiuretic hormone secretion after pituitary surgery. Endocrinol Nutr. 2014 Apr;61(4):e15–24. Epub 2014 Mar 1. English, Spanish.

III.54. Answer b.

This patient has the signs and symptoms of long-standing acromegaly, including obstructive sleep apnea, hypertension, diabetes mellitus, carpal tunnel syndrome, skin tags, and enlarged hands and feet. Measuring IGF-1 is the most appropriate initial test to diagnose acromegaly, but the most appropriate next steps are to administer a random cortisol test and IV corticosteroids. This patient has refractory hypotension, which requires pressure support, and mildly low Na^+ and high-normal potassium levels. These signs suggest adrenal insufficiency. In addition, he has a headache, ophthalmoplegia, and a decreased level of consciousness with a pituitary tumor. These signs and symptoms are consistent with pituitary apoplexy, which is suggested by the fluid-fluid level. His risk factors for pituitary apoplexy include hypertension, anticoagulation, and an underlying pituitary adenoma. Although pituitary apoplexy is considered a surgical emergency, the resultant adrenal insufficiency must be addressed immediately. Expansion of the sella compresses the left cavernous sinus and leads to cranial nerve deficits. Although measuring the HbA_{1c} level would be helpful for assessing the patient's metabolic status, the cause of his blurred vision is not metabolic.

Capatina C, Inder W, Karavitaki N, Wass JA. Management of endocrine disease: pituitary tumour apoplexy. Eur J Endocrinol. 2015 May;172(5):R179–90. Epub 2014 Dec 1.

Katznelson L, Laws ER Jr, Melmed S, Molitch ME, Murad MH, Utz A, et al; Endocrine Society. Acromegaly: an Endocrine Society clinical practice guideline. J Clin Endocrinol Metab. 2014 Nov;99(11):3933–51. Epub 2014 Oct 30.

III.55. Answer b.

The patient is a 45-year-old man with hypopituitarism who was admitted with sepsis due to left lower lobe pneumonia and evidence of adrenal insufficiency, hypotension, and hyponatremia. For this patient, a stress dose of corticosteroid is required and should be administered. The measured cortisol concentration (15 mcg/dL) reflects the hydrocortisone dose that the patient received before admission. Although this cortisol concentration is in the reference range, the patient's current regimen may not provide sufficient supplementation during critical illness. In patients with secondary hypothyroidism, thyrotropin levels can be low, low normal, or occasionally mildly elevated. Therefore, a low thyrotropin level is not useful for assessing adequate thyroid hormone replacement, and this patient's low thyrotropin level does not indicate exogenous excess. Instead, adequate replacement can be assessed only by measuring free thyroxine. Thyroid hormone replacement is administered orally or through a nasogastric tube. Typically, 70% to 80% of oral levothyroxine is absorbed. IV levothyroxine can be administered if oral administration is not possible, but the dose needs to be decreased to appropriately account for maximal absorption when administered IV.

Jonklaas J, Bianco AC, Bauer AJ, Burman KD, Cappola AR, Celi FS, et al; American Thyroid Association Task Force on Thyroid Hormone Replacement. Guidelines for the treatment of hypothyroidism: prepared by the American Thyroid Association Task Force on Thyroid Hormone Replacement. Thyroid. 2014 Dec;24(12):1670–751.

Yamada M, Mori M. Mechanisms related to the pathophysiology and management of central hypothyroidism. Nat Clin Pract Endocrinol Metab. 2008 Dec;4(12):683–94. Epub 2008 Oct 21.

III.56. Answer d.

On admission, this patient had severe hypoglycemia and hypotension, and she could not lactate after childbirth. In addition, she recently had a complicated delivery with bleeding and required blood transfusions. The patient's presentation and history are suggestive of Sheehan syndrome, which is postpartum ischemic necrosis of the pituitary. Her symptoms of fatigue, nausea, and dizziness suggest adrenal insufficiency, which was confirmed by the low random cortisol level with an inappropriately normal corticotropin level. Hypoglycemia is also a rare manifestation of adrenal insufficiency in adults and is a stress response; therefore, she does not require an 8 am cortisol test, which would be expected to show an elevated level after she received a stress dose of corticosteroid. During the insulin tolerance test, induced hypoglycemia should result in the release of corticotropin. When the patient presented with hypoglycemia, her random cortisol level was low, which is consistent with adrenal insufficiency.

The patient's inability to lactate suggests that she cannot produce prolactin. Laboratory test results show central hypothyroidism with low thyrotropin and free thyroxine levels, thereby providing additional evidence of anterior pituitary hormone dysfunction. Although MRI should be performed to confirm the absence of a mass lesion causing panhypopituitarism, treatment with a stress dose of corticosteroid is required. Thyroid hormone replacement should be administered only after corticosteroid administration because thyroid hormone replacement can increase cortisol metabolism and worsen adrenal insufficiency.

Capatina C, Wass JA. Hypopituitarism: growth hormone and corticotropin deficiency. Endocrinol Metab Clin North Am. 2015 Mar;44(1):127–41. Epub 2014 Nov 6.

Kilicli F, Dokmetas HS, Acibucu F. Sheehan's syndrome. Gynecol Endocrinol. 2013 Apr;29(4):292–5. Epub 2012 Dec 18.

III.57. Answer b.

Hyponatremia is common in myxedema coma and may be related to decreased free water excretion or relative adrenal insufficiency. Hypoglycemia is also common and may result from adrenal insufficiency or decreased gluconeogenesis. Hypoventilation can occur with a decreased respiratory drive. Hypothermia (*not* hyperthermia) is a feature of myxedema coma and is caused by decreased cellular metabolism that results from low levels of T_4 and T_3.

Hampton J. Thyroid gland disorder emergencies: thyroid storm and myxedema coma. AACN Adv Crit Care. 2013 Jul-Sep;24(3):325–32.

III.58. Answer b.

In patients with thyroid storm, β-blockers are initially administered to treat hyperadrenergic symptoms such as tachycardia, and they may help to inhibit T_4-to-T_3 conversion. Bile acid sequestrants decrease enterohepatic thyroid hormone recirculation, which decreases serum hormone levels. Glucocorticoid administration may inhibit T_4-to-T_3 conversion and help treat underlying autoimmune disease. However, a thionamide agent must be administered before iodine-containing solutions because the thionamide agent blocks iodine from being used to create new thyroid hormone. An iodine-containing solution, such as strong iodine (Lugol) solution, blocks T_4 and T_3 release from the thyroid gland.

Nayak B, Burman K. Thyrotoxicosis and thyroid storm. Endocrinol Metab Clin North Am. 2006 Dec;35(4):663–86.

III.59. Answer a.

In differentiating stress hyperglycemia from previously undiagnosed diabetes mellitus in hyperglycemic and critically ill patients, inpatient studies have shown that treatment of hyperglycemia can potentially affect morbidity and mortality regardless of whether patients have received a diagnosis of diabetes. It is clear that the lack of a definitive diagnosis of diabetes mellitus should not preclude aggressive glycemic management, especially for patients with acute neurologic injury. Although poor glycemic control in critical care patients carries a worse prognosis, IIT provides no mortality benefit and carries a higher risk of hypoglycemia and associated adverse effects. Bolus administration of insulin and glucose solutions should be strictly avoided.

Egi M, Bellomo R, Stachowski E, French CJ, Hart GK, Hegarty C, et al. Blood glucose concentration and outcome of critical illness: the impact of diabetes. Crit Care Med. 2008 Aug;36(8):2249–55.

Robba C, Bilotta F. Admission hyperglycemia and outcome in ICU patients with sepsis. J Thorac Dis. 2016 Jul;8(7):E581–3.

III.60. Answer c.

The NICE-SUGAR trial (published in 2009) showed that a higher percentage of ICU patients who received IIT (compared with the control group) had cardiovascular-related death (by 5.8%); an increased absolute risk of death at 90 days (by 2.6%, with a number needed to harm of 38); and a higher rate of severe hypoglycemia (6.8% vs 0.5%). In that trial, moderate blood glucose control (goal, 140-180 mg/dL) was associated with lower mortality and a lower risk of hypoglycemia compared to tight control. Another study of neurocritically ill patients (published in 2012) found no benefit when IIT was compared with intermediate glycemic targets (110-180 mg/dL), suggesting that IIT benefits were derived from minimizing secondary injury by keeping glycemic levels less than 180 mg/dL.

NICE-SUGAR Study Investigators, Finfer S, Chittock DR, Su SY, Blair D, Foster D, Dhingra V, et al. Intensive versus conventional glucose control in critically ill patients. N Engl J Med. 2009 Mar 26;360(13):1283–97. Epub 2009 Mar 24.

Kramer AH, Roberts DJ, Zygun DA. Optimal glycemic control in neurocritical care patients: a systematic review and meta-analysis. Crit Care. 2012 Oct 22;16(5):R203.

III.61. Answer d.

This patient meets the criteria for severe sepsis. Early IV antibiotics to decrease mortality are indicated (as recommended by the Surviving Sepsis Campaign); the patient should initially receive appropriate IV fluids resuscitation. The role of low-dose corticosteroids in sepsis is controversial, and they may worsen uncontrolled hyperglycemia. The CORTICUS study did not find that corticosteroid treatment improved mortality among patients with sepsis.

Lipiner-Friedman D, Sprung CL, Laterre PF, Weiss Y, Goodman SV, Vogeser M, et al; CORTICUS Study Group. Adrenal function in sepsis: the retrospective CORTICUS cohort study. Crit Care Med. 2007 Apr;35(4):1012–8.

Marik PE, Pastores SM, Annane D, Meduri GU, Sprung CL, Arlt W, et al; American College of Critical Care Medicine. Recommendations for the diagnosis and management of corticosteroid insufficiency in critically ill adult patients: consensus statements from an international task force by the American College of Critical Care Medicine. Crit Care Med. 2008 Jun;36(6):1937–49.

III.62. Answer d.

Optimal glycemic control includes an insulin infusion protocol that is reliable, is based on frequent blood glucose monitoring, avoids fingerstick glucose testing through the use of arterial or venous glucose samples, uses appropriate monitoring to avoid dangerous hypoglycemia, and provides appropriate nutritional support. The essential components of an insulin infusion system include a validated insulin titration program, appropriate staffing resources, accurate monitoring technology, standardized approaches to infusion preparation, and consistent provision of carbohydrates, calories, and nutritional support with dextrose replacement for preventing and treating hypoglycemia. Quality improvement of glycemic management programs should include analyzing hypoglycemia rates and maintaining charts of glucose values between 140 and 180 mg/dL.

A major concern with IIT for neurocritically ill patients is the danger of neuroglycopenia because brain glucose uptake and metabolism are essentially supply driven. Although some data suggest that IIT does not improve outcomes among neurologic patients and may be deleterious, other data indicate that IIT may deter neurologic complications. In neurocritically ill patients, mild levels of hypoglycemia should be avoided, and severe ranges of hypoglycemia (<70 mg/dL) should be absolutely avoided.

Bilotta F, Rosa G. Optimal glycemic control in neurocritical care patients. Crit Care. 2012 Oct 30;16(5):163.
Krinsley J, Schultz MJ, Spronk PE, van Braam Houckgeest F, van der Sluijs JP, Melot C, et al. Mild hypoglycemia is strongly associated with increased intensive care unit length of stay. Ann Intensive Care. 2011 Nov 24;1:49.

III.63. Answer a.

The diagnosis of AI in critically ill patients remains controversial. The ACCM in 2008 created the term *CIRCI* to identify dysfunction of the HPA axis during critical illness, particularly sepsis and ARDS. Clinical signs that suggest AI include hypotension that is resistant to fluid resuscitation and vasopressors, high cardiac output with low systemic vascular resistance, emesis, diarrhea, weakness, eosinophilia, metabolic acidosis, hyponatremia with hyperkalemia, hypoglycemia, decreased mental status, and fever of unknown origin. Testing for AI remains controversial, but a serum cortisol level less than 10 mcg/dL or an increase in serum cortisol level of less than 9 mcg/dL after giving 250 mcg cosyntropin is a diagnostic criterion recommended by the ACCM. Variables that affect both parameters include the following: the high degree of binding of cortisol to serum albumin and cortisol-binding globulin and the reduction in total cortisol when those transport proteins are low; the limited availability of testing of free cortisol as the hormone's biologically active form; continued discussion about the cosyntropin dose for stimulation testing (high dose [250 mcg] vs low dose [1 mcg]); and the role of cytokines in the deficiency syndrome.

Marik PE, Pastores SM, Annane D, Meduri GU, Sprung CL, Arlt W, et al; American College of Critical Care Medicine. Recommendations for the diagnosis and management of corticosteroid insufficiency in critically ill adult patients: consensus statements from an international task force by the American College of Critical Care Medicine. Crit Care Med. 2008 Jun;36(6):1937–49.

III.64. Answer d.

Etomidate is a sedative with few adverse cardiovascular effects and no effect on intracranial pressure with maintenance of cerebral perfusion pressure. It has a rapid onset (5-15 seconds) and a relatively short duration of action (5-14 minutes). However, it blocks conversion of 11-deoxycortisol into cortisol. Studies have shown that after a single dose, the cortisol blood concentration is decreased and the response to cosyntropin stimulation is decreased for up to 24 hours (or possibly longer). Patients with sepsis appear to be particularly affected. Some data show associations with an increased vasopressor requirement, increased mortality, longer hospital stay, longer ICU stay, and more ventilator days.

Bornstein SR. Predisposing factors for adrenal insufficiency. N Engl J Med. 2009 May 28;360(22):2328–39.

III.65. Answer c.

This patient has multiple risk factors for AI. She has stress from her recent trauma and surgical intervention, and it might be assumed that she was taking corticosteroids for her rheumatoid arthritis. Suggestive signs and symptoms include hypotension unresponsive to fluid replacement and vasopressors, hyponatremia, and hypoglycemia. When diagnostic confirmation is desired, dexamethasone may be given to allow physiologic stabilization while testing proceeds with the recommended high dose of cosyntropin. If initiation of emergency IV corticosteroids is not required and appropriate diagnostic tests have been implemented, IV hydrocortisone can be administered. Fludrocortisone has a special role in treating severely hyponatremic patients, but it is not the usual initial therapy.

Marik PE, Varon J. Requirement of perioperative stress doses of corticosteroids: a systematic review of the literature. Arch Surg. 2008 Dec;143(12):1222–6.
Yong SL, Marik P, Esposito M, Coulthard P. Supplemental perioperative steroids for surgical patients with adrenal insufficiency. Cochrane Database Syst Rev. 2009 Oct 7;(4):CD005367. Update in: Cochrane Database Syst Rev. 2012;12:CD005367.

Gastrointestinal Disorders

III.66. Answer c.

Stress-related mucosal damage results most commonly in shallow, oozing ulcerations in the fundus of the stomach and is thought to be due to a disruption in the balance between gastric acid production and mucosal protection. Major risk factors for stress ulceration include mechanical ventilation longer than 48 hours and coagulopathy, defined as a platelet count less than 50×10^9/L or an INR of more than 1.5. Other risk factors include multiple trauma, major burns, shock, traumatic central nervous system injury, and high-dose glucocorticoid therapy. Options for prophylaxis include proton pump inhibitors, histamine$_2$-receptor blockers, antacids, and sucralfate. These treatments may be associated with higher rates of nosocomial pneumonia and *Clostridium difficile*–associated diarrhea.

Buendgens L, Bruensing J, Matthes M, Duckers H, Luedde T, Trautwein C, et al. Administration of proton pump inhibitors in critically ill medical patients is associated with increased risk of developing *Clostridium difficile*-associated diarrhea. J Crit Care. 2014 Aug;29(4):696.e11–5. Epub 2014 Mar 7.
Cook DJ, Fuller HD, Guyatt GH, Marshall JC, Leasa D, Hall R, et al. Risk factors for gastrointestinal bleeding in critically ill patients. Canadian Critical Care Trials Group. N Engl J Med. 1994 Feb 10;330(6):377–81.

III.67. Answer d.

This patient presents with symptoms of upper gastrointestinal bleeding. The most common cause of upper gastrointestinal bleeding is peptic ulcer disease; therefore, initiation of therapy with a proton pump inhibitor is appropriate pending a definitive diagnosis of the cause of bleeding. If bleeding is determined to not be caused by an ulcer, then therapy with the high-dose proton inhibitor should be discontinued. The patient's history makes variceal hemorrhage very likely; therefore, pharmacologic treatment aimed at reducing variceal hemorrhage should include octreotide. Octreotide, a somatostatin analogue, has been shown to improve hemostasis during acute variceal hemorrhage when used in combination with endoscopic therapy. Although correction of coagulopathy would be appropriate regardless of the cause of the upper gastrointestinal bleeding, red cell transfusion threshold should be a hemoglobin level less than 9 mg/dL, and possibly less than 7 mg/dL. The PT and INR do not reliably predict bleeding risk in patients with cirrhosis, and platelet transfusions are generally recommended for a platelet level less than 50×10^9/L, active bleeding, or recent use of antiplatelet medications. Excessive transfusion in patients with hypervolemic cirrhosis may cause further complications such as pulmonary edema, transfusion-related acute lung injury, or even increased surface tension within the varices. Short-term antibiotic prophylaxis increases survival in patients with cirrhosis and gastrointestinal hemorrhage.

Banares R, Albillos A, Rincon D, Alonso S, Gonzalez M, Ruiz-del-Arbol L, et al. Endoscopic treatment versus endoscopic plus pharmacologic treatment for acute variceal bleeding: a meta-analysis. Hepatology. 2002 Mar;35(3):609–15.

Barkun AN, Bardou M, Kuipers EJ, Sung J, Hunt RH, Martel M, et al; International Consensus Upper Gastrointestinal Bleeding Conference Group. International consensus recommendations on the management of patients with nonvariceal upper gastrointestinal bleeding. Ann Intern Med. 2010 Jan 19;152(2):101–13.

de Franchis R. Evolving consensus in portal hypertension: report of the Baveno IV consensus workshop on methodology of diagnosis and therapy in portal hypertension. J Hepatol. 2005 Jul;43(1):167–76. Erratum in: J Hepatol. 2005 Sep;43(3):547.

Villanueva C, Colomo A, Bosch A, Concepcion M, Hernandez-Gea V, Aracil C, et al. Transfusion strategies for acute upper gastrointestinal bleeding. N Engl J Med. 2013 Jan 3;368(1):11–21. Erratum in: N Engl J Med. 2013 Jun 13;368(24):2341.

III.68. Answer a.

Variceal bleeding persists despite endoscopic and pharmacologic treatment in 10% to 20% of patients. Rescue therapies include both temporizing measures and shunt therapies. Balloon tamponade is used to stabilize patients until more definitive therapy can be performed and can be effective for achieving short-term hemostasis in more than 80% of patients. Complications from esophagogastric balloons can include esophageal necrosis and rupture. Shunt therapies include placement of transjugular intrahepatic portosystemic shunts or surgical shunt therapy. The selection of shunt therapy depends on local expertise and availability. Whether balloon tamponade or shunt therapy is chosen next, strong consideration should be given to endotracheal intubation to decrease the risk of aspiration. Recombinant factor VIIa has not been shown to provide improvement in the clinical end points of hemostasis or death due to variceal bleeding and cannot yet be recommended.

Avgerinos A, Armonis A. Balloon tamponade technique and efficacy in variceal haemorrhage. Scand J Gastroenterol Suppl. 1994;207:11–6.

Bendtsen F, D'Amico G, Rusch E, de Franchis R, Andersen PK, Lebrec D, et al. Effect of recombinant Factor VIIa on outcome of acute variceal bleeding: an individual patient based meta-analysis of two controlled trials. J Hepatol. 2014 Aug;61(2):252–9. Epub 2014 Apr 5.

III.69. Answer c.

This patient presents with melena and symptoms of anemia, and the source of bleeding is unknown. His vital signs are suggestive of hypovolemia because the presence of tachycardia and mild hypotension indicates a 15% to 30% intravascular volume loss. Appropriate initial steps in management should include establishing adequate IV access, restoration of intravascular volume, and ensuring appropriate oxygen delivery. Hemoglobin level, by itself, may not be a surrogate of the adequacy of resuscitation. Additional end points such as HR, BP, lactate level, or pH should also be used to guide initial stabilization. After stability is achieved, further diagnostic and therapeutic measures can be undertaken.

Baradarian R, Ramdhaney S, Chapalamadugu R, Skoczylas L, Wang K, Rivilis S, et al. Early intensive resuscitation of patients with upper gastrointestinal bleeding decreases mortality. Am J Gastroenterol. 2004 Apr;99(4):619–22.

Committee on Trauma. Advanced trauma life support program for doctors: ATLS. 6th ed. Chicago (IL): American College of Surgeons; c1997. p. 103–12.

III.70. Answer b.

In this patient, acute gastrointestinal hemorrhage has developed from a previously unrecognized source, such as a peptic ulcer, arteriovenous malformation, or occult malignancy. She still has circulating heparin, which has a 90-minute half-life, and this should be urgently reversed to minimize ongoing hemorrhage. Protamine sulfate at a dose of 1 mg/100 units of heparin should be administered, although this dose should not exceed 50 mg in any 10-minute interval. Idarucizumab is a monoclonal antibody that binds to dabigatran and its metabolites. Prothrombin complex concentrate has a rapid onset of action and contains vitamin K-dependent clotting factors. Although the primary role of prothrombin complex concentrate is the reversal of VKAs, data are mixed regarding the efficacy for reversing direct factor Xa inhibitors and direct thrombin inhibitors. Provision of fresh frozen plasma is not necessary at this time because 1 dose of warfarin is unlikely to inhibit vitamin K-dependent clotting factors sufficiently to cause a coagulopathy. Likewise, given the lack of qualitative or quantitative platelet dysfunction, there is no role for platelet transfusion. Platelet and plasma transfusions may be indicated later if the patient requires more than 4 units of red blood cells and coagulopathy associated with massive transfusion develops. After hemostasis is obtained, consideration will need to be given to the patient's candidacy for an IVC filter or repeat challenge with anticoagulation.

Holcomb JB, Tilley BC, Baraniuk S, Fox EE, Wade CE, Podbielski JM, et al; PROPPR Study Group. Transfusion of plasma, platelets, and red blood cells in a 1:1:1 vs a 1:1:2 ratio and mortality in patients with severe trauma: the PROPPR randomized clinical trial. JAMA. 2015 Feb 3;313(5):471–82.

Siegal DM. Managing target-specific oral anticoagulant associated bleeding including an update on pharmacological reversal agents. J Thromb Thrombolysis. 2015 Apr;39(3):395–402.

III.71. Answer d.

The patient presents with sepsis, likely from spontaneous bacterial peritonitis. Treatment for sepsis followed widely accepted guidelines: volume resuscitation, cultures, broad-spectrum antibiotics, initial and follow-up tests for lactate levels, and additional verification of adequate volume resuscitation with focused bedside echocardiography. Spontaneous bacterial peritonitis is a well-known risk factor for ileus because inflammation of the peritoneal cavity stimulates and alters intrinsic and extrinsic mediators such as vasoactive intestinal peptide, cholecystokinin, mast cells, macrophages, and vagal nerve stimulation. Plain anteroposterior and lateral radiography is the initial first step in assessment of suspected clinical status of ileus. It can detect both catastrophic issues such as free air indicating ruptured viscus and air-fluid levels and indicate the region most affected: gastric, small bowel, or colon. If there are further questions or unclear abnormalities on plain radiography, then CT of the abdomen and pelvis is appropriate. Placement of a nasogastric tube in a patient without emesis is not advocated at this time. Antiemetics will be more helpful. Placing a nasogastric tube can disrupt the need for air-fluid interaction for peristalsis to be stimulated or initiated. Methylnaltrexone is the second medication approved by the US Food and Drug Administration to treat opioid-induced constipation. The fact that the patient was given narcotics on the same day that ileus was identified points in another direction as the cause of ileus. However, methylnaltrexone might reduce the additional negative impact that the narcotics have on the enteric system.

Mehta N, O'Connell K, Giambrone GP, Baqai A, Diwan S. Efficacy of methylnaltrexone for the treatment of opioid-induced constipation: a meta-analysis and systematic review. Postgrad Med. 2016;128(3):282–9. Epub 2016 Feb 23.

Nuvials X, Palomar M, Alvarez-Lerma F, Olaechea P, Catalan M, Gimeno R, et al; ENVIN-HELICS. Adherence to surviving sepsis campaign recommendations in patients admitted to

ICU: 2013 ENVIN-HELICS Registry Data [abstract]. Intensive Care Med. 2014 Oct;40(Suppl 1):S211.

III.72. Answer b.

Certainly, all of the options can be done, but evidence clearly shows that, after a reasonable period of conservative treatment for Ogilvie syndrome, neostigmine, 2 mg IV, is effective for resolving colonic pseudo-obstruction. Much attention is needed to exclude obstruction, pneumatosis intestinalis, ischemia, or infarction of the bowel. CT with contrast will certainly help exclude these conditions. The gastrointestinal team can help you in decompressing the part of the colon that is accessible to them. Management of insufflation after a critical point of maximal distention can have an increased risk of perforation, and the scenario then becomes an emergency. A rectal tube will help decompress the rectum and perhaps part of the descending or sigmoid colon, but it will not totally address the current problem. Enemas have a similar effect as suppositories for local stimulation, but serial insertions increase the risk of local perforation and thus are not advised. Although not enough information was provided to calculate the Model for End-Stage Liver Disease score, the patient has known cirrhosis and AKI, and thus the score is likely increased. In such instances, surgery is not advised unless the situation is an emergency, which is not the case.

Cho HC, Jung HY, Sinn DH, Choi MS, Koh KC, Paik SW, et al. Mortality after surgery in patients with liver cirrhosis: comparison of Child-Turcotte-Pugh, MELD and MELDNa score. Eur J Gastroenterol Hepatol. 2011 Jan;23(1):51–9.

Ponec RJ, Saunders MD, Kimmey MB. Neostigmine for the treatment of acute colonic pseudo-obstruction. N Engl J Med. 1999 Jul 15;341(3):137–41.

III.73. Answer b.

In general, patients with acute liver failure do not have established portal hypertension, and the consequences thereof, including varices, are uncommon. Cerebral edema is a frequent and concerning complication, particularly associated with high-grade encephalopathy. Multiorgan failure, including kidney failure and vasodilatory hypotension, is common.

Bernal W, Wendon J. Acute liver failure. N Engl J Med. 2013 Dec 26;369(26):2525–34.

European Association for the Study of the Liver. EASL Clinical Practical Guidelines on the Management of Acute (Fulminant) Liver Failure. J Hepatol. 2017 May;66(5):1047–81.

III.74. Answer d.

The patient has findings consistent with grade 3 hepatic encephalopathy. In patients with acute liver failure, this is an indication for intubation and mechanical ventilation. There is a substantial risk of cerebral edema in this population, frequent neurologic monitoring is appropriate, and CT of the head may be useful in evaluation, but airway and ventilatory management should not be delayed for this. If not already initiated, *N*-acetylcysteine therapy is indicated, but it is not the most urgent concern.

Lee WM, Larson AM, Stravitz RT. AASLD positon paper: the management of acute liver failure: update 2011 [Internet]. American Association for the Study of Liver Diseases. c2011 [cited 2016 Nov 22]. Available from: https://www.aasld.org/sites/default/files/ guideline_documents/alfenhanced.pdf.

Wijdicks EFM. Hepatic encephalopathy. N Engl J Med. 2016 Oct 27;375(17):1660–70.

III.75. Answer c.

Obliteration of liver dullness to percussion results from peritoneal air, which is an objective sign of hollow viscus perforation.

Squires R, Carter SN, Postier RG. Acute abdomen. In: Townsend CM, Beauchamp RD, Evers BM, Mattox KL, editors. Sabiston textbook of surgery. 20th ed. Philadelphia (PA): Elsevier; c2017. p. 1120–38.

III.76. Answer b.

Extraluminal air may not be demonstrable if the perforation is very small, self-sealed, or well contained by adjacent organs. Alternatively, the reported sensitivity for the detection of extraluminal air on plain radiography is 50% to 70%. If spillage is exposed in the retroperitoneal or extraperitoneal space, there should be no free air in the abdominal cavity. Surgical consultation would be appropriate, but there is no indication for urgent operative management.

Cho KC, Baker SR. Extraluminal air: diagnosis and significance. Radiol Clin North Am. 1994 Sep;32(5):829–44.

Furukawa A, Sakoda M, Yamasaki M, Kono N, Tanaka T, Nitta N, et al. Gastrointestinal tract perforation: CT diagnosis of presence, site, and cause. Abdom Imaging. 2005 Sep-Oct;30(5):524–34.

Ghahremani GG. Radiologic evaluation of suspected gastrointestinal perforations. Radiol Clin North Am. 1993 Nov;31(6):1219–34.

III.77. Answer d.

If there are any suspicions about compartment syndrome, it is important to measure intra-abdominal pressure with a Foley catheter. Normally, intra-abdominal pressure in critically ill patients is considered to be 5 to 7 mm Hg. Intra-abdominal pressure may increase as a result of many disorders or treatment: peritonitis, intestinal obstruction, ileus, cirrhosis with ascites, pancreatitis, after massive resuscitation or massive transfusions, sepsis, acidosis, or respiratory failure that requires high positive end-expiratory pressure levels for treatment.

Malbrain ML. Abdominal pressure in the critically ill: measurement and clinical relevance. Intensive Care Med. 1999 Dec;25(12):1453–8.

III.78. Answer d.

The manifestations and septic complications that result are highly variable and depend on the character and location of the perforated hollow organ, duration since the injury, the diameter of the spillage, the volume and chemical content of substance coming from the perforated organ, the abilities of neighboring tissues to resorb those contents, and the underlying comorbidities that may affect the patient's immune response to the injury and functional reserve.

Moore LJ, Moore FA. Early diagnosis and evidence-based care of surgical sepsis. J Intensive Care Med. 2013 Mar-Apr;28(2):107–17. Epub 2011 Jul 11.

III.79. Answer d.

If investigations show duodenal ulcer perforation with minimal free air and fluid in the abdomen without signs of generalized peritonitis, conservative treatment may be attempted (nasogastric tube and permanent suction). When gastrointestinal perforations are localized or successfully treated with endoscopic closure and physical examinations show visceral peritoneal irritation resulting from pneumoperitoneum, image-guided paracentesis is recommended. Traditionally, gastrointestinal perforation with diffuse pneumoperitoneum has been treated with surgical exploration. Surgical treatment of intra-abdominal perforations may be accomplished by endoscopy, laparoscopy, or open surgery. If bedside endoscopy shows acute gastrointestinal perforation without considerably inflamed edges (diameter <1 cm), primary endoscopic closure of the defect may be performed by suturing or using endoscopic clips. In case of failure of endoscopic technique, laparoscopy or laparotomy is recommended.

Dascalescu C, Andriescu L, Bulat C, Danila R, Dodu L, Acornicesei M, et al. Taylor's method: a therapeutic alternative for perforated gastroduodenal ulcer. Hepatogastroenterology. 2006 Jul-Aug;53(70):543–6.

Haito-Chavez Y, Law JK, Kratt T, Arezzo A, Verra M, Morino M, et al. International multicenter experience with an over-the-scope clipping device for endoscopic management of GI defects (with video). Gastrointest Endosc. 2014 Oct;80(4):610–22. Epub 2014 Jun 5.

Siu WT, Leong HT, Law BK, Chau CH, Li AC, Fung KH, et al. Laparoscopic repair for perforated peptic ulcer: a randomized controlled trial. Ann Surg. 2002 Mar;235(3):313–9.

Weaver TL, Goldberg RF, Stauffer JA, Frey ES. Needle before the knife: nonoperative management of pneumoperitoneum with image-guided aspiration after gastrointestinal perforation. Surg Laparosc Endosc Percutan Tech. 2014 Apr;24(2):e74–6. Erratum in: Surg Laparosc Endosc Percutan Tech. 2014 Jun;24(3):282.

III.80. Answer b.

The differential diagnosis for any patient with lower abdominal pain and bright red rectal bleeding should include ischemic colitis. This diagnosis should especially be considered after an aortic aneurysm repair, in which the inferior mesenteric artery is usually sacrificed. It is most common in elderly patients. However, ischemic colitis can develop in patients of any age who also have polyarteritis nodosa, lupus, rheumatoid arthritis, scleroderma, or polycythemia vera.

In ischemic colitis, the vascular insult mainly involves the small arterioles, sparing the major colonic vessels. It is more common in the splenic flexure and distal sigmoid colon "watershed areas," even though ischemia can affect any part of the colon. Endoscopy with biopsies for histopathologic evaluation establishes the diagnosis and assists in ruling out other causes. In addition, the classic thumbprinting of the bowel wall can be seen on barium enema examination. However, these diagnostic methods are contraindicated, and urgent laparotomy is diagnostic and therapeutic if perforation is suspected. Conservative management is a key in ischemic colitis, because ischemia typically improves over several days with appropriate hydration and management of other comorbidities. Surgical intervention is reserved for other complications, including peritonitis and stricture development.

Brandt LJ, Feuerstadt P, Longstreth GF, Boley SJ; American College of Gastroenterology. ACG clinical guideline: epidemiology, risk factors, patterns of presentation, diagnosis, and management of colon ischemia (CI). Am J Gastroenterol. 2015 Jan;110(1):18–44. Epub 2014 Dec 23.

III.81. Answer d.

The most common cause of acute occlusion of the superior mesenteric artery is arterial emboli. The heart is the most common source of these emboli, either from a mural thrombus after MI or from the atria in patients with atrial fibrillation. Also, PFO is a potential cause of arterial occlusion through paradoxical embolism. The initial presentation includes severe abdominal pain that is out of proportion to the findings on physical examination. The physical finding of peritonitis implies transmural ischemia and thus is a late stage in the evolution of the process. Acute occlusion of the superior mesenteric artery does not result in complete foregut infarction because the proximal jejunum is typically spared in the case of embolic disease.

Clair DG, Beach JM. Mesenteric ischemia. N Engl J Med. 2016 Mar 10;374(10):959–68.

Wyers MC. Acute mesenteric ischemia: diagnostic approach and surgical treatment. Semin Vasc Surg. 2010 Mar;23(1):9–20.

III.82. Answer d.

Intra-abdominal hypertension leads to obstruction of the IVC and reduces venous return from the lower extremities. In addition, cephalad deviation of the diaphragm produces a mechanical narrowing of the vena cava through the diaphragmatic crura. In ACS, although the diaphragm is in direct contact with the right ventricle, direct pressure of the diaphragm on the aorta or right or left side of the heart is not the main cardiovascular change. In contrast, an increase in intrathoracic pressure with cephalad deviation of the diaphragm and direct pressure on the IVC are the hallmark cardiovascular changes.

Cullen DJ, Coyle JP, Teplick R, Long MC. Cardiovascular, pulmonary, and renal effects of massively increased intra-abdominal pressure in critically ill patients. Crit Care Med. 1989 Feb;17(2):118–21.

III.83. Answer b.

Recommended treatment in patients with primary ACS is prompt surgical decompression. Although the effect of decompressive laparotomy on organ function is not uniform, improvement in oxygenation indexes and urinary output seem to be the most pronounced effects of decompressive laparotomy. A tight abdomen is a specific sign. Measurement of intra-abdominal pressure with standardized technique should be the diagnostic method of choice. According to previous data, patients with intra-abdominal pressure exceeding 25 mm Hg within the first 4 days after disease onset might be good candidates for surgical decompression. Failure of other measures to control intra-abdominal pressure portends the risk of delayed surgical intervention.

De Waele JJ, Hoste EA, Malbrain ML. Decompressive laparotomy for abdominal compartment syndrome: a critical analysis. Crit Care. 2006;10(2):R51.

Renal Disorders

III.84. Answer c.

This patient most likely has AIN from use of pantoprazole at admission. Eosinophiluria (>1% eosinophils in urine) and white cell casts can be found in patients with AIN. Muddy-brown or granular casts are typically found in patients with ATN, and hyaline casts are usually found in states of hypovolemia.

Brewster UC, Perazella MA. Proton pump inhibitors and the kidney: critical review. Clin Nephrol. 2007 Aug;68(2):65–72.

Leonard CE, Freeman CP, Newcomb CW, Reese PP, Herlim M, Bilker WB, et al. Proton pump inhibitors and traditional nonsteroidal anti-inflammatory drugs and the risk of acute interstitial nephritis and acute kidney injury. Pharmacoepidemiol Drug Saf. 2012 Nov;21(11):1155–72. Epub 2012 Aug 9.

III.85. Answer c.

This patient has stage III AKI due to likely sepsis-associated ATN. Her potassium and HCO_3^- levels are acceptable, as are her oxygen requirements; therefore, she currently has no indication for immediate dialysis. High-dose loop diuretics can be used to manage hypervolemia, but there is no benefit from converting nonoliguric AKI to oliguric AKI. Because her oxygen requirements are minimal, there is no need for high-dose loop diuretics at this time.

Ho KM, Sheridan DJ. Meta-analysis of frusemide to prevent or treat acute renal failure. BMJ. 2006 Aug 26;333(7565):420. Epub 2006 Jul 21.

Sampath S, Moran JL, Graham PL, Rockliff S, Bersten AD, Abrams KR. The efficacy of loop diuretics in acute renal failure: assessment using Bayesian evidence synthesis techniques. Crit Care Med. 2007 Nov;35(11):2516–24.

III.86. Answer b.

This patient has stage III AKI with hyperkalemia refractory to medical therapy, and thus initiation of dialysis is warranted. Intermittent hemodialysis treatments increase the brain water content, an effect that increases intracranial pressure. Hemodialysis leads to a rapid increase in the serum HCO_3^- level, but HCO_3^- cannot readily pass across the blood-brain barrier. Carbon dioxide, however, diffuses rapidly across the blood-brain barrier; the result is intracellular acidosis, which causes breakdown of intracellular proteins to create idiogenic osmoles. Thus, an osmotic gradient is created for water movement into the brain, which leads to an increase in intracranial pressure and reduction in cerebral perfusion pressure. Because these changes are much more gradual during continuous renal replacement therapy, it is the method of choice for patients with cerebral edema or at risk for cerebral edema.

Davenport A. Renal replacement therapy in the patient with acute brain injury. Am J Kidney Dis. 2001 Mar;37(3):457–66.

Kumar A, Cage A, Dhar R. Dialysis-induced worsening of cerebral edema in intracranial hemorrhage: a case series and clinical perspective. Neurocrit Care. 2015 Apr;22(2):283–7.

III.87. Answer a.

ATN is characterized by muddy-brown or granular casts in the urine sediment. The results of renal ultrasonography are usually normal in patients with ATN, but high resistive indices can be found and are also nonspecific findings. Red cell casts are a hallmark of glomerulonephritis and should prompt further evaluation for the cause of the same. The FeNa is usually more than 1% in patients with ATN. FeNa less than 1% typically is found in patients with prerenal azotemia.

Perazella MA, Coca SG, Kanbay M, Brewster UC, Parikh CR. Diagnostic value of urine microscopy for differential diagnosis of acute kidney injury in hospitalized patients. Clin J Am Soc Nephrol. 2008 Nov;3(6):1615–9. Epub 2008 Sep 10.

III.88. Answer a.

Recent studies have shown that the incidence of both dialysis-requiring and nondialysis-requiring AKI is increasing in developed countries. Therefore, answer *a* is correct.

Hsu RK, McCulloch CE, Dudley RA, Lo LJ, Hsu CY. Temporal changes in incidence of dialysis-requiring AKI. J Am Soc Nephrol. 2013 Jan;24(1):37–42. Epub 2012 Dec 6.

Kolhe NV, Muirhead AW, Wilkes SR, Fluck RJ, Taal MW. The epidemiology of hospitalised acute kidney injury not requiring dialysis in England from 1998 to 2013: retrospective analysis of hospital episode statistics. Int J Clin Pract. 2016 Apr;70(4):330–9. Epub 2016 Jan 22.

III.89. Answer b.

Multiple studies have shown good correlation of pH, P_{CO_2}, HCO_3^-, and base excess levels between venous and ABG results. However, venous blood gas results have slightly lower pH (0.03-0.04) and slightly higher P_{CO_2} (4-6 mm Hg). Hypoxemia cannot be diagnosed on the basis of the venous P_{O_2} because the arterial P_{O_2} is typically 36.9 mm Hg more than the venous P_{O_2} and has considerable variability.

Byrne AL, Bennett M, Chatterji R, Symons R, Pace NL, Thomas PS. Peripheral venous and arterial blood gas analysis in adults: are they comparable? A systematic review and meta-analysis. Respirology. 2014 Feb;19(2):168–75. Epub 2014 Jan 3.

Koul PA, Khan UH, Wani AA, Eachkoti R, Jan RA, Shah S, et al. Comparison and agreement between venous and arterial gas analysis in cardiopulmonary patients in Kashmir valley of the Indian subcontinent. Ann Thorac Med. 2011 Jan;6(1):33–7.

III.90. Answer a.

The results of ABG testing show an uncompensated metabolic acidosis with an anion gap of 25 mmol/L. Lactic acidosis, salicylate toxicity, and methanol ingestion will cause an increase in unmeasured anions and, therefore, a widening of the anion gap. Renal tubular acidosis is due to HCO_3^- loss in the kidneys and manifests as non-anion gap metabolic acidosis.

Gunnerson KJ, Kellum JA. Acid-base and electrolyte analysis in critically ill patients: are we ready for the new millennium? Curr Opin Crit Care. 2003 Dec;9(6):468–73.

Kaplan LJ, Kellum JA. Fluids, pH, ions and electrolytes. Curr Opin Crit Care. 2010 Aug;16(4):323–31.

III.91. Answer c.

The following principles make a drug more likely to be dialyzed: small molecular size, low protein binding, low volume of distribution, high water solubility, and high renal clearance component of plasma clearance. Choice *a* can be an attractive distractor, but a medication with low lipid solubility has higher water solubility and, therefore, would likely be eliminated by hemodialysis. Choices *b* and *d* are listed in the properties of dialyzable drugs above and in the reading. Choice *c* is the correct answer because medications that are predominantly cleared via mechanisms other than renal clearance (nonrenal plasma clearance) are generally not removed via hemodialysis.

Bailie GR, Mason NA. Bailie and Mason's 2016 dialysis of drugs [Internet]. Renal Pharmacy Consultants, LLC. c2013 [cited 2017 Nov 15]. Available from: http://renalpharmacyconsultants.com/.

Smyth B, Jones C, Saunders J. Prescribing for patients on dialysis. Aust Prescr. 2016 Feb;39(1):21–4. Epub 2016 Feb 1.

III.92. Answer a.

Medications with a narrow therapeutic index require additional monitoring in patients with renal dysfunction. Gentamicin is the correct answer because the therapeutic window for this medication is relatively small with peak levels of 6 to 12 mcg/mL depending on the infection source and trough levels less than 1.5 mcg/mL to prevent kidney toxicity and ototoxicity from developing. Both meropenem and ceftriaxone are β-lactam antibiotics and, therefore, have a wide therapeutic index and do not require therapeutic drug monitoring. Meropenem does require adjustment in patients with renal dysfunction because a large percentage (about 70%) is excreted unchanged in the urine, a common characteristic for intermediate and wide therapeutic index medications requiring dosage adjustment. Levofloxacin is another antibiotic that requires adjustment in renal dysfunction, but it does not have a narrow therapeutic index.

Doogue MP, Polasek TM. Drug dosing in renal disease. Clin Biochem Rev. 2011 May;32(2):69–73.

Micromedex [Internet]. Truven Health Analytics. c2017 [cited 2017 Nov 15]. Available from: http://www.micromedexsolutions.com/ home/dispatch.

III.93. Answer b.

Amalgamation does not occur during renal replacement therapy. Convection, the movement of water across the semipermeable membrane bringing with it dissolved solutes, is the primary mechanism of solute clearance in hemofiltration. Adsorption, the adherence of molecules to the surface of the membrane, removes molecules from the circulation, providing clearance. Diffusion, the movement of molecules across the semipermeable membrane driven by concentration gradients, is the primary mechanism of solute removal in hemodialysis.

Cerda J, Ronco C. Modalities of continuous renal replacement therapy: technical and clinical considerations. Semin Dial. 2009 Mar-Apr;22(2):114–22.

Ricci Z, Romagnoli S, Ronco C. Renal replacement therapy. F1000Res. 2016 Jan 25;5. pii: F1000 Faculty Rev-103.

III.94. Answer c.

Hemodiafiltration combines the clearances of diffusion and convection. There are no clinical data to suggest that it is better than either hemodialysis or hemofiltration relative to patient outcomes. It can be more expensive than hemodialysis because 2 fluids are needed, both dialysis fluid and replacement fluid, and thus costs are increased. It does not eliminate the need for dialysis fluid.

Cerda J, Ronco C. Modalities of continuous renal replacement therapy: technical and clinical considerations. Semin Dial. 2009 Mar-Apr;22(2):114–22.

Ricci Z, Romagnoli S, Ronco C. Renal replacement therapy. F1000Res. 2016 Jan 25;5. pii: F1000 Faculty Rev-103.

III.95. Answer d.

The right internal jugular vein site is preferred for a dialysis catheter. Subclavian catheters are discouraged because of the high incidence of subclavian vein stenosis. Because the left internal jugular vein site requires a long catheter and the catheter has to bend twice for proper placement, the risk of poor catheter flow rates is increased. Femoral catheters also need to be long and are in a relatively low-flow vessel, factors that may increase recirculation and lead to reduced clearances.

Frankel A. Temporary access and central venous catheters. Eur J Vasc Endovasc Surg. 2006 Apr;31(4):417–22. Epub 2005 Dec 19.

III.96. Answer c.

MDMA, also known as ecstasy, has been shown to cause serious hyponatremia. This is due to the direct effect of the drug on stimulation of arginine vasopressin secretion and thirst. The arginine vasopressin secretion leads to avid water reabsorption in the renal tubule, and polydipsia increases free water intake. The increased water reabsorption and polydipsia present clinically with euvolemic hypo-osmolar hyponatremia. Diaphoresis and fever can increase salt and water losses, but typically the losses are hypotonic and result in hypernatremia. Moreover, a urine Na^+ level of more than 10 mEq/L argues against a hypovolemic state. Psychogenic polydipsia would be associated with a low urine osmolality. This occurs due to washing out of the interstitial medullary concentration gradient. Acute alcohol intoxication typically presents with hypernatremia during the diuresis phase. Chronic alcohol intake is classically associated with hyponatremia.

Campbell GA, Rosner MH. The agony of ecstasy: MDMA (3,4-methylenedioxymethamphetamine) and the kidney. Clin J Am Soc Nephrol. 2008 Nov;3(6):1852–60. Epub 2008 Aug 6.

van Dijken GD, Blom RE, Hene RJ, Boer WH; NIGRAM Consortium. High incidence of mild hyponatraemia in females using ecstasy at a rave party. Nephrol Dial Transplant. 2013 Sep;28(9):2277–83. Epub 2013 Mar 8.

III.97. Answer a.

The patient is hypotensive, and the clinical picture is consistent with hypovolemic hypernatremia. Treatment of hypovolemic hypernatremia is dependent on restoration of volume status with isotonic saline. Choice *b* is incorrect because administering 5% dextrose in water without correcting the hypovolemia will not correct this patient's salt losses and, with his disoriented state, his oral intake of solute will likely be minimal. Choice *c* is incorrect because 0.45% saline will not correct his hypovolemic state in a timely manner. Choice *d* is incorrect because it is unlikely that the patient will be able to ingest an adequate amount of fluid or solute to replete his deficits.

Muhsin SA, Mount DB. Diagnosis and treatment of hypernatremia. Best Pract Res Clin Endocrinol Metab. 2016 Mar;30(2):189–203. Epub 2016 Mar 4.

Rose BD, Post TW. Clinical physiology of acid-base and electrolyte disorders. 5th ed. New York (NY): McGraw-Hill; c2001. 992 p.

III.98. Answer d.

The patient presents with symptomatic hyponatremia. Therefore, the treatment approach must be geared toward management of acute symptoms. The only treatment approach that will rapidly correct serum sodium is 3% saline. Therefore choices *b* and *c* are incorrect. One liter of hypertonic saline will increase serum sodium level by an estimate of 13 mEq. The rate of correction in a patient with a high likelihood of chronic hyponatremia should not exceed 4 to 6 mEq in the first 24 hours. With use of the Adrogue-Madias formula to predict change in Na^+, the predicted change in Na^+ based on this patient's total body water is approximately 11 mEq in 1 L of 3% saline. For a goal of 4 mEq change in serum Na^+, 364 mL of 3% normal saline is used, which is 61 mL per hour during the first 6 hours.

Adrogue HJ, Madias NE. The challenge of hyponatremia. J Am Soc Nephrol. 2012 Jul;23(7):1140–8. Epub 2012 May 24.

Sterns RH, Silver SM. Complications and management of hyponatremia. Curr Opin Nephrol Hypertens. 2016 Mar;25(2):114–9.

III.99. Answer a.

Cerebral salt wasting and the syndrome of inappropriate secretion of antidiuretic hormone present alike. The core underlying pathophysiologic state is hypovolemic hyponatremia in cerebral salt wasting and euvolemia and sometimes hypervolemia in the syndrome of inappropriate secretion of antidiuretic hormone. Factors that are consistent with the hypovolemic state include low central venous pressure and a high hematocrit level. Urine osmolality and uric acid level are similar in both cerebral salt wasting and the syndrome of inappropriate secretion of antidiuretic hormone. The urine Na^+ level can be high in both conditions.

Spasovski G, Vanholder R, Allolio B, Annane D, Ball S, Bichet D, et al; Hyponatraemia Guideline Development Group. Clinical practice guideline on diagnosis and treatment of hyponatraemia. Nephrol Dial Transplant. 2014 Apr;29 Suppl 2:i1–i39. Epub 2014 Feb 25. Erratum in: Nephrol Dial Transplant. 2014 Jun;40(6):924.

Yee AH, Burns JD, Wijdicks EF. Cerebral salt wasting: pathophysiology, diagnosis, and treatment. Neurosurg Clin N Am. 2010 Apr;21(2):339–52.

III.100. Answer c.

This patient has manifestations of osmotic demyelination syndrome, which developed because of rapid correction of hyponatremia. Na^+ corrected by 11 mEq over 24 hours. For patients with risk factors of this syndrome, the recommendation is to not exceed more than 6 mEq of Na^+ correction during the first 24 hours. The patient has several risk factors for chronic hyponatremia and osmotic demyelination syndrome, including chronic alcohol use, hypokalemia, and low urine osmolality. Low urine osmolality is suggestive of a low-solute diet and can occur in patients with higher fluid to solute intake. The most appropriate treatment approach is to slow the correction rate by administering desmopressin and D5W to bring the Na^+ level to 115 mEq or less. Choice *a* is incorrect because the patient's symptoms are due to osmotic demyelination syndrome and not to hyponatremia. Replacing potassium chloride will further increase the serum Na^+ level. Half-normal saline will decrease the Na^+ level, but the response will be slow.

Mount DB. The brain in hyponatremia: both culprit and victim. Semin Nephrol. 2009 May;29(3):196–215.

Sterns RH, Thomas DJ, Herndon RM. Brain dehydration and neurologic deterioration after rapid correction of hyponatremia. Kidney Int. 1989 Jan;35(1):69–75.

Hematologic and Inflammatory Disorders

III.101. Answer a.

In cases of ongoing ischemia or other symptoms, the hemoglobin level should be maintained at 10 g/dL or more. In a pilot trial of 110 patients with ACS, a threshold hemoglobin level of 10 g/dL was safer. Also, transfusion to a level of 10 g/dL or more (liberal strategy) was associated with greater survival at 30 days (98%) than transfusion to a level less than 8 g/dL (87%).

Carson JL, Brooks MM, Abbott JD, Chaitman B, Kelsey SF, Triulzi DJ, et al. Liberal versus restrictive transfusion thresholds for patients with symptomatic coronary artery disease. Am Heart J. 2013 Jun;165(6):964–971.e1. Epub 2013 Apr 8.

Hebert PC, Wells G, Blajchman MA, Marshall J, Martin C, Pagliarello G, et al; Transfusion Requirements in Critical Care Investigators, Canadian Critical Care Trials Group. A multicenter, randomized, controlled clinical trial of transfusion requirements in critical care. N Engl J Med. 1999 Feb 11;340(6):409–17. Erratum in: N Engl J Med 1999 Apr 1;340(13):1056.

Robertson CS, Hannay HJ, Yamal JM, Gopinath S, Goodman JC, Tilley BC; Epo Severe TBI Trial Investigators, Baldwin A, Rivera Lara L, Saucedo-Crespo H, Ahmed O, Sadasivan S, Ponce L, et al. Effect of erythropoietin and transfusion threshold on neurological recovery after traumatic brain injury: a randomized clinical trial. JAMA. 2014 Jul 2;312(1):36–47.

III.102. Answer b.

This patient is at risk for development of tumor lysis syndrome, which occurs soon after chemotherapy for high-grade hematologic cancer. All the answers are correct, but given the imminent progression of ECG changes and potential life-threatening arrhythmias, the treatment of hyperkalemia must be the first priority.

Hande KR, Garrow GC. Acute tumor lysis syndrome in patients with high-grade non-Hodgkin's lymphoma. Am J Med. 1993 Feb;94(2):133–9.

Jasek AM, Day HJ. Acute spontaneous tumor lysis syndrome. Am J Hematol. 1994 Oct;47(2):129–31.

III.103. Answer a.

Cardiac toxicity can occur at any time after treatment. The typical risks include older age and previous heart disease or ventricular dysfunction. The classic chemotherapy drugs doxorubicin and cyclophosphamide can cause more permanent dysfunction, whereas new biological agents such as trastuzumab can cause temporary dysfunction. Monitoring of cardiac function is important in patients receiving drugs known to have potential cardiac toxicity.

Ewer MS, Vooletich MT, Durand JB, Woods ML, Davis JR, Valero V, et al. Reversibility of trastuzumab-related cardiotoxicity: new insights based on clinical course and response to medical treatment. J Clin Oncol. 2005 Nov 1;23(31):7820–6.

Sawaya H, Sebag IA, Plana JC, Januzzi JL, Ky B, Cohen V, et al. Early detection and prediction of cardiotoxicity in chemotherapy-treated patients. Am J Cardiol. 2011 May 1;107(9):1375–80. Epub 2011 Mar 2.

III.104. Answer d.

The clinical scenario shows evidence of multiorgan involvement with many plausible explanations and initial treatments. However, given the striking levels of leukocytosis and the presence of myeloblasts in peripheral blood, the patient is very likely to have leukostasis with organ dysfunction caused by WBC plugs and increased blood viscosity. Urgent leukapheresis and consultation with a hematologist for prompt chemotherapy are indicated.

Daver N, Kantarjian H, Marcucci G, Pierce S, Brandt M, Dinardo C, et al. Clinical characteristics and outcomes in patients with acute promyelocytic leukaemia and hyperleucocytosis. Br J Haematol. 2015 Mar;168(5):646–53. Epub 2014 Oct 14.

Porcu P, Cripe LD, Ng EW, Bhatia S, Danielson CM, Orazi A, et al. Hyperleukocytic leukemias and leukostasis: a review of pathophysiology, clinical presentation and management. Leuk Lymphoma. 2000 Sep;39(1–2):1–18.

III.105. Answer b.

Patients who are recipients of hematopoietic stem cell transplants are likely to have a particular set of noninfectious complications that follow a timeline for presentation. The patient described above has the typical presentation of engraftment syndrome within the first month of transplant, coinciding with the recovery of the WBC count. Fever, rash, and gastrointestinal and pulmonary manifestations are common. Engraftment syndrome has mostly a good prognosis and is responsive to steroids.

Chi AK, Soubani AO, White AC, Miller KB. An update on pulmonary complications of hematopoietic stem cell transplantation. Chest. 2013 Dec;144(6):1913–22.

Lucena CM, Torres A, Rovira M, Marcos MA, de la Bellacasa JP, Sanchez M, et al. Pulmonary complications in hematopoietic SCT: a prospective study. Bone Marrow Transplant. 2014 Oct;49(10):1293–9. Epub 2014 Jul 21.

Spitzer TR. Engraftment syndrome: double-edged sword of hematopoietic cell transplants. Bone Marrow Transplant. 2015 Apr;50(4):469–75. Epub 2015 Jan 12.

III.106. Answer d.

The clinical probability scoring system assessment should be performed immediately. For patients with an intermediate to high probability of HIT, use of heparin (or LMWH) should be discontinued and a nonheparin anticoagulant given because of the risk of thrombosis (HIT with thrombosis). For low-risk patients, heparin use may be continued because HIT is unlikely. Thrombosis is a risk for all patients with HIT regardless of the degree of thrombocytopenia. No heparin or LMWH should be given because of the risk of thrombosis and the presence of cross-reactivity. Great caution must be used in transitioning to warfarin. The platelet count must be back in the normal range, warfarin should be given at a low dosage, and use of the nonheparin anticoagulant should be continued until the INR is in the therapeutic range. Follow special specific recommendations for transitioning to warfarin from argatroban, because argatroban also increases the INR and thus complicates monitoring of warfarin.

Cuker A, Crowther MA. 2013 Clinical Practice Guideline on the Evaluation and Management of Adults with Suspected Heparin-Induced Thrombocytopenia (HIT). Washington (DC): American Society of Hematology; c2013.

Marder VJ, Aird WC, Bennett JS, Schulman S, White GC II, editors. Hemostasis and thrombosis: basic principles and clinical practice. 6th ed. Philadelphia (PA): Wolters Kluwer Health/Lippincott Williams & Wilkins; c2013. p. 751–828.

III.107. Answer a.

ITP is a diagnosis of exclusion. Thrombocytopenia and bleeding symptoms (if present) are isolated. Generally, there are no constitutional symptoms, such as weight loss, bone pain, or night sweats, and no hepatosplenomegaly, lymphadenopathy, or signs of congenital conditions on physical examination. A bone marrow examination may be considered in older adults if abnormalities are found in the WBCs or on the peripheral blood smear. All adults with newly diagnosed ITP should be tested for hepatitis C and HIV.

American Society of Hematology. 2011 Clinical Practice Guideline on the Evaluation and Management of Immune Thrombocytopenia (ITP). Washington (DC): American Society of Hematology; c2011.

Marder VJ, Aird WC, Bennett JS, Schulman S, White GC II, editors. Hemostasis and thrombosis: basic principles and clinical practice. 6th ed. Philadelphia (PA): Wolters Kluwer Health/Lippincott Williams & Wilkins; c2013. p. 751–828.

III.108. Answer d.

Prompt initiation of therapeutic plasma exchange with plasma blood products has reduced mortality from 80% to 20%. Testing for ADAMTS13 activity and percentage inhibition is useful but is not commonly available, and results may not be available for several hours to days. If the ADAMTS13 activity is in the normal range, therapeutic plasma exchange can be discontinued. Review of the peripheral blood smear will show the presence of increased numbers of schistocytes (and some spherocytes). The schistocytes, increased lactate dehydrogenase level, and the low hemoglobin and platelet counts, in addition to the patient's history, make TTP highly likely. Because pregnancy can often be a precipitating factor for TTP, a pregnancy test might be considered. TTP is actually not a congenital platelet disorder, and this patient's history is not suggestive of a congenital platelet disorder. Thus, next-generation sequencing for this patient is not the best use of resources. Congenital TTP may present in infancy or childhood as chronic relapsing TTP, but sometimes it presents in adults. If the family history is positive, the patient has relapses, or the ADAMTS13 levels do not return to normal after recovery, congenital TTP may be of greater concern. Splenectomy is of no benefit in TTP.

Kitchens CS, Kessler CM, Konkle BA, editors. Consultative hemostasis and thrombosis [electronic resource]. 3rd ed. Philadelphia (PA): Elsevier/Saunders; c2013. p. 103–49.

Marder VJ, Aird WC, Bennett JS, Schulman S, White GC II, editors. Hemostasis and thrombosis: basic principles and clinical practice. 6th ed. Philadelphia (PA): Wolters Kluwer Health/Lippincott Williams & Wilkins; c2013. p. 751–828.

III.109. Answer b.

Unlike thrombocytopenia associated with infectious diseases, the platelet count in patients with drug-induced thrombocytopenia tends to rebound quickly after stopping use of the medication (after use of gold salts, platelets can take much longer to recover). Many nutritional supplements and over-the-counter herbal remedies affect the platelets; food and drinks may also. Ginkgo biloba, garlic, ginseng, acai berry, valerian, and St. John's wort are all known to affect platelet function and sometimes platelet number. Quinine is the most commonly reported cause of drug-induced thrombocytopenia, but many people do not consider it a drug when providing a medication history. Quinine is present in tonic water and some nutritional supplements. Cases of drug-induced thrombocytopenia are thought to be largely underreported, especially if the effects are mild to moderate or the patient has multiple comorbidities. Chronic use of large amounts of alcohol can cause mild to severe depression of megakaryocytopoiesis selectively. Vitamin deficiency related to alcohol intake, splenomegaly, and cirrhosis can also lower platelet counts. Abstinence from alcohol for a few weeks usually results in a return to normal platelet counts. Moderate thrombocytopenia can persist in some patients after stopping alcohol ingestion. Preformed antibodies can recognize platelets coated with a medication and cause platelet destruction within hours. Abciximab causes a decrease in platelets within 6 to 12 hours in 2% of patients exposed for the first time and a higher percentage in subsequent exposures. The mechanism may involve antibodies to murine peptide sequences in the abciximab Fab fragment.

Kitchens CS, Kessler CM, Konkle BA, editors. Consultative hemostasis and thrombosis [electronic resource]. 3rd ed. Philadelphia (PA): Elsevier/Saunders; c2013. p. 103–49.

Marder VJ, Aird WC, Bennett JS, Schulman S, White GC II, editors. Hemostasis and thrombosis: basic principles and clinical practice. 6th ed. Philadelphia (PA): Wolters Kluwer Health/Lippincott Williams & Wilkins; c2013. p. 751–828.

III.110. Answer c.

Because the patient's own platelets are decreased in number or are dysfunctional in congenital platelet disorders, platelet transfusions are indicated for active bleeding to supply normally functioning and adequate numbers of platelets. Congenital platelet disorders are rare, and acquired thrombocytopenias are much more common. Platelet disorders tend to cause mucocutaneous bleeding (nose, mouth, gastrointestinal tract, genitourinary tract, skin) rather than muscle and joints, as in coagulation factor deficiencies. Postoperative bleeding is immediate with platelet disorders because the platelets are involved in the first step of clotting (primary hemostasis). During very severe bleeding, it may be difficult to differentiate whether the origin is a problem with the platelets or the coagulation factors, or both. Mild congenital platelet disorders may not be recognized until adulthood and are frequently confused with ITP. Patients with ITP who are not responsive to glucocorticoids, rituximab, or even splenectomy should be considered for a congenital platelet disorder work-up, including an examination of the peripheral blood smear for unusually large platelets, lack of platelet granules, and WBC inclusions (Döhle-like bodies) and platelet function testing as part of the initial work-up. A family history of a low platelet count or consanguinity may be ascertained and a physical examination performed to look for other associated abnormalities such as hearing loss, skeletal deformities, and renal dysfunction. Classification of some platelet disorders may be accomplished with available testing (platelet function testing, peripheral blood smear review, flow cytometry, electron microscopy, genetic mutational analysis). However, for many patients, congenital thrombocytopenia cannot be readily classified; next-generation sequencing of platelet disorders may improve future diagnosis, treatment, and understanding.

Kitchens CS, Kessler CM, Konkle BA, editors. Consultative hemostasis and thrombosis [electronic resource]. 3rd ed. Philadelphia (PA): Elsevier/Saunders; c2013. p. 103–49.

Marder VJ, Aird WC, Bennett JS, Schulman S, White GC II, editors. Hemostasis and thrombosis: basic principles and clinical practice. 6th ed. Philadelphia (PA): Wolters Kluwer Health/ Lippincott Williams & Wilkins; c2013. p. 751–828.

III.111. Answer a.

DIC is a systemic process with the potential for causing thrombosis and hemorrhage. The International Society on Thrombosis and Haemostasis defines DIC as an acquired syndrome with intravascular activation of coagulation that may be due to different causes. It can be initiated from damage to microvasculature and, in turn, cause damage to microvasculature, which, if sufficiently severe, can lead to organ dysfunction. Also known as consumption coagulopathy or defibrination syndrome, DIC is characterized by abnormal activation of coagulation cascade that results in formation of widespread microthrombi in small blood vessels, disrupting normal hemostasis by depletion of clotting factors and platelets. DIC, typically occurring in patients with critical illness, can manifest as an acute, life-threatening emergency or as a chronic, subclinical process, depending on the influence of morbidity from the underlying cause.

Matsuda T. Clinical aspects of DIC: disseminated intravascular coagulation. Pol J Pharmacol. 1996 Jan-Feb;48(1):73–5.

Taylor FB Jr, Toh CH, Hoots WK, Wada H, Levi M; Scientific Subcommittee on Disseminated Intravascular Coagulation (DIC) of the International Society on Thrombosis and Haemostasis (ISTH). Towards definition, clinical and laboratory criteria, and a scoring system for disseminated intravascular coagulation. Thromb Haemost. 2001 Nov;86(5):1327–30.

III.112. Answer c.

Acute DIC, typically occurring in patients with trauma, sepsis, hemolytic reaction, or HELLP syndrome, occurs when blood is exposed to substantial amounts of TF or other procoagulant substances over a brief period with substantial generation of thrombin. This process leads to rapid consumption of coagulation factors that exceeds their synthesis. However, in chronic DIC, such as in patients with myeloproliferative disorders, blood constantly (or intermittently) is exposed to smaller quantities of TF or other procoagulant substances. Although coagulation factors and platelets are also consumed in chronic DIC, their production is compensated and the liver is able to clear the FDPs.

Gordon SG, Mielicki WP. Cancer procoagulant: a factor X activator, tumor marker and growth factor from malignant tissue. Blood Coagul Fibrinolysis. 1997 Mar;8(2):73–86.

Levi M, Ten Cate H. Disseminated intravascular coagulation. N Engl J Med. 1999 Aug 19;341(8):586–92.

III.113. Answer d.

DIC is initiated by exposure of blood to a procoagulant such as TF, but it is less likely due to prekallikrein. In hemolysis-related DIC, coagulation is activated by a combination of processes including TF release, generation of cytokines including interleukin-1 and tumor necrosis factor, and reduced nitric oxide function. NETs are highly procoagulant and activate the clotting cascade, influencing primary and secondary hemostasis through several mechanisms, including delivery of TF, activation of the contact phase of coagulation by cell-free DNA (which activates cell-surface toll-like receptors), induction of platelet aggregation, and proteolytic degradation of anticoagulants such as TF pathway inhibitor through neutrophil elastase.

Liaw PC, Ito T, Iba T, Thachil J, Zeerleder S. DAMP and DIC: the role of extracellular DNA and DNA-binding proteins in the pathogenesis of DIC. Blood Rev. 2016 Jul;30(4):257–61. Epub 2015 Dec 31.

Martinod K, Wagner DD. Thrombosis: tangled up in NETs. Blood. 2014 May 1;123(18):2768–76. Epub 2013 Dec 23.

III.114. Answer d.

No single laboratory test can accurately confirm or eliminate the diagnosis of DIC. Increased D-dimer level, prolonged PT or aPTT, low fibrinogen level, and thrombocytopenia are sensitive, but not specific, for DIC. It is imperative to note that several conditions other than DIC, such as recent surgery, trauma, or venous thromboembolism, can be associated with an increased level of FDPs. The natural anticoagulants such as protein C and antithrombin are often decreased in DIC, and these also have been shown to have prognostic significance.

Levi M, Toh CH, Thachil J, Watson HG; British Committee for Standards in Haematology. Guidelines for the diagnosis and management of disseminated intravascular coagulation. Br J Haematol. 2009 Apr;145(1):24–33. Epub 2009 Feb 12.

Mesters RM, Mannucci PM, Coppola R, Keller T, Ostermann H, Kienast J. Factor VIIa and antithrombin III activity during severe sepsis and septic shock in neutropenic patients. Blood. 1996 Aug 1;88(3):881–6.

III.115. Answer d.

In patients with DIC, blood product transfusion includes fresh frozen plasma, platelets, and fibrinogen replacement in the form of cryoprecipitate or fibrinogen concentrates. Platelet transfusion may be needed if the patient has bleeding and the platelet count is less than 50×10^9/L, whereas a lower threshold of 20 to 30×10^9/L may be used in patients without bleeding. The threshold for platelet transfusion should be dependent on the clinical situation and the descending trend of platelets. In DIC, the natural anticoagulant AT is depleted early during the disproportionately high thrombin generation. A low AT level is known to be a prognosticator of poor clinical outcome in patients with sepsis and an independent marker of mortality in DIC. However, AT treatment for DIC is not yet approved worldwide, although a tailored AT dosing has been approved in Japan. Hyperfibrinolysis, a common phenomenon in DIC, is a natural reactionary process to deal with the uncontrolled thrombin generation. Thus, inhibiting excessive fibrinolysis with antifibrinolytic agents such as ε-aminocaproic acid, tranexamic acid, or aprotinin may be harmful for patients with DIC. Soluble thrombomodulin has less bleeding risk than the other anticoagulants such as activated protein C, because its anticoagulant property is dependent on the extent of thrombin generated. It is currently being evaluated in clinical trials.

CRASH-2 trial collaborators, Shakur H, Roberts I, Bautista R, Caballero J, Coats T, Dewan Y, et al. Effects of tranexamic acid on death, vascular occlusive events, and blood transfusion in trauma patients with significant haemorrhage (CRASH-2): a randomised, placebo-controlled trial. Lancet. 2010 Jul 3;376(9734):23–32. Epub 2010 Jun 14.

Gando S, Wada H, Thachil J; Scientific and Standardization Committee on DIC of the International Society on Thrombosis and Haemostasis (ISTH). Differentiating disseminated intravascular coagulation (DIC) with the fibrinolytic phenotype from coagulopathy of trauma and acute coagulopathy of trauma-shock (COT/ACOTS). J Thromb Haemost. 2013 May;11(5):826–35.

Wada H, Thachil J, Di Nisio M, Mathew P, Kurosawa S, Gando S, et al; The Scientific Standardization Committee on DIC of the International Society on Thrombosis Haemostasis. Guidance for diagnosis and treatment of DIC from harmonization of the recommendations from three guidelines. J Thromb Haemost. 2013 Feb 4. [Epub ahead of print]

III.116. Answer b.

A prolonged PT or aPTT may reflect either a coagulation factor deficiency or the presence of an inhibitor. The way to distinguish between them is to perform a mixing study with normal pooled plasma. Correction of the prolonged clotting time suggests a coagulation factor deficiency, whereas failure to correct the prolonged clotting time suggests the presence of an inhibitor.

Kamal AH, Tefferi A, Pruthi RK. How to interpret and pursue an abnormal prothrombin time, activated partial thromboplastin time, and bleeding time in adults. Mayo Clin Proc. 2007 Jul;82(7):864–73.

Kitchens CS. Prolonged activated partial thromboplastin time of unknown etiology: a prospective study of 100 consecutive cases referred for consultation. Am J Hematol. 1988 Jan;27(1):38–45.

III.117. Answer d.

The normal platelet count excludes a quantitative platelet disorder, and normal PT and aPTT exclude a coagulation factor deficiency (DIC) or inhibitor (against factor VIII and V). Mild to moderate deficiencies of von Willebrand factor do not affect the PT or aPTT and, given that the patient has a monoclonal protein disorder, acquired von Willebrand syndrome is the most likely explanation.

Kamal AH, Tefferi A, Pruthi RK. How to interpret and pursue an abnormal prothrombin time, activated partial thromboplastin time, and bleeding time in adults. Mayo Clin Proc. 2007 Jul;82(7):864–73.

III.118. Answer a.

This patient has an underlying autoimmune disorder (systemic lupus erythematosus) and has now presented with new onset of hemorrhage. On laboratory testing, the PT is normal, but the aPTT is prolonged and inhibited. Therefore, the patient has a factor VIII inhibitor coagulopathy. Factor V inhibitors prolong both the PT and aPTT; therefore, that answer choice is not likely in this situation. DIC is a consumptive coagulopathy and, therefore, may prolong both the PT and aPTT. However, both will correct on mixing study. Although an acquired von Willebrand syndrome has possibly developed, deficiencies of von Willebrand factor generally do not prolong the aPTT.

Kamal AH, Tefferi A, Pruthi RK. How to interpret and pursue an abnormal prothrombin time, activated partial thromboplastin time, and bleeding time in adults. Mayo Clin Proc. 2007 Jul;82(7):864–73.

III.119. Answer c.

In this urgent situation, plasma transfusion would not be the optimal approach to reverse the effect of warfarin. However, it may be considered if factor concentrates, such as 4F-PCC, are not available. With an INR between 4 and 6, the appropriate 4F-PCC dosing is 35 IU/kg. To sustain the effects and promote activation of vitamin K-dependent factors, supplemental vitamin K should be administered. IV administration offers a more rapid response than oral (equivalent by 24 hours) and subcutaneous administration. Vitamin K is a fat-soluble vitamin, and subcutaneous administration for rapid reversal of VKAs is not recommended.

Holbrook A, Schulman S, Witt DM, Vandvik PO, Fish J, Kovacs MJ, et al. Evidence-based management of anticoagulant therapy: antithrombotic therapy and prevention of thrombosis, 9th ed: American College of Chest Physicians Evidence-Based Clinical Practice Guidelines. Chest. 2012 Feb;141(2 Suppl):e152S–e84S.

Sarode R, Milling TJ Jr, Refaai MA, Mangione A, Schneider A, Durn BL, et al. Efficacy and safety of a 4-factor prothrombin complex concentrate in patients on vitamin K antagonists presenting with major bleeding: a randomized, plasma-controlled, phase IIIb study. Circulation. 2013 Sep 10;128(11):1234–43. Epub 2013 Aug 9.

III.120. Answer d.

In this patient, the presence of antiphospholipid antibodies results in ex vivo prolongation of the aPTT, which is evident in the patient's baseline laboratory result and is contrary to the clinical thrombophilia. Using a fixed ratio of the patient's baseline aPTT (choice *a*) or the normal UFH therapeutic range (choice *b*) would be inappropriate for this patient. There is no evidence for selecting a higher aPTT range (choice *c*). A UFH concentration of more than 1.0 U/mL is supratherapeutic and may increase the risk of bleeding. For this patient, the best method to monitor UFH therapy is with the anti-Xa assay with the goal of 0.3 to 0.7 U/mL.

Bates SM, Weitz JI. Coagulation assays. Circulation. 2005 Jul 26;112(4):e53–60.

Vandiver JW, Vondracek TG. Antifactor Xa levels versus activated partial thromboplastin time for monitoring unfractionated heparin. Pharmacotherapy. 2012 Jun;32(6):546–58. Epub 2012 Apr 24.

III.121. Answer b.

Because of the acute retroperitoneal hemorrhage and concurrent anticoagulation with UFH, the effect of the UFH should be reversed. Because the patient was receiving a continuous heparin infusion for the past 2 to 2.5 hours at 1,260 U/h, the patient should receive approximately 30 mg of protamine sulfate IV. UFH has a half-life of 60 to 90 minutes, and 12 mg would neutralize only the UFH given within the past hour. However, too much protamine may result in increased anticoagulation. Plasma is not indicated for reversing heparin and may worsen the anticoagulant effect of UFH.

Garcia DA, Baglin TP, Weitz JI, Samama MM. Parenteral anticoagulants: antithrombotic therapy and prevention of thrombosis, 9th ed: American College of Chest Physicians Evidence-Based Clinical Practice Guidelines. Chest. 2012 Feb;141(2 Suppl):e24S–e43S. Errata in: Chest. 2012 May;141(5):1369. Chest. 2013 Aug;144(2):721.

Jobes DR, Aitken GL, Shaffer GW. Increased accuracy and precision of heparin and protamine dosing reduces blood loss and transfusion in patients undergoing primary cardiac operations. J Thorac Cardiovasc Surg. 1995 Jul;110(1):36–45.

III.122. Answer d.

Dabigatran is the first DOAC to have a specific reversal agent approved by the US Food and Drug Administration. Idarucizamab should be administered according to the manufacturer's recommendation (5 g). Although dabigratran is dialyzable, data are limited, and this is not the optimal treatment option for this patient.

Pollack CV Jr, Reilly PA, Eikelboom J, Glund S, Verhamme P, Bernstein RA, et al. Idarucizumab for dabigatran reversal. N Engl J Med. 2015 Aug 6;373(6):511–20. Epub 2015 Jun 22.

Pradaxa [package insert]. Ridgefield (CT): Boehringer Ingelheim Pharmaceuticals, Inc; c2017. [cited 2017 Jan 3]. Available from: http://docs.boehringer-ingelheim.com/Prescribing%20Information/PIs/Pradaxa/Pradaxa.pdf.

III.123. Answer d.

Although a reversal agent for direct Xa inhibitors is not available for clinical use, one advantage of the DOACs is the short half-life, barring hepatic or renal dysfunction. DOACs usually do not require monitoring, and routine laboratory testing is not readily available by most laboratories. Rivaroxaban has a half-life of 5 to 9 hours, and after 30 hours and without hepatic or kidney dysfunction, a considerable amount of drug has been metabolized. At this time, the best treatment management is frequent monitoring and transfusion support. Routine laboratory testing has variable sensitivities to DOACs and is unreliable for determining subtherapeutic, therapeutic, or supratherapeutic levels, especially because the therapeutic ranges are not established for any DOACs. If life-threatening or uncontrolled bleeding occurs with recent administration of a DOAC, a specific reversal agent is not currently available. However, factor concentrates such as nonactivated or activated prothrombin complex concentrate may be considered.

Connolly SJ, Milling TJ Jr, Eikelboom JW, Gibson CM, Curnutte JT, Gold A, et al; ANNEXA-4 Investigators. Andexanet alfa for acute major bleeding associated with factor Xa inhibitors. N Engl J Med. 2016 Sep 22;375(12):1131–41. Epub 2016 Aug 30.

Cuker A, Siegal D. Monitoring and reversal of direct oral anticoagulants. Hematology Am Soc Hematol Educ Program. 2015;2015:117–24.

III.124. Answer d.

Plasma is used as the replacement fluid when treating TTP because it is a source of the missing enzyme ADAMTS13, and it maintains clotting factors because exchanges must be performed daily. Patients who cannot participate in their care (fist pumping and remaining still) should receive central venous catheters for vascular access. The apheresis instrument requires anticoagulation to prevent clotting in the circuit.

Sanford KW, Balogun RA. Therapeutic apheresis in critically ill patients. J Clin Apher. 2011;26(5):249–51. Epub 2011 Aug 10.

Schwartz J, Padmanabhan A, Aqui N, Balogun RA, Connelly-Smith L, Delaney M, et al. Guidelines on the use of therapeutic apheresis in clinical practice-evidence-based approach from the Writing Committee of the American Society for Apheresis: The seventh special issue. J Clin Apher. 2016 Jun;31(3):149–62.

III.125. Answer a.

The American College of Chest Physicians evidence-based clinical practice guidelines for the treatment and prevention of HIT recommend short-term use of heparin during cardiac surgery over nonheparin anticoagulants in patients with a history of HIT who do not have demonstrable heparin antibodies. In this setting, TPE is not indicated because the pathogenic antibody is no longer present in the patient's plasma.

Linkins LA, Dans AL, Moores LK, Bona R, Davidson BL, Schulman S, et al. Treatment and prevention of heparin-induced thrombocytopenia: Antithrombotic Therapy and Prevention of Thrombosis, 9th ed: American College of Chest Physicians Evidence-Based Clinical Practice Guidelines. Chest. 2012 Feb;141(2 Suppl):e495S–e530S. Erratum in: Chest. 2015 Dec;148(6):1529.

Pham HP, Schwartz J. New apheresis indications in hematological disorders. Curr Opin Hematol. 2016 Nov;23(6):581–7.

III.126. Answer a.

Identification of gout crystals on aspiration does not eliminate the possibility of septic arthritis, particularly in a patient with aspiration pneumonia. Other risk factors for septic arthritis include this patient's age and diabetes mellitus. Antibiotics should cover both gram-positive and gram-negative organisms in the setting of a hospitalized patient with diabetes mellitus. Nonsteroidal anti-inflammatory drugs such as indomethacin (choice *a*) can be used for an acute gout flare. However, septic arthritis has not been ruled out in this patient. Further, his creatinine level is increased to 2.3, and thus nonsteroidal anti-inflammatory drugs would not be ideal. Choice *c* is an option for treatment for acute gout flare. If infection were to be excluded with culture, then this may be an ideal option for treatment because there would be minimal systemic effect. However, until septic arthritis is excluded, this treatment should be deferred. Colchicine (choice *d*) is another option for treatment of acute gout flare. It is most successful when given as soon as possible after the flare. It can be a good option because it is not immunosuppressive, in comparison with corticosteroids, in a patient such as this who also has pneumonia. However, with the patient's increased creatinine level, this treatment would increase the toxicity associated with colchicine. Further, there must be caution with drug-drug interactions with colchicine. In this example, colchicine can increase the myopathic risk of simvastatin.

Khanna D, Khanna PP, Fitzgerald JD, Singh MK, Bae S, Neogi T, et al; American College of Rheumatology. 2012 American College of Rheumatology guidelines for management of gout. Part 2: therapy and antiinflammatory prophylaxis of acute gouty arthritis. Arthritis Care Res (Hoboken). 2012 Oct;64(10):1447–61.

Margaretten ME, Kohlwes J, Moore D, Bent S. Does this adult patient have septic arthritis? JAMA. 2007 Apr 4;297(13):1478–88.

III.127. Answer a.

Because of the vision loss, the patient should receive high-dose corticosteroids. Because of a high level of concern for giant cell arteritis, therapy should not be delayed for the temporal artery biopsy. If the biopsy is completed within a few weeks of therapy, the yield of the biopsy should not be substantially affected. Ideally the biopsy would be done within a week of the start of corticosteroid therapy, and, depending on the results, the dosage of corticosteroids decreased (if biopsy is positive for giant cell arteritis) to 80 to 100 mg/day orally if the visual symptoms are present or 40 to 60 mg/day if they are not present. Choice *b* is not a good choice; because of the high clinical concern in the setting of transient vision loss, scalp tenderness, polymyalgia rheumatica–like symptoms (difficulty getting up from the chair to the bed because of pain), and increased levels of inflammatory markers, treatment should not be delayed for the purposes of the biopsy. The goal of treatment with high-dose corticosteroids is to prevent vision loss, which is the result of ischemia of the optic nerve due to involvement of posterior ciliary arteries. Once vision loss occurs, it can be permanent. Prednisone, 15 mg daily (choice *c*) is an appropriate dose if the concern is that the patient has polymyalgia rheumatica in isolation. However, it would be insufficient to treat giant cell arteritis, particularly in a patient who has already had an episode of transient visual loss. Choice *d* is not the correct answer because of both the low dose of prednisone and the timing of the biopsy in relation to treatment initiation.

Dasgupta B, Borg FA, Hassan N, Alexander L, Barraclough K, Bourke B, et al; BSR and BHPR Standards, Guidelines and Audit Working Group. BSR and BHPR guidelines for the management of giant cell arteritis. Rheumatology (Oxford). 2010 Aug;49(8):1594–7. Epub 2010 Apr 5.

Dejaco C, Singh YP, Perel P, Hutchings A, Camellino D, Mackie S, et al; European League Against Rheumatism; American College of Rheumatology. 2015 recommendations for the management of polymyalgia rheumatica: a European League Against

Rheumatism/American College of Rheumatology collaborative initiative. Arthritis Rheumatol. 2015 Oct;67(10):2569–80.

Sepsis and Other Infectious Diseases

III.128. Answer d.

Multiple diagnostic tests are available for diagnosis of *C difficile* infections. To avoid overdiagnosis and unnecessary treatment, testing for *C difficile* is recommended only for patients who have active diarrhea or in the setting of suspected ileus caused by *C difficile* infection (choice *c*). An important part of treatment is to stop risk factors for *C difficile* infection (ie, stopping use of unnecessary antibiotics, choice *a*) and to start adequate antimicrobial therapy depending on whether the infection is mild, moderate, or severe. Current guidelines recommend the use of vancomycin for episodes of severe *C difficile* infections (choice *b*). Metronidazole can be useful for mild or moderate infections. Test of cure is not recommended at the completion of treatment (choice *d*).

Cohen SH, Gerding DN, Johnson S, Kelly CP, Loo VG, McDonald LC, et al; Society for Healthcare Epidemiology of America; Infectious Diseases Society of America. Clinical practice guidelines for *Clostridium difficile* infection in adults: 2010 update by the Society for Healthcare Epidemiology of America (SHEA) and the Infectious Diseases Society of America (IDSA). Infect Control Hosp Epidemiol. 2010 May;31(5):431–55.

III.129. Answer c.

A urinary catheter should be placed only in patients with clear indications (eg, urinary retention, close urine output monitoring) to prevent catheter-related urinary tract infections. The presence of pyuria will not help distinguish asymptomatic bacteriuria from urinary tract infection. Soon after placement, urinary catheters become colonized by bacteria. This is the reason that urine cultures are recommended only in patients with clinical findings suggestive of catheter-related urinary tract infections with fever only by virtue of the underlying conditions specified in choice *c*. With rare exceptions, asymptomatic bacteriuria, catheter associated or not, does not need to be treated; exceptions include late stages of pregnancy and immediately before a procedural intervention that could obstruct the renal collection system. The presence of pyuria is not a reliable parameter for differentiating asymptomatic bacteriuria from catheter-related urinary tract infection (choice *b*).

Hooton TM, Bradley SF, Cardenas DD, Colgan R, Geerlings SE, Rice JC, et al; Infectious Diseases Society of America. Diagnosis, prevention, and treatment of catheter-associated urinary tract infection in adults: 2009 International Clinical Practice Guidelines from the Infectious Diseases Society of America. Clin Infect Dis. 2010 Mar 1;50(5):625–63.

III.130. Answer d.

Of the listed options, only daily chlorhexidine baths have shown benefit for preventing central line–associated bloodstream infections. Central lines should not be routinely cultured unless clinically indicated (choice *a*). If a central line was exchanged over a guidewire and the catheter tip culture is positive, thus indicating catheter exit-site infection, then discontinuation of the exchanged line and placement of a new catheter at a different site is indicated.

Mermel LA, Allon M, Bouza E, Craven DE, Flynn P, O'Grady NP, et al. Clinical practice guidelines for the diagnosis and management of intravascular catheter-related infection: 2009 update by the Infectious Diseases Society of America. Clin Infect Dis. 2009 Jul 1;49(1):1–45. Errata in: Clin Infect Dis. 2010 Apr 1;50(7):1079. Clin Infect Dis. 2010 Feb 1;50(3):457.

Miller SE, Maragakis LL. Central line-associated bloodstream infection prevention. Curr Opin Infect Dis. 2012 Aug;25(4):412–22.

III.131. Answer d.

Although the most common microorganisms for catheter-related bloodstream infections are gram positive (ie, *Staphylococcus aureus*, coagulase-negative staphylococci), as a group the next most common pathogens are the aerobic gram-negative bacteria followed by *Candida*. Brain MRI is not indicated at this time because his status epilepticus has been controlled and no new neurologic symptoms have developed. Continuing the same antibiotic therapy and adding only gram-negative coverage may be insufficient to adequately treat the sepsis in this patient.

Mermel LA, Allon M, Bouza E, Craven DE, Flynn P, O'Grady NP, et al. Clinical practice guidelines for the diagnosis and management of intravascular catheter-related infection: 2009 update by the Infectious Diseases Society of America. Clin Infect Dis. 2009 Jul 1;49(1):1–45. Errata in: Clin Infect Dis. 2010 Apr 1;50(7):1079. Clin Infect Dis. 2010 Feb 1;50(3):457.

III.132. Answer d.

This patient is experiencing a severe, complicated *C difficile* infection (which is defined as leukocytosis with a WBC count $\geq 15\times10^9$/L or a serum creatinine level 1.5 times or more the premorbid level) associated with hypotension or shock, ileus, or megacolon. Both oral vancomycin and IV metronidazole are indicated. Rapid surgical evaluation is recommended because early intervention (if indicated) can reduce mortality. Finally, his clinical course is consistent with transmural polymicrobial infection of the bowel wall and septic shock complicating *C difficile* colitis.

Bagdasarian N, Rao K, Malani PN. Diagnosis and treatment of *Clostridium difficile* in adults: a systematic review. JAMA. 2015 Jan 27;313(4):398–408.

Cohen SH, Gerding DN, Johnson S, Kelly CP, Loo VG, McDonald LC, et al; Society for Healthcare Epidemiology of America; Infectious Diseases Society of America. Clinical practice guidelines for *Clostridium difficile* infection in adults: 2010 update by the Society for Healthcare Epidemiology of America (SHEA) and the Infectious Diseases Society of America (IDSA). Infect Control Hosp Epidemiol. 2010 May;31(5):431–55.

III.133. Answer c.

All of the above options are usually effective against *E faecalis*. Unfortunately, cephalosporins (all generations) are not effective against *Enterococcus* spp as monotherapy, with the exception of the fifth-generation ceftaroline, which has some activity.

Sanford Guide to Antimicrobial Therapy [Internet]. Antibacterial agents; mobile device application. [cited 2016 Oct 27]. Available from: https:// store.sanfordguide.com/antimicrobial-therapy-cross-platform-app-subscriptionp93.aspx?gclid=EAIaIQobChMIk9_Qo6PQ1wIVBTFpCh1m-RAJDEAAYAiAAEgI36fD_BwE.

III.134. Answer a.

All of the above options are active against MSSA, but the treatments of choice for *S aureus* microorganisms are the antistaphylococcal penicillins (eg, nafcillin, oxacillin). Ceftriaxone can be effective against MSSA but is inferior to nafcillin. Vancomycin is effective against MSSA and MRSA, but it is also inferior against antistaphylococcal penicillins. Linezolid is also effective against MSSA and MRSA, but the already established efficacy of antistaphylococcal and the concern of toxicity-related adverse effects (eg, myelosuppression) do not make it the best choice.

Baddour LM, Wilson WR, Bayer AS, Fowler VG Jr, Tleyjeh IM, Rybak MJ, et al; American Heart Association Committee on Rheumatic Fever, Endocarditis, and Kawasaki Disease of the Council on Cardiovascular Disease in the Young, Council on Clinical Cardiology, Council on Cardiovascular Surgery and Anesthesia, and Stroke Council. Infective endocarditis in adults: diagnosis, antimicrobial therapy, and management of complications: a scientific statement for healthcare professionals from the American Heart Association. Circulation. 2015 Oct 13;132(15):1435–86. Epub 2015 Sep 15. Errata in: Circulation. 2015 Oct 27;132(17):e215. Circulation. 2016 Aug 23;134(8):e113.

Murray BE, Arias CA, Nannini EC. Glycopeptides (vancomycin and teicoplanin), streptogramins (quinupristin-dalfopristin), lipopeptides (daptomycin), and lipoglycopeptides (telavancin). In: Bennett JE, Dolin R, Blaser MJ, editors. Mandell, Douglas, and Bennett's principles and practice of infectious diseases. 8th ed. Vol. 1. Philadelphia (PA): Elsevier/ Saunders; c2015. p. 377–400.

Petri WA Jr. Penicillins, cephalosporins, and other β-lactam antibiotics. In: Brunton LL, editor. Goodman & Gilman's: the pharmacological basis of therapeutics. 12th ed. New York (NY): McGraw- Hill Medical; c2011. p. 1477–1503.

III.135. Answer d.

All of the listed regimens can potentially be used in the management of infections due to *P aeruginosa*, with the exception of cefotaxime. Unfortunately, *P aeruginosa* can be a multidrugresistant microorganism and develop resistance to one or many of the known agents against *P aeruginosa*. Ceftolozane/tazobactam is a newly developed agent that may be used for treatment of multidrug-resistant *P aeruginosa*.

Viale P, Giannella M, Tedeschi S, Lewis R. Treatment of MDR-gram negative infections in the 21st century: a never ending threat for clinicians. Curr Opin Pharmacol. 2015 Oct;24:30–7. Epub 2015 Jul 24.

III.136. Answer b.

All of the options are effective for the treatment of infections due to *Candida* spp. The microorganism involved in this case is susceptible to all antifungal agents. For management of CNS infections, consideration has to be given to drugs with adequate tissular penetration. Echinocandins (eg, caspofungin) are well distributed throughout the body with the exception of the CNS, eye, and urine.

Pappas PG, Kauffman CA, Andes DR, Clancy CJ, Marr KA, Ostrosky-Zeichner L, et al. Clinical Practice Guideline for the Management of Candidiasis: 2016 update by the Infectious Diseases Society of America. Clin Infect Dis. 2016 Feb 15;62(4):e1–50. Epub 2015 Dec 16.

III.137. Answer b.

This patient is experiencing a brain abscess possibly related to the recent immunosuppression from steroid use. Blood culture results indicate a multidrug- resistant *P aeruginosa* (thus, the likely cause of the brain abscess). The microorganism carries the presence of an extended- spectrum β-lactamase which would preclude the use of all β-lactam antibiotics with the exclusion of the carbapenems, which have excellent CNS penetration. The patient has been admitted for recent new- onset seizures, imipenem use would not be an appropriate choice because of its epileptogenic potential. Ertapenem lacks coverage for *P aeruginosa*.

Doi Y, Chambers HF. Penicillins and β-lactamase inhibitors. In: Bennett JE, Dolin R, Blaser MJ, editors. Mandell, Douglas, and Bennett's principles and practice of infectious diseases. 8th ed. Vol. 1. Philadelphia (PA): Elsevier/Saunders; c2015. p. 263–77.

Petri WA Jr. Penicillins, cephalosporins, and other β-lactam antibiotics. In: Brunton LL, editor. Goodman & Gilman's: the pharmacological basis of therapeutics. 12th ed. New York (NY): McGraw-Hill Medical; c2011. p. 1477–1503.

III.138. Answer c.

Prompt early recognition of a patient who has signs of sepsis is key to improving morbidity and mortality. Rapid identification of patients with infection who are at risk for sepsis can be accomplished with the quick SOFA assessment:

BP ≤100 mm Hg: 1 point
Respiratory rate ≥22 breaths/min: 1 point
Altered mentation: 1 point

A quick SOFA score of 2 or more is associated with higher mortality and need for intensive care. The patient described has risk factors, including age and being African-American and a smoker, and he has several comorbidities that can increase the infection risk. In addition, investigations to find and control a source are crucial; this patient has a colonic abscess that will need intervention. The Surviving Sepsis Campaign recommends prompt administration of antibiotics within 1 hour of recognition because each hour of delay increases mortality.

Seymour CW, Liu VX, Iwashyna TJ, Brunkhorst FM, Rea TD, Scherag A, et al. Assessment of clinical criteria for sepsis: for the Third International Consensus Definitions for Sepsis and Septic Shock (Sepsis-3). JAMA. 2016 Feb 23;315(8):762–74. Erratum in: JAMA. 2016 May 24–31;315(20):2237.

Singer M, Deutschman CS, Seymour CW, Shankar-Hari M, Annane D, Bauer M, et al. The Third International Consensus Definitions for Sepsis and Septic Shock (Sepsis-3). JAMA. 2016 Feb 23;315(8):801–10.

III.139. Answer d.

The INR (derived measure of PT) is not part of the SOFA score. Coagulation is represented by the platelet count, and liver function is represented by the bilirubin level. Measures of oxygenation (the Pao_2/Fio_2 ratio), cardiovascular function (mean arterial pressure), GCS score, and renal function are also included.

Quick sepsis related organ failure assessment (qSOFA) [Internet]. [cited 2017 Nov 22]. Available from: http://www.qsofa.org/.

III.140. Answer b.

Institution of protocols for sepsis management beginning at recognition of a patient at risk is essential to improving morbidity and mortality. Airway management, circulation optimization with resuscitation fluids and potentially vasoactive medications, obtaining blood culture specimens, administering broad-spectrum antibiotics, and establishing a source are all essential and are normally performed with a team approach. Morbidity and mortality will most improve with source control. If this is delayed, shock will worsen despite all the appropriate therapies. If a source is unknown and clinical deterioration is progressive, consider immediate CT.

ProCESS Investigators, Yealy DM, Kellum JA, Huang DT, Barnato AE, Weissfeld LA, Pike F, et al. A randomized trial of protocol-based care for early septic shock. N Engl J Med. 2014 May 1;370(18):1683–93. Epub 2014 Mar 18.

Rhodes A, Evans LE, Alhazzani W, Levy MM, Antonelli M, Ferrer R, et al. Surviving Sepsis Campaign: International Guidelines for Management of Sepsis and Septic Shock: 2016. Intensive Care Med. 2017 Mar;43(3):304–377. Epub 2017 Jan 18.

III.141. Answer d.

Clinical trials have shown that the administration of benzodiazepines accelerates the onset or intensity of sepsis-associated encephalopathy and delirium overall in the ICU and increases mortality. Benzodiazepines are usually reserved for patients who cannot tolerate the hemodynamic effects of dexmedetomidine, propofol, or, rarely, ketamine, have a worsening acidosis and lipid panel results concerning for propofol infusion syndrome, or require a more profound level of sedation for ventilator-synchrony in ARDS management.

Barr J, Fraser GL, Puntillo K, Ely EW, Gelinas C, Dasta JF, et al; American College of Critical Care Medicine. Clinical practice guidelines for the management of pain, agitation, and delirium in adult patients in the intensive care unit. Crit Care Med. 2013 Jan;41(1):263–306.

Pandharipande PP, Pun BT, Herr DL, Maze M, Girard TD, Miller RR, et al. Effect of sedation with dexmedetomidine vs lorazepam on acute brain dysfunction in mechanically ventilated patients: the MENDS randomized controlled trial. JAMA. 2007 Dec 12;298(22):2644–53.

Zampieri FG, Park M, Machado FS, Azevedo LC. Sepsis-associated encephalopathy: not just delirium. Clinics (Sao Paulo). 2011;66(10):1825–31.

Dermatologic Concerns

III.142. Answer a.

The most common causes of drug hypersensitivity syndrome include antiepileptic drugs and sulfonamides.

Tas S, Simonart T. Drug rash with eosinophilia and systemic symptoms (DRESS syndrome). Acta Clin Belg. 1999 Aug;54(4):197–200.

Tas S, Simonart T. Management of drug rash with eosinophilia and systemic symptoms (DRESS syndrome): an update. Dermatology. 2003;206(4):353–6.

III.143. Answer d.

The severity-of-illness score for toxic epidermal necrolysis is based on criteria for age, HR, malignancy, extent of epidermal detachment, SUN, serum glucose, and serum HCO_3^-. Serum aspartate aminotransferase is not a prognostic factor.

Bastuji-Garin S, Fouchard N, Bertocchi M, Roujeau JC, Revuz J, Wolkenstein P. SCORTEN: a severity-of-illness score for toxic epidermal necrolysis. J Invest Dermatol. 2000 Aug;115(2):149–53.

Harr T, French LE. Toxic epidermal necrolysis and Stevens-Johnson syndrome. Orphanet J Rare Dis. 2010 Dec 16;5:39.

Trauma and Burns

III.144. Answer d.

This patient has a multisystem injury with evidence of severe traumatic brain injury and shock, likely due to intra-abdominal hemorrhage. He has multiple problems that are immediately life threatening and must be addressed in a short amount of time: a threatened airway, inadequate respirations, active bleeding, decreased mental status, and open fractures. Advanced Trauma Life Support guidelines help direct the team as to the order of interventions that should be performed when multiple team members are not available to perform simultaneous interventions. In this patient, the most pressing need is for definitive airway control with an endotracheal tube because loss of airway and hypoxemia would result in the most rapid death of this patient.

In an ideal situation, however, multiple team members would be available to care for this patient, and intubation could be accomplished simultaneously with chest tube placement (if needed), blood product infusion, direct pressure or tourniquet application to control extremity bleeding, and mobilization to the operating room for intra-abdominal hemorrhage control.

American College of Surgeons, Committee on Trauma. Advanced trauma life support: student course manual. 9th ed. Chicago (IL): American College of Surgeons; c2012. 366 p.

Codner PA, Brasel KJ. Initial assessment and management. In: Mattox KL, Moore EE, Feliciano DV, editors. Trauma. 7th ed. New York (NY): McGraw-Hill Medical; c2013. p. 154–66.

III.145. Answer a.

The primary survey is a quick assessment of the most immediate threats to a patient's life: ABCDE. Adjuncts to the primary survey are measures taken to aid in diagnosis and to prevent further complications, such as urinary and gastric catheter placement, FAST, chest radiography, and ECG. Nasogastric tube placement is considered an adjunct to the primary survey because gastric decompression could help decrease the risk of aspiration and could help identify upper gastrointestinal tract hemorrhage from a traumatic cause. Nasogastric tube placement is not required for all patients, but it is recommended for any patient with decreased level of consciousness, endotracheal intubation, or active vomiting. Airway examination is part of the primary survey; AMPLE history is part of the secondary survey; and a tetanus booster is not considered an adjunct to the primary or secondary survey, but it should be considered for patients with open wounds who are not current on immunizations or whose immunization status is unknown.

American College of Surgeons, Committee on Trauma. Advanced trauma life support: student course manual. 9th ed. Chicago (IL): American College of Surgeons; c2012. 366 p.

Codner PA, Brasel KJ. Initial assessment and management. In: Mattox KL, Moore EE, Feliciano DV, editors. Trauma. 7th ed. New York (NY): McGraw-Hill Medical; c2013. p. 154–66.

III.146. Answer a.

This patient has multisystem trauma with delayed physiologic decompensation. Any of his injuries could be driving the sudden change in status, and any of the options outlined above may be an appropriate treatment plan. The ABCDE approach to trauma patient evaluation and management is a useful way to identify and treat the new developments regardless of the location of the patient or the time from the initial presentation.

American College of Surgeons, Committee on Trauma. Initial assessment and management. In: Advanced trauma life support: student course manual. 9th ed. Chicago (IL): American College of Surgeons; c2012. p. 2–28.

Codner PA, Brasel KJ. Initial assessment and management. In: Mattox KL, Moore EE, Feliciano DV, editors. Trauma. 7th ed. New York (NY): McGraw-Hill Medical; c2013. p. 154–66.

III.147. Answer c.

In this critically injured patient, ECG would be the best indicator of cardiac complications of blunt chest injury. Assessment of potential blunt cardiac injury should include both ECG and troponin levels. With ectopic beats on cardiac telemetry during the initial evaluation, ECG would be the top priority. Physicians should have a low threshold for ordering formal echocardiography if a patient has abnormal hemodynamics, and the patient should be monitored with telemetry. If a patient has hemodynamic instability, use of inotropes is indicated. Extracorporeal support is reserved for the most severe cases.

Mattox KL, Moore EE, Feliciano DV, editors. Trauma. 7th ed. New York (NY): McGraw-Hill Medical; c2013. 1224 p.

Tieu B, Schipper P, Sukumar M, Mayberry JC. Pertinent surgical anatomy of the thorax and mediastinum. In: Asensio JA, Trunkey DD, editors. Current therapy of trauma and surgical critical care. 2nd ed. Philadelphia (PA): Elsevier; c2016. p. 205–28.

III.148. Answer d.

Nonoperative management of splenic injury has failed. Clinicians should have a high degree of awareness for delayed splenic bleeding in conservatively managed patients. In this hemodynamically unstable patient with known splenic injury, emergent splenectomy is indicated. A follow-up FAST is a useful and expeditious bedside method to confirm the diagnosis, whether at the bedside in the ICU or in the ED.

Mattox KL, Moore EE, Feliciano DV, editors. Trauma. 7th ed. New York (NY): McGraw-Hill Medical; c2013. 1224 p.

Tieu B, Schipper P, Sukumar M, Mayberry JC. Pertinent surgical anatomy of the thorax and mediastinum. In: Asensio JA, Trunkey DD, editors. Current therapy of trauma and surgical critical care. 2nd ed. Philadelphia (PA): Elsevier; c2016. p. 205–28.

III.149. Answer c.

This patient is not yet fully resuscitated as evidenced by the serum lactate of 4.8 mmol/L, so the most appropriate next step is damage control orthopedics with irrigation and débridement of the open fractures, external fixation of the lower extremity long-bone fractures, and splinting of the upper extremity fracture. Although intramedullary nailing of the lower extremity long-bone fractures (choices *a* and *b*) will be the ultimate treatment, it is not appropriate when a patient is in unstable condition and needs further resuscitation. Splinting alone of lower extremity long-bone fractures (choice *d*) does not provide adequate stabilization compared with external fixation.

Pape HC, Tornetta P 3rd, Tarkin I, Tzioupis C, Sabeson V, Olson SA. Timing of fracture fixation in multitrauma patients: the role of early total care and damage control surgery. J Am Acad Orthop Surg. 2009 Sep;17(9):541–9.

Turen CH, Dube MA, LeCroy MC. Approach to the polytraumatized patient with musculoskeletal injuries. J Am Acad Orthop Surg. 1999 May-Jun;7(3):154–65.

III.150. Answer c.

Although all the choices are signs and symptoms of compartment syndrome, the most important symptom of impending compartment syndrome is pain out of proportion for the injury. For most patients, pain decreases after a fracture is reduced and immobilized. Patients who require increasing doses of pain medications for uncontrolled pain should be examined closely for possible compartment syndrome. Paresthesia (choice *a*), pulselessness (choice *b*), and paralysis (choice *d*) are all indicators of compartment syndrome, but they are often late findings and are less sensitive indicators than pain.

Whitesides TE, Heckman MM. Acute compartment syndrome: update on diagnosis and treatment. J Am Acad Orthop Surg. 1996 Jul;4(4):209–18.

Willis RB, Rorabeck CH. Treatment of compartment syndrome in children. Orthop Clin North Am. 1990 Apr;21(2):401–12.

III.151. Answer c.

ABC assessment is always the first step in burn management. Inhalational injury can occur with most burn patients, and this patient, who was rescued from a house fire with facial burns, is at risk for airway compromise. Airway inflammation can progress rapidly, leading to difficulty in endotracheal intubation and the need for a surgical airway. Evaluation for other injuries, assessment of the extent of the burn, and initiation of appropriate fluid resuscitation are important early steps. Local cooling should be instituted early to prevent expansion of burn injury, and analgesia should be addressed, but ABC assessment has primacy.

Allison K, Porter K. Consensus on the prehospital approach to burns patient management. Emerg Med J. 2004 Jan;21(1):112–4.

III.152. Answer a.

The main criticism of the Parkland formula is the risk of overadministration of fluid. The consequences can include abdominal compartment syndrome. For this reason, other protocols use lower initial fluid rates. Regardless of the approach, the response to resuscitation should be monitored and therapy adjusted appropriately. The formula makes no assumptions about circulating volume. Although colloids are included in some protocols, the role of colloids in burn resuscitation is controversial.

Alvarado R, Chung KK, Cancio LC, Wolf SE. Burn resuscitation. Burns. 2009 Feb;35(1):4–14. Epub 2008 Jun 9.

Tricklebank S. Modern trends in fluid therapy for burns. Burns. 2009 Sep;35(6):757–67. Epub 2009 May 30.

Cardiothoracic Critical Care

III.153. Answer c.

Acute MI is the most common cause of cardiogenic shock even after CABG surgery. All the choices may give clues and confirmation of ongoing cardiac ischemia, but echocardiography (either transesophageal or transthoracic) is the most specific and sensitive test to help diagnose cardiac ischemia.

Mark JB. Multimodal detection of perioperative myocardial ischemia. Tex Heart Inst J. 2005;32(4):461–6.

III.154. Answer b.

All the choices would be correct management strategies for this cardiothoracic surgical patient except maintaining the systolic BP greater than 110 mm Hg. Systolic BP should be no higher than 100 to 110 mm Hg, and higher pressures may contribute to more bleeding. All postoperative care should include correction of hypothermia and acidosis, especially for bleeding cardiac surgical patients. Standard care in blood component therapy includes maintaining a higher fibrinogen level (>150 mg/dL) and hemoglobin level (>8 g/dL).

Perkins JG, Cap AP, Weiss BM, Reid TJ, Bolan CD. Massive transfusion and nonsurgical hemostatic agents. Crit Care Med. 2008 Jul;36(7 Suppl):S325–39. Erratum in: Crit Care Med. 2008 Sep;36(9):2718.

Sivarajan M, Amory DW, Everett GB, Buffington C. Blood pressure, not cardiac output, determines blood loss during induced hypotension. Anesth Analg. 1980 Mar;59(3):203–6.

III.155. Answer a.

The mean transvalvular gradient, the pressure difference across the aortic valve, is considered one of the most important echocardiographic parameters for deciding whether to replace the aortic valve. The systolic pulmonary artery pressure (choice *b*), ejection fraction (choice *c*), and left ventricular end-diastolic pressure (choice *d*) are not used in making a decision about replacing the aortic valve.

Nishimura RA, Otto CM, Bonow RO, Carabello BA, Erwin JP 3rd, Guyton RA, et al; American College of Cardiology/American Heart Association Task Force on Practice Guidelines. 2014 AHA/ACC guideline for the management of patients with valvular heart disease: executive summary: a report of the American College of Cardiology/American Heart Association Task Force on Practice Guidelines. J Am Coll Cardiol. 2014 Jun 10;63(22):2438–88. Epub 2014 Mar 3. Erratum in: J Am Coll Cardiol. 2014 Jun 10;63(22):2489.

III.156. Answer a.

Low pH and low $Paco_2$ are associated with metabolic acidosis with respiratory compensation (choice *b*). High pH and high $Paco_2$ are associated with metabolic alkalosis with respiratory compensation (choice *c*). Low pH and high $Paco_2$ are associated with respiratory acidosis (choice *d*). This patient most likely has PE due to DVT. Characteristically, PE causes hypoxia and respiratory alkalosis. Older age, immobilization, and recent open heart surgery are all risk factors for DVT in this patient. Symptoms include pleuritic chest pain, sudden-onset dyspnea, cough, anxiety, low-grade fever, and hemoptysis. Tachypnea, hypoxia, and tachycardia may be present on physical examination, and another sign of DVT is a swollen, erythematous, and warm lower extremity. Classically, PE increases the dead space, resulting in ventilation-perfusion mismatch, and blood is redistributed in the lungs, limiting the ventilation-perfusion match and gas exchange. Consequently, pulmonary vascular resistance increases, elevating pulmonary arterial pressure.

Tapson VF. Acute pulmonary embolism. N Engl J Med. 2008 Mar 6;358(10):1037–52.

III.157. Answer c.

This patient has clear signs of pericardial tamponade. Common risk factors for cardiac tamponade after cardiothoracic surgery include reoperative sternotomy, repair of a previously repaired valve, kidney failure, diabetes mellitus, prolonged bypass time, hypothermia, and long-term use of corticosteroids. The diagnosis is clinical but can be aided with echocardiography. The clinical diagnosis includes sinus tachycardia, elevated jugular venous pressure, pulsus paradoxus, and pericardial rub. The patient in the question has signs of hypotension, equalization of cardiac chamber pressures, and low chest tube output, which are all signs that may suggest cardiac tamponade. An echocardiographic diagnosis of acute pericardial tamponade is based on the presence of a pericardial effusion, a plethoric IVC, end-diastolic collapse or compression of the right atrium, and early diastolic collapse of the right ventricular free wall. Management strategies include keeping the heart "fast, full, and tight" by giving fluids to maintain preload, avoiding bradycardia, avoiding vasodilators, and attempting to maintain sympathetic tone. Treatment is pericardiocentesis either by needle or through the open chest with evacuation.

Chandraratna PA, Mohar DS, Sidarous PF. Role of echocardiography in the treatment of cardiac tamponade. Echocardiography. 2014 Aug;31(7):899–910. Epub 2014 Apr 4.

III.158. Answer d.

Sepsis, adrenal insufficiency, and anaphylaxis cause a high flow rate. Saddle PE causes obstructive shock, resulting in low flow to the LVAD.

Sen A, Larson JS, Kashani KB, Libricz SL, Patel BM, Guru PK, et al. Mechanical circulatory assist devices: a primer for critical care and emergency physicians. Crit Care. 2016 Jun 25;20(1):153.

Slaughter MS, Pagani FD, Rogers JG, Miller LW, Sun B, Russell SD, et al; HeartMate II Clinical Investigators. Clinical management of continuous-flow left ventricular assist devices in advanced heart failure. J Heart Lung Transplant. 2010 Apr;29(4 Suppl):S1–39. Epub 2010 Feb 24.

III.159. Answer c.

If a patient has been taking warfarin, therapy should include 4F-PCC. Tranexamic acid is beneficial only if the bleeding occurred after administration of tissue plasminogen activator; idarucizumab is used for dabigatran reversal. Dabigatran and the other non–vitamin K antagonist oral anticoagulants are not approved for use in patients with devices. Platelets are a possibility if patients are receiving aspirin, but the efficacy of platelets is questionable, and their use should be considered only if a neurosurgical procedure is a possibility.

Backes D, van den Bergh WM, van Duijn AL, Lahpor JR, van Dijk D, Slooter AJ. Cerebrovascular complications of left ventricular assist devices. Eur J Cardiothorac Surg. 2012 Oct;42(4):612–20. Epub 2012 Jun 1.

Kato TS, Schulze PC, Yang J, Chan E, Shahzad K, Takayama H, et al. Pre-operative and post-operative risk factors associated with neurologic complications in patients with advanced heart failure supported by a left ventricular assist device. J Heart Lung Transplant. 2012 Jan;31(1):1–8. Epub 2011 Oct 8.

III.160. Answer d.

In a patient with severe ARDS, pulmonary vascular resistance often increases and results in PH that may convert a left-to-right shunt into a right-to-left shunt. During VV ECMO, normal intracardiac blood flows are maintained; with anticoagulation, spontaneous intracardiac thrombus formation is highly unlikely. During VV ECMO, the aorta is not cannulated.

Sidebotham D, McGeorge A, McGuinness S, Edwards M, Willcox T, Beca J. Extracorporeal membrane oxygenation for treating severe cardiac and respiratory failure in adults: part 2-technical considerations. J Cardiothorac Vasc Anesth. 2010 Feb;24(1):164–72. Epub 2009 Oct 28.

III.161. Answer b.

NSE levels have been validated in ECMO for prognostication of poor neurologic outcomes. The cutoff of greater than 100 mcg/L is higher than was found for cardiac arrest patients without ECMO (>33 mcg/L). NSE appears to have excellent specificity but only modest sensitivity (and positive predictive value) for poor neurologic outcomes during ECMO.

Floerchinger B, Philipp A, Foltan M, Keyser A, Camboni D, Lubnow M, et al. Neuron-specific enolase serum levels predict severe neuronal injury after extracorporeal life support in resuscitation. Eur J Cardiothorac Surg. 2014 Mar;45(3):496–501. Epub 2013 Jul 21.

Ramont L, Thoannes H, Volondat A, Chastang F, Millet MC, Maquart FX. Effects of hemolysis and storage condition on neuron-specific enolase (NSE) in cerebrospinal fluid and serum: implications in clinical practice. Clin Chem Lab Med. 2005;43(11):1215–7.

Reisinger J, Hollinger K, Lang W, Steiner C, Winter T, Zeindlhofer E, et al. Prediction of neurological outcome after cardiopulmonary resuscitation by serial determination of serum neuron-specific enolase. Eur Heart J. 2007 Jan;28(1):52–8. Epub 2006 Oct 23.

III.162. Answer a.

If a patient's lungs are dysfunctional during VA ECMO, any blood pumped through the lungs and out the left ventricle into the proximal aorta may be hypoxemic. This patient had severe pulmonary edema, and her right hand pulse oximetry readings were consistent with proximal aortic arch hypoxemia. The hypoxic blood was likely also perfusing the carotid and vertebral branches of the aorta, thus leading to anoxic injury. The more distal aorta, including the left subclavian artery, was likely perfused with well-oxygenated blood pumped from the ECMO cannula in the femoral artery (ABG analysis from the left arm showed normal $Paco_2$ and good oxygenation).

Hoeper MM, Tudorache I, Kuhn C, Marsch G, Hartung D, Wiesner O, et al. Extracorporeal membrane oxygenation watershed. Circulation. 2014 Sep 2;130(10):864–5.

III.163. Answer b.

Normal cerebral autoregulation is vulnerable to some of the events preceding ECMO and the physiologic disturbances caused by ECMO. Cerebral autoregulation is impaired for several hours after respiratory or cardiac arrest, even after restoration of normal pulsatile blood flow and normalization of ABGs. Furthermore, nonpulsatile flow, such as during VA ECMO, interferes with normal cerebral autoregulation.

Cornwell WK 3rd, Tarumi T, Aengevaeren VL, Ayers C, Divanji P, Fu Q, et al. Effect of pulsatile and nonpulsatile flow on cerebral perfusion in patients with left ventricular assist devices. J Heart Lung Transplant. 2014 Dec;33(12):1295–303. Epub 2014 Aug 28.

Ono M, Joshi B, Brady K, Easley RB, Kibler K, Conte J, et al. Cerebral blood flow autoregulation is preserved after continuous-flow left ventricular assist device implantation. J Cardiothorac Vasc Anesth. 2012 Dec;26(6):1022–8.

Tweed A, Cote J, Lou H, Gregory G, Wade J. Impairment of cerebral blood flow autoregulation in the newborn lamb by hypoxia. Pediatr Res. 1986 Jun;20(6):516–9.

III.164. Answer a.

The examination findings are consistent with compartment syndrome in the lower extremity (pallor, pulselessness, and paresthesia). From his history, the patient was likely sedated during the early stages of compartment syndrome. Peripheral VA ECMO with femoral arterial cannulation carries a higher risk of distal limb ischemia, particularly if an antegrade reperfusion catheter is not inserted in the superficial femoral artery distal to the ECMO cannula. The cannula or an associated hematoma could compress the femoral nerve near the cannulation site, but in this situation motor strength and sensation from the sciatic nerve distribution would be intact.

Cheng R, Hachamovitch R, Kittleson M, Patel J, Arabia F, Moriguchi J, et al. Complications of extracorporeal membrane oxygenation for treatment of cardiogenic shock and cardiac arrest: a meta-analysis of 1,866 adult patients. Ann Thorac Surg. 2014 Feb;97(2):610–6. Epub 2013 Nov 8.

Hund E. Neurological complications of sepsis: critical illness polyneuropathy and myopathy. J Neurol. 2001 Nov;248(11):929–34.

Kutlesa M, Santini M, Krajinovic V, Raffanelli D, Barsic B. Acute motor axonal neuropathy associated with pandemic H1N1 influenza A infection. Neurocrit Care. 2010 Aug;13(1):98–100.

Rastan AJ, Dege A, Mohr M, Doll N, Falk V, Walther T, et al. Early and late outcomes of 517 consecutive adult patients treated with extracorporeal membrane oxygenation for refractory postcardiotomy cardiogenic shock. J Thorac Cardiovasc Surg. 2010 Feb;139(2):302–11.

III.165. Answer d.

The patient has pericardial symptoms and pulsus paradoxus on examination, indicating cardiac tamponade, which is most likely due to perforation caused by a pacing lead. This will be immediately confirmed and treated with urgent echocardiography and then pericardiocentesis. The pleuritic nature of the chest pain indicates that it is not caused by ischemia, so coronary angiography is not indicated. The ECG shows that the pacing leads are capturing, so no changes in pacing output are needed. Repositioning the pacing lead may be required, but the most urgent intervention is echocardiography and pericardiocentesis.

Labovitz AJ, Noble VE, Bierig M, Goldstein SA, Jones R, Kort S, et al. Focused cardiac ultrasound in the emergent setting: a consensus statement of the American Society of Echocardiography and American College of Emergency Physicians. J Am Soc Echocardiogr. 2010 Dec;23(12):1225–30.

Schwerg M, Stockburger M, Schulze C, Bondke H, Poller WC, Lembcke A, et al. Clinical, anatomical, and technical risk factors for postoperative pacemaker or defibrillator lead perforation with particular focus on myocardial thickness. Pacing Clin Electrophysiol. 2014 Oct;37(10):1291–6. Epub 2014 May 30.

III.166. Answer d.

Pause-dependent polymorphic ventricular tachycardia with a prolonged QT interval (torsades de pointes), which is shown on the ECG strip, is best treated with temporary pacing while awaiting the effects of QT-prolonging medications to subside. Renal transplant patients are at particular risk for QT prolongation, often requiring multiple QT-prolonging medications. Certain antibiotics, antifungals, tacrolimus, and other medications in addition to electrolyte fluctuations increase the risk of QT prolongation. While amiodarone is the treatment of choice for cardiac arrest in patients with ventricular fibrillation resistant to defibrillation, antiarrhythmic medications have an unclear role in the treatment of drug-induced polymorphic ventricular tachycardia, and the use of QT-prolonging antiarrhythmics such as sotalol should be avoided. QT prolongation is associated with hypokalemia, not hyperkalemia, so giving insulin and glucose to cause an intracellular shift of potassium would not be indicated. IV magnesium and isoproterenol are effective, but temporary transvenous pacing is the most effective treatment. ICDs should not be implanted for reversible causes of ventricular arrhythmias.

Drew BJ, Ackerman MJ, Funk M, Gibler WB, Kligfield P, Menon V, et al; American Heart Association Acute Cardiac Care Committee of the Council on Clinical Cardiology, the Council on Cardiovascular Nursing, and the American College of Cardiology Foundation. Prevention of torsade de pointes in hospital settings: a scientific statement from the American Heart Association and the American College of Cardiology Foundation. Circulation. 2010 Mar 2;121(8):1047–60. Epub 2010 Feb 8. Erratum in: Circulation. 2010 Aug 24;122(8):e440.

Kay GN, Plumb VJ, Arciniegas JG, Henthorn RW, Waldo AL. Torsade de pointes: the long-short initiating sequence and other clinical features: observations in 32 patients. J Am Coll Cardiol. 1983 Nov;2(5):806–17.

III.167. Answer a.

This patient has recurrent bacteremia despite appropriate antibiotic therapy. Therefore, changing antibiotics is not indicated.

The only way that the source of infection will be cleared is to remove all potentially infected hardware, even if no vegetations are noted on transesophageal echocardiography. Lead vegetation is seen on transesophageal echocardiography in 62% of patients with systemic infections. Follow-up transesophageal echocardiography is not indicated. Removal of the pulse generator only would not clear the infection. The patient has underlying complete heart block, so he will require a temporary pacemaker while waiting for the infection to clear.

Golzio PG, Fanelli AL, Vinci M, Pelissero E, Morello M, Grosso Marra W, et al. Lead vegetations in patients with local and systemic cardiac device infections: prevalence, risk factors, and therapeutic effects. Europace. 2013 Jan;15(1):89–100. Epub 2012 Sep 11.

Wilkoff BL, Love CJ, Byrd CL, Bongiorni MG, Carrillo RG, Crossley GH 3rd, et al; Heart Rhythm Society; American Heart Association. Transvenous lead extraction: Heart Rhythm Society expert consensus on facilities, training, indications, and patient management: this document was endorsed by the American Heart Association (AHA). Heart Rhythm. 2009 Jul;6(7):1085–104. Epub 2009 May 22.

III.168. Answer d.

At this point in the patient's evaluation, it is unclear whether he received appropriate or inappropriate shocks. However, the shocks have been frequent. The immediate step should be to place a magnet over the device and then interrogate the device. The electrograms during the shock episodes will indicate whether the shock was appropriate (leading to antiarrhythmic therapy) or inappropriate (leading to chest radiography to evaluate the integrity of the defibrillator lead). From the clinical history, he has remained conscious during all the episodes; therefore, he will likely be hemodynamically stable during further investigation. The most important intervention is to prevent him from receiving another inappropriate shock, and this is immediately prevented with application of a magnet. Even a normally functioning device must be interrogated after magnet application because of a small risk that the tachycardia therapies would remain suspended after magnet removal.

Jacob S, Panaich SS, Maheshwari R, Haddad JW, Padanilam BJ, John SK. Clinical applications of magnets on cardiac rhythm management devices. Europace. 2011 Sep;13(9):1222–30. Epub 2011 May 26.

Porres JM, Lavineta E, Reviejo C, Brugada J. Application of a clinical magnet over implantable cardioverter defibrillators: is it safe and useful? Pacing Clin Electrophysiol. 2008 Dec;31(12):1641–4.

III.169. Answer c.

Because the patient is pacemaker dependent, by definition his ventricular escape will be less than 30 bpm if he has a ventricular escape rhythm after pacing is turned off. Therefore, his hemodynamic status will change considerably if his pacing is turned off; he may even become asystolic. Defibrillation functions can be inactivated with no clinically significant change in his clinical status. A magnet will inhibit only defibrillation functions and have no effect on pacing. Because withdrawing a device intervention is ethically identical to not initiating it, inactivating the pacemaker is not ethically the same as physician-assisted suicide, where an intervention is given to hasten death.

Lampert R, Hayes DL, Annas GJ, Farley MA, Goldstein NE, Hamilton RM, et al; American College of Cardiology; American Geriatrics Society; American Academy of Hospice and Palliative Medicine; American Heart Association; European Heart Rhythm Association; Hospice and Palliative Nurses Association. HRS Expert Consensus Statement on the Management of Cardiovascular Implantable Electronic Devices (CIEDs) in patients nearing end of life or requesting withdrawal of therapy. Heart Rhythm. 2010 Jul;7(7):1008–26. Epub 2010 May 14.

Mueller PS, Hook CC, Hayes DL. Ethical analysis of withdrawal of pacemaker or implantable cardioverter-defibrillator support at the end of life. Mayo Clin Proc. 2003 Aug;78(8):959–63.

Transplant Critical Care

III.170. Answer d.

Preexisting PH in the recipient is an important risk factor for graft failure after heart transplant. The patient must be thoroughly evaluated before transplant, and PH must be included in the risk stratification. If the transpulmonary gradient is greater than 15 mm Hg, is relatively fixed, and is not responsive to vasodilators, patients may benefit from a LVAD as a bridge to heart transplant; over time the device should alleviate PH. Immediately after transplant, a high CVP with low mixed venous oxygen saturation and decreased carbon monoxide suggests right-sided heart failure and should be aggressively treated with inotropes, pulmonary vasodilators, and diuretics. In severe cases, VA ECMO is needed as a rescue therapy.

Stobierska-Dzierzek B, Awad H, Michler RE. The evolving management of acute right-sided heart failure in cardiac transplant recipients. J Am Coll Cardiol. 2001 Oct;38(4):923–31.

III.171. Answer b.

The intrinsic HR after heart transplant is around 100 bpm. This is related to cardiac denervation, and patients do benefit hemodynamically from a slightly higher HR postoperatively. A slower HR can be treated with either isoproterenol or cardiac pacing. Epinephrine, dobutamine, and other β_2-agonists sometimes also help to maintain an HR around 100 bpm. Atropine is not effective in heart transplant recipients because of the cardiac denervation, and atropine has been shown to cause fatal arrhythmia in these patients, so it should not be used.

Brunner-La Rocca HP, Kiowski W, Bracht C, Weilenmann D, Follath F. Atrioventricular block after administration of atropine in patients following cardiac transplantation. Transplantation. 1997 Jun 27;63(12):1838–9.

Liem LB, DiBiase A, Schroeder JS. Arrhythmias and clinical electrophysiology of the transplanted human heart. Semin Thorac Cardiovasc Surg. 1990 Jul;2(3):271–8.

III.172. Answer c.

Reperfusion injury occurs in the first 72 hours after lung transplant. Severe noncardiogenic pulmonary edema is characteristic, as in ARDS. Meticulous supportive care should include lung-protective ventilation with volume restriction. Rarely, a patient may have severe acute rejection (usually after 2-3 weeks), cytomegalovirus pneumonia (around 2-3 months), or pulmonary contusions (focal and typically resolving without much impairment in gas exchange rather than worsening).

Christie JD, Carby M, Bag R, Corris P, Hertz M, Weill D; ISHLT Working Group on Primary Lung Graft Dysfunction. Report of the ISHLT Working Group on Primary Lung Graft Dysfunction part II: definition: a consensus statement of the International Society for Heart and Lung Transplantation. J Heart Lung Transplant. 2005 Oct;24(10):1454–9. Epub 2005 Jun 4.

III.173. Answer b.
AKI can result from an elevated tacrolimus level (which causes afferent arteriolar constriction) particularly in the immediate recovery phase, when fluid restriction is often implemented. The sudden increase in the tacrolimus level is from a drug-to-drug interaction, where diltiazem suppresses the hepatic cytochrome P450 3A4 isozyme and leads to delayed tacrolimus metabolism and clearance. In addition to monitoring daily drug levels, the clinical team must be cognizant of pharmacokinetic interactions between tacrolimus and other medications and make necessary dose adjustments to minimize adverse effects and complications.

Knoop C, Haverich A, Fischer S. Immunosuppressive therapy after human lung transplantation. Eur Respir J. 2004 Jan;23(1):159–71.

III.174. Answer c.
A persistently high lactate level may indicate poor initial graft function. Lactate is converted to pyruvate in the liver, so if the lactate level does not decrease, it may indicate that the liver is not functioning well enough to clear the lactate.

Randall HB, Klintmalm GB. Postoperative intensive care unit management: adult liver transplant recipients. In: Busuttil RW, Klintmalm GB, editors. Transplantation of the liver. 2nd ed. Philadelphia (PA): Elsevier/Saunders; c2005. p. 833–51.

III.175. Answer a.
Patients with acute liver failure, hepatopulmonary syndrome, or portopulmonary hypertension may require care in the ICU longer than other transplant patients.

Keegan MT, Kramer DJ. Perioperative care of the liver transplant patient. Crit Care Clin. 2016 Jul;32(3):453–73.

III.176. Answer b.
Any recipient of a transplanted kidney has a high risk of graft loss due to arterial or venous thrombosis, which is usually diagnosed with Doppler ultrasonographic evaluation of flows in the transplanted kidney. Both arterial and venous flows can be assessed. For this patient, the concern is for renal vein thrombosis. CT and MRI are unnecessary unless the Doppler evaluation is nondiagnostic. Urinalysis results would have limited value.

Kawano PR, Yamamoto HA, Gerra R, Garcia PD, Contti MM, Nga HS, et al. A case report of venous thrombosis after kidney transplantation. We can save the graft? Time is the success factor. Int J Surg Case Rep. 2017;36:82–5. Epub 2017 May 19.

Rodgers SK, Sereni CP, Horrow MM. Ultrasonographic evaluation of the renal transplant. Radiol Clin North Am. 2014 Nov;52(6):1307–24. Epub 2014 Sep 4.

III.177. Answer d.
Calcineurin inhibitors, PRES, and sepsis are all associated with neurologic complications in a kidney transplant recipient. Subarachnoid hemorrhage is uncommon unless the patient had a history of polycystic kidney disease and concomitant cerebral aneurysm.

Bechstein WO. Neurotoxicity of calcineurin inhibitors: impact and clinical management. Transpl Int. 2000;13(5):313–26.

Hinchey J, Chaves C, Appignani B, Breen J, Pao L, Wang A, et al. A reversible posterior leukoencephalopathy syndrome. N Engl J Med. 1996 Feb 22;334(8):494–500.

III.178. Answer c.
The most common reason for small bowel transplant is short gut syndrome. Failure of home TPN due to an inability to absorb essential nutrients (because of problems such as recurrent infection and deep vein thrombosis) is another indication for transplant. Transplant can also be offered to patients with recurrent pseudo-obstruction. Metastatic tumors, however, are a contraindication.

Khan FA, Selvaggi G. Overview of intestinal and multivisceral transplantation. In: Robson KM, editor. UpToDate. Waltham (MA): UpToDate; c2016.

Sudan D. The current state of intestine transplantation: indications, techniques, outcomes and challenges. Am J Transplant. 2014 Sep;14(9):1976–84. Epub 2014 Aug 6.

III.179. Answer c.
Most patients with intestinal transplant have a higher incidence of neurologic complications. If patients have short gut syndrome preoperatively, they may be predisposed to vitamin deficiencies and metabolic disturbances, which can persist or recur after transplant and lead to metabolic encephalopathy. Also, because of the lymphoid tissue in the small intestine, higher immunosuppressive doses are needed. This can lead to increased risk of drug toxicity causing neurologic sequelae and to the possibility of infectious neurologic complications. The anesthetic agent is not a specific cause of neurologic complications in these patients.

Jacewicz M, Marino CR. Neurologic complications of pancreas and small bowel transplantation. Handb Clin Neurol. 2014;121:1277–93.

Patchell RA. Neurological complications of organ transplantation. Ann Neurol. 1994 Nov;36(5):688–703.

Toxicity and Toxins

III.180. Answer c.
Choice *a* lists features of anticholinergic toxicity. Choice *b* lists features of hypersympathetic conditions that may occur with ingestion of cocaine, amphetamines, PCP, or a mixture of these drugs and may overlap with serotonin toxicity. Choice *d* lists features of dopamine depletion (neuroleptic malignant syndrome).

Klaassen CD, editor. Casarett and Doull's toxicology: the basic science of poisons. 8th ed. New York (NY): McGraw-Hill Education/Medical; c2013. 1,454 p.

Wang RZ, Vashistha V, Kaur S, Houchens NW. Serotonin syndrome: preventing, recognizing, and treating it. Cleve Clin J Med. 2016 Nov;83(11):810–817.

III.181. Answer c.
Choice *c* is the outlier because only current amphetamine use, sleep aids (eg, mirtazapine or trazodone), antiepileptics (eg, valproate and possibly carbamazepine or lamotrigine), and antineuropathy medications (eg, tapentadol, SNRIs or TCAs) should have direct or indirect serotonergic activity. Levofloxacin is less likely than ciprofloxacin to slow the metabolism of serotonin. In choice *a*, an SSRI with a long half-life may have potentiated serotonergic activity in a patient with diffuse brain injury who may have additional mixed serotonin agonism from opiates (especially fentanyl and meperidine). In choice *b*, the effects of serotonin agonists

(eg, TCAs, triptans, ginseng, St John's wort, and yohimbine) are multiplied by the addition of a drug with monoamine oxidase inhibitor activity (eg, linezolid, tedizolid, or cycloserine). In choice *d*, the patient receives new medications (fluconazole and erythromycin) that indirectly inhibit peripheral serotonin breakdown and promote synaptic serotonin availability for implicated 5-HT receptor subtypes (metoclopramide, ondansetron, and granisetron) in a patient already taking 3 weakly serotonergic medications.

Iqbal MM, Basil MJ, Kaplan J, Iqbal MT. Overview of serotonin syndrome. Ann Clin Psychiatry. 2012 Nov;24(4):310–8.

Pedavally S, Fugate JE, Rabinstein AA. Serotonin syndrome in the intensive care unit: clinical presentations and precipitating medications. Neurocrit Care. 2014 Aug;21(1):108–13.

III.182. Answer c.

Diagnostic criteria for NMS include hyperthermia, muscle rigidity, increased CK level, and altered mental status.

Adnet P, Lestavel P, Krivosic-Horber R. Neuroleptic malignant syndrome. Br J Anaesth. 2000 Jul;85(1):129–35.

American Psychiatric Association. Diagnostic and statistical manual of mental disorders. 5th ed. Arlington (VA): American Psychiatric Association; c2013. 947 p.

III.183. Answer d.

A genetic predisposition from a defect in the sarcolemma predisposes patients to NMS, and family history is the strongest risk factor. The use of anxiolytics or SSRIs is not a risk factor, but the use of multiple neuroleptics is. Hyperthermia and dehydration are other risk factors.

Cox B, Kerwin R, Lee TF. Dopamine receptors in the central thermoregulatory pathways of the rat. J Physiol. 1978 Sep;282:471–83.

Hermesh H, Aizenberg D, Lapidot M, Munitz H. Risk of malignant hyperthermia among patients with neuroleptic malignant syndrome and their families. Am J Psychiatry. 1988 Nov;145(11):1431–4.

III.184. Answer b.

Marijuana is the most commonly used illicit drug (77% of current users of illicit drugs report use of marijuana). Approximately 10% of the US population reports being a current user of illicit drugs (defined as use within the past 30 days). Synthetic cannabinoids, especially newer variants, are associated with psychomotor agitation, seizures, AKI, acute stroke, ACS, and death. US deaths from prescription opioids have quadrupled since 1999; opioid use now exceeds motor vehicle accidents as a cause of unintentional death in the United States.

Azofeifa A, Mattson ME, Schauer G, McAfee T, Grant A, Lyerla R. National estimates of marijuana use and related indicators: National Survey on Drug Use and Health, United States, 2002–2014. MMWR Surveill Summ. 2016 Sep 2;65(11):1–28.

National Institute on Drug Abuse: Advancing Addiction Science [Internet]. National Survey of Drug Use and Health. Rockville (MD): National Institute on Drug Abuse (NIDA). c2016 [cited 2016 Sep 29]. Available from: https://www.drugabuse.gov/national-survey-drug-use-health.

III.185. Answer a.

The patient presents with evidence of a classic opioid toxidrome. The CT scan does not show cerebral edema suggestive of anoxic injury or evidence of other causes for the clinical presentation. Despite receiving a higher dose of naloxone, the patient does not respond appropriately. Effects from heroin would be expected to improve with a low dose of naloxone. A patient who used marijuana would not present with this toxidrome. A patient who used cocaine would present with a sympathomimetic toxidrome, although CNS depression may occur with acute intracranial hemorrhage. Therapy for nonpharmaceutical fentanyls may require a considerably higher dose of naloxone to achieve the desired clinical response.

Boyer EW. Management of opioid analgesic overdose. N Engl J Med. 2012 Jul 12;367(2):146–55.

Lozier MJ, Boyd M, Stanley C, Ogilvie L, King E, Martin C, et al. Acetyl fentanyl, a novel fentanyl analog, causes 14 overdose deaths in Rhode Island, March-May 2013. J Med Toxicol. 2015 Jun;11(2):208–17.

III.186. Answer c.

The patient presented after she had a seizure at an electronic dance festival. Although she does have some elements of a sympathomimetic toxidrome, she has profound hyponatremia and cerebral edema, classic findings for MDMA toxicity. α-PVP toxicity may resemble a sympathomimetic toxidrome, but patients typically present with psychomotor agitation. Nonpharmaceutical fentanyls cause a typical opiate toxidrome, and ketamine, which acts as a dissociative agent, does not typically cause cerebral edema or hyponatremia.

Farah R, Farah R. Ecstasy (3,4-methylenedioxymethamphetamine)-induced inappropriate antidiuretic hormone secretion. Pediatr Emerg Care. 2008 Sep;24(9):615–7.

Moritz ML, Kalantar-Zadeh K, Ayus JC. Ecstacy-associated hyponatremia: why are women at risk? Nephrol Dial Transplant. 2013 Sep;28(9):2206–9. Epub 2013 Jun 26.

III.187. Answer d.

The patient is 1 of many critically ill patients from a deliberate chemical mass exposure with sarin. Lack of decontamination of a patient in extremis has resulted in off-gassing from a volatile agent and secondary contamination of medical staff. Signs and symptoms are consistent with a cholinergic toxidrome. Eye pain is a prominent finding of fixed, extreme miosis and was the most common complaint during the Tokyo sarin attack. Lewisite would cause blistering injuries, and phosgene would cause delayed pulmonary injury. Cyanide might result in a patient presenting in extremis, but it would not result in a cholinergic toxidrome through secondary contamination.

Okumura T, Suzuki K, Fukuda A, Kohama A, Takasu N, Ishimatsu S, et al. The Tokyo subway sarin attack: disaster management, Part 1: Community emergency response. Acad Emerg Med. 1998 Jun;5(6):613–7.

Tomassoni AJ, French RN, Walter FG. Toxic industrial chemicals and chemical weapons: exposure, identification, and management by syndrome. Emerg Med Clin North Am. 2015 Feb;33(1):13–36. Epub 2014 Nov 15.

III.188. Answer b.

The patient has signs and symptoms of pneumonic plague (*Yersinia pestis*), an unusual form of naturally occurring plague but expected to be common with deliberate aerosolized dissemination. Patchy infiltrates and normal mediastinum in a critically ill patient exclude pneumonic anthrax, and the lack of pustules excludes smallpox. Ebola virus disease, a viral hemorrhagic fever, is associated with copious, bloody body fluids.

Adalja AA, Toner E, Inglesby TV. Clinical management of potential bioterrorism-related conditions. N Engl J Med. 2015 Mar 5;372(10):954–62.

Breman JG, Henderson DA. Diagnosis and management of smallpox. N Engl J Med. 2002 Apr 25;346(17):1300–8. Epub 2002 Mar 28.

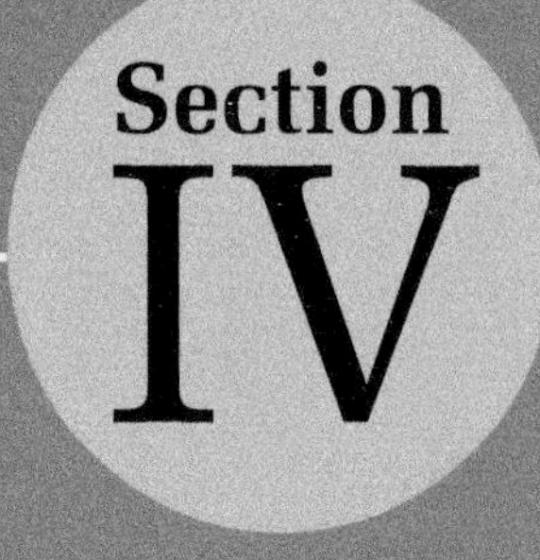

Neurocritical Illness

Acute Cerebrovascular Disorders

78 Diagnosis and Management of Hemispheric Infarction

SANJEET S. GREWAL, MD; BENJAMIN L. BROWN, MD

Goals

- Recognize ischemic infarction of large-artery territories (eg, hemispheric infarction of the middle cerebral artery territory).
- Stategize and implement medical management of hemispheric and large-artery infarctions.
- Understand which patients may benefit from decompressive hemicraniectomy, and know when to seek consultation or to refer such patients to a neurosurgical center where this surgery is performed.

Introduction

Hemispheric infarction is a major cause of morbidity and death among patients with acute stroke. The infarcts involve the entire territory of the middle cerebral artery (MCA) and may involve other territories according to the location of the clot. The rapid swelling and deterioration distinguish this group from many other types of stroke. These patients must receive a timely diagnosis and treatment for the best outcomes. Treatment is often multimodal and requires close and meaningful communication with the patient and family about management options and the risks and benefits of each.

Diagnosis

Definition

The classification of hemispheric infarction is based on a combination of clinical and radiologic localization. Typically, patients with hemispheric infarction have a National Institutes of Health Stroke Scale (NIHSS) score greater than 15 and imaging findings that are consistent with infarction due to occlusion of the internal carotid artery (ICA) or MCA. With the involvement of other vascular territories, such as infarctions of the anterior cerebral artery and MCA territories that occur with a carotid terminus occlusion, the risk of hemispheric infarction and subsequent cerebral edema is even greater. Patients with multiple vascular territory infarctions typically present with clinical features such as hemiplegia, gaze preference, aphasia, and hemibody neglect. An investigative approach that includes both imaging and clinical findings is critical for prompt diagnosis of hemispheric infarctions.

Imaging

The initial imaging for a patient with acute stroke is computed tomography (CT) without contrast medium to exclude structural lesions and to evaluate for hemorrhagic conversion. CT findings predictive for progression to "malignant" hemispheric infarction and cerebral edema with uncal herniation include hyperdensity of the MCA or hypodensity involving at least one-third of the MCA territory. More subtle signs of progressive edema and increased intracranial pressure (ICP) include increased midline shift at the septum pellucidum and effacement of the ipsilateral sulci and lateral ventricles.

Early use of magnetic resonance imaging can also be helpful in predicting which patients will have a more fulminant course. Diffusion-weighted imaging lesion volumes greater than 80 mL have been predictive of a rapid progression of infarction and subsequent malignant edema.

Other potential imaging studies include CT angiography, cerebral perfusion imaging, and transcranial Doppler imaging, but data are limited for their use in hemispheric infarction. However, with the increased use of thrombectomy for large-vessel occlusions, CT angiography has been useful for localizing the thrombus. Perfusion imaging can be used to distinguish the penumbra and potentially salvageable tissue from infarcted tissue.

The initial workup for hemispheric infarction may identify patients who have clinical signs of hemispheric dysfunction but have large-vessel occlusions that have not yet progressed to hemispheric infarction.

Endovascular Management of Large-Vessel Occlusion

With the advancements in endovascular techniques and devices, mechanical thrombectomy has become a viable option for patients who have large-vessel occlusion and acute hemispheric ischemia. Five landmark trials were published in 2015: 1) the Multicenter Randomized Clinical Trial of Endovascular Treatment for Acute Ischemic Stroke in the Netherlands (MR CLEAN); 2) the Endovascular Treatment for Small Core and Anterior Circulation Proximal Occlusion With Emphasis on Minimizing CT to Recanalization Times (ESCAPE) trial; 3) the Extending the Time for Thrombolysis in Emergency Neurological Deficits—Intra-Arterial (EXTEND-IA) trial; 4) the Solitaire FR With the Intention for Thrombectomy as Primary Endovascular Treatment for Acute Ischemic Stroke (SWIFT PRIME) trial; and 5) the Randomized Trial of Revascularization With Solitaire FR Device Versus Best Medical Therapy in the Treatment of Acute Stroke Due to Anterior Circulation Large Vessel Occlusion Presenting Within Eight Hours of Symptom Onset (REVASCAT). All these studies showed that endovascular thrombectomy was more beneficial than intravenous (IV) tissue plasminogen activator therapy alone for treating large-vessel occlusions with hemispheric infarctions. Shortly after these trials were published, the American Stroke Association published new guidelines supporting the role of endovascular therapy. Patients with large-vessel occlusion who do not benefit from IV tissue plasminogen activator therapy or mechanical thrombectomy tend to progress to hemispheric infarction. Its management is discussed below.

Management of Hemispheric Infarction

Effective treatment of hemispheric infarctions requires monitoring several patient variables. Widespread edema shifts tissue and causes a deterioration of consciousness and, eventually, a change in pupillary responses. Patient monitoring often requires serial CT scanning in the first 24 to 48 hours.

Medical

No data support routine ICP monitoring in patients with hemispheric infarcts. These patients typically do not have globally increased ICP until late in the disease process after additional injury to viable brain tissue has already occurred. Clinical deterioration often results from a mass effect and a midline shift and precedes an elevation in ICP, which occurs with either a progressive loss of function, as defined by midposition (pontine) pupils, or a worsening motor response. If the elevation in ICP is more sudden, the patient may have a unilaterally dilated "blown" pupil and a worsening of the motor response.

Medical management of clinical deterioration should proceed with a stepwise approach. Mild hyperventilation should be promoted to cause cerebral vasoconstriction. Mannitol or hypertonic saline can be used to decrease the mass effect; the serum sodium level should be 145 to 155 mmol/L. Serum osmolarity should be maintained at less than 320 mOsm/L to prevent renal toxicity from mannitol. The head of the patient's bed should be elevated more than 30° to promote venous drainage and decrease edema. Corticosteroids have not improved mortality or functional outcomes. Similarly, few data support the use of therapeutic cooling for large infarctions, but its potential has not been studied sufficiently.

Surgical

Four large, prospective randomized controlled trials have assessed decompressive hemicraniectomy in patients with supratentorial hemispheric infarction: 1) the Sequential-Design, Multicenter, Randomized, Controlled Trial of Early Decompressive Craniectomy in Malignant Middle Cerebral Artery Infarction (DECIMAL); 2) the Decompressive Surgery for the Treatment of Malignant Infarction of the Middle Cerebral Artery (DESTINY) trial; 3) the Hemicraniectomy After Middle Cerebral Artery Infarction With Life-Threatening Edema Trial (HAMLET); and 4) a multicenter, open, randomized trial that assessed the use of early (<48 hours) decompressive surgery in patients younger than 60 years. A pooled analysis of the DECIMAL, DESTINY, and HAMLET trials included 93 patients younger than 60 years and showed that more patients in the decompressive surgery group than in the control group, respectively, had a modified Rankin scale (mRS) score of 4 or less (75% vs 24%), had an mRS score of 3 or less (43% vs 21%), and survived (78% vs 29%); the number needed to treat (NNT) for survival with an mRS of 3 or less is 4 patients and the NNT for any survival benefit is 2 patients.

These initial trials were limited to patients younger than 60 years, but many septuagenarians and octogenarians have malignant cerebral infarctions. Until recently, only minimal data were available on the treatment of elderly patients. The DESTINY II trial, published in 2014, assessed decompression in patients 61 to 82 years old. This study showed a survival benefit with surgery (67% vs 30%), but no patients were living independently after hemispheric stroke, regardless of the intervention.

The timing of surgery is controversial, although a marked decrease in neurologic status (eg, a decrease in the Glasgow Coma Scale score of ≥2 points) despite aggressive medical management is reasonable to use as a trigger. Surgical intervention is deemed a lifesaving procedure, and families should be counseled about the goals of surgery, with an explanation that it is lifesaving without markedly altering the overall functional outcome.

Airway

Intubation may be necessary if the level of consciousness decreases. Indications for endotracheal intubation are persistent hypoxemia, upper airway obstruction, apneic episodes, and the development of hypoxemic or hypercarbic respiratory failure; secondary reasons include generalized seizures or aspiration. After intubation, the PaCO_2 should be corrected to normocapnia; no benefit has been shown with prophylactic hyperventilation. The use of short-acting anesthetics (eg, propofol) is appropriate to help the patient be more comfortable with the ventilator and avoid unnecessary agitation and hypertension, with a resultant increase in ICP.

Hemodynamics

The use of hypo-osmolar agents should be avoided. Maintenance fluids should include either isotonic saline or mildly hypertonic saline. No data support the use of prophylactic hypertonic solutions, and no specific sodium goals have been identified. Our goal is normonatremia unless the patient shows signs of increased ICP.

Cardiac arrhythmias are usually self-limited in patients with hemispheric stroke. However, atrial fibrilliation with a rapid ventricular response should be pharmacologically managed with IV agents to obtain rate control.

A patient with an acute infarct may lose blood pressure autoregulation. The ideal blood pressure guidelines for patients with hemispheric infarcts are controversial. Blood pressure tends to increase and perfuse the penumbra, but hypertension with a systolic blood pressure greater than 220 mm Hg or a diastolic pressure greater than 105 mm Hg has been associated with an increased risk of hemorrhagic transformation and should be treated.

Temperature

The use of therapeutic hypothermia in hemispheric infarction is not supported with level 1 evidence. Neurogenic fevers (central fevers) are less likely in patients with ischemic stroke; therefore, an early fever should be evaluated and treated appropriately. Our goal is to maintain euthermia with early treatment of any fever without the use of hypothermia.

Glucose

An optimal range for glucose control has not been identified. Hyperglycemia is an independent risk factor for death and poor functional outcomes after acute ischemic stroke. Multiple theories describe the mechanism of hyperglycemia in acute stroke. Most involve activation of the hypothalamic-pituitary-adrenal axis resulting in increased cortisol production and subsequent glycogenolysis and gluconeogenesis. Hyperglycemia probably leads to poor outcomes because of its role in impairing recanalization (it contributes to a thrombogenic state), decreasing reperfusion (it limits the ability of the vasculature to dilate), and increasing reperfusion injury (it increases oxidative stress and inflammation). However, tight glycemic control has not been shown to be beneficial, and, according to the results of a randomized trial, it can even contribute to enlarging an infarct.

Summary

- Proximal MCA or ICA occlusion can progress rapidly to a hemispheric swelling with uncal herniation. Therefore, a high degree of clinical awareness or use of CT angiography can be helpful in diagnosing the condition.
- Initial medical management of hemispheric and large-artery infarction involves osmotherapy (mannitol or hypertonic saline), elevation of the head of the bed, prevention of aspiration, and intubation with mechanical ventilation if needed.
- In patients younger than 60 years, decompressive hemicraniectomy decreases mortality and morbidity according to results of 4 randomized trials. Therefore, proper selection of patients is critical.

SUGGESTED READING

Bardutzky J, Schwab S. Antiedema therapy in ischemic stroke. Stroke. 2007 Nov;38(11):3084–94. Epub 2007 Sep 27.

Berkhemer OA, Fransen PS, Beumer D, van den Berg LA, Lingsma HF, Yoo AJ, et al; MR CLEAN Investigators. A randomized trial of intraarterial treatment for acute ischemic stroke. N Engl J Med. 2015 Jan 1;372(1):11–20. Epub 2014 Dec 17. Erratum in: N Engl J Med. 2015 Jan 22;372(4):394.

Berrouschot J, Rossler A, Koster J, Schneider D. Mechanical ventilation in patients with hemispheric ischemic stroke. Crit Care Med. 2000 Aug;28(8):2956–61.

Bruno A, Levine SR, Frankel MR, Brott TG, Lin Y, Tilley BC, et al; NINDS rt-PA Stroke Study Group. Admission glucose level and clinical outcomes in the NINDS rt-PA Stroke Trial. Neurology. 2002 Sep 10;59(5):669–74.

Campbell BC, Mitchell PJ, Kleinig TJ, Dewey HM, Churilov L, Yassi N, et al; EXTEND-IA Investigators. Endovascular therapy for ischemic stroke with perfusion-imaging selection. N Engl J Med. 2015 Mar 12;372(11):1009–18. Epub 2015 Feb 11.

de Courten-Myers GM, Kleinholz M, Holm P, DeVoe G, Schmitt G, Wagner KR, et al. Hemorrhagic infarct conversion in experimental stroke. Ann Emerg Med. 1992 Feb;21(2):120–6.

Gilmore RM, Stead LG. The role of hyperglycemia in acute ischemic stroke. Neurocrit Care. 2006;5(2):153–8.

Goyal M, Demchuk AM, Menon BK, Eesa M, Rempel JL, Thornton J, et al; ESCAPE Trial Investigators. Randomized assessment of rapid endovascular treatment of ischemic stroke. N Engl J Med. 2015 Mar 12;372(11):1019–30. Epub 2015 Feb 11.

Greer DM, Funk SE, Reaven NL, Ouzounelli M, Uman GC. Impact of fever on outcome in patients with stroke and neurologic injury: a comprehensive meta-analysis. Stroke. 2008 Nov;39(11):3029–35. Epub 2008 Aug 21.

Hacke W, Schwab S, Horn M, Spranger M, De Georgia M, von Kummer R. 'Malignant' middle cerebral artery territory infarction: clinical course and prognostic signs. Arch Neurol. 1996 Apr;53(4):309–15.

Hofmeijer J, Kappelle LJ, Algra A, Amelink GJ, van Gijn J, van der Worp HB; HAMLET investigators. Surgical decompression for space-occupying cerebral infarction (the Hemicraniectomy After Middle Cerebral Artery Infarction With Life-threatening Edema Trial [HAMLET]): a multicentre, open, randomised trial. Lancet Neurol. 2009 Apr;8(4):326–33. Epub 2009 Mar 5.

Jovin TG, Chamorro A, Cobo E, de Miquel MA, Molina CA, Rovira A, et al; REVASCAT Trial Investigators. Thrombectomy within 8 hours after symptom onset in ischemic stroke. N Engl J Med. 2015 Jun 11;372(24):2296–306. Epub 2015 Apr 17.

Juttler E, Schwab S, Schmiedek P, Unterberg A, Hennerici M, Woitzik J, et al; DESTINY Study Group. Decompressive Surgery for the Treatment of Malignant Infarction of the Middle Cerebral Artery (DESTINY): a randomized, controlled trial. Stroke. 2007 Sep;38(9):2518–25. Epub 2007 Aug 9.

Juttler E, Unterberg A, Woitzik J, Bosel J, Amiri H, Sakowitz OW, et al; DESTINY II Investigators. Hemicraniectomy in older patients with extensive middle-cerebral-artery stroke. N Engl J Med. 2014 Mar 20;370(12):1091–100.

Kasner SE, Demchuk AM, Berrouschot J, Schmutzhard E, Harms L, Verro P, et al. Predictors of fatal brain edema in massive hemispheric ischemic stroke. Stroke. 2001 Sep;32(9):2117–23.

Kruyt ND, Biessels GJ, Devries JH, Roos YB. Hyperglycemia in acute ischemic stroke: pathophysiology and clinical management. Nat Rev Neurol. 2010 Mar;6(3):145–55. Epub 2010 Feb 16.

Manno EM, Nichols DA, Fulgham JR, Wijdicks EF. Computed tomographic determinants of neurologic deterioration in patients with large middle cerebral artery infarctions. Mayo Clin Proc. 2003 Feb;78(2): 156–60.

Mlynash M, Lansberg MG, De Silva DA, Lee J, Christensen S, Straka M, et al; DEFUSE-EPITHET Investigators. Refining the definition of the malignant profile: insights from the DEFUSE-EPITHET pooled data set. Stroke. 2011 May;42(5):1270–5. Epub 2011 Apr 7.

Nagai M, Hoshide S, Kario K. The insular cortex and cardiovascular system: a new insight into the brain-heart axis. J Am Soc Hypertens. 2010 Jul-Aug;4(4):174–82.

Pallesen LP, Barlinn K, Puetz V. Role of decompressive craniectomy in ischemic stroke. Front Neurol. 2019 Jan 9;9:1119.

Rosso C, Corvol JC, Pires C, Crozier S, Attal Y, Jacqueminet S, et al. Intensive versus subcutaneous insulin in patients with hyperacute stroke: results from the randomized INSULINFARCT trial. Stroke. 2012 Sep;43(9):2343–9. Epub 2012 Jun 14.

Sandercock PA, Soane T. Corticosteroids for acute ischaemic stroke. Cochrane Database Syst Rev. 2011 Sep 7;(9):CD000064.

Saver JL, Goyal M, Bonafe A, Diener HC, Levy EI, Pereira VM, et al; SWIFT PRIME Investigators. Stent-retriever thrombectomy after intravenous t-PA vs. t-PA alone in stroke. N Engl J Med. 2015 Jun 11;372(24):2285–95. Epub 2015 Apr 17.

Schwarz S, Georgiadis D, Aschoff A, Schwab S. Effects of hypertonic (10%) saline in patients with raised intracranial pressure after stroke. Stroke. 2002 Jan;33(1): 136–40.

Vahedi K, Hofmeijer J, Juettler E, Vicaut E, George B, Algra A, et al; DECIMAL, DESTINY, and HAMLET investigators. Early decompressive surgery in malignant infarction of the middle cerebral artery: a pooled analysis of three randomised controlled trials. Lancet Neurol. 2007 Mar;6(3):215–22.

Vahedi K, Vicaut E, Mateo J, Kurtz A, Orabi M, Guichard JP, et al; DECIMAL Investigators. Sequential-design, multicenter, randomized, controlled trial of early decompressive craniectomy in malignant middle cerebral artery infarction (DECIMAL Trial). Stroke. 2007 Sep;38(9):2506–17. Epub 2007 Aug 9.

79 Basilar Artery Occlusion

MICHAEL R. PICHLER, MD; JENNIFER E. FUGATE, DO

Goals

- Understand that recognition of the clinical signs of basilar artery occlusion is critical for early intervention.
- Advanced imaging is needed, to determine whether the posterior circulation vascular anatomy is occluded and to determine the extent of brainstem and thalamic injury.
- Recognize locked-in syndrome as a manifestation of acute basilar artery occlusion.

Introduction

Basilar artery occlusion (BAO), a type of posterior circulation stroke, refers to occlusion of the basilar artery at any point along its course. The singular basilar artery arises at the pontomedullary junction from the joining of the vertebral arteries. The basilar trunk directly provides deep penetrating median and paramedian arteries and short and long circumferential arteries, which supply the main body of the pons. The basilar artery terminates in bilateral posterior cerebral arteries, which give off penetrating arteries to the midbrain and thalamus, course around the cerebral peduncles, and perfuse the occipital lobes and inferior and medial temporal lobes. The basilar artery can be arbitrarily divided into proximal, middle, and distal segments with the anterior inferior cerebellar artery and superior cerebellar artery as boundaries. Basilar artery anatomy is shown in Figure 79.1. Patients with BAO can present in many ways, depending on the location of the occlusion and the collateral blood supply.

Approximately 20% of all strokes affect the posterior circulation, with BAO accounting for around 1% of ischemic strokes overall. Occlusion of the basilar artery most often results from large-artery atherosclerotic disease affecting the vertebrobasilar system or from a cardioembolic source. Important considerations, especially in young patients, are emboli and extension of thrombus from vertebral dissection. Less common causes include basilar artery dissection, hereditary connective tissue disease and arteriopathies (eg, Ehlers-Danlos syndrome and Marfan syndrome), meningitis, arteritis, and compression from severe cervical rheumatoid arthritis. The cause is cryptogenic in up to one-third of patients.

Clinical Features

Patients with posterior circulation or basilar artery ischemic disease may present with various clinical signs and symptoms (Table 79.1), which are different from those of classic anterior circulation disease. Atherosclerotic transient ischemic attacks involving the posterior circulation may precede BAO by several days to weeks. In patients with prodromal symptoms, nausea and vomiting may precede head or neck pain. Transient motor deficits, bulbar symptoms, diplopia, and convulsive-like movements may also occur. In contrast, sudden embolic or thrombotic occlusions are more likely to cause sudden, severe symptoms due to extensive infarction with potentially devastating outcomes. Although coma does not typically occur in patients with ischemic stroke, acute BAO should be considered whenever a patient is acutely comatose, particularly if the patient has associated brainstem abnormalities or extensor posturing on examination. Acute BAO presents with posterior circulation findings that begin with the letter *D*: depressed level of consciousness, dysarthria, diplopia, dysphagia, and dysconjugate gaze. Hemiparesis can occur with either anterior or posterior circulation events and with hemisensory findings. Hemianopia could occur with large middle cerebral artery infarction, but bilateral blindness should be a clue of acute BAO with bilateral posterior cerebral artery involvement.

Locked-in syndrome, a relatively rare but serious complication of BAO, is caused by ischemia in the ventral

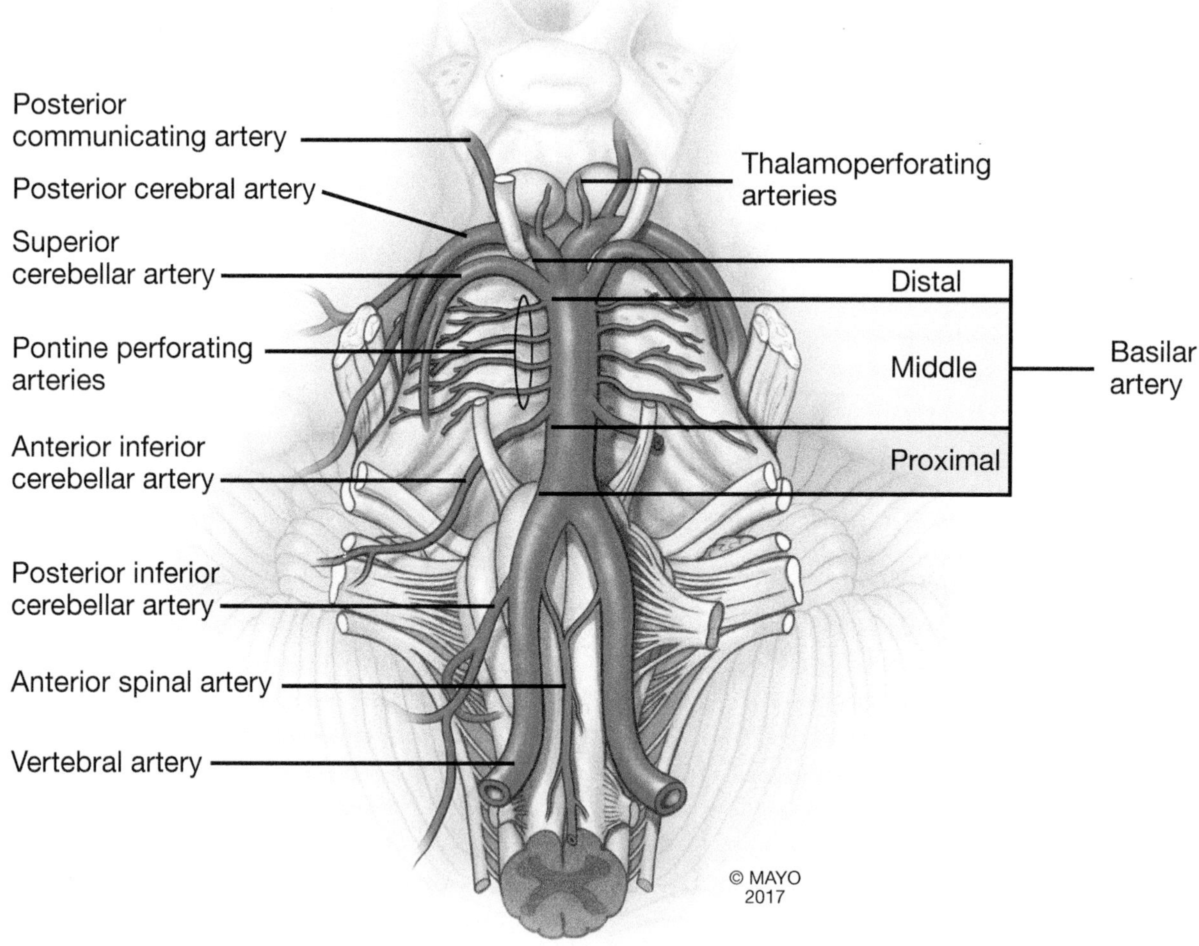

Figure 79.1. Posterior Circulation to the Brain. Many perforators enter the brainstem, and other important branches lead to the cerebellum and thalamus.

pons (proximal and middle segments of the basilar artery). Clinically, locked-in syndrome may appear similar to coma or vegetative state. Symptoms include quadriplegia, anarthria, dysphagia, facial diplegia, and impaired horizontal eye movements. If damage is confined to the pons and spares the midbrain tegmentum, vertical eye movements and blinking are retained, providing a possible method of communication. These features may be an important clue to the diagnosis in what appears to be an otherwise unresponsive patient. Patients with locked-in syndrome are awake and alert, but this state may not be recognized because of their limited means of communication. If patients have a less extensive infarct in the distribution of the proximal or middle segments of the basilar artery, they may have incomplete locked-in syndrome with various degrees of dysarthria, dysphagia, decreased consciousness, horizontal gaze paresis, and cranial nerve impairment.

The "top of the basilar" syndrome occurs with occlusion of the upper basilar circulation, including the thalamoperforatorsand may include the posterior cerebral arteries. Top of the basilar syndrome is a well-described syndrome characterized by oculomotor, visual, and behavioral abnormalities, with or without motor involvement (Figure 79.2). Ocular abnormalities result from ischemia in the midbrain tegmentum and may include impaired

Table 79.1 • Potential Clinical Manifestations of Basilar Artery Occlusion

Symptom by Segment of Basilar Artery Occlusion	Anatomical Correlate
Proximal basilar artery	
Depressed level of consciousness and weakness (hemiparesis to quadriplegia)	Corticospinal tracts and medial lemniscus pathways (via anteromedial penetrating basilar arteries at pontomedullary junction)
Sensory loss to vibration and light touch	
Mid basilar artery (locked-in syndrome)	
Weakness (hemiparesis to quadriplegia) and extensor plantar response	Corticospinal tracts in pons or cerebral peduncles
Sensory loss	Medial lemniscus and spinothalamic tracts
Horizontal gaze palsy	Abducens nerve nuclei, medial longitudinal fasciculus, and paramedian pontine reticular formation
Anarthria and dysphagia	Corticobulbar tracts
Incontinence	Pontine micturition center and connections from parasympathetic hypothalamic nuclei
Vertigo and vestibular dysfunction	Cerebellum and cerebellar peduncles
Hearing loss	Inner ear and vestibulocochlear nerve or nucleus (via branches of anterior inferior cerebellar artery)
Distal basilar artery (top of the basilar syndrome)	Unilateral or bilateral occipital lobes
Hemianopia or cortical blindness	Midbrain tegmentum
	Medial longitudinal fasciculus
Vertical gaze paresis	
Internuclear ophthalmoplegia	
Third nerve palsy	Third nerve nucleus and fascicle
Pupillary abnormalities	Edinger-Westphal nuclei and diencephalon
Somnolence or coma	Midbrain reticular formation and bilateral thalami
Disorientation and memory impairment	Thalamic nuclei and medial temporal lobes
Ataxia, tremor, and dysarthria	Cerebellum (via superior cerebellar artery)
Sensory loss	Medial lemniscus, spinothalamic tracts, and thalamic nuclei

vertical gaze, convergence dysfunction, and skew deviation. If the area of infarct extends more caudally in the midbrain, ventral to the aqueduct, it may affect the medial longitudinal fasciculus (causing internuclear ophthalmoplegia) or the nuclei of cranial nerve III (causing nuclear third nerve palsy). Other findings associated with midbrain lesions include the Collier sign (elevation and retraction of the upper eyelids) and intermittent eccentric positioning of the iris. Depending on whether the occlusion is unilateral or bilateral, deficits can include hemianopia, cortical blindness, aspects of Balint syndrome, amnesia, or agitation. Behavioral abnormalities in patients with top of the basilar syndrome can include hypersomnolence due to infarcts in the bilateral thalami or the reticular formation of the midbrain. With thalamic involvement, marked fluctuations in the level of alertness are common. Visual hallucinations and bizarre behaviors have also been reported.

Imaging

Advanced neuroimaging, such as computed tomographic angiography (CTA) and magnetic resonance angiography (MRA) have become essential in the diagnosis of acute BAO because of the lack of sensitivity of noncontrast computed tomography (CT), in diagnosing BAO due to vertebrobasilar calcifications in older patients. Noncontrast CT, however, is often the initial imaging study used to evaluate patients for acute stroke. CT is also poor for detection of ischemia of the brainstem (dark with low Hounsfield unit values), although hyperdensity of the basilar artery may provide a clue to diagnosis (Figure 79.3). Hyperdensity of the basilar artery has been found in 60% to 70% of patients with BAO. In patients with a high pretest probability of posterior circulation stroke, the presence of the hyperdense basilar artery sign is an accurate predictor of thrombosis. With its rapid acquisition time, CTA is often the initial diagnostic study of choice for pathologic confirmation of the vertebrobasilar circulation since it is usually easier to perform at most hospitals because use of magnetic resonance imaging (MRI) requires a questionnaire related to magnetic fields and concerns about metallic implants and pacemakers. Unless a family is available to fill out an MRI questionnaire for a comatose patient, CTA is easier and faster for demonstrating BAO; renal function is the main concern with intravenous contrast administration.

Compared with CT, MRI is superior for the detection of acute ischemia. Within minutes to hours after vessel

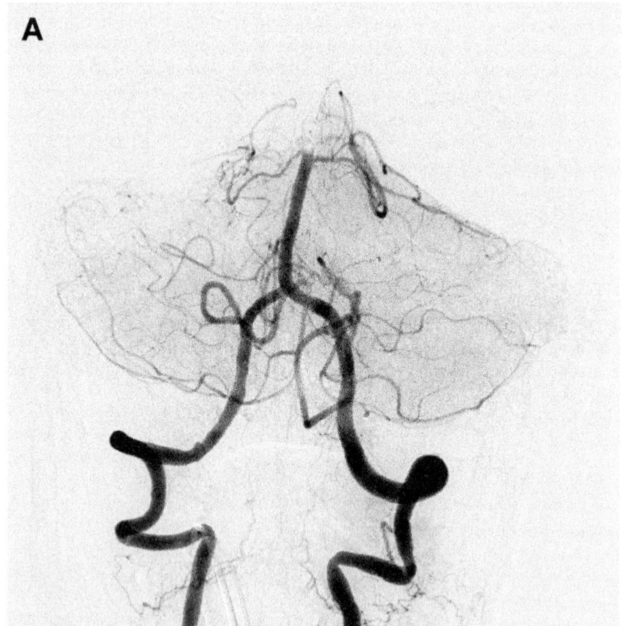

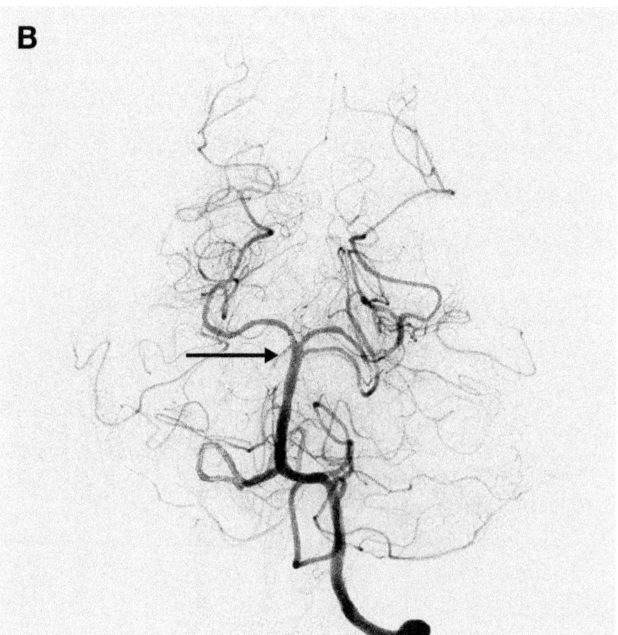

Figure 79.2. Top of the Basilar Syndrome. A 64-year-old man with severe coronary artery disease and chronic systolic heart failure presented to the emergency department for decreased consciousness and inability to speak. While there, he became comatose with pupillary asymmetry and extensor posturing of his arms. Computed tomography (CT) did not show evidence of acute ischemia, and CT angiography showed occlusion of the distal basilar artery. He underwent emergent endovascular treatment. A, Both proximal posterior cerebral artery segments were occluded, and the right superior cerebellar artery (SCA) had diminished flow. B, Recanalization was successful after mechanical thrombectomy and intra-arterial thrombolysis, although slow flow persisted in the right SCA (arrow). Magnetic resonance imaging showed infarct bilaterally in the occipital lobes, medial temporal lobes, thalami, pons, and superior aspects of the cerebellum. The patient gradually awoke from coma and followed simple commands, but he died of cardiac complications within 2 weeks after presentation.

occlusion, cytotoxic edema from acute infarct may appear in diffusion-weighted imaging and in apparent diffusion coefficient sequences. Loss of flow void on fluid-attenuated inversion recovery images may signify BAO, but magnetic resonance angiography is used to confirm occlusion by showing a filling defect in the basilar artery. Preferences for MRI and MRA compared with CT and CTA vary depending on the hospital and stroke interventional team. Given these concerns, advanced CT and MRA with angiography are most useful for patients with acute basilar circulation strokes. For most patients with acute BAO and long times to presentation, MRI can also help define the extent of areas already infarcted.

Transcranial Doppler ultrasonography provides limited penetration and identification of the basilar artery. Transcranial color-coded duplex sonography improves the echogenicity of blood with intravenous contrast agents, increasing identification of the basilar artery to more than 90% in some cases, but the methods vary with the user, so it cannot be used to rule out BAO with absolute certainty. Four-vessel digital subtraction angiography (DSA) is considered the gold standard for the diagnosis of BAO (as for other large-vessel intracranial occlusions) since it subtracts areas that could be artifacts on CT or MRI. DSA, however, is an invasive procedure with a low risk (2%) of ischemic stroke from atherosclerotic plaque or arterial dissection. Initial imaging is typically performed with CTA or MRA; DSA is performed if the diagnosis remains uncertain or if acute endovascular therapy is needed.

Treatment

Early recognition of acute BAO is essential to provide appropriate therapies aimed at vessel recanalization and restoration of perfusion. Without successful recanalization, the likelihood of death or a poor outcome exceeds 90%. The best method for recanalization for acute BAO has not been clearly defined in randomized trials since most have focused on anterior circulation large-vessel occlusion. Randomized prospective studies have clearly shown a benefit with administration of intravenous and intra-arterial recombinant tissue plasminogen activator (tPA) in acute ischemic stroke regardless of anterior or

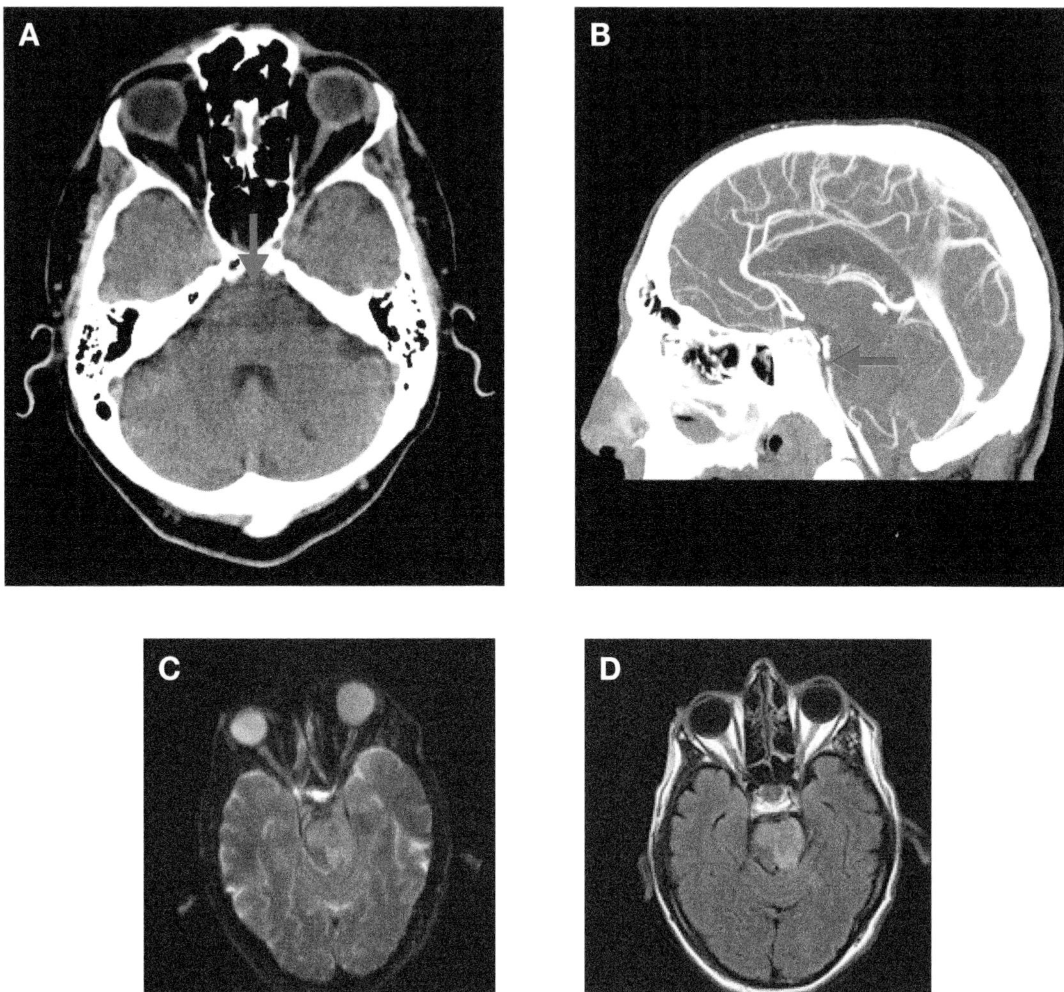

Figure 79.3. Acute Vertebral Artery Dissection With Distal Basilar Artery Occlusion. A 60-year-old man with dominant vertebral artery dissection and distal embolism to the upper third of his basilar artery presented with a depressed level of consciousness, tetraparesis, dysphagia, and dysconjugate gaze. On initial examination, the patient had locked-in syndrome and could only move his eyes upward and blink. He was intubated for airway protection. A, Noncontrast computed tomography of the head shows a hyperdense basilar artery sign (arrow). B, Computed tomographic angiography of the head (saggital view) shows occlusion in the upper third of the basilar artery (arrow). C and D, Diffusion-weighted magnetic resonance image of the head (C) and fluid-attenuated inversion recovery sequence (D) show bipontine infarction. The patient eventually received an antithrombotic regimen (aspirin and clopidogrel), tracheostomy, and percutaneous gastrostomy tube, and he was transferred to rehabilitation after motor function returned to the right side of his face and to his arm and leg.

posterior circulation origin, but those studies included few, if any, patients with BAO because of its lower incidence.

Early studies investigating intravenous thrombolysis (IVT) and intra-arterial thrombolysis showed mixed results among patients with BAO, and interpretations were limited by small sample size or retrospective design. The Basilar Artery International Cooperation Study (BASICS) was the largest prospective, observational registry of consecutive cases of acute BAO. BASICS was designed to collect preliminary data on treatment options and patient characteristics in 3 treatment groups: 1) only antiplatelet drugs or anticoagulation; 2) IVT with or without intra-arterial thrombolysis; and 3) intra-arterial therapy, which comprised thrombolysis, mechanical thrombectomy, or stenting alone or in combination. Overall, 68% of patients had a poor outcome at 1 month (death or a modified Rankin scale of 4 or 5). No treatment strategy provided a statistically significant benefit, but patients with severe deficits (coma, locked-in syndrome, or tetraplegia) had a lower risk of poor outcome with IVT or intra-arterial therapy.

In 2015, multiple prospective clinical trials were published that changed the initial management of anterior circulation ischemic stroke due to intracranial large-vessel occlusion. Those studies showed the benefit of IVT in combination with mechanical thrombectomy in eligible patients. Better patient selection, use of IVT in combination with endovascular mechanical thrombectomy, and improved recanalization rates with newer devices most likely contributed to the positive results in these trials compared with earlier studies. The results of these anterior circulation large-vessel occlusion trials were applied to the management of BAO, largely in restrospective studies that showed benefit compared with medical management alone. In light of all available evidence, the current standard for management of BAO is to provide IVT to eligible patients and then provide intra-arterial thrombolysis.

Time to treatment is one of the most important predictors of outcome for patients with ischemic stroke, and early recanalization is the primary objective. However, the time cutoff for treatment is not as well defined for acute BAO as it is for large-vessel occlusion in the anterior circulation. In general, for acute anterior circulation ischemic stroke, intravenous tPA is given within 4.5 hours in eligible patients and can be combined with endovascular treatment for up to 6 hours with improved outcomes (as in the Multicenter Randomized Clinical Trial of Endovascular Treatment for Acute Ischemic Stroke in the Netherlands [MR CLEAN]). No randomized trial for acute BAO has compared IVT alone with IVT and intra-arterial thrombectomy or other therapy, such as retrievable stents as used in MR CLEAN and anterior circulation large-vessel occlusion trials. Progressive BAO symptoms may relate to the persistent occlusion of penetrating arteries rather than to failing collateral flow or to thalamic or scattered brainstem infarctions. In patients without established brainstem infarct, reperfusion therapy should still be considered hours after symptom onset, especially given the dismal prognosis if recanalization is not achieved.

Antithrombotic therapy (eg, aspirin or anticoagulation) should be started as soon as possible depending on the stroke mechanism, but it should be delayed 24 hours after administration of intravenous tPA because of concern for an increased risk of intracranial and systemic bleeding. According to American Stroke Association guidelines, anticoagulation is not recommended for management of acute stroke during the early phase of ischemic stroke (<7 days) because of the risk of hemorrhagic conversion. However, it could be considered if there is a compelling indication for anticoagulation and a low risk of intracranial bleeding (eg, mechanical heart valve in the mitral position with concomitant atrial fibrillation). Even in these circumstances, though, the most common recommendation is to use antiplatelet therapy to bridge toward anticoagulation after the risk of intracranial bleeding lessens (after 7-14 days). Subcutaneous heparin (5,000 units every 8 hours) can also be used for deep vein thrombosis prevention and adds negligible intracranial bleeding risk even when used with aspirin. This combination therapy was used in the Chinese Acute Stroke Trial (CAST) and prevented some recurrent stroke. The most common recommendation is to discontinue use of aspirin after full anticoagulation is started unless it is indicated because of a mechanical heart value. When a patient's condition worsens or within 24 hours after intervention, follow-up CT or MRI should be performed to evaluate for hemorrhagic complications and to evaluate the extent of ischemia. If not already completed, diagnostic evaluation for causes of occlusion should be pursued and tailored to the patient profile.

Patients with BAO should be monitored in an intensive care unit or a stroke unit and undergo frequent neurologic examinations. Sedating medications should be avoided because of the potential to mask clinical worsening. Short-term permissive hypertension is allowed for maximizing collateral perfusion. If thrombolytics are given or if mechanical recanalization is achieved, most stroke units adhere to permissive hypertension for the first 24 hours and do not treat it unless the systolic pressure exceeds 185 mm Hg or the diastolic pressure exceeds 110 mm Hg. Normothermia and euglycemia should be maintained. Patients often require intubation and mechanical ventilation because of decreased consciousness and respiratory compromise. With prolonged intubation or aspiration from severe bulbar function and lack of airway protection, tracheostomy may be required. Physical, occupational, and speech rehabilitation services should be initiated when the patient is medically stable.

Outcome

IVT can be used if acute BAO is diagnosed within 4.5 hours after onset and if the typical tPA inclusion-exclusion criteria are met; it can be used in conjunction with endovascular

Box 79.1 • Predictors of Poor Outcome for Patients With Basilar Artery Occlusion

Patient characteristics
- Older age
- Presence of comorbid conditions such as chronic kidney disease and heart failure

Clinical presentation
- Coma or severely decreased consciousness
- Need for mechanical ventilation
- Higher score on National Institutes of Health Stroke Scale
- Longer time to treatment
- Unsuccessful vessel recanalization
- Associated symptomatic intracerebral hemorrhage

Neuroimaging
- Large established infarct on initial imaging
- Extensive thrombus involving multiple segments of the basilar artery and vertebral artery

clot retrieval to achieve recanalization if the patient can be evaluated at an endovascular center. After such selection, recanalization can be achieved in about 80% of patients. However, even with newer treatment options, mortality from BAO still exceeds 30%. In addition, an embolus from tandem vertebral artery lesions is associated with a worse clinical outcome despite successful recanalization. Several factors have been linked to patient outcomes, and most reflect the severity of symptoms or ischemia (Box 79.1). Coma or severely decreased consciousness, need for prolonged mechanical ventilation, presence of a large brainstem infarct on initial imaging, higher National Institutes of Health Stroke Scale score, and symptomatic intracerebral hemorrhage are all associated with worse outcomes. The segment of the basilar artery that is occluded also affects outcomes, and extensive thrombus or occlusion of multiple segments signifies a worse prognosis. Patient age is often taken into account when deciding on aggressive interventions. However, more than 20% of patients older than 75 years, if identified early enough with intervention, have a good functional outcome; so age itself should not be a discriminating factor for limiting treatment.

Summary

- Patients with acute BAO can present with various clinical signs and symptoms depending on the extent of the infarct and the anatomical region affected.
- Posterior circulation ischemia in acute BAO often presents with findings that begin with *D*: depressed level of consciousness, dysarthria, diplopia, dysphagia, and dysconjugate gaze.
- Acute tetraparesis with coexisting extraocular movement abnormalities, ataxia, or decreased alertness should increase suspicion for BAO or posterior circulation ischemia.
- Recanalization of an acute BAO is an important predictor for outcomes because without recanalization in a patient with severe clinical signs, death or severe disability is almost certain.
- Little prospective evidence is available to guide the immediate management of BAO, but generally intravenous tPA is used for eligible patients, and then patients undergo evaluation for endovascular thrombectomy if BAO or posterior circulation large-vessel occlusion is noted on CTA or MRA.

SUGGESTED READING

Allen LM, Hasso AN, Handwerker J, Farid H. Sequence-specific MR imaging findings that are useful in dating ischemic stroke. Radiographics. 2012 Sep-Oct;32(5):1285–97.

Archer CR, Horenstein S. Basilar artery occlusion: clinical and radiological correlation. Stroke. 1977 May-Jun;8(3):383–90.

Arnold M, Nedeltchev K, Schroth G, Baumgartner RW, Remonda L, Loher TJ, et al. Clinical and radiological predictors of recanalisation and outcome of 40 patients with acute basilar artery occlusion treated with intra-arterial thrombolysis. J Neurol Neurosurg Psychiatry. 2004 Jun;75(6):857–62.

Baik SH, Park HJ, Kim JH, Jang CK, Kim BM, Kim DJ. Mechanical thrombectomy in subtypes of basilar artery occlusion: relationship to recanalization rate and clinical outcome. Radiology. 2019 Mar 26:181924. [Epub ahead of print]

Brandt T, Knauth M, Wildermuth S, Winter R, von Kummer R, Sartor K, et al. CT angiography and Doppler sonography for emergency assessment in acute basilar artery ischemia. Stroke. 1999 Mar;30(3):606–12.

Brandt T, von Kummer R, Muller-Kuppers M, Hacke W. Thrombolytic therapy of acute basilar artery occlusion: variables affecting recanalization and outcome. Stroke. 1996 May;27(5):875–81.

Caplan LR. Caplan's stroke: a clinical approach. 4th ed. Philadelphia (PA): Elsevier/Saunders; c2009.

Caplan LR. "Top of the basilar" syndrome. Neurology. 1980 Jan;30(1):72–9.

Chen CJ, Ding D, Starke RM, Mehndiratta P, Crowley RW, Liu KC, et al. Endovascular vs medical management of acute ischemic stroke. Neurology. 2015 Dec 1;85(22):1980–90. Epub 2015 Nov 4.

Donnan GA, Baron JC, Ma H, Davis SM. Penumbral selection of patients for trials of acute stroke therapy. Lancet Neurol. 2009 Mar;8(3):261–9.

Ernst M, Romero JM, Buhk JH, Cheng B, Herrmann J, Fiehler J, et al. Sensitivity of hyperdense basilar artery sign on non-enhanced computed tomography. PLoS One. 2015 Oct 19;10(10):e0141096.

Ferbert A, Bruckmann H, Drummen R. Clinical features of proven basilar artery occlusion. Stroke. 1990 Aug;21(8):1135–42.

Goldmakher GV, Camargo EC, Furie KL, Singhal AB, Roccatagliata L, Halpern EF, et al. Hyperdense basilar artery sign on unenhanced CT predicts thrombus and outcome in acute posterior circulation stroke. Stroke. 2009 Jan;40(1):134–9. Epub 2008 Nov 26.

Gory B, Eldesouky I, Sivan-Hoffmann R, Rabilloud M, Ong E, Riva R, et al. Outcomes of stent retriever thrombectomy in basilar artery occlusion: an observational study and systematic review. J Neurol Neurosurg Psychiatry. 2016 May;87(5):520–5. Epub 2015 May 18.

Greving JP, Schonewille WJ, Wijman CA, Michel P, Kappelle LJ, Algra A; BASICS Study Group. Predicting outcome after acute basilar artery occlusion based on admission characteristics. Neurology. 2012 Apr 3;78(14):1058–63. Epub 2012 Mar 21.

Hacke W, Kaste M, Bluhmki E, Brozman M, Davalos A, Guidetti D, et al; ECASS Investigators. Thrombolysis with alteplase 3 to 4.5 hours after acute ischemic stroke. N Engl J Med. 2008 Sep 25;359(13):1317–29.

Jauch EC, Saver JL, Adams HP Jr, Bruno A, Connors JJ, Demaerschalk BM, et al; American Heart Association Stroke Council; Council on Cardiovascular Nursing; Council on Peripheral Vascular Disease; Council on Clinical Cardiology. Guidelines for the early management of patients with acute ischemic stroke: a guideline for healthcare professionals from the American Heart Association/American Stroke Association. Stroke. 2013 Mar;44(3):870–947. Epub 2013 Jan 31.

Jung S, Mono ML, Fischer U, Galimanis A, Findling O, De Marchis GM, et al. Three-month and long-term outcomes and their predictors in acute basilar artery occlusion treated with intra-arterial thrombolysis. Stroke. 2011 Jul;42(7):1946–51. Epub 2011 May 5.

Kermer P, Wellmer A, Crome O, Mohr A, Knauth M, Bahr M. Transcranial color-coded duplex sonography in suspected acute basilar artery occlusion. Ultrasound Med Biol. 2006 Mar;32(3):315–20.

Israeli-korn SD, Schwammenthal Y, Yonash-Kimchi T, Bakon M, Tsabari R, Orion D, et al. Ischemic stroke due to acute basilar artery occlusion: proportion and outcomes. Isr Med Assoc J. 2010 Nov;12(11):671–5.

Lindsberg PJ, Mattle HP. Therapy of basilar artery occlusion: a systematic analysis comparing intra-arterial and intravenous thrombolysis. Stroke. 2006 Mar;37(3):922–8. Epub 2006 Jan 26.

Lindsberg PJ, Soinne L, Tatlisumak T, Roine RO, Kallela M, Happola O, et al. Long-term outcome after intravenous thrombolysis of basilar artery occlusion. JAMA. 2004 Oct 20;292(15):1862–6.

Mak CH, Ho JW, Chan KY, Poon WS, Wong GK. Intra-arterial revascularization therapy for basilar artery occlusion: a systematic review and analysis. Neurosurg Rev. 2016 Oct;39(4):575–80. Epub 2016 Jan 25.

Meyding-Lamade U, Rieke K, Krieger D, Forsting M, Sartor K, Sommer C, et al. Rare diseases mimicking acute vertebrobasilar artery thrombosis. J Neurol. 1995 May;242(5):335–43.

National Institute of Neurological Disorders and Stroke rt-PA Stroke Study Group. Tissue plasminogen activator for acute ischemic stroke. N Engl J Med. 1995 Dec 14;333(24):1581–7.

Patterson JR, Grabois M. Locked-in syndrome: a review of 139 cases. Stroke. 1986 Jul-Aug;17(4):758–64.

Ruecker M, Furtner M, Knoflach M, Werner P, Gotwald T, Chemelli A, et al. Basilar artery dissection: series of 12 consecutive cases and review of the literature. Cerebrovasc Dis. 2010 Aug;30(3):267–76. Epub 2010 Jul 24.

Sairanen T, Strbian D, Soinne L, Silvennoinen H, Salonen O, Artto V, et al; Helsinki Stroke Thrombolysis Registry (HSTR) Group. Intravenous thrombolysis of basilar artery occlusion: predictors of recanalization and outcome. Stroke. 2011 Aug;42(8):2175–9. Epub 2011 Jul 7.

Schonewille WJ, Wijman CA, Michel P, Algra A, Kappelle LJ; BASICS Study Group. The basilar artery international cooperation study (BASICS). Int J Stroke. 2007 Aug;2(3):220–3.

Schonewille WJ, Wijman CA, Michel P, Rueckert CM, Weimar C, Mattle HP, et al; BASICS study group. Treatment and outcomes of acute basilar artery occlusion in the Basilar Artery International Cooperation Study (BASICS): a prospective registry study. Lancet Neurol. 2009 Aug;8(8):724–30. Epub 2009 Jul 3.

Smith E, Delargy M. Locked-in syndrome. BMJ. 2005 Feb 19;330(7488):406–9.

Strbian D, Sairanen T, Silvennoinen H, Salonen O, Kaste M, Lindsberg PJ. Thrombolysis of basilar artery occlusion: impact of baseline ischemia and time. Ann Neurol. 2013 Jun;73(6):688–94. Epub 2013 Jul 8.

Tatu L, Moulin T, Bogousslavsky J, Duvernoy H. Arterial territories of human brain: brainstem and cerebellum. Neurology. 1996 Nov;47(5):1125–35.

Turney TM, Garraway WM, Whisnant JP. The natural history of hemispheric and brainstem infarction in Rochester, Minnesota. Stroke. 1984 Sep-Oct;15(5):790–4.

van Houwelingen RC, Luijckx GJ, Mazuri A, Bokkers RP, Eshghi OS, Uyttenboogaart M. Safety and outcome of intra-arterial treatment for basilar artery occlusion. JAMA Neurol. 2016 Oct 1;73(10):1225–30.

Vergouwen MD, Algra A, Pfefferkorn T, Weimar C, Rueckert CM, Thijs V, et al; Basilar Artery International Cooperation Study (BASICS) Study Group. Time is brain(stem) in basilar artery occlusion. Stroke. 2012 Nov;43(11):3003–6. Epub 2012 Sep 18.

Vergouwen MD, Compter A, Tanne D, Engelter ST, Audebert H, Thijs V, et al. Outcomes of basilar artery occlusion in patients aged 75 years or older in the Basilar Artery International Cooperation Study. J Neurol. 2012 Nov;259(11):2341–6. Epub 2012 Apr 18.

Voetsch B, DeWitt LD, Pessin MS, Caplan LR. Basilar artery occlusive disease in the New England Medical Center Posterior Circulation Registry. Arch Neurol. 2004 Apr;61(4):496–504.

Warach S, Chien D, Li W, Ronthal M, Edelman RR. Fast magnetic resonance diffusion-weighted imaging of acute human stroke. Neurology. 1992 Sep;42(9):1717–23. Erratum in: Neurology 1992 Nov;42(11):2192.

Weimar C, Goertler M, Harms L, Diener HC. Distribution and outcome of symptomatic stenoses and occlusions in patients with acute cerebral ischemia. Arch Neurol. 2006 Sep;63(9):1287–91.

Wijdicks EF, Nichols DA, Thielen KR, Fulgham JR, Brown RD Jr, Meissner I, et al. Intra-arterial thrombolysis in acute basilar artery thromboembolism: the initial Mayo Clinic experience. Mayo Clin Proc. 1997 Nov;72(11):1005–13.

80 Carotid Artery Disease[a]

NNENNA MBABUIKE, MD; RABIH G. TAWK, MD

Goals

- Recognize the clinical manifestations of carotid artery disease.
- Define the medical, surgical, and endovascular management options for symptomatic carotid artery disease.
- Recognize the medical management options for asymptomatic carotid artery disease.

Introduction

Carotid artery disease is a common source of ischemic stroke due to ulcerated or hemorrhagic plaque. Risk factors for carotid artery disease include typical atherosclerotic disease risk factors, such as smoking, hyperlipidemia, and diabetes mellitus. This chapter reviews the diagnostic approach to symptomatic carotid artery disease (including stroke and transient ischemic attacks), the overall management approach for symptomatic carotid artery disease (including endovascular and open carotid endarterectomy), and medical management options for asymptomatic carotid artery disease. Perioperative management after carotid artery intervention is discussed.

Pathophysiology

Carotid artery disease can lead to transient ischemic attacks (TIAs) or stroke when arterial narrowing or thromboembolism from an atheromatous plaque results in low flow into distal intracranial vessels. Atherosclerotic changes often occur at the carotid bifurcation, at the outer wall (a region of low shear stress), or in the internal carotid artery (ICA) just past the bifurcation of the common carotid artery or near the carotid siphon or the intracranial carotid artery. Regardless of their location, the presence of carotid plaques increases the incidence of stroke and cerebral infarction.

A high-grade stenosis (70%-99%) of the ICA can lead to a *critical stenosis*, which causes a precipitous decrease in the cerebral blood flow rate and can result in a TIA or stroke with failure of the distal collateral circulation across the posterior and anterior communicating arteries. Thromboembolism of carotid plaque may occlude intracranial arteries, and the resulting cerebral ischemia or infarction and clinical syndrome depends on the corresponding cerebrovascular territory involved. TIAs that result from low flow tend to be brief and repetitive, but TIAs that result from embolism tend to be singular and involve a vascular territory, most commonly of the middle cerebral artery.

Patients with carotid artery stenosis can have symptomatic disease or asymptomatic disease. A carotid bruit that is focal, high-pitched, and long correlates with moderate to severe carotid artery stenosis. Signs and symptoms of symptomatic ICA disease include hemiparesis and hemisensory loss. They can also include contralateral visual loss if infarction involves the middle cerebral artery and if the temporal lobe (Meyer loop) or deeper parietal vision fibers are affected. *Amaurosis fugax*, transient or permanent monocular blindness due to ischemia of the ipsilateral ophthalmic artery, is a specific syndrome of typically high-grade ICA stenosis.

The specific characteristics of carotid plaques are thought to contribute to the risk of symptoms from carotid

[a] Portions of text from Kernan WN, Ovbiagele B, Black HR, Bravata DM, Chimowitz MI, Ezekowitz MD, et al; American Heart Association Stroke Council, Council on Cardiovascular and Stroke Nursing, Council on Clinical Cardiology, and Council on Peripheral Vascular Disease. Guidelines for the prevention of stroke in patients with stroke and transient ischemic attack: a guideline for healthcare professionals from the American Heart Association/American Stroke Association. Stroke. 2014 Jul;45(7):2160-236. Epub 2014 May 1. Erratum in: Stroke. 2015 Feb;46(2):e54; used with permission.

Table 80.1 • Diagnostic Imaging Methods for the Carotid Artery

Imaging Method	Advantages	Disadvantages
Carotid duplex ultrasonography	Noninvasive Readily accessible No radiation Low cost	Operator dependent Decreased sensitivity with calcified vessels and tortuosity
Magnetic resonance angiography	Noninvasive No radiation Intracranial and cervical imaging of the artery	May not be available at small centers Decreased sensitivity with calcified vessels and tortuosity Relative contraindications with poor kidney function
Computed tomographic angiography	Noninvasive Readily accessible Allows evaluation of relationship between carotid artery and surrounding structures	Exposure to radiation Decreased sensitivity with calcified vessels Relative contraindications with poor kidney function
Digitial subtraction angiography	2- and 3-dimensional imaging Allows visualization of collateral circulation Allows visualization of eccentric and concentric stenosis Diagnostic and therapeutic (with carotid angioplasty and stenting)	Minimally invasive Relative contraindications with poor kidney function, allergy to dye, vasculopathy resulting in poor peripheral access, tortuous anatomy making proximal access difficult, or patient's inability to lie flat

artery disease. Plaque ulceration, intraplaque hemorrhage, and plaque emboli occur more often in symptomatic carotid artery disease.

Evaluation and Diagnosis

Carotid artery stenosis can be diagnosed with the use of carotid duplex ultrasonography, magnetic resonance angiography (MRA), computed tomographic angiography (CTA), and digital subtraction angiography (DSA) (Table 80.1). These methods of imaging can be used to measure the stenosis with equations developed in studies on the efficacy of carotid endarterectomy (CEA) in preventing stroke (Box 80.1).

B-mode ultrasonography is used in combination with Doppler imaging to record the velocity of blood flow. The combination is mostly suitable for screening because it is fast, noninvasive, and broadly available with a high specificity and sensitivity in high-grade stenosis (70%-99%).

Box 80.1 • Two Methods for Measuring Carotid Artery Stenosis

North American Symptomatic Carotid Endarterectomy Trial (NASCET) method: (1–N/D) × 100

European Carotid Surgery Trial (ECST) method: (1–N/B) × 100

Abbreviations: B, estimated size of the carotid bulb; D, diameter of the normal distal cervical internal carotid artery; N, narrowest diameter of the internal carotid artery.

However, it is operator dependent, its interpretation can vary, and it is less sensitive for calcified vessels. It also has limitations related to tortuosity and large body habitus, and its use is restricted to the cervical carotid arteries.

MRA uses time-of-flight and contrast-enhanced techniques to generate 2- and 3-dimensional images of the carotid arteries. Contrast-enhanced MRA is less susceptible to artifacts than time-of-flight MRA, and it provides more accurate representation of the vessels. Both techniques have good sensitivity and specificity in high-grade stenosis, but the accuracy decreases with moderate stenosis. With MRA, the degree of stenosis tends to be overestimated, and MRA is contraindicated if a patient has a pacemaker or a metallic implant. To avoid the use of gadolinium as a contrast agent in patients with kidney impairment, newer contrast agents (eg, ferumoxytol) can be used safely in selected patients.

CTA produces contrast-enhanced 2- and 3-dimensional images of the carotid arteries and intracranial circulation that show the carotid arteries in relation to the cervical spine. CTA provides excellent representation of the arterial lumen in tortuous carotids and has a high sensitivity and specificity for detection of high-grade stenosis and nearly complete occlusion. However, CTA has limitations in patients with kidney dysfunction or calcifications at the bifurcation.

DSA produces 2- and 3-dimensional images of the extracranial and intracranial segments of the carotid artery and is considered the gold standard for evaluation of carotid artery stenosis. In addition, DSA provides information about collateral circulation and other vessels contributing to the revascularization of a compromised carotid artery. Rotational angiography allows the assessment of eccentric, irregular, and nonconcentric lesions causing the stenosis. Furthermore, after cerebral angiography, endovascular treatment can be provided when indicated. However, DSA is invasive, and the risks include dislodging atherosclerotic plaque and causing ischemic stroke. Other drawbacks are that DSA is not readily available at all centers, it is time consuming, it is more expensive than other methods, and it has limitations if patients have kidney dysfunction precluding the use of an iodinated contrast agent, allergy to dye, or vasculopathy with poor vascular access. During DSA, patients must cooperate for an extended time, which can be challenging for certain patients.

Overall, carotid ultrasonography is a good screening tool and is reliable for identifying a high-grade stenosis. Before considering any treatment, the stenosis can be confirmed with a noninvasive test (either CTA or contrast-enhanced MRA). DSA can be used as a last resource for confirming conflicting results from noninvasive methods and before treatment.

Therapy

The most dreaded risk of carotid artery disease is ischemic stroke, and the main challenge, especially with modern medical management, is related to the uncertainty of not knowing in which patients stroke will occur. Although stroke can be devastating, medical and interventional options also have associated risks. Thus, options must be carefully considered for each patient and management options must be weighed against the natural history of the disease.

Medical Management

Medical management of carotid artery disease centers on modifying risk factors, decreasing serum levels of cholesterol, treating hypertension and diabetes mellitus, and providing antiplatelet therapy. Advances in medical therapy led to the reevaluation of the management of asymptomatic stenosis in the second Carotid Revascularization and Medical Management for Asymptomatic Carotid Stenosis Trial (CREST-2), a prospective randomized study comparing medical management with the use of endarterectomy or stenting.

Statins decrease serum cholesterol levels, decrease the risk of ischemic stroke, decrease vessel inflammation, stabilize plaque, and thereby slow the progression of arterial disease. The American Heart Association (AHA)/American Stroke Association (ASA) guidelines recommend tight control of glycemia and hypertension and lifestyle modifications that include smoking cessation, weight reduction, regular physical activity and exercise, and diet modification.

Antiplatelet therapy and antithrombotic therapy have been studied in various trials for prevention of stroke. Patients with noncardioembolic ischemic stroke or TIA should receive antiplatelet therapy rather than oral anticoagulation. After TIA or ischemic stroke, initial therapy for prevention of future stroke should include aspirin alone (50-325 mg daily) or aspirin 325 mg once daily in combination with extended-release dipyridamole 200 mg twice daily. Clopidogrel (75 mg) is a reasonable option for secondary prevention of stroke as monotherapy (instead of aspirin) or in combination with aspirin and dipyridamole.

Carotid Endarterectomy

CEA involves the open surgical removal of plaque to restore normal blood flow through the artery (Figure 80.1). It has been well studied in prospective randomized trials for symptomatic and asymptomatic disease. According to the North American Symptomatic Carotid Endarterectomy Trial (NASCET), for every 6 patients treated with CEA, 1 major stroke would be prevented at 2 years in symptomatic patients with a 70% to 99% stenosis. For asymptomatic patients, as with any prophylactic operation, careful evaluation of the relative benefits and risks is required on an individual basis. Perioperative CEA risks for combined 30-day mortality and stroke risk should be less than 3% for asymptomatic patients and 6% or less for symptomatic patients. High-risk factors for CEA are listed in Box 80.2.

Three large trials compared CEA with medical therapy in symptomatic patients (Table 80.2). A pooled analysis of the trials concluded that 1) CEA provided no significant benefit if the ICA was nearly occluded, and 2) CEA was beneficial if patients had a 50% to 69% symptomatic stenosis.

Carotid Angioplasty and Stenting

Carotid angioplasty and stenting (CAS) is a minimally invasive treatment alternative to CEA especially for high-risk patients (Figure 80.2). Despite recent advances in endovascular treatment, the improvements in medical management have led to reevaluation of all treatment methods (medical, endovascular, and surgical) in asymptomatic stenosis, and CREST-2, when completed, may provide valuable answers.

Four trials compared the outcomes between CEA and CAS for symptomatic carotid disease (Table 80.2). The current AHA/ASA guidelines are as follows:

- For patients with TIA or ischemic stroke within 6 months and ipsilateral severe stenosis (70%-99%), CEA is recommended if the perioperative morbidity and mortality risk is <6%. For patients with moderate stenosis (50%-69%), CEA is recommended, depending on patient-specific factors such as age, sex, and comorbidities. For patients with stenosis <50%, CEA and CAS are not recommended.
- When revascularization is indicated, it is reasonable to perform the procedure within 2 weeks if the patient has no contraindications to early revascularization.

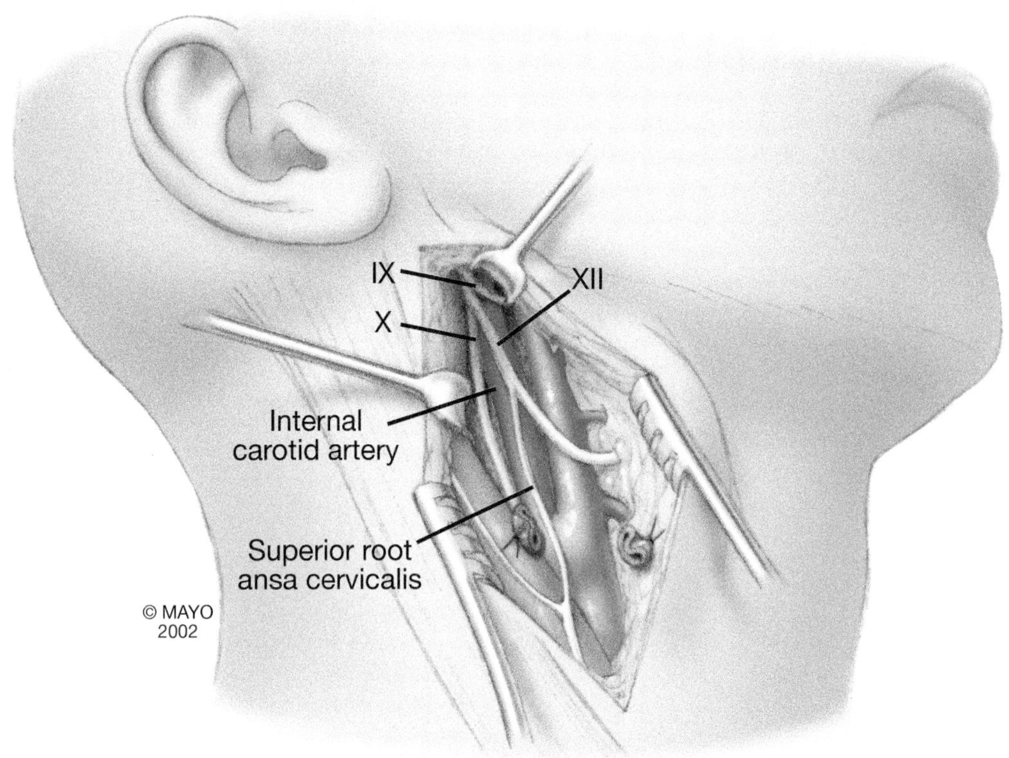

Figure 80.1. Carotid Endarterectomy. Carotid endarterectomy requires 2 to 3 hours (average cross-clamping time, 30-40 minutes). The proximity of the cranial nerves (indicated with roman numerals) predisposes them to injury during carotid exposure.

(From Wijdicks EFM. The clinical practice of critical care neurology. 2nd ed. Oxford (UK): Oxford University Press; c2003. Chapter 27, Carotid endarterectomy; p. 439-53; used with permission of Mayo Foundation for Medical Education and Research.)

Box 80.2 • High-Risk Factors for Cartoid Endarterectomy

- Age 80 y or older
- Class III or IV congestive heart failure
- Class III or IV angina pectoris
- Left main or multivessel coronary artery disease
- Need for open heart surgery within 30 d
- Left ventricular ejection fraction of 30% or less
- Recent heart attack (within 30 d)
- Severe lung disease or chronic obstructive pulmonary disease
- Severe renal disease
- High cervical (C2) or intrathoracic lesion
- Previous radical neck surgery or radiotherapy
- Contralateral carotid artery occlusion
- Previous ipsilateral carotid endarterectomy
- Contralateral laryngeal nerve injury
- Tracheostomy

- CAS is indicated as an alternative to CEA for symptomatic patients at average or low risk for complications associated with endovascular intervention when the ICA diameter is decreased by >70% according to noninvasive imaging; >50% according to catheter angiography; or >50% according to noninvasive imaging with corroboration, and the expected perioperative morbidity and mortality risk is <6%.
- For patients older than 70 years, CEA may be associated with improved outcome compared with CAS, particularly when the arterial anatomy is unfavorable for endovascular intervention. For younger patients, CAS is equivalent to CEA in terms of risk for periprocedural complications (ie, stroke, myocardial infarction, or death) and long-term risk for ipsilateral stroke.
- CAS is reasonable for symptomatic severe stenosis (>70%) in patients with anatomical or medical conditions that increase the risk of surgery or in patients with radiation-induced stenosis or restenosis after CEA.

Table 80.2 • Randomized, Prospective, Multicenter Controlled Trials for Symptomatic and Asymptomatic Carotid Artery Disease

Study[a]	Comments
North American Symptomatic Carotid Endarterectomy Trial (NASCET)	Studied patients with 70%-99% ipsilateral symptomatic stenosis undergoing CEA Recruited 659 patients with hemispheric or retinal TIAs or a nondisabling stroke within 180 d CEA was highly beneficial for patients with recent TIA or nondisabling stroke with 70%-99% ipsilateral stenosis and moderately beneficial for patients with 50%-69% symptomatic ipsilateral stenosis Older patients (≥75 y) with 50%-99% stenosis benefited more from CEA than younger patients did
European Carotid Surgery Trial (ECST)	Included 2,518 patients with a nondisabling ischemic stroke, TIA, or retinal infarct due to ipsilateral stenosis Randomly assigned to medical therapy with aspirin or CEA CEA was beneficial for symptomatic stenosis of 80%-99%
Veterans Affairs Cooperative Study (VACS)	Randomly assigned 444 men with 50%-99% asymptomatic stenosis to receive CEA in combination with medical management or to receive medical management alone After 4 y of follow-up, the stroke rate was lower in the CEA group (8.6% vs 12.4%) When all strokes or perioperative events were considered, results were no different between the CEA group and the medical management group
International Carotid Stenting Study (ICSS)	Enrolled >1,700 adults (age >40 y) with recently symptomatic carotid stenosis (>50%) who were randomly assigned to receive CEA or CAS Cumulative 5-y risk of fatal or disabling stroke was similar for CAS and CEA groups Risk of any stroke was significantly higher for CAS group (absolute risk difference, 5.8%)
Stent-Protected Angioplasty Versus Carotid Endarterectomy (SPACE)	Randomly assigned 1,183 patients with severe symptomatic stenosis to undergo CAS or CEA; excluded high-risk patients with uncontrolled hypertension, severe concomitant disease, or a poor prognosis At 2 y, results were not significantly different between CAS and CEA groups in the composite end point of any periprocedural stroke or death and ipsilateral ischemic stroke
Endarterectomy Versus Angioplasty in Patients With Symptomatic Severe Carotid Stenosis (EVA-3S)	Randomly assigned 527 patients with severe symptomatic stenosis to undergo CAS or CEA Incidence of any stroke or death at 30 d was significantly higher with CAS than with CEA
Carotid Revascularization Endarterectomy Versus Stenting Trial (CREST)	Randomly assigned 2,502 asymptomatic and symptomatic patients to undergo CEA or CAS Primary end point (stroke, MI, or death in ≤30 d after treatment and any ipsilateral stroke during 10-y follow-up) was similar for CAS and CEA groups For patients 70 y or older, the rate of the primary end point and adverse events favored CEA over CAS Rate of stroke or death in ≤30 d was significantly higher with CAS than with CEA (4.4% vs 2.3%) Frequency of MI in ≤30 d was significantly less in the CAS group (1.1% vs 2.3%)

Abbreviations: CAS, carotid artery stenting; CEA, carotid endarterectomy; MI, myocardial infarction; TIA, transient ischemic attack.
[a] See Suggested Reading.

- CEA and CAS in the above settings should be performed by operators with established periprocedural patient morbidity and mortality rates of <6% (as in trials comparing CEA with medical therapy).
- Optimal medical therapy, including antiplatelet therapy, statins, and modification of risk factors, is recommended for all patients with carotid artery stenosis and TIA or stroke.

Asymptomatic Carotid Artery Disease

The treatment of asymptomatic carotid artery disease is controversial. Treatment often revolves around recommendations for intensive medical therapy, revascularization of high-grade stenosis (70%-99%), or revascularization of high-grade stenosis and modification of risk factors. Medical management includes statins, antiplatelets, antihypertensive agents, smoking cessation, and control of diabetes mellitus. In a systematic review of prospective data, annual stroke rates decreased after 1980 among patients who received medical intervention alone. However, revascularization techniques have improved, and the CREST-2 trial is comparing the effectiveness of medical management with the effectiveness of CEA and CAS.

Three large randomized trials have compared CEA with medical management in patients with asymptomatic carotid artery disease (Table 80.3). However, a patient must live

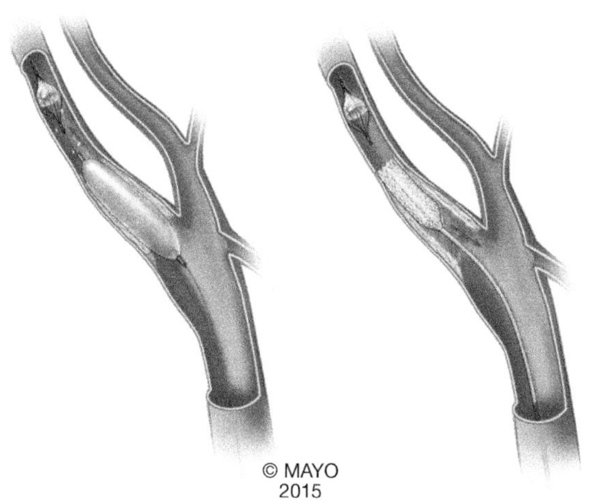

Figure 80.2. Carotid Angioplasty and Stenting. Carotid angioplasty and stenting involves balloon dilatation (left) and subsequent stent placement (right).

(Modified from Lanzino G, Rabinstein AA, Brown RD Jr. Treatment of carotid artery stenosis: medical therapy, surgery, or stenting? Mayo Clin Proc. 2009 Apr;84(4):362–87; used with permission of Mayo Foundation for Medical Education and Research.)

for years before the postoperative risks are outweighed by the decreased risk of stroke, death, and other problems. Therefore, additional factors must be considered, and long-term survival for patients with asymptomatic stenosis may need further consideration during decisions about prophylactic procedures. Risks of complications from CEA or CAS include older age at operation, diabetes mellitus, cardiac disease, previous vascular surgery, and other medical comorbidities.

Overall, the risk of stroke in the territory of an asymptomatic carotid artery is substantially less than the risk of stroke in the territory of a symptomatic artery with a similar stenosis. In addition, the risk of stroke in the territory of an asymptomatic artery peaks at high degrees of stenosis and decreases with nearly complete occlusion. This phenomenon has been observed in symptomatic patients. Other factors that must be considered include the perioperative risks at specific institutions and with specific surgeons because CEA should be performed only at institutions where the perioperative stroke rate and death rate are less than 3% for the patient to benefit from surgical intervention. Furthermore, current management decisions are guided primarily by the degree of stenosis and without accounting for plaque composition and biological activity.

Table 80.3 • Randomized Controlled Trials for Asymptomatic Carotid Artery Disease

Study[a]	Comments
Veterans Affairs Cooperative Study (VACS)	Randomly assigned 444 men with 50%-99% asymptomatic stenosis to receive aspirin alone or aspirin in combination with CEA Compared with the aspirin group, the surgical group had a lower incidence of stroke or TIA (8% vs 20.6%); relative risk reduction, 0.38 (95% CI, 0.22-0.67) The combined stroke and death rate was not different between the groups at 30 d or 48 mo (41% vs 44%)
Asymptomatic Carotid Atherosclerosis Study (ACAS)	Randomly assigned 1,662 patients with 60%-99% stenosis to receive aspirin (325 mg daily) in combination with CEA or to receive aspirin alone The incidence of ipsilateral stroke and perioperative stroke or death was significantly less in the surgical group than in the aspirin group (5% vs 11%); relative risk reduction, 0.53 (95% CI, 0.22-0.72) The incidence of major ipsilateral stroke and major perioperative stroke and death was nonsignificantly less in the surgical group (3.4% vs 6%)
Asymptomatic Carotid Surgery Trial (ACST)	Randomly assigned 3,120 patients with ≥60% asymptomatic stenosis to undergo CEA immediately or to defer CEA until a definite indication occurred The net 5-y risk of stroke or perioperative death for the immediate CEA group was nearly half the risk for the deferred CEA group (6.4% vs 11.8%; 95% CI, 2.96%-7.75%) The immediate CEA group had a perioperative risk of stroke or death of 3.1% within 30 d after surgery The immediate CEA group had a worse event-free survival compared with the deferred CEA group until just before 2 y after surgery, when the immediate CEA group had a better outcome
Stenting and Angioplasty With Protection in Patients at High Risk for Endarterectomy (SAPPHIRE)	Randomly assigned 334 patients to either CAS or CEA; symptomatic patients had ≥50% stenosis and asymptomatic patients had ≥80% stenosis (70% had asymptomatic carotid disease) The nonsignificant difference in the primary composite end point of a major cardiovascular event at 1 y for CAS compared with CEA was 12.2% vs 20.1% (absolute difference, 7.9%; 95% CI, -0.7% to 16.4%)
Carotid Revascularization Endarterectomy Versus Stenting Trial (CREST)	The proportion of enrolled patients with asymptomatic carotid artery disease was 47% (53% had symptomatic disease) The overall effectiveness and safety of the 2 procedures (CAS and CEA) were similar, and the benefits were equal for men and women and for patients with asymptomatic or symptomatic carotid artery disease

Abbreviations: CAS, carotid artery stenting; CEA, carotid endarterectomy; TIA, transient ischemic attack.

[a] See Suggested Reading.

High-resolution magnetic resonance imaging (MRI) can be used to detect characteristics of the vulnerable plaque (eg, a thin or ruptured fibrous cap, a large lipid or necrotic core, and intraplaque hemorrhage [IPH]) and to examine plaque regression and progression. MRI and positron emission tomography can be used to evaluate inflammation within the plaque and to help understand the risk of ipsilateral cerebrovascular events in asymptomatic disease since IPH confers additional risk in symptomatic and asymptomatic patients. Conversely, patients without IPH remain asymptomatic, and the absence of IPH may be a reassuring marker of plaque stability and a lower risk of thromboembolism.

A few randomized trials have included both asymptomatic and symptomatic patients (Table 80.3). Overall, the current AHA/ASA guidelines for patients with asymptomatic carotid artery disease are the following:

- Patients with asymptomatic carotid artery stenosis should be prescribed daily aspirin and a statin with institution of appropriate lifestyle changes and medical therapy.
- CEA is a reasonable consideration for asymptomatic patients with a high-grade stenosis (>70%) if the risk of perioperative stroke, myocardial infarction, and death is low (<3%).
- Patients scheduled to undergo CEA should receive aspirin perioperatively and postoperatively unless contraindicated.
- Prophylactic CAS may be considered for highly selected patients who have asymptomatic carotid artery stenosis (≥60% with angiography or ≥70% with validated Doppler ultrasonography), but its effectiveness compared with medical therapy alone in this situation is not well established.

Conclusions

Recent advances in medical management, imaging modalities, and endovascular and surgical techniques have revolutionized the management of carotid artery disease for preventing its progression and decreasing the risk of ischemic stroke. Various imaging methods can be used to further analyze the characteristics of each lesion and provide individualized care. Medical management is the mainstay of treatment regardless of the symptoms. Revascularization with CEA or CAS requires an individualized decision based on the AHA/ASA guidelines. The goal of ongoing clinical trials is to answer questions about best practice in specific populations, including patients with asymptomatic carotid artery disease.

Summary

- Carotid artery disease leads to luminal narrowing from typical atherosclerotic risk factors.
- Clinically symptomatic carotid artery disease usually leads to anterior circulation neurologic deficits (eg, aphasia, right hemiparesis, sensory loss from left middle cerebral artery ischemia, and monocular blindness [amaurosis fugax]).
- Medical management includes decreasing patient risk factors through steps such as smoking cessation, hyperlipidemia management, control of diabetes mellitus, and use of antiplatelet agents such as aspirin.
- For patients with symptomatic ICA stenosis, surgical options such as stenting or CEA are weighed against the patient's operative risks and the severity of the neurologic deficits.

SUGGESTED READING

Abbott AL. Medical (nonsurgical) intervention alone is now best for prevention of stroke associated with asymptomatic severe carotid stenosis: results of a systematic review and analysis. Stroke. 2009 Oct;40(10):e573–83. Epub 2009 Aug 20.

Altaf N, Morgan PS, Moody A, MacSweeney ST, Gladman JR, Auer DP. Brain white matter hyperintensities are associated with carotid intraplaque hemorrhage. Radiology. 2008 Jul;248(1):202–9.

Babikian VL, Hyde C, Pochay V, Winter MR. Clinical correlates of high-intensity transient signals detected on transcranial Doppler sonography in patients with cerebrovascular disease. Stroke. 1994 Aug;25(8):1570–3.

Brott TG, Hobson RW 2nd, Howard G, Roubin GS, Clark WM, Brooks W, et al; CREST Investigators. Stenting versus endarterectomy for treatment of carotid-artery stenosis. N Engl J Med. 2010 Jul 1;363(1):11–23. Epub 2010 May 26. Errata in: N Engl J Med. 2010 Jul 8;363(2):198. N Engl J Med. 2010 Jul 29;363(5):498.

Caplan LR. Caplan's stroke: a clinical approach. 4th ed. Philadelphia (PA): Elsevier/Saunders; c2009. Chapter 3, Diagnosis and the clinical encounter; p. 64–86.

Debrey SM, Yu H, Lynch JK, Lovblad KO, Wright VL, Janket SJ, et al. Diagnostic accuracy of magnetic resonance angiography for internal carotid artery disease: a systematic review and meta-analysis. Stroke. 2008 Aug;39(8):2237–48. Epub 2008 Jun 12.

Eliasziw M, Smith RF, Singh N, Holdsworth DW, Fox AJ, Barnett HJ; North American Symptomatic Carotid Endarterectomy Trial (NASCET) Group. Further comments on the measurement of carotid stenosis from angiograms. Stroke. 1994 Dec;25(12):2445–9.

European Carotid Surgery Trialists' Collaborative Group. MRC European Carotid Surgery Trial: interim results for symptomatic patients with severe (70-99%) or with mild (0-29%) carotid stenosis. Lancet. 1991 May 25;337(8752):1235–43.

Executive Committee for the Asymptomatic Carotid Atherosclerosis Study. Endarterectomy for asymptomatic carotid artery stenosis. JAMA. 1995 May 10;273(18):1421–8.

Fisher M, Paganini-Hill A, Martin A, Cosgrove M, Toole JF, Barnett HJ, et al. Carotid plaque pathology: thrombosis, ulceration, and stroke pathogenesis. Stroke. 2005 Feb;36(2):253–7. Epub 2005 Jan 13. Erratum in: Stroke. 2005 Oct;36(10):2330.

Galyfos G, Sachsamanis G, Anastasiadou C, Sachmpazidis I, Kikiras K, Kastrisios G, et al. Carotid endarterectomy versus carotid stenting or best medical treatment in asymptomatic patients with significant carotid stenosis: a meta-analysis. Cardiovasc Revasc Med. 2018 Jul 6. pii: S1553-8389(18)30278-1. [Epub ahead of print]

Halliday A, Mansfield A, Marro J, Peto C, Peto R, Potter J, et al; MRC Asymptomatic Carotid Surgery Trial (ACST) Collaborative Group. Prevention of disabling and fatal strokes by successful carotid endarterectomy in patients without recent neurological symptoms: randomised controlled trial. Lancet. 2004 May 8;363(9420):1491–502. Erratum in: Lancet. 2004 Jul 31;364(9432):416.

Hobson RW 2nd, Weiss DG, Fields WS, Goldstone J, Moore WS, Towne JB, et al; The Veterans Affairs Cooperative Study Group. Efficacy of carotid endarterectomy for asymptomatic carotid stenosis. N Engl J Med. 1993 Jan 28;328(4):221–7.

Hollander M, Bots ML, Del Sol AI, Koudstaal PJ, Witteman JC, Grobbee DE, et al. Carotid plaques increase the risk of stroke and subtypes of cerebral infarction in asymptomatic elderly: the Rotterdam study. Circulation. 2002 Jun 18;105(24):2872–7.

Hosseini AA, Kandiyil N, Macsweeney ST, Altaf N, Auer DP. Carotid plaque hemorrhage on magnetic resonance imaging strongly predicts recurrent ischemia and stroke. Ann Neurol. 2013 Jun;73(6):774–84. Epub 2013 Jun 4.

International Carotid Stenting Study investigators, Ederle J, Dobson J, Featherstone RL, Bonati LH, van der Worp HB, de Borst GJ, et al. Carotid artery stenting compared with endarterectomy in patients with symptomatic carotid stenosis (International Carotid Stenting Study): an interim analysis of a randomised controlled trial. Lancet. 2010 Mar 20;375(9719):985–97. Epub 2010 Feb 25. Erratum in: Lancet. 2010 Jul 10;376(9735):90.

Jones DW, Brott TG, Schermerhorn ML. Trials and frontiers in carotid endarterectomy and stenting. Stroke. 2018 Jul;49(7):1776–83. Epub 2018 Jun 4.

Kernan WN, Ovbiagele B, Black HR, Bravata DM, Chimowitz MI, Ezekowitz MD, et al; American Heart Association Stroke Council, Council on Cardiovascular and Stroke Nursing, Council on Clinical Cardiology, and Council on Peripheral Vascular Disease. Guidelines for the prevention of stroke in patients with stroke and transient ischemic attack: a guideline for healthcare professionals from the American Heart Association/American Stroke Association. Stroke. 2014 Jul;45(7):2160–236. Epub 2014 May 1. Erratum in: Stroke. 2015 Feb;46(2):e54.

Kistler JP, Ropper AH, Heros RC. Therapy of ischemic cerebral vascular disease due to atherothrombosis (1). N Engl J Med. 1984 Jul 5;311(1):27–34.

Marcucci G, Accrocca F, Antonelli R, Giordano AG, Gabrielli R, Mounayergi F, et al. High-risk patients for carotid endarterectomy: turned down cases are rare. J Cardiovasc Surg (Torino). 2012 Jun;53(3):333–43.

Mas JL, Trinquart L, Leys D, Albucher JF, Rousseau H, Viguier A, et al; EVA-3S investigators. Endarterectomy Versus Angioplasty in Patients with Symptomatic Severe Carotid Stenosis (EVA-3S) trial: results up to 4 years from a randomised, multicentre trial. Lancet Neurol. 2008 Oct;7(10):885–92. Epub 2008 Sep 5.

Mayberg MR, Wilson SE, Yatsu F, Weiss DG, Messina L, Hershey LA, et al; Veterans Affairs Cooperative Studies Program 309 Trialist Group. Carotid endarterectomy and prevention of cerebral ischemia in symptomatic carotid stenosis. JAMA. 1991 Dec 18;266(23):3289–94.

North American Symptomatic Carotid Endarterectomy Trial. Methods, patient characteristics, and progress. Stroke. 1991 Jun;22(6):711–20.

Rothwell PM, Eliasziw M, Gutnikov SA, Fox AJ, Taylor DW, Mayberg MR, et al; Carotid Endarterectomy Trialists' Collaboration. Analysis of pooled data from the randomised controlled trials of endarterectomy for symptomatic carotid stenosis. Lancet. 2003 Jan 11;361(9352):107–16.

Rothwell PM, Gibson RJ, Slattery J, Sellar RJ, Warlow CP; European Carotid Surgery Trialists' Collaborative Group. Equivalence of measurements of carotid stenosis: a comparison of three methods on 1001 angiograms. Stroke. 1994 Dec;25(12):2435–9.

Sadat U, Teng Z, Young VE, Graves MJ, Gillard JH. Three-dimensional volumetric analysis of atherosclerotic plaques: a magnetic resonance imaging-based study of patients with moderate stenosis carotid artery disease. Int J Cardiovasc Imaging. 2010 Dec;26(8):897–904. Epub 2010 Jun 8.

Singh N, Moody AR, Gladstone DJ, Leung G, Ravikumar R, Zhan J, et al. Moderate carotid artery stenosis: MR imaging-depicted intraplaque hemorrhage predicts risk of cerebrovascular ischemic events in asymptomatic men. Radiology. 2009 Aug;252(2):502–8. Epub 2009 Jun 9.

SPACE Collaborative Group, Ringleb PA, Allenberg J, Bruckmann H, Eckstein HH, Fraedrich G, Hartmann M, et al. 30 day results from the SPACE trial of stent-protected angioplasty versus carotid endarterectomy in symptomatic patients: a randomised non-inferiority trial. Lancet. 2006 Oct 7;368(9543):1239–47. Erratum in: Lancet. 2006 Oct 7;368(9543):1238.

Suwanwela N, Can U, Furie KL, Southern JF, Macdonald NR, Ogilvy CS, et al. Carotid Doppler ultrasound criteria for internal carotid artery stenosis based on residual lumen diameter calculated from en bloc carotid endarterectomy specimens. Stroke. 1996 Nov;27(11):1965–9.

Wardlaw JM, Chappell FM, Best JJ, Wartolowska K, Berry E; NHS Research and Development Health Technology Assessment Carotid Stenosis Imaging Group. Non-invasive imaging compared with intra-arterial angiography in the diagnosis of symptomatic carotid stenosis: a meta-analysis. Lancet. 2006 May 6;367(9521):1503–12.

Yadav JS, Wholey MH, Kuntz RE, Fayad P, Katzen BT, Mishkel GJ, et al; Stenting and Angioplasty with Protection in Patients at High Risk for Endarterectomy Investigators. Protected carotid-artery stenting versus endarterectomy in high-risk patients. N Engl J Med. 2004 Oct 7;351(15):1493–501.

Adult Primary Central Nervous System Vasculitis

CARLO SALVARANI, MD; ROBERT D. BROWN JR, MD, MPH; GENE G. HUNDER, MD

Goals

- Describe the clinical features and diagnostic criteria of primary central nervous system vasculitis.
- Describe the most appropriate diagnostic tests for primary central nervous system vasculitis.
- Describe the rationale for an aggressive treatment approach for primary central nervous system vasculitis.

Introduction

Primary central nervous system vasculitis (PCNSV) is an infrequent and not well understood form of vasculitis that is limited to the brain and spinal cord. However, PCNSV is the most frequent vasculitis involving the central nervous system (CNS). Recognition of this vasculitis as a separate entity began in the mid-1950s, when Cravioto and Feigin described several cases of a "noninfectious granulomatous angiitis" with a predilection for the nervous system. In a study from Olmsted County, Minnesota, the incidence rate for PCNSV was calculated as 2.4 cases per 1,000,000 person-years. Men and women are similarly affected, and the median age at diagnosis is approximately 50 years.

Diagnosis

Diagnostic Criteria

Criteria for diagnosing PCNSV were proposed by Calabrese and Mallek in 1988. A diagnosis of PCNSV can be made if the following 3 criteria are satisfied: 1) history or clinical findings of an acquired neurologic deficit unexplained after a thorough initial basic evaluation; 2) cerebral angiogram with typical features of vasculitis or a CNS biopsy showing vasculitis; and 3) no evidence of systemic vasculitis or another condition that could account for the angiographic or pathologic features.

It is very likely that CNS vasculitis has been overdiagnosed, with many patients presenting with reversible cerebral vasoconstriction syndrome. This syndrome, reported over the years under many different names (postpartum angiopathy, migrainous vasospasm, drug-induced cerebral vasculopathy, and benign angiopathy of the CNS), is characterized by severe headaches, often thunderclap in nature, with or without other symptoms, and with segmental constriction of cerebral arteries on arterial imaging that resolves within 3 months. Approximately 60% of patients present in the postpartum period or after exposure to adrenergic or serotonergic drugs. The course is usually uniphasic. Diagnosis requires the identification of multifocal segmental cerebral artery vasoconstriction on cerebral angiography or magnetic resonance angiography (MRA), with complete or nearly complete resolution on subsequent examination within 12 weeks after onset. The treatment is calcium channel blockers and not immunosuppression.

Angiography

Angiographic findings suggestive of vasculitis include segments of intracranial arterial stenosis or occlusion, sometimes with intervening focal areas of dilatation. The findings typically involve several arterial segments (Figure 81.1A); findings in a single artery would be uncommon and should prompt other diagnostic considerations.

For patients with the usual clinical findings, cerebral angiography may provide strong support for the diagnosis, but certainty would require a CNS biopsy. Common

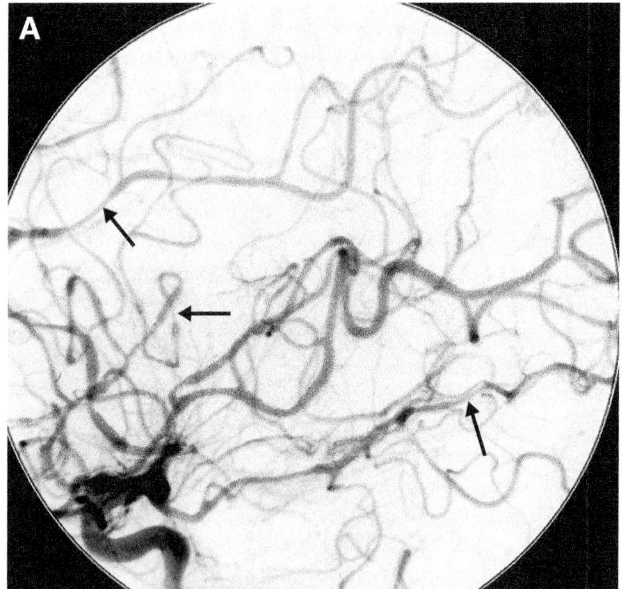

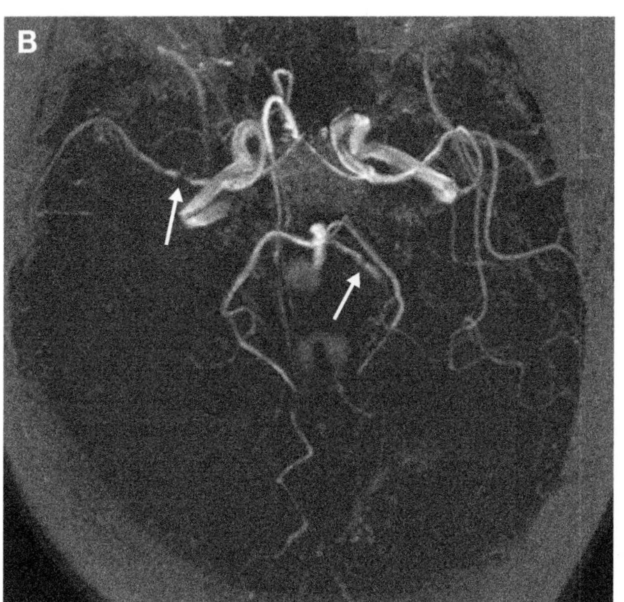

Figure 81.1. Imaging From Patients With Primary Central Nervous System Vasculitis (PCNSV). A, Cerebral angiogram shows alternating stenosis and dilatation consistent with PCNSV (arrows). B, Magnetic resonance angiography of the brain shows stenosis of the left posterior cerebral artery and the right middle cerebral artery (arrows).

angiographic diseases that mimic PCNSV include reversible cerebral vasoconstriction syndrome, atherosclerosis, emboli to cerebral arteries, infection, lymphoma, and vasospasm. Some patients with biopsy-proven PCNSV have normal cerebral angiographic findings, suggesting small-artery involvement that is beyond the resolution of angiography.

The sensitivity of angiography is 30% to 50%, and the specificity is about 30%. A cerebral angiogram with findings strongly suggestive of PCNSV should be considered in the context of magnetic resonance imaging (MRI) findings, the clinical presentation, and other laboratory assessment given that other disorders may show similar angiographic abnormalities. MRA and computed tomographic angiography (CTA) are less sensitive than standard angiography in the more distal intracranial arteries, but MRA (Figure 81.1B) and CTA can be helpful in the initial arterial imaging assessment of patients with possible PCNSV. If MRA findings are normal, but the patient has a typical clinical presentation for PCNSV and supporting laboratory abnormalities (ie, from MRI and cerebrospinal fluid [CSF]), cerebral angiography should be performed.

Magnetic Resonance Imaging

Most patients with PCNSV have abnormal MRI findings, but the findings are not specific for PCNSV. These

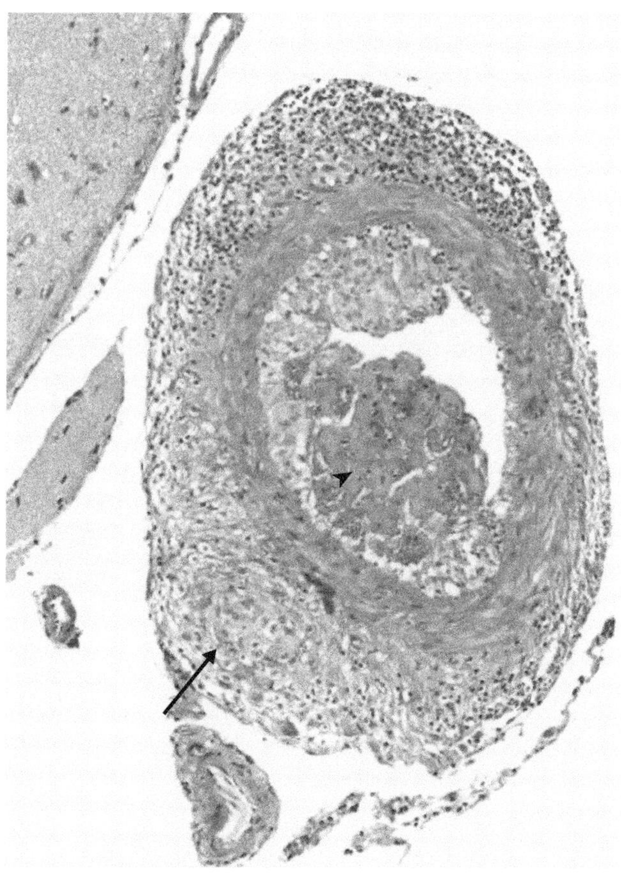

Figure 81.2. Histopathology of Granulomatous Primary Central Nervous System Vasculitis. This specimen shows leptomeningeal artery involvement with transmural inflammation, prominent mononuclear and granulomatous adventitial inflammation (arrow), and fibrin-rich thrombus formation (arrowhead) (hematoxylin-eosin, original magnification ×20).

findings may include multiple areas of increased T2-signal intensity or increased fluid-attenuated inversion recovery (FLAIR) signal subcortically, cerebral infarctions in cortical or subcortical locations, parenchymal and leptomeningeal enhancement, intracerebral and subarachnoid hemorrhage, and a tumorlike mass. Arterial wall thickening with contrast enhancement and perivascular enhancement may also be seen. On MRI, disorders that mimic PCNSV may have different vessel wall enhancement characteristics, such as the following: atherosclerosis tends to be eccentric, PCNSV tends to be concentric, and reversible cerebral vasoconstriction syndrome is associated with minimal enhancement.

Biopsy

A diagnosis of PCNSV can be made with certainty from cerebral and meningeal biopsy specimens. Although the risk from biopsy is low, serious complications occur in about 1% of patients. Biopsy findings suggesting vasculitis include transmural arterial inflammation in small and medium-sized leptomeningeal and parenchymal arteries. A granulomatous pattern occurs in about 60% of patients (Figure 81.2), a lymphocytic pattern in 30%, and a necrotizing pattern in 10%. The granulomatous pattern may be associated with β4-amyloid in about half the patients, but it is uncommon in other pathologic subtypes. In necrotizing vasculitis, the acute necrotizing inflammation

Table 81.1 • Clinical Manifestations at Presentation

Characteristic	All Patients (N=101), No. (%)	Diagnosis From Biopsy (n=31), No. (%)	Diagnosis From Angiography (n=70), No. (%)
Headache	64 (63)	16 (52)	48 (69)
Altered cognition	50 (50)	22 (71)	28 (40)
Hemiparesis	44 (44)	6 (19)	38 (54)
Persistent neurologic deficit or stroke	40 (40)	8 (26)	32 (46)
Aphasia	28 (28)	11 (36)	17 (24)
Transient ischemic attack	28 (28)	5 (16)	23 (33)
Ataxia	19 (19)	5 (16)	14 (20)
Seizure	16 (16)	2 (7)	14 (20)
Visual symptom (any kind)	42 (42)	9 (29)	33 (47)
Visual field defect	21 (21)	5 (16)	16 (23)
Diplopia (persistent or transient)	16 (16)	5 (16)	11 (16)
Blurred vision or decreased visual acuity	11 (11)	0 (0)	11 (16)
Monocular visual symptoms or amaurosis fugax	1 (1)	0 (0)	1 (1)
Papilledema	5 (5)	2 (7)	3 (4)
Intracranial hemorrhage	8 (8)	2 (7)	6 (9)
Amnestic syndrome	9 (9)	4 (13)	5 (7)
Paraparesis or quadriparesis	7 (7)	4 (13)	3 (4)
Parkinsonism or extrapyramidal sign	1 (1)	0 (0)	1 (1)
Prominent constitutional symptom	9 (9)	4 (13)	5 (7)
Fever	9 (9)	4 (13)	5 (7)
Nausea or vomiting	25 (25)	6 (19)	19 (27)
Vertigo or dizziness	9 (9)	3 (10)	6 (9)
Dysarthria	15 (15)	2 (7)	13 (19)
Unilateral numbness	13 (13)	0 (0)	13 (19)

Modified from Salvarani C, Brown RD Jr, Calamia KT, Christianson TJ, Weigand SD, Miller DV, et al. Primary central nervous system vasculitis: analysis of 101 patients. Ann Neurol. 2007 Nov;62(5):442–51; used with permission.

with transmural fibrinoid necrosis may mimic the findings in patients with polyarteritis nodosa. Since PCNSV may not affect all arteries in a diffuse manner, normal biopsy findings do not rule out the diagnosis. The likelihood of a biopsy providing a specific PCNSV diagnosis may be as high as 78% if the specimen is from an area of imaging abnormality; the likelihood is low without such imaging guidance.

Clinical Manifestations

The clinical symptoms and signs at the time of PCNSV diagnosis are summarized in Table 81.1. Most patients have several of these manifestations. While symptoms can have a sudden onset, most are slowly progressive. The most common manifestation is headache of various types and character; cognitive concerns are the next most common. Frequent focal symptoms include weakness, aphasia, ataxia, and visual deficit. More generalized symptoms such as fever and weight loss are uncommon. Paraparesis or quadriparesis, suggesting a spinal cord disorder, is infrequent.

Laboratory Testing

Laboratory testing can support a diagnosis of PCNSV. CSF assessment should be used to rule out infection or malignancy. On analysis of CSF, about 80% of patients have a

Table 81.2 • Characteristics and Outcome of Different PCNSV Subsets

Subset	Findings	Outcome
Angiography negative for PCNSV and PCNSV with prominent leptomeningeal enhancement: vasculitis of small vessels beyond the resolution of conventional angiography	Rapid clinical onset, frequently with a cognitive dysfunction Elevated CSF protein level Negative for PCNSV on angiography or MRA association with CAA Lesions with meningeal or parenchymal enhancment on MRI	Relapsing disease is frequent Favorable response to glucocorticoid therapy with rapid clinical improvement and favorable outcome
PCNSV with CAA: about 25% of patients with biopsy positive for PCNSV have evidence of cerebral amyloid vascular deposition (ABRA)	Patients are older than those with PCNSV without CAA but younger than those with CAA with no inflammation Cognitive dysfunction or seizures or spells at presentation Elevated CSF protein level Enhancing leptomeningeal lesions on MRI; negative on angiography or MRA Cerebral biopsy: granulomatous vasculitis and deposits of amyloid-β	Therapeutic response, survival, and outcome resemble those of PCNSV without CAA
Rapidly progressive PCNSV	Rapidly progressive course Bilateral, multiple, large cerebral vessel lesions on angiography and multiple bilateral cerebral infarctions on MRI Histopathologic pattern: granulomatous or necrotizing (or both)	Poor therapeutic response with rapidly progressive course and fatal outcome
PCNSV with spinal cord involvement	5% of patients Usually associated with cerebral involvement Predominantly affects the thoracic spinal cord	Frequent relapses, but response to therapy and outcome are usually favorable
PCNSV with intracranial hemorrhage	12% of patients Intracerebral hemorrhage is more common than subarachnoid hemorrhage, which is rare Altered cognition and persistent neurologic deficit are uncommon Evidence of cerebral infarction on MRI is uncommon Necrotizing vasculitis is the predominant histopathologic pattern	Therapeutic response and outcome are favorable, resembling those of patients without intracranial hemorrhage
PCNSV with tumorlike mass lesion	About 4% of patients Association with CAA in 29% of patients	Excision of the lesion may be curative Aggressive immunosuppressive therapy may obviate the need for surgery

Abbreviations: ABRA, amyloid-β–related angiitis; CAA, cerebral amyloid angiopathy; CSF, cerebrospinal fluid; MRA, magnetic resonance angiography; MRI, magnetic resonance imaging; PCNSV, primary central nervous system vasculitis.

Box 81.1 • Differential Diagnosis for Primary CNS Vasculitis

- Vasoconstriction syndromes
  - Reversible cerebral vasoconstriction syndrome (postpartum angiopathy, migrainous vasospasm, benign angiopathy of the CNS)
  - Drug-induced CNS vasculopathy (cocaine, amphetamine, ephedrine, and phenylpropanolamine)
- Secondary CNS vasculitis
  - Viral infections
    - Varicella-zoster virus
    - Human immunodeficiency virus
    - Hepatitis C virus
    - Cytomegalovirus
    - Parvovirus B19
  - Bacterial infections
    - *Treponema pallidum*
    - *Borrelia burgdorferi*
    - *Mycobacterium tuberculosis*
    - *Mycoplasma pneumoniae*
    - *Bartonella henselae*
    - *Rickettsia*
  - Fungal infections
    - Aspergillosis
    - Mucormycosis
    - Coccidioidomycosis
    - Candidiasis
  - Parasitic infections
    - Cysticercosis
  - Systemic vasculitides
    - Granulomatosis with polyangiitis
    - Churg-Strauss syndrome
    - Behçet disease
    - Polyarteritis nodosa
    - Henoch-Schönlein purpura
    - Kawasaki disease
    - Giant cell arteritis
    - Takayasu arteritis
  - Connective tissue diseases
    - Systemic lupus erythematosus
    - Rheumatoid arthritis
    - Sjögren syndrome
    - Dermatomyositis
    - Mixed connective tissue disease
  - Miscellaneous
    - Antiphospholipid antibody syndrome
    - Hodgkin lymphoma and non-Hodgkin lymphoma
    - Neurosarcoidosis
    - Inflammatory bowel disease
    - Graft-vs-host disease
    - Bacterial endocarditis
    - Acute bacterial meningitis

Abbreviation: CNS, central nervous system.

mild increase in the protein level or the white blood cell count (usually leukocytes). Blood test abnormalities, such as an elevated erythrocyte sedimentation rate or an elevated C-reactive protein level, occur in less than a third of patients.

PCNSV Subtypes and Differential Diagnosis

Several PCNSV subgroups have been suggested. Most likely, they differ in prognosis and management (Table 81.2).

The differential diagnosis includes 1) common diseases that mimic PCNSV and 2) secondary causes of CNS vasculitis (Box 81.1).

Treatment and Outcome

No randomized therapeutic trials for PCNSV have been reported, but a reasonable algorithm for PCNSV management based on practice experience is provided in Figure 81.3. Patients with inflammation restricted to small cortical and leptomeningeal vessels typically have a more benign course and generally respond favorably to glucocorticoid treatment with an initial dose of prednisone (1 mg/kg daily, or the equivalent). If a patient does not have a prompt response, oral or intravenous pulse cyclophosphamide, which has proved to be effective for other vasculitides, should be added. Less toxic drugs, such as azathioprine or mycophenolate mofetil, may be used instead of cyclophosphamide, but the data are limited on the efficacy of those treatment options. Patients with involvement of a large or proximal artery or rapidly progressive disease are typically treated with high doses of intravenous methylprednisolone (1,000 mg daily for 3-5 days) and cyclophosphamide. After that initial aggressive treatment, another immunosuppressive agent, such as azathioprine or mycophenolate mofetil, may be used to sustain remission. The treatment course is typically 12 to 18 months. If a patient has serious adverse effects or a lack of response to cyclophosphamide, tumor necrosis factor α blockers or rituximab may be considered.

The risk of glucocorticoid-related osteoporosis is reduced with the use of calcium (1,000-1,500 mg daily) and vitamin D (800 international units daily). Weekly bisphosphonate therapy should be added for postmenopausal women and for men older than 50 years. The risk of *Pneumocystis jiroveci* infection is lessened with trimethoprim-sulfamethoxazole (800/160 mg on alternate days or 400/80 mg daily) and is

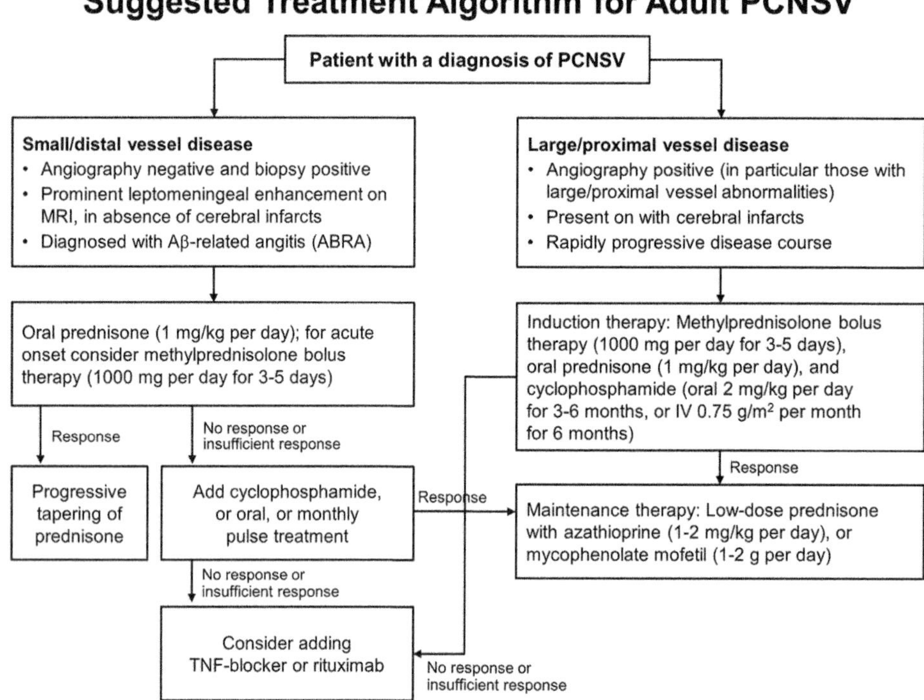

Figure 81.3. Suggested Treatment Algorithm for Adults With Primary Central Nervous System Vasculitis (PCNSV). ABRA indicates amyloid-β–related angiitis; IV, intravenously; MRI, magnetic resonance imaging; TNF, tumor necrosis factor. *(From Salvarani C, Brown RD Jr, Christianson T, Miller DV, Giannini C, Huston J 3rd, et al. An update of the Mayo Clinic cohort of patients with adult primary central nervous system vasculitis: description of 163 patients. Medicine [Baltimore]. 2015 May;94[21]:e738; used with permission.)*

recommended for patients receiving cyclophosphamide and rituximab.

Even though therapy is helpful and may be lifesaving, patients with PCNSV have an increased mortality rate. The higher rates of mortality and disability are usually associated with characteristics related to involvement of larger arteries (Table 81.2).

Summary

- The gold standard for the diagnosis of PCNSV is a brain or spinal cord biopsy.
- A cerebral angiogram with findings strongly suggestive of PCNSV should be considered in the context of MRI findings, the clinical presentation, and other laboratory assessments.
- The prognosis and most effective management differ according to the subgroup of PCNSV.
- Early diagnosis and therapy may lessen the likelihood of an adverse outcome.
- The majority of patients show improvement after receiving glucocorticoids alone or in combination with cyclophosphamide.

SUGGESTED READING

Byram K, Hajj-Ali RA, Calabrese L. CNS vasculitis: an approach to differential diagnosis and management. Curr Rheumatol Rep. 2018 May 30;20(7):37.

Calabrese LH, Mallek JA. Primary angiitis of the central nervous system: report of 8 new cases, review of the literature, and proposal for diagnostic criteria. Medicine (Baltimore). 1988 Jan;67(1):20–39.

Cravioto H, Feigin I. Noninfectious granulomatous angiitis with a predilection for the nervous system. Neurology. 1959 Sep;9:599–609.

Duna GF, Calabrese LH. Limitations of invasive modalities in the diagnosis of primary angiitis of the central nervous system. J Rheumatol. 1995 Apr;22(4):662–7.

Dutra LA, de Souza AW, Grinberg-Dias G, Barsottini OG, Appenzeller S. Central nervous system vasculitis in adults: an update. Autoimmun Rev. 2017 Feb;16(2):123–31. Epub 2017 Jan 11.

Giannini C, Salvarani C, Hunder G, Brown RD. Primary central nervous system vasculitis: pathology and mechanisms. Acta Neuropathol. 2012 Jun;123(6):759–72. Epub 2012 Mar 16.

John S, Hajj-Ali RA. CNS vasculitis. Semin Neurol. 2014 Sep;34(4):405–12. Epub 2014 Nov 4.

Kadkhodayan Y, Alreshaid A, Moran CJ, Cross DT 3rd, Powers WJ, Derdeyn CP. Primary angiitis of the central nervous system at conventional angiography. Radiology. 2004 Dec;233(3):878–82. Epub 2004 Oct 21.

Limaye K, Samaniego EA, Adams HP Jr. Diagnosis and treatment of primary central nervous system angiitis. Curr Treat Options Neurol. 2018 Aug 4;20(9):38.

Miller DV, Salvarani C, Hunder GG, Brown RD, Parisi JE, Christianson TJ, et al. Biopsy findings in primary angiitis of the central nervous system. Am J Surg Pathol. 2009 Jan;33(1):35–43.

Molloy ES, Singhal AB, Calabrese LH. Tumour-like mass lesion: an under-recognised presentation of primary angiitis of the central nervous system. Ann Rheum Dis. 2008 Dec;67(12):1732–5. Epub 2008 Jul 14.

Moore PM. Diagnosis and management of isolated angiitis of the central nervous system. Neurology. 1989 Feb;39(2 Pt 1):167–73.

Obusez EC, Hui F, Hajj-Ali RA, Cerejo R, Calabrese LH, Hammad T, et al. High-resolution MRI vessel wall imaging: spatial and temporal patterns of reversible cerebral vasoconstriction syndrome and central nervous system vasculitis. AJNR Am J Neuroradiol. 2014 Aug;35(8):1527–32. Epub 2014 Apr 10.

Salvarani C, Brown RD Jr, Calamia KT, Christianson TJ, Weigand SD, Miller DV, et al. Primary central nervous system vasculitis: analysis of 101 patients. Ann Neurol. 2007 Nov;62(5):442–51.

Salvarani C, Brown RD Jr, Christianson TJ, Huston J 3rd, Giannini C, Miller DV, et al. Adult primary central nervous system vasculitis treatment and course: analysis of one hundred sixty-three patients. Arthritis Rheumatol. 2015 Jun;67(6):1637–45.

Salvarani C, Pipitone N, Hunder GG. Management of primary and secondary central nervous system vasculitis. Curr Opin Rheumatol. 2016 Jan;28(1):21–8.

Younger DS. Treatment of vasculitis of the nervous system. Neurol Clin. 2019 May;37(2):399–423. Epub 2019 Mar 18.

82 Intracerebral and Intraventricular Hemorrhage

OANA DUMITRASCU, MD; MARIA I. AGUILAR, MD

Goals

- Recognize the types of intracerebral hemorrhage according to their location and possible pathogenesis.
- Review the medical management of intracerebral hemorrhage and intraventricular hemorrhage, including reversal of anticoagulation.
- Review the indications for neurosurgical treatment of intracerebral hemorrhage and intraventricular hemorrhage.

Introduction

Intraparenchymal cerebral hemorrhage and intraventricular hemorrhage are common cerebrovascular emergencies with various causes and prognoses. Rapid triage and individualized management are required because appropriate critical care management improves morbidity and mortality. A multidisciplinary approach for diagnosis and treatment is recommended.

Epidemiology of Intracerebral Hemorrhage

Intracerebral hemorrhage (ICH), also termed *intraparenchymal hemorrhage,* is defined as bleeding into the cerebrum. The incidence of spontaneous nontraumatic ICH is 12 to 15 cases per 100,000 per year and is highest among Japanese and African Americans. ICH risk factors are shown in Box 82.1. Among the types of ICH, 35% to 70% are deep (ie, in the basal ganglia), whereas 5% to 10% occur in the posterior fossa (brainstem and cerebellum). Lobar hemorrhages (15%-30% of cases) occur in cortical-subcortical areas within the cerebral lobes, and 12% to 14% of ICH cases are associated with vitamin K antagonists (VKAs). The use of direct oral anticoagulants (DOACs) presents lower ICH relative risks than VKAs.

Pathophysiology of ICH

Spontaneous noncoagulopathic ICH results from rupture of small penetrating arteries (Charcot-Bouchard microaneurysms and lipohyalinosis). The mechanical effect to brain parenchyma causes primary ICH injury. Secondary injury occurs from perihemorrhagic inflammation, blood breakdown products, and perihematomal edema. Coagulopathic ICH expands for up to 24 hours; noncoagulopathic ICH, for up to 6 hours. According to magnetic resonance (MR) imaging, most ICH edema is cytotoxic. Aggressive lowering of systolic blood pressure (BP) (to <120 mm Hg) could induce perihematomal ischemia, microvasculopathy, and increased intracranial pressure (ICP).

Amyloid deposition within meningeal and cortical capillaries, arterioles, and vessel walls of small arteries causes cerebral amyloid angiopathy (CAA). Vascular amyloid is similar to that in brain plaques in Alzheimer disease but different from that in systemic amyloidosis. Congophilic material induces perivascular inflammation, microaneurysms, and fibrinoid necrosis.

ICH after administration of intravenous (IV) recombinant tissue plasminogen activator (rtPA) is caused by breakdown of the blood-brain barrier and lingering effects of the rtPA.

Differential Diagnosis of ICH

Determining the cause of ICH requires a critical clinical review of historical factors, a thorough physical examination, a review of the patient's current medications, and

Box 82.1 • Risk Factors for Intracerebral Hemorrhage (ICH)

- Hypertension—mainly for deep ICH (ie, in the basal ganglia)
- Cerebral amyloid angiopathy—mainly for lobar ICH (ie, in cortical-subcortical areas within the central lobes)
- Advanced age—higher incidence among persons older than 85 years
- Anticoagulation intensity
- Leukoaraiosis or white matter disease
- Previous stroke or ICH
- Hematologic abnormalities
  - Anticoagulant-induced coagulopathy
  - Use of antiplatelet agents
  - Congenital and acquired factor deficiencies
  - Thrombocytopenic or thrombocytopathic disorders
  - Lymphoproliferative disorders
- Chronic kidney disease
- Trauma and falls
- Aneurysm or vascular malformations
- Alcohol consumption
- Drug abuse—amphetamine, cocaine, heroin, and ecstasy

Box 82.2 • Differential Diagnosis of Intracerebral Hemorrhage

- Hypertensive—most commonly basal ganglia, internal capsule, pons, and cerebellum
- Cerebral amyloid angiopathy—commonly lobar and in older patients
- Arteriovenous malformation
- Cavernous malformation
- Aneurysmal rupture—can result in both subarachnoid hemorrhage and intraparenchymal cerebral hemorrhage
- Primary central nervous system tumor
- Metastatic tumor—renal cell carcinoma, melanoma, lung cancer, and choriocarcinoma
- Bleeding diathesis—low platelet count and disseminated intravascular coagulation
- Hemorrhagic conversion of ischemic stroke
- Venous hypertension and infarction—typically cortical
- Traumatic contusion—usually frontal pole and tip of temporal lobe
- Medications—sympathomimetics, thrombolytics, and warfarin
- Moyamoya disease—typically basal ganglia
- Vasculitis

neuroimaging. The differential diagnosis of ICH is shown in Box 82.2. Hypertensive ICHs are located deep (in descending order of frequency: basal ganglia, subcortical white matter, cerebellum, thalamus, and pons) and attributed to degenerative changes in the vessel wall associated with age, hypertension, and diabetes mellitus. CAA is the most common cause of lobar ICH in the elderly. Patients with CAA have a high risk of recurrent ICH, especially with apolipoprotein E ε2 or ε4 alleles, which may constitute a hereditary form of CAA. Coagulopathy-associated ICH is lobar more often than deep and is associated with larger bleeding volumes and higher mortality. ICHs after IV rtPA are lobar and multifocal, with blood-plasma or fluid-fluid levels on computed tomography (CT) and less perihematomal edema.

Clinical Presentation of ICH

Patients with ICH present with abrupt-onset strokelike symptoms and focal neurologic deficits that correspond to neuroanatomical localization and progress over minutes to hours. These patients are more likely to have headache, nausea, and vomiting than patients with ischemic stroke, and they are more likely to have a depressed level of consciousness (LOC) due to elevated ICP, obstructive or nonobstructive hydrocephalus, brainstem compression or herniation, convulsive or nonconvulsive seizures, or a postictal state.

Diagnostic Evaluation of ICH

The first diagnostic step is to quickly ascertain medical history, current medications, history of trauma, malignancy, brain vascular malformations or aneurysms, recent neurosurgical procedures, and use of alcohol or illicit drugs. Additional clues are seizure at onset, coagulopathy risk factors (eg, use of VKAs or DOACs), liver disease, and hematologic disorders (eg, thrombocytopenia or leukemia).

Physical Examination

In addition to evaluation of vital signs, an examination should proceed quickly from head to toe with assessment for signs of trauma to the head, neck, or body that might suggest the need for immobilization of the cervical spine. In lieu of a standard neurologic examination, the Glasgow Coma Scale (GCS) score is determined for assessing airway protection. The National Institutes of Health Stroke Scale is sometimes used to grade the severity of ICH-related deficits in conjunction with medical measures for stabilizing the patient's condition. The Full Outline of Unresponsiveness (FOUR), another useful LOC scale, has 4 components (each is scored from 0-4): eye response, motor response, brainstem reflexes, and respiration. The FOUR is validated and superior to the GCS because a FOUR score of zero is equivalent to brain death criteria, the FOUR score is used to assess brainstem function that can deteriorate with herniation, and the FOUR score remains testable in intubated patients. Lower FOUR scores predict higher in-hospital mortality compared with GCS scores.

Diagnostic Testing

Patients with ICH should have a complete blood cell count, coagulation tests (prothrombin time [PT], international normalized ratio [INR], and activated partial thromboplastin time [aPTT]), measurement of blood glucose level, and electrocardiography (ECG). Urgent noncontrast CT of the head is performed to diagnose acute ICH, which appears as a hyperdense area (ie, bright or white). Hyperdensity that is consistent with blood is apparent immediately after the onset of an ICH. Isodense blood products that are less bright on CT are seen when patients have anemia and fluid-fluid levels in coagulopathic ICH. On CT, the appearance of subacute to chronic ICH (≥6 weeks) changes from hyperdense to isodense to, finally, hypodense fluid cavities.

ICH volume, estimated with the ABC/2 method (Figure 82.1), is a predictor of 30-day mortality. Another CT finding is the *black hole sign*, which is a relatively hypoattenuated area that is encapsulated within the hyperattenuating hematoma and is not connected with the adjacent brain tissue.

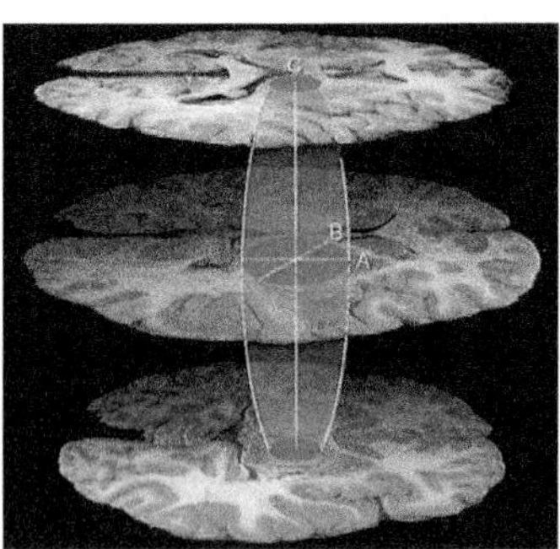

Figure 82.1. Calculation of Intracerebral Hemorrhage (ICH) by the ABC/2 Method. The computed tomographic (CT) slice with the largest area of hematoma is identified. The largest diameter of ICH in that slice, measured in centimeters, is A. B *is the largest diameter of ICH 90° to* A. *The number of vertical CT slices in which ICH is seen is* C. C *is multiplied by slice thickness. For example, if* A *and* B *are each 3 cm, and if* C *is 3 slices and each CT slice is 5 mm,* (A×B×C)/2 = (3 cm × 3 cm × 3 × 0.5 cm)/2 = 6.75 cm^3 = 6.75 mL.
(From Freeman WD, Aguilar MI. Intracranial hemorrhage: diagnosis and management. Neurol Clin. 2012 Feb;30[1]:211–40; used with permission.)

The black hole sign has 31.9% sensitivity and 94.1% specificity when used to predict hematoma growth.

CT angiography of the head and contrast-enhanced CT should be used to identify patients at risk for ICH related to aneurysm or vascular malformation and to look for the *spot sign* (leakage of contrast material within the hematoma), which, as a predictor of hematoma expansion (HE), has 51% sensitivity and 85% specificity. The HE prediction score is an accurate predictor of the probability of substantial HE (defined as an absolute increase in ICH volume >6 mL or an increase >33% on follow-up CT). The ratio of initial ICH volume to the onset-to-imaging time can also be used to predict HE and outcome.

When clinical or radiologic suspicion exists, CT or MR venography and MR angiography are useful for evaluating underlying structural lesions (eg, vascular malformations or multifocal segmental cerebral vasoconstriction). Contrast-enhanced MR imaging of the brain is useful for identifying posterior fossa hemorrhages or underlying structural abnormalities (tumors) and for determining the timing of ICH. Gradient ultrasonography is used to identify silent microhemorrhages in CAA or cavernous malformations.

Catheter angiography should be performed if suspicion is high for an intracranial aneurysm or arteriovenous malformation (in lobar hemorrhages) or for an atypically located ICH. Catheter angiography is also useful for young patients who have ICH and the cause is not obvious.

Management of ICH

Management of ICH begins with triage by using an LOC scale (eg, FOUR or GCS). Rapid-sequence intubation is suggested for patients with severely depressed LOC, no airway protection (GCS score ≤8 and no gag or cough response), or respiratory failure.

Medical Monitoring

Most patients with ICH are admitted to a neurosciences intensive care or stroke unit for close monitoring of impending neurologic deterioration. Blood glucose levels should be kept in the normoglycemic range (140-180 mg/dL). Normothermia is the goal (36.6°C-37°C). Acetaminophen and topical cooling methods are indicated for fever. Fever should prompt a workup for sepsis (eg, aspiration pneumosepsis or urosepsis), and administration of antibiotics should be timely.

BP Control

The optimal BP goal is controversial despite 2 landmark trials (Antihypertensive Treatment of Acute Cerebral Hemorrhage II [ATACH-2] trial and Intensive Blood Pressure Reduction in Acute Cerebral Hemorrhage Trial [INTERACT]). In the absence of contraindications to decreasing the BP, current guidelines suggest that if systolic BP is 150 to 220 mm Hg, it can be decreased to 140 mm Hg safely and effectively to improve functional outcome without increasing the risk of death or serious complications. Recommended antihypertensive agents include labetalol (5- to 20-mg bolus every 15 minutes or 2 mg/min); nicardipine (5-15 mg/h); enalapril (1.25-5 mg IV every 6 hours as needed); hydralazine (5-10 mg every 30 minutes as needed or 1.5-5 mcg/kg/min); and sodium nitroprusside (0.1-10 mcg/kg/min). At most medical centers, sodium nitroprusside is not given because it may increase ICP (it is a nonselective arteriovenous dilator) and cause cyanide toxicity with long-term use.

Seizure Control

Prophylactic antiseizure medication is recommended for patients who had a seizure at the onset of the ICH, but its routine use is not recommended in the absence of symptomatic ICH-related seizures. Patients with depressed LOC or coma have a higher risk for subclinical or purely electrographic seizures and can be evaluated with electroencephalography (EEG) before administration of antiseizure medication. Prolonged EEG monitoring has a higher yield when patients have depressed LOC that is out of proportion to the degree of brain injury seen on imaging because electrographic seizures may be intermittent.

Thromboprophylaxis for Deep Vein Thrombosis and Pulmonary Embolism

Patients with ICH have high thromboembolic risk due to immobility, hospitalization, and the inflammatory state. Intermittent pneumatic compression for prevention of deep vein thrombosis (DVT) and pulmonary embolism (PE) should start on the day of hospital admission. Graduated compression stockings are not recommended. The early use of a prophylactic dose of enoxaparin on postadmission days 1 through 6 decreases the risk of PE, decreases the risk of death (but not statistically significantly), and provides no difference for DVT or HE, but its use can be considered if the findings on neuroimaging are stable. Use of systemic anticoagulation for 7 to 14 days is considered for selected patients with symptomatic DVT or PE and stabilized ICH after having a neurosurgical consultation and weighing the risk-benefit ratio if ICH recurs. Inferior vena cava filters are temporary measures that only prevent major saddle PE. They should be used in conjunction with medical anticoagulation and removed after 3 months of anticoagulation if the DVT has resolved.

Coagulopathy Management

The first steps in coagulopathy management are to identify patients at risk who are taking VKAs or DOACs, have an increased PT or aPTT, and are not receiving anticoagulation or having sudden thrombocytopenia. A hematologist should be consulted. For known coagulation factor deficiencies or platelet disorders, replacement with the appropriate factors or platelets is indicated. For patients receiving IV heparin infusion, IV protamine sulfate should be given immediately (1 mg/100 units heparin, up to a maximum of 50 mg). A similar dose of protamine sulfate can be administered for low-molecular-weight heparinoids, but its reversal effects will be only partial. For ICH patients receiving antiplatelet agents, the usefulness of platelet transfusion is controversial according to the results of the Platelet Transfusion Versus Standard Care After Acute Stroke Due to Spontaneous Cerebral Hemorrhage Associated With Antiplatelet Therapy (PATCH) trial and others that identified medical complications in patients receiving platelet transfusion.

Management With VKAs and DOACs

The use of VKAs should be discontinued immediately, and the INR emergently corrected if it is greater than 1.5. DOACs are newer anticoagulants that include dabigatran (a direct thrombin inhibitor) and the factor Xa inhibitors apixaban, rivaroxaban, and edoxaban. Anticoagulant and antithrombotic-related ICH guidelines are summarized in Box 82.3.

Restarting anticoagulation is individualized and depends on the cause of ICH. Resuming anticoagulation in warfarin-associated ICH increases the risk of traumatic ICH and extracranial hemorrhage. In deep or hypertensive ICH, anticoagulation should be resumed after weighing the embolic risk-factors against the risk of death from recurrent ICH. If an ICH poses a high risk of embolism (eg, the patient has a prosthetic heart valve or a high risk for cardioembolic stroke due to atrial fibrillation), discontinuation of warfarin therapy for 1 to 2 weeks carries a comparatively low probability of an embolic event, and ICH recurrence that soon is exceedingly uncommon.

Surgical Treatment

The classic indications for neurosurgical evacuation are 1) lobar hematomas within 1 cm of the surface and larger than 30 mL and 2) cerebellar hemorrhages (typically >3 cm) in patients with neurologic deterioration, brainstem compression, or hydrocephalus from ventricular obstruction.

For patients with supratentorial ICH, randomized trials that compared surgery performed early in the course of ICH with conservative treatment found no significant difference in mortality or 6-month functional outcome. Meta-analysis showed that surgical treatment in combination with medical treatment is associated with a significant decrease in mortality or dependency at final follow-up. Surgical timing is controversial. Ultra-early craniotomy (ie, within 4 hours) increased the risk of rebleeding, whereas patients who underwent craniotomy within 8 hours had improved outcomes. The Minimally Invasive

Box 82.3 • Guidelines for Use of Anticoagulant Reversal Agents for Symptomatic Patients With ICH

Warfarin and other VKAs

The goal is to decrease the INR to at least 1.5.

For ICH that is considered a medical or surgical emergency, 5 to 10 mg vitamin K (phytonadione) should be administered IV slowly. The onset of action is within 2 hours and is maximal by 24 hours if hepatic function is normal. Vitamin K is insufficient for reversal of warfarin or VKA in the first few hours because it does not fully correct the INR until about 24 hours through production of synthetic factors.

FFP is often given also, but it takes up to 24 hours to correct the INR (partially because of FFP thawing time and proper blood bank crossmatching). FFP may require a large intravascular volume (eg, 2 L), which can lead to cardiovascular volume overload, pulmonary edema, and hypoxemia. FFP carries a small risk of allergic and infectious transfusion reactions (eg, TRALI).

PCC is a smaller, more concentrated human coagulation factor concentrate that can be given faster than FFP. If given quickly (up to 150 IU/min), 25 to 50 IU/kg PCC usually normalizes the INR within 30 to 60 minutes. Although no trials have directly compared different PCC products for clinical outcomes, because PCC has fewer overall complications and corrects INR faster, PCC should be considered over FFP whenever PCC is available.

rFVIIa works quickly, safely decreasing the INR within 15 minutes, but it does not replace all the vitamin K cofactors of factors II, VII, IX, and X. rFVIIa was studied in the FAST trial of warfarin-associated ICH, but rFVIIa did not improve outcomes, and it increased thromboembolic complications. rFVIIa is not recommended for VKA reversal unless it is for ICH associated with hemophilia.

Dabigatran

Dabigatran is the only DOAC that has an FDA-approved agent for reversal. Idarucizumab (a humanized monoclonal antibody fragment) 5 g IV reverses dabigatran-related coagulopathy within minutes and induces normal hemostasis without safety concerns.

Immediate discontinuation of dabigatran and use of activated charcoal are recommended if the most recent dose was taken within the previous 2 hours. Hemodialysis was reported in severe systemic bleeding for dabigatran, but its practicality is uncertain now that idarucizumab is available. Before idarucizumab, the use of anti-inhibitor coagulant complex or rFVIIa showed minimal efficacy.

Factor Xa inhibitors

Andexanet alfa is given as a 400-mg bolus over 15 minutes, and the infusion dose is 480 mg.

PCC has a partial effect.

FFP and vitamin K are ineffective in reversing any DOAC.

Heparinoids: UFH and LMWH

Ciraparantag (formerly known as aripazine) is a synthetic cationic molecule that binds to UFH, LMWH, edoxaban, rivaroxaban, apixaban, and dabigatran.

If protamine sulfate is given (1 mg/100 units heparin, up to a maximum of 50 mg), a high dose should be administered cautiously to avoid hypotension.

The reversal of heparinoids is still being studied.

IV rtPA

Reversal agents are cryoprecipitate (6-8 units) and ε-aminocaproic acid (4-5 g IV and then 1 g orally or IV hourly until bleeding is controlled). Fibrinogen should be rechecked every 4 hours and cryoprecipitate transfused as needed to maintain fibrinogen levels greater than 150 mg/dL.

Control BP according to rtPA guidelines and BP management in postthrombolysis ICH.

Abbreviations: BP, blood pressure; DOAC, direct oral anticoagulant; FAST, Factor Seven for Acute Hemorrhagic Stroke; FDA, US Food and Drug Administration; FFP, fresh frozen plasma; ICH, intracerebral hemorrhage; INR, international normalized ratio; IU, international units; IV, intravenous; LMWH, low-molecular-weight heparin; PCC, prothrombin complex concentrate; rFVIIa, recombinant factor VIIa; rtPA, recombinant tissue plasminogen activator; TRALI, transfusion-related acute lung injury; UFH, unfractionated heparin; VKA, vitamin K antagonist.

Surgery Plus rtPA for ICH Evacuation (MISTIE) trial aimed to determine the safety of minimally invasive surgery in combination with rtPA and found a significant decrease in perihematomal edema with hematoma evacuation and a trend toward improved outcomes. Meta-analysis suggested that minimally invasive surgery may be superior to larger craniotomy, but results from the MISTIE III trial (best medical management vs a minimally invasive approach) were essentially negative with no improvement in outcome. The benefit of neurosurgical treatment of deeper ICH 30 mL or larger has not been determined, but the Early Minimally Invasive Removal of Intracerebral Hemorrhage (ENRICH) trial is comparing minimally invasive neurosurgical therapy with conservative management.

ICP Monitoring and Treatment

Measurement of ICP requires placement of an ICP probe or ventricular drain even if clinical signs suggest that the patient has an increased ICP or herniation. Indications for placement of an ICP monitor include patients not expected to die soon who have a GCS score of 8 or less, transtentorial herniation, clinically significant intraventricular hemorrhage (IVH), and hydrocephalus. After the ICP monitor has been placed, the target cerebral perfusion pressure should be 50 to 70 mm Hg. Interventions for decreasing ICP include elevating the head of the patient's bed 30° to 45°; mannitol (0.25 to 1 g/kg IV as needed); hypertonic saline 3% as an infusion (30-60 mL/h) or hypertonic saline 23.4% as a bolus (15- to 30-mL boluses) while monitoring sodium levels every 4 to 6 hours (target, 145-155 mmol/L); sedation; intubation; mechanical ventilation; and paralytic agents. Corticosteroids are not indicated because most ICH edema is cytotoxic rather than vasogenic. Ventricular drainage can be used for symptomatic hydrocephalus.

Outcomes of ICH

The most powerful predictors of poor outcome are ICH volume greater than 60 mL and a GCS score of less than 8. Additional predictors are deep location, intraventricular extension, time to presentation, withdrawal of medical support, and do-not-attempt-resuscitation orders on the first day of hospitalization.

Intraventricular Hemorrhage

IVH is bleeding within the cerebrospinal fluid (CSF)-filled ventricles. IVH can be primary (ie, isolated bleeding within 1 or more ventricles) or secondary (ie, ICH extension from the parenchyma into 1 or more ventricles). The differential diagnosis is shown in Box 82.4. IVH occurs in 45% to 50% of patients with spontaneous ICH and independently correlates with poor outcome and higher mortality. IVH volume is an independent predictor of mortality. Traumatic IVH is considered when the history or findings support trauma.

Box 82.4 • Differential Diagnosis of Intraventricular Hemorrhage (IVH)

Primary IVH—cerebral aneurysm, arteriovenous malformation, trauma, coagulopathy, choroid plexus tumor, and ependymal lesion

Secondary IVH—spontaneous intracerebral hemorrhage with IVH extension (45%-50% of patients) or aneurysm (10%-30% of patients)

Standard treatment of IVH with acute obstructive hydrocephalus includes placement of a CSF drain through an external ventriculostomy. Meta-analysis of patients with secondary IVH treated with either a ventricular catheter (VC) or a VC in combination with intraventricular fibrinolysis found that the patients treated with urokinase had a significant decrease in mortality with similar complications. Patients treated with intraventricular rtPA had significantly lower ICP and fewer VC obstructions and a nonsignificantly shorter requirement for VC in the Clot Lysis Evaluation of Accelerated Resolution of Intraventricular Hemorrhage (CLEAR) III trial. The CLEAR III trial did not show improved outcomes with intraventricular rtPA compared with saline irrigation every 8 hours; in a subanalysis, intraventricular rtPA worked best for patients with a high IVH score and considerable IVH in all ventricles.

Summary

- *Intracranial hemorrhage* is defined as any bleeding within the intracranial vault and includes ICH and IVH.
- Most ICH is associated with chronic hypertension, which is a risk factor for deep (ie, basal ganglia) ICH; superficial ICH in elderly patients is often associated with CAA.
- Immediate reversal of anticoagulation and moderate BP control with medical management are the standard of care for patients with ICH or IVH.
- In patients who have ICH or IVH with symptomatic hydrocephalus, an external ventricular drain for CSF diversion can be considered.
- ICH has only certain neurosurgical indications, including an ICH larger than 3 cm in the posterior fossa and symptomatic hydrocephalus from IVH.

SUGGESTED READING

Aguilar MI, Brott TG. Update in intracerebral hemorrhage. Neurohospitalist. 2011 Jul;1(3):148–59.

Chatterjee S, Sardar P, Biondi-Zoccai G, Kumbhani DJ. New oral anticoagulants and the risk of intracranial hemorrhage: traditional and Bayesian meta-analysis and mixed treatment comparison of randomized trials of new oral anticoagulants in atrial fibrillation. JAMA Neurol. 2013 Dec;70(12):1486–90.

Claassen DO, Kazemi N, Zubkov AY, Wijdicks EF, Rabinstein AA. Restarting anticoagulation therapy after warfarin-associated intracerebral hemorrhage. Arch Neurol. 2008 Oct;65(10):1313–8.

Demchuk AM, Dowlatshahi D, Rodriguez-Luna D, Molina CA, Blas YS, Dzialowski I, et al; PREDICT/Sunnybrook ICH CTA study group. Prediction of haematoma growth and outcome in patients with intracerebral haemorrhage using the CT-angiography spot sign (PREDICT): a prospective observational study. Lancet Neurol. 2012

Apr;11(4):307–14. Epub 2012 Mar 8. Erratum in: Lancet Neurol. 2012 Jun;11(6):483.

Freeman WD, Aguilar MI. Intracranial hemorrhage: diagnosis and management. Neurol Clin. 2012 Feb;30(1):211–40.

Frontera JA, Lewin JJ 3rd, Rabinstein AA, Aisiku IP, Alexandrov AW, Cook AM, et al. Guideline for reversal of antithrombotics in intracranial hemorrhage: a statement for healthcare professionals from the Neurocritical Care Society and Society of Critical Care Medicine. Neurocrit Care. 2016 Feb;24(1):6–46.

Gaberel T, Magheru C, Parienti JJ, Huttner HB, Vivien D, Emery E. Intraventricular fibrinolysis versus external ventricular drainage alone in intraventricular hemorrhage: a meta-analysis. Stroke. 2011 Oct;42(10):2776–81. Epub 2011 Aug 4.

Gross BA, Jankowitz BT, Friedlander RM. Cerebral intraparenchymal hemorrhage: a review. JAMA. 2019 Apr 2;321(13):1295–1303.

Hallevi H, Albright KC, Aronowski J, Barreto AD, Martin-Schild S, Khaja AM, et al. Intraventricular hemorrhage: anatomic relationships and clinical implications. Neurology. 2008 Mar 11;70(11):848–52.

Hanley DF, Thompson RE, Rosenblum M, Yenokyan G, Lane K, McBee N, et al; MISTIE III Investigators. Efficacy and safety of minimally invasive surgery with thrombolysis in intracerebral haemorrhage evacuation (MISTIE III): a randomised, controlled, open-label, blinded endpoint phase 3 trial. Lancet. 2019 Mar 9;393(10175):1021–32. Epub 2019 Feb 7. Erratum in: Lancet. 2019 Apr 20;393(10181):1596.

Hemphill JC 3rd, Greenberg SM, Anderson CS, Becker K, Bendok BR, Cushman M, et al; American Heart Association Stroke Council; Council on Cardiovascular and Stroke Nursing; Council on Clinical Cardiology. Guidelines for the management of spontaneous intracerebral hemorrhage: a guideline for healthcare professionals from the American Heart Association/American Stroke Association. Stroke. 2015 Jul;46(7):2032–60. Epub 2015 May 28.

Kothari RU, Brott T, Broderick JP, Barsan WG, Sauerbeck LR, Zuccarello M, et al. The ABCs of measuring intracerebral hemorrhage volumes. Stroke. 1996 Aug;27(8):1304–5.

Li N, Worthmann H, Heeren M, Schuppner R, Deb M, Tryc AB, et al. Temporal pattern of cytotoxic edema in the perihematomal region after intracerebral hemorrhage: a serial magnetic resonance imaging study. Stroke. 2013 Apr;44(4):1144–6. Epub 2013 Feb 7.

Mayer SA, Brun NC, Begtrup K, Broderick J, Davis S, Diringer MN, et al; FAST Trial Investigators. Efficacy and safety of recombinant activated factor VII for acute intracerebral hemorrhage. N Engl J Med. 2008 May 15;358(20):2127–37.

Mendelow AD, Gregson BA, Fernandes HM, Murray GD, Teasdale GM, Hope DT, et al; STICH investigators. Early surgery versus initial conservative treatment in patients with spontaneous supratentorial intracerebral haematomas in the International Surgical Trial in Intracerebral Haemorrhage (STICH): a randomised trial. Lancet. 2005 Jan 29-Feb 4;365(9457):387–97.

Morgan T, Awad I, Keyl P, Lane K, Hanley D. Preliminary report of the clot lysis evaluating accelerated resolution of intraventricular hemorrhage (CLEAR-IVH) clinical trial. Acta Neurochir Suppl. 2008;105:217–20.

Mould WA, Carhuapoma JR, Muschelli J, Lane K, Morgan TC, McBee NA, et al; MISTIE Investigators. Minimally invasive surgery plus recombinant tissue-type plasminogen activator for intracerebral hemorrhage evacuation decreases perihematomal edema. Stroke. 2013 Mar;44(3):627–34. Epub 2013 Feb 7.

Mowzoon N, Flemming KD, editors. Neurology board review: an illustrated study guide. Rochester (MN): Mayo Clinic Scientific Press; c2007. 1003 p.

O'Carroll CB, Aguilar MI. Management of postthrombolysis hemorrhagic and orolingual angioedema complications. Neurohospitalist. 2015 Jul;5(3):133–41.

Phan TG, Koh M, Wijdicks EF. Safety of discontinuation of anticoagulation in patients with intracranial hemorrhage at high thromboembolic risk. Arch Neurol. 2000 Dec;57(12):1710–3.

Prasad K, Mendelow AD, Gregson B. Surgery for primary supratentorial intracerebral haemorrhage. Cochrane Database Syst Rev. 2008 Oct 8;(4):CD000200.

Rodriguez-Luna D, Rubiera M, Ribo M, Coscojuela P, Pineiro S, Pagola J, et al. Ultraearly hematoma growth predicts poor outcome after acute intracerebral hemorrhage. Neurology. 2011 Oct 25;77(17):1599–604. Epub 2011 Oct 12.

Schechter MA, Shah AA, Englum BR, Williams JB, Ganapathi AM, Davies JD, et al. Prolonged postoperative respiratory support after proximal thoracic aortic surgery: is deep hypothermic circulatory arrest a risk factor? J Crit Care. 2016 Feb;31(1):125–9. Epub 2015 Nov 6.

Yao X, Xu Y, Siwila-Sackman E, Wu B, Selim M. The HEP score: a nomogram-derived hematoma expansion prediction scale. Neurocrit Care. 2015 Oct;23(2):179–87.

Zhou X, Chen J, Li Q, Ren G, Yao G, Liu M, et al. Minimally invasive surgery for spontaneous supratentorial intracerebral hemorrhage: a meta-analysis of randomized controlled trials. Stroke. 2012 Nov;43(11):2923–30. Epub 2012 Sep 18.

Aneurysmal Subarachnoid Hemorrhage

GIUSEPPE LANZINO, MD; BIAGIA LA PIRA, MD

Goals

- Define the risk factors for aneurysmal subarachnoid hemorrhage, including typical age and incidence.
- Recognize the clinical presentation of patients who have aneurysmal subarachnoid hemorrhage (eg, sudden severe headache, seizure, or loss of consciousness).
- Recognize the diagnostic imaging features of aneurysmal subarachnoid hemorrhage, including the characteristic pattern of subarachnoid blood on noncontrast computed tomography of the head and confirmation of the aneurysm with computed tomographic angiography or formal cerebral angiography.
- Recognize that in delayed presentations of aneurysmal subarachnoid hemorrhage, a lumbar puncture can be helpful diagnostically if the initial computed tomographic findings are negative for subarachnoid hemorrhage.
- Review the management of subarachnoid hemorrhage with acute aneurysm repair to prevent further rebleeding, to monitor and manage vasospasm, and to prevent other systemic complications.

Introduction

The term *subarachnoid hemorrhage* (SAH) refers to extravasation of blood into the subarachnoid space. The term *spontaneous* is used to distinguish causes other than traumatic. The characteristic SAH pattern of most aneurysmal causes is SAH blood in the basal cisterns or around the circle of Willis. In traumatic SAH, blood tends to be in the sulci or the tentorium. This chapter focuses on *aneurysmal SAH* (*aSAH*) related to rupture of an intracranial aneurysm. A medical and neurosurgical emergency, aSAH is associated with a 1-month mortality as high as 40%, and survivors have considerable morbidity and persisting neurologic deficits. Early recognition and management of aSAH are critical to optimizing outcomes.

Epidemiology

The incidence of aSAH varies geographically. It is higher in Japan and Finland than in the United States, where the annual incidence is estimated to be 6.9 to 9.4 per 100,000. In the United States, Hispanics and African Americans have higher incidence rates than other ethnic groups. Although the incidence of aSAH has been relatively constant over the years, the incidence seems to be decreasing in the Western world in a trend that is probably related to decreased rates of smoking and better control of hypertension. The incidence of aSAH increases with older age, and aSAH is generally more common in women than in men (2:1), but the distribution between sexes varies between age groups.

Established modifiable risk factors for aSAH include smoking and hypertension. Current smokers have a higher risk than former smokers, but the evidence is weaker for other modifiable risk factors such as alcohol consumption and hormonal factors. The risk of aSAH is higher for women who are current smokers than for men who are current smokers. Smoking in combination with hypertension carries a risk that is higher than the increased risk ascribed to either factor alone. This observation suggests that smoking and hypertension have an additive effect on the risk of aSAH.

Clinical Presentation

An instantaneously maximal, excruciating headache is the clinical hallmark of aSAH. Even patients with migraine headaches distinguish the severity and suddenness of an aSAH compared with a typical migraine. The onset of aSAH is so sudden and distinctive that it is described as a "thunderclap" headache like the shock wave of sound that occurs after a bolt of lightning. Patients may report nausea, vomiting, and brief loss of consciousness. Associated signs (eg, nuchal rigidity) may take hours to develop while aSAH blood moves down toward the cervical spine and eventually the lumbosacral region. Loss of consciousness may be brief or prolonged in relation to the intensity of the hemorrhage and sudden spike in intracranial pressure (ICP).

Seizures and seizure-like movements (*convulsive syncope*) are common at the onset of aSAH and are related to the sudden increase in ICP, lower cerebral perfusion pressure (CPP), and transient decrease in cerebral blood flow (CBF). In patients with severe aSAH, low intracranial CBF and CPP from elevated ICP or hydrocephalus can decrease the level of consciousness until an external ventricular drain (EVD) is placed and CPP and CBF are restored. In other patients with severe aSAH, a diffuse ischemic vascular injury may impair consciousness even after an EVD is placed 1 or more days later. A gradual decrease in the level of consciousness within the first few hours or days after the initial onset of aSAH is typical of progressive hydrocephalus that requires cerebrospinal fluid (CSF) diversion with an EVD.

The diagnosis of aSAH can be challenging if the patient has a history of headaches, especially if the history of thunderclap onset is not obtainable from an unresponsive patient. After a patient has a headache that is described as the worst or the first, noncontrast computed tomography (CT) is the first-line test within the first few days because it has high sensitivity for detection of blood in acute SAH. The differentiation between spontaneous and traumatic aSAH can be challenging in some contexts because a patient with an aSAH can initially collapse and fall, resulting in secondary head trauma. In contrast, a patient with traumatic head injury can initially have torn cortical vessels and a cortical SAH bleeding pattern with secondary loss of consciousness. Trauma may be suspected as the primary cause if a witness provides a detailed history of events that involve trauma or if signs of trauma are evident. If a patient presents with the classic thunderclap headache with a CT aSAH pattern around the basal cisterns, the astute clinician should have a high degree of suspicion for ruptured aneurysm and perform CT angiography (CTA) immediately. If a patient's history suggests that trauma was the primary cause, such as a motor vehicle collision, and the CT pattern suggests a traumatic blood pattern, aSAH should be considered less likely. However, since aSAH can cause loss of consciousness while driving, aSAH should be considered a primary event with a secondary motor vehicle collision. When the cause is uncertain, excluding an aSAH as the primary cause can be useful because an aSAH dictates different management steps to secure the aneurysm in addition to the typical procedures for management after trauma.

The patient's initial clinical condition is the most important predictor of final clinical outcome. Several scales, such as the Glasgow Coma Scale (GCS), are incorporated into the World Federation of Neurosurgical Societies (WFNS) grading scale, which ranges from 0 (severe headache, a GCS score of 15 at presentation, and no major focal deficit) to 5 (GCS score of 3-6 with or without major deficit). The initial clinical state, however, can be affected by factors such as untreated increased ICP from hydrocephalus that may improve with rapid placement of an EVD. Increasing evidence suggests that WFNS grading after systemic and neurologic stabilization occurs is more important in predicting the final prognosis within the first 24 hours.

Table 83.1 • Grading Scales for Subarachnoid Hemorrhage

Grade	Hunt and Hess	WFNS[a]
1	Asymptomatic or mild headache; slight nuchal rigidity	15
2	CN palsy (eg, CN III or IV); moderate to severe headache; nuchal rigidity	13-14 without focal deficit
3	Mild focal deficit; lethargy or confusion	13-14 with focal deficit
4	Stupor; moderate to severe hemiparesis; early decerebrate rigidity	7-12
5	Deep coma; decerebrate rigidity; moribund appearance	3-6

Abbreviations: CN, cranial nerve; WFNS, World Federation of Neurosurgical Societies.
[a] Numbers refer to Glasgow Coma Scale score.

While numerous clinical grading scales have been used over the years in predicting outcome, the WFNS and the Hunt and Hess grading scales continue to be strongly predictive of aSAH outcome and are used in clinical practice (Table 83.1). Although not perfect, these scales are easy to remember or find on the Internet. These scales are also useful since they have good interobserver reliability and can be used to communicate with other medical providers. Emergency department and neurosurgical clinicians often dichotomize SAH according to the initial score on the WFNS or Hunt and Hess scale as *good grade* (grades 1-3) or *poor grade* (grades 4 and 5) depending on the probability of a good or poor outcome.

Diagnosis

An immediate noncontrast CT of the head is the first-line diagnostic study for confirming an aSAH. The sensitivity of noncontrast CT of the head is close to 100% in the first few hours after onset and progressively decreases over the first week. If CT performed within 6 hours after onset is interpreted by a board-certified neuroradiologist as negative for aSAH, a lumbar puncture (LP) may not be necessary. However, because of the potentially catastrophic consequences of missing a potential ruptured aneurysm and "sentinel leak," LP is indicated in the presence of high clinical suspicion for aSAH even if CT is negative for the typical aSAH blood pattern. A sentinel leak is a small-volume aSAH that is unseen on 5-mm CT sections. An abrupt aneurysmal wall change may be associated with a thunderclap headache pattern, and in patients who present days after thunderclap onset, a useful indirect sign of isodense subacute blood in the subarachnoid space may be the lack of sulci or lack of visualization of the sylvian fissure on CT of the head. In such patients, LP shows xanthochromia (ie, yellow CSF) with similar quantities of red blood cells (RBCs) in tubes 1 and 4. With traumatic LPs, the number of RBCs typically decreases from tubes 1 to 4, whereas with aSAH, the RBC quantities are similar in tubes 1 and 4 (typically, 1,000-100,000/mcL). The following formula is used to correct CSF white blood cell (WBC) counts after traumatic LP:

$$\text{Corrected CSF WBC} = \text{CSF WBC} - [(\text{Serum WBC} \times \text{CSF RBC}) / \text{Serum RBC}].$$

If serum WBC and RBC counts are relatively normal, a mental calculation can be used: Subtract 1 WBC from the CSF WBC count for every 750 CSF RBCs.

Magnetic resonance imaging (MRI) has a limited role in the diagnosis of acute SAH, although specific sequences such as fluid-attenuated inversion recovery and gradient-echo MRI are helpful in identifying subarachnoid blood if CT was negative but the clinical suspicion for SAH is strong, especially for a sentinel leak with a small amount of SAH blood. However, CTA is usually faster than MRI for the diagnosis of intracranial aneurysms that are at least 2 to 4 mm. CTA is commonly the first-line method for identifying aneurysms in patients presenting with aSAH.

Catheter-based digital subtraction angiography (DSA) is the gold standard for the diagnosis of all intracranial aneurysms, especially when an aSAH is not apparent on CTA but yet a high degree of clinical suspicion exists. Also, DSA is usually used if an aSAH has been coiled or secured from active bleeding. Therefore, DSA is useful both diagnostically and therapeutically. Further, because DSA allows visualization of the external carotid arteries, it can sometimes be used to detect a nidal aneurysm within a dural arteriovenous fistula, which can occasionally cause an aSAH that is not a pure intracranial aneurysm.

Subsequent DSA is indicated within 1 to 2 weeks if the initial DSA was negative for aneurysm and a pattern of diffuse aneurysmal bleeding was apparent on the initial CT. Subsequent angiography is not necessary for patients with nonaneurysmal perimesencephalic SAH (Figure 83.1)

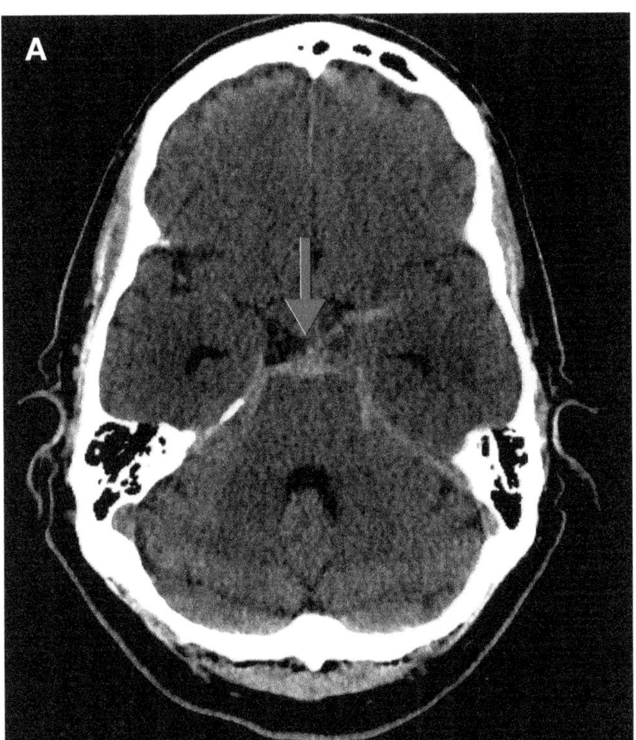

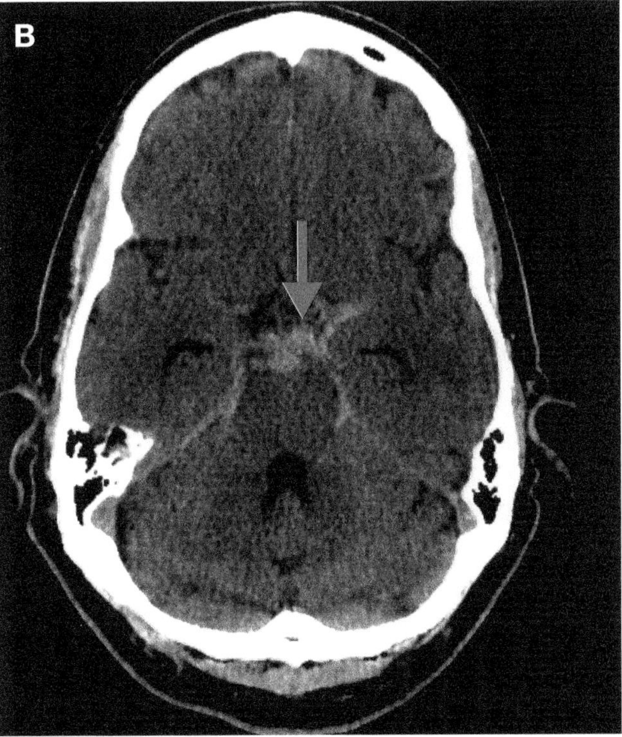

Figure 83.1. Nonaneurysmal Perimesencephalic Subarachnoid Hemorrhage. A and B, Noncontrast computed tomography of the head shows a typical pattern for nonaneurysmal perimesencephalic subarachnoid hemorrhage, with a thick area of blood in the prepontine cistern (red arrows) and a faint extension of subarachnoid blood into the proximal third of the sylvian fissure.

whose first catheter angiogram was negative for aneurysm. In older patients with diffuse atherosclerosis, CTA may be a substitute for catheter angiography. If endovascular therapy is indicated, aCTA results may be used (like a road map) to guide selective catheter angiography, so that catheterization of only the target vessel is necessary for treatment of the aneurysm.

Treatment

Treatment of aSAH has 3 primary goals: 1) Optimize CPP, which is the difference between mean arterial pressure and ICP. This is accomplished by decreasing systolic blood pressure (SBP) to less than 160 mm Hg (to prevent aneurysm rerupture) and by placing an EVD (to decrease ICP if hydrocephalus is suspected) or giving mannitol (or both). 2) Secure the aneurysm to minimize rebleeding because rebleeding is associated with a stepwise decrease from the initial WFNS grade to worse outcomes. 3) Prevent secondary acute or subacute neurologic and systemic injuries, such as delayed cerebral ischemia or vasospasm, which typically occur from days 4 through 14 after initial aSAH bleeding; prevent systemic complications, such as aspiration pneumonia or ventilator-associated pneumonia; and aggressively evaluate and treat fever (central fever or fever from a systemic cause) and hyponatremia, which occur commonly with aSAH.

Prevention of Rebleeding

Aneurysmal rebleeding is the most feared complication. It is common (occurring in up to 15% of patients within the first 24 hours after initial aSAH) and potentially lethal. For centers without a neurosurgeon who could secure the aneurysm, tranexamic acid, an antifibrinolytic agent, was shown to provide a statistically significant decrease in the risk of aneurysmal rebleeding in a randomized trial. Prolonged use of antifibrinolytics (for more than 4-14 days after aSAH) is no longer recommended because of a higher incidence of thrombotic complications. Clinically, aneurysmal rebleeding is often associated with a sudden increase in SBP, bradycardia (Cushing reflex), a sudden neurologic deterioration from baseline, and sometimes an apparently tonic-clonic seizure or an event that resembles a seizure. A tonic-clonic seizure in a patient with an unsecured ruptured aneurysm should prompt suspicion of aneurysmal rebleeding unless proved otherwise with subsequent imaging.

The most effective intervention to prevent rebleeding is securing the ruptured aneurysm during DSA, which is now performed in about 80% of patients through endovascular coil embolization and is a valid alternative to surgical clipping. Current evidence indicates that endovascular treatment should be pursued if an aneurysm is suitable according to its dome to neck ratio, geometry, and other factors (Figure 83.2). In young patients (<40 years old) with anterior circulation aneurysms (Figure 83.3), surgical clip ligation may be preferable because of better durability and the low risk after surgical treatment. The use of newer endovascular techniques, such as stent-assisted coiling and flow diverter devices, is typically discouraged immediately

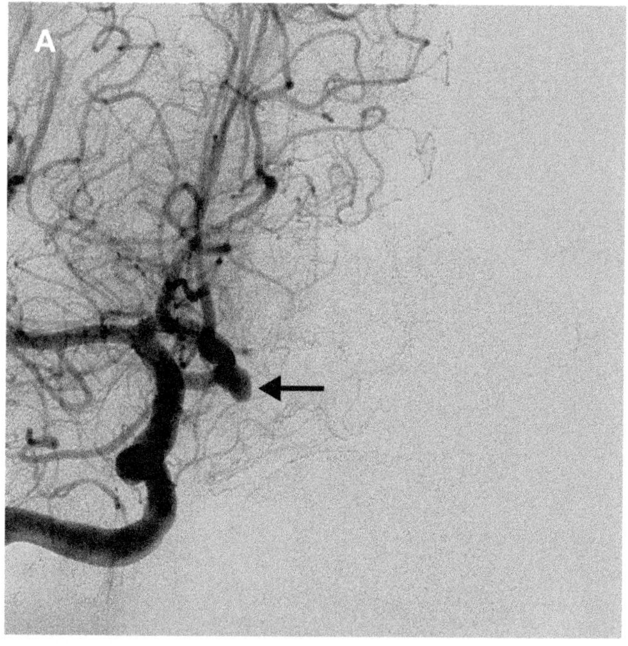

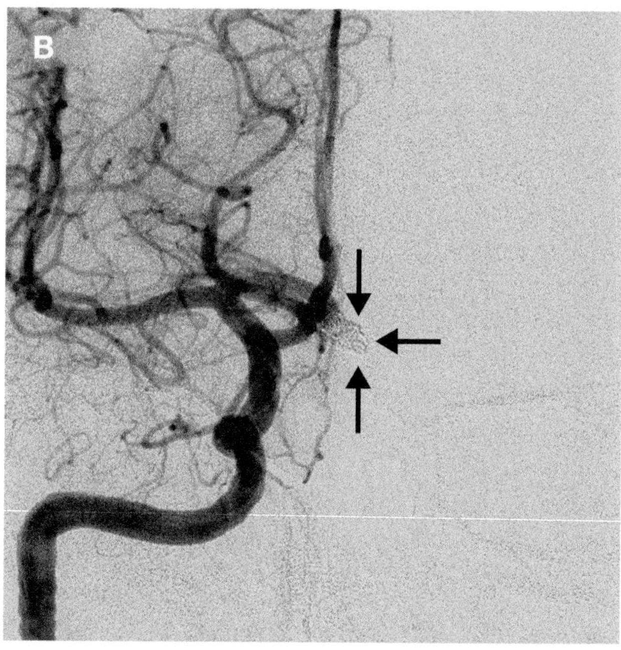

Figure 83.2. Aneurysmal Subarachnoid Hemorrhage (aSAH). A, A 60-year-old man presented with aSAH from a ruptured aneurysm of the anterior communicating artery (arrow). B, The aneurysm was successfully treated with coil embolization (arrows).

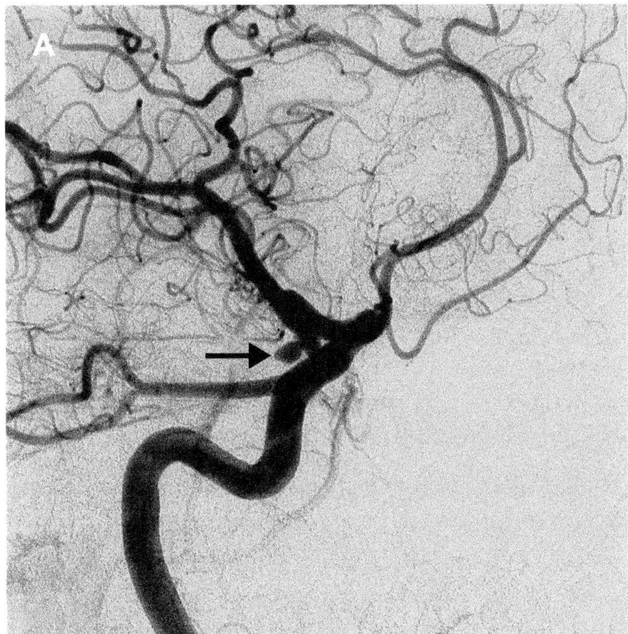

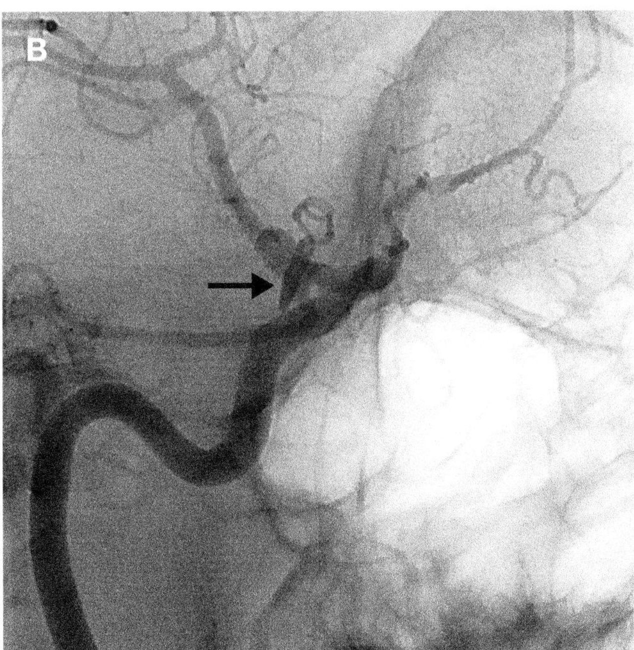

Figure 83.3. Anterior Circulation Aneurysmal Subarachnoid Hemorrhage (aSAH). A, A 39-year-old patient presented with a good-grade aSAH from a small aneurysm of the posterior communicating artery (arrow) with a relatively broad neck. Surgical clip ligation was the preferred treatment because of the patient's young age, the anterior circulation location of the aneurysm, and the relatively unfavorable geometry of the aneurysm. B, A postoperative angiogram provided confirmation that clip exclusion of the aneurysm was complete (arrow).

after aSAH and is reserved for selected high-risk patients because these stent devices require dual antiplatelet therapy (eg, aspirin and clopidogrel) for 1 to 3 months. Dual antiplatelet therapy may pose an additional risk of bleeding (eg, intracranial bleeding around the EVD site or stress ulcer bleeding in the gastrointestinal tract) or complicate ventriculoperitoneal shunt planning because holding dual antiplatelet agents can cause stroke from stent thrombosis.

Delayed Cerebral Ischemia and Vasospasm

The terms *delayed cerebral ischemia* (DCI) and *vasospasm* are often used interchangeably to describe delayed vascular complications that peak 4 to 14 days after aSAH. DCI is apparent as ischemic changes on CT or MRI that occur after aSAH, resemble ischemic stroke changes, and are not due to other causes or procedural complications. Vasospasm, however, is apparent as vascular narrowing on CTA, magnetic resonance angiography (MRA), DSA, or transcranial Doppler ultrasonography (TCD) and is related to the blood vessel narrowing. Risk of DCI and vasospasm can be stratified on initial noncontrast CT of the head with the modified Fisher scale, which linearly correlates scale grades 1 through 4 with symptomatic vasospasm risk (grade 1, 10% risk; grade 2, 20%; grade 3, 30%; and grade 4, 40%). Symptomatic vasospasm must be distinguished from radiographic vasospasm. While one-third of aSAH patients with a modified Fisher grade 3 blood pattern have symptomatic vasospasm neurologic deficits, two-thirds of the patients have radiologic vasospasm on some form of neuroimaging (TCD, CTA, MRA, or DSA) by 2 weeks. The neurologic examination is by far the most important and reliable monitor for development of symptomatic vasospasm (eg, patients with symptomatic middle cerebral artery [MCA] vasospasm and patients with an acute MCA ischemic syndrome have similar clinical signs and symptoms).

After aneurysm treatment, intubated patients should be extubated as soon as safely possible and monitored by nurses trained in neurologic examination. Use of narcotics for pain control should be minimized because they may mask early signs and symptoms of symptomatic vasospasm. Gabapentin, a nonnarcotic medication, has been found to be safe and tolerable in decreasing meningismus pain in combination with standard pain medications.

TCD is a noninvasive imaging tool that can be used at the bedside. Progressively elevated MCA velocities (eg, >120 cm/s, mild; >150 cm/s, moderate; and >200 cm/s, severe) should alert the clinician to be especially vigilant for potentially symptomatic vasospasm. The Lindegaard ratio is the hemispheric ratio of the mean velocity in the ipsilateral MCA to the mean velocity in the internal carotid artery and is useful when a patient has a hyperdynamic hemodynamic state (eg, from use of inotropes that increase cardiac output). The Lindegaard ratio is discussed in more detail in Chapter 129 ("Transcranial Doppler Ultrasonography").

During the vasospasm risk period, an adequate circulating blood volume or hydration status must be maintained to meet the goal of euvolemia and to avoid hypotension and dehydration. After several randomized trials in the 1980s, nimodipine, an L-type calcium channel blocker, was proved to improve neurologic outcomes compared with placebo despite conflicting data on angiographic or radiographic vasospasm. Nimodipine (60 mg enterally every 4 hours for 21 days) should be administered as soon as the diagnosis of aSAH is confirmed. Symptomatic vasospasm is a diagnosis of exclusion for a patient with aSAH who presents with new or worsening neurologic deficits. Thus, potentially correctable causes of rapid neurologic deterioration, including high fever, hypoglycemia, hyponatremia, hydrocephalus, and cerebral edema, should be excluded quickly with bedside examination and laboratory tests before proceeding to symptomatic vasospasm management.

The triple therapy of induced hypertension, induced hypervolemia, and hemodilution (so-called HHH) was previously recommended for medical management of symptomatic vasospasm. However, considerable evidence has reduced HHH to induced hypertension and judicious hypervolemia (net fluid balance, 500 mL). Extreme hemodilution can decrease delivery of oxygen and was thought, in theory, to decrease blood viscosity. Marked hypervolemia (eg, a positive fluid balance of several liters) can cause respiratory failure, congestive heart failure, and pulmonary edema.

Therefore, induced hypertension is first-line treatment in symptomatic patients along with maintenance of an adequate volume status by increasing SBP 10 to 20 mm Hg from baseline with judicious use of crystalloids, colloids, or vasopressors (individually or in combination). If patients have no response to induced hypertension, angiographic vasospasm may need to be confirmed with imaging studies such as CTA (with or without perfusion) or DSA. In refractory cases, pharmacologic angioplasty (through intra-arterial injection of vasodilatative agents) or mechanical angioplasty (with endovascular balloons) can alleviate symptomatic vasospasm. Prophylactic HHH and angioplasty are not recommended. A euvolemic fluid balance should be maintained when a patient is asymptomatic, however, especially during cerebral salt wasting (CSW), which can be challenging.

Hydrocephalus

Acute hydrocephalus and increased ICP are common in patients with aSAH. Although ventricular size is commonly used in clinical practice as a surrogate for hydrocephalus and the potential need for CSF diversion, ventriculomegaly is not always associated with increased ICP. Patients with poor-grade aSAH (WFNS grade 4 or 5) may also have markedly increased ICP without a corresponding increase in ventricular size and require EVD placement for diagnostic and therapeutic (CSF drainage) purposes.

CSF diversion is indicated for patients with a compromised level of consciousness or progressively worsening neurologic condition because of acute hydrocephalus or increased ICP. For these patients, CSF diversion usually involves placement of an EVD. Dual drainage with both an EVD and a lumbar drain in patients with symptomatic hydrocephalus may improve outcomes if placed early (within the first 24 hours).

In addition to acute hydrocephalus, patients with aSAH are at risk for delayed communicating hydrocephalus, which is probably related to a dysfunction in CSF reabsorption. Risk factors for delayed hydrocephalus include older age, higher subarachnoid blood burden, and associated intraventricular hemorrhage. These patients benefit from permanent CSF diversion through placement of a ventriculoperitoneal shunt after the vasospasm period has passed.

Systemic Complications

Systemic complications are common after aSAH, and the risks are higher for patients with poorer grade aSAH. Complications can affect most organ systems, such as the lungs (aspiration, pneumonia, and pulmonary edema), heart (takotsubo cardiomyopathy and troponin leak), and gastrointestinal tract (Cushing ulcer). Arrhythmias and electrocardiographic changes are also common at aSAH presentation because of increased catecholamine release from aSAH with or without underlying coronary pathology.

Electrolyte imbalances (especially hyponatremia from CSW) are common. The urine output of a patient with CSW can be quite high (up to 1 L/h if left unchecked), as in diabetes insipidus, and lead to hypovolemia. The management of CSW is outside the scope of this chapter and is discussed elsewhere. However, the general approach for managing fluid balance and electrolytes starts with a baseline history to screen for endocrine disorders and with measurements of thyrotropin and free thyroxine to ensure a normal euthyroid state. Several laboratory findings are useful for distinguishing CSW from other neuroendocrine disturbances (Table 83.2). Although the mechanism of CSW is unknown, diabetes insipidus occurs from central depletion of antidiuretic hormone with pituitary stalk surgery or injury. Like CSW, diabetes insipidus is characterized by large volumes of dilute urine with a low specific gravity (about 1.000 instead of 1.020).

Diabetes insipidus is treated with desmopressin (Chapter 34, "Diabetes Insipidus"). CSW is usually managed with crystalloid fluid volume replacement (0.9% normal saline), 5% albumin replacement every 8 hours, and

Table 83.2 • Neuroendocrine Disturbances After Aneurysmal Subarachnoid Hemorrhage

Feature	SIADH	CSW	DI
Volume status[a]	↑	↓	↓
Serum sodium	↓	Normal or ↓	↑↑
Urine output	↓	↑↑	↑↑
Urine color	Dark yellow (concentrated)	Clear	Clear
Urine sodium	Normal	↑	↓
Urine specific gravity	↑	↓	↓

Abbreviations: CSW, cerebral salt wasting; DI, diabetes insipidus; SIADH, syndrome of inappropriate secretion of antidiuretic hormone; ↓, decreased; ↑, increased; ↑↑, greatly increased.

[a] Intravascular volume status reflects fluid balance (input and output), daily weight, and central venous pressure (if applicable).

fludrocortisone (0.1-0.2 mg twice daily) while monitoring potassium and electrolyte concentrations. After the aneurysm is secured, the use of deep vein thrombosis prophylaxis, with sequential compression devices immediately and chemical thromboprophylaxis later (eg, subcutaneous heparin 5,000 units every 8 to 12 hours), should be discussed with the neurosurgeon, especially for patients with impaired mobility.

Outcome and Follow-up

The historical mortality associated with aSAH (10%-40%) has decreased over time to about 10% at most high-volume centers because of improved care. An estimated 35% to 55% of aSAH survivors have good functional outcome at follow-up (modified Rankin scale score, 1-3). Patients who survive aSAH without residual physical deficits commonly complain of cognitive dysfunction, such as short-term memory loss or mood and sleep disorders that affect their overall quality of life. Patients with aSAH are at risk for future aneurysm and aSAH and should be monitored for aneurysm recurrence. Younger age at the first aSAH, current smoking, and family history are associated with a higher risk of recurrent aSAH. Follow-up with patients after aSAH is typically within the first few months and then every 6 months to 1 year. If the patient's status is stable, the follow-up interval can be extended, and noninvasive brain imaging (eg, CTA or MRA) can be used to detect *de novo* or recurrent brain aneurysm. If an aneurysm recurs or an unstable area of the previous aneurysm is visualized during follow-up, outpatient treatment with DSA or open neurosurgery may be discussed.

Summary

- Most commonly, aSAH occurs from a ruptured intracranial saccular aneurysm, with the immediate complications being a severe first headache or the worst headache of one's life, with or without loss of consciousness, seizure, increased ICP, and hydrocephalus.
- Initial management of aSAH includes CPP optimization until aneurysm repair and use of an EVD for hydrocephalus if present.
- Delayed vasospasm peaks 7 to 14 days after initial aSAH bleeding and can lead to new neurologic deficits (delayed cerebral ischemia or symptomatic vasospasm) and neuronal damage.
- Nimodipine (60 mg enterally every 4 hours for 21 days) improves aSAH outcomes in randomized trials; if a patient becomes hypotensive, the dose should be decreased (to 30 mg every 2 hours).
- Management of aSAH involves monitoring, early recognition, fluid management, induced hypertension, and, if needed, endovascular therapies such as balloon angioplasty or intra-arterial verapamil.

SUGGESTED READING

Al-Mufti F, Amuluru K, Damodara N, El-Ghanem M, Nuoman R, Kamal N, et al. Novel management strategies for medically-refractory vasospasm following aneurysmal subarachnoid hemorrhage. J Neurol Sci. 2018 Jul 15;390:44–51. Epub 2018 Feb 23.

Burrell C, Avalon NE, Siegel J, Pizzi M, Dutta T, Charlesworth MC, et al. Precision medicine of aneurysmal subarachnoid hemorrhage, vasospasm and delayed cerebral ischemia. Expert Rev Neurother. 2016 Nov;16(11):1251–62. Epub 2016 Jul 11.

Connolly ES Jr, Rabinstein AA, Carhuapoma JR, Derdeyn CP, Dion J, Higashida RT, et al; American Heart Association Stroke Council; Council on Cardiovascular Radiology and Intervention; Council on Cardiovascular Nursing; Council on Cardiovascular Surgery and Anesthesia; Council on Clinical Cardiology. Guidelines for the management of aneurysmal subarachnoid hemorrhage: a guideline for healthcare professionals from the American Heart Association/American Stroke Association. Stroke. 2012 Jun;43(6):1711–37. Epub 2012 May 3.

Dhakal LP, Hodge DO, Nagel J, Mayes M, Richie A, Ng LK, et al. Safety and tolerability of gabapentin for aneurysmal subarachnoid hemorrhage (SAH) headache and meningismus. Neurocrit Care. 2015 Jun;22(3):414–21. Erratum in: Neurocrit Care. 2015 Jun;22(3):422.

Frontera JA, Claassen J, Schmidt JM, Wartenberg KE, Temes R, Connolly ES Jr, et al. Prediction of symptomatic vasospasm after subarachnoid hemorrhage: the modified Fisher scale. Neurosurgery. 2006 Jul;59(1):21–7.

Hillman J, Fridriksson S, Nilsson O, Yu Z, Saveland H, Jakobsson KE. Immediate administration of tranexamic acid and reduced incidence of early rebleeding after aneurysmal subarachnoid hemorrhage: a prospective randomized study. J Neurosurg. 2002 Oct;97(4):771–8.

Klimo P Jr, Kestle JR, MacDonald JD, Schmidt RH. Marked reduction of cerebral vasospasm with lumbar drainage of cerebrospinal fluid after subarachnoid hemorrhage. J Neurosurg. 2004 Feb;100(2):215–24.

Kongable GL, Lanzino G, Germanson TP, Truskowski LL, Alves WM, Torner JC, et al. Gender-related differences in aneurysmal subarachnoid hemorrhage. J Neurosurg. 1996 Jan;84(1):43–8.

Lawton MT, Vates GE. Subarachnoid hemorrhage. N Engl J Med. 2017 Jul 20;377(3):257–66.

Loan JJM, Wiggins AN, Brennan PM. Medically induced hypertension, hypervolaemia and haemodilution for the treatment and prophylaxis of vasospasm following aneurysmal subarachnoid haemorrhage: systematic review. Br J Neurosurg. 2018 Apr;32(2):157–64. Epub 2018 Jan 17.

Medscape. CSF WBC correction in blood contaminated CSF calculator [Internet]. MedCalc 3000. c1998–2011 Foundation Internet Services [cited 2018 Aug 9]. Available from: https://reference.medscape.com/calculator/csf-wbc-blood-correction.

Nesvick CL, Oushy S, Rinaldo L, Wijdicks EF, Lanzino G, Rabinstein AA. Clinical complications and outcomes of angiographically negative subarachnoid hemorrhage. Neurology. 2019 Apr 17. pii: 10.1212/WNL.0000000000007501. [Epub ahead of print]

Nimodipine [package insert]. Atlanta (GA): Arbor Pharmaceuticals, Inc; 2013. Available from: https://www.accessdata.fda.gov/ drugsatfda_docs/label/2013/203340lbl.pdf.

Rabinstein AA, Bruder N. Management of hyponatremia and volume contraction. Neurocrit Care. 2011 Sep;15(2):354–60.

Rabinstein AA, Lanzino G. Aneurysmal subarachnoid hemorrhage: unanswered questions. Neurosurg Clin N Am. 2018 Apr;29(2):255–62.

Schievink WI, Wijdicks EF. Origin of pretruncal nonaneurysmal subarachnoid hemorrhage: ruptured vein, perforating artery, or intramural hematoma? Mayo Clin Proc. 2000 Nov;75(11):1169–73.

Vergouwen MD, Vermeulen M, van Gijn J, Rinkel GJ, Wijdicks EF, Muizelaar JP, et al. Definition of delayed cerebral ischemia after aneurysmal subarachnoid hemorrhage as an outcome event in clinical trials and observational studies: proposal of a multidisciplinary research group. Stroke. 2010 Oct;41(10):2391–5. Epub 2010 Aug 26.

Wijdicks EF, Kallmes DF, Manno EM, Fulgham JR, Piepgras DG. Subarachnoid hemorrhage: neurointensive care and aneurysm repair. Mayo Clin Proc. 2005 Apr;80(4):550–9.

84 Intracranial Arteriovenous Malformations[a]

KELLY D. FLEMMING, MD; MICHAEL J. LINK, MD

Goals

- Recognize the clinical features of intracranial arteriovenous malformations at presentation.
- Recognize the radiologic features of arteriovenous malformations.
- Review the 4 main management approaches to patients with arteriovenous malformation: medical management, open neurosurgical approach (after assessment of operative risk with the Spetzler-Martin grading system), stereotactic radiosurgery, and endovascular approaches.

Introduction

Intracranial arteriovenous malformations (AVMs) are a type of intracranial vascular malformation that consists of an abnormal connection of arteries and veins without intervening capillary beds. AVMs may come to medical attention because of seizure, intracranial hemorrhage, or incidental radiographic findings in a patient undergoing brain imaging for a different indication. This chapter focuses on the epidemiology, natural history, diagnosis, and management of intracranial AVMs.

Definition

Intracranial AVMs are fistulous connections of cerebral arteries and veins without a normal intervening capillary bed. These connections create high-flow shunts where arterial blood flows directly into the venous system. This direct transmission of arterial pressure to venous structures results in dilatation, tortuosity, and arterialization of the draining vein(s). Venous hypertension may result. The tortuous vessels connecting the feeding arteries to the draining veins are commonly referred to as the *nidus*. The nidus may be compact or diffuse. Pathologically, residua from previous hemorrhage (eg, calcification and hemosiderin) may surround the AVM. Histologically, macrophages are often laden with hemosiderin.

Pathogenesis

In the past, AVMs were thought to be congenital lesions. However, accumulating evidence indicates that AVMs are acquired lesions that form at other times during life. De novo lesions have been described, and AVMs are rarely found *in utero* or in infants. In addition, recurrent AVMs have been documented after resection and negative angiography, particularly in children and young adults. Examples like these support the possibility that abnormalities in venous outflow, hormonal influences, or angiogenic humoral factors are involved in the pathogenesis and formation of AVMs during life.

AVMs are typically sporadic, although a rare, familial form exists. AVMs may occur with other vascular malformations or be part of a syndrome. For example, AVMs and other intracranial vascular malformations are common in patients with hereditary hemorrhagic telangiectasia, Cobb syndrome, capillary malformation–arteriovenous malformation syndrome (from mutation of the *RASA-1* gene), and Wyburn-Mason syndrome.

[a] Portions of text from Flemming KD, Brown RD Jr. The natural history of intracranial vascular malformations. In: Winn HR, editor. Youmans neurological surgery. 6th ed. 4-Volume set. Philadelphia (PA): Elsevier/Saunders; c2011. p. 4016-33; used with permission.

Epidemiology

The exact incidence and prevalence of AVM are unknown. In population-based studies, the estimated sex- and age-adjusted annual incidence is 0.51 to 1.34 per 100,000 persons. Autopsy and magnetic resonance imaging (MRI) studies suggest a prevalence of 0.2% to 1.0%. In autopsy studies, about 15% of cases had findings related to an AVM. Among patients aged 15 to 45 years presenting with intracerebral hemorrhage, 38% have AVMs.

AVMs are typically diagnosed when patients are 20 to 40 years old. Common in men and women, AVMs may have a slight male predominance. Most AVMs are supratentorial and solitary, but rarely patients have had multiple AVMs. In the posterior fossa, the cerebellum is the most common site. Many AVMs are situated at the border zone areas of the anterior, middle, and posterior cerebral arteries. They are often pyramidal with the base parallel to the cortex and the apex pointing inward toward the ventricle.

Clinical Features

Incidental AVM

With the increased availability of brain imaging since the 1990s, an increasing number of patients have presented with an *incidental AVM*—that is, an AVM that is not related to the symptoms that led to the brain imaging being performed. Autopsy studies suggest that the majority of patients with AVM are asymptomatic. However, clinical studies suggest that in 10% to 40% of patients with an AVM, the AVM is an incidental finding.

Hemorrhage

Many patients with AVM initially present for medical care because of intracranial hemorrhage. Clinical studies suggest that approximately 50% of patients (range, 30%-70%) present with hemorrhage. Intraparenchymal hemorrhage is the most common, but intraventricular hemorrhage, subarachnoid hemorrhage, and, very rarely, subdural hemorrhage may also occur.

Certain radiologic features from conventional angiography are predictors of initial presentation with hemorrhage in patients with AVM, but the features do not necessarily correspond with subsequent rehemorrhage. The risk factors that are useful for predicting presentation with hemorrhage include small size, exclusive deep venous drainage, deep location, posterior fossa location, association with an aneurysm, and venous ectasia. Radiologic risk factors must be interpreted cautiously because certain biases may affect angiography in the early phase. In addition, in studies of populations after hemorrhage, patients with early death were excluded; this may be a source of bias. Hemorrhage at presentation may be associated with morbidity of 20% to 30% and mortality of 10% to 40%.

Seizures

Approximately 15% to 35% of patients with AVMs first present with a seizure. Seizures may result from an associated hemorrhage or from a mass effect with cortical irritation or flow characteristics leading to steal, ischemia, and neuronal damage. Seizures are most commonly focal (simple or partial complex) but may also be generalized.

Most of the seizures (90%) occur in patients with a supratentorial AVM. Other AVM characteristics in patients who are more likely to present with seizure include superficial or cortical location and frontal or temporal location.

Focal Neurologic Deficits and Headaches

A small percentage of patients (<10%) may present with neurologic deficits. These patients may have transient, permanent, or progressive focal neurologic deficits that are not a result of hemorrhage or seizure. Mechanisms for this type of presentation may include *vascular steal phenomena* (ie, ischemia due to a high-flow AVM diverting ["stealing"] blood from local tissue), recurrent small hemorrhages, local pressure or mass effect from the AVM, or accompanying hydrocephalus.

Patients may also present with headaches without hemorrhage. Determining whether the headaches are related to the AVM or to a primary headache disorder can be difficult. A patient with a large AVM may have ipsilateral headaches that resemble migraine. One hypothesis is that headaches occur because of long-standing meningeal artery involvement and recruitment of blood supply by the AVM. Another hypothesis is that headaches may result from venous outflow obstruction.

Diagnostic Imaging

Computed Tomography

Computed tomography (CT) of the brain is often the first diagnostic test a patient undergoes after presenting with seizure or focal neurologic deficit. CT is helpful for assessing for hemorrhage from the AVM. Spinal fluid testing (for red blood cell count and xanthochromia) may be required if a patient presents with a thunderclap headache with a known or suspected AVM on imaging but without obvious hemorrhage on CT. If a patient has intraparenchymal hemorrhage, the underlying AVM may not be visible on CT alone and a diagnosis may require MRI of the brain, CT angiography, magnetic resonance angiography (MRA), or conventional angiography. With larger AVMs, focal areas of spiculated calcification may be present in 20% to 30% of patients, so that additional imaging (MRI, noninvasive angiography, or conventional angiography) is necessary to confirm an AVM. When contrast medium is administered with CT, AVMs may appear as a serpiginous, enhancing lesion, but very small AVMs may not be readily visible.

Magnetic Resonance Imaging

MRI of the brain is superior to CT for identifying an AVM. MRI can aid in determining the size and location of the AVM. T1-weighted and T2-weighted MRI may show areas of flow voids suggestive of an AVM (Figure 84.1). Fluid-attenuated inversion recovery MRI may be useful for identifying mass effect, edema, and ischemic changes in surrounding brain tissue. In addition, MRI of the brain with hemosiderin-sensitive sequences may show evidence of previous asymptomatic hemorrhage or subclinical hemorrhage. Functional MRI and tractography may be useful in preoperative planning when needed.

Angiography

Noninvasive angiography can be useful in the diagnosis of AVM; however, cerebral angiography is superior for assessing the angioarchitecture of the AVM. The characteristic finding is the pial arterial supply with arteriovenous shunting and early filling of veins. The nidus is the tortuous coil of vessels, which may be compact or diffuse, that connects the arteries to the draining veins. Angiography is useful for determining the size of the AVM, the compactness of the nidus, and the feeding arteries and draining veins. In addition, it is helpful for establishing whether there are any associated aneurysms (of the feeding artery or nidus).

Natural History

Brain hemorrhage or rehemorrhage is a feared complication in patients with AVM because of its associated potential morbidity and mortality. Natural history studies have attempted to determine the risk of bleeding from intracranial AVM, but these calculated risks have inherent biases. Some studies have calculated the risk of hemorrhage retrospectively. *Retrospective risk* is calculated as follows: exposure from birth to hemorrhage or intervention (in person-years) divided by the number of patients with hemorrhage. Retrospective risk is based on the assumption that the lesion is congenital and has a constant risk over time, which may not be accurate. *Prospective risk* may be more useful; however, surgical selection and referral bias are common. Specifically, natural history studies may include patients who have high-grade AVMs and asymptomatic patients, and the overall risk does not apply to an individual. Previous studies have also had inconsistent follow-up and variability in adjudicating symptomatic hemorrhage.

Despite those limitations, several natural history studies, meta-analyses, and a single clinical trial have estimated that the overall risk of hemorrhage for patients with AVMs is 2% to 4% per year. Some have suggested assessing the lifetime risk of rupture in patients with the following formula: Lifetime Risk = 1 – (Risk of No Hemorrhage) expected years of life, which can be simplified to Lifetime Risk = 105 – Age.

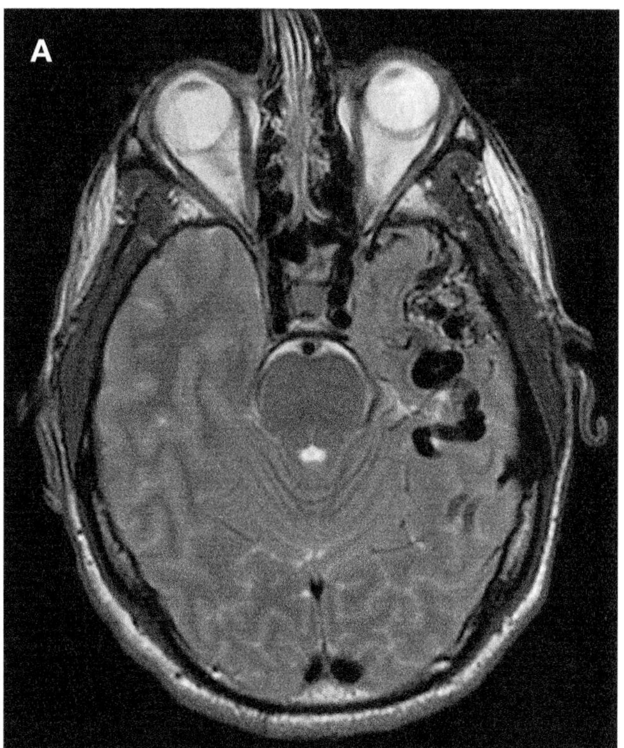

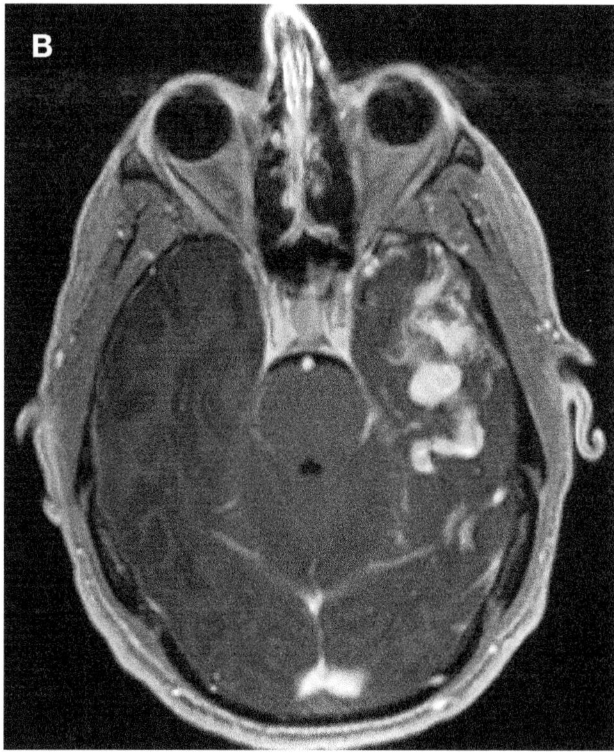

Figure 84.1. Arteriovenous Malformation. A, Axial T2-weighted magnetic resonance imaging (MRI) of the brain shows numerous flow voids in the left temporal region suggestive of an underlying arteriovenous malformation (AVM). B, Axial T1-weighted MRI with gadolinium contrast medium shows contrast enhancement of the abnormal vessels. C, Conventional angiography shows an AVM fed by a branch of the middle cerebral artery.

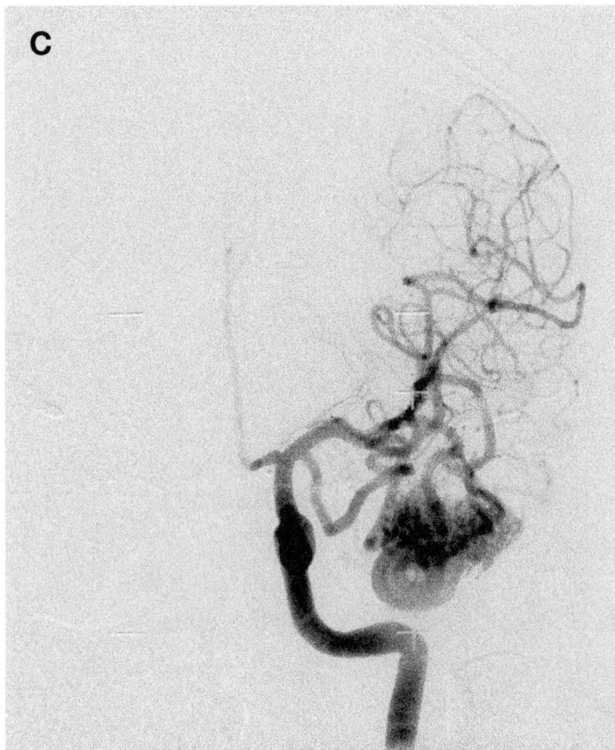

Figure 84.1. Continued

These formulas assume a constant rate of hemorrhage over time and do not take into account individual differences.

An individual's risk, however, depends on multiple factors and can range from low (<1% for patients with low-risk features who are asymptomatic) to high (>20% for patients with high-risk features who have bled). The strongest and most consistent predictor of hemorrhage is prior hemorrhage. Thus, patients who present initially because of hemorrhage have a high risk of rebleeding (as high as 20%-40%). Rebleeding is most common within the first year after an initial hemorrhage. In 1 study, the bleeding rate in those who presented with hemorrhage initially was higher in the first year (15.4%), decreasing to 5.3% in the next 4 years and 1.7% after 5 years. Other clinical risk factors for predicting hemorrhage identified in some studies (not consistently in all studies) were age, sex, and radiologic findings that included deep location with exclusive deep venous drainage and large size. The natural history is not affected by partial treatment of the AVM.

Acute Care

Emergency Medical Care

Patients presenting with sudden focal neurologic deficits, acute thunderclap headache, or seizure require immediate care and standard measures for assessment of airway, breathing, and circulation, including initial blood pressure measurement (Figure 84.2). The patient should be intubated if the Glasgow Coma Scale score is 8 or less. The emergency personnel should notify the emergency department and transport the patient to a stroke center if possible. If seizure is suspected, the seizure protocol should be initiated in the field.

Seizure

If patients present with an isolated seizure, CT of the brain should be performed to rule out associated brain hemorrhage as a precipitant of the seizure. If hemorrhage is absent, the patient should receive antiseizure medications and be evaluated further as an outpatient for long-term seizure and AVM management (see Treatment section below). If the patient had multiple seizures within several hours or is in status epilepticus, further inpatient treatment and monitoring are necessary.

Intraventricular and Intraparenchymal Hemorrhage

Upon arrival at a stroke center, a patient with a focal neurologic deficit or thunderclap headache should immediately undergo imaging of the brain. Imaging will aid in establishing whether brain hemorrhage has occurred and in determining whether the patient has any associated mass effect or hydrocephalus. Many patients have brain hemorrhage but do not have an AVM. An AVM should be considered as a possible cause of brain hemorrhage in patients younger than 40 years, especially if the hemorrhage is in a lobar location. An AVM should also be considered if patients have isolated interventricular blood, if patients are older and have hemorrhage but no typical risk factors such as hypertension, or if blood is in an atypical location. If AVM is suspected, consideration should be given to noninvasive angiography (eg, CT angiography or MRA), which may be especially helpful for planning purposes if the patient may require urgent hematoma evacuation. If an AVM is discovered, conventional angiography would be needed for a more detailed evaluation.

Hydrocephalus and mass effect require immediate attention because they can markedly increase morbidity and mortality. Hydrocephalus often accompanies intraventricular extension of hemorrhage. Use of an external ventricular drain may need to be considered. Management of increased intracranial pressure (ICP) with medications or surgery (or both) should be considered. The reason to perform surgery early in patients with life-threatening bleeding or increased ICP is to remove enough of the hematoma to decrease the ICP. The AVM, however, is typically not resected at the same time unless it is small and superficial.

After their condition is stabilized, patients with intracranial hemorrhage related to AVM should be hospitalized in a neurosciences intensive care unit. Standard intracerebral hemorrhage management should be followed to

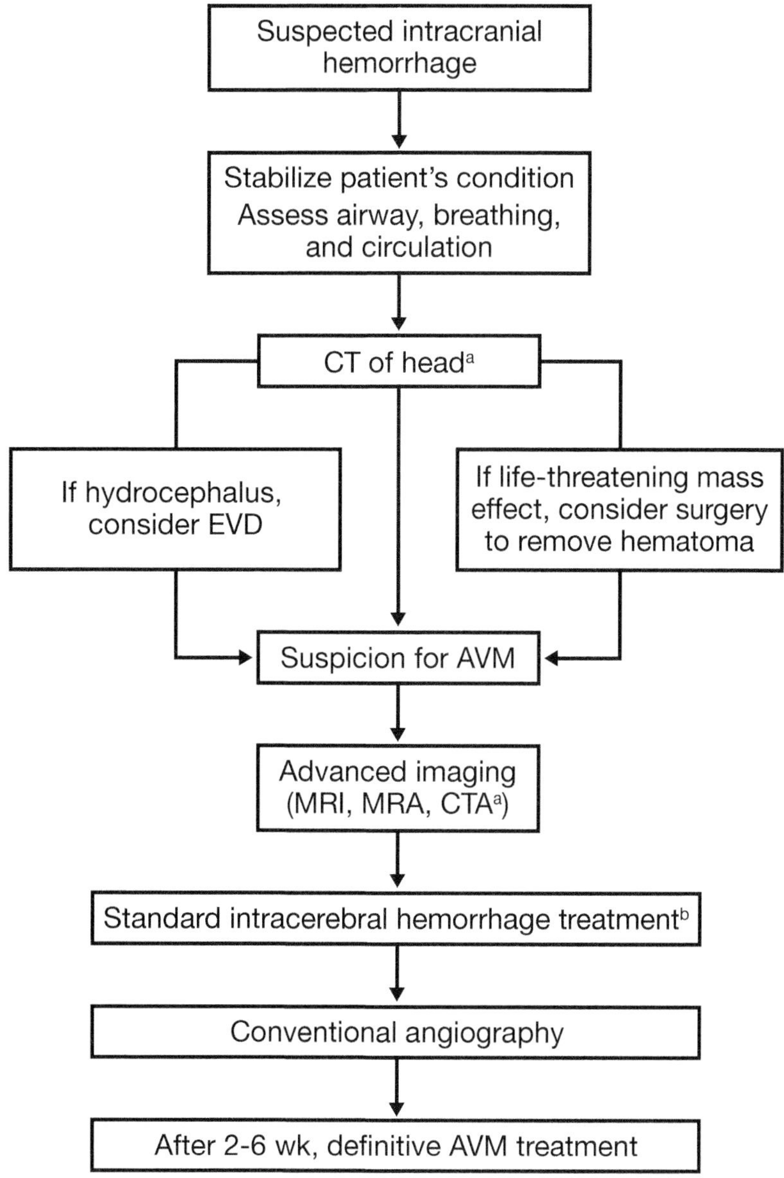

Figure 84.2. Acute Care for Patients With Suspected Intracranial Hemorrhage. Superscript a indicates that if surgery is planned to remove a hematoma, computed tomographic angiography (CTA) may be performed earlier. Superscript b *indicates that guidelines for the management of acute intracerebral hemorrhage have been published by the American Heart Association. AVM indicates arteriovenous malformation; CT, computed tomography; EVD, external ventricular drain; MRA, magnetic resonance angiography; MRI, magnetic resonance imaging.*

correct coagulopathies, hyperthermia, and hyperglycemia. Analgesia should be considered for pain. Seizure prophylaxis is not required, but seizure medications should be instituted if the patient presented with seizure or if seizure is a concern. An exact blood pressure goal is not clear, but the general recommendation is to maintain a systolic pressure of 140 mm Hg or less while maintaining cerebral perfusion pressure between 60 and 80 mm Hg according to data extrapolated from the Intensive Blood Pressure Reduction in Acute Cerebral Hemorrhage Trial (INTERACT). Invasive monitoring of ICP may be required if the patient has hydrocephalus or is comatose.

Securing the AVM

If an AVM has ruptured and the risk of recurrent hemorrhage is high, the AVM should be secured. Surgery is generally preferred to stereotactic radiosurgery because of the immediacy of decreasing recurrent hemorrhage (see

Treatment section below). However, many patient and AVM features must be considered to determine the appropriate treatment.

Conventional angiography is usually performed to assess the AVM in more detail. In certain situations, a feeding artery aneurysm may be coiled during cerebral angiography, especially if it is larger than 7 mm or appears to be the source of bleeding. Additionally, transarterial embolization of some of the feeding arteries can be performed to aid in future AVM removal. If surgery is considered, it is often delayed by 2 to 6 weeks to allow edema to resolve (so it does not obscure and compress the AVM) and to allow the hematoma to liquefy (to allow for a better dissection plane).

After AVM surgical treatment, a patient should be admitted to the neurosciences intensive care unit for 24 hours. Treatment goals should include normotension and euvolemia. A postoperative angiogram is recommended to ensure complete obliteration of the AVM.

Treatment

Overview

The 4 approaches to treatment are medical or conservative management, open neurosurgery, endovascular neurosurgery, and radiosurgery. More than 1 may be used for a complex AVM (eg, endovascular neurosurgery before radiosurgery or open surgery). Recommendations for management of AVM are from natural history cohorts, 1 clinical trial, surgical series, expert reviews, and the 2001 American Heart Association guidelines. The goals of treating an AVM are to decrease the risk of hemorrhage, prevent seizures, and, in some patients, palliate symptoms (eg, headache and focal neurologic deficit). Options for treatment include 1 or more of the following: microvascular surgery, stereotactic radiosurgery, and endovascular embolization. A multidisciplinary team should determine the type of intervention for each patient with AVM and assess the risk of AVM rupture, the surgical or intervention risk due to the AVM location and other comorbidities, and the patient's preferences. If intervention is recommended, the appropriate timing must be considered. Medical management of symptoms and observation of the AVM may be warranted. Observation may be especially appropriate if the patient is asymptomatic and the AVM has low-risk features.

Patients with AVM presenting with intracranial hemorrhage have a high risk of morbidity, death, and future bleeding, so they require definitive treatment to decrease the risk of future hemorrhage. When possible, surgical intervention is preferred for recent hemorrhage because it can be curative immediately, whereas radiosurgery decreases the hemorrhage rate after 2 to 3 years, which is the time it takes for the AVM to involute and be obliterated.

Less certain is the management of unruptured AVMs. A Randomized Trial of Unruptured Brain Arteriovenous Malformations (ARUBA) randomly assigned patients to 1) medical management and observation or 2) medical management and AVM intervention (the type of intervention was at the discretion of the treating team). The treating teams had to accept that a patient could be randomly assigned to either group in the trial, the patient had to agree to random assignment, and the AVM needed to be one that could be obliterated by intervention. The main outcome measure was death or symptomatic stroke. The study had a planned enrollment of 400 patients, but the trial was stopped after 226 were entered because the outcomes in the medical group were superior to those in the intervention group, which had a significant increased risk of death or stroke. The study had many criticisms and left further questions about treatment of patients with unruptured AVM. The most common concerns included selection bias, low enrollment rate, choice of outcome measures, heterogeneity of patients, short follow-up, and lack of standard intervention.

Microvascular Neurosurgery

Microsurgical AVM resection with complete removal of the AVM has a curative rate of 94% to 100%. Definitive removal of the AVM eliminates the risk of future hemorrhage immediately. Postoperative angiography is often performed to show the successful complete resection. When surgery is performed because of intractable seizures, up to 60% to 80% of patients may become seizure-free in 2 to 3 years.

The Spetzler-Martin AVM grading system is commonly used to assess surgical risk (Table 84.1). In the original grading system, points were assigned for AVM size, presence of deep venous drainage, and eloquence of the AVM location, resulting in 5 AVM grades. A higher Spetzler-Martin grade indicates higher surgical risk. Various modifications of this scoring system have been proposed, including the 3-tier Spetzler-Ponce classification (Table 84.2). With this AVM classification, Spetzler-Martin grades I and II are grouped into class A, which includes AVMs for which surgical resection is generally recommended. Spetzler-Martin grade III AVMs are grouped into class B; multimodal treatment is generally recommended for class B AVMs. Spetzler-Martin grades IV and V are grouped into class C; in general, conservative management is recommended for these AVMs. If patients have recurrent hemorrhage, progressive neurologic deficits, or intractable seizures and a class C AVM, intervention could be considered.

Over the years, morbidity and mortality from surgery have decreased because of the use of numerous tools, including functional imaging and tractography for preoperative planning, green indocyanine intraoperatively to ensure complete obliteration of the AVM, and newer surgical instruments. Despite these advances, surgery still

Table 84.1 • Spetzler-Martin Grading System for Intracranial AVMs

Feature	Points[a]
Size of nidus, cm	
<3	1
3-6	2
>6	3
Eloquence[b]	
No	0
Yes	1
Pattern of venous drainage	
Superficial	0
Deep	1

Abbreviation: AVM, arteriovenous malformation.

[a] Grade is determined from the sum of the points for each of the 3 features, from grade I (1 point) to grade V (5 points).

[b] Eloquent brain areas: sensorimotor, language, and visual areas of the cerebral cortex; hypothalamus and thalamus; brainstem; cerebellar nuclei; and regions immediately adjacent to these structures.

From Spetzler RF, Martin NA. A proposed grading system for arteriovenous malformations. J Neurosurg. 1986 Oct;65(4):476–83; used with permission.

carries risks, including intraoperative rupture, feeding vessel thrombosis, and edema, and the location and diffuse angioarchitecture of an AVM can limit surgical accessibility. Surgical morbidity and mortality vary considerably because of these factors and others, but in general, estimates of risk range from 2% to 8%.

Stereotactic Radiosurgery

Stereotactic radiosurgery (eg, Gamma Knife, linear accelerator, and proton beam therapy) is also a consideration for the treatment of AVMs. It uses multiple focused beams of radiation aimed at the nidus of the AVM. With this technique, radiation results in proliferation of smooth muscle in the vessel wall with subsequent involution and obliteration or thrombosis of the AVM, which takes approximately 2 to 3 years. During that time, the patient remains at risk for hemorrhage. For this reason, surgery is generally preferred if an AVM has already hemorrhaged and is surgically accessible. Among patients who have had seizures and undergo radiosurgery, 50% to 60% achieve seizure freedom, depending on the size of the AVM and other characteristics.

Stereotactic radiosurgery is most successful in patients with small lesions and a compact nidus. In approximately 80% of patients with AVMs smaller than 3 cm in greatest diameter, radiosurgery results in complete obliteration of the AVM after 3 years. Patients with larger AVMs may have lower obliteration rates, a higher risk of radiation-related complications, or a need for staged radiosurgery (ie, multiple treatment sessions). Patients with a large, diffuse AVM nidus are less favorable candidates for stereotactic radiosurgery. The risk of subsequent radiation necrosis is approximately 1% to 3% and depends on the dose delivered and the volume treated.

Table 84.2 • Spetzler-Ponce 3-Tier Classification for Intracranial AVMs

Class	Spetzler-Martin Grade	Suggested Treatment
A	I and II	Surgical resection
B	III	Multimodality treatment
C	IV and V	No treatment

Abbreviation: AVM, arteriovenous malformation.

From Spetzler RF, Ponce FA. A 3-tier classification of cerebral arteriovenous malformations: clinical article. J Neurosurg. 2011 Mar;114(3):842–9. Epub 2010 Oct 8; used with permission.

Endovascular Embolization and Treatment

Endovascular embolization is a common adjunct to surgical treatment of AVMs and may be curative, in isolation, in less than 10% of patients. Endovascular embolization of arterial feeders can be useful for decreasing nidal size and vascularity before resection. In addition, endovascular treatment of associated aneurysms is often considered. In some patients, embolization is used for palliation of symptoms (eg, headache and focal neurologic deficit) when an AVM is not amenable to radiosurgery or excision. Superselective catheterization and occlusion of arterial feeders with metallic coils or liquid embolic material (eg, ethylene vinyl alcohol copolymer or *N*-butyl cyanoacrylate) can be performed to reduce high-flow shunts, to decrease AVM nidus size, and, rarely, to obliterate intranidal aneurysms that may have bled.

By performing embolization before surgery, the size and vascularity of the AVM can be decreased, potentially decreasing blood loss and surgical complications in complex AVMs. Preoperative embolization is rarely used before stereotactic radiosurgery (to decrease the size of the AVM); no evidence exists that this approach is effective, and in many studies, outcomes have actually been worse after radiosurgery on previously embolized AVMs.

Although an endovascular approach is less invasive than surgery, complications can occur. In a large meta-analysis (Gross and Du, 2013; see Suggested Reading), complication rates were 5% to 22%, with permanent morbidity and death occurring in approximately 6%. Risks can include embolization of arteries supplying healthy brain tissue; perforation of arterial feeders, resulting in hemorrhage; occlusion of draining veins before obliterating arterial inflow, with a resultant increase in intranidal pressure and a potential for catastrophic hemorrhage; and incomplete embolization.

Summary

- Intracranial AVMs are high-flow shunts from arteries to veins without intervening parenchyma.
- Patients with intracranial AVMs most commonly present emergently because of brain hemorrhage (50% of patients), seizures (15%-35%), neurologic deficits (<10%), or headache, or an intracranial AVM may be an incidental finding on an imaging study performed for an unrelated reason.
- Patients with intracranial AVMs who present with brain hemorrhage have a high risk of morbidity and death.
- Urgent diagnosis and treatment of associated hydrocephalus, seizures, and mass effect are important.
- The natural history of the AVM and the risk of future hemorrhage for each patient should be weighed against the risk of treatment to determine the best management approach to minimize the risk of morbidity and death.
- Securing the AVM itself is often performed 2 to 6 weeks post hemorrhage.
- The Spetzler-Martin AVM grading systemand careful consideration of patient factors and angioarchitectural features of the AVM can aid practitioners in decision making for treatment of ruptured AVM.

SUGGESTED READING

Albert P. Personal experience in the treatment of 178 cases of arteriovenous malformations of the brain. Acta Neurochir (Wien). 1982;61(1-3):207–26.

Anderson CS, Heeley E, Huang Y, Wang J, Stapf C, Delcourt C, et al; INTERACT2 Investigators. Rapid blood-pressure lowering in patients with acute intracerebral hemorrhage. N Engl J Med. 2013 Jun 20;368(25):2355–65. Epub 2013 May 29.

Aoki N. Do intracranial arteriovenous malformations cause subarachnoid haemorrhage? Review of computed tomography features of ruptured arteriovenous malformations in the acute stage. Acta Neurochir (Wien). 1991;112(3-4):92–5.

Aoun SG, Bendok BR, Batjer HH. Acute management of ruptured arteriovenous malformations and dural arteriovenous fistulas. Neurosurg Clin N Am. 2012 Jan;23(1):87–103.

Awad IA, Robinson JR Jr, Mohanty S, Estes ML. Mixed vascular malformations of the brain: clinical and pathogenetic considerations. Neurosurgery. 1993 Aug;33(2):179–88.

Braksick SA, Fugate JE. Management of brain arteriovenous malformations. Curr Treat Options Neurol. 2015 Jul;17(7):358.

Brown RD Jr, Wiebers DO, Torner JC, O'Fallon WM. Incidence and prevalence of intracranial vascular malformations in Olmsted County, Minnesota, 1965 to 1992. Neurology. 1996 Apr;46(4):949–52.

Crawford PM, West CR, Chadwick DW, Shaw MD. Arteriovenous malformations of the brain: natural history in unoperated patients. J Neurol Neurosurg Psychiatry. 1986 Jan;49(1):1–10.

Crawford PM, West CR, Shaw MD, Chadwick DW. Cerebral arteriovenous malformations and epilepsy: factors in the development of epilepsy. Epilepsia. 1986 May-Jun;27(3):270–5.

Forster DM, Steiner L, Hakanson S. Arteriovenous malformations of the brain: a long-term clinical study. J Neurosurg. 1972 Nov;37(5):562–70.

Fults D, Kelly DL Jr. Natural history of arteriovenous malformations of the brain: a clinical study. Neurosurgery. 1984 Nov;15(5):658–62.

Goldberg J, Raabe A, Bervini D. Natural history of brain arteriovenous malformations: systematic review. J Neurosurg Sci. 2018 Aug;62(4):437–43. Epub 2018 Mar 28.

Gonzalez LF, Bristol RE, Porter RW, Spetzler RF. De novo presentation of an arteriovenous malformation: case report and review of the literature. J Neurosurg. 2005 Apr;102(4):726–9.

Guidetti B, Delitala A. Intracranial arteriovenous malformations: conservative and surgical treatment. J Neurosurg. 1980 Aug;53(2):149–52.

Hartmann A, Mohr JP. Acute management of brain arteriovenous malformations. Curr Treat Options Neurol. 2015 May;17(5):346.

Jomin M, Lesoin F, Lozes G. Prognosis for arteriovenous malformations of the brain in adults based on 150 cases. Surg Neurol. 1985 Apr;23(4):362–6.

Kader A, Young WL, Pile-Spellman J, Mast H, Sciacca RR, Mohr JP, et al. The influence of hemodynamic and anatomic factors on hemorrhage from cerebral arteriovenous malformations. Neurosurgery. 1994 May;34(5):801–7.

Kalimo H, Katse M, Haltia M. Vascular diseases. In: Graham DI, Lantos PL, editors. Greenfield's neuropathology. 6th ed. Vol. 1. London (UK): Arnold; New York (NY): Oxford University Press; c1991. p. 345–7.

Khaw AV, Mohr JP, Sciacca RR, Schumacher HC, Hartmann A, Pile-Spellman J, et al. Association of infratentorial brain arteriovenous malformations with hemorrhage at initial presentation. Stroke. 2004 Mar;35(3):660–3. Epub 2004 Jan 29.

Laakso A, Hernesniemi J. Arteriovenous malformations: epidemiology and clinical presentation. Neurosurg Clin N Am. 2012 Jan;23(1):1–6.

Langer DJ, Lasner TM, Hurst RW, Flamm ES, Zager EL, King JT Jr. Hypertension, small size, and deep venous drainage are associated with risk of hemorrhagic presentation of cerebral arteriovenous malformations. Neurosurgery. 1998 Mar;42(3):481–6.

Lasjaunias P, Piske R, Terbrugge K, Willinsky R. Cerebral arteriovenous malformations (C. AVM) and associated arterial aneurysms (AA): analysis of 101 C. AVM cases, with 37 AA in 23 patients. Acta Neurochir (Wien). 1988;91(1-2):29–36.

Magro E, Gentric J-C, Darsaut TE, Ziegler D, Bojanowski MW, Raymond J. Responses to ARUBA: a systematic review and critical analysis for the design of future arteriovenous malformation trials. J Neurosurg. 2017 Feb;126(2):486–94. Epub 2016 Apr 29.

Mahajan A, Manchandia TC, Gould G, Bulsara KR. De novo arteriovenous malformations: case report and review of the literature. Neurosurg Rev. 2010 Jan;33(1):115–9. Epub 2009 Sep 29.

McCormick WF. The pathology of vascular ("arteriovenous") malformations. J Neurosurg. 1966 Apr;24(4):807–16.

Michelsen WJ. Natural history and pathophysiology of arteriovenous malformations. Clin Neurosurg. 1979;26:307–13.

Mohr JP, Moskowitz AJ, Stapf C, Hartmann A, Lord K, Marshall SM, et al. The ARUBA trial: current status, future hopes. Stroke. 2010 Aug;41(8):e537–40. Epub 2010 Jul 15.

Morello G, Borghi GP. Cerebral angiomas: a report of 154 personal cases and a comparison between the results of surgical excision and conservative management. Acta Neurochir (Wien). 1973;28(3):135–55.

Novakovic RL, Lazzaro MA, Castonguay AC, Zaidat OO. The diagnosis and management of brain arteriovenous malformations. Neurol Clin. 2013 Aug;31(3):749–63. Epub 2013 Apr 17.

Ogilvy CS, Stieg PE, Awad I, Brown RD Jr, Kondziolka D, Rosenwasser R, et al; Special Writing Group of the Stroke Council, American Stroke Association. AHA Scientific Statement: recommendations for the management of intracranial arteriovenous malformations: a statement for healthcare professionals from a special writing group of the Stroke Council, American Stroke Association. Stroke. 2001 Jun;32(6):1458–71.

Ondra SL, Troupp H, George ED, Schwab K. The natural history of symptomatic arteriovenous malformations of the brain: a 24-year follow-up assessment. J Neurosurg. 1990 Sep;73(3):387–91.

Perret G, Nishioka H. Report on the cooperative study of intracranial aneurysms and subarachnoid hemorrhage. Section VI. Arteriovenous malformations: an analysis of 545 cases of cranio-cerebral arteriovenous malformations and fistulae reported to the cooperative study. J Neurosurg. 1966 Oct;25(4):467–90.

Pollock BE, Flickinger JC, Lunsford LD, Bissonette DJ, Kondziolka D. Factors that predict the bleeding risk of cerebral arteriovenous malformations. Stroke. 1996 Jan;27(1):1–6.

Redekop G, TerBrugge K, Montanera W, Willinsky R. Arterial aneurysms associated with cerebral arteriovenous malformations: classification, incidence, and risk of hemorrhage. J Neurosurg. 1998 Oct;89(4):539–46.

Sorenson TJ, Brinjikji W, Bortolotti C, Kaufmann G, Lanzino G. Recurrent brain arteriovenous malformations (avms): a systematic review. World Neurosurg. 2018 Aug;116:e856–66. Epub 2018 May 26.

Spetzler RF, Hargraves RW, McCormick PW, Zabramski JM, Flom RA, Zimmerman RS. Relationship of perfusion pressure and size to risk of hemorrhage from arteriovenous malformations. J Neurosurg. 1992 Jun;76(6):918–23.

Spetzler RF, Martin NA. A proposed grading system for arteriovenous malformations. J Neurosurg. 1986 Oct;65(4):476–83.

Spetzler RF, Ponce FA. A 3-tier classification of cerebral arteriovenous malformations: clinical article. J Neurosurg. 2011 Mar;114(3):842–9. Epub 2010 Oct 8.

Starke RM, Komotar RJ, Hwang BY, Fischer LE, Garrett MC, Otten ML, et al. Treatment guidelines for cerebral arteriovenous malformation microsurgery. Br J Neurosurg. 2009 Aug;23(4):376–86.

Stefani MA, Porter PJ, terBrugge KG, Montanera W, Willinsky RA, Wallace MC. Angioarchitectural factors present in brain arteriovenous malformations associated with hemorrhagic presentation. Stroke. 2002 Apr;33(4):920–4.

Wu EM, El Ahmadieh TY, McDougall CM, Aoun SG, Mehta N, Neeley OJ, et al. Embolization of brain arteriovenous malformations with intent to cure: a systematic review. J Neurosurg. 2019 Feb 1:1–12. [Epub ahead of print]

85 Cerebral Venous and Dural Sinus Thrombosis

SARA E. HOCKER, MD

Goals

- Describe the diagnosis of cerebral venous and dural sinus thrombosis.
- Review early interventions for patients with cerebral venous thrombosis.
- Review the management of clinical complications of cerebral venous and dural sinus thrombosis.
- Review recommendations for prevention of recurrence of cerebral venous and dural sinus thrombosis.

Introduction

Cerebral venous and dural sinus thrombosis (CVDST) is a rare cause of stroke that accounts for only 0.5% to 1% of all strokes. Diagnosis is challenging because of the diverse spectrum of clinical presentations. Onset is usually acute or subacute, but symptoms may be subtle, and neurologic examination findings may be normal. When a stroke occurs, it is often a hemorrhagic infarct. Therefore, to make a timely diagnosis, a high degree of awareness is required when at-risk patients present with neurologic symptoms or signs.

Clinical Presentation

Headache is present in 90% of patients with CVDST. Patients commonly present with a subacute-onset headache that may occur in combination with 1 or more of the following: encephalopathy, focal deficits, or seizures. Seizures, which may be focal or generalized, occur in approximately 40% of patients. Signs and symptoms suggestive of increased intracranial pressure may also be present. These include intermittent visual obscurations, garbled speech, or diplopia. If intracranial hypertension is suspected, supportive evidence may include papilledema or sixth nerve palsies. Stupor or coma rarely occurs at hospital admission, and often patients have extensive thrombosis or involvement of the deep venous system with bilateral thalamic lesions.

Uncommon presentations include isolated thunderclap headache, transient ischemic attack, isolated or multiple cranial nerve palsies, cavernous sinus syndrome, tinnitus, or psychiatric symptoms. The combination of orbital pain, chemosis, proptosis, and oculomotor palsies points to a cavernous sinus syndrome; aphasia may suggest transverse sinus involvement on the dominant side; and a combination of sensorimotor deficits and focal seizures may suggest cortical vein thrombosis.

Risk Factors and Pathophysiology

The symptoms and signs of CVDST arise from intracranial hypertension resulting from impaired venous drainage and focal brain injury from venous ischemia, infarction, or hemorrhage. Causes are related to stasis of blood flow, hypercoagulability, and endothelial injury to the vessel wall, and acquired or genetic risks may be present. Clinicians should inquire about historical features, including a personal or family history of venous thromboembolism, systemic inflammatory disease, or malignancy; recent head trauma; use of exogenous hormones or puerperal status; recent or ongoing parameningeal or central nervous system infections (otitis media, sinusitis, or mastoiditis); and dehydration (eg, from recent severe vomiting or diarrhea). Several causes and tests are helpful in defining the risk of recurrence (Box 85.1). The most common associated risk factor is oral contraceptive use. The next most common risk factors are prothrombotic conditions (eg, antithrombin III deficiency, protein C or S deficiency, and

Box 85.1 • Risk Factors and Related Tests for Defining Risk of CVDST Recurrence

- Acquired risks
  - Medications
    - Inquire about oral contraceptive use
    - Drug of abuse screen
  - Recent head trauma
  - Dehydration
    - History of vomiting or diarrhea
    - Serum urea nitrogen concentration
    - Hemoconcentration
  - Infection or inflammatory disease
    - Inquire about infectious symptoms, including ear or tooth pain and sinus tenderness
    - Chest radiograph, urinalysis, blood cultures, ESR, stool studies, lumbar puncture, otoscopic examination, or CT of maxillofacial structures as indicated according to clinical history
  - Pregnancy
    - Serum or urine hCG test
  - Malignancy
    - History of fever, night sweats, weight loss
    - Consider CT of chest and abdomen
- Genetic risks
  - Thrombophilia evaluation
    - Prothrombin time
    - Activated prothrombin time
    - Protein C and S deficiencies[a]
    - Prothrombin G20210A (homozygous or heterozygous)
    - Factor V Leiden (homozygous or heterozygous)
    - Antithrombin III deficiency[a]
    - Antiphospholipid antibody syndrome (lupus anticoagulant, anticardiolipin antibody, and anti-β2 glycoprotein 1)
    - Increased factor VIII
    - Hyperhomocysteinemia
  - Systemic diseases
    - Systemic lupus erythematosus
    - Inflammatory bowel disease
    - Sarcoidosis
    - Behçet disease

Abbreviations: CT, computed tomography; CVDST, cerebral venous and dural sinus thrombosis; ESR, erythrocyte sedimentation rate; hCG, human chorionic gonadotropin.

[a] Testing should be deferred until 2 to 4 weeks after completion of anticoagulation.

antiphospholipid antibody syndrome); pregnancy or puerperium; and parameningeal infections. Many uncommon associations have also been reported, and approximately 12% of patients have no identifiable risk factor.

Diagnosis

When CVDST is suspected, the initial test is computed tomography (CT). Although CT of the head may show no abnormalities for 25% to 50% of patients, CT is necessary because a diagnosis of CVDST is supported by identification of infarctions in nonarterial distributions near the sinuses, bilateral thalamic infarctions, and thrombosed veins that appear as hyperdense lesions close to the skull. Approximately 30% to 40% of patients with CVDST present with intracranial hemorrhage that is most commonly intraparenchymal but may be subarachnoid (Figure 85.1). Confirmation can be achieved with imaging of the cerebral veins and sinuses with a CT venogram (CTV) or magnetic resonance venogram (MRV). Figure 85.2 shows the cerebral venous system and the most frequent locations of cerebral venous and sinus thrombosis. Cerebral 4-vessel digital subtraction angiography is recommended when patients have inconclusive CTV or MRV findings and clinical suspicion remains high.

Initial Treatment

The American Heart Association and American Stroke Association have developed an algorithm for the diagnosis and management of patients with CVDST (Figure 85.3). Current recommendations include the use of dose-adjusted intravenous heparin (targeting an activated partial thromboplastin time that is twice the control) or weight-adjusted subcutaneous low-molecular-weight heparin. The evidence for this practice is based predominantly on small trials and systematic reviews; however, anticoagulation is clearly favored for all patients with CVDST, including those with intracranial hemorrhage. Outcomes are better for patients receiving anticoagulation overall and are not worse for patients receiving anticoagulation. Some evidence suggests that hematoma enlargement is related to clot propagation rather than to anticoagulation itself.

After hydration and anticoagulation, patients should be followed with serial neurologic examinations and CT of the head whenever examination findings change. In addition, the patient's vision should be examined, and those with papilledema or visual blurring may benefit from lumbar puncture. Progressive loss of vision, as measured by serial perimetry, may require optic nerve fenestration for correction.

Deterioration From CVDST

If patients have persistent or evolving symptoms, follow-up CT of the head and either CTV or MRV are recommended. Of the potential causes of deterioration in patients with CVDST (Box 85.2), the most concerning initially is propagation of thrombus despite adequate anticoagulation. Propagation of thrombus may lead to additional venous

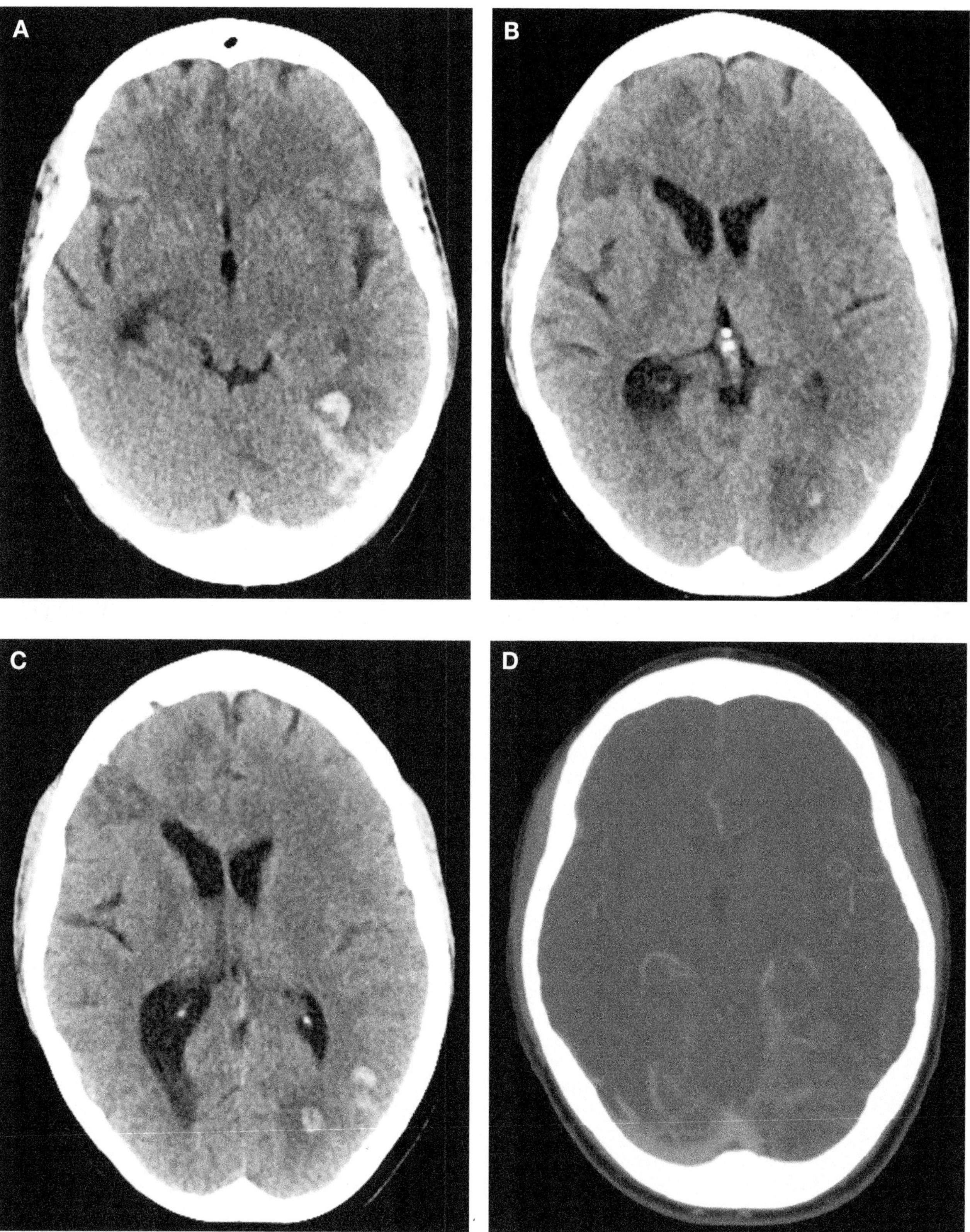

Figure 85.1. Computed Tomography (CT) of the Head Showing Hematoma and Thrombosis. A and B, Axial slices show acute left parietooccipital intraparenchymal hematoma. C, A spontaneous hyperdensity of the left transverse sinus is apparent. B and C, CT shows associated edema and mass effect on the brain parenchyma with effacement of the temporal horn of the left lateral ventricle. D, CT venogram of the head with intravenous contrast agent shows occlusive venous sinus thrombosis within the left transverse sinus.

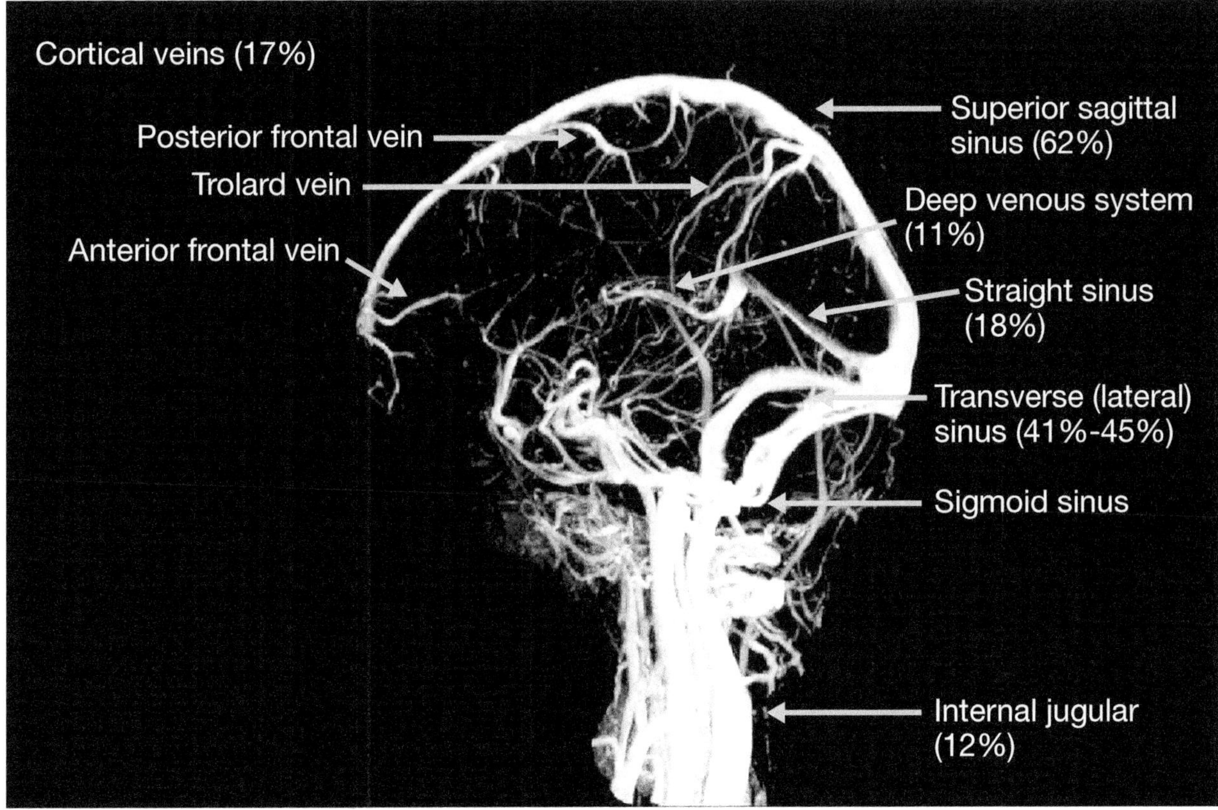

Figure 85.2. Magnetic Resonance Venogram of Cerebral Venous System and Most Frequent Locations of Cerebral Venous and Sinus Thrombosis. Percentages indicate frequencies from a sample of 624 patients.

(From Saposnik G, Barinagarrementeria F, Brown RD Jr, Bushnell CD, Cucchiara B, Cushman M, et al; American Heart Association Stroke Council and the Council on Epidemiology and Prevention. Diagnosis and management of cerebral venous thrombosis: a statement for healthcare professionals from the American Heart Association/American Stroke Association. Stroke. 2011 Apr;42[4]:1158-92. Epub 2011 Feb 3; used with permission. Data for figure from: Ferro JM, Canhao P, Stam J, Bousser MG, Barinagarrementeria F; ISCVT Investigators. Prognosis of cerebral vein and dural sinus thrombosis: results of the International Study on Cerebral Vein and Dural Sinus Thrombosis [ISCVT]. Stroke. 2004 Mar;35[3]:664-70. Epub 2004 Feb 19.)

infarctions, hemorrhagic transformation of infarcted brain, and worsening cerebral edema. Endovascular therapy may be considered for these patients and may involve catheter-directed local administration of thrombolytics with or without mechanical clot disruption. These techniques have been shown to be reasonably safe. Systemic thrombolysis has also been attempted in this situation, but the evidence is not as robust as it is for endovascular therapy.

Progressive cerebral edema or an enlarging hematoma may produce tissue shift leading to brainstem compression. Hyperosmolar therapy with or without sedation is indicated; however, it may be less effective in patients with an impaired blood-brain barrier. When clinical and radiographic herniation occurs despite these measures, decompressive craniectomy to evacuate the hematoma or allow the edematous brain to swell away from the brainstem may be needed.

A decreasing level of consciousness with no change on CT may indicate intracranial hypertension, expected fluctuations due to thalamic lesions, or nonconvulsive seizures. Seizures occur in 10% to 37% of patients with CVDST and are most commonly focal. Prophylactic antiseizure drugs are not recommended; however, if patients have a single seizure, initiation of an antiseizure drug to prevent subsequent seizures is appropriate.

Long-term Management

If a patient's condition remains stable or improves after anticoagulation, therapy should be transitioned to an oral anticoagulant for 3 to 6 months or life, depending on the underlying cause of thrombosis. Consultation with a physician with expertise in thrombosis may be useful to assist in the prothrombotic testing and determination of duration of anticoagulation therapy. Patients with provoked CVDST (ie, associated with a transient risk factor such as pregnancy or head trauma) are treated with vitamin K antagonists for 3 to 6 months, and those with unprovoked CVDST

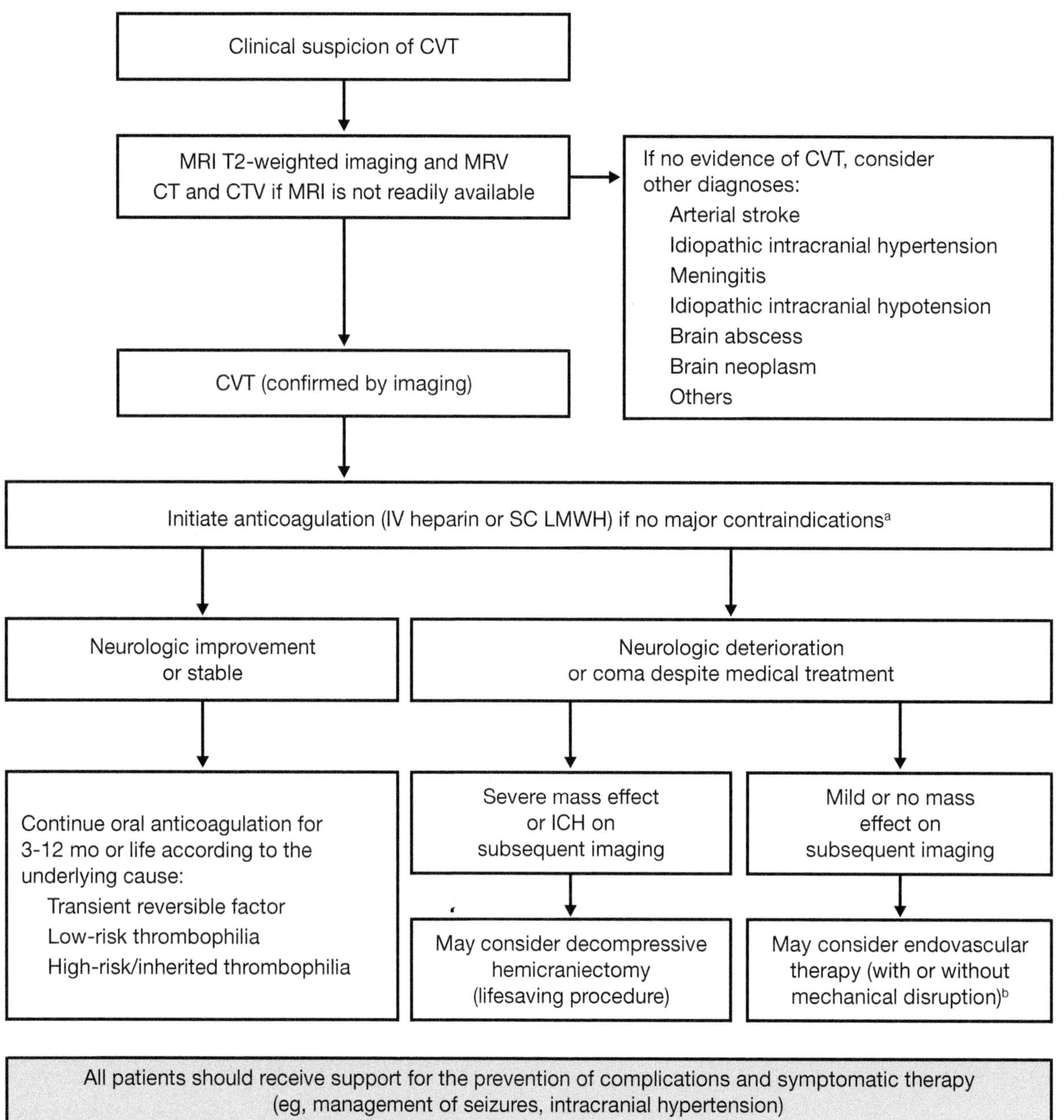

Figure 85.3. Algorithm for the Initial Management of Cerebral Venous Thrombosis (CVT). Anticoagulation is the principal therapy and is aimed at preventing thrombus propagation and increasing recanalization, but treatment must be individualized. (For details, see Saposnik et al, 2011; see Suggested Reading.) Superscript a *indicates that intracranial hemorrhage that occurred as a consequence of cerebral venous and sinus thrombosis is not a contraindication for anticoagulation. Superscript* b *indicates that endovascular therapy may be considered if the patient has absolute contraindications for anticoagulation therapy or if initial therapeutic doses of anticoagulant therapy failed. CT indicates computed tomography; CTV, computed tomographic venography; ICH, intracerebral hemorrhage; IV, intravenous; LMWH, low-molecular-weight heparin; MRI, magnetic resonance imaging; MRV, magnetic resonance venography; SC subcutaneous.*

(From Saposnik G, Barinagarrementeria F, Brown RD Jr, Bushnell CD, Cucchiara B, Cushman M, et al; American Heart Association Stroke Council and the Council on Epidemiology and Prevention. Diagnosis and management of cerebral venous thrombosis: a statement for healthcare professionals from the American Heart Association/American Stroke Association. Stroke. 2011 Apr;42[4]:1158-92. Epub 2011 Feb 3; used with permission.)

Box 85.2 • Causes of Deterioration in Patients With Cerebral Venous and Dural Sinus Thrombosis

Propagation of thrombus
Venous infarction
Hemorrhagic transformation of venous infarctions
Brainstem compression from an enlarging hematoma
Cerebral edema
Seizures (convulsive or nonconvulsive)
Pulmonary emboli from thrombosed jugular veins or deep vein thrombosis associated with immobilization

From Wijdicks EFM, Rabinstein AA, Hocker SE, Fugate JE. Neurocritical care. 2nd ed. New York (NY): Oxford University Press; c2016. Chapter 11, Cerebral venous thrombosis not responding to anticoagulation; p. 77-84. (What do I do now? series); used with permission of Mayo Foundation for Medical Education and Research.

are treated for 6 to 12 months (target international normalized ratio, 2-3). Anticoagulation may be considered for an indefinite duration if patients have recurrent CVDST, venous thromboembolism after an episode of CVDST, or a first episode of CVDST with severe thrombophilia (ie, homozygous prothrombin G20210A, homozygous factor V Leiden, antithrombin III deficiency, combined thrombophilia defects, antiphospholipid antibody syndrome, or deficiency of protein C or S). Follow-up vascular imaging (CTV or MRV) is recommended after 3 to 6 months of treatment to assess for recanalization of the occluded veins or sinuses. For patients without thrombophilia, the timing and risks of discontinuing anticoagulation are unknown.

Outcome

Outcome is favorable overall with an in-hospital mortality rate of 2% and long-term death and dependency rates of 15%. Predictors of poor outcome include hydrocephalus, extensive parenchymal brain lesions, central nervous system infections, and coma at presentation; however, exceptions exist and should not preclude aggressive treatment.

Summary

- A high degree of awareness is required when patients at risk for CVDST present with headache, because examination and neuroimaging findings may initially be normal.
- Full anticoagulation is the standard of care even if patients have intracranial hemorrhage.
- Patients who have clot propagation despite anticoagulation may benefit from endovascular therapy.
- Decompressive craniectomy or hematoma evacuation (or both) may be lifesaving for patients who have mass effect from stroke.
- Risk of recurrence must be estimated to determine duration of anticoagulation.

SUGGESTED READING

Bousser MG, Ferro JM. Cerebral venous thrombosis: an update. Lancet Neurol. 2007 Feb;6(2):162–70.

Chen C, Li X, Huang L, Zhang J, Chen S, Ye H, et al. Mechanical thrombectomy with intraoperative local thrombolysis versus mechanical thrombectomy with continuous thrombolysis for treatment of cerebral venous sinus thrombosis: a systematic review of 82 cases. World Neurosurg. 2019 Jan 17. pii: S1878-8750(19)30067-1. [Epub ahead of print]

Dmytriw AA, Song JSA, Yu E, Poon CS. Cerebral venous thrombosis: state of the art diagnosis and management. Neuroradiology. 2018 Jul;60(7):669–85. Epub 2018 May 11.

Einhaupl K, Stam J, Bousser MG, De Bruijn SF, Ferro JM, Martinelli I, et al; European Federation of Neurological Societies. EFNS guideline on the treatment of cerebral venous and sinus thrombosis in adult patients. Eur J Neurol. 2010 Oct;17(10):1229–35.

Einhaupl KM, Villringer A, Meister W, Mehraein S, Garner C, Pellkofer M, et al. Heparin treatment in sinus venous thrombosis. Lancet. 1991 Sep 7;338(8767):597–600. Erratum in: Lancet 1991 Oct 12;338(8772):958.

Ferro JM, Canhao P, Stam J, Bousser MG, Barinagarrementeria F; ISCVT Investigators. Prognosis of cerebral vein and dural sinus thrombosis: results of the International Study on Cerebral Vein and Dural Sinus Thrombosis (ISCVT). Stroke. 2004 Mar;35(3):664–70. Epub 2004 Feb 19.

Liberman AL, Gialdini G, Bakradze E, Chatterjee A, Kamel H, Merkler AE. Misdiagnosis of cerebral vein thrombosis in the emergency department. Stroke. 2018 Jun;49(6):1504–6.

Nasr DM, Brinjikji W, Cloft HJ, Saposnik G, Rabinstein AA. Mortality in cerebral venous thrombosis: results from the national inpatient sample database. Cerebrovasc Dis. 2013;35(1):40–4. Epub 2013 Feb 14.

Saposnik G, Barinagarrementeria F, Brown RD Jr, Bushnell CD, Cucchiara B, Cushman M, et al; American Heart Association Stroke Council and the Council on Epidemiology and Prevention. Diagnosis and management of cerebral venous thrombosis: a statement for healthcare professionals from the American Heart Association/American Stroke Association. Stroke. 2011 Apr;42(4):1158–92. Epub 2011 Feb 3.

Siddiqui FM, Dandapat S, Banerjee C, Zuurbier SM, Johnson M, Stam J, et al. Mechanical thrombectomy in cerebral venous thrombosis: systematic review of 185 cases. Stroke. 2015 May;46(5):1263–8. Epub 2015 Apr 21.

Silvis SM, de Sousa DA, Ferro JM, Coutinho JM. Cerebral venous thrombosis. Nat Rev Neurol. 2017 Sep;13(9):555–65.

Viegas LD, Stolz E, Canhao P, Ferro JM. Systemic thrombolysis for cerebral venous and dural sinus thrombosis: a systematic review. Cerebrovasc Dis. 2014;37(1):43–50. Epub 2013 Dec 18.

Zubkov AY, McBane RD, Brown RD, Rabinstein AA. Brain lesions in cerebral venous sinus thrombosis. Stroke. 2009 Apr;40(4):1509–11. Epub 2009 Jan 29.

86 Cervical Arterial Dissection

BART M. DEMAERSCHALK, MD

Goals

- Recognize the clinical signs of spontaneous and traumatic arterial dissections.
- Review the neuroradiology of arterial dissections.
- Review the management of neurovascular arterial dissections.

Introduction

Cervical arterial dissections (CDs) are among the most common causes of stroke in young and middle-aged adults. CD is most prevalent in the upper cervical spine and may involve either the vertebral arteries (VAs) or the carotid arteries. Mechanical forces can lead to intimal injuries of the cervical arteries and result in CD.

Patients with CD can present with unilateral headache, posterior cervical spine pain, or retinal and cerebral ischemia from artery-to-artery embolization, cranial nerve palsies, oculosympathetic palsy, or pulsatile tinnitus. The diagnosis of CD requires a heightened suspicion, a thorough history and physical examination, and selected ancillary tests. Disability related to CD varies from relatively minor (more commonly) to severe neurologic disability or death (less commonly). Emergency treatment of ischemic stroke related to CD may include intravenous alteplase and endovascular management. Antiplatelet and anticoagulant medications are used for prevention of stroke related to CD. Follow-up neuroimaging is generally achieved with noninvasive methods.

Epidemiologic Factors

Although CD accounts for only 2% of all cases of ischemic stroke, it is responsible for 8% to 25% of all ischemic strokes in patients younger than 45 years. The chance of an ischemic stroke being caused by CD is higher for young adults who do not have vascular risk factors. The annual incidence of carotid artery dissection is approximately 3 per 100,000 persons, and the annual incidence of VA dissection is approximately 1 per 100,000. CDs appear to have a slight male predominance (55% vs 45%).

Etiologic Factors

The underlying pathogenesis for CD is unknown, but factors associated with CD are numerous (Box 86.1). CD may be either spontaneous or traumatic. The traumatic event may have been severe (eg, a high-speed collision) or mild (eg, coughing, heavy lifting, or yoga) and blunt or penetrating. The prevalence of CD from trivial trauma is as high as approximately 30%; the prevalence from blunt cervical trauma is approximately 2%. CD may also occur with minor trauma associated with cervical spine hyperextension, rotation, and lateroversion. Cervical manipulative therapy (CMT) is associated with CD.

Anatomical Factors

Internal carotid arteries (ICAs) are more mobile than VAs and so are thought to be less likely to be involved in CD due to CMT. ICA dissections generally begin a few centimeters rostral to the bifurcation and may extend to or beyond the petrous canal. CD may affect both extracranial and intracranial segments of the ICAs and VAs. ICA dissections are less likely than VA dissections to extend intracranially.

In CD, a defect in the intimal layer of the arterial wall allows blood to flow from the lumen into the vessel wall. An intramural hematoma, or false lumen, may exist in the tunica media of the vessel. Several complications may arise: The intramural hematoma may compress the true lumen, resulting in a flow-limiting stenosis, an occlusion, or a near occlusion (angiographically appearing as a string sign). At the proximal end, these stenoses have a markedly

Box 86.1 • Factors Associated With Cervical Arterial Dissection

Alpha$_1$-antitrypsin deficiency
Arterial hypertension
Autosomal dominant polycystic kidney disease
Current use of oral contraceptives
Cystic medial necrosis
Familial cases
Fibromuscular dysplasia
Hereditary hemochromatosis
Hyperhomocysteinemia
Infections
Intercellular adhesion molecule (ICAM)-1 E4690K genetic polymorphism
Lentiginosis
Major and minor cervical trauma
Marfan syndrome
Methylenetetrahydrofolate reductase (MTHFR) C677T genotype
Migraine
Moyamoya disease
Osteogenesis imperfecta type I
Styloid process length
Trauma
Turner syndrome
Ultrastructural connective tissue abnormalities
Vascular subtype of Ehlers-Danlos syndrome
Vessel redundancies
Williams syndrome
Young age

tapered appearance; at the distal end, the lumen may be abruptly reformed. The pathologic constituents of a tapered arterial occlusion result in the classic angiographic appearance of a candle flame. A false lumen may reconnect more distally with the true lumen, creating a double-barreled appearance. The intramural hematoma may traverse into the vessel adventitia and form a dissecting aneurysm or an aneurysmal pouch.

Clinical Features

The typical clinical presentation of an ICA dissection is unilateral pain in the head, face, or neck accompanied by ipsilateral partial Horner syndrome. Pain is usually the initial manifestation, and retinal or cerebral ischemia occurs hours or days later. The neck pain is located in the upper anterolateral neck and may be accompanied by facial, dental, or orbital pain. Headache is typically in the frontotemporal area, and the onset is occasionally like that of a thunderclap headache but is most commonly gradual. The severity of the headache and neck pain is variable. The average time from onset of pain to the appearance of neurologic symptoms is 9 days. Horner syndrome, when present, is partial. Facial anhidrosis is not a feature because the facial sweat glands are innervated by the sympathetic plexus surrounding the external carotid artery, not the ICA. Cranial nerve palsies can be detected in approximately 12% of patients with ICA dissection. The lower cranial nerves are most commonly affected, particularly the hypoglossal nerve. Pulsatile tinnitus may be reported, and a bruit may be present on auscultation. Cerebral or retinal ischemic symptoms are reported in over half of patients with ICA dissection.

The typical clinical presentation of a VA dissection is pain in the posterior neck or head initially and posterior circulation ischemia later. The pain, when unilateral, is ipsilateral to the dissected VA. The average interval between the onset of neck pain and the appearance of ischemic symptoms is approximately 14 days. Among posterior circulation ischemic syndromes related to VA dissection, the lateral medullary syndrome is commonly recognized. Transient ischemic attacks are reported less frequently after VA dissection than after ICA dissection. Subarachnoid hemorrhage is uncommon and occurs only with dissections that extend intracranially.

Diagnosis

Establishing a definitive diagnosis of CD necessitates a comprehensive history, a physical examination, and focused diagnostic testing. Diagnostic considerations include having a high level of awareness in the appropriate clinical context, excluding other arteriopathies (eg, atherosclerosis), viewing no particular test as an absolute gold standard, imaging the arterial wall and the lumen, and recognizing that additional imaging may be required.

Ultrasonography (US) is useful because it is noninvasive, affordable, and broadly available. The direct features of CD on US are stenosis, occlusion, echolucent vessel hematoma, and double lumen. The indirect features are a pulsatility alteration and collateral or retrograde flow. For CD, the sensitivity of US depends on the severity of the stenosis and ranges from 100% in severe stenosis or occlusion to 40% in mild stenosis. Technical proficiency and experience are necessary for identification of the more subtle US findings and may limit its use.

The benefits of computed tomographic (CT) angiography are spatial resolution, rapid image acquisition, broad availability, noninvasiveness, and lower cost compared with the alternatives of magnetic resonance angiography (MRA) and digital subtraction angiography (DSA). Contraindications to CT angiography include poor kidney function, allergy to iodinated contrast, and pregnancy. The disadvantages of CT angiography, compared with magnetic resonance imaging (MRI), include radiation exposure and reduced sensitivity for detection of acute ischemic stroke. The main benefit of MRI for CD is the high sensitivity of diffusion-weighted imaging sequences for detection of acute ischemic stroke. MRA, especially with a gadolinium contrast bolus, has superior spatial resolution and is not affected by bony artifact. This feature is especially relevant in the V3 and V4 segments of the VA and in the ICA because MRA penetrates the skull base. Contraindications and disadvantages of MRI and MRA include pacemakers, ferromagnetic metallic implants and prosthetic appliances, greater expense, prolonged scanning time, claustrophobic conditions, large body habitus and mass, and susceptibility to motion artifacts.

DSA has been called the gold standard for imaging arterial lumens; however, imaging of the vessel wall in CD with new US, CT, and MRI diagnostic techniques has shown that false-negative results with DSA are as high as 17%. The DSA features of CD are pseudoaneurysm, intimal flap, double lumen, and a smooth or irregularly shaped tapering or occlusion. Concerns over DSA include time, cost, technical proficiency, contrast administration, invasiveness, and radiation exposure, and with the sensitive, noninvasive imaging available at most centers, the use of DSA has been limited.

Management

No randomized trials have specifically evaluated the management or prevention of CD. Thrombolysis with intravenous alteplase is reasonably safe if given to patients within 4.5 hours after an acute ischemic stroke caused by CD. For patients with transient ischemic attack or ischemic stroke resulting from CD, administration of antiplatelet therapy or anticoagulant therapy for 3 to 6 months is reasonable. Endovascular therapy may be considered for patients with CD who have had definite recurrent cerebral ischemic events while receiving appropriate antithrombotic therapy. Rarely, stenting is used to open critically stenotic carotid arteries if there are no other options for recanalization. Otherwise, antithrombotic therapy is the mainstay of CD management.

Overall, the majority of patients with CD have good outcomes as measured with the modified Rankin Scale. Factors associated with poor clinical outcome include stroke with an initially high severity, high severity of arterial stenosis and occlusion, and absence of sufficient collaterals. Generally the neurologic outcome depends on the stroke location and severity. Recovery of arterial patency is approximately 75%. Factors associated with an improved likelihood of recanalization include having a spontaneous (nontraumatic) dissection, having a stenotic (not occluded) vessel, being a nonsmoker, and being female. The antithrombotic selection does not appear to influence the timing or degree of recanalization. The timing of recanalization is generally within 6 months (median, approximately 4 months). The cumulative rate of dissection recurrence is approximately 2% in 1 month, 3% in 2 years, 5% in 5 years, and 12% in 10 years; therefore, the rate of recurrence is approximately 1% per year.

Summary

- CD, a commonly recognized cause of ischemic stroke in young and middle-aged patients, is most commonly identified in the upper cervical spine and may involve a VA or an ICA.
- CD can occur spontaneously or from trauma.
- Management of CD is predicated on the diagnosis and typically the use of antithrombotics (eg, aspirin for naive patients); in severe cases, neuroendovascular evaluation is indicated.
- Disability after CD varies, and the majority of patients have good outcomes, but some have serious neurologic disability or die.

SUGGESTED READING

Biousse V, D'Anglejan-Chatillon J, Touboul PJ, Amarenco P, Bousser MG. Time course of symptoms in extracranial carotid artery dissections: a series of 80 patients. Stroke. 1995 Feb;26(2):235–9.

Derex L, Nighoghossian N, Turjman F, Hermier M, Honnorat J, Neuschwander P, et al. Intravenous tPA in acute ischemic stroke related to internal carotid artery dissection. Neurology. 2000 Jun 13;54(11):2159–61.

English SW, Passe TJ, Lindell EP, Klaas JP. Multiple cranial neuropathies as a presentation of spontaneous internal carotid artery dissection: a case report and literature review. J Clin Neurosci. 2018 Apr;50:129–31.

Hakimi R, Sivakumar S. Imaging of carotid dissection. Curr Pain Headache Rep. 2019 Jan 19;23(1):2.

Narula N, Kadian-Dodov D, Olin JW. Fibromuscular dysplasia: contemporary concepts and future directions. Prog Cardiovasc Dis. 2018 Mar -Apr;60(6):580–5. Epub 2018 Mar 10.

Ortiz J, Ruland S. Cervicocerebral artery dissection. Curr Opin Cardiol. 2015 Nov;30(6):603–10.

Robertson JJ, Koyfman A. Cervical artery dissections: a review. J Emerg Med. 2016 Nov;51(5):508–18. Epub 2016 Sep 12.

Schievink WI. Spontaneous dissection of the carotid and vertebral arteries. N Engl J Med. 2001 Mar 22;344(12):898–906.

Schievink WI, Wijdicks EF, Michels VV, Vockley J, Godfrey M. Heritable connective tissue disorders in cervical artery dissections: a prospective study. Neurology. 1998 Apr;50(4):1166–9.

Traumatic Brain and Spine Injury

87 Traumatic Brain Injury and Spinal Cord Injury

MAYA A. BABU, MD

Goals

- Understand the different types of major traumatic brain injuries and how to identify them clinically and radiologically.
- Recognize the neuroimaging modalities for identifying major traumatic brain injury.
- Be able to use the American Spinal Injury Association impairment scale to classify acute spinal cord injury.
- Review the approach to management of traumatic brain injury and spinal cord injury.

Introduction

Traumatic brain injury (TBI) is one of the most common global disorders leading to neurologic morbidity, especially in young adults. Spinal cord injury (SCI) can also occur with trauma and lead to paraparesis, tetraparesis, or paralysis with lifelong disability. This chapter is a basic overview of TBI and SCI, the initial approach to management and stabilization, and recent guidelines.

Traumatic Brain Injury

TBI is one of the most devastating forms of acute brain disease. It carries high morbidity and mortality rates in addition to high societal costs for survivors. The most common causes of TBI are motor vehicle accidents and violence among younger patients, but falls are an increasingly common cause among the elderly. TBI comprises different pathophysiologic injuries reflecting the magnitude and acceleration of the trauma, including direct injury to the brain parenchyma, diffuse axonal injury (DAI), and bleeding, such as epidural hematomas (EDHs), subdural hematomas (SDHs), parenchymal contusions, and subarachnoid hemorrhage (SAH). Other chapters in this book address additional aspects of TBI diagnosis and management.

Diffuse Axonal Injury

High-velocity injury, such as high-speed travel in a vehicle that suddenly decelerates, can result in DAI, which occurs when shearing forces sever axons and vessels diffusely. Immediately after a rapid-deceleration TBI, imaging studies such as computed tomography (CT) of the head may not show any evidence of a mass lesion. However, abnormal neurologic examination findings may seem inconsistent with the CT images, which do not shown an obvious intracranial mass effect or lesion. The prognosis for patients with DAI is generally poor, especially when the DAI affects the corpus callosum and brainstem and the diffuse reticular activating system projection fibers to the cortex. When the reticular activating system has been disrupted, DAI can result in chronic alterations of consciousness, such as persistent vegetative state (PVS) or minimally conscious state. If imaging does not show a mass lesion, but the patient's neurologic status is poor, management often consists of monitoring intracranial pressure (ICP) or close monitoring of the patient's neurologic status in addition to supportive care, including hyperosmolar therapy. In the absence of focal mass effect or hematoma, surgical intervention is typically not recommended. However, TBI patients with refractory intracranial hypertension may benefit from bilateral decompressive craniectomy to aid survival, but the prognosis for such patients is guarded.

Magnetic resonance imaging (MRI) of the brain with gradient-recalled echo (GRE) sequencing (or a similar technique) is one of the most sensitive imaging modalities for making the diagnosis. It shows several areas of small

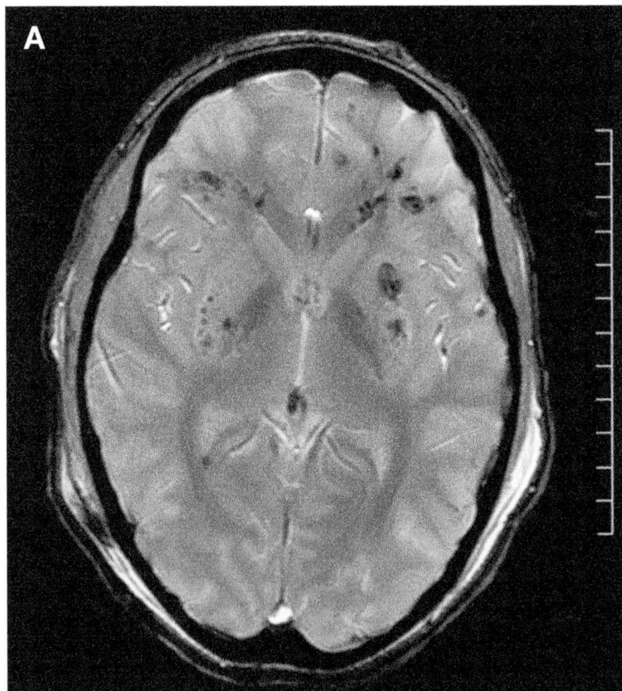

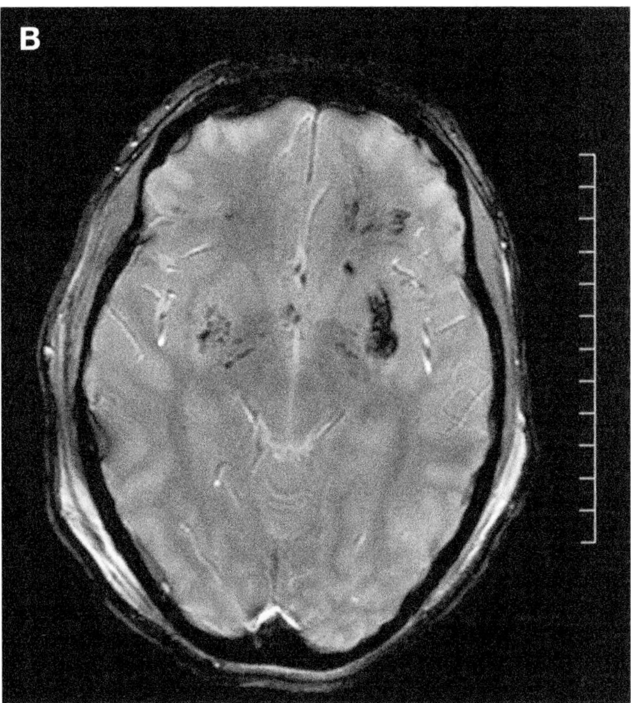

Figure 87.1. Magnetic Resonance Imaging of the Brain (Gradient-Recalled Echo Sequence). A and B, Images show diffuse, scattered punctate areas of microhemorrhage consistent with diffuse axonal injury and petechial microhemorrhage.
(From Kabbani Y, Tarabishy AR. CDEM Curriculum: brain imaging [Internet]. [cited 2018 Jun 21]. Available from: https://cdemcurriculum.com/brain-imaging/; used with permission.)

hemorrhages or microhemorrhages in the white matter tracts, such as the corpus callosum (Figure 87.1). Diffusion tensor imaging is a newer MRI method used to assess the degree of preservation of connecting tracts; this technique is promising for assisting with prognostication for patients with DAI, but its use is still investigational.

Epidural Hematoma

EDHs result from a high-velocity impact injury or blunt force trauma to the head. Classically, patients with EDH have a transient *lucid interval*, in which they may first lose consciousness but regain it transiently and verbalize and seem appropriate immediately after the injury. However, these patients have a rapid neurologic decline after the lucid interval because brain compression and herniation cause the EDH to increase in volume. EDHs are typically caused by an arterial tear in the middle meningeal artery and an associated skull fracture along its course in the temple.

Initially, the clinical evaluation of EDH should be like that of a neurosurgical emergency that may involve a craniotomy or craniectomy for EDH evacuation and relief of the mass effect. Since EDH blood products are external to the dura, the dura need not be incised. However, after trauma, a concomitant SDH may be present, so that opening the dura and investigating the subdural space surgically may be advisable. If small EDHs cause negligible brain compression, nonsurgical treatment may include serial scans and close monitoring of neurologic status with frequent examinations (every 1 or 2 hours). Radiographically, EDH has a classic lens shape and typically stays within intracranial suture lines. Because of the high arterial pressure, bleeding from the middle meningeal artery, and the potential for rapid deterioration, mortality from EDH has been reported to be as high as 25% (Figure 87.2). The surgical approach to EDH is discussed in Chapter 88 ("Traumatic Epidural and Subdural Hematomas").

Subdural Hematoma

Traumatic SDHs are caused by tears in bridging veins between the cerebral veins and the dural venous sinus connections. SDHs are associated with different velocities of trauma or blunt force injury. With aging, the brain becomes smaller (through atrophy), resulting in increased space between the brain and the bridging veins. Therefore, SDHs often occur in elderly patients after minor trauma or falls or with the use of anticoagulants or similar drugs, which magnify the SDH bleeding. In younger patients, SDH often occurs in combination with other TBI mechanisms of injury such as DAI, intraparenchymal contusion,

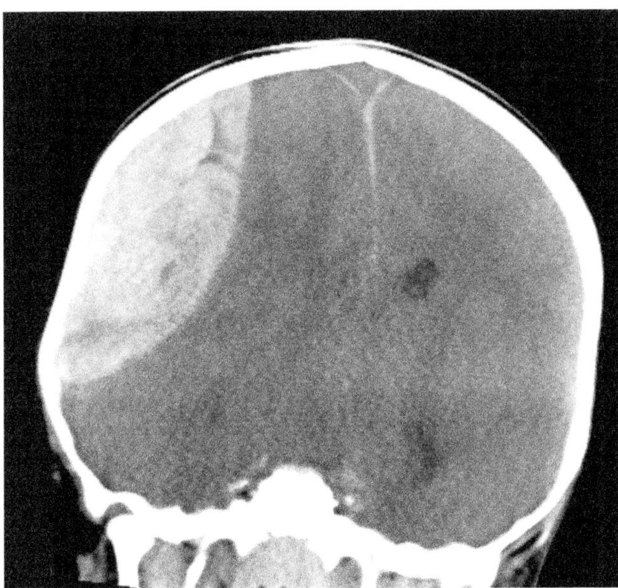

Figure 87.2. Computed Tomographic Scan of the Head. Image shows a large, right-sided epidural hematoma.
(From University of North Dakota. Fogarty EF. Teaching files: epidural hematoma [pediatric] [Internet]. [cited 2018 Jun 21]. Available from: http://med.und.edu/radiology/teaching-files/epidural-hematoma.cfm; used with permission.)

subarachnoid bleeding, or EDH due to rapid–acceleration-deceleration injury. Given low-pressure venous bleeding, patients with SDH typically present with acute or subacute progressive neurologic symptoms, such as progressive headache, before focal neurologic deficits become apparent. Exceptions to this subacute clinical presentation include patients receiving warfarin or anticoagulants who present with uncontrolled SDH expansion that causes a rapid decline in neurologic status (like in EDH), but imaging shows a hemispheric convex pattern or a crescent-shaped bleeding pattern consistent with SDH. Acute SDH medical and surgical management is discussed in Chapter 88 ("Traumatic Epidural and Subdural Hematomas").

Intraparenchymal Hemorrhage and Contusion

Intraparenchymal hemorrhagic (IPH) contusions also result from blunt force brain injury. The putative mechanism of traumatic IPH is shearing of the small parenchymal and cortical pial vessels with resultant punctate bleeding. Initial CT of the head often shows findings of DAI and petechial IPH. However, if the patient's condition appears consistent with DAI and coma, MRI of the brain with GRE sequences may show DAI and numerous small, scattered IPHs if the initial CT does not. Sometimes CT of the head shows these IPH "blossoming" artifacts on subsequent CT scans 24 to 48 hours later. Most commonly, IPH contusions occur near brain-calvarial locations of acceleration-deceleration injury in the brain, (including the anterior and posterior temporal lobes and inferior frontal lobes), near dura mater (eg, the tentorium or falx cerebri), or in combination with EDH or SDH. High-velocity TBI injuries and bleeding often occur with a linear deceleration pattern known as *coup and contre-coup* injury, with 1 side of the head sustaining the direct impact while the opposite side of the brain sustains a deceleration injury within the skull compartment. IPH contusions can expand and cause mass effect and brain compression. Therefore, subsequent CT imaging for any change in neurologic status or for signs of uncal hernation (dilated, fixed pupil) may be required to detect this expansion, which warrants medical management with or without operative neurosurgical intervention.

Decompressive hemicraniectomy or bifrontal craniectomy with or without clot evacuation may be considered for midline shift or refractory increased ICP. However, in the Decompressive Craniectomy (DECRA) trial, bifrontal craniectomy for severe TBI patients with refractory increased ICP shortened the length of stay in the intensive care unit but was associated with worse outcomes.

Subarachnoid Hemorrhage

Traumatic SAH occurs in approximately 35% of traumatic head injuries and likely results from shearing of small cortical pial vessels or vessels near areas with parenchymal cerebrospinal fluid such as near the brainstem and basal cisterns. In severe TBI, the traumatic SAH pattern can mimic the star pattern of aneurysmal SAH, but CT angiography does not show any large-artery aneurysms. SAH may also be present in the cerebral sulci and near adjacent skull fractures. CT of the head is the best imaging modality for assessing patients for traumatic SAH. Serial CT imaging may not be useful for traumatic SAH unless abrupt neurologic changes occur. If the traumatic SAH is diffuse or results in a thick layering hematoma, oxyhemoglobin may cause vasospasm as in aneurysmal SAH; nimodipine has been used, but according to the results of a meta-analysis, its clinical benefit is questionable in patients with TBI and traumatic SAH. Similarly, TBI with traumatic SAH in patients who are expected to recover may cause intraventricular hemorrhage with subsequent progressive communicating hydrocephalus that may warrant cerebrospinal fluid diversion with an external ventricular drain.

Medical Management of Severe TBI

TBI is associated with several forms of brain injury (DAI, traumatic EDH, traumatic SDH, and traumatic SAH). Despite considerable research, no neuroprotectant is known to reverse these forms of primary brain injury that occur near the time of onset. Therefore, the mainstay of medical management is avoidance of secondary brain injury caused by systemic or intracranial hypotension (cerebral perfusion pressure [CPP] <55 mm Hg), hypoxemia (<92%), fever (>38.5°C), and prevention of extremes in serum glucose (ie, glucose <120 mg/dL or >180 mg/dL). Clinicians prefer to use an ICP monitor if a patient is comatose (Glasgow Coma Scale [GCS] score, 3-8) or has abnormalities on CT that are consistent with increased ICP. However, surveys of level I trauma centers in the United States have shown marked underuse of ICP monitoring. ICP monitoring allows calculation of CPP, which is the brain's end-organ perfusion pressure. In normal brain states, autoregulation of CPP controls cerebral blood flow (CBF):

CPP = MAP − ICP, where MAP is mean arterial pressure.
CBF = CPP/CVR, where CVR is cerebrovascular resistance.

In TBI, autoregulation of cerebrovascular pressure becomes decoupled or unregulated, and CBF becomes linearly related to CPP. A decrease in CPP to less than 55 mm Hg can cause critical ischemia and oligemia resulting in secondary brain ischemia. Some clinicians use additional invasive monitoring (eg, with brain tissue oxygen monitors).

In the Brain Oxygen Optimization in Severe Traumatic Brain Injury Phase-II (BOOST-II) trial, early goal-directed therapy (EGDT) increased brain tissue oxygenation during a crisis with a trend toward improved outcomes compared with therapy directed toward only ICP. A randomized multicenter phase 3 trial is evaluating whether monitoring brain tissue oxygen for EGDT improves clinical outcomes.

While it is technically possible to use multimodal monitoring (MMM) to measure CPP "optimal values" for each patient, single-center data for MMM CPP optimal values show worse outcomes with lower CPP optimal values. No multicenter randomized trial data have confirmed the benefit of CPP optimal values or how to apply them outside major academic centers.

Monitoring of ICP and CPP is generally recommended for severe TBI to reduce 2-week mortality (according to the fourth edition of the Brain Trauma Foundation [BTF] guidelines for managing severe TBI). Advanced MMM has insufficient evidence to recommend its use outside research. Similarly, the BTF guidelines no longer advise use of corticosteroids and hypothermia for ICP or cerebral edema.

Medical Complications

Patients with severe TBI are at risk for typical hospital-acquired nosocomial infections and for medical and systemic complications, such as aspiration pneumonia, ventilator-associated pneumonia, and venous thromboembolism. Chemical thromboprophylaxis for deep vein thrombosis should be started when feasible. BTF guidelines suggest the use of sequential compression devices if the patient does not have any long bone fractures of the legs; if neuroimaging findings are stable, without concern of ongoing bleeding, subcutaneous unfractionated heparin may be considered for prevention of deep vein thrombosis.

Paroxysmal sympathetic hyperactivity (PSH) ("autonomic storms") is a common complication after severe TBI. It is characterized by acute episodes of tachycardia, tachypnea, and hypertension that occur especially with tactile or other forms of stimulation. PSH can also occur spontaneously. Patients with PSH may have central fever, spells of diaphoresis, and episodes of dystonic posturing. PSH episodes gradually lessen over time but can be challenging in the first few weeks because of patient ventilator desynchrony, the degree of nursing care required for vital sign fluctuations and dystonic episodes, and the family and caregiver distress that arises during the episodes. PSH is typically refractory to various medications and historically responds best to short-term intravenous boluses of morphine sulfate or fentanyl as needed. The fluctuations in PSH episodes may be lessened with the use of long-acting β-blockers (eg, propranolol 10 mg 2 times daily), clonidine 0.1 mg as needed, dexmedetomidine infusions, and gabapentin titrated up to 3 times daily. Initially, PSH may be confused with seizure, but electroencephalography can exclude this possibility with the lack of epileptiform discharges during an episode.

Prognosis

The prognosis for patients with TBI has been addressed in large cohort studies that have provided robust data on overall short-term mortality risks (eg, the Corticosteroid Randomization After Significant Head Injury [CRASH] score and the International Mission for Prognosis and Analysis of Clinical Trials in Traumatic Brain Injury [IMPACT] score). However, long-term TBI prognostication (eg, survival at 1 year with functional outcomes) is challenging. Many neurosurgeons are reluctant to use the CRASH and IMPACT prognostic algorithms when patients are young, have brain injury without brainstem involvement, or may undergo neurosurgical intervention. If a hospital lacks appropriate resources, TBI patients should be referred to a high-volume trauma center for care and prognostication if their condition is stable enough to allow for transport.

Spinal Cord Injury

SCI occurs commonly with mechanisms similar to TBI, including motor vehicle collisions (46%), falls (22%), assaults (16%), and sports injuries (12%). Each year, 17,000 new SCIs occur in the United States, and an estimated 282,000 US residents (80% male) are living with an SCI. The prognosis varies with the location of the injury within the spinal cord, the severity of the SCI, and whether the injury disrupted sensation, motor function, or autonomic spinal cord areas of control. After a severe SCI resulting in paraparesis (leg weakness), tetraparesis, or paralysis, the most common causes of death are related to pulmonary, cardiac, or infectious problems such as sepsis.

Pathophysiology

The 4 mechanisms for primary SCI are 1) impact with continued compression, such as in burst fractures with retropulsion of bone; 2) impact with transient compression; 3) transection or laceration of the spinal cord due to penetrating injury or severe dislocation; and 4) distraction leading to spinal cord stretch injury. Infarction or hemorrhage may result from disrupted blood vessels. After the primary SCI, a secondary cascade may include hemorrhage within the central gray matter of the spinal cord, which can lead to ischemia, cord edema, and cellular apoptosis. Neuronal and astrocyte demise involves free radicals, calcium-mediated intracellular shifts, mitochondrial dysfunction, cellular metabolism abnormalities, and neurotransmitter release. Neurogenic shock can occur if the SCI involves the thoracic sympathetic nervous system. Neurogenic shock resembles distributive septic shock because of the loss of autonomic tone after SCI and the reduced systemic vascular resistance, which causes abrupt hypotension. Systemic hypotension can exacerbate primary SCI and result in a secondary ischemic cascade.

Long-term management of SCI involves adequate pulmonary function and pulmonary toileting, clearance of secretions, and management of swallowing and nutrition with short-term use of an enteral tube or a percutaneous endoscopic gastrostomy tube. SCI patients also need specialized rehabilitation and occupational therapy, including training in bowel and bladder care, inspection of assistive wheelchairs, and wound care to prevent autonomic dysreflexia syndrome due to unrecognized skin or bone lesions that precipitate attacks. Most SCI patients are followed in a specialized rehabilitation center to track and prevent these secondary complications. Use of high-dose corticosteroids, historically studied for patients with SCI, has fallen out of favor and is not advised because of the risks of systemic complications.

Neurologic Presentation

The spinal cord consists of tracts that transmit motor (descending) and sensory (ascending) signals. The corticospinal tracts are located anteriorly within the spinal cord and are descending motor axons extending from the cerebral cortex to motor neurons in the ventral horn. The corticospinal tract crosses (*decussates*) in the medulla. The dorsal columns transmit ascending sensory information (including light touch, vibration, and proprioception) from sensory fibers in the extremities to the sensory cerebral cortex. The lateral spinothalamic tracts transmit pain and temperature information from the extremities. The anterior spinothalamic tract transmits light touch.

Injury to the corticospinal tracts and dorsal columns can lead to ipsilateral paralysis and loss of light touch sensation, vibratory sensation, and proprioception. Injury to the lateral spinothalamic neuronal pathway causes loss of pain and temperature in the contralateral extremity. Injury to the anterior spinothalamic tract can lead to loss of vibratory sensation and proprioception, with incomplete loss of light touch sensation. Hemisection of the spinal cord may result in ipsilateral loss of proprioception and motor control and contralateral loss of pain and temperature sensation (*Brown-Séquard syndrome*). Cervical injuries may cause a central cord syndrome (man-in-the-barrel syndrome) characterized by motor weakness that is more profound in the upper extremities than in the lower extremities and is often accompanied by sacral sensory sparing. *Conus medullaris syndrome* is characterized by loss of reflexive control of the bowel and bladder and may also include weakness in the lower extremities. In some situations, the bulbocavernous and micturition reflexes are spared. *Cauda equina syndrome* is caused by injury to the lumbosacral nerve roots and is characterized by loss of bowel or bladder control, with motor weakness or sensory loss, typically in a radicular pattern.

Classification

Various clinical SCI syndromes may develop depending on the type of SCI injury and secondary injury. The simplest method for classifying SCI is based on American Spinal Injury Association (ASIA) terminology: A *complete* injury is characterized by both motor and sensory paralysis at a certain spinal cord level (eg, C6), and an *incomplete* SCI is characterized by motor paralysis at a certain level, but sensation may be intact at a level lower than that of the injury. The ASIA scale was developed to help categorize spinal cord injuries (Figure 87.3).

Tetraplegia describes weakness in all 4 extremities and is associated with injuries to the cervical spinal cord. *Paraplegia* describes weakness in the lower extremities and is associated with injuries to the thoracic or upper lumbar spinal cord. In patients with tetraplegia, C5 tends to be the most common level of injury. In patients with paraplegia, T12-L1 tends to be the most common level of injury.

Respiratory function of the diaphragm is innervated through the phrenic nerve, which emanates from cervical spinal cord levels C3 through C5 (hence, the mnemonic "C3, 4, and 5 keep the diaphragm alive"). Therefore, involvement of these cervical levels complicates SCI management because respiratory failure may result from insufficient tidal volumes and minute ventilation. For patients with unstable fractures of the cervical spine, fiberoptic intubation is advised along with mechanical ventilation until after the initial SCI is stabilized and the patient is weaned from the ventilator to determine whether the patient will continue to need a ventilator. Some patients with high cervical injury require tracheostomy.

Medical Issues Immediately After an SCI

Immediately after an SCI, several conditions may be observed. *Neurogenic shock* (described above) is the constellation of loss of sympathetic tone causing hypotension, bradycardia, and peripheral vasodilatation. *Spinal shock*, however, refers to a temporary physiologic reflex depression of the anterior spinal cord, which can include the loss of reflexes and rectal tone (initially resembling a lower motor neuron disorder until the emergence of upper motor neuron signs, such as spasticity and hyperreflexia). After SCI, a physiologic stress response causes a surge in catecholamines, which can be associated with an initial increase in blood pressure that is followed by hypotension. The patient may have flaccid paralysis of the extremities at or below the level of the SCI and, in certain situations, priapism from unopposed parasympathetic function of the penis.

Immediate management revolves around maintaining adequate spinal cord perfusion pressure (SCPP):

$$SCPP = MAP - ITP,$$

where ITP is intrathecal pressure. Systemic blood pressure (MAP) may need to be augmented and unstable spinal fractures stabilized. Patients should be protected with full spinal precautions (spinal cervical immobilization collar or similar thoracic or lumbar braces) and logrolled carefully (until the spine is stabilized surgically) or turned by other methods approved by the neurosurgeon.

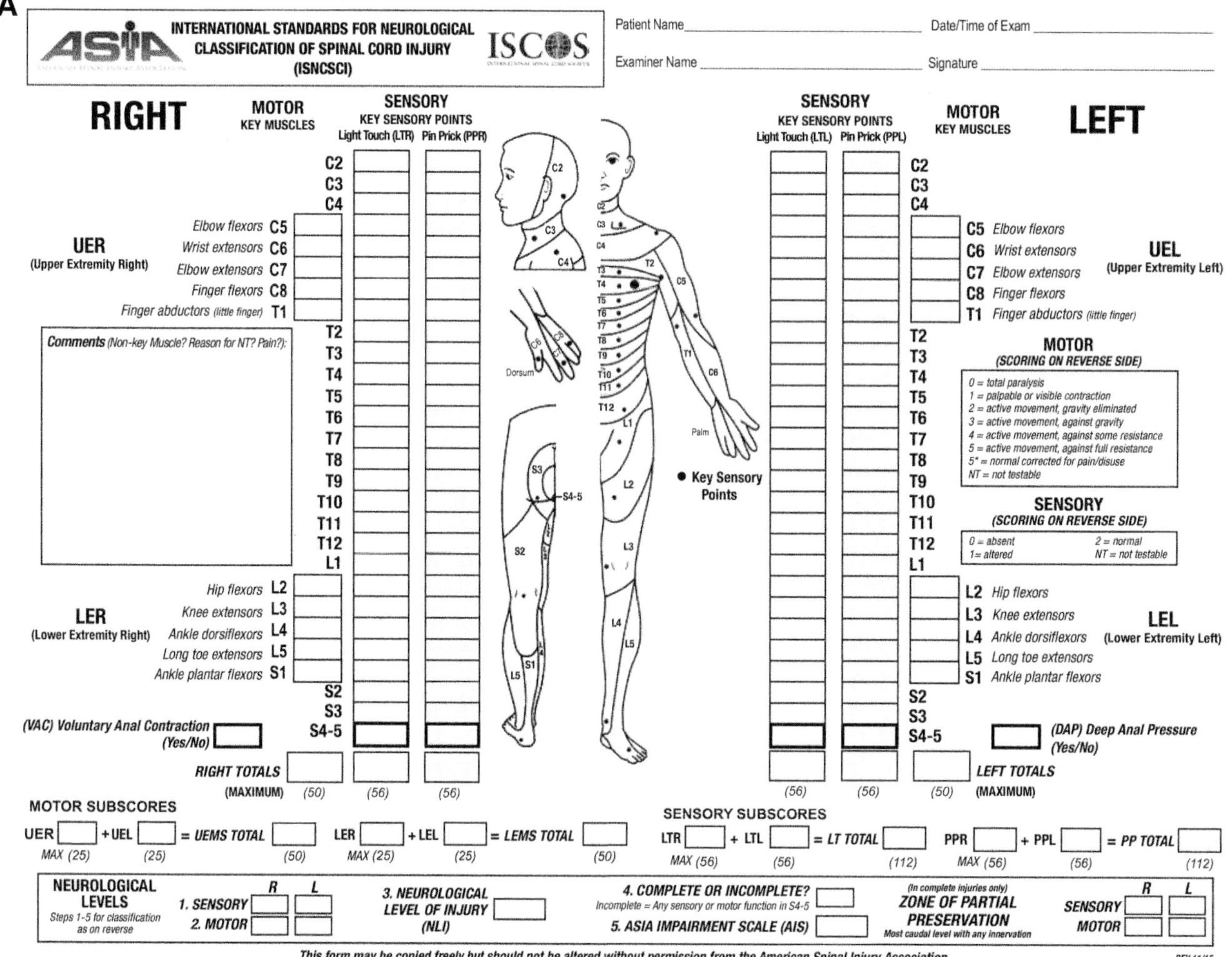

A

ASIA — INTERNATIONAL STANDARDS FOR NEUROLOGICAL CLASSIFICATION OF SPINAL CORD INJURY (ISNCSCI) — ISCOS

Patient Name ______ Date/Time of Exam ______

Examiner Name ______ Signature ______

RIGHT — MOTOR: KEY MUSCLES — SENSORY: KEY SENSORY POINTS, Light Touch (LTR), Pin Prick (PPR)

C2, C3, C4

UER (Upper Extremity Right): Elbow flexors C5; Wrist extensors C6; Elbow extensors C7; Finger flexors C8; Finger abductors (little finger) T1

Comments (Non-key Muscle? Reason for NT? Pain?):

T2, T3, T4, T5, T6, T7, T8, T9, T10, T11, T12, L1

LER (Lower Extremity Right): Hip flexors L2; Knee extensors L3; Ankle dorsiflexors L4; Long toe extensors L5; Ankle plantar flexors S1

S2, S3, S4-5

(VAC) Voluntary Anal Contraction (Yes/No)

RIGHT TOTALS (MAXIMUM) (50) (56) (56)

LEFT — SENSORY: KEY SENSORY POINTS, Light Touch (LTL), Pin Prick (PPL) — MOTOR: KEY MUSCLES

C2, C3, C4

UEL (Upper Extremity Left): C5 Elbow flexors; C6 Wrist extensors; C7 Elbow extensors; C8 Finger flexors; T1 Finger abductors (little finger)

T2, T3, T4, T5, T6, T7, T8, T9, T10, T11, T12, L1

MOTOR (SCORING ON REVERSE SIDE)
0 = total paralysis
1 = palpable or visible contraction
2 = active movement, gravity eliminated
3 = active movement, against gravity
4 = active movement, against some resistance
5 = active movement, against full resistance
5* = normal corrected for pain/disuse
NT = not testable

SENSORY (SCORING ON REVERSE SIDE)
0 = absent
1 = altered
2 = normal
NT = not testable

LEL (Lower Extremity Left): L2 Hip flexors; L3 Knee extensors; L4 Ankle dorsiflexors; L5 Long toe extensors; S1 Ankle plantar flexors

S2, S3, S4-5

(DAP) Deep Anal Pressure (Yes/No)

LEFT TOTALS (MAXIMUM) (56) (56) (50)

MOTOR SUBSCORES

UER ___ + UEL ___ = UEMS TOTAL ___ LER ___ + LEL ___ = LEMS TOTAL ___

MAX (25) (25) (50) MAX (25) (25) (50)

SENSORY SUBSCORES

LTR ___ + LTL ___ = LT TOTAL ___ PPR ___ + PPL ___ = PP TOTAL ___

MAX (56) (56) (112) MAX (56) (56) (112)

NEUROLOGICAL LEVELS (Steps 1-5 for classification as on reverse) — R L — 1. SENSORY; 2. MOTOR

3. NEUROLOGICAL LEVEL OF INJURY (NLI)

4. COMPLETE OR INCOMPLETE? (Incomplete = Any sensory or motor function in S4-5)

5. ASIA IMPAIRMENT SCALE (AIS)

(In complete injuries only) ZONE OF PARTIAL PRESERVATION (Most caudal level with any innervation) — R L — SENSORY; MOTOR

This form may be copied freely but should not be altered without permission from the American Spinal Injury Association.

REV 11/15

Figure 87.3. American Spinal Injury Association Impairment Scale for Spinal Cord Injuries. The evaluation form (A) is completed according to the grading instructions (B).

B

Muscle Function Grading

0 = total paralysis
1 = palpable or visible contraction
2 = active movement, full range of motion (ROM) with gravity eliminated
3 = active movement, full ROM against gravity
4 = active movement, full ROM against gravity and moderate resistance in a muscle specific position
5 = (normal) active movement, full ROM against gravity and full resistance in a functional muscle position expected from an otherwise unimpaired person
5* = (normal) active movement, full ROM against gravity and sufficient resistance to be considered normal if identified inhibiting factors (i.e. pain, disuse) were not present
NT = not testable (i.e. due to immobilization, severe pain such that the patient cannot be graded, amputation of limb, or contracture of > 50% of the normal ROM)

Sensory Grading

0 = Absent
1 = Altered, either decreased/impaired sensation or hypersensitivity
2 = Normal
NT = Not testable

When to Test Non-Key Muscles:

In a patient with an apparent AIS B classification, non-key muscle functions more than 3 levels below the motor level on each side should be tested to most accurately classify the injury (differentiate between AIS B and C).

Movement	Root level
Shoulder: Flexion, extension, abduction, adduction, internal and external rotation **Elbow:** Supination	C5
Elbow: Pronation **Wrist:** Flexion	C6
Finger: Flexion at proximal joint, extension. **Thumb:** Flexion, extension and abduction in plane of thumb	C7
Finger: Flexion at MCP joint **Thumb:** Opposition, adduction and abduction perpendicular to palm	C8
Finger: Abduction of the index finger	T1
Hip: Adduction	L2
Hip: External rotation	L3
Hip: Extension, abduction, internal rotation **Knee:** Flexion **Ankle:** Inversion and eversion **Toe:** MP and IP extension	L4
Hallux and Toe: DIP and PIP flexion and abduction	L5
Hallux: Adduction	S1

ASIA Impairment Scale (AIS)

A = Complete. No sensory or motor function is preserved in the sacral segments S4-5.

B = Sensory Incomplete. Sensory but not motor function is preserved below the neurological level and includes the sacral segments S4-5 (light touch or pin prick at S4-5 or deep anal pressure) AND no motor function is preserved more than three levels below the motor level on either side of the body.

C = Motor Incomplete. Motor function is preserved at the most caudal sacral segments for voluntary anal contraction (VAC) OR the patient meets the criteria for sensory incomplete status (sensory function preserved at the most caudal sacral segments (S4-S5) by LT, PP or DAP), and has some sparing of motor function more than three levels below the ipsilateral motor level on either side of the body.
(This includes key or non-key muscle functions to determine motor incomplete status.) For AIS C – less than half of key muscle functions below the single NLI have a muscle grade ≥ 3.

D = Motor Incomplete. Motor incomplete status as defined above, with at least half (half or more) of key muscle functions below the single NLI having a muscle grade ≥ 3.

E = Normal. If sensation and motor function as tested with the ISNCSCI are graded as normal in all segments, and the patient had prior deficits, then the AIS grade is E. Someone without an initial SCI does not receive an AIS grade.

Using ND: To document the sensory, motor and NLI levels, the ASIA Impairment Scale grade, and/or the zone of partial preservation (ZPP) when they are unable to be determined based on the examination results.

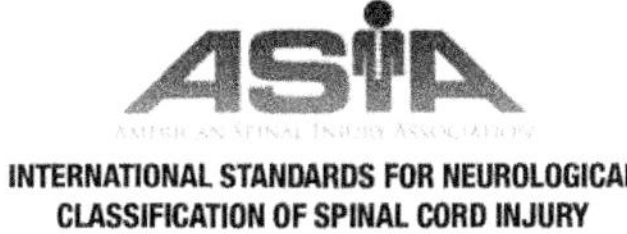

INTERNATIONAL STANDARDS FOR NEUROLOGICAL CLASSIFICATION OF SPINAL CORD INJURY

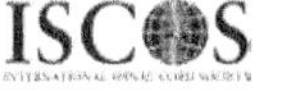

Steps in Classification

The following order is recommended for determining the classification of individuals with SCI.

1. Determine sensory levels for right and left sides.
The sensory level is the most caudal, intact dermatome for both pin prick and light touch sensation.

2. Determine motor levels for right and left sides.
Defined by the lowest key muscle function that has a grade of at least 3 (on supine testing), providing the key muscle functions represented by segments above that level are judged to be intact (graded as a 5).
Note: in regions where there is no myotome to test, the motor level is presumed to be the same as the sensory level, if testable motor function above that level is also normal.

3. Determine the neurological level of injury (NLI)
This refers to the most caudal segment of the cord with intact sensation and antigravity (3 or more) muscle function strength, provided that there is normal (intact) sensory and motor function rostrally respectively.
The NLI is the most cephalad of the sensory and motor levels determined in steps 1 and 2.

4. Determine whether the injury is Complete or Incomplete.
(i.e. absence or presence of sacral sparing)
If voluntary anal contraction = ***No*** *AND all S4-5 sensory scores =* ***0***
AND deep anal pressure = ***No,*** *then injury is* ***Complete.***
Otherwise, injury is ***Incomplete.***

5. Determine ASIA Impairment Scale (AIS) Grade:

Is injury Complete? **If YES, AIS=A** and can record ZPP (lowest dermatome or myotome on each side with some preservation)

NO

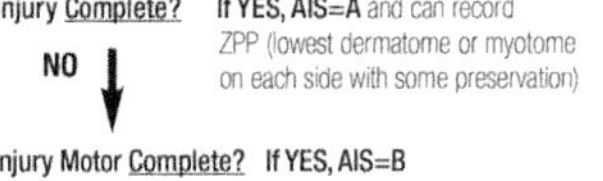

Is injury Motor Complete? **If YES, AIS=B**

NO (No=voluntary anal contraction OR motor function more than three levels below the motor level on a given side, if the patient has sensory incomplete classification)

Are at least half (half or more) of the key muscles below the neurological level of injury graded 3 or better?

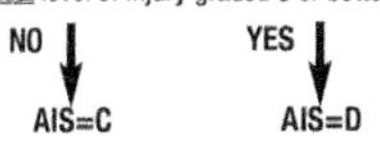

NO → **AIS=C**   **YES** → **AIS=D**

If sensation and motor function is normal in all segments, AIS=E
Note: AIS E is used in follow-up testing when an individual with a documented SCI has recovered normal function. If at initial testing no deficits are found, the individual is neurologically intact; the ASIA Impairment Scale does not apply.

Figure 87.3. Continued

Immobility may lead to additional complications, such as deep vein thrombosis (resulting in pulmonary embolism with acute tachycardia), hypoxemia, hypotension, and cardiac arrest. Pulmonary issues are discussed above. Patients with decubitus or pressure ulcers in insensate areas after SCI require turning every 2 hours, careful positioning, and skin integrity monitoring along with appropriate nutrition and specialized beds that alternate pressure on the sacral area. Infected ulcers can lead to skin breakdown and transgression of bacteria into the bloodstream, causing sepsis and death. Daily wound care and inspection of areas of the body that the patient cannot feel are important for prevention of wounds and sepsis.

Summary

- *TBI* is an overall term for various mechanisms of primary brain injury, which include DAI, IPH or contusions, SDH, EDH, and SAH.
- TBI pathophysiologic mechanisms are due to rapid acceleration and deceleration of the brain within the skull compartment.
- Secondary brain injury occurs from systemic hypotension, increased ICP that compromises CPP and cerebral blood flow, and secondary injury caused by metabolic neuronal insults from hypoglycemia or hyperglycemia, infection, and fever.
- For patients with severe TBI and coma (GCS score, 3-8), BTF guidelines suggest ICP and CPP monitoring for the first 14 days to optimize outcomes.
- Corticosteroids and hypothermia are no longer advised for control of ICP or cerebral edema in patients with TBI, and corticosteroids are no longer advised for patients with SCI.
- Patients with TBI or SCI require neurocritical or intensive care until their condition is stabilized, and each patient has unique and inherent neuromedical complications that require monitoring and managing

until the patient reaches a stable rehabilitation phase of recovery.

SUGGESTED READING

Abou El Fadl MH, O'Phelan KH. Management of traumatic brain injury: an update. Neurosurg Clin N Am. 2018 Apr;29(2):213–21.

Baptiste DC, Fehlings MG. Pharmacological approaches to repair the injured spinal cord. J Neurotrauma. 2006 Mar-Apr;23(3-4):318–34.

Bonner S, Smith C. Initial management of acute spinal cord injury. CEACCP. 2013 Dec;13(6):224–31.

Bullock MR, Chesnut R, Ghajar J, Gordon D, Hartl R, Newell DW, et al; Surgical Management of Traumatic Brain Injury Author Group. Surgical management of acute subdural hematomas. Neurosurgery. 2006 Mar;58(3 Suppl):S16–24.

Carney N, Totten AM, O'Reilly C, Ullman JS, Hawryluk GWJ, Bell MJ, et al. Guidelines for the management of severe traumatic brain injury, 4th edition [Internet]. [cited 2018 Oct 16]. Brain Trauma Foundation; Sept 2016. Available from: https://braintrauma.org/uploads/03/12/ Guidelines_for_Management_of_Severe_TBI_4th_Edition.pdf.

Carney N, Totten AM, O'Reilly C, Ullman JS, Hawryluk GWJ, Bell MJ, et al. Guidelines for the management of severe traumatic brain injury, fourth edition [Internet]. [cited 2018 Oct 16]. Neurosurgery. 2016;0(0):1–10. Available from: https://braintrauma.org/uploads/07/04/Guidelines_for_the_Management_of_Severe_Traumatic.97250__2_.pdf.

Chesnut RM, Temkin N, Carney N, Dikmen S, Rondina C, Videtta W, et al; Global Neurotrauma Research Group. A trial of intracranial-pressure monitoring in traumatic brain injury. N Engl J Med. 2012 Dec 27;367(26):2471–81. Epub 2012 Dec 12. Erratum in: N Engl J Med. 2013 Dec 19;369(25):2465.

Cooper DJ, Rosenfeld JV, Murray L, Arabi YM, Davies AR, D'Urso P, et al; DECRA Trial Investigators; Australian and New Zealand Intensive Care Society Clinical Trials Group. Decompressive craniectomy in diffuse traumatic brain injury. N Engl J Med. 2011 Apr 21;364(16):1493–502. Epub 2011 Mar 25. Erratum in: N Engl J Med. 2011 Nov 24;365(21):2040.

Donnelly J, Czosnyka M, Adams H, Robba C, Steiner LA, Cardim D, et al. Pressure reactivity-based optimal cerebral perfusion pressure in a traumatic brain injury cohort. Acta Neurochir Suppl. 2018;126:209–12.

Dumont RJ, Okonkwo DO, Verma S, Hurlbert RJ, Boulos PT, Ellegala DB, et al. Acute spinal cord injury, part I: pathophysiologic mechanisms. Clin Neuropharmacol. 2001 Sep-Oct;24(5):254–64.

Eisenberg HM, Gary HE Jr, Aldrich EF, Saydjari C, Turner B, Foulkes MA, et al. Initial CT findings in 753 patients with severe head injury: a report from the NIH Traumatic Coma Data Bank. J Neurosurg. 1990 Nov;73(5):688–98.

Eum SW, Lim DJ, Kim BR, Cho TH, Park JY, Suh JK, et al. Prognostic factors in patients with diffuse axonal injury. J Korean Neurosurg Soc. 1998 Dec;27:1668–74.

Furlan JC, Fehlings MG. Cardiovascular complications after acute spinal cord injury: pathophysiology, diagnosis, and management. Neurosurg Focus. 2008;25(5):E13.

Gan Y-C, Choksey MS. Rebleed in traumatic subarachnoid haemorrhage. Injury Extra. 2006;37:484–6.

Ganz JC. The lucid interval associated with epidural bleeding: evolving understanding. J Neurosurg. 2013 Apr;118(4):739–45. Epub 2013 Jan 18.

Geeraerts T, Velly L, Abdennour L, Asehnoune K, Audibert G, Bouzat P, et al; French Society of Anaesthesia; Intensive Care Medicine; in partnership with Association de neuro-anesthésie-réanimation de langue française (Anarlf); French Society of Emergency Medicine (Société Française de Médecine d'urgence [SFMU]; Société française de neurochirurgie (SFN); Groupe francophone de réanimation et d'urgences pédiatriques (GFRUP); Association des anesthésistes-réanimateurs pédiatriques d'expression française (Adarpef). Management of severe traumatic brain injury (first 24 hours). Anaesth Crit Care Pain Med. 2018 Apr;37(2):171–86. Epub 2017 Dec 27.

Haselsberger K, Pucher R, Auer LM. Prognosis after acute subdural or epidural haemorrhage. Acta Neurochir (Wien). 1988;90(3-4):111–6.

Ivamoto HS, Lemos HP Jr, Atallah AN. Surgical treatments for chronic subdural hematomas: a comprehensive systematic review. World Neurosurg. 2016 Feb;86:399–418. Epub 2015 Oct 17.

Kim CH, Lee HK, Koh YC, Hwang DY. Clinical analysis of diffuse axonal injury (DAI) diagnosed with magnetic resonance image (MRI) J Korean Neurosurg Soc. 1997 Feb;26(2):241–8.

Kim HJ, Park IS, Kim JH, Kim KJ, Hwang SH, Kim ES, et al. Clinical analysis of the prognosis of the patients with cerebral diffuse axonal injuries, based on gradient-echo MR imaging. J Korean Neurosurg Soc. 2001 Feb;30(2):168–72.

Lo V, Esquenazi Y, Han MK, Lee K. Critical care management of patients with acute spinal cord injury. J Neurosurg Sci. 2013 Dec;57(4):281–92.

Martin RM, Wright MJ, Lutkenhoff ES, Ellingson BM, Van Horn JD, Tubi M, et al. Traumatic hemorrhagic brain injury: impact of location and resorption on cognitive outcome. J Neurosurg. 2017 Mar;126(3):796–804. Epub 2016 May 27.

Mirvis SE, Shanmuganathan K. Trauma radiology: Part IV. Imaging of acute craniocerebral trauma. J Intensive Care Med. 1994 Nov-Dec;9(6):305–15.

Moen KG, Skandsen T, Folvik M, Brezova V, Kvistad KA, Rydland J, et al. A longitudinal MRI study of traumatic axonal injury in patients with moderate and severe traumatic brain injury. J Neurol Neurosurg Psychiatry. 2012 Dec;83(12):1193–200. Epub 2012 Aug 29.

Okonkwo DO, Shutter LA, Moore C, Temkin NR, Puccio AM, Madden CJ, et al. Brain oxygen optimization in severe traumatic brain injury phase-II: a phase II randomized trial. Crit Care Med. 2017 Nov;45(11):1907–14.

Popa C, Popa F, Grigorean VT, Onose G, Sandu AM, Popescu M, et al. Vascular dysfunctions following spinal cord injury. J Med Life. 2010 Jul-Sep;3(3):275–85.

Stratman RC, Wiesner AM, Smith KM, Cook AM. Hemodynamic management after spinal cord injury. Orthopedics. 2008 Mar;31(3):252–5.

Talbott JF, Gean A, Yuh EL, Stiver SI. Calvarial fracture patterns on CT imaging predict risk of a delayed epidural hematoma following decompressive craniectomy for traumatic brain injury. AJNR Am J Neuroradiol. 2014 Oct;35(10):1930–5. Epub 2014 Jun 19.

Vergouwen MD, Vermeulen M, Roos YB. Effect of nimodipine on outcome in patients with traumatic subarachnoid haemorrhage: a systematic review. Lancet Neurol. 2006 Dec;5(12):1029–32.

Wardlaw JM, Statham PF. How often is haemosiderin not visible on routine MRI following traumatic intracerebral haemorrhage? Neuroradiology. 2000 Feb;42(2):81–4.

Wei SC, Ulmer S, Lev MH, Pomerantz SR, Gonzalez RG, Henson JW. Value of coronal reformations in the CT evaluation of acute head trauma. AJNR Am J Neuroradiol. 2010 Feb;31(2):334–9. Epub 2009 Oct 1.

Wu Z, Li S, Lei J, An D, Haacke EM. Evaluation of traumatic subarachnoid hemorrhage using susceptibility-weighted imaging. AJNR Am J Neuroradiol. 2010 Aug;31(7):1302–10. Epub 2010 Feb 25.

Zacharia TT, Nguyen DT. Subtle pathology detection with multidetector row coronal and sagittal CT reformations in acute head trauma. Emerg Radiol. 2010 Mar;17(2):97–102. Epub 2009 Oct 7.

88 Traumatic Epidural and Subdural Hematomas

PATRICK R. MALONEY, MD; MICHELLE J. CLARKE, MD

Goals

- Distinguish epidural hematoma from subdural hematoma on computed tomographic images.
- Recognize acute, subacute, and chronic subdural hematoma on computed tomographic images.
- Review the medical and surgical management of epidural hematomas as well as acute and chronic subdural hematomas.
- Review the management of medical complications, such as seizures, that occur with epidural and subdural hematomas.

Introduction

Traumatic brain injury (TBI) and spinal cord injury are primarily discussed in Chapter 87 ("Traumatic Brain Injury and Spinal Cord Injury"). TBI, however, is a broad topic and encompasses a spectrum of pathophysiologic disorders that result in increased intracranial pressure (ICP), cerebral edema, bleeding, mass effect, cerebral herniation, and death. Traumatic epidural hematoma (EDH) and subdural hematoma (SDH) are the focus of this chapter. EDH and SDH are intracranial blood collections that have mass effect within the intracranial vault (Figure 88.1) for which operative and nonoperative management criteria are established.

Traumatic EDH

Traumatic EDH occurs after acute head trauma that causes either arterial or venous bleeding into the epidural space. Skull fractures, specifically temporal bone fractures, are commonly associated with EDH. Overall, arterial bleeding is responsible for 85% of EDHs. The middle meningeal artery is commonly involved, often producing a lenticular (ie, convex or lens-shaped) extra-axial hyperdense lesion on computed tomography (CT) in the middle fossa. One-third of patients have other intracranial traumatic lesions, such as intraparenchymal hemorrhage, contusion, SDH, and cerebral edema.

EDH often produces clinical signs of increased ICP. The classic description of EDH in clinical vignettes is a patient with a blow to the head who has a period of unconsciousness and then a brief lucid interval before sudden and rapid neurologic decline and herniation. This presentation is not overly common but may occur in less than a third of patients. Like in patients with any TBI, a brief loss of consciousness after the initial impact is hypothesized to occur because of a transient loss of neuronal function. The lucid interval is thought to be caused by arteriovenous shunting in the epidural space before the critical volume of the EDH causes symptomatic brain compression. Also, serious head blows can cause transient loss of consciousness without subsequent development of EDH.

Progressive enlargement of EDH causes 1) rapid neurologic decline with ipsilateral hemispheric dysfunction; 2) brainstem compression manifested by ipsilateral pupillary dilatation (ie, uncal herniation from compression of the ipsilateral cranial nerve III) (Figure 88.2); 3) contralateral hemiparesis (due to compression of the upper third of the pontine corticospinal tract fibers that cross to the other side); and 4) language dysfunction (if the dominant hemisphere is affected, which is the left hemisphere in most persons). A false localizing sign, the *Kernohan notch phenomenon*, can occur from diagonal brainstem shift across to the contralateral tentorium cerebelli or dural edge, which compresses the contralateral cerebral peduncle and cranial nerve III, resulting in hemiparesis ipsilateral to the side of the lesion.

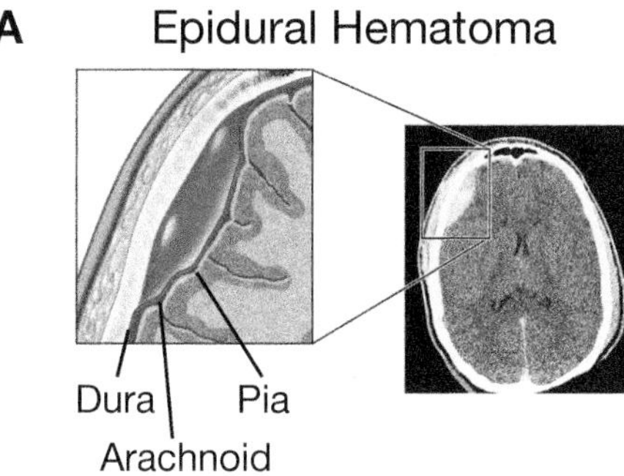

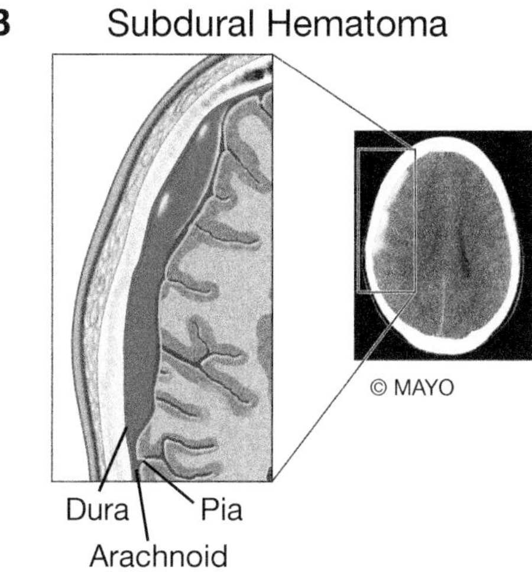

Figure 88.1. Comparison of Epidural Hematoma and Subdural Hematoma. A drawing (left) and a computed tomographic image (right) are shown for each. A, Epidural hematoma is hemorrhage between the skull and the dura. B, Subdural hematoma is hemorrhage between the dura and the arachnoid.

(Used with permission of Mayo Foundation for Medical Education and Research.)

Initial Management of EDH

Emergency medical systems personnel, emergency medicine clinicians, and intensivists should rapidly perform an initial neurologic examination at baseline and use a coma scale (eg, Glasgow Coma Scale [GCS] or Full Outline of Unresponsiveness [FOUR] score) in case the patient's neurologic status rapidly deteriorates. Also, baseline GCS or FOUR scores are useful if the patient later requires airway protection (eg, GCS score ≤8). In parallel with rapid clinical evaluation, emergent noncontrast CT of the head should be performed if the patient was involved with a high-impact force (eg, high-speed motor vehicle collision with loss of consciousness). Also, rapid determination of baseline laboratory values for a complete blood cell count is suggested, especially if the patient has had polytrauma to other organs or is at risk for systemic bleeding or exsanguination, in addition to determination of coagulation parameters, especially for patients receiving antithrombotics according to their history and medication list. CT sequences of the brain should be studied closely at the base of the skull for identifying fractures and for defining the extent of the lesion, mass effect on the brain, herniation, and associated lesions (eg, skull fractures). If patients have signs of herniation, such as dilated and unreactive pupil, mannitol (0.25-1.5 g/kg) is given as an intravenous piggyback until a surgical decision is made.

Reversal of concurrent anticoagulant medications such as warfarin may complicate the timing of emergent neurosurgical operative management of traumatic EDH. If the international normalized ratio (INR) exceeds 2.0, warfarin anticoagulation is usually reversed rapidly with a combination of prothombin complex concentrate and intravenous vitamin K (5-10 mg as a slow infusion) to an INR of less than 1.5; INR is then checked every 6 hours postoperatively for 24 hours and then daily for 3 days to ensure adequate hemostasis. Direct oral anticoagulants, such as rivaroxaban and apixaban, can be reversed with a US Food and Drug Administration–approved agent, andexanet alfa.

Bleeding diatheses must be diagnosed and corrected for optimal surgical and medical management. The recommended laboratory workup includes INR or prothrombin time, activated partial thromboplastin time for coagulopathy detection, and complete blood cell count and thromboelastogram for platelet count and function.

No randomized controlled trials have compared surgical treatment with nonoperative or medical management for patients with EDH. However, accepted neurosurgical criteria for emergent surgical treatment of acute EDH include hematoma volume greater than 30 mL regardless of the patient's GCS score. EDH can be managed nonoperatively with serial CT scanning and close neurologic observation in a neurosurgical center if the patient has a midline shift less than 5 mm, EDH maximum axial clot thickness less than 15 mm, and a GCS score greater than 8 without a focal neurologic deficit, such as hemiparesis or pupillary dilatation.

Surgical removal of EDH involves open craniotomy to remove the blood products causing mass effect and cauterization to stop the active bleeding. The timing of surgical evacuation in relation to the timing of neurologic deterioration is critical for successful treatment of EDH. Similarly, the Surgical Management of TBI Author Group (Bullock et al, 2006; see Suggested Reading) strongly recommended that patients with acute EDH, a GCS score of 9 or less, and pupillary anisocoria should have evacuation as soon as possible because outcomes are worse when evacuation is performed more than 70 minutes after the onset of pupillary dilatation than when it is performed sooner. Clinicians

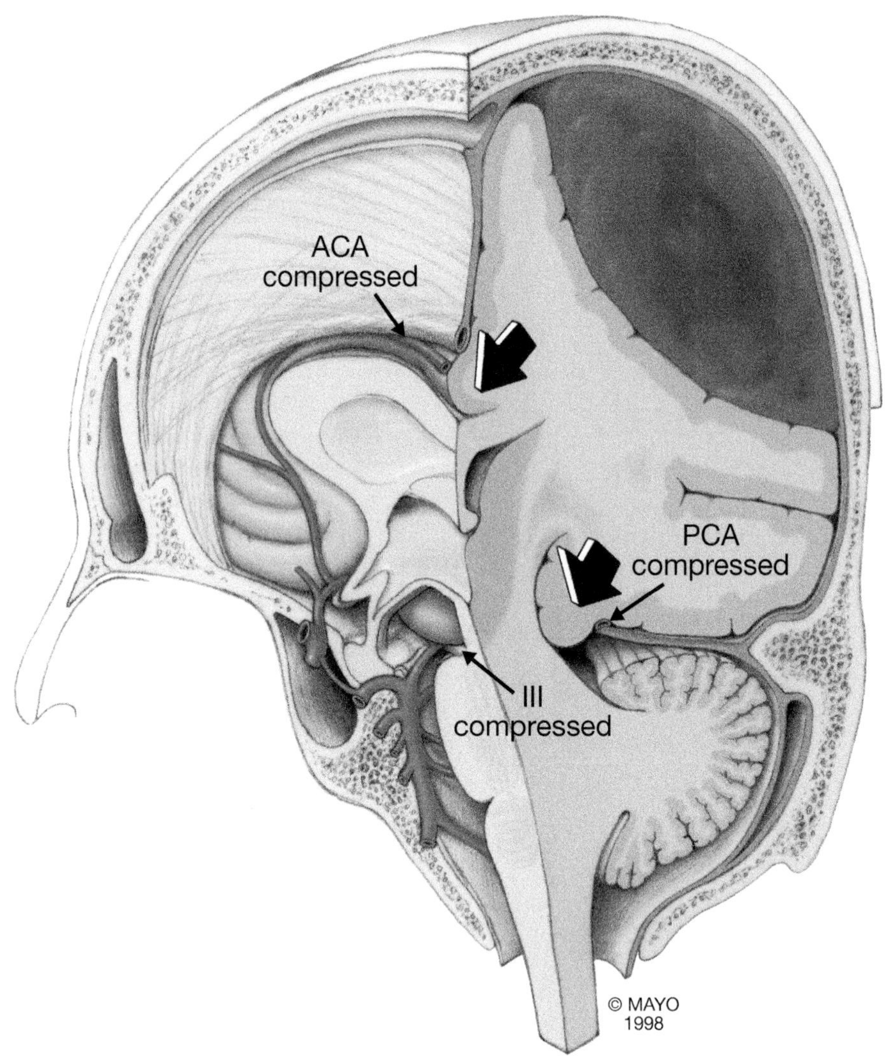

Figure 88.2. *Subdural Hematoma Herniation. The posterior cerebral artery (PCA) and cranial nerve III (III) are compressed as the uncus of the temporal lobe herniates around the tentorium cerebelli (lower arrow). The upper arrow indicates brain herniating under the falx cerebri with compression of the anterior cerebral artery (ACA).*

(From Wijdicks EFM. Catastrophic neurologic disorders in the emergency department. 2nd ed. Oxford [UK]: Oxford University Press; c2004. Chapter 8, Altered arousal and coma; p. 53-93; used with permission of Mayo Foundation for Medical Education and Research.)

should have a low threshold for surgical management if a patient's condition deteriorates.

Traumatic SDH

SDH (Figure 88.3) is classified according to duration, which can be inferred from the radiologic appearance (Table 88.1 and Figure 88.4). On CT, *acute* traumatic SDHs are visualized as hyperdense or bright white compared with brain (which is gray) and cerebrospinal fluid (which is black or hypodense). As the clot evolves, it liquefies and passes through a *subacute* phase, in which the SDH is isodense or gray like brain parenchyma on CT. An isodense SDH clinical vignette may be shown with an image that requires careful examination for the brain cortical sulci and gyri on the normal side compared with their absence on the other side with the isodense SDH. A *chronic* SDH is hypodense, with a CT density resembling that of cerebrospinal fluid or water. This classification is useful in the medical and operative management of SDH disease.

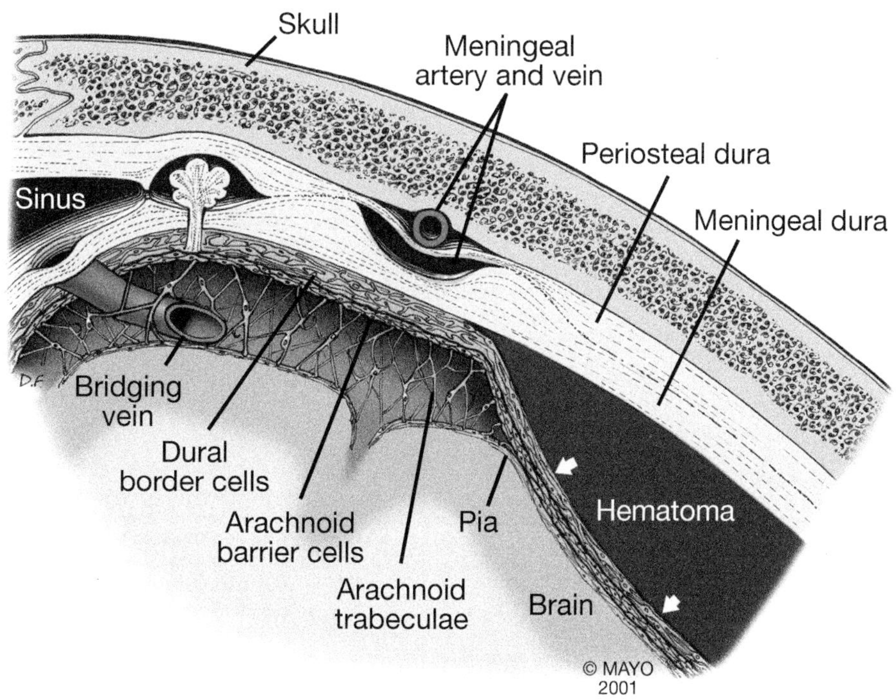

Figure 88.3. Anatomy of a Subdural Hematoma.
(Modified from Atkinson JLD. Subdural hematoma and variations. In: Batjer HH, Loftus CM, editors. Textbook of neurological surgery: principles and practice. Philadelphia [PA]: Lippincott Williams & Wilkins; c2003. p. 2830-40; used with permission of Mayo Foundation for Medical Education and Research.)

Acute SDH

Acute SDH usually results from head trauma occurring within the previous 4 days. The usual mechanism is 1) the tearing of cerebral veins, which become more vulnerable because of parenchymal atrophy with advancing age and alcoholism, or 2) the extension or extravasation of an intracerebral hemorrhage. Unlike patients with EDH, patients with acute traumatic SDH typically have a higher rate of underlying parenchymal brain injury with concomitant cerebral edema, so the neurologic recovery is difficult to predict, even after evacuation or stabilization of the lesion. Part of this uncertainty arises because after evacuation, brain re-expansion is variable.

Imaging characteristics of SDHs vary with the age of the lesion, but an SDH typically forms a crescent that crosses suture lines. SDHs are found less commonly in the interhemispheric fissure and along the tentorium cerebelli. If the hemorrhage is rapid and ongoing, a *swirl sign* may be present on CT. Fluid-fluid levels, similar to swirl signs, are heterogeneous densities within the clot, which can also be seen if a patient has been receiving anticoagulants or has an intrinsic coagulopathy or disseminated intravascular coagulation.

Table 88.1 • Classification of SDH Duration According to Density on CT

Duration of SDH	Approximate Age of SDH Since Initial Bleeding	Density of SDH on CT
Acute	1-4 d	Hyperdense (>65 and <200 HU)
Subacute	>3 d to 2 wk	Isodense (about 40-65 HU)
Chronic	>3 wk	Hypodense (mixed density can be seen with chronic membranes) (<40 HU)

Abbreviations: CT, computed tomography; HU, Hounsfield units; SDH, subdural hematoma.

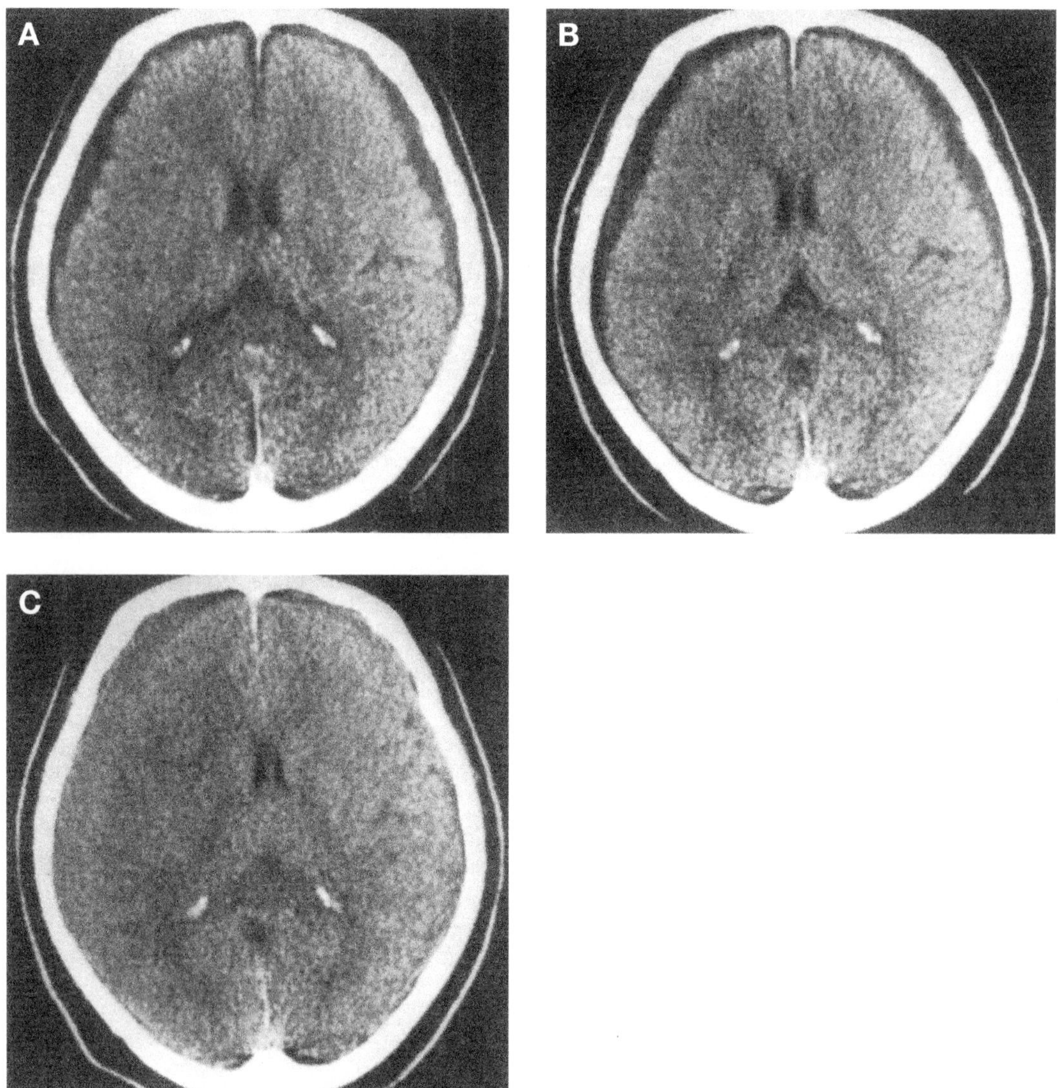

Figure 88.4. Chronicity of Subdural Hematomas by Hounsfield Density on Computed Tomography. A, Acute. B, Subacute. C, Chronic.

(From Ohno K, Suzuki R, Masaoka H, Matsushima Y, Inaba Y, Monma S. Chronic subdural haematoma preceded by persistent traumatic subdural fluid collection. J Neurol Neurosurg Psychiatry. 1987 Dec;50[12]:1694-7; used with permission.)

Indications for surgery for SDHs are more complex than for EDHs. Because many SDHs are small and slow forming, patient age, baseline neurologic function, comorbidities, and SDH location should all be considered before the patient is offered surgery. The Surgical Management of TBI Author Group also suggested that surgery is indicated for a midline shift greater than 5 mm and a maximum clot thickness of more than 10 mm regardless of the GCS score (most SDHs are measured in the axial plane on CT imaging). They also suggested that all patients with SDH and coma with a GCS score of 9 or less should undergo ICP monitoring. Surgical candidates also include comatose SDH patients whose GCS score decreased by 2 or more points from the score at admission who have asymmetric or fixed and dilated pupils or ICP of 20 mm Hg or more.

SDH evacuation involves a craniotomy with or without bone flap removal and duroplasty to remove SDH blood products and to find and repair the lacerated vein. If the patient has a large associated parenchymal injury with cerebral swelling at the time of the operation, leaving the bone flap off (like in a hemicraniectomy) can allow room for cerebral edema and brain expansion and potentially accommodate malignant intracranial hypertension that may peak 3 to 5 days after the injury. Mortality from acute SDH is high (58%-90%), with higher rates typically correlated with older age and anticoagulation therapy.

Chronic SDH

Unlike acute SDHs, chronic SDHs are generally several weeks old (or at least 14 days old) for blood products to liquefy sufficiently and become hypodense to brain parenchyma on CT of the head (Table 88.1). Patients with chronic SDH tend to have a more insidious course and a history of remote minor or moderate trauma. Chronic SDH can also result from the evolution of a medically managed acute SDH that liquefied and redistributed over time. Chronic SDHs are more common in older patients (average age, 62-65 years).

Patients with chronic SDH can present with headaches, nausea and vomiting, seizures, and subtle localizing signs, such as aphasia and mild hemiparesis that may lead to gait instability. Confusion and mild encephalopathy can also occur. However, many patients with chronic SDH may be asymptomatic, and SDH may be an incidental finding when brain imaging is performed for other reasons.

Surgical evacuation of chronic SDH is indicated when patients have focal neurologic deficits attributable to the mass lesion and when the maximal diameter of the collection is 1 cm or more (not measured at the vertices of the skull). Although many techniques have been described for evacuating a chronic SDH, most practitioners favor the least invasive burr-hole method with the use of a subdural drain. A closed-system drain has been shown to decrease the recurrence rate by as much as 10%.

Fibroblasts are responsible for generating chronic SDH membranes that can form immature capillaries. This neovascularization can lead to recurrent microhemorrhages and reaccumulation or even expansion of the chronic SDH. This is a reason why the recurrence rate for chronic SDH can be as high as 20%.

Medical Management of EDH and SDH

Evaluation of acute SDH or EDH should be a multipronged effort with a focus on 1) a rapid, global neurologic assessment with the GCS or FOUR score to assess whether airway, breathing, and circulatory issues must be managed and 2) a rapid history and laboratory assessment of anticoagulation or antiplatelet agent use. Symptomatic patients or those with declining neurologic status who are receiving warfarin or similar anticoagulant drugs should be treated with fresh frozen plasma or prothrombin complex concentrates and a slow intravenous infusion of 5 to 10 mg vitamin K to decrease the INR to 1.5 until the patient's long-term risks (eg, atrial fibrillation risk) can be reassessed. For patients who are neurologically asymptomatic except for headache, most neurosurgeons and clinicians advise stopping oral anticoagulation but monitoring the patient's neurologic status every 1 to 2 hours (ie, at a neurocritical or intensive care level) unless the patient becomes symptomatic rapidly and requires emergent anticoagulation reversal. Oral atorvastatin was shown to decrease the volume of chronic subdural hematomas in a randomized, placebo-controlled trial, the Effect of Atorvastatin on Chronic Subdural Hematoma (ATOCH).

Operative factors for SDH decompression should be individualized according to the patient's age and overall medical condition and according to the size of the SDH (maximal thickness ≥1 cm), and the presence or absence of midline shift. For example, for a 65-year-old patient with an SDH who has a GCS score of 15 and a maximal axial thickness of 8 mm with no midline shift, clinical observation may be acceptable if the patient does not have neurologic deficits. However, craniotomy and SDH evacuation would benefit a 25-year-old TBI patient with a right-sided SDH (maximal thickness, 1 cm) who is symptomatic, has a GCS score of 9 (previously the GCS score was 15), has a 5-mm midline shift, and was otherwise in good clinical condition,

Patients with SDH or EDH are at increased risk for seizures, both clinical and subclinical, and seizures may be more common after craniotomy. Thus, a reasonable approach is to treat patients with a prophylactic antiseizure medication and to perform electroencephalography if the examination findings do not correlate well with the radiologic findings. Also, for severe TBI (GCS score ≤8), general TBI guidelines suggest 1 week of phenytoin for seizure prophylaxis. However, prophylaxis for more than 1 week is not advised unless the patient had a history of symptomatic seizures at onset or had other reasons for continuing the medication.

Seizure prophylaxis for patients with chronic SDH is a matter of debate. From the results of some studies, prophylaxis is favored for high-risk patients. Such patients can have events that resemble transient ischemic attack or seizure. Electroencephalography can be helpful to determine whether epileptiform activity is present and to guide management especially if seizures are present. Some patients with chronic SDH appear to respond to antiseizure medication and can pose vexing clinical challenges because hemosiderin and iron products on the surface of the cerebral cortex may cause cortical irritation.

Summary

- Patients with traumatic EDH or SDH and TBI with loss of consciousness should undergo rapid assessment of their baseline neurologic state with the GCS or FOUR score, baseline laboratory testing (complete blood cell count and coagulation profile), and noncontrast CT of the head.
- Patients with traumatic EDH may have a transient lucid interval before their status rapidly deteriorates.
- SDH and EDH can rapidly become neurosurgical emergencies with herniation, coma, and death.

- Patients with SDH or EDH who have a decline in motor response or new focal signs should have the hematoma evacuated unless the patients have major comorbid factors or their families will not consent.
- Patients with acute SDH have a high rate of underlying brain injury, which results in high morbidity and mortality, especially in older patients who have other comorbidities. The outcome is worse for comatose patients who are older than 80 years and have an acute SDH with a volume larger than 50 mL.
- Patients with chronic SDH may be largely asymptomatic and may require radiologic monitoring unless they become neurologically symptomatic.
- Seizures are prevalent in patients with acute SDH and EDH and in patients with severe TBI with coma; 1 week of seizure prophylaxis is generally recommended but not continued unless the patient had a history of seizures at onset or seizures persist during hospitalization.

SUGGESTED READING

Alford EN, Rotman LE, Erwood MS, Oster RA, Davis MC, Pittman HBC, et al. Development of the Subdural Hematoma in the Elderly (SHE) score to predict mortality. J Neurosurg. 2019 Apr 12:1–7. [Epub ahead of print]

Bezircioglu H, Ersahin Y, Demircivi F, Yurt I, Donertas K, Tektas S. Nonoperative treatment of acute extradural hematomas: analysis of 80 cases. J Trauma. 1996 Oct;41(4):696–8.

Bokka S, Trivedi A. Histopathological study of the outer membrane of the dura mater in chronic sub dural hematoma: its clinical and radiological correlation. Asian J Neurosurg. 2016 Jan-Mar;11(1):34–8.

Bullock MR, Chesnut R, Ghajar J, Gordon D, Hartl R, Newell DW, et al; Surgical Management of Traumatic Brain Injury Author Group. Surgical management of acute epidural hematomas. Neurosurgery. 2006 Mar;58(3 Suppl):S7–15.

Bullock MR, Chesnut R, Ghajar J, Gordon D, Hartl R, Newell DW, et al; Surgical Management of Traumatic Brain Injury Author Group. Surgical management of traumatic parenchymal lesions. Neurosurgery. 2006 Mar;58(3 Suppl):S25–46.

Carney N, Totten AM, O'Reilly C, Ullman JS, Hawryluk GW, Bell MJ, et al. Guidelines for the management of severe traumatic brain injury, fourth edition. Neurosurgery. 2017 Jan 1;80(1):6–15.

Driver J, DiRisio AC, Mitchell H, Threlkeld ZD, Gormley WB. Non-electrographic seizures due to subdural hematoma: a case series and review of the literature. Neurocrit Care. 2018 Feb 23. [Epub ahead of print]

Ducruet AF, Grobelny BT, Zacharia BE, Hickman ZL, DeRosa PL, Andersen KN, et al. The surgical management of chronic subdural hematoma. Neurosurg Rev. 2012 Apr;35(2):155–69. Epub 2011 Sep 10. Erratum in: Neurosurg Rev. 2015 Oct;38(4):771.

Fomchenko EI, Gilmore EJ, Matouk CC, Gerrard JL, Sheth KN. Management of subdural hematomas: Part II. Surgical management of subdural hematomas. Curr Treat Options Neurol. 2018 Jul 18;20(8):34.

Ganz JC. The lucid interval associated with epidural bleeding: evolving understanding. J Neurosurg. 2013 Apr;118(4):739–45. Epub 2013 Jan 18.

Grande P-O, Juul N. Comparative analysis of various guidelines for treatment of severe TBI. In: Sundstrom T, Grande P-O, Juul N, Kock-Jensen C, Romner B, Wester K, editors. Management of severe traumatic brain injury: evidence, tricks, and pitfalls. Heidelberg (Berlin): Springer; c2012. p. 267–72.

Huang KT, Bi WL, Abd-El-Barr M, Yan SC, Tafel IJ, Dunn IF, et al. The neurocritical and neurosurgical care of subdural hematomas. Neurocrit Care. 2016 Apr;24(2):294–307.

Jones NR, Molloy CJ, Kloeden CN, North JB, Simpson DA. Extradural haematoma: trends in outcome over 35 years. Br J Neurosurg. 1993;7(5):465–71.

Nakaguchi H, Tanishima T, Yoshimasu N. Factors in the natural history of chronic subdural hematomas that influence their postoperative recurrence. J Neurosurg. 2001 Aug;95(2):256–62.

Schaumann A, Klene W, Rosenstengel C, Ringel F, Tuttenberg J, Vajkoczy P. COXIBRAIN: results of the prospective, randomised, phase II/III study for the selective COX-2 inhibition in chronic subdural haematoma patients. Acta Neurochir (Wien). 2016 Nov;158(11):2039–44. Epub 2016 Sep 7. Erratum in: Acta Neurochir (Wien). 2016 Nov 9.

Siddiqui FM, Bekker SV, Qureshi AI. Neuroimaging of hemorrhage and vascular defects. Neurotherapeutics. 2011 Jan;8(1):28–38.

Warkentin AE, Donadini MP, Spencer FA, Lim W, Crowther M. Bleeding risk in randomized controlled trials comparing warfarin and aspirin: a systematic review and meta-analysis. J Thromb Haemost. 2012 Apr;10(4):512–20.

Wijdicks EFM. The practice of emergency and critical care neurology. New York (NY): Oxford University Press; c2016. 915 p.

Yoo WK, Kim DS, Kwon YH, Jang SH. Kernohan's notch phenomenon demonstrated by diffusion tensor imaging and transcranial magnetic stimulation. J Neurol Neurosurg Psychiatry. 2008 Nov;79(11):1295–7.

Unstable Spinal Fractures

WILLIAM E. CLIFTON III, MD; MARK A. PICHELMANN, MD

Goals

- Review the anatomical basis for spinal stability.
- Identify the priorities for assessment of spinal stability in patients who may have unstable spinal fractures.
- Review different types of bony and ligamentous disruption at different levels of the spine and their optimal treatment.
- Outline the management of spinal fractures to prevent traumatic spinal cord injury.

Introduction

Traumatic spinal injuries occur relatively frequently, with an incidence of about 12,000 patients per year in the United States. Modern advances in critical care management of patients with spinal injuries and spinal cord injuries have greatly decreased mortality. Therefore, the prevalence in the United States is more than 200,000 patients per year. The importance of early diagnosis and proper management of acute spinal fractures cannot be understated. This chapter reviews the different types of bony and ligamentous disruption in the cervical, thoracic, lumbar, and sacral spine that can lead to new or worsened neurologic injury if left untreated.

Definition of Spinal Stability

A working definition of *spinal stability* is the ability of the spine to resist changes in its natural structure when disruptive mechanical forces are introduced. In essence, the elasticity of the bony and ligamentous structures ensures that the sensitive neural elements are not damaged during periods of mechanical stress. Any damage to these protective elements that does not allow for elastic correction with active movement is considered *unstable*. Not all bony fractures are unstable, and not all instability is accompanied by a bony fracture.

Relevant Anatomy

The occipitocervical (OC) junction provides the most rotational capability of the head. The atlantoaxial joint is also key in this movement. The atlas (C1) is a ring-shaped vertebra that connects the base of the skull to the remainder of the neuraxis by 2 joints on either side. Several key ligaments connect the atlas to the dens of the axis ventrally. The vertebrae of the subaxial cervical spine are linked together by axially situated joints on either side of the posterior elements. The cervical bodies are connected to the posterior elements by thin pedicles. The thoracic vertebrae have coronally facing joints and thick pedicles connecting the vertebral bodies to the posterior elements. The lumbar vertebrae also generally have large pedicles with joints oriented in the sagittal plane. Knowledge of the anatomy and function of the facet joints at the cervical, thoracic, and lumbar levels is important for understanding the effects of trauma at each level.

Denis 3-Column Model

In the Denis 3-column model, the spine is divided into 3 columns when viewed in the sagittal plane: 1) The *anterior column* contains the anterior two-thirds of the vertebral body and disk and the anterior longitudinal ligament. 2) The *middle column* contains the posterior one-third of the vertebral body and disk and the posterior longitudinal ligament. 3) The *posterior column* contains the lamina, spinous process, and posterior ligamentous complex. The modern classification systems of spinal fractures hinge on an understanding of the contents of each of these 3 columns.

Assessment of Patients With Spinal Injury

The initial assessment of a trauma patient should begin with the ABC approach (airway, breathing, and circulation). The patient's vital signs and hemodynamic status may alert the examiner to associated vascular injury that should take priority over the neurologic assessment. Any suspected or imaged OC-atlantoaxial injuries or 3-column injuries in the cervical or thoracic spine should prompt additional vascular imaging with magnetic resonance angiography or computed tomographic (CT) angiography as part of the initial evaluation. After the initial trauma assessment, the neurologic assessment should begin with the American Spinal Injury Association Impairment Scale to determine whether the patient has a spinal cord injury. In the absence of a focal deficit, palpation of the spinal axis and passive and active movement of the patient's neck will aid in determining whether ligamentous injuries are present. Infection and neoplasia may also be associated with compression or burst fractures, and a comprehensive workup should include appropriate studies if these processes are suspected clinically or if the patient has a relevant previous history.

Radiologic Analysis

Flexion-extension plain radiography is used when conscious patients do not have neurologic deficits but do have suspected subaxial cervical spine disease. Anterior or posterior subluxation of vertebrae is a sign of instability on movement images, but patients with acute ligamentous injury have a high rate of false-negative results due to muscle spasm. Radiographic views should include the following: swimmer's (thoracolumbar junction), open-mouth (OC and atlantoaxial joints), lateral, oblique, flexion, and extension. Motion studies should be performed if OC-atlantoaxial injury or subaxial instability is suspected clinically from the type of neurologic signs, because mobilization may worsen the neurologic injury.

CT offers a fast and inexpensive method of evaluating the spine for bony injury. Ligamentous injury may be inferred from the imaging results, but CT does not allow visualization of the spinal canal or neural elements as well as magnetic resonance imaging (MRI).

MRI is the diagnostic choice for assessment of ligamentous and neurologic injury. Disadvantages include prolonged examination times and inferior bony imaging compared with CT.

Pathology and Instability of the Spine

OC Junction

OC dislocation is characterized by separation of the occipital condyles from the superior facets of the atlas. It is relatively uncommon and is often quickly fatal. Other complications include lower cranial nerve palsy and vertebral artery injury. All OC dislocations are considered unstable and are treated with open reduction and fusion as indicated. Radiographic analysis consists of measuring the atlantodental interval (reference range: <3 mm in adults; >5 mm in children). The Powers ratio is calculated as the distance from the lower edge of the clivus (ie, the basion) to the posterior arch of C1 divided by the distance from the posterior lip of the foramen magnum (ie, the opisthion) to the anterior arch of C1. A Powers ratio greater than 1 indicates dislocation.

The Tuli classification of occipital condylar fractures recognizes 3 types: Type 1 is a nondisplaced fracture with no slippage on imaging; type 2A, a displaced fracture with no slippage on imaging; and type 2B, a displaced or nondisplaced fracture with movement or slippage on imaging.

The treatment of OC fractures is widely debated and not extensively studied because OC fractures are rare. As with any unstable spinal column fracture, types 2A and 2B should be treated with a halo vest or open surgical fixation.

Atlas

Fractures of C1 can occur in conjunction with OC fractures, but more commonly they are isolated. Transverse ligament disruption is the main factor in stability assessment. Neurologic symptoms are rare. Three types of isolated atlas fractures occur (Figure 89.1): *Posterior arch fractures* are usually not unstable. Treatment consists of bracing if neck pain is severe. The likelihood of union is high with conservative therapy. *Lateral mass fractures* are unilateral or bilateral without ligamentous disruption. They may be treated with bracing. Halo fixation is indicated for comminuted fractures or ligamentous instability. *Burst (Jefferson) fractures* are classified according to the rule of Spence: An overhang of the lateral mass on C2 that is more than 7 mm indicates transverse ligament disruption, and the fracture is considered unstable. For unstable fractures, halo fixation or C1-C2 fusion is indicated.

Axis

The 2 anatomical weak points in the axis are the pars interarticularis and the odontoid process. Fractures of C2 are divided into 2 groups: pars (hangman's) fractures (from hyperextension injuries) and odontoid fractures (from hyperflexion injuries).

Pars fractures are divided into 3 types (Figure 89.2) according to the amount of subluxation between C2 and C3 as described by Effendi et al (1981) (see Suggested Reading): *Type I* is a vertical fracture with subluxation of less than 3 mm. If the patient is neurologically stable, treatment is with a hard cervical collar. *Type IA* is an oblique fracture that carries a higher risk of neurologic injury. If the patient is neurologically stable, treatment is with a halo; otherwise treatment is surgical fixation.

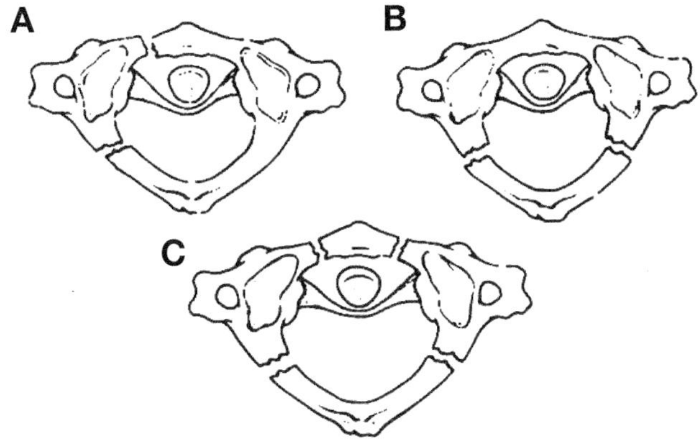

Figure 89.1. Types of C1 Ring Fractures. A, Lateral mass fracture. B, Posterior arch fracture. C, Burst (Jefferson) fracture. (Modified from Oner FC. Spinal injury classification systems. In: Jallo J, Vaccaro AR, editors. Neurotrauma and critical care of the spine. New York [NY]: Thieme Medical Publishers. 2009. p. 45-67; used with permission.)

Type II is a vertical fracture with subluxation of more than 3 mm. Treatment is with closed reduction and use of a halo or collar. *Type IIA* is an oblique fracture with angulation. Treatment consists of open reduction or fixation (no traction). *Type III* is a vertical fracture with facet involvement. Treatment consists of open reduction or fixation (no traction).

Odontoid fractures can be divided into 3 types (Figure 89.3): *Type I* is a fracture through the tip of the odontoid. If the patient is neurologically stable, treatment is with a hard cervical collar. *Type II* is a fracture through the base. Unstable, displaced fractures have a high rate of nonunion with halo immobilization. Treatment is with a trial of halo immobilization or surgical fixation. *Type III* is a fracture through the body of C2. Treatment is with a cervical collar if the patient is neurologically stable; otherwise, halo immobilization should be used. With any OC, C1, or C2 fracture in a patient who presents with neurologic deficits, the fracture must be reduced and stabilized promptly.

Subaxial Cervical Spine

Injury to the subaxial cervical spine can take many forms. Generally, these injuries are classified according to the column of the spine involved (as in the Denis 3-column model) or the mechanism of the disruptive force.

Compression fractures occur in the anterior column only, and patients generally do not present with neurologic deficits; bracing is used for pain.

Burst fractures occur in the anterior and middle columns; surgery is reserved for patients with neurologic deficits, and bracing is used as indicated for pain.

Flexion and compression (teardrop) injuries can appear misleadingly benign on CT or plain radiographs; however, anterior and posterior ligamentous disruption is common with serious neurologic sequelae. Surgical intervention is warranted.

Unilateral and bilateral facet dislocations (rotation injury) are treated with open or closed reduction (after MRI) or with fixation (or with both), depending on concomitant pathology.

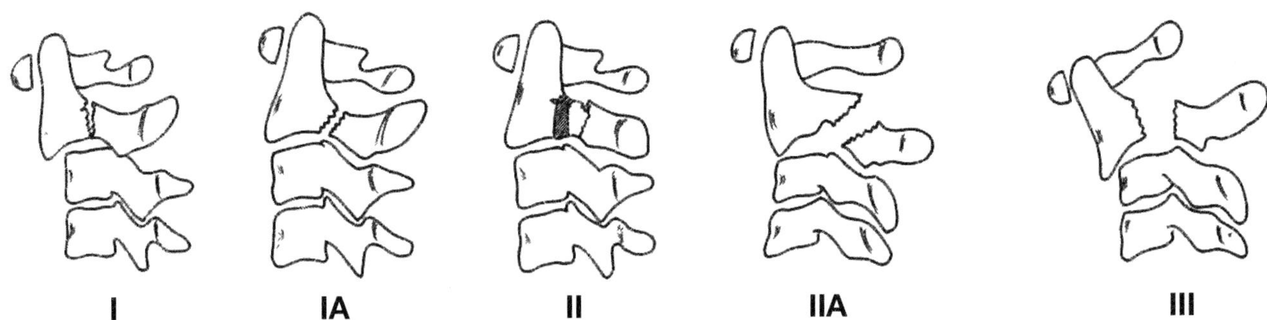

Figure 89.2. Types of C2 Pars Fractures. Roman numerals indicate the type. (Modified from Oner FC. Spinal injury classification systems. In: Jallo J, Vaccaro AR, editors. Neurotrauma and critical care of the spine. New York [NY]: Thieme Medical Publishers. 2009. p. 45-67; used with permission.)

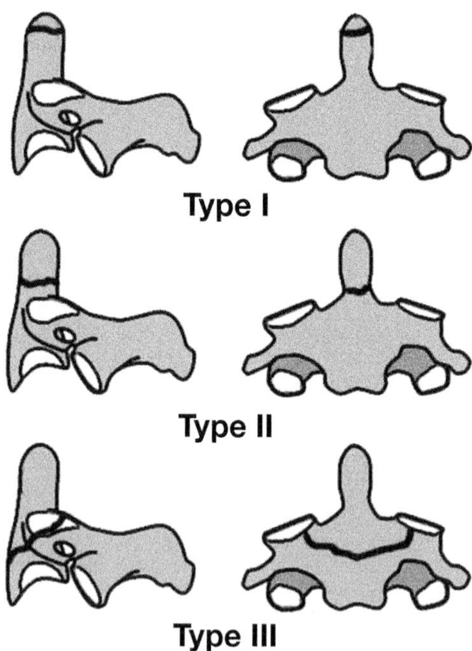

Figure 89.3. Types of Odontoid Fractures.
(Modified from Oner FC. Spinal injury classification systems. In: Jallo J, Vaccaro AR, editors. Neurotrauma and critical care of the spine. New York [NY]: Thieme Medical Publishers. 2009. p. 45-67; used with permission.)

Flexion, extension, and distraction (whiplash) injuries are characterized by ligamentous disruption rather than bony disruption. Instability occurs with disruption of the posterior longitudinal ligament, and surgery is indicated.

Thoracolumbar Spine

Fractures of the thoracolumbar vertebrae have been classified several ways. The most modern and applicable is the thoracolumbar injury classification and severity (TLICS) score (Table 89.1). This system uses 3 components: morphology of the injury, ligamentous injury status, and neurologic involvement. If the patient has more than 1 injury, the most severe injury is scored. A total score of 3 or less indicates that nonoperative treatment is warranted; patients with a score of 4 may need either nonoperative or operative treatment; and a score of 5 or more indicates the need for operative treatment with open surgery and fixation.

Compression fractures are usually stable and have a high rate of spontaneous healing with bracing and expectant management. The most common cause is osteoporosis, but neoplastic metastases are frequent causes. If conservative treatment is insufficient, kyphoplasty or vertebroplasty may be used for pain control, but malignancy must be ruled out with a biopsy first.

Table 89.1 • Thoracolumbar Injury Classification and Severity Scoring

Description	Points
Morphology	
Compression fracture	1
Burst fracture	2
Translational/rotational	3
Distraction	4
Posterior ligamentous complex	
Intact	0
Indeterminate	2
Injured	3
Neurologic involvement	
Intact	0
Nerve root	2
Spinal cord, conus medullaris	
Complete	3
Incomplete	2
Cauda equine	3

From Lee JY, Vaccaro AR, Lim MR, Oner FC, Hulbert AJ, Hedlund R, et al. Thoracolumbar injury classification and severity score: a new paradigm for the treatment of thoracolumbar spine trauma. J Orthop Sci. 2005 Nov;10(6):671-5; used with permission.

Burst fractures may be stable or unstable. If they ae unstable, they should be treated with decompression surgery or fixation. Stable burst fractures in patients with no neurologic signs or symptoms will heal with conservative therapy as well as with surgery (level of evidence: I).

Flexion, distraction, and translational injuries are 3-column injuries that disrupt the posterior ligamentous complex. They are always unstable, and the incidence of complete cord lesions is high. Open surgery is indicated.

Sacral Spine

Traumatic sacral fractures are rare and have not been studied extensively. In general, they are classified into 3 types according to the relationship of the fracture to the dorsal neural foramina: *Type 1* is lateral, *type 2* is through the neural foramen, and *type 3* is through the central canal. Treatment is determined according to the extent of neurologic injury and spinopelvic deformity.

Summary

- Traumatic spinal injuries are caused by motor vehicle collisions, falls, and other trauma.
- A systematic approach with history, radiographs, and CT of the spine can be helpful in identifying spinal fractures and potential instability.
- Classification of spinal fractures is based on the spinal elements involved and the level of the fracture.

- MRI should be used if ligamentous injury or soft tissue injury is suspected when CT of the spine is inconclusive.
- Early identification of a spinal fracture and potential instability is the key to preventing instability and spinal cord injury.
- A hard cervical collar should be used for immobilization when instability is suspected and intubation is needed, with in-line stabilization and advanced airway management (eg, fiberoptic intubation).

SUGGESTED READING

Anderson PA, Montesano PX. Morphology and treatment of occipital condyle fractures. Spine (Phila Pa 1976). 1988 Jul;13(7):731–6.

Baaj AA, Uribe JS, Nichols TA, Theodore N, Crawford NR, Sonntag VK, et al. Health care burden of cervical spine fractures in the United States: analysis of a nationwide database over a 10-year period. J Neurosurg Spine. 2010 Jul;13(1):61–6.

Denis F. Spinal instability as defined by the three-column spine concept in acute spinal trauma. Clin Orthop Relat Res. 1984 Oct;(189):65–76.

Effendi B, Roy D, Cornish B, Dussault RG, Laurin CA. Fractures of the ring of the axis: a classification based on the analysis of 131 cases. J Bone Joint Surg Br. 1981;63–B(3):319–27.

Frangen TM, Zilkens C, Muhr G, Schinkel C. Odontoid fractures in the elderly: dorsal C1/C2 fusion is superior to halo-vest immobilization. J Trauma. 2007 Jul;63(1):83–9.

Greene KA, Dickman CA, Marciano FF, Drabier JB, Hadley MN, Sonntag VK. Acute axis fractures: analysis of management and outcome in 340 consecutive cases. Spine (Phila Pa 1976). 1997 Aug 15;22(16):1843–52.

Hadley MN, Browner C, Sonntag VK. Axis fractures: a comprehensive review of management and treatment in 107 cases. Neurosurgery. 1985 Aug;17(2):281–90.

Hadley MN, Fitzpatrick BC, Sonntag VK, Browner CM. Facet fracture-dislocation injuries of the cervical spine. Neurosurgery. 1992 May;30(5):661–6.

Omeis I, Duggal N, Rubano J, Cerabona F, Abrahams J, Fink M, et al. Surgical treatment of C2 fractures in the elderly: a multicenter retrospective analysis. J Spinal Disord Tech. 2009 Apr;22(2):91–5.

Pearson AM, Martin BI, Lindsey M, Mirza SK. C2 vertebral fractures in the medicare population: incidence, outcomes, and costs. J Bone Joint Surg Am. 2016 Mar 16;98(6):449–56.

Roy-Camille R, Bleynie JF, Saillant G, Judet T. [Odontoid process fractures associated with fractures of the pedicles of the axis (author's transl)]. Rev Chir Orthop Reparatrice Appar Mot. 1979 Oct-Nov;65(7):387–91. French.

Santos-Nunez G, Lo HS, Kotecha H, Jose J, Abayazeed A. Imaging of spine fractures with emphasis on the craniocervical junction. Semin Ultrasound CT MR. 2018 Aug;39(4):324–35. Epub 2018 Apr 16.

Sonntag VK, Hadley MN. Nonoperative management of cervical spine injuries. Clin Neurosurg. 1988;34:630–49.

Spetzler RF, Hadley MN, Sonntag VK. The transoral approach to the anterior superior cervical spine: a review of 29 cases. Acta Neurochir Suppl (Wien). 1988;43:69–74.

Tong Y, Wu Q. Thoracolumbar injury classification and severity score. J Neurosurg Spine. 2015 Apr;22(4):444–5.

Acute Central Nervous System Infections

90 Encephalitis

ALLEN J. AKSAMIT JR, MD

Goals

- Discuss the most common forms of encephalitis.
- Understand the diagnosis and management of the main types of viral encephalitis.
- Recognize the overlap between viral and autoimmune encephalitis.

Introduction

Encephalitis is an inflammatory process affecting the parenchyma of the brain, most commonly diffusely, and therefore leading to a clouding of consciousness early in its course. At a gross pathologic level, encephalitis is generally nonpurulent and is distinguished from cerebritis, which tends to be overtly purulent on gross inspection. *Encephalitis* is the preferred term for viral or autoimmune inflammation of the brain.

Definitions

Viral encephalitis is encephalitis caused by direct parenchymal infection from a virus. A classic example is herpes simplex encephalitis (HSE), which is most often caused by herpes simplex virus (HSV) type 1 (HSV-1).

Postinfectious encephalitis is inflammation of the brain gray matter due to an immunologic reaction after systemic infection. When inflammation is present while the infection is occurring but without viral invasion of the brain, the condition is sometimes referred to as *parainfectious encephalitis*. Another form of postinfectious encephalitis is *acute disseminated encephalomyelitis*, where the immune reaction is directed at central nervous system white matter more than gray matter. This condition should be in a separate disease category with other acute demyelinating disorders.

Autoimmune encephalitis is a primary autoimmune reaction against the brain without a preceding infection. When the reaction occurs with systemic cancer, the condition is called *paraneoplastic encephalitis*. Typical syndromes include an immune reaction that is triggered by a systemic cancer but is directed against neural antigens, as in limbic encephalitis. This is typical for a neoplasm-associated, antigen-driven immune response, such as voltage-gated potassium channel–complex encephalitis associated with cancer, which typically injures the limbic structures of the brain. However, autoimmune encephalitis can be a primary autoimmune reaction against the brain. Anti–*N*-methyl-D-aspartate (NMDA) receptor encephalitis is an example of an autoimmune response against central nervous system antigens that may occur without precipitating preexisting cancer or infection. However, paraneoplastic and postinfectious forms of anti-NMDA receptor encephalitis exist. Another example is Hashimoto encephalitis, sometimes called steroid-responsive encephalopathy associated with autoimmune thyroiditis (SREAT). This condition is associated with autoimmune thyroid antibodies, but the antibodies are a marker of systemic autoimmunity, which is associated with but not directly caused by the antibodies against the thyroid gland.

Epidemiology

Details of the epidemiology of encephalitis are challenging to ascertain. The burden of encephalitis associated with hospitalizations in the United States results in substantial use of medical resources. One study evaluated encephalitis in the United States between 1998 and 2010, when an estimated 263,000 encephalitis-associated hospitalizations occurred (an average of >20,000 cases of encephalitis each year). Fatality was estimated at 15,000 deaths for the entire period (approximately 6% of patients). A specific cause of the encephalitis was identified in an estimated 50% of patients; for 20% of the entire study group, the cause was viral. An unspecified cause was recorded for 50% of patients.

Several studies have tried to characterize the frequency of infectious, autoimmune, and unknown causes of encephalitis (Table 90.1). In aggregate, these studies indicate that the ability to identify the cause of infectious and autoimmune encephalitis is improving because of advancing technology and the discovery of novel forms of encephalitis that are increasingly associated with biomarkers.

Overlap Between Viral and Autoimmune Encephalitis

In a study by the California Encephalitis Project, 761 patients had encephalitis from an uncertain cause. When a reference laboratory provided autoimmunity data for those patients, anti-NMDA receptor encephalitis was most common and was identified 4 times as frequently as encephalitis caused by HSV-1, West Nile virus, or varicella-zoster virus. Enterovirus was identified in 30 patients, HSV-1 in 7 patients, and varicella-zoster virus and West Nile virus in 5 patients each. For 32 patients, test results were positive for anti-NMDA receptor encephalitis. In that study, magnetic resonance imaging (MRI) was helpful for distinguishing HSV encephalitis from anti-NMDA receptor encephalitis; the typical localization associated with HSE was present in all patients, whereas only 14% of patients with anti-NMDA receptor encephalitis had imaging abnormality in the temporal lobe. Fever was not a distinguishing factor. Unlike viral encephalitis, most anti-NMDA receptor encephalitis (65%) occurred in patients younger than 18 years, and it occurred in more female patients than male patients. Psychoses and autonomic instability were also more common in anti-NMDA receptor encephalitis. Electroencephalographic and cerebrospinal fluid (CSF) findings were not distinctive.

Other studies have looked at imaging more thoroughly and compared HSV with autoimmune encephalitis. In those studies, MRI results were essentially always abnormal for patients with HSV but were abnormal for only 60% of patients with autoimmune encephalitis, and the findings were less regionally specific.

Viral Encephalitis

Agents causing viral encephalitis are arboviruses, herpesviruses, enteroviruses, human immunodeficiency virus (HIV), retrovirus, and miscellaneous viruses (eg, rabies virus) (Box 90.1). The principal arthropod-borne encephalitis viruses are the flaviviruses, bunyaviruses, and alphaviruses. Among herpesviruses, the most common is HSV-1. Occasionally, HSV type 2 (HSV-2) causes encephalitis. Others in this category include cytomegalovirus, varicella-zoster virus, Epstein-Barr virus, and human herpesvirus 6. Encephalitis can also be caused by enteroviruses, including coxsackievirus, echovirus, poliovirus, enterovirus D68, and enterovirus 71.

Herpes Simplex Encephalitis

HSV (mostly HSV-1) causes 10% of encephalitis cases in children and adults in the United States. HSE is the most common cause of an identifiable, sporadic form of viral encephalitis. Before antivirals were discovered for this disorder, 70% of patients died. With acyclovir treatment, mortality has decreased considerably, to 15%, but patients still have considerable morbidity (<20% can return to work).

HSE often starts with fever, subacute decline in cognitive function, personality changes, focal signs, and

Table 90.1 • Causes of Encephalitis

Source	Years of Study	Population	Cause: Infectious	Cause: Inflammatory/ Autoimmune	Cause: Unknown
Singh et al, 2015	2000-2012	Adults (N=198); USA	48%	22%	30%
Granerod et al, 2010	2005-2006	Children and adults (N=203); England	42% (TB included)	21%	37%
Mailles et al, 2009	2007	Children and adults (N=253); France	52% (TB and *Listeria* included)	Not determined	48%
Glaser et al, 2006	1998-2005	Children and adults (N=1,570); USA	16% (TB, bacterial, fungal, prion, and parasitic included)	8%	76%

Abbreviation: TB, tuberculosis; USA, United States of America.

Box 90.1 • Causes of Viral Encephalitis

- Arboviruses (arthropod borne)
  - Flaviviruses
    - St Louis encephalitis virus
    - West Nile virus
    - Zika virus
    - Japanese encephalitis virus
    - Powassan virus (tick borne)
    - European tick-borne encephalitis virus, Siberian tick-borne encephalitis virus, and Far Eastern tick-borne encephalitis virus
  - Bunyaviruses
    - La Crosse (California encephalitis) virus
  - Alphaviruses
    - Eastern equine encephalitis virus
    - Western equine encephalitis virus
    - Chikungunya virus
- Herpesviruses
  - Herpes simplex virus type 1 (occasionally type 2)
  - Cytomegalovirus
  - Varicella-zoster virus
  - Epstein-Barr virus
  - Human herpesvirus 6
- Enteroviruses
  - Poliovirus types 1, 2, and 3
  - Coxsackievirus group A (serotypes 2, 6, 7, and 9) and group B (serotypes 1-6)
  - Echovirus 6 and 9
  - Enterovirus 71
  - Enterovirus D68
- Others
  - HIV encephalitis
  - Rabies virus
  - JC virus (PML)

Abbreviations: HIV, human immunodeficiency virus; PML, progressive multifocal leukoencephalopathy.

seizures. Most people receive medical attention within 3 days after the onset of symptoms. HSV-1 has a strong predilection for the medial temporal lobes (limbic structures) and the inferior frontal lobes. In suspected cases, MRI of the brain is the most valuable test. It shows focal involvement with increased T2 signal involving the mesial temporal cortex and hippocampal structures, the inferior frontal and orbital frontal cortical areas, and the insular cortex (Figure 90.1). When findings are bilateral, they are typically asymmetric. MRI may show gadolinium enhancement. The thalamus is involved in 25% of patients.

In a study that compared HSE with similar diseases, bilateral, symmetric temporal lobe involvement suggested autoimmune forms of encephalitis, and lesions outside the temporal lobe, cingulate, or insula suggested non-HSE or an autoimmune cause. Contrast enhancement is not useful in discriminating the cause. Hemorrhage, although previously considered useful for identifying HSE, is infrequent and not specific for HSE.

Evaluation of HSE requires polymerase chain reaction (PCR) analysis of CSF to identify the virus. PCR is the most sensitive and specific test for HSE. Sensitivity, although originally thought to be 98%, may be as low as 80% with only 1 CSF sample. Therefore, when HSE is suspected from imaging findings, PCR should be performed on the CSF. CSF typically shows modest elevation of protein, lymphocytic pleocytosis, and a normal glucose level. Red blood cells are variably present in the CSF, and their presence does not distinguish HSE from similar diseases.

For patients with HSE, initiation of intravenous (IV) acyclovir is strongly associated with better outcomes. Thus, IV acyclovir should be started immediately when HSE is suspected. How quickly antiviral treatment influences PCR CSF results is unknown. A second CSF examination should be performed if PCR results are negative when HSE is suspected. Acyclovir dosing is 10 mg/kg IV every 8 hours for 14 to 21 days. Although trials were done with 14 days of therapy, expert opinion suggests that patients with severe forms of encephalitis or with profound neurologic deficits should be treated preferentially with IV acyclovir for 21 days. If patients have renal impairment, the acyclovir dose must be adjusted. The value of IV corticosteroid therapy in addition to acyclovir is unproven.

Spatially limited and nonnecrotizing HSE, confirmed with HSV PCR, may be associated with clinical symptoms previously thought to be too mild for HSE but now supporting the notion of a spectrum of clinical presentations. On the severe end of the spectrum, older age, worse Glasgow Coma Scale score, and delay in initiating acyclovir therapy are correlated with greater morbidity and mortality. Cognitive sequelae are common. In a study of relatively high-functioning HSE survivors, an additional 3-month course of oral valacyclovir did not provide additional benefit as measured with neuropsychological testing 12 months later.

HSE-Triggered Anti-NMDA Receptor Encephalitis

A relapsing form of encephalitis has been identified in patients who have had confirmed HSE that seems to relapse clinically but yields PCR results that are negative for HSV. Typically, these patients have psychiatric and behavioral symptoms or refractory status epilepticus with a mean latency of 30 days after the original episode of HSE. The relapse has been associated with the presence of anti-NMDA receptor antibodies in the CSF, suggesting an

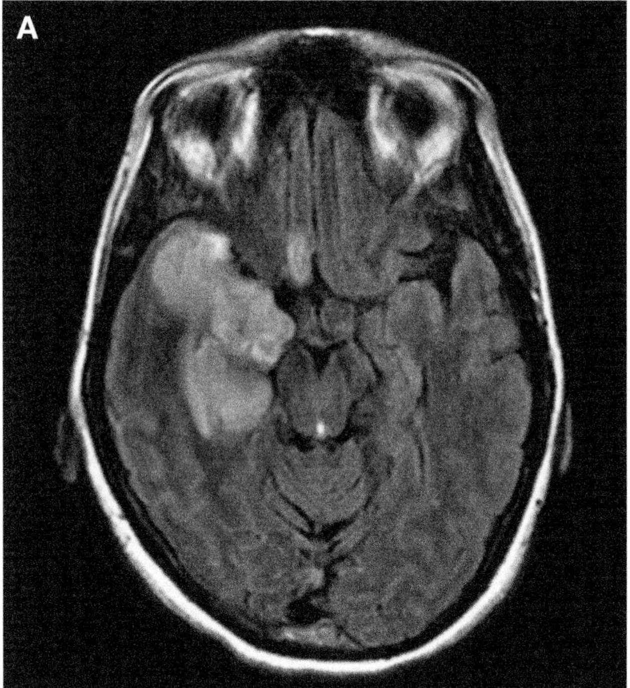

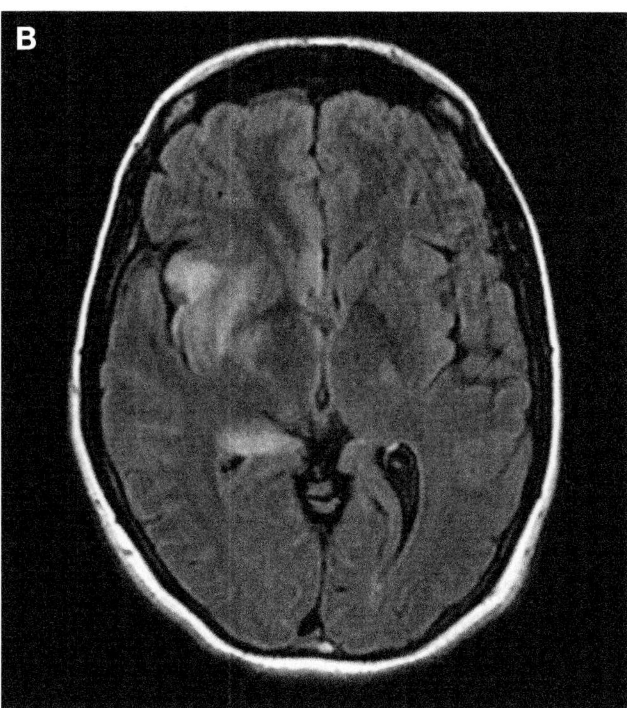

Figure 90.1. Magnetic Resonance Imaging of the Head in a Patient With Herpes Simplex Encephalitis (HSE). A and B, T2-weighted fluid-attenuated inversion recovery images from a patient with HSE show increased signal involving the right anterior and mesial temporal cortex, hippocampal area, inferior frontal anterior cingulate cortex, and insular cortex. These areas are typically involved in patients with HSE.

autoimmune injury to the nervous system after HSV infection. In most of these patients, MRI of the brain shows new areas of contrast enhancement and mass effect with swelling that responds to immunotherapy with high doses of corticosteroids.

Similarly, a relapse may occur in children, who are typically younger than 2 years. After an initial bout of HSE, they may have choreoathetosis and a decreased level of consciousness associated with anti-NMDA receptor antibodies in the CSF or with other neuronal autoantibodies. Treatment is with IV methylprednisolone, oral corticosteroids, IV immunoglobulin, or plasma exchange.

West Nile Virus

West Nile virus has become a common cause of encephalitis epidemics in the United States since its appearance in 1999. Its natural hosts are birds, and the usual route of transmission between bird hosts is through mosquitoes. Most people infected with West Nile virus are asymptomatic, but in 10% to 20%, fever, rash, or gastrointestinal tract symptoms develop without any neurologic syndrome. Serologic studies suggest that neurologic disease from neuroinvasion occurs in approximately 1 in 150 infected patients. Death from meningoencephalitis is most common in people older than 60 years. Immunosuppression may increase the potential for morbidity and mortality. Most commonly, patients with encephalitis have normal MRI findings, but occasionally MRI shows T2 hyperintensities in the brainstem in particular but also in the basal ganglia. Treatment is supportive.

Presenting symptoms of patients with neuroinvasion include fever, headache, nausea, vomiting, and stiff neck. When encephalitis occurs, it is often brainstem encephalitis, and a reduced level of consciousness occurs early in the course of the disease. Epidemics continue to occur in the United States, as they did with high incidences in 2002 and 2003 and again in 2012, with fewer cases in the intervening years. Neuroinvasive disease is reportable to the Centers for Disease Control and Prevention (CDC), which maintains an active US epidemiologic map during the mosquito season with recorded cases of both seropositive disease and neuroinvasive disease.

Encephalitis is the most common form of neuroinvasive disease. Next is meningitis and a rare form of acute anterior horn cell disease, now called acute flaccid myelitis, which is considered "the new polio" because it selectively infects the anterior horn cell, causing rapid, flaccid paralysis. It is distinct from Guillain-Barré syndrome. Older patients and immunosuppressed hosts are more vulnerable to neuroinvasive disease.

Up to 50% of patients with West Nile encephalitis have a high incidence of polymorphonuclear cell predominance in the CSF at presentation. The diagnostic test of choice for central nervous system infection is CSF immunoglobulin (Ig)M antibody. False-negative results for CSF IgM may occur if the CSF is collected within 8 days after the onset of symptoms; after 7 days, however, most patients have positive IgM in the CSF and by 14 days virtually all patients are seropositive. This means that CSF antibody results may be falsely negative at presentation. The patient's immune status also may influence these test results. PCR is available for West Nile virus, but the likelihood of detecting the virus is relatively low: Sensitivity is estimated to be about 55% within the first 5 days after neuroinvasion and only about 10% with blood samples. Specificity, though, is high.

No effective treatment exists for West Nile encephalitis. No vaccine is available for human use.

St Louis Encephalitis Virus

Before the emergence of West Nile virus in the United States, St Louis encephalitis virus was the country's most common cause of epidemic, mosquito-borne encephalitis. In 2002, 28 cases were reported from various states, particularly Texas. Many lulls in outbreaks of St Louis encephalitis have occurred between outbreaks, and concurrent outbreaks of St Louis encephalitis and West Nile disease have occurred in Arizona.

Serologic cross-reactivity between West Nile virus and St Louis encephalitis virus makes the distinction of these viral infections challenging. Confirmatory, neutralizing antibody testing in public health laboratories is required for distinguishing between these 2 flaviviruses.

Chikungunya Virus

Chikungunya virus is a reemerging, mosquito-borne alphavirus. Outbreaks have occurred in Africa, Asia, Europe, and on islands in the Indian and Pacific Oceans. In late 2013 the chikungunya virus was found in the Americas for the first time (on islands in the Caribbean). In 2014 the first locally acquired cases of chikungunya infection were reported in Florida. Those cases were thought to be the first instances of mosquitoes spreading the virus to nontravelers in the continental United States. Americans can be infected while traveling in the Caribbean, South America, and the Pacific Islands and bring the virus with them when they return.

Small studies on chikungunya-associated encephalitis have been published. The estimated case fatality rate in 1 study was 16%.

Enterovirus D68

In 2014 a nationwide outbreak of enterovirus D68 in the United States caused severe respiratory illness. From August 2014 to January 2015, the CDC and public health laboratories confirmed that at least 1,000 people in 49 states had respiratory illness caused by this virus.

Temporal association with acute flaccid myelitis was identified among children in several states, including Colorado, Missouri, and Illinois. The children tended to be younger than 15 years (mean age, 7 years). At least 75% of the patients had CSF pleocytosis. MRI showed increased signal in spinal cord gray matter, and pathology results showed anterior horn cell disease, but enterovirus D68 was not successfully isolated.

Table 90.2 • Testing CSF for Viral Encephalitis

Virus	Disease	CSF Test	Comment
West Nile virus	West Nile encephalitis	IgM	. . .
HSV type 1	Herpes simplex encephalitis	PCR	Sensitive (80%-90%) and specific
HSV type 2	Primary or recurrent meningitis; rarely encephalitis	PCR	Sensitive and specific in first 4 d
VZV	Meningoencephalitis	PCR	Confirmatory when used with CSF findings
Enterovirus	Meningoencephalitis and meningitis	PCR	Sensitive and specific
EBV	EBV encephalitis	PCR	Suggests viral invasion of CNS; false-positive results can occur
JC virus	Progressive multifocal leukoencephalopathy	PCR	Diagnostic but incompletely sensitive (70%-75%)
CMV	CMV ventriculitis	PCR	Sensitive and specific

Abbreviations: CMV, cytomegalovirus; CNS, central nervous system; CSF, cerebrospinal fluid; EBV, Epstein-Barr virus; HSV, herpes simplex virus; Ig, immunoglobulin; PCR, polymerase chain reaction; VZV, varicella-zoster virus.

Acute flaccid myelitis was also detected in California from 2012 to 2015. Enteroviruses were the most frequently detected pathogens in the nasopharynx, stool specimens, and serum samples, but no pathogens were isolated from the CSF. All the patients had acute flaccid paralysis associated with fever, and most also had respiratory or gastrointestinal tract illness.

Zika Virus

Zika virus, a flavivirus, was first isolated in 1948 in Africa. In 2007 human outbreaks were first detected in the Yap Islands in Micronesia; in 2013 outbreaks of Zika virus were associated with Guillain-Barré syndrome in French Polynesia. Infection spread to the Americas, initially to Brazil, associated with fetal congenital infection and microcephaly. Scattered among those congenital infection outbreaks in Brazil were cases of Zika virus–associated Guillain-Barré syndrome in adults first in Brazil, then Colombia, and finally the Caribbean. Outbreaks were well studied in Colombia in 2015 and in Puerto Rico in 2016.

The relationship between this mosquito-borne virus and encephalitis is yet to be clarified. Rare, isolated cases of encephalitis or myelitis, with virus isolated from the CSF, have been identified but are dwarfed by the number of patients with parainfectious Guillain-Barré syndrome and congenital Zika virus infection of the fetal brain with resulting postnatal microcephaly.

Zika virus is best detected serologically but cross-reactivity occurs between Zika virus and dengue virus, which is found where Zika virus is endemic. In the United States, cases of Zika virus infection have occurred in Florida and Texas, presumably from mosquito-borne infection. Its clinical spectrum and association with encephalitis have not yet been defined.

Testing CSF for Viral Encephalitis

The use of PCR on CSF to test for viruses has become commonplace, and PCR is the principal method for detecting recognizable viruses in the CSF. However, the sensitivity of the assays varies considerably depending on the agent involved (Table 90.2). The most important exception to the use of PCR for viral encephalitis is West Nile virus because identification of IgM antibodies against West Nile virus in the CSF is the diagnostic microbiologic test of choice. In other types of viral encephalitis, the presence or absence of viral DNA or RNA in CSF is identified with PCR techniques.

Both HSV-1 and HSV-2 are detectable with PCR. Distinguishing HSV-1 from HSV-2 requires the additional step of PCR amplification for genes specific to the individual viruses. Detection of HSV-1 in CSF is highly specific for HSE, and the sensitivity is 80% to 90%. HSV-2 testing is sensitive and specific for HSE in the first 4 days of infection. Varicella-zoster virus, another herpesvirus, is easily detectable in CSF with PCR but its sensitivity is less well defined. Epstein-Barr virus has been associated with encephalitis, and PCR is the diagnostic test for detecting it in the CSF. However, because Epstein-Barr virus can colonize B cells in immunosuppressed hosts without viral disease, PCR on CSF may yield false-positive results in patients without evident neuroinvasive virus.

Among the RNA viruses that cause meningoencephalitis and meningitis, enteroviruses are common agents. PCR of CSF has largely replaced culture of CSF as the best test for the enterovirus group. Because so many subtypes of enterovirus exist, PCR detection uses genes shared by the enterovirus group.

Cytomegalovirus is particularly associated with ventriculitis in patients who have AIDS or ascending polyradiculopathy. PCR is sensitive and specific for that virus, but, because of the rarity of the disease, its sensitivity has not been well defined.

JC virus, the cause of progressive multifocal leukoencephalopathy, is also detected with PCR of the CSF. With a positive result, the test is diagnostic, but the test is sensitive for only 70% to 75% of cases. Therefore, if PCR is negative, but progressive multifocal leukoencephalopathy is still suspected, follow-up testing can be beneficial.

A commercial CSF panel has been developed to identify multiple causes of viral encephalitis. The 16-target meningitis and encephalitis panel provides results for many viruses, including cytomegalovirus, enterovirus, Epstein-Barr virus, HSV-1, HSV-2, human herpesvirus 6, parechovirus, and varicella-zoster virus. Additionally, *Cryptococcus* and 6 bacteria are examined. The laboratory panel may be useful for detecting infection when meningitis or encephalitis is suspected.

Summary

- HSE is the most common identifiable cause of viral encephalitis and is treatable. Better outcomes depend on early treatment.
- HSE can be complicated by postinfectious anti-NMDA receptor encephalitis that is treatable.
- West Nile virus encephalitis is a common epidemic viral encephalitis in the United States that is diagnosed with IgM antibodies in the CSF, but treatment is supportive.
- New viruses that cause encephalitis, like chikungunya and Zika viruses, are likely to continue to emerge.
- Multiagent PCR studies of CSF to test for multiple infectious organisms are available and rapid.

SUGGESTED READING

Armangue T, Leypoldt F, Malaga I, Raspall-Chaure M, Marti I, Nichter C, et al. Herpes simplex virus encephalitis is a trigger of brain autoimmunity. Ann Neurol. 2014 Feb;75(2):317–23. Epub 2014 Feb 25.

Britton PN, Eastwood K, Paterson B, Durrheim DN, Dale RC, Cheng AC, et al; Australasian Society of Infectious Diseases (ASID); Australasian College of Emergency Medicine (ACEM); Australian and New Zealand Association of Neurologists (ANZAN); Public Health Association of Australia (PHAA). Consensus guidelines for the investigation and management of encephalitis in adults and children in Australia and New Zealand. Intern Med J. 2015 May;45(5):563–76.

Castillo P, Woodruff B, Caselli R, Vernino S, Lucchinetti C, Swanson J, et al. Steroid-responsive encephalopathy associated with autoimmune thyroiditis. Arch Neurol. 2006 Feb;63(2):197–202.

Chan BK, Wilson T, Fischer KF, Kriesel JD. Deep sequencing to identify the causes of viral encephalitis. PLoS One. 2014 Apr 3;9(4):e93993.

Chow FC, Glaser CA, Sheriff H, Xia D, Messenger S, Whitley R, et al. Use of clinical and neuroimaging characteristics to distinguish temporal lobe herpes simplex encephalitis from its mimics. Clin Infect Dis. 2015 May 1;60(9):1377–83. Epub 2015 Jan 30.

Cinque P, Cleator GM, Weber T, Monteyne P, Sindic CJ, van Loon AM. The role of laboratory investigation in the diagnosis and management of patients with suspected herpes simplex encephalitis: a consensus report: the EU concerted action on virus meningitis and encephalitis. J Neurol Neurosurg Psychiatry. 1996 Oct;61(4):339–45.

Gable MS, Sheriff H, Dalmau J, Tilley DH, Glaser CA. The frequency of autoimmune *N*-methyl-D-aspartate receptor encephalitis surpasses that of individual viral etiologies in young individuals enrolled in the California Encephalitis Project. Clin Infect Dis. 2012 Apr;54(7):899–904. Epub 2012 Jan 26.

Gerardin P, Couderc T, Bintner M, Tournebize P, Renouil M, Lemant J, et al; Encephalchik Study Group. Chikungunya virus-associated encephalitis: a cohort study on La Reunion Island, 2005–2009. Neurology. 2016 Jan 5;86(1):94–102. Epub 2015 Nov 25.

Glaser CA, Honarmand S, Anderson LJ, Schnurr DP, Forghani B, Cossen CK, et al. Beyond viruses: clinical profiles and etiologies associated with encephalitis. Clin Infect Dis. 2006 Dec 15;43(12):1565–77. Epub 2006 Nov 8.

Gnann JW Jr, Skoldenberg B, Hart J, Aurelius E, Schliamser S, Studahl M, et al; National Institute of Allergy and Infectious Diseases Collaborative Antiviral Study Group. Herpes simplex encephalitis: lack of clinical benefit of long-term valacyclovir therapy. Clin Infect Dis. 2015 Sep 1;61(5):683–91. Epub 2015 May 8. Erratum in: Clin Infect Dis. 2016 Feb 15;62(4):530.

Granerod J, Ambrose HE, Davies NW, Clewley JP, Walsh AL, Morgan D, et al; UK Health Protection Agency (HPA) Aetiology of Encephalitis Study Group. Causes of encephalitis and differences in their clinical presentations in England: a multicentre, population-based prospective study. Lancet Infect Dis. 2010 Dec;10(12):835–44. Epub 2010 Oct 15. Erratum in: Lancet Infect Dis. 2011 Feb;11(2):79.

Hawkes MA, Carabenciov ID, Wijdicks EFM, Rabinstein AA. Critical West Nile neuroinvasive disease. Neurocrit Care. 2018 Aug;29(1):47–53.

Hawkes MA, Carabenciov ID, Wijdicks EFM, Rabinstein AA. Outcomes in patients with severe West Nile neuroinvasive disease. Crit Care Med. 2018 Sep;46(9):e955–8.

Keating MR. Antiviral agents for non-human immunodeficiency virus infections. Mayo Clin Proc. 1999 Dec;74(12):1266–83.

Leber AL, Everhart K, Balada-Llasat JM, Cullison J, Daly J, Holt S, et al. Multicenter evaluation of biofire filmarray meningitis/encephalitis panel for detection of bacteria, viruses, and yeast in cerebrospinal fluid specimens. J Clin Microbiol. 2016 Sep;54(9):2251–61. Epub 2016 Jun 22.

Leypoldt F, Titulaer MJ, Aguilar E, Walther J, Bonstrup M, Havemeister S, et al. Herpes simplex virus-1 encephalitis can trigger anti-NMDA receptor encephalitis: case report. Neurology. 2013 Oct 29;81(18):1637–9. Epub 2013 Oct 2.

Lim HK, Seppanen M, Hautala T, Ciancanelli MJ, Itan Y, Lafaille FG, et al. TLR3 deficiency in herpes simplex encephalitis: high allelic heterogeneity and recurrence risk. Neurology. 2014 Nov 18;83(21):1888–97. Epub 2014 Oct 22.

Mailles A, Stahl JP; Steering Committee and Investigators Group. Infectious encephalitis in France in 2007: a national prospective study. Clin Infect Dis. 2009 Dec 15;49(12):1838–47.

Martinez-Torres F, Menon S, Pritsch M, Victor N, Jenetzky E, Jensen K, et al; GACHE Investigators. Protocol for German trial of acyclovir and corticosteroids in Herpes-simplex-virus-encephalitis (GACHE): a multicenter, multinational, randomized, double-blind, placebo-controlled German, Austrian and Dutch trial [ISRCTN45122933]. BMC Neurol. 2008 Oct 29;8:40.

Naccache SN, Peggs KS, Mattes FM, Phadke R, Garson JA, Grant P, et al. Diagnosis of neuroinvasive astrovirus infection in an immunocompromised adult with encephalitis by unbiased next-generation sequencing. Clin Infect Dis. 2015 Mar 15;60(6):919–23. Epub 2015 Jan 7.

Oyanguren B, Sanchez V, Gonzalez FJ, de Felipe A, Esteban L, Lopez-Sendon JL, et al. Limbic encephalitis: a clinical-radiological comparison between herpetic and autoimmune etiologies. Eur J Neurol. 2013 Dec;20(12):1566–70. Epub 2013 Aug 14.

Singh TD, Fugate JE, Rabinstein AA. The spectrum of acute encephalitis: causes, management, and predictors of outcome. Neurology. 2015 Jan 27;84(4):359–66. Epub 2014 Dec 24.

Skoldenberg B, Aurelius E, Hjalmarsson A, Sabri F, Forsgren M, Andersson B, et al. Incidence and pathogenesis of clinical relapse after herpes simplex encephalitis in adults. J Neurol. 2006 Feb;253(2):163–70. Epub 2005 Oct 17.

Skoldenberg B, Forsgren M, Alestig K, Bergstrom T, Burman L, Dahlqvist E, et al. Acyclovir versus vidarabine in herpes simplex encephalitis: randomised multicentre study in consecutive Swedish patients. Lancet. 1984 Sep 29;2(8405):707–11.

Stahl JP, Mailles A. Herpes simplex virus encephalitis update. Curr Opin Infect Dis. 2019 Mar 27. [Epub ahead of print]

Steiner I, Budka H, Chaudhuri A, Koskiniemi M, Sainio K, Salonen O, et al. Viral meningoencephalitis: a review of diagnostic methods and guidelines for management. Eur J Neurol. 2010 Aug;17(8):999–e57. Epub 2010 Mar 3.

Venkat H, Krow-Lucal E, Hennessey M, Jones J, Adams L, Fischer M, et al. Concurrent outbreaks of St Louis encephalitis virus and West Nile virus disease: Arizona, 2015. MMWR Morb Mortal Wkly Rep. 2015 Dec 11;64(48):1349–50.

Venkatesan A, Tunkel AR, Bloch KC, Lauring AS, Sejvar J, Bitnun A, et al; International Encephalitis Consortium. Case definitions, diagnostic algorithms, and priorities in encephalitis: consensus statement of the international encephalitis consortium. Clin Infect Dis. 2013 Oct;57(8):1114–28. Epub 2013 Jul 15.

Vora NM, Holman RC, Mehal JM, Steiner CA, Blanton J, Sejvar J. Burden of encephalitis-associated hospitalizations in the United States, 1998–2010. Neurology. 2014 Feb 4;82(5):443–51. Epub 2014 Jan 2.

Whitley RJ, Alford CA, Hirsch MS, Schooley RT, Luby JP, Aoki FY, et al. Vidarabine versus acyclovir therapy in herpes simplex encephalitis. N Engl J Med. 1986 Jan 16;314(3):144–9.

Whitley RJ, Kimberlin DW. Herpes simplex encephalitis: children and adolescents. Semin Pediatr Infect Dis. 2005 Jan;16(1):17–23.

Wilson MR, Naccache SN, Samayoa E, Biagtan M, Bashir H, Yu G, et al. Actionable diagnosis of neuroleptospirosis by next-generation sequencing. N Engl J Med. 2014 Jun 19;370(25):2408–17. Epub 2014 Jun 4.

Zhang SY, Jouanguy E, Ugolini S, Smahi A, Elain G, Romero P, et al. TLR3 deficiency in patients with herpes simplex encephalitis. Science. 2007 Sep 14;317(5844):1522–7.

91 Acute Bacterial Meningitis

EELCO F. M. WIJDICKS, MD, PhD

Goals

- Recognize the clinical features of acute bacterial meningitis.
- Discuss the priorities for managing bacterial meningitis to optimize outcomes.
- Identify prognostic indicators of severe meningitis.

Introduction

Meningitis, an infection of the meninges and subarachnoid space, is a syndrome involving the cortex and vasculature that leads to vasculitis and secondary infarctions. The cerebral venous system is involved in severe cases. Acute bacterial meningitis usually results from community-acquired infections, but when it occurs in hospitalized patients (ie, *nosocomial* bacterial meningitis), it is usually due to invasive procedures. In the United States, acute bacterial meningitis is caused mostly by *Streptococcus pneumoniae; Neisseria meningitidis* is a far less common cause because of aggressive vaccination programs. Pneumococcal meningitis occurs more frequently in young children and the elderly, but pneumococcal vaccines have decreased its prevalence. Pneumococcal meningitis is also more common in patients who have a poor nutritional state or alcoholism (or both). Factors that increase the risk of community-acquired meningitis include the immunocompromised state, human immunodeficiency virus infections, asplenia, and genetic factors such as complement factor deficiencies. In most adults with acute bacterial meningitis, a normal state of health is first interrupted by an upper respiratory tract infection or an ear infection that does not improve with antibiotic therapy. The potential source for acute bacterial meningitis, such as pneumonia, paranasal sinusitis, or middle ear infection, should be sought.

Pathophysiology

At autopsy, the only evidence of bacterial meningitis may be purulent meningitis with pus and yellow and green deposits on the leptomeninges. Generally, the pus follows the distribution of the meningeal blood vessels. Microscopic features are neutrophils (Figure 91.1) and fibrin in the subarachnoid space with macrophages. Arteritis is recognized as one of the most important secondary complications leading to ischemic strokes and a worse outcome. *Fulminant meningitis*, defined as meningitis with rapid-onset coma, may occur with cerebral edema and little exudate, but there have been no systematic pathology studies of adult bacterial meningitis.

Usually the infection starts with mucosal colonization in the nasopharynx, and meningeal invasion occurs only after bacteremia disrupts the blood–cerebrospinal fluid (CSF) barrier. The host defenses in the CSF are marginal, and bacteria easily multiply. Leukocyte infiltration into the brain parenchyma may also involve the arteries, causing luminal narrowing, cerebral hypoperfusion, and infarction.

In patients with acute bacterial meningitis, increased intracranial pressure can result from multiple mechanisms. Occasionally it results from acute hydrocephalus and hemorrhagic infarctions associated with cerebral venous thrombosis, but usually it results from diffuse cerebral edema (Figure 91.2). High mortality among patients with bacterial meningitis can result from diffuse cerebral edema, but more commonly it results from septic shock. Management of septic shock is equally important in reducing mortality.

Clinical Presentation

The clinical features of acute bacterial meningitis have a recognizable pattern, which often includes a history of myalgias, ear pain, sore throat, joint stiffness, and fatigue occurring several days before major clinical deterioration.

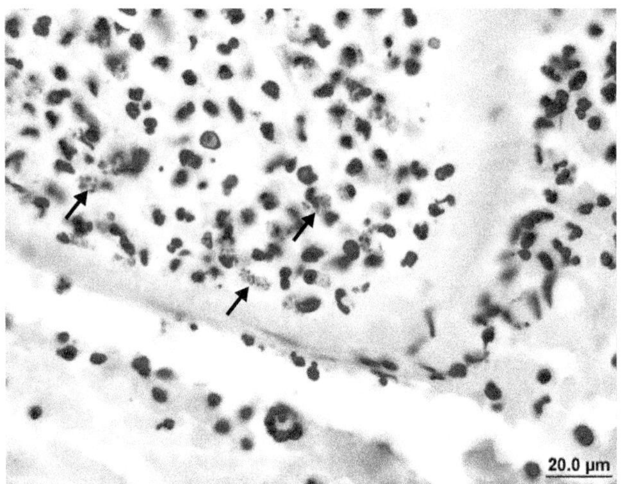

Figure 91.1. Inflammatory Response in Meningitis. Arrows indicate neutrophils (Gram stain).

Fever and vomiting are the most constant early signs, present in more than three-fourths of the patients, without much variation between age groups. Headache, often described as "bursting" and "splitting," is severe enough that most commonly prescribed medications do not relieve it. Altered consciousness is characteristic but may vary from delirium to drowsiness and stupor. Acute agitation in a febrile elderly patient should always prompt consideration of acute bacterial meningitis, and symptoms should not be assumed to have resulted from a trivial pneumonia or urinary tract infection. More than 75% of patients with bacterial meningitis are confused, irritable, or stuporous. Most patients can be roused with a forcible command or painful stimulus. The degree of fever in bacterial meningitis may vary, but the temperature is usually constantly elevated.

Patients with meningeal irritation present with neck stiffness and Brudzinski and Kernig signs. A Brudzinski sign is present when neck flexion results in flexion of the knees and hips (a hand is used to prevent the patient from rising) (Figure 91.3A). The Kernig sign is present when flexion of the neck or passive extension of the knees with the hips flexed at 90° results in pain, opening of the eyes, a verbal response, and occasionally combative behavior (Figure 91.3B). Kernig and Brudzinski signs have high specificity but poor sensitivity for bacterial meningitis.

In the early stages of bacterial meningitis, papilledema is unusual, but it may occur with an evolving sagittal sinus thrombosis or progressive brain edema. Papilledema is most often present with fulminant bacterial meningitis in a comatose patient.

At initial presentation, focal neurologic findings are uncommon (eg, aphasia, hemiparesis, or cranial nerve palsies). Cranial nerves are generally not affected in patients with acute bacterial meningitis, but if they are (most commonly the oculomotor nerves), tuberculosis, syphilis, or carcinomatous meningitis should be considered. Cranial nerve involvement may include abducens nerve palsy as a false localizing sign of increased intracranial pressure or facial nerve palsy associated with mastoiditis.

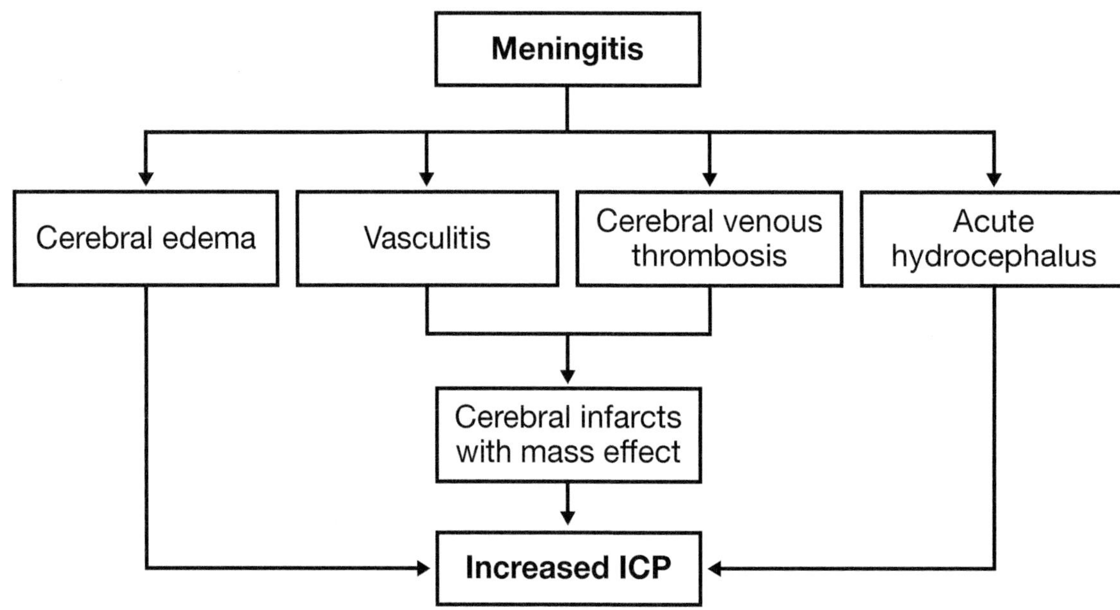

Figure 91.2. Pathophysiology of Bacterial Meningitis. Various mechanisms can result in increased intracranial pressure (ICP).

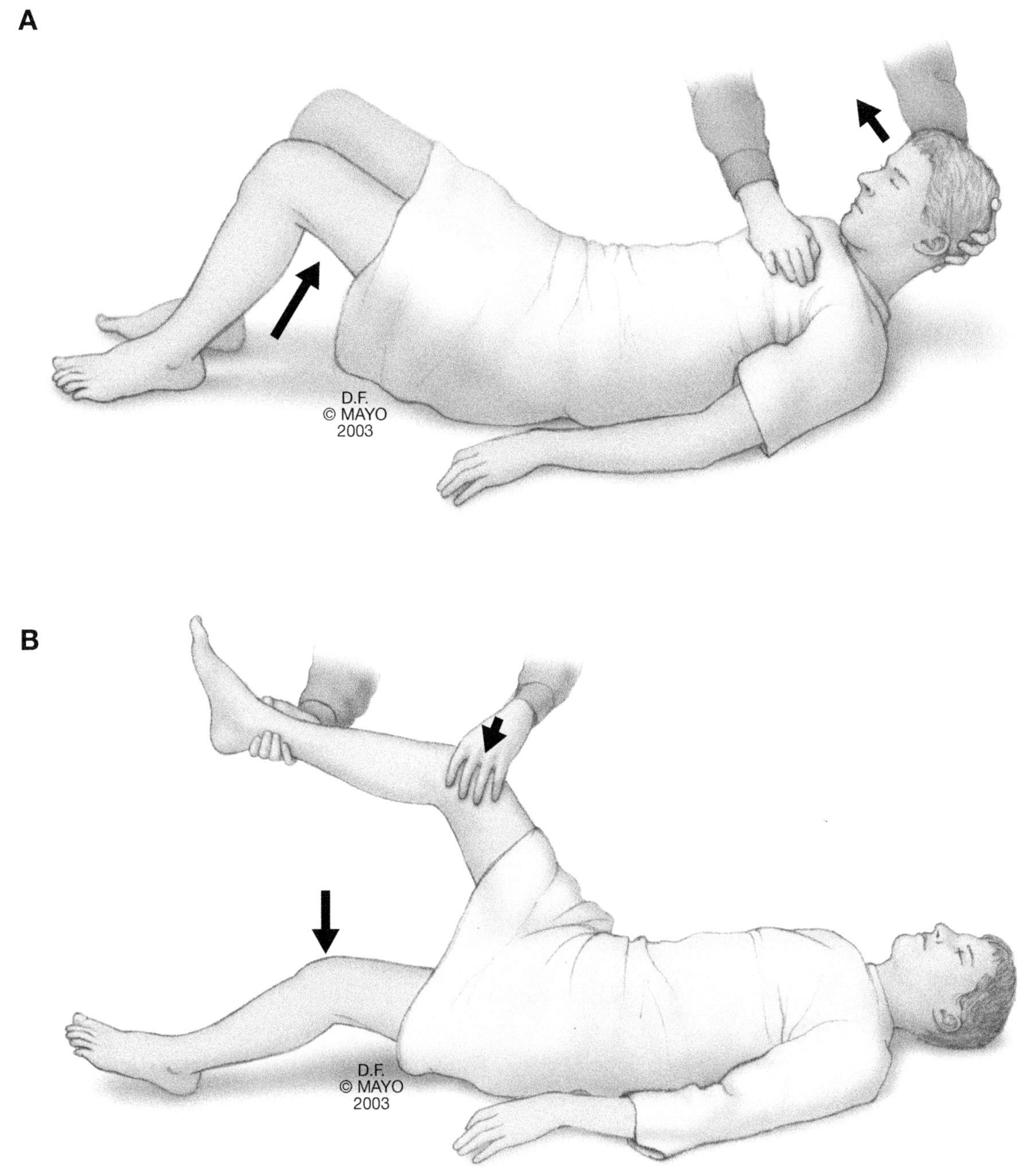

Figure 91.3. *Signs of Meningitis. A, Brudzinski sign. B, Kernig sign.*
(A and B from Wijdicks EFM. Catastrophic neurologic disorders in the emergency department. 2nd ed. Oxford [United Kingdom]: Oxford University Press; c2004. Chapter 8, Altered arousal and coma; p. 53-93; used with permission of Mayo Foundation for Medical Education and Research.)

Seizures may occur in up to 15% of adults. Seizures, particularly focal seizures, can be attributed to focal edema, early cortical venous thrombosis, and cerebral infarction from occlusion of penetrating branches encased by the basal purulent exudate. Focal or generalized tonic-clonic seizures should prompt consideration of extension of bacterial meningitis to the parenchyma. Persistent generalized or focal seizures may also occur in patients with subdural empyema, a disorder associated with sinusitis or mastoiditis that strongly resembles acute bacterial meningitis but may be reliably documented only with magnetic resonance imaging.

Rapidly developing coma with pathologic motor responses is uncommon in adults, but its presence signals a fulminant variant with diffuse cerebral edema or multiple cerebral infarcts from secondary inflammatory vasculitis. Increased intracranial pressure occurs in approximately 10% of patients. Rarely, meningeal veins become necrotic or thrombosed, a condition leading to extensive hemorrhagic cortical infarction and bihemispheric swelling. Transverse sinus thrombosis is a possible consequence of bacterial meningitis in patients with mastoiditis, and the clot may propagate to the sagittal sinus.

Septic shock arises more frequently in meningitis from *N meningitidis* or *Staphylococcus aureus*, but it can be caused by any severe bacterial meningitis. Meningococcal meningitis may progress to shock from adrenal hemorrhage. Petechiae, widespread purpuric rash with patches of necrotic skin, conjunctival hemorrhage, and punctate lesions inside the mouth and on the lips occur with shock, profound hyponatremia and hyperkalemia (Addison disease), and laboratory evidence of intravascular coagulation.

Rashes are not specific for any cause, nor is there any characteristic distribution. Petechiae and erythematous rashes may occur with Rocky Mountain spotted fever, West Nile fever, and echovirus 9 infection. A maculopapular rash, however, may suggest acute bacterial meningitis caused by *S pneumoniae* or *S aureus*. A limited petechial rash may occur with *S aureus* meningitis, *N meningitidis* meningitis, or any viral meningitis.

Diagnostic Investigations

CSF examination is important for diagnosis, but it is not essential for initial management. Delayed recognition of bacterial meningitis and management with antibiotics is a common problem that has been identified as a top health concern in bacterial meningitis guidelines. Any patient with suspected bacterial meningitis should have blood drawn for cultures, receive antibiotics and corticosteroids, and undergo computed tomography (CT) and, eventually, CSF examination. Blood cultures can be positive for two-thirds of patients, but sensitivity may be lower if patients have previously received antibiotics. The CSF glucose concentration, which is normally 70% of the serum glucose value, may be normal or decreased (ie, <50% of the serum glucose value) in acute bacterial meningitis. (The CSF glucose to serum glucose ratio may be less useful if patients have had a recent infusion of glucose-containing fluids; 2 hours are required for equilibration.) Protein values are usually more than 100 mg/dL and may be less useful for discriminating between viral meningitis and bacterial meningitis.

Contraindications for CSF examination include a preexisting bleeding disorder resulting from sepsis or clear evidence of diffuse cerebral edema on CT. CSF examination typically shows pleocytosis with polymorphic leukocytes, low glucose concentration, low CSF glucose to blood glucose ratio, and increased protein levels. The CSF lactate level is higher in bacterial meningitis than in viral meningitis. Gram stain may indicate the cause of meningitis: CSF Gram staining for bacteria has a yield of up to 90% in pneumococcal meningitis and meningococcal meningitis, and the sensitivity is not substantially influenced by previous antibiotic exposure. Low CSF leukocyte counts (eg, <500 cells/mcL) are associated with meningitis-related intracranial complications and worse outcomes.

Polymerase chain reaction has been used increasingly for diagnosis of bacterial meningitis, with reported sensitivity of 79% to 100% for *S pneumoniae* meningitis and 91% to 100% for *N meningitidis* meningitis.

Management

Initial management consists primarily of emergent antibiotic therapy, usually ceftriaxone in combination with vancomycin (Table 91.1). Vancomycin is necessary to cover for *Staphylococcus* and penicillin-resistant *Streptococcus* until susceptibility test results are available. For *Listeria monocytogenes*, which is common in adults older than 50 years, alcoholics, and immunosuppressed patients, treatment should include ampicillin empirically.

Several studies have shown that the early use of corticosteroids with dexamethasone has improved outcomes. Current guidelines recommend administering dexamethasone with antibiotic treatment, but a 4-hour delay is acceptable. For adults, the dexamethasone dose is 10 mg intravenously every 6 hours for 4 days.

Seizures can be focal or generalized tonic-clonic seizures. Nonconvulsive status epilepticus occasionally complicates bacterial meningitis, but it is recognized only with prolonged electroencephalographic recordings. Seizure management is the same as for seizures from a different cause.

The development of hemodynamic compromise requires treatment with adequate fluid replacement and with vasopressors to maintain adequate mean arterial blood pressure. Norepinephrine should be started early in sepsis, and a second vasopressor, usually vasopressin, should be added to treat hypotension adequately. Phenylephrine is not an optimal drug because it has only α-adrenergic action, which may decrease cardiac output and subsequently impair tissue blood flow. There is no evidence that corticosteroids improve outcomes for patients who have sepsis, and standard guidelines for sepsis management should be followed.

Patients with bacterial meningitis have a high fatality rate, particularly if cerebral edema is present on CT. In some patients, CT shows cortical and sylvian fissure effacement, compression of ventricles, and, eventually, obliteration of basal cisterns. It is unclear whether placement of intracranial pressure monitors and the subsequent use of osmotic therapy (20% mannitol or hypertonic saline) affect outcomes, but for comatose patients with early cerebral edema, this is a common approach. Hypertonic saline may also control the

Table 91.1 • Antibiotics for Presumed Bacterial Meningitis

Demographic or Risk Factor	Bacterial Pathogens	Empirical Therapy
Community-acquired infection Age >50 y	*Streptococcus pneumoniae* *Neisseria meningitidis* *Listeria monocytogenes* Aerobic gram-negative bacilli	Vancomycin *and* ampicillin *and* a third-generation cephalosporin (either cefotaxime or ceftriaxone)
Immunocompromised state	*S pneumoniae* *N meningitidis* *L monocytogenes* *Staphylococcus aureus* *Salmonella* species Aerobic gram-negative bacilli (including *Pseudomonas aeruginosa*)	Vancomycin *and* ampicillin *and* either cefepime or meropenem

Abbreviation: HIV, human immunodeficiency virus.

Modified from van de Beek D, Brouwer MC, Thwaites GE, Tunkel AR. Advances in treatment of bacterial meningitis. Lancet. 2012 Nov 10;380(9854):1693-702; used with permission.

commonly observed hyponatremia. In other patients, serial CT shows worsening hydrocephalus, and a ventriculostomy can then be used for monitoring intracranial pressure.

Outcome

Prediction of outcome for patients with severe meningitis is aided considerably by the use of the Full Outline of Unresponsiveness (FOUR) score, which provides a better evaluation of the brainstem reflexes and respiration status. In 1 study, no patients with bacterial meningitis survived if their FOUR score was less than 5. Mortality among patients with streptococcal meningitis ranges from 20% to 30% in Western countries to 50% in developing countries. Patients with bacterial meningitis commonly have neurologic sequelae, including hearing loss, epilepsy, and cognitive impairment. However, patients with fulminant meningitis and even patients with early cerebral edema, may improve with aggressive antibiotic and supportive treatment.

Summary

- Acute bacterial meningitis is a neurocritical illness that may become critical illness due to sepsis.
- For all patients, blood cultures and empirical intravenous antibiotics should be started and CT performed before CSF examination.
- A fulminant variant of meningitis occurs with diffuse cerebral edema or multiple cerebral infarcts from secondary inflammatory vasculitis.
- Many patients have a good outcome if the diagnosis and treatment are early.

SUGGESTED READING

Adriani KS, Brouwer MC, van der Ende A, van de Beek D. Bacterial meningitis in adults after splenectomy and hyposplenic states. Mayo Clin Proc. 2013 Jun;88(6):571–8. Epub 2013 Apr 28.

Griffiths MJ, McGill F, Solomon T. Management of acute meningitis. Clin Med (Lond). 2018 Mar;18(2):164–9.

Kastenbauer S, Pfister HW. Pneumococcal meningitis in adults: spectrum of complications and prognostic factors in a series of 87 cases. Brain. 2003 May;126(Pt 5):1015–25.

van de Beek D, Brouwer M, Hasbun R, Koedel U, Whitney CG, Wijdicks E. Community-acquired bacterial meningitis. Nat Rev Dis Primers. 2016 Nov 3;2:16074.

van Ettekoven CN, Brouwer MC, Bijlsma MW, Wijdicks EFM, van de Beek D. The FOUR score as predictor of outcome in adults with bacterial meningitis. Neurology. In Press

van Ettekoven CN, van de Beek D, Brouwer MC. Update on community-acquired bacterial meningitis: guidance and challenges. Clin Microbiol Infect. 2017 Sep;23(9):601–6. Epub 2017 May 3.

Wall EC, Ajdukiewicz KM, Bergman H, Heyderman RS, Garner P. Osmotic therapies added to antibiotics for acute bacterial meningitis. Cochrane Database Syst Rev. 2018 Feb 6;2:CD008806.

Brain Abscess and Spinal Epidural Abscess

SELBY G. CHEN, MD

Goals

- Describe the most common clinical manifestations and causes of brain abscesses and spinal epidural abscesses.
- Identify adequate antibiotic therapy for brain abscesses and spinal epidural abscesses.
- Recognize the indications for surgical treatment of brain abscesses and spinal epidural abscesses.

Introduction

Two infections of the brain are relatively common. Patients with brain abscess are often critically ill and have a high mortality rate. The reported incidence of brain abscesses ranges from 0.4 to 0.9 per 100,000 people. In contrast, spinal epidural abscess (SEA), an infection of the epidural space, has increased in incidence from approximately 0.2 to 1.2 per 10,000 hospital admissions in the mid-1970s to a currently estimated 2.0 to 12.5 per 10,000 admissions. The higher incidence most likely reflects an aging population, increased use of spinal instrumentation, and increased use of intravenous drugs. Both disorders are now more easily detected with magnetic resonance imaging (MRI), and this has improved early management, but clinical recognition is still a challenge for many physicians.

Brain Abscess

Infectious Agents

Immunosuppression is often a predisposing factor in brain abscess, whether it is related to viral infection (eg, human immunodeficiency virus [HIV]) or immunosuppressive medications (eg, in posttransplant patients) (Table 92.1).

Posttransplant patients receiving long-term immunosuppression often have tuberculous or fungal infections, whereas postsurgical patients often have infections caused by skin-colonizing bacteria (eg, *Staphylococcus aureus* or *Staphylococcus epidermidis*) or gram-negative bacilli.

Infection may spread directly from contiguous sources (eg, sinusitis, mastoiditis, or surgical site infection) or hematogenously from systemic sources (eg, endocarditis). Contiguous sources account for approximately half of all brain abscesses, hematogenous spread accounts for one-third, and unknown sources account for the rest. Contiguous sources often involve streptococcal species, but staphylococcal and polymicrobial infections occur frequently as well.

Clinical Presentation

The specific presenting signs and symptoms of patients with brain abscess depend primarily on the location of the abscess itself, although most often patients present with headache as a result of increased intracranial pressure. Frontal or temporal abscesses may lead to personality changes. Posterior fossa abscesses may lead to ataxia, cranial nerve dysfunction, or signs of obstructive hydrocephalus, such as increased lethargy.

Diagnosis

Noncontrast computed tomography (CT) of the head is a quick and effective screening tool when a patient presents with concerns related to intracranial pathology. When an abscess is suspected, contrast-enhanced CT can be performed to better delineate the mass, or contrast-enhanced MRI with diffusion-weighted and apparent diffusion coefficient images may be used instead. Peripheral enhancement with perilesional edema is a characteristic finding. Restricted diffusion helps in differentiating an abscess from other lesions, such as necrotic glial tumors or metastases (Figure 92.1). For detection of brain abscesses, diffusion-weighted imaging has 96% sensitivity and specificity (positive predictive value, 98%; negative predictive value, 92%).

Table 92.1 • Predisposing Conditions and Microbial Isolates in Patients With Brain Abscess

Predisposing Condition	Common Microbial Isolates
Immunocompromise	
HIV infection	*Toxoplasma gondii* *Nocardia* species and *Mycobacterium* species *Listeria monocytogenes* *Cryptococcus neoformans*
Neutropenia	Aerobic gram-negative bacilli *Aspergillus* species Mucorales *Candida* species and *Scedosporium* species
Transplant	*Aspergillus* species and *Candida* species Mucorales *Scedosporium* species Enterobacteriaceae[a] *Nocardia* species *T gondii* *Mycobacterium tuberculosis*
Contiguous spread of bacteria	
Penetrating trauma or neurosurgery	*Staphylococcus aureus* *Staphylococcus epidermidis* *Streptococcus* species (anaerobic and aerobic) Enterobacteriaceae[a] *Clostridium* species
Otitis media or mastoiditis	*Streptococcus* species (anaerobic and aerobic) *Bacteroides* species and *Prevotella* species Enterobacteriaceae[a]
Paranasal sinusitis	*Streptococcus* species (anaerobic and aerobic) *Bacteroides* species Enterobacteriaceae[a] *S aureus* *Haemophilus* species
Hematogenous spread of bacteria	
Lung abscess, empyema, bronchiectasis	*Fusobacterium* *Actinomyces* *Bacteroides* *Prevotella* *Nocardia* *Streptococcus* species
Bacterial endocarditis	*S aureus* *Streptococcus* species
Congenital heart disease	*Streptococcus* species *Haemophilus* species
Dental infection	Mixed infection with *Fusobacterium, Prevotella, Actinomyces, Bacteroides,* and *Streptococcus* species (anaerobic and aerobic)

Abbreviation: HIV, human immunodeficiency virus.

[a] The Enterobacteriaceae family includes *Escherichia coli, Enterobacter, Klebsiella, Proteus,* and *Salmonella.*

From Brouwer MC, Tunkel AR, McKhann GM 2nd, van de Beek D. Brain abscess. N Engl J Med. 2014 Jul 31;371(5):447-56; used with permission.

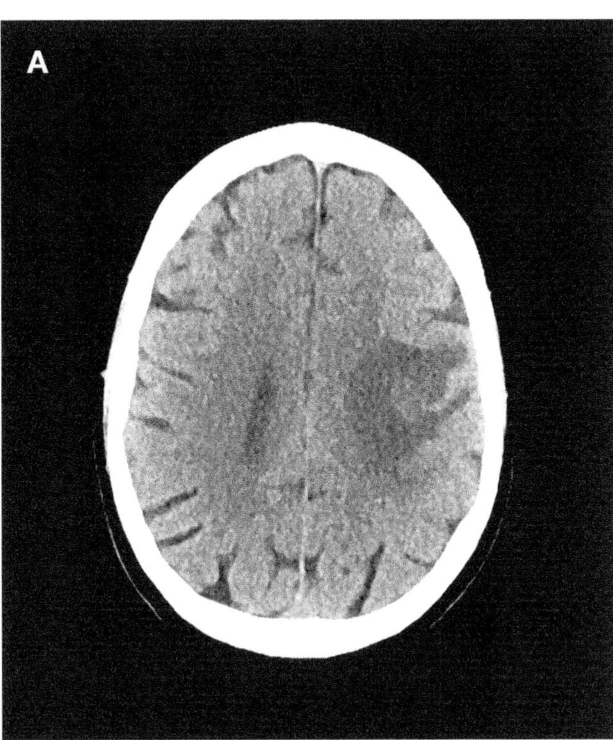

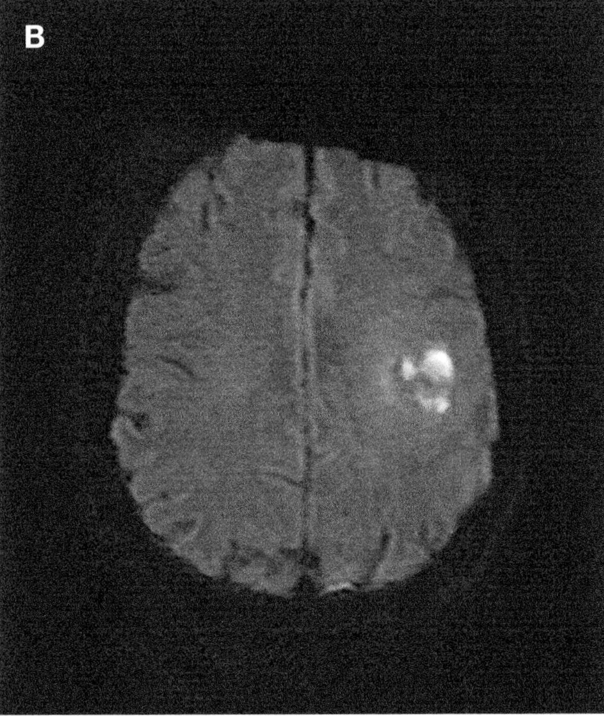

Figure 92.1. Nocardia *Brain Abscess. A, Computed tomographic scan. B, Magnetic resonance image. Diffusion-weighted imaging shows increased restriction.*

With blood cultures and cerebrospinal fluid cultures, the specific microbe can be identified in approximately 25% of cases. However, the benefits of a lumbar puncture should be weighed against the risks of downward herniation, especially because the diagnostic yield is lower if patients do not have signs or symptoms of meningitis. Aspiration of the abscess itself is the gold standard for diagnosis.

Management

Neurosurgical

Neurosurgical intervention is often warranted for both diagnostic and therapeutic purposes. Stereotactic aspiration of the abscess itself is needed to identify the infectious pathogen if other diagnostic measures have not been useful (eg, if results are negative from blood cultures or for serum markers such as anti-*Toxoplasma* immunoglobulin [Ig]G antibodies). If a specific pathogen has been identified, indications for stereotactic drainage depend on the size of the abscess and the patient's signs and symptoms. Large lesions with a mass effect resulting in symptomatic brain compression merit surgical drainage. Some have proposed 2.5 cm as a threshold for operative intervention, but this is not a universally accepted standard. In patients with multiple brain abscesses, the largest abscess should be aspirated for diagnostic purposes. If an abscess is abutting but has not yet ruptured into the ventricles, drainage may prevent rupture and resultant ventriculitis.

Stereotactic MRI, or stereotactic CT merged with MRI, should be performed for preoperative planning. A target point should be set within the center of the abscess, and a path should be selected that avoids traversing through eloquent brain, sulci, or the ventricular system. Aspirated samples should be evaluated with Gram stain and aerobic and anaerobic cultures as a standard part of any infectious workup. If patients are immunocompromised, smears and cultures should be evaluated for mycobacteria, *Nocardia* species, and fungi; polymerase chain reaction (PCR) assay should be performed for *Toxoplasma gondii*. If culture results are negative, PCR-based 16S ribosomal DNA sequencing may provide a definitive diagnosis.

Medical

Antimicrobial therapy should be initiated as soon as specimens have been obtained for bacterial analysis. Usually broad-spectrum antibiotic therapy is begun to cover gram-positive, gram-negative, and anaerobic microbes. Antifungals, such as voriconazole, can be added if fungal infection may be involved (depending on the patient's risk factors). Empirical therapy can be tailored to the patient's predisposing conditions. Transplant patients should receive treatment with a third-generation cephalosporin (ceftriaxone or cefotaxime) *and* metronidazole, trimethoprim-sulfamethoxazole *or* trimethoprim-sulfadiazine to cover for *Nocardia*, and voriconazole to cover for fungal species (Table 92.2). HIV-infected patients with anti-*Toxoplasma* IgG antibodies should also receive agents targeting *Toxoplasma* (pyrimethamine and sulfadiazine). For patients who have known risk factors for tuberculosis, appropriate treatment may include antitubercular medications (isoniazid, rifampin, pyrazinamide, and ethambutol). Postneurosurgical patients often receive vancomycin, cefepime, and metronidazole. Patients with contiguous spread from a nearby area of infection are usually treated with ceftriaxone or cefotaxime in combination with metronidazole.

When the infectious agent has been identified, antimicrobial susceptibilities should be determined and antibiotic therapy tailored accordingly (Table 92.2). If blood cultures show only 1 microbe, broad-spectrum antibiotics are advised until the results of the abscess culture are finalized because 27% of brain abscesses are polymicrobial. Glucocorticoid therapy is often used to decrease perilesional edema. However, glucocorticoids should be used judiciously because they may decrease the passage of antimicrobial agents into the brain.

Traditionally, the duration of intravenous antimicrobial therapy in patients with bacterial brain abscess has been 6 to 8 weeks. Serial MRI is often performed biweekly for up to 3 months until clinical recovery is evident. One follow-up MRI 6 to 12 weeks after completion of antibiotic therapy is standard.

Prognosis

The prognosis for patients with a cerebral abscess has improved dramatically. Today the fatality rate is approximately 10%, whereas 50 years ago, it was 40%. Additionally, 70% of patients make a good recovery with minimal or no neurologic sequelae. The better prognosis reflects improved imaging techniques, use of minimally invasive neurosurgical techniques, and better antimicrobial protocols.

Spinal Epidural Abscess

Infectious Agents

The most common SEA pathogens in blood or tissue cultures are methicillin-sensitive *S aureus* (38.9%) and methicillin-resistant *S aureus* (19.9%) (Table 92.3). Antibiotic management should be tailored to the specific antimicrobial susceptibilities.

Clinical Presentation

Historically, the thoracic spine was the most common site of SEA (50% of patients), the lumbar region (35%) was the second most common (35%), and the cervical spine was the third (15%). Now, however, probably because more lumbar instrumented fusions are performed, the lumbar

Table 92.2 • Antimicrobial Therapy for Patients With Brain Abscess

Type of Treatment	Therapy
Empirical	
Standard	Cefotaxime or ceftriaxone *and* metronidazole; alternatively, meropenem (add vancomycin if infecting pathogen may be *Staphylococcus aureus*, pending organism identification and in vitro susceptibility testing)
For transplant recipients	Cefotaxime or ceftriaxone *and* metronidazole, voriconazole, and trimethoprim-sulfamethoxazole *or* trimethoprim-sulfadiazine
For patients with human immunodeficiency virus infection	Cefotaxime or ceftriaxone *and* metronidazole, pyrimethamine, and sulfadiazine; consider isoniazid, rifampin, pyrazinamide, and ethambutol to cover possible tuberculosis infection
Based on isolated pathogen	
Bacteria	
Actinomyces species	Penicillin G
Bacteroides fragilis	Metronidazole
Enterobacteriaceae	Cefotaxime or ceftriaxone
Fusobacterium species	Metronidazole
Haemophilus species	Cefotaxime or ceftriaxone
Listeria monocytogenes	Ampicillin or penicillin G
Mycobacterium tuberculosis	Isoniazid, rifampin, pyrazinamide, and ethambutol
Nocardia species	Trimethoprim-sulfamethoxazole *or* trimethoprim-sulfadiazine
Prevotella melaninogenica	Metronidazole
Pseudomonas aeruginosa	Ceftazidime or cefepime
Methicillin-sensitive *S aureus*	Nafcillin or oxacillin
Methicillin-resistant *S aureus*	Vancomycin
Streptococcus anginosus group and other streptococcal species	Penicillin G
Fungi	
Aspergillus species	Voriconazole
Candida species	Amphotericin B preparation
Cryptococcus neoformans	Amphotericin B preparation
Mucorales	Amphotericin B preparation
Scedosporium apiospermum	Voriconazole
Protozoa	
Toxoplasma gondii	Pyrimethamine *and* sulfadiazine

From Brouwer MC, Tunkel AR, McKhann GM 2nd, van de Beek D. Brain abscess. N Engl J Med. 2014 Jul 31;371(5):447-56; used with permission.

Table 92.3 • Spinal Epidural Abscess Pathogens

Pathogen	Patients, %
Methicillin-sensitive *Staphylococcus aureus*	39
Methicillin-resistant *S aureus*	20
Gram-negative bacteria	8
Coagulase-negative *Staphylococcus*	7
Streptococcus species	7
Polymicrobial infection	5
None	14

From Arko L 4th, Quach E, Nguyen V, Chang D, Sukul V, Kim BS. Medical and surgical management of spinal epidural abscess: a systematic review. Neurosurg Focus. 2014 Aug;37(2):E4; used with permission.

spine is the most common site (48%), the thoracic spine is second (31%), and the cervical spine is third (24%).

The average age of patients with SEA reported in the literature ranges from 45 to 65 years, with a slight preponderance among men. Patients presenting with SEA often have predisposing conditions, including chronic conditions, such as diabetes mellitus (27% of SEA patients), hepatic disease (14%), renal failure (12%), and cardiac dysfunction (12%). Other prevalent risk factors are intravenous drug use (22% of SEA patients), alcoholism (13%), and trauma (12%), including spinal surgery. Cardiac valve vegetations must be considered because nearly 30% of all spinal infections arising from hematogenous spread are associated with bacterial endocarditis.

The most common presenting symptom is severe back pain with tenderness on palpation. Radicular symptoms can be present from nerve root irritation or compression. Neurologic findings include bowel or bladder dysfunction, sensory abnormalities, and focal weakness, progressing to paraplegia or quadriplegia if the cervical spine is involved. Patients may also have signs of meningitis (neck stiffness or photosensitivity). Systemic symptoms, such as fevers, chills, and night sweats, are often present.

Diagnosis

If SEA is suspected, the diagnostic test of choice is contrast-enhanced MRI. Osteomyelitis and diskitis are common associated findings. T1-weighted imaging shows a hypointense or isointense epidural mass. T2-weighted images show a hyperintense mass. Contrast enhancement is often present, although the pattern may be homogeneous, heterogeneous, or rim enhancing (Figure 92.2). In the early stages of abscess formation, enhancement may not be apparent if granulation tissue has not yet formed.

Laboratory findings are consistent with an acute infection: increased white blood cell count (although it may be normal with a chronic infection), increased erythrocyte sedimentation rate (ESR), and increased C-reactive protein (CRP) level. For vertebral osteomyelitis, reported specificity is 98% for CRP and 100% for ESR. Blood cultures should be used to assess for bacteremia and to identify the pathogenic organism when possible. When blood culture results are negative, tissue biopsy is needed to identify the infectious organism. In patients with diskitis or osteomyelitis, a CT-guided biopsy can be performed. For an epidural abscess without bony or soft tissue infection, a needle biopsy is often difficult and possibly dangerous; open surgical biopsy is preferred. Tissue should be collected for aerobic, anaerobic, fungal, and acid-fast bacilli cultures. If the patient is hemodynamically stable, antibiotics should be withheld until culture results are available because the yield decreases from 80% to 48% after antibiotic therapy has been initiated.

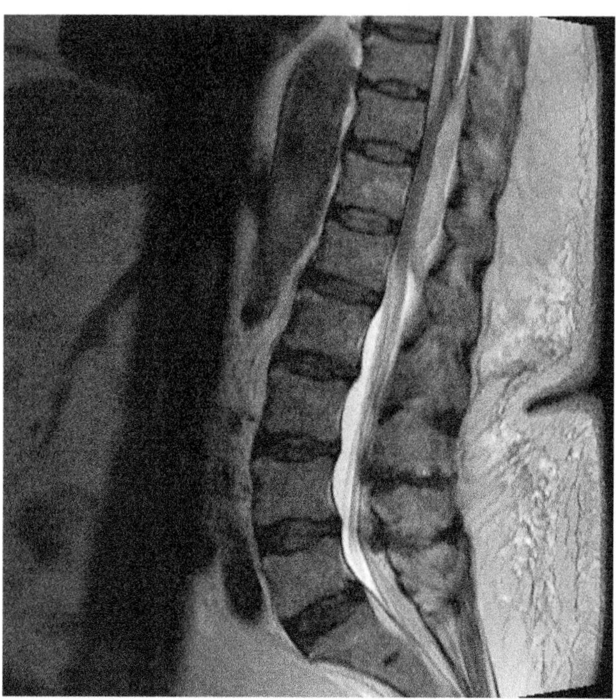

Figure 92.2. Spinal Epidural Abscess. Sagittal thoracic magnetic resonance image shows pockets of pus.

Management

Earlier detection of SEA with MRI has led to a shift away from early surgical intervention because patients often present without any neurologic deficits, and successful outcomes have resulted with nonoperative medical treatment alone. Medical management is indicated when a patient does not have neurologic deficits. Surgical treatment (ie, decompression and abscess evacuation) is mandated when a patient has weakness due to neural compression. If a patient has substantial canal compromise without neurologic deficits, the risk of deterioration is high and surgery can be considered. Many authors have advocated more aggressive surgical management of cervical and thoracic epidural abscesses, because the spinal canal has less room at these levels, and small increases in the size of the abscess can lead to precipitous deterioration in neurologic status.

One literature review found that current practices include medical management for 40% of patients with SEA (compared with 12.7% historically) and that most studies found no significant difference in clinical outcome between medical and surgical treatment cohorts. However, 1 study did find that medical treatment failed in 49% of patients, who then required surgical treatment. Risk factors for needing surgical management included diabetes mellitus, CRP level greater than 115 mg/L, leukocytosis (white blood cells $>12\times10^9$/L), positive blood culture results, age older than 65 years, methicillin-resistant *S aureus*, and advanced neurologic deficit.

The specifics of surgical management depend on the surgical goals. If diagnosis is the only goal, CT-guided biopsy of the adjacent disk or vertebra may be sufficient because spinal epidural abscesses often involve surrounding structures. If decompression is the primary objective, often a laminectomy without fusion will suffice. However, if the infection crosses the cervicothoracic or thoracolumbar junction, a laminectomy alone may result in instability, and instrumented fusion is indicated. Additionally, if corpectomy is needed to adequately decompress the spinal canal anteriorly, fusion is needed for stabilization. Corpectomies often require a strut graft. Autograft is the preferred bone graft of choice, but long strut grafts have often led to long-term pain at the donor site. Allografts are considered acceptable. Use of titanium cages has gained favor and has had a low rate of chronic infection or rejection. Anterior decompressions are usually supplemented with a posterior instrumented fusion for added stability.

Prognosis

Regardless of whether surgery is part of the clinical management, use of appropriate antibiotic treatment for several weeks is the mainstay of therapy. Multiple studies have shown that antibiotic treatment for at least 4 weeks affords a cure rate of 88% to 91%. Therefore, if the diagnosis is made early in the disease process, the prognosis is good.

Summary

- A brain abscess can mimic a brain tumor.
- With MRI, a glioma can be reliably distinguished from an infection.
- SEA is commonly misdiagnosed because patients may present with sepsis syndrome.
- Antibiotic treatment is the first course of action, but surgical débridement is needed in some patients.

SUGGESTED READING

Al Masalma M, Armougom F, Scheld WM, Dufour H, Roche PH, Drancourt M, et al. The expansion of the microbiological spectrum of brain abscesses with use of multiple 16S ribosomal DNA sequencing. Clin Infect Dis. 2009 May 1;48(9):1169–78.

Arko L 4th, Quach E, Nguyen V, Chang D, Sukul V, Kim BS. Medical and surgical management of spinal epidural abscess: a systematic review. Neurosurg Focus. 2014 Aug;37(2):E4.

Bodilsen J, Brouwer MC, Nielsen H, Van De Beek D. Anti-infective treatment of brain abscess. Expert Rev Anti Infect Ther. 2018 Jul;16(7):565–78. Epub 2018 Jul 5.

Brouwer MC, Tunkel AR, McKhann GM 2nd, van de Beek D. Brain abscess. N Engl J Med. 2014b Jul 31;371(5):447–56.

Brouwer MC, van de Beek D. Management of bacterial central nervous system infections. Handb Clin Neurol. 2017;140:349–64.

Cornett CA, Vincent SA, Crow J, Hewlett A. Bacterial spine infections in adults: evaluation and management. J Am Acad Orthop Surg. 2016 Jan;24(1):11–8.

Curry WT Jr, Hoh BL, Amin-Hanjani S, Eskandar EN. Spinal epidural abscess: clinical presentation, management, and outcome. Surg Neurol. 2005 Apr;63(4):364–71.

Kim SD, Melikian R, Ju KL, Zurakowski D, Wood KB, Bono CM, et al. Independent predictors of failure of nonoperative management of spinal epidural abscesses. Spine J. 2014 Aug 1;14(8):1673–9. Epub 2013 Oct 30.

Liu J, Bai R, Li Y, Staedtke V, Zhang S, van Zijl PCM, et al. MRI detection of bacterial brain abscesses and monitoring of antibiotic treatment using bacCEST. Magn Reson Med. 2018 Aug;80(2):662–71. Epub 2018 Mar 25.

Mamelak AN, Mampalam TJ, Obana WG, Rosenblum ML. Improved management of multiple brain abscesses: a combined surgical and medical approach. Neurosurgery. 1995 Jan;36(1):76–85.

Patel AR, Alton TB, Bransford RJ, Lee MJ, Bellabarba CB, Chapman JR. Spinal epidural abscesses: risk factors, medical versus surgical management, a retrospective review of 128 cases. Spine J. 2014 Feb 1;14(2):326–30. Epub 2013 Nov 12.

Reddy JS, Mishra AM, Behari S, Husain M, Gupta V, Rastogi M, et al. The role of diffusion-weighted imaging in the differential diagnosis of intracranial cystic mass lesions: a report of 147 lesions. Surg Neurol. 2006 Sep;66(3):246–50.

Acute Neuromuscular Disorders

93 Myasthenia Gravis

MAXIMILIANO A. HAWKES, MD; EELCO F. M. WIJDICKS, MD, PhD

Goals

- Introduce general concepts about myasthenia gravis.
- Define myasthenic crisis.
- Discuss the criteria for admission of patients with myasthenia gravis to the intensive care unit.
- Review the initial triage, work-up, and treatment of myasthenia gravis in the intensive care unit.

Introduction

Myasthenia gravis (MG) is a well-characterized B-cell–mediated disease caused by autoantibodies against targets located in the postsynaptic end plate of the neuromuscular junction. Fluctuating weakness and fatigability are clinical hallmarks of this disease. MG can be divided into subgroups based on the age at onset, serum antibodies, and thymic tumor, and different clinical courses can be anticipated with each.

This chapter describes general concepts about MG, focusing on the triage, work-up, and management of severe myasthenic exacerbation (crisis).

Pathophysiology

As a consequence of the nerve action potential, calcium influx to the nerve terminal triggers the release of acetylcholine (ACh) into the synaptic cleft. ACh binds to postsynaptic receptors (AChR), and this binding causes sodium channels to open, muscle depolarization, and subsequent muscle contraction.

The muscle-specific tyrosine kinase (MuSK) and its coreceptor, the low-density lipoprotein receptor-related protein 4 (LRP4), are activated by agrin, which is also secreted by the nerve terminal. The interaction of MuSK-LRP4-agrin results in clustering of AChR and conformational change of the neuromuscular junction. When antibodies react against any of these targets, the neuromuscular transmission is affected, and the fluctuating weakness and fatigability of MG result.

The rapid diffusion of ACh out of the synaptic cleft and its inactivation by the enzyme acetylcholinesterase terminate the effect of nerve depolarization. This enzyme is a therapeutic target, given that its pharmacologic inhibition increases the levels of ACh in the synaptic fissure.

Epidemiology

MG affects 4 to 12 persons per 1 million per year and has an estimated prevalence of 150 to 250 cases per 1 million in the general population. Except for a subset of early-onset MG, known as juvenile MG, which predominates in Asia, there is little geographic variation. AChR-associated MG subtype affects about 80% of patients and has a bimodal incidence in the fourth and sixth decades of life. Seronegative (5%), MuSK-associated (4%), and LRP4-associated (2%) MG follow in frequency.

The discovery of new antibodies, widespread antibody testing, and the decrease in mortality due to better recognition and treatment of exacerbations and crisis explain the increasing prevalence of MG in recent reports.

Classification

MG can be divided into several variants on the basis of age at symptom onset, target molecule of antibodies, thymic status, and clinical phenotype.

AChR Antibodies–Associated MG

- Early onset.
  - Onset of symptoms before age 50 y.
  - Female preponderance (3:1).
  - Frequently associated with thymic follicular hyperplasia.
  - Good response to thymectomy.
- Late onset.
  - Onset of symptoms after age 50 y.
  - Slight male preponderance.
  - Low incidence of thymic hyperplasia.
  - Poor response to thymectomy.

Thymoma-Associated MG

- Almost all patients have AChR antibodies and generalized disease.
- Thymoma is found in 10%-15% of patients. (MG will develop in about 30% of patients with a thymoma.)

MuSK-Associated MG

- Negative for AChR antibodies.
- Predominates in adults.
- Neither thymic abnormality nor response to thymectomy.
- Prominent cranial and bulbar muscle involvement and ventilatory insufficiency.

LRP4-Associated MG

- Female preponderance.
- Associated with ocular or mild generalized forms.

Antibody-Negative Generalized MG

- Heterogeneous group with no clear distinctive features.
- Low-affinity antibodies not detectable in routine assays are present in 20%-50% of patients.

Ocular MG

- Among patients with MG, 20% have this form.
- Restricted ocular muscle involvement.
- Only 10% of patients who have restricted ocular weakness for 2 years will have development of generalized weakness.
- AChR antibodies are found in 50% of patients.

Clinical Presentation

The hallmark of MG is fatigable weakness. Symptoms fluctuate during the day depending on physical activity and typically worsen in the evening.

Around 60% of patients initially present with ptosis or diplopia (or both). The compromise of external eye muscles is usually asymmetric, whereas limb weakness is symmetric and mostly proximal.

When the ventilatory muscles are affected, the most feared complication is respiratory failure. The weakness of bulbar muscles compromises upper airway patency and clearance of secretions. The need for positive pressure ventilation, invasive or not, defines the myasthenic crisis. Crises are more common within the first few years after disease onset and are usually precluded by gradual exacerbation of symptoms. Before the availability of effective immunosuppressive treatments, up to 30% of patients experienced a crisis within 2 years after symptom onset. Less frequently, crises are the first event leading to the diagnosis of the disease. Common triggers for myasthenic crises are infections (especially pneumonia), surgery, and discontinuation of MG medications. Some medications can interfere with neuromuscular transmission and potentially trigger myasthenic crises (Box 93.1). Of note, these associations are based on anecdotal reports, case reports, or in vitro studies, and their clinical relevance is largely undetermined. In 30% of myasthenic crises, a trigger cannot be identified, and this lack of association may be related to the fluctuating character of the disease.

Increasing doses of pyridostigmine, usually prescribed to improve the worsening symptoms, can produce cholinergic hyperactivity. Remarkably, cholinergic crises are rare in the absence of underlying myasthenic crisis.

Although AChR, MuSK, and LRP4 antibodies do not cross-react with the heart muscle, cardiac function can be affected in patients with MG. Thus, monitoring of heart function is recommended during severe MG exacerbations and crisis.

Diagnosis

Most patients admitted to the intensive care unit (ICU) with a myasthenic crisis have a prior known diagnosis of MG. Patients admitted because of neuromuscular respiratory failure of unknown cause will especially benefit from a detailed anamnesis, physical examination, and complementary neurophysiologic studies.

Anamnesis

Questions should inquire about fluctuating weakness, fatigability, ptosis, diplopia, head drop, voice changes, and dysphagia. Worsening of symptoms with high temperatures and at the end of the day are also important clues.

Patients with a known diagnosis of MG should be asked about compliance with MG medications, ingestion of new drugs (prescribed or over-the-counter), recent infections, and recently increased doses of pyridostigmine. Symptoms of cholinergic overactivity should also be investigated.

Box 93.1 • Drugs to Avoid or Use With Caution in Patients with MG

- Telithromycin: antibiotic for community-acquired pneumonia. The FDA has designated a black box warning for this drug in MG. Should not be used in MG
- Fluoroquinolones (eg, ciprofloxacin, moxifloxacin, and levofloxacin): commonly prescribed broad-spectrum antibiotics that are associated with worsening MG. The FDA has designated a black box warning for these agents in MG. Use cautiously, if at all
- Botulinum toxin: avoid
- D-Penicillamine: used for Wilson disease and rarely for rheumatoid arthritis. Strongly associated with causing MG. Avoid
- Quinine: occasionally used for leg cramps. Use prohibited except in malaria in US
- Magnesium: potentially dangerous if given intravenously (ie, for eclampsia during late pregnancy or for hypomagnesemia). Use only if absolutely necessary and observe for worsening
- Macrolide antibiotics (eg, erythromycin, azithromycin, clarithromycin): commonly prescribed antibiotics for gram-positive bacterial infections. May worsen MG. Use cautiously, if at all
- Aminoglycoside antibiotics (eg, gentamicin, neomycin, tobramycin): used for gram-negative bacterial infections. May worsen MG. Use cautiously if no alternative treatment available
- Corticosteroids: a standard treatment for MG, but may cause transient worsening within the first 2 weeks. Monitor carefully for this possibility
- Procainamide: used for irregular heart rhythm. May worsen MG. Use with caution
- Desferoxamine: chelating agent used for hemochromatosis. May worsen MG
- β-Blockers: commonly prescribed for hypertension, heart disease, and migraine but potentially dangerous in MG. May worsen MG. Use cautiously
- Statins (eg, atorvastatin, pravastatin, rosuvastatin, simvastatin): used to reduce serum cholesterol. May worsen or precipitate MG. Use cautiously if indicated and at lowest dose needed
- Iodinated radiologic contrast agents: older reports document increased MG weakness, but modern contrast agents appear safer. Use cautiously and observe for worsening

Abbreviations: MG, myasthenia gravis; US, United States; FDA, US Food and Drug Administration.

From Mehrizi M, Fontem RF, Gearhart TR, Pascuzzi RM. Medications and myasthenia gravis (a reference for health care professionals) [Internet]. New York (NY): Myasthenia Gravis Foundation of America [cited 2018 Sep 20]; used with permission.

Physical Examination

Fluctuating weakness and signs of cholinergic excess must be carefully examined. Signs of impending respiratory failure and inability to protect the airway must be particularly investigated. MuSK-associated MG usually shows a heightened sensitivity to cholinergic effects.

Specific findings are as follows:

- Muscular weakness, especially of neck flexors and proximal limbs.
  - Arm outstretched at 90° for 90 seconds.
  - Head lift 45° supine for 120 seconds.
  - Legs outstretched supine at 45° for 10 seconds.
- Bulbar muscles dysfunction: drooling, nasal voice, choking, and frequent, although ineffective, cough.
- Fatigability of ocular and bulbar muscles.
  - Sustained upgaze for 60 seconds to look for development of ptosis (Figure 93.1).
  - Extraocular muscle movements after prolonged and forced eye closure.
  - Ability to maintain a tongue depressor between posterior teeth after a prolonged bite.
  - Dysarthria during or after counting from 1 to 50.
- The ice test evaluates for relief of eyelid ptosis after applying ice over a closed eye. Its sensitivity and specificity are 0.94 and 0.97 for ocular myasthenia and 0.82 and 0.96 for generalized myasthenia.
- Central atrophy of the tongue has been described in anti-MuSK myasthenia gravis.
- Signs of respiratory failure are forehead sweating, staccato speech, inability to count aloud from 1 to 20 after a single maximal breath, and abdominal paradox.
- Signs of cholinergic overactivity are diarrhea, abdominal cramps, urinary incontinence, miosis, bradycardia, emesis, lacrimation, increased oral and bronchial secretions, and, rarely, muscle fasciculations.

Ancillary Tests

Serologic and electrophysiologic studies are necessary only when the diagnosis of MG is uncertain. Cases in which the history and physical examination are highly suggestive of MG can be confirmed with serologic testing. However, in the ICU, electrophysiologic tests are faster to obtain and particularly useful when antibodies are negative. Decremental response to repetitive nerve stimulation is characteristic of MG. Increased jitter on single-fiber electromyography is more sensitive, but testing for this finding may be difficult in the ICU. A therapeutic trial with a short-acting ACh inhibitor such as edrophonium is another rapid method to diagnose MG and to differentiate it from Lambert-Eaton myasthenic syndrome. Currently, it is

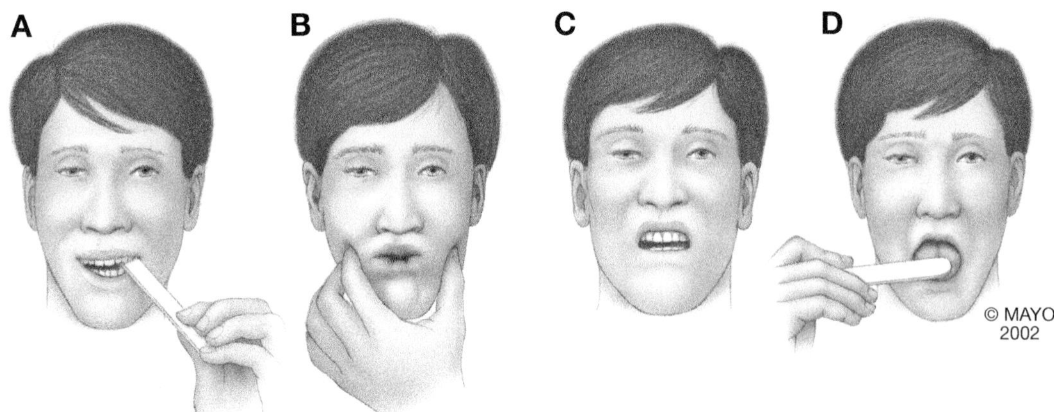

Figure 93.1. Clinical Examination of Pertinent Features in Myasthenia Gravis. A, Biting on tongue depressor to test for masseter weakness. B, Puffing out cheeks and resisting pressure from examiner's fingers. C, Ptosis and typical snarl of bifacial weakness. D, Pushing away tongue depressor with tongue to test force.

(From Wijdicks EFM. The clinical practice of critical care neurology. 2nd ed. Oxford [UK]: Oxford University Press; c2003. Chapter 26, Myasthenia gravis; p. 422–36; used with permission of Mayo Foundation for Medical Education and Research.)

not commonly used given the widespread availability of electrophysiologic tests.

Patients with a new diagnosis of MG, especially early-onset AChR-associated MG, should be studied with computed tomography or magnetic resonance imaging of the chest to exclude thymoma. Contrast agent administration is necessary to optimize the sensitivity of these imaging studies. Yet, several reports have found an association between iodine and myasthenic crisis. Even more rarely, myasthenia exacerbation has also been reported after gadolinium administration. For this reason, it is reasonable to avoid contrast agent administration in patients with unstable myasthenia.

Myasthenic exacerbations with bulbar and respiratory compromise should be studied with chest radiography to detect early complications such as aspiration pneumonia or atelectasis. Arterial blood gas tests are also useful, but results must be carefully interpreted within the clinical context (see Chapter 15, "Neuromuscular Respiratory Failure").

Pulmonary function tests may be useful to monitor progression of weakness in patients with myasthenic crisis. However, clear cutoff values have not been clearly established, probably because the fluctuating nature of weakness results in unpredictable measurements with serial spirometry.

Initial Triage and Management

Myasthenic exacerbations and crisis treatment are treated with immunomodulation. The 2 available therapeutic options are plasma exchange (PLEX) and intravenous immunoglobulin (IVIg). These interventions are not immediately effective; typically, the onset of the response is not until 2 to 5 days from the initiation of therapy. Thus, early intensive care with respiratory support and prevention and treatment of complications are critical. Patients with bulbar weakness must have a formal swallowing evaluation, and a nasogastric tube should be placed if there are concerns for aspiration.

In this regard, patients who need ICU levels of care should be rapidly identified (Figure 93.2). This approach has decreased the mortality rate of myasthenic crisis from 50% to less than 5%.

All patients with severe weakness and respiratory distress or bulbar compromise with a high risk of aspiration should be admitted to the ICU. Early initiation of noninvasive ventilation can prevent intubation in almost 50% of patients. Avoiding invasive ventilation decreases pulmonary complications and length of ICU and hospital stays. If oral secretions can be managed with proper oral suctioning and local anticholinergics, even patients with severe oropharyngeal weakness can tolerate noninvasive ventilation. The management of patients with MG being treated with noninvasive ventilation must be nuanced. The dose of pyridostigmine may need to be carefully reduced when there are clear signs of cholinergic excess, but use of the medication should not be stopped. Initiating or increasing the dose of corticosteroids should be done cautiously because one-third to one-half of patients will experience considerable worsening of weakness within a few days of these interventions. Therapy with PLEX or IVIg must be initiated as soon as possible.

Severe hypoxemia and abundant secretions are indications for invasive ventilation. Also, patients with profound hypercapnia and atelectasis should be considered

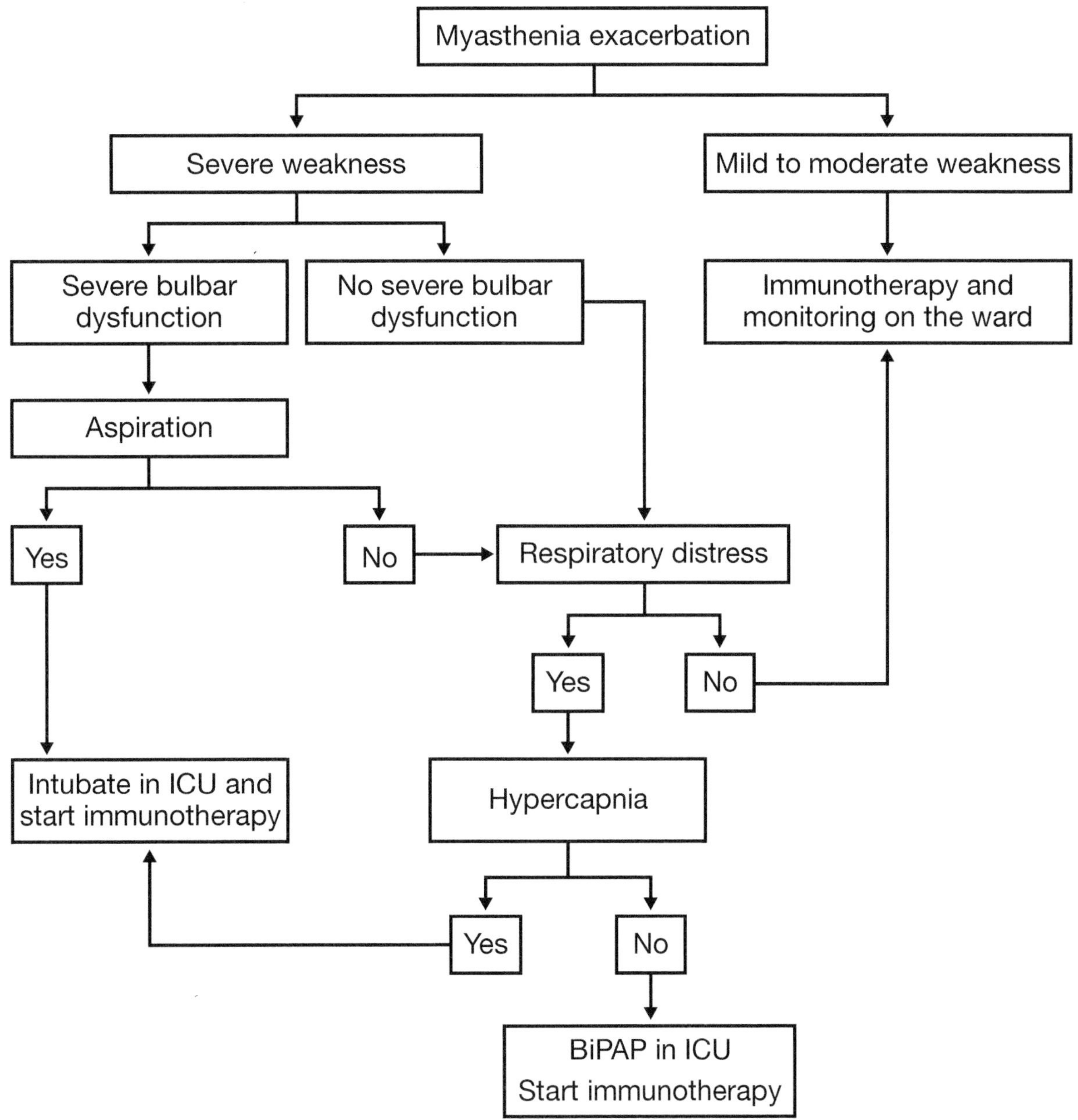

Figure 93.2. Algorithm for Triage and Management of Myasthenic Crisis. BiPAP indicates bilevel positive airway pressure; ICU, intensive care unit.

(From Rabinstein AA. Practical management of Guillain-Barré syndrome and myasthenic crisis. In: Manno EM, editor. Emergency management in neurocritical care. Chichester [United Kingdom]: Wiley-Blackwell; c2012. p. 141–51. [Neurology in practice series]; used with permission.)

candidates for intubation because both conditions predict failure to a trial of noninvasive ventilation. Once a patient is intubated, high-dose corticosteroids can be given and use of anticholinergics discontinued without concerns for further deterioration. Regardless of whether a patient is managed with noninvasive or invasive ventilation, therapy with PLEX or IVIg must be initiated as soon as possible.

Pharmacologic Treatment

The ideal pharmacologic treatment of myasthenic exacerbations and crisis is the combination of immunomodulatory, immunosuppressive, and acetylcholinesterase enzyme inhibitor agents. Immunomodulatory options, IVIg and PLEX, are equally effective for accelerating recovery in myasthenic exacerbations. Because patients with myasthenic crises were underrepresented in clinical trials, data about the effectiveness of IVIg and PLEX for decreasing the duration of invasive ventilation are lacking, and their use in this setting is mostly based on clinical experience. There are no data supporting that the combination of both treatments is superior to either alone. Nonetheless, using a second alternative should be considered in patients not responding to the first choice. The selection of the treatment should be tailored to a patient's characteristics, adverse effects profile, availability, and experience of the center. IVIg is easy to administer and it has been associated with lower admission costs. However, PLEX might have a faster effect and may be more effective in patients with MuSK-associated MG. Box 93.2 lists the adverse effect profile of both treatments.

In the context of a surgery, either IVIg or PLEX can be used preoperatively in patients with MG who have respiratory or bulbar weakness.

High-dose corticosteroids can be added when patients are not improving. Even though their optimal route of administration and dose are not well established, prednisone 1 mg/kg of ideal body weight is usually prescribed. Given their retarded onset of action, corticosteroid-sparing immunosuppressive drugs (azathioprine, mycophenolate, and cyclophosphamide) should be given or maximized early during the admission to ensure long-term stability.

Rituximab, an anti-CD20 B-lymphocyte–receptor monoclonal antibody, may be a valuable option in patients with MuSK antibodies. In fact, recent data show that it is effective in more than 80% of patients with refractory MG regardless of the antibody subtype. The onset of actions is slower than that of other immunomodulatory agents, but its effect can last for 6 to 12 months.

Acetylcholinesterase inhibitors are used for symptomatic relief. Doses vary greatly depending on individual response, previous use, and cholinergic adverse effects. Oral pyridostigmine is most commonly prescribed. It can be administered through a nasogastric tube in patients with severe dysphagia. Intravenous neostigmine is a useful option for patients with gastrointestinal diseases that prevent the use of the enteral route. Edrophonium is a short-acting agent, useful only for diagnostic purposes. Glycopyrrolate or hyoscyamine can be safely administered when patients have excessive oral and respiratory secretions. Loperamide should be considered in patients with profuse diarrhea. Long-term treatment may include prednisone and thymectomy both for thymoma and nonthymomatous disease; 2 recent clinical trials found benefit at 3 to 5 years.

Box 93.2 • Adverse Effect Profile of Immunomodulatory Treatments

- Plasma exchange
  - Venous catheter-related
    - Infection
    - Pneumothorax
    - Local hematoma
  - Hemodynamic instability (hypotension)
  - Hemoconcentration
  - Coagulopathy (mild)
  - Hypocalcemia
  - Removal of highly protein-bound drugs
  - Transfusion reaction (including TRALI)
- Intravenous immunoglobulin
  - Infusion-related
    - Headache
    - Shivering
    - Myalgias
  - Chest pain
  - Hyperviscosity (risk of thrombosis, including arterial events)
  - Aseptic meningitis
  - Acute kidney injury
  - Anaphylaxis (if IgA deficiency)
  - Transfusion reaction (including TRALI)

Abbreviations: IgA, immunoglobulin A; TRALI, transfusion-related acute lung injury.

From Rabinstein AA. Acute neuromuscular respiratory failure. Continuum (Minneap Minn). 2015 Oct;21(5 Neurocritical Care):1324–45; used with permission.

Weaning From Mechanical Ventilation

Once intubated, most patients will usually need invasive ventilation for about 10 days. Weaning them from invasive ventilation can be challenging. Extubation failure can be expected in up to 40% of patients, especially in older men with prolonged intubation (>10 days) and atelectasis. Reinitiation or introduction of a cholinerase inhibitor is indicated before initiating weaning to optimize respiratory muscles strength; titration should be gradual to avoid excessive secretions that can complicate the process of extubation. Extubation of patients to bilateral positive airway pressure can prevent reintubation and should be particularly considered during the first night after extubation.

Summary

- MG is a B-cell–mediated autoimmune disease caused by autoantibodies against the postsynaptic end plate characterized by fluctuating weakness and fatigability.
- Myasthenic crisis is defined by the need for ventilatory support.
- Infections are the principal cause of myasthenic crisis. A cause for the crisis cannot be identified in 1 of 3 patients.

- Patients with myasthenic crises and severe bulbar weakness should be triaged early to the ICU.
- Early initiation of noninvasive ventilation can prevent intubation in almost 50% of patients.
- Severe hypoxemia, profound hypercapnia, copious oral secretions, and atelectasis are indications for intubation.
- Bedside pulmonary function tests should be used to monitor patients with MG, but clear cutoff values for intubation are not well established.
- IVIg and PLEX are equally effective to accelerate recovery in myasthenic exacerbations and crises. The combination of both treatments is not superior to either alone.
- Extubation to bilateral positive airway pressure should be considered to prevent reintubation.

SUGGESTED READING

Barth D, Nabavi Nouri M, Ng E, Nwe P, Bril V. Comparison of IVIg and PLEX in patients with myasthenia gravis. Neurology. 2011 Jun 7;76(23):2017–23. Epub 2011 May 11.

Benatar M. A systematic review of diagnostic studies in myasthenia gravis. Neuromuscul Disord. 2006 Jul;16(7):459–67. Epub 2006 Jun 21.

Cabrera Serrano M, Rabinstein AA. Usefulness of pulmonary function tests and blood gases in acute neuromuscular respiratory failure. Eur J Neurol. 2012 Mar;19(3):452–6. Epub 2011 Oct 4.

Gajdos P, Chevret S, Toyka KV. Intravenous immunoglobulin for myasthenia gravis. Cochrane Database Syst Rev. 2012 Dec 12;12:CD002277.

Gilhus NE. Myasthenia gravis. N Engl J Med. 2016 Dec 29;375(26):2570–81.

Gilhus NE, Romi F, Hong Y, Skeie GO. Myasthenia gravis and infectious disease. J Neurol. 2018 Jun;265(6):1251–8. Epub 2018 Jan 25.

Gilhus NE, Verschuuren JJ. Myasthenia gravis: subgroup classification and therapeutic strategies. Lancet Neurol. 2015 Oct;14(10):1023–36.

Kalita J, Kohat AK, Misra UK. Predictors of outcome of myasthenic crisis. Neurol Sci. 2014 Jul;35(7):1109–14. Epub 2014 Feb 5.

Mandawat A, Kaminski HJ, Cutter G, Katirji B, Alshekhlee A. Comparative analysis of therapeutic options used for myasthenia gravis. Ann Neurol. 2010 Dec;68(6):797–805.

Mehrizi M, Fontem RF, Gearhart TR, Pascuzzi RM. Medications and myasthenia gravis (a reference for health care professionals) [Internet]. New York (NY): Myasthenia Gravis Foundation of America; August c2012 [cited 2018 Jan 31]. Available from: http://www.myasthenia.org/portals/0/draft_medications_and_myasthenia_gravis_for_MGFA_website_8%2010%2012.pdf.

Nicolle MW. Myasthenia gravis and Lambert-Eaton myasthenic syndrome. Continuum (Minneap Minn). 2016 Dec;22(6, Muscle and Neuromuscular Junction Disorders):1978–2005.

Rabinstein AA. Acute neuromuscular respiratory failure. Continuum (Minneap Minn). 2015 Oct;21(5 Neurocritical Care):1324–45.

Rabinstein AA. Practical management of Guillain-Barré syndrome and myasthenic crisis. In: Manno EM, editor. Emergency management in neurocritical care. Chichester (United Kingdom): Wiley-Blackwell; c2012. p. 141–51. (Neurology in practice series).

Sanders DB, Wolfe GI, Benatar M, Evoli A, Gilhus NE, Illa I, et al. International consensus guidance for management of myasthenia gravis: executive summary. Neurology. 2016 Jul 26;87(4):419–25. Epub 2016 Jun 29.

Seneviratne J, Mandrekar J, Wijdicks EF, Rabinstein AA. Noninvasive ventilation in myasthenic crisis. Arch Neurol. 2008 Jan;65(1):54–8.

Seneviratne J, Mandrekar J, Wijdicks EF, Rabinstein AA. Predictors of extubation failure in myasthenic crisis. Arch Neurol. 2008 Jul;65(7):929–33.

Skeie GO, Apostolski S, Evoli A, Gilhus NE, Illa I, Harms L, et al; European Federation of Neurological Societies. Guidelines for treatment of autoimmune neuromuscular transmission disorders. Eur J Neurol. 2010 Jul;17(7):893–902. Epub 2010 Apr 12.

Thomas CE, Mayer SA, Gungor Y, Swarup R, Webster EA, Chang I, et al. Myasthenic crisis: clinical features, mortality, complications, and risk factors for prolonged intubation. Neurology. 1997 May;48(5):1253–60.

Wijdicks EFM. The practice of emergency and critical care neurology. 2nd ed. New York (NY): Oxford University Press; c2016. Chapter 43, Myasthenia gravis; p. 608–25.

Wolfe GI, Kaminski HJ, Aban IB, Minisman G, Kuo HC, Marx A, et al; MGTX Study Group. Long-term effect of thymectomy plus prednisone versus prednisone alone in patients with non-thymomatous myasthenia gravis: 2-year extension of the MGTX randomised trial. Lancet Neurol. 2019 Mar;18(3):259–68. Epub 2019 Jan 25.

94 Guillain-Barré Syndrome

EELCO F. M. WIJDICKS, MD, PhD

Goals

- Describe the pathophysiology of Guillain-Barré syndrome and mechanisms underlying its treatment.
- Describe neuromuscular respiratory failure in Guillain-Barré syndrome.
- Describe intensive care in Guillain-Barré syndrome.

Introduction

The incidence of Guillain-Barré syndrome (GBS) is about 1 case per 100,000 per year, but it is twice that in elderly persons. Multiple antecedent events have been reported. Its association with infections is established in not only *Campylobacter jejuni*, cytomegalovirus, Epstein-Barr virus, influenza A, *Mycoplasma pneumoniae*, and *Haemophilus influenzae* but also hepatitis (A, B, and E). Outbreaks are very rare but may have occurred in the wake of previous vaccination programs or, more currently, as a result of the Zika virus epidemic.

GBS can become a major neurocritical illness. Admission to the intensive care unit is expected in 1 of 5 patients with GBS. Rapidly progressive limb weakness may extend to the oropharyngeal muscles or diaphragm, an effect that often leads to intubation and mechanical ventilation.

There are several major clinical issues with GBS: early recognition of progression and potential for respiratory compromise, recognition of dysautonomia, recognition of available specific immunotherapy, and long-term rehabilitation.

Pathophysiology

GBS is often a postinfectious, immune-mediated nerve injury. Four phenotypes are likely: 1) mainly demyelinating, 2) mainly axonal, and 3) demyelinating with axonal involvement, and 4) several variants, including Miller Fisher variant. The immunopathogenesis of GBS is depicted in Figure 94.1. Current understanding holds that GBS is antibody-mediated. Auto-antibodies binding to GM_1 or GD_{1a} gangliosides (at nodes of Ranvier) activate complement, and this activation results in myelin destruction. Complement-cascade activation is mediated by binding antibodies to Schwann cells and results in vesicular myelin degeneration. The proclivity of motor axonal involvement has led to the designation acute motor axonal neuropathy. *C jejuni* infection is the prototype of this mechanism, and molecular mimicry has been found between terminal structures of *C jejuni* and GM_1 and GD_{1a}. The target molecule in purely demyelinating disease is yet unknown.

Plasma exchange and intravenous immunoglobulin (IVIg) are currently the 2 main therapeutic options. Plasma exchange removes antibodies and other inflammatory components such as complement and also may improve T-cell suppressor function. IVIg is pooled donor IgG, but its mechanism of action may be due to neutralization of antibodies or Fc receptor blockade, or there may be an indirect effect on B- or T-cell function.

Clinical Presentation

Symptoms and signs usually progress within 1 to 2 weeks. The diagnosis of GBS is fairly typical, and differential diagnosis is narrow (eg, spinal cord lesion, toxicity). The typical presenting symptoms are severe back pain and distal limb paresthesias that cause a "tight band" feeling. The paresthesias gradually move proximally over the limbs. Muscle weakness starts more proximally, most notably 1 or 2 days after the onset of paresthesias. Patients describe difficulty with climbing stairs and rising from a chair. Symmetrically weak muscles are accompanied by depressed or absent deep tendon reflexes. Legs are more typically involved than arms, a feature that creates the clinical impression of an ascending paralysis. In half of patients, facial and oropharyngeal muscles are affected.

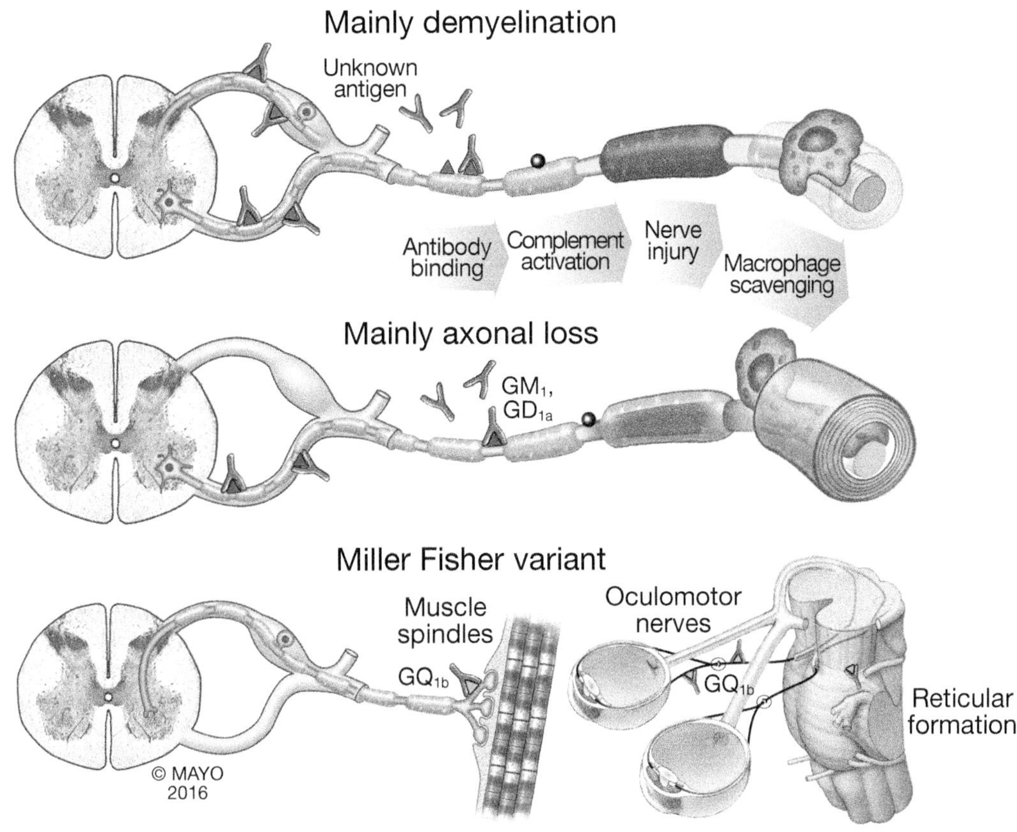

Figure 94.1. *Current Understanding of the Pathogenesis and Clinical Variants of Guillain-Barré Syndrome (GBS). In demyelinating GBS, unequivocal antigens have yet to be identified but are inferred by complement activation, myelin destruction, and cleanup by macrophages. In axonal variant and Miller Fisher variant, gangliosides GM_1, GD_{1A}, and GQ_{1b} are targeted by immunoglobulins and share antigenic epitopes with various bacterial and viral antigens. These antigenic targets are at nodal structures, at roots, and at the end organs. In Miller Fisher variant, the GQ_{1b} antigen also exists within the brainstem. In this variant, the macrophages clean up the axon debris and come in from the nodes.*

(From Wijdicks EF, Klein CJ. Guillain-Barré syndrome. Mayo Clin Proc. 2017 Mar;92[3]:467–79; used with permission of Mayo Foundation for Medical Education and Research.)

The initial manifestation of GBS may be weakness of these muscle groups (Figure 94.2). Variants of GBS are more difficult to recognize and include Miller Fisher syndrome (oculomotor weakness, ataxia, and areflexia), paraparesis alone, pharyngeal-cervical-brachial weakness, bilateral facial palsy, and bilateral lumbar polyradiculopathy.

Neuromuscular respiratory failure is a worrisome development, and it remains difficult for clinicians to appreciate its seriousness. Clinically, respiratory muscle weakness leads to low tidal volume ("shallow" breathing) and poor gas exchange, which, in turn, lead to tachypnea and later hypercapnia. Affected patients also have increased dead space ventilation in addition to their elevated respiratory drive. The rapid breathing is the result of signals to the respiratory center from the abnormal, weak respiratory muscles. Usually. the arterial Pco_2 decreases because of this rapid breathing; however, when respiratory muscle strength is more than 25% of normal, Pco_2 remains in normal range. When respiratory weakness is severe, paradoxic breathing, also called thoracoabdominal asynchrony, occurs. Clinically, it is apparent by a rocking horse–type movement of the chest (outward) and abdomen (inward) and may occur with each breath.

Another manifestation of a developing neurocritical illness is dysautonomia, recognized by extreme blood pressure fluctuations and exaggerated drug responses, cardiac arrhythmias, hypersecretions, gastrointestinal dysfunction, and bladder dysfunction. Baroreflex abnormality, altered as a result of vagal nerve demyelination, may cause the blood pressure fluctuations. Moreover, because sympathetic nerves have less myelin, a sympathetic overdrive may occur. Dysfunction of afferent input from atrial stretch receptors could also influence blood pressure swings.

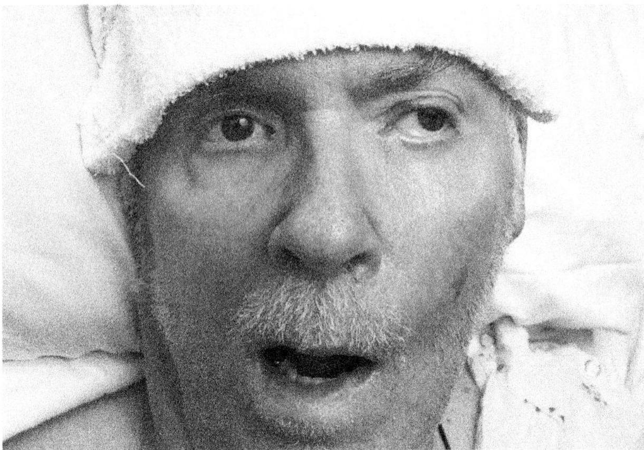

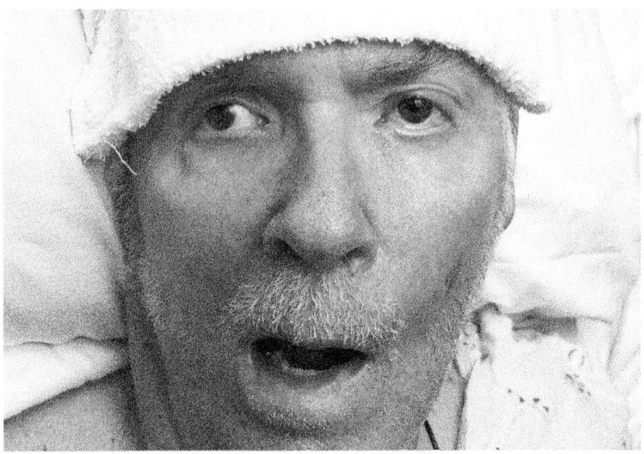

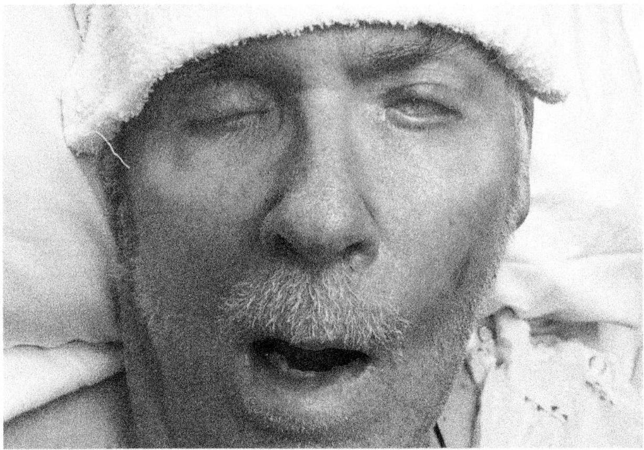

Figure 94.2. Patient With Severe Ptosis, Bifacial Palsy, and Ophthalmoparesis.

Laboratory Tests

On cerebrospinal fluid analysis, typically the protein level is high and the white blood cell count is normal (the classic albuminocytologic dissociation). Although unusual, the white blood cell count may be more than 10×10^9/L, but this value is more common in associated disorders such as Lyme disease, sarcoidosis, and AIDS.

Electrophysiologic studies are far more useful for diagnosis. Demyelination is seen as conduction block or increased conduction velocities. For proximal nerve involvement that occurs early in the disease course, specific tests include recording of F waves and abnormalities such as dispersion or dropout in F-wave signal. Prolonged F waves may be the only confirmatory finding if the patient is tested early.

Bedside pulmonary function tests are useful. Patients with diaphragmatic weakness have decreased vital capacity when supine, but the decrease must be more than 25% from baseline to be called abnormal. Conversely, a normal vital capacity while supine makes inspiratory muscle weakness highly unlikely. The maximal inspiratory pressure has the advantage that recoil of the chest wall contributes to the value. A high maximal inspiratory pressure (>80 cm H_2O), particularly in combination with vital capacity, makes neuromuscular respiratory failure unlikely. Respiratory function tests are usually reliable, but not in severe facial weakness; this limitation can be easily overcome using mask spirometry. Pulse oximetry is important in any patient with neuromuscular respiratory disease, but, obviously, it does not identify CO_2 retention. Rapid, shallow breathing leads to chronic hypercapnia in patients with neuromuscular disease. It markedly decreases total volume, shortens inspiratory time, and truncates vital capacity, resulting in hypercarbia. Overnight monitoring by pulse oximetry is essential because nocturnal hypoventilation indicates respiratory muscle weakness in the appropriate setting.

Arterial blood gas measurements can be informative. In many patients, diaphragm failure is noted by normal $Paco_2$ with increased respiratory rate. The diaphragm weakness results in failure to blow off CO_2, and the expected hypocapnia does not occur with tachypnea (Figure 94.3). Results may show hypoxemic, hypercapnic respiratory failure in a patient in obvious respiratory distress. Hypercapnia is a late feature in acute neuromuscular failure. Poor diaphragmatic function leads to poor ventilation due to alveolar collapse, which results in hypoxemia.

Management

Many patients with GBS become bed-bound, and this immobilization requires expert nursing care. Skin, eye, and mouth care is crucial to the comfort of quadriplegic patients. Cramping pain is common and can be relieved by narcotics or nonsteroidal anti-inflammatory drugs. Carbamazepine or increasing doses of gabapentin or pregabalin may be helpful.

Preventive measures are important. A bedside test for swallowing dysfunction is essential, and aspiration of thin liquid resulting in spontaneous cough during this test greatly increases the risk of aspiration. Enteral nutrition may be necessary in most patients. Subcutaneous heparin is required in addition to intermittent pneumatic compression devices. However, in some patients with GBS, these

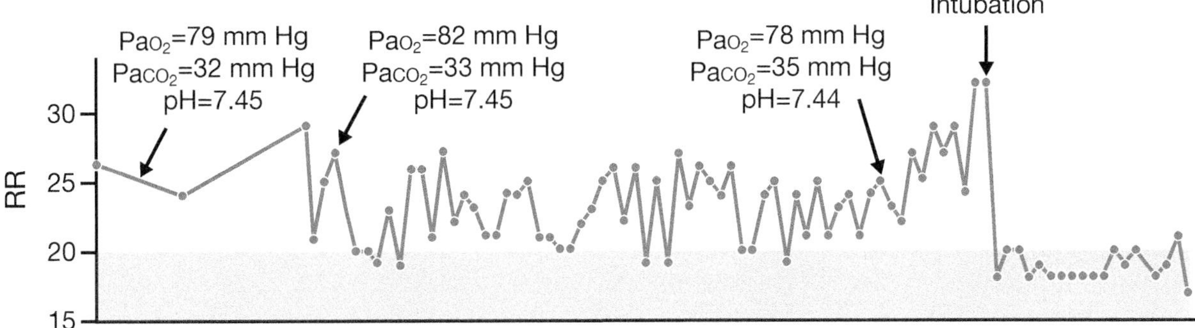

Figure 94.3. Relatively Normal P_{CO_2} as a Sign of Diaphragm Weakness Until Intubation. RR indicates respiratory rate (breaths per minute).

high-frequency devices cause discomfort. It is important to start physical therapy with passive range of motion in paralyzed limbs early.

The main treatment in acute GBS is 5 courses of plasma exchange or IVIg (0.4 g/kg per day) for 5 days. For nonambulatory patients with GBS who present within 4 weeks of disease onset, both of these are recommended. The effectiveness of plasma exchange in GBS has been established in large multicenter trials. This therapy is most effective when started within 7 days of symptom onset. With plasma exchange, clinical improvement occurs earlier, the need for mechanical ventilation is reduced, and recovery is faster. Two plasma exchanges are superior to none in mild GBS, and 4 exchanges are superior to 2 in moderately severe GBS. However, 6 exchanges are not superior to 4 in severe GBS requiring mechanical ventilation.

For the treatment of GBS, IVIg has not been compared with placebo in randomized trials, but IVIg has been shown to be as effective as plasma exchange. In analysis of disability scores at 4 weeks, plasma exchange and IVIg were not significantly different, but improvement was faster with plasma exchange. The dose of IVIg may be insufficient for some patients and has led to a practice of repeating the treatment, but there is no evidence that this improves outcomes or the pace of recovery. Likewise, combining IVIg with plasma exchange has no proven benefit. The use of corticosteroids alone has no substantial benefit. Intravenous methylprednisolone used in combination with IVIg may hasten recovery but does not affect long-term outcome or neuropathic pain.

Any patient with worsening weakness, specifically early oropharyngeal weakness, on initial evaluation or presentation will need to be admitted to and observed in an intensive care unit (Figure 94.4). However, only 1 in 3 patients will deteriorate enough to mandate further or prolonged close monitoring and possibly endotracheal intubation.

Respiratory failure associated with GBS can be assessed clinically, but pulmonary function tests of forced maximal inspiratory and expiratory pressures and vital capacity can be useful. A decrease in vital capacity to 20 mL/kg, decrease of maximal inspiratory pressure to -30 cm H_2O, and decrease of maximal expiratory pressure to 40 cm H_2O (the 20–30–40 rule) are critical values warranting intubation. Some researchers have found the time between onset of weakness and hospital admission, the presence of facial weakness or oropharyngeal dysfunction, and the severity of limb weakness, as assessed by the Medical Research Council score, to be useful predictors of respiratory failure and the need for intubation.

Mechanical ventilation is often prolonged in GBS. Generally, weaning from mechanical ventilation should be guided by improvement in diaphragm strength and normalization of values on serial pulmonary function tests. In GBS, diaphragmatic weakness may resolve before extremity weakness; thus, the timing of weaning should not be gauged solely by recovery of extremity muscle strength. There are several conditions to consider before even attempting to wean a patient from the ventilator. In addition, the patient should have no evidence of atelectasis, pleural effusion, or marked difficulty handling secretions. Secretion volume, whether the patient is comfortable with a T-piece trial, and completely normal results on chest radiography offer accurate predictive value for successful extubation in any patient with acute neuromuscular respiratory failure. Results of pulmonary function tests can predict successful weaning to some extent, but they are far from reliable. The maximal expiratory pressure, which indicates the ability to cough up secretions, and thus abdominal musculature strength, might be the best predictor of successful weaning.

Weaning trials can begin when the following conditions are met: 1) vital capacity is more than 15 mL/kg, 2) maximal inspiratory pressure is more than -30 cm H_2O, and 3) oxygenation is sufficient with a fraction of inspired oxygen of 40% or less. Weaning should begin as early as possible because prolonged intubation is related to several complications. The treating physician can determine whether the intermittent mandatory ventilation rate or pressure-support level can be reduced as weaning approaches.

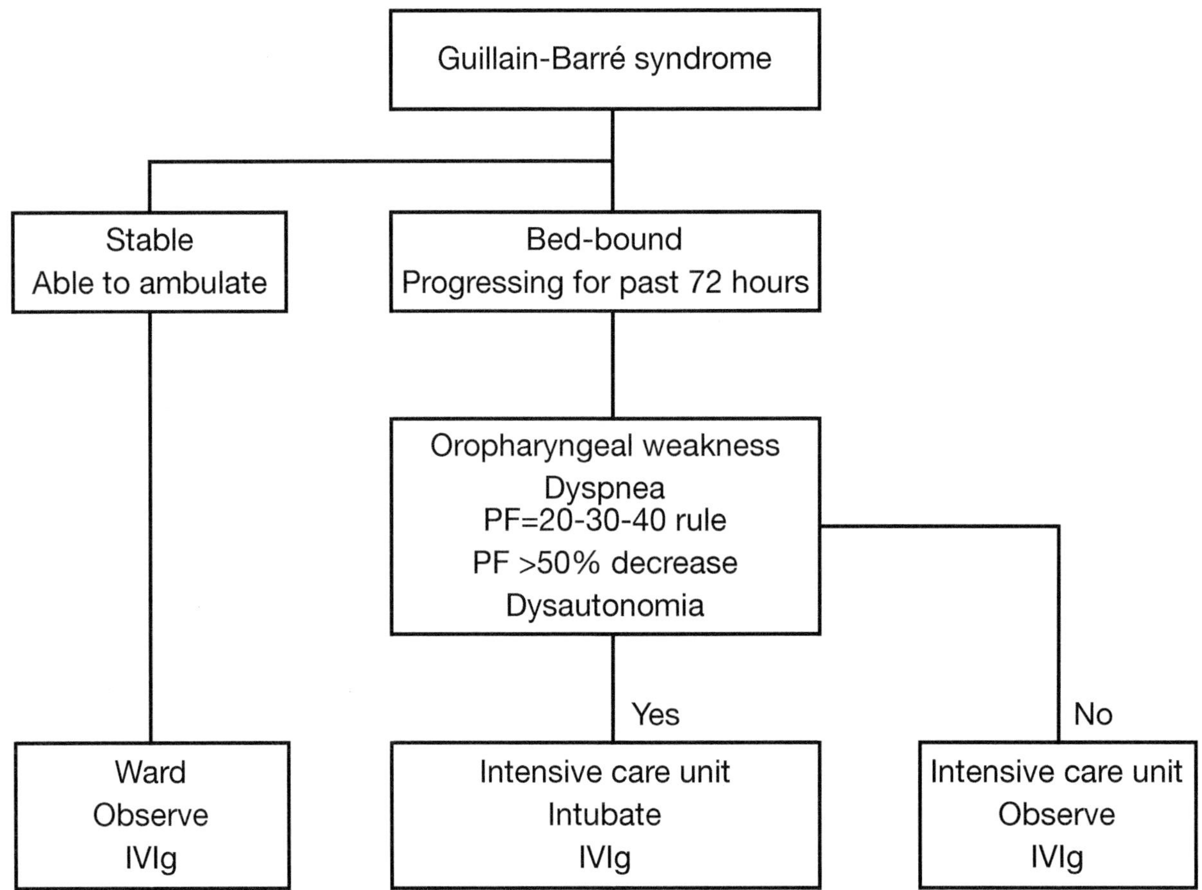

Figure 94.4. *Triage Algorithm for Patients With Guillain-Barré Syndrome. IVIg indicates intravenous immunoglobulin; PF, pulmonary function test results.*

(From Wijdicks EF, Klein CJ. Guillain-Barré syndrome. Mayo Clin Proc. 2017 Mar;92[3]:467–79; used with permission of Mayo Foundation for Medical Education and Research.)

Outcome

Supportive care, which may include critical care of acute respiratory failure and dysautonomia, remains the main treatment. Plasma exchange or IVIg is recommended for nonambulatory patients with GBS who present early in disease onset. A combination of both treatments has been considered in more severe cases, but its efficacy is unproved, and the same is true of later immunomodulating treatments. One in 3 patients will deteriorate enough to require prolonged intensive care monitoring and, possibly, mechanical ventilation. Full recovery occurs frequently in severe cases, but 10% of patients may retain some disability indefinitely. Most patients do regain the ability to walk. Progress has been made in intensive care support and rehabilitation.

Summary

- Admission to the intensive care unit is warranted for patients with GBS who are unable to walk and have oropharyngeal weakness.
- Diaphragmatic weakness may progress rapidly, and many patients require long-term mechanical ventilation.
- Dysautonomia is underappreciated but is life-threatening because of wide swings in blood pressure and cardiac arrhythmias.

SUGGESTED READING

Brown WF, Feasby TE. Conduction block and denervation in Guillain-Barré polyneuropathy. Brain. 1984 Mar;107 (Pt 1):219–39.

Burns TM, Lawn ND, Low PA, Camilleri M, Wijdicks EF. Adynamic ileus in severe Guillain-Barré syndrome. Muscle Nerve. 2001 Jul;24(7):963–5.

Derenne JP, Macklem PT, Roussos C. The respiratory muscles: mechanics, control, and pathophysiology. Part I. Am Rev Respir Dis. 1978 Jul;118(1):119–33.

Derenne JP, Macklem PT, Roussos C. The respiratory muscles: mechanics, control, and pathophysiology. Part II. Am Rev Respir Dis. 1978 Aug;118(2):373–90.

Derenne JP, Macklem PT, Roussos C. The respiratory muscles: mechanics, control, and pathophysiology. Part III. Am Rev Respir Dis. 1978 Sep;118(3):581–601.

Edmundson C, Bird SJ. Acute manifestations of neuromuscular disease. Semin Neurol. 2019 Feb;39(1):115–24. Epub 2019 Feb 11.

Flachenecker P, Hartung HP, Reiners K. Power spectrum analysis of heart rate variability in Guillain-Barré syndrome: a longitudinal study. Brain. 1997 Oct;120 (Pt 10):1885–94.

Henderson RD, Lawn ND, Fletcher DD, McClelland RL, Wijdicks EF. The morbidity of Guillain-Barré syndrome admitted to the intensive care unit. Neurology. 2003 Jan 14;60(1):17–21.

Jacobs BC, Rothbarth PH, van der Meche FG, Herbrink P, Schmitz PI, de Klerk MA, et al. The spectrum of antecedent infections in Guillain-Barré syndrome: a case-control study. Neurology. 1998 Oct;51(4):1110–5.

Lichtenfeld P. Autonomic dysfunction in the Guillain-Barré syndrome. Am J Med. 1971 Jun;50(6):772–80.

Liu S, Dong C, Ubogu EE. Immunotherapy of Guillain-Barré syndrome. Hum Vaccin Immunother. 2018;14(11): 2568–79. Epub 2018 Jul 12.

Rabinstein AA, Wijdicks EF. Warning signs of imminent respiratory failure in neurological patients. Semin Neurol. 2003 Mar;23(1):97–104.

Ropper AH. Unusual clinical variants and signs in Guillain-Barré syndrome. Arch Neurol. 1986 Nov;43(11): 1150–2.

Ropper AH, Wijdicks EF. Blood pressure fluctuations in the dysautonomia of Guillain-Barré syndrome. Arch Neurol. 1990 Jun;47(6):706–8.

Ropper AH, Wijdicks EFM, Truax BT. Guillain-Barré syndrome. Philadelphia (PA): F.A Davis; c1991. 369 p.

Tham SL, Prasad K, Umapathi T. Guillain-Barré syndrome mimics. Brain Behav. 2018 Apr 10;8(5):e00960.

Truax BT. Autonomic disturbances in the Guillain-Barré syndrome. Semin Neurol. 1984;4:462–8.

van den Berg B, Fokke C, Drenthen J, van Doorn PA, Jacobs BC. Paraparetic Guillain-Barré syndrome. Neurology. 2014 Jun 3;82(22):1984–9. Epub 2014 May 7.

Willison HJ, Jacobs BC, van Doorn PA. Guillain-Barré syndrome. Lancet. 2016 Aug 13;388(10045):717–27. Epub 2016 Mar 2.

Yuki N, Taki T, Inagaki F, Kasama T, Takahashi M, Saito K, et al. A bacterium lipopolysaccharide that elicits Guillain-Barré syndrome has a GM1 ganglioside-like structure. J Exp Med. 1993 Nov 1;178(5):1771–5.

Zaeem Z, Siddiqi ZA, Zochodne DW. Autonomic involvement in Guillain-Barré syndrome: an update. Clin Auton Res. 2018 Jul 17. [Epub ahead of print]

Zochodne DW. Autonomic involvement in Guillain-Barré syndrome: a review. Muscle Nerve. 1994 Oct;17(10):1145–55.

95 Amyotrophic Lateral Sclerosis

JENNIFER M. MARTINEZ-THOMPSON, MD; NATHAN P. STAFF, MD, PhD

Goals

- Learn how to identify amyotrophic lateral sclerosis in the intensive care unit.
- Review the diagnostic evaluation of amyotrophic lateral sclerosis.
- Review the respiratory and nutritional management of amyotrophic lateral sclerosis.

Introduction

Amyotrophic lateral sclerosis (ALS) is a rare, progressive neurodegenerative disorder with both upper and lower motor neuron involvement. It presents with weakness, muscle wasting, spasticity involving the limbs, bulbar dysfunction, and, typically later in the disease, respiratory involvement. Up to 20% of patients may also have a frontotemporal-type dementia. Average duration of survival is 2 to 4 years from symptom onset, and the peak incidence is between the ages of 50 and 75 years. Only 10% of patients have familial forms, and the remainder have sporadic ALS.

ALS typically presents with disability involving 1 segment of the body and contiguously spreads to other segments as the disease progresses. Eighty percent of patients present with asymmetric limb weakness, either painless footdrop or hand dysfunction. These patients do not present to the intensive care unit (ICU) until the late stages of disease. Bulbar-onset ALS with prominent dysarthria and dysphagia occurs in 15% to 20% of cases and has a faster progression. With this form, the median duration of survival is 2 years from the time of symptom onset. Other less common presentations include axial-onset weakness manifesting with a head drop or generalized bulbar and limb weakness in fulminant cases. Rarely is the initial presentation neuromuscular respiratory failure (1%-3% of cases). When it is, the diagnosis has likely been established late. Most patients with diaphragmatic involvement have clinical signs indicating an advanced stage.

The diagnosis and management of ALS are complex, more so with atypical presentations. This chapter outlines the approach to recognizing ALS in the intensive care unit, reviews symptom management, and focuses on respiratory and nutrition management.

Clinical Features

Patients in the ICU in whom ALS has not been diagnosed typically have 1 or a combination of the following presentations: 1) acute neuromuscular respiratory failure, 2) rapidly progressive bulbar-onset ALS with severe bulbar weakness and secretions resulting in an inability to protect the airway, and 3) generalized weakness in fulminant disease. A limited clinical examination for a patient in whom ALS is suspected should attempt to look for findings expected in any of these presentations. Frequently, patients are intubated for hypercapnic hypoxemic respiratory failure, and this may hinder a full examination.

If the patient is not intubated at the time of evaluation, the initial focus should be on the respiratory evaluation. Patients with signs of impending neuromuscular respiratory failure may be unable to complete full sentences in a single breath (staccato speech). Accessory muscle use and a paradoxic breathing pattern may be present. Assessment of respiratory function is difficult in the setting of endotracheal intubation, but patients with neuromuscular respiratory weakness may fail multiple weaning attempts from the ventilator. With targeted questioning, there is often a history of respiratory insufficiency of at least several months before the decompensation that prompted hospitalization. Often, the decompensation is triggered by a respiratory infection or aspiration event.

The examination should then focus on establishing the presence of both upper and lower motor neuron signs and muscle weakness in the segments that can be assessed clinically (bulbar, cervical, and lumbosacral segments). Upper motor neuron signs that are more reliably determined in the ICU setting include limb spasticity, jaw or limb hyperreflexia, and extensor plantar responses. Limited lower motor neuron evaluation includes inspection of the tongue and limbs for atrophy and fasciculations. This assessment may be difficult in an intubated patient, although profound tongue fasciculations and atrophy can be expected. Sensory loss or eye movement abnormalities are not expected in ALS. Neuromuscular weakness that does not have a mixed upper and lower motor neuron pattern should prompt consideration of ALS mimickers, such as compressive myelopathies or more rare genetic disorders (Table 95.1).

Table 95.1 • Mimickers of Amyotrophic Lateral Sclerosis in the Intensive Care Unit

		Motor Neuron Involvement			
Diagnosis	**Weakness**	**Upper**	**Lower**	**Upper and Lower**	**Defining Characteristics**
Kennedy disease	Yes	No	Yes	No	X-linked Perioral fasciculations Gynecomastia Peripheral neuropathy
SMA	Yes	No	Yes	No	Onset >30 years old Axial > limb weakness Abdominal cramps
PLS	Yes	Yes	No	No	Slow progression of UMN findings before respiratory failure
Infectious myelitis, WNV, coxsackievirus B, enterovirus, poliovirus	Yes	No	Yes	No	Seasonal exposure Subacute presentation
AIDP and variants	Yes	No	Yes	No	Ascending sensorimotor symptoms Diffuse hyporeflexia Diplopia (Miller Fisher)
Demyelinating disease	Yes	Yes	No	Yes	Saccadic abnormalities (INO) Bowel or bladder dysfunction
Hyperparathyroidism	Yes	No	No	Yes	Proximal > distal symmetric weakness Sensory loss, ataxia
Myeloradiculopathy Cervical spondylosis Copper deficiency	Yes	Yes	Yes	Yes	Sensory loss, ataxia Focal reflex loss
Lymphoma	Yes	No	Yes	Yes (rare)	± Cranial neuropathies Leg weakness (lumbar polyradiculopathy)
Paraneoplastic ANNA-1 (SCLC) ANNA-2 (BRCA) MaTa (Hodgkin, NHL)	Yes	Yes	Yes	Yes	± Encephalitis PLS- or SMA-like presentation
Myasthenia gravis	Yes	No	No	No	Diplopia, ptosis Fluctuating weakness
Myopathy IBM Acid-maltase deficiency NAM	Yes	No	No	No	Proximal > distal symmetric weakness CK variable, >10× ULN in NAM

Abbreviations: AIDP, acute inflammatory demyelinating polyradiculoneuropathy; ANNA-1, ANNA-2, antineuronal nuclear antibodies; BRCA, breast cancer; CK, creatine kinase; IBM, inclusion body myositis; INO, internuclear ophthalmoplegia; NAM, necrotizing autoimmune myopathy; NHL, Non-Hodgkin lymphoma; PLS, primary lateral sclerosis; SCLC, small cell lung cancer; SMA, spinal muscular atrophy; ULN, upper limit of normal; UMN, upper motor neuron; WNV, West Nile virus; ±, with or without.

Diagnostic Tests

The diagnosis of ALS is clinical, complemented by electromyography to establish the extent of lower motor neuron involvement. The results of sensory and motor nerve conduction studies are typically normal in ALS, but motor nerve conduction studies recorded over severely atrophic muscles may show low-amplitude responses. Needle electromyography shows signs of acute denervation in affected segments, which include fibrillations, positive sharp waves, and fasciculation potentials. There is evidence of chronic denervation and reinnervation with large, complex motor unit potentials with reduced recruitment and considerable instability. In cases of isolated respiratory failure, needle electromyography of the diaphragm shows similar changes. These changes are not specific to ALS but are helpful when found in multiple segments in the appropriate clinical context.

Neuroimaging can be considered to exclude ALS mimickers from a structural cause. Lower motor neuron findings in the limbs may prompt use of cervical and lumbar spine magnetic resonance imaging to exclude substantial spine or root compression as the cause of the findings. With isolated bulbar symptoms, brain magnetic resonance imaging should be considered. With upper motor neuron findings, magnetic resonance imaging should cover the segments rostral to the clinical findings. Although resulsts of magnetic resonance imaging are typically normal in ALS, signal can be increased within the corticospinal tracts on T2-weighted imaging. Similar T2 changes and contrast enhancement of the ventral lumbar roots have also been reported.

To evaluate for ALS mimickers, laboratory evaluation in the ICU may include routine complete blood count with differential, electrolytes including calcium and parathyroid hormone, liver and thyroid function, inflammatory markers, vitamin B_{12}, copper, zinc, serum electrophoresis with immunofixation, HIV screening, creatine kinase, and ganglioside and paraneoplastic antibodies. The creatine kinase level can be increased up to 1,000 U/L in ALS because of muscle denervation. In patients with bulbar dysfunction, acetylcholine receptor antibodies and muscle-specific kinase antibodies to evaluate for myasthenia gravis can be considered. A lumbar puncture with cytologic analysis can be considered in subacutely progressive motor neuron disorders as part of the evaluation for systemic malignancy or infectious myelitis.

Respiratory Management

ALS affects all components of the mechanical respiratory system. Upper airway muscle weakness results in inadequate handling of secretions and increases the risk for aspiration. Extensive involvement of the expiratory muscles leads to cough impairment. Inspiratory muscle weakness results in restrictive lung disease with eventual carbon dioxide retention and hypercarbic respiratory failure. Primary oxygenation issues are uncommon in ALS until the late stages of the disease. As a result, oxygen as a primary therapy for this type of respiratory insufficiency is not recommended unless it is being used to manage dyspnea at the end of life.

Good respiratory management addresses all components of the mechanical respiratory system. Salivary secretions can be minimized through the use of anticholinergic agents (amitriptyline, glycopyrrolate, sublingual atropine, and scopolamine patches). For refractory cases, nonpharmacologic strategies such as salivary gland onabotulinum A toxin injections or irradiation are logistically difficult and without immediate effect in the ICU setting. Use of suction devices is also helpful. Cough function can be augmented by manual cough assist and with the use of mechanical insufflation-exsufflation devices as long as the patient has adequate bulbar function to maintain a seal on the mouthpiece. The American Academy of Neurology practice parameters recommend using these strategies to augment cough when the peak cough expiratory flow is less than 270 L/min.

Respiratory failure from inspiratory muscle weakness can be difficult to predict in patients who have ALS, but this scenario is likely in the ICU. If the patient is not intubated and does not have severe bulbar involvement, bedside spirometry is used to measure the forced vital capacity, maximal inspiratory pressure, and maximal expiratory pressure. Oxygen saturation and arterial blood gases should also be tested. Factors indicating respiratory failure are listed in Box 95.1. Importantly, a forced vital capacity less than 50% of predicted should lead to a discussion with the patient

Box 95.1 • Factors Suggesting Respiratory Failure in Motor Neuron Disease[a]

- FVC <50% of predicted
- FVC <80% of predicted with symptoms of respiratory failure
- MIP <40 cm H_2O
- MIP <65 cm H_2O (men) or <55 cm H_2O (women) and respiratory symptoms
- Rate of MIP decrease over 3 months is >10 cm H_2O with repeated testing
- Daytime arterial CO_2 of ≥45 mm Hg
- Daytime O_2 saturations of ≤94%
- Nocturnal episodes of hypercapnia or hypoxia

Abbreviatons: FVC, forced vital capacity; MIP, maximal inspiratory pressure.

[a] These laboratory assessments are typically obtained in ambulatory patients. In hospitalized patients, FVC, MIP, and maximal expiratory pressure are assessed at the bedside (for comparison and more details, see Chapter 93, "Myasthenia Gravis," and Chapter 94, "Guillain-Barré Syndrome").

and family about the use of noninvasive ventilation through bilevel positive airway pressure (BiPAP) according to the most recent American Academy of Neurology practice guidelines and about patient-specific preferences for invasive ventilation if there is further decompensation. BiPAP should be considered to treat respiratory insufficiency, both to lengthen survival and to provide comfort. If patients are intubated, weaning from the ventilator can be attempted after reversible causes of acute respiratory failure have been treated and with the immediate transition to continuous BiPAP and use of mechanical insufflation-exsufflation devices to minimize respiratory muscle fatigue.

In the outpatient setting, BiPAP is typically initiated at night because of the high frequency of sleep-disordered breathing, and use is increased during the day as the disease progresses. Once bulbar function is severe enough, the discussion must shift to considering invasive ventilation (endotracheal intubation and tracheostomy) as an option for continued survival given the risk of aspiration pneumonia and the lack of protection afforded by BiPAP in this regard. In the United States, few patients with ALS choose tracheostomy as an option when this option is discussed before the onset of acute respiratory failure; most instances of invasive ventilation occur in the emergency setting in the absence of advanced planning.

The available evidence suggests that BiPAP use prolongs survival and improves quality of life in patients with ALS who have milder bulbar involvement. Maintenance of quality of life has also been reported with unplanned tracheostomy placement, but patients older than 60 years tend to do poorly. This result should factor into discussions at a point of transition of care in elderly patients.

Nutritional Management

Progressive dysphagia and bulbar weakness in ALS affect adequate oral intake, resulting in substantial weight loss and dehydration. The American Academy of Neurology practice parameters recommend considering gastrostomy tube placement when a patient's nutritional status is compromised by dysphagia, weight loss of 5% to 10% of the premorbid body weight has occurred, or when the body mass index is less than 20 kg/m^2. The procedure is preferably performed while the patient's forced vital capacity is more than 50% of predicted because the complication rates are higher and survival times shorter in patients with extensive respiratory compromise. Placement is considered hazardous once the forced vital capacity is less than 30% of predicted and is generally not recommended.

Currently, percutaneous endoscopic gastrostomy (PEG) and percutaneous radiologic gastrostomy (PRG) tube placement are the main options for patients with ALS in the United States. There is conflicting evidence on which method is safer. Several studies have shown an increased rate of gastrostomy tube-related complications in patients undergoing PRG tube placement, presumably due to tube migration or dislodgment because the tubes are less securely fixed than tubes inserted by PEG. Higher risk of aspiration with sedation use has been reported during PEG placement without a substantial difference in postprocedural mortality compared with that in PRG. BiPAP support during PEG placement has been suggested as a safe alternative to endotracheal intubation in patients with ALS who have extensive respiratory compromise, but no formal studies have compared the safety between the 2. Overall, PEG placement is suggested as the optimal method when respiratory function is relatively unimpaired, and PRG is considered once respiratory function is substantially compromised. For safety, outpatients can be monitored in the hospital setting after the procedure to ensure there are no immediate complications.

The rationale for early gastrostomy tube placement is not solely to avoid respiratory complications but to optimize a patient's potential for weight gain postprocedurally. Studies have shown that patients with loss of more than 10% of their premorbid body weight at the time of gastrostomy tube placement do not regain their weight and often continue to lose weight after gastrostomy because of a hypermetabolic state. Evidence is mixed regarding survival benefits of nutrition through gastrostomy. In general, it is not thought to confer a long-term survival benefit despite stabilization of weight loss but can help patients stay hydrated and be used as a conduit for medications to manage symptoms.

Treatment of Other Associated Symptoms

Other issues that may be relevant in the ICU setting include spasticity, cramps, and laryngospasm. Spasticity and cramps can be a source of pain in patients with ALS. Common medications used to treat spasticity include baclofen, tizanidine, benzodiazepines, and dantrolene. Cramps are often treated with antiseizure medications (gabapentin) or mexiletine. Laryngospasm usually lasts for seconds with inspiratory stridor due to forceful contraction of the laryngeal adductors. Episodes can be triggered by contact of saliva or refluxed stomach acid with the larynx. This condition is best managed by placing the patient's upper body in the upright position and having the patient inhale through the nose and exhale through pursed lips with attempted swallows in between. With frequent episodes, low-dose benzodiazepines can be used. Many additional symptoms are experienced by patients with ALS during their disease course, but these are best managed in the outpatient setting and are beyond the scope of this discussion.

Counseling and Palliation

Because ALS is a fatal disorder, it is important to establish goals of care and advance directives for patients in the ICU. Patients and families may have already had these discussions, but in many cases they need to be initiated within the ICU setting. It is also important to determine whether a patient has concomitant frontotemporal dementia (which can be challenging in anarthric or systemically ill patients) within the context of these discussions.

Baseline testing that can help guide discussions include videofluoroscopic swallow evaluations, bedside spirometry, and overnight oximetry. Decrease in the maximal inspiratory pressure, decrease in the forced vital capacity, or a suggestion of sleep-disordered breathing based on the overnight oximetry results should prompt discussion about initiating noninvasive ventilation. Evidence of aspiration on the swallow evaluation may initiate discussion about gastrostomy placement, the timing of which is guided by a patient's current respiratory function. If patients are failing, the discussion about noninvasive ventilation should focus on invasive ventilation with the goal of tracheostomy if it is in line with a patient's wishes. The goal is to stabilize the patient for eventual transition to the outpatient setting under the care of an ALS multidisciplinary clinic. Families can consult the ALS Association website (http://www.alsa.org) to identify local resources and additional educational materials.

Most often, patients will be in the ICU at the late stages of disease. The discussions focus on similar topics, only patients may be too late in their presentation for interventions to have benefit. At this stage, patients are often eligible for hospice with a shift toward end-of-life symptom management.

Summary

- An ALS diagnosis requires combined upper and lower motor neuron involvement in multiple body segments. ALS mimickers should be considered in the absence of mixed findings.
- Initial respiratory assessment includes bedside spirometry, overnight oximetry, and initiation of BiPAP.
- Noninvasive ventilation should be considered preferentially over invasive ventilation when the forced vital capacity is less than 50% of predicted or the patient has respiratory symptoms.
- PEG tube placement should be considered with substantial dysphagia, body weight decrease of 5% to 10% of premorbid weight, or a body mass index less than 20 kg/m^2.

SUGGESTED READING

Allen JA, Chen R, Ajroud-Driss S, Sufit RL, Heller S, Siddique T, et al. Gastrostomy tube placement by endoscopy versus radiologic methods in patients with ALS: a retrospective study of complications and outcome. Amyotroph Lateral Scler Frontotemporal Degener. 2013 May;14(4):308–14. Epub 2013 Jan 4.

Bach JR, Sinquee DM, Saporito LR, Botticello AL. Efficacy of mechanical insufflation-exsufflation in extubating unweanable subjects with restrictive pulmonary disorders. Respir Care. 2015 Apr;60(4):477–83. Epub 2014 Dec 9.

Benditt JO, Boitano L. Respiratory treatment of amyotrophic lateral sclerosis. Phys Med Rehabil Clin N Am. 2008 Aug;19(3):559–72.

Bourke SC, Tomlinson M, Williams TL, Bullock RE, Shaw PJ, Gibson GJ. Effects of non-invasive ventilation on survival and quality of life in patients with amyotrophic lateral sclerosis: a randomised controlled trial. Lancet Neurol. 2006 Feb;5(2):140–7.

Cabrera Serrano M, Rabinstein AA. Causes and outcomes of acute neuromuscular respiratory failure. Arch Neurol. 2010 Sep;67(9):1089–94.

Chio A, Logroscino G, Hardiman O, Swingler R, Mitchell D, Beghi E, et al; Eurals Consortium. Prognostic factors in ALS: a critical review. Amyotroph Lateral Scler. 2009 Oct-Dec;10(5–6):310–23.

de Carvalho M, Dengler R, Eisen A, England JD, Kaji R, Kimura J, et al. Electrodiagnostic criteria for diagnosis of ALS. Clin Neurophysiol. 2008 Mar;119(3):497–503. Epub 2007 Dec 27.

Dorst J, Ludolph AC, Huebers A. Disease-modifying and symptomatic treatment of amyotrophic lateral sclerosis. Ther Adv Neurol Disord. 2017 Oct 9;11:1756285617734734.

Hobson EV, McDermott CJ. Supportive and symptomatic management of amyotrophic lateral sclerosis. Nat Rev Neurol. 2016 Sep;12(9):526–38. Epub 2016 Aug 12.

Jackson CE, McVey AL, Rudnicki S, Dimachkie MM, Barohn RJ. Symptom management and end-of-life care in amyotrophic lateral sclerosis. Neurol Clin. 2015 Nov;33(4):889–908.

Krivickas LS. Amyotrophic lateral sclerosis and other motor neuron diseases. Phys Med Rehabil Clin N Am. 2003 May;14(2):327–45.

Miller RG, Jackson CE, Kasarskis EJ, England JD, Forshew D, Johnston W, et al; Quality Standards Subcommittee of the American Academy of Neurology. Practice parameter update: the care of the patient with amyotrophic lateral sclerosis: drug, nutritional, and respiratory therapies (an evidence-based review): report of the Quality Standards Subcommittee of the American Academy of Neurology. Neurology. 2009 Oct 13;73(15):1218–26. Errata in: Neurology. 2010 Mar 2;74(9):781. Neurology. 2009 Dec 15;73(24):2134.

Mitsumoto H, Rabkin JG. Palliative care for patients with amyotrophic lateral sclerosis: "prepare for the worst and hope for the best." JAMA. 2007 Jul 11;298(2):207–16.

Niedermeyer S, Murn M, Choi PJ. Respiratory failure in amyotrophic lateral sclerosis. Chest. 2019 Feb;155(2):401–8. Epub 2018 Jul 7.

Petrov D, Mansfield C, Moussy A, Hermine O. ALS clinical trials review: 20 years of failure. Are we any closer to registering a new treatment? Front Aging Neurosci. 2017 Mar 22;9:68.

Rabinstein AA. Noninvasive ventilation for neuromuscular respiratory failure: when to use and when to avoid. Curr Opin Crit Care. 2016 Apr;22(2):94–9.

Radunovic A, Annane D, Rafiq MK, Mustfa N. Mechanical ventilation for amyotrophic lateral sclerosis/motor neuron disease. Cochrane Database Syst Rev. 2013 Mar 28;(3):CD004427. Update in: Cochrane Database Syst Rev. 2017 Oct 06;10:CD004427.
Russ KB, Phillips MC, Wilcox CM, Peter S. Percutaneous endoscopic gastrostomy in amyotrophic lateral sclerosis. Am J Med Sci. 2015 Aug;350(2):95–7.
Traynor BJ, Codd MB, Corr B, Forde C, Frost E, Hardiman O. Amyotrophic lateral sclerosis mimic syndromes: a population-based study. Arch Neurol. 2000 Jan;57(1):109–13.
Tripodoro VA, De Vito EL. What does end stage in neuromuscular diseases mean? Key approach-based transitions. Curr Opin Support Palliat Care. 2015 Dec;9(4):361–8.
Vianello A, Arcaro G, Palmieri A, Ermani M, Braccioni F, Gallan F, et al. Survival and quality of life after tracheostomy for acute respiratory failure in patients with amyotrophic lateral sclerosis. J Crit Care. 2011 Jun;26(3):329.e7–14. Epub 2010 Jul 23.
Vajda A, McLaughlin RL, Heverin M, Thorpe O, Abrahams S, Al-Chalabi A, et al. Genetic testing in ALS: a survey of current practices. Neurology. 2017 Mar 7;88(10):991–9. Epub 2017 Feb 3.

Rhabdomyolysis and Toxic Myopathies

JUSTIN C. KAO, MB, ChB; MARGHERITA MILONE, MD, PhD

Goals

- Describe major primary myopathies in the intensive care unit.
- Describe myotoxic drugs.
- Describe diagnosis and management of rhabdomyolysis.

Introduction

Myopathies in patients in the intensive care unit are comparatively rare and often are due to critical illness (rhabdomyolysis, critical illness myopathy). Rhabdomyolysis is commonly a consequence of continuous muscle activity, such as in status epilepticus and serotonin syndrome. Toxic myopathies are caused by drug exposure. Recognition and management of these 2 major myopathies are discussed.

Rhabdomyolysis

Rhabdomyolysis is a potentially life-threatening condition that is due to acute muscle fiber necrosis and leaking of its contents, including electrolytes, myoglobin, and other sarcoplasmic proteins such as creatine kinase (CK), into the bloodstream. Rhabdomyolysis is defined as an acute increase of the serum CK level accompanied by acute onset of 1 or more of the following clinical features: myalgia, muscle edema, muscle weakness, worsening of preexisting weakness, and myoglobinuria (pigmenturia without hematuria). Rhabdomyolysis is followed by clinical improvement and return of the CK level to baseline. Although there is no consensus on the cutoff CK value for defining an episode of rhabdomyolysis, the most recent literature suggests a serum CK level of 10 times more than baseline or higher.

Epidemiology

Information is limited on the incidence of rhabdomyolysis in the general population. Mild cases of rhabdomyolysis probably pass unrecognized. A study of military trainees at Lackland Air Force Base in the southern United States suggested an incidence of 22.2 cases per 100,000 trainees per year, but that study targeted a very select population, used a much lower CK cutoff value than that in other studies (5 times greater than the upper limit of normal), and did not investigate the possibility of underlying inherited myopathies. The incidence in the intensive-care-unit population is unknown.

Pathophysiology

The cause of rhabdomyolysis is heterogeneous, but the final common pathway is the result of either direct injury to the sarcolemma or depletion of adenosine triphosphate (ATP) within the myofibers. The latter causes dysfunction of the Na^+/K^+ ATPase and Ca^{2+}ATPase pumps, which normally maintain a low level of sarcoplasmic calcium at rest. Dysfunction of such pumps results in sarcoplasmic hypercalcemia and persistent muscle fiber contraction with further energy depletion. The downstream effect is activation of calcium-dependent proteases and phospholipases. This leads to cytoskeletal and membrane protein destruction, lysosomal digestion of the myofiber contents, and, ultimately, death of the myofiber. When trauma is a major factor in rhabdomyolysis, ischemia and subsequent reperfusion also contribute to muscle necrosis.

Clinical Features and Laboratory Tests

Rhabdomyolysis is characterized by acute onset of muscle pain, weakness, or swelling. Myoglobinuria may lead to cola- or tea-colored urine, and this finding often corresponds with a CK level of about 100,000 U/L. If the

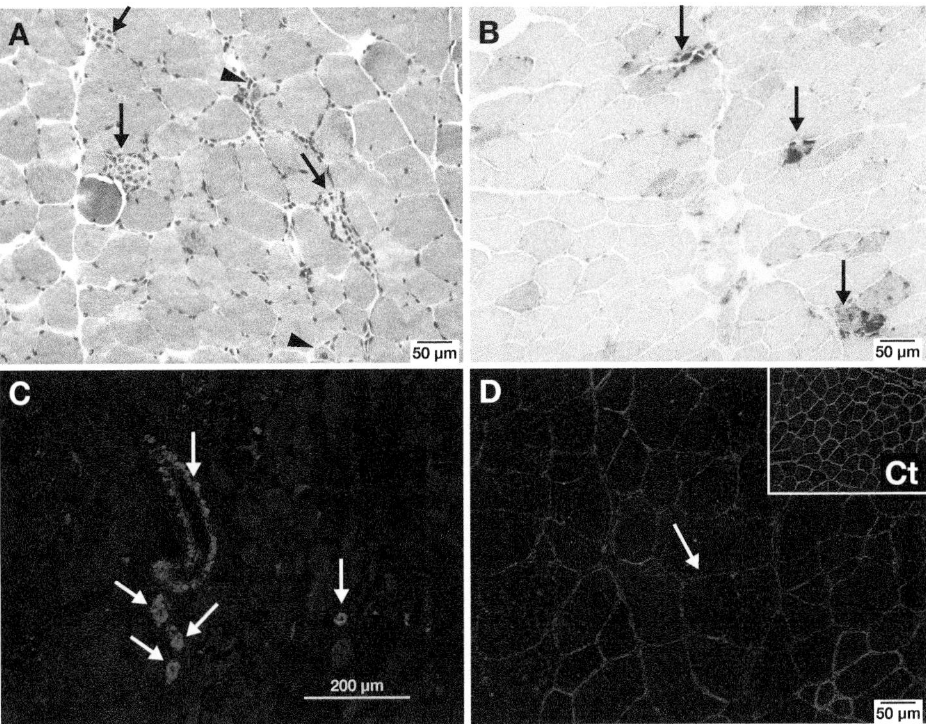

Figure 96.1. Photomicrographs of Muscle Biopsy Specimens From Patients With Rhabdomyolysis. A and B, Specimen obtained a few days after the onset of rhabdomyolysis shows numerous necrotic muscle fibers (arrows) and scattered regenerating fibers (arrowheads) (A, hematoxylin-eosin). Macrophages invading necrotic muscle fibers stain red in acid phosphatase (B). C, Amyloid deposits (arrows) are present within the wall of intramuscular blood vessels of a patient with muscular dystrophy due to anoctamin-5 mutations who had manifestations of rhabdomyolysis (Congo red, viewed under rhodamine optics). D, Sarcolemmal immunoreactivity for α-dystroglycan is reduced (arrow) compared with control (Ct, insert) in a patient with muscular dystrophy due to α-dystroglycanopathy who had an episode of rhabdomyolysis in association with baseline mild weakness.

rhabdomyolysis is mild or the urine myoglobin content is less than 100 mg/dL, urine discoloration may be absent and myoglobinuria may pass undetected. Rhabdomyolysis can occur once in a lifetime in otherwise healthy persons or recur. Recurrent rhabdomyolysis suggests an underlying myopathy. In such cases, patients may be asymptomatic between episodes of rhabdomyolysis or have baseline myopathic symptoms. When patients have baseline weakness and hyperCKemia due to a chronic myopathy (eg, muscular dystrophy), acute exacerbation of the known weakness and further increase of CK values (more than 10 times the baseline value) define rhabdomyolysis.

In addition to CK, other muscle enzymes, including aldolase, lactate dehydrogenase, alanine aminotransferase, and aspartate aminotransferase, increase in serum during rhabdomyolysis. A normal serum γ-glutamyltransferase value in association with increased values for CK, aspartate aminotransferase, and alanine aminotransferase suggests a myopathic origin of the increases in aspartate aminotransferase and alanine aminotransferase and is not suggestive of and an associated hepatopathy.

Needle electromyography shows myopathic changes (early recruitment, low-amplitude and short-duration motor unit potentials) with abnormal spontaneous muscle activity (fibrillation potentials and positive sharp waves).

Muscle biopsy shows scattered necrotic muscle fibers and, depending on the stage of rhabdomyolysis, a variable number of regenerating fibers (Figure 96.1). A few inflammatory cells can be observed, often in the vicinity of necrotic fibers. However, muscle biopsy is usually not helpful in the acute phase, and at least a month should pass from the time of rhabdomyolysis before performing biopsy. In the acute phase, extensive muscle necrosis may obscure underlying structural abnormalities that might indicate the cause of rhabdomyolysis. In addition, biochemical studies to search for enzyme deficiency that may be responsible for a metabolic myopathy (eg, carnitine palmitoyltransferase 2), are more reliable outside the acute phase of rhabdomyolysis.

Etiology

The cause of rhabdomyolysis is heterogeneous and can be acquired or inherited. An acquired factor causes the

Table 96.1 • Acquired Causes of Rhabdomyolysis

Cause	Example
Intense exertion	Marathon running, military training, status epilepticus, tetanus
Trauma	Crush syndrome, prolonged muscle pressure, burns, hypothermia
Ischemia	Arterial embolism or occlusion, compartment syndrome, sickle cell disease, DIC
Endocrine, metabolic, electrolyte defects	Hypothyroidism; hypokalemia, hypophosphatemia, hyponatremia, or hypernatremia associated with underlying endocrinopathy; acquired or inherited renal tubular dysfunction resulting in profound hypokalemia
Infections	Bacterial (*Escherichia coli, Salmonella, Streptococcus, Staphylococcus,* tetanus, vibrio, *Listeria, Leptospira, Legionella, Coxiella, Brucella, Mycoplasma*) Viral (adenovirus, CMV, coxsackievirus, enterovirus, EBV, HIV, HSV, influenza, measles, VZV) Others (*Plasmodium*)
Drugs and toxins	Statins, alone or in combination with other drugs (eg, fibrates, amiodarone, macrolide antibiotics, protease inhibitors, colchicine, daptomycin, fluconazole, tacrolimus, or cyclosporine) Antidepressants: tricyclic, venlafaxine, sertraline, escitalopram Antipsychotics: aripriprazole, clozapine, haloperidol, risperidone, quetiapine Antiretrovirals: tenofovir/abacavir, raltegavir Aminocaproic acid Colchicine + clarithromycin, colchicine + tacrolimus Daptomycin Interferon alpha Illicit drugs including amphetamines, heroin, cocaine, LSD, ecstasy Venoms: snake, spider, and others
Inflammatory, autoimmune	Myositis, paraneoplastic, necrotizing autoimmune myopathy

Abbreviations: CMV, cytomegalovirus; DIC, disseminated intravascular coagulation; EBV, Epstein-Barr virus; HSV, herpes simplex virus; LSD, lysergic acid diethylamide; VZV, varicella zoster virus.

rhabdomyolysis in more than 75% of cases, and more than 1 acquired trigger is identified in about 60% of cases. Also, acquired and inherited causes can coexist in a patient and be responsible for the muscle necrosis.

Acquired Causes

The acquired causes of rhabdomyolysis are summarized in Table 96.1. Muscle trauma from crush injuries, prolonged pressure, or intense exertion can lead to rhabdomyolysis. Trauma can cause direct muscle injury from rupture of the sarcolemma and consequent entry of ionized calcium into the sarcoplasm. Physical exertion can be involuntary, as in status epilepticus.

Drug exposure, including prescribed medications and illicit substances, can cause rhabdomyolysis. In several studies, alcohol and illicit drugs were identified as triggers for rhabdomyolysis in 30% to 35% of patients hospitalized for rhabdomyolysis.

Among prescribed medications, statins can trigger rhabdomyolysis. Statins are widely prescribed and, although minor adverse effects such as myalgias are common, only rarely (approximately 1 in 10,000 treated persons per year) do they cause serious muscle damage manifesting with weakness and an increased CK level. Statin-induced rhabdomyolysis occurs at an estimated rate of 0.4 per 10,000 person-years. Its risk can increase in association with hypothyroidism (which itself can trigger rhabdomyolysis), adjunctive treatment with other cholesterol-lowering agents (especially fibrates), coexisting therapy with other medications metabolized by the cytochrome P450 isozyme 3A4, or predisposing genetic background. Statin-induced rhabdomyolysis is self-limiting and should be distinguished from the less frequent statin-associated necrotizing autoimmune myopathy, which does not resolve with discontinuation of drug use and requires aggressive immunotherapy. Measurement of antibodies directed against 3-hydroxy-3-methylglutaryl-coenzyme A reductase may be helpful for differentiating between the 2 conditions. Their presence suggests necrotizing autoimmune myopathy, but their absence does not exclude it.

Numerous other prescription medications have been implicated in rhabdomyolysis. Antipsychotic and antidepressant drugs, especially selective serotonin reuptake inhibitors, can cause rhabdomyolysis in neuroleptic malignant syndrome and serotonin syndrome, respectively. Exposure to anesthetic agents can cause malignant hyperthermia with rhabdomyolysis in patients with specific underlying genetic defects.

Inherited Causes

In an otherwise asymptomatic patient with an isolated episode of rhabdomyolysis, especially if the acquired trigger is identified, no further investigations are usually needed, and the risk of recurrence is low. Inherited causes should be considered in cases of 1) recurrent rhabdomyolysis; 2) rhabdomyolysis provoked by minimal exertion, fever, heat exposure, or fasting; 3) a personal or family history of malignant hyperthermia; 4) symptoms suggestive of myopathy outside the episode of rhabdomyolysis, including exertional myalgia, muscle cramps, muscle weakness, muscle atrophy, or hypertrophy and baseline hyperCKemia; 5) a personal history of nonischemic cardiomyopathy; and 6) a family history of inherited myopathy. The presence of any of these features should trigger a diagnostic workup for an inherited myopathy, even in the presence of an external trigger for the rhabdomyolysis.

Inherited myopathies manifesting with rhabdomyolysis and clinical features that may serve as clues to the diagnosis are summarized in Table 96.2. In addition to metabolic myopathies and mitochondrial disorders, rhabdomyolysis

Table 96.2 • Inherited Myopathies Causing Rhabdomyolysis and Clues to Diagnosis

Disorder	Clinical Clues	Serum[a] and Urine Biomarkers	Muscle Biopsy Findings
Disorders of glycogen/glucose metabolism Myophosphorylase (McArdle disease, GSD V), phosphofructokinase (Tarui disease, GSD VII) Phosphorylase b kinase (GSD IXa1) Phosphoglycerate kinase (GSD IX) Phosphoglycerate mutase (GSD X), lactate DH (GSD XI) Phosphoglucomutase 1 deficiency (GSD XIV)	Rhabdomyolysis triggered by brief, intense activity; second-wind phenomenon McArdle disease: exercise-induced, electrically silent cramps Tarui disease: hemolytic anemia and arthritic gout Lactate DH deficiency: obstetric complications due to uterine stiffness requiring cesarean section	McArdle disease, Tarui disease, and phosphorylase b kinase deficiency: CK often increased Tarui disease: increased bilirubin, haptoglobin, reticulocyte count, and uric acid	McArdle disease: absent myophosphorylase reactivity Tarui disease: glycogen accumulation, ± polyglucosan bodies Phosphoglycerate mutase deficiency: tubular aggregates
Disorders of lipid metabolism Carnitine palmitoyltransferase II; very long, long, medium, short, multiple-chain acyl-coenzyme A DH; carnitine; electron transfer flavoprotein and flavoprotein DH; trifunctional enzyme deficiency	Rhabdomyolysis triggered by prolonged exercise, fasting or febrile illness Short-chain acyl-coenzyme A DH deficiency: PEO, ptosis, facial weakness	CK normal between attacks, except in multiple-chain acyl-coenzyme A DH deficiency Abnormal plasma acylcarnitines and urine organic acids	Normal or increased lipid content
Mitochondrial myopathies Defects in mitochondrial DNA or nuclear genes affecting mitochondrial function	PEO, peripheral neuropathy, strokelike events, seizures, SN hearing loss	CK normal or mildly increased Lactate normal or increased	Ragged red fibers, ragged blue fibers, cytochrome c oxidase–negative fibers
Muscular dystrophies Dystrophin, α-dystroglycan, anoctamin-5, caveolin-3, calpain-3, sarcoglycanopathies	Dystrophinopathy: calf hypertrophy, cardiomyopathy Anoctamin-5 myopathy: inability to walk on toes Caveolin-3 myopathy: rippling muscle	CK increased	Often dystrophic features Anoctamin-5 myopathy: interstitial amyloid Caveolin-3 myopathy: no caveolin-3 sarcolemmal immunoreactivity
Ryanodine receptor 1 myopathies	Malignant hyperthermia	CK normal or increased	Central cores, multiple minicores, or normal
Lipin 1 myopathy	Recurrent rhabdomyolysis in children, onset before age 6 y Fever and fasting common triggers		Lipid droplets

Abbreviations: CK, creatine kinase; DH, dehydrogenase; GSD, glycogen storage disease; PEO, progressive external ophthalmoplegia; SN, sensorineural; ±, with or without.

[a] The creatine kinase value refers to measurement between episodes of rhabdomyolysis.

can occur in certain muscular dystrophies. In general, a normal CK value between episodes of rhabdomyolysis indicates a metabolic myopathy over a muscular dystrophy, but persistent hyperCKemia is often detected in McArdle disease (myophosphorylase deficiency). Fixed weakness and other clinical features, such as calf muscle enlargement, calf muscle weakness, muscle rippling, or muscle biopsy findings, can help with diagnosis of the specific underlying myopathy, although often biochemical and genetic studies are needed.

Ryanodine receptor 1 is a gene known to cause a congenital myopathy called central core disease and malignant hyperthermia. Mutations in this gene are increasingly recognized as a cause of isolated rhabdomyolysis and may account for up to a third of otherwise unexplained cases. Patients may or may not have a history of malignant hyperthermia. In myopathy caused by this gene, rhabdomyolysis can be unprovoked or occur after intense exercise. When associated with exercise, it is often delayed by more than 24 hours from the time of physical exertion.

Diagnosis

The combination of acute muscle weakness, myalgia, muscle edema, and increased CK level suggests rhabdomyolysis. The most useful biochemical marker of rhabdomyolysis is a CK value more than 10 times the upper limit of normal, with or without myoglobinuria. The serum myoglobin level increases rapidly after muscle injury, but it has a very short half-life of 2 to 3 hours. It is cleared rapidly through renal excretion and catabolism to bilirubin. Indeed, a normal myoglobin level can be reestablished within 24 hours of muscle injury, and most patients with rhabdomyolysis do not seek medical attention during this time frame. Urine myoglobin, however, can pass undetected if the rhabdomyolysis is mild and the urine myoglobin level does not exceed 100 mg/dL.

In contrast, serum CK has a much longer half-life of 36 hours. The CK level starts to increase 2 to 12 hours after muscle injury and peaks at day 3 to 5 before declining over the subsequent days. Thus, it is a more useful and reliable biochemical marker of muscle injury and severity.

Measurement of other serum and urine biomarkers can be helpful for identifying the cause of rhabdomyolysis (Table 96.2).

Management

The immediate management of rhabdomyolysis is largely directed at preventing its complications. The most concerning complication is acute renal failure, which negatively affects prognosis. Other potential complications of rhabdomyolysis include electrolyte imbalance, particularly hyperkalemia; compartment syndrome; and disseminated intravascular coagulation.

Muscle necrosis results in third spacing and hypovolemia, which in turn contribute to the development of renal failure. The precipitation of myoglobin in distal renal tubules can cause obstruction, contributing further to renal injury. The mainstay of acute management is early intravascular volume expansion with aggressive fluid replacement. This remains the only intervention of clinically proven benefit to date. Fluids, typically 0.9% saline intravenously, should be given at the rate of 1.5 L/h and titrated with the goal of maintaining a urine output of 200 to 300 mL/h. Fluid requirements may be as high as 10 L per day, depending on the severity of rhabdomyolysis. Fluid administration should be continued until the CK level has decreased substantially.

Electrolytes should be carefully monitored. Hyperkalemia, which can occur early and even precede the development of kidney injury, must be treated aggressively because of the risk of cardiac arrhythmias. In addition, monitoring for metabolic acidosis is essential to prevent worsening of the hyperkalemia. Hypocalcemia usually does not require treatment unless it is symptomatic or associated with severe hyperkalemia. However, hypercalcemia during improvement of the kidney function is suggestive of acute injury secondary to rhabdomyolysis and is mainly due to mobilization of calcium accumulated in muscle and correction of the hyperphosphatemia. Hyperkalemia may have to be treated with diuretics, insulin with glucose, and calcium gluconate.

Supportive renal replacement therapy may be necessary for severe kidney injury accompanied by severe hyperkalemia, acidosis, or volume overload. Because of the small size of myoglobin, conventional dialysis is not very effective for its removal. Moreover, there are no data to suggest that removing myoglobin with conventional dialysis or continuous hemofiltration is of clinical benefit.

When there is concern about compartment syndrome, early orthopedic consultation and monitoring of compartment pressures are helpful. Decompressive fasciotomy should be considered when intramuscular pressures exceed 50 mm Hg or are consistently around 30 to 50 mm Hg for longer than 6 hours.

The benefit of urine alkalization with sodium bicarbonate to a target pH of 6.5 is not well established. Although urine alkalization may have been beneficial in a subgroup of patients with CK levels more than 30,000 U/L, it did not prevent renal failure, need for dialysis, or death in 1 large study of trauma-associated rhabdomyolysis.

The use of diuretics, including mannitol, is likewise controversial, and their benefits have not been established in clinical trials. If mannitol is administered, plasma osmolality should be closely monitored and use of the drug discontinued if the osmolal gap increases to more than 55 mOsm per kilogram. Loop diuretics should be used similarly to what is recommended for acute renal failure due to other causes.

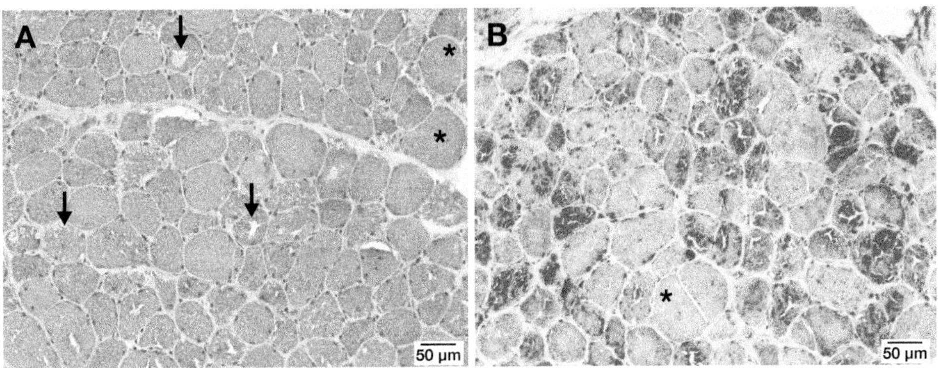

Figure 96.2. Muscle Biopsy Specimens From Patients With Myopathy Due to Hydroxychloroquine Toxicity. A, The majority of muscle fibers harbor multiple vacuoles (arrows), which are not present in the few normal muscle fibers (asterisks) (hematoxylin-eosin). B, The vacuoles overreact for acid phosphatase, staining bright red (asterisk indicates normal muscle fibers).

Toxic Myopathies

Many substances, including prescribed medications, can have adverse effects on muscle. Drugs can cause myotoxicity after a few weeks of treatment or as a result of cumulative effect. Statins are known to cause toxic necrotizing myopathy that, in severe cases, can be complicated by myoglobinuria. The immunophilins tacrolimus and cyclosporine can also cause a similar toxic myopathy. Hypertrophic cardiomyopathy can rarely accompany tacrolimus-induced myopathy. The myopathy develops within a few months of starting therapy with tacrolimus and cyclosporine, whereas it can develop years after therapy with statins.

Corticosteroids are common causes of myopathy through impaired protein synthesis or increased catabolism. The risk of corticosteroid-induced myopathy is greatest with chronic, high-dose exposure (prednisone dose 30 mg/day or more), but the myopathy can also occur within weeks of starting treatment. Normal CK level and lack of abnormal spontaneous electromyographic muscle activity in a patient taking corticosteroids and new weakness, or worsening baseline weakness, favor corticosteroid-induced myopathy.

Chloroquine, hydroxychloroquine, amiodarone, and colchicine can cause myopathy or neuromyopathy. In the presence of coexisting peripheral neuropathy, electromyography will show myopathic changes in proximal muscles and neurogenic changes distally (Figure 96.2). Chloroquine and hydroxychloroquine can also cause cardiomyopathy.

The antiretroviral azidothymidine, also called zidovudine, can induce a mitochondrial myopathy, but it is now less frequent with newer antiretroviral therapy. Unlike HIV-associated myositis, muscle biopsy shows no inflammation, but signs of mitochondrial dysfunction are suggested by the presence of ragged red, ragged blue, and cytochrome c oxidase–negative fibers.

Clinical and Laboratory Features

The symptoms of a toxic myopathy are generally indistinguishable from those of other myopathies. Therefore, a careful review of the medication history and attention to the temporal relationship between symptom onset and introduction of the drug is crucial for diagnosis.

CK levels can be normal or increased. Electromyography shows myopathic changes with or without fibrillation potentials. Detection of an associated peripheral neuropathy may signal associated peripheral nerve toxicity (eg, amiodarone). Muscle histopathologic findings can shed light on the offending drug.

Treatment

Often, muscle strength gradually improves after discontinuing use of the offending agent, but improvement may take many months. In corticosteroid-induced myopathy, dose reduction and alternate-day regimen, of the drug and exercise are helpful.

Summary

- Rhabdomyolysis is acute muscle fiber necrosis, characterized by acute onset of muscle pain, weakness, swelling, and increased CK level to more than 10 times the upper limit of normal, with or without myoglobinuria.
- Because of its longer half-life, CK is a more reliable biochemical marker of muscle injury than myoglobin.
- The cause of rhabdomyolysis is heterogeneous and can be acquired or inherited.

- Recurrent rhabdomyolysis suggests an underlying inherited myopathy.
- Muscular dystrophies and congenital myopathies, in addition to metabolic myopathies, can manifest with rhabdomyolysis.
- Acute renal injury and hyperkalemia are the most serious acute complications from rhabdomyolysis. Early intravascular volume expansion with aggressive fluid replacement is the mainstay of management.
- Toxic myopathies caused by prescribed medications generally improve with discontinuation of use of the medication, although improvement can take many months.
- Statin-triggered rhabdomyolysis must be distinguished from statin-associated necrotizing autoimmune myopathy, which requires aggressive immunotherapy.

SUGGESTED READING

Alpers JP, Jones LK Jr. Natural history of exertional rhabdomyolysis: a population-based analysis. Muscle Nerve. 2010 Oct;42(4):487–91.

Bosch X, Poch E, Grau JM. Rhabdomyolysis and acute kidney injury. N Engl J Med. 2009 Jul 2;361(1):62–72. Erratum in: N Engl J Med. 2011 May 19;364(20):1982.

Dlamini N, Voermans NC, Lillis S, Stewart K, Kamsteeg EJ, Drost G, et al. Mutations in RYR1 are a common cause of exertional myalgia and rhabdomyolysis. Neuromuscul Disord. 2013 Jul;23(7):540–8. Epub 2013 Apr 28.

Giannoglou GD, Chatzizisis YS, Misirli G. The syndrome of rhabdomyolysis: pathophysiology and diagnosis. Eur J Intern Med. 2007 Mar;18(2):90–100.

Kassardjian CD, Lennon VA, Alfugham NB, Mahler M, Milone M. Clinical features and treatment outcomes of necrotizing autoimmune myopathy. JAMA Neurol. 2015 Sep;72(9):996–1003.

Katzberg HD, Kassardjian CD. Toxic and endocrine myopathies. Continuum (Minneap Minn). 2016 Dec;22(6, Muscle and Neuromuscular Junction Disorders):1815–28.

Lahoria R, Milone M. Rhabdomyolysis featuring muscular dystrophies. J Neurol Sci. 2016 Feb 15;361:29–33. Epub 2015 Dec 10.

Liewluck T, Tian X, Wong LJ, Pestronk A. Dystrophinopathy mimicking metabolic myopathies. Neuromuscul Disord. 2015 Aug;25(8):653–7. Epub 2015 Apr 11.

Lilleker JB, Keh YS, Roncaroli F, Sharma R, Roberts M. Metabolic myopathies: a practical approach. Pract Neurol. 2018 Feb;18(1):14–26. Epub 2017 Dec 9.

Mackay MT, Kornberg AJ, Shield LK, Dennett X. Benign acute childhood myositis: laboratory and clinical features. Neurology. 1999 Dec 10;53(9):2127–31.

Mathews KD, Stephan CM, Laubenthal K, Winder TL, Michele DE, Moore SA, et al. Myoglobinuria and muscle pain are common in patients with limb-girdle muscular dystrophy 2I. Neurology. 2011 Jan 11;76(2):194–5.

Nance JR, Mammen AL. Diagnostic evaluation of rhabdomyolysis. Muscle Nerve. 2015 Jun;51(6):793–810. Epub 2015 Mar 14.

Pinal-Fernandez I, Casal-Dominguez M, Mammen AL. Immune-mediated necrotizing myopathy. Curr Rheumatol Rep. 2018 Mar 26;20(4):21.

Pasnoor M, Barohn RJ, Dimachkie MM. Toxic myopathies. Neurol Clin. 2014 Aug;32(3):647–70.

Perreault S, Birca A, Piper D, Nadeau A, Gauvin F, Vanasse M. Transient creatine phosphokinase elevations in children: a single-center experience. J Pediatr. 2011 Oct;159(4):682–5. Epub 2011 May 17.

Scalco RS, Gardiner AR, Pitceathly RD, Hilton-Jones D, Schapira AH, Turner C, et al. CAV3 mutations causing exercise intolerance, myalgia and rhabdomyolysis: expanding the phenotypic spectrum of caveolinopathies. Neuromuscul Disord. 2016 Aug;26(8):504–10. Epub 2016 May 11.

Tobon A. Metabolic myopathies. Continuum (Minneap Minn). 2013 Dec;19(6 Muscle Disease):1571–97.

Warren JD, Blumbergs PC, Thompson PD. Rhabdomyolysis: a review. Muscle Nerve. 2002 Mar;25(3):332–47.

Zutt R, van der Kooi AJ, Linthorst GE, Wanders RJ, de Visser M. Rhabdomyolysis: review of the literature. Neuromuscul Disord. 2014 Aug;24(8):651–9. Epub 2014 May 21.

Myopathy and Neuropathy Acquired in the Intensive Care Unit

PRIYA S. DHAWAN, MD; JENNIFER A. TRACY, MD

Goals

- Discuss the clinical features of critical illness polyneuropathy and critical illness myopathy.
- Discuss the evaluation and differential diagnosis of critical illness polyneuropathy and critical illness myopathy.
- Discuss concepts of pathophysiology of critical illness polyneuropathy and critical illness myopathy.
- Discuss the management and outcome of critical illness polyneuropathy and critical illness myopathy.

Introduction

Acquired weakness in critically ill patients is common, affecting between one-third to one-half of patients in the intensive care unit (ICU). Exposure to simultaneous stressors such as metabolic derangements, fluid and electrolyte shifts, infection, catabolic stress, and medications put patients in the ICU at risk for damage to both nerve and skeletal muscle with substantial and often lasting morbidity. It is typically after medical stabilization however, as weaning from mechanical ventilation or sedative medications is attempted, that weakness is appreciated.

Critical illness polyneuropathy (CIP) is a length-dependent, axonal peripheral neuropathy occurring in patients in the ICU and unrelated to the primary illness. Critical illness myopathy (CIM) is an ICU-associated muscle disorder occurring independently of denervation and uniquely identified by electrophysiologic and histologic characteristics. CIM can occur alone or in concert with CIP; the latter condition is commonly called critical illness neuromyopathy (CINM). Respiratory status can often be compromised in these conditions, and the severity of diaphragm involvement is not always commensurate with the severity of limb involvement.

Increased ICU survival rates have unmasked the high incidence of CIM and CIP as more patients graduate from ICUs to rehabilitation units. Weakness in the ICU is 2 to 3 times more likely to be from CINM than from primary neuromuscular disorders such as Guillain-Barré syndrome or motor neuron disease. In 1 study, women were 3 to 4 times as likely as men to have development of CINM, possibly as a result of smaller baseline muscle mass. Survivors of critical illness often have weakness for months to years after discharge, and many of these have persistent impairments.

Critical Illness Polyneuropathy

Clinical Features

CIP is a symmetric, length-dependent, axonal, sensorimotor peripheral neuropathy causing limb weakness (distal greater than proximal) and affecting respiratory function. The clinical presentation varies from mild to severe and may be predominantly respiratory failure (ie, failure to wean from mechanical ventilation). Facial muscles are affected in only very severe cases, and extraocular muscles are spared. Limb weakness typically is more severe in the lower extremities, and sensory abnormalities are often subclinical. Large and small sensory fibers are affected with length-dependent defects to pain, temperature, light touch, and vibration. Deep tendon reflexes may be present initially but ultimately will be reduced to absent.

In the encephalopathic or sedated patient for whom sensory examination is challenging, compression of a nail bed may elicit a grimace, but without limb withdrawal, as typically occurs with noxious stimuli. However, severe weakness can also contribute to these reduced physical manifestations of pain. Electrodiagnostic testing is often required to establish sensory involvement and classify the weakness as neuropathic.

Limb strength is quantified by bedside manual muscle testing or handgrip dynamometry, and respiratory muscle strength is quantified by maximal inspiratory pressure, maximal expiratory pressure, and vital capacity. Low respiratory scores typically correlate with limb muscle weakness and are associated with increases in both mortality and long-term morbidity. CIP is an independent risk factor for failure to wean from a ventilator and prolonged mechanical ventilation, but diaphragm weakness occurs frequently in any mechanically ventilated patient.

Electrodiagnostic Studies

Nerve conduction studies should include examination of upper and lower limb motor and sensory nerves. Nerve conduction protocols may vary, but typical motor studies include peroneal, tibial, and ulnar nerves, and sensory nerve evaluation includes sural nerve and at least 1 upper extremity sensory study (commonly median or ulnar). Repetitive stimulation studies should be considered when neuromuscular junction disease is suspected as an alternative cause. Phrenic nerve conduction studies should be considered when respiratory involvement is suspected; however, ultrasonography of the diaphragm to evaluate for thickness and excursion is also a good option as a noninvasive, informative, and technically less challenging evaluation of the diaphragm. Special attention should be given to ensuring that a patient's temperature is normalized, as decreased body temperature can alter the results of nerve conduction studies. Another technical issue can be an apparent reduction in motor and sensory conduction amplitudes from edema rather than true nerve dysfunction.

In CIP, nerve conduction studies generally show reduction in compound motor action potential and sensory nerve action potential amplitudes, consistent with an axonal process, with preservation (or minimal slowing) of conduction velocity and distal and peak latencies. Amplitudes may be minimally to considerably reduced or absent depending on severity. Absence of demyelinating features and length-dependent electromyographic abnormalities, minimal or no facial weakness, and normal cerebrospinal fluid protein levels are useful for distinguishing weakness of CIP from that of acute inflammatory demyelinating polyradiculoneuropathy or Guillain-Barré syndrome. Importantly, the duration of the compound motor action potential is normal in CIP without accompanying CIM.

Results of needle examination at rest may be normal, particularly early on in the disease process. However, varying degrees of fibrillation potentials are not uncommon. Examination of voluntary motor units, which requires active patient cooperation, is often compromised by a patient's ability to participate in the ICU setting, often related to sedation or encephalopathy. In the earliest phase of a neurogenic process, the primary finding on needle electromyography is reduced recruitment, but motor units ultimately become polyphasic and larger in amplitude and duration as denervation and reinnervation take place. Fibrillation potentials may decrease and motor unit duration may increase as a nerve recovers over time.

Histopathology

Autopsy studies in patients with CIP have shown evidence of axonal degeneration in distal motor and sensory nerves. Nerve biopsies are typically not indicated when CIP is suspected because results may be normal early in the disease course or show varying degrees of axonal loss without considerable interstitial abnormalities. The main indication for nerve biopsy when CIP is suspected is a strong suspicion for an alternative cause for the observed neuropathy (eg, inflammatory-immune or neoplastic or lymphomatous). There is some evidence of reduced intraepidermal nerve fiber density on serial skin biopsies in critically ill patients, supporting a degree of small nerve fiber dysfunction as well. The only central nervous system manifestation is that of anterior horn cell chromatolysis, a consequence of distal axonal damage.

Critical Illness Myopathy

Clinical Features

CIM may present identically to CIP, that is, failure to wean from the ventilator and flaccid limb weakness after removal of sedation. Deep tendon reflexes are generally reduced but present, and results of sensory examination are normal. Electrodiagnostic evaluation is often required to distinguish CIM from CIP. The importance of this distinction is that CIM, in the absence of diffuse muscle fiber necrosis, has a much more favorable prognosis than CIP, and patients often have complete recovery.

Rhabdomyolysis may rarely occur, presenting with flaccid weakness, marked increase in creatine kinase level, myoglobinuria, and muscle biopsy with minimal to moderate fiber necrosis. The prognosis is favorable. However, rarely, patients may present with a diffuse necrotizing myopathy, in which case they fare poorly with prolonged impairments in limb and respiratory function.

Immobility alone (often proportionate to days with mechanical ventilation) results in diffuse muscle wasting and compounds the severity of weakness in patients in the ICU. In this case, results of electromyography and the creatine kinase level are typically normal, and muscle biopsy shows minimal abnormalities or type II fiber atrophy.

Electrodiagnostic Studies

Nerve conduction studies show low-amplitude compound motor action potential with prolongation of its duration, often by 2 to 3 times that of healthy controls. Temporal dispersion, conduction block, and other features of demyelination are absent. Needle examination shows a sparse to moderate degree of fibrillation potentials and small, myopathic motor units. These features improve as a patient improves clinically. As noted under the discussion for CIP, diaphragm evaluation may also be very important from a myopathy standpoint, with use of the same techniques as outlined above.

Histopathology

Muscle biopsy results may be normal in mild cases of ICU-acquired weakness. Patients who are severely affected will have characteristic focal loss of thick (myosin) filaments in nonatrophic fibers, best appreciated on adenosine triphosphate–reaction sections (Figure 97.1). Varying degrees of muscle fiber necrosis may be present, and diffuse necrosis occurs much less commonly. Type II fiber atrophy often accompanies the myopathy. The increase in the creatine kinase level is typically proportional to the degree of muscle fiber necrosis, and thus the level is normal to mildly increased in most cases. When there is an additional component of CIP, features of denervation atrophy (angular, atrophic fibers both histochemically type I and II, atrophic fibers overreacting for nonspecific esterase, target formations, pyknotic clumps of nuclei) may be present on muscle biopsy.

Risk Factors for CIP and CIM

The risk factors for development of CIP and CIM are listed in Box 97.1.

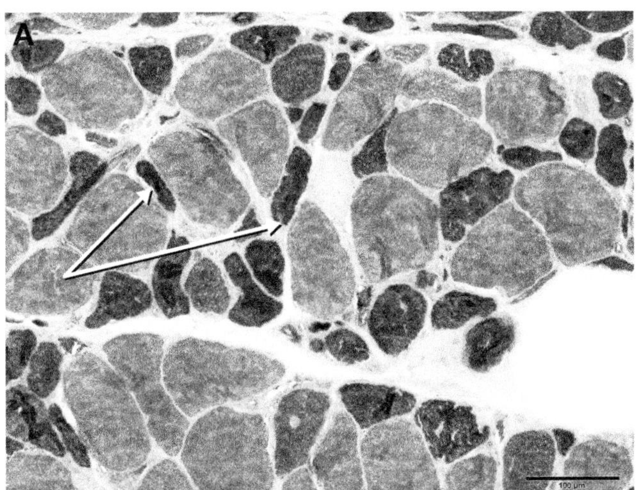

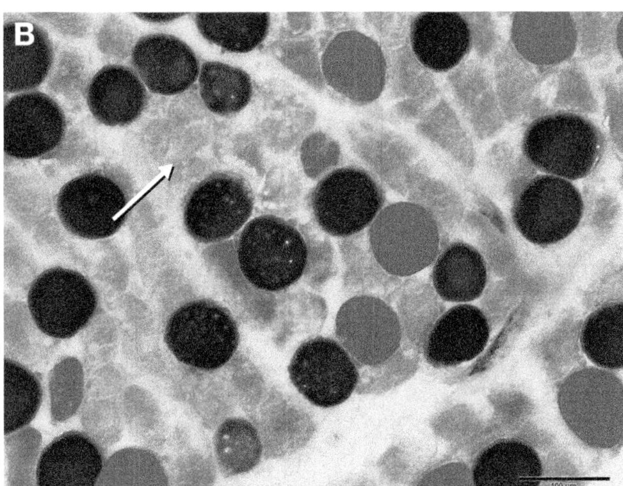

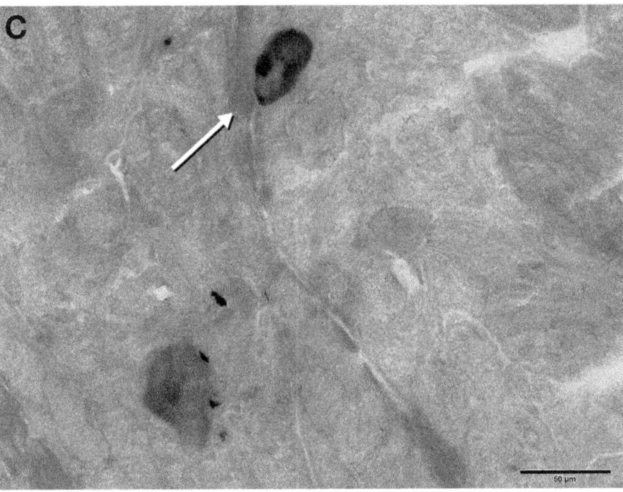

Figure 97.1. Muscle Histopathologic Findings in Critical Illness Myopathy. A, Severe type II atrophy (pH 9.4 adenosine triphosphate reaction). Dark fibers indicate type II fibers. B, Several fibers with total absence of reactivity, intermingled with normally staining type I (brown) and type II (pink) fibers (pH 4.3 adenosine triphosphate reaction). C, Focal loss of myosin staining in a type I fiber (pH 4.3 adenosine triphosphate reaction).

(Courtesy of A. G. Engel, MD, Mayo Clinic, Rochester, Minnesota; used with permission.)

Box 97.1 • Risk Factors for Development of Critical Illness Polyneuropathy and Myopathy

Sepsis
Systemic inflammatory response syndrome
Multiple (>2) organ failure
Glucocorticoid treatment[a]
Prolonged mechanical ventilation (4-7 days)
Prolonged stay in the intensive care unit (>1 wk)
Increased duration and severity of illness
Nondepolarizing neuromuscular blocking agents[a,b]
Immobility
Female sex
Renal failure and renal replacement therapy
Hyperosmolality
Parenteral nutrition
Low serum albumin

[a] The literature has some contradictory data; they may be related to timing, type, and total amount of medication use.

[b] Use of cisatracurium besylate improves survival and reduces ventilation time in patients with acute respiratory distress syndrome.

Pathophysiology of CIP and CIM

Mechanisms behind CIM are widely hypothesized but incompletely understood. The rapid onset and, in many cases, reversibility of deficits, often in the setting of normal histologic appearance, have suggested a functional rather than structural cause for nerve and muscle failure. CIP and CIM are thought to be a consequence of the larger process leading to multiorgan dysfunction and, as a result, are ischemic, cellular, and metabolic in origin.

Impaired muscle and nerve microcirculation during sepsis and multiorgan failure has been suggested as a contributing mechanism in CIM and CIP. Expression of E-selectin (marker of endothelial activation) is increased in epineurial and endoneurial vessels in patients with CIP, and activation of endoneurial leukocytes in association with cytokine production is proposed to cause increased vascular permeability, endoneurial edema, and ischemic hypoxia. Density of perfused versus nonperfused muscle capillaries is reduced in patients with sepsis, a finding that resolves in patients who survive.

Mitochondrial impairment is a known cause of organ damage in critical illness; the resulting reduction in adenosine triphosphate synthesis and generation of energy lead to hypoxia due to damage at the cellular level. The resultant cytopathic hypoxia may contribute to muscle and nerve failure in CINM. Metabolic derangements such as stress hormone secretion with subsequent insulin resistance and hyperglycemia exacerbate endoneurial edema. Intensive glycemic control, although it increases mortality in the ICU, is known to reduce the incidence of CIP.

Early activation of the ubiquitin-proteasome pathway in muscle causing selective myosin loss has been suggested as a relevant mechanism in CIM. Rat models have suggested that an acquired sodium channelopathy, causing both muscle and nerve hypoexcitability, may contribute to functional impairments in CIP and CIM. Depolarized resting membrane potentials and impaired rapid inactivation of sodium channels cause alteration in voltage dependence toward negative potentials.

Diagnostic Approach to CIP and CIM

The diagnostic approach to CIP and CIM is shown in Figure 97.2.

Differential Diagnosis of CIP and CIM

The differential diagnosis for CIP and CIM is listed in Box 97.2.

Management and Prognosis of CIP and CIM

No treatment, aside from intensive glycemic control, which is avoided because of increased mortality in the ICU, has been shown to reduce the incidence or severity of CIM or CIP.

Prevention and management of weakness in critically ill patients are largely supportive and require a paradigm shift from more conventional ideas about the care of patients in the ICU. Previously held beliefs regarding artificially supporting immobilized patients for as long as possible have given way to attempts at earlier weaning of artificial hemodynamic and ventilatory support to allow earlier recovery of a patient's own organ system function. During the past few decades, implementation of early mobilization and physical therapy (even before a patient is clinically stable), daily sedation vacations, regular trials of spontaneous breathing without the ventilator, and intense neurorehabilitation after discharge has gone a long way toward improving outcomes in critically ill patients.

Patients with severe CIP, diffuse necrotizing CIM, or advanced age typically have a poor prognosis, whereas those with rhabdomyolysis, muscle wasting, and the more common thick filament myopathy have a much better prognosis. Improvements can be slow. One study showed that,

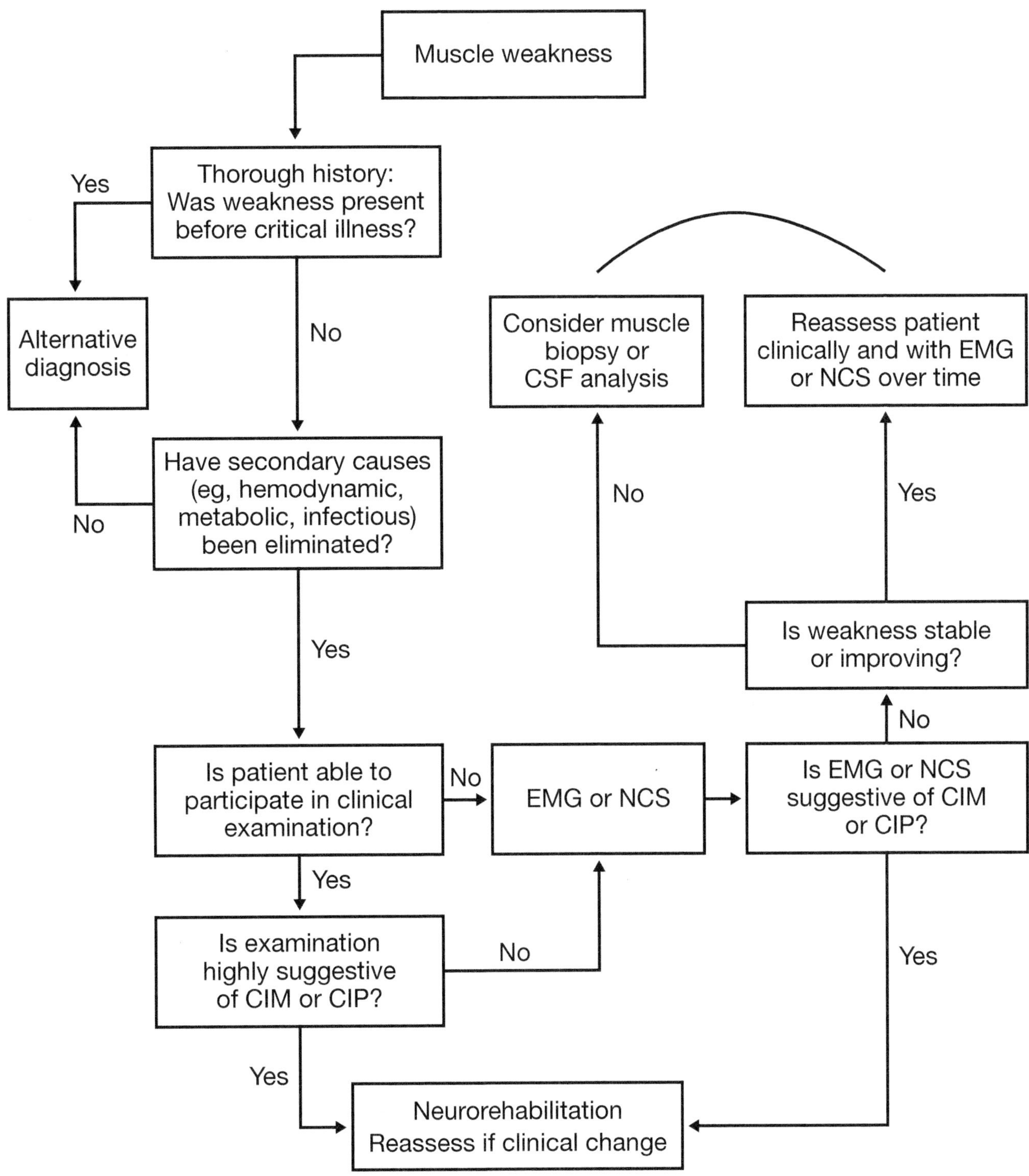

Figure 97.2. Diagnostic Approach to Critical Illness Polyneuropathy (CIP) and Critical Illness Myopathy (CIM). CSF indicates cerebrospinal fluid; EMG, electromyography; NCS, nerve conduction study.

of 15 patients with CIM, CIP, or a combination thereof, by 3 months one-third had normalized muscle strength and two-thirds still had considerable weakness. Patients with isolated CIM had better recovery than those with CIP or combined CIM and CIP. Another study showed that by 12 months after ICU discharge, 88% of patients with CIM and 55% of those with CIM and CIP had normal electrophysiologic findings, but only 50% of the CIM group and

Box 97.2 • Differential Diagnosis for Critical Illness Polyneuropathy and Myopathy

- Guillian-Barré syndrome
- Myasthenic crisis
- Motor neuron disease
- Postsurgical inflammatory neuropathy (many patients in the intensive care unit have had surgery)
- Axial myopathies (ie, adult-onset acid maltase deficiency)
- Metabolic myopathy (ie, hypokalemia, hypophosphatemia)
- Hypermagnesemia causing impaired neuromuscular transmission
- Neuromuscular blocking agents
- Drug-induced myopathies (ie, statins, antiretrovirals, chloroquine)
- Propofol infusion syndrome causing organ failure and rhabdomyolysis or necrotizing myopathy

27% of the CIM and CIP group were determined to have normal physical capacity.

Summary

- CIP and CIM are common causes of muscle weakness in critically ill patients.
- CIP and CIM are important to recognize because they can affect ability to wean from assisted ventilation, duration of ICU stay, and prognosis.
- Clinical and electrophysiologic examinations are important for differentiating CIP and CIM from mimickers that would require other forms of treatment.

SUGGESTED READING

Ali NA, O'Brien JM Jr, Hoffmann SP, Phillips G, Garland A, Finley JC, et al; Midwest Critical Care Consortium. Acquired weakness, handgrip strength, and mortality in critically ill patients. Am J Respir Crit Care Med. 2008 Aug 1;178(3):261–8. Epub 2008 May 29.

Bolton CF. Neuromuscular complications of sepsis. Intensive Care Med. 1993;19 Suppl 2:S58–63.

Bolton CF. Neuromuscular manifestations of critical illness. Muscle Nerve. 2005 Aug;32(2):140–63.

Bolton CF, Laverty DA, Brown JD, Witt NJ, Hahn AF, Sibbald WJ. Critically ill polyneuropathy: electrophysiological studies and differentiation from Guillain-Barré syndrome. J Neurol Neurosurg Psychiatry. 1986 May;49(5):563–73.

Boon AJ, Sekiguchi H, Harper CJ, Strommen JA, Ghahfarokhi LS, Watson JC, et al. Sensitivity and specificity of diagnostic ultrasound in the diagnosis of phrenic neuropathy. Neurology. 2014 Sep 30;83(14):1264–70. Epub 2014 Aug 27.

Bunnell A, Ney J, Gellhorn A, Hough CL. Quantitative neuromuscular ultrasound in intensive care unit-acquired weakness: a systematic review. Muscle Nerve. 2015 Nov;52(5):701–8. Epub 2015 Sep 21.

De Backer D, Ospina-Tascon G, Salgado D, Favory R, Creteur J, Vincent JL. Monitoring the microcirculation in the critically ill patient: current methods and future approaches. Intensive Care Med. 2010 Nov;36(11):1813–25. Epub 2010 Aug 6.

De Jonghe B, Bastuji-Garin S, Durand MC, Malissin I, Rodrigues P, Cerf C, et al; Groupe de Reflexion et d'Etude des Neuromyopathies en Reanimation. Respiratory weakness is associated with limb weakness and delayed weaning in critical illness. Crit Care Med. 2007 Sep;35(9):2007–15.

De Jonghe B, Bastuji-Garin S, Sharshar T, Outin H, Brochard L. Does ICU-acquired paresis lengthen weaning from mechanical ventilation? Intensive Care Med. 2004 Jun;30(6):1117–21. Epub 2004 Feb 6.

De Jonghe B, Sharshar T, Lefaucheur JP, Authier FJ, Durand-Zaleski I, Boussarsar M, et al; Groupe de Reflexion et d'Etude des Neuromyopathies en Reanimation. Paresis acquired in the intensive care unit: a prospective multicenter study. JAMA. 2002 Dec 11;288(22):2859–67.

Dettling-Ihnenfeldt DS, Wieske L, Horn J, Nollet F, van der Schaaf M. Functional recovery in patients with and without intensive care unit-acquired weakness. Am J Phys Med Rehabil. 2017 Apr;96(4):236–42.

Fenzi F, Latronico N, Refatti N, Rizzuto N. Enhanced expression of E-selectin on the vascular endothelium of peripheral nerve in critically ill patients with neuromuscular disorders. Acta Neuropathol. 2003 Jul;106(1):75–82. Epub 2003 Apr 16.

Goodman BP, Harper CM, Boon AJ. Prolonged compound muscle action potential duration in critical illness myopathy. Muscle Nerve. 2009 Dec;40(6):1040–2.

Guarneri B, Bertolini G, Latronico N. Long-term outcome in patients with critical illness myopathy or neuropathy: the Italian multicentre CRIMYNE study. J Neurol Neurosurg Psychiatry. 2008 Jul;79(7):838–41. Epub 2008 Mar 13.

Helliwell TR, Wilkinson A, Griffiths RD, McClelland P, Palmer TE, Bone JM. Muscle fibre atrophy in critically ill patients is associated with the loss of myosin filaments and the presence of lysosomal enzymes and ubiquitin. Neuropathol Appl Neurobiol. 1998 Dec;24(6):507–17.

Hermans G, De Jonghe B, Bruyninckx F, Van den Berghe G. Interventions for preventing critical illness polyneuropathy and critical illness myopathy. Cochrane Database Syst Rev. 2009 Jan 21;(1):CD006832. Update in: Cochrane Database Syst Rev. 2014;1:CD006832.

Hermans G, Wilmer A, Meersseman W, Milants I, Wouters PJ, Bobbaers H, et al. Impact of intensive insulin therapy on neuromuscular complications and ventilator dependency in the medical intensive care unit. Am J Respir Crit Care Med. 2007 Mar 1;175(5):480–9. Epub 2006 Nov 30.

Hough CL, Steinberg KP, Taylor Thompson B, Rubenfeld GD, Hudson LD. Intensive care unit-acquired neuromyopathy and corticosteroids in survivors of persistent ARDS. Intensive Care Med. 2009 Jan;35(1):63–8. Epub 2008 Oct 23.

Jolley SE, Bunnell AE, Hough CL. ICU-Acquired weakness. Chest. 2016 Nov;150(5):1129–40. Epub 2016 Apr 7.

Jung B, Moury PH, Mahul M, de Jong A, Galia F, Prades A, et al. Diaphragmatic dysfunction in patients with ICU-acquired weakness and its impact on extubation failure.

Intensive Care Med. 2016 May;42(5):853–61. Epub 2015 Nov 16.

Koch S, Wollersheim T, Bierbrauer J, Haas K, Morgeli R, Deja M, et al. Long-term recovery in critical illness myopathy is complete, contrary to polyneuropathy. Muscle Nerve. 2014 Sep;50(3):431–6. Epub 2014 Jul 14.

Kress JP, Hall JB. ICU-acquired weakness and recovery from critical illness. N Engl J Med. 2014 Apr 24;370(17):1626–35.

Lachmann G, Morgeli R, Kuenz S, Piper SK, Spies C, Kurpanik M, et al; BIOCOG Consortium. Perioperatively acquired weakness. Anesth Analg. 2019 Mar 4. [Epub ahead of print]

Lacomis D, Giuliani MJ, Van Cott A, Kramer DJ. Acute myopathy of intensive care: clinical, electromyographic, and pathological aspects. Ann Neurol. 1996 Oct;40(4):645–54.

Lacomis D, Zochodne DW, Bird SJ. Critical illness myopathy. Muscle Nerve. 2000 Dec;23(12):1785–8.

Latronico N, Bertolini G, Guarneri B, Botteri M, Peli E, Andreoletti S, et al. Simplified electrophysiological evaluation of peripheral nerves in critically ill patients: the Italian multi-centre CRIMYNE study. Crit Care. 2007;11(1):R11.

Latronico N, Bolton CF. Critical illness polyneuropathy and myopathy: a major cause of muscle weakness and paralysis. Lancet Neurol. 2011 Oct;10(10):931–41.

Latronico N, Fenzi F, Recupero D, Guarneri B, Tomelleri G, Tonin P, et al. Critical illness myopathy and neuropathy. Lancet. 1996 Jun 8;347(9015):1579–82.

Latronico N, Herridge M, Hopkins RO, Angus D, Hart N, Hermans G, et al. The ICM research agenda on intensive care unit-acquired weakness. Intensive Care Med. 2017 Sep;43(9):1270–81. Epub 2017 Mar 13.

Maramattom BV, Wijdicks EF. Acute neuromuscular weakness in the intensive care unit. Crit Care Med. 2006 Nov;34(11):2835–41.

Novak KR, Nardelli P, Cope TC, Filatov G, Glass JD, Khan J, et al. Inactivation of sodium channels underlies reversible neuropathy during critical illness in rats. J Clin Invest. 2009 May;119(5):1150–8.

Neviere R, Mathieu D, Chagnon JL, Lebleu N, Millien JP, Wattel F. Skeletal muscle microvascular blood flow and oxygen transport in patients with severe sepsis. Am J Respir Crit Care Med. 1996 Jan;153(1):191–5.

Papazian L, Forel JM, Gacouin A, Penot-Ragon C, Perrin G, Loundou A, et al; ACURASYS Study Investigators. Neuromuscular blockers in early acute respiratory distress syndrome. N Engl J Med. 2010 Sep 16;363(12):1107–16.

Piper RD, Pitt-Hyde M, Li F, Sibbald WJ, Potter RF. Microcirculatory changes in rat skeletal muscle in sepsis. Am J Respir Crit Care Med. 1996 Oct;154(4 Pt 1):931–7.

Puthucheary ZA, Phadke R, Rawal J, McPhail MJ, Sidhu PS, Rowlerson A, et al. Qualitative ultrasound in acute critical illness muscle wasting. Crit Care Med. 2015 Aug;43(8):1603–11.

Qaseem A, Humphrey LL, Chou R, SnowV, Shekelle P; Clinical Guidelines Committee of the American College of Physicians. Use of intensive insulin therapy for the management of glycemic control in hospitalized patients: a clinical practice guideline from the American College of Physicians. Ann Intern Med. 2011 Feb 15;154(4):260–7.

Rich MM, Pinter MJ. Crucial role of sodium channel fast inactivation in muscle fibre inexcitability in a rat model of critical illness myopathy. J Physiol. 2003 Mar 1;547(Pt 2):555–66. Epub 2003 Jan 24.

Rossignol B, Gueret G, Pennec JP, Morel J, Giroux-Metges MA, Talarmin H, et al. Effects of chronic sepsis on the voltage-gated sodium channel in isolated rat muscle fibers. Crit Care Med. 2007 Feb;35(2):351–7.

Showalter CJ, Engel AG. Acute quadriplegic myopathy: analysis of myosin isoforms and evidence for calpain-mediated proteolysis. Muscle Nerve. 1997 Mar;20(3):316–22.

Sibbald WJ, Messmer K, Fink MP. Roundtable conference on tissue oxygenation in acute medicine, Brussels, Belgium, 14–16 March 1998. Intensive Care Med. 2000 Jun;26(6):780–91.

Singer M, De Santis V, Vitale D, Jeffcoate W. Multiorgan failure is an adaptive, endocrine-mediated, metabolic response to overwhelming systemic inflammation. Lancet. 2004 Aug 7–13;364(9433):545–8.

Skorna M, Kopacik R, Vlckova E, Adamova B, Kostalova M, Bednarik J. Small-nerve-fiber pathology in critical illness documented by serial skin biopsies. Muscle Nerve. 2015 Jul;52(1):28–33. Epub 2015 May 29.

Supinski GS, Morris PE, Dhar S, Callahan LA. Diaphragm dysfunction in critical illness. Chest. 2018 Apr;153(4):1040–51. Epub 2017 Sep 5.

Van den Berghe G, Schoonheydt K, Becx P, Bruyninckx F, Wouters PJ. Insulin therapy protects the central and peripheral nervous system of intensive care patients. Neurology. 2005 Apr 26;64(8):1348–53.

Visser LH. Critical illness polyneuropathy and myopathy: clinical features, risk factors and prognosis. Eur J Neurol. 2006 Nov;13(11):1203–12.

Zochodne DW, Bolton CF, Wells GA, Gilbert JJ, Hahn AF, Brown JD, et al. Critical illness polyneuropathy: a complication of sepsis and multiple organ failure. Brain. 1987 Aug;110(Pt 4):819–41.

Miscellaneous Disorders of Acute Brain Injury

Status Epilepticus

CHRISTOPHER P. ROBINSON, DO, MS; SARA E. HOCKER, MD

Goals

- Review the classification of status epilepticus and its clinical manifestations.
- Review the initial diagnostic approach to a patient in status epilepticus.
- Review the initial management of status epilepticus.
- Review the management of refractory states of status epilepticus.

Introduction

Status epilepticus (SE) is a medical and neurologic emergency defined as persistent seizure activity lasting longer than 5 minutes or recurrent seizure activity without return to baseline between events. Several classifications exist. The Neurocritical Care Society recommends a simplified classification in which SE is dichotomized as *convulsive* or *nonconvulsive*, with nonconvulsive status epilepticus (NCSE) further stratified as *focal* or *generalized*. The International League Against Epilepsy refined the classification of SE (Box 98.1).

Convulsive SE and NCSE can be focal or generalized. Causes include intracranial hemorrhage, intracranial mass lesions, cerebral infarction, diffuse metabolic disturbance, and medication toxicity. Differentiation depends on clinical presentation and is discussed below in further detail.

Myoclonic SE is generally associated with anoxic ischemic injury (after cardiorespiratory arrest, hanging, or drowning) and is described clinically as brief jerking movements involving the extremities, face, and trunk.

Epilepsia partialis continua (EPC) is usually a consequence of focal cerebral lesions and manifests as continuous clonic movements of 1 body area with preserved consciousness. EPC is frequently resistant to treatment. *Refractory status epilepticus* (RSE) and *super-refractory status epilepticus* (SRSE) are defined clinically by their resistance to pharmacologic interventions: RSE is resistant to 2 antiseizure medications, and SRSE is continuous or recurrent seizures occurring 24 hours or more after the initiation of anesthetic antiepileptic medications.

Convulsive SE is a medical and neurologic emergency associated with high morbidity and mortality. Neurologic complications include irreversible cortical damage with resultant focal deficits and cognitive dysfunction. Medical complications include a wide array of cardiopulmonary complications, acid-base imbalances, musculoskeletal injuries, rhabdomyolysis, and renal failure. Such complications therefore require prompt diagnosis and adequate clinical intervention. Morbidity with NCSE is less clear because NCSE is a heterogeneous group of disorders with highly variable outcomes. The following review discusses the pathophysiology, epidemiology, diagnosis, management, and outcomes of SE.

Epidemiology

SE is a relatively common clinical condition. The overall annual incidence varies between Europe (10-16 per 100,000) and the United States (18-41 per 100,000). In the United States, minority populations have an increased incidence (57 per 100,000) compared with the overall population. The majority of patients with SE (54%) do not have a known history of epilepsy, and in patients who do have epilepsy, SE typically occurs soon after epilepsy is diagnosed. The age distribution of patients with SE is bimodal, with peaks in the first year of life and after age 60 years. NCSE, which is often underrecognized, is estimated to occur in 10% to 15% of patients who have altered mental status and are admitted to the hospital. In the only

Box 98.1 • Classification of Status Epilepticus (SE)

A. With prominent motor symptoms

A.1. Convulsive SE (CSE) (synonym: tonic-clonic SE)
- A.1.a. Generalized CSE
- A.1.b. Focal onset evolving into bilateral CSE
- A.1.c. Unknown whether focal or generalized

A.2. Myoclonic SE (prominent epileptic myoclonic jerks)
- A.2.a. With coma
- A.2.b. Without coma

A.3. Focal motor
- A.3.a. Repeated focal motor seizures (Jacksonian)
- A.3.b. Epilepsia partialis continua (EPC)
- A.3.c. Adversive status
- A.3.d. Oculoclonic status
- A.3.e. Ictal paresis (ie, focal inhibitory SE)

A.4. Tonic status

A.5. Hyperkinetic SE

B. Without prominent motor symptoms (ie, nonconvulsive SE [NCSE])

B.1. NCSE with coma (including "subtle" SE)

B.2. NCSE without coma
- B.2.a. Generalized
  - B.2.a.a. Typical absence status
  - B.2.a.b. Atypical absence status
  - B.2.a.c. Myoclonic absence status
- B.2.b. Focal
  - B.2.b.a. Without impairment of consciousness (aura continua, with autonomic, sensory, visual, olfactory, gustatory, emotional/psychic/experiential, or auditory symptoms)
  - B.2.b.b. Aphasic status
  - B.2.b.c. With impaired consciousness
- B.2.c. Unknown whether focal or generalized
  - B.2.c.a. Autonomic SE

From Trinka E, Cock H, Hesdorffer D, Rossetti AO, Scheffer IE, Shinnar S, et al. A definition and classification of status epilepticus: report of the ILAE Task Force on Classification of Status Epilepticus. Epilepsia. 2015 Oct;56(10):1515-23. Epub 2015 Sep 4; used with permission.

prospective study to date, RSE occurred in 23% of patients with SE, and SRSE occurred in 9%; a retrospective analysis suggested that 31% to 43% of SE episodes are refractory.

Morbidity and mortality related to SE vary according to chronicity and known predictors of outcome. Two scores have been developed for estimating prognosis and outcome for patients with SE: the Status Epilepticus Severity Score (STESS) and the Epidemiology-Based Mortality Score in Status Epilepticus (EMSE). Predictors of severity include age, history of previous seizures, potentially fatal causes, medical comorbidities, electroencephalographic (EEG) findings, level of consciousness on presentation, and seizure type.

Pathophysiology

SE has a unique quality of self-perpetuation. The initial phase of a seizure involves a cascade of molecular modifications, including the inactivation of ion channels and receptor phosphorylation leading to desensitization. These changes allow for signal propagation and spread of an epileptic focus. In the first minutes after modification, abnormal receptor trafficking ensues. Endocytotic internalization of the inhibitory γ-aminobutyric acid type A ($GABA_A$) receptors occurs in concert with externalization of the excitatory α-amino-3-hydroxy-5-methyl-4-isoxazolepropionic acid (AMPA) and *N*-methyl-D-aspartate (NMDA) receptors, leading to an enhanced glutamatergic response (Figure 98.1). This process allows for increased cortical excitability and self-propagation of a stimulus. In the first hours after seizure onset, the process features increased expression of proconvulsive neuropeptides, including substance P and neurokinin B, and depletion of inhibitory neuropeptides, including dynorphin and somatostatin. In the first days to weeks after the onset of SE, the final pathologic modifications that occur are changes in gene expression. The change in neuronal gene expression in these patients results in a chronic proepileptic state commonly characterized by recurrence of SE and seizures.

Clinical Presentation

Convulsive SE

Convulsive SE is classically defined as a prolonged tonic phase and a violent convulsive or clonic phase. As the seizure progresses, the clonic movements disperse and the tonic phase shortens. Cessation of the tonic-clonic movements can occur during either termination of the event or evolution into NCSE. Convulsive SE is associated with overt sympathetic hyperactivity manifested by pupillary dilatation, hypertension, tachycardia, tachypnea, increased cerebral perfusion, and an increased concentration of serum lactate.

Nonconvulsive Status Epilepticus

Generalized NCSE can be difficult to interpret because it can occur as several different semiologic variants. Patients with NCSE may present with or without coma. In patients

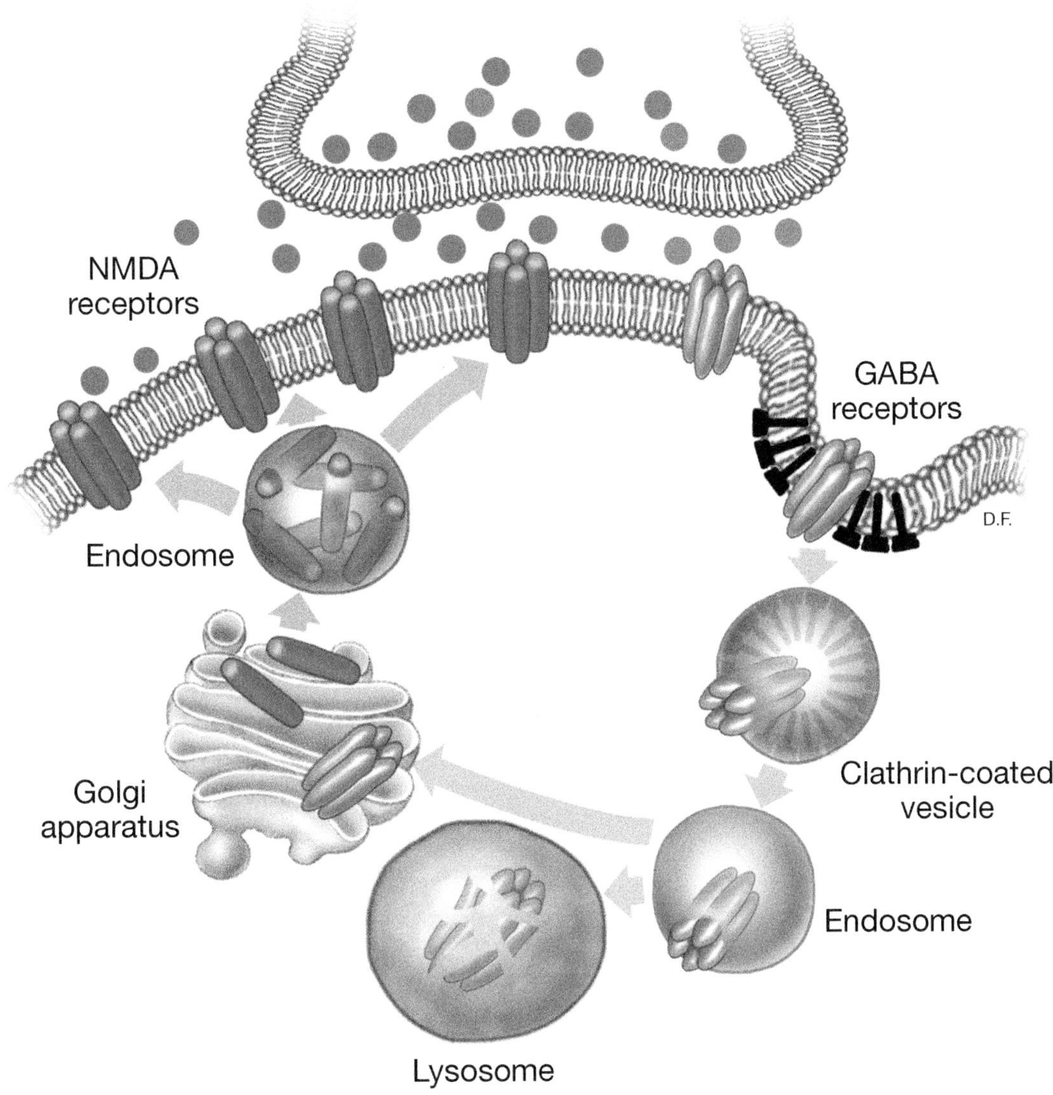

Figure 98.1. Receptor Trafficking During Transition of a Single Seizure to Status Epilepticus. See text for details. GABA indicates γ-aminobutyric acid; NMDA, N*-methyl-*D*-aspartate.*

(From Wijdicks EFM. Handling difficult situations. Oxford [UK]; New York [NY]: Oxford University Press; c2014. Chapter 2, When seizures continue; p. 17-29. [Core principles of acute neurology series]; used with permission of Mayo Foundation for Medical Education and Research as modified from Mazarati AM, Liu H, Naylor DE, Suchomelova L, Thompson KW, Pereira de Vasconselos A, et al. Self-containing status epilepticus. In: Wasterlain CG, Treiman DM, editors. Status epilepticus: mechanisms and management. Cambridge [MA]: MIT Press; c2006. p. 209-28; used with permission.)

with coma, NCSE can develop without antecedent convulsive activity, or it can occur after an episode of convulsive SE characterized by persistent electrographic seizure activity after cessation of clinical features (also termed *subtle SE*). NCSE without coma can be focal or generalized. Patients with focal NCSE typically present with preserved consciousness; objective findings include speech arrest, automatisms, encephalopathy, and eye deviation. Patients may be found wandering and confused. If untreated, focal NCSE may progress to stupor or coma as the seizure becomes generalized. When clinical suspicion is high, critically ill patients should undergo routine EEG monitoring to assess for the possibility of NCSE. If epileptic activity is occurring, the patient should undergo continuous monitoring and receive a trial of a short-acting intravenous (IV) antiseizure medication to assess for resolution.

Focal Motor SE

Focal motor SE can be categorized into several variants, including repeated focal motor seizures, EPC, adversive SE, oculoclonic SE, and ictal paresis. *Focal motor SE* can be defined clinically as rhythmic, focal jerking of a single group of muscles, a limb, a digit, or a group of facial muscles that can be incited by motor or sensory stimulus and may continue for hours or days.

Myoclonic SE

Myoclonic SE varies clinically according to the cortical structures involved. A simple clinical definition of *myoclonic SE* is myoclonus that occurs every 10 to 60 seconds continually for 10 to 30 minutes and is confirmed electrographically. Myoclonic SE occurs virtually always in comatose patients, and the myoclonus can involve the limbs, trunk, and face. It should be distinguished from *action myoclonus*, which occurs in awake patients and is associated with movement.

Evaluation and Management

Initial evaluation and treatment of SE must occur in parallel. The underlying cause must be identified expeditiously during treatment to decrease the possibility of neuronal and systemic damage. Because both evaluation and management are important and complex, they are discussed individually below.

Evaluation

The initial evaluation of a patient with SE includes immediate assessment of the patient's oxygenation, ventilation, and hemodynamic status (Box 98.2). A detailed history should be obtained in combination with the examination while simultaneously initiating appropriate clinical interventions. Urgent noncontrast computed tomography of the head should be performed to rule out acute hemorrhage or localization-related changes from previous disease involving the nervous system. Routine laboratory evaluation, including arterial blood gas analysis and toxicology, is necessary to rule out metabolic abnormalities, acid-base deficiencies, multisystem organ failure, and intoxication. If the patient has a history of seizures, antiepileptic drug levels should be determined. For any patient (with or without a known history of seizure), lumbar puncture can be considered. A strong argument can be made that lumbar puncture should be performed for all patients presenting with fever, prior infectious symptoms, unexplained focal neurologic deficits, or known immunosuppression. The patient's medications must be identified to exclude those that lower the seizure threshold. Emergent EEG can be used to assess for treatment-related failure; if persistent epileptic activity is found, continuous EEG is indicated (Box 98.3). Finally, the patient should be transferred to a neurointensive care unit for medical management.

Box 98.2 • Initial Evaluation of Patients With Status Epilepticus

- Laboratory tests
  - Electrolytes
  - Magnesium
  - Calcium
  - Serum urea nitrogen and creatinine
  - Lactate
  - Phosphorus
  - Arterial blood gas
  - Blood glucose
  - Transaminases
  - Ammonia
  - Alcohol
  - Urine toxicology
  - Creatine kinase
  - Troponin
  - Antiepileptic drug levels (if indicated)
- Imaging
  - Chest radiography
  - Noncontrast computed tomography of the head
- Evaluation of organ systems
  - Physical examination
  - Urine output
  - Oxygenation
  - Ventilation
  - Hemodynamic status
  - Electrocardiogram
- Cerebrospinal fluid analysis (if indicated)
  - Cell count
  - Glucose
  - Protein
  - Gram stain
  - Culture
  - Herpes simplex polymerase chain reaction
  - Other serologies as indicated, including autoantibody panels (eg, *N*-methyl-D-aspartate)

Management

Treatment of SE must proceed urgently to prevent neuronal injury, medical complications, and development of refractoriness. Published guidelines tend to divide treatment protocols into 3 stages that are discussed below in further detail.

First-Line Treatment

First-line treatment of SE should encompass all elements of critical care, including vital sign monitoring,

Box 98.3 • Indications for Continuous Electroencephalography

Clinical seizure or status epilepticus without return to cognitive baseline at 10 minutes

Epileptic activity or epileptic discharges on routine 30-minute electroencephalography

Suspected nonconvulsive status epilepticus in patients with persistent altered mental status

Anoxia or hypoxia after cardiac arrest

Persistent coma without a definable cause

Intracranial hemorrhage, including subarachnoid hemorrhage, traumatic brain injury, and intracerebral hemorrhage

peripheral IV access, basic laboratory evaluation, airway maintenance, vasopressor support if needed, fever management, and initial antiseizure therapy. From randomized controlled trial data, benzodiazepines have been well established as the initial treatment of choice in SE. The Veterans Affairs Status Epilepticus Cooperative Study trial compared 4 treatments: lorazepam, phenobarbital, phenytoin, and phenytoin *and* diazepam. IV lorazepam was significantly more likely to terminate SE compared with phenytoin alone, and IV lorazepam was as effective as phenobarbital and phenytoin *and* diazepam with fewer associated complications and easier administration. In a later trial, both diazepam and lorazepam were superior to placebo, with SE stopping in 43% of patients receiving diazepam, in 59% of patients receiving lorazepam, and in 21% of patients receiving placebo. In further investigations comparing the efficacy of specific benzodiazepines in the treatment of SE, lorazepam was preferred for IV administration, midazolam for intramuscular administration, and diazepam for rectal administration.

Second-Line Treatment

Second-line therapy, which is provided after the administration of benzodiazepines, is necessary for all patients presenting in SE. The 2 objectives are clear: 1) If SE is terminated with benzodiazepines, urgent second-line antiepileptic therapy is indicated for secondary seizure prevention. 2) If SE is not terminated with benzodiazepines, second-line therapy is aimed at termination of further epileptic activity. Although some data are conflicting, urgent second-line therapy should include the use of IV fosphenytoin (or phenytoin) or IV valproate sodium. Some authors also suggest the use of phenobarbital, levetiracetam, or continuous infusion of midazolam as alternative second-line agents. At this stage, preparations should be made for endotracheal intubation if necessary, and initiation of continuous EEG monitoring should be considered because titration of medications may be warranted if SE becomes refractory.

Refractory SE

SE is considered *refractory* after failure of 2 antiseizure drugs. At this stage, a third-line agent is warranted. The general consensus is that the preferred treatment of convulsive SE is an anesthetic agent, including midazolam, propofol, or a barbiturate infusion (pentobarbital or thiopental). Third-line treatment of NCSE, myoclonic SE, and EPC is less well established and should be determined on an individual basis, taking into account the patient's level of consciousness, age, comorbidities, and prognosis.

When anesthetic drug therapy is initiated, urgent continuous EEG should be used to titrate the anesthetic agent to cessation of electrographic seizures or burst suppression. No guidelines exist for duration of therapy; however, experts generally agree that electrographic seizure control should be maintained for 24 to 48 hours before weaning the patient from the anesthetic drug. During weaning, both the patient and the EEG should be observed frequently to assess for recurrence of seizures. If seizures recur during anesthetic weaning, or if seizure control is not achieved with anesthesia, SE is considered SRSE.

Super-Refractory SE

For SRSE or malignant SE, treatment options include the use of IV ketamine, halogenated inhalational anesthetics, or adjunctive therapies such as a ketogenic diet, hypothermia, or electrical stimulation therapies. Interventions at this stage are unproven, although limited evidence does exist for ketamine and for a ketogenic diet.

Outcome

Outcomes related to SE are influenced by type of SE, level of consciousness at onset, patient age, cause of SE, refractoriness of the seizures, and associated comorbidities. The overall mortality of nonrefractory SE is generally reported as 20%; however, further delineation confers a mortality of 9% to 21% for convulsive SE and 18% to 52% for NCSE. Studies have also shown that the use of anesthetics to induce coma is associated with higher risk of death, increased infection rates, and longer hospital stays; however, this association may disappear when seizure refractoriness is accounted for.

Patients with RSE or SRSE have an increased overall mortality compared with patients with nonrefractory SE; however, good outcomes are possible and duration of coma is not clearly associated with outcome. Factors associated with increased morbidity and refractoriness in RSE and SRSE include older age, severely impaired consciousness, and a cryptogenic cause.

Summary

- SE is a medical and neurologic emergency.
- *SE* is defined as persistent seizure activity lasting longer than 5 minutes or recurrent seizure activity without a clear return to cognitive baseline between events.
- Initial management of SE should follow a stepwise evidence-based approach aimed at seizure termination.
- Management of RSE and SRSE has a limited evidence base but may include the use of anesthetic medications and perhaps adjunctive measures, including a ketogenic diet, hypothermia, or electrical stimulation therapies.
- Mortality for patients with SE increases progressively with increasing refractoriness.

SUGGESTED READING

Alvarez V, Lee JW, Westover MB, Drislane FW, Novy J, Faouzi M, et al. Therapeutic coma for status epilepticus: differing practices in a prospective multicenter study. Neurology. 2016 Oct 18;87(16):1650–9. Epub 2016 Sep 24.

Brophy GM, Bell R, Claassen J, Alldredge B, Bleck TP, Glauser T, et al; Neurocritical Care Society Status Epilepticus Guideline Writing Committee. Guidelines for the evaluation and management of status epilepticus. Neurocrit Care. 2012 Aug;17(1):3–23.

Chakraborty T, Hocker S. The clinical spectrum of new-onset status epilepticus. Crit Care Med. 2019 Apr 5. [Epub ahead of print]

Chen JW, Wasterlain CG. Status epilepticus: pathophysiology and management in adults. Lancet Neurol. 2006 Mar;5(3):246–56.

Das AS, Lee JW, Rosenthal ES, Vaitkevicius H. Successful wean despite emergence of ictal-interictal EEG patterns during the weaning of prolonged burst-suppression therapy for super-refractory status epilepticus. Neurocrit Care. 2018 Dec;29(3):452–62. Epub 2018 Jun 8.

Hawkes MA, Hocker SE. Systemic complications following status epilepticus. Curr Neurol Neurosci Rep. 2018 Feb 7;18(2):7.

Hocker S, Tatum WO, LaRoche S, Freeman WD. Refractory and super.refractory status epilepticus: an update. Curr Neurol Neurosci Rep. 2014 Jun;14(6):452.

Pichler M, Hocker S. Management of status epilepticus. Handb Clin Neurol. 2017;140:131–51.

Rai S, Drislane FW. Treatment of refractory and super-refractory status epilepticus. Neurotherapeutics. 2018 Jul;15(3):697–712. Epub 2018 Jun 19.

Rossetti AO, Logroscino G, Milligan TA, Michaelides C, Ruffieux C, Bromfield EB. Status Epilepticus Severity Score (STESS): a tool to orient early treatment strategy. J Neurol. 2008 Oct;255(10):1561–6. Epub 2008 Sep 3.

Rossetti AO, Trinka E, Stahli C, Novy J. New ILAE versus previous clinical status epilepticus semiologic classification: analysis of a hospital-based cohort. Epilepsia. 2016 Jul;57(7):1036–41. Epub 2016 Jun 1.

Shorvon S, Ferlisi M. The treatment of super-refractory status epilepticus: a critical review of available therapies and a clinical treatment protocol. Brain. 2011 Oct;134(Pt 10):2802–18. Epub 2011 Sep 13.

Treiman DM, Meyers PD, Walton NY, Collins JF, Colling C, Rowan AJ, et al; Veterans Affairs Status Epilepticus Cooperative Study Group. A comparison of four treatments for generalized convulsive status epilepticus. N Engl J Med. 1998 Sep 17;339(12):792–8.

Trinka E, Cock H, Hesdorffer D, Rossetti AO, Scheffer IE, Shinnar S, et al. A definition and classification of status epilepticus: report of the ILAE Task Force on Classification of Status Epilepticus. Epilepsia. 2015 Oct;56(10):1515–23. Epub 2015 Sep 4.

99 Posterior Reversible Encephalopathy Syndrome

SUDHIR V. DATAR, MBBS; JENNIFER E. FUGATE, DO

Goals

- Describe the clinical presentation of posterior reversible encephalopathy syndrome.
- Describe the neuroimaging characteristics of posterior reversible encephalopathy syndrome.
- Describe the clinical evaluation to identify the cause of posterior reversible encephalopathy syndrome.

Introduction

Posterior reversible encephalopathy syndrome (PRES), previously known as *hypertensive encephalopathy*, is a clinicoradiologic entity manifesting as acute onset of headache, encephalopathy, seizures, and vision abnormalities. The characteristic clinical features and predominantly posterior cerebral edema were first described by Hinchey and colleagues in 1996. Since then, many conditions have been associated with PRES. Predisposing factors frequently associated with PRES include severe hypertension, eclampsia, immunotherapy, cytotoxic drugs, and bone marrow and organ transplant (Box 99.1).

Neuroimaging studies usually show signal intensity changes in the subcortical white matter preferentially distributed in the parietooccipital regions but also involving other cortical and deep gray matter structures, such as the brainstem and cerebellum. The diagnosis is usually established with clinical history and imaging findings.

Epidemiology

The true incidence of PRES in the general population is unknown because the published studies are almost exclusively retrospective. The incidence of PRES in intensive care unit (ICU) settings is also unknown, but more patients seem to be recognized who have an altered mental status or seizures and hypertensive urgency. PRES appears to have a female predominance. The syndrome is common in young to middle-aged patients, although PRES can affect patients in all age groups, including infancy. It may be less common in children, and in a retrospective review of 2,588 pediatric ICU admissions, the incidence of PRES was about 0.4% (10 patients). The reported incidence after allogenic bone marrow transplant varies from 2.5% to 25%. In a UK study evaluating the incidence of PRES in patients undergoing bone marrow transplant for hemoglobinopathies, the incidence was 19% during the 2 months after transplant.

Clinical Features

Typical neurologic manifestations include a combination of acute encephalopathy, visual disturbances, headache, seizures, and, sometimes, focal neurologic deficits. Acute onset of headache and encephalopathy are the most common manifestations at presentation. The headache is usually dull and global with a gradual onset. Acute onset of thunderclap headache would signal either an alternative diagnosis, such as subarachnoid hemorrhage, or an associated reversible cerebral vasoconstriction syndrome, a syndrome with severe vasospasm possibly causing infarction. The degree of impaired consciousness is variable, and patients can present with confusion, drowsiness, and hallucinations or, in severe cases, stupor and coma. If hypertension is the predisposing factor, the symptoms usually develop quickly (in 24-48 hours) and are often associated with rapid fluctuations in blood pressure. Patients often have a severe increase in blood pressure when they first receive medical care, which is typically in the emergency department. The absolute blood pressure may be less important than the change above the patient's baseline

Box 99.1 • Disorders Precipitating Posterior Reversible Encephalopathy Syndrome

- Severe hypertension or marked blood pressure fluctuations
  - Essential hypertension
  - Secondary hypertension
  - Autonomic dysreflexia due to spinal cord injury
  - Dysautonomia due to Guillain-Barré syndrome or other causes
  - Induced hypertension for hemodynamic augmentation
- Immunosuppression
  - Calcineurin inhibitors (eg, cyclosporine and tacrolimus)
  - Angiogenesis inhibitors (eg, bevacizumab)
  - Combination chemotherapy
  - Methotrexate
- Eclampsia or preeclampsia
- Sepsis or septic shock
- Autoimmune disorders
  - Thrombotic thrombocytopenic purpura
  - Hemolytic uremic syndrome
  - Inflammatory bowel disease (eg, Crohn disease or ulcerative colitis)
  - Vasculitis (eg, polyarteritis nodosa and cryoglobulinemia)
  - Connective tissue disorders (eg, systemic lupus erythematosus, Sjögren disease, and scleroderma)
  - Hashimoto thyroiditis
  - Primary sclerosing cholangitis
- Metabolic disorders
  - Porphyria
  - Ornithine transcarbamylase deficiency

blood pressure. For example, a mean arterial pressure of 100 mm Hg is quite high for a patient with a baseline of 70 mm Hg.

Seizures, either focal or generalized tonic-clonic, have been reported to occur in 60% to 80% of patients. Status epilepticus may also occur, so electroencephalography is often appropriate to exclude ongoing seizures especially if patients present with altered consciousness.

Patients typically have vision abnormalities because of vasogenic edema in the occipital areas; the abnormalities may range from visual blurring to visual hallucinations to visual field deficits and, in severe manifestations, cortical blindness. On funduscopic examination, hypertensive retinopathy may be apparent. Focal neurologic deficits (eg, motor weakness or language disturbances) are relatively uncommon, but they have been reported to occur in 5% to 15% of patients.

Results of blood tests are generally nonspecific and nondiagnostic. Patients may have a variable degree of leukocytosis, especially after seizures. Renal failure (acute, acute on chronic, or chronic) is a characteristic predisposing factor that is present in about half the patients with PRES. With prolonged seizures, patients may present with lactic acidosis and rhabdomyolysis. Lumbar puncture is not necessary for a diagnosis of PRES in most patients; however, it may be needed if patients have atypical features or if other diagnoses (eg, meningitis or encephalitis) need to be ruled out. This is particularly true for patients who are receiving immunosuppressive therapy or who have malignancies. Expected cerebrospinal fluid findings in patients with PRES include a normal leukocyte count and a mildly elevated protein level (usually not >100 mg/dL). When patients are receiving immunosuppressive drugs (eg, tacrolimus or cyclosporine), serum levels may be used to evaluate for supratherapeutic values, but serial values are more important than absolute values.

Neuroimaging

Imaging of the brain is crucial because the clinical symptoms of PRES, while characteristic, are not specific. Imaging typically shows bilateral, predominantly posterior vasogenic edema primarily involving white matter (Figure 99.1). In association with the white matter involvement, the cerebral cortex may be involved.

Magnetic resonance imaging is preferable to computed tomography because of its higher sensitivity. Fluid-attenuated inversion recovery sequences are often useful for identifying areas of vasogenic edema; diffusion-weighted imaging and the apparent diffusion coefficient are used to identify areas of infarction; and a susceptibility-weighted sequence, such as gradient echo imaging, can be used to look for cerebral microhemorrhages or small sulcal subarachnoid hemorrhages.

Although classically described with lesions in the parietooccipital region, vasogenic edema is often found in other brain areas: the frontal and temporal lobes in up to 75% of patients, the cerebellum in up to 50%, and the brainstem and basal ganglia in up to 33%. In most patients, even when PRES involves atypical regions, such as the brainstem and basal ganglia, concomitant involvement of the parietooccipital regions is also apparent (Figure 99.2). Edema can occur asymmetrically, but strictly unilateral involvement or isolated edema in the brainstem or cerebellum is uncommon.

The 3 patterns described for PRES occur in up to 70% of patients: 1) the parietooccipital pattern, 2) the holohemispheric watershed pattern, and 3) the superior frontal sulcus pattern. These patterns are not pathognomonic for PRES, although they are supportive of the diagnosis in the appropriate clinical setting. Notably, the severity of the

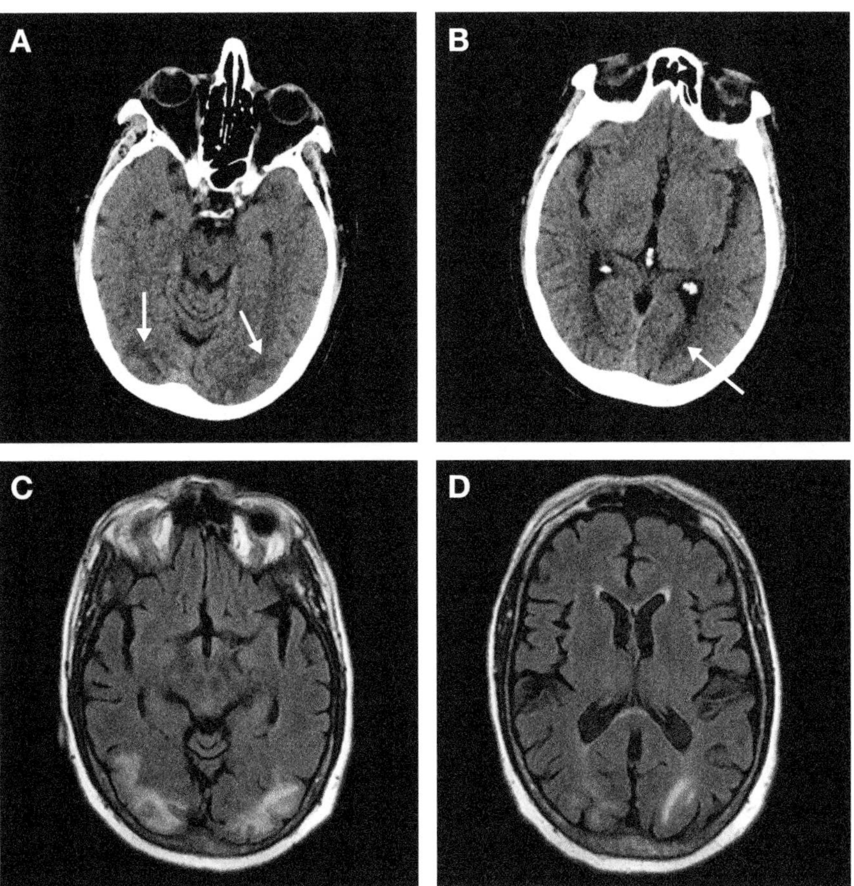

Figure 99.1. Characteristic Imaging Findings in Posterior Reversible Encephalopathy Syndrome. A and B, Axial noncontrast computed tomography shows hypodensity involving the posterior subcortical white matter (arrows). C and D, Axial fluid-attenuated inversion recovery sequences from magnetic resonance imaging of the brain in the same patient showed vasogenic edema posteriorly.

clinical presentation does not correlate with the extent or distribution of vasogenic edema.

In observational PRES studies, diffusion restriction has been reported to occur in 15% to 30% of patients. Areas of restricted diffusion tend to be punctate or small and often occur within larger regions of vasogenic edema. Uncommonly, large homogeneous regions of restricted diffusion may be present, and these can be difficult to distinguish from ischemic brain infarctions. Although isolated cases of reversible restricted diffusion lesions have been reported, they are exceptional. In general, the presence of restricted diffusion is associated with irreversible structural injury and, depending on the brain region involved, may be associated with incomplete clinical recovery.

Intracranial hemorrhage (ICH) occurs in about 10% to 20% of patients with PRES and ranges in size from microhemorrhage to large lobar ICH. Intraparenchymal hemorrhage is the most common pattern (Figure 99.3), and convexal (or sulcal) subarachnoid hemorrhage is the next most common. About 20% of patients with ICH in PRES have both intraparenchymal and subarachnoid involvement. Unsurprisingly, ICH in PRES is associated with coagulopathy, anticoagulant use, and thrombocytopenia.

The percentage of patients receiving a contrast agent, and therefore the reported frequency of contrast enhancement, is quite variable. However, enhancement—most likely reflecting disruption of the blood-brain barrier—can be seen in up to 20% to 25% of patients after administration of gadolinium.

When vascular imaging studies are performed, vasoconstriction has been reported to be present in a small proportion of patients in a pattern similar to what is observed with reversible cerebral vasoconstriction syndrome. This similarity suggests that the 2 disorders overlap in a pathophysiologic continuum.

Treatment

The most important aspect of PRES treatment is quick recognition of the syndrome so that the precipitating cause can be promptly removed or treated. Admission to the ICU

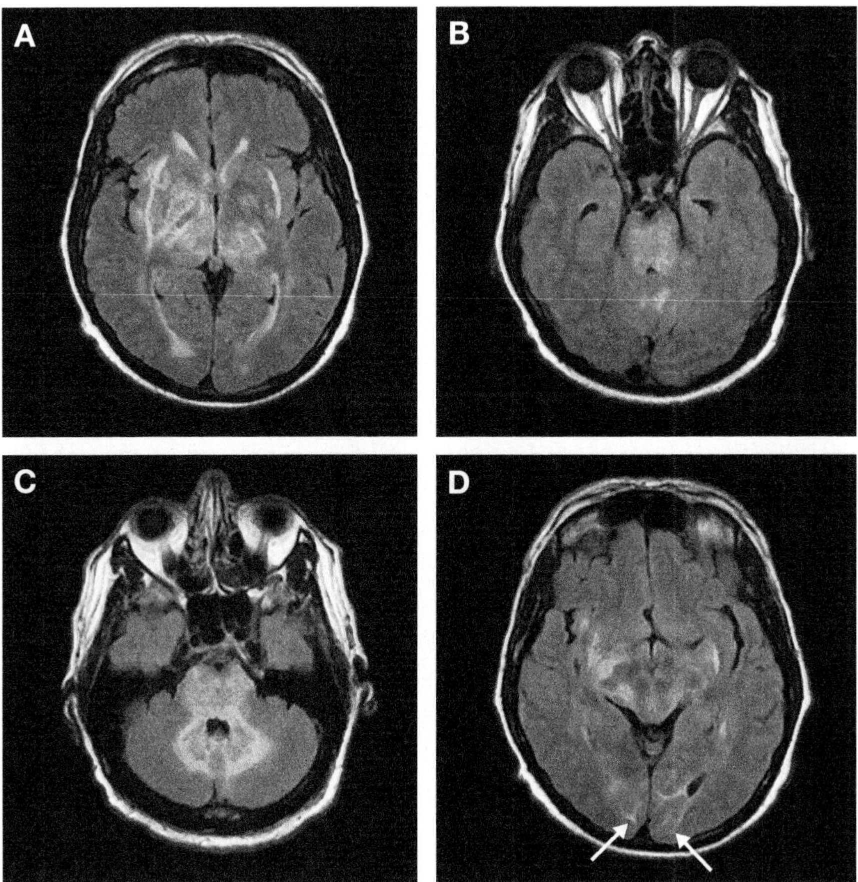

Figure 99.2. Atypical Pattern of Posterior Reversible Encephalopathy Syndrome With Predominant Involvement of the Basal Ganglia and Brainstem. Axial fluid-attenuated inversion recovery sequences from magnetic resonance imaging of the brain show that while the predominant signal abnormality involves the basal ganglia (A), brainstem (B), and cerebellum (C), the bilateral occipital white matter (D) is also involved (arrows).

is often warranted to treat severe hypertension. Large fluctuations in blood pressure should be avoided, and most experts recommend that the blood pressure should not be decreased by more than 25% within the first several hours to reduce the risk of cerebral ischemia, renal ischemia, and acute coronary syndrome.

Use of a continuous antihypertensive infusion is usually the best way to provide smooth control of the blood pressure. Commonly available options include intravenous nicardipine, labetalol, hydralazine, and sodium nitroprusside. The choice of agent is largely guided by physician preference and individual patient characteristics (eg, heart rate, treatment resistance, and underlying comorbidities). An arterial catheter is often necessary for close monitoring of blood pressure during titration of the infusions, and mean arterial pressure is more accurate than systolic blood pressure. Although intravenous infusions are used for immediate control of blood pressure, patients usually begin use of oral medication and are gradually weaned from the infusion.

Depending on their level of consciousness and their ability to protect their airway, patients may need endotracheal intubation. Frequently, patients who need large doses of benzodiazepines for controlling seizures or anesthetic drips for status epilepticus also need intubation and mechanical ventilation. If intubation is purely for airway protection, sedation should be minimized or avoided if possible to allow frequent neurologic evaluation.

Frequent seizures or status epilepticus is another common indication for ICU admission for PRES patients. Antiseizure medications and route of administration are selected as they would be for treating seizures from other causes. Patients in status epilepticus may need infusion of anesthetics, but super-refractory status epilepticus is uncommon. Patients are often monitored with continuous video electroencephalography to detect subclinical epileptiform activity and to guide treatment. Bilateral occipital sharp waves have been frequently reported, although they are not pathognomonic for PRES. A reasonable approach is to consider discontinuation of antiseizure medications

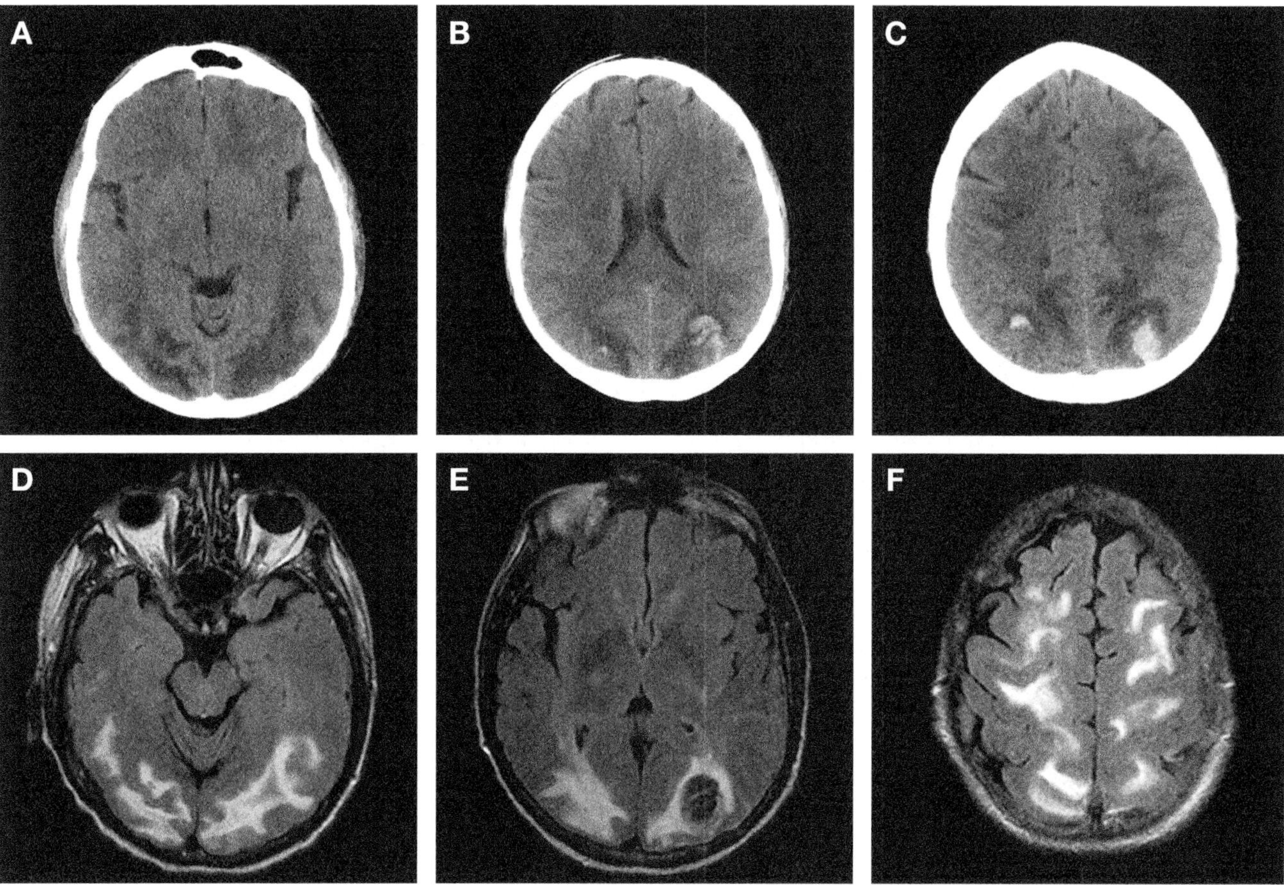

Figure 99.3. Intracranial Hemorrhage (ICH) in Posterior Reversible Encephalopathy Syndrome. A, Axial noncontrast computed tomography of the head shows characteristic hypodensity in the bilateral parietooccipital brain regions. B and C, Areas of ICH are seen within the region of vasogenic edema. D and E, Corresponding axial fluid-attenuated inversion recovery sequences on magnetic resonance imaging (MRI) confirm vasogenic edema (D) and hemorrhage (E). F, Also better seen on MRI more superiorly is holohemispheric watershed involvement, a pattern described in the radiology literature.

when imaging findings of PRES have resolved and underlying risk factors have been adequately controlled. This usually occurs within a few weeks after the onset. No prospective studies provide specific guidance for the total duration of treatment with antiseizure medications.

If the seizures occur with eclampsia, magnesium sulfate infusion is the treatment of choice. This medication is usually administered as a continuous infusion while serum magnesium levels and deep tendon reflexes are monitored; the loss of deep tendon reflexes is usually the first sign of magnesium toxicity. Calcium gluconate may be administered to counteract magnesium toxicity. Whether magnesium sulfate should be used for treating seizures other than those due to eclampsia is unknown.

If PRES is attributed to cytotoxic or immunosuppressive drugs, consideration should be given to stopping use of the offending medication at the earliest opportunity. The literature is sparse on the best approach after PRES has been controlled (ie, whether to resume the same medication at the previous dose or at a lower dose or to switch to another agent). It is reasonable to use the same medication at a lower dose if the levels were in the toxic or supratherapeutic range before the onset of PRES. However, some data indicate that PRES may recur after the same cytotoxic drug is resumed, so if an alternative exists, it should be considered. Rarely, cerebellar or brainstem edema may cause obstructive hydrocephalus from compression of the fourth ventricle, and an external ventricular drain may be necessary until the edema resolves. PRES is usually reversible, so long-term placement of a ventriculoperitoneal shunt is almost never necessary.

Outcome

In most patients, PRES is reversible and outcomes are favorable. However, permanent neurologic sequelae and even death can occur with PRES. Mortality rates of 3% to 6% have been reported in some case series. Death can result from catastrophic ICH, brainstem compression from posterior fossa edema, massive edema, hydrocephalus, or systemic causes. When long-term neurologic sequelae occur, they are usually attributed to regions of cerebral infarction or cerebral hemorrhage. Recurrent PRES, reported to occur in up to 10% of patients, is more common when the precipitating cause is uncontrolled hypertension. Recurrent seizures occur in 10% to 15% of patients during the first few years after PRES. In a majority of those patients, the seizures can be attributed to provoking factors such as recurrent PRES or metabolic disturbances rather than to the development of epilepsy (estimated risk, 1%-2%).

Summary

- PRES is a clinical syndrome characterized by encephalopathy, seizures, headache, vision disturbances, and, less commonly, focal neurologic deficits.
- PRES is associated with fluctuations in blood pressure, severe hypertension, kidney failure, chemotherapeutics, immunosuppressive medications, eclampsia, and autoimmune conditions.
- Magnetic resonance imaging is the best neuroimaging tool and is needed to exclude other diagnoses because the clinical symptoms of PRES are nonspecific.
- PRES can be severe, and patients may need care in the ICU for seizures, status epilepticus, control of severe hypertension, ICH, hydrocephalus, or massive brain edema.
- Outcomes for patients with PRES are usually favorable; however, the rate of long-term morbidity or mortality is approximately 10% to 15%.

SUGGESTED READING

Bartynski WS. Posterior reversible encephalopathy syndrome, part 1: fundamental imaging and clinical features. AJNR Am J Neuroradiol. 2008 Jun;29(6):1036–42. Epub 2008 Mar 20.

Bartynski WS, Boardman JF. Distinct imaging patterns and lesion distribution in posterior reversible encephalopathy syndrome. AJNR Am J Neuroradiol. 2007 Aug;28(7):1320–7.

Bastide L, Legros B, Rampal N, Gilmore EJ, Hirsch LJ, Gaspard N. Clinical correlates of periodic discharges and nonconvulsive seizures in posterior reversible encephalopathy syndrome (PRES). Neurocrit Care. 2018 Dec;29(3):481–90. Epub 2018 Jun 8.

Brady E, Parikh NS, Navi BB, Gupta A, Schweitzer AD. The imaging spectrum of posterior reversible encephalopathy syndrome: a pictorial review. Clin Imaging. 2018 Jan-Feb;47:80–9. Epub 2017 Aug 30.

Datar S, Singh T, Rabinstein AA, Fugate JE, Hocker S. Long-term risk of seizures and epilepsy in patients with posterior reversible encephalopathy syndrome. Epilepsia. 2015 Apr;56(4):564–8. Epub 2015 Feb 18.

Datar S, Singh TD, Fugate JE, Mandrekar J, Rabinstein AA, Hocker S. Albuminocytologic dissociation in posterior reversible encephalopathy syndrome. Mayo Clin Proc. 2015 Oct;90(10):1366–71. Epub 2015 Sep 5.

Fugate JE, Claassen DO, Cloft HJ, Kallmes DF, Kozak OS, Rabinstein AA. Posterior reversible encephalopathy syndrome: associated clinical and radiologic findings. Mayo Clin Proc. 2010 May;85(5):427–32.

Fugate JE, Rabinstein AA. Posterior reversible encephalopathy syndrome: clinical and radiological manifestations, pathophysiology, and outstanding questions. Lancet Neurol. 2015 Sep;14(9):914–25. Epub 2015 Jul 13. Erratum in: Lancet Neurol. 2015 Sep;14(9):874.

Hage P, Kseib C, Hmaimess G, Jaoude PA, Noun P. Recurrent posterior reversible encephalopathy syndrome with cerebellar involvement leading to acute hydrocephalus. Clin Neurol Neurosurg. 2018 Sep;172:120–3. Epub 2018 Jul 5.

Hinchey J, Chaves C, Appignani B, Breen J, Pao L, Wang A, et al. A reversible posterior leukoencephalopathy syndrome. N Engl J Med. 1996 Feb 22;334(8):494–500.

Kozak OS, Wijdicks EF, Manno EM, Miley JT, Rabinstein AA. Status epilepticus as initial manifestation of posterior reversible encephalopathy syndrome. Neurology. 2007 Aug 28;69(9):894–7.

Lee VH, Wijdicks EF, Manno EM, Rabinstein AA. Clinical spectrum of reversible posterior leukoencephalopathy syndrome. Arch Neurol. 2008 Feb;65(2):205–10.

Rabinstein AA, Mandrekar J, Merrell R, Kozak OS, Durosaro O, Fugate JE. Blood pressure fluctuations in posterior reversible encephalopathy syndrome. J Stroke Cerebrovasc Dis. 2012 May;21(4):254–8. Epub 2011 May 4.

Vaughan CJ, Delanty N. Hypertensive emergencies. Lancet. 2000 Jul 29;356(9227):411–7.

Demyelinating Disorders of the Central Nervous System

AURELIA A. SMITH, MD; BRIAN G. WEINSHENKER, MD

Goals

- Discuss major demyelinating disorders that require intensive care.
- Discuss the differential diagnosis and appropriate tests for demyelinating disorders.
- Discuss immunotherapy indications for patients with demyelinating disorders.

Introduction

Patients with central nervous system (CNS) inflammatory demyelinating disease (IDD) usually have acute relapses of neurologic symptoms that frequently remit spontaneously or after corticosteroid administration; they may also present with a progressive neurodegenerative condition, either de novo or after 1 or more acute relapses. Most patients with acute relapses of demyelinating disease do not have severe disability and can be treated as outpatients. Most hospitalizations for patients with multiple sclerosis (MS), for instance, are for reasons unrelated to MS, such as infection. However, patients with CNS IDD occasionally present with serious, emergent complications caused directly by CNS inflammation or indirectly by secondary complications, either of which can require critical care management.

Clinical Features and Spectrum of Disorders

Several important disorders include CNS IDD: MS, acute disseminated encephalomyelitis (ADEM), neuromyelitis optica spectrum disorder (NMOSD), tumefactive MS, and other rarer disorders such as Baló concentric sclerosis and Marburg variant of MS.

The hallmark of MS is dissemination of demyelinating disease over time as manifested by multiple distinct clinical attacks or by a single clinical attack with radiologic evidence of dissemination later. When the criteria are not fully met at the initial presentation, the first episodes are often referred to as clinically isolated syndromes. Patients with acute focal demyelinating lesions in the brainstem or the high cervical spinal cord are most likely to require critical care management.

ADEM is typically a monophasic illness, most commonly occurring in children days to weeks after a viral illness or immunization, but ADEM also occurs in adults in association with anti-myelin oligodendrocyte glycoprotein antibodies. Antecedent infections linked to ADEM include herpesvirus infection, influenza, rubella, mumps, and human immunodeficiency virus infection. Immunizations linked to ADEM include vaccines for human papillomavirus, varicella virus, influenza virus, diphtheria and tetanus toxoids, poliovirus, and rabies virus. ADEM is typically polysymptomatic, resulting in encephalopathy, but it also results in transverse myelitis, optic neuritis, and other symptoms. Encephalopathy has been considered a required characteristic, but encephalopathy by itself is not pathognomonic and it may not be absolutely required in the presence of other characteristics or pathologic findings of ADEM.

Patients with NMOSD typically have longitudinally extensive transverse myelitis (ie, lesions on magnetic resonance imaging [MRI] extending over ≥3 vertebral segments) or optic neuritis (or both) and other well-described syndromes, including intractable nausea and emesis or intractable hiccups from an area postrema lesion and acute narcolepsy from hypothalamic lesions. The majority of patients with NMOSD have positive results for anti–aquaporin-4 autoantibodies in the serum, but approximately 30% of patients are seronegative. Relapses of NMOSD are typically more severe than MS relapses.

Tumefactive MS refers to CNS demyelination associated with lesions larger than 2.0 cm in diameter, vasogenic edema, mass effect, and partially open ring enhancement on MRI. Tumefactive MS may be considered a characteristic of a lesion in certain patients rather than a disease, and tumefactive MS may occur in patients with prototypic MS, neuromyelitis optica, or certain variants of demyelinating disease (eg, Baló concentric sclerosis). Clinical manifestations may include cortical syndromes that are atypical for MS, such as apraxia, aphasia, and cortical blindness. The lesions may be difficult to distinguish from malignant lesions, such as high-grade glioma, metastatic disease, or primary CNS lymphoma. A biopsy is often required, especially with isolated lesions, unless the lesion has a highly specific appearance (eg, Baló concentric sclerosis) or coexisting lesions are suggestive of MS. Caution is required to avoid misdiagnosing the lesions as brain tumor, which can occur with pathologic misdiagnosis of highly cellular lesions; in the past, radiotherapy for presumed malignancy was thought to worsen demyelinating disease, but the risks may be lower than expected. Although patients with tumefactive MS present with more severe deficits than patients with general MS, long-term follow-up has shown that their average disability due to demyelinating disease is less, so that aggressive therapy for acute disease is justified.

Disorders that mimic CNS IDD include vasculitis or noninflammatory vasculopathy, tumors, infections, toxic exposure, mitochondrial disorders, and other systemic inflammatory diseases (Box 100.1). Red flags that should prompt consideration of a diagnosis other than CNS IDD include a documented history of malignancy or systemic autoimmune disease (although NMOSD frequently coexists with systemic autoimmune diseases); symptoms atypical for demyelinating disease (eg, hearing loss in Susac syndrome); systemic symptoms suggesting another cause (eg, mouth ulcers or splinter hemorrhages); and imaging findings such as a prominent mass effect, homogenous enhancement, or lack of enhancement of the acute symptomatic lesion.

Box 100.1 • Differential Diagnosis of Acute Inflammatory Demyelinating Disease

Inflammatory (eg, sarcoidosis, systemic autoimmunity, and drug-induced demyelination)

Ischemic or vascular (eg, vasculopathy, vasculitis, thromboembolic, and venous infarct)

Metabolic or nutritional (eg, vitamin B_{12} or copper deficiency and mitochondrial disease)

Infectious (eg, abscess, encephalitis, PML, HIV infection, and neurosyphilis)

Postinfectious

Radiation induced

Toxic exposure (eg, chemotherapy, solvents, lead, and carbon monoxide)

Genetic (eg, CADASIL syndrome and mitochondrial encephalopathy)

Oncologic (eg, glioma, primary CNS lymphoma, intravascular lymphoma, and paraneoplastic conditions)

Miscellaneous (eg, PRES and CLIPPERS)

Abbreviations: CADASIL, cerebral autosomal dominant arteriopathy with subcortical infarcts and leukoencephalopathy; CLIPPERS, chronic lymphocytic inflammation with pontine perivascular enhancement responsive to steroids; CNS, central nervous system; HIV, human immunodeficiency virus; PML, progressive multifocal leukoencephalopathy; PRES, posterior reversible encephalopathy syndrome.

Modified from Bunyan RF, Tang J, Weinshenker B. Acute demyelinating disorders: emergencies and management. Neurol Clin 2012 Feb;30(1):285–307; used with permission.

Laboratory Tests

The most important (and usually the first) diagnostic procedure is contrast MRI of the brain, cervical spine, and thoracic spine. MRI may provide valuable clues about the cause from characteristics of spinal cord lesions. Non-MRI evaluation may be helpful in ruling out conditions that resemble CNS IDD, and those tests should be performed selectively as indicated (Table 100.1). Empirical treatment with corticosteroids, which have relatively few contraindications, is appropriate until the results of the tests are available. If a patient's condition is rapidly deteriorating or is refractory to treatment, brain biopsy may be required for definitive diagnosis if the lesion is safely accessible and, preferably, gadolinium enhancing.

Treatment

Symptoms due to CNS IDD are frequently reversible, and aggressive supportive care is indicated. Therapy targeting the acute inflammatory attack begins with intravenous corticosteroids, typically given as high doses of intravenous methylprednisolone (1 g daily) for 5 consecutive days. Corticosteroids begin to decrease inflammation within hours of administration, and the clinical response is often rapid. Depending on the clinical situation, empirical treatment with corticosteroids may need to begin before a definitive diagnosis is reached.

If symptoms are refractory to corticosteroids, the recommendation is to proceed with plasmapheresis. Both the American Academy of Neurology and the American Society for Apheresis agree that plasmapheresis is appropriate for the treatment of acute fulminant CNS demyelinating disease. A randomized controlled trial showed class I evidence of significant benefit from plasmapheresis, and other uncontrolled or retrospective studies have also confirmed its efficacy. The mechanism of action is thought to be removal of humoral circulating factors (including anti–aquaporin-4

Table 100.1 • Tests for Investigation of Leukoencephalopathy

Test	Examples of Conditions With Positive Results
CSF oligoclonal bands and IgG index	CNS IDD, SSPE, HIV infection, and other infections
CSF antibody titers or PCR	Specific infections
CSF lactate or pyruvate level	Mitochondrial disorders
Echocardiography	Endocarditis, other cardioembolism, and paradoxical embolism
Ophthalmologic examination (including fluorescein angiography) for vasculitis or uveitis	Retinal vasculitis, sarcoidosis, and lymphoma
CT of the chest, abdomen, and pelvis	Sarcoidosis and metastatic disease
Cerebral angiography or black-blood MRI	Vasculitis, vasculopathy, venous sinus thrombosis, and atheroembolism
Non-CNS biopsy (eg, conjunctiva, skin)	Sarcoidosis, systemic lupus erythematous, vasculitis, and CADASIL
CNS biopsy	Neoplastic disease and tumefactive demyelination

Abbreviations: CADASIL, cerebral autosomal dominant arteriopathy with subcortical infarcts and leukoencephalopathy; CNS, central nervous system; CSF, cerebrospinal fluid; CT, computed tomography; HIV, human immunodeficiency virus; IDD, inflammatory demyelinating disease; Ig, immunoglobulin; MRI, magnetic resonance imaging; PCR, polymerase chain reaction; SSPE, subacute sclerosing panencephalitis.

Modified from Bunyan RF, Tang J, Weinshenker B. Acute demyelinating disorders: emergencies and management. Neurol Clin 2012 Feb;30(1):285–307; used with permission.

autoantibody), although some evidence suggests that T-cell behavior may also be altered. The recommended course of plasmapheresis is removal of 1.0 to 1.5 plasma volumes per exchange, with 7 treatments administered over a 2-week period. The major risks of plasmapheresis are hypotension, which is usually easily managed, and complications related to catheter insertion and infection.

Cyclophosphamide has been used as rescue therapy for refractory, severe attacks of demyelinating disease, but its use has not been studied prospectively. In retrospective studies, it has been beneficial for transverse myelitis.

Intravenous immunoglobulin has provided some benefit to children with steroid-refractory ADEM. The recommended regimen is 1 to 2 g/kg given in 1 dose or divided over 3 to 5 days.

Complications of CNS IDD

Emergency complications of CNS IDD may result from deficits related to the unique location of the lesion, the complications of severe inflammation, or the unique pathophysiologic effects of certain illnesses (Box 100.2).

Large lesions (as in tumefactive MS) or many multifocal lesions (as in ADEM) may cause elevated intracranial pressure and herniation syndromes. Management includes elevation of the head of the bed, hyperventilation, and mannitol or other hypertonic solutions with or without hypothermia. In refractory cases, hemicraniectomy has been a successful lifesaving measure.

Respiratory failure can occur in patients with CNS IDD if they have acute lesions involving the brain or cervical spinal cord (more commonly in patients with NMOSD than with MS). In patients with chronic progressive MS, respiratory failure is more likely to result from aspiration pneumonia than from an acute brainstem lesion.

Acute medullary lesions in the nucleus tractus solitarius have been reported to cause neurogenic pulmonary edema in isolation or with other signs of medullary dysfunction,

Box 100.2 • Emergency Complications of CNS IDD

Elevated intracranial pressure
Cerebral herniation
Neurogenic pulmonary edema
Myocardial dysfunction
Posterior reversible encephalopathy syndrome
Hypothermia

Abbreviations: CNS, central nervous system; IDD, inflammatory demyelinating disease.

Modified from Bunyan RF, Tang J, Weinshenker B. Acute demyelinating disorders: emergencies and management. Neurol Clin 2012 Feb;30(1):285–307; used with permission.

such as rotary nystagmus, hemifacial numbness, or unilateral soft palate paralysis.

Acute heart failure, a rare complication of CNS IDD, may cause pulmonary edema or cardiogenic shock. An increase in sympathetic tone is a potential explanation for this phenomenon. It is likely similar to stress cardiomyopathy in pathogenesis and may be treated similarly.

Posterior reversible encephalopathy syndrome (PRES) has been reported to occur in patients with NMOSD. PRES probably results from loss of aquaporin-4 channels, which leads to altered water regulation in the brain. Treatment is with supportive care and corticosteroids to decrease the inflammation from NMOSD.

In patients with advanced, chronic forms of MS, severe hypothermia may develop and cause episodic encephalopathy, which is not usually caused by an acute inflammatory attack. MRI sometimes shows lesions within the hypothalamus. This diagnosis requires a thermometer that can accurately measure core temperatures as low as 29°C. Systemic symptoms, including thrombocytopenia, coagulopathy, or bradycardia, may also be present. Patients typically respond well to rewarming within 48 hours.

Summary

- Common CNS IDDs include MS, NMOSDs, ADEM, and tumefactive MS.
- Many disorders may mimic CNS IDD, and if patients have clinical features such as a history of malignancy or systemic autoimmune disease, or if they have systemic symptoms, other causes should be considered.
- Ancillary studies that may be useful for the differential diagnosis include CSF analysis, echocardiography, ophthalmologic evaluation, CT of the body, cerebral angiography, and biopsies.
- Initial treatment of CNS IDD is with high doses of intravenous corticosteroids.
- Refractory disease often responds to plasmapheresis.
- Emergency complications of CNS IDD include elevated intracranial pressure, neurogenic pulmonary edema, myocardial dysfunction, PRES, and hypothermia.

SUGGESTED READING

Bunyan RF, Tang J, Weinshenker B. Acute demyelinating disorders: emergencies and management. Neurol Clin. 2012 Feb;30(1):285–307.

Crawley F, Saddeh I, Barker S, Katifi H. Acute pulmonary oedema: presenting symptom of multiple sclerosis. Mult Scler. 2001 Feb;7(1):71–2.

de Seze J. [Multiple sclerosis: clinical aspects, acute disseminated encephalomyelitis, neuromyelitis optica and other inflammatory variants]. Rev Neurol (Paris). 2007 Jun;163(6–7):647–50. French.

Gentiloni N, Schiavino D, Della Corte F, Ricci E, Colosimo C. Neurogenic pulmonary edema: a presenting symptom in multiple sclerosis. Ital J Neurol Sci. 1992 Jun;13(5):435–8.

Greenberg BM, Thomas KP, Krishnan C, Kaplin AI, Calabresi PA, Kerr DA. Idiopathic transverse myelitis: corticosteroids, plasma exchange, or cyclophosphamide. Neurology. 2007 May 8;68(19):1614–7.

Hinson SR, Pittock SJ, Lucchinetti CF, Roemer SF, Fryer JP, Kryzer TJ, et al. Pathogenic potential of IgG binding to water channel extracellular domain in neuromyelitis optica. Neurology. 2007 Dec 11;69(24):2221–31. Epub 2007 Oct 10.

Huhn K, Lee DH, Linker RA, Kloska S, Huttner HB. Pneumococcal-meningitis associated acute disseminated encephalomyelitis (ADEM): case report of effective early immunotherapy. Springerplus. 2014 Aug 8;3:415.

Jarius S, Paul F, Aktas O, Asgari N, Dale RC, de Seze J, et al. MOG encephalomyelitis: international recommendations on diagnosis and antibody testing. J Neuroinflammation. 2018 May 3;15(1):134.

Keegan M, Konig F, McClelland R, Bruck W, Morales Y, Bitsch A, et al. Relation between humoral pathological changes in multiple sclerosis and response to therapeutic plasma exchange. Lancet. 2005 Aug 13–19;366(9485):579–82.

Kjellman UW, Hallgren P, Bergh CH, Lycke J, Oldfors A, Wiklund L. Weaning from mechanical support in a patient with acute heart failure and multiple sclerosis. Ann Thorac Surg. 2000 Feb;69(2):628–30.

Krupp LB, Banwell B, Tenembaum S; International Pediatric MS Study Group. Consensus definitions proposed for pediatric multiple sclerosis and related disorders. Neurology. 2007 Apr 17;68(16 Suppl 2):S7–12.

Lennon VA, Kryzer TJ, Pittock SJ, Verkman AS, Hinson SR. IgG marker of optic-spinal multiple sclerosis binds to the aquaporin-4 water channel. J Exp Med. 2005 Aug 15;202(4):473–7. Epub 2005 Aug 8.

Linker RA, Mohr A, Cepek L, Gold R, Prange H. Core hypothermia in multiple sclerosis: case report with magnetic resonance imaging localization of a thalamic lesion. Mult Scler. 2006 Feb;12(1):112–5.

Llufriu S, Castillo J, Blanco Y, Ramio-Torrenta L, Rio J, Valles M, et al. Plasma exchange for acute attacks of CNS demyelination: predictors of improvement at 6 months. Neurology. 2009 Sep 22;73(12):949–53.

Lucchinetti CF, Gavrilova RH, Metz I, Parisi JE, Scheithauer BW, Weigand S, et al. Clinical and radiographic spectrum of pathologically confirmed tumefactive multiple sclerosis. Brain. 2008 Jul;131(Pt 7):1759–75. Epub 2008 Jun 5.

Marchioni E, Marinou-Aktipi K, Uggetti C, Bottanelli M, Pichiecchio A, Soragna D, et al. Effectiveness of intravenous immunoglobulin treatment in adult patients with steroid-resistant monophasic or recurrent acute disseminated encephalomyelitis. J Neurol. 2002 Jan;249(1):100–4.

Mariano R, Flanagan EP, Weinshenker BG, Palace J. A practical approach to the diagnosis of spinal cord lesions. Pract Neurol. 2018 Jun;18(3):187–200. Epub 2018 Mar 2.

Marrie RA, Elliott L, Marriott J, Cossoy M, Blanchard J, Tennakoon A, et al. Dramatically changing rates and reasons for hospitalization in multiple sclerosis. Neurology. 2014 Sep 2;83(10):929–37. Epub 2014 Aug 1.

Melin J, Usenius JP, Fogelholm R. Left ventricular failure and pulmonary edema in acute multiple sclerosis. Acta Neurol Scand. 1996 May;93(5):315–7.

Menge T, Hemmer B, Nessler S, Wiendl H, Neuhaus O, Hartung HP, et al. Acute disseminated encephalomyelitis: an update. Arch Neurol. 2005 Nov;62(11):1673–80.

Miller RC, Lachance DH, Lucchinetti CF, Keegan BM, Gavrilova RH, Brown PD, et al. Multiple sclerosis, brain radiotherapy, and risk of neurotoxicity: the Mayo Clinic experience. Int J Radiat Oncol Biol Phys. 2006 Nov 15;66(4):1178–86. Epub 2006 Sep 11.

Murthy SN, Faden HS, Cohen ME, Bakshi R. Acute disseminated encephalomyelitis in children. Pediatrics. 2002 Aug;110(2 Pt 1):e21.

Pittock SJ, Weinshenker BG, Wijdicks EF. Mechanical ventilation and tracheostomy in multiple sclerosis. J Neurol Neurosurg Psychiatry. 2004 Sep;75(9):1331–3.

Pradhan S, Gupta RP, Shashank S, Pandey N. Intravenous immunoglobulin therapy in acute disseminated encephalomyelitis. J Neurol Sci. 1999 May 1;165(1):56–61.

Nilsson P, Larsson EM, Kahlon B, Nordstrom CH, Norrving B. Tumefactive demyelinating disease treated with decompressive craniectomy. Eur J Neurol. 2009 May;16(5):639–42. Epub 2009 Mar 20.

Ramanathan S, Dale RC, Brilot F. Anti-MOG antibody: the history, clinical phenotype, and pathogenicity of a serum biomarker for demyelination. Autoimmun Rev. 2016 Apr;15(4):307–24. Epub 2015 Dec 17.

Simon RP, Gean-Marton AD, Sander JE. Medullary lesion inducing pulmonary edema: a magnetic resonance imaging study. Ann Neurol. 1991 Nov;30(5):727–30.

Sonneville R, Klein I, de Broucker T, Wolff M. Post-infectious encephalitis in adults: diagnosis and management. J Infect. 2009 May;58(5):321–8. Epub 2009 Apr 14.

Tenembaum S, Chitnis T, Ness J, Hahn JS; International Pediatric MS Study Group. Acute disseminated encephalomyelitis. Neurology. 2007 Apr 17;68(16 Suppl 2):S23–36.

Torisu H, Okada K. Vaccination-associated acute disseminated encephalomyelitis. Vaccine. 2019 Feb 14;37(8):1126–9. Epub 2019 Jan 23.

Weinshenker BG. Tumefactive demyelinating lesions: characteristics of individual lesions, individual patients, or a unique disease entity? Mult Scler. 2015 Nov;21(13):1746–7. Epub 2015 Sep 11.

Weinshenker BG, Lucchinetti CF. Acute leukoencephalopathies: differential diagnosis and investigation. Neurologist. 1998 May;4(3):148–66.

Weinshenker BG, O'Brien PC, Petterson TM, Noseworthy JH, Lucchinetti CF, Dodick DW, et al. A randomized trial of plasma exchange in acute central nervous system inflammatory demyelinating disease. Ann Neurol. 1999 Dec;46(6):878–86.

Weiss N, Hasboun D, Demeret S, Fontaine B, Bolgert F, Lyon-Caen O, et al. Paroxysmal hypothermia as a clinical feature of multiple sclerosis. Neurology. 2009 Jan 13;72(2):193–5.

White KD, Scoones DJ, Newman PK. Hypothermia in multiple sclerosis. J Neurol Neurosurg Psychiatry. 1996 Oct;61(4):369–75.

Wingerchuk DM, Banwell B, Bennett JL, Cabre P, Carroll W, Chitnis T, et al; International Panel for NMO Diagnosis. International consensus diagnostic criteria for neuromyelitis optica spectrum disorders. Neurology. 2015 Jul 14;85(2):177–89. Epub 2015 Jun 19.

Wingerchuk DM, Hogancamp WF, O'Brien PC, Weinshenker BG. The clinical course of neuromyelitis optica (Devic's syndrome). Neurology. 1999 Sep 22;53(5):1107–14.

Young NP, Weinshenker BG, Lucchinetti CF. Acute disseminated encephalomyelitis: current understanding and controversies. Semin Neurol. 2008 Feb;28(1):84–s94.

Rapidly Progressive Dementia and Coma

PRASUNA KAMIREDDI, MBBS; JASON L. SIEGEL, MD;
DENNIS W. DICKSON, MD

Goals

- Describe the causes of rapidly progressive dementia in patients admitted to the intensive care unit.
- Describe the classification of prion disease.
- Describe the risks with prion disease.

Introduction

In most patients with dementia, the clinical signs and symptoms progress gradually over many years. However, neurointensivists may encounter patients who have rapidly progressive dementia (RPD). Often these patients need to be admitted to the intensive care unit for management of status epilepticus, agitation, or ventilation in coma. Although the prototype of RPD is Creutzfeldt-Jakob disease (CJD), this chapter reviews other common causes of RPD. An established definition of RPD does not exist, but in this chapter *RPD* refers to the loss of more than 1 cognitive domain and functional ability, usually occurring over a few months.

Epidemiology

The prevalence and incidence of RPD are unknown. In studies from high-volume centers, the most common cause of RPD is prion diseases, of which sporadic CJD (sCJD) is the most common (sCJD is more common than all nonprion causes of RPD combined). Other causes of RPD are the more common dementias and neurodegenerative diseases (including Alzheimer disease, dementia with Lewy bodies, frontotemporal dementia, and corticobasal degeneration). These diseases were reported to account for 26% to 60% of all nonprion RPD, but the percentages are less now because of advances in the diagnosis of nonprion disease, particularly recognition of autoimmune encephalitis.

Clinical Features

The most common symptom in patients with RPD is a rapid loss of executive function. Special attention should be paid to symptom onset (acute or insidious); time course; type of progression (fluctuating, stepwise, or unremitting steady decline); domains of cognition (memory, language, executive function, and disinhibition); motor findings (myoclonus, extrapyramidal signs, and ataxia); and other signs and symptoms related to nonneurologic disease (eg, unexplained weight loss, night sweats, chronic cough, nagging abdominal pain, and heart disease).

Table 101.1 lists common causes of nonprion RPD with clinical characteristics, and Table 101.2 outlines the first- and second-line tests in the diagnostic workup of patients with RPD.

Prion Diseases

Prion diseases, or transmissible spongiform encephalopathies, are fatal neurodegenerative diseases caused by a posttranslational conversion of the normal cellular prion protein (PrP^C) into the abnormal scrapie form (PrP^{Sc}). Neuronal loss is considered the principal cause of clinical symptoms in prion disease. One theory, which is controversial, is that neurodegeneration is triggered by the loss of the neuroprotective function of PrP^C or by the effect of toxic properties on conversion into PrP^{Sc}. Human prion diseases are classified into 3 etiologic groups: sporadic, genetic or familial, and acquired (Table 101.3).

Sporadic Creutzfeldt-Jakob Disease

The most common type of prion disease is sCJD (accounting for about 85% of all CJD), with an annual worldwide incidence of 1 to 2 cases per 1 million population. It occurs with equal frequency in both sexes, and the peak

Table 101.1 • Nonprion and Potentially Reversible Causes of Rapidly Progressive Dementia

Cause	Clinical Features	Investigational Features
Autoimmune		
Acute disseminated encephalomyelitis	Subacute onset Fluctuating course Tremor Headache Personal or family history of autoimmunity History of neoplasia	CSF: elevated protein, pleocytosis, oligoclonal bands, elevated CSF index MRI: mesial temporal or other regional hyperintensities on T2-weighted images, hypometabolism on functional imaging
Antibody-mediated encephalopathy		Detection of neural antibody
Paraneoplastic diseases (eg, limbic encephalopathy)		Paraneoplastic blood tests: positive results
Hashimoto encephalopathy	Symptoms of hypothyroidism Past history of hypothyroidism or autoimmune thyroiditis	Corticosteroid responsive Antithyroglobulin and antithyroperoxidase antibodies
Neurodegenerative		
Alzheimer disease	Older age at onset Memory impairment: common and a prominent initial symptom	MRI: medial temporal lobe atrophy FDG-PET: hypoperfusion in hippocampus, lateral parietal cortex, and posterior cortex CSF: decreased Aβ42; increased total tau or phosphorylated tau
Dementia with Lewy bodies	Early impairment in attention, visuospatial function, and execution Cognitive fluctuation Visual hallucinations Parkinsonism	SPECT and PET: hypoperfusion in occipital regions
Frontotemporal degeneration	Early prominent behavioral features Primary progressive aphasia	Functional imaging: hypoperfusion at regions specific to symptoms
Progressive supranuclear palsy	Supranuclear ophthalmoparesis Parkinsonism Postural instability	CT or MRI: hummingbird sign (also called penguin sign) due to midbrain atrophy
Neurofilament inclusion body disease	Prominent features: early falling and mutism Rapid progression in loss of mobility	MRI: frontal, temporal, and caudate atrophy
Corticobasal degeneration	Progressive asymmetric movement disorder with akinesia, rigidity, focal myoclonus, ideomotor apraxia, and alien limb phenomena Resistant to levodopa	Imaging: asymmetrical cortical atrophy, focal atrophy of the posterior frontal and parietal regions, asymmetrical ventricles, and atrophy of the corpus collosum
Vascular		
Multi-infarct, thalamic infarct, callosum infarct	Acute onset or stepwise progression Unilateral upper motor neuron weakness Aphasia	Diffusion-weighted imaging: restricted diffusion
Cerebral amyloid angiopathy	Older patients Insidious	Gradient-echo MRI: hypointensities consistent with lobar and cortical hemosiderin deposition
Dural arteriovenous fistulas	Headache Seizure Aphasia	Noninvasive angiography or venography: vascular abnormalities
Venous thrombosis	Acute Headache Seizure Increased ICP Coma	MRI: edema and venous infarction
Cerebroretinal microangiopathy with calcifications and cysts	Children	CT: multiple calcifications
Posterior reversible encephalopathy syndrome	Headache, vision changes, high blood pressure, renal failure, transplant patients	Noncontrast CT of the head: subcortical and cortical hypodensities (vasogenic edema) T2-weighted FLAIR MRI of the brain: hyperintensities typically in the occipital lobes

(*continued next page*)

Table 101.1 • Continued

Cause	Clinical Features	Investigational Features
Infectious		
Viral encephalitis	Meningismus Fever Leukocytosis Headache	PCR: HSV, VZV, and West Nile virus
HIV dementia	History of HIV infection Recurrent infections Low CD4 count	HIV serology Viral DNA CD4 counts
Progressive multifocal leukoencephalopathy	History of immunosuppression (including immunosuppressive drugs)	PCR: JC virus
Neurosyphilis	History of syphilis Meningitis Cranial neuropathies Concomitant uveitis, vitreitis, and retinitis Genital lesions	CSF VDRL test FTA-ABS test
Lyme disease	Target rash Tick exposure Arthralgias	Lyme disease antibody test
Whipple disease	Cognitive and psychiatric dysfunction Hemiparesis, seizures, and ataxia Oculomasticatory myorhythmia	PCR: *Tropheryma whipplei* Duodenal biopsy: acid-fast bacilli
Subacute sclerosing panencephalitis	Unvaccinated children (measles)	Measles serology
Amebic infection (*Balamuthia mandrillaris*)	Meningoencephalitis Cutaneous lesions (may or may not be present), ranging from ecthymalike lesions to erythematous plaques	Immunofluorescent assays Skin biopsy: trophozoites
Toxic or metabolic		
Metal toxicity	History of exposure Lithium: encephalopathy Inorganic mercury: tremor and psychological disturbance Organic mercury: triad of concentric visual field loss, paresthesia, and cerebellar ataxia without tremor Bismuth: cognitive dysfunction, tremor, ataxia, dysarthria, and myoclonus	Urine heavy metal screen
Vitamin deficiencies	Vitamin B_{12}: peripheral neuropathies, myelopathy (loss of dorsal columns), and subacute combined degeneration Niacin: diarrhea, dementia, and dermatitis Vitamin B_1: symptoms of Wernicke encephalopathy (confusion, ophthalmoplegia, and ataxia)	Serum vitamin levels Increased methylmalonic acid levels MRI: mammillary body changes
Endocrinologic abnormalities	Symptoms and signs of thyroid hormone or cortisol abnormalities	Thyroid function tests Corticotropin level Cortisol level
Metabolic abnormalities	History of diabetes mellitus, renal or liver disease, or infections Symptoms and signs indicating liver or renal disease	Electrolyte disturbances Hypoxia Hypoglycemia or hyperglycemia Abnormal results on liver function tests Hyperammonemia Uremia Electrolyte abnormalities

Table 101.1 • Continued

Cause	Clinical Features	Investigational Features
Malignancy		
Metastases to brain	History of neoplasia elsewhere in the body	MRI or CT: mass lesions Biopsy needed for diagnosis
Primary CNS tumors (eg, CNS lymphoma, lymphomatoid granulomatosis, and gliomatosis cerebri)	Symptoms and signs of mass effect or increased ICP due to obstruction	MRI or CT: mass lesions Biopsy needed for diagnosis
Epilepsy	History of seizures or convulsions	EEG: epileptic discharges Nonconvulsive status epilepticus
Iatrogenic	Medication history (eg, lithium, methotrexate, or chemotherapy) Illicit drug use	Urine toxicology screen Drug levels
Systemic		
Sarcoidosis	Pulmonary symptoms, fever, weight loss, and erythema nodosum	Chest radiography: bilateral hilar lymphadenopathy Increased ACE levels
Mitochondrial disease (eg, MELAS syndrome)	Myopathies History of strokelike episodes	Lactic acidosis MRI: lesions do not follow vascular territories
Delirium	Acute fluctuations in alertness, inattention, and disorganized thinking A secondary syndrome due to a systemic, infectious, metabolic, or medication- or drug-induced process Reverses with correction of primary illness Higher lifetime risk for true dementia	Metabolic and systemic derangements EEG: slow delta and theta waves; triphasic waves

Abbreviations: Aβ42, β-amyloid 42; ACE, angiotensin-converting enzyme; CNS, central nervous system; CSF, cerebrospinal fluid; CT, computed tomography; EEG, electroencephalography; FDG, fludeoxyglucose F18-labeled; FLAIR, fluid-attenuated inversion recovery; FTA-ABS, fluorescent treponemal antibody absorption; HIV, human immunodeficiency virus; HSV, herpes simplex virus; ICP, intracranial pressure; MELAS, mitochondrial encephalopathy, lactic acidosis, and strokelike episodes; MRI, magnetic resonance imaging; PCR, polymerase chain reaction; PET, positron emission tomography; SPECT, single-photon emission computed tomography; VZV, varicella zoster virus.

age at onset is 60 to 69 years. The disease carries an 85% to 90% 1-year mortality rate and a mean survival of about 6 months.

On the basis of the methionine (M) and valine (V) polymorphism in the prion gene at codon 129 and the molecular weight of protease-resistant protein fragments, sCJD is further classified into 6 types (Table 101.3).

sCJD can mimic several neurologic or psychiatric conditions (Table 101.3). Behavioral abnormalities may be the first symptom in 20% of patients; 5% to 10% may have initial or early sensory symptoms. About one-third of patients have prodromal features such as asthenia or fatigue, headache, malaise, vertigo or dizziness, altered sleep and eating patterns, and unexplained weight loss.

Tissue sampling (brain biopsy or autopsy) is the gold standard for diagnosis of any prion disease. Gross pathology is usually normal with age-appropriate changes, but histopathologic examination shows nerve cell loss, gliosis, and vacuolation (also called *spongiform change*) (Figure 101.1).

Tissue analysis is highly invasive, yields false-negative results, and exposes the surgical team to pathogenic transmission. Thus, noninvasive tests should be completed first. In about two-thirds of patients, electroencephalography shows 1- to 2-Hz periodic sharp-wave complexes (Figure 101.1 A and B). These abnormalities usually do not appear until the disease is quite advanced. Magnetic resonance imaging (MRI) diffusion-weighted imaging and apparent diffusion coefficient sequences show restricted diffusion in the cortical or subcortical gray matter. MRI has high diagnostic utility, with sensitivity and specificity greater than 90%. Results from cerebrospinal fluid (CSF) analysis are usually normal with the exception of a mildly elevated protein level (usually <100 mg/dL). CSF S-100-β biomarkers such

Table 101.2 • Diagnostic Tests for Evaluation of Rapidly Progressive Dementia

Category	First-Line Tests	Second-Line Tests
Blood tests	Routine hematology Basic metabolic panel Liver function tests Calcium and magnesium levels Thyroid function tests Vitamin B_{12} Inflammatory markers (eg, ESR and CRP) Serum ammonia Drug levels (as appropriate)	Blood smear Coagulation profile and hypercoagulability testing Homocysteine and methylmalonic acid levels Additional endocrinology tests Lymphoma markers
Serology	ANA ANCA Voltage-gated potassium channel antibodies NMDA receptor antibodies RPR TPHA (for neurosyphilis) HIV (ELISA)	Serology for specific infections (eg, Lyme disease) Paraneoplastic antibodies Antithyroglobulin and antithyroperoxidase antibodies Other rheumatologic tests (eg, anti-Smith antibody, rheumatoid factor, and complement components C3 and C4)
Imaging	MRI of the brain, including diffusion-weighted axial images, FLAIR, hemosiderin sequence, and postgadolinium imaging	Angiography (for vasculitis, dural arteriovenous fistula, and intravascular lymphoma) Cancer screening: CT of the whole body, FDG-PET, testicular or pelvic ultrasonography, and mammography Carotid ultrasonography and echocardiography
CSF	Cell counts, biochemistry, and oligoclonal bands Gram stain, acid-fast stain, fungal stains and culture, and cryptococcal antigen 14-3-3 protein, S-100-β protein, RT-QuIC assay, Aβ42, total tau	CSF serology for NMDA receptor encephalitis Measles serology PCR for JC virus and for viruses associated with other encephalitides PCR for Whipple disease Phosphorylated tau, Aβ42 β2 Microglobulin
Genetics	*PRNP* analysis	Dementia gene panel
Urine	Urinanalysis and culture Urine toxicology screen	Heavy metal screen
Other tests	EEG	Electromyography and nerve conduction studies Brain biopsy Autopsy

Abbreviations: Aβ42, β-amyloid 42; ANA, antinuclear antibody; ANCA, antineutrophil cytoplasmic antibody; CRP, C-reactive protein; CSF, cerebrospinal fluid; CT, computed tomography; EEG, electroencephalography; ELISA, enzyme-linked immunosorbent assay; ESR, erythrocyte sedimentation rate; FDG, fludeoxyglucose F18-labeled; FLAIR, fluid-attenuated inversion recovery; HIV, human immunodeficiency virus; MRI, magnetic resonance imaging; NMDA, *N*-methyl-D-aspartate; PCR, polymerase chain reaction; PET, positron emission tomography; *PRNP*, prion protein gene; RPR, rapid plasma regain; RT-QuIC, real-time quaking-induced conversion; TPHA, *Treponema pallidum* hemagglutination assay.

as 14-3-3 protein, S-100-β protein, neuron-specific enolase, and total tau indicate neuronal injury, but their sensitivity and specificity are controversial. Real-time quaking-induced conversion, which detects prions by amplifying them into amyloid fibrils, has been shown to have modest sensitivity (77%-92%) but very high specificity (99%-100%).

Management

No cure for CJD has been discovered, and management consists mainly of treating various symptoms, preventing infections, and addressing metabolic derangements. The National Prion Disease Pathology Surveillance Center can be consulted to confirm the diagnosis, register patients, and provide the specific genotype. The disease progresses rapidly, so palliative care should be initiated for the patient's comfort.

Transmission Risk

Prion diseases are not known to be transmitted by typical social or clinical contact. Highly infective tissues are brain, dura mater, spinal cord, eye, and cornea. CSF, liver, lymph node, kidney, lung, and spleen carry a low risk of infection, and other human tissues have no infective potential. Hospitalized patients need not be kept in isolation, but standard precautions should be taken. Gloves should be worn when handling bodily secretions, and tissue

Table 101.3 • Clinical Characteristics of Prion Diseases

Type	Occurrence	Age at Onset, y[a]	Duration of Illness[b]	Clinical Features
sCJD	85% of CJD			
MM1/MV1	60%-70%	65 (42-91)	4 (1-18) mo	Cognitive impairment, myoclonus, ataxia, visual impairment, unilateral signs at onset In patients with MV1, ataxia and sensory defects are more common at onset
VV2	14%	60 (41-81)	6 (3-18) mo	Ataxia at onset, late dementia, myoclonus and pyramidal signs, no aphasia or apraxia
MV2	9%	60 (40-81)	17 (5-72) mo	Ataxia, late dementia, myoclonus and pyramidal signs, aphasia or apraxia, long duration
MM2 Cortical	2%-8%	65 (49-77)	16 (9-36) mo	Progressive dementia and then aphasia Eventually myoclonus and pyramidal signs Parkinsonism, apraxia, and seizures in 30% of patients
MM2 Thalamic	2%	50 (36-70)	24 (15-53) mo	Ataxia, visual signs, and cognitive impairment Most patients have insomnia, dementia, and motor signs, including ataxia, dysarthria, tremor, myoclonus, and spasticity
VV1	1%	39 (24-49)	15 (14-16) mo	Young age at onset Progressive dementia, mainly frontotemporal type Myoclonus and pyramidal signs eventually appear
VPSPr	35 cases reported worldwide	. . .	>2 y	Predominantly psychiatric symptoms and then rapid cognitive decline with aphasia, ataxia, and parkinsonism
Genetic				
Genetic CJD	5%-15% of CJD	30-55	4 mo to 4 y	Similar to sCJD except that personality changes occur early in patients with the T183A-129M haplotype
GSS	1 per 100 million per year	30-60	3.5-9.5 y	Ataxic or motor symptoms and then dementia
FFI	100 cases in 40 families	36-62	12 mo	Insomnia, sleep fragmentation, altered arousal, and dreamlike automatism during the day with dysautonomia
Acquired	<1% of CJD			
Kuru	. . .	4-60	12 mo	Incubation period, 4.5-40 y Prodrome of headache and joint pain and then cerebellar ataxic syndrome (stages progress from ambulatory to sedentary to recumbent) Other common features: horizontal convergent strabismus, nystagmus, facial spasm, and palsy
Variant CJD	. . .	29 (16-39)	14 mo	Begins with psychiatric prodrome about 6 mo before onset of neurologic symptoms Cognitive dysfunction, dysesthesia, cerebellar dysfunction, and involuntary movements
Iatrogenic CJD	. . .	. . .	6-12 mo	Resembles kuru when spread from human growth hormone Resembles sCJD when linked to dura mater grafts

Abbreviations: CJD, Creutzfeldt-Jakob disease; FFI, fatal familial insomnia; GSS, Gerstmann-Sträussler-Scheinker syndrome; M, methionine; sCJD, sporadic Creutzfeldt-Jakob disease; V, valine; VPSPr, variably protease-sensitive prionopathy.

[a] Values are mean (range) or range.

[b] Values are mean, mean (range), or range.

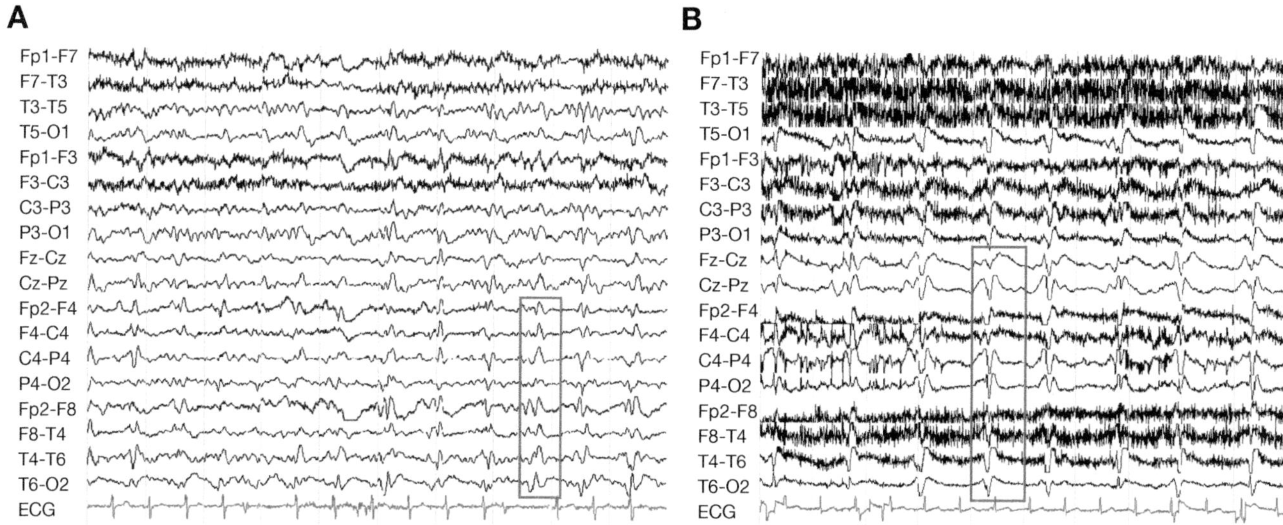

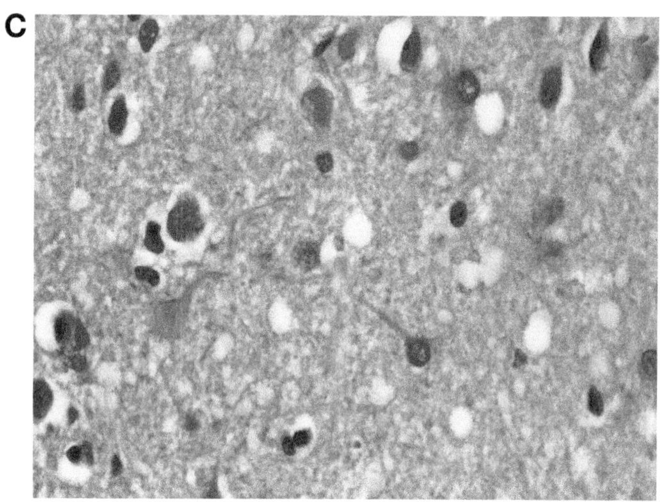

Figure 101.1. Sporadic Creutzfeldt-Jakob Disease. The patient presented with diplopia and ataxia, but the disease progressed to aphasia, mutism, right hemiparesis, coma, and death within 7 months. A, Electroencephalogram (EEG) at presentation showed sharp waves predominantly over the right hemisphere (red rectangle). ECG indicates electrocardiogram. B, EEG 1 week later showed evolution of periodic sharp-wave complexes (red rectangle). C, Histopathologic examination showed spongiform changes (small, round, oval vacuoles in the neuropil), pyknosis, and gliosis (hematoxylin-eosin).

samples should be labeled *Biohazard* and *Suspected CJD.* Equipment that was in contact with high-risk tissue should be sterilized by autoclave at 134°C for more than 18 minutes in a prevacuum sterilizer (or at 121°C-132°C for 1 hour in a gravity displacement sterilizer), discarded, or cleaned with bleach (1:10 dilution).

Summary

- CJD is the prototype of RPD.
- The most common subtype of CJD is sCJD, constituting 85% of all CJD cases.
- The initial symptoms of sCJD include cognitive deficits, myoclonus, cerebellar ataxia, and behavioral changes.
- MRI, electroencephalography, and CSF biomarkers in combination with the clinical picture can be helpful in making a diagnosis of probable CJD, but tissue analysis is required for confirmation.
- Treatment of prion disease is mainly supportive and palliative because no cure is known.
- Brain, spinal cord, and eye tissues are highly infective, and special precautions should be taken to avoid exposure to them; CSF carries a low risk of infection.

SUGGESTED READING

Appleby BS, Yobs DR. Symptomatic treatment, care, and support of CJD patients. Handb Clin Neurol. 2018;153:399–408.

Armstrong MJ, Litvan I, Lang AE, Bak TH, Bhatia KP, Borroni B, et al. Criteria for the diagnosis of corticobasal degeneration. Neurology. 2013 Jan 29;80(5):496–503.

Belay ED. Transmissible spongiform encephalopathies in humans. Annu Rev Microbiol. 1999;53:283–314.

Boeve BF. Progressive supranuclear palsy. Parkinsonism Relat Disord. 2012 Jan;18 Suppl 1:S192–4.

Bueler H, Fischer M, Lang Y, Bluethmann H, Lipp HP, DeArmond SJ, et al. Normal development and behaviour of mice lacking the neuronal cell-surface PrP protein. Nature. 1992 Apr 16;356(6370):577–82.

Chen C, Dong XP. Epidemiological characteristics of human prion diseases. Infect Dis Poverty. 2016 Jun 2;5(1):47.

Chitravas N, Jung RS, Kofskey DM, Blevins JE, Gambetti P, Leigh RJ, et al. Treatable neurological disorders misdiagnosed as Creutzfeldt-Jakob disease. Ann Neurol. 2011 Sep;70(3):437–44. Epub 2011 Jun 14.

Gambetti P, Kong Q, Zou W, Parchi P, Chen SG. Sporadic and familial CJD: classification and characterisation. Br Med Bull. 2003;66:213–39.

Geschwind MD. Prion diseases. Continuum (Minneap Minn). 2015 Dec;21(6 Neuroinfectious Disease):1612–38.

Geschwind MD. Rapidly progressive dementia. Continuum (Minneap Minn). 2016 Apr;22(2 Dementia):510–37.

Geschwind MD, Shu H, Haman A, Sejvar JJ, Miller BL. Rapidly progressive dementia. Ann Neurol. 2008 Jul;64(1):97–108.

Haik S, Brandel JP. Infectious prion diseases in humans: cannibalism, iatrogenicity and zoonoses. Infect Genet Evol. 2014 Aug;26:303–12. Epub 2014 Jun 20.

Hur K, Kim JI, Choi SI, Choi EK, Carp RI, Kim YS. The pathogenic mechanisms of prion diseases. Mech Ageing Dev. 2002 Nov;123(12):1637–47.

Imran M, Mahmood S. An overview of human prion diseases. Virol J. 2011 Dec 24;8:559.

Josephs KA, Ahlskog JE, Parisi JE, Boeve BF, Crum BA, Giannini C, et al. Rapidly progressive neurodegenerative dementias. Arch Neurol. 2009 Feb;66(2):201–7.

Josephs KA, Holton JL, Rossor MN, Braendgaard H, Ozawa T, Fox NC, et al. Neurofilament inclusion body disease: a new proteinopathy? Brain. 2003 Oct;126(Pt 10):2291–303. Epub 2003 Jul 22.

Kim MO, Geschwind MD. Clinical update of Jakob-Creutzfeldt disease. Curr Opin Neurol. 2015 Jun;28(3):302–10.

Manson JC, Clarke AR, Hooper ML, Aitchison L, McConnell I, Hope J. 129/Ola mice carrying a null mutation in PrP that abolishes mRNA production are developmentally normal. Mol Neurobiol. 1994 Apr-Jun;8(2–3):121–7.

McKeith IG, Dickson DW, Lowe J, Emre M, O'Brien JT, Feldman H, et al; Consortium on DLB. Diagnosis and management of dementia with Lewy bodies: third report of the DLB Consortium. Neurology. 2005 Dec 27;65(12):1863–72. Epub 2005 Oct 19. Erratum in: Neurology. 2005 Dec 27;65(12):1992.

McKeon A. Autoimmune encephalopathies and dementias. Continuum (Minneap Minn). 2016 Apr;22(2 Dementia):538–58.

McKhann GM, Knopman DS, Chertkow H, Hyman BT, Jack CR Jr, Kawas CH, et al. The diagnosis of dementia due to Alzheimer's disease: recommendations from the National Institute on Aging-Alzheimer's Association workgroups on diagnostic guidelines for Alzheimer's disease. Alzheimers Dement. 2011 May;7(3):263–9. Epub 2011 Apr 21.

Poser S, Mollenhauer B, Kraubeta A, Zerr I, Steinhoff BJ, Schroeter A, et al. How to improve the clinical diagnosis of Creutzfeldt-Jakob disease. Brain. 1999 Dec;122 (Pt 12):2345–51.

Prusiner SB. Prions. Proc Natl Acad Sci U S A. 1998 Nov 10;95(23):13363–83.

Prusiner SB. The prion diseases. Brain Pathol. 1998 Jul;8(3):499–513.

Rutala WA, Weber DJ. Creutzfeldt-Jakob disease: recommendations for disinfection and sterilization. Clin Infect Dis. 2001 May 1;32(9):1348–56. Epub 2001 Apr 10.

Saa P, Harris DA, Cervenakova L. Mechanisms of prion-induced neurodegeneration. Expert Rev Mol Med. 2016 Apr 8;18:e5.

Sandberg MK, Al-Doujaily H, Sharps B, Clarke AR, Collinge J. Prion propagation and toxicity in vivo occur in two distinct mechanistic phases. Nature. 2011 Feb 24;470(7335):540–2.

Sandberg MK, Al-Doujaily H, Sharps B, De Oliveira MW, Schmidt C, Richard-Londt A, et al. Prion neuropathology follows the accumulation of alternate prion protein isoforms after infective titre has peaked. Nat Commun. 2014 Jul 9;5:4347.

Schafer KR, Shah N, Almira-Suarez MI, Reese JM, Hoke GM, Mandell JW, et al. Disseminated Balamuthia mandrillaris infection. J Clin Microbiol. 2015 Sep;53(9):3072–6. Epub 2015 Jul 1.

Studart Neto A, Soares Neto HR, Simabukuro MM, Solla DJF, Goncalves MRR, Fortini I, et al. Rapidly progressive dementia: prevalence and causes in a neurologic unit of a tertiary hospital in Brazil. Alzheimer Dis Assoc Disord. 2017 Jul-Sep;31(3):239–43.

Tee BL, Longoria Ibarrola EM, Geschwind MD. Prion diseases. Neurol Clin. 2018 Nov;36(4):865–97.

Warren JD, Rohrer JD, Rossor MN. Frontotemporal dementia. BMJ. 2013 Aug 6;347:f4827.

Will RG, Ironside JW. Sporadic and infectious human prion diseases. Cold Spring Harb Perspect Med. 2017 Jan 3;7(1). pii: a024364.

Yuan J, Xiao X, McGeehan J, Dong Z, Cali I, Fujioka H, et al. Insoluble aggregates and protease-resistant conformers of prion protein in uninfected human brains. J Biol Chem. 2006 Nov 17;281(46):34848–58. Epub 2006 Sep 20.

Neuro-oncology

Brain and Spine Tumors

MITHUN SATTUR, MBBS; MATTHEW E. WELZ, MS;
BERNARD R. BENDOK, MD

Goals

- Discuss the classification of brain tumors.
- Discuss management and surgical treatment of the manifestations of brain and spine tumors.
- Discuss postoperative complications of brain and spine tumors.

Introduction

Despite advances in imaging methods, neurosurgical techniques, adjuvant radiation, radiosurgery, and chemotherapy, neurocritical care of the patient with neuraxial tumors is an important component of care. Treatment of these tumors may include management of refractory (often focal) seizures and treatment of mass effect and shift from associated edema. This chapter outlines the important pathophysiologic concepts behind the clinical presentation, neurosurgical management, and perioperative intensive care of patients who have these tumors.

Brain Tumors

Epidemiology

In the United States, primary brain tumors have an annual incidence of nearly 14.8 per 100,000 and a male predominance. Malignant primary brain tumors occur at a rate of 4.1 to 5.8 per 100,000 per year and are diagnosed in more than 20,000 patients annually. As expected, metastases form a higher proportion of the population with intracranial tumors, occurring in up to 43,000 patients per year. Not all brain tumors are malignant. Of the benign tumors, meningiomas are most common. Meningiomas are far from "benign" and may require complicated and risky neurosurgical extirpation. Commonly associated risk factors for brain tumors include exposure to high-dose radiation, presence of certain hereditary syndromes, and increasing age; many other putative factors have very weak to poor strength of association.

Types

The recent World Health Organization classification of brain tumors highlights the evolving landscape of neuro-oncology given the rapid knowledge of tumor genes and molecular markers. The broad headings under which brain tumors are classified are as follows:

1. Diffuse astrocytic and oligodendroglial tumors (glioblastoma, astrocytoma)
2. Other astrocytic tumors (pilocytic astrocytoma)
3. Ependymal tumors (ependymoma)
4. Other gliomas (choroid glioma)
5. Choroid plexus tumors
6. Meningiomas
7. Mesenchymal, nonmeningothelial tumors (hemangioblastoma)
8. Neuronal and mixed neuronal-glial tumors (ganglioglioma)
9. Tumors of the pineal region (pineoblastoma)
10. Embryonal tumors (medulloblastoma)
11. Tumors of cranial and paraspinal nerves (schwannoma)
12. Melanocytic tumors
13. Lymphomas
14. Histiocytic tumors (Langerhans cell histiocytosis)
15. Germ cell tumors (yolk sac tumor, germinoma)
16. Tumors of sellar region (craniopharyngioma)
17. Metastatic tumors

Clinical Manifestations

Increased Intracranial Pressure

The most common clinical correlate of increased intracranial pressure (ICP) is headaches that classically are present on awakening from sleep or awaken a patient from sleep, worsened by lying down and Valsalva maneuvers, relieved by the head-up position, and associated with vomiting and blurred vision from papilledema.

In the initial phase of an enlarging mass lesion, the ICP increase is minimal until a point beyond which even small increases in tumor size may lead to dramatic intracranial hypertension. This is due to the nature of the compliance curve. Often, a secondary insult such as intratumoral hemorrhage or seizure-related edema tilts the balance. The pace of intracranial volume increase is also important, as exemplified by the difference in presentation between a malignant tumor such as glioblastoma and a slower-growing meningioma. Increased intracranial hypertension may also be a consequence of obstructive hydrocephalus that develops with infratentorial tumors. In a given patient, the ICP increases from a brain tumor may be severe enough to reduce cerebral perfusion pressure to the point of causing transient visual obscurations or even inducing syncope.

Herniation

The most important herniation syndrome to recognize with a unilateral supratentorial brain tumor is the uncal transtentorial type because it causes catastrophic midbrain compression if left untreated. Recognition is particularly important with temporal lobe tumors because of anatomical proximity to the midbrain. The presence of pupillary dilatation ipsilateral to the tumor in a progressively obtunded patient is an indication to rush a patient to the operating room for decompression. Posterior cerebral artery infarctions as a result of compression of the enlarging tumor can occur. Tonsillar herniation is potentially fatal because of direct medulla oblongata compression. The risk of sudden death is very high with infratentorial tumors, and the threshold to intervene neurosurgically is much lower. Superior cerebellar artery infarction can occur in this instance. Acute obstructive hydrocephalus can result in central downward herniation.

Seizures

Seizures can occur in both intra-axial (within brain parenchyma such as gliomas) and extra-axial tumors (meningiomas) from cortical irritation. The pattern of seizure (may range from focal seizures (far more common) to status epilepticus (unusual). The incidence of seizures is less than 50% in glioblastoma to as high as 85% with low-grade glioma. Seizures can occur in up to 30% of patients with meningiomas and more than 10% of patients with brain metastases. Seizures per se can result in magnetic resonance imaging changes on T2 and fluid-attenuated inversion recovery sequences. Clinically, a seizure can prove devastating by increasing ICP acutely in a patient with a large tumor with poor intracranial compliance. Perioperative antiepileptic drugs are standard at most centers.

Focal Signs

The specific neurologic function affected by the presence of a mass lesion depends on its location along the neuraxis and forms the basis of clinical localization from the history and examination. Commonly, cranial nerve deficits are produced by extra-axial lesions along the skull base or intra-axial tumors within the brainstem. Pituitary tumors and others in the sellar-suprasellar areas (craniopharyngioma) typically impact vision from anterior optic pathway (optic nerves and chiasm, optic tracts) involvement. Hypothalamic dysfunction can also occur from large suprasellar masses and manifest with anorexia, temperature dysregulation, and diabetes insipidus. Hemispheric supratentorial tumors produce typical clinical syndromes depending on their location in the dominant or nondominant frontal, temporal, parietal, or occipital lobes. Various combinations of speech difficulty, cognitive issues, higher mental function execution, and motor and sensory deficits may be evident. Posterior fossa tumors usually have some component of cerebellar dysfunction.

Endocrinopathy is an important clinical presentation in pituitary tumors and other lesions in the area, producing either hyperfunction (Cushing disease, acromegaly) or hypofunction (hypopituitarism) that has implications for perioperative management.

Treatment

Comprehensive Approach

Depending on tumor type, brain tumor management broadly is a comprehensive approach involving neurosurgical resection or biopsy, stereotactic radiosurgery, radiation therapy, and chemotherapy. Tumors that are benign and in an accessible location, such as a convexity meningioma, can be definitively treated with microsurgical resection alone. Stereotactic radiosurgery has specific indications such as for upfront therapy or postoperative boost for brain metastases and small skull base tumors such as acoustic neuromas and for postsurgical treatment of recurrent or residual meningioma, pituitary adenoma, or acoustic neuroma. Malignant tumors such as glioblastoma require surgery followed by radiation and chemotherapy. Sometimes aggressive tumor removal is not feasible and surgery is restricted to stereotactic biopsy to diagnose tumor type and direct further therapy. Yet an increasing number of novel treatments are being delivered to deep-seated lesions through stereotactic neurosurgical techniques. Delivery of chemotherapy agents through a stereotactically placed catheter and stereotactic laser ablation are examples of innovative procedures for malignant glioma. Endovascular neurosurgical techniques are indicated in certain instances, such as preoperative tumor embolization in meningiomas. For hydrocephalus, a temporary ventriculostomy may be placed with close monitoring of cerebrospinal fluid drainage and pressure, and for permanent diversion a ventriculoperitoneal shunt or endoscopic third ventriculostomy may be performed.

Resection

Diligent preoperative preparation and planning, careful surgical technique, and close postoperative monitoring are key. Patients with substantial brain edema are usually given dexamethasone. Almost all brain tumor resections are performed with neuronavigation guidance and planning. Antibiotics are standard at induction of general anesthesia. Positioning for optimal tumor exposure may require unique configurations such as the park-bench, sitting, or lateral position with attention to pressure-point padding and neutral neck alignment. Anesthetic techniques to provide brain relaxation are paramount and involve controlled hyperventilation, reverse Trendelenberg position, osmotic agents (mannitol and hypertonic saline), and corticosteroids. One of the major goals is to resect the tumor while avoiding damage to critical areas, and neurosurgeons are aided by intraoperative neuromonitoring with somatosensory evoked potentials and motor evoked potentials and by cranial nerve monitoring when indicated. Awake craniotomy is indicated for supratentorial tumor removal when mapping of motor and language areas is essential to avoiding neurologic deficit. The surgical microscope is indispensable for safe tumor removal, and other adjuncts include ultrasonic aspirator, irrigating bipolar forceps, microdissectors, and indocyanine-green angiography. Tumor resection is followed by meticulous hemostasis because a postoperative hematoma can be devastating. Postoperatively, patients are closely observed and managed for edema, seizures, fluid and electrolyte balance, and wound care.

Perioperative Neurocritical Care Management

With large vascular tumors, cerebral autoregulation may be interrupted postoperatively. In turn, this change may lead to erratic swings in cerebral blood flow with changes in blood pressure and potentially catastrophic manifestations. Therefore, maintenance of a stable blood pressure is important after craniotomy for brain tumor resection. Most neurosurgeons (and this is our practice) recommend maintaining systolic blood pressure lower than 160 mm Hg to prevent postoperative hematoma while also preserving cerebral perfusion pressure. Hypotonic maintenance intravenous fluids such as lactated Ringer solution should be avoided; instead, 0.9% normal saline should be administered to prevent exacerbation of edema.

Dilutional hyponatremia worsens cerebral edema and can result in seizures or altered sensorium. The risk is higher in patients who are confused or obtunded at baseline, and sodium levels need to be monitored regularly in such cases. The risk is also higher in patients with sellar-suprasellar tumors. Correction should not be so rapid as to risk myelinolysis. Similar diligence is necessary to detect and manage hypernatremia, including management of diabetes insipidus.

Corticosteroids are first-line agents to control the vasogenic edema from brain tumors. The most widely used agent is dexamethasone, and it is used in both parenteral and oral forms. The usual initial dose is 10 mg, followed by 4 mg every 6 hours and then a taper depending on clinical response. Doses as high as 100 mg per day have been used in the acute period. Most of the concerns with high-dose corticosteroid administration in the acute phase are related to ulcer prophylaxis and control of hyperglycemia. Chronic corticosteroid therapy is associated with hyperglycemia, hypertension, peptic ulcers, poor wound healing, immunosuppression, and myopathy. Corticosteroids can produce irritability, insomnia, and even psychosis.

Osmotic agents are commonly used to treat cerebral edema. Mannitol (20%) is typically given as a bolus infusion of 0.5 to 1.0 g/kg. Hyperosmolarity, dehydration, and acute kidney injury are main concerns. Hypertonic saline (3%, 7.5%, or 23.4%) is another valuable osmotic agent that maintains intravascular volume. It can be given as a bolus or continuous infusion. Serum sodium level and osmolality are monitored every 4 to 6 hours, and dose adjustments are made accordingly.

In patients who are intubated, hyperventilation for short periods (P_{CO_2} about 30 mm Hg) is a useful technique to control ICP. In addition, sedation and analgesia are indispensable for preventing ICP spikes in such patients. Other simple measures include keeping the head end of the bed elevated to 30°. In cases of refractory intracranial hypertension, ipsilateral decompressive hemicraniectomy can be invaluable. Indeed, in certain cases, when extensive hemispheric edema is expected postoperatively, the bone opening may be extended and the craniotomy flap left out to accommodate swelling without increased ICP.

Hydrocephalus associated with tumors is usually managed with perioperative ventriculostomy placement and cerebrospinal fluid drainage (external ventricular drainage). A drain "challenge" is typically instituted to attempt to wean patients from the drainage. If it is unsuccessful, a shunt is placed or, alternatively in some cases, an endoscopic third ventriculostomy may be indicated.

Prophylactic anticonvulsant therapy in a seizure-naive patient is controversial and not recommended. However, seizures can precipitate edema, which can be problematic preoperatively, during tumor resection, and postoperatively. Therefore, the use of antiepileptic drugs for prevention of seizures perioperatively is preferred by most neurosurgery centers. The preferred agent is levetiracetam, and administration is continued postoperatively for 1 to 2 weeks. Patients with seizures caused by a tumor typically are maintained with medication for 2 to 4 years.

Perioperative seizures can be difficult to recognize. There may be subtle clues such as eyelid fluttering or brief tonic deviation of the neck or gaze. Continuous electroencephalographic monitoring will detect nonconvulsive status epilepticus, but it has to be differentiated from tumor-associated interictal discharges.

Strict use of compression stockings and early ambulation are important. The most common pharmacologic or chemical prophylaxis used is subcutaneous unfractionated heparin or low-molecular-weight heparin, although the evidence is controversial. Typically, we start therapy with subcutaneous unfractionated heparin 24 to 48 hours after an uncomplicated craniotomy, except in specific cases such as a documented postoperative hematoma. Low-molecular-weight heparin such as enoxaparin is also an option, but the effects of the drug cannot be fully reversed if needed.

Postoperative Neurosurgical Care

Regular inspection of the surgical site cannot be overemphasized. Repeated surgery, chronic use of corticosteroids, malnutrition, and impaired mobility are considerable risk factors for wound complications. Unfortunately, these factors can be common in patients with recurrent malignant glioma or brain metastases. It is important to recognize signs of cerebrospinal fluid leak or cerebrospinal fluid collection under the scalp incision (pseudomeningocele) because they may indicate underlying hydrocephalus. A wound that is leaking cerebrospinal fluid should be treated as an emergency in order to prevent meningitis. Table 102.1

Table 102.1 • Complications of Brain Tumor Surgery and Their Management

Complication	Presentation	Investigation	Management
Hemorrhage in residual tumor or tumor bed	Acute decline in level of consciousness Seizures Focal deficit or worsening of existing deficit Worsening headache	CT of head Coagulation: prothrombin time, partial thromboplastin time Platelet count	Reverse coagulopathy Systolic BP <140-160 mm Hg Control seizure Edema control Evacuation
CSF leak	Drainage noted from incision or nose or ear Low-pressure headaches (orthostatic)	CT for hydrocephalus	Bed rest IV antibiotics (second- or third-generation cephalosporin or vancomycin) Re-exploration of incision CSF diversion with ventricular drain or shunt or endoscopy
Seizure	Staring Eye deviation Tonic-clonic spasm Clonic twitching in limb	cEEG Serum sodium CT of head	Anticonvulsants May escalate to IV anesthetics if prognosis allows
Progressive brain edema	Drowsiness Focal deficit of gradual onset Seizure	CT or MRI of head Serum sodium	IV corticosteroids Hypertonic saline Mannitol Correct sodium
Hydrocephalus	Drowsiness Wound bulge or CSF leak	CT or MRI of head	Ventriculostomy if reversible cause or as temporizing Shunt placement Endoscopic third ventriculostomy
Infection	Wound discharge Meningitis Brain abscess	CT or MRI of head Lumbar puncture, if safe Culture wound	IV antibiotics with appropriate coverage Exploration and débridement
General surgical complications	UTI Pneumonia Superficial thrombophlebitis	Investigate and treat appropriately	Investigate and treat appropriately
Deep venous thrombosis or pulmonary embolism	DVT: often asymptomatic and requires surveillance Doppler ultrasonography PE: acute tachycardia and hypoxemia (increased A-a gradient)	Ultrasonography CT angiography of chest	Anticoagulation in pulmonary embolus Vena cava filter placement

Abbreviations: BP, blood pressure; cEEG, continuous electroencephalography; CSF, cerebrospinal fluid; CT, computed tomography; DVT, deep vein thrombosis; IV, intravenous; MRI, magnetic resonance imaging; PE, pulmonary embolism; UTI, urinary tract infection.

summarizes the major concerns associated with postoperative care of patients with brain tumors.

Spine Tumors

Spine tumors are a broad category of lesions that may be classified as follows (with examples):

1. Tumors involving the vertebral column (axial skeleton): metastasis, myeloma, osteoma
2. Extradural tumors: metastasis, lymphoma
3. Intradural extramedullary tumors: meningioma, neurofibroma
4. Intramedullary (spinal cord) tumors: astrocytoma, ependymoma

As with cranial tumors, neurosurgical management includes multiple strategies with surgical resection, radiation and radiosurgery, and chemotherapy, alone or in combination, depending on the disease. Preoperative tumor embolization is performed in certain cases to limit operative blood loss or as therapy. Additional considerations in spine tumors include attention to spine stability and requirement of spine stabilization with instrumentation and graft options. Cement injection through vertebroplasty or kyphoplasty is a minimally invasive technique indicated for stabilization and pain control.

Surgical Approaches

Spine tumors are accessed by various strategic approaches in the cervical, thoracic, and lumbosacral regions. These are broadly divided into anterior and posterior approaches. Table 102.2 summarizes the unique complications associated with each. Any spine tumor resection has the potential for neurologic injury (spinal cord or nerve roots), instability, and instrumentation-related complications. Extensive approaches that involve multilevel fixation have a risk of impressive fluid shifts and anemia.

Table 102.2 • Approaches for Spine Surgery and Their Complications

Region of Spine	Approach	Complication
Cervical	Anterior transcervical	Tense neck hematoma causing airway obstruction Esophageal perforation and mediastinitis Vertebral artery injury
Thoracic	Anterior transthoracic	Chest tube maintenance Lung collapse, pneumonia Venous or aortic injury Pain
	Costotransversectomy lateral extracavitary	Pneumothorax or chest tube maintenance Lung collapse, pneumonia
Lumbar	Anterior: retroperitoneal or transperitoneal	Ileus, intestinal perforation, peritonitis Iliac or aortic injury Inferior vena cava injury Ureteric injury
	Posterior approach: all levels	Pain and spasm from muscle dissection

Relevant Neurocritical Care Management

Pain control is an important postoperative concern and requires therapy with opioids (fentanyl, hydromorphone, and morphine), acetaminophen, and diazepam for spasms. Nonsteroidal anti-inflammatory drugs are not preferred if stabilization has been performed with bone grafting because of the reduction of fusion rates. Prior extensive opioid use may be common in some patient subsets, especially those with metastases, and pain control can be particularly challenging. Ketamine infusion is also used in select cases. Prevention of deep vein thrombosis, mechanically and chemically, is paramount, especially in patients who have limited mobility due to paresis or pain issues. For other considerations such as prevention and management of pulmonary complications, nutrition, infection prevention, and miscellaneous medical complications, standard practice guidelines are followed.

Summary

- Postoperative neurocritical care of patients with brain tumors involves management of brain edema and seizures and close electrolyte and fluid management.
- Ventriculostomy may be needed for a compressive brain tumor.
- Surgery for spine tumors requires close monitoring for deep venous thrombosis and avoidance of cerebrospinal fluid leakage.

SUGGESTED READING

Amar AP, Hage ZA, Bendok BR, Prestigiacomo CJ, Boulos AS, Lavine SD, et al. Comments on: Gore P, Theodore N, Brasiliense L, Kim LJ, Garrett M, Nakaji P, et al. The utility of onyx for preoperative embolization of cranial and spinal tumors. Neurosurgery. 2008 Jun;62(6):1204–11.

Ansell JE, Laulicht BE, Bakhru SH, Hoffman M, Steiner SS, Costin JC. Ciraparantag safely and completely reverses the anticoagulant effects of low molecular weight heparin. Thromb Res. 2016 Oct;146:113–8. Epub 2016 Jul 18.

Batchelor T, DeAngelis LM. Medical management of cerebral metastases. Neurosurg Clin N Am. 1996 Jul;7(3):435–46.

Bondy ML, Scheurer ME, Malmer B, Barnholtz-Sloan JS, Davis FG, Il'yasova D, et al; Brain Tumor Epidemiology Consortium. Brain tumor epidemiology: consensus from the Brain Tumor Epidemiology Consortium. Cancer. 2008 Oct 1;113(7 Suppl):1953–68.

Brophy GM, Bell R, Claassen J, Alldredge B, Bleck TP, Glauser T, et al; Neurocritical Care Society Status Epilepticus Guideline Writing Committee. Guidelines for the evaluation and management of status epilepticus. Neurocrit Care. 2012 Aug;17(1):3–23.

Bruce JN, Fine RL, Canoll P, Yun J, Kennedy BC, Rosenfeld SS, et al. Regression of recurrent malignant gliomas with convection-enhanced delivery of topotecan. Neurosurgery. 2011 Dec;69(6):1272–9.

Carabenciov ID, Buckner JC. Controversies in the therapy of low-grade gliomas. Curr Treat Options Oncol. 2019 Mar 14;20(4):25.

Cloughesy TF, Landolfi J, Hogan DJ, Bloomfield S, Carter B, Chen CC, et al. Phase 1 trial of vocimagene amiretrorepvec and 5-fluorocytosine for recurrent high-grade glioma. Sci Transl Med. 2016 Jun 1;8(341):341ra75.

Cohen-Inbar O, Lee CC, Sheehan JP. The contemporary role of stereotactic radiosurgery in the treatment of meningiomas. Neurosurg Clin N Am. 2016 Apr;27(2):215–28. Epub 2016 Feb 18.

Cote DJ, Dawood HY, Smith TR. Venous thromboembolism in patients with high-grade glioma. Semin Thromb Hemost. 2016 Nov;42(8):877–83. Epub 2016 Aug 30.

Devin CJ, McGirt MJ. Best evidence in multimodal pain management in spine surgery and means of assessing postoperative pain and functional outcomes. J Clin Neurosci. 2015 Jun;22(6):930–8. Epub 2015 Mar 9.

Dietrich J, Rao K, Pastorino S, Kesari S. Corticosteroids in brain cancer patients: benefits and pitfalls. Expert Rev Clin Pharmacol. 2011 Mar;4(2):233–42.

Englot DJ, Magill ST, Han SJ, Chang EF, Berger MS, McDermott MW. Seizures in supratentorial meningioma: a systematic review and meta-analysis. J Neurosurg. 2016 Jun;124(6):1552–61. Epub 2015 Dec 4.

Espay AJ. Neurologic complications of electrolyte disturbances and acid-base balance. Handb Clin Neurol. 2014;119:365–82.

Fox BD, Cheung VJ, Patel AJ, Suki D, Rao G. Epidemiology of metastatic brain tumors. Neurosurg Clin N Am. 2011 Jan;22(1):1–6.

Fuller KL, Wang YY, Cook MJ, Murphy MA, D'Souza WJ. Tolerability, safety, and side effects of levetiracetam versus phenytoin in intravenous and total prophylactic regimen among craniotomy patients: a prospective randomized study. Epilepsia. 2013 Jan;54(1):45–57. Epub 2012 Jun 27.

Gelb AW, Craen RA, Rao GS, Reddy KR, Megyesi J, Mohanty B, et al. Does hyperventilation improve operating condition during supratentorial craniotomy? A multicenter randomized crossover trial. Anesth Analg. 2008 Feb;106(2):585–94.

Gemma M, Cozzi S, Tommasino C, Mungo M, Calvi MR, Cipriani A, et al. 7.5% hypertonic saline versus 20% mannitol during elective neurosurgical supratentorial procedures. J Neurosurg Anesthesiol. 1997 Oct;9(4):329–34.

Gerszten PC, Monaco EA 3rd. Complete percutaneous treatment of vertebral body tumors causing spinal canal compromise using a transpedicular cavitation, cement augmentation, and radiosurgical technique. Neurosurg Focus. 2009 Dec;27(6):E9.

Gould MK, Garcia DA, Wren SM, Karanicolas PJ, Arcelus JI, Heit JA, et al. Prevention of VTE in nonorthopedic surgical patients: antithrombotic therapy and prevention of thrombosis, 9th ed: American College of Chest Physicians Evidence-Based Clinical Practice Guidelines. Chest. 2012 Feb;141(2 Suppl):e227S-77S. Erratum in: Chest. 2012 May;141(5):1369.

Hamilton MG, Yee WH, Hull RD, Ghali WA. Venous thromboembolism prophylaxis in patients undergoing cranial neurosurgery: a systematic review and meta-analysis. Neurosurgery. 2011 Mar;68(3):571–81.

Hervey-Jumper SL, Berger MS. Evidence for improving outcome through extent of resection. Neurosurg Clin N Am. 2019 Jan;30(1):85–93. Epub 2018 Nov 1.

Hormigo A, Liberato B, Lis E, DeAngelis LM. Nonconvulsive status epilepticus in patients with cancer: imaging abnormalities. Arch Neurol. 2004 Mar;61(3):362–5.

Kim DJ, Czosnyka Z, Kasprowicz M, Smieleweski P, Baledent O, Guerguerian AM, et al. Continuous monitoring of the Monro-Kellie doctrine: is it possible? J Neurotrauma. 2012 May 1;29(7):1354–63. Epub 2011 Nov 4.

Kocher M, Soffietti R, Abacioglu U, Villa S, Fauchon F, Baumert BG, et al. Adjuvant whole-brain radiotherapy versus observation after radiosurgery or surgical resection of one to three cerebral metastases: results of the EORTC 22952–26001 study. J Clin Oncol. 2011 Jan 10;29(2):134–41. Epub 2010 Nov 1.

Ledbetter LN, Leever JD. Imaging of intraspinal tumors. Radiol Clin North Am. 2019 Mar;57(2):341–57. Epub 2018 Dec 3.

Lote K, Stenwig AE, Skullerud K, Hirschberg H. Prevalence and prognostic significance of epilepsy in patients with gliomas. Eur J Cancer. 1998 Jan;34(1):98–102.

Louis DN, Perry A, Reifenberger G, von Deimling A, Figarella-Branger D, Cavenee WK, et al. The 2016 World Health Organization classification of tumors of the central nervous system: a summary. Acta Neuropathol. 2016 Jun;131(6):803–20. Epub 2016 May 9.

Malzkorn B, Reifenberger G. Practical implications of integrated glioma classification according to the World Health Organization classification of tumors of the central nervous system 2016. Curr Opin Oncol. 2016 Nov;28(6):494–501.

Mathiesen O, Dahl B, Thomsen BA, Kitter B, Sonne N, Dahl JB, et al. A comprehensive multimodal pain treatment reduces opioid consumption after multilevel spine surgery. Eur Spine J. 2013 Sep;22(9):2089–96. Epub 2013 May 17.

Mikkelsen T, Paleologos NA, Robinson PD, Ammirati M, Andrews DW, Asher AL, et al. The role of prophylactic anticonvulsants in the management of brain metastases: a systematic review and evidence-based clinical practice guideline. J Neurooncol. 2010 Jan;96(1):97–102. Epub 2009 Dec 3.

Mitra S, Sinatra RS. Perioperative management of acute pain in the opioid-dependent patient. Anesthesiology. 2004 Jul;101(1):212–27.

Mohammadi AM, Hawasli AH, Rodriguez A, Schroeder JL, Laxton AW, Elson P, et al. The role of laser interstitial thermal therapy in enhancing progression-free survival of difficult-to-access high-grade gliomas: a multicenter study. Cancer Med. 2014 Aug;3(4):971–9. Epub 2014 May 9.

Nathan JK, Brezzell AL, Kim MM, Leung D, Wilkinson DA, Hervey-Jumper SL. Early initiation of chemoradiation following index craniotomy is associated with decreased survival in high-grade glioma. J Neurooncol. 2017 Nov;135(2):325–33. Epub 2017 Jul 25.

Rades D, Schiff D. Epidural and intramedullary spinal metastasis: clinical features and role of fractionated radiotherapy. Handb Clin Neurol. 2018;149:227–38.

Ryken TC, McDermott M, Robinson PD, Ammirati M, Andrews DW, Asher AL, et al. The role of steroids in the management of brain metastases: a systematic review and evidence-based clinical practice guideline. J Neurooncol. 2010 Jan;96(1):103–14. Epub 2009 Dec 3.

Salmaggi A, Simonetti G, Trevisan E, Beecher D, Carapella CM, DiMeco F, et al. Perioperative thromboprophylaxis in patients with craniotomy for brain tumours: a systematic review. J Neurooncol. 2013 Jun;113(2):293–303. Epub 2013 Mar 30.

Schumacher AJ, Lall RR, Lall RR, Iii AN, Ayer A, Sejpal S, et al. Low-dose gamma knife radiosurgery for vestibular schwannomas: tumor control and cranial nerve function preservation after 11 Gy. J Neurol Surg B Skull Base. 2017 Feb;78(1):2–10. Epub 2016 May 31.

Singh G, Rees JH, Sander JW. Seizures and epilepsy in oncological practice: causes, course, mechanisms and treatment. J Neurol Neurosurg Psychiatry. 2007 Apr;78(4):342–9.

Sirven JI, Wingerchuk DM, Drazkowski JF, Lyons MK, Zimmerman RS. Seizure prophylaxis in patients with brain tumors: a meta-analysis. Mayo Clin Proc. 2004 Dec;79(12):1489–94.

Soustiel JF, Mahamid E, Chistyakov A, Shik V, Benenson R, Zaaroor M. Comparison of moderate hyperventilation and mannitol for control of intracranial pressure control in patients with severe traumatic brain injury: a study of cerebral blood flow and metabolism. Acta Neurochir (Wien). 2006 Aug;148(8):845–51. Epub 2006 Jun 12.

Strozzi I, Nolan SJ, Sperling MR, Wingerchuk DM, Sirven J. Early versus late antiepileptic drug withdrawal for people with epilepsy in remission. Cochrane Database Syst Rev. 2015 Feb 11;(2):CD001902.

Thiex R, Harris MB, Sides C, Bono CM, Frerichs KU. The role of preoperative transarterial embolization in spinal tumors: a large single-center experience. Spine J. 2013 Feb;13(2):141–9. Epub 2012 Dec 6.

Todd MM, Tommasino C, Moore S. Cerebral effects of isovolemic hemodilution with a hypertonic saline solution. J Neurosurg. 1985 Dec;63(6):944–8.

Tremont-Lukats IW, Ratilal BO, Armstrong T, Gilbert MR. Antiepileptic drugs for preventing seizures in people with brain tumors. Cochrane Database Syst Rev. 2008 Apr 16;(2):CD004424.

Wu AS, Trinh VT, Suki D, Graham S, Forman A, Weinberg JS, et al. A prospective randomized trial of perioperative seizure prophylaxis in patients with intraparenchymal brain tumors. J Neurosurg. 2013 Apr;118(4):873–83. Epub 2013 Feb 8.

Wu CL, Cohen SR, Richman JM, Rowlingson AJ, Courpas GE, Cheung K, et al. Efficacy of postoperative patient-controlled and continuous infusion epidural analgesia versus intravenous patient-controlled analgesia with opioids: a meta-analysis. Anesthesiology. 2005 Nov;103(5):1079–88.

103 Neoplastic Meningitis

ALYX B. PORTER, MD

Goals

- Describe clinical recognition of cancer-related meningitis.
- Describe chemotherapy and radiation options for cancer-related meningitis.
- Describe outcome expectations for cancer-related meningitis.

Introduction

Neoplastic meningitis (NM), also known as carcinomatous meningitis or leptomeningeal metastases, is usually a late-stage complication of cancer. This complication occurs in approximately 5% of patients with cancer, but the incidence in autopsy studies is 3 times higher. Cases of NM are increasing because of increased use of advanced imaging techniques. Breast, lung, and melanoma are the most common solid tumor malignancies leading to this complication, and leukemia and lymphoma are the most common hematologic malignancies. (NM may present as the initial presentation of cancer).

Clinical Manifestations

Clinical manifestations are based on the level of the neuraxis affected. Headache and gait apraxia from meningeal involvement and acute hydrocephalus are common clinical findings. Most prominent is a history (and clinical confirmation) of cognitive decline with memory difficulties and impaired executive function. Other central nervous system symptoms include confusion, nausea, vomiting, dizziness, dysphagia, seizures, hemiparesis, and cranial nerve dysfunction. A patient who presents with peripheral nervous system dysfunction may experience lower motor neuron pattern weakness, reflex asymmetry, dermatomal sensory loss, or bowel or bladder dysfunction. The nuchal rigidity that is typical with infectious meningitides is rarely apparent (approximately 15% of patients).

Laboratory Tests

Gadolinium-enhanced magnetic resonance imaging is more sensitive than computed tomography for the detection of meningeal metastases and is considered the standard imaging technique to aid in diagnosis (Figure 103.1). Results of magnetic resonance imaging with contrast are abnormal in approximately 70% of patients with NM. To ensure appropriate evaluation of the meninges of the spine, high-resolution magnetic resonance imaging with fat suppression is needed. Enhancement and clumping of nerve roots of the cauda equina, conus medullaris, and surface of the spinal cord can be noted, and thickened areas or frank tumor nodules appear at seemingly sporadic locations along the neuraxis. Findings may also include patchy, asymmetric leptomeningeal enhancement over the cerebral convexities and sulci, basilar cisterns and insular regions, pituitary stalk, cranial nerve roots, and cerebellar folia. There may be communicating hydrocephalus with bilateral transependymal edema in the periventricular white matter of the cerebral hemispheres.

Hydrocephalus may be found in patients with NM. Results of cerebrospinal fluid (CSF) studies are abnormal in 30% to 70% of patients. The most common sites of blockage include the skull base, spinal canal, and cerebral convexities. Patients with interruption of CSF flow have decreased survival.

CSF examination, however, will prove the diagnosis, but nearly 45% of patients with NM will have negative cytologic results on initial examination. For that reason, at least 2 large-volume spinal fluid analyses are recommended. With this approach, the likelihood of a positive cytologic result increases to 77% to 100%. For consideration of lymphomatous meningitis, flow cytometry is recommended.

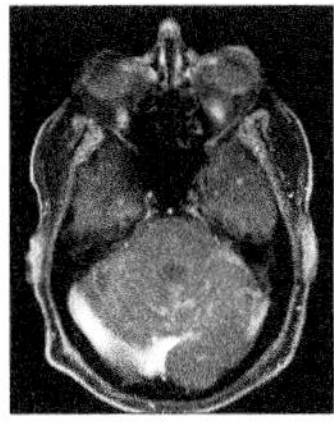

Figure 103.1. Magnetic Resonance Imaging Results for 67-Year-Old Man With Metastatic Melanoma. T1-weighted image with contrast shows intraparenchymal and leptomeningeal metastases with layering of cancer deposits within the cerebellar folia.

Treatment and Outcome

The median duration of survival of untreated patients is between 4 and 6 weeks. Treatment may prolong survival to 4 to 6 months and improve performance status. The surgical management of NM is primarily limited to 1) meningeal biopsy for diagnosis, 2) placement of intraventricular (eg, Ommaya) reservoirs for CSF access, and 3) CSF diversionary procedures (eg, ventriculoperitoneal shunts). The reservoir allows repeated access to the CSF and is associated with decreased discomfort compared with the discomfort resulting from lumbar puncture. In addition, patients seem to better tolerate the repetitive treatments necessary for intrathecal chemotherapy induction (initially, often 2 or more treatments per week) with intraventricular devices than with intralumbar treatments. There is also evidence that intraventricular administration results in improved drug distribution within the CSF pathways compared with intralumbar administration.

Historically, craniospinal irradiation was the primary treatment for NM, and it still is indicated as first-line treatment in certain circumstances, such as treatment of poor-risk medulloblastoma and pineoblastoma or as salvage therapy when initial intrathecal or systemic treatment for leukemic meningitis has failed. Typical radiation dosing is on the order of 30 Gy in 10 fractions. One potential negative effect of craniospinal irradiation is permanent hematologic toxicity, which often impedes the future provision of therapeutic doses of systemic therapy for systemic disease relapse. Nevertheless, palliative benefit is achievable and potentially more rapid with radiotherapy than with other treatments, and thus each case needs to be approached uniquely.

Many patients are too ill to receive aggressive therapy and opt for supportive or hospice care. However, there remains a subset of patients who might otherwise be reasonable candidates for chemotherapy. These patients are generally younger, have a better performance status, and often have controlled systemic disease and a life expectancy of more than 3 months. Drug therapy is a consideration for these select patients. In theory, agents that are capable of producing adequate CSF concentrations after systemic (oral or intravenous) administration also have potential to provide benefit to patients with NM while avoiding the need for invasive intrathecal or intraventricular therapy.

Table 103.1 • Intrathecal Chemotherapy for Neoplastic Meningitis

Drug	Half-Life	Dose Schedule
Methotrexate	4.5-8 h	10-15 mg twice weekly
Cytarabine (ara-C)	3-4 h	25-100 mg twice weekly
Sustained-release ara-C	100-263 h	50 mg every other week
Thiotepa	<4 h	10 mg twice weekly
Mafosfamide	<20 min	3-5 mg twice weekly
Topotecan	2-3 h	0.4 mg twice weekly
Interferon alfa	<10 min	1×10^6 U 3 times weekly
Etoposide	3-12 h	0.5 mg 5 days per week
Rituximab	11-104 h	25 mg 3 times weekly

Agents that are currently available for intrathecal use in the United States include methotrexate, cytarabine (ara-C), sustained-release ara-C, thiotepa, mafosfamide, etoposide, rituximab-interferon alpha, and topotecan. The first 4 of these agents have been used most often in clinical practice. Some of the more frequent doses and schedules that have been reported are listed in Table 103.1. Importantly, none of these agents are approved by the US Food and Drug Administration for this specific indication (intrathecal treatment of NM from solid tumors). Sustained-release ara-C has received conditional approval for treatment of lymphomatous meningitis, and methotrexate and ara-C are indicated for treatment of lymphomatous and leukemic meningitis. Results of randomized controlled clinical trials and promising studies using newer agents are summarized in Tables 103.2 and 103.3.

Summary

- NM is a late complication of systemic cancer and is associated with substantial neurologic morbidity and mortality.
- All patients in whom central nervous system metastasis is suspected should have 1 or 2 lumbar punctures (flow cytometry if lymphoma or leukemia is suspected) and contrast-enhanced neuroimaging of the brain and spine. Radioisotope flow studies are done for patients who are good candidates for therapy.
- Treatment decisions may vary based on tumor type and the performance status of the patient. Options

Table 103.2 • Randomized Clinical Trials of Intrathecal Chemotherapies for Neoplastic Meningitis

Author (Year)	Design	Response	Toxicity
Hitchins et al (1987)	N=44 Nonleukemic malignancy IT MTX vs MTX + ara-C	RR[a]: 61% vs 45% MS[a]: 12 vs 7 wk	N or V: 35% vs 50% Pancytopenia: 9% vs 10% Mucositis: 14% vs 10%
Grossman et al (1993)	N=59 Nonleukemic malignancy IT MTX vs thiotepa 2×/wk	No neurologic improvements MS: 15.9 vs 14.1 wk	Mucositis and neurologic complications more frequent in the MTX group
Glantz et al (1999)	N=61 Solid tumors SR ara-C vs MTX	RR[a]: 26% vs 20% OS[a]: 105 vs 78 d TTP: 58 vs 30 d	Altered mental status: 5% vs 2% Headache: 4% vs 2%
Glantz et al (1999)	N=28 Lymphoma SR ara-C vs ara-C	TTP[a]: 78.5 vs 42 d OS[a]: 99.5 vs 63 d RR: 71% vs 15%	Headache: 27% vs 2% Nausea: 9% vs 2% Fever: 8% vs 4%
Boogerd et al (2004)	N=35 Breast cancer MTX or ara-C (n=17) vs no IT treatment (n=18)	TTP[a]: 23 vs 24 wk MS: 18.3 vs 30 wk	Neurologic complications: 47% vs 6%
Shapiro et al (2006)	N=128 Solid tumors (n=103) Lymphoma (n=25) SR ara-C vs ara-C, MTX, or ara-C + MTX	SR ara-C vs MTX and ara-C PFS[a]: 35 vs 43 d SR ara-C vs MTX PFS: 35 vs 37.5 d SR ara-C vs ara-C PFS: 34 vs 50 d	SR ara-C vs MTX and ara-C Drug-related AEs: 48% vs 60% Serious AEs: 86% vs 77%

Abbreviations: AE, adverse events; ara-C, cytarabine; IT, intrathecal; MS, median survival; MTX, methotrexate; N or V, nausea or vomiting; OS, overall survival; PFS, progression-free survival; RR, relapse rate; SR, sustained-release; TTP, time to progression; Tx, treatment.

[a] No significant difference between groups.

Modified from Porter AB, Jaeckle KA. Neoplastic meningitis. In: Winn RH, editor. Youmans neurological surgery. 6th ed. Philadelphia: Elsevier Saunders; 2011. p.1529-33.

Table 103.3 • Phase I and II Studies of Newer Agents Used in the Treatment of Neoplastic Meningitis

Author (Year)	Agent	Dose	Response	Toxicity
Groves et al (2008), phase II	Topotecan N=62	0.4 mg biweekly × 6 wk	30% 13-wk PFS 19% 6-mo PFS 15-wk MS	32% mild arachnoiditis
Kramer et al (2007), phase I	Iodine I 131 monoclonal antibody N=13	MTD 10 mCi × single dose	23% CSF or MRI responses	Self-limited headache, fever, vomiting
Chamberlain et al (2006), phase II	Etoposide N=27	0.5 mg daily × 5 d every other week × 8 wk	11% 6-mo PFS 4% 1-y survival	18% mild arachnoiditis
Wong et al (2006), phase I	Iodine I 131-sodium iodide N=31	120 mCi × single dose; MTD not reached	29% CSF clearance	All less than grade 2
Blaney et al (2005), phase I	Mafosfamide 1: N=30 2: N=25	1: 5 mg biweekly × 4 wk 2: 14 mg biweekly × 6 wk	1: 43% response or SD	1: headache and neck pain 2: mild irritability

Abbreviations: CSF, cerebrospinal fluid; MRI, magnetic resonance imaging; MS, median survival; MTD, maximal tolerated dose; PFS, progression-free survival; SD, stable disease.

Modified from Porter AB, Jaeckle KA. Neoplastic meningitis. In: Winn RH, editor. Youmans neurological surgery. 6th ed. Philadelphia: Elsevier Saunders; 2011. p.1529-33.

may include craniospinal irradiation, systemic chemotherapy, or intrathecal chemotherapy.

- If a patient's performance status is poor and there is evidence of uncontrolled systemic disease, palliation and hospice are more appropriate.

SUGGESTED READING

Franzoi MA, Hortobagyi GN. Leptomeningeal carcinomatosis in patients with breast cancer. Crit Rev Oncol Hematol. 2019 Mar;135:85–94. Epub 2019 Feb 1.

Le Rhun E, Galanis E. Leptomeningeal metastases of solid cancer. Curr Opin Neurol. 2016 Dec;29(6):797–805.

Nayar G, Ejikeme T, Chongsathidkiet P, Elsamadicy AA, Blackwell KL, Clarke JM, et al. Leptomeningeal disease: current diagnostic and therapeutic strategies. Oncotarget. 2017 Aug 16;8(42):73312–28.

Pellerino A, Bertero L, Ruda R, Soffietti R. Neoplastic meningitis in solid tumors: from diagnosis to personalized treatments. Ther Adv Neurol Disord. 2018 Mar 7;11:1756286418759618.

Rigakos G, Liakou CI, Felipe N, Orkoulas-Razis D, Razis E. Clinical presentation, diagnosis, and radiological findings of neoplastic meningitis. Cancer Control. 2017 Jan;24(1):9–21.

Taillibert S, Chamberlain MC. Leptomeningeal metastasis. Handb Clin Neurol. 2018;149:169–204.

Taylor G, Karlin N, Halfdanarson TR, Coppola K, Grothey A. Leptomeningeal carcinomatosis in colorectal cancer: the Mayo Clinic experience. Clin Colorectal Cancer. 2018 Jun;17(2):e183–7. Epub 2017 Nov 21.

Volkov AA, Filis AK, Vrionis FD. Surgical treatment for leptomeningeal disease. Cancer Control. 2017 Jan;24(1):47–53.

Wang N, Bertalan MS, Brastianos PK. Leptomeningeal metastasis from systemic cancer: review and update on management. Cancer. 2018 Jan 1;124(1):21–35. Epub 2017 Nov 22.

104 Autoimmune Encephalitis

ESLAM SHOSHA, MB, BCh; SEAN J. PITTOCK, MD

Goals

- Understand the clinical features and laboratory test results that aid in the diagnosis of autoimmune encephalitis.
- Discuss appropriate antibody testing and imaging for the diagnosis of autoimmune encephalitis.
- Discuss immunotherapy for autoimmune encephalitis.

Introduction

Autoimmune encephalitis is an increasingly recognized, life-threatening disorder that, because of its variable clinical presentations, poses a diagnostic challenge in the intensive care setting.

The increased recognition of this potentially immunotherapy-responsive disorder is facilitated by a dramatic increase in cerebrospinal fluid (CSF) neural antibody biomarkers of central nervous system autoimmunity, testing for which is now readily available through commercial laboratories and can be performed on both serum and CSF.

Patients with autoimmune encephalitis often need to be in an intensive care unit for management of life-threatening complications commonly related to multifocal nervous system involvement that includes status epilepticus, cognitive decline and behavioral changes, psychosis, and autonomic instability.

Clinical Features

Many patients present with a symptom complex, including the following:

- Acute onset or fluctuating course of a decline in consciousness; profound personality changes and new psychotic breaks; new onset of seizures, status epilepticus, or generalized myoclonus; dysautonomic fluctuation in heart rate, blood pressure, or central hypoventilation; and abnormal movement or posture (eg, opsoclonus myoclonus).
- A history of concurrent malignancy or a personal or family history of an organ-specific or non–organ-specific autoimmune disorder may serve as a diagnostic clue (eg, thyroid disease such as Hashimoto disease or Graves disease, Sjögren syndrome, systemic lupus erythematosus, vitiligo).

Some patients present with a characteristic syndromic presentation, whereas others have atypical or multifocal presentations that do not fit within any predefined entity or neural antibody–associated phenotype. According to Dalmau's working group, the diagnosis of anti-*N*-methyl-D-aspartate (NMDA) encephalitis should be highly suspected with the following clinical presentation:

1. Rapid onset (<3 months) of at least 4 of the 6 following major groups of symptoms:
   - Abnormal (psychiatric) behavior or cognitive dysfunction.
   - Speech dysfunction (pressured speech, verbal reduction, mutism).
   - Seizures.
   - Movement disorder, dyskinesias, or rigidity or abnormal postures.
   - Decreased level of consciousness.
   - Autonomic dysfunction or central hypoventilation.
2. At least 1 of the following laboratory study results:
   - Abnormal electroencephalographic results (focal or diffuse slow or disorganized activity, epileptic activity, or extreme delta brush).
   - CSF with pleocytosis or oligoclonal bands.

(Data in numbers 1 and 2 modified from Graus F, Titulaer MJ, Balu R, Benseler S, Bien CG, Cellucci T, et al. A clinical approach to diagnosis of autoimmune encephalitis. Lancet

Neurol. 2016 Apr;15(4):391-404. Epub 2016 Feb 20; used with permission.)

The diagnosis can also be made in the presence of 3 of the 6 groups of symptoms accompanied by a systemic teratoma or with 1 or more of the 6 major groups of symptoms and NMDA-receptor antibodies detected in CSF (higher specificity than serum).

Laboratory Tests

In serum, nonneural antibodies, both organ-specific (eg, thyroperoxidase) and non–organ-specific (eg, antinuclear antibody, Sjögren syndrome-related antibody, antiphospholipid), indicate a predisposition to autoimmunity and may be associated with neural autoimmunity.

CSF examination may show a mild to moderate lymphocytic pleocytosis (<100 leukocytes/mm^3, in 60%-80% of patients), increased protein level, oligoclonal bands (>4 CSF-specific), and increased immunoglobulin G index. Even mild leukocyte increases of 5 to 10/mm^3 are considered supportive of an autoimmune cause.

An example of abnormal results on magnetic resonance imaging of the brain is shown in Figure 104.1, and imaging findings are summarized as follows:

- Many patients with autoimmune encephalitis may have normal results on magnetic resonance imaging.
- On T2-fluid attenuated inversion recovery hyperintensities in the mesiotemporal region, basal ganglia, cortex, or cerebellum, with or without enhancement.
- Other possible findings: nonspecific leukoaraiosis, posterior reversible encephalopathy syndrome, focal hemorrhage, and necrosis.
- Positron emission tomography shows focal hypometabolism or hypermetabolism in limbic or other cortical regions.

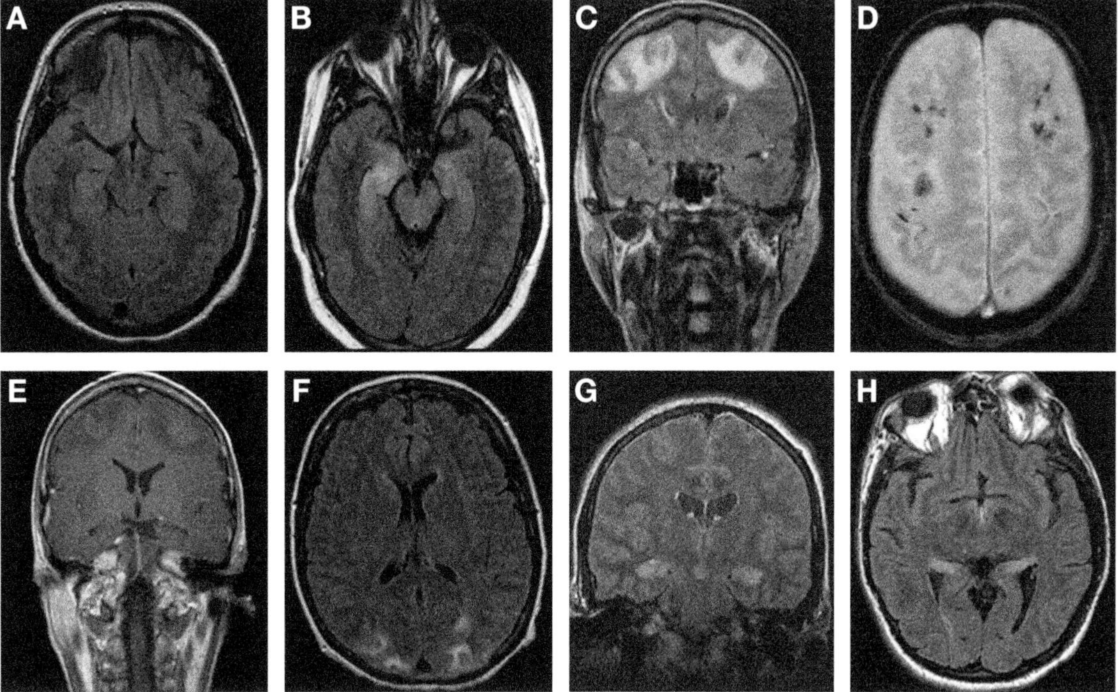

Figure 104.1. Selected Magnetic Resonance Images (MRI) of Head From Patients With Autoimmune Encephalitis Managed in the Neuroscience Intensive Care Unit. MRI sequences were fluid attenuated inversion recovery (axial [A, B, F, and H] or coronal [C and G]), susceptibility-weighted (axial, D), and T1, post-gadolinium (coronal, E). A, Patient with N-methyl-D-aspartate–receptor encephalitis had normal findings, but disease was fatal. B, Patient with Ma1 and Ma2 antibodies had classic limbic encephalitic-appearing hyperintense mesial temporal lobes bilaterally. C-E, Patient had negative results for encephalitis antibody but had diffuse front parietal white matter abnormalities (C), hypointensities consistent with hemorrhage (D), and enhancement (E). F, Patient had parietal and occipital T2 hyperintensities consistent with posterior reversible encephalopathy syndrome. G and H, Patient had abnormal hippocampal T2 signal (G) that extended posteriorly (H).

(From Mittal MK, Rabinstein AA, Hocker SE, Pittock SJ, Wijdicks EF, McKeon A. Autoimmune encephalitis in the ICU: analysis of phenotypes, serologic findings, and outcomes. Neurocrit Care. 2016 Apr;24[2]:240-50; used with permission.)

Electroencephalography is essential, often with continuous monitoring. Many patients have seizures and often are in convulsive or nonconvulsive status epilepticus. Occasionally, electroencephalographic abnormalities point to a specific autoimmune cause (eg, NMDA-receptor encephalitis and extreme delta brush).

Detection of a neural-specific autoantibody supports a diagnosis of an autoimmune neurologic disorder and may aid in identification of a paraneoplastic cause. A comprehensive autoimmune encephalopathy evaluation for neural-specific autoantibodies is shown in Figure 104.2. Generally, antibodies targeting intracellular nuclear and cytoplasmic (including enzymes, transcription factors, and RNA-binding proteins) proteins, including antineuronal nuclear antibody-1 and collapsin response-mediator protein 5-immunoglobulin G, serve as markers of peptide-specific, cytotoxic T-cell–mediated injury. These disorders are usually poorly responsive to immunotherapy (classic paraneoplastic syndromes). Antibodies targeting plasma membrane (neurotransmitter receptors, ion channels, water channels, and channel-complex proteins) proteins, including NMDA receptor and leucine-rich, glioma-inactivated 1 antibodies, are pathogenic. These disorders are generally immunotherapy-responsive.

Classification of antibodies is helpful for guiding a targeted cancer work-up and treatment strategies (Tables 104.1 and 104.2). A negative autoantibody profile does not exclude paraneoplastic or idiopathic neurologic autoimmunity. Importantly, there is considerable overlap of clinical phenotype resulting from immunoglobulin Gs targeting various neural receptors and channels. For example, in many patients, limbic encephalitis associated with antibodies targeting NMDA-receptor, leucine-rich glioma-inactivated 1, γ-aminobutyric acid-B, contactin-associated protein-like 2, paraneoplastic antigen Ma2, and collapsin response-mediator protein-5 may be clinically and radiologically similar. Thus, comprehensive autoantibody testing is advisable. Antibody tests performed on serum alone are often sufficiently informative, but CSF testing sometimes increases the diagnostic yield. In the case of NMDA-receptor antibodies, CSF is frequently more informative than serum. The opposite is true for voltage-gated potassium channel–complex (leucine-rich glioma-inactivated 1 and contactin-associated protein-like 2) and aquaporin-4 antibodies, which (almost always) are more readily detectable in serum than in CSF.

Because neoplasms associated with autoimmunity are often detected early, they are commonly limited and may be difficult to identify on conventional imaging. Subtle imaging abnormalities should be investigated further. Common cancers associated with paraneoplastic disease are listed in Tables 104.1 and 104.2. The following tests can be considered:

- General malignancy screening: Computed tomography (CT) of chest, abdomen, and pelvis with contrast agent.
- Thymoma: chest CT with contrast agent.
- Upper endoscopy (esophagogastroduodenoscopy) and colonoscopy.
- Children: 50% of children presenting with opsoclonus myoclonus syndrome (erratic eye movements, startle or myoclonus, ataxia) have neuroblastoma. Chest and abdominal CT or magnetic resonance imaging and urine testing for homovanillic acid metabolites should be undertaken in children in whom neuroblastoma is suspected.
- Adolescents or young females: A major search for an ovarian teratoma is needed, especially with NMDA-receptor encephalitis (psychosis, behavioral changes, movement disorder, seizures, hypoventilation, coma). In women, transvaginal ultrasonography is done, if possible. Breast mammography or magnetic resonance imaging should be performed.
- Young males: A major search for seminoma is needed, especially with Ma2 antibodies (limbic encephalitis, brainstem encephalitis, hypothalamic dysfunction). Ultrasonography of the testicles is needed, as is CT of the chest because seminoma can be found in the thorax.
- Positron emission tomography, alone or in combination with anatomical data (positron emission tomography-CT), increases the cancer diagnostic yield by 20% when all standard evaluations (eg, whole-body CT) have been uninformative. However, positron emission tomography is not helpful for detecting gonadal tumors (ovary or testis), neuroblastoma, or thymoma.

Management

Immunotherapies are recommended to maximize reversibility.

- Immunotherapy (Table 104.3): intravenous corticosteroids, intravenous immunoglobulin G, and plasmapharesis, single or combined, are first-line therapies. Immunosuppression with rituximab or cyclophosphamide is considered if initial treatment fails, but there is no evidence against using them as first-line agents.
- Refractory seizures, status epilepticus, abnormal movements; sympathetic hyperactivity; or agitation: management is according to standard therapies for each.
- Concomitant oncologic therapy: For patients proved to have paraneoplastic disease, standard oncologic therapy (eg, teratoma removal in NMDA encephalitis) is recommended.

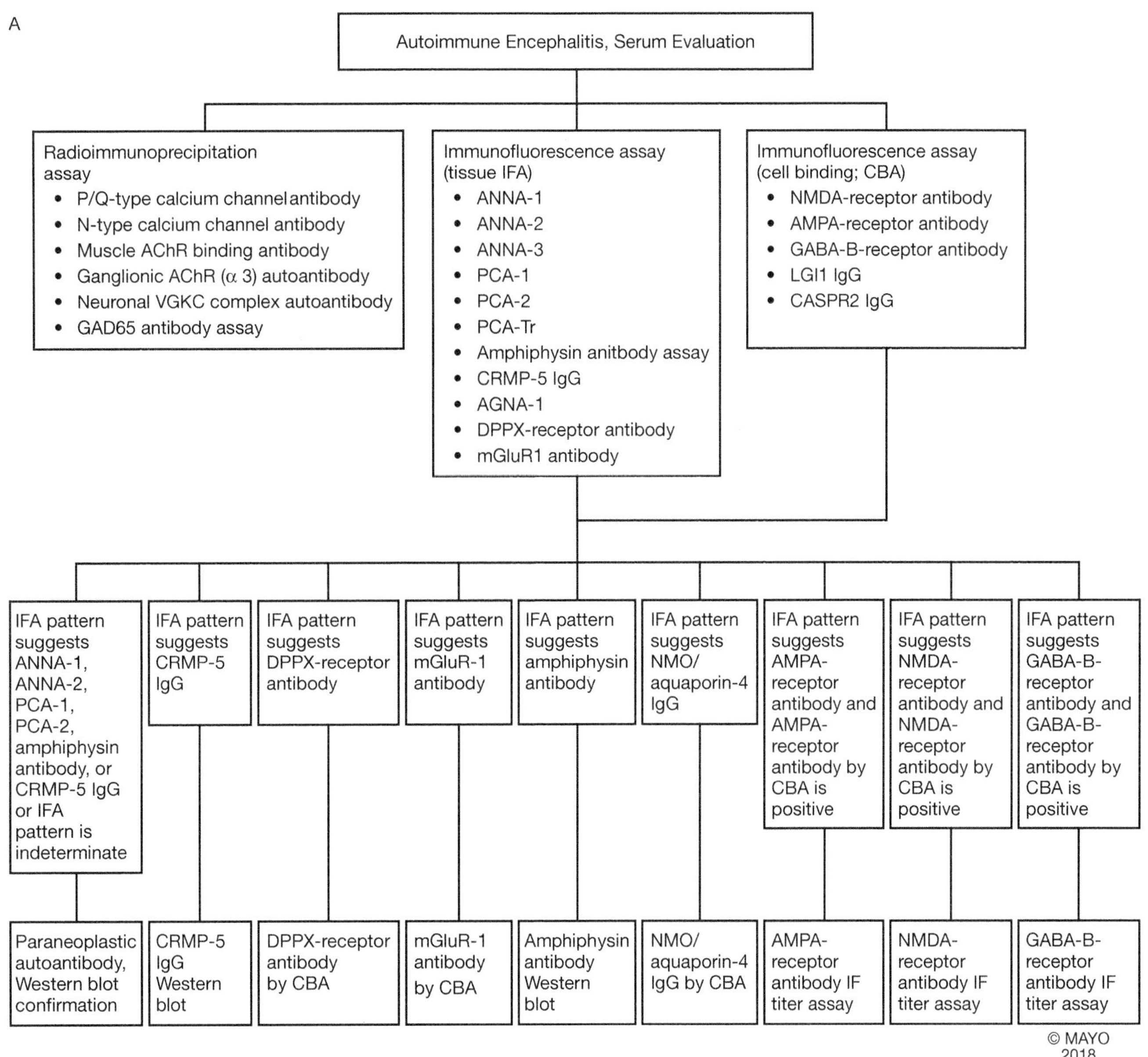

Figure 104.2. Algorithms for Evaluation for Autoimmune Encephalitis. A, Serum.
(Modified from Linnoila J, Pittock SJ. Autoantibody-associated central nervous system neurologic disorders. Semin Neurol. 2016 Aug;36[4]:382-96. Epub 2016 Sep 19; used with permission of Mayo Foundation for Medical Education and Research.)
B, Spinal fluid. AChR indicates acetylcholine receptor; AGNA-1, antiglial nuclear antibody type 1; AMPA, α-amino-3-hydroxy-5-methyl-4-isoxazole propionic acid; ANNA, antineuronal nuclear antibody (type 1, 2, or 3); CASPR2, contactin-associated protein-like 2; CRMP-5, collapsin response-mediator protein-5; DPPX, dipeptidyl-peptidase–like protein-6; GABA-B, α-aminobutyric acid; GAD65, glutamic acid decarboxylase; IF, immunofluorescence; IgG, immunoglobulin G; LGI1, leucine-rich glioma-inactivated 1; mGluR1, metabotropic glutamate receptor 1; NMDA, N-methyl-D-aspartate; *NMO, neuromyelitis optica; PCA, Purkinje cell cytoplasmic antibody (type 1, 2, or Tr); VGKC, voltage-gated potassium channel complex.*
(Used with permission of Mayo Foundation for Medical Education and Research.)

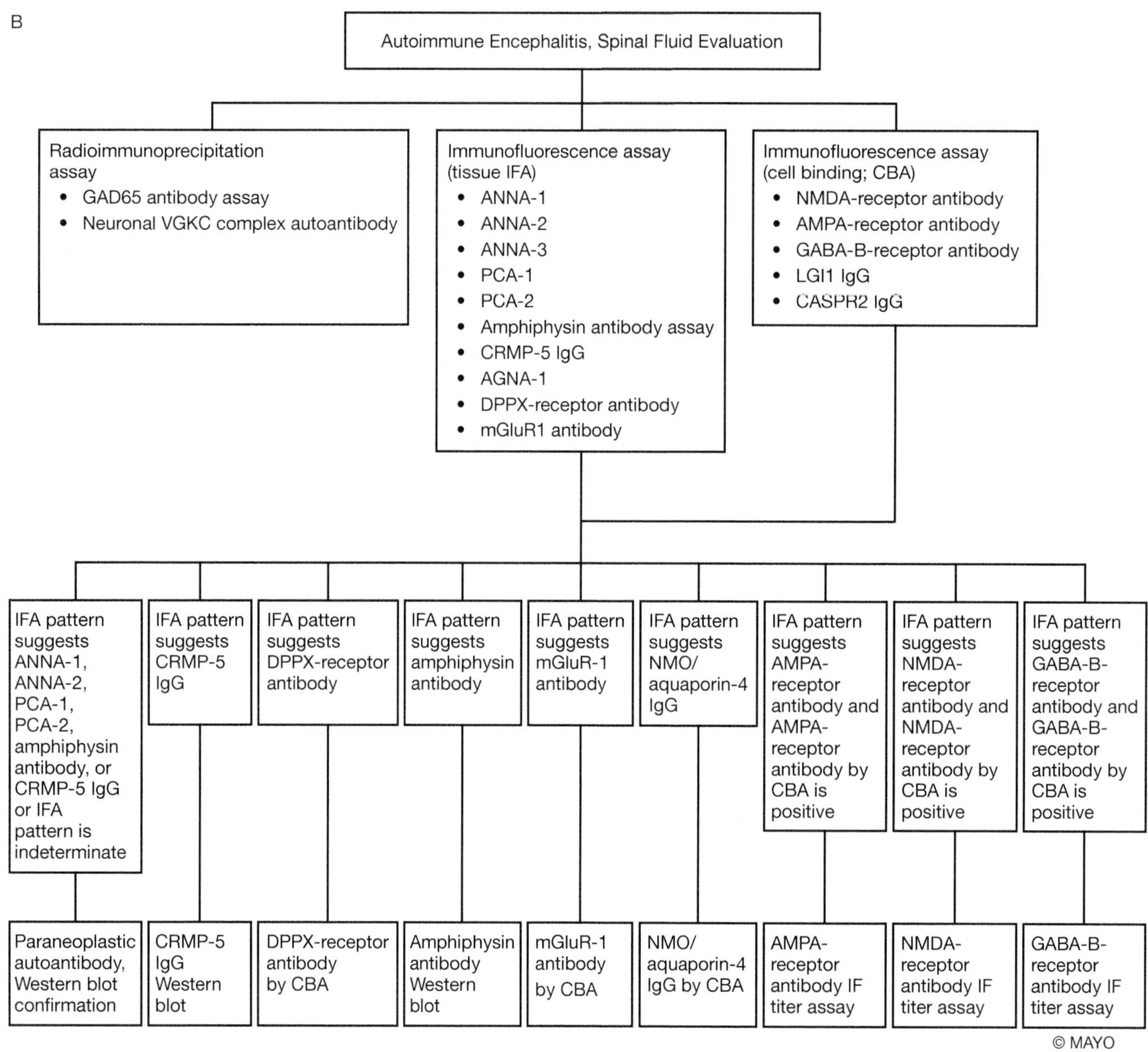

Figure 104.2. Continued

- Coexisting conditions: Treatment of herpes encephalitis could precede or accompany that of NMDA encephalitis.

Outcome

Early and aggressive treatment is important. Admission to an intensive care unit by itself is a risk factor for increased morbidity and mortality. Patients can die of severe brainstem or limbic encephalitis, superrefractory status epilepticus, metastatic cancer, and other intensive care unit–associated medical morbidities. The NEOS score predicts 1-year functional status in patients with anti-NMDA-receptor encephalitis. Young patients can do well.

Summary

- Autoimmune encephalitis can be characterized and several tests for underlying cancer (particularly ovarian teratoma) are needed.
- Treatment with corticosteroids and immunotherapy has improved outcome.

Table 104.1 • Oncologic and Neurologic Accompaniments of Neural Nuclear and Cytoplasmic Antibodies in the Intensive Care Unit

Antigen	Clinical Features	Associated Tumors[a]
AGNA (SOX1)	Limbic encephalitis	Highly associated with small cell lung cancer
Amphiphysin	Wide clinical spectrum: limbic encephalitis, encephalomyelitis, PERM	About 85% (breast, small cell lung cancer[b])
ANNA-1 (anti-Hu)	Wide clinical spectrum: limbic encephalitis, encephalomyelitis, status epilepticus, autonomic dysfunction, opsoclonus myoclonus	About 80% (small cell lung cancer, neuroblastoma, prostate cancer)
ANNA-2 (Anti-Ri)	Opsoclonus myoclonus, brainstem encephalitis, laryngospasm	About 60% (breast, gynecologic, lung,[b] bladder cancer)
ANNA-3	Encephalomyelitis	About 60% (lung cancer[b])
CRMP5 (anti-CV2)	Wide clinical spectrum: limbic encephalitis, chorea, encephalomyelitis	About 75% (small cell lung cancer, thymoma)
GAD-65	Usually >20 nM (normal ≤0.02 nM) Wide clinical spectrum: encephalitis, stiff person syndrome, seizure disorder	<10% (lung cancer,[b] neuroendocrine tumor, thymoma, breast cancer)
Anti-PNMa1 and anti-PNMa2 (anti-Ma)	Anti-Ma: cerebellar and brainstem dysfunction	Breast, colon, parotid, non–small cell lung cancer
Anti-PNMa2 only (anti-Ta)	Limbic encephalitis, hypothalamic dysfunction, brainstem encephalitis	Germ cell testicular
PCA-2 (anti Map1B)	Encephalomyelitis	About 90% (lung cancer[b])
GFAPα-IgG	Meningoencephalitis	22%, diverse (ovarian teratoma most common)

Abbreviations: AGNA, antiglial nuclear antibody; ANNA, antineuronal nuclear antibody; CAR, cancer associated retinopathy; CRMP5, collapsin response-mediator protein 5; GAD-65, glutamic acid decarboxylase; GFAPα-IgG, glial febrillary acidic protein immunoglobulin G; MAP1B, microtubule-associated protein 1B; PCA, Purkinje cell cytoplasmic antibody; PERM, progressive encephalomyelitis with rigidity and myoclonus; PNMa1, paraneoplastic Ma1; PNMa2, paraneoplastic Ma2; SOX1, sex-determining region Y box 1 transcription factor.

[a] Percentages are percentage of patients with particular antibody who also have malignancy.

[b] Lung cancer includes both small cell and non–small cell lung cancer, unless otherwise specified. Percentage refers to percentage of patients with particular antibody that also have malignancy.

Modified from Linnoila J, Pittock SJ. Autoantibody-associated central nervous system neurologic disorders. Semin Neurol. 2016 Aug;36(4):382-96. Epub 2016 Sep 19; used with permission.

Table 104.2 • Oncologic and Neurologic Accompaniments of Neural Cell Surface Autoantibodies in the Intensive Care Unit

Antigen	Clinical Features	Associated Tumors[a]
AMPAR	Limbic encephalitis, may occur with pure psychiatric manifestations, relapses common	About 70% (lung, breast, thymoma)
CASPR2	Encephalitis, Morvan syndrome, relapses of encephalitis common	0%-40% (thymoma)
DPPX	Encephalitis with CNS hyperexcitability: confusion, psychiatric manifestations, myoclonus, PERM-like symptoms	Rare B-cell neoplasms reported
GABA-A receptor	Refractory seizures, status epilepticus, or epilepsia partialis continua	Infrequent
GABA-B receptor	Limbic encephalitis, status epilepticus	About 50% (lung, neuroendocrine)
GlyαR	Wide clinical spectrum: stiff person syndrome, limbic encephalitis, PERM	Infrequent
LGI-1	Limbic encephalitis, dystonic faciobrachial seizures, REM sleep behavior disorder, myoclonus, about 60% with hyponatremia	<10% (smallcell lung cancer, thymoma)
mGluR5	Ophelia syndrome: limbic encephalitis, myoclonus; few cases	Hodgkin lymphoma; may occur without tumor

(*continued next page*)

Table 104.2 • Continued

Antigen	Clinical Features	Associated Tumors[a]
NMDA receptor (GluN1)	NMDA receptor encephalitis: progression through psychiatric manifestations, insomnia, reduced verbal output, seizures, amnesia, movement disorders, catatonia, hypoventilation, autonomic instability, coma	Age-dependent: 10%-45%, most often ovarian teratomas, rarely carcinomas; rare in children
VGCC (P/Q and N-type)	Variable; includes encephalopathy, seizures, LEMS	LEMS: about 50% (small cell lung cancer) <10% have prospectively identified cancer

Abbreviations: AMPAR, α-amino-3-hydroxy-5-methyl-4-isoxazolepropionic acid receptor; CASPR2, contactin-associated protein-like 2; CNS, central nervous system; DPPX, dipeptidyl-peptidase–like protein-6; GABA, γ-aminobutyric acid; GluN1, ionotropic NMDA glutamate receptor; GlyαR, glycine α receptor; LEMS, Lambert-Eaton myasthenic syndrome; LGI-1, leucine-rich, glioma-inactivated 1; mGluR, metabotropic glutamate receptor; NMDA, *N*-methyl-D-aspartate; PERM, progressive encephalomyelitis with rigidity and myoclonus; REM, rapid eye movement; VGCC, voltage-gated calcium channel.
[a] Percentages are percentage of patients with particular antibody who also have malignancy.

Modified from Linnoila J, Pittock SJ. Autoantibody-associated central nervous system neurologic disorders. Semin Neurol. 2016 Aug;36(4):382-96. Epub 2016 Sep 19; used with permission.

Table 104.3 • Treatment Options, Adverse Effects, and Monitoring of Some Commonly Used Immunotherapies in the Intensive Care Unit

Medication	Dose	Route	Frequency	Adverse Effect	Suggested Monitoring, Other Advice
Methyl-prednisolone	1 g	IV	Daily × 3-5, then weekly × 6, then every other wk × 6	Insomnia, increased appetite, psychosis, Cushing syndrome, diabetes mellitus, cataracts, osteoporosis, hip avascular necrosis, skin thinning	Check hCG before starting; monitor glucose, blood pressure; avoid live vaccines; osteoporosis prophylaxis with 1,500 mg calcium and 1,000 international units vitamin D daily; *Pneumocystis carinii* prophylaxis with TMP-SMX DS 1 pill Mon, Wed, Fri; gastritis prophylaxis with proton pump inhibitor or H_2-blocker
Immunoglobulin	0.4-1 g/kg	IV	Daily × 3-5, then weekly × 6, then every other wk × 6	Aseptic meningitis, deep venous thrombosis, headache, anaphylaxis, renal failure	Check IgA before starting, and if low consider other therapy; monitor for anaphylaxis, rash, and clots
Rituximab	1 g, repeat in 2 wk	IV	Every 6 mo	Infusion reactions, edema, hypertension, fever, fatigue, chills, headache, insomnia, rash, pruritus, nausea, diarrhea, weight gain, cytopenia, neutropenic fever, liver toxicity, hepatitis B reactivation	Check hepatitis B and tuberculosis before starting; monitor CBC
Cyclophos-phamide	500-1,000 mg/m² per mo OR 1-2 mg/kg per d	IV PO	Monthly Two daily divided doses	Chronic infertility, alopecia, mucositis, hemorrhagic cystitis, myelotoxicity	Check hCG before starting; use mesna and hydration for cystitis prophylaxis; monitor creatinine, CBC, LFT results; avoid live vaccines

Abbreviations: CBC, complete blood count; DS, double strength; H_2, histamine receptor 2; hCG, human chorionic gonadotropin; IgA, immunoglobulin A; IV, intravenous; LFT, liver function test; Mon, Wed, Fri, Monday, Wednesday, Friday; PO, by mouth; TMP-SMX, trimethoprim-sulfamethoxazole.

Modified from Linnoila J, Pittock SJ. Autoantibody-associated central nervous system neurologic disorders. Semin Neurol. 2016 Aug;36(4):382-96. Epub 2016 Sep 19; used with permission.

SUGGESTED READING

Balu R, McCracken L, Lancaster E, Graus F, Dalmau J, Titulaer MJ. A score that predicts 1-year functional status in patients with anti-NMDA receptor encephalitis. Neurology. 2019 Jan 15;92(3):e244–52. Epub 2018 Dec 21.

Dalmau J, Graus F. Antibody-mediated encephalitis. N Engl J Med. 2018 Mar 1;378(9):840–51.

Daneshmand A, Goyal G, Markovic S, Zekeridou A, Wijdicks EFM, Hocker SE. Autoimmune encephalitis secondary to melanoma. Ann Intern Med. 2019 Feb 12. [Epub ahead of print]

Harutyunyan G, Hauer L, Dunser MW, Karamyan A, Moser T, Pikija S, et al. Autoimmune encephalitis at the neurological intensive care unit: etiologies, reasons for admission and survival. Neurocrit Care. 2017 Aug;27(1):82–9.

Irani SR, Alexander S, Waters P, Kleopa KA, Pettingill P, Zuliani L, et al. Antibodies to Kv1 potassium channel-complex proteins leucine-rich, glioma inactivated 1 protein and contactin-associated protein-2 in limbic encephalitis, Morvan's syndrome and acquired neuromyotonia. Brain. 2010 Sep;133(9):2734–48. Epub 2010 Jul 27.

Lai M, Huijbers MG, Lancaster E, Graus F, Bataller L, Balice-Gordon R, et al. Investigation of LGI1 as the antigen in limbic encephalitis previously attributed to potassium channels: a case series. Lancet Neurol. 2010 Aug;9(8):776–85. Epub 2010 Jun 28.

Mittal MK, Rabinstein AA, Hocker SE, Pittock SJ, Wijdicks EF, McKeon A. Autoimmune encephalitis in the ICU: analysis of phenotypes, serologic findings, and outcomes. Neurocrit Care. 2016 Apr;24(2):240–50.

Neyens RR, Gaskill GE, Chalela JA. Critical care management of anti-N-methyl-D-aspartate receptor encephalitis. Crit Care Med. 2018 Sep;46(9):1514–21.

Pittock SJ, Palace J. Paraneoplastic and idiopathic autoimmune neurologic disorders: approach to diagnosis and treatment. Handb Clin Neurol. 2016;133:165–83.

Rubin DB, Batra A, Vodopivec I, Vaitkevicius H. Autoimmune encephalitis in critical care: optimizing immunosuppression. Semin Respir Crit Care Med. 2017 Dec;38(6):807–20. Epub 2017 Dec 20.

Titulaer MJ, McCracken L, Gabilondo I, Armangue T, Glaser C, Iizuka T, et al. Treatment and prognostic factors for long-term outcome in patients with anti-NMDA receptor encephalitis: an observational cohort study. Lancet Neurol. 2013 Feb;12(2):157–65. Epub 2013 Jan 3.

Titulaer MJ, McCracken L, Gabilondo I, Iizuka T, Kawachi I, Bataller L, et al. Late-onset anti-NMDA receptor encephalitis. Neurology. 2013 Sep 17;81(12):1058–63. Epub 2013 Aug 14.

105 Radiation Therapy

SAMEER R. KEOLE, MD

Goals

- Understand the principles of radiation oncology.
- Discuss the planning of radiation therapy.
- Discuss neurologic conditions requiring emergency radiation therapy.

Introduction

Radiation oncology is the specialty of medicine in which ionizing radiation is used to treat both malignant and benign conditions. The term *radiation therapy* (RT) is used, in part, as a differentiator from *diagnostic radiation*. In radiation oncology, treatment is provided with a team-based approach by physicians, nurses, physicists, dosimetrists, and radiation therapists. Dosimetrists perform the initial planning and mapping of the radiation fields. Radiation therapists deliver the treatment with external beam radiation therapy machines.

RT operates on the electromagnetic spectrum (EMS) with short wavelengths and therefore high frequencies because these 2 factors are inversely proportional. Energy is directly related to frequency by the Planck constant. Therefore, RT uses higher-energy radiation than diagnostic x-rays (eg, radiographs and computed tomograms [CT]). Proton beam therapy is charged-particle RT and is not on the electromagnetic spectrum, although its result is the deposition of sparsely ionizing RT. Proton beams differ from x-rays in that they can stop on the axis of travel. The distance proton beams travel depends on the energy imparted on the hydrogen packets. Proton beam therapy centers are relatively rare and deliver less than 1% of RT in the United States.

Principles

Radiation oncology is diverse in terms of the therapeutic options available. RT has 4 main categories:

1. External beam radiation therapy (EBRT)
2. Brachytherapy (BT)
3. Radioisotope therapy
4. Radionuclide therapy

The majority of treatments administered by a radiation oncology team are EBRT x-ray with a linear accelerator. Other EBRT delivery methods include cobalt-60–based units and proton beam. Because most RT is delivered as EBRT, this chapter focuses on this delivery method.

Decisions about RT modality, target volume, and dose need to be determined. These decisions are based on several factors, including, but not limited to, tumor histologic features and the radiation tolerance of adjacent or nearby normal structures.

RT needs to be delivered with the patient in a comfortable and reproducible position. Patients receiving RT above the clavicles (brain, head, neck) are usually placed in some type of immobilization device to keep this area still. Usually, a mask is made for the patient that can be attached to the treatment table. Once the patient is positioned on the CT table in the immobilization device, the patient is scanned in the treatment position. The CT images are then transferred to a treatment planning system. RT planning is almost always done on a CT scan (gamma knife radiosurgery is the notable exception); however, this imaging modality is often not optimal to define target volumes and normal structures. To aid the radiation oncologist, a magnetic resonance imaging scan can be obtained of the target volume, preferably in treatment position, and fused to the planning CT scan in the treatment planning system.

The radiation oncologist is responsible for contouring the target volume and critical structures. The initial volume is called the gross tumor volume (GTV), defined as the visible disease in intact disease or as the resected tumor bed in the postoperative setting. A margin is often applied to account for suspected but not visualized disease to create the clinical target volume (CTV). The CTV respects anatomical boundaries of spread and is not uniform. For example, a 5-mm CTV expansion (in addition to the GTV volume) for a posterior fossa tumor would not be allowed to extend into the supratentorial area of the brain, brainstem, or bone unless there was evidence of direct extension into such an area. Finally, a uniform expansion is applied for setup uncertainties to create the planning target volume (PTV). For central nervous system targets, the PTV is often 3 mm or less because immobilization and daily reproducibility of this area are excellent with modern RT techniques. In summary, the GTV is created first, followed by the CTV and finally the PTV. Prescription doses are usually to the PTV.

The treatment planning process is a team approach performed by the radiation oncologist, dosimetrist, and medical physicist. After the target volumes (GTV, CTV, PTV) are agreed on, the optimal radiation plan unique to the patient is created. Once this is done and reviewed, quality assurance is performed, either virtually or in water phantom on the actual treatment machine, before the RT plan is delivered to the patient.

Stereotactic radiosurgery (SRS) is a form of EBRT. Although it would be rarely used in the acute setting, it is a common RT approach used in the management of intracranial tumors, benign or malignant. Frameless SRS has allowed this process to extend to as many as 5 days. Generally, SRS refers to high-dose radiation delivered in 1 to 5 RT sessions.

BT refers to "short-distance" radiation. BT is rarely used in central nervous system applications. The most common indications for BT are prostate, cervical, and endometrial cancers. BT has been used to boost postoperative tumor bed cavities, most notably in patients with glioblastoma multiforme.

Indications

In patients with spinal cord compression, level 1 data favor neurosurgical decompression over RT in terms of overall survival and function. However, many patients presenting with spinal cord compression also have considerable comorbidities and may not be suitable candidates for surgery. Radiation dose and fractionation schedules have ranged from 50.4 Gy in 28 fractions to 8 Gy in 1 fraction. A single fraction of RT and a slightly longer course of 10 days of RT may be equivalent in terms of overall survival. When RT is used for spinal cord compression, it is often because the patient is not a surgical candidate and has a poor performance status. The duration of RT should be determined on the basis of patient factors and disease burden. A course as short as 8 Gy in a single day can be used. A course longer than 30 Gy in 10 fractions is rare (Table 105.1).

For intracranial RT, the most common indication is brain metastases. Of cancers that metastasize to the brain, lung cancer is the most common (more than 70% of cases). Of primary brain tumors, the most common histologic type is high-grade glioma, specifically glioblastoma (grade 4). SRS is now becoming the most common method of addressing intracranial metastases. Whole-brain RT is still used, especially for patients with multiple brain metastases or poor performance status. SRS is an outpatient procedure and almost never performed as an inpatient procedure because of the additional time needed for treatment simulation, planning, and quality assurance. EBRT is used for inpatient emergency central nervous system RT, to either brain or spinal sites. For gliomas, surgical resection remains the cornerstone of therapy. Depending on the extent of resection and grade of tumor, postoperative RT may be indicated, to doses between 50 and 60 Gy in 25 to 33 fractions. In older patients with high-grade gliomas, mild hypofractionation regimens that reduce the length of treatment to 10 to 15 fractions (2-3 weeks) have been proved effective in prospective trials.

When patients present with neurologic symptoms from brain metastases, if there is a single dominant mass, surgical decompression is often indicated, even when multiple brain metastases are present. Postoperative radiation therapy is often used. It can be either single-fraction SRS or longer courses of fractionated RT. In the past 10 years, the RT trend has been toward SRS, except where there is an overwhelming burden of intracranial metastases. When patients should be converted from SRS to conventionally

Table 105.1 • Indications for Emergency Radiotherapy

CNS Emergency	Management
Spinal cord compression	If surgery is an option, then use postoperative RT. If surgery is not an option, then consider RT (dose ranges from 8 Gy in 1 fraction-30 Gy in 10 fractions)
Brain metastases	Neurosurgical removal of dominant mass, if feasible. Consider postoperative RT to tumor bed or residual tumor, with either outpatient SRS or inpatient or outpatient external beam RT. If the number of brain metastases is large, then whole-brain RT may be an option (30 Gy in 10 fractions is the most common regimen). For patients with many metastases, palliative care consult and best supportive care may be the best options.

Abbreviations: CNS, central nervous system; RT, radiation therapy; SRS, stereotactic radiosurgery.

Table 105.2 • Complications of Radiotherapy

Area Irradiated	Adverse Effect or Complication	Management
Visual pathways	Blindness	None. Prevent with proper RT dose to retina, optic nerves, and optic chiasm
Cochlea	Hearing deficits or loss	Cochlear implants sometimes effective. Prevent with proper dose to cochlea and middle ear
Pituitary	Endocrinopathies	Supplementation. Prevent with avoidance when possible
Brain tissue	Necrosis	Corticosteroids, hyperbaric oxygen, bevacizumab. Rare with doses <60 Gy, but higher volume of irradiation lowers threshold dose or increases risk

Abbreviation: RT, radiation therapy.

fractionated RT is not fully resolved, but 10 metastases is a reasonable number. When emergency inpatient intracranial RT is required, simpler EBRT techniques are used (Table 105.1).

Other RT emergencies, although not all specific to neurologic conditions, include superior vena cava syndrome, acute nerve root compression, painful metastases, acute hemorrhage, and acute airway obstruction due to tumor.

Complications

Radiation-induced adverse effects are commonly divided into 2 distinct categories, acute and late, 90 days post-RT being the delineation. In terms of acute central nervous system RT effects, intracranial RT can lead to nausea and vomiting, although the incidence is low. In terms of late central nervous system RT effects, necrosis of the brain tissue can occur in extreme cases. Although this is rare, management is challenging if it occurs. Corticosteroids are the most common initial management for symptoms. Other approaches used for managing RT-related central nervous system necrosis include hyperbaric oxygen and bevacizumab. Other potential late adverse effects of radiation are largely dependent on the area of the brain irradiated (Table 105.2).

Summary

- SRS is mostly reserved for treatment of intracranial metastases.
- In spinal cord compression, outcome and survival are better with neurosurgical decompression than with RT.
- With a single large mass and multiple brain metastases, surgical decompression is often indicated, followed by RT.
- Cranial RT leads infrequently to nausea and vomiting early. Corticosteroids are effective.
- In extreme cases, late RT effect includes necrosis of brain tissue. Hyperbaric oxygen and bevacizumab may be needed for treatment.

SUGGESTED READING

Badiyan SN, Regine WF, Mehta M. Stereotactic radiosurgery for treatment of brain metastases. J Oncol Pract. 2016 Aug;12(8):703–12.

Delishaj D, Ursino S, Pasqualetti F, Cristaudo A, Cosottini M, Fabrini MG, et al. Bevacizumab for the treatment of radiation-induced cerebral necrosis: a systematic review of the literature. J Clin Med Res. 2017 Apr;9(4):273–80. Epub 2017 Feb 21.

Khuntia D. Contemporary review of the management of brain metastasis with radiation. Adv Neurosci. 2015;2015:Article ID 372856. 13 p.

Li J, Brown PD. The diminishing role of whole-brain radiation therapy in the treatment of brain metastases. JAMA Oncol. 2017 Aug 1;3(8):1023–4.

Mahajan A, Ahmed S, McAleer MF, Weinberg JS, Li J, Brown P, et al. Post-operative stereotactic radiosurgery versus observation for completely resected brain metastases: a single-centre, randomised, controlled, phase 3 trial. Lancet Oncol. 2017 Aug;18(8):1040–8. Epub 2017 Jul 4.

Mainwaring W, Bowers J, Pham N, Pezzi T, Shukla M, Bonnen M, et al. Stereotactic radiosurgery versus whole brain radiation therapy: a propensity score analysis and predictors of care for patients with brain metastases from breast cancer. Clin Breast Cancer. 2019 Apr;19(2):e343–e351. Epub 2018 Nov 12.

Mitera G, Swaminath A, Wong S, Goh P, Robson S, Sinclair E, et al. Radiotherapy for oncologic emergencies on weekends: examining reasons for treatment and patterns of practice at a Canadian cancer centre. Curr Oncol. 2009 Aug;16(4):55–60.

Rades D, Schiff D. Epidural and intramedullary spinal metastasis: clinical features and role of fractionated radiotherapy. Handb Clin Neurol. 2018;149:227–38.

Vellayappan B, Tan CL, Yong C, Khor LK, Koh WY, Yeo TT, et al. Diagnosis and management of radiation necrosis in patients with brain metastases. Front Oncol. 2018 Sep 28;8:395.

Zhuang H, Shi S, Yuan Z, Chang JY. Bevacizumab treatment for radiation brain necrosis: mechanism, efficacy and issues. Mol Cancer. 2019 Feb 7;18(1):21.

Postoperative Neurosurgery

106 Intensive Care After Spinal Surgery

CLARENCE B. WATRIDGE, MD

Goals

- Discuss the appropriate priorities for critical care after spinal surgery.
- Recognize the main complications of spinal surgery according to the surgical approach.
- Identify the most common systemic complications after spinal surgery.

Introduction

Spinal surgery is a relatively common surgical procedure in the United States. More than 600,000 spinal operations are performed each year, and many are performed as outpatient procedures. Although only a small percentage of spinal surgery patients require intensive care unit (ICU) admission, spinal surgery does carry a risk of death. In addition, the neurologic recovery is often limited by the nature of the condition, and surgical outcomes can be adversely affected postoperatively. In 2012, the mortality was 1.8% for 108,419 surgical patients in the Scoliosis Research Society Morbidity and Mortality Database. In descending order, the causes of death were respiratory or pulmonary causes, cardiac causes, sepsis, stroke, and surgical blood loss.

Spinal fusion is being performed more frequently because techniques and technology are evolving, patients are aging and wanting to remain active, and modern imaging techniques are being used to help define anatomical abnormalities. However, morbidity and mortality are considerable for patients undergoing spinal fusion. The different surgical approaches carry different risks of complications. Morbidity and mortality are highest with the combination of anterior and posterior approaches, second highest with the anterior approach, and lowest with the posterior approach.

Patients undergoing surgical procedures on the spinal canal, spinal nerves, and spinal cord have a relatively high risk for death and morbidity because even well-performed spinal operations can create unstable cardiopulmonary and neurologic states that increase the risk of complications. Postoperative care in the ICU for particularly high-risk patients and patients with serious comorbidities is necessary to minimize the risk of complications, death, and neurologic morbidity. The risks are particularly high because the spinal cord and spinal nerves tolerate injury poorly, and their recovery can be limited or delayed. ICU personnel and resources can provide the safest postoperative care for many of these patients. Patient characteristics identified as significantly increasing the risk of having at least 1 minor or major complication after spinal surgery are female sex, body mass index, arthrodesis procedure, diabetes mellitus, chronic obstructive pulmonary disease, cardiac conditions, renal insufficiency, preoperative neurologic abnormalities, previous wound infection, corticosteroid use, history of sepsis, American Society of Anesthesiologists classification greater than 2, preoperative albumin level less than 3 g/dL, older age, and longer operative times. Therefore, optimal postoperative care is necessary to decrease morbidity and mortality among spinal surgery patients (Box 106.1).

Surgical Approaches

Spinal disorders require surgical approaches that allow an optimal ability to visualize and modify the anatomy with the least risk to the neurologic structures. Those factors, along with risk to other anatomical structures, are the reasons that certain approaches are used. Anterior, posterior, lateral, and posterolateral approaches, alone or in combination, each have certain advantages and disadvantages. Other body systems besides the nervous system must also be considered in determining the safest approach.

Box 106.1 • Basic Goals of Postoperative Care for Spinal Surgery Patients

Provide a safe transition from the surgical and anesthetic status.

Ensure a proper hemodynamic, intravascular volume, and electrolyte status.

Pay meticulous attention to the airway and pulmonary status.

Treat coagulopathy and blood clotting disorders (maintain the INR <1.5 and the platelet count >50×10^9/L).

Manage comorbid conditions (eg, COPD and CAD).

Assess neurologic function carefully and frequently.

Use appropriate monitors (eg, cardiac, Spo_2, blood pressure, and fluid and drain monitoring).

Know the patient's medical and neurologic status preoperatively.

Know the neurologic condition being treated (eg, spinal cord compression or spinal deformity) to prevent neurologic decline or radiculopathy.

Identify preoperative comorbid conditions.

Know the surgical positioning and how it affects pulmonary, eye, and wound care.

Be aware of relevant details related to the surgical procedure:

- Neurologic injury or changes in neurologic function during monitoring
- Intraoperative blood loss (some surgeons use perioperative antifibrinolytics)
- Hemodynamic state throughout the procedure
- Pulmonary conditions before, during, and immediately after the procedure
- Anesthetic technique and duration of procedure and anesthesia

Abbreviations: CAD, coronary artery disease; COPD, chronic obstructive pulmonary disease; INR, international normalized ratio; Spo_2, oxygen saturation by pulse oximetry.

Anterior Cervical

The anterior approach to the cervical spine is most commonly used for degenerative disk disease and spinal stenosis. The spinal cord cannot be retracted from side to side, so removal of a mass, such as a ruptured disk or a bone spur, to relieve pressure on neural elements can be optimized with use of the anterior cervical approach. Through this approach, compressing structures are removed to relieve pressure on neurologic structures and anatomical reconstruction proceeds with bone products and cages, plates, and screws.

Structures of importance in the anterior cervical approach include the spinal cord, esophagus, airway, carotid sheath (which includes the carotid artery, vagus nerve, and jugular vein), superior and recurrent laryngeal nerves, hypoglossal nerve, sympathetic trunk, and thoracic duct (on the left side). Although permanent injury to these structures is uncommon, surgical manipulation of them may produce transient dysfunction that can lead to new problems with oxygenation, swelling, dysphagia, hoarseness, and pain.

Potential complications related to the anterior cervical approach include 1) spinal cord injury, with new weakness and sensory loss, and hypoventilation (when the cord damage is higher than C5 because the phrenic nerves that innervate the diaphragm are formed from branches of the C3 to C5 roots); 2) esophageal perforation; 3) carotid damage, which can result in stroke (from cerebral embolism or local compromise of blood flow), and bleeding complications; and 4) hematomas in the surgical site, which can produce life-threatening airway compromise. After an anterior cervical surgical procedure, if a patient has a sense of impending doom because of difficulty breathing, the cause may be a retropharyngeal hematoma, which must be treated emergently to establish or maintain an airway. Treatment may require immediate opening of the surgical site to remove the hematoma, additional surgery, and reintubation (which may be impossible) or tracheostomy.

Less severe complications include cerebrospinal fluid (CSF) leak, dysphagia, hoarseness due to recurrent laryngeal injury, and Horner syndrome. Other potentially adverse consequences are certainly possible but are beyond the purview of intensive care.

Posterior Cervical

Many cervical conditions requiring surgery are optimally approached posteriorly. The most common is multilevel cervical spondylosis with stenosis. The posterior approach is useful for tumors, both intradural and extradural, and stabilization.

The advantage of the posterior approach is that the anterior cervical structures do not need to be exposed, so risks and complications of injury to them are eliminated. The disadvantage, however, is that more muscle dissection is required and surgical site pain is greater in the immediate postoperative period.

Combination of Anterior and Posterior Cervical

Some spinal disorders require both anterior and posterior approaches to appropriately manage the condition. These approaches can be performed during the same anesthetic session, or they can be staged, depending on the duration of the procedure, the complexity of the case, and blood and fluid management. Ordinarily these operations require removal of structures and subsequent stabilization in the front and back of the spinal cord and nerves. The use of both approaches carries all the risks of both anterior and posterior approaches and a higher risk of complications.

Posterior and Posterolateral Thoracic

Posterior surgical approaches to the thoracic spine are the most common. These approaches are standard for intradural spinal cord tumors and for spinal deformity corrective surgery. Major concerns include postoperative pain management and spinal cord or nerve root function. The blood supply to the higher thoracic spinal cord segments is provided by the anterior spinal artery, which arises from the vertebral artery and spinal segmental arteries. The lower thoracic cord is supplied primarily by the artery of Adamkiewicz, which typically arises from a left posterior intercostal artery between T8 and L1, although many anatomical variations exist. Much of the midthoracic spinal cord is a watershed area of this arterial supply and is vulnerable to ischemic injury from hypotension or decreased perfusion due to compression. Other risks include postoperative bleeding or hematoma formation, CSF leak, and infections. Management priorities are blood pressure management, pulmonary function optimization, maintenance of adequate fluid status and electrolytes, deep vein thrombosis (DVT) prophylaxis, bracing, and mobilization.

Posterolateral approaches can be used when the patient has anterior spinal cord pathology or needs an osteotomy to correct a scoliosis deformity. Postoperative management is similar to that for posterior procedures with the added risk of pleural exposure and the potential for pneumothorax. Terms that describe a posterolateral approach to the spinal canal include *transpedicular* and *costotransversectomy*. Posterolateral approaches allow access to the spinal canal without retracting the spinal cord. Retraction on the spinal cord for removal of masses such as a thoracic disk herniation can be complicated by a high incidence of new paraparesis or paraplegia, most likely related to the watershed nature of the thoracic spinal cord blood supply.

Median Sternotomy

Surgical approaches for conditions involving levels from C7 to T4 pose special challenges. From a surgical exposure standpoint, this region may be considered no-man's-land because it is difficult to address anterior spinal lesions from posterior or posterolateral approaches. This location may require the use of a sternal splitting procedure to gain access to the anterior spine. Surgeons who operate on spines typically rely on cardiovascular expertise for such approaches. Cardiopulmonary management is of great importance postoperatively.

Transthoracic

Some thoracic spinal conditions require approaching the spine from a lateral direction. This requires entry into the pleural space and special pulmonary management. Commonly a double-lumen endotracheal tube is used during the procedure with collapse of the lung on the side of the approach. Midline calcified thoracic disk herniations are amenable to completion of anterior spinal canal decompression through the chest. Additionally, many vertebral tumors affecting the vertebral bodies require this approach for an en block resection. Reconstruction with bone grafts, cages, and metal plates is commonly required because resection of the vertebral body can destabilize the spine. Most procedures are performed from the left side to manipulate the aorta and to avoid the liver. If the spine is approached from the right, the thoracic duct is at risk and visualizing it is difficult. Unrecognized trauma to the thoracic duct can produce chylothorax and the need for reexploration and ligation of the duct.

Combined Thoracic

Complex spinal conditions may require a combined thoracic approach. Decompression may be performed better from a lateral approach, but stabilization with metal rods and screws is optimally done posteriorly. These operations are complex, and the risks of using the anterior (lateral) approach in combination with the posterior approach require that utmost attention be given to the patient's cardiopulmonary function, fluid balance, and hematologic status.

Posterior and Lateral Lumbar

The majority of lumbar spine surgical procedures are performed with a posterior approach. Normally the spinal cord ends at T12-L1; therefore, the spinal cord is not at risk unless the procedures extend up to or above those levels. The cauda equina is more amenable to mobilization than the cervical and thoracic spinal cord, which tolerates retraction and mobilization poorly. After most posterior procedures, including multilevel operations with or without stabilization procedures, patients can be hospitalized without admission to the ICU. Patients with clinically significant comorbidities (eg, unstable hypertension, pulmonary insufficiency, or brittle diabetes mellitus alone or in combination) may be optimally treated in the ICU during short stays because the trauma of surgery can challenge the stability of chronic illnesses. Most interventions should be directed toward prevention of decompensation, management of wound drains, bracing, mobilization, fluid and electrolyte balance, monitoring of blood loss, and DVT prophylaxis. Neurologic function should be monitored so that interventions can be initiated if the patient's neurologic status worsens.

The lateral lumbar approach facilitates vertebral body access and intervertebral disk removal and manipulation. However, the lateral approach puts the lumbar plexus and nerves at risk for stretch or injury as the dissection progresses through the psoas muscle. The levels of the lumbar spine that can be approached reasonably well through the lateral approach are L1 through L4. L5 is not easily approached laterally because of the pelvic bones. Sometimes L1 and L2 require a transthoracic approach.

Anterior Lumbar

The lower lumbar spine can be approached through the abdomen. Midline and paramedian (retroperitoneal) approaches provide exposure for removal of disks and vertebrae and subsequent stabilization. The major risk with these approaches is injury to the vascular structures. In addition, the sympathetic and sacral nerves are at risk, and their injury can produce erectile dysfunction, bladder emptying abnormalities, and retrograde ejaculation.

Management of Specific Variables and Comorbidity in the ICU

Fluid Balance

After spinal surgery, patients generally benefit from normalization of fluid status. Normal blood pressure with avoidance of hypotension ensures adequate perfusion of the neural elements of the spine. Prevention of hypertension may reduce postoperative bleeding with resultant spinal or wound hematomas. Hypo-osmolarity should be avoided because it may exacerbate spinal swelling or edema.

Anemia

Profound anemia (hemoglobin <7 g/dL) from blood loss may compromise spinal cord and systemic tissue oxygenation and provoke hemodynamic instability. Patients undergoing spinal surgery typically have their red blood cells typed and crossmatched before surgery in case they need transfusion of packed red blood cells. Most hemoglobin transfusion thresholds reflect the presence or absence of known coronary artery disease and active ischemia (if known). For patients with coronary artery disease, the threshold to transfuse is a hemoglobin level less than 7 g/dL compared with the usual transfusion strategy of targeting 10 g/dL as a threshold. In a recent randomized trial, tranexamic acid provided no benefit to patients undergoing minor lumbar decompressive surgery; the medication has been beneficial, though, in case-control studies of patients undergoing fusion surgery.

Hyperglycemia

Hyperglycemia may contribute to postoperative complications, including infection. Maintenance of normoglycemia (ie, 140-180 mg/dL) is the goal according to the Normoglycemia in Intensive Care Evaluation—Survival Using Glucose Algorithm Regulation (NICE-SUGAR) trial. Setting a goal of tight glucose control (<100-140 mg/dL) may be complicated by symptomatic hypoglycemia, which offsets benefits for many patients when compared with a goal of 140 to 180 mg/dL. With the stresses of prolonged surgical procedures, postoperative pain, fluid management, perioperative use of corticosteroids, and exacerbation of blood glucose management, diabetic patients may require the temporary use of insulin drips with adjustment of the patient's long-term insulin and diabetic medication regimen to maintain blood glucose at 140 to 180 mg/dL.

Surgical Site Infection

Surgical site infection is uncommon; however, the development of a parameningeal infection can cause neurologic deterioration and even death. Careful surveillance for surgical site infection is crucial because early detection and treatment may prevent death and neurologic morbidity.

Pulmonary Atelectasis

Pulmonary atelectasis can occur in patients undergoing spinal surgery with a long operation time (eg, 12 hours in the operating room). After extubation, careful attention to pulmonary hygiene ("pulmonary toilet") (eg, incentive spirometry and cough assistance) is required because pain may cause shallow breathing. Postoperative pain, narcotics, and lack of early mobilization issues contribute to atelectasis and relative hypoxemia, but incentive spirometry and other measures of respiratory therapy can enhance postoperative lung recovery and help prevent morbidity.

Assessment of Neurologic Function

Postsurgical bleeding can lead to spinal epidural hematomas that require emergent surgery, hypotensive states can lead to poor spinal cord perfusion in watershed areas, and malpositioned surgical hardware may require revision. Many spinal surgical procedures require exposure, mobilization, or manipulation of major vascular structures, and ischemic injury to the spinal cord or brain may produce new neurologic deficits.

Anticoagulation

Anticoagulation after spinal surgery must be considered for every patient. DVT prophylaxis is advisable if patients do not have other complications. DVT and pulmonary embolism occur more frequently with surgical procedures for spinal deformity and trauma. Sequential compression devices and prophylactic subcutaneous heparin or low-molecular-weight heparin are indicated, with prophylaxis usually started 24 hours after surgery. Full anticoagulation with intravenous unfractionated heparin, low-molecular-weight heparin, warfarin, or a direct oral anticoagulant, however, has led to hemorrhagic complications in the first 30 days after spinal surgery. For patients with hypercoagulable states, bare metal stents, or prosthetic heart valves, the risks and benefits must be considered for each patient. After spinal surgery, an alternative for patients who have postoperative DVT may be placement of a temporary inferior vena cava filter if therapeutic anticoagulation would not be safe. However, anticoagulation should be started sometime as the definitive treatment, and the inferior vena cava filter should be removed. Anticoagulation is needed to dissolve the DVT because inferior vena cava filters prevent only massive saddle emboli and not smaller pulmonary emboli. Patients with cardiac ischemia may need therapeutic anticoagulation; however, close neurologic assessment and short-acting or reversible heparinoids could be used to minimize the incidence of operative site hemorrhage.

Wound Care

Wound care requires careful attention. In the early postoperative period, surgical sites must be kept clean and dry and covered with a clean dressing or an adhesive clear cover. Wounds that become soiled should be cleaned with antiseptic as quickly as possible. Immobility due to pain and movement restriction can result in prolonged pressure on the skin and an increased risk of skin breakdown. Even immobilized patients who are restricted to bed can be rolled from side to side to prevent prolonged skin pressure. Nursing care should include turning the patient every 2 hours and monitoring the skin over the sacrum and other vulnerable sites. Providing wound care nursing, specialized beds or wound prevention pads, and optimal nutrition can also assist in preventing decubitus ulcers.

Wound Drains

Surgeons may leave a wound drain in place to evacuate postoperative bleeding and oozing. These drains can usually be removed within 24 hours, but continued output through the drain may require keeping it in place longer. There is no consensus on whether prophylactic antibiotics should be administered to patients who have a wound drain. Antibiotic prophylaxis is usually favored, however, for procedures requiring extensive exposures, instrumentation, and a drain. Antibiotics to prevent surgical site wound infection are generally given within 1 hour before the incision and discontinued within 23 hours after surgery. Patients who have undergone prolonged surgical procedures and procedures with extensive tissue dissection and hardware implantation may receive longer courses of prophylactic antibiotics, but there is no level 1 evidence to support a specific approach.

Braces

Braces are frequently used to immobilize the spine for stabilization of the new fusion constructs. The decision on how long to use the brace should be based on the patient's comfort, protection of the surgical reconstruction, skin care, and compromise of airway and swallowing.

CSF Drainage

Anterior and posterior approaches for spinal procedures may be complicated by opening of the dural sac and the resultant CSF drainage. This is always the case with removal of an intradural mass. The usual volume of CSF in adults is approximately 150 mL. CSF is formed primarily by the choroid plexus of the ventricular system at a rate of about 0.5 mL/min (approximately 500-720 mL in 24 hours). Postoperative management of the dural opening can include placement of a lumbar drain and controlled CSF drainage to facilitate closure of the dural defect by decreasing the pressure on the dural closure. Excessive drainage should be avoided. Patients usually tolerate CSF diversion best if the continuous drainage rate is no more than 10 mL/h. An alternative is to drain 30 to 40 mL every 4 hours under direct control to avoid the possibility of excessive drainage in the unattended patient.

Pain Control

Pain control is crucial after extensive spinal procedures. Consultation with a specialist in anesthesia or pain medicine may be required to determine the need for appropriate synergistic drug regimens, regional blocks, and epidural administration of local anesthetic-narcotic combinations, particularly in the initial 48 to 72 hours postoperatively. Pain control with oral analgesics, along with a decreasing need for parenteral narcotic medications, should be expected for 3 to 4 days after surgery.

Nausea, Vomiting, and Bowel Hypomotility

Patients may have marked nausea and vomiting, and some may have postoperative bowel hypomotility. Treatment of these conditions improves patient comfort and nutrition and protects recent spinal reconstructions. Minimizing the administration of narcotics and using a bowel regimen with a cathartic (eg, sennosides) in combination with stool softeners is advised to prevent these complications. Mobilization and physical therapy should be discussed with the surgeon. Assistive spinal braces, if needed, can help several postoperative factors, including preventing DVT, decreasing atelectasis, improving pulmonary function, and improving bowel motility by ambulating and getting out of bed.

Bladder Management

Foley catheters are routinely used for long surgical procedures to allow for bladder emptying, accurate output assessment, and avoidance of urinary retention. The catheters should be removed at the earliest opportunity. Nursing protocols with ultrasonographic monitoring for retention of urine in the bladder can be used to minimize the risk of urinary tract infection.

Mobilization

Mobilization of patients after spinal surgery has evolved with the invention and use of modern spinal fixation devices. Keeping patients immobilized in bed increases the risk of complications, including skin breakdown, atelectasis, DVT, and delayed recovery. The use of external braces or orthoses is determined according to the surgeon's preference. Although special circumstances may limit early mobilization (eg, poor bone quality, insecure spinal fixation, or neurologic instability), most spinal surgery patients are mobilized out of bed within 24 hours after surgery. Active physical therapy is started early to improve body mechanics, mobilization, gait stability, and muscle strengthening and thereby enhance patient recovery and decrease complications.

Summary

- Spinal disease and spinal surgery are increasingly common indications for postoperative monitoring in the ICU.
- The number of complex, long anterior-posterior and combination operations is increasing because the aging population has more spinal deformities.
- Perioperative spinal surgery management is focused on managing comorbidities and preventing complications of pulmonary atelectasis, preventing myocardial stress in patients with coronary artery disease (if known), preventing DVT, and optimizing bowel and bladder function by mobilizing patients as soon as feasible postoperatively.
- Blood glucose goals are typically between 140 and 180 mg/dL.
- Postoperative hemoglobin goals are typically restrictive (>7 g/dL) except in specific situations.

SUGGESTED READING

Barnes B, Alexander JT, Branch CL Jr. Postoperative Level 1 anticoagulation therapy and spinal surgery: practical guidelines for management. Neurosurg Focus. 2004 Oct 15;17(4):E5.

Cheng JS, Arnold PM, Anderson PA, Fischer D, Dettori JR. Anticoagulation risk in spine surgery. Spine (Phila Pa 1976). 2010 Apr 20;35(9 Suppl):S117–24.

Elmose S, Andersen MO, Andresen EB, Carreon LY. Double-blind, randomized controlled trial of tranexamic acid in minor lumbar spine surgery: no effect on operative time, intraoperative blood loss, or complications. J Neurosurg Spine. 2019 Apr 12:1–7. [Epub ahead of print]

Farrokhi MR, Ghaffarpasand F, Khani M, Gholami M. An evidence-based stepwise surgical approach to cervical spondylotic myelopathy: a narrative review of the current literature. World Neurosurg. 2016 Oct;94:97–110. Epub 2016 Jul 5.

Hebert PC, Carson JL. Transfusion threshold of 7 g per deciliter: the new normal. N Engl J Med. 2014 Oct 9;371(15):1459–61. Epub 2014 Oct 1.

Hebert PC, Wells G, Blajchman MA, Marshall J, Martin C, Pagliarello G, et al; Transfusion Requirements in Critical Care Investigators, Canadian Critical Care Trials Group. A multicenter, randomized, controlled clinical trial of transfusion requirements in critical care. N Engl J Med. 1999 Feb 11;340(6):409–17. Erratum in: N Engl J Med 1999 Apr 1;340(13):1056.

Kobayashi K, Imagama S, Sato K, Kato F, Kanemura T, Yoshihara H, et al. Postoperative complications associated with spine surgery in patients older than 90 years: a multicenter retrospective study. Global Spine J. 2018 Dec;8(8):887–91. Epub 2018 Apr 19.

Lu VM, Ho YT, Nambiar M, Mobbs RJ, Phan K. The perioperative efficacy and safety of antifibrinolytics in adult spinal fusion surgery: a systematic review and meta-analysis. Spine (Phila Pa 1976). 2018 Aug;43(16):E949–E58.

Memtsoudis SG, Vougioukas VI, Ma Y, Gaber-Baylis LK, Girardi FP. Perioperative morbidity and mortality after anterior, posterior, and anterior/posterior spine fusion surgery. Spine (Phila Pa 1976). 2011 Oct 15;36(22):1867–77.

NICE-SUGAR Study Investigators, Finfer S, Chittock DR, Su SY, Blair D, Foster D, Dhingra V, et al. Intensive versus conventional glucose control in critically ill patients. N Engl J Med. 2009 Mar 26;360(13):1283–97. Epub 2009 Mar 24.

Schoenfeld AJ, Ochoa LM, Bader JO, Belmont PJ Jr. Risk factors for immediate postoperative complications and mortality following spine surgery: a study of 3475 patients from the National Surgical Quality Improvement Program. J Bone Joint Surg Am. 2011 Sep 7;93(17):1577–82.

Shriver MF, Zeer V, Alentado VJ, Mroz TE, Benzel EC, Steinmetz MP. Lumbar spine surgery positioning complications: a systematic review. Neurosurg Focus. 2015 Oct;39(4):E16.

Smith JS, Saulle D, Chen CJ, Lenke LG, Polly DW Jr, Kasliwal MK, et al. Rates and causes of mortality associated with spine surgery based on 108,419 procedures: a review of the Scoliosis Research Society Morbidity and Mortality Database. Spine (Phila Pa 1976). 2012 Nov 1;37(23):1975–82.

Snell RS. Clinical neuroanatomy. 7th ed. Philadelphia (PA): Wolters Kluwer Health/Lippincott Williams & Wilkins; c2010. 542 p.

Swann MC, Hoes KS, Aoun SG, McDonagh DL. Postoperative complications of spine surgery. Best Pract Res Clin Anaesthesiol. 2016 Mar;30(1):103–20. Epub 2016 Jan 19.

Intensive Care After Craniotomy

KELLY GASSIE, MD; BELINDA G. BRADLEY, APRN;
ROBERT E. WHAREN JR, MD; BETTY Y. S. KIM, MD, PhD

Goals

- Discuss risk factors associated with postoperative complications in patients after craniotomy, and provide guidance for consideration of their admission to the intensive care unit.
- Provide monitoring strategies, and discuss general postoperative care of patients after craniotomy.
- Recognize the signs and symptoms of common postoperative complications in patients after craniotomy, and discuss the optimal management of those complications.

Introduction

Technologic advances and a better understanding of the pathophysiologic basis of neurologic diseases have greatly improved the care of critically ill patients after neurosurgical procedures. Essential to the success has been the multidisciplinary model of coordinated care. Despite those improvements, in a review of approximately 38,000 patients undergoing intracranial procedures, the overall complication rate was 24%. Risk factors for the development of adverse events have been identified, and early identification and treatment of complications are essential. This chapter provides an overview of the initial evaluation of patients for intensive care unit (ICU) admission after intracranial procedures, general care of those patients, and specific management strategies for early detection and treatment of complications.

Indications for Postoperative ICU Admission

After noncerebrovascular intracranial operations, only 15% of neurosurgical patients require ICU admission for more than 1 day. The majority of those patients require close observation rather than active therapy. Since most postoperative intracranial hemorrhages occur within the first 6 hours after surgery, all patients should be closely monitored in the immediate postoperative period. Patients who require neurologic examinations with adequate cardiovascular and respiratory stabilization are monitored in the intermediate care unit. For patients with risk factors for postoperative complications (Box 107.1), direct ICU admission should be considered (Figure 107.1).

Postoperative Monitoring

Clinical Monitoring

Most clinical deterioration occurs before changes in other physiologic parameters alert the care provider. Therefore, frequent neurologic examination is essential for all neurosurgical patients because early identification of complications may avoid long-term neurologic sequelae. A focused neurologic examination should include the Glasgow Coma Scale score, cranial nerve function (including pupillary responses), and motor and sensory examination of the limbs. A surgery-specific, focused neurologic examination may also be considered (which would include evaluation of speech, visual fields, and bulbar function). Bedside assessments are performed in accordance with standards of ICU nursing care. New focal deficits, decreased level of consciousness, altered content of consciousness (eg, confusion or agitation), unilateral pupillary dilatation, and hypertension with bradycardia are among the signs that warrant immediate investigation. Urgent brain imaging (usually with computed tomography [CT]) is indicated in all instances of unexpected clinical deterioration. Importantly, the use of narcotics or hypnotics may mask focal neurologic deterioration or decreased level of consciousness; therefore, the use of those agents should be minimized.

Box 107.1 • Risk Factors That May Prompt Intensive Care Unit (ICU) Admission

- Inability to maintain the airway or unsuccessful tracheal extubation in the operating room
- Patient has a high risk for clinical deterioration (eg, bleeding, swelling, or seizure)
- Dysfunction of the lower cranial nerves
  - Decreased cough or swallowing reflexes
  - Brainstem compression
- Posterior fossa surgery
- Depressed level of consciousness (preoperative Glasgow Coma Scale score ≤8)
- Increased risk of catastrophic intracranial hemorrhage
- Difficult airway in patient
  - High body mass index
  - Previous neck radiotherapy
- Surgery duration more than 6 h
- Severe comorbidities (eg, cardiac disease) that require postoperative monitoring in the ICU

Hemodynamic and Respiratory Monitoring

The best neurologic monitoring involves frequent clinical assessments, but continued cardiovascular and respiratory monitoring is also critical. Given that the brain is exquisitely sensitive to physiologic alterations, even short episodes of hypoxia and hypotension can be detrimental to neurologic recovery. Cerebral blood flow, which is dependent on $Paco_2$ and Pao_2, is autoregulated; however, this regulation mechanism can be abnormal in injured or postoperative patients.

Neurosurgical patients have unique direct and indirect influences on regulation of the autonomic nervous system, so maintaining tight control of postoperative hemodynamics may be difficult. For example, autonomic regulators that maintain cardiovascular and hemodynamic stability include the brainstem and cortical and subcortical structures (hypothalamus, insula, anterior cingulate gyrus, and amygdala). Commonly observed hemodynamic changes after neurologic procedures include hypertension or hypotension, electrocardiographic alterations with myocardial failure (catecholaminergic cardiomyopathy and arrhythmias), and neurogenic pulmonary edema. The use of continuous monitoring of oxygen saturation with cardiac and blood pressure monitoring is therefore advised. Maintenance of the cerebral perfusion pressure (mean arterial pressure minus intracranial pressure) within the range of 70 to 110 mm Hg is recommended, but individual targets may differ.

In patients with preexisting cardiopulmonary disease, additional invasive monitoring may be helpful (eg, central venous catheter or pulmonary artery catheter). Pain, shivering, hypercarbia, and bladder distention must also be excluded in all patients after craniotomy. Maintenance of euthermia is particularly important because fever and shivering due to hypothermia are associated with increased oxygen consumption.

Postoperative hypertension has been associated with intracranial bleeding and should be avoided. Control of arterial blood pressure is dependent on the preoperative baseline blood pressure. Severe hypertension can be treated with a short-acting antihypertensive (eg, labetalol 0.15 mg/kg as an intravenous [IV] push bolus or later as an IV drip as tolerated) or with a calcium channel blocker (eg, nicardipine 0.5-1 mg as a bolus and then as an infusion at 5-15 mg/h) to maintain predetermined blood pressure parameters. Labetolol is a mixed α- and β-blockade agent; because it is a β-adrenergic antagonist, it must be used with caution in patients who have asthma. Similarly, use of nicardipine should be avoided in patients with aortic stenosis. A secondary sudden, refractory increase in blood pressure can be an early sign of an intracranial process with mass effect; therefore, if the cause is unknown, investigation should proceed with brain imaging.

Hypotension is less common after craniotomy. Its development may be due to sepsis, cardiac failure, or excessive use of vasodilators or sedatives. Isotonic or hypertonic fluids or vasopressors (eg, norepinephrine) can be used for treatment.

Intracranial Pressure Monitoring

Untreated increased intracranial pressure (ICP) can be detrimental. Signs of increased ICP include altered mental status, severe onset of headaches, nausea, vomiting, and pupillary changes. The Cushing triad is a constellation of hypertension, bradycardia, and respiratory changes that may signify increased ICP. ICP monitoring after craniotomy is rarely necessary if the patient's postoperative course is routine. Risk factors for increased ICP include high-grade glioma surgery, duration of surgery exceeding 6 hours, and multiple operations.

Treatment of increased ICP includes immediately elevating the head of the patient's bed to at least 30° and assessing the neck for extrinsic factors that may impede venous outflow. Infusion of 20% mannitol (0.25-1 g/kg as an IV bolus) can be initiated. With central line access, 30 mL of 23% hypertonic saline can be infused over 10 to 20 minutes. If hydrocephalus is present, an external ventricular drainage catheter should be inserted urgently at the bedside for therapy and diagnosis (as an ICP monitor). If the ICP remains elevated (>20 mm Hg) despite these measures, hyperventilation is used to temporarily decrease the $Paco_2$ level and vasoconstrict the blood vessels, although central perfusion pressure may be compromised. Analgesia, sedation, and neuromuscular blockade are secondary options for ICP management. A decompressive hemicraniectomy may be considered if other treatment is not successful.

Admission after neurosurgery

↓

Ward	Intermediate care unit	ICU
Uncomplicated surgery Small supratentorial lesions Transphenoidal surgery Needle biopsy Surgery not involving the brain parenchyma CSF diversion Ventriculoperitoneal shunt or Ommaya reservoir Endoscopic third ventriculostomy	Surgery >6 h Blood loss >300 mL Age >70 y Severe postoperative pain or nausea	Preoperative comorbidities Moderate-severe hypertension and hypoxemia Postoperative neurologic deficit or seizures Posterior fossa surgery (cranial nerves IX-XII) Skull base procedures Risk factors for increased ICP External ventricular drain Cerebrovascular procedures

↓

General care		Specific care	
Analgesics	Acetaminophen 1 g every 6 h IV with or without opioids	**Corticosteroids**	Dexamethasone 4 mg every 6 h IV for 24 h; then tapered accordingly
Antiemetics	Ondansetron 4-8 mg every 6-8 h IV	**Antiepileptics**	Levetiracetam 500 mg every 12 h IV or phenytoin 100 mg every 8 h IV
Antibiotics	Vancomycin 1 g every 12 h IV	**Hormone replacement**	Accordingly after pituitary or craniopharyngioma surgery
Thromboprophylaxis	SCD/TEDS, low-dose heparin SC		

↓

Neurologic deterioration

↓

CT of the brain	
Intracranial hemorrhage	Consider reoperation ICU admission and ICP management Frequent neurologic checks CBC, hemoglobin, platelet count, coagulation tests
Hydrocephalus	ICP management
Malignant cerebral edema	Corticosteroids 10 mg IV ICP management
Tension pneumocephalus	Nonrebreather mask treatment ICP management

Blood	
Hyponatremia	Electrolytes
Hypoxemia	Arterial blood gas CBC, hemoglobin
Infection	Blood cultures if indicated Consider lumbar puncture
Drug toxicity	AED levels Liver and kidney profiles Minimize the use of sedating drugs
Coagulation profile	INR, PTT, platelets

EEG	
Seizures	Loading of AED Consider continuous EEG monitoring Rule out subclinical seizures Rule out status epilepticus

Figure 107.1. Overview of Patient Care After Neurosurgery. AED indicates antiepileptic drug; CBC, complete blood cell count; CSF, cerebrospinal fluid; CT, computed tomography; EEG, electroencephalography; GCS, Glasgow Coma Scale; ICP, intracranial pressure; ICU, intensive care unit; INR, international normalized ratio; IV, intravenously; PTT, partial thromboplastin time; SC, subcutaneously; SCD, sequential compression device; TEDS, thromboembolic deterrent stockings.

(Modified from Velly L, Simeone P, Bruder N. Postoperative care of neurosurgical patients. Curr Anesthesiol Rep. 2016 Sep;6[3]:257-66; used with permission.).

General Care

Nausea and Vomiting

Postoperative nausea and vomiting (PONV) is a frequent complication for craniotomy patients. Postoperative nausea occurs in approximately 50% of patients, and vomiting occurs in 40%. In an observational study of 519 neurosurgery patients undergoing elective spinal and intracranial procedures at Mayo Clinic, young women with a history of PONV and infratentorial or posterior fossa surgery were most likely to have PONV. Treatment includes IV administration of ondansetron (4-8 mg every 6-8 hours), promethazine (6.25-25 mg every 6-8 hours; marked sedation may occur), and dexamethasone. Persistent PONV may be a sign of increased ICP and should prompt immediate brain imaging.

Postoperative Analgesia

The main goal with postoperative analgesia management is to provide patient comfort while maintaining the ability to perform an accurate neurologic assessment. Thus, the use of sedating agents must be limited. Analgesic requirements should be anticipated before patients awaken, especially if patients receive intraoperative ultra–short-acting opioids, such as remifentanil. Dissection of the temporalis or posterior cervical musculature can further exacerbate pain due to muscle spasms.

Common analgesics after craniotomy include IV acetaminophen (500-1,000 mg every 6 hours); its use requires caution or reduced dosing in patients with hepatic impairment. Although opiates can cause excessive sedation and can occasionally increase ICP, their use has been effective and safe after craniotomy. IV options include fentanyl (12.5-50 mcg every 1-2 hours as needed or as a continuous infusion), morphine (1-2 mg every 2-4 hours), and hydromorphone (0.5-1 mg every 1-4 hours). Oral options include oxycodone or hydrocodone every 4 to 6 hours. Analgesics can be combined with muscle relaxants, such as methocarbamol (500-1,000 mg every 8 hours as needed). Intraoperative subcutaneous scalp infiltration has been shown to decrease postoperative pain scores for approximately 2 hours postoperatively, and formal scalp blocks have been shown to decrease the requirements for other analgesic needs over a longer period.

Thromboprophylaxis

Several risk factors are associated with the development of venous thromboembolism (VTE) in neurosurgical patients (Table 107.1). Thromboemboli limited to the calf are associated with low morbidity; however, 30% to 50% of them subsequently extend into the proximal deep veins and half of those embolize or produce postphlebetic syndrome. If VTE develops during the first postoperative week, the cause of death is more likely to be pulmonary embolism than bleeding even if the patient was receiving anticoagulation (26% vs 6% of total deaths).

Prophylactic measures include passive range of motion exercises, early ambulation, and the use of mechanical aids such as sequential compression devices and graduated compression (thromboembolic deterrent) stockings, which should be used until the patient can ambulate more than 4 hours daily. Chemical methods include the use of low-dose unfractionated heparin (5,000 units subcutaneously every 8-12 hours) and low-molecular-weight heparin. The benefits of chemical prophylaxis must be carefully considered because of increased risks of symptomatic intracranial hemorrhage. The addition of enoxaparin on postoperative day 1 has been shown to decrease the

Table 107.1 • Risk and Prophylaxis of DVT in Neurosurgical Patients

Risk Group	Estimated Risk of Calf DVT, %	Neurosurgical Patient Characteristics	Treatment
Low	<10	Age <40 y General anesthesia <30 min	None
Moderate	10-40	Age ≥40 y Malignancy Prolonged bed rest Extensive surgery Varicose veins Obesity Subarachnoid hemorrhage	TEDS/SCD *or* Low-dose heparin
High	>40-80	History of DVT or PE Limb paralysis Brain tumor (especially meningioma or high-grade glioma)	TEDS/SCD *and* Low-dose heparin

Abbreviations: DVT, deep vein thrombosis; PE, pulmonary embolism; SCD, sequential compression device; TEDS, thromboembolic deterrent stockings.

From Greenberg MS. Handbook of neurosurgery. 8th ed. New York (NY): Thieme; c2016. Chapter 9, Hematology; p. 153-73; used with permission.

development of VTE with a trend toward increased bleeding events postoperatively.

Management of Common Complications

Cerebral Edema

Cerebral edema after tumor resection or cerebrovascular surgery can be pronounced. Risk factors include prolonged brain retraction, multiple operations, and surgical duration of more than 6 hours. Corticosteroids are the treatment of choice for decreasing vasogenic edema surrounding brain tumors, but they have minimal effect on cytotoxic or interstitial edema. Dexamethasone, with its low mineralocorticoid activity, has become the main therapy for the management of cerebral edema in patients with brain tumor (Table 107.2). Typically, a 10-mg bolus of IV dexamethasone is given intraoperatively, and a maintenance dose of 4 mg is given every 6 hours (16 mg daily) in the ICU. Although a higher dose of short-term (1-2 days) dexamethasone therapy (6-10 mg every 6 hours) can be considered if a patient has a focal neurologic deficit, the goal with corticosteroid therapy should be to decrease the corticosteroid dose as quickly as possible. Adverse effects from corticosteroids are dependent on the cumulative dose and duration. During the postoperative period, adverse effects include hyperglycemia, psychiatric disorders, hypokalemia, and impaired wound healing. In particular, hyperglycemia is associated with longer ICU stays, increased infection rates, and poor outcomes. Although the end points of glycemic control are controversial, a range of 100 to 180 mg/dL is generally recommended.

Seizures

Seizures during the immediate postoperative period are associated with serious complications such as intracranial bleeding, hypoxemia, and pulmonary aspiration. However, according to recommendations from the American Academy of Neurology Quality Standards Subcommittee and others, the routine and prophylactic use of antiepileptic drugs (AEDs) should be avoided. If they are used, AEDs should be discontinued during the first week if patients do not have a past history of seizures. A reasonable alternative to phenytoin may be levetiracetam, which has a more favorable profile of adverse effects. Patients receiving AED therapy preoperatively should continue with their maintenance dose. AEDs are not recommended after posterior fossa surgery because seizures rarely occur. When seizures or status epilepticus do occur, they should be managed according to usual standards.

Table 107.2 • Equivalent Corticosteroid Dosing

Corticosteroid	Equivalent Dose, mg	Mineralocorticoid Potency
Cortisone	25	2+
Hydrocortisone	20	2+
Prednisone	5	1+
Methylprednisolone	4	0
Dexamethasone	0.75	0

Modified from Greenberg MS. Handbook of neurosurgery. 8th ed. New York (NY): Thieme; c2016. Chapter 8, Endocrinology; p. 144-52; used with permission.

Intracranial Hemorrhage

Postoperative symptomatic intracranial hemorrhage is associated with poor outcomes. The reported rates of intracranial hemorrhage vary from 0.8% to 2.2%. Risk factors include preoperative coagulation disorders, platelet count less than 100×10^9/L, preoperative use of anticoagulation, and history of amyloid angiopathy. In the immediate postoperative period, a hyperemic response from hypertension at awakening may exceed the limits of autoregulation and result in intracranial hemorrhage or cerebral edema. The decision to reoperate must be individualized depending on the patient's age, neurologic condition, and size and location of hemorrhage. Emergent evacuation should be considered for symptomatic hemorrhage associated with rapid deterioration, brainstem compression, or refractory intracranial hypertension. Platelet and hemoglobin levels and the coagulation profile should be checked immediately. For asymptomatic hemorrhage, patients should be closely monitored in the ICU. Involvement of the posterior fossa carries a lower threshold for surgical intervention.

Tension Pneumocephalus

Although rare, symptomatic *pneumocephalus* (ie, the presence of gas within an intracranial compartment) may occur with signs of increased ICP and severe restlessness or seizures and may be a life-threatening emergency. On CT, the classic *Mount Fuji sign* for tension pneumocephalus is created by the presence of subdural air compressing the frontal lobes and producing a widened interhemispheric space between the tips of the frontal lobes (Figure 107.2) with scattered air bubbles within the cisterns (*air bubble sign*). Pneumocephalus may result in headache, nausea and vomiting, seizures, dizziness, or altered neurologic status. Rapid treatment of symptomatic tension pneumocephalus is recommended with supplemental 100% oxygen with a nonrebreather mask. In rare circumstances, a frontal burr hole is required to rapidly release the trapped subdural air.

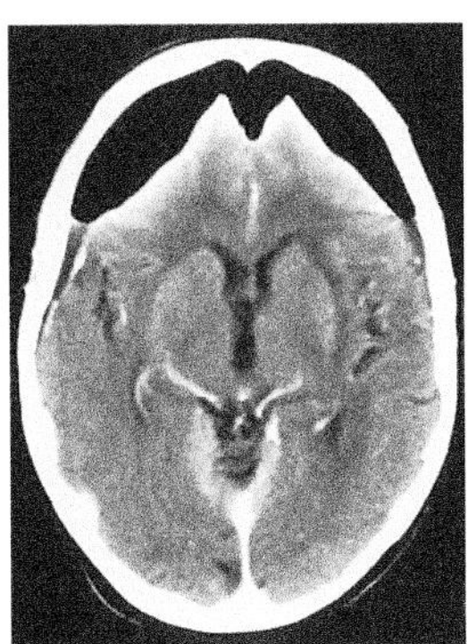

Figure 107.2. *Mount Fuji Sign. Unenhanced axial computed tomography of the brain shows bifrontal subdural hypoattentuation with compression of the frontal poles.* (From Heckmann JG, Ganslandt O. The Mount Fuji sign. N Engl J Med. 2004 Apr 29;350[18]:1881; used with permission.)

Hyponatremia and Other Electrolyte Abnormalities

Hyponatremia is the most common electrolyte disorder encountered in patients after craniotomy, with an incidence as high as 50%. Complications from severe hyponatremia include cerebral edema, confusion, seizures, coma, and death. The most common mechanisms in neurosurgery patients include syndrome of inappropriate secretion of antidiuretic hormone (SIADH) and cerebral salt wasting (CSW). SIADH is differentiated from CSW on the basis of intravascular volume status. Serum sodium and fluid balance should be closely monitored as sodium is repleted.

Sodium repletion in patients with SIADH or CSW includes salt tablets (3-6 g daily) and hypertonic saline (2%-3% infusion) with or without fludrocortisone acetate (2 mg orally or IV twice daily). The use of 3% hypertonic saline (approximately 1 mL/kg) increases the serum sodium concentration by 1 mmol/L. When hyponatremia is chronic, the sodium level should not be increased by more than 8 to 10 mmol/L over 24 hours to prevent the risk of osmotic demyelination (also known as central pontine myelinolysis and extrapontine myelinolysis).

Hypokalemia and hypomagnesemia are also relatively common postoperative findings. They require correction to avoid deleterious consequences, such as cardiac dysrhythmias.

Prophylaxis and Nutrition

In critically ill patients, hypercatabolic states can result from inflammatory mediators, sympathetic nervous system hyperactivity, and dysregulation of glucose metabolism. Early introduction of nutrition has been associated with fewer complications and improved recovery. Although research is unclear about caloric consumption, each patient should receive individualized care from nutritionists and a multidisciplinary team. After craniotomy, patients who are able to eat should be encouraged to do so. If swallowing or mental status prevents oral intake, gastric access should be obtained to initiate enteral nutrition.

Summary

- Postoperative care of patients after craniotomy is based on knowing their preoperative neurologic deficits, examining the patients for postoperative deficits, and identifying and managing comorbidities in the ICU.
- After craniotomy, normotension (systolic blood pressure <140 mm Hg) is typical with some exceptions, such as patients with severe, poorly controlled, chronic hypertension.
- Postoperative complications in patients with sudden neurologic deterioration after craniotomy include postoperative bleeding, intracranial hematoma and uncal herniation, postoperative seizures, and cerebral edema.
- Postoperative headaches after craniotomy may result from the surgery itself or from involvement of the superficial nerves near the incision site or the masticatory muscles. Headaches and facial swelling may worsen during the first 24 hours but gradually lessen.
- When pneumocephalus occurs after craniotomy, normobaric hyperoxia can be used for 12 to 24 hours in alternating or continuous fashion to alleviate headache and intracranial air.
- Mobilization and nutrition should be individualized according to the complexity and risks of dysphagia.
- Nasogastric tubes (or other nasal tubes) and continuous positive airway pressure are not used in patients after transsphenoidal surgery because of the ethmoidal/nasal disruption and the risk of intracranial air entrainment.

SUGGESTED READING

Ayoub C, Girard F, Boudreault D, Chouinard P, Ruel M, Moumdjian R. A comparison between scalp nerve block and morphine for transitional analgesia after remifentanil-based anesthesia in neurosurgery. Anesth Analg. 2006 Nov;103(5):1237–40.

Basali A, Mascha EJ, Kalfas I, Schubert A. Relation between perioperative hypertension and intracranial hemorrhage after craniotomy. Anesthesiology. 2000 Jul;93(1):48–54.

Chughtai KA, Nemer OP, Kessler AT, Bhatt AA. Postoperative complications of craniotomy and craniectomy. Emerg Radiol. 2019 Feb;26(1):99–107. Epub 2018 Sep 25.

Cote LP, Greenberg S, Caprini JA, Stone J, Arcelus JI, Lopez-Jimenez L, et al; RIETE Investigators. Outcomes in neurosurgical patients who develop venous thromboembolism: a review of the RIETE registry. Clin Appl Thromb Hemost. 2014 Nov;20(8):772–8. Epub 2014 May 5.

Dabdoub CB, Salas G, Silveira Edo N, Dabdoub CF. Review of the management of pneumocephalus. Surg Neurol Int. 2015 Sep 29;6:155.

Glantz MJ, Cole BF, Forsyth PA, Recht LD, Wen PY, Chamberlain MC, et al. Practice parameter: anticonvulsant prophylaxis in patients with newly diagnosed brain tumors: report of the Quality Standards Subcommittee of the American Academy of Neurology. Neurology. 2000 May 23;54(10):1886–93.

Gottschalk A, Berkow LC, Stevens RD, Mirski M, Thompson RE, White ED, et al. Prospective evaluation of pain and analgesic use following major elective intracranial surgery. J Neurosurg. 2007 Feb;106(2):210–6.

Greenberg MS. Handbook of neurosurgery. 8th ed. New York (NY): Thieme; c2016. 1661 p.

Heckmann JG, Ganslandt O. The Mount Fuji sign. N Engl J Med. 2004 Apr 29;350(18):1881.

Hellickson JD, Worden WR, Ryan C, Miers AG, Benike DA, Frank SP, et al. Predictors of postoperative nausea and vomiting in neurosurgical patients. J Neurosci Nurs. 2016 Dec;48(6):352–7.

Hockey B, Leslie K, Williams D. Dexamethasone for intracranial neurosurgery and anaesthesia. J Clin Neurosci. 2009 Nov;16(11):1389–93. Epub 2009 Aug 7.

Lin N, Han R, Zhou J, Gelb AW. Mild sedation exacerbates or unmasks focal neurologic dysfunction in neurosurgical patients with supratentorial brain mass lesions in a drug-specific manner. Anesthesiology. 2016 Mar;124(3):598–607.

Mayer SA, Chong JY. Critical care management of increased intracranial pressure. J Intensive Care Med. 2002 Mar 1;17(2):55–67.

Pfister D, Strebel SP, Steiner LA. Postoperative management of adult central neurosurgical patients: systemic and neuro-monitoring. Best Pract Res Clin Anaesthesiol. 2007 Dec;21(4):449–63.

Pulman J, Greenhalgh J, Marson AG. Antiepileptic drugs as prophylaxis for post-craniotomy seizures. Cochrane Database Syst Rev. 2013 Feb 28;(2):CD007286. Update in: Cochrane Database Syst Rev. 2015;(3):CD007286.

Ragland J, Lee K. Critical care management and monitoring of intracranial pressure. J Neurocrit Care. 2016;9(2):105–12.

Rolston JD, Han SJ, Lau CY, Berger MS, Parsa AT. Frequency and predictors of complications in neurological surgery: national trends from 2006 to 2011. J Neurosurg. 2014 Mar;120(3):736–45. Epub 2013 Nov 22.

Salmaggi A, Simonetti G, Trevisan E, Beecher D, Carapella CM, DiMeco F, et al. Perioperative thromboprophylaxis in patients with craniotomy for brain tumours: a systematic review. J Neurooncol. 2013 Jun;113(2):293–303. Epub 2013 Mar 30.

Samuels MA. The brain-heart connection. Circulation. 2007 Jul 3;116(1):77–84.

Soros P, Hachinski V. Cardiovascular and neurological causes of sudden death after ischaemic stroke. Lancet Neurol. 2012 Feb;11(2):179–88.

Suarez JI, Zaidat OO, Suri MF, Feen ES, Lynch G, Hickman J, et al. Length of stay and mortality in neurocritically ill patients: impact of a specialized neurocritical care team. Crit Care Med. 2004 Nov;32(11):2311–7.

Velly L, Simeone P, Bruder N. Postoperative care of neurosurgical patients. Curr Anesthesiol Rep. 2016 Sep;6(3):257–66.

Ziai WC, Varelas PN, Zeger SL, Mirski MA, Ulatowski JA. Neurologic intensive care resource use after brain tumor surgery: an analysis of indications and alternative strategies. Crit Care Med. 2003 Dec;31(12):2782–7.

Intensive Care After Neuroendovascular Procedures

MITHUN SATTUR, MBBS; CHANDAN KRISHNA, MD;
BERNARD R. BENDOK, MD; BRIAN W. CHONG, MD

Goals

- Understand the indications for neuroendovascular interventions.
- Understand the options in endovascular tumor embolization.
- Understand the postoperative care of patients who have had an intracranial aneurysm treated with endovascular techniques.
- Discuss the endovascular options for treating cerebral vasospasm.
- Describe the endovascular techniques used to treat acute stroke, and understand the management issues that arise after clot retrieval.

Introduction

Endovascular therapy for cerebrovascular disease is widespread. Patients with brain aneurysms, acute stroke, brain vascular malformations, and tumors are treated with endovascular techniques primarily or in conjunction with other traditional surgical and medical approaches. Postprocedural concerns unique to endovascular treatment include complications related to access or arterial puncture, contrast nephrotoxicity, and radiation dose complications (eg, alopecia and skin burns). Other complications, such as stroke and hemorrhage, that are not unique are discussed below.

General Considerations

Complications related to arterial puncture are recognized postoperatively by loss of pulse or hemorrhage and are accentuated by anticoagulation and thrombolytics, which are often required for prevention or treatment of stroke during the procedure. Clinical surveillance during recovery focuses on documenting the presence of pulses at and distal to the puncture sites, clinical signs of hematoma, and laboratory evidence of blood loss. Imaging with ultrasonography and computed tomography (CT) can help identify a dissection or a hemorrhage site.

Hemorrhage into the retroperitoneal cavity may be a cause of hypotension and the sudden appearance of marked anemia. Monitoring for increasing levels of serum creatinine, decreasing estimated glomerular filtration rate, and oliguria is routine (Box 108.1).

Tumor Embolization

Preoperative embolization of an intracranial tumor is most commonly performed for meningioma. The decision to embolize a meningioma is typically dependent on the preference of the neurosurgical team and in general is considered when the tumor is large and is hypervascular with a dural vascular supply that is relatively inaccessible (as in skull base tumors). External carotid artery feeders are invariably targeted. Penetration of the tumor mass with embolic material can decrease intraoperative bleeding and surgical time.

Typical embolization agents are polyvinyl alcohol particles (100-300 μm), which have reasonably good distal penetration while preventing dangerous distal penetration, cranial nerve deficits, or postembolization hemorrhage. Other agents of choice are a liquid embolic agent (ethylene vinyl alcohol copolymer) or *N*-butyl-2-cyanoacrylate glue for more controlled penetration. Tumor resection usually proceeds within the following week. Most teams wait at

Box 108.1 • Monitoring for Complications in Endovascular Therapy

Key points

- Immediately check pulses at the access site and distal to it.
- Check for hematoma and monitor the hemoglobin level.
- Monitor for nephrotoxicity (oliguria, serum creatinine, and estimated glomerular filtration rate).

Troubleshooting

- If dissection or hematoma is suspected, Doppler ultrasonography or computed tomography should be performed immediately.

least 48 to 96 hours to allow the tumor to soften. A longer interval before surgery may result in worsening edema that leads to clinical deterioration or, in some instances, formation of new collateral vessels.

The main feared complication is postembolization tumor hemorrhage (risk, 3.2%-5% in large series), which may necessitate emergency surgical resection (Box 108.2). Another possible complication is cranial nerve deficits due to occlusion of the cranial nerve blood supply (risk, 3.7%-6% in major series). The risk of cranial neuropathy may be decreased with the use of careful technique (eg, avoiding dangerous external carotid–internal carotid anastomoses at the skull base, using slow injection to avoid reflux, and carefully monitoring the patient's neurologic status during the intervention).

Box 108.2 • Brain Tumor Embolization

Key points

- Immediately check neurologic status, including cranial nerves, and the access site.
- Monitor for worsening edema (headaches, neurologic deficits, and seizures).
- Monitor for tumor hemorrhage (acute deterioration in neurologic status).
- Monitor neurovascular status at the site and side of access.

Troubleshooting

- If worsening edema or bleeding is a concern, perform computed tomography of the head immediately.
- Treatment of bleeding includes detecting and reversing coagulopathy, blood pressure control, and surgery.
- Treatment of edema includes intravenous corticosteroids, mannitol, and hypertonic saline and surgery.
- Treatment of seizures includes intravenous lorazepam and a loading dose of levetiracetam or fosphenytoin.

Occlusion of an Unruptured Aneurysm

Endovascular occlusion of an unruptured intracranial aneurysm is usually an elective procedure. One of the following techniques may be used: 1) coiling of the aneurysm sac; 2) stent-assisted coiling (SAC) (the stent is deployed in the parent artery permanently); 3) balloon-assisted coiling (BAC) (temporary balloon inflation at the neck of the aneurysm); and 4) flow diversion from deployment of special stents in the parent artery.

The technique depends on the morphology of the aneurysm. Narrow-necked aneurysms are amenable to straightforward coiling alone, whereas wide-necked lesions require SAC or BAC to prevent the coils from prolapsing into the parent artery. Fusiform aneurysms with wide or poorly defined necks are selected for flow diversion. SAC and flow diversion require platelet inhibition with dual antiplatelet therapy before the procedure to prevent acute in-stent thrombosis. Many centers perform tests for platelet inhibition preoperatively to assess the efficacy of antiplatelet drug therapy.

The procedure is usually performed under general anesthesia because of the requirements for delicate microcatheter manipulation of the aneurysm sac. Access is usually through the femoral artery. After the guide sheath is placed, therapeutic heparinization with intravenous (IV) heparin is administered at 70 to 100 international units/kg to achieve an activated clotting time of 250 to 300 seconds. At the conclusion of the procedure, the devices are withdrawn and the vascular sheath is either left in situ for later removal or withdrawn after compression of the artery or placement of a vascular closure device. Heparinization is typically not reversed, so a closure device is preferred if the sheath is not left in situ.

Intraoperative complications of greatest concern are aneurysm rupture (risk, 2%) and thromboembolic phenomena related to device placement or stent occlusion (risk, 7.3%) (Box 108.3). Aneurysm rupture is particularly hazardous because the patient is fully heparined and often the platelets are inhibited. Potential steps include 1 or more of the following: continued coil placement to seal the rupture site (through the same or a second microcatheter), temporary balloon occlusion at the neck, or injection of a liquid embolic agent into the aneurysm sac. With massive hemorrhage, therapy may include immediate reversal of anticoagulation, ventriculostomy, and possibly craniotomy. Monitoring for vasospasm is necessary (as it is when patients present with subarachnoid hemorrhage [SAH]).

Box 108.3 • Embolization of Unruptured Aneurysm

Key points

- Immediately check baseline neurologic status and the access site.
- Maintain adequate cerebral perfusion pressure (SBP >120 mm Hg and <180 mm Hg) to maintain perfusion and prevent SAH and ICH.
- Monitor for thromboembolic signs, including new neurologic deficits.
- Monitor for coagulopathy-related ICH: headache or acute deterioration in neurologic status.
- Monitor neurovascular status at the site and side of access.

Troubleshooting

- If bleeding is a concern, perform CT of the head immediately.
- Treatment of bleeding includes detecting and reversing coagulopathy, blood pressure control, and surgery.
- Treatment of thromboembolism includes performing angiography and CT angiography immediately, increasing SBP, and initiating heparinization and abciximab infusion.
- Treatment of seizures includes intravenous lorazepam and a loading dose of levetiracetam or fosphenytoin.

Abbreviations: CT, computed tomography; ICH, intracerebral hemorrhage; SAH, subarachnoid hemorrhage; SBP, systolic blood pressure.

Thromboembolic phenomena are another dreaded complication of neuroendovascular procedures. When they are recognized intraoperatively, abciximab bolus infusion is immediately administered intra-arterially or IV. Abciximab infusion is considered only in the acute intraoperative or perioperative phase when the thrombus is platelet rich. Otherwise, mechanical thrombectomy or intra-arterial tissue plasminogen activator (tPA) may be considered. Concomitant heparin infusion is to be avoided because of the synergistic effect with abciximab.

Subarachnoid Hemorrhage

Immediate occlusion of the aneurysm is the goal after aneurysmal rupture and SAH. Endovascular coiling or open craniotomy and clipping are indicated. The therapy chosen usually depends on the clinical grade, aneurysm morphology, coexisting large parenchymal hematoma, and institutional preference and expertise. Coiling of ruptured intracranial aneurysms (RIAs) has high rates of aneurysm occlusion and low rates of rerupture. Endovascular occlusion uses coiling alone or remodeling techniques such as coiling with assistance of balloon or stent remodeling (BAC or SAC, as described above for unruptured aneurysms). Use of remodeling techniques results in better anatomical results without increasing the periprocedural hemorrhage rate. To prevent thrombosis of the stent with SAC, patients should be premedicated with dual antiplatelet therapy, which can be a concern if the patient requires ventriculostomy placement, because studies have documented a higher rate of hemorrhage with dual antiplatelet therapy. However, some reports relate the trepidation of full antiplatelet therapy for SAH to a higher incidence of thromboembolic phenomena. Procedure-related complications of greatest importance are intraoperative rupture (reported risk, 5.4%) and thromboembolic events (reported risk, 13.3%) (Box 108.4).

The critical care of a patient who has undergone coiling of an RIA consists of managing cerebral vasospasm and other complications of SAH such as seizures, hydrocephalus, and hyponatremia.

Box 108.4 • Subarachnoid Hemorrhage and Embolization of Ruptured Aneurysm

Key points

- Immediately check baseline neurologic status and the access site.
- Maintain adequate cerebral perfusion pressure (SBP up to 160-180 mm Hg) to maintain perfusion.
- If patient has a stent, monitor for thromboembolic signs, such as a new neurologic deficit (vasospasm may be more common, depending on the time course).
- Monitor for coagulopathy-related ICH or rerupture: headache or acute deterioration in neurologic status.
- Monitor neurovascular status at the site and side of access.
- Monitor cardiac status closely.

Troubleshooting

- If rerupture or ICH is a concern, perform CT of the head immediately.
- Treatment of bleeding includes detecting and reversing coagulopathy, blood pressure control, and ventriculostomy.
- Treatment of thromboembolism includes performing angiography and CT angiography immediately and initiating abciximab infusion.
- Treatment of seizures includes intravenous lorazepam and a loading dose of levetiracetam or fosphenytoin.

Abbreviations: CT, computed tomography; ICH, intracerebral hemorrhage; SBP, systolic blood pressure.

Monitoring and Treatment of Cerebral Vasospasm

Vasospasm with delayed ischemic neurologic deficit is a highly morbid accompaniment of SAH and usually peaks on posthemorrhage days 7 through 10. Prevention involves maintaining normal volume status and electrolyte levels. Nimodipine (a selective cerebrovascular calcium channel blocker) is considered standard of care in SAH (enteral dose, 60 mg every 4 hours), despite the lack of conclusive evidence that it prevents vasospasm (clinical or angiographic), because it has been consistently shown to improve outcomes. Reduction in systemic blood pressure is possible with nimodipine and may necessitate the use of a dose that is lower or spread out (30 mg orally every 2 hours), along with aggressive hemodynamic management to maintain systolic blood pressure up to 160 mm Hg (depending on the baseline blood pressure). An important and validated tool in monitoring for vasospasm is transcranial Doppler (TCD) ultrasonography; elevation of flow velocity is indicative of vasospasm, and the degree is proportional to the severity of vasospasm. Periodic bedside TCD ultrasonographic monitoring is critical in detecting vasospasm and monitoring the response to therapy. Other forms of imaging that have been investigated are CT angiography, magnetic resonance perfusion, and angiography itself. Each has specific limitations, so that TCD ultrasonography continues to be an attractive tool.

Patients with symptomatic vasospasm have a deterioration in the sensorium, the appearance of new focal deficits, or the worsening of an existing deficit. These changes can be subtle initially, but they are evident in 20% to 30% of patients with SAH, in contrast to a much higher percentage in patients with angiographic vasospasm (≥70%). In a patient whose RIA is secured, the first step in treating clinical vasospasm is to induce hypertension and mild hypervolemia (previously termed triple-*H* therapy when hemodilution was considered to be a third component) to increase cerebral perfusion pressure. The systolic blood pressure goal is typically higher than 180 mm Hg and requires use of inotropes (phenylephrine, norepinephrine, or dopamine). Cardiac status must be monitored closely (Box 108.5).

Endovascular strategies in treating symptomatic vasospasm involve performing cerebral angiography and vasodilator infusion into affected territories. Various agents have been used, but the most common are verapamil and nicardipine. This strategy is most effective for vasospasm in smaller arteries. For symptomatic vasospasm in large intracranial arteries, intraluminal balloon angioplasty is effective in reversing vasospasm. Medical therapy may be used in combination with intraluminal balloon angioplasty.

Monitoring for seizures and treating them is important, especially in patients with high-grade SAH because of the high risk for nonconvulsive status epilepticus. Continuous electroencephalographic monitoring is indicated for patients treated with sedation and ventilation. Typical agents used to control seizures are levetiracetam and fosphenytoin.

Hydrocephalus should be carefully monitored with frequent imaging as indicated clinically, and symptomatic patients should be treated with ventriculostomy. For patients with a ventricular drain, standard drain maintenance precautions apply. Other issues that frequently arise include sodium disturbances, fever, and medical complications. Chemical prophylaxis for deep vein thrombosis may be initiated when the aneurysm is secure, but controversies vis-à-vis ventriculostomy placement exist.

Box 108.5 • Vasospasm After Aneurysm Occlusion in Subarachnoid Hemorrhage

Key points

- Nimodipine is standard of care.
- Maintain euvolemia.
- Make frequent transcranial Doppler ultrasonographic velocity assessments.
- Perform CT as needed for hydrocephalus.
- Monitor sodium level and treat as needed.
- For symptomatic vasospasm
  - Maintain perfusion (SBP >180 mm Hg) and administer inotropes as needed.
  - Maintain euvolemia or mild hypervolemia.
  - Closely monitor cardiac status.
  - Perform CT to monitor for hydrocephalus, and treat with ventriculostomy if needed.
  - Perform continuous EEG monitoring for seizures, and treat with levetiracetam or fosphenytoin if needed.

Troubleshooting

- If the patient's neurologic status continues to deteriorate, perform CT to rule out an established infarct and angiography to document and treat vasospasm (and treat with vasodilators or balloon angioplasty or both).
- Persistent neurologic deterioration should carry a low threshold for proceeding to aggressive measures in rapid sequence.

Abbreviations: CT, computed tomography; EEG, electroencephalographic; SBP, systolic blood pressure.

Endovascular Thrombectomy in Acute Stroke

Current guidelines recommend urgent endovascular intervention for clot retrieval in patients who have acute stroke caused by a proximal arterial occlusion in the anterior circulation, who receive IV tPA in standard fashion, and who can receive groin puncture within 6 hours of the initial

CT. An important prerequisite for such therapy is a high Alberta Stroke Program Early CT Score (ASPECTS) (≥6). Therefore, a typical endovascular candidate would have received tPA in the 4.5-hour window and would not have a large area of established infarction.

The use of IV tPA within hours before a scheduled endovascular retrieval can be questioned because dispersion of the clot (in about 15% of patients) may increase the difficulty of retrieval and the duration of the procedure. While this dilemma is being studied, standard treatment is to use IV tPA in the absence of contraindications.

Recanalization is typically achieved with suction aspiration in combination with deployment of a stent retriever. In practice, thrombectomy is being used more often to treat patients, including those who have a contraindication to IV tPA, those who are beyond the 6-hour CT-to-groin window, and those who have a more distal occlusion (eg, the M2 segment of the middle cerebral artery). Successful recanalization rates ranged from 59% to 86% in the landmark randomized trials that established endovascular thrombectomy as a durable procedure. All those studies identified a statistically significant increase in the number of patients who had good modified Rankin scores indicating functional independence. In a subset of patients, however, endovascular stent retriever deployment or suction aspiration is technically not feasible. Intra-arterial tPA administration is an option for those patients (with or without IV tPA).

Postprocedurally patients are closely monitored in the intensive care unit with the specific aim of early detection of reperfusion hemorrhage and progression of severe ischemic brain edema causing a shift and a decline in consciousness (Box 108.6). Spontaneous intracerebral hemorrhage (sICH) with IV tPA (reperfusion hemorrhage) is reported to occur in 6% to 8% of patients (Box 108.4). With use of a stent retriever, sICH rates are not increased. sICH carries high morbidity, and detection and treatment are crucial. Acute neurologic deterioration raises suspicion of this complication; after confirmation with CT, sICH should be treated aggressively with cryoprecipitate and platelet infusions. Milder oozing from sites such as IV lines and groin puncture sites usually abate spontaneously.

If patients with proximal arterial occlusion do not have adequate reperfusion and if the penumbra tissue is not salvaged despite IV tPA or endovascular therapies (or both), the risk for progressive edema and malignant infarction increases. Clues include the presence of a large infarct (more than two-thirds of the territory on CT or >145 cc diffusion restriction on magnetic resonance imaging) and early mass effect. Affected patients require aggressive management of intracranial pressure with hypertonic saline or mannitol and early consideration of decompressive craniectomy. Early seizures in patients with proximal infarcts are rare (<6% in most series), and prophylaxis is not indicated routinely. Continuous electroencephalographic monitoring may be indicated if patients have progressive edema.

Box 108.6 • Acute Stroke and Endovascular Thrombectomy

Key points

- Immediately check baseline neurologic status and the access site.
- Maintain adequate cerebral perfusion pressure (SBP up to 160-180 mm Hg) to maintain perfusion.
- Monitor for tPA-related ICH: headache or acute deterioration in neurologic status.
- Monitor neurovascular status at the site and side of access.
- Monitor for edema: gradual deterioration in neurologic status.

Troubleshooting

- If ICH is a concern, perform CT of the head immediately.
- Treatment of bleeding includes reverse coagulopathy with tranexamic acid, cryoprecipitate and platelets, blood pressure control, and craniotomy.
- Treatment of edema includes hypertonic saline, elevating the head of the bed 30°, mannitol, and early decompressive craniectomy.
- Treatment of seizures includes intravenous lorazepam, a loading dose of levetiracetam or fosphenytoin, CT, and continuous EEG monitoring.

Abbreviations: CT, computed tomography; EEG, electroencephalographic; ICH, intracerebral hemorrhage; tPA, tissue plasminogen activator.

Embolization of Brain Arteriovenous Malformations and Dural Arteriovenous Fistulas

Endovascular therapy for brain arteriovenous malformations or dural arteriovenous fistulas most commonly consists of embolization of the lesion with a liquid embolic agent under general anesthesia. Sometimes coils are used, particularly if a transvenous route is undertaken for embolization.

The most serious postoperative complications after embolization of brain arteriovenous malformations include hemorrhage and stroke, which occur in up to 14% of patients. These complications are uncommon after embolization of dural arteriovenous fistulas; that treatment can also lead to cranial neuropathy due to nontarget embolization of cranial nerve nuclei supplied by branches of the external carotid artery. Otherwise, postoperative concerns are similar to those with other endovascular procedures already discussed.

Summary

- In proximal arterial occlusions, successful recanalization rates were high (failure rate, 15%-40%) in randomized trials that established endovascular thrombectomy as a durable procedure for stroke.
- Endovascular treatment of cerebral vasospasm includes angioplasty or intra-arterial verapamil.
- Endovascular treatment of intracranial aneurysms (ruptured or unruptured) is now the preferred approach, and clipping is reserved for complex aneurysms that cannot be treated with an embolization device.

SUGGESTED READING

Carli DF, Sluzewski M, Beute GN, van Rooij WJ. Complications of particle embolization of meningiomas: frequency, risk factors, and outcome. AJNR Am J Neuroradiol. 2010 Jan;31(1):152–4. Epub 2009 Sep 3.

Chong BW. Current issues in endovascular surgical neuroradiology. Semin Neurol. 2007 Sep;27(4):385–92.

Cognard C, Pierot L, Anxionnat R, Ricolfi F; Clarity Study Group. Results of embolization used as the first treatment choice in a consecutive nonselected population of ruptured aneurysms: clinical results of the Clarity GDC study. Neurosurgery. 2011 Oct;69(4):837–41.

Connolly ES Jr, Rabinstein AA, Carhuapoma JR, Derdeyn CP, Dion J, Higashida RT, et al; American Heart Association Stroke Council; Council on Cardiovascular Radiology and Intervention; Council on Cardiovascular Nursing; Council on Cardiovascular Surgery and Anesthesia; Council on Clinical Cardiology. Guidelines for the management of aneurysmal subarachnoid hemorrhage: a guideline for healthcare professionals from the American Heart Association/American Stroke Association. Stroke. 2012 Jun;43(6):1711–37. Epub 2012 May 3.

Hong Y, Wang YJ, Deng Z, Wu Q, Zhang JM. Stent-assisted coiling versus coiling in treatment of intracranial aneurysm: a systematic review and meta-analysis. PLoS One. 2014 Jan 15;9(1):e82311.

Lin Y, Schulze V, Brockmeyer M, Parco C, Karathanos A, Heinen Y, et al. Endovascular thrombectomy as a means to improve survival in acute ischemic stroke: a meta-analysis. JAMA Neurol. 2019 Apr 8. [Epub ahead of print]

Pandey AS, Elias AE, Chaudhary N, Thompson BG, Gemmete JJ. Endovascular treatment of cerebral vasospasm: vasodilators and angioplasty. Neuroimaging Clin N Am. 2013 Nov;23(4):593–604. Epub 2013 May 24.

Pierot L, Spelle L, Vitry F; ATENA Investigators. Immediate clinical outcome of patients harboring unruptured intracranial aneurysms treated by endovascular approach: results of the ATENA study. Stroke. 2008 Sep;39(9):2497–504. Epub 2008 Jul 10.

Pierot L, Wakhloo AK. Endovascular treatment of intracranial aneurysms: current status. Stroke. 2013 Jul;44(7):2046–54.

Powers WJ, Derdeyn CP, Biller J, Coffey CS, Hoh BL, Jauch EC, et al; American Heart Association Stroke Council. 2015 American Heart Association/American Stroke Association focused update of the 2013 guidelines for the early management of patients with acute ischemic stroke regarding endovascular treatment: a guideline for healthcare professionals from the American Heart Association/American Stroke Association. Stroke. 2015 Oct;46(10):3020–35. Epub 2015 Jun 29.

Powers WJ, Rabinstein AA, Ackerson T, Adeoye OM, Bambakidis NC, Becker K, et al; American Heart Association Stroke Council. 2018 Guidelines for the early management of patients with acute ischemic stroke: a guideline for healthcare professionals from the American Heart Association/American Stroke Association. Stroke. 2018 Mar;49(3):e46-e110. Epub 2018 Jan 24. Errata in: Stroke. 2018 Mar;49(3):e138. Stroke. 2018 Apr 18.

Rahman WT, Griauzde J, Chaudhary N, Pandey AS, Gemmete JJ, Chong ST. Neurovascular emergencies: imaging diagnosis and neurointerventional treatment. Emerg Radiol. 2017 Apr;24(2):183–93. Epub 2016 Oct 7.

Ryu CW, Park S, Shin HS, Koh JS. Complications in stent-assisted endovascular therapy of ruptured intracranial aneurysms and relevance to antiplatelet administration: a systematic review. AJNR Am J Neuroradiol. 2015 Sep;36(9):1682–8. Epub 2015 Jul 2.

Wang A, Abramowicz AE. Endovascular thrombectomy in acute ischemic stroke: new treatment guide. Curr Opin Anaesthesiol. 2018 Aug;31(4):473–80.

Zacharia BE, Vaughan KA, Jacoby A, Hickman ZL, Bodmer D, Connolly ES Jr. Management of ruptured brain arteriovenous malformations. Curr Atheroscler Rep. 2012 Aug;14(4):335–42.

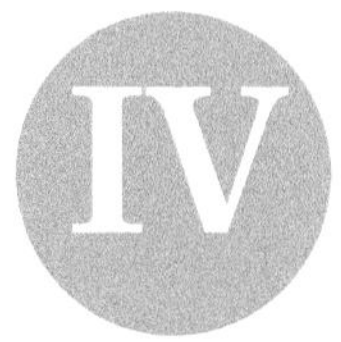

Questions and Answers

Abbreviations Used

ADEM	acute disseminated encephalomyelitis
AICA	anterior inferior cerebellar artery
AMPA	α-amino-3-hydroxy-5-methyl-4-isoxazolepropionic acid
ANNA-1 (-2)	antineuronal nuclear antibody type 1 (or 2)
aPTT	activated partial thromboplastin time
aSAH	aneurysmal subarachnoid hemorrhage
ASIA	American Spinal Injury Association
AST	aspartate transaminase
AVM	arteriovenous malformation
BAVM	brain arteriovenous malformation
BP	blood pressure
CAS	carotid artery stenting
CEA	carotid endarterectomy
CIM	critical illness myopathy
CINM	critical illness neuromyopathy
CIP	critical illness polymyopathy
CJD	Creutzfeldt-Jakob disease
CK	creatine kinase
CLEAR	Clot Lysis Evaluation of Accelerated Resolution of Intraventricular Hemorrhage
CMAP	compound motor action potential
CNS	central nervous system
CRP	C-reactive protein
CSF	cerebrospinal fluid
CT	computed tomographic
CTA	computed tomographic angiography
CTV	computed tomographic venography
CVDST	cerebral venous and dorsal sinus thrombosis
DAI	diffuse axonal injury
DAVF	dural arteriovenous fistula
DHC	decompressive hemicraniectomy
DTI	diffusion tensor imaging
DWI	diffusion-weighted imaging
ED	emergency department
EDH	epidural hematoma
EEG	electroencephalography
FFP	fresh frozen plasma
FLAIR	fluid-attenuated inversion recovery
FVC	forced vital capacity
GABA	γ-aminobutyric acid
GBS	Guillain-Barré syndrome
GCS	Glasgow Coma Scale
GRE	gradient-recalled echo
HER2	human epidermal growth factor receptor 2
HMGCR	anti-3-hydroxy-3-methylgluteryl-coenzyme A reductase
HSE	herpes simplex encephalitis
HSV	herpes simplex virus
ICA	internal carotid artery
ICH	intracerebral hemorrhage
ICP	intracranial pressure
ICU	intensive care unit
IDD	inflammatory demyelinating disease
INR	international normalized ratio
ISAT	International Subarachnoid Aneurysm Trial
IV	intravenous
IVH	intraventricular hemorrhage
IVIG	intravenous immunoglobulin
MG	myasthenia gravis
MISTIE	Minimally Invasive Surgery Plus rtPA for Intracerebral Hemorrhage Evacuation
MR	magnetic resonance
MRA	magnetic resonance angiography
MRI	magnetic resonance imaging
MRSA	methicillin-resistant *Staphylococcus aureus*
MS	multiple sclerosis
NIV	noninvasive ventilation

NMDA	*N*-methyl-D-aspartate
NMOSD	neuromyelitis optica spectrum disorder
NSAID	nonsteroidal anti-inflammatory drug
PCA	posterior cerebral artery
PCNSV	primary central nervous system vasculitis
PCA-1	Purkinje cell cytoplasmic antibody type 1
PCR	polymerase chain reaction
PEG	percutaneous endoscopic gastrostomy
PEmax	maximal expiratory pressure
PET	positron emission tomography
PImax	maximal inspiratory pressure
PLEX	plasma exchange
PRES	posterior reversible encephalopathy syndrome
PSWC	periodic sharp-wave complexes
PTT	partial thromboplastin time
RCVS	reversible cerebral vasoconstriction syndrome
rtPA	recombinant tissue plasminogen activator
SAH	subarachnoid hemorrhage
sCJD	sporadic Creutzfeldt-Jakob disease
SDH	subdural hematoma
SE	status epilepticus
SIADH	syndrome of inappropriate secretion of antidiuretic hormone
SPECT	single-photon emission computed tomography
SVR	systemic vascular resistance
TBI	traumatic brain injury
TCD	transcranial Doppler
TIA	transient ischemic attack
TRALI	transfusion-related lung injury

Questions

Multiple Choice (choose the best answer)

Acute Cerebrovascular Disorders

IV.1. A 55-year-old woman, found 24 hours after she was last observed to be acting normally, has aphasia and right hemiplegia. She is found to have a left terminal ICA occlusion, dense left middle cerebral artery sign, and an early left hemispheric infarction and midline shift. For this patient, which of the following best describes DHC?

a. DHC does not decrease mortality.
b. DHC decreases mortality but does not change the underlying morbidity of the ischemic stroke and associated deficits.
c. DHC decreases mortality and improves stroke deficits compared with results for the nonsurgical groups in randomized trials.
d. DHC is no longer recommended for large, dominant left hemispheric infarcts.

IV.2. A 45-year-old man has a left ICA dissection with occlusion and a large left hemispheric infarction. The radiologist reading the CT scan reports a large area of left hemispheric hypodensity and cerebral edema. Which of the following best describes cerebral edema and large hemispheric infarction?

a. Corticosteroids are effective in decreasing cerebral edema after cerebral infarcts and should be given immediately to prevent herniation.
b. Corticosteroids have not been studied in patients with cerebral infarction, so the risk-benefit ratio is unknown.
c. Osmotherapy (mannitol and hypertonic saline), rather than corticosteroids, is advised for symptomatic patients with cerebral edema (ie, clinical deterioration with radiographic herniation).
d. Decompressive hemicraniectomy decreases cerebral edema.

IV.3. Which of the following is most likely to be preserved in patients with locked-in syndrome?

a. Facial strength
b. Vertical eye movements and blinking
c. Horizontal eye movements
d. Swallowing

IV.4. Which of the following vessels arises from the main trunk of the basilar artery?

a. Anterior spinal artery
b. Posterior inferior cerebellar arteries
c. AICAs
d. Posterior communicating arteries

IV.5. Which brain structure is supplied by branches off the PCAs?

a. Thalamus
b. Caudate
c. Medulla
d. Pons

IV.6. Which of the following has the largest effect on patient outcomes in acute basilar artery occlusion?

a. Patient age
b. Duration of symptoms before treatment
c. Recanalization and reperfusion
d. IV thrombolysis

IV.7. A 53-year-old woman presents to the ED after her neighbor found her minimally responsive and confused. She opens her eyes only to sternal rub and is not oriented or able to provide a clear history. She withdraws all extremities to nail bed pressure. Which of the following additional findings should raise concern for posterior circulation ischemia?

a. Fever
b. Dysconjugate gaze and anisocoria
c. Forced gaze deviation
d. Wide pupils

IV.8. Which of the following is consistent with an carotid TIA?

a. Dysarthria, diplopia, and dysphagia
b. Vision loss in a bilateral homonymous pattern
c. Sudden coma with locked-in state
d. Light-sensitive amaurosis fugax

IV.9. A right-handed patient has been followed by his primary care physician for an asymptomatic left carotid stenosis (70%) for a few years with ultrasonography. The patient has a period of inability to speak and a transient (<5 minutes) loss of control of his right arm. A family member also observed a right facial droop. After a workup for stroke, no other cause is identified. What should be the plan of action?

a. Because his symptoms resolved, the patient has asymptomatic ICA disease, so start aspirin therapy and monitor for future symptoms that would require further intervention.
b. Perform EEG to exclude seizure.
c. Do not start medical therapy, but refer the patient for urgent CEA.
d. If the patient is not taking aspirin, he should begin taking 325 mg daily, and he should be referred to a vascular specialist (a neurosurgeon or vascular surgeon) for evaluation for CEA or CAS as soon as possible.

IV.10. A 26-year-old woman was brought to the ED with a 3-day history of confusion, agitation, and acute-onset headache, which the patient described as the worst pain in her life. She was 2 weeks post partum. The headache was bilateral, recurrent, and intense, peaking in less than 1 minute. Results from laboratory tests, including coagulation and immunologic studies, were normal. Two days after admission, right leg weakness developed. Results from CSF examination were normal. MRI showed multiple acute infarcts. Cerebral angiography showed diffuse multiple segmental stenoses and dilatations affecting several intracerebral vessels. Findings on chest radiography, transesophageal echocardiography, and carotid duplex ultrasonography were unremarkable. What is the diagnosis for this patient?

a. PCNSV
b. Postpartum angiopathy
c. RCVS
d. Severe migraine

IV.11. A 47-year-old man presented with lethargy and progressive right hemiparesis. Results were normal for acute inflammatory markers (erythrocyte sedimentation rate, 3 mm/h; reference range, 0-22 mm/h), and coagulation and immunologic studies. Viral and fungal serologies were negative. CSF findings included protein 69 mg/dL (reference range, 14-45 mg/dL); erythrocyte count 528/mcL; and white blood cell count 22/mcL (85% lymphocytes, 14% monocytes, and 1% neutrophils). MRI showed multiple bilateral infarcts, and MRA showed multifocal arterial narrowing. Cerebral angiography also showed narrowing in the distributions of the left anterior cerebral artery, right and left middle cerebral arteries, and the left PCA. No abnormalities were apparent on chest radiography or transesophageal echocardiography. The diagnosis was PCNSV. Which treatment should be recommended?

a. Oral prednisone and mycophenolate mofetil
b. Oral prednisone and azathioprine
c. Methylprednisolone pulses and then oral prednisone
d. Methylprednisolone pulses and then oral prednisone and IV cyclophosphamide

IV.12. A 64-year-old woman presented with a 1.5-month history of headache, confusion, personality change, and progressive cognitive decline. Laboratory assessment results, including those for inflammatory markers, were negative. CSF findings included protein 97 mg/dL (reference range, 14-45 mg/dL); erythrocyte count 50/mcL; and white blood cell count 23/mcL (90% lymphocytes and 10% monocytes). Cytologic results were normal. CSF cultures were negative. No abnormalities were apparent on chest radiography or transesophageal echocardiography. MRI showed multifocal cerebral infarctions with leptomeningeal enhancement involving the cerebrum and the cerebellum bilaterally. Cerebral angiography did not show any abnormalities. Brain biopsy findings included granulomatous involvement of the leptomeningeal and intraparenchymal arteries, with intra-arterial deposition of β4-amyloid that was consistent with cerebral amyloid angiopathy. These findings were consistent with PCNSV associated with cerebral amyloid angiopathy. Management included oral prednisone (initial dosage, 60 mg daily) and monthly pulse IV cyclophosphamide (1.7 g monthly). What other medications should be administered?

a. Bisphosphonate
b. Calcium and vitamin D supplementation
c. Trimethoprim-sulfamethoxazole
d. Bisphosphonate, calcium, vitamin D supplementation, and trimethoprim-sulfamethoxazole

IV.13. A 29-year-old left-handed woman with no remarkable past medical history presents with sudden-onset right arm and leg weakness and sensory deficits, global aphasia, and confusion. BP is 140/90 mm Hg. The other vital signs are normal. Urinalysis is negative for toxins. Noncontrast CT of the head shows hemorrhage in the left frontal lobe. Noncontrast MRI of the brain confirms the hematoma and is negative for other findings. What diagnostic study should be performed next?

a. CT angiography of the head
b. MRI of the brain with contrast agent
c. Digital subtraction angiography
d. Lumbar puncture

IV.14. A 65-year-old man who has a history of atrial fibrillation and has been taking rivaroxaban for about 6 months presents with left-sided deficits and neglect that are associated with vomiting and altered mentation. He was last seen appearing normal by a family member 12 hours ago, when he had his latest dose of rivaroxaban. Noncontrast CT of the head shows a right temporoparietal lobar hemorrhage. PTT is 40 seconds. What should be your management strategy?

a. Administer activated charcoal.
b. Administer prothrombin complex concentrate.
c. Administer andexanet alfa.
d. Administer idarucizumab.

IV.15. Which statement describes IVH?

a. Patients treated with intrathecal rtPA need a ventricular catheter for a much shorter period.
b. Intraventricular administration of urokinase is associated with decreased mortality.
c. IVH occurs in approximately 80% of patients with spontaneous ICH and is not associated with a poor outcome.
d. CSF drain placement for obstructive hydrocephalus due to IVH is not generally recommended.

IV.16. A 71-year-old man presents with sudden-onset aphasia, confusion, headache, and nausea. Emergency noncontrast CT of the head shows a 25-mL temporal lobe hematoma located 1.2 cm from the cortex. Which of the following statements is true?

a. Emergent surgical evacuation is indicated.
b. Minimally invasive surgery in combination with rtPA may be safe and superior to craniotomy alone according to a phase 3 research trial.
c. If a patient's condition is deteriorating, hematoma evacuation should be considered as a lifesaving measure.
d. Surgical evacuation in combination with medical therapy increases the odds of the patient dying soon or being dependent.

IV.17. Which of the following can be used to assess patients at risk for hematoma expansion?

a. The presence of the spot sign on CTA, which has a sensitivity of 90%
b. Ultra-early hematoma growth as determined with the ratio of the onset-to-imaging time to the initial ICH volume
c. The hematoma expansion prediction score, which is an accurate predictor of the probability of substantial hematoma expansion
d. The 24-point BRAIN score, which includes the ICH location

IV.18. Which of the following is a modifiable risk factor for aSAH?

a. High body mass
b. Elevated creatinine level
c. Hypertension
d. Diabetes mellitus

IV.19. Before the aneurysm is secured in a patient with aSAH, short-term treatment with antifibrinolytic drugs is a reasonable medical measure to decrease the incidence of rebleeding if the patient does *not* have which of the following comorbidities?

a. Obstructive lung disease
b. Liver dysfunction
c. Coronary artery disease
d. Thrombocytosis

IV.20. What is the first line of treatment in a normotensive patient with a developing mild neurologic deficit related to vasospasm?
a. Induced hypertension
b. Early mechanical angioplasty
c. Hemodilution
d. Elevation of the head of the bed

IV.21. A 60-year-old patient presents with a good-grade aSAH from a 7-mm basilar bifurcation aneurysm with a small neck. According to current evidence, what is the best treatment?
a. Surgical clip ligation
b. Flow diversion
c. Aneurysm trapping and bypass
d. Coil embolization

IV.22. Seven days after undergoing successful coil embolization of a ruptured anterior communicating artery, a 58-year-old patient has mild weakness in the right lower extremity. His serum sodium level is 135 mmol/L; he is afebrile and CT of the head does not show any evidence of new bleeding or hydrocephalus. What is the most common diagnosis?
a. Cerebral edema
b. Symptomatic vasospasm
c. Rebleeding
d. Seizures

IV.23. In a patient with intracranial AVM, which of the following is associated with an increased risk of hemorrhage?
a. Presentation with seizure
b. AVM larger than 6 cm
c. Diffuse nidus
d. Previous intracranial hemorrhage

IV.24. Besides intracranial AVMs being found incidentally, what is the most common reason that patients present with AVM?
a. Seizures
b. Intracranial hemorrhage
c. SAH
d. Focal neurologic deficits due to the vascular steal phenomena

IV.25. For what purpose is the Spetzler-Martin grade useful?
a. To determine the risk of future rupture of an AVM
b. To assess the risk of complications from radiosurgery
c. To describe the nidus of an AVM
d. To determine the risk of complications from surgical excision

IV.26. Which of the following statements is true about stereotactic radiosurgery for AVM?
a. It results in gradual involution of an AVM over 2 to 3 years.
b. It can be performed only in patients who can undergo preplanning MRI.
c. It is useful only for AVMs smaller than 3 cm.
d. It is a favored procedure for immediately decreasing the risk of rehemorrhage.

IV.27. For which patients is seizure medication indicated?
a. Those presenting with intracranial hemorrhage
b. Those with a cortically based AVM
c. Those with a single seizure from an AVM
d. Those who are comatose from a ruptured AVM

IV.28. What should be the initial therapy for patients presenting with bithalamic hemorrhage due to deep venous sinus thrombosis?
a. Catheter-directed thrombolysis
b. Mechanical thrombectomy
c. Anticoagulation
d. Hydration

IV.29. A patient is admitted with a transverse venous sinus occlusion and a recent small intracerebral hematoma. After therapy is started with IV heparin, the patient complains of more headaches. CTV shows no appreciable enlargement. What would be the best next step?
a. Consider endovascular treatment.
b. Stop the heparin infusion.
c. Give a heparin bolus.
d. Observe closely, measure anti–factor Xa levels frequently, and repeat the CTV.

IV.30. Which of the following is the typical clinical presentation of cervical arterial dissection of the ICA?
a. Contralateral pain of the head, face, and neck and ipsilateral Horner syndrome with ischemia contralaterally
b. Ipsilateral pain in the head, face, or neck accompanied by ipsilateral partial Horner syndrome and then retinal or cerebral ischemia hours or days later
c. Neck pain only in addition to Horner syndrome
d. Chest pain that ascends as the dissection goes up into the neck and then neck pain

IV.31. Which of the following is the typical angiographic appearance of a cervical ICA dissection?
a. Stump
b. Bifurcation
c. Rose petal
d. Candle flame

Traumatic Brain and Spine Injury

IV.32. Which imaging modality is most accurate for detecting DAI?
a. CT of the head with 1-mm sections
b. MRI of the brain with GRE sequences
c. PET of the brain with fludeoxyglucose F18 tracer
d. SPECT of the brain to look for the “hollow skull” sign

IV.33. What percentage of traumatic head injuries are associated with SAH?
a. 25%
b. 35%
c. 45%
d. 50%

IV.34. Which of the following statements characterizes neurogenic shock after spinal cord injury?
a. It manifests with tachycardia.
b. It manifests with peripheral vasoconstriction.
c. It is due to hypotension.
d. It leads to loss of vascular tone.

IV.35. Which of the following imaging modalities has the highest resolution for identifying tiny intraparenchymal hematomas and contusions?
a. CT of the head
b. MRI of the brain with FLAIR sequencing
c. MRI of the brain with GRE sequencing
d. MRI of the brain with DTI

IV.36. A patient with a traumatic spinal cord injury has no feeling or motor function from the umbilicus level (T10) down. On examination, the patient has no response to pinprick from the T10 level down to the toes, and the legs have a motor function grade of zero on the Medical Research Council scale. What is the patient’s grade on the ASIA Impairment Scale?
a. C, T10
b. B, T10
c. E, T10
d. A, T10

IV.37. Which of the following is a radiologic feature that would particularly suggest an underlying extrinsic or intrinsic coagulation disorder in a patient with an acute SDH?
- a. Volume of the clot
- b. Maximal diameter of the clot
- c. Degree of midline shift
- d. Presence of fluid levels

IV.38. What pathophysiologic mechanism is responsible for the false localization of a hemispheric mass lesion?
- a. Compression of the ipsilateral cerebral peduncle from midline shift against the tentorial edge
- b. Compression of the contralateral cerebral peduncle from midline shift against the tentorial edge
- c. Compression of the ipsilateral third nerve
- d. Compression of the contralateral third nerve

IV.39. A 65-year-old man who sustained a motor vehicle collision with TBI arrives in the ED. He has a GCS score of 14. CT of the head shows an EDH with maximal thickness of 5 mm and no midline shift. He has no pupillary asymmetry. The patient is taking warfarin, and his INR is 1.5. Which of the following is the best course of action for EDH according to the Surgical Management of TBI Author Group?
- a. Discharge from the ED.
- b. Consult the neurosurgery service for emergency neurosurgical decompression now given the present lucid interval and the expected neurologic decline.
- c. Admit to the neurocritical ICU for serial observation, and perform CT if the GCS score decreases 2 points or more from baseline or if anisocoria develops.
- d. Emergently reverse the INR with FFP.

IV.40. An alcoholic man is found lying in the street and is brought into the ED. On CT, he has a 5-mm thick isodense SDH with no midline shift. His GCS score is 14 for confusion, and he has no anisocoria. Which of the following best describes the age of the SDH?
- a. Acute
- b. Subacute
- c. Chronic
- d. Indeterminate according to the CT findings

IV.41. What does a swirl sign indicate when it is seen on CT of a patient with EDH?
- a. The patient was involved in high-velocity trauma.
- b. The patient has active bleeding in the EDH blood collection, which may portend rapid neurologic decline.
- c. The swirl sign indicates radiologic stability of the EDH blood.
- d. The swirl sign indicates anticoagulation.

IV.42. A 45-year-old man presents to the ED after a motor vehicle accident. Upon arrival, he is ambulatory, and his ASIA score is E. He has pain on flexion of his neck and tenderness to palpation along his cervical spinous processes. His vital signs are stable. What should be the next step in management?
- a. Plain radiographs
- b. Flexion-extension radiographs
- c. CT
- d. MRI

IV.43. A 78-year-old man is brought to the ED by emergency medical services after he fell at home. He states that he had transient paresthesia in his hands bilaterally, but that has since resolved. His ASIA score is E. CT shows a nondisplaced type II odontoid fracture. What is the next step in management, and, if the next step is nonoperative, what is the rate of nonunion?
- a. Halo fixation; 90%
- b. Halo fixation; 60%
- c. Hard collar; 20%
- d. Urgent surgery

IV.44. A 56-year-old woman with a history of Sjögren syndrome and rheumatoid arthritis presents to the ED with a complaint of acute difficulty moving her hands after a minor motor vehicle accident on her way to work. On examination, she has signs of bilateral upper extremity myelopathy. She does not have any neck pain. What tests or imaging should be performed, what is the suspected condition, and what is the most appropriate treatment option?
- a. CT; tumor; transoral approach
- b. Plain radiography; degenerative arthritis; bracing
- c. MRI; inflammatory pannus; posterior approach
- d. Flexion-extension radiography; degenerative arthritis; hard collar

Acute Central Nervous System Infections

IV.45. Which of the following would best distinguish HSE from autoimmune encephalitis?
- a. Fever
- b. Seizures
- c. Asymmetric temporal lobe on MRI
- d. Lymphocytic pleocytosis in CSF

IV.46. Which dose of IV acyclovir provides the best outcome in the treatment of HSE if it is given every 8 hours for 14 to 21 days?
- a. 1 mg/kg
- b. 10 mg/kg
- c. 30 mg/kg
- d. 30 mg/kg *and* a prolonged course of oral valacyclovir

IV.47. What is the mean latency of anti-NMDA receptor encephalitis after an episode of HSE?
- a. 7 days
- b. 14 days
- c. 30 days
- d. 3 months

IV.48. What distinguishes patients with West Nile encephalitis from patients with other arboviral causes of encephalitis?
- a. Polymorphonuclear pleocytosis in the CSF
- b. Normal MRI findings
- c. High sensitivity with PCR of the CSF
- d. Headache and stiff neck

IV.49. With which of the following is Zika virus adult neurologic disease most commonly associated?
- a. Anterior horn cell infection
- b. Encephalitis
- c. Seizures
- d. GBS

IV.50. Which clinical sign or symptom is *least* common in patients presenting with acute bacterial meningitis?
- a. Headache
- b. Confusion or stupor
- c. Seizures
- d. Neck stiffness

IV.51. What is the most common organism involved in acute bacterial meningitis in immunosuppressed patients?
- a. *Neisseria meningitidis*
- b. *Listeria monocytogenes*
- c. *Haemophilus influenzae* type b
- d. *Escherichia coli*

IV.52. What is the best therapy for increased ICP in patients with bacterial meningitis?
- a. Corticosteroids and osmotherapy
- b. Hypothermia
- c. Frequent CSF taps
- d. Decompressive craniotomy

IV.53. Which condition increases the risk of acute bacterial meningitis?
a. Hypovitaminosis
b. TBI
c. Asplenia
d. Corticosteroids

IV.54. Which factor is prognostic for patients with acute bacterial meningitis?
a. High CSF protein level
b. Low CSF leukocyte count
c. Young age
d. Seizures

IV.55. For detection of brain abscesses, what is the sensitivity and specificity of DWI MRI?
a. Greater than 95%
b. 90% to 94%
c. 85% to 59%
d. 80% to 84%

IV.56. In postneurosurgical patients with a brain abscess at the surgical site, which of the following is *not* a part of standard empirical therapy?
a. Vancomycin
b. Voriconazole
c. Cefepime
d. Metronidazole

IV.57. What is the fatality rate among patients with a brain abscess?
a. 5%
b. 10%
c. 20%
d. 40%

IV.58. Which of the following is *not* a risk factor for failure of medical management in patients with spinal epidural abscess?
a. Age older than 65 years
b. CRP greater than 115 mg/L
c. Fever greater than 40°C
d. Bacteremia

IV.59. Which of the following is *not* a definitive indication for surgical intervention in patients with spinal epidural abscess?
a. Mild neurologic deficit
b. Spinal instability
c. Failure of antibiotic therapy to clear infection
d. Severe spinal cord compression in the cervical or thoracic spine

Acute Neuromuscular Disorders

IV.60. Which of the following defines a myasthenic crisis?
a. The need for mechanical ventilation
b. The need for immunomodulatory treatment (IVIG or PLEX)
c. The need for positive pressure ventilation
d. The need for hospital admission

IV.61. Which of the following statements about the treatment of a myasthenic crisis is true?
a. PLEX has been shown to be superior to IVIG for liberating patients from mechanical ventilation.
b. As soon as NIV is started, use of acetylcholine esterase inhibitors should be stopped to minimize the burden of oral secretions.
c. In nonintubated patients, corticosteroids should be carefully titrated to avoid worsening of muscular weakness.
d. In patients requiring NIV, continuous positive airway pressure is the mode of choice.

IV.62. Which of the following is *not* an adverse effect of PLEX?
a. Aseptic meningitis
b. Hypocalcemia
c. Removal of highly protein-bound drugs
d. Transfusion reaction (including TRALI)

IV.63. Which of the following increases the risk of extubation failure?
a. Advanced age
b. Atelectasis
c. Prolonged intubation
d. All are correct

IV.64. Patients receiving anti-acetylcholinesterase inhibitors should be questioned and examined for signs of cholinergic overactivity. Which of the following signs is not produced by cholinergic overactivity?
a. Diarrhea
b. Urinary incontinence
c. Mydriasis
d. Bradycardia

IV.65. The diagnosis of GBS is likely with which of the following?
a. Tingling, areflexia, and acute weakness
b. Initial presentation of oropharyngeal weakness
c. Ophthalmoparesis and ptosis
d. Dysautonomia

IV.66. Which disorder mimics GBS most frequently?
a. Hyponatremia
b. MG
c. Spinal cord disorder
d. Brainstem stroke

IV.67. Intubation is most likely required with which of the following pulmonary function test results?
a. PImax 50 cm H_2O
b. PEmax 50% decrease
c. Vital capacity <1 L
d. >50% reduction of PImax, vital capacity, and PEmax

IV.68. In GBS, what is the median duration for mechanical ventilation?
a. 6 months
b. 2 weeks
c. 1 month
d. 3 months

IV.69. What is the most common form of early dysautonomia with GBS?
a. Tachycardia
b. Hypertension
c. Ileus
d. Wide swings in BP

IV.70. A 63-year-old man is admitted to the ICU for management of acute respiratory failure. An NIV device was placed without sedation. Results of arterial blood gas analysis before device placement were a Pao_2 of 85 mm Hg and a $Paco_2$ of 70 mm Hg. Examination shows paradoxic breathing when the NIV mask is removed. He is unable to describe his symptoms in much detail because of the dyspnea, but he has had trouble with breathing after mild exertion for the past 6 months. He has moderate neck flexor weakness and upper limb weakness that is greater on the right. Fasciculations are present in several muscle groups of both upper limbs and in the right leg. Reflexes are brisk in the right arm and leg, and there is an extensor plantar response on the right. Sensation is intact. What is the best next step to assist with the diagnosis?
a. MRI of the cervical spine
b. Head CT
c. Electromyography with nerve conduction studies
d. Lumbar puncture

IV.71. When should the use of NIV be considered for a patient with a diagnosis of amyotrophic lateral sclerosis?
  a. The FVC is less than 50% of predicted for the patient's height and weight.
  b. The FVC is 90% of predicted, and the patient endorses dyspnea with mild exertion.
  c. The Pimax is 50 cm H_2O with an FVC of 85% of predicted in an asymptomatic patient.
  d. The Pemax is 50 cm H_2O with an FVC of 85% of predicted in an asymptomatic patient.

IV.72. A 68-year-old woman with a recent diagnosis of bulbar-onset amyotrophic lateral sclerosis was admitted for management of pneumonia. She required NIV initially on admission, but with treatment of the infection this was weaned over a few days. On bedside spirometry, the FVC was 53%, Pimax was 50 cm H_2O, and Pemax was 40 cm H_2O. The patient has been concerned about her oral intake because of her dysphagia and asks whether PEG tube placement is appropriate. What is the best response?
  a. PEG is not an option at this point given her FVC.
  b. PEG can be considered with her current FVC.
  c. PEG tube should be placed given her issues with dysphagia.
  d. PEG needs to be done in combination with a tracheostomy.

IV.73. Which of the following has been associated with poor ability to gain weight after PEG tube placement?
  a. Loss of more than 10% of premorbid body weight at the time of PEG placement
  b. Body mass index of less than 22 kg/m^2 at the time of PEG tube placement
  c. Age older than 60 years at the time of PEG tube placement
  d. Female sex

IV.74. A patient with amyotrophic lateral sclerosis was admitted to the ICU because of recurrent episodes of sudden-onset shortness of breath without associated oxygen desaturations. Several episodes within the first half hour of admission were witnessed. These consisted of inspiratory stridor and noisy breathing after a coughing fit lasting up to a minute. What is the best next treatment for this patient?
  a. Conservative management only with patient repositioning and guided breathing
  b. Scopolamine patch to decrease salivary secretions
  c. Use of NIV during the episodes
  d. Scheduled use of benzodiazepines

IV.75. What is the best serum biomarker of rhabdomyolysis?
  a. CK level
  b. Aldolase level
  c. AST level
  d. Myoglobin level

IV.76. What is the best time to do a diagnostic muscle biopsy after rhabdomyolysis?
  a. 2 days
  b. 1 week
  c. 1 month
  d. 6 months

IV.77. What is suggested by the detection of serum HMGCR antibodies?
  a. Statin toxic myopathy
  b. Statin-associated necrotizing autoimmune myopathy
  c. Amiodarone toxic myopathy
  d. Hydroxychloroquine toxic myopathy

IV.78. Which of the following characteristics can distinguish CIM from CIP?
  a. Prolonged CMAP duration in CIM
  b. Increased protein level in CSF
  c. Prolonged CMAP duration in CIP
  d. Nerve conduction studies suggesting demyelination

IV.79. Which of the following is the worst prognostic factor in patients with ICU-associated weakness?
  a. Young age
  b. Rhabdomyolysis
  c. CIP
  d. CIM

Miscellaneous Disorders of Acute Brain Injury

IV.80. An adult with a recent diagnosis of refractory convulsive SE is receiving 2 antiseizure medications (fosphenytoin and levetiracetam). EEG continues to show generalized SE. What should be the next intervention?
  a. Isoflurane anesthesia
  b. IV lorazepam
  c. Ketogenic diet
  d. IV midazolam infusion

IV.81. A patient presents to the ED in generalized convulsive SE. What is the most appropriate and urgent first intervention?
  a. IV fosphenytoin
  b. IV lorazepam
  c. Intranasal midazolam
  d. Primary survey including airway, breathing, and circulation

IV.82. Which of the following is required for a clinical diagnosis of refractory SE?
  a. Seizure lasting longer than 1 hour but less than 6 hours
  b. Seizure lasting longer than 6 hours but less than 12 hours
  c. Recurrent SE that occurs after weaning from IV anesthetics
  d. SE refractory to 2 antiseizure medications

IV.83. Which of the following describes the self-perpetuation of SE?
  a. The internalization of NMDA and AMPA receptors induces excitation.
  b. Initial activation of ion channels allows for receptor sensitization.
  c. Internalization of GABA receptors aids in the propagation of cortical signals.
  d. Antiepileptic peptide expression increases, allowing further signal propagation.

IV.84. A patient who presents to the ED in convulsive SE is given 0.1 mg/kg lorazepam IV in divided doses. The seizures do not resolve, and the patient is intubated. What is the most appropriate next step?
  a. Urgent EEG
  b. Initiation of hypothermia
  c. IV fosphenytoin or valproate sodium
  d. Use of an anesthetic agent, including midazolam or propofol

IV.85. Which of the following is *not* a characteristic clinical feature of PRES?
  a. Acute encephalopathy
  b. Headache
  c. Seizures
  d. Asterixis

IV.86. Which of the following MRI findings would *not* be seen in a patient with PRES?
a. Vasogenic edema
b. Cytotoxic edema
c. Cerebral hemorrhage
d. Ring enhancement with central necrosis

IV.87. Which of the following is the most common precipitating factor for PRES?
a. Hypertension
b. Cytotoxic drugs
c. Eclampsia
d. Systemic lupus erythematosus

IV.88. Which of the following statements is true about PRES?
a. Patients with PRES usually present with isolated brainstem or cerebellar vasogenic edema.
b. By definition, PRES is always reversible.
c. Seizures are reported to occur in up to 60% to 80% of patients with PRES.
d. CT of the brain is the preferred imaging modality.

IV.89. For a patient with PRES due to eclampsia, what is the recommended first-line therapy for seizure control?
a. Lamotrigine
b. Carbamazepine
c. Magnesium sulphate
d. Valproic acid

IV.90. A 5-year-old boy had vision loss, right hemibody weakness, ataxia, and confusion approximately 10 days after receiving an immunization. He later received a diagnosis of ADEM. Which of the following vaccines would be *least* likely to have provoked his illness?
a. Hepatitis A
b. Influenza virus
c. Pneumococcal conjugate
d. Human papillomavirus

IV.91. A 29-year-old woman presents with acute onset of complete paralysis, sphincter dysfunction, and sensory loss below the T4 dermatome. MRI of the spinal cord shows a longitudinally extensive enhancing lesion extending from T4 through T11. The patient is treated with high doses of IV methylprednisolone for 5 days, but her condition does not improve. What treatment should be considered next?
a. Plasmapheresis
b. Cyclophosphamide
c. Interferon beta-1a
d. IVIG

IV.92. A 35-year-old woman with relapsing-remitting MS has rotary nystagmus, hemifacial numbness, and unilateral soft palate paralysis. MRI shows an enhancing lesion in the nucleus tractus solitarius. What emergency complication of demyelinating disease is most likely to develop?
a. Neurogenic pulmonary edema
b. PRES
c. Brainstem herniation
d. Elevated ICP

IV.93. A 60-year-old man with secondary progressive MS, who has been wheelchair bound for the past 10 years, presents with encephalopathy that progresses to a comatose state. He has bradycardia, thrombocytopenia, and an elevated INR. What complication of demyelinating disease is most likely?
a. A new lesion in the medulla at the nucleus tractus solitarius
b. Elevated ICP
c. Hypothermia
d. PRES

IV.94. A 34-year-old man presents with rapidly worsening right hemiparesis and apraxia. MRI shows a large left frontal lesion with mass effect and a partial open ring enhancement. His mental status deteriorates and he becomes comatose. Which of the following treatment options should you be *avoided*?
a. High doses of IV corticosteroids
b. Radiotherapy to the lesion
c. Hemicraniectomy
d. Mannitol

IV.95. In patients with sCJD, MRI is useful for showing changes in which of the following?
a. Brainstem
b. Vascular territories
c. White matter
d. Gray matter

IV.96. A patient who is suspected of having sCJD has MRI changes that are compatible with CJD, EEG results that show PSWC changes, and positive results for 14-3-3 protein. The patient is now comatose (GCS score, 9). Which of the following is recommended?
a. Quinine therapy
b. Consultation with the National Prion Disease Pathology Surveillance Center resources
c. Hospice care
d. Intubation and aggressive SE management of EEG PSWC changes

Neuro-oncology

IV.97. A 50-year-old man is admitted from the ED after worsening headache of 2 days. He has been experiencing headaches for 2 months and has also noticed subtle difficulty with hand dexterity. MRI of the brain shows a large right frontal glioblastoma with mass effect and early hemorrhage. What is the best course of action?
a. Admission to the neurocritical care unit and therapy with high-dose dexamethasone
b. Emergency surgery
c. Palliation
d. Radiation

IV.98. An 18-year-old woman presents with severe headaches and ataxia and is found to have an astrocytoma of the vermis with obstructive hydrocephalus. She is awaiting surgery but is admitted on an emergency basis after she was noted to be more drowsy acutely. What is the plan of action?
a. Start therapy with mannitol.
b. Start therapy with high-dose corticosteroids.
c. Ventriculostomy should be placed on an urgent basis.
d. Perform CSF diversion with concurrent tumor surgery.

IV.99. During resection of a large left temporal glioblastoma, intraoperative edema was severe and the patient was transferred from the operating room to the neurocritical care unit and intubated. Which of the following measures is *not* appropriate for managing intracranial hypertension?
a. Hypertonic saline
b. Sustained hyperventilation
c. CSF drainage with a ventriculostomy catheter
d. Mannitol

IV.100. A 60-year-old man undergoes resection of a T9 vertebral body metastasis and spinal instrumentation. Which of the following is *not* appropriate for postoperative pain management?
a. Single-agent opioid infusion
b. Combination opioid therapy
c. IV acetaminophen
d. NSAIDs

IV.101. A 69-year-old man with a history of non–small cell adenocarcinoma of the lung and uncontrolled systemic disease is brought to the ED by emergency medical services after being found on the floor by family members. On the basis of the clinical assessment, the patient is determined to be in nonconvulsive SE. Noncontrast CT of the head shows hydrocephalus. After the patient has been stabilized neurologically, what is the best next step?
 a. MRI with and without contrast
 b. Lumbar puncture
 c. Craniospinal radiation
 d. Intrathecal chemotherapy

IV.102. A 44-year-old woman with triple-negative breast cancer now has diplopia and dysphagia. MRI of the brain shows diffuse leptomeningeal enhancement, but she has had negative results from 3 lumbar punctures. What is the next appropriate step?
 a. Watchful waiting with serial MRI
 b. Imaging the remaining neuraxis in preparation for radiation therapy
 c. Intrathecal trastuzamab
 d. A fourth lumbar puncture with flow cytometry

IV.103. A 23-year-old female flight attendant was brought to the ED with diminshed comprehension and paraphasic errors and a 2-day history of fever and flu. MRI of the head showed subtle T2-signal abnormality in the left temporal lobe, and CSF analysis confirmed HSV encephalitis (PCR was positive for HSV). The patient received a course of IV acyclovir, made a good recovery, and was discharged. Three weeks later, she started to have abnormal orofacial movements. Her colleagues noticed bizarre behavior and distorted thinking during flight hours. She had a witnessed generalized seizure and was again brought to the ED. She was admitted to the ICU for management after she had 2 more seizures in the ED. MRI of the brain showed marked swelling of the left more than the right mesial temporal lobe. What test is most likely to confirm the diagnosis?
 a. CT of the abdomen and pelvis
 b. EEG
 c. Serum testing for NMDA receptor antibody
 d. CSF testing for NMDA receptor antibody

IV.104. A 48-year-old businessman was admitted to the ICU with SE. His spouse reported that he had been having difficulties at work and with managing their finances and had become increasingly forgetful during the preceding 2 months. He required a propofol drip for management of his SE. MRI of the head showed a mild CSF pleocytosis and high T2 and FLAIR signal intensity over both medial temporal lobes. Oncology screening showed a mass in his left testis.What is the most likely neural antibody to be detected on paraneoplastic serum evaluation?
 a. ANNA-1 (anti-Hu)
 b. ANNA-2 (anti-Ri)
 c. Anti-Ma2
 d. PCA-1 (anti-Yo)

IV.105. For what neurologic emergency is radiation therapy an option?
 a. Newly diagnosed glioblastoma
 b. Spinal cord compression
 c. Trigeminal neuralgia
 d. AVM

IV.106. What is the most common indication for intracranial radiation therapy?
 a. Ependymoma
 b. Meningioma
 c. Pituitary adenoma
 d. Brain metastases

IV.107. What is the most common intervention for symptoms due to radiation therapy?
 a. Corticosteroids
 b. Mannitol
 c. Flat body position and bed rest
 d. NSAIDs

Postoperative Neurosurgery

IV.108. Which surgical approach to the spine carries the greatest risk for morbidity or death?
 a. Anterior cervical
 b. Thoracolumbar
 c. Lateral lumbar
 d. Combination of anterior and posterior

IV.109. If a patient has undergone a procedure through an anterior cervical surgical approach and is restless and breathless and has a sense of impending doom, which of the following complications must be considered?
 a. Retropharyngeal hematoma and airway compromise
 b. Perforated esophagus
 c. Spinal cord compression
 d. Primary anxiety disorder

IV.110. Where is the least robust spinal cord blood supply?
 a. Cervical spine
 b. Thoracic spine
 c. Conus medullaris
 d. Lumbar spine

IV.111. Which of the following does *not* increase the risk of spinal surgery morbidity and death?
 a. Respiratory failure
 b. Cardiac instability
 c. Combination of anterior and posterior surgical approaches
 d. Blood glucose level of 175 mg/dL

IV.112. A patient who has undergone a corrective procedure for a long-segment spinal deformity now has deep vein thrombosis and pulmonary embolism. What may be the safest treatment?
 a. Therapeutic anticoagulation
 b. Subcutaneous heparin with a prophylactic dose regimen
 c. Early mobilization
 d. Temporary inferior vena cava filter and discussion with the surgeon about the use of heparinoids when safe (from a spinal hemostasis standpoint)

IV.113. A patient in the ICU has elevated BP (180/110 mm Hg) after undergoing a right frontal craniotomy for tumor 6 hours ago. Which of the following is the most appropriate next step?
 a. Administer a muscle relaxant.
 b. Administer an analgesic.
 c. Administer a short-acting antihypertensive IV as needed to decrease the systolic BP to less than 140 mm Hg, and reassess in 15 minutes.
 d. Administer an antiepileptic drug.

IV.114. Which of the following is *not* included in the management of increased ICP?
 a. Raise the head of the bed at least 30°.
 b. Use hyperventilation to increase the $Paco_2$.
 c. Administer 20% mannitol IV.
 d. Insert an external ventricular drainage catheter.

IV.115. How is SIADH best differentiated from cerebral salt wasting?
 a. Urine osmolality
 b. Serum osmolality
 c. Intravascular volume status according to body weight
 d. Serum sodium concentration

IV.116. Which of the following is true about preoperative embolization of tumors, such as meningiomas?
   a. Waiting more than 96 hours to resect the tumor could result in excessive swelling, which may lead to clinical deterioration.
   b. Postembolization hemorrhage is not a concern because it is unlikely after the feeding arteries have been occluded during embolization.
   c. The tumor should be resected within 48 hours after embolization (before the tumor softens).
   d. Fever and pain are common after embolization of meningiomas.

IV.117. Which of the following is true about elective coiling of unruptured cerebral aneurysms?
   a. Stroke secondary to thromboembolism is more common than aneurysm rupture.
   b. Ventriculostomies should always be placed before treatment because patients receive anticoagulation for the aneurysm repair.
   c. If intraoperative stroke occurs, rtPA should be given immediately and heparinization should be reversed.
   d. If intraoperative stroke occurs, abciximab should be given along with heparin.

IV.118. Cerebral vasospasm related to aneurysm rupture carries high morbidity. Which of the following is *false*?
   a. Endovascular therapy for refractory vasospasm consists of balloon angioplasty of medium-sized to large intracranial arteries with or without intra-arterial infusion of calcium channel blockers (eg, verapamil).
   b. Induced hypertension and mild hypervolemia (but not hemodilution) are standards of prophylaxis for vasospasm.
   c. TCD, CTA, MRA, and angiography are used to monitor for vasospasm.
   d. The clinical examination is the best tool for detection of early vasospasm.

IV.119. Which statement correctly describes endovascular treatment of acute stroke?
   a. Endovascular treatment with thombectomy is not advised if the patient receives IV rtPA.
   b. Suction aspiration of the clot is used in combination with mechanical removal with a stent retriever.
   c. Endovascular therapy is contraindicated if the patient has received aspirin or clopidogrel.
   d. The risk of intracranial hemorrhage is markedly increased with endovascular therapy compared with use of IV rtPA alone.

IV.120. Which of the following statements is *false*?
   a. Hemorrhage occurs in up to 14% of patients undergoing embolization of a BAVM or DAVF.
   b. Liquid embolic agents and coils are usually used in combination for endovascular therapy for BAVMs or DAVFs.
   c. Postoperative stroke, hemorrhage, and cranial neuropathy are the most common complications after embolization of BAVMs or DAVFs.
   d. Seizure and cerebral edema are less common clinical concerns after embolization of BAVMs or DAVFs.

Answers

Acute Cerebrovascular Disorders

IV.1. Answer b.

DHC decreases mortality but does not change the underlying cerebral infarct damage and associated neurologic deficits. In randomized trials, DHC has not improved stroke deficits, but it may improve functional outcomes. Although considerable debate is ongoing about dominant hemispheric strokes compared with nondominant hemispheric strokes, DHC can be used for either hemisphere.

Gupta A, Sattur MG, Aoun RJN, Krishna C, Bolton PB, Chong BW, et al. Hemicraniectomy for ischemic and hemorrhagic stroke: facts and controversies. Neurosurg Clin N Am. 2017 Jul;28(3):349–60.

Wijdicks EF, Sheth KN, Carter BS, Greer DM, Kasner SE, Kimberly WT, et al; American Heart Association Stroke Council. Recommendations for the management of cerebral and cerebellar infarction with swelling: a statement for healthcare professionals from the American Heart Association/American Stroke Association. Stroke. 2014 Apr;45(4):1222–38. Epub 2014 Jan 30.

IV.2. Answer c.

Corticosteroids are not advised for the management of ischemic stroke or hemispheric infarction, which is cytotoxic not vasogenic. Osmotherapy is considered first-line medical management for patients whose clinical condition is deteriorating from cerebral edema. Studies on the use of corticosteroids showed that the adverse effects outweighed the potential benefit. DHC changes the Monro-Kellie pressure-volume relationship by changing the intracranial volume but not the infarcted cerebral tissue edema.

Norris JW. Steroid therapy in acute cerebral infarction. Arch Neurol. 1976 Jan;33(1):69–71.

Wijdicks EF, Sheth KN, Carter BS, Greer DM, Kasner SE, Kimberly WT, et al; American Heart Association Stroke Council. Recommendations for the management of cerebral and cerebellar infarction with swelling: a statement for healthcare professionals from the American Heart Association/American Stroke Association. Stroke. 2014 Apr;45(4):1222–38. Epub 2014 Jan 30.

IV.3. Answer b.

Locked-in syndrome results from damage to the ventral pons. Clinical features may include quadriplegia, anarthria, dysphagia, facial diplegia, and impaired horizontal eye movements. If damage spares the midbrain tegmentum, vertical eye movements and blinking are retained, providing a possible method of communication.

Smith E, Delargy M. Locked-in syndrome. BMJ. 2005 Feb 19;330(7488):406–9.

IV.4. Answer c.

The paired AICAs and superior cerebellar arteries are the largest branches from the basilar trunk before it terminates as the PCAs. The AICAs supply the inferior pons and middle cerebellar peduncles. The AICAs also typically give rise to the internal auditory and labyrinthine arteries. The anterior spinal artery and posterior inferior cerebellar arteries arise from the vertebral arteries, before the origin of the basilar artery. The posterior communicating arteries arise from the PCAs and connect the anterior and posterior circulation.

Caplan LR. Caplan's stroke: a clinical approach. 4th ed. Philadelphia (PA): Elsevier/Saunders; c2009.

Tatu L, Moulin T, Bogousslavsky J, Duvernoy H. Arterial territories of human brain: brainstem and cerebellum. Neurology. 1996 Nov;47(5):1125–35.

IV.5. Answer a.

Thalamogeniculate arteries arise from the PCAs and supply the thalamus. Top of the basilar syndrome can result from bilateral thalamic infarcts due to occlusion of the PCAs.

Caplan LR. Caplan's stroke: a clinical approach. 4th ed. Philadelphia (PA): Elsevier/Saunders; c2009.

IV.6. Answer c.

Although all the items listed have been linked to patient outcomes, recanalization and reperfusion are the most important. Without recanalization, mortality may exceed 90%, regardless of other factors.

Brandt T, von Kummer R, Muller-Kuppers M, Hacke W. Thrombolytic therapy of acute basilar artery occlusion: variables affecting recanalization and outcome. Stroke. 1996 May;27(5):875–81.

Schonewille WJ, Wijman CA, Michel P, Rueckert CM, Weimar C, Mattle HP, et al; BASICS study group. Treatment and outcomes of acute basilar artery occlusion in the Basilar Artery International Cooperation Study (BASICS): a prospective registry study. Lancet Neurol. 2009 Aug;8(8):724–30. Epub 2009 Jul 3.

IV.7. Answer b.

Somnolence and confusion can result from infectious, metabolic, toxic, or ischemic causes. The presence of additional deficits localizing to the posterior circulation (eg, dysconjugate gaze) should prompt the use of head and vascular imaging for further evaluation. Forced gaze deviation would be suggestive of either seizure activity or anterior circulation ischemia involving the frontal eye fields. Fever would support an infectious cause of presenting symptoms. Wide pupils are a nonspecific finding and would not help in establishing a diagnosis.

Mattle HP, Arnold M, Lindsberg PJ, Schonewille WJ, Schroth G. Basilar artery occlusion. Lancet Neurol. 2011 Nov;10(11):1002–14.

IV.8. Answer d.

Answer choices *a*, *b*, and *c* are consistent with a posterior circulation syndrome such as basilar occlusion instead of an anterior circulation syndrome from ICA disease. Light-sensitive amaurosis fugax is highly sensitive to high-grade ICA arterial narrowing or low flow, which is also called the Whisnant phenomenon.

Brown RD Jr, Rocca WA. Jack P. Whisnant, MD, FAAN (1924–2015). Neurology. 2015 Nov 24;85(21):1832–3.

Hurwitz BJ, Heyman A, Wilkinson WE, Haynes CS, Utley CM. Comparison of amaurosis fugax and transient cerebral ischemia: a prospective clinical and arteriographic study. Ann Neurol. 1985 Dec;18(6):698–704.

Wilson LA, Russell RW. Amaurosis fugax and carotid artery disease: indications for angiography. Br Med J. 1977 Aug 13;2(6084):435–7.

IV.9. Answer d.

The patient has symptomatic ICA disease. EEG is not indicated given the history and findings, which are consistent with a TIA likely involving the left ICA or middle cerebral artery. After symptomatic ICA disease has occurred, the patient's risk is higher for stroke and more severe anterior circulation stroke deficits. The best plan would include starting aspirin medical therapy immediately and having the patient evaluated as a possible candidate for CEA surgery or CAS.

Abbott AL, Paraskevas KI, Kakkos SK, Golledge J, Eckstein HH, Diaz-Sandoval LJ, et al. Systematic review of guidelines for the management of asymptomatic and symptomatic carotid stenosis. Stroke. 2015 Nov;46(11):3288–301. Epub 2015 Oct 8.

Howard VJ, Meschia JF, Lal BK, Turan TN, Roubin GS, Brown RD Jr, et al; CREST-2 Study Investigators. Carotid revascularization and medical management for asymptomatic carotid stenosis: protocol of the CREST-2 clinical trials. Int J Stroke. 2017 Oct;12(7):770–8. Epub 2017 May 2.

IV.10. Answer c.

RCVS is a disease that may mimic PCNSV, so differentiation is crucial because immunosuppressive therapy is not warranted for syndromes caused by vasoconstriction. In PCNSV, precipitating factors are absent, the onset is more insidious, the headache is not usually the thunderclap type, and CSF results are usually abnormal. In RCVS, CSF results are usually normal.

Hammad TA, Hajj-Ali RA. Primary angiitis of the central nervous system and reversible cerebral vasoconstriction syndrome. Curr Atheroscler Rep. 2013 Aug;15(8):346.

IV.11. Answer d.

PCNSV occasionally presents with rapidly progressive neurologic symptoms and signs. Angiography may show bilateral, diffuse involvement of the large cerebral arteries, and MRI may show multifocal cerebral infarctions in the cortical and subcortical areas of the brain. The diagnosis of PCNSV in the described patient is supported by the clinical presentation, angiographic findings, and CSF results. The past medical history did not indicate use of any medications that are typically involved with RCVS. The optimal treatment would include urgent use of IV methylprednisolone and then oral prednisone and cyclophosphamide.

Kadkhodayan Y, Alreshaid A, Moran CJ, Cross DT 3rd, Powers WJ, Derdeyn CP. Primary angiitis of the central nervous system at conventional angiography. Radiology. 2004 Dec;233(3):878–82. Epub 2004 Oct 21.

Zuccoli G, Pipitone N, Haldipur A, Brown RD Jr, Hunder G, Salvarani C. Imaging findings in primary central nervous system vasculitis. Clin Exp Rheumatol. 2011 Jan-Feb;29(1 Suppl 64):S104–9. Epub 2011 May 11.

IV.12. Answer d.

To prevent glucocorticoid-induced osteoporosis, calcium (1,000-1,500 mg daily) and vitamin D (800 international units daily) should be started with any dose or duration of glucocorticoid therapy. Bisphosphonate should be added for postmenopausal women and for men older than 50 years who are starting glucocorticoid therapy with an expected glucocorticoid duration of at least 3 months. Prophylaxis against infection with *Pneumocystis jiroveci* with trimethoprim-sulfamethoxazole (800/160 mg on alternate days or 400/80 mg daily) should be started in all patients receiving cyclophosphamide and rituximab. Therefore, this patient should receive bisphosphonate, calcium, vitamin D supplementation, and trimethoprim-sulfamethoxazole with the immunosuppressive treatment.

Salvarani C, Brown RD Jr, Hunder GG. Adult primary central nervous system vasculitis: an update. Curr Opin Rheumatol 2012; 24:46–52.

IV.13. Answer c.

Young patients with no other apparent risk factors who present with a lobar hemorrhage and have no microbleeds or other findings on MRI of the brain should undergo conventional angiography for further investigation of a possible underlying vascular malformation or vascular pathology.

Aguilar MI, Demaerschalk BM. Intracerebral hemorrhage. Semin Neurol. 2007 Sep;27(4):376–84.

IV.14. Answer b.

Prothrombin complex concentrate has been used for ICH associated with factor Xa inhibitors; however, andexanet alfa is costly. Vitamin K, FFP, and recombinant factor VIIa are not suggested for rivaroxaban-induced ICH. Idarucizumab is the antidote of choice for ICH associated with direct-thrombin inhibitors (eg, dabigatran) but not for ICH due to factor Xa inhibitors. Activated charcoal may be useful if the latest dose of rivaroxaban was taken within the previous 2 hours, so it may not be effective in this patient.

Kaatz S, Kouides PA, Garcia DA, Spyropolous AC, Crowther M, Douketis JD, et al. Guidance on the emergent reversal of oral thrombin and factor Xa inhibitors. Am J Hematol. 2012 May;87 Suppl 1:S141–5. Epub 2012 Apr 4. Erratum in: Am J Hematol. 2012 Jul;87(7):748.

Tummala R, Kavtaradze A, Gupta A, Ghosh RK. Specific antidotes against direct oral anticoagulants: a comprehensive review of clinical trials data. Int J Cardiol. 2016 Jul 1;214:292–8. Epub 2016 Mar 28.

IV.15. Answer a.

Intraventricular administration of urokinase was associated with decreased mortality in early clinical studies. However, urokinase studies were discontinued because of drug manufacturing problems, and subsequent research shifted to rtPA, which is less applicable for general clinical practice. Subsequent trials (CLEAR phase 2 and phase 3 trials) compared the administration of intraventricular rtPA with placebo (saline irrigation). The other statements are incorrect: Patients treated with rtPA had a nonsignificantly shorter requirement for a ventricular catheter. IVH occurs in about 45% to 50% of patients with spontaneous ICH and is associated with poorer outcomes. CSF drain placement for obstructive hydrocephalus is suggested for patients who are not expected to die soon or whose hydrocephalic obtundation could be treated medically and surgically. Ventricular catheters, however, do not reverse underlying ICH parenchymal neurologic deficits.

Gaberel T, Magheru C, Parienti JJ, Huttner HB, Vivien D, Emery E. Intraventricular fibrinolysis versus external ventricular drainage alone in intraventricular hemorrhage: a meta-analysis. Stroke. 2011 Oct;42(10):2776–81. Epub 2011 Aug 4.

Hallevi H, Albright KC, Aronowski J, Barreto AD, Martin-Schild S, Khaja AM, et al. Intraventricular hemorrhage: anatomic relationships and clinical implications. Neurology. 2008 Mar 11;70(11):848–52.

Morgan T, Awad I, Keyl P, Lane K, Hanley D. Preliminary report of the clot lysis evaluating accelerated resolution of intraventricular hemorrhage (CLEAR-IVH) clinical trial. Acta Neurochir Suppl. 2008;105:217–20.

IV.16. Answer c.

Minimally invasive surgery in combination with rtPA may be safe and superior to craniotomy according to the MISTIE II trial and a published meta-analysis of select ICH cases. However, phase 3 trial (MISTIE III) results showed no benefit. Surgical evacuation is not indicated for lobar hematomas deeper than 1 cm and with volumes 30 mL or smaller according to the ICH guidelines. The best timing of evacuation is uncertain (early hematoma evacuation is not clearly beneficial compared with hematoma evacuation when a patient's condition deteriorates). If a patient's condition is deteriorating, evacuation must be considered as a lifesaving measure. Surgical evacuation in combination with medical therapy decreases the odds of the patient dying soon or being dependent.

Morgenstern LB, Hemphill JC 3rd, Anderson C, Becker K, Broderick JP, Connolly ES Jr, et al; American Heart Association Stroke Council and Council on Cardiovascular Nursing. Guidelines for the management of spontaneous intracerebral hemorrhage: a guideline for healthcare professionals from the American Heart Association/American Stroke Association. Stroke. 2010 Sep;41(9):2108–29. Epub 2010 Jul 22.

Mould WA, Carhuapoma JR, Muschelli J, Lane K, Morgan TC, McBee NA, et al; MISTIE Investigators. Minimally invasive surgery plus recombinant tissue-type plasminogen activator for intracerebral hemorrhage evacuation decreases perihematomal edema. Stroke. 2013 Mar;44(3):627–34. Epub 2013 Feb 7.

IV.17. Answer c.

The hematoma expansion prediction score is an accurate predictor of the probability of substantial hematoma expansion. As a predictor of hematoma expansion, the CTA spot sign has a sensitivity of 51% and a specificity of 85%. Ultra-early hematoma growth is determined with the ratio of initial ICH volume to the onset-to-imaging time. The 24-point BRAIN score is based on ICH volume, recurrent ICH, anticoagulation with warfarin at the onset, intraventricular extension, and number of hours to baseline CT from symptom onset.

Demchuk AM, Dowlatshahi D, Rodriguez-Luna D, Molina CA, Blas YS, Dzialowski I, et al; PREDICT/Sunnybrook ICH CTA study group. Prediction of haematoma growth and outcome in patients with intracerebral haemorrhage using the CT-angiography spot sign (PREDICT): a prospective observational study. Lancet Neurol. 2012 Apr;11(4):307–14. Epub 2012 Mar 8. Erratum in: Lancet Neurol. 2012 Jun;11(6):483.

Rodriguez-Luna D, Rubiera M, Ribo M, Coscojuela P, Pineiro S, Pagola J, et al. Ultraearly hematoma growth predicts poor outcome after acute intracerebral hemorrhage. Neurology. 2011 Oct 25;77(17):1599–604. Epub 2011 Oct 12.

Wang X, Arima H, Al-Shahi Salman R, Woodward M, Heeley E, Stapf C, et al; INTERACT Investigators. Clinical prediction algorithm (BRAIN) to determine risk of hematoma growth in acute intracerebral hemorrhage. Stroke. 2015 Feb;46(2):376–81. Epub 2014 Dec 11.

Yao X, Xu Y, Siwila-Sackman E, Wu B, Selim M. The HEP score: a nomogram-derived hematoma expansion prediction scale. Neurocrit Care. 2015 Oct;23(2):179–87.

IV.18. Answer c.

Hypertension is a well-established modifiable risk factor for aSAH. Evidence for the role of other risk factors is less robust.

Feigin VL, Rinkel GJ, Lawes CM, Algra A, Bennett DA, van Gijn J, et al. Risk factors for subarachnoid hemorrhage: an updated systematic review of epidemiological studies. Stroke. 2005 Dec;36(12):2773–80. Epub 2005 Nov 10.

Sandvei MS, Romundstad PR, Muller TB, Vatten L, Vik A. Risk factors for aneurysmal subarachnoid hemorrhage in a prospective population study: the HUNT study in Norway. Stroke. 2009 Jun;40(6):1958–62. Epub 2009 Feb 19.

IV.19. Answer c.

Randomized studies in the 1980s showed that antifibrinolytic drugs administered IV and continuously for several days decreased the incidence of rebleeding but increased the risk of delayed cerebral ischemia from vasospasm and hydrocephalus without improving the overall outcome. However, in a more recent multicenter study in Sweden, the incidence of rebleeding decreased significantly after administration of a short course of tranexamic acid (1 g every 6 hours up to 72 hours) starting immediately after aSAH was diagnosed. Antifibrinolytic drugs may increase the likelihood of thromboembolic complications, so their use should be avoided in patients with a history of coronary artery disease.

Connolly ES Jr, Rabinstein AA, Carhuapoma JR, Derdeyn CP, Dion J, Higashida RT, et al; American Heart Association Stroke Council; Council on Cardiovascular Radiology and Intervention; Council on Cardiovascular Nursing; Council on Cardiovascular Surgery and Anesthesia; Council on Clinical Cardiology. Guidelines for the management of aneurysmal subarachnoid hemorrhage: a guideline for healthcare professionals from the American Heart Association/American Stroke Association. Stroke. 2012 Jun;43(6):1711–37. Epub 2012 May 3.

IV.20. Answer a.

Although no randomized trials support the value of induced hypertension as the first line of medical therapy against new neurologic deficits, enough evidence has been collected to suggest that it is a reasonable option. Because of the complications associated with hypervolemia, many medical centers no longer use it; instead, the goal should be to maintain euvolemia and replace any fluid losses. Although theoretically appealing, hemodilution is no longer used to counteract the effects of vasospasm.

Connolly ES Jr, Rabinstein AA, Carhuapoma JR, Derdeyn CP, Dion J, Higashida RT, et al; American Heart Association Stroke Council; Council on Cardiovascular Radiology and Intervention; Council on Cardiovascular Nursing; Council on Cardiovascular Surgery and Anesthesia; Council on Clinical Cardiology. Guidelines for the management of aneurysmal subarachnoid hemorrhage: a guideline for healthcare professionals from the American Heart Association/American Stroke Association. Stroke. 2012 Jun;43(6):1711–37. Epub 2012 May 3.

Macdonald RL, Schweizer TA. Spontaneous subarachnoid haemorrhage. Lancet. 2017 Feb 11;389(10069):655–66. Epub 2016 Sep 13.

IV.21. Answer d.

In controlled clinical trials (primarily the ISAT), patients undergoing coil embolization rather than clip ligation have had a better functional outcome at 1 year. Therefore, if an aneurysm is amenable to either surgical or endovascular treatment, coil embolization is preferred. The exception may be young patients with anterior circulation aneurysms that are amenable to safe surgical treatment.

Lanzino G, Murad MH, d'Urso PI, Rabinstein AA. Coil embolization versus clipping for ruptured intracranial aneurysms: a meta-analysis of prospective controlled published studies. AJNR Am J Neuroradiol. 2013 Sep;34(9):1764–8. Epub 2013 Apr 11.

Molyneux AJ, Kerr RS, Birks J, Ramzi N, Yarnold J, Sneade M, et al; ISAT Collaborators. Risk of recurrent subarachnoid haemorrhage, death, or dependence and standardised mortality ratios after clipping or coiling of an intracranial aneurysm in the International Subarachnoid Aneurysm Trial (ISAT): long-term follow-up. Lancet Neurol. 2009 May;8(5):427–33. Epub 2009 Mar 28.

IV.22. Answer b.

Vasospasm peaks from days 7 through 14 and, if severe enough, results in symptomatic vasospasm, which may cause delayed cerebral ischemia. Vasospasm is a diagnosis of exclusion, and other potential causes of neurologic deterioration must be excluded or considered insufficient to explain the neurologic deterioration.

Macdonald RL, Schweizer TA. Spontaneous subarachnoid haemorrhage. Lancet. 2017 Feb 11;389(10069):655–66. Epub 2016 Sep 13.

IV.23. Answer d.

In observational studies, previous intracranial hemorrhage increased risk of hemorrhage more than the other risk factors.

Mast H, Young WL, Koennecke HC, Sciacca RR, Osipov A, Pile-Spellman J, et al. Risk of spontaneous haemorrhage after diagnosis of cerebral arteriovenous malformation. Lancet. 1997 Oct 11;350(9084):1065–8.

IV.24. Answer b.

Intracranial hemorrhage is the most common reason that patients present with an otherwise asymptomatic AVM. On average, intracranial hemorrhage occurs in about 50% of patients with AVM; seizures occur in 15% to 35%, and focal neurologic deficits occur in less than 10%.

Forster DM, Steiner L, Hakanson S. Arteriovenous malformations of the brain: a long-term clinical study. J Neurosurg. 1972 Nov;37(5):562–70.

IV.25. Answer d.

The Spetzler-Martin grading system is used to weigh the operative risk of open craniotomy and AVM surgery.

Spetzler RF, Martin NA. A proposed grading system for arteriovenous malformations. J Neurosurg. 1986 Oct;65(4):476–83.

IV.26. Answer a.

Radiosurgery does not cause an immediate change. AVM involution occurs in 2 to 3 years.

Ogilvy CS, Stieg PE, Awad I, Brown RD Jr, Kondziolka D, Rosenwasser R, et al; Special Writing Group of the Stroke Council, American Stroke Association. AHA Scientific Statement: recommendations for the management of intracranial arteriovenous malformations: a statement for healthcare professionals from a special writing group of the Stroke Council, American Stroke Association. Stroke. 2001 Jun;32(6):1458–71.

IV.27. Answer c.

Patients who present with a seizure are at increased risk for the AVM causing subsequent seizures. Prophylactic medication should be considered for those patients in the context of AVM treatment options (such as medical management and observation) or higher risk options (such as operative neurosurgery, an endovascular approach, or radiosurgery).

Ogilvy CS, Stieg PE, Awad I, Brown RD Jr, Kondziolka D, Rosenwasser R, et al; Special Writing Group of the Stroke Council, American Stroke Association. AHA Scientific Statement: recommendations for the management of intracranial arteriovenous malformations: a statement for healthcare professionals from a special writing group of the Stroke Council, American Stroke Association. Stroke. 2001 Jun;32(6):1458–71.

IV.28. Answer c.

Although hydration is important, the mechanism of clinical deterioration is impaired venous drainage due to venous sinus thrombosis, which must be treated promptly with IV heparinization (to an aPTT that is twice the control) or with weight-adjusted subcutaneous low-molecular-weight heparin. The evidence favors anticoagulation for all patients with CVDST, including those with hemorrhagic transformation of venous infarctions. Endovascular therapy is reserved for patients who have clot propagation despite adequate anticoagulation.

Einhaupl KM, Villringer A, Meister W, Mehraein S, Garner C, Pellkofer M, et al. Heparin treatment in sinus venous thrombosis. Lancet. 1991 Sep 7;338(8767):597–600. Erratum in: Lancet 1991 Oct 12;338(8772):958.

Saposnik G, Barinagarrementeria F, Brown RD Jr, Bushnell CD, Cucchiara B, Cushman M, et al; American Heart Association Stroke Council and the Council on Epidemiology and Prevention. Diagnosis and management of cerebral venous thrombosis: a statement for healthcare professionals from the American Heart Association/American Stroke Association. Stroke. 2011 Apr;42(4):1158–92. Epub 2011 Feb 3.

IV.29. Answer d.

The pressure to provide additional therapy because this patient is not improving should be resisted. Endovascular thrombolysis should be considered only if the patient has clot propagation despite adequate anticoagulation. Critical monitoring of anticoagulation status and repeating CTV to evaluate for propagation of the clot would be the best course of action for this patient.

Bousser MG, Ferro JM. Cerebral venous thrombosis: an update. Lancet Neurol. 2007 Feb;6(2):162–70.

Saposnik G, Barinagarrementeria F, Brown RD Jr, Bushnell CD, Cucchiara B, Cushman M, et al; American Heart Association Stroke Council and the Council on Epidemiology and Prevention. Diagnosis and management of cerebral venous thrombosis: a statement for healthcare professionals from the American Heart Association/American Stroke Association. Stroke. 2011 Apr;42(4):1158–92. Epub 2011 Feb 3.

IV.30. Answer b.

ICA dissection causes referred pain to the forehead, face, or neck, often with ipsilateral Horner syndrome, and later retinal or cerebral ischemia.

Robertson JJ, Koyfman A. Cervical artery dissections: a review. J Emerg Med. 2016 Nov;51(5):508–18. Epub 2016 Sep 12.

Schievink WI. Spontaneous dissection of the carotid and vertebral arteries. N Engl J Med. 2001 Mar 22;344(12):898–906.

IV.31. Answer d.

On angiography, the pathologic constituents of a dissection have a characteristically tapered appearance resembling a candle flame.

Robertson JJ, Koyfman A. Cervical artery dissections: a review. J Emerg Med. 2016 Nov;51(5):508–18. Epub 2016 Sep 12.

Schievink WI. Spontaneous dissection of the carotid and vertebral arteries. N Engl J Med. 2001 Mar 22;344(12):898–906.

Traumatic Brain and Spine Injury

IV.32. Answer b.

MRI with GRE sequences is the most sensitive for DAI. The CT "stealth" or brain laboratory protocol with 1-mm sections is for stereotactic 3-dimensional operating room navigation; the images may appear grainy compared with standard 5-mm sections. PET imaging can show global brain hypermetabolism and hypometabolism, but it is not the tool for diagnosing DAI. The SPECT hollow skull sign is seen in brain death because the entire brain does not pick up the SPECT signal, so SPECT is not advised for DAI.

Beretta L, Gemma M, Anzalone N. The value of MR imaging in posttraumatic diffuse axonal injury. J Emerg Trauma Shock. 2008 Jul;1(2):126–7.

IV.33. Answer b.

Traumatic SAH occurs in about 35% of traumatic head injuries. Some variation exists, depending on factors such as the severity of the TBI, use of antithrombotic agents, and coagulation parameters.

Zasler ND, Katz DI, Zafonte RD, editors. Brain injury medicine: principles and practice. New York (NY): Demos; c2007. 1275 p.

IV.34. Answer d.

Loss of sympathetic nervous system tone causes loss of SVR from the thoracic sympathetic ganglia. Patients present with hypotension due to SVR and potentially bradycardia due to loss of sympathetic tone to the heart. Tachycardia is a compensatory response to decreased SVR, but it may not occur with sympathetic spinal cord injury.

Hagen EM. Acute complications of spinal cord injuries. World J Orthop. 2015 Jan 18;6(1):17–23.

IV.35. Answer c.

MRI with GRE sequencing is one of the most sensitive techniques for detection of small petechiae and tiny areas of parenchymal contusion since blood appears as a "blossoming" artifact on GRE sequencing, which makes hematomas and contusions appear larger than their actual size. DTI is useful for detection of white matter tracts that may have been disrupted in TBI but not for detection of small hemorrhages. CT is the fastest way to detect macrohemorrhages, but it may not show tiny parenchymal hemorrhages seen with GRE MRI sequences. FLAIR sequencing is commonly used in MRI for detecting various abnormalities (old stroke, fluid, and protein or injury) but not specifically microhemorrhages.

Heit JJ, Iv M, Wintermark M. Imaging of intracranial hemorrhage. J Stroke. 2017 Jan;19(1):11–27. Epub 2016 Dec 12.

IV.36. Answer d.

Complete loss of motor and sensory functioin at and below a specific level is graded *A*. Grades *B, C*, and *D* indicate various incomplete levels of sensory or motor function. Grade *E* indicates normal motor and sensory function.

Roberts TT, Leonard GR, Cepela DJ. Classifications in brief: American Spinal Injury Association (ASIA) impairment scale. Clin Orthop Relat Res. 2017 May;475(5):1499–1504. Epub 2016 Nov 4.

IV.37. Answer d.

Fluid levels and a different density within the acute clot suggest the possibility of an underlying coagulopathy, such as warfarin anticoagulation. Although coagulopathy may be associated with a larger, actively bleeding SDH, the other answer choices do not discriminate between patients with and without an underlying coagulopathy.

Siddiqui FM, Bekker SV, Qureshi AI. Neuroimaging of hemorrhage and vascular defects. Neurotherapeutics. 2011 Jan;8(1):28–38.

Wijdicks EFM. The practice of emergency and critical care neurology. New York (NY): Oxford University Press; c2016. 915 p.

IV.38. Answer b.

Large midline shift of the brainstem against the contralateral tentorial edge compresses the contralateral cerebral peduncle and produces hemiparesis ipsilateral to the side of the lesion, a false localizing sign known as the Kernohan notch phenomenon.

Wijdicks EFM. The practice of emergency and critical care neurology. New York (NY): Oxford University Press; c2016. 915 p.

Yoo WK, Kim DS, Kwon YH, Jang SH. Kernohan's notch phenomenon demonstrated by diffusion tensor imaging and transcranial magnetic stimulation. J Neurol Neurosurg Psychiatry. 2008 Nov;79(11):1295–7.

IV.39. Answer c.

Observation is advised for this patient's EDH. However, if the GCS score decreases by at least 2 points (from a baseline of 14 to 12 or less), CT should be performed and the neurosurgeon alerted for probable neurosurgical intervention for a growing EDH. The patient's INR is already 1.5, which should be sufficient if the patient needs surgery. Also, FFP is unlikely to decrease the INR from 1.5 to 1.0 and would be an additional fluid load.

Holland LL, Brooks JP. Toward rational fresh frozen plasma transfusion: the effect of plasma transfusion on coagulation test results. Am J Clin Pathol. 2006 Jul;126(1):133–9.

IV.40. Answer b.

The SDH is subacute since the hematoma is isodense (ie, about 40-60 Hounsfield units). Therefore, the SDH developed at least several days ago rather than within the past 24 hours.

Ohno K, Suzuki R, Masaoka H, Matsushima Y, Inaba Y, Monma S. Chronic subdural haematoma preceded by persistent traumatic subdural fluid collection. J Neurol Neurosurg Psychiatry. 1987 Dec;50(12):1694–7.

IV.41. Answer b.

The swirl sign is concerning for active bleeding in an EDH and could indicate that the patient's neurologic status will soon rapidly deteriorate. In SDH, the swirl sign may resemble fluid-fluid levels radiologically, but in EDH, the swirl sign is typically due to arterial bleeding rather than venous bleeding. Anticoagulation status should be checked at baseline if the swirl sign or fluid-fluid levels are present in SDH or EDH, especially if the patient has a history of anticoagulation, which may require emergent reversal.

Guo C, Liu L, Wang B, Wang Z. Swirl sign in traumatic acute epidural hematoma: prognostic value and surgical management. Neurol Sci. 2017 Dec;38(12):2111–6. Epub 2017 Sep 11.

IV.42. Answer c.

CT is warranted because the patient has neck pain after trauma. Immediately after an injury, plain radiographs have a high rate of false-negative results because muscle spasm restricts motion on flexion-extension views.

Walters BC, Hadley MN, Hurlbert RJ, Aarabi B, Dhall SS, Gelb DE, et al; American Association of Neurological Surgeons; Congress of Neurological Surgeons. Guidelines for the management of acute cervical spine and spinal cord injuries: 2013 update. Neurosurgery. 2013 Aug;60(Suppl 1):82–91.

IV.43. Answer c.

Nondisplaced odontoid fractures in the elderly may be treated with a trial of bracing with a hard collar for 10 to 12 weeks. Halo fixation is also an option. Surgical management is definitive for fixation. The rate of nonunion with conservative management of type II odontoid fractures is 20% to 30%.

Sonntag VK, Hadley MN. Nonoperative management of cervical spine injuries. Clin Neurosurg. 1988;34:630–49.

IV.44. Answer c.

C1-C2 anterior pannus with cord compression should be suspected because of the patient's history of autoimmune conditions. Surgical treatment is warranted. The anterior transoral approach is associated with considerable morbidity and must be combined with posterior fusion. Posterior decompression of C1-C2 with fixation is the preferred option because anterior pannus generally resolves over time with fixation of the joint.

Zhang S, Wadhwa R, Haydel J, Toms J, Johnson K, Guthikonda B. Spine and spinal cord trauma: diagnosis and management. Neurol Clin. 2013 Feb;31(1):183–206.

Acute Central Nervous System Infections

IV.45. Answer c.

Fever, seizures, and lymphocytic pleocytosis are common among all forms of encephalitis. Although autoimmune limbic encephalitis causes temporal lobe imaging abnormalities, the characteristic asymmetric pattern is helpful for distinguishing HSE from it and others.

Chow FC, Glaser CA, Sheriff H, Xia D, Messenger S, Whitley R, et al. Use of clinical and neuroimaging characteristics to distinguish temporal lobe herpes simplex encephalitis from its mimics. Clin Infect Dis. 2015 May 1;60(9):1377–83. Epub 2015 Jan 30.

IV.46. Answer b.
Higher dosing or a prolonged course of oral valacyclovir has not been proved to result in a better outcome.

Gnann JW Jr, Skoldenberg B, Hart J, Aurelius E, Schliamser S, Studahl M, et al; National Institute of Allergy and Infectious Diseases Collaborative Antiviral Study Group. Herpes simplex encephalitis: lack of clinical benefit of long-term valacyclovir therapy. Clin Infect Dis. 2015 Sep 1;61(5):683–91. Epub 2015 May 8. Erratum in: Clin Infect Dis. 2016 Feb 15;62(4):530.

Whitley RJ, Alford CA, Hirsch MS, Schooley RT, Luby JP, Aoki FY, et al. Vidarabine versus acyclovir therapy in herpes simplex encephalitis. N Engl J Med. 1986 Jan 16;314(3):144–9.

IV.47. Answer c.
Clinical relapse thought to be related to NMDA receptor antibodies occurs usually 1 month after the original episode of HSE.

Armangue T, Moris G, Cantarin-Extremera V, Conde CE, Rostasy K, Erro ME, et al; Spanish Prospective Multicentric Study of Autoimmunity in Herpes Simplex Encephalitis. Autoimmune post-herpes simplex encephalitis of adults and teenagers. Neurology. 2015 Nov 17;85(20):1736–43. Epub 2015 Oct 21.

IV.48. Answer a.
Patients with West Nile encephalitis frequently present with polymorphonuclear pleocytosis in the CSF.

Tyler KL, Pape J, Goody RJ, Corkill M, Kleinschmidt-DeMasters BK. CSF findings in 250 patients with serologically confirmed West Nile virus meningitis and encephalitis. Neurology. 2006 Feb 14;66(3):361–5. Epub 2005 Dec 28.

IV.49. Answer d.
Although microcephaly is associated with congenital infection and direct brain infection in utero, in adults Zika virus may be associated with parainfectious immune-mediated GBS. Encephalitis occurs rarely.

Parra B, Lizarazo J, Jimenez-Arango JA, Zea-Vera AF, Gonzalez-Manrique G, Vargas J, et al. Guillain-Barré syndrome associated with Zika virus infection in Colombia. N Engl J Med. 2016 Oct 20;375(16):1513–23. Epub 2016 Oct 5.

IV.50. Answer c.
A fully alert patient with bacterial meningitis would most likely have neck stiffness. Seizures occur in 15% of patients and are not common at presentation.

Zoons E, Weisfelt M, de Gans J, Spanjaard L, Koelman JH, Reitsma JB, et al. Seizures in adults with bacterial meningitis. Neurology. 2008 May 27;70(22 Pt 2):2109–15. Epub 2008 Feb 27.

IV.51. Answer b.
Listeria monocytogenes is the most common. Treatment requires ampicillin.

van de Beek D, Brouwer M, Hasbun R, Koedel U, Whitney CG, Wijdicks E. Community-acquired bacterial meningitis. Nat Rev Dis Primers. 2016 Nov 3;2:16074.

IV.52. Answer a.
High doses of corticosteroids and frequent administration of mannitol or hypertonic saline may counter severe cerebral edema; the use of osmotic agents is supported with a low level of evidence.

van de Beek D, Brouwer M, Hasbun R, Koedel U, Whitney CG, Wijdicks E. Community-acquired bacterial meningitis. Nat Rev Dis Primers. 2016 Nov 3;2:16074.

Wall EC, Ajdukiewicz KM, Bergman H, Heyderman RS, Garner P. Osmotic therapies added to antibiotics for acute bacterial meningitis. Cochrane Database Syst Rev. 2018 Feb 6;2:CD008806.

IV.53. Answer c.
Loss of splenic function or splenectomy results in increased susceptibility to pneumococcal infections.

Adriani KS, Brouwer MC, van der Ende A, van de Beek D. Bacterial meningitis in adults after splenectomy and hyposplenic states. Mayo Clin Proc. 2013 Jun;88(6):571–8. Epub 2013 Apr 28.

IV.54. Answer b.
Prognostication of bacterial meningitis is very difficult and should be generally avoided while awaiting the effect of aggressive antibiotic and corticosteroid treatment. Only a few factors are associated with less likelihood of a poor outcome, and low CSF leukocyte counts have been associated with worse outcomes.

Kastenbauer S, Pfister HW. Pneumococcal meningitis in adults: spectrum of complications and prognostic factors in a series of 87 cases. Brain. 2003 May;126(Pt 5):1015–25.

IV.55. Answer a.
MRI is an important diagnostic test for any brain mass and may help in the differential diagnosis of a mass. DWI MRI has a sensitivity and specificity of 96% for the diagnosis of brain abscesses.

Reddy JS, Mishra AM, Behari S, Husain M, Gupta V, Rastogi M, et al. The role of diffusion-weighted imaging in the differential diagnosis of intracranial cystic mass lesions: a report of 147 lesions. Surg Neurol. 2006 Sep;66(3):246–50.

IV.56. Answer b.
Vancomycin is indicated for coverage of gram-positive bacteria, including MRSA, cefepime for coverage of gram-negative bacteria, and metronidazole for coverage of anaerobes. Fungal coverage with voriconazole is indicated only for immunocompromised patients.

Brouwer MC, Tunkel AR, McKhann GM 2nd, van de Beek D. Brain abscess. N Engl J Med. 2014 Jul 31;371(5):447–56.

IV.57. Answer b.
Mortality among patients with a brain abscess has changed. The fatality rate is now about 10% (historically it was about 40%).

Brouwer MC, Coutinho JM, van de Beek D. Clinical characteristics and outcome of brain abscess: systematic review and meta-analysis. Neurology. 2014 Mar 4;82(9):806–13. Epub 2014 Jan 29.

IV.58. Answer c.
Severity of fever has not been shown to be a risk factor for failure of medical management of spinal epidural abscess.

Kim SD, Melikian R, Ju KL, Zurakowski D, Wood KB, Bono CM, et al. Independent predictors of failure of nonoperative management of spinal epidural abscesses. Spine J. 2014 Aug 1;14(8):1673–9. Epub 2013 Oct 30.

Patel AR, Alton TB, Bransford RJ, Lee MJ, Bellabarba CB, Chapman JR. Spinal epidural abscesses: risk factors, medical versus surgical management, a retrospective review of 128 cases. Spine J. 2014 Feb 1;14(2):326–30. Epub 2013 Nov 12.

IV.59. Answer a.
Observation may be best for a patient with a mild (nondisabling) neurologic deficit. Spinal epidural abscess may be managed medically unless any of the other answer choices is part of the clinical picture. Cord compression in the cervical or thoracic spine, which can lead to neurologic impairment, is a definite indication for aggressive intervention (at least decompressive surgery).

Cornett CA, Vincent SA, Crow J, Hewlett A. Bacterial spine infections in adults: evaluation and management. J Am Acad Orthop Surg. 2016 Jan;24(1):11–8.

Acute Neuromuscular Disorders

IV.60. Answer c.
The need for positive pressure ventilation treatment, invasive or not, defines a mysthenic crisis and differentiates it from a myasthenic exacerbation. Noninvasive ventilation is useful to avoid intubation in half of patients with neuromuscular respiratory failure due to MG.

Gilhus NE. Myasthenia gravis. N Engl J Med. 2016 Dec 29;375(26):2570–81.
Gilhus NE, Verschuuren JJ. Myasthenia gravis: subgroup classification and therapeutic strategies. Lancet Neurol. 2015 Oct;14(10):1023–36.

IV.61. Answer c.
IVIG and PLEX are equally effective for accelerating recovery in myasthenic exacerbations. The dose of acetylcholinesterase inhibitors should be carefully decreased in patients with abundant oral secretions to avoid worsening weakness and deterioration requiring mechanical ventilation. The starting dose of corticosteroids should be low, and the dose should be slowly increased because up to half of patients will experience considerable worsening of weakness within a few days of these interventions. In a patient with myasthenic crisis, this worsening may lead to intubation. Neuromuscular respiratory failure leads to hypoventilation. Thus, bilevel positive pressure ventilation is the mode of choice for respiratory support.

IV.62. Answer a.
Headache is a common adverse effect in patients receiving IVIG. In a minority of patients, headache can be caused by aseptic meningitis and venous sinus thrombosis. Hypocalcemia, removal of highly protein-bound drugs, and transfusion reactions are adverse effects of plasmapheresis.

IV.63. Answer d.
In up to 40% of patients with myasthenic crisis, extubation fails. Being elderly, being intubated for more than 10 days, and atelectasis on chest radiography are the most common risk factors.

IV.64. Answer d.
Acetylcholinesterase inhibitors increase the levels of acetylcholine in the neuromuscular junction of the iris sphincter muscle. The excess of acetylcholine leads to muscle contraction producing miosis. Alternatively, anticholinergics (eg, atropine) and drugs that boost sympathetic transmission (eg, phenylephrine, cocaine) cause mydriasis.

IV.65. Answer a.
GBS is usually easy to diagnose. In most patients, GBS starts with tingling and weakness and then rapidly progresses. Areflexia is a key finding. When less obvious presentations occur, the diagnosis becomes more difficult. Other presentations are rare variants.

Ropper AH, Wijdicks EFM, Truax BT. Guillain-Barré syndrome. Philadelphia (PA): F.A Davis; c1991. 369 p.

IV.66. Answer c.
Spinal cord disease (compressive, inflammatory, or autoimmune) is commonly not considered in patients with GBS. All the other disorders mentioned have other more characteristic manifestations (eg, fatigable weakness).

Ropper AH, Wijdicks EFM, Truax BT. Guillain-Barré syndrome. Philadelphia (PA): F.A Davis; c1991. 369 p.

IV.67. Answer d.
All variables of pulmonary function tests should be considered, not just a single value. A decrease of more than 50% is important. The 20-30-40 rule is a useful clinical guide for endotracheal intubation.

Rabinstein AA, Wijdicks EF. Warning signs of imminent respiratory failure in neurological patients. Semin Neurol. 2003 Mar;23(1):97–104.

IV.68. Answer c.
All other options are outliers.

Henderson RD, Lawn ND, Fletcher DD, McClelland RL, Wijdicks EF. The morbidity of Guillain-Barré syndrome admitted to the intensive care unit. Neurology. 2003 Jan 14;60(1):17–21.
Hughes RA, Cornblath DR. Guillain-Barré syndrome. Lancet. 2005 Nov 5;366(9497):1653–66.

IV.69. Answer a.
All other answers are severe manifestations.

Truax BT. Autonomic disturbances in the Guillain-Barré syndrome. Semin Neurol. 1984;4:462–8.

IV.70. Answer c.
The patient has signs of neuromuscular respiratory weakness with secondary hypercarbic respiratory failure resulting in admission to the ICU. Examination shows evidence of both upper and lower motor neuron involvement of the cranial, cervical, and lumbosacral segments, concerning for amyotrophic lateral sclerosis. Electromyography and nerve conduction studies would confirm the extent of lower motor neuron involvement in contiguous segments. Neuroimaging could be considered in the setting of isolated findings to exclude a structural abnormality but would not help with the diagnosis. Lumbar puncture would be reserved for cases of subacutely progressive predominantly lower motor neuron syndromes concerning for an underlying inflammatory or paraneoplastic process.

de Carvalho M, Dengler R, Eisen A, England JD, Kaji R, Kimura J, et al. Electrodiagnostic criteria for diagnosis of ALS. Clin Neurophysiol. 2008 Mar;119(3):497–503. Epub 2007 Dec 27.
Krivickas LS. Amyotrophic lateral sclerosis and other motor neuron diseases. Phys Med Rehabil Clin N Am. 2003 May;14(2):327–45.

IV.71. Answer a.
The American Academy of Neurology practice parameters recommend considering NIV when the FVC is less than 50% of predicted. Additionally, NIV can be considered in the setting of FVC or Pımax abnormalities if the patient is endorsing respiratory symptoms related to the neuromuscular respiratory weakness.

Benditt JO, Boitano L. Respiratory treatment of amyotrophic lateral sclerosis. Phys Med Rehabil Clin N Am. 2008 Aug;19(3):559–72.
Miller RG, Jackson CE, Kasarskis EJ, England JD, Forshew D, Johnston W, et al; Quality Standards Subcommittee of the American Academy of Neurology. Practice parameter update: the care of the patient with amyotrophic lateral sclerosis: drug, nutritional, and respiratory therapies (an evidence-based

review): report of the Quality Standards Subcommittee of the American Academy of Neurology. Neurology. 2009 Oct 13;73(15):1218–26. Errata in: Neurology. 2010 Mar 2;74(9):781. Neurology. 2009 Dec 15;73(24):2134.

IV.72. Answer b.

The American Academy of Neurology considers PEG tube placement safe when the FVC is more than 50%. The tube can be placed with respiratory precautions when the FVC is less than this threshold but is not recommend once the FVC is less than 30%. Artificial nutrition can be considered with prominent dysphagia symptoms, but other nutritional and respiratory parameters should be considered before proceeding because treatment may be futile.

Allen JA, Chen R, Ajroud-Driss S, Sufit RL, Heller S, Siddique T, et al. Gastrostomy tube placement by endoscopy versus radiologic methods in patients with ALS: a retrospective study of complications and outcome. Amyotroph Lateral Scler Frontotemporal Degener. 2013 May;14(4):308–14. Epub 2013 Jan 4.

Miller RG, Jackson CE, Kasarskis EJ, England JD, Forshew D, Johnston W, et al; Quality Standards Subcommittee of the American Academy of Neurology. Practice parameter update: the care of the patient with amyotrophic lateral sclerosis: drug, nutritional, and respiratory therapies (an evidence-based review): report of the Quality Standards Subcommittee of the American Academy of Neurology. Neurology. 2009 Oct 13;73(15):1218–26. Errata in: Neurology. 2010 Mar 2;74(9):781. Neurology. 2009 Dec 15;73(24):2134.

IV.73. Answer a.

Patients with loss of more than 10% of their premorbid body weight at the time of PEG tube placement typically do not regain their weight and may continue losing weight. Body mass index is considered when making a decision about timing of PEG tube placement but has not been directly associated with inability to gain weight postprocedurally. Age and sex have also not been directly associated with weight gain outcomes after PEG tube placement.

Allen JA, Chen R, Ajroud-Driss S, Sufit RL, Heller S, Siddique T, et al. Gastrostomy tube placement by endoscopy versus radiologic methods in patients with ALS: a retrospective study of complications and outcome. Amyotroph Lateral Scler Frontotemporal Degener. 2013 May;14(4):308–14. Epub 2013 Jan 4.

Russ KB, Phillips MC, Wilcox CM, Peter S. Percutaneous endoscopic gastrostomy in amyotrophic lateral sclerosis. Am J Med Sci. 2015 Aug;350(2):95–7.

IV.74. Answer d.

The patient's episodes are consistent with recurrent laryngospasm. Given the frequency of the episodes, conservative management with guided breathing is unlikely to help on its own. Low-dose benzodiazepines can be used for frequent episodes. NIV is unlikely to resolve the episodes and may create anxiety if the device is placed during an episode. Anticholinergic agents such as scopolamine can be used to manage secretions (a frequent trigger of laryngospasm), but on their own they would not prevent the laryngospasm.

Benditt JO, Boitano L. Respiratory treatment of amyotrophic lateral sclerosis. Phys Med Rehabil Clin N Am. 2008 Aug;19(3):559–72.

Hobson EV, McDermott CJ. Supportive and symptomatic management of amyotrophic lateral sclerosis. Nat Rev Neurol. 2016 Sep;12(9):526–38. Epub 2016 Aug 12.

IV.75. Answer a.

Because of its half-life of about 36 hours, CK is a better indicator of rhabdomyolysis than serum myoglobin, which has a shorter half-life. Aldolase, AST, and troponin, although present in muscle, in addition to other tissues, are less sensitive.

Giannoglou GD, Chatzizisis YS, Misirli G. The syndrome of rhabdomyolysis: pathophysiology and diagnosis. Eur J Intern Med. 2007 Mar;18(2):90–100.

Zutt R, van der Kooi AJ, Linthorst GE, Wanders RJ, de Visser M. Rhabdomyolysis: review of the literature. Neuromuscul Disord. 2014 Aug;24(8):651–9. Epub 2014 May 21.

IV.76. Answer c.

Muscle biopsy is usually not helpful in the acute phase of rhabdomyolysis because the necrotic findings are nonspecific. It is advisable to wait at least 1 month from the time of rhabdomyolysis before performing biopsy. In the acute phase, extensive muscle necrosis may obscure the underlying structural abnormalities that might indicate the cause of the rhabdomyolysis. In addition, biochemical studies to search for enzyme deficiency that may be responsible for a metabolic myopathy (eg, carnitine palmitoyltransferase 2) are more reliable outside the setting of acute rhabdomyolysis.

Nance JR, Mammen AL. Diagnostic evaluation of rhabdomyolysis. Muscle Nerve. 2015 Jun;51(6):793–810. Epub 2015 Mar 14.

Zutt R, van der Kooi AJ, Linthorst GE, Wanders RJ, de Visser M. Rhabdomyolysis: review of the literature. Neuromuscul Disord. 2014 Aug;24(8):651–9. Epub 2014 May 21.

IV.77. Answer b.

Anti-HMGCR antibodies are associated with an immune-mediated myopathy in patients with a history of statin exposure or in statin-naive patients. Contrary to statin- or other drug-induced toxic myopathies, necrotizing autoimmune myopathy requires immune therapy.

Christopher-Stine L, Basharat P. Statin-associated immune-mediated myopathy: biology and clinical implications. Curr Opin Lipidol. 2017 Apr;28(2):186–92.

Kassardjian CD, Lennon VA, Alfugham NB, Mahler M, Milone M. Clinical features and treatment outcomes of necrotizing autoimmune myopathy. JAMA Neurol. 2015 Sep;72(9):996-1003.

Mammen AL. Statin-associated autoimmune myopathy. N Engl J Med. 2016 Feb 18;374(7):664–9.

IV.78. Answer a.

CMAP duration is prolonged in CIM but not in CIP, a characteristic used to differentiate the 2 conditions and aid in prognostication. The mechanism for prolonged CMAP duration in CIM is unclear; reduced muscle membrane excitability has been suggested. The protein level in CSF is typically normal in both CIM and CIP, and demyelinating features are not found. Both of these features differentiate CIP from acute inflammatory demyelinating polyneuropathy, another potential cause of respiratory failure and limb weakness in the ICU.

Goodman BP, Harper CM, Boon AJ. Prolonged compound muscle action potential duration in critical illness myopathy. Muscle Nerve. 2009 Dec;40(6):1040–2.

Rich MM, Pinter MJ. Crucial role of sodium channel fast inactivation in muscle fibre inexcitability in a rat model of critical illness myopathy. J Physiol. 2003 Mar 1;547(Pt 2):555–66. Epub 2003 Jan 24.

IV.79. Answer c.

CIP has a worse prognosis than CIM; axonal loss, particularly when severe, is not as amenable to recovery as muscle. Patients with the typical muscle changes of CIM (thick filament myopathy and type II atrophy) typically recover well. Patients with rhabdomyolysis as a presentation of CIM also have a favorable prognosis; however, those with a diffuse necrotizing myopathy do not. Patients with CINM at an advanced age have a worse outcome than younger patients.

Bolton CF. Neuromuscular manifestations of critical illness. Muscle Nerve. 2005 Aug;32(2):140–63.

Latronico N, Bolton CF. Critical illness polyneuropathy and myopathy: a major cause of muscle weakness and paralysis. Lancet Neurol. 2011 Oct;10(10):931–41.

Miscellaneous Disorders of Acute Brain Injury

IV.80. Answer d.

Present evidence is based on expert consensus, and current guidelines recommend the initiation of anesthetic agents as third-line therapy. Propofol and midazolam are the most widely accepted agents. Therapy should be individualized according to the patient's age, comorbidities, and prognosis.

Shorvon S, Ferlisi M. The treatment of super-refractory status epilepticus: a critical review of available therapies and a clinical treatment protocol. Brain. 2011 Oct;134(Pt 10):2802–18. Epub 2011 Sep 13.

Thakur KT, Probasco JC, Hocker SE, Roehl K, Henry B, Kossoff EH, et al. Ketogenic diet for adults in super-refractory status epilepticus. Neurology. 2014 Feb 25;82(8):665–70. Epub 2014 Jan 22.

IV.81. Answer d.

Generalized SE is a neurologic and medical emergency. Systemic complications of SE include respiratory failure, cardiovascular collapse, acidosis, and renal failure. On initial presentation, assessment and treatment of physiologic variables should be undertaken to ensure that safe, prompt neurologic management can be instituted.

Alldredge BK, Gelb AM, Isaacs SM, Corry MD, Allen F, Ulrich S, et al. A comparison of lorazepam, diazepam, and placebo for the treatment of out-of-hospital status epilepticus. N Engl J Med. 2001 Aug 30;345(9):631–7. Erratum in: N Engl J Med 2001 Dec 20;345(25):1860.

Treiman DM, Meyers PD, Walton NY, Collins JF, Colling C, Rowan AJ, et al; Veterans Affairs Status Epilepticus Cooperative Study Group. A comparison of four treatments for generalized convulsive status epilepticus. N Engl J Med. 1998 Sep 17;339(12):792–8.

IV.82. Answer d.

Refractory SE and super-refractory SE are defined clinically by their resistance to pharmacologic interventions. Specifically, refractory SE is classified as failure of 2 antiseizure medications.

Brophy GM, Bell R, Claassen J, Alldredge B, Bleck TP, Glauser T, et al; Neurocritical Care Society Status Epilepticus Guideline Writing Committee. Guidelines for the evaluation and management of status epilepticus. Neurocrit Care. 2012 Aug;17(1):3–23.

Trinka E, Cock H, Hesdorffer D, Rossetti AO, Scheffer IE, Shinnar S, et al. A definition and classification of status epilepticu: report of the ILAE Task Force on Classification of Status Epilepticus. Epilepsia. 2015 Oct;56(10):1515–23. Epub 2015 Sep 4.

IV.83. Answer c.

SE has a unique quality of self-perpetuation. In the initial minutes after seizure onset, endocytotic internalization of the inhibitory GABA type A receptors occurs in concert with externalization of the excitatory AMPA and NMDA receptors, leading to an enhanced glutamatergic response.

Chen JW, Naylor DE, Wasterlain CG. Advances in the pathophysiology of status epilepticus. Acta Neurol Scand Suppl. 2007;186:7–15.

Chen JW, Wasterlain CG. Status epilepticus: pathophysiology and management in adults. Lancet Neurol. 2006 Mar;5(3):246–56.

IV.84. Answer c.

Second-line therapy, which is provided after the administration of benzodiazepines, is necessary for all patients presenting in SE. Although conflicting data exist and much of the protocol is driven by expert opinion, urgent second-line therapy should include the use of IV fosphenytoin (or phenytoin) or IV valproate sodium. With second-line intervention, the goals are to terminate an existing seizure focus and to prevent further seizure activity.

Agarwal P, Kumar N, Chandra R, Gupta G, Antony AR, Garg N. Randomized study of intravenous valproate and phenytoin in status epilepticus. Seizure. 2007 Sep;16(6):527–32. Epub 2007 Jul 9.

Treiman DM, Meyers PD, Walton NY, Collins JF, Colling C, Rowan AJ, et al; Veterans Affairs Status Epilepticus Cooperative Study Group. A comparison of four treatments for generalized convulsive status epilepticus. N Engl J Med. 1998 Sep 17;339(12):792–8.

IV.85. Answer d.

Characteristic clinical features of PRES are acute encephalopathy, headache, seizures, and visual disturbances. Asterixis is more specific for uremic or hepatic encephalopathy.

Bartynski WS. Posterior reversible encephalopathy syndrome, part 1: fundamental imaging and clinical features. AJNR Am J Neuroradiol. 2008 Jun;29(6):1036–42. Epub 2008 Mar 20.

Fugate JE, Rabinstein AA. Posterior reversible encephalopathy syndrome: clinical and radiological manifestations, pathophysiology, and outstanding questions. Lancet Neurol. 2015 Sep;14(9):914–25. Epub 2015 Jul 13. Erratum in: Lancet Neurol. 2015 Sep;14(9):874.

IV.86. Answer d.

Ring enhancement with central necrosis is typically seen in patients with brain abscess or an aggressive tumor. Vasogenic edema, cytotoxic edema or infarction, and cerebral hemorrhage can all be seen in patients with PRES.

Kastrup O, Schlamann M, Moenninghoff C, Forsting M, Goericke S. Posterior reversible encephalopathy syndrome: the spectrum of MR imaging patterns. Clin Neuroradiol. 2015 Jun;25(2): 161–71. Epub 2014 Feb 20.

Lamy C, Oppenheim C, Meder JF, Mas JL. Neuroimaging in posterior reversible encephalopathy syndrome. J Neuroimaging. 2004 Apr;14(2):89–96.

IV.87. Answer a.

Hypertension is the most common precipitating factor (reported to occur in up to 80%-90% of patients). The second most common is immunosuppression (usually after solid organ transplant).

Bartynski WS. Posterior reversible encephalopathy syndrome, part 1: fundamental imaging and clinical features. AJNR Am J Neuroradiol. 2008 Jun;29(6):1036–42. Epub 2008 Mar 20.

Fugate JE, Rabinstein AA. Posterior reversible encephalopathy syndrome: clinical and radiological manifestations, pathophysiology, and outstanding questions. Lancet Neurol. 2015 Sep;14(9):914–25. Epub 2015 Jul 13. Erratum in: Lancet Neurol. 2015 Sep;14(9):874.

IV.88. Answer c.

Seizures (both focal and generalized tonic-clonic) have been reported to occur in 60% to 80% of patients. Isolated brainstem or cerebellar vasogenic edema is uncommon in patients with PRES and should prompt a search for another diagnosis. PRES is not always reversible and has been associated with morbidity and mortality in 10% to 15% of patients. CT of the brain is not sensitive for detecting vasogenic edema and is positive for edema in less than 50% of patients. MRI of the brain is more sensitive for detection of vasogenic edema and is helpful in evaluation of the differential diagnosis.

Fugate JE, Rabinstein AA. Posterior reversible encephalopathy syndrome: clinical and radiological manifestations, pathophysiology, and outstanding questions. Lancet Neurol. 2015 Sep;14(9):914–25. Epub 2015 Jul 13. Erratum in: Lancet Neurol. 2015 Sep;14(9):874.

Li Y, Gor D, Walicki D, Jenny D, Jones D, Barbour P, et al. Spectrum and potential pathogenesis of reversible posterior leukoencephalopathy syndrome. J Stroke Cerebrovasc Dis. 2012 Nov;21(8):873–82. Epub 2011 Jun 23.

IV.89. Answer c.

Magnesium sulfate infusion is the recommended first-line therapy for seizure control in patients with eclampsia. Lamotrigine is not available IV and takes a long time to reach therapeutic blood levels because the medication is usually titrated starting from a small dose because of the risk of Stevens-Johnson syndrome if it is started at a high dose. Carbamazepine and valproic acid are not recommended for pregnant patients because of the risk of fetal toxicity and teratogenicity.

Brewer J, Owens MY, Wallace K, Reeves AA, Morris R, Khan M, et al. Posterior reversible encephalopathy syndrome in 46 of 47 patients with eclampsia. Am J Obstet Gynecol. 2013 Jun;208(6):468.e1–6. Epub 2013 Feb 7.

Cozzolino M, Bianchi C, Mariani G, Marchi L, Fambrini M, Mecacci F. Therapy and differential diagnosis of posterior reversible encephalopathy syndrome (PRES) during pregnancy and postpartum. Arch Gynecol Obstet. 2015 Dec;292(6):1217–23. Epub 2015 Jun 30.

IV.90. Answer c.

In a case review, the most common causes of postvaccination CNS IDD were influenza, human papillomavirus, and hepatitis vaccines. No cases have been reported of pneumococcal vaccination leading to ADEM, although pneumococcal meningitis itself can lead to ADEM.

Huhn K, Lee DH, Linker RA, Kloska S, Huttner HB. Pneumococcal-meningitis associated acute disseminated encephalomyelitis (ADEM): case report of effective early immunotherapy. Springerplus. 2014 Aug 8;3:415.

IV.91. Answer a.

Class I evidence supports the use of plasmapheresis for corticosteroid-refractory acute demyelinating disease, such as this patient's possible NMOSD. Cyclophosphamide and IVIG may be considered as options for severely refractory disease, but these treatments lack class I evidence. No evidence supports the use of interferons in acute illness, and they may worsen NMOSD.

Weinshenker BG, O'Brien PC, Petterson TM, Noseworthy JH, Lucchinetti CF, Dodick DW, et al. A randomized trial of plasma exchange in acute central nervous system inflammatory demyelinating disease. Ann Neurol. 1999 Dec;46(6):878–86.

IV.92. Answer a.

Medullary lesions in the nucleus tractus solitarius can cause neurogenic pulmonary edema even in the absence of other symptoms. PRES most commonly occurs as a complication of NMOSD. Brainstem herniation and elevated ICP are more likely in lesions with a mass effect such as tumefactive MS.

Crawley F, Saddeh I, Barker S, Katifi H. Acute pulmonary oedema: presenting symptom of multiple sclerosis. Mult Scler. 2001 Feb;7(1):71–2.

Gentiloni N, Schiavino D, Della Corte F, Ricci E, Colosimo C. Neurogenic pulmonary edema: a presenting symptom in multiple sclerosis. Ital J Neurol Sci. 1992 Jun;13(5):435–8.

IV.93. Answer c.

Hypothermia can occur in patients with advanced MS and can be related to hypothalamic lesions. Patients respond well to rewarming. A medullary lesion could lead to neurogenic pulmonary edema. Elevated ICP is typically present in patients with tumefactive lesions or ADEM rather than progressive MS. PRES occurs in patients with NMOSD.

Weiss N, Hasboun D, Demeret S, Fontaine B, Bolgert F, Lyon-Caen O, et al. Paroxysmal hypothermia as a clinical feature of multiple sclerosis. Neurology. 2009 Jan 13;72(2):193–5.

IV.94. Answer b.

The imaging findings are suggestive of tumefactive MS (open ring enhancement), and radiotherapy may worsen the underlying demyelinating disease. High doses of corticosteroids may help to improve edema associated with a tumor and to treat demyelinating disease; they are not contraindicated for this patient. Mannitol, hyperventilation, and hemicraniectomy are all used to treat elevated ICP associated with tumefactive demyelinating lesions and to treat elevated ICP from other causes.

Miller RC, Lachance DH, Lucchinetti CF, Keegan BM, Gavrilova RH, Brown PD, et al. Multiple sclerosis, brain radiotherapy, and risk of neurotoxicity: the Mayo Clinic experience. Int J Radiat Oncol Biol Phys. 2006 Nov 15;66(4):1178–86. Epub 2006 Sep 11.

IV.95. Answer d.

In patients with sCJD, MRI of the brain typically shows changes involving the gray matter (cortex and basal ganglia).

Geschwind MD. Rapidly progressive dementia. Continuum (Minneap Minn). 2016 Apr;22(2 Dementia):510–37.

Imran M, Mahmood S. An overview of human prion diseases. Virol J. 2011 Dec 24;8:559.

IV.96. Answer b

National Prion Disease Pathology Surveillance Center resources are helpful for confirming and registering cases of CJD and for providing the specific genotype. The resources also include informational handouts for family members. Quinine is not an effective therapy for CJD. Aggressive management of PSWC changes is not advised because PSWC changes are merely signals of progressive CJD brain disease. Hospice care may ultimately be considered after a diagnosis of CJD is confirmed.

Case Western Reserve University. Prion center: National Prion Disease Pathology Surveillance Center [Internet]. Cleveland (OH): Case Western Reserve University [cited 2018 Oct 4].

Neuro-oncology

IV.97. Answer a.

A patient whose ICP has increased to the point of producing acute worsening of headache may rapidly become comatose. Such patients should be admitted, be given high-dose corticosteroids, and undergo operation on the next immediately available schedule. Diagnosis is needed before the next course of action.

Dietrich J, Rao K, Pastorino S, Kesari S. Corticosteroids in brain cancer patients: benefits and pitfalls. Expert Rev Clin Pharmacol. 2011 Mar;4(2):233–42.

IV.98. Answer d.

Rapid CSF drainage in a patient with a posterior fossa tumor risks upward herniation. After the procedure, CSF drainage should be gradual, and the drainage chamber should be leveled to at least 20 cm H_2O. Tumor resection proceeds immediately.

Cuneo RA, Caronna JJ, Pitts L, Townsend J, Winestock DP. Upward transtentorial herniation: seven cases and a literature review. Arch Neurol. 1979 Oct;36(10):618–23.

IV.99. Answer b.

Carbon dioxide is a potent vasodilator of the cerebral arterioles and thus directly affects autoregulation. Hyperventilation and resultant decrease in Pco_2 can effectively reduce ICP by reducing cerebral blood flow. However, if it is prolonged, it can lead to cerebral ischemia. To be effective and safe, hyperventilation should be used for short periods with a Pco_2 goal of 32 to 34 mm Hg.

Soustiel JF, Mahamid E, Chistyakov A, Shik V, Benenson R, Zaaroor M. Comparison of moderate hyperventilation and mannitol for control of intracranial pressure control in patients with severe traumatic brain injury: a study of cerebral blood flow and metabolism. Acta Neurochir (Wien). 2006 Aug;148(8):845–51. Epub 2006 Jun 12.

IV.100. Answer d.

Some studies have shown that NSAIDs impair bony fusion rates after spine surgery. Some spine neurosurgeons recommend using methyl methacrylate instead of bone for grafting in cases of metastatic spine disease (if life expectancy is very short), and in such patients NSAID use may be considered.

Lumawig JM, Yamazaki A, Watanabe K. Dose-dependent inhibition of diclofenac sodium on posterior lumbar interbody fusion rates. Spine J. 2009 May;9(5):343–9. Epub 2008 Sep 14.

IV.101. Answer a.

Lumbar puncture could be dangerous if the cause of the hydrocephalus has not been identified. Craniospinal radiation may be appropriate, but it would be given after advanced neuroimaging. Few data suggest that immediate use of intrathecal chemotherapy would improve this patient's neurologic status.

Clarke JL. Leptomeningeal metastasis from systemic cancer. Continuum (Minneap Minn). 2012 Apr;18(2):328–42.

Clarke JL, Perez HR, Jacks LM, Panageas KS, Deangelis LM. Leptomeningeal metastases in the MRI era. Neurology. 2010 May 4;74(18):1449–54.

IV.102. Answer b.

Given the significance of the clinical and radiographic findings, this patient would benefit from treatment, and watchful waiting is not an option. Intrathecal trastuzamab is an option only if the patient had HER2-positive disease. A fourth lumbar puncture with flow cytometry is most useful for the diagnosis of lymphoma. There is no strong evidence that clinically useful information is identified after the third lumbar puncture.

Brower JV, Saha S, Rosenberg SA, Hullett CR, Ian Robins H. Management of leptomeningeal metastases: prognostic factors and associated outcomes. J Clin Neurosci. 2016 May;27:130–7. Epub 2016 Jan 8.

Chang EL, Maor MH. Standard and novel radiotherapeutic approaches to neoplastic meningitis. Curr Oncol Rep. 2003 Jan;5(1):24–8.

IV.103. Answer d.

Preceding infections (from mycoplasma, varicella-zoster virus, and HSV) have been suspected to have a role in cases of non-paraneoplastic, presumed autoimmune anti-NMDA receptor encephalitis. In a case series of 44 patients with HSV encephalitis, 33% had NMDA receptor antibodies. Antibody-positive sera resulted in downregulation of synaptic marker proteins in hippocampal neurons, a suggestion of a pathogenic effect. Subsequent reports have provided further support for a link between relapsing symptoms after post-HSV encephalitis and antibodies directed against synaptic proteins, mainly the NMDA receptor. In all reported patients, relapsing symptoms have presented 2 to 6 weeks after the initial viral infection. The role of HSV encephalitis as a trigger for development of NMDA receptor antibodies was shown in a series of patients with antibody-negative serum and CSF at the time of HSV encephalitis infection who had seroconversion to positive NMDA receptor antibodies a few weeks later in the setting of relapsing symptoms. In the case of NMDA receptor antibodies, CSF is frequently more informative (more sensitive and specific) than serum.

Armangue T, Leypoldt F, Malaga I, Raspall-Chaure M, Marti I, Nichter C, et al. Herpes simplex virus encephalitis is a trigger of brain autoimmunity. Ann Neurol. 2014 Feb;75(2):317–23. Epub 2014 Feb 25.

IV.104. Answer c.

The neurologic manifestations in patients with anti-Ma2 (anti-Ta)–associated encephalitis are generally restricted to the limbic areas, diencephalon, and brainstem. MRI abnormalities are frequent in these brain regions, and inflammatory changes are typically present in the CSF. Testicular germ cell tumors are the most common associated neoplasm. Patients typically require aggressive therapy with IV corticosteroid and monthly IV or daily oral cyclophosphamide. The other antibodies are associated with different malignancies and neurologic phenotypes.

Voltz R, Gultekin SH, Rosenfeld MR, Gerstner E, Eichen J, Posner JB, et al. A serologic marker of paraneoplastic limbic and brain-stem encephalitis in patients with testicular cancer. N Engl J Med. 1999 Jun 10;340(23):1788–95.

IV.105. Answer b.

The most common neurologic condition requiring emergency radiation therapy is spinal cord compression. Multidisciplinary evaluation with neurosurgery is required. When surgical resection is feasible, this approach is generally preferred.

Mitera G, Swaminath A, Wong S, Goh P, Robson S, Sinclair E, et al. Radiotherapy for oncologic emergencies on weekends: examining reasons for treatment and patterns of practice at a Canadian cancer centre. Curr Oncol. 2009 Aug;16(4):55–60.

IV.106. Answer d.

The most common indication for radiation therapy is brain metastases. Other tumors require neurosurgical resection.

Khuntia D. Contemporary review of the management of brain metastasis with radiation. Adv Neurosci. 2015;2015:Article ID 372856. 13 p.

Li J, Brown PD. The diminishing role of whole-brain radiation therapy in the treatment of brain metastases. JAMA Oncol. 2017 Aug 1;3(8):1023-4.

Mahajan A, Ahmed S, McAleer MF, Weinberg JS, Li J, Brown P, et al. Post-operative stereotactic radiosurgery versus observation for completely resected brain metastases: a single-centre, randomised, controlled, phase 3 trial. Lancet Oncol. 2017 Aug;18(8):1040–8. Epub 2017 Jul 4.

IV.107. Answer a.

Corticosteroids are the most common initial management for symptoms. Other approaches used for managing radiotherapy-related CNS necrosis include hyperbaric oxygen and bevacizumab.

Patel U, Patel A, Cobb C, Benkers T, Vermeulen S. The management of brain necrosis as a result of SRS treatment for intracranial tumors. Transl Cancer Res. 2014 Aug;3(4):373–82.

Postoperative Neurosurgery

IV.108. Answer d.

The combination of anterior and posterior approaches presents risks from both procedures. The anterior procedure, especially in the cervical region, involves anterior neck structures and increases the risk of injury to the vagus nerve, swallowing dysfunction, and anterior airway swelling and compromise.

Farrokhi MR, Ghaffarpasand F, Khani M, Gholami M. An evidence-based stepwise surgical approach to cervical spondylotic myelopathy: a narrative review of the current literature. World Neurosurg. 2016 Oct;94:97–110. Epub 2016 Jul 5.

Memtsoudis SG, Vougioukas VI, Ma Y, Gaber-Baylis LK, Girardi FP. Perioperative morbidity and mortality after anterior, posterior, and anterior/posterior spine fusion surgery. Spine (Phila Pa 1976). 2011 Oct 15;36(22):1867–77.

IV.109. Answer a.

The patient has an airway compromise, which is one reason that a patient may require care in the ICU (ie, for difficult airway considerations). Anxiety, although common after any kind of operation, should be a diagnosis of exclusion after anterior cervical surgery. Evidence of esophageal perforation may appear more slowly as neck pain, dysphagia, odynophagia, and sepsis (if infection ensues).

Schoenfeld AJ, Ochoa LM, Bader JO, Belmont PJ Jr. Risk factors for immediate postoperative complications and mortality following spine surgery: a study of 3475 patients from the National Surgical Quality Improvement Program. J Bone Joint Surg Am. 2011 Sep 7;93(17):1577–82.

Smith JS, Saulle D, Chen CJ, Lenke LG, Polly DW Jr, Kasliwal MK, et al. Rates and causes of mortality associated with spine surgery based on 108,419 procedures: a review of the Scoliosis Research Society Morbidity and Mortality Database. Spine (Phila Pa 1976). 2012 Nov 1;37(23):1975–82.

IV.110. Answer b.

The artery of Adamkiewicz is considered a vulnerable vascular territory in the thoracic region.

Snell RS. Clinical neuroanatomy. 7th ed. Philadelphia (PA): Wolters Kluwer Health/Lippincott Williams & Wilkins; c2010. 542 p.

IV.111. Answer d.

A blood glucose level of 175 mg/dL, which is in the goal range of 140 to 180 mg/dL, does not increase the risk of morbidity and death after spinal surgery. The other answer choices do increase the risk.

Schoenfeld AJ, Ochoa LM, Bader JO, Belmont PJ Jr. Risk factors for immediate postoperative complications and mortality following spine surgery: a study of 3475 patients from the National Surgical Quality Improvement Program. J Bone Joint Surg Am. 2011 Sep 7;93(17):1577–82.

IV.112. Answer d.

Anticoagulation is the preferred treatment of acute deep vein thrombosis and pulmonary embolism, but after neuraxial spinal surgery, epidural or intra-axial hemorrhage is a risk. Therefore, the surgeon should discuss the safety of full anticoagulation with the patient. In some situations, an inferior vena cava filter can prevent fatal saddle pulmonary embolism if used in conjunction with short-term and long-term anticoagulation (eg, heparinoids).

Barnes B, Alexander JT, Branch CL Jr. Postoperative Level 1 anticoagulation therapy and spinal surgery: practical guidelines for management. Neurosurg Focus. 2004 Oct 15;17(4):E5.

IV.113. Answer c.

Postoperative pain can induce acute on chronic hypertension, which should be treated with an antihypertensive. Use of a muscle relaxant should be avoided because it may interfere with the neurologic examination. An analgesic is not preferred unless the patient's elevated BP is due to severe pain, which is not the cause in this patient. An antiepileptic drug is not preferred because it will not primarily treat the underlying hypertension.

Mayer SA, Chong JY. Critical care management of increased intracranial pressure. J Intensive Care Med. 2002 Mar 1;17(2):55–67.

IV.114. Answer b.

Hyperventilation decreases the level of carbon dioxide and does not increase the $Paco_2$. The other 3 interventions decrease ICP.

Ragland J, Lee K. Critical care management and monitoring of intracranial pressure. J Neurocrit Care. 2016;9(2):105–12.

IV.115. Answer c.

SIADH is best differentiated from cerebral salt wasting on the basis of intravascular volume status. In SIADH, the concentration of urine is increased (increased urine osmolality), whereas cerebral salt wasting typically causes high output of urine that is less concentrated according to urine specific gravity and osmolality. Numerous factors such as IV fluid rates and the patient's oral intake must be considered in the context of any urine laboratory and output values.

Velly L, Simeone P, Bruder N. Postoperative care of neurosurgical patients. Curr Anesthesiol Rep. 2016 Sep;6(3):257–66.

IV.116. Answer a.

Hemorrhage into the tumor is a concern because it occurs in up to 5% of patients and may necessitate surgical intervention. Softening of the tumor is desirable before resection, so the operation is often delayed for 48 to 96 hours after embolization. Fever and pain are not common features after meningioma embolization.

Eskey CJ, Meyers PM, Nguyen TN, Ansari SA, Jayaraman M, McDougall CG, et al; American Heart Association Council on Cardiovascular Radiology and Intervention and Stroke Council. Indications for the performance of intracranial endovascular neurointerventional procedures: a scientific statement from the American Heart Association. Circulation. 2018 May 22;137(21):e661–89. Epub 2018 Apr 19.

IV.117. Answer a.

Stroke occurs in approximately 7% of patients, whereas aneurysm rupture occurs in 2% of patients. Ventriculostomies are not placed prophylactically in patients with unruptured aneurysms, so choice *b* is incorrect. If intraoperative stroke or large-vessel occlusion occurs, abciximab (intra-arterial bolus with no drip) is preferred, and heparin should be stopped (because of the synergistic effect of heparin and the increased risk of bleeding), so choices *c* and *d* are incorrect.

Eskey CJ, Meyers PM, Nguyen TN, Ansari SA, Jayaraman M, McDougall CG, et al; American Heart Association Council on Cardiovascular Radiology and Intervention and Stroke Council. Indications for the performance of intracranial endovascular neurointerventional procedures: a scientific statement from the American Heart Association. Circulation. 2018 May 22;137(21):e661–89. Epub 2018 Apr 19.

IV.118. Answer d.

Clinical examination findings are often nonfocal and subtle (eg, confusion, agitation, abulia) and are therefore not very specific. Many symptoms can be caused by worsening hydrocephalus (commonly) or nonconvulsive status epilepticus (not commonly).

Chong BW. Current issues in endovascular surgical neuroradiology. Semin Neurol. 2007 Sep;27(4):385–92.

IV.119. Answer b.

Endovascular therapy is advised for a large-vessel occlusion even if the patient receives IV rtPA. Furthermore, there is no increased risk of intracranial hemorrhage compared with use of IV rtPA. Endovascular therapy should begin within 6 hours after stroke onset, but many centers have extended the therapeutic window according to imaging features (perfusion on CT or MRI). Use of aspirin or clopidogrel is not considered an absolute contraindication to endovascular therapy.

Eskey CJ, Meyers PM, Nguyen TN, Ansari SA, Jayaraman M, McDougall CG, et al; American Heart Association Council on Cardiovascular Radiology and Intervention and Stroke Council. Indications for the performance of intracranial endovascular neurointerventional procedures: a scientific statement from the American Heart Association. Circulation. 2018 May 22;137(21):e661–89. Epub 2018 Apr 19.

IV.120. Answer a.

After treatment of BAVMs, hemorrhage occurs in up to 14% of patients, but hemorrhage is uncommon after embolization of DAVFs.

Zacharia BE, Vaughan KA, Jacoby A, Hickman ZL, Bodmer D, Connolly ES Jr. Management of ruptured brain arteriovenous malformations. Curr Atheroscler Rep. 2012 Aug;14(4):335–42.

Section

V

Imaging in Critical Illness

109 Radiography and Computed Tomography of the Chest

BARBARA L. MCCOMB, MD

Goals

- Review an approach to the interpretation of chest radiographs.
- Discuss the imaging assessment of pulmonary edema, pneumonia, aspiration, atelectasis, and pleural disease in the intensive care unit.
- Discuss the imaging evaluation of pneumothorax, pneumomediastinum, and pneumopericardium.
- Review common radiographic findings in thoracic injuries.
- Discuss the role of chest radiography in the assessment of common support devices.

Introduction

A portable chest radiograph frequently complements the clinical evaluation of a patient in the intensive care unit (ICU). Standard posteroanterior (PA) chest radiographs are obtained from a distance of 72 inches with the patient erect and facing the detector. The x-ray tube is behind the patient, and the beam passes from posterior to anterior. In the ICU, the PA radiograph is replaced by the portable anteroposterior (AP) radiograph, which is obtained from a 40-inch distance with the tube in front of the patient and the patient supine or semierect. Because tissues attenuate x-rays to various degrees, different densities are shown on radiographs. Air-containing lungs appear relatively lucent because of low attenuation, whereas the mediastinum and soft tissues have intermediate levels of attenuation and are represented by various shades of gray and white. Bones highly attenuate x-rays and appear opaque, and metals are extremely opaque.

Guidelines by the American College of Radiology recommend chest radiography for a change in the clinical condition of a patient and after the placement of tubes, catheters, and other life-saving support devices. Routine daily radiographs are not recommended. Although the relative radiation level associated with portable chest radiography in an adult is deemed low (<0.1 mSv), repeated imaging can substantially increase radiation dose to a patient. A systematic approach to interpretation of a chest radiograph (Table 109.1), and comparison with prior examinations, can help facilitate early detection of pathologic features. Correlation between radiographic and clinical findings is also very important, as is good communication between the clinical team and radiology personnel; both steps will optimize image quality and interpretation.

Interpretation of an ICU chest radiograph can be challenging despite the benefit of different tissue densities. Limitations of the supine position include low lung volumes, redistribution of blood flow, widening of the superior mediastinum and cardiac silhouette, limited differentiation of viscera from overlying soft tissue, and reduced bony detail. Devices can also obscure portions of the thorax, and layering pleural effusion and rising pleural air can be difficult to identify. Nevertheless, the ICU chest radiograph can provide a wealth of valuable information.

Computed tomography (CT) requires greater radiation exposure than chest radiography and sometimes necessitates an intravenous contrast agent. However, if it is feasible to transfer a patient from the ICU to the CT suite, CT can be particularly useful in certain situations, such as to evaluate complex or otherwise puzzling radiographic presentations. Ultrasonography has also been increasingly used in the ICU to evaluate the thorax. It can be quickly performed at the bedside and does not involve radiation. Common uses include assessment of pleural effusion, pneumothorax, and pericardial effusion and intervention guidance.

Table 109.1 • Approach to Interpretation of a Chest Radiograph in the ICU[a]

Item or Area Reviewed	Characteristics Reviewed
1. **A**ssessment of quality	Patient information (name, ID); right vs left accuracy; PA or AP, position (supine, semierect, or erect), inspiration (5-6 anterior ribs, 10-11 posterior ribs), ventilator, exposure, rotation
2. **D**evices	Track from proximal to distal
3. **C**ardiac silhouette	Size, cardiothoracic ratio, effect of positioning and level of inspiration
4. Mediastinum (**G**reat vessels)	Contours, width, density, shift; follow tracheobronchial tree
5. **H**ila	Contours, density, size, and position
6. Lungs (**F**ields and fissures)	Lung volumes, density, symmetry, pulmonary vessels including redistribution and visibility through diaphragms and cardiac silhouette, parenchymal opacities and type, bronchial cuffing, fissural displacement and thickening
7. Pleura (**E**ffusion)	Effusions (correlate with supine or erect patient position), thickening, nodules, air collections
8. **B**ones, soft tissues, artifacts	Chest wall, neck, diaphragm, upper abdomen (eg, fractures, degenerative changes, lytic or sclerotic lesions, soft tissue edema or mass, breast tissue, skin lesions, diaphragm contours, abdominal mass or calcifications, clothing artifact)

Abbreviations: AP, anteroposterior; ICU, intensive care unit; ID, identification; PA, posteroanterior.

[a] The alphabetic mnemonic ABCDEFGH may be helpful for recalling the list; however, order used above is suggested for review of radiographs.

This chapter reviews common indications for thoracic imaging in the ICU, including the evaluation of pulmonary edema, pneumonia, aspiration, atelectasis, pleural disease, intrathoracic air, and device placement and complications. Thoracic imaging for trauma detection and characterization is also described.

Pulmonary Edema

The conventional chest radiograph has endured as a frontline imaging tool to assess pulmonary edema. Well-documented appearances correlate with hydrostatic interstitial and air space edema, for which heart failure is the most common cause. Interstitial edema has been reported at a transmural arterial pressure from 15 to 25 mm Hg. Radiographic findings include ill-defined perihilar vessels, peribronchial cuffing, interlobular septal (Kerley) lines, and pleural effusion. Air space filling at pressures more than 25 mm Hg may present as ill-marginated opacities or coalescent consolidation concentrated in dependent regions. The dependent location of parenchymal and pleural disease may be best appreciated with the patient in the erect position. Parenchymal opacification becomes increasingly homogeneous and bilateral as air space edema worsens, and air-filled bronchi (air bronchograms) may be seen. The classic bat-wing pattern (Figure 109.1) of edema on a chest radiograph is uncommon and often associated with rapid development, as in massive myocardial infarction or papillary muscle rupture. Pulmonary edema can rarely present as unilateral or lobar opacification. Radiographic findings of hydrostatic edema do not necessarily correlate temporally with capillary wedge pressures or patient symptoms. Wedge pressures may increase before radiographic findings present, and radiographic findings may lag behind wedge pressure improvement. Interstitial edema may present radiographically well before symptoms develop.

Differentiation of hydrostatic edema from permeability edema with diffuse alveolar damage can be important for a patient in the ICU (Table 109.2). Acute respiratory

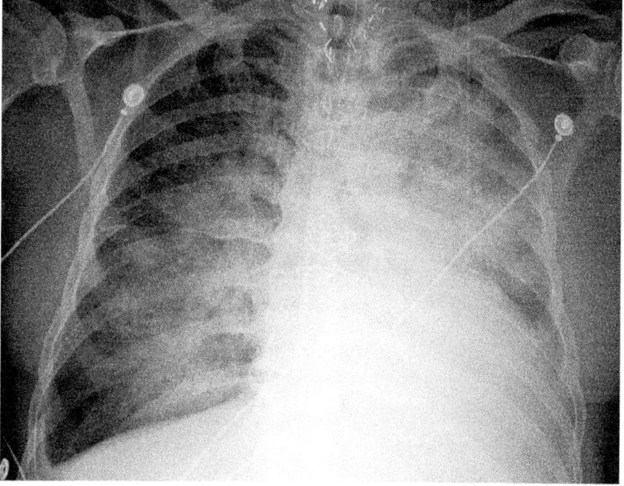

Figure 109.1. Chest Radiograph of Pulmonary Air Space Edema (Bat-Wing Pattern) With Air Bronchograms. On right, note fissural thickening and Kerley lines of interstitial edema in addition to small meniscus from effusion at the lateral costophrenic sulcus. On left, note retrocardiac opacification with loss of the hemidiaphragm margin (silhouette sign) due to edema, atelectasis, and effusion in this case. Endotracheal tube is also seen.

Table 109.2 • Radiographic Features of Cardiogenic Edema and Acute Respiratory Distress Syndrome

Radiographic Feature	Cardiogenic Edema	Acute Respiratory Distress Syndrome
Cardiac silhouette size	Often enlarged	Usually not enlarged
Vascular pedicle[a]	Widened	Not widened
Blood flow distribution	Inverted	Balanced
Septal lines	Common	Uncommon
Peribronchial thickening	Common	Uncommon
Air bronchograms	Uncommon	Common
Distribution	Symmetric, central or dependent	Multifocal, peripheral, may spare costophrenic angles

[a] Wang H, Shi R, Mahler S, Gaspard J, Gorchynski J, D'Etienne J, et al. Vascular pedicle width on chest radiograph as a measure of volume overload: meta-analysis. West J Emerg Med. 2011 Nov;12(4):426-32.

Modified from Milne ENC. A physiological approach to reading critical care unit films. J Thorac Imag. 1986;1(3):60-90; used with permission.

distress syndrome (ARDS) is a common cause of permeability edema with diffuse alveolar damage. Interstitial disease can reflect its early exudative stage, but it may not necessarily be captured radiographically because it is rapidly followed by diffuse or multifocal air space opacification. ARDS can also coexist with hydrostatic edema. ARDS is favored over hydrostatic edema when Kerley lines, peribronchial thickening, mediastinal widening, and cardiac silhouette enlargement are absent. The air space pattern in the later exudative stage of ARDS may simulate cardiogenic edema, pulmonary hemorrhage, diffuse aspiration, and various other causes of air space disease. Both ARDS and hydrostatic edema can have a perihilar distribution early on and a diffuse distribution later, and both may show a gravitational gradient. Pleural effusions are uncommon on chest radiographs in ARDS, although they may be present on CT. Cardiogenic edema typically has more fluctuation in appearance than ARDS on short-interval radiographs. Recurrent exudative episodes of ARDS can complicate its appearance. ARDS may appear more heterogeneous in the proliferative phase, and distortion and cystic lesions may develop in the fibrotic phase.

Permeability edema without diffuse alveolar damage presents with various degrees of peribronchial cuffing, ill-defined vacularity, and multifocal parenchymal opacification. For example, the radiographic appearance of high-altitude edema can differ considerably depending on the degree of hypoxia. When radiographic findings are not associated with other complications (eg, aspiration or renal insufficiency), they may regress over a short interval.

Mixed hydrostatic and permeability edema often presents with air space opacities that range from heterogeneous to homogeneous, and it may be difficult to distinguish from other lung abnormalities (eg, fluid overload, aspiration, hemorrhage, and pneumonia). The diagnosis is often one of exclusion, although certain radiographic patterns have a greater association with certain causes. For example, neurogenic edema may predominate in the upper zones, whereas edema from air embolism is frequently in lower zones. Reexpansion edema predominates in previously collapsed areas. Temporal differences can sometimes aid in distinguishing causes. Neurogenic edema may present within minutes to hours of a severe central nervous system event; alternatively, its onset may be delayed hours to days. Edema after lung transplant may present within 48 hours, continue to increase to day 5, and then improve over 2 weeks. Reexpansion edema may worsen radiographically over 24 to 48 hours and then resolve over 5 to 7 days.

Pneumonia, Aspiration, and Atelectasis

Chest radiographs can help confirm or exclude parenchymal disease in the setting of suspected pneumonia, assess the distribution and extent of involvement, gauge response to antimicrobial therapy, and detect other disease. They are helpful in the diagnosis of pleural effusions and other complications (eg, adenopathy, cavitation, pneumothorax, empyema, bronchopleural fistula, chest wall invasion). Early cavitation and abscess formation can sometimes be subtle, particularly on a supine portable radiograph, although an erect or decubitus radiograph may show an air-fluid level not seen on a supine image. Care must also be taken not to overdiagnose cavities, because they can be simulated by areas of aerated lung amid multifocal parenchymal or pleural disease. When clinically indicated and feasible to perform, CT can be a useful adjunct to conventional radiography. In particular, it can improve the assessment of complex radiographic presentations and help select sites for biopsy or pleural drainage when necessary.

Table 109.3 • Imaging Clues to Pneumonias

Finding	Associated Organisms
Lobar or multilobar consolidation	*Streptococcus pneumoniae, Klebsiella pneumoniae* (expansile), *Legionella pneumophila, Haemophilus influenzae, Mycoplasma pneumoniae*
Peribronchial opacities	*Staphylococcus aureus, H influenzae, K pneumoniae, Pseudomonas aeruginosa, Aspergillus fumigatus, Mycoplasma pneumoniae, L pneumophila*, mycobacteria, anaerobes
Interstitial thickening	Viruses, *M pneumoniae, Pneumocystis jirovecii*
Nodular opacities	Mycobacteria, fungi, viruses, *Nocardia asteroides, M pneumoniae, L pneumophila, A fumigatus*; (CT Halo=invasive *Aspergillus*, Zygomycetes, *Candida, Coccidioides, Cryptococcus, Pseudomonas*, viruses)
Cavities, abscesses	*S aureus, K pneumoniae, P aeruginosa, Actinomyces, N asteroides, Burkholderia pseudomallei, Rhodococcus equi, Aspergillus, Actinomyces israelii, N asteroides*, mycobacteria, anaerobes, fungi
Pneumatoceles	*S aureus, P jirovecii*
Lymphadenopathy	*M pneumoniae, Mycobacterium tuberculosis*
Empyema	*S pneumoniae, S aureus, M tuberculosis*, gram-negative bacteria
Chest wall invasion	*A israelii, N asteroides, M tuberculosis*, fungi

Pneumonias express a wide range of radiographic appearances, although some are more characteristic of certain organisms (Table 109.3). For example, streptococcal pneumonia often presents as lobar consolidation with air bronchograms. *Klebsiella* infection should be considered when there is associated lobar expansion producing a bulging fissure sign. *Staphylococcus aureus* infection commonly produces multifocal peribronchial opacities characteristic of bronchopneumonia and may be accompanied by abscess formation. *Pseudomonas* infection may present as a reticular pattern of interstitial thickening and is sometimes associated with pneumatoceles.

Cardiogenic edema, ARDS, and other air space diseases sometimes obscure developing pneumonia on a chest radiograph. The pneumonia may ultimately be recognized by a gradual worsening of an area of opacification on serial radiographs in the setting of other stable or fluctuating abnormalities. Chronic diseases can also simulate pneumonia on a single radiograph, and comparison or follow-up radiographs can help distinguish such abnormalities. Multifocal opacities that persist as acute pneumonia resolves may raise concern for underlying causes, such as metastases, vasculitis, or granulomatous disease.

The radiographic presentation of aspiration can vary with the quantity, pH, and type of aspirate; patient hydration; and ability to mount an inflammatory response. Aspiration of low-pH gastric contents in Mendelson syndrome can evoke a rapid, diffuse chemical pneumonitis and pulmonary edema pattern. It can be difficult to distinguish radiographically from other abnormality (eg, ARDS, pneumonia, hemorrhage, and cardiogenic air space edema), but it characteristically develops rapidly and clears rapidly unless complicated by ARDS or infectious pneumonia. Aspiration can also produce focal opacities; in particular, the bilateral upper lobe posterior segments and lower lobe superior and posterior basal segments may be involved in a patient in the supine position, or the lower lobes, middle lobe, and lingula may be involved in a patient who is erect. Posterior basal lower lobe involvement can be difficult to visualize through the hemidiaphragms and cardiac silhouette on a frontal radiograph, and a lateral or oblique radiograph can be helpful. The gradual development of focal opacification over a period of days suggests pneumonia. CT can be useful to evaluate equivocal or complex radiographic findings, identify an aspirated foreign body or type of aspirated material, and assess a febrile neutropenic patient who has nonspecific radiographic findings.

Atelectasis can have various radiographic appearances and may exist alone or in conjunction with other processes, including aspiration and pneumonia. It frequently presents as linear or platelike opacities that cross fissural boundaries, although the presentation can range from ill-defined opacities to segmental, lobar, or multilobar involvement. In addition, there are atypical manifestations. In the ICU, atelectasis is particularly common in the lower lobes, especially the left lower lobe. It may project through the cardiac silhouette and hemidiaphragms and be difficult to distinguish from pneumonia except by rapid fluctuation on serial studies in some cases. If associated with a large central mucous plug, bronchial cutoff may be seen. Prior comparison radiographs can help exclude preexisting volume loss, which might indicate the need for a work-up to exclude an obstructive lesion that preceded the presentation to the ICU (Figure 109.2).

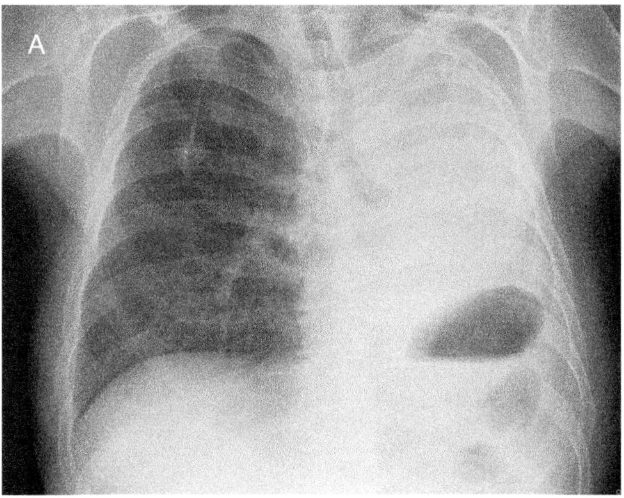

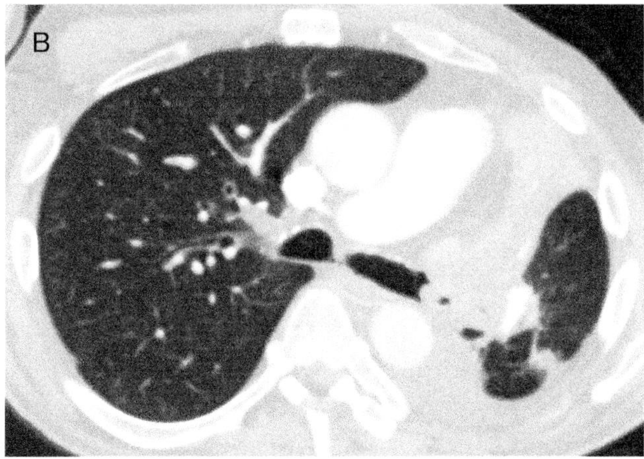

Figure 109.2. Chest Radiograph and Computed Tomography Scan of Endobronchial Mass. A, Chest radiograph on admission. Bronchial cutoff sign in left main bronchus in association with left lung collapse, left hemidiaphragm elevation, and ipsilateral mediastinal shift. Note also right infusion-port catheter. B, Comparison contrast-enhanced computed tomography image obtained 1 month earlier (lung window). Left hilar mass with endobronchial component and lingular collapse. Note also left pleural effusion and left lower lobe nodule.

Pleural Disease

In the initial imaging evaluation of pleural disease, the chest radiograph provides a survey of the entire thorax. PA and lateral radiographs are preferable to AP radiographs, and AP radiographs obtained with the patient erect are preferable to those with the patient supine. Decubitus radiographs were used for many years to assess the degree to which an effusion was free-flowing, although ultrasonography has now supplanted decubitus imaging in some centers. Reviewing prior comparison studies is important to help assess the chronicity of pleural disease.

Pleural effusion typically presents as a relatively homogeneous area of opacification on a chest radiograph. Its appearance can vary with several factors, including volume and viscosity, presence of loculations, and patient position. In the absence of adhesions, pleural effusion typically accumulates in a dependent location near the hemidiaphragms in an erect patient and along the posterior thorax in a supine patient. In an erect patient, a 75-mL effusion can occupy a subpulmonic location between the lung and diaphragm and produce a posterior costophrenic sulcus meniscus, whereas a 175-mL or greater effusion may extend into the lateral costophrenic sulcus. With increasing size, an effusion may obscure, or silhouette (Figure 109.1), the margin of the diaphragm and other normal anatomical structures. Massive effusion can completely opacify a thorax, invert the diaphragm, and shift the mediastinum to the contralateral side. A diaphragm may appear denser than normal in the case of subpulmonic effusion, and its apex can appear to be shifted laterally (Figure 109.3A). The gastric bubble may be inferiorly displaced with a large left effusion. Loculated pleural effusion can also present as an incompletely circumscribed masslike opacity with a circumscribed margin when viewed in tangent and as an ill-defined appearance when viewed en face.

In some cases, pleural effusion can be difficult to recognize on an AP radiograph obtained with a patient supine or semierect. A small effusion may not produce costophrenic sulcus blunting, and the degree of opacification it produces may not even be sufficient to distinguish it from normal. With a patient in the semierect position, effusion may present as veillike opacification at the base of the thorax that gradually diminishes superiorly. The costophrenic angle may or may not show a meniscus. With a patient in the supine position, the same veillike effect may extend more superiorly, and effusion may produce an apical cap that disappears when reimaging is done with the patient erect. In both the semierect and supine positions, effusion may course into fissures and sometimes produce a biconvex masslike opacity, or "pseudotumor," which can simulate a lung lesion. A large effusion that produces a wide area of opacification can be challenging to distinguish from extensive air space disease; however, pulmonary vessels are generally visible and air bronchograms are generally absent with effusion unless there is associated volume loss or consolidation. If the clinical condition permits, a radiograph obtained with a patient in the decubitus position may help gauge the relative amounts of effusion and lung disease contributing to the opacification of the thorax.

Transthoracic ultrasonography can also assist in the evaluation and management of pleural disease. Advantages over chest radiography include increased sensitivity in detection of pleural fluid, portability, real-time imaging, and absence of radiation. Ultrasonography is typically performed through an intercostal space using a curvilinear array transducer of 2 to 5 MHz. A higher-frequency transducer (7.5-10 MHz) can improve resolution, although penetration is decreased, especially in patients with thick chest walls. Doppler ultrasonography is not mandatory for portable ultrasonographic procedures, but it can help differentiate effusion from solid mass and identify blood vessels along the potential path of a needle.

Ultrasonography is more sensitive than conventional radiography for detecting effusion. Simple pleural effusions are generally anechoic or hypoechoic relative to the liver (Figure 109.3C), although ultrasonography cannot always definitively distinguish transudate from exudate. Septations are often better seen than with noncontrast CT, but the full extent and complexity of pleural disease may be better seen on CT. Hemothorax and empyema are often echogenic, and sometimes isoechoic, compared with the liver on ultrasonography. Malignant effusion may be associated with floating echogenic material and pleural thickening or nodularity. The likelihood of pneumothorax during thoracentesis under ultrasonographic guidance is low. An ultrasound transducer can be directed in various planes through an intercostal space to assist in the selection of a high-yield location for intervention.

CT has an improved ability over ultrasonography to show the full extent of pleural disease, particularly areas that may not be accessible with ultrasonography. CT is generally performed at a single breath hold and displayed at 1- to 3-mm intervals in the axial plane. Coronal and sagittal reconstructions can also be performed.

Very small amounts of pleural fluid in the range of 2 to 10 mL can be detected by CT, although attenuation values may not reliably distinguish a transudate from an exudate. CT can improve the evaluation of loculated fluid and air collections, parenchymal consolidations, and destructive chest wall lesions. It can help distinguish empyema from lung abscess; identify a bronchopleural fistula; show mediastinal, diaphragmatic, and upper abdominal abnormalities; and guide interventions. Thickened, enhanced visceral and parietal pleura separated by a lenticular fluid collection produces the split pleura sign (Figure 109.4), which may represent empyema in the appropriate clinical setting. The presence of air is virtually pathognomonic of empyema in the absence of an alternative cause.

Hemothorax may produce relatively high attenuation fluid that exceeds 35 Hounsfield units (HU) when acute and reaches 70 HU when clotted, whereas reactive effusion is in the range of 15 HU. In some cases, a hematocrit level may also be present, produced by higher-attenuation sedimented blood products and a lower-attenuation supernatant. Active bleeding can have attenuation values similar to those of adjacent enhanced vessels on contrast CT. The density of an effusion can also vary with amounts of cholesterol, fat, and protein content. Chylothorax and pseudochylothorax may even present with negative attenuation values. Although often not feasible to perform on a critically ill patient, magnetic resonance imaging can potentially differentiate exudates and transudates and assess hemothorax age.

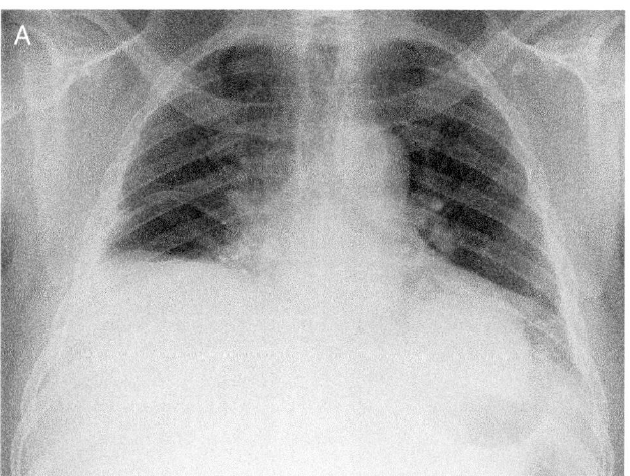

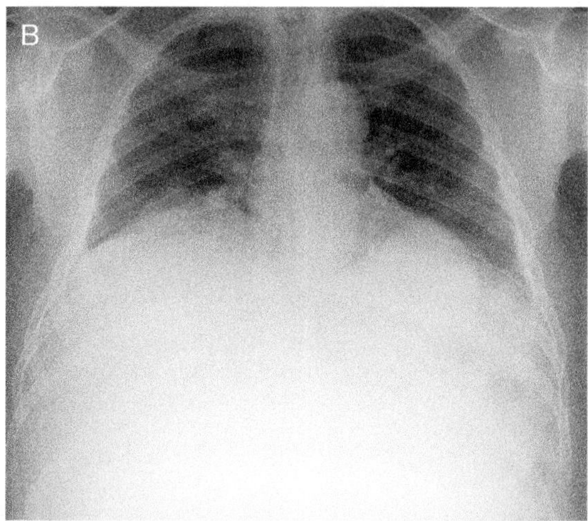

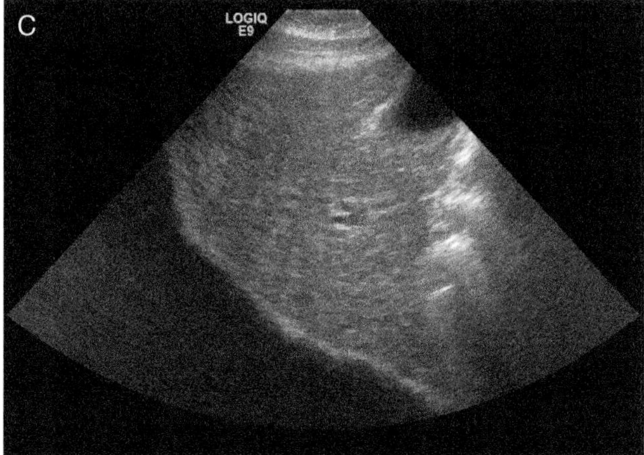

Figure 109.3. Chest Radiograph and Sonogram of Subpulmonic Pleural Effusion. A, Chest radiograph shows right subpulmonic effusion, manifested as increased density of the right hemidiaphragm with the apparent dome also shifted laterally. B, Chest radiograph obtained 1 month earlier did not show right subpulmonic effusion. Dome is more medial than in A, and pulmonary vessels are better visualized through the dome than in A. C, Sonogram obtained at time of radiograph in A shows anechoic right effusion. Echogenic hemidiaphragm separates effusion from liver.

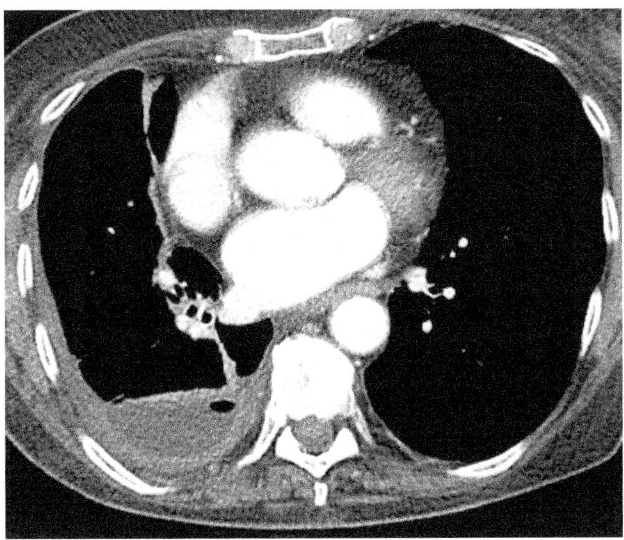

Figure 109.4. Contrast-Enhanced Computed Tomography Scan of Empyema. Empyema is seen in posterior right hemithorax with split pleura sign and tiny anechoic air collection (no history of thoracentesis).

Box 109.1 • Radiographic Findings of Pneumothorax in a Supine Patient

Relative lucency of involved hemithorax

Visualization of visceral pleura (search multiple locations: apicolateral, anteromedial, subpulmonic, and posteromedial)

Increased sharpness of margins of cardiac silhouette and superior mediastinum

Increased sharpness of margin of descending aorta or costovertebral sulcus

Increased sharpness of margin of hemidiaphragm

Widening of lateral costophrenic sulcus (deep sulcus sign)

Visualization of anterior and posterior diaphragm (double diaphragm sign)

Depression of diaphragm or shift mediastinal structures (tension pneumothorax)

Data from Ho M-L, Gutierrez FR. Chest radiography in thoracic polytrauma. AJR Am J Roentgenol. 2009 Mar;192(3):599-612 and Tocino IM. Pneumothorax in the supine patient: radiographic anatomy. Radiographics. 1985 Jul;5(4):557-86.

Pneumothorax, Pneumomediastinum, and Pneumopericardium

Conventional chest radiography is the first-line imaging study for pneumothorax. The appearance of pneumothorax is influenced by various factors, including patient position, anatomy, gravity, and lung recoil. The normal visceral pleura is typically identified as a thin white line outlined by both aerated lung and air in the pleural space. With a patient in the erect position, pleural air tends to collect in an apicolateral location, and as little as 50 mL can be visible on a frontal chest radiograph. In many cases, lung is not seen peripheral to a visualized visceral pleural line in pneumothorax, although its presence does not exclude pneumothorax; differences in lung recoil and limitations of the 2-dimensional projection of the chest radiograph can sometimes account for such an appearance. Skin folds can mimic pneumothorax, although frequently they are multiple and extend beyond the thoracic cavity over the ribs, mediastinum, or diaphragm. In addition, they present as an edge, rather than a line, accompanied by a negative Mach band on the lateral side and relatively increased opacification on the medial side.

For the detection of pneumothorax, a radiograph obtained with a patient supine is not as sensitive as one obtained with a patient in the lateral decubitus position. For the latter, with the side in question placed nondependently, as little as 5 mL of air has been reported to be detected. With a patient in the supine position (Box 109.1), pneumothorax tends to rise to the anteromedial part of the thorax and into the subpulmonic space. It has been reported that at least 200 mL of air must be present for a definitive diagnosis of pneumothorax in a supine patient.

In some cases, a subtle sign of pneumothorax is increased lucency of one hemithorax relative to the other. In the upper part of the chest, anteromedial pneumothorax may sharply delineate mediastinal contours, including the superior vena cava and azygous vein, left subclavian artery, and anterior junction line. In the lower part of the chest, the heart, paracardiac fat, and inferior vena cava may be outlined. Subpulmonic pneumothorax may outline the anterior and posterior aspects of the hemidiaphragms (double diaphragm sign) or produce a widened costophrenic sulcus (deep sulcus sign) (Figure 109.5). Posterior pneumothorax may extend into the azygoesophageal recess on the right or along the descending aorta and paraspinal line on the left and is typically a left-sided abnormality seen in the setting of left lower lobe volume loss or consolidation. Signs of tension pneumothorax include hyperlucency, diaphragmatic depression, widened intercostal spaces, and contralateral mediastinal shift, which has been reported in the range of 300 to 500 mL of air. In some cases, tension pneumothorax may be reflected as only a subtle shift of a posterior or anterior structure, such as the azygoesophageal recess reflection or anterior junction line, or as lung collapse without expected ipsilateral shift of the mediastinum.

Ultrasonography is also used to evaluate pneumothorax emergently at the bedside. Typically, imaging is done with the transducer directed into the third or fourth intercostal

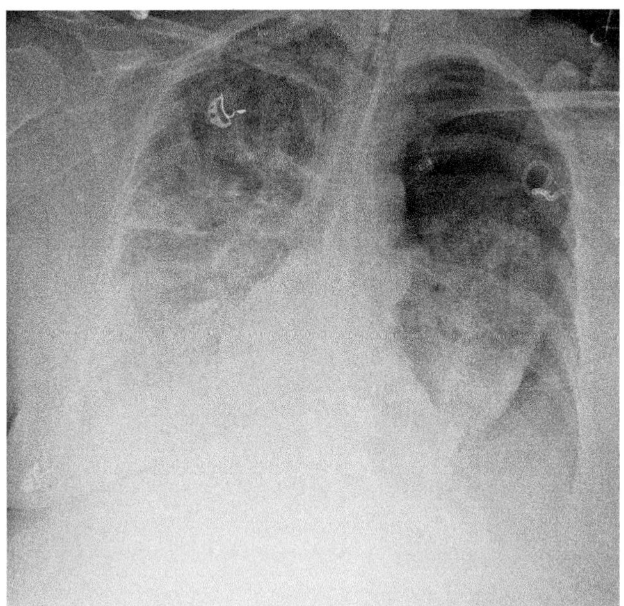

Figure 109.5. Chest Radiograph of Tension Pneumothorax. Tension pneumothorax on left in acute respiratory distress syndrome with deep sulcus sign (subpulmonic component of pneumothorax), partial lung collapse, and contralateral shift of the cardiac silhouette despite pleural pigtail catheter. Note also endotracheal tube, feeding tube, and right peripherally inserted central catheter.

space along the parasternal or midclavicular line. If a patient can be moved to the CT suite, CT is particularly useful to evaluate for air collections in locations difficult to access with ultrasonography and to evaluate complex abnormality that may include various combinations of air, fluid, hemorrhage, adhesions, and pleural thickening or nodularity.

Differentiating medial pneumothorax from pneumomediastinum can be challenging on a radiograph in a supine patient. If repositioning of the patient is possible, an erect or decubitus position can be helpful. Pneumomediastinum often appears as low-density streaks or bands that track along communicating spaces and vascular sheaths and rupture through fascial planes into adjacent anatomical compartments. It can outline anatomical structures (eg, aorta, pulmonary arteries, superior vena cava) and dissect into soft tissues outside the thorax to produce subcutaneous emphysema. If posterior, it may follow the course of the esophagus. It may also extend into a costovertebral sulcus or along the hemidiaphragms and inferior to the cardiac silhouette (continuous diaphragm sign).

In contrast to the streaks of pneumomediastinum, pneumopericardium is usually visible as a single lucent band of air around the heart. It may extend into pericardial recesses, and it stops superiorly at the level of the ascending aorta and main pulmonary artery. In tension pneumopericardium, the heart may be compressed and the cardiothoracic ratio reduced. Air that outlines the aortic arch, distal left pulmonary artery, or superior vena cava above the azygos vein is pneumomediastinum. On CT, the presence of connective tissue septae in pneumomediastinum can also help distinguish it from pneumopericardium.

Trauma

Compared with chest radiography, CT offers improved detection and characterization of many thoracic injuries. However, AP supine chest radiography is often by necessity the first-line imaging examination in trauma. Despite its limitations, chest radiography can provide a wealth of valuable information quickly. For example, it can help quickly include or exclude pneumothorax, pneumomediastinum, massive hemothorax, and many skeletal injuries. Mediastinal widening, opacification, contour irregularity, and mass effect may also be shown and indicate the presence of hemorrhage and other abnormalities.

Results of chest radiography may be normal or nearly normal in up to 7% of cases of acute traumatic aortic injury, although radiographs can provide valuable clues to diagnosis in many cases. Direct signs include an abnormal aortic contour and sudden change in aortic caliber. Indirect signs include mediastinal widening; obscuration or irregularity of the aortic margin; loss of the aortic-pulmonic window; rightward tracheal, esophageal, or nasogastric tube deviation; left main bronchus depression; paraspinal line widening; and left apical capping or dependent effusion. Aortic dissection can occasionally be suggested on a chest radiograph by discontinuous or displaced calcification at the knob; alternatively, CT can better identify and characterize dissection and many other abnormalities, including hemopericardium, aneurysm and pseudoaneurysm, cardiac rupture, vessel avulsion, and minimal aortic injury. Traditional axial CT images are often accompanied by multiplanar reformations in the evaluation of acute traumatic aortic injury.

Pericardial effusion can have various presentations on an AP chest radiograph. It may not be recognizable in some cases, whereas other cases may show cardiac silhouette enlargement (Figure 109.6), the differential density sign, or widening of the carinal angle. A lateral radiograph has been reported to improve detection. Ultrasonography is a valuable imaging tool for pericardial effusion and can quickly assess for pericardial tamponade. Benefits of CT include the ability to show injuries to adjacent structures and a tract in the setting of a penetrating injury.

Pulmonary contusion may not be visible on a chest radiograph for the first 6 hours, although CT may detect it within that time frame. CT can also better localize areas involved, quantify the extent of contusion, and act as a prognosticator of morbidity and mortality. Contusion may be conspicuous on chest radiography by 24 hours, after which time the development of parenchymal opacification should

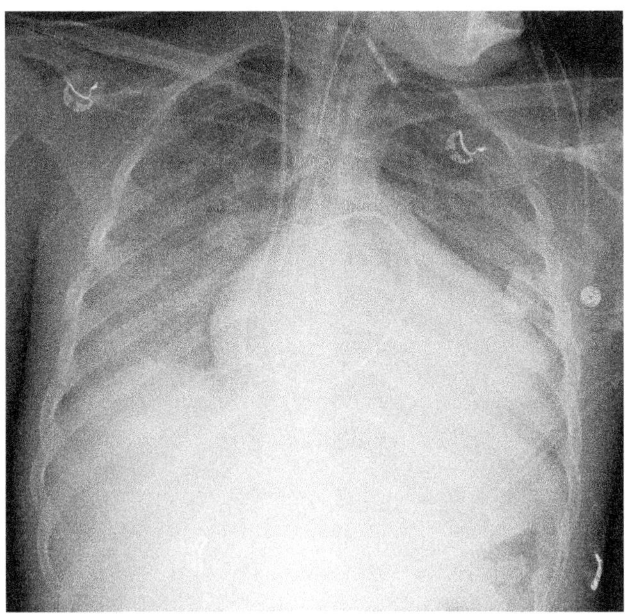

Figure 109.6. Chest Radiograph of Pericardial Effusion. Effusion produced enlarged cardiac silhouette with a water-bottle configuration. Note also bilateral pulmonary edema pattern, endotracheal tube, Swan-Ganz catheter, feeding tube, and right peripherally inserted central catheter.

raise the possibility of another diagnosis, such as aspiration, fat embolism, or pneumonia. If uncomplicated, pulmonary contusion may begin resolving by 24 to 48 hours, and complete resolution may occur within 3 to 14 days.

Small pulmonary lacerations are better identified by CT than chest radiography, although opacities and air collections that accompany lacerations can be seen on chest radiographs in some cases. Subcutaneous hematoma is sometimes easy to recognize on a chest radiograph by opacification that projects outside the bony thorax. However, if it projects over the lung or mediastinum on a single-view AP image, it can be difficult to distinguish its extrathoracic location from an intrathoracic one.

Tracheal rupture can sometimes be suggested on chest radiography by endotracheal tube balloon overdistension or herniation. Persistent pneumothorax after chest tube placement may also signify tracheobronchial injury. On occasion, in the case of bronchial transection, lung may be displaced from the hilum into the dependent hemithorax to produce the fallen lung sign. Both tracheal disruption and esophageal injury can produce pneumomediastinum and mediastinal widening. Esophageal injury may also be associated with pleural effusion.

The radiographic appearances of pneumothorax and pneumopericardium have been previously discussed. Air embolism caused by organ rupture or penetrating trauma can also present on chest radiography as hyperlucent areas, in this case in the right side of the heart, pulmonary arteries, and systemic veins. Right-sided heart failure, pulmonary oligemia, and pulmonary edema may also be present. Air in small distal pulmonary vessels is not generally visible. CT is more sensitive than radiography for the detection of small amounts of intravascular air. Transesophageal echocardiography has better resolution than transthoracic echocardiography and can detect microbubbles of air.

Diaphragmatic rupture has various presentations on a chest radiograph, ranging from normal to new subtle irregularity of the diaphragm contour to conspicuous diaphragm elevation and intrathoracic abdominal contents. CT with multiplanar reformations has improved sensitivity compared with chest radiography. Diaphragm discontinuity, waistlike stricturing of herniated abdominal contents (collar sign), or viscera along the dependent thoracic wall (dependent viscera sign) might be seen on CT. Associated findings can include lower rib fractures, basilar opacification, pneumothorax, and pneumoperitoneum. Several conditions can also mimic or obscure diaphragmatic rupture, among them diaphragmatic paralysis and eventration, subpulmonic effusion, basilar atelectasis, and congenital diaphragmatic hernia.

Sternal fractures can be difficult to identify on AP chest radiographs, and detection may require a lateral view, oblique sternal view, or CT. The fractures can also be subtle on axial CT and better appreciated on sagittal or coronal reformations. Accompanying anterior mediastinal hemorrhage typically leaves a preserved fat plane with the aorta, unlike in acute traumatic aortic injury. Reduction in bony detail on supine AP radiographs can challenge the ability to detect clavicular and shoulder fractures and dislocations. Lower ribs can also be obscured by diaphragms on an AP view in some cases, and posterior ribs may be better seen than anterior ribs. Nondisplaced or minimally displaced rib fractures can be difficult to identify, particularly where there is overlap of ribs. Costochondral cartilage is not visible unless sufficiently calcified. Careful assessment of the chest radiograph can be needed to detect evidence of flail chest when rib fracture displacement is not conspicuous. Spinal deformities may also be easily missed on an AP chest radiograph. A lateral view can be helpful, although CT with reformations is generally the preferred method of imaging unless there is indication for emergency magnetic resonance imaging, such as in the setting of a progressive neurologic deficit.

Devices

The chest radiograph continues to play a key role in assessing the placement of various support devices used in the ICU and the potential complications associated with them. Examples of complications of line placement include malpositioning, pneumothorax, mediastinal hematoma, and pleural effusion.

Recognition of the proper positioning of tubes and lines on an AP radiograph is facilitated by an understanding of anatomy. In a well-positioned patient, the cavoatrial junction can be approximated as the vicinity of the distal bronchus intermedius. This knowledge can aid in assessing the proper placement of a central venous catheter in the superior vena cava between the most central valve of the subclavian or jugular vein and the right atrium. A pulmonary artery catheter should take a smooth curved course, and its tip should ideally reside just proximal to a right or left interlobar pulmonary artery. It should also generally be seen no more than 1 cm lateral to the mediastinum. Because the complication rate is reduced with the balloon inflated only during insertion and pressure measurement, the chest radiograph should depict the location of the catheter tip with the balloon deflated; the catheter will advance several centimeters when the balloon is inflated and the catheter is wedged. Pulmonary infarction may present radiographically with volume loss or a wedge-shaped or rounded peripheral opacity distal to the tip. A spectrum of findings for pulmonary infarction may be seen on CT.

Chest radiographs can help assess pacemaker placement and complications, including malpositioning, lead fracture, pneumothorax, perforation, and hemothorax. Thin epicardial wires can sometimes be difficult to visualize. However, transvenous implantable cardioverter-defibrillators may show 1 or 2 thickened metal shock coils, which should project in the regions of the brachiocephalic vein-superior vena cava junction and right ventricle. An AP view should show the lead electrode of a subcutaneous implantable cardioverter-defibrillator running parallel to and 1 to 2 cm to the left of the midsternum, whereas a lateral view best assesses the anteroposterior position of the pulse generator. A lateral radiograph also best depicts the proper anterior course of an electrode directed into the right atrial appendage. A coronary sinus lead will appear to be directed across the heart on an AP view. It should course posteriorly relative to the heart on a lateral view. Transcutaneous pacing pads can be radiopaque and may partially obscure underlying devices and anatomical structures.

An intra-aortic balloon pump is seen as a lucent fusiform structure over the aortic shadow if captured inflated in diastole. When deflated in systole, only the tip should be visible as a 3- to 4-mm metallic density in the descending aorta distal to the region of the left subclavian artery. The aortic knob is typically used as a landmark for proper positioning, although some authors have advocated positioning the intra-aortic balloon pump tip 2 cm above the carina to more reliably avoid a location too close to the left subclavian artery.

A correctly placed endotracheal tube terminates in the middle third of the trachea, about 3 to 7 cm above the carina with the head in neutral position. Placement in this location allows for safe excursion of the tube with flexion and extension of the neck. Considerable movement of an endotracheal tube occurs with neck flexion and extension and to a lesser degree with neck rotation. Maximal movement has been reported in the range of one-third to one-fourth the length of the trachea. When neck position is not readily apparent on the chest radiograph, the position of the chin relative to the vertebral bodies can be helpful. The chin typically projects over the C5 or C6 vertebra in neutral position, over the T1 or T2 vertebra in flexion, and above the C4 vertebra in extension. If the carina is not easily visible, its location may be estimated by following the medial margins of the main bronchi centrally. The carina typically projects from the C5 to C7 level, and a tube tip at the C3 or C4 level is generally satisfactorily positioned. A tip 3.4 to 5.0 cm above a line drawn tangentially to the right from the inferior aortic margin in a supine patient has also been reported as sufficiently positioned in 95% of patients.

Positioning an endotracheal tube too low may result in right main bronchus intubation, right lung overinflation, and left lung atelectasis (Figure 109.7). Malpositioning too high can place the patient at risk for laryngeal injury, aspiration, and spontaneous extubation. Esophageal intubation and tracheal rupture are potentially serious complications of intubation. Radiographic signs of esophageal intubation include overdistension of the stomach and esophagus, projection of the endotracheal tube lateral to the tracheal air

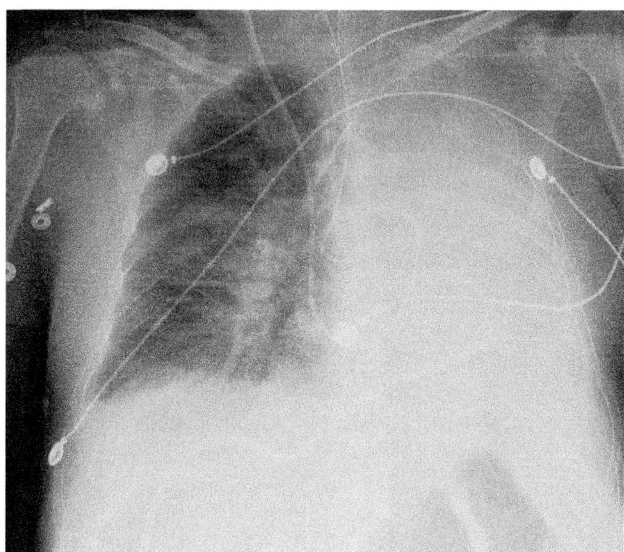

Figure 109.7. Chest Radiograph of Malpositioned Endotracheal Tube in Right Main Bronchus. It is associated with left lung collapse with ipsilateral mediastinal shift and obscured diaphragm margin. Abdominal drain placed from right upper quadrant terminates higher than expected, consistent with elevated left diaphragm. Also, malpositioned Swan-Ganz catheter is looped back on itself in the right pulmonary artery. Nasogastric tube is looped in stomach, and left internal jugular line is in superior vena cava. Pulmonary edema pattern is seen in right lung.

column, and displacement of the trachea by the inflated cuff. Radiographic findings of tracheal rupture can include mediastinal and subcutaneous emphysema, cuff overinflation with distal tube orientation to the right relative to the tracheal lumen, and balloon migration toward the tip. A tracheostomy tube should terminate over the T3 to T4 level about halfway between the stoma and carina. The width of the tube should be about two-thirds that of the trachea, and the cuff should not overly distend the tracheal lumen. Unlike an endotracheal tube, a tracheostomy tube should maintain its position with the neck flexed or extended.

A thoracostomy tube, or intercostal drainage tube, is frequently seen coursing through the fourth to fifth intercostal space. The proximal side hole can be identified by an interruption in the radiopaque line visible along the tube and should always project inside the confines of the ribs. The tube should not be angulated. It may be directed anterosuperiorly in the case of pneumothorax or posterosuperiorly in the case of effusion, although it can sometimes be difficult on a single AP radiograph to distinguish an anterior from a posterior course or a malpositioned intrafissural or intraparenchymal location. Additional projections may be necessary, and CT may be required in some cases.

A correctly placed nasoenteric tube takes a direct vertical course through the esophagus in the midline or just to the left of it. It should not be seen to be directed into either of the main bronchi below the level of the carina. The distal tube should cross the diaphragm and terminate in the range of 10 cm or more beyond the level of the gastroesophageal junction. If the tube is intended to be placed in the small bowel, an abdominal radiograph may be needed to see the tip in some cases.

Management of hydrocephalus may require the use of a cerebrospinal fluid shunt. The chest radiograph is part of a series taken for shunt evaluation, which also includes radiographs of the skull and abdomen. Because the entire length of a shunt must be imaged, overlapping radiographs may be needed. Radiography can help assess the course and status of a shunt, including for fractures, disconnections, and distal catheter migration. The presence of hydrothorax can also be assessed in the case of a ventriculopleural shunt. When feasible to obtain, PA radiographs reduce eye exposure and position a tunneled shunt closer to the image detector than AP radiographs.

Summary

- The American College of Radiology recommends chest radiography to assess a change in clinical condition or evaluate placement of a tube, catheter, and other life-saving support device. Routine chest radiography is not recommended.
- Well-documented chest radiographic appearances correlate with the presence of interstitial and air space pulmonary edema.
- Pleural effusion may have various presentations on portable radiographs and may be difficult to differentiate from air space disease in some cases.
- In a supine patient, pneumothorax tends to rise to the anteromedial part of the thorax and into the subpulmonic space.
- Signs of tension pneumothorax include hyperlucency, diaphragmatic depression, widened intercostal spaces, and contralateral mediastinal shift.
- There are both direct and indirect radiographic signs of acute traumatic aortic injury. Chest radiographic results have been reported as normal or nearly normal in up to 7% of cases.
- The chest radiograph has a key role in the assessment of support devices in patients in the ICU.
- Ultrasonography is a valuable tool for the bedside evaluation of several thoracic abnormalities and for bedside intervention.
- CT can improve the assessment of complex or otherwise puzzling radiographic presentations.

SUGGESTED READING

Abramowitz Y, Simanovsky N, Goldstein MS, Hiller N. Pleural effusion: characterization with CT attenuation values and CT appearance. AJR Am J Roentgenol. 2009 Mar;192(3):618–23.

Baber CE, Hedlund LW, Oddson TA, Putman CE. Differentiating empyemas and peripheral pulmonary abscesses: the value of computed tomography. Radiology. 1980 Jun;135(3):755–8.

Battle C, Hayward S, Eggert S, Evans PA. Comparison of the use of lung ultrasound and chest radiography in the diagnosis of rib fractures: a systematic review. Emerg Med J. 2019 Mar;36(3):185–90. Epub 2018 Nov 23.

Bejvan SM, Godwin JD. Pneumomediastinum: old signs and new signs. AJR Am J Roentgenol. 1996 May;166(5):1041–8.

Bergin D, Ennis R, Keogh C, Fenlon HM, Murray JG. The "dependent viscera" sign in CT diagnosis of blunt traumatic diaphragmatic rupture. AJR Am J Roentgenol. 2001 Nov;177(5):1137–40.

Borasio P, Ardissone F, Chiampo G. Post-intubation tracheal rupture: a report on ten cases. Eur J Cardiothorac Surg. 1997 Jul;12(1):98–100.

Brander L, Ramsay D, Dreier D, Peter M, Graeni R. Continuous left hemidiaphragm sign revisited: a case of spontaneous pneumopericardium and literature review. Heart. 2002 Oct;88(4):e5.

Conrardy PA, Goodman LR, Lainge F, Singer MM. Alteration of endotracheal tube position: flexion and extension of the neck. Crit Care Med. 1976 Jan-Feb;4(1):8–12.

Davis SD, Henschke CI, Yankelevitz DF, Cahill PT, Yi Y. MR imaging of pleural effusions. J Comput Assist Tomogr. 1990 Mar-Apr;14(2):192–8.

Eisenhuber E, Schaefer-Prokop CM, Prosch H, Schima W. Bedside chest radiography. Respir Care. 2012 Mar;57(3):427–43.

Franquet T. Imaging of pneumonia: trends and algorithms. Eur Respir J. 2001 Jul;18(1):196–208.

Gluecker T, Capasso P, Schnyder P, Gudinchet F, Schaller MD, Revelly JP, et al. Clinical and radiologic features of pulmonary edema. Radiographics. 1999 Nov-Dec;19(6):1507–31.

Goodman A, Perera P, Mailhot T, Mandavia D. The role of bedside ultrasound in the diagnosis of pericardial effusion and cardiac tamponade. J Emerg Trauma Shock. 2012 Jan;5(1):72–5.

Gordon CE, Feller-Kopman D, Balk EM, Smetana GW. Pneumothorax following thoracentesis: a systematic review and meta-analysis. Arch Intern Med. 2010 Feb 22;170(4):332–9.

Gordon R. The deep sulcus sign. Radiology. 1980 Jul;136(1):25–7.

Gurney JW. Atypical manifestations of pulmonary atelectasis. J Thorac Imaging. 1996 Summer;11(3):165–75.

Han D, Lee KS, Franquet T, Muller NL, Kim TS, Kim H, et al. Thrombotic and nonthrombotic pulmonary arterial embolism: spectrum of imaging findings. Radiographics. 2003 Nov-Dec;23(6):1521–39.

Haus BM, Stark P, Shofer SL, Kuschner WG. Massive pulmonary pseudotumor. Chest. 2003 Aug;124(2):758–60.

He H, Stein MW, Zalta B, Haramati LB. Pulmonary infarction: spectrum of findings on multidetector helical CT. J Thorac Imaging. 2006 Mar;21(1):1–7.

Hew M, Tay TR. The efficacy of bedside chest ultrasound: from accuracy to outcomes. Eur Respir Rev. 2016 Sep;25(141):230–46.

Ho AM, Ling E. Systemic air embolism after lung trauma. Anesthesiology. 1999 Feb;90(2):564–75.

Ho ML, Gutierrez FR. Chest radiography in thoracic polytrauma. AJR Am J Roentgenol. 2009 Mar;192(3):599–612.

Jalli R, Sefidbakht S, Jafari SH. Value of ultrasound in diagnosis of pneumothorax: a prospective study. Emerg Radiol. 2013 Apr;20(2):131–4. Epub 2012 Nov 21.

Kesieme EB, Dongo A, Ezemba N, Irekpita E, Jebbin N, Kesieme C. Tube thoracostomy: complications and its management. Pulm Med. 2012;2012:256878. Epub 2011 Oct 16.

Ketai LH, Godwin JD. A new view of pulmonary edema and acute respiratory distress syndrome. J Thorac Imaging. 1998 Jul;13(3):147–71.

Kim JT, Lee JR, Kim JK, Yoon SZ, Jeon Y, Bahk JH, et al. The carina as a useful radiographic landmark for positioning the intraaortic balloon pump. Anesth Analg. 2007 Sep;105(3):735–8.

Koh DM, Burke S, Davies N, Padley SP. Transthoracic US of the chest: clinical uses and applications. Radiographics. 2002 Jan-Feb;22(1):e1.

Kuhlman JE, Singha NK. Complex disease of the pleural space: radiographic and CT evaluation. Radiographics. 1997 Jan-Feb;17(1):63–79.

Kundel HL, Seshadri SB, Langlotz CP, Lanken PN, Horii SC, Nodine CF, et al. Prospective study of a PACS: information flow and clinical action in a medical intensive care unit. Radiology. 1996 Apr;199(1):143–9.

LeBlang SD, Dolich MO. Imaging of penetrating thoracic trauma. J Thorac Imaging. 2000 Apr;15(2):128–35.

Mayo PH, Goltz HR, Tafreshi M, Doelken P. Safety of ultrasound-guided thoracentesis in patients receiving mechanical ventilation. Chest. 2004 Mar;125(3):1059–62.

Miller PR, Croce MA, Bee TK, Qaisi WG, Smith CP, Collins GL, et al. ARDS after pulmonary contusion: accurate measurement of contusion volume identifies high-risk patients. J Trauma. 2001 Aug;51(2):223–8.

Mirvis SE, Shanmuganagthan K. Imaging hemidiaphragmatic injury. Eur Radiol. 2007 Jun;17(6):1411–21. Epub 2007 Feb 17.

Oh KS, Fleischner FG, Wyman SM. Characteristic pulmonary finding in traumatic complete transection of a mainstem bronchus. Radiology. 1969 Feb;92(2):371–2.

Pappas JN, Goodman PC. Predicting proper endotracheal tube placement in underexposed radiographs: tangent line of the aortic arch. AJR Am J Roentgenol. 1999 Nov;173(5):1357–9.

Rollins RJ, Tocino I. Early radiographic signs of tracheal rupture. AJR Am J Roentgenol. 1987 Apr;148(4):695–8.

Schmidt AJ, Stark P. Radiographic findings in *Klebsiella* (Friedlander's) *pneumonia*: the bulging fissure sign. Semin Respir Infect. 1998 Mar;13(1):80–2.

Sharma S, Maycher B, Eschun G. Radiological imaging in pneumonia: recent innovations. Curr Opin Pulm Med. 2007 May;13(3):159–69.

Steenburg SD, Ravenel JG, Ikonomidis JS, Schonholz C, Reeves S. Acute traumatic aortic injury: imaging evaluation and management. Radiology. 2008 Sep;248(3):748–62.

Suh RD, Genshaft SJ, Kirsch J, Kanne JP, Chung JH, Donnelly EF, et al. ACR Appropriateness Criteria® intensive care unit patients. J Thorac Imaging. 2015 Nov;30(6):W63–5.

Tehranzadeh J, Kelley MJ. The differential density sign of pericardial effusion. Radiology. 1979 Oct;133(1):23–30.

Tocino IM. Pneumothorax in the supine patient: radiographic anatomy. RadioGraphics. 1985 Jul;5(4):557–86.

Tsujimoto N, Saraya T, Light RW, Tsukahara Y, Koide T, Kurai D, et al. A simple method for differentiating complicated parapneumonic effusion/empyema from parapneumonic effusion using the split pleura sign and the amount of pleural effusion on thoracic CT. PLoS One. 2015 Jun 15;10(6):e0130141.

Tulay CM, Yaldız S, Bilge A. Oblique chest x-ray: an alternative way to detect pneumothorax. Ann Thorac Cardiovasc Surg. 2018 Jun 20;24(3):127–30. Epub 2018 Mar 16.

Wallace AN, McConathy J, Menias CO, Bhalla S, Wippold FJ 2nd. Imaging evaluation of CSF shunts. AJR Am J Roentgenol. 2014 Jan;202(1):38–53.

Wanek S, Mayberry JC. Blunt thoracic trauma: flail chest, pulmonary contusion, and blast injury. Crit Care Clin. 2004 Jan;20(1):71–81.

Winkler MH, Touw HR, van de Ven PM, Twisk J, Tuinman PR. Diagnostic accuracy of chest radiograph, and when concomitantly studied lung ultrasound, in critically ill patients with respiratory symptoms: a systematic review and meta-analysis. Crit Care Med. 2018 Jul;46(7):e707–14.

Wolverson MK, Crepps LF, Sundaram M, Heiberg E, Vas WG, Shields JB. Hyperdensity of recent hemorrhage at body computed tomography: incidence and morphologic variation. Radiology. 1983 Sep;148(3):779–84.

Woodring JH. Recognition of pleural effusion on supine radiographs: how much fluid is required? AJR Am J Roentgenol. 1984 Jan;142(1):59–64.

Abdominal Radiography

JOSEPH G. CERNIGLIARO, MD; DAVID J. DISANTIS, MD

Goals

- Describe how to distinguish a normal bowel gas pattern from bowel obstruction, ileus, or mural pneumatosis on abdominal radiographs.
- Know where to look for extraluminal gas on a supine frontal abdominal radiograph.
- Understand that abdominal radiographs can provide clues to a wide range of abnormalities, including bowel ischemia, pancreatitis, ascites, and aneurysms.

Introduction

Hospitalized patients in a critical care environment are at risk for adverse intra-abdominal events involving bowel, solid organs, and vasculature. For assessment of hospitalized patients with abdominal pain, a thorough history and physical examination should precede indicated laboratory testing and imaging studies.

One expedient means of evaluation is abdominal radiography. In very ill patients, it can be performed at the bedside. The American College of Radiology Appropriateness Criteria assign abdominal radiography a middling grade of 5 (on a scale of 1-9, 9 being most appropriate) for acute, nonlocalized abdominal pain. With the exception of suspected cholecystitis (for which ultrasonography is the initial study of choice), computed tomography (CT) of the abdomen and pelvis with oral and intravenous contrast material is the preferred examination. Because of its ready availability and occasional definitive diagnostic information, however, abdominal radiography often is the first imaging study performed. Ideally, a supine frontal image is supplemented with an upright or left lateral decubitus (left-side down) frontal view.

Bowel Gas Pattern

In the acute care setting, an orderly approach to evaluation of an abdominal radiograph is fundamental. Analysis begins with the bowel gas pattern. Small bowel generally occupies the central aspect of the abdomen, and the colon is along the periphery (Figure 110.1). The small bowel folds normally are thin and traverse the entire lumen, whereas the colonic haustral folds are thicker and do not traverse the lumen. Small bowel is considered dilated when its diameter exceeds 3 cm.

The most common cause of small bowel obstruction (SBO) is postsurgical adhesions. Internal or body wall hernia, volvulus, mass, inflammatory bowel disease, impacted gallstone, and ingested foreign body are rarer causes.

The radiographic hallmark of SBO is dilated, gas-filled small bowel not accompanied by colonic dilatation (Figure 110.2), whereas both small bowel and colon typically are dilated in hypodynamic ileus (Figure 110.3). With SBO, air-fluid levels in the small bowel lumen often are visible on upright (Figure 110.2 B) or decubitus (left-side down) views. Levels 2.5 cm or longer particularly suggest obstruction, as do air-fluid levels of different heights in the same small bowel segment (Figure 110.2B). A less common sign of SBO is tiny bubbles of gas trapped by mucosal folds, arrayed along the small bowel lumen on upright or decubitus views, known metaphorically as the string of pearls (Figure 110.4).

Occasionally, abdominal radiographs show discrepant small bowel caliber (dilated proximal to the obstruction, nondilated distally), a clue to the level of obstruction (Figure 110.5).

The reported accuracy of radiographs for the diagnosis of SBO varies widely, from 50% to 86%. A source of error is dilated small bowel filled with fluid but not gas,

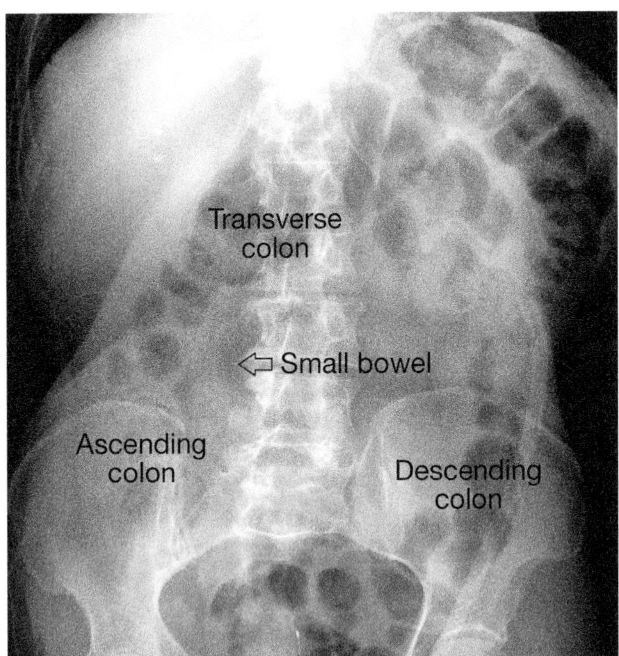

Figure 110.1. Normal Bowel Gas Pattern. Most bowel gas is colonic, in the periphery of the abdomen. Little gas is located centrally in small bowel.

a feature escaping radiographic detection. Focal inflammatory processes (pancreatitis, abscess) can cause a localized ileus with potentially confusing dilatation of immediately adjacent small bowel. Conversely, distal colon obstruction can mimic ileus if gaseous distention extends proximally to involve the small bowel. Sigmoid volvulus is a type of distal colonic obstruction that is often visible radiographically (Figure 110.6).

Bowel Wall

Small bowel folds should have a maximum thickness of about 3 mm, and colonic haustra, no more than 1 cm. Small bowel wall thickening has a broad differential diagnosis. In the intensive care unit, edema (eg, with hypoproteinemia and fluid overload) or hemorrhage (anticoagulants, disseminated intravascular coagulation) are leading considerations (Figure 110.7).

Colonic haustral thickening likewise is nonspecific, but *Clostridium difficile* colitis should be highly suspected in hospitalized patients (Figure 110.8). Rarely, inflammatory or infectious colitides give rise to toxic megacolon: thin friable wall, gaseous colonic distention (particularly the transverse colon in supine patients), and a nodular mucosal contour (Figure 110.9). Affected patients are acutely ill and often have peritoneal signs.

Radiographic findings of mesenteric or intestinal ischemia generally are nonspecific: mild to moderate bowel

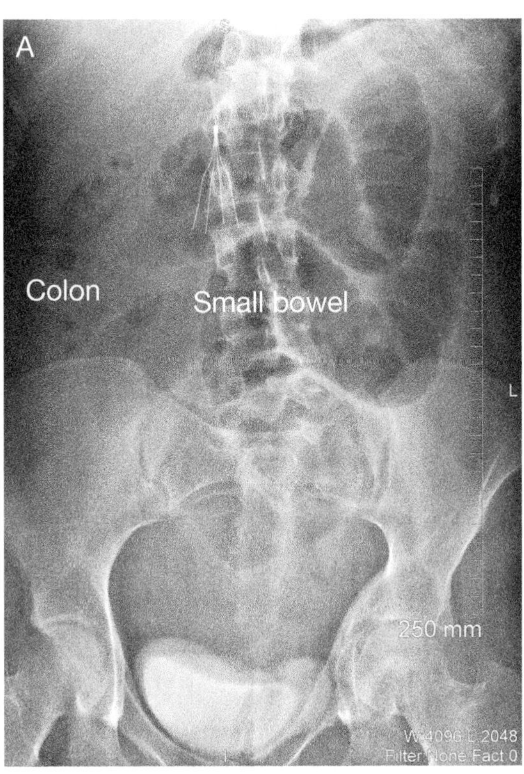

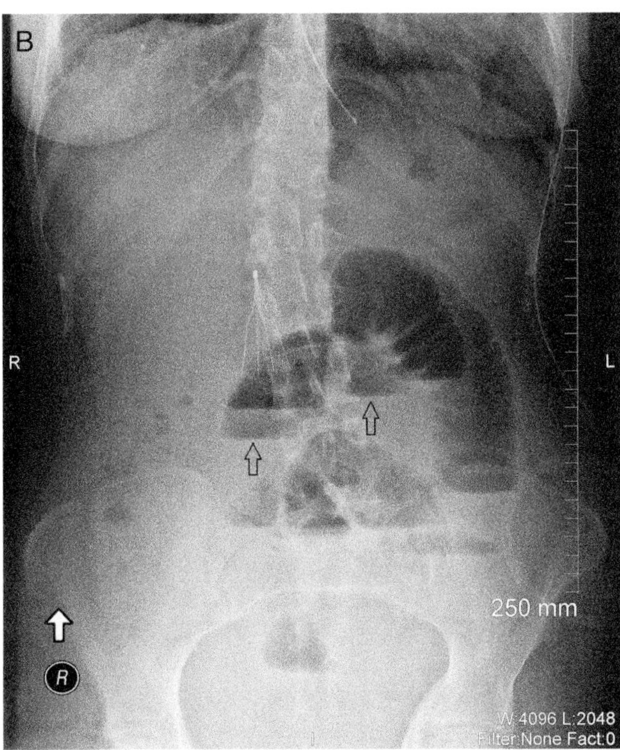

Figure 110.2. Small Bowel Obstruction. A, Dilated, gas-filled small bowel in the midabdomen. Normal colon caliber. B, Upright view. Small bowel obstruction is indicated by air-fluid levels in dilated small bowel. Black arrows highlight fluid levels at different heights in the same loop. L indicates left; R, right.

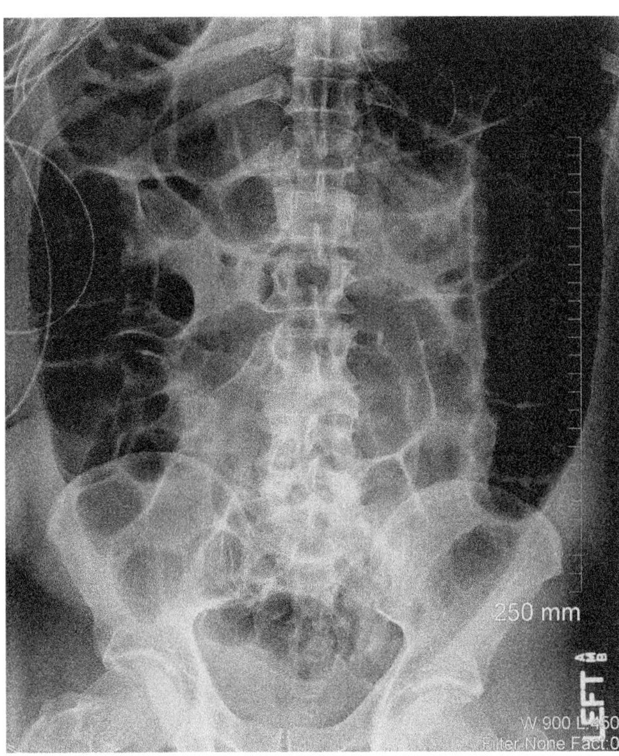

Figure 110.3. Hypodynamic Ileus. Note gas-filled small bowel in the midabdomen, accompanied by gas-filled colon along the periphery.

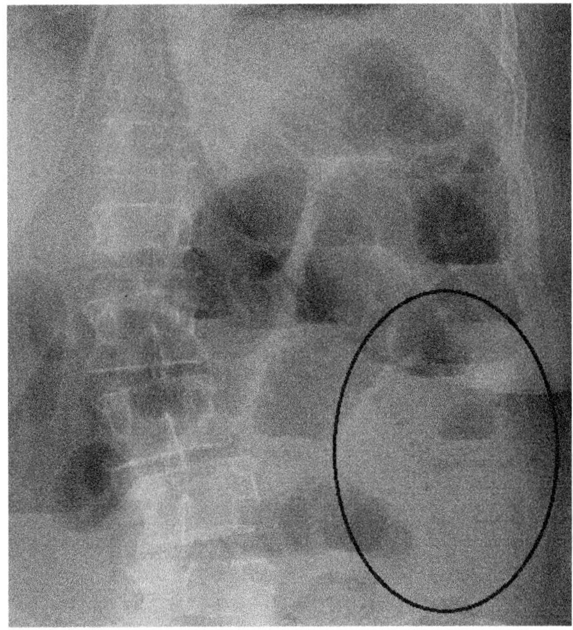

Figure 110.4. Small Bowel Obstruction With the String-of-Pearls Sign (oval): Tiny gas bubbles are trapped along the folds in fluid-filled small bowel. Upright view.

(From Burgess LK, Lee JT, DiSantis DJ. The string of pearls sign. Abdom Radiol [NY]. 2016 Jul;41[7]:1435-6; used with permission.)

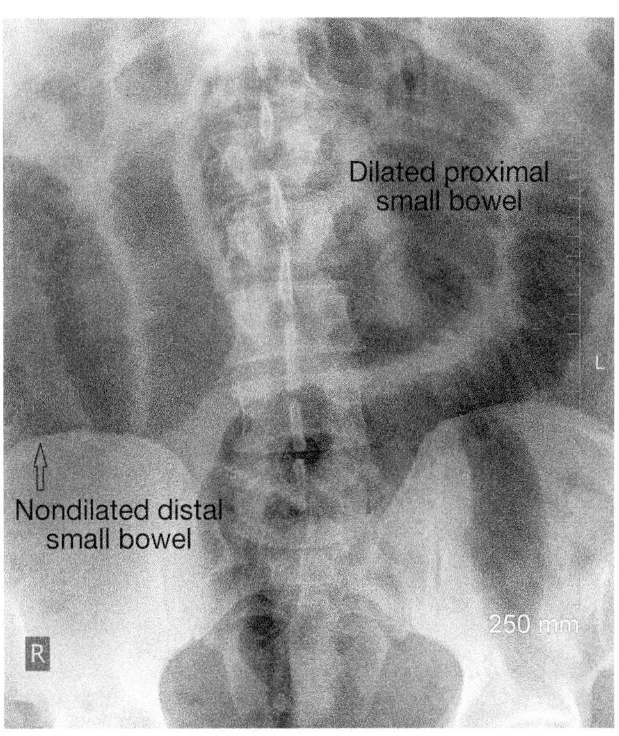

Figure 110.5. Mid to Distal Small Bowel Obstruction. Proximal mid small bowel is gas-filled and dilated, whereas the distal ileum is of normal caliber. L indicates left.

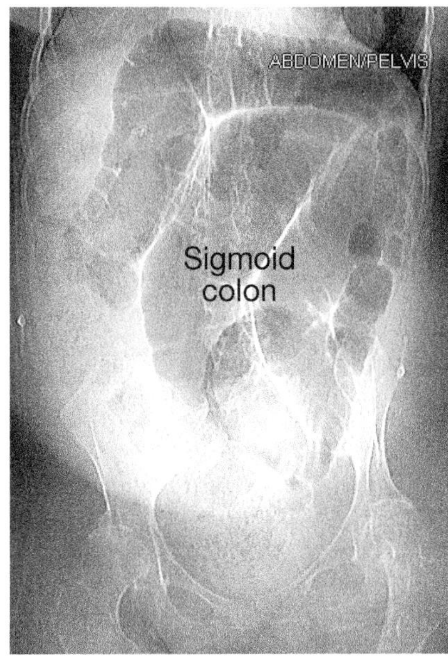

Figure 110.6. Sigmoid Volvulus. Computed tomographic scout view shows gas-filled, dilated colon, particularly in the sigmoid portion.

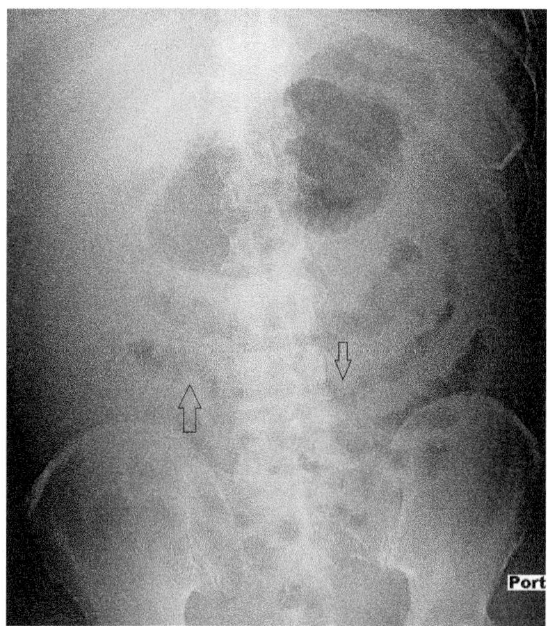

Figure 110.7. Small Bowel Wall Thickening and Nodularity (arrows) in a Patient With Bowel Mural Edema.
(Courtesy of C. O. Menias, MD, Mayo Clinic, Scottsdale, Arizona; used with permission.)

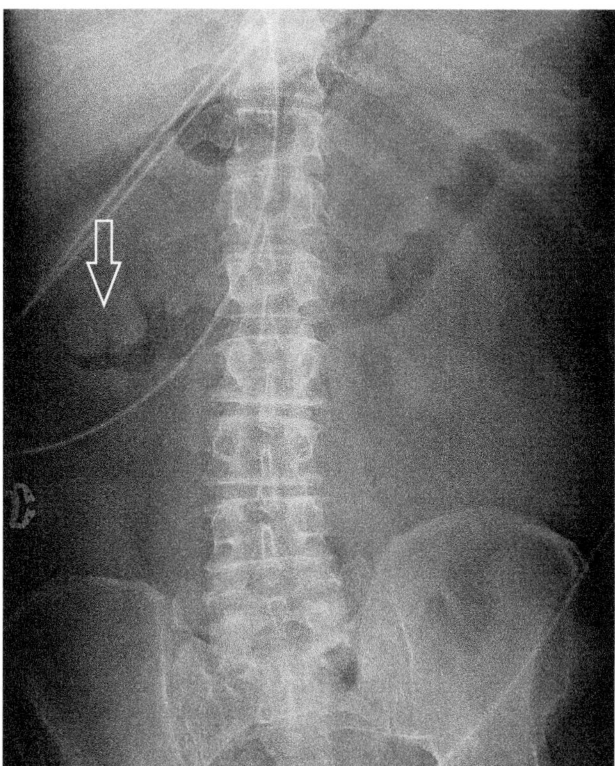

Figure 110.8. Marked Haustral Thickening (arrow) Due to Clostridium difficile *Colitis.*

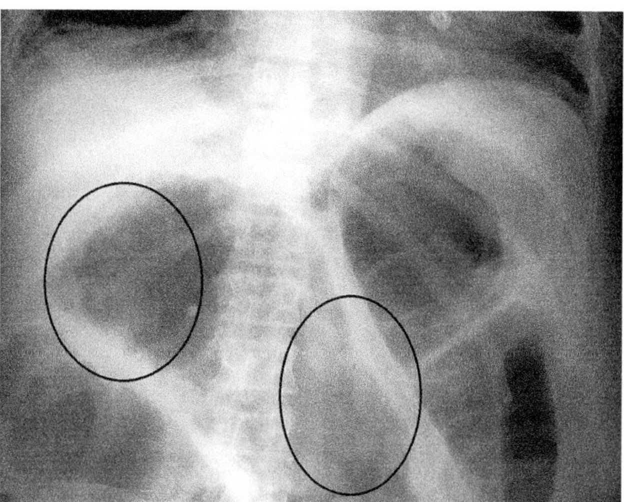

Figure 110.9. Toxic Megacolon. Gaseous colonic distention, particularly in the transverse portion. Nodular mucosal contour (ovals) represents inflammatory pseudopolyps due to extensive ulceration.

dilatation, air-fluid levels, or mural thickening. Less frequently, abdominal radiographs show the more ominous and specific findings of gas in the bowel wall (mural pneumatosis) or in the portal venous system (Figure 110.10). Suspicion of bowel vascular compromise should prompt emergency CT (preferably including CT angiography).

Pneumoperitoneum

Recognizing the radiographic signs of pneumoperitoneum is essential. Free intraperitoneal gas collects beneath the hemidiaphragms on an upright abdominal view (Figure 110.11A) and lateral to the liver on a left lateral decubitus view (Figure 110.11B). The left-side-down view is preferable because gas is more easily discerned adjacent to the liver.

For very ill patients in the intensive care unit, abdominal radiography might be limited to a supine frontal abdominal view; detection of pneumoperitoneum is more difficult and generally requires a large volume of free gas. Various sizes of gas collections in the right upper quadrant, adjacent to or overlying the liver, are most frequent (Figure 110.12). Gas outlining both sides of the bowel wall (Rigler sign) is the next most common clue to pneumoperitoneum on a supine frontal view (Figure 110.13).

Detection of pneumoperitoneum should prompt a thorough review of a patient's history for potential causes. Recent surgery, peritoneal dialysis, or percutaneous enteric tube placement, for example, cause temporary free intraperitoneal gas. A history of any procedure that might be

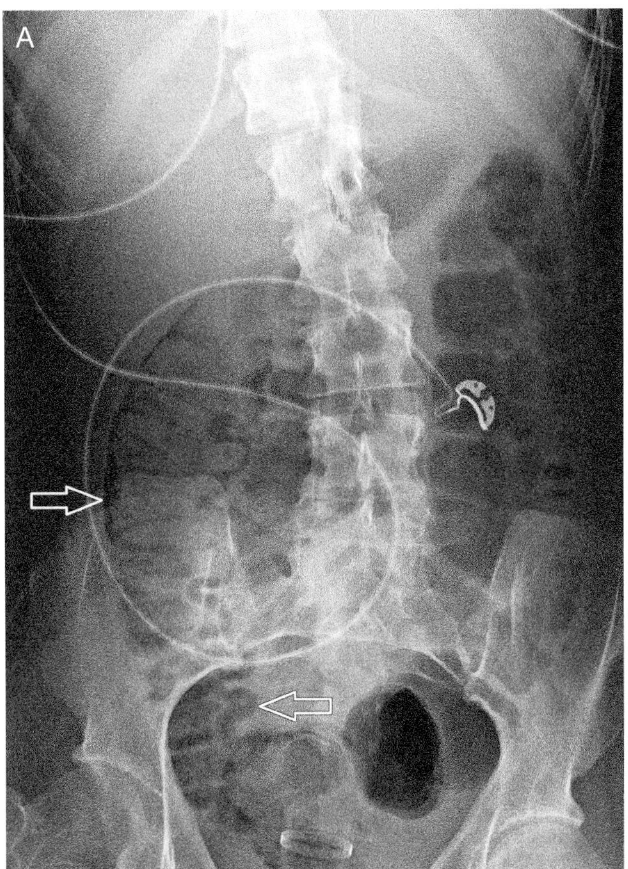

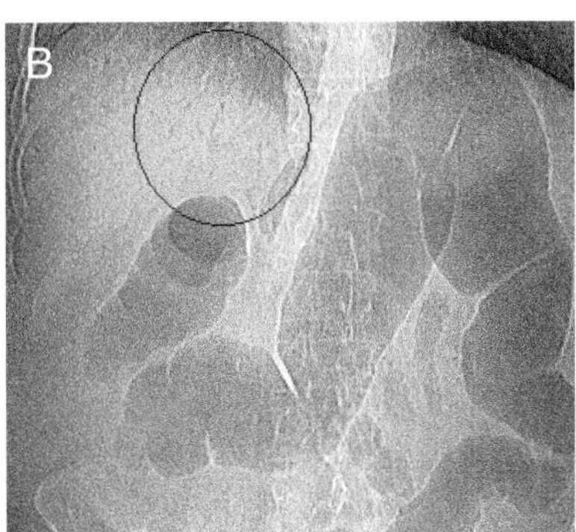

Figure 110.10. *Findings of Bowel Ischemia. A, Bowel mural pneumatosis. Gas in the ascending colon wall (arrows) is due to ischemic colitis. B, Portal venous gas. Computed tomographic scout image. Branching radiolucent (dark) structures reach to the periphery of the liver (circle).*

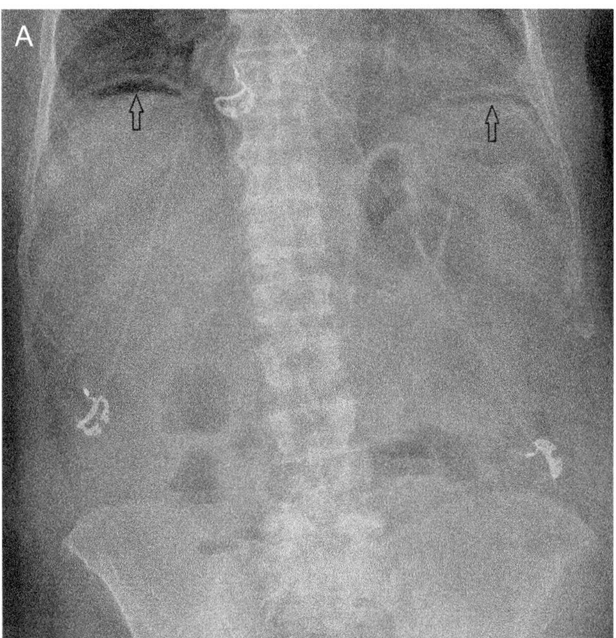

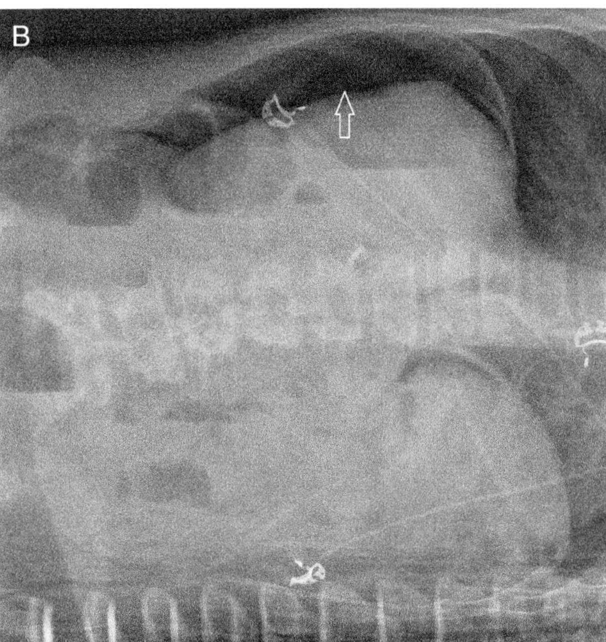

Figure 110.11. *Pneumoperitoneum. A, On upright view, pneumoperitoneum is seen with gas collecting beneath the hemidiaphragms (arrows). B, On left-side-down decubitus view, pneumoperitoneum with free gas (arrow) is seen between the liver and adjacent body wall.*

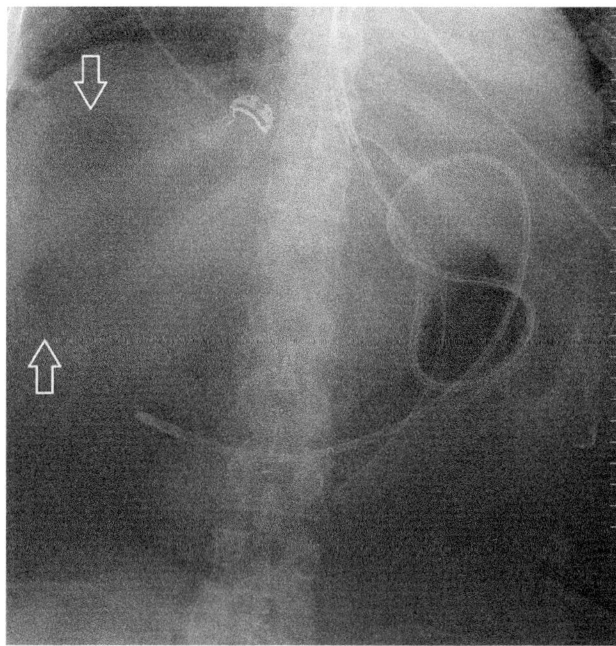

Figure 110.12. Pneumoperitoneum With Gas Accumulating Ventral to the Liver (arrows).

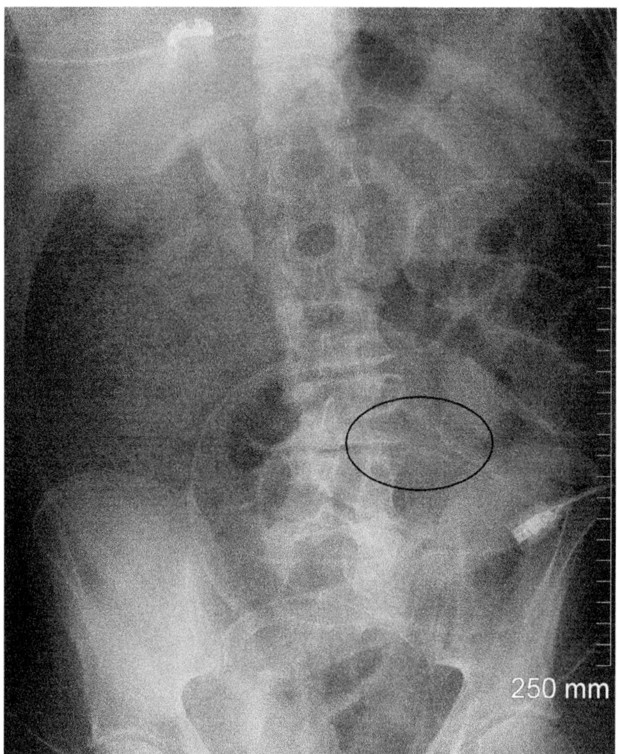

Figure 110.13. Rigler Sign of Pneumoperitoneum. Gas is visible outlining both inside and outside of the bowel walls (oval).

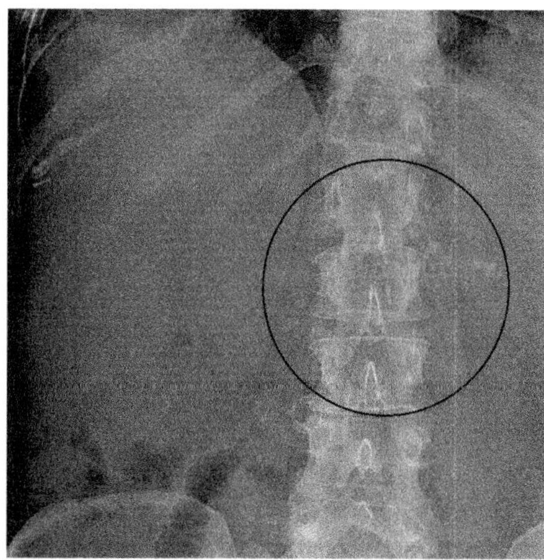

Figure 110.14. Chronic Calcific Pancreatitis. Coarse, heterogeneous calcifications in the midabdomen (circle).

complicated by perforated viscus (such as endoscopy, particularly with biopsy or polypectomy) or known ulcer disease is particularly germane.

Signs of Other Diagnoses

Calcifications visible on abdominal radiographs can provide clues to the diagnosis of cholelithiasis, chronic calcific pancreatitis (Figure 110.14), and urinary tract calculi. Atherosclerotic calcification can indicate mesenteric vascular disease and aneurysms (Figure 110.15).

With large-volume ascites, gas-filled bowel floats near the midline, the flanks bulge, and the abdomen shows overall hazy increased opacity. Bladder distention, hepatosplenomegaly (Figure 110.16), and sizable abdominal or pelvic masses (Figure 110.17) can be identified by their increased opacity or mass effect displacing adjacent bowel. Vigilance for unexpected radiopaque material, such as surgically related paraphernalia, is needed.

Although abdominal radiography can provide valuable diagnostic clues in the acute care setting, CT is more often definitive. Pneumoperitoneum, signs of bowel ischemia, site of bowel obstruction, architecture of the solid organs, and intra-abdominal inflammation are better depicted by CT. If abdominal radiographs obtained in the intensive care unit fail to explain the clinical findings, CT is considered the appropriate next imaging study.

Summary

- For the patient in the intensive care unit, abdominal radiographs can aid in the diagnosis of bowel abnormalities, extraluminal gas, and occasionally vascular and inflammatory abnormalities.
- If abdominal radiography provides no definitive answer, CT is the appropriate next imaging study.

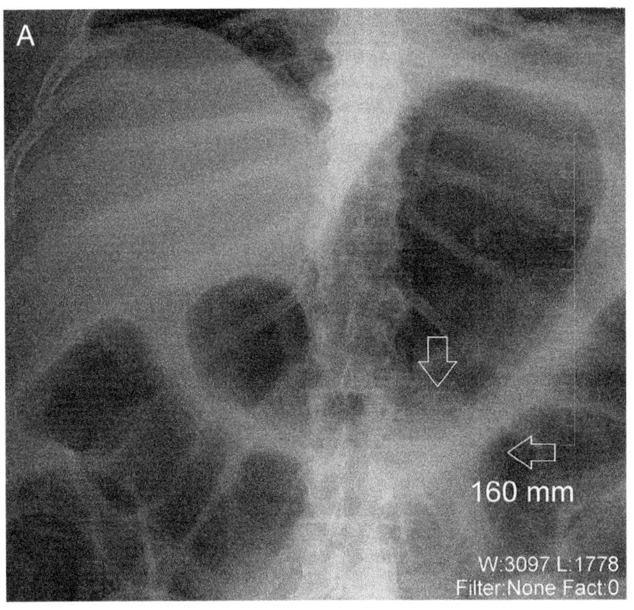

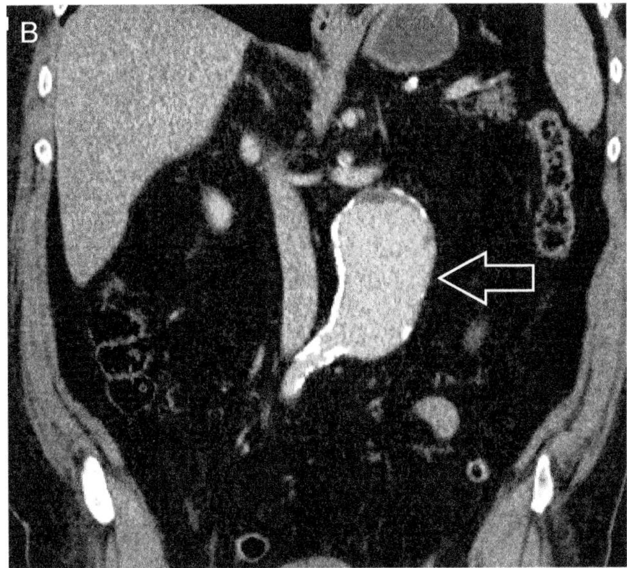

Figure 110.15. Calcified Abdominal Aortic Aneurysm. A, Findings on abdominal radiography (arrows). B, Corresponding contrast-enhanced coronal computed tomographic view depicts the aneurysm (arrow).

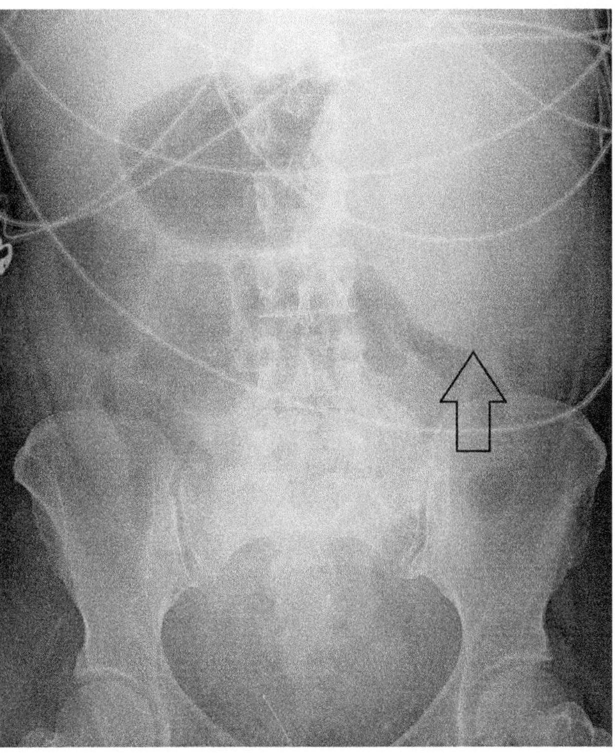

Figure 110.16. Splenomegaly (arrow) Displacing Adjacent Gas-filled Bowel.

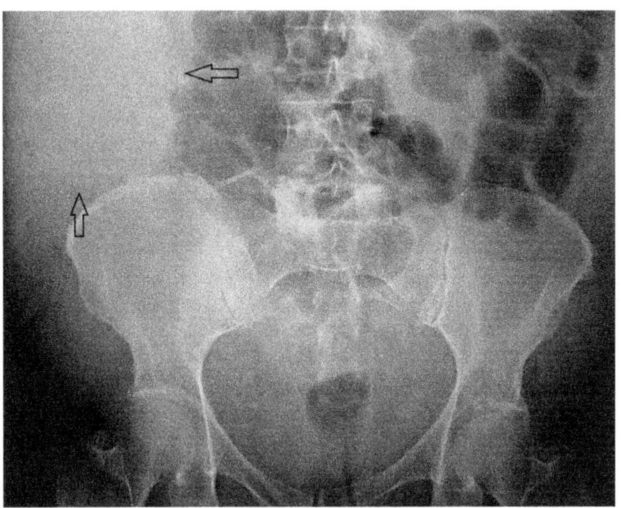

Figure 110.17. Extraperitoneal Hematoma (arrows).

SUGGESTED READING

American College of Radiology ACR Appropriateness Criteria [Internet]. Acute (nonlocalized) abdominal pain and fever or suspected abdominal abscess. [cited 2018 Mar 1]. Available from: https://acsearch.acr.org/docs/69467/Narrative/.

Bertin CL, Ponthus S, Vivekanantham H, Poletti PA, Kherad O, Rutschmann OT. Overuse of plain abdominal radiography in emergency departments: a retrospective cohort study. BMC Health Serv Res. 2019 Jan 14; 19(1):36.

Chawla A, Peh WCG. Abdominal radiographs in the emergency department: current status and controversies. J Med Radiat Sci. 2018 Dec;65(4):250–1.

Egri C, Darras KE, Scali EP, Harris AC. Classification of error in abdominal imaging: pearls and pitfalls for radiologists. Can Assoc Radiol J. 2018 Nov;69(4):409–16. Epub 2018 Oct 11.

Fernandez M, Craig S. Appropriateness of adult plain abdominal radiograph requesting in a regional emergency department. J Med Imaging Radiat Oncol. 2019 Apr;63(2):175–82. Epub 2019 Jan 10.

Geng WZM, Fuller M, Osborne B, Thoirs K. The value of the erect abdominal radiograph for the diagnosis of mechanical bowel obstruction and paralytic ileus in adults presenting with acute abdominal pain. J Med Radiat Sci. 2018 Dec;65(4):259–66. Epub 2018 Jul 23.

Levine MS, Scheiner JD, Rubesin SE, Laufer I, Herlinger H. Diagnosis of pneumoperitoneum on supine abdominal radiographs. AJR Am J Roentgenol. 1991 Apr;156(4):731–5.

MacKersie AB, Lane MJ, Gerhardt RT, Claypool HA, Keenan S, Katz DS, et al. Nontraumatic acute abdominal pain: unenhanced helical CT compared with three-view acute abdominal series. Radiology. 2005 Oct;237(1):114–22.

Nevitt PC. The string of pearls sign. Radiology. 2000 Jan;214(1):157–8.

Paulson EK, Thompson WM. Review of small-bowel obstruction: the diagnosis and when to worry. Radiology. 2015 May;275(2):332–42.

Stoker J, van Randen A, Lameris W, Boermeester MA. Imaging patients with acute abdominal pain. Radiology. 2009 Oct;253(1):31–46.

Fluoroscopy: Principles and Safety

DAVID M. SELLA, MD; GLENN M. STURCHIO, PhD;
BETH A. SCHUELER, PhD

Goals

- Understand the basic components of fluoroscopic imaging systems.
- Discuss ways to minimize fluoroscopic dose to patients.
- Discuss ways to minimize personnel exposure when operating fluoroscopic equipment.

Introduction

Fluoroscopy is a valuable tool that can be used in critically ill patients. Detrimental effects on a patient physiologically and on hospital resources from unnecessary transport can be minimized with bedside procedures performed by an appropriately trained team. Operators must understand the basics of fluoroscopic imaging systems, radiation dose, and the ways in which exposure can be limited to both patients and personnel to avoid undesirable effects.

Fluoroscopic Imaging Systems

Fluoroscopic systems include an x-ray tube, generator, image receptor, and video system for image display and recording (Figure 111.1). A collimator defines the shape of the x-ray beam, automatically limiting the x-ray beam to the image receptor field of view; manual adjustment allows a smaller field. Fluoroscopy is performed with either continuous x-ray generation or x-ray pulses with frame rates ranging from 1 to 30 frames per second. Pulsed fluoroscopy is useful for examining moving structures by reducing the motion blur that occurs within each image as a result of the shorter acquisition time. Higher-dose image acquisition can consist of a single exposure or a series at frame rates ranging from 1 to 30 frames per second.

Both image intensifiers and flat-panel detectors are used for fluoroscopy image receptors. Image intensifiers convert x-rays into light, and a video camera captures the output image and displays it on a monitor. Flat-panel detectors are solid-state devices that produce a digital electronic signal.

Radiation Dose

Patient Exposure

For monitoring radiation dose to patients, fluoroscopy systems display the entrance-skin air kerma in milligrays during the procedure. Air kerma rates for an average-sized adult abdomen range from 20 to 60 mGy/min. Radiation effects include both tissue damage and increased cancer risk. Transient erythema requires a threshold dose of 2,000 mGy, and more severe effects (eg, epilation and desquamation) result from higher doses. Cancer induction is thought to have no threshold dose. As a result, care must be taken to minimize radiation exposure when performing fluoroscopic procedures.

Fluoroscopic dose can be reduced by minimizing beam-on time. Moreover, fluoroscopy should not be used if the operator is not looking at the image display. In addition, last-image–hold should be used for review and stored for image archive as an alternative to an additional acquired image. Fluoroscopy systems typically have several dose rate modes available for selection. Using low dose rate and low frame rate pulsed fluoroscopy mode minimizes radiation dose. Collimator blades should be adjusted to include only the area of clinical interest to reduce patient dose by reducing exposed tissue.

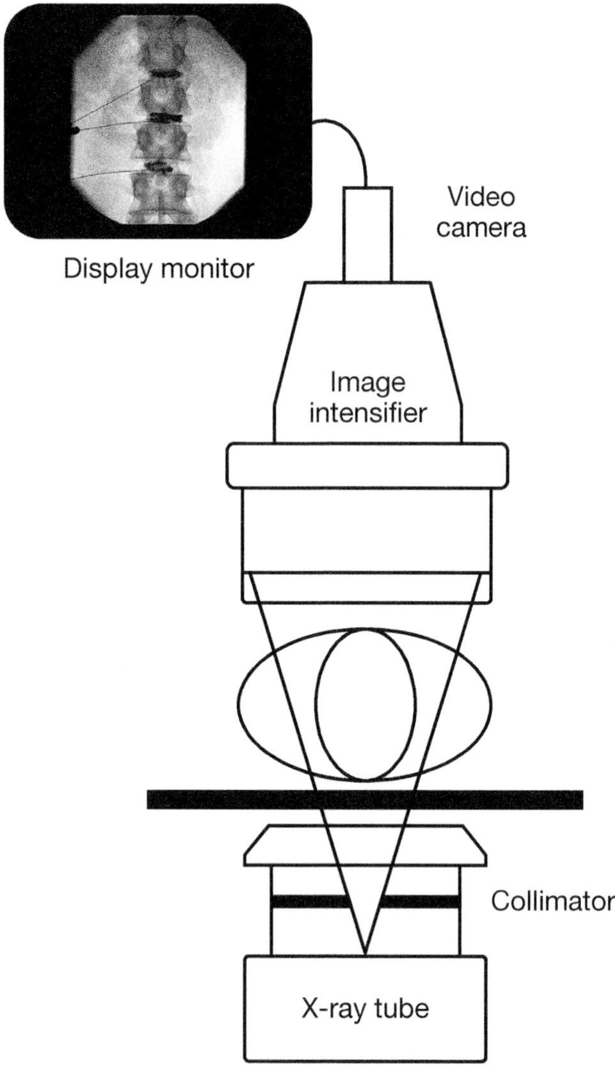

Figure 111.1. Components of a Fluoroscopic System.

When the patient is positioned for fluoroscopy, the entrance skin surface should be positioned as far as possible from the x-ray tube. Also, the image receptor should be as close as possible to the exit surface. Both of these actions result in lower patient dose. Because the dose rate typically increases as magnification increases, magnification modes should be used only when necessary. The fluoroscopy operator should use the displayed patient air kerma value to monitor the delivered dose throughout the procedure.

Personnel Exposure

Monitoring radiation to personnel is essential to ensure worker safety. Specific protocols are determined by the radiation safety officer. For reliable tracking of occupational dose, dosimeters must be worn consistently. The recommended annual dose limit for personnel is 50 mSv to the whole body and 150 mSv to the lens of the eye.

Scattered x-rays from the patient are the major source of personnel radiation exposure. These x-rays travel in all directions, originating from the patient with dose rates typically from 1 to 10 mGy/h at the operator's position. Because scatter x-ray dose is generally proportional to patient dose, implementation of the patient dose reduction techniques described above decrease personnel radiation dose proportionally.

Figure 111.2 shows a scatter isodose plot for a C-arm fluoroscopy configuration with an under-table x-ray tube. The scatter radiation intensity for a lateral projection is shown in Figure 111.3. When possible, personnel move back from the exposed area of the patient because the scatter levels decrease rapidly. For C-arm fluoroscopy systems, the x-ray tube should be placed under the patient table. When the C-arm is angled or positioned horizontally, personnel should stand nearest the image receptor. For stationary over-table x-ray tube fluoroscopy systems, the highest intensity of scatter radiation is directed toward the upper body and head of an operator.

Radiation shielding devices include aprons, thyroid shields, leaded eyewear, and mobile shields mounted on the floor, ceiling, or procedure table. Because these devices generally block more than 90% of incident radiation, they are useful for reducing personnel exposure.

Thyroid shields are recommended for personnel whose collar radiation monitors indicate more than 4 mSv per month. These shields are less critical for personnel older than 40 years because their risk of radiation-induced thyroid cancer is reduced considerably.

Similarly, leaded eyewear is recommended when collar readings exceed 4 mSv per month. Investigations on the radiosensitivity of the eye indicate that the threshold dose may be lower, and current dose-limit recommendations are being reassessed. Careful attention must be given to radiation protection of the eye, especially for personnel routinely using over-table x-ray tube systems. Ceiling-suspended shields can also provide substantial eye protection to fluoroscopy operators.

All personnel present in the procedure room during fluoroscopy must have knowledge of safe operating procedures in a radiation environment. Those performing the procedure must be thoroughly familiar with the particular fluoroscopic equipment used and dose-reduction and image-quality optimization principles.

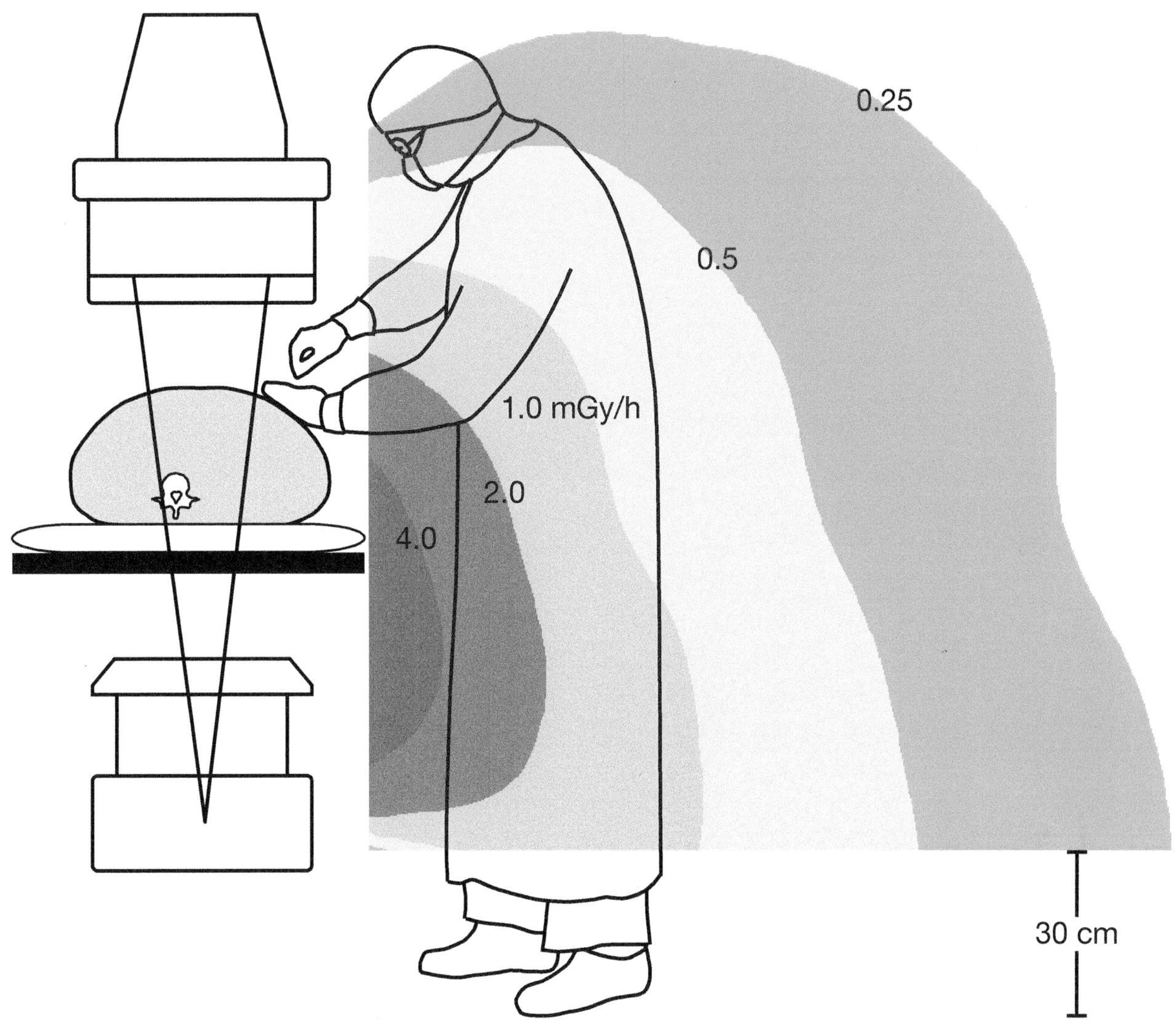

Figure 111.2. Scatter Radiation Isodose Plot for a C-arm Fluoroscopy System With Undertable X-Ray Tube and Overtable Image Receptor.

(From Schueler BA, Vrieze TJ, Bjarnason H, Stanson AW. An investigation of operator exposure in interventional radiology. Radiographics. 2006 Sep-Oct;26[5]:1533-41; used with permission.)

Summary

- Monitoring radiation dose with fluoroscopy is important because undesired radiation effects include both tissue damage and increased cancer risk.
- Fluoroscopic dose can be reduced by appropriate patient positioning, minimizing beam-on time, use of low-dose rate and low-frame-rate pulsed fluoroscopy mode, collimator blades, and last-image–hold for archiving.
- Radiation exposure to personnel can be minimized by implementing dose-reduction techniques and use of radiation shielding devices.

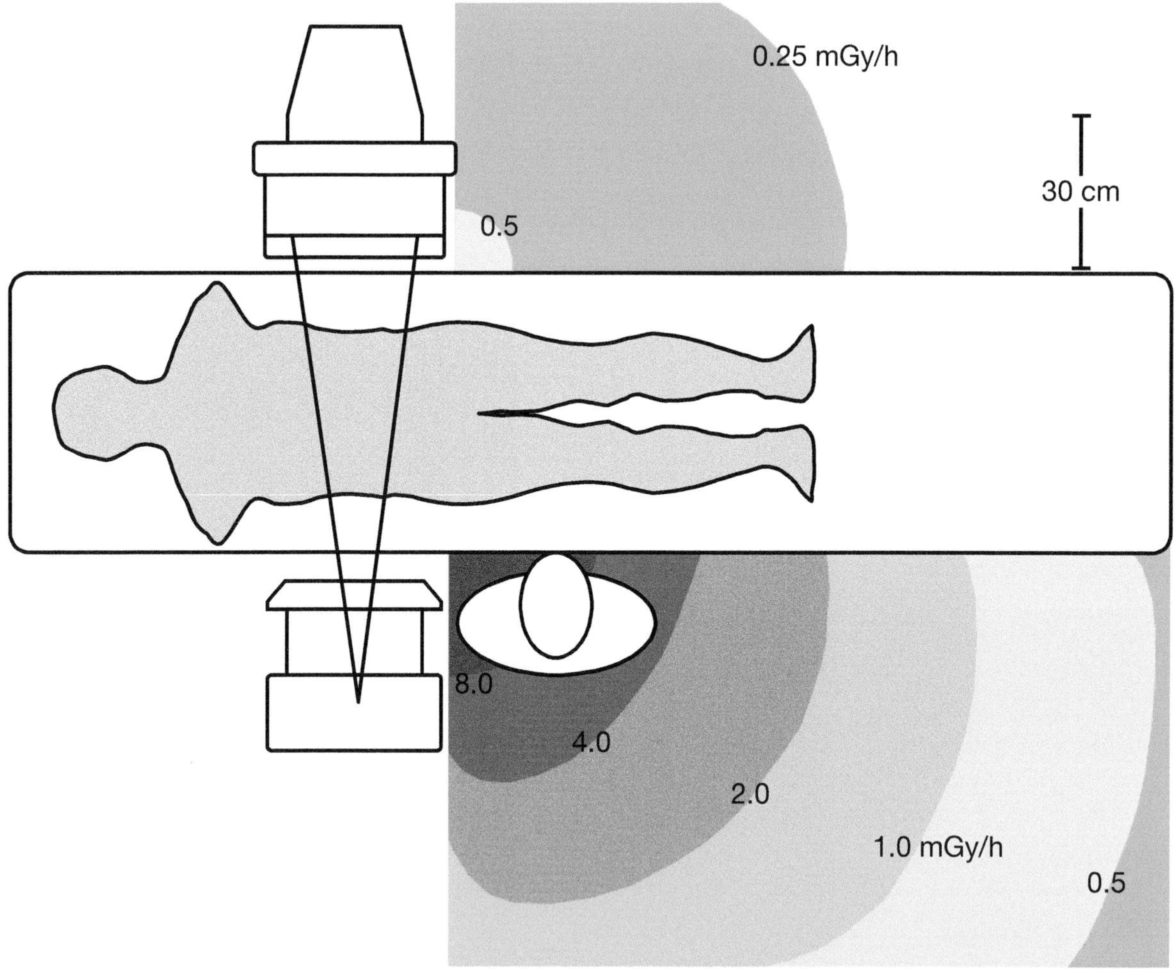

Figure 111.3. *Scatter Radiation Isodose Plot for a C-arm Fluoroscopy System in a Lateral Projection.*
(From Schueler BA. Operator shielding: how and why. Tech Vasc Interv Radiol. 2010 Sep;13[3]:167-71; used with permission.)

SUGGESTED READING

Crowhurst J, Whitby M. Lowering fluoroscopy pulse rates to reduce radiation dose during cardiac procedures. J Med Radiat Sci. 2018 Dec;65(4):247–9.

Fiorilli PN, Kobayashi T, Giri J, Hirshfeld JW Jr. Strategies for radiation exposure-sparing in fluoroscopically guided invasive cardiovascular procedures. Catheter Cardiovasc Interv. 2019 Apr 13. [Epub ahead of print]

International Commission on Radiological Protection (ICRP). 2012 ICRP statement on tissue reactions/early and late effects of radiation in normal tissues and organs: threshold doses for tissue reactions in a radiation protection context [Internet]. ICRP Publication 118. Ann. ICRP 41(1/2); c2012. Available from: http://www.icrp.org/publication.asp?id=ICRP%20Publication%20118.

Kinnin J, Hanna TN, Jutras M, Hasan B, Bhatia R, Khosa F. Top 100 cited articles on radiation exposure in medical imaging: a bibliometric analysis. Curr Probl Diagn Radiol. 2018 Mar 20. pii: S0363-0188(18)30016-1. [Epub ahead of print]

Mettler FA Jr. Medical radiation exposure in the United States: 2006-2016 trends. Health Phys. 2019 Feb;116(2):126–8.

National Council on Radiation Protection and Measurements (NCRP). Limitation of exposure to ionizing radiation [Internet]. NCRP Report No. 116. Bethesda (MD): National Council on Radiation Protection and Measurements; c1993. Available from: https://ncrponline.org/publications/reports/ncrp-reports-116/.

Schueler BA. Operator shielding: how and why. Tech Vasc Interv Radiol. 2010 Sep;13(3):167–71.

Schueler BA, Vrieze TJ, Bjarnason H, Stanson AW. An investigation of operator exposure in interventional radiology. Radiographics. 2006 Sep-Oct;26(5):1533–41.

Urakov TM. Practical assessment of radiation exposure in spine surgery. World Neurosurg. 2018 Dec;120:e752–4. Epub 2018 Aug 30.

Wagner LK, Archer BR. Minimizing risks from fluoroscopic X-rays: bioeffects, instrumentation, and examination. 4th ed. The Woodlands (TX): Partners in Radiation Management; c2004.

112 Ultrasonography

SANTIAGO NARANJO-SIERRA, MD; LAUREN K. NG TUCKER, MD

Goals

- Describe the usefulness of ultrasonography in the intensive care unit.
- Describe the applications of ultrasonography in the intensive care unit.
- Describe the limitations of ultrasonography in the intensive care unit.

Introduction

Ultrasonography is the use of sound waves to create images and is used mainly for diagnostic purposes and for real-time guidance during procedures. The use of ultrasonography by nonradiologist physicians began in the 1950s, and now its use extends to many areas of medicine. Point-of-care ultrasonography is widely used in fields such as anesthesia, critical care, and emergency medicine, in which it is becoming an important part of the current standard of care because of its ability to provide accurate visual information about a patient, either to rapidly evaluate clinical status or to provide guidance for procedures, without requiring transfers to other areas. For patients in an intensive care unit, focused ultrasonography has been reported to result in management changes in more than 50%. However, rigorous studies that show improved outcomes are still lacking.

Applications of Bedside Ultrasonography in Critical Care Medicine

Procedural Guidance

Vascular Access

The standard of care for placing invasive vascular access in the intensive care unit involves real-time ultrasound guidance instead of landmark guidance. International evidence-based guidelines recommend continuous visualization of the needle during its trajectory (in-plane technique) when the major cannulation risk is penetrating the posterior wall of the vein, but a transverse view is recommended in the setting of small target vessels or when vital structures are near the target vessel. The current Guidelines for the Appropriate Use of Bedside General and Cardiac Ultrasonography in the Evaluation of Critically Ill Patients highlights that the short-axis view is used during insertion to improve the success rate.

Other Procedures

The same evidence-based guidelines recommend ultrasound guidance for paracentesis and thoracentesis.

Focused Cardiac Ultrasonography

Focused critical care echocardiography is defined as a time-sensitive examination performed by noncardiologists that can be done serially to evaluate circulatory or respiratory failure. The number of possible diagnoses that can be investigated is limited (eg, tamponade, hypovolemic shock, and severe ventricular dysfunction), and several anatomical areas can be evaluated, including the abdomen, thorax, and central veins. The definition emphasizes that the examination is not intended to replace a comprehensive echocardiographic examination.

Current evidence suggests that nonradiologists can perform and interpret focused echocardiography, and emergency physicians, trauma surgeons, and intensivists are increasingly doing so. The cardiac ultrasound transducer has a small footprint to create acoustic windows through intercostal spaces, and firmly pressing the probe to the skin (on which conductive gel is placed) is essential to obtain adequate views. The transducer should be held like a pen for all views except the subcostal view, for which it should instead be gripped from the top. The indicator on the transducer corresponds to the marker on the side of the ultrasound sector on the monitor. The procurement of echocardiographic views with focused cardiac ultrasonography is summarized in Table 112.1.

Table 112.1 • Characteristics of Focused Cardiac Ultrasonography

View	Location of Transducer	Probe Orientation Marker	Depth, cm	Helpful Tips
Subcostal	2-3 cm below xyphoid process or RUQ if chest tubes are placed	About 2- to 3-o'clock	20-25	Hold the transducer from the top; apply angulations between 10° and 40° Supine position
Subcostal: IVC	From the previous view, rotate the transducer 90° counterclockwise	About 12 o'clock	15-20	Keep right atrium to IVC junction on the screen. Need to see the IVC merging into right atrium
Apical	Point of maximal impulse if feasible, or start anterior axillar line toward the nipple using a zigzag movement and maintain a 60° angle with thoracic wall. Under the breast crease in female patients	About 3 o'clock	15-20	Ensure good contact with the rib (gentle pressure) and maintain a 60° angle with chest wall
Parasternal: long-axis	3rd-4th intercostal space	About 10- to 11-o'clock	12-20 (up to 24 if pleural-pericardial effusion)	Try in supine position first. If any difficulty, then proceed with left lateral decubitus position
Parasternal: short-axis	Rotate 90° clockwise from the parasternal long-axis view	About 2-o'clock	12-16	With "tilting" movement of the probe Aortic valve level: the transducer faces slightly upward toward the patient's right shoulder Mitral valve level: the transducer is perpendicular to chest wall Papillary muscle level: the transducer faces slightly downward toward patient's left flank

Abbreviations: IVC, inferior vena cava; RUQ, right upper quadrant.

From Ratzlaff RA, Builes A, Diaz-Gomez JL. Current practical applications of ultrasonography in surgical anesthesia. Adv Anesth. 2015;33:129-55; used with permission.

Focused cardiac ultrasonography is not only important for evaluating of cardiac structure (enlargement, hypertrophy) and estimating ventricular function but also helpful for recognizing pericardial effusion and cardiac tamponade and assessing volume status. Volume status is assessed by visualizing the inferior vena cava (IVC) and measuring the collapsibility index (patients with spontaneous breathing) or the distensibility index (patients receiving mechanical ventilatory support). To calculate the distensibility index, the following formula is used:

$$\text{distensibility index} = (\text{IVC maximal diameter [end inspiration]} - \text{IVC minimal diameter [end exhalation]} / \text{IVC minimal diameter [end exhalation]}) \times 100 (\text{expressed as percentage}).$$

A distensibility index of more than 18% predicts fluid responsiveness with a positive predictive value of 93% and a negative predictive value of 92%. The index was validated in mechanically ventilated patients in sinus rhythm with tidal volumes ranging from 8 to 15 mL/kg of ideal body weight. A small tidal volume can lead to false-negative results, whereas an excessive tidal volume can lead to false-positive results and right ventricular failure. A left ventricular end-diastolic area less than 5.5 cm^2 is also highly suggestive of intravascular volume-depletion status.

Pericardial effusions can be visualized, but it is important to evaluate them in several views. Occasionally, a swinging heart can be seen within an effusion, but it is not very common. Special care must be taken for patients who have had cardiothoracic surgery because they sometimes have posterior pericardial effusions that can be seen only with a transesophageal study. Some findings such as the inversion or collapse of structures of the right side of the heart (right atrium during systole, more sensitive; right ventricle during diastole, more specific) or distended (noncompliant) IVC can suggest that the physiologic events of tamponade are occurring. Right ventricular collapse may not be seen in conditions such as right ventricular hypertrophy or pulmonary hypertension.

For patients who have had cardiac arrest and return of spontaneous circulation, an evidence-based recommendation is to use ultrasonography to look for segmental wall motion abnormalities and rule out coronary artery disease as the cause for arrest. Evaluation of segmental wall motion abnormalities and some conditions such as endocarditis requires a high level of training and, therefore, echocardiographers should always be involved in the diagnostic process. According to the current guidelines, transesophageal echocardiography should be performed in all cases of suspected infective endocarditis.

Lung Ultrasonography

The accuracy of lung ultrasound is good for identifying pleural entities such as pneumothorax or pleural effusion and parenchymal conditions such as pulmonary edema or pneumonia. In addition, the use of ultrasonography for evaluation of respiratory failure has been described.

For ultrasonography of the lungs, the chest wall can be divided into quadrants. Because patients receiving critical care are mainly in the supine position, the examination emphasizes the anterior aspect of the thorax, where the linear probe should be longitudinally applied perpendicular to the wall for all quadrants. After that, the examination requires use of the phased-array transducer to evaluate the deeper tissues. Diagnosis from results of lung ultrasonography is based on recognition of patterns that are suggestive of associated diseases.

Sliding of the visceral and parietal pleura during respiration produces the finding of lung sliding, which indicates that both surfaces are intact. A-lines are a normal finding produced by reverberation artifacts of parietal pleural reflections. B-lines (lung comets) are also artifacts produced when ultrasound waves interact with small air-fluid interfaces, as in alveolar interstitial syndrome. The presence of lung sliding and B-lines rules out a pneumothorax, and ultrasonography seems to be superior to chest radiography for detecting it.

The International Consensus Conference on Lung Ultrasound standardized lung ultrasonographic signs and suggested a sequential approach for lung ultrasonography.

Integration of Cardiac and Lung Ultrasonography

For evaluation of patients with circulatory or respiratory failure, a combination of cardiac and lung ultrasonography is crucial. For example, it can facilitate characterization of pulmonary edema, differentiating hydrostatic from nonhydrostatic pulmonary edema. A sequence for a focused assessment is shown in Figure 112.1. Algorithms for echocardiographic assessment of unstable patients in the intensive care unit have been published. The algorithm in Figure 112.1 is a focused, methodical approach to a patient in shock. An algorithm for focused lung and cardiac ultrasonography perioperatively for a patient in shock is shown in Figure 112.2.

Abdominal Ultrasonography

Abdominal ultrasonography is recommended when acalculous cholecystitis is suspected, to exclude mechanical causes of acute renal failure, and to evaluate ascites. In the trauma setting, abdominal ultrasonography is used to establish the presence of free fluid (which indicates bleeding) with the focused assessment with sonography for trauma protocol. Abdominal ultrasonography also has other potential applications, such as ruling out free air suggestive of hollow viscus rupture, evaluating the abdominal aorta to detect aneurysm rupture or dissection, observing gut peristalsis, and assessing gastric volume.

Vascular Ultrasonography of the Lower Extremities

Acute thromboembolic disease is a common cause of acute respiratory failure in patients in critical care units. Vascular bedside ultrasonography is a reliable tool that may provide a prompt diagnosis of deep vein thrombosis and could be helpful when pulmonary embolism is suspected, particularly in combination with cardiac and lung ultrasonography.

Evidence shows that critical care physicians can rapidly and accurately diagnose lower extremity proximal deep vein thrombosis using compression ultrasonography at the bedside.

Optic Nerve Ultrasonography

Measurement of optic nerve sheath diameter with ultrasonography has good accuracy for detection of intracranial hypertension, an advantage that allows for early management of intracranial hypertension, especially when

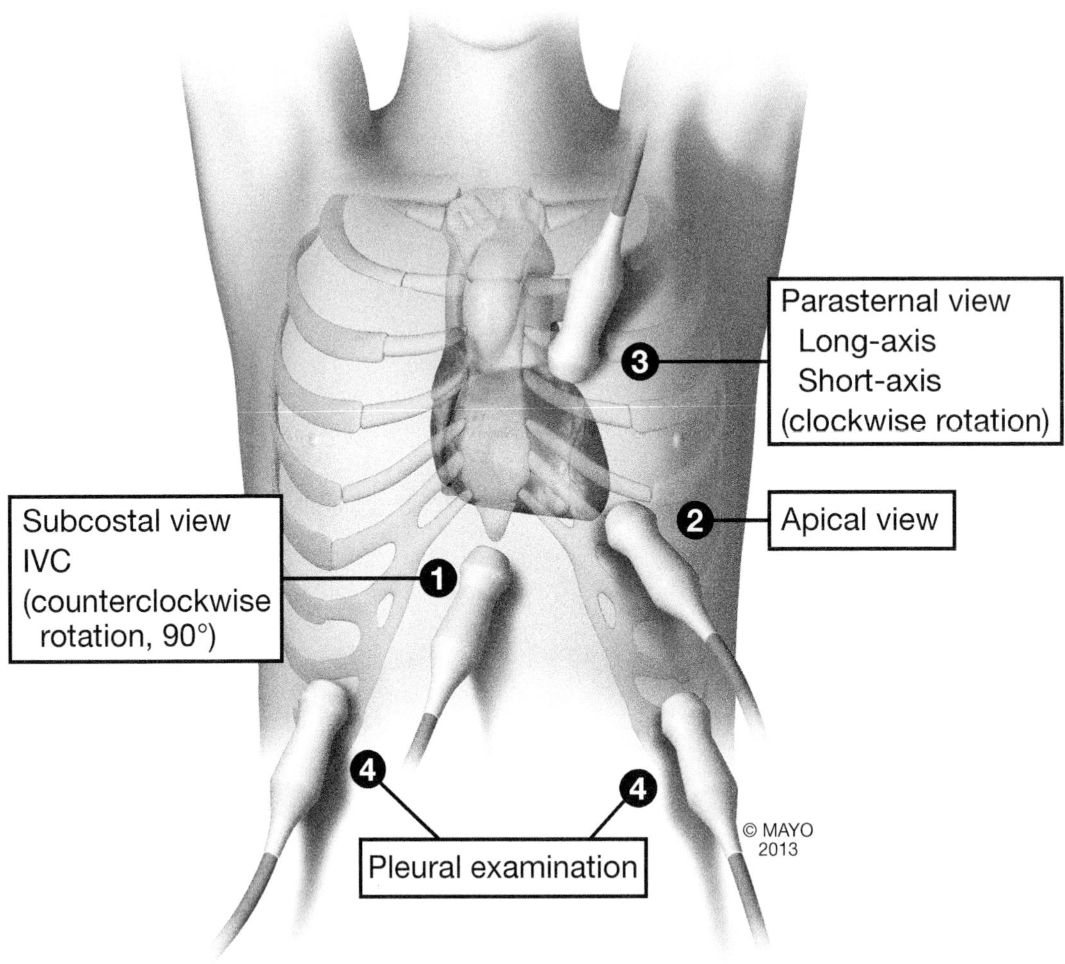

Figure 112.1. The Focused Assessment With Transthoracic Echocardiography Protocol. IVC indicates inferior vena cava. (From Ratzlaff RA, Builes A, Diaz-Gomez JL. Current practical applications of ultrasonography in surgical anesthesia. Adv Anesth. 2015;33:129-55; used with permission of Mayo Foundation for Medical Education and Research.)

intracranial pressure monitoring is unavailable or contraindicated. Although it is a useful tool, invasive intracranial devices remain the standard for intracranial pressure monitoring. Also, optic nerve sonography has no agreed-on thresholds, and its accuracy is influenced by operator expertise.

Limitations

The limitations of ultrasonography performed in the intensive care unit are related to the current lack of formal training for physicians and to patient characteristics. For example, suboptimal positioning; the presence of edema, subcutaneous emphysema, severe chronic lung disease, mechanical ventilator, chest wall deformity, and even fatty tissue; and the postoperative state can often interfere with image acquisition. In most patients, at least 1 "good" view can be obtained, and often it can be enough to provide helpful information for the diagnostic and therapeutic approaches.

The main problem with this powerful tool is its dependence on operator skill. Acquiring the expertise needed to perform ultrasound studies requires time and practice, and misdiagnosis resulting from incorrect interpretation of the data can lead to wrong decisions.

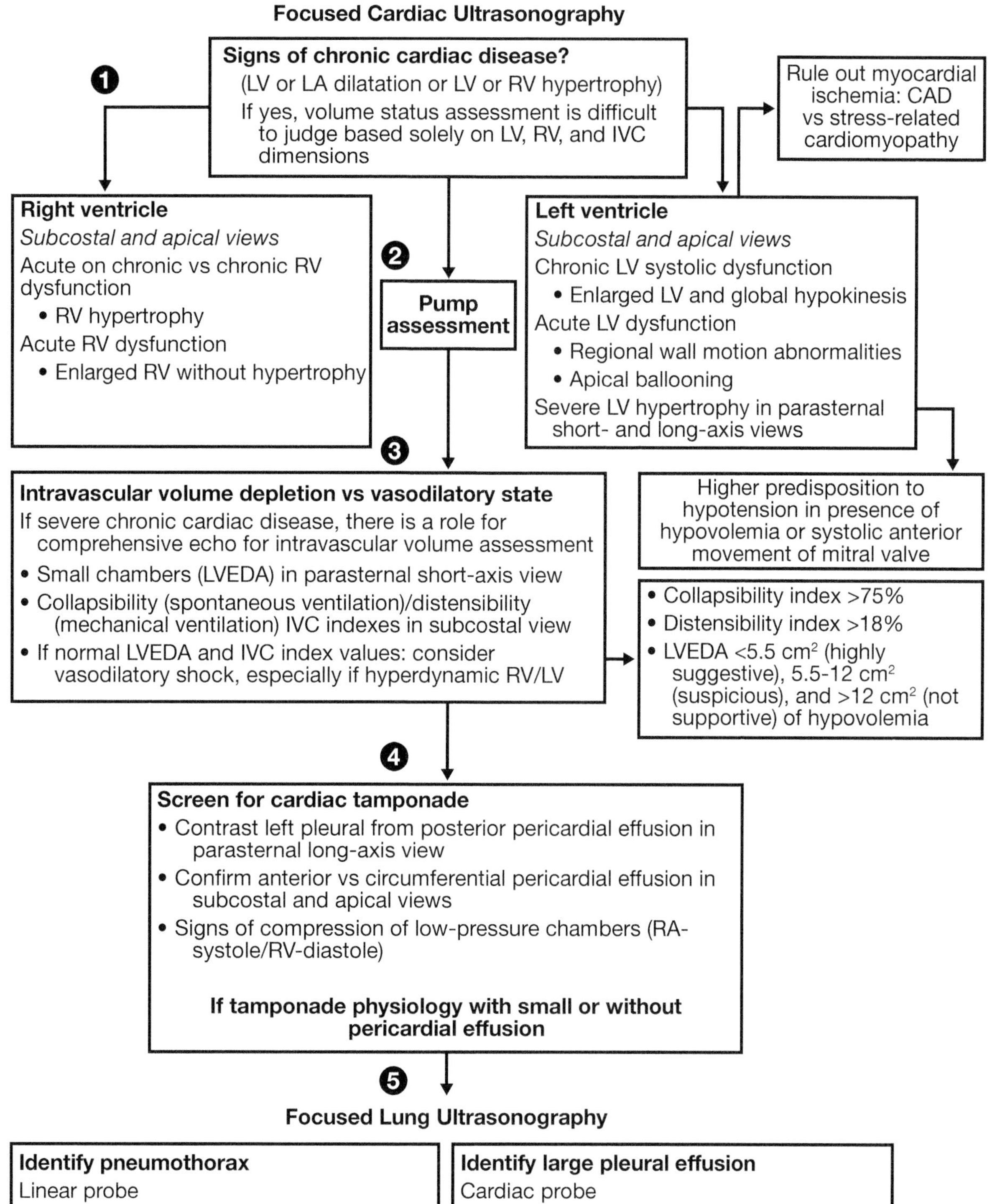

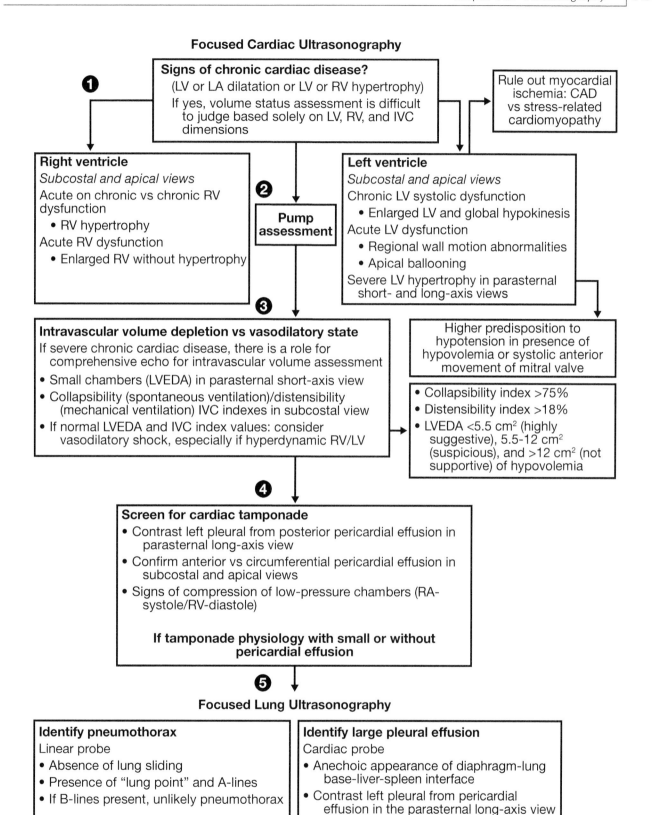

Figure 112.2. Practical and Methodical Approach to Shock With Focused Cardiac and Lung Ultrasonography. The examinations should be conducted in sequence, as numbered. CAD indicates coronary artery disease; echo, echocardiography; IVC, inferior vena cava; LA, left atrium; LV, left ventricle; LVEDA, left ventricular end-diastolic area; RA, right atrium; RV, right ventricle.

(From Diaz-Gomez JL, Via G, Ramakrishna H. Focused cardiac and lung ultrasonography: implications and applicability in the perioperative period. Rom J Anaesth Intensive Care. 2016 Apr;23[1]:41-54; used with permission of Mayo Foundation for Medical Education and Research.)

Training and Certification

Current opinion recommends that advanced training is necessary to achieve the goals for use of ultrasonography, particularly in the intensive care unit. As such, awareness of the key role of formal training and of mentored or proctored review of images is increasing in the medical community around the world. Guidelines for training and competency have already been published, and most experts believe that formal training should include examination interpretation, performing supervised studies, and theoretical competencies. European and American groups are moving toward establishing a certification process for critical care ultrasonography.

Summary

- Ultrasonography is a useful diagnostic and procedural instrument in the intensive care unit because of its noninvasiveness, safety, and lack of radiation.
- Ultrasonography performed in intensive care units can assist the decision-making process by improving diagnostic accuracy, facilitating therapeutic interventions, and evaluating the response to changes in management.

SUGGESTED READING

Baddour LM, Wilson WR, Bayer AS, Fowler VG Jr, Tleyjeh IM, Rybak MJ, et al; American Heart Association Committee on Rheumatic Fever, Endocarditis, and Kawasaki Disease of the Council on Cardiovascular Disease in the Young, Council on Clinical Cardiology, Council on Cardiovascular Surgery and Anesthesia, and Stroke Council. Infective endocarditis in adults: diagnosis, antimicrobial therapy, and management of complications: a scientific statement for healthcare professionals from the American Heart Association. Circulation. 2015 Oct 13;132(15):1435–86. Epub 2015 Sep 15. Errata in: Circulation. 2015 Oct 27;132(17):e215. Circulation. 2016 Aug 23;134(8):e113.

Barbier C, Loubieres Y, Schmit C, Hayon J, Ricome JL, Jardin F, et al. Respiratory changes in inferior vena cava diameter are helpful in predicting fluid responsiveness in ventilated septic patients. Intensive Care Med. 2004 Sep;30(9):1740–6. Epub 2004 Mar 18.

Breitkreutz R, Walcher F, Seeger FH. Focused echocardiographic evaluation in resuscitation management: concept of an advanced life support-conformed algorithm. Crit Care Med. 2007 May;35(5 Suppl):S150–61.

Campbell SJ, Bechara R, Islam S. Point-of-care ultrasound in the intensive care unit. Clin Chest Med. 2018 Mar;39(1):79–97.

Cowie B. Three years' experience of focused cardiovascular ultrasound in the peri-operative period. Anaesthesia. 2011 Apr;66(4):268–73. Epub 2011 Feb 24.

Diaz-Gomez JL, Via G, Ramakrishna H. Focused cardiac and lung ultrasonography: implications and applicability in the perioperative period. Rom J Anaesth Intensive Care. 2016 Apr;23(1):41–54.

Dubourg J, Javouhey E, Geeraerts T, Messerer M, Kassai B. Ultrasonography of optic nerve sheath diameter for detection of raised intracranial pressure: a systematic review and meta-analysis. Intensive Care Med. 2011 Jul;37(7):1059–68. Epub 2011 Apr 20.

Edler I, Hertz CH. The use of ultrasonic reflectoscope for the continuous recording of the movements of heart walls. 1954. Clin Physiol Funct Imaging. 2004 May;24(3):118–36.

Expert Round Table on Ultrasound in ICU. International expert statement on training standards for critical care ultrasonography. Intensive Care Med. 2011 Jul;37(7):1077–83. Epub 2011 May 26.

Frankel HL, Kirkpatrick AW, Elbarbary M, Blaivas M, Desai H, Evans D, et al. Guidelines for the appropriate use of bedside general and cardiac ultrasonography in the evaluation of critically ill patients-Part I: general ultrasonography. Crit Care Med. 2015 Nov;43(11):2479–502.

Hamada SR, Garcon P, Ronot M, Kerever S, Paugam-Burtz C, Mantz J. Ultrasound assessment of gastric volume in critically ill patients. Intensive Care Med. 2014 Jul;40(7):965–72. Epub 2014 May 20.

Jensen MB, Sloth E, Larsen KM, Schmidt MB. Transthoracic echocardiography for cardiopulmonary monitoring in intensive care. Eur J Anaesthesiol. 2004 Sep;21(9):700–7.

Kory PD, Pellecchia CM, Shiloh AL, Mayo PH, DiBello C, Koenig S. Accuracy of ultrasonography performed by critical care physicians for the diagnosis of DVT. Chest. 2011 Mar;139(3):538–42. Epub 2010 Oct 28.

Lamperti M, Bodenham AR, Pittiruti M, Blaivas M, Augoustides JG, Elbarbary M, et al. International evidence-based recommendations on ultrasound-guided vascular access. Intensive Care Med. 2012 Jul;38(7):1105–17. Epub 2012 May 22.

Levitov A, Frankel HL, Blaivas M, Kirkpatrick AW, Su E, Evans D, et al. Guidelines for the appropriate use of bedside general and cardiac ultrasonography in the evaluation of critically ill patients-Part II: cardiac ultrasonography. Crit Care Med. 2016 Jun;44(6):1206–27.

Lichtenstein DA, Meziere GA, Lagoueyte JF, Biderman P, Goldstein I, Gepner A. A-lines and B-lines: lung ultrasound as a bedside tool for predicting pulmonary artery occlusion pressure in the critically ill. Chest. 2009 Oct;136(4):1014–20.

Lichtenstein DA, Meziere GA. Relevance of lung ultrasound in the diagnosis of acute respiratory failure: the BLUE protocol. Chest. 2008 Jul;134(1):117–25. Epub 2008 Apr 10. Erratum in: Chest. 2013 Aug;144(2):721.

Manno E, Navarra M, Faccio L, Motevallian M, Bertolaccini L, Mfochive A, et al. Deep impact of ultrasound in the intensive care unit: the "ICU-sound" protocol. Anesthesiology. 2012 Oct;117(4):801–9.

Oren-Grinberg A, Talmor D, Brown SM. Focused critical care echocardiography. Crit Care Med. 2013 Nov;41(11):2618–26.

Orme RM, Oram MP, McKinstry CE. Impact of echocardiography on patient management in the intensive care unit: an audit of district general hospital practice. Br J Anaesth. 2009 Mar;102(3):340–4. Epub 2009 Jan 18.

Perera P, Mailhot T, Riley D, Mandavia D. The RUSH exam: Rapid Ultrasound in SHock in the evaluation of the critically Ill. Emerg Med Clin North Am. 2010 Feb;28(1):29–56.

Scalea TM, Rodriguez A, Chiu WC, Brenneman FD, Fallon WF Jr, Kato K, et al. Focused Assessment with Sonography for Trauma (FAST): results from an international consensus conference. J Trauma. 1999 Mar;46(3):466–72.

Sekiguchi H, Schenck LA, Horie R, Suzuki J, Lee EH, McMenomy BP, et al. Critical care ultrasonography differentiates ARDS, pulmonary edema, and other causes in the early course of acute hypoxemic respiratory failure. Chest. 2015 Oct;148(4):912–8.

Spodick DH. Acute cardiac tamponade. N Engl J Med. 2003 Aug 14;349(7):684–90.

Via G, Hussain A, Wells M, Reardon R, ElBarbary M, Noble VE, et al; International Liaison Committee on Focused Cardiac UltraSound (ILC-FoCUS); International Conference on Focused Cardiac UltraSound (IC-FoCUS): international evidence-based recommendations for focused cardiac ultrasound. J Am Soc Echocardiogr. 2014 Jul;27(7):683.e1–33.

Volpicelli G, Elbarbary M, Blaivas M, Lichtenstein DA, Mathis G, Kirkpatrick AW, et al; International Liaison Committee on Lung Ultrasound (ILC-LUS) for International Consensus Conference on Lung Ultrasound (ICC-LUS). International evidence-based recommendations for point-of-care lung ultrasound. Intensive Care Med. 2012 Apr;38(4):577–91. Epub 2012 Mar 6.

Wallbridge P, Steinfort D, Tay TR, Irving L, Hew M. Diagnostic chest ultrasound for acute respiratory failure. Respir Med. 2018 Aug;141:26–36. Epub 2018 Jun 19.

113 Transesophageal Echocardiography

RYAN C. CRANER, MD; FAROUK MOOKADAM, MB, BCh;
HARISH RAMAKRISHNA, MD

Goals

- Know the indications for use of transesophageal echocardiography in the intensive care unit.
- Review the contraindications to transesophageal echocardiography.
- Learn the complications associated with transesophageal echocardiography.
- Learn the strengths and weaknesses of transesophageal echocardiography compared with transthoracic echocardiography in the intensive care unit.

Introduction

The use of ultrasound has revolutionized care in the intensive care unit (ICU). The use of critical care echocardiography, including transthoracic echocardiography (TTE), has become commonplace in ICUs worldwide. In North America, however, intensivists rarely perform transesophageal echocardiography (TEE) unless they have anesthesiology training or have received specialized training to be competent in TEE. In Europe and Australia, TEE is used frequently in the ICU, and TEE training is often completed during fellowship training. In many centers, neurology critical care is provided within the general ICU, and many tertiary-care centers have a dedicated ICU for specialized cases that require advanced and intensive neurologic care.

Certification in TEE

Mastery of critical care TEE requires understanding of the cognitive elements of the procedure, image acquisition, and interpretation elements that require training by faculty skilled at TEE. The American Society of Echocardiography and the Society of Cardiovascular Anesthesiologists established joint guidelines regarding the training of and maintenance of competence by physicians performing TEE. The National Board of Echocardiography, in collaboration with these 2 societies, offers 3 pathways for certification in perioperative TEE: general diagnostic echocardiography, advanced perioperative TEE, and basic perioperative TEE. The technical skills needed for advanced-level TEE include more specific assessment of valvular disease, pathologic conditions of the heart (hypertrophic cardiomyopathy, aneurysm, and dissections), placement of mechanical circulatory support devices, and evaluation of congenital heart lesions.

Echocardiography in the Critical Care Setting

TTE has many benefits, but its use in the ICU has some limitations. In up to half of patients who are mechanically ventilated, adequate images cannot be obtained with TTE. This drawback may be due to poor acoustic windows caused by body habitus, mechanical ventilation with high positive end-expiratory pressure, surgical dressings, and tubes. The American College of Cardiology/American Heart Association/American Society of Echocardiography guidelines offer indications for the use of TEE as an initial diagnostic test. These include a high likelihood of nondiagnostic TTE due to patient characteristics, suspected aortic abnormality, suspected prosthetic valve dysfunction, diagnosis of or evaluation for complications of endocarditis, evaluation for a cardiovascular source of embolus, and an aid for clinical decision making in patients with atrial fibrillation (Box 113.1).

In the ICU, TEE may more thoroughly investigate the abnormality in certain situations, including unexplained hypotension or hypoxia, suspected complications after acute myocardial infarction, chest trauma, and evaluation of volume status.

Box 113.1 • Criteria for Use of Transesophageal Echocardiography as an Initial or Supplemental Test

When there is a high likelihood of nondiagnostic transthoracic echocardiography because of patient characteristics or inadequate visualization of relevant structures

Suspected acute aortic abnormality, including but not limited to dissection or transection

To diagnose infective endocarditis with a low pretest probability (eg, transient fever, known alternative source of infection, or negative blood cultures or atypical pathogen for endocarditis)

To diagnose infective endocarditis with a moderate or high pretest probability (eg, *Staphylococcus* bacteremia, fungemia, prosthetic heart valve, or intracardiac device)

Evaluation for cardiovascular source of embolus with no identified noncardiac source

Evaluation to facilitate clinical decision making with regard to anticoagulation, cardioversion, or radiofrequency ablation in patients with atrial fibrillation

Modified from American College of Cardiology Foundation Appropriate Use Criteria Task Force; American Society of Echocardiography; American Heart Association; American Society of Nuclear Cardiology; Heart Failure Society of America; Heart Rhythm Society; Society for Cardiovascular Angiography and Interventions; Society of Critical Care Medicine; Society of Cardiovascular Computed Tomography; Society for Cardiovascular Magnetic Resonance; American College of Chest Physicians, Douglas PS, Garcia MJ, Haines DE, Lai WW, Manning WJ, Patel AR, et al. ACCF/ASE/AHA/ASNC/HFSA/HRS/SCAI/SCCM/SCCT/SCMR 2011 Appropriate Use Criteria for Echocardiography. A report of the American College of Cardiology Foundation Appropriate Use Criteria Task Force, American Society of Echocardiography, American Heart Association, American Society of Nuclear Cardiology, Heart Failure Society of America, Heart Rhythm Society, Society for Cardiovascular Angiography and Interventions, Society of Critical Care Medicine, Society of Cardiovascular Computed Tomography, Society for Cardiovascular Magnetic Resonance, American College of Chest Physicians. J Am Soc Echocardiogr. 2011 Mar;24(3):229-67; used with permission.

Box 113.2 • Common Problems That Can Be Diagnosed With Transesophageal Echocardiography in Neurosurgical Patients

Venous air embolism and paradoxical air embolism

Identification of hemodynamic instability perioperatively

Cardiac manifestation of intracranial hemorrhage

Positioning of ventriculoatrial shunt and complications related to it

Positioning of a right atrial catheter

Percutaneous placement of a ventriculoatrial shunt

Modified from Choudhury M. Transoesophageal echocardiography: what a neuroanaesthesiologist should know? J Neuroanaesthesiol Crit Care. 2015 Jan-Apr;2(1):3–14; used with permission.

TEE is more than just a monitor; it is also an excellent diagnostic tool in life-threatening situations that present perioperatively. Prompt recognition and treatment of venous air embolism and determination of the cause of major cardiovascular instability in the operating room and in the ICU are key factors in limiting associated morbidity and mortality in patients undergoing neurosurgical procedures (Box 113.2).

The advantages of sitting and semi-sitting positions during neurosurgical procedures are well known; however, these positions are not risk-free. Feared complications of head-up positioning are air embolism and the potential for central nervous system dysfunction. The incidence of venous air embolism ranges from 1.6% to 76% depending on both patient and surgical factors. These include the presence of an intracardiac shunt (atrial septal defect or patent foramen ovale) and surgery done with the patient in a sitting or semi-sitting position.

Preoperative examination with TEE or TTE during a Valsalva maneuver and with an intravenous echocardiographic contrast agent can help to diagnose only the presence of an intracardiac shunt with high sensitivity. Unfortunately, this knowledge may not aid in the management of a patient in whom a venous air embolism has already occurred. Intraoperatively, visualization of air bubbles in the major vessels or cardiac chambers on TEE has to be considered an indicator of possible venous air embolism. Should air bubbles arise, necessary steps such as ensuring tight connections on intravenous lines and adequate volume resuscitation, possible interruption of surgical manipulation, and quick closure of venous system leaks should be completed.

To assess for the presence of a patent foramen ovale or atrial septal defect, standard 2-dimensional TEE midesophageal 4-chamber and bicaval views should be obtained. From these views, the intra-atrial septum should be the focal point. Interrogation of the intra-atrial septum with color flow Doppler imaging with a low Nyquist limit can be used to look for blood flow crossing the intra-atrial septum. If the result of color flow Doppler imaging is negative, agitated saline can be injected intravenously and, within moments, saline bubbles will appear in the right atrium and right ventricle. If an intracardiac shunt is present, the left chambers will also show the appearance of saline bubbles within 4 beats (Figure 113.1 and Figure 113.2).

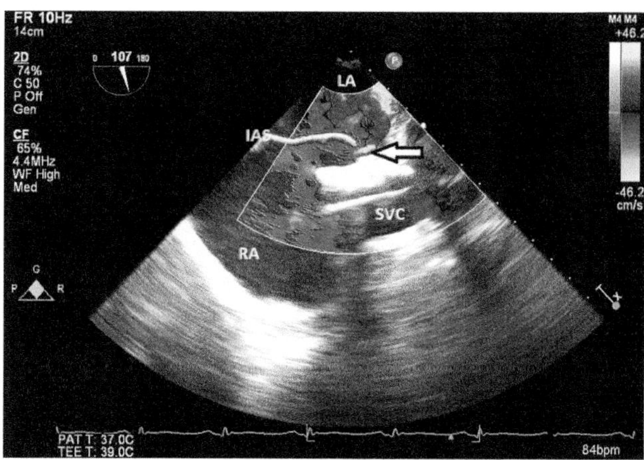

Figure 113.1. Color Flow Doppler Transesophageal Echocardiogram. Bicaval view; arrow indicates atrial septal defect. IAS indicates interatrial septum; LA, left atrium; RA right atrium; SVC, superior vena cava.

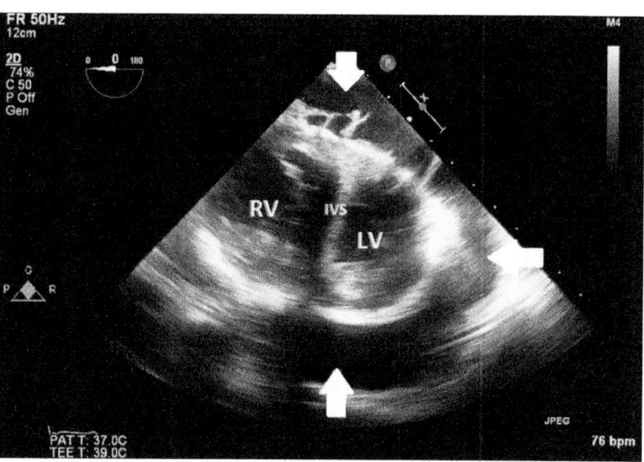

Figure 113.3. Transesophageal Echocardiogram. Transgastric short-axis view shows a large, circumferential pericardial effusion (arrows). IVS indicates intraventricular septum; LV, left ventricle; RV, right ventricle.

Use of TEE for Identification of Cardiovascular Instability in the Operating Room and ICU

Intracranial hemorrhage may also present with cardiac manifestations that alter inpatient outcomes and pose a challenge for neurointensivists. Cardiac involvement may vary from minor changes on electrocardiography to myocardial ischemia and infarction, ventricular dysfunction, congestive heart failure, and Takotsubo cardiomyopathy. Takotsubo cardiomyopathy is a condition in which echocardiography is key for establishing the diagnosis.

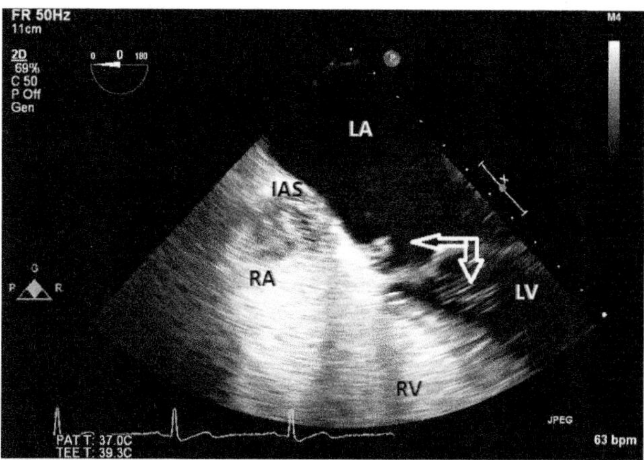

Figure 113.2. Transesophageal Echocardiogram. Four-chamber view shows bubbles opacifying right atrium (RA) and right ventricle (RV) and flow into left atrium (LA) (arrow) and left ventricle (LV) (arrow). IAS indicates interatrial septum.

Subarachnoid hemorrhage due to aneurysmal disease often presents with hemodynamic instability and pulmonary edema requiring vasoactive medications for hemodynamic support. This situation is often accompanied by severe left ventricular dysfunction and associated hemodynamic consequences. Differentiating a stress cardiomyopathy from an acute coronary syndrome is vital for guiding optimal management. The differential diagnosis of hemodynamic compromise perioperatively is vast, and appropriate use of TEE can assist in diagnosis. Myocardial ischemia with ST-segment changes can occur during aneurysm clipping but also at any time perioperatively, and use of TEE to evaluate for the presence of regional wall motion abnormalities can guide further steps to optimize myocardial oxygen consumption and assist in guiding therapy should further cardiovascular interventions be warranted. Assessment for pericardial effusion and subsequent tamponade physiology and evaluation for hypovolemia from acute blood loss after serious vascular injury or during major spine surgery can be done by evaluating preload, contractility, and afterload from basic TEE windows (Figure 113.3).

Ventriculoatrial shunt placement is a common neurosurgical procedure and is indicated for the treatment of hydrocephalus. Ensuring correct positioning of the distal end of the catheter in the right atrium is key for monitoring shunt patency and reducing the incidence of ventriculoatrial shunt–related complications. TEE can be helpful for guiding final placement of the catheter.

Probe Manipulation

Once the TEE probe is placed, different windows are used to obtain images. Four of the most common windows are named according to the position of the probe within the

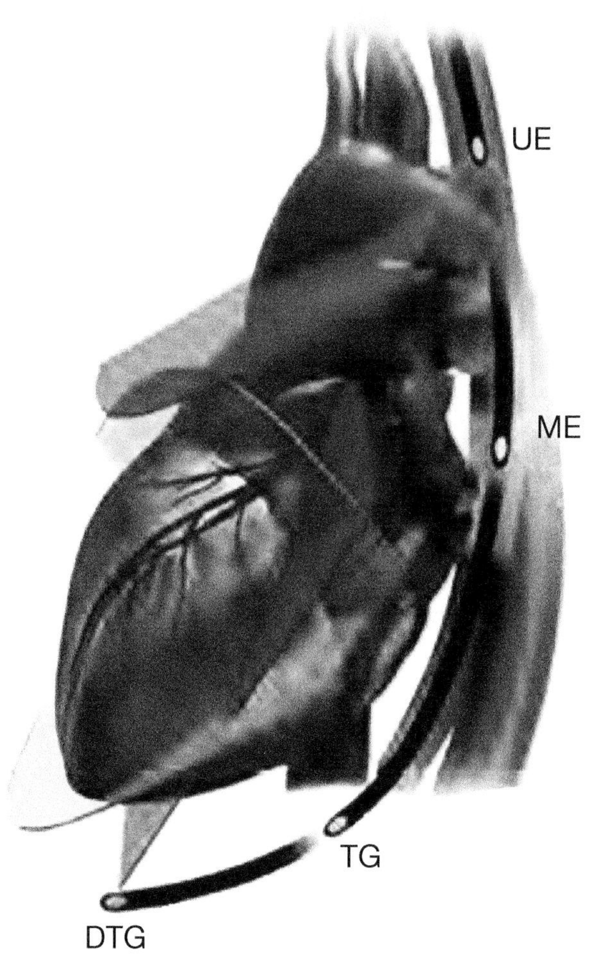

Figure 113.4. Transesophageal Echocardiographic Windows. DTG indicates deep transgastric; ME, midesophageal; TG, transgastric; UE, upper esophageal.

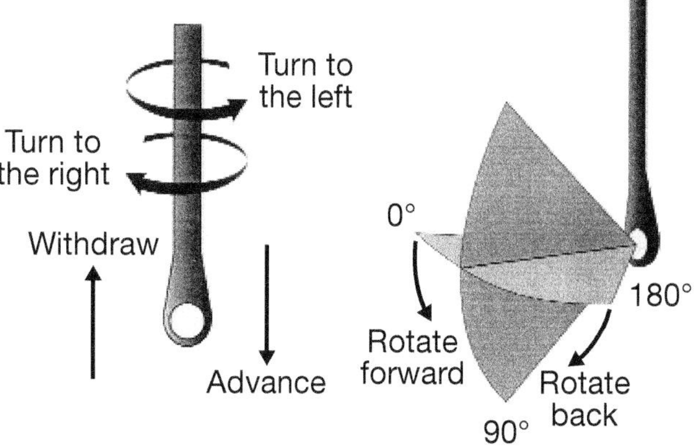

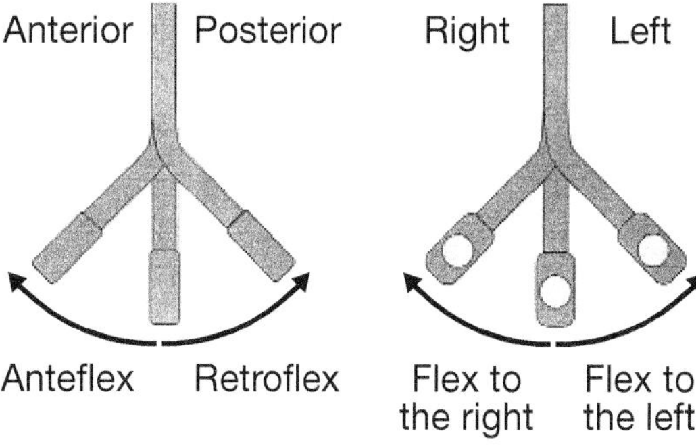

Figure 113.5. Probe Positions for Transesophageal Echocardiographic Manipulation.

esophagus. These include the upper esophageal, midesophageal, transgastric, and deep transgastric windows (Figure 113.4).

Within each of these windows, various cardiac structures can be visualized by manipulating the position of the ultrasound transducer. Basic probe movements include advancement or withdrawal of the probe, turning of the probe to the right or left, anteflexion (flexion of the probe toward the sternum), retroflexion (flexion of the probe toward the spine), and lateral flexion of the probe tip to the left or right (Figure 113.5). This omniplane feature enables the echocardiographer to visualize cardiac structures in multiple planes from the same anatomical window (Figure 113.6).

Indications for TEE

Aortic Disease

The proximity of the esophagus and thoracic aorta permits excellent evaluation of the aorta from its root to the abdominal aorta, with the exception of the distal ascending aorta and aortic arch because of the interposition of the trachea and right main-stem bronchus, respectively. Aortic atherosclerosis is readily identifiable on TEE from thick plaques (>4 mm) or from the presence of mobile lesions associated with a high embolic risk, especially in patients with severe aortic atherosclerosis who undergo invasive procedures such as cardiac catheterization or intra-aortic balloon placement.

In several studies, TEE has been validated to be both sensitive (86%-100%) and specific (90%-100%) for the diagnosis of aortic dissection. In addition to identifying the location and extent of the dissection, TEE can be used to assist in differentiation of the intimal flap and true and false lumens, measure flow dynamics, and determine the presence of thrombus. Important perioperative considerations include assessment of global cardiac function, evaluation of possible aortic valve and annular involvement in the dissection, and assess for the presence or absence of pericardial fluid in patients who are hemodynamically unstable.

Valvular Disease

TEE is useful for obtaining an unobstructed view of cardiac structure and function. It provides an unobstructed view of

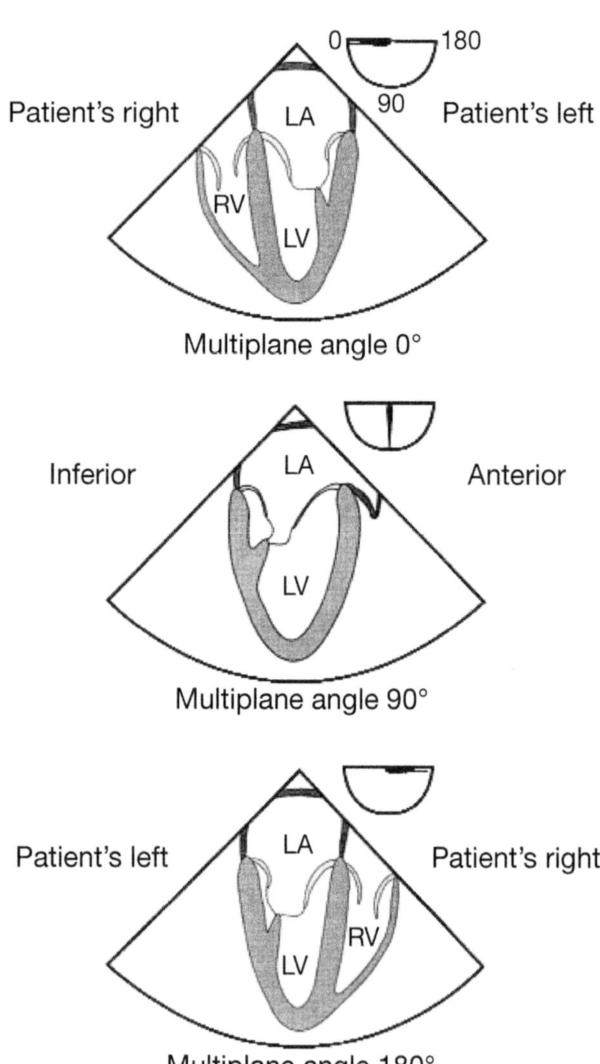

Figure 113.6. Omniplane Feature of Transesophageal Echocardiography. Cardiac structures in multiple planes can be visualized from same anatomical window. LA indicates left atrium; LV, left ventricle; RV, right ventricle.

the cardiac valves and is the imaging method of choice for suspected prosthetic valve dysfunction because reverberation artifact and shadowing can limit TTE imaging. Many echocardiographic techniques have been reported and are available to characterize and assess the severity of valvular lesions, although a review of these methods is beyond the scope of this text. TEE is an important tool in the identification of regurgitant and stenotic lesions and dynamic left ventricular outflow tract obstruction and can assist in management.

The ability to identify clinically significant regurgitant lesions is a basic skill for anyone using echocardiography to care for critically ill patients. Color flow Doppler imaging is suggested as a basic screening tool to aid in detection of these lesions. One method of quantifying the severity of a regurgitant lesion is the vena contracta method, in which, with color flow Doppler imaging, the most narrow central flow region of a jet at or just downstream of the orifice of a regurgitant valve is identified. The vena contracta width should be measured in at least 2 anatomically orthogonal views. In mitral regurgitant lesions, a vena contracta width more than 0.8 cm usually indicates severe mitral regurgitation and a width less than 0.3 cm is usually associated with mild mitral regurgitation. For vena contracta widths between these values or in mitral regurgitation with multiple jets, other techniques of quantification should be used. The same technique can be applied to aortic insufficiency, in which a vena contracta width more than 0.6 indicates severe regurgitation and a width less than 0.3 cm indicates trivial insufficiency. Color flow Doppler imaging alone is a good guide for semiquantitative assessment of valvular regurgitant lesions. It is also helpful for assessing intracardiac shunts or fistulas, and appropriate lower velocity settings are used for lower flow assessment. Overgain, artifact from mechanical devices, may affect color Doppler assessment considerably. The ease of quantitative Doppler assessment is therefore necessary to quantify regurgitation severity. Meticulous quantification allows for serial assessment of valvular lesions. Color flow Doppler imaging is extremely helpful for assessing perivalvular leaks and annular dehiscence severity, in both 2-dimensional mode and 3-dimensional mode with color.

TEE is also useful for identifying and quantifying stenotic valvular disease. The valve in question should be investigated 2-dimensionally. Findings such as calcific annulus, thickened leaflets, or cusps with restricted motion are invaluable clues to aid in diagnosis. An efficient and relatively simple technique to quantify the severity of any stenotic valve is the application of continuous-wave Doppler through the valve orifice. The mean and peak pressure gradients can readily be obtained with the software available on most TEE platforms (using the modified Bernoulli equation), and these can be related to the severity of stenosis of a specific valve. In mitral stenosis, several nonvalvular features can assist in diagnosis, including 1) atrial dilatation, 2) left-to-right bowing of the atrial septum, 3) spontaneous echo contrast (very slow moving blood) in the left atrium, and 4) the presence of left atrial thrombus. Precise assessment of all of the hemodynamic or anatomical specifics of each valve is not necessary to answer all clinical questions in the ICU; however, the ability to obtain the appropriate views and correctly assess the hemodynamic implications can assist in appropriate patient management.

Dynamic left ventricular outflow tract obstruction is due to a narrowing of the distance between the anterior leaflet of the mitral valve and the interventricular septum during systole. This may be due to hypertrophy of the left ventricle (hypertensive heart disease or hypertrophic cardiomyopathy) or to systolic anterior motion of the anterior leaflet of the mitral valve after mitral valve repair. Dynamic left ventricular outflow tract obstruction is worsened by hypovolemia, decreased afterload, or positive inotropy, all of which are common conditions in patients in the ICU. In addition to the spike-and-dome configuration of the arterial line tracing, characteristic TEE findings include visulization of the anterior leaflet of the mitral valve into the left ventricular outflow tract with resultant mitral regurgitation. Therapy should be instituted with volume resuscitation and an afterload-increasing agent such as phenylephrine. Careful administration of β-adrenergic blockers could be considered to reduce inotropy and heart rate if initial therapy is unsuccessful.

Cardiac Source of Embolism

In patients who are at risk for or have already experienced embolic strokes, the roles of echocardiography are to establish the source of emboli, determine whether the source is a plausible cause of systemic embolism, and guide therapy. Several conditions are known to lead to systemic embolization, and they are divided into a high-risk and a low-risk group depending on their embolic potential (Box 113.3).

From a practical standpoint, echocardiography has a crucial role in the evaluation, diagnosis, and management of cardiac and aortic sources of embolism. Determination of the appropriate use of TTE vs TEE is sometimes unclear, depending on patient circumstances. Anterior cardiac structures are better visualized with TTE, and it may provide more information about structures not visualized well by TEE, including left ventricular thrombus. In contrast, TEE excels in imaging of posterior cardiac structures and the ascending and descending thoracic aorta. In summary, TEE is not indicated when TTE findings are diagnostic, but it may be used as an initial or supplemental test for evaluation of a potential source of embolus with no identified noncardiac source, in patients with a moderate or high pretest probability of infective endocarditis (IE), or as an initial test to determine clinical treatment regarding anticoagulation, cardioversion, or possible radiofrequency ablation for atrial fibrillation.

Box 113.3 • Classification of Cardiac Sources of Embolism

- High embolic potential
  - Intracardiac thrombi
  - Atrial arrhythmias
  - Valvular atrial fibrillation
  - Nonvalvular atrial fibrillation
  - Atrial flutter
  - Ischemic heart disease
  - Recent myocardial infarction
  - Chronic myocardial infarction, especially with LV aneurysm
  - Nonischemic cardiomyopathies
  - Prosthetic valves and devices
  - Intracardiac vegetations
  - Native valve endocarditis
  - Prosthetic valve endocarditis
  - Nonvalvular endocarditis
  - Intracardiac tumors
  - Myxoma
  - Papillary fibroelastoma
  - Other tumors
  - Aortic atheroma
  - Thromboembolism
  - Cholesterol crystal emboli
- Low embolic potential
  - Potential precursors of intracardiac thrombi
  - SEC (in the absence of atrial fibrillation)
  - LV aneurysm without a clot
  - Mitral valve prolapse
  - Intracardiac calcifications
  - Mitral annular calcification
  - Calcific aortic stenosis
  - Valvular anomalies
  - Fibrin strands
  - Giant Lambl excrescences
  - Septal defects and anomalies
  - Patent foramen ovale
  - Atrial septal aneurysm
  - Atrial septal defect

Abbreviations: LV, left ventricular; SEC, spontaneous echo contrast.

Endocarditis

IE is a life-threatening disease that continues to be associated with a high mortality rate as a result of its various complications, including embolic events, perivalvular extension, and valvular destruction with development of acute heart failure. Echocardiography, both transthoracic and transesophageal, has a key role in the diagnosis of IE (Figure 113.7).

Major echocardiographic criteria for the diagnosis of IE include the presence of vegetations, abscess, or new dehiscence of a prosthetic valve. TEE also has increased sensitivity for detecting each of these phenomenon

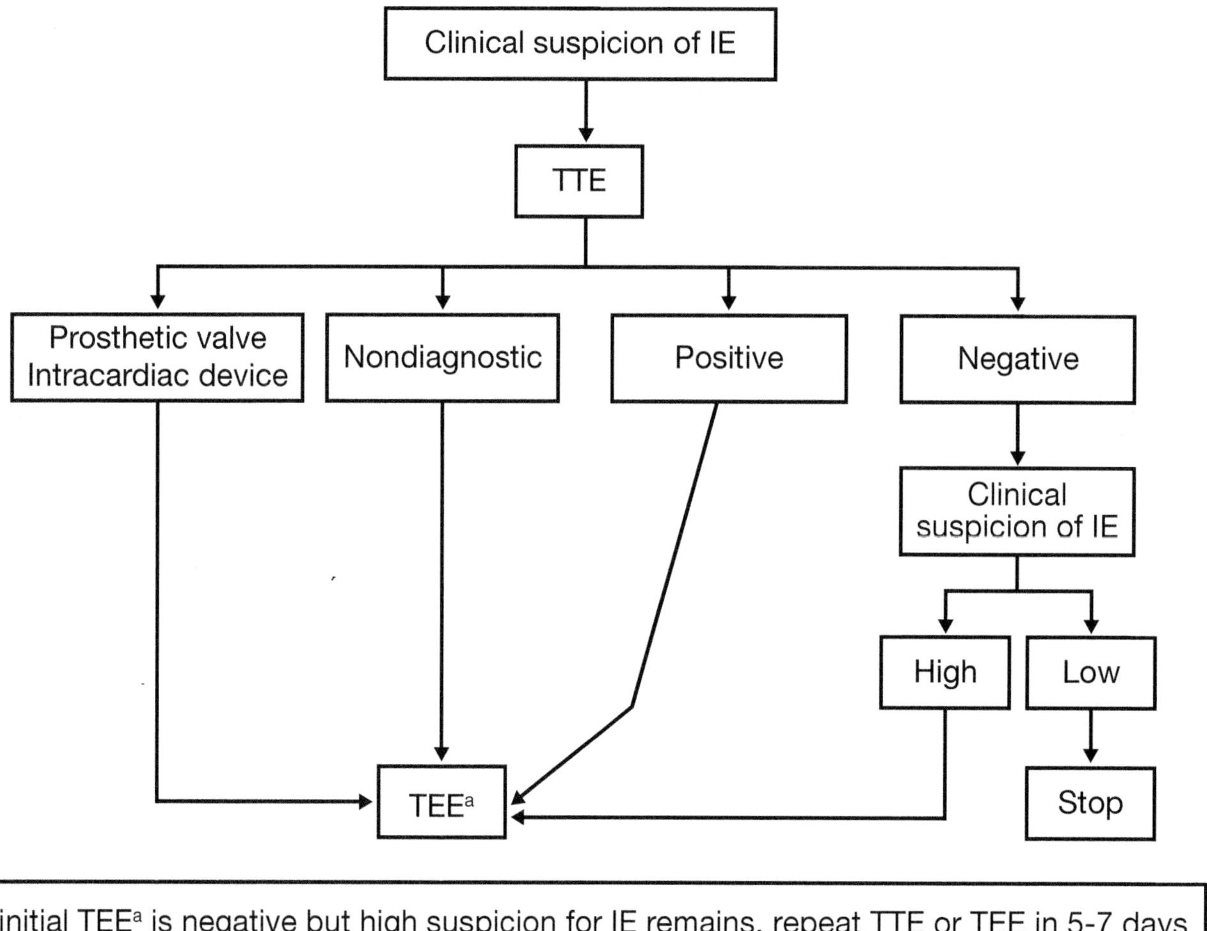

Figure 113.7. Indications for Echocardiography When Infective Endocarditis (IE) Is Suspected. TEE indicates transesophageal echocardiography; TTE, transthoracic echocardiography.

[a] *TEE is not mandatory in isolated right-sided native-valve IE with good-quality TEE examination and unequivocal echocardiographic findings.*

(From Habib G, Lancellotti P, Antunes MJ, Bongiorni MG, Casalta JP, Del Zotti F, et al; ESC Scientific Document Group. 2015 ESC guidelines for the management of infective endocarditis: The Task Force for the Management of Infective Endocarditis of the European Society of Cardiology [ESC]. Endorsed by: European Association for Cardio-Thoracic Surgery [EACTS], the European Association of Nuclear Medicine [EANM]. Eur Heart J. 2015 Nov 21;36[44]:3075-128; used with permission.)

compared with TTE. Other echocardiographic findings of IE may be present but are not main criteria for, but merely suggestive of, the diagnosis. These include valve destruction, perforation, or new prolapse or aneurysm (Figure 113.8).

Despite the benefits of echocardiography, its diagnostic capability has some limitations. Echocardiography is not 100% sensitive or specific for the diagnosis of endocarditis, especially early in the disease process or in patients with preexisting severe valvular lesions. In addition, a diagnosis of IE may be false when it is difficult to differentiate between actual IE vegetations and thrombi, myxomatous changes, or noninfective vegetations.

Hemodynamic Assessment

Until recently, the pulmonary artery catheter was considered the standard for assessment of central hemodynamics in critically ill patients. The routine placement of a pulmonary artery catheter in critically ill patients has decreased significantly because of questions about the invasiveness of the device and interpretation of the data it provides. Several studies have evaluated the risk-benefit profile of this device. Echocardiography has been rapidly gaining acceptance as a minimally invasive approach to determine a patient's hemodynamic profile at the bedside.

Use of TEE in skilled hands can provide hemodynamic parameters such as volumes and pressures and direct

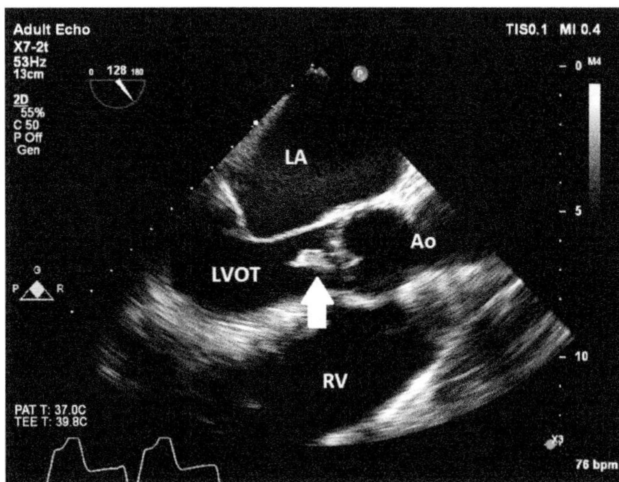

Figure 113.8. Transesophageal Echocardiogram. Upper esophageal view of the aortic valve in long axis with large vegetation (arrow). Ao indicates aorta; LA, left atrium; LVOT, left ventricular outflow tract; RV, right ventricle.

visualization of the ventricular size and function to evaluate for myocardial ischemia.

Cardiac output can be calculated by echo across any structure where one can measure the velocity of blood flow, known as the velocity time integral, and the cross-sectional area of that structure. The product of the velocity time integral and the cross-sectional area of the conduit where the measurement was obtained (cm^2) provides the estimated stroke volume, and stroke volume multiplied by heart rate results in the cardiac output. The pulmonary artery in the midesophageal short-axis view is the most convenient echo window to obtain the diameter of the pulmonary artery and flow signals using continuous- or pulsed-wave Doppler imaging. The ascending aorta may also be used for velocity time integral measurement after advancing the TEE probe to the deep transgastric window to allow alignment of the ultrasound beam and blood flow. Cardiac output obtained with Doppler was found to have close agreement with thermodilution cardiac output in an intraoperative TEE study.

In addition to direct measurement of cardiac output, TEE provides information about other indicators of volume status. One of these is the left ventricular end-diastolic area. When studied in cardiac surgical patients, left ventricular end-diastolic area decreased linearly in response to acute blood volume deficits; however, in patients with sepsis it was a poor indicator of volume responsiveness. Dynamic tests of volume responsiveness have consistently shown that the magnitude of respiratory variation of surrogates of stroke volume accurately predicts fluid responsiveness. These surrogates include arterial pulse pressure variation and many other devices that incorporate some type of arterial waveform analysis. TEE evaluation using pulsed-wave Doppler to evaluate respiratory variation of the aortic flow has also been studied. In patients with septic shock, TEE was performed, and the velocity time integral of blood flow was obtained in the left ventricular outflow tract over a single respiratory cycle. Patients with a change in peak blood velocity of more than 12% during respiration were found to be responsive to volume expansion.

In addition to variations in aortic blood flow, evaluation of the respirophasic change in diameter of the inferior vena cava with TTE has been shown to assist in determination of volume responsiveness in mechanically ventilated patients. Instead of visualizing the inferior vena cava with TEE, a collapsibility index of the superior vena cava (maximal diameter at expiration – minimal diameter at inspiration/maximal diameter at expiration) of more than 36% was associated with volume responsiveness with a sensitivity and specificity of 90% and 87%, respectively.

Mechanical Support Devices

The variety and use of mechanical circulatory devices for short-term mechanical circulatory support have increased substantially in the past decade. An analysis of the National (Nationwide) Inpatient Sample suggests that use of extracorporeal membrane oxygenation increased 433% from 2006 to 2011 and that use of percutaneous devices for short-term mechanical circulatory support increased by 1,511% from 2007 to 2011. Many of the percutaneous devices are placed in the cardiac catheterization suite under direct fluoroscopic guidance. Unfortunately, they are often subject to migration or displacement during transport or continued ICU care. Plain chest radiography, although useful for verification of initial placement on arrival in the ICU, can be burdensome if further manipulation is needed.

TEE can assist in real-time confirmation of device placement and in repositioning, if needed. In addition, color flow Doppler imaging can be useful for verifying device location and function (Figures 113.9 and 113.10).

Complications of TEE

The incidence of complications with use of TEE is low, both in the outpatient setting and in the operating room and ICU. In 7,200 patients who had cardiac surgery, the TEE-associated morbidity and mortality were 0.2% and 0%, respectively, and the most common complication was odynophagia (0.1%). The incidence of other reported complications was also low, including dental injury (0.03%), endotracheal tube malpositioning (0.03%), upper gastrointestinal bleeding (0.03%), and esophageal perforation (0.01%). In a review of more than 2,500 TEE examinations in the ICU, the complication rate was 2.6%, and there was no examination-related mortality. The most frequent occurrence was dislodgment of the nasogastric or nasojejunal feeding tube (8.7%), and other complications included

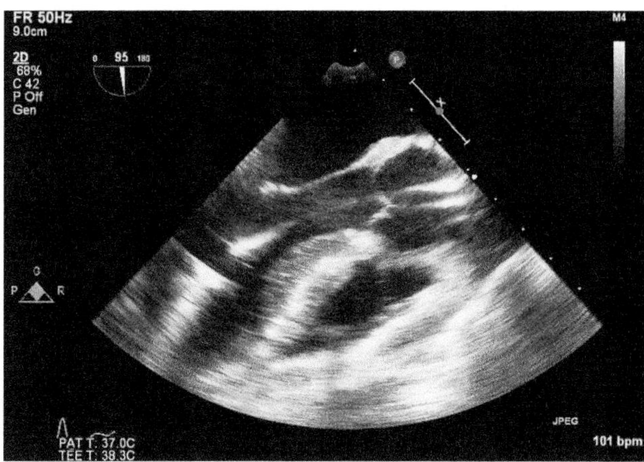

Figure 113.9. Transesophageal Echocardiogram. Upper esophageal aortic valve in long axis shows heart pump across the aortic valve.

mucosal lesions (0.7%), hypotension (0.6%), and coughing (0.3%).

Despite the low incidence of complications, there are several contraindications to the use of TEE. They include esophageal strictures, tracheoesophageal fistula, post-esophageal surgery, and recent esophageal trauma. There is no clear evidence about other esophageal abnormalities, including Barrett esophagus, hiatal hernia, large descending aortic aneurysm, and unilateral vocal cord paralysis. A few small trials suggest that TEE may be safely used in patients with grade 1 or 2 esophageal varices. Ultimately, TEE may be used with caution in patients with oral, esophageal, or gastric disease if the expected benefit outweighs the potential risk.

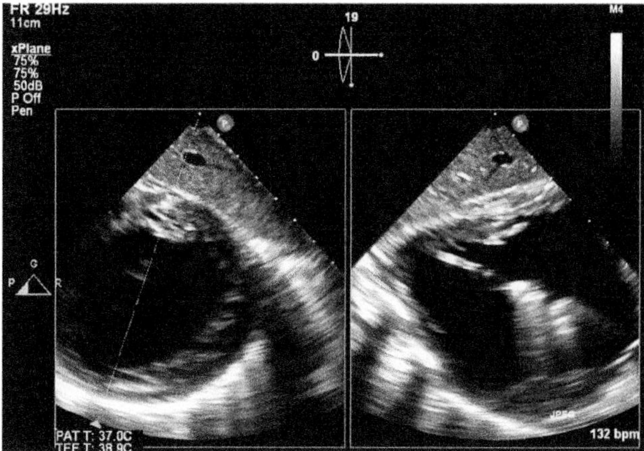

Figure 113.10. Transesophageal Echocardiogram. Transgastric short-axis view with concurrent x-plane shows a heart pump within the left ventricle.

Conclusion

The use of traditional TTE in critically ill patients is invaluable, but it is not without limitation. TEE can overcome some of these limitations and, although it is not entirely without risk, it can assist the intensivist in real-time diagnosis, decision making, and treatment in critically ill patients and provide real-time feedback regarding the response to therapy at the bedside.

Summary

- The use of ultrasonography in the ICU has revolutionized patient care and is continuing to evolve as new tools are developed. The use of TEE offers additional information when use of TTE may be limited.
- Mastery of TEE requires mastery of the cognitive elements and tactile skill for obtaining and interpreting images.
- TEE in skilled hands can offer answers to many clinical questions, including source of potential arterial embolism, evaluation of aortic disease, nature and severity of cardiac valvular disease, assessment of cardiac function, verification of cardiac support devices, and estimation of circulating volume.

SUGGESTED READING

American College of Cardiology Foundation Appropriate Use Criteria Task Force; American Society of Echocardiography; American Heart Association; American Society of Nuclear Cardiology; Heart Failure Society of America; Heart Rhythm Society; Society for Cardiovascular Angiography and Interventions; Society of Critical Care Medicine; Society of Cardiovascular Computed Tomography; Society for Cardiovascular Magnetic Resonance; American College of Chest Physicians, Douglas PS, Garcia MJ, Haines DE, Lai WW, Manning WJ, Patel AR, et al. ACCF/ASE/AHA/ASNC/HFSA/HRS/SCAI/SCCM/SCCT/SCMR 2011 Appropriate Use Criteria for Echocardiography. A Report of the American College of Cardiology Foundation Appropriate Use Criteria Task Force, American Society of Echocardiography, American Heart Association, American Society of Nuclear Cardiology, Heart Failure Society of America, Heart Rhythm Society, Society for Cardiovascular Angiography and Interventions, Society of Critical Care Medicine, Society of Cardiovascular Computed Tomography, Society for Cardiovascular Magnetic Resonance, American College of Chest Physicians. J Am Soc Echocardiogr. 2011 Mar;24(3):229–67.

American Society of Anesthesiologists and Society of Cardiovascular Anesthesiologists Task Force on Transesophageal Echocardiography. Practice guidelines for perioperative transesophageal echocardiography: an updated report by the American Society of Anesthesiologists and the Society of Cardiovascular Anesthesiologists Task Force on

Transesophageal Echocardiography. Anesthesiology. 2010 May;112(5):1084–96.
Black S, Muzzi DA, Nishimura RA, Cucchiara RF. Preoperative and intraoperative echocardiography to detect right-to-left shunt in patients undergoing neurosurgical procedures in the sitting position. Anesthesiology. 1990 Mar;72(3):436–8.
Cheung AT, Savino JS, Weiss SJ, Aukburg SJ, Berlin JA. Echocardiographic and hemodynamic indexes of left ventricular preload in patients with normal and abnormal ventricular function. Anesthesiology. 1994 Aug;81(2):376–87.
Cucchiara RF, Seward JB, Nishimura RA, Nugent M, Faust RJ. Identification of patent foramen ovale during sitting position craniotomy by transesophageal echocardiography with positive airway pressure. Anesthesiology. 1985 Jul;63(1):107–9.
Daniel WG, Erbel R, Kasper W, Visser CA, Engberding R, Sutherland GR, et al. Safety of transesophageal echocardiography: a multicenter survey of 10,419 examinations. Circulation. 1991 Mar;83(3):817–21.
Daniel WG, Mugge A, Grote J, Hausmann D, Nikutta P, Laas J, et al. Comparison of transthoracic and transesophageal echocardiography for detection of abnormalities of prosthetic and bioprosthetic valves in the mitral and aortic positions. Am J Cardiol. 1993 Jan 15;71(2):210–5.
Durack DT, Lukes AS, Bright DK. New criteria for diagnosis of infective endocarditis: utilization of specific echocardiographic findings. Duke Endocarditis Service. Am J Med. 1994 Mar;96(3):200–9.
Evangelista A, Avegliano G, Aguilar R, Cuellar H, Igual A, Gonzalez-Alujas T, et al. Impact of contrast-enhanced echocardiography on the diagnostic algorithm of acute aortic dissection. Eur Heart J. 2010 Feb;31(4):472–9. Epub 2009 Dec 25.
Evangelista A, Gonzalez-Alujas MT. Echocardiography in infective endocarditis. Heart. 2004 Jun;90(6):614–7.
Fathi AR, Eshtehardi P, Meier B. Patent foramen ovale and neurosurgery in sitting position: a systematic review. Br J Anaesth. 2009 May;102(5):588–96. Epub 2009 Apr 4.
Feigl GC, Decker K, Wurms M, Krischek B, Ritz R, Unertl K, et al. Neurosurgical procedures in the semisitting position: evaluation of the risk of paradoxical venous air embolism in patients with a patent foramen ovale. World Neurosurg. 2014 Jan;81(1):159–64. Epub 2013 Jan 4.
Feissel M, Michard F, Mangin I, Ruyer O, Faller JP, Teboul JL. Respiratory changes in aortic blood velocity as an indicator of fluid responsiveness in ventilated patients with septic shock. Chest. 2001 Mar;119(3):867–73.
Flachskampf FA, Decoodt P, Fraser AG, Daniel WG, Roelandt JR; Subgroup on Transesophageal Echocardiography and Valvular Heart Disease; Working Group on Echocardiography of the European Society of Cardiology. Guidelines from the working group: recommendations for performing transesophageal echocardiography. Eur J Echocardiogr. 2001 Mar;2(1):8–21.
French Study of Aortic Plaques in Stroke Group, Amarenco P, Cohen A, Hommel M, Moulin T, Leys D, Bousser M-G. Atherosclerotic disease of the aortic arch as a risk factor for recurrent ischemic stroke. N Engl J Med. 1996 May 9;334(19):1216–21.
Habib G, Lancellotti P, Antunes MJ, Bongiorni MG, Casalta JP, Del Zotti F, et al; ESC Scientific Document Group. 2015 ESC guidelines for the management of infective endocarditis: The Task Force for the Management of Infective Endocarditis of the European Society of Cardiology (ESC). Endorsed by: European Association for Cardio-Thoracic Surgery (EACTS), the European Association of Nuclear Medicine (EANM). Eur Heart J. 2015 Nov 21;36(44):3075–128. Epub 2015 Aug 29.
Habib G. Embolic risk in subacute bacterial endocarditis: determinants and role of transesophageal echocardiography. Curr Infect Dis Rep. 2005 Jul;7(4):264–71.
Hahn RT, Abraham T, Adams MS, Bruce CJ, Glas KE, Lang RM, et al. Guidelines for performing a comprehensive transesophageal echocardiographic examination: recommendations from the American Society of Echocardiography and the Society of Cardiovascular Anesthesiologists. J Am Soc Echocardiogr. 2013 Sep;26(9):921–64.
Hall SA, Brickner ME, Willett DL, Irani WN, Afridi I, Grayburn PA. Assessment of mitral regurgitation severity by Doppler color flow mapping of the vena contracta. Circulation. 1997 Feb 4;95(3):636–42.
Harvey S, Harrison DA, Singer M, Ashcroft J, Jones CM, Elbourne D, et al; PAC-Man study collaboration. Assessment of the clinical effectiveness of pulmonary artery catheters in management of patients in intensive care (PAC-Man): a randomised controlled trial. Lancet. 2005 Aug 6–12;366(9484):472–7.
Hasbun R, Vikram HR, Barakat LA, Buenconsejo J, Quagliarello VJ. Complicated left-sided native valve endocarditis in adults: risk classification for mortality. JAMA. 2003 Apr 16;289(15):1933–40.
Hoen B, Alla F, Selton-Suty C, Beguinot I, Bouvet A, Briancon S, et al; Association pour l'Etude et la Prevention de l'Endocardite Infectieuse (AEPEI) Study Group. Changing profile of infective endocarditis: results of a 1-year survey in France. JAMA. 2002 Jul 3;288(1):75–81.
Huttemann E, Schelenz C, Kara F, Chatzinikolaou K, Reinhart K. The use and safety of transoesophageal echocardiography in the general ICU: a minireview. Acta Anaesthesiol Scand. 2004 Aug;48(7):827–36.
Jadik S, Wissing H, Friedrich K, Beck J, Seifert V, Raabe A. A standardized protocol for the prevention of clinically relevant venous air embolism during neurosurgical interventions in the semisitting position. Neurosurgery. 2009 Mar;64(3):533–8.
Kallmeyer I, Morse DS, Body SC, Collard CD. Case 2–2000: transesophageal echocardiography-associated gastrointestinal trauma. J Cardiothorac Vasc Anesth. 2000 Apr;14(2):212–6.
Konstadt SN, Reich DL, Quintana C, Levy M. The ascending aorta: how much does transesophageal echocardiography see? Anesth Analg. 1994 Feb;78(2):240–4.
Kowalczyk AK, Mizuguchi KA, Couper GS, Wang JT, Fox AA. Use of intraoperative transesophageal echocardiography to evaluate positioning of TandemHeart percutaneous right ventricular assist device cannulae. Anesth Analg. 2014 Jan;118(1):72–5.
Luckner G, Margreiter J, Jochberger S, Mayr V, Luger T, Voelckel W, et al. Systolic anterior motion of the mitral valve with left ventricular outflow tract obstruction: three cases of acute perioperative hypotension in noncardiac surgery. Anesth Analg. 2005 Jun;100(6):1594–8.
Mahjoub H, Pibarot P, Dumesnil JG. Echocardiographic evaluation of prosthetic heart valves. Curr Cardiol Rep. 2015 Jun;17(6):48.

Mayo PH, Beaulieu Y, Doelken P, Feller-Kopman D, Harrod C, Kaplan A, et al. American College of Chest Physicians/La Societe de Reanimation de Langue Francaise statement on competence in critical care ultrasonography. Chest. 2009 Apr;135(4):1050–60. Epub 2009 Feb 2.

Meredith EL, Masani ND. Echocardiography in the emergency assessment of acute aortic syndromes. Eur J Echocardiogr. 2009 Jan;10(1):i31–9.

Muratsu A, Muroya T, Kuwagata Y. Takotsubo cardiomyopathy in the intensive care unit. Acute Med Surg. 2019 Mar 1;6(2):152–7.

Pantham G, Waghray N, Einstadter D, Finkelhor RS, Mullen KD. Bleeding risk in patients with esophageal varices undergoing transesophageal echocardiography. Echocardiography. 2013 Nov;30(10):1152–5. Epub 2013 Jun 6.

Parker MM, Cunnion RE, Parrillo JE. Echocardiography and nuclear cardiac imaging in the critical care unit. JAMA. 1985 Nov 22–29;254(20):2935–9.

Parra V, Fita G, Rovira I, Matute P, Gomar C, Pare C. Transoesophageal echocardiography accurately detects cardiac output variation: a prospective comparison with thermodilution in cardiac surgery. Eur J Anaesthesiol. 2008 Feb;25(2):135–43. Epub 2007 Aug 2.

Patel KM, Sherwani SS, Baudo AM, Salvacion A, Herborn J, Soong W, et al. Echo rounds: the use of transesophageal echocardiography for confirmation of appropriate Impella 5.0 device placement. Anesth Analg. 2012 Jan;114(1):82–5. Epub 2011 Oct 24.

Pepi M, Evangelista A, Nihoyannopoulos P, Flachskampf FA, Athanassopoulos G, Colonna P, et al; European Association of Echocardiography. Recommendations for echocardiography use in the diagnosis and management of cardiac sources of embolism: European Association of Echocardiography (EAE) (a registered branch of the ESC). Eur J Echocardiogr. 2010 Jul;11(6):461–76.

Pretorius M, Hughes AK, Stahlman MB, Saavedra PJ, Deegan RJ, Greelish JP, et al. Placement of the TandemHeart percutaneous left ventricular assist device. Anesth Analg. 2006 Dec;103(6):1412–3.

Quinones MA, Douglas PS, Foster E, Gorcsan J 3rd, Lewis JF, Pearlman AS, et al; American College of Cardiology; American Heart Association; American College of Physicians; American Society of Internal Medicine Task Force on Clinical Competence. American College of Cardiology/American Heart Association clinical competence statement on echocardiography: a report of the American College of Cardiology/American Heart Association/American College of Physicians: American Society of Internal Medicine Task Force on Clinical Competence. Circulation. 2003 Feb 25;107(7):1068–89.

Quinones MA, Otto CM, Stoddard M, Waggoner A, Zoghbi WA; Doppler Quantification Task Force of the Nomenclature and Standards Committee of the American Society of Echocardiography. Recommendations for quantification of Doppler echocardiography: a report from the Doppler Quantification Task Force of the Nomenclature and Standards Committee of the American Society of Echocardiography. J Am Soc Echocardiogr. 2002 Feb;15(2):167–84.

Roldan CA, Shively BK, Crawford MH. Valve excrescences: prevalence, evolution and risk for cardioembolism. J Am Coll Cardiol. 1997 Nov 1;30(5):1308–14.

Saric M, Armour AC, Arnaout MS, Chaudhry FA, Grimm RA, Kronzon I, et al. Guidelines for the use of echocardiography in the evaluation of a cardiac source of embolism. J Am Soc Echocardiogr. 2016 Jan;29(1):1–42.

Sauer CM, Yuh DD, Bonde P. Extracorporeal membrane oxygenation use has increased by 433% in adults in the United States from 2006 to 2011. ASAIO J. 2015 Jan-Feb;61(1):31–6.

Shanewise JS, Cheung AT, Aronson S, Stewart WJ, Weiss RL, Mark JB, et al. ASE/SCA guidelines for performing a comprehensive intraoperative multiplane transesophageal echocardiography examination: recommendations of the American Society of Echocardiography Council for Intraoperative Echocardiography and the Society of Cardiovascular Anesthesiologists Task Force for Certification in Perioperative Transesophageal Echocardiography. J Am Soc Echocardiogr. 1999 Oct;12(10):884–900.

Vieillard-Baron A, Chergui K, Rabiller A, Peyrouset O, Page B, Beauchet A, et al. Superior vena caval collapsibility as a gauge of volume status in ventilated septic patients. Intensive Care Med. 2004 Sep;30(9):1734–9. Epub 2004 Jun 26.

Vignon P, Mentec H, Terre S, Gastinne H, Gueret P, Lemaire F. Diagnostic accuracy and therapeutic impact of transthoracic and transesophageal echocardiography in mechanically ventilated patients in the ICU. Chest. 1994 Dec;106(6):1829–34.

Willett DL, Hall SA, Jessen ME, Wait MA, Grayburn PA. Assessment of aortic regurgitation by transesophageal color Doppler imaging of the vena contracta: validation against an intraoperative aortic flow probe. J Am Coll Cardiol. 2001 Apr;37(5):1450–5.

Zoghbi WA, Enriquez-Sarano M, Foster E, Grayburn PA, Kraft CD, Levine RA, et al; American Society of Echocardiography. Recommendations for evaluation of the severity of native valvular regurgitation with two-dimensional and Doppler echocardiography. J Am Soc Echocardiogr. 2003 Jul;16(7):777–802.

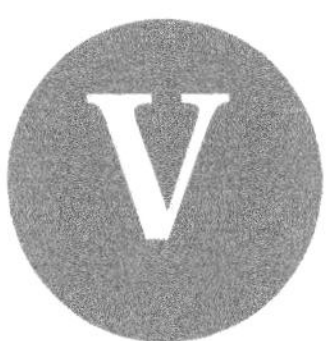

Questions and Answers

Abbreviations Used

ARDS acute respiratory distress syndrome
CT computed tomography
ICU intensive care unit
TEE transesophageal echocardiography
TTE transthoracic echocardiography

Questions

Multiple Choicc (choose the best answer)

V.1. Which of the following is *incorrect* about pneumothorax in a supine patient?
  a. The deep sulcus sign is associated with a subpulmonic pneumothorax.
  b. Tension pneumothorax does not always shift the mediastinum.
  c. Anteromedial pneumothorax can produce increased sharpness of the border of the cardiac silhouette or superior mediastinum.
  d. The double diaphragm sign refers to pneumothorax in the lateral costophrenic sulcus.

V.2. Which of the following is true about radiographic presentations of pulmonary edema?
  a. Well-documented appearances correlate with interstitial and air space edema.
  b. Air bronchograms are a sign of interstitial edema.
  c. The bat-wing pattern of pulmonary edema is common.
  d. ARDS never demonstrates an interstitial pattern.

V.3. Which of the following is *incorrect* about the radiographic presentation of aspiration?
  a. Low-pH gastric contents can evoke a rapid chemical pneumonitis and produce an extensive parenchymal edema pattern.
  b. Opacities from aspiration can be difficult to differentiate from ARDS, pneumonia, and pulmonary hemorrhage.
  c. Posterior lower lobe opacification from aspiration may be difficult to detect on a frontal radiograph because of projection through the hemidiaphragms and cardiac silhouette.
  d. Common locations for opacities from aspiration in a supine patient are the lingula and right middle lobe.

V.4. Which of the following is true regarding the split pleura sign?
  a. It is seen in the setting of pneumothorax on a chest radiograph.
  b. It is a CT sign associated with pneumomediastinum.
  c. It is a CT sign that refers to thickening of the visceral and parietal pleura separated by fluid.
  d. It is a CT finding associated with a pleural tear in the setting of a displaced rib fracture.

V.5. On a supine frontal radiograph of the abdomen, where is free intra-abdominal gas most often identified?
  a. The cul-de-sac
  b. The perinephric space
  c. The lesser sac
  d. The right upper quadrant

V.6. If abdominal radiographs do not explain the source of a patient's acute abdominal pain, what is the appropriate next imaging examination?
  a. Magnetic resonance imaging
  b. Ultrasonography
  c. Barium enema
  d. CT

V.7. Which of the following patient skin injuries due to overexposure during a fluoroscopic x-ray procedure is matched with the correct single-dose threshold?
  a. Erythema (single-dose threshold, 2,000 mGy)
  b. Epilation (single-dose threshold, 1,000 mGy)
  c. Moist desquamation (single-dose threshold, 9,000 mGy)
  d. Secondary ulceration (single-dose threshold, 30,000 mGy)

V.8. To minimize the patient radiation dose, which of the following techniques can be used to minimize the patient skin dose?
  a. Position the patient as far as reasonable from the image receptor (reduces dose rate).
  b. Position the patient as close to the x-ray tube as feasible (reduces dose rate).
  c. Use fluoroscopy sparingly and use last-image–hold for review (reduces irradiation time).
  d. Use pulsed fluoroscopy in as high a frame rate as practicable (reduces irradiation time).

V.9. During a nightshift, you are asked to evaluate a 63-year-old man who is a current smoker with a 50-pack-year history. He presented to the hospital with pain and swelling in his left leg. He remembers that a couple of days ago he injured his leg with a chair. His body temperature is 38°C, the edema in the calf is evident, the lower extremity pulses are normal, and testing for Homans sign is negative. What is the next step in evaluating this patient?
  a. Obtain a venogram of the leg as soon as possible.
  b. Obtain an echocardiogram performed by a cardiologist.
  c. Perform a focused assessment with sonography for trauma.
  d. Perform bedside vascular ultrasonography of the lower extremities immediately.

V.10. A 30-year-old man is transferred from the emergency department to the ICU after the activation of a sepsis code. He presented with high fever of 39.5°C, tachycardia, and normal blood pressure. He is awake but confused. During the physical examination, you find nontender hemorrhagic macular lesions of a few millimeters in diameter on the soles of his feet and a new diastolic aortic murmur. After you stabilize the patient, which of the following is the most appropriate diagnostic step?
a. Consult the cardiology service for a TEE as soon as possible.
b. Perform focused cardiac ultrasonography at the bedside.
c. Evaluate the inferior vena cava with ultrasonography to calculate the distensibility index.
d. Perform rescue TEE before transferring the patient to the ICU.

V.11. While making rounds on the hospital service, the resident informs you about a 49-year-old woman who came to the emergency department because of progressive dyspnea at rest during the past few days. Her past medical history includes metastatic breast cancer that was treated with chemotherapy and radiation. On physical examination, you find remarkable jugular venous distention and pulsus paradoxus. The electrocardiogram shows sinus tachycardia and alternation of the QRS complex amplitude. Which of the following is *not* an echocardiographic sign that you expect to find in the physiologic features of cardiac tamponade?
a. Right atrial collapse extending into ventricular systole
b. Right ventricular early diastolic collapse
c. Swinging of the heart within the effusion
d. Left atrial late diastolic collapse

V.12. Which of the following is *not* a reason to use TEE instead of TTE in patients in an ICU?
a. Morbid obesity
b. Improved diagnostic accuracy
c. Presence of surgical dressings
d. Increased patient safety

V.13. Which of the following is the most common complication of TEE in patients undergoing bedside TEE in the ICU?
a. Esophageal perforation
b. Dental injury
c. Dislodgment of nasogastric or nasojejunal feeding tubes
d. Odynophagia

V.14. Which of the following is *not* a contraindication to TEE placement?
a. Esophageal strictures
b. Tracheoesophageal fistula
c. Postesophageal surgery
d. Grade 1 esophageal varices

V.15. TEE provides excellent visualization of many cardiac structures because of the proximity of the esophagus to the heart and great vessels. In a normal TEE, the view of which of the following structures is impeded?
a. Aortic valve
b. Aortic root
c. Aortic arch
d. Descending thoracic aorta

V.16. Which of the following is *not* classified as having a high embolic potential?
a. Giant Lambl excrescences
b. Native valve endocarditis
c. Cardiac myxoma
d. Aortic atherosclerotic plaque

Answers

V.1. Answer d.

The deep sulcus sign can be seen with subpulmonic pneumothorax and is produced by air collecting inferiorly and laterally in the thorax in a supine patient. In some cases, tension pneumothorax may not shift the mediastinum or may produce only very subtle shift of mediastinal lines. The double diaphragm sign refers to an appearance produced by air along the anterior and posterior hemidiaphragms.

Gordon R. The deep sulcus sign. Radiology. 1980 Jul;136(1):25–7.

Ho ML, Gutierrez FR. Chest radiography in thoracic polytrauma. AJR Am J Roentgenol. 2009 Mar;192(3):599–612.

Tocino IM. Pneumothorax in the supine patient: radiographic anatomy. RadioGraphics. 1985 Jul;5(4):557–86.

V.2. Answer a.

Interstitial and air space patterns have distinct radiographic appearances. Air bronchograms are a sign of air space disease; Kerley lines are an example of a sign of interstitial thickening. The classic bat-wing pattern of edema is uncommon. Early ARDS may produce an interstitial pattern in some cases.

Gluecker T, Capasso P, Schnyder P, Gudinchet F, Schaller MD, Revelly JP, et al. Clinical and radiologic features of pulmonary edema. Radiographics. 1999 Nov-Dec;19(6):1507–31.

Ketai LH, Godwin JD. A new view of pulmonary edema and acute respiratory distress syndrome. J Thorac Imaging. 1998 Jul;13(3):147–71.

V.3. Answer d.

The middle lobe and lingula are common locations for aspiration in an erect, not a supine, patient. In a supine patient, the lower lobe superior and posterior basal segments and upper lobe posterior segments commonly show opacities from aspiration. The other statements are true.

Gurney JW. Atypical manifestations of pulmonary atelectasis. J Thorac Imaging. 1996 Summer;11(3):165–75.

Mendelson CL. The aspiration of stomach contents into the lungs during obstetric anesthesia. Am J Obstet Gynecol. 1946 Aug;52:191–205.

V.4. Answer c.

The split pleura sign may be seen with empyema and certain other cases of chronic exudative effusion, such as metastatic disease. The sign helps distinguish empyema from a peripheral lung abscess. The other statements are false.

Kuhlman JE, Singha NK. Complex disease of the pleural space: radiographic and CT evaluation. Radiographics. 1997 Jan-Feb;17(1):63–79.

Tsujimoto N, Saraya T, Light RW, Tsukahara Y, Koide T, Kurai D, et al. A simple method for differentiating complicated parapneumonic effusion/empyema from parapneumonic effusion using the split pleura sign and the amount of pleural effusion on thoracic CT. PLoS One. 2015 Jun 15;10(6):e0130141.

V.5. Answer d.

Free intraperitoneal gas most often is visible in the right upper quadrant, overlying or adjacent to the liver.

Levine MS, Scheiner JD, Rubesin SE, Laufer I, Herlinger H. Diagnosis of pneumoperitoneum on supine abdominal radiographs. AJR Am J Roentgenol. 1991 Apr;156(4):731–5.

V.6. Answer d.

CT frequently provides a more specific diagnosis.

MacKersie AB, Lane MJ, Gerhardt RT, Claypool HA, Keenan S, Katz DS, et al. Nontraumatic acute abdominal pain: unenhanced helical CT compared with three-view acute abdominal series. Radiology. 2005 Oct;237(1):114–22.

V.7. Answer a.

It is important to understand basic single-dose thresholds for potential effects on skin from fluoroscopy. These include early transient erythema at 2,000 mGy, epilation at 3,000 mGy, moist desquamation at 18,000 mGy, and secondary ulceration at 24,000 mGy.

Balter S, Miller DL. Patient skin reactions from interventional fluoroscopy procedures. AJR Am J Roentgenol. 2014 Apr;202(4):W335–42.

Wagner L. Radiation injury is a potentially serious complication to fluoroscopically-guided complex interventions. Biomed Imaging Interv J. 2007 Apr;3(2):e22. Epub 2007 Apr 1.

V.8. Answer c.

Multiple strategies can be used to minimize a patient's skin dose. The dose rate can be reduced by positioning the patient as close as reasonable to the image receptor and as far from the x-ray tube as feasible. The irradiation time can be reduced by use of fluoroscopy sparingly, use of last-image–hold for review, and use of pulsed fluoroscopy in as low a frame rate as practicable. Collimating the area of interest reduces the irradiated tissue volume.

Miller DL, Balter S, Schueler BA, Wagner LK, Strauss KJ, Vano E. Clinical radiation management for fluoroscopically guided interventional procedures. Radiology. 2010 Nov;257(2):321–32.

National Council on Radiation Protection and Measurements (NCRP). Radiation dose management for fluoroscopically guided interventional medical procedures [Internet]. NCRP Report No. 168. Bethesda (MD): National Council on Radiation Protection and Measurements; c2010. Available at: https://ncrponline.org/publications/reports/ncrp-report-168/.

V.9. Answer d.

In this case, there is a high level of clinical suspicion for deep vein thrombosis of the left leg. Accurate and prompt diagnosis of proximal lower extremity deep vein thrombosis can be realized by intensivists performing compression ultrasonography at the bedside, and this testing is recommended by the current evidence-based guidelines.

Frankel HL, Kirkpatrick AW, Elbarbary M, Blaivas M, Desai H, Evans D, et al. Guidelines for the appropriate use of bedside general and cardiac ultrasonography in the evaluation of critically ill patients-Part I: general ultrasonography. Crit Care Med. 2015 Nov;43(11):2479–502.

Kory PD, Pellecchia CM, Shiloh AL, Mayo PH, DiBello C, Koenig S. Accuracy of ultrasonography performed by critical care physicians for the diagnosis of DVT. Chest. 2011 Mar;139(3):538–42. Epub 2010 Oct 28.

V.10. Answer a.

In this case, the clinical suspicion is infective endocarditis. Echocardiographic evaluation of conditions such as endocarditis, in which comprehensive evaluation of details is needed, requires a higher level of training, and therefore echocardiographers should always be involved in the diagnostic process. TEE is more sensitive than TTE for the diagnosis of endocarditis, and the current guidelines recommend that TEE should be performed in all cases of suspected infective endocarditis. Rescue TEE is a diagnostic test performed in patients experiencing substantial hemodynamic instability, mainly in the intraoperative setting, and is not indicated in this case.

Baddour LM, Wilson WR, Bayer AS, Fowler VG Jr, Tleyjeh IM, Rybak MJ, et al; American Heart Association Committee on Rheumatic Fever, Endocarditis, and Kawasaki Disease of the

Council on Cardiovascular Disease in the Young, Council on Clinical Cardiology, Council on Cardiovascular Surgery and Anesthesia, and Stroke Council. Infective endocarditis in adults: diagnosis, antimicrobial therapy, and management of complications: a scientific statement for healthcare professionals from the American Heart Association. Circulation. 2015 Oct 13;132(15):1435–86. Epub 2015 Sep 15. Errata in: Circulation. 2015 Oct 27;132(17):e215. Circulation. 2016 Aug 23;134(8):e113.

V.11. Answer c.

In this case, the clinical suspicion is cardiac tamponade from pericardial metastases. Cardiac tamponade occurs when fluid (eg, blood) compresses the heart in the pericardial space and jeopardizes cardiac output. Echocardiographic signs are present when the intrapericardial pressure exceeds the cardiac chamber pressure and partial collapse of the chamber results. Usually, the sign that occurs first, and is sensitive but not specific, is right atrial collapse. If that persists into ventricular systole or lasts at least 30% of the cardiac cycle, it is a more specific sign. Conversely, right ventricular early diastolic collapse requires more pressure and is less sensitive but more specific. In about 25% of patients, the left atrium also collapses and is a highly specific sign. Occasionally, it is possible to see the swinging heart within the effusion, but it does not indicate cardiac tamponade.

Spodick DH. Acute cardiac tamponade. N Engl J Med. 2003 Aug 14;349(7):684–90.

V.12. Answer d.

TTE is estimated to be inadequate in 50% of patients receiving mechanical ventilation and in 60% of all patients in an ICU. Acoustic windows are frequently suboptimal in patients who are morbidly obese, have multiple chest tubes, have dressings, or are receiving mechanical ventilation. TEE also is superior to TTE in the ability to answer clinical questions in patients in shock. Although severe complications associated with TEE are rare at less than 3%, they are still present, and TTE has virtually no risk while the study is conducted.

Huttemann E, Schelenz C, Kara F, Chatzinikolaou K, Reinhart K. The use and safety of transoesophageal echocardiography in the general ICU: a minireview. Acta Anaesthesiol Scand. 2004 Aug;48(7):827–36.

Parker MM, Cunnion RE, Parrillo JE. Echocardiography and nuclear cardiac imaging in the critical care unit. JAMA. 1985 Nov 22–29;254(20):2935–9.

Vignon P, Mentec H, Terre S, Gastinne H, Gueret P, Lemaire F. Diagnostic accuracy and therapeutic impact of transthoracic and transesophageal echocardiography in mechanically ventilated patients in the ICU. Chest. 1994 Dec;106(6):1829–34.

V.13. Answer c.

In a review of 2,500 TEE examinations in the ICU, dislodgment of feeding tubes was most common (8.7%), and other complications included mucosal lesions, hypotension, and coughing (0.3%-0.7%). In a separate review in patients in the operating room, esophageal perforation occurred in 0.01% of cases. In the operating room, TEE is also safe and effective. In a case series of 7,200 patients who had cardiac surgery, the incidence of TEE-associated morbidity was 0.2% and that of mortality was 0%.

Huttemann E, Schelenz C, Kara F, Chatzinikolaou K, Reinhart K. The use and safety of transoesophageal echocardiography in the general ICU: a minireview. Acta Anaesthesiol Scand. 2004 Aug;48(7):827–36.

Kallmeyer IJ, Collard CD, Fox JA, Body SC, Shernan SK. The safety of intraoperative transesophageal echocardiography: a case series of 7,200 cardiac surgical patients. Anesth Analg. 2001 May;92(5):1126–30.

V.14. Answer d.

Blind placement of any device into the esophagus of patients with a stricture or a fistula or postoperative status could be associated with a risk of perforation. A small study evaluated the use of TEE in patients with grade 1 or grade 2 esophageal varices and found no adverse outcomes.

American Society of Anesthesiologists and Society of Cardiovascular Anesthesiologists Task Force on Transesophageal Echocardiography. Practice guidelines for perioperative transesophageal echocardiography: an updated report by the American Society of Anesthesiologists and the Society of Cardiovascular Anesthesiologists Task Force on Transesophageal Echocardiography. Anesthesiology. 2010 May;112(5):1084–96.

Pantham G, Waghray N, Einstadter D, Finkelhor RS, Mullen KD. Bleeding risk in patients with esophageal varices undergoing transesophageal echocardiography. Echocardiography. 2013 Nov;30(10):1152–5. Epub 2013 Jun 6.

V.15. Answer c.

The distal ascending aorta and aortic arch are often obscured from visualization with TEE because of the interposition of the trachea and the right main-stem bronchus.

Flachskampf FA, Decoodt P, Fraser AG, Daniel WG, Roelandt JR; Subgroup on Transesophageal Echocardiography and Valvular Heart Disease; Working Group on Echocardiography of the European Society of Cardiology. Guidelines from the working group: recommendations for performing transesophageal echocardiography. Eur J Echocardiogr. 2001 Mar;2(1):8–21.

Konstadt SN, Reich DL, Quintana C, Levy M. The ascending aorta: how much does transesophageal echocardiography see? Anesth Analg. 1994 Feb;78(2):240–4.

V.16. Answer a.

Lambl excrescences or strands are filiform structures less than 2 mm wide and between 3 and 10 mm in length localized to the line of leaflet closure. In a prospective study, strands were found with TEE in 40% to 50% of all patients and were not related to systemic embolic events. Each of the other abnormalities is associated with a high embolic potential.

Roldan CA, Shively BK, Crawford MH. Valve excrescences: prevalence, evolution and risk for cardioembolism. J Am Coll Cardiol. 1997 Nov 1;30(5):1308–14.

Saric M, Armour AC, Arnaout MS, Chaudhry FA, Grimm RA, Kronzon I, et al. Guidelines for the use of echocardiography in the evaluation of a cardiac source of embolism. J Am Soc Echocardiogr. 2016 Jan;29(1):1–42.

Procedures

Airway Procedures and Modes of Ventilation

Basics of Airway and Oxygen Delivery Devices

ANDREW W. MURRAY, MD

Goals

- Describe airway anatomy pertinent to intubation.
- Discuss the evaluation of natural airway adequacy.
- Discuss the device options for noninvasive oxygen therapy.

Introduction

One of the greatest responsibilities in managing an airway is to maintain a continuously patent airway. Any loss of patency of the patient's airway is critical, and if the ability to provide ventilatation is lost, brain damage can rapidly develop potentially lead to brain death.

Maintenance of an adequate airway can be compromised by injury, infection, loss of consciousness, respiratory failure, and medication. Allowing the patient to wake up and resume spontaneous ventilation is not necessarily applicable in the intensive care unit (ICU). Also, when anesthesia is induced for intubation, especially in obese or morbidly obese patients, the patients may recover from neuromuscular blockade without recovering responsiveness and ventilator response before life-threatening hypoxemia occurs.

The definition of *difficult airway* is not standardized in the anesthesiology literature, but Apfelbaum and colleagues have described it as the situation when "a conventionally trained anesthesiologist experiences difficulty with facemask ventilation of the upper airway, difficulty with tracheal intubation, or both." Managing a difficult airway requires the ability to recognize when a patient may present challenges with either ventilation or intubation (or both). The American Society of Anesthesiologists (ASA) difficult airway algorithm (Figure 114.1) is an excellent resource for decisions that need to be made to avoid difficulties and for an algorithmic guide on how to address the problems of difficult intubation and ventilation. The guidelines are clearly directed toward induction of anesthesia and surgery, but they may be applied to other situations or specialties.

Anatomical Considerations

A thorough understanding of airway anatomy is necessary to be able to predict which patients will present difficulty in intubation. The ASA difficult airway algorithm (Figure 114.1) has been used extensively to attempt risk stratification for difficult ventilation or intubation (Table 114.1). Studies have shown that use of only 1 item is a poor measure of predicting difficult intubation and that anesthesiologists should use combinations of tests to assess risk. In a meta-analysis, the combination of the Mallampati score and the thyromental distance was most likely to be useful in predicting a difficult intubation.

If a patient has a prior history of difficulty related to managing the patient's airway, the practitioner should pause and carefully assess the airway.

The goal of airway manipulation in preparation for intubation is to align 3 axes to facilitate both ventilation and intubation: the oral axis, the pharyngeal axis, and the laryngeal axis. Traditionally the so-called sniffing position has been considered the goal for alignment of those axes. However, a study performed with magnetic resonance imaging (but without any form of laryngoscopy) showed that those axes cannot be fully aligned in awake patients, although the angle between the line of vision and the laryngeal axis did improve (Figure 114.2).

1. Assess the likelihood and clinical impact of basic management problems
   Difficulty with patient cooperation or consent
   Difficult mask ventilation
   Difficult supraglottic airway placement
   Difficult laryngoscopy
   Difficult intubation
   Difficult surgical airway access
2. Actively pursue opportunities to deliver supplemental oxygen throughout the process of difficult airway management
3. Consider the relative merits and feasibility of basic management choices
   Awake intubation vs intubation after induction of general anesthesia
   Noninvasive technique vs invasive techniques for the initial approach to intubation
   Video-assisted laryngoscopy as an initial approach to intubation
   Preservation vs ablation of spontaneous ventilation
4. Develop primary and alternative strategies

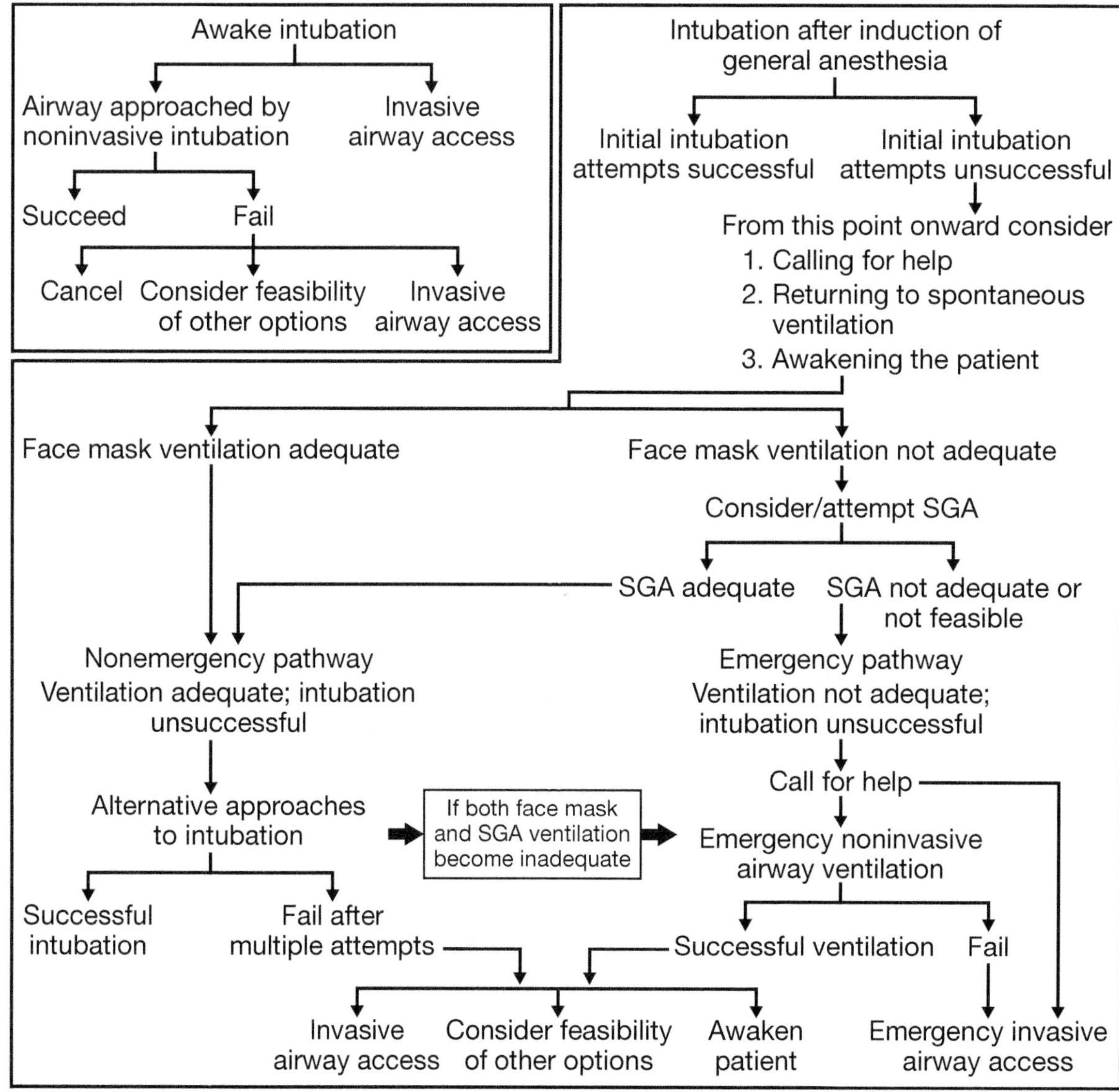

Figure 114.1. American Society of Anesthesiologists Difficult Airway Algorithm. SGA indicates supraglottic airway. (From Apfelbaum JL, Hagberg CA, Caplan RA, Blitt CD, Connis RT, Nickinovich DG, et al; American Society of Anesthesiologists Task Force on Management of the Difficult Airway. Practice guidelines for management of the difficult airway: an updated report by the American Society of Anesthesiologists Task Force on Management of the Difficult Airway. Anesthesiology. 2013 Feb;118[2]:251-70; used with permission.)

Table 114.1 • Elements of the Airway Examination

Examination Finding	Nonreassuring Finding
Length of incisors	Relatively long
Relative position of mandibular and maxillary incisors with jaw relaxed	Overbite
Relative position of mandibular and maxillary incisors with jaw protruded	Overbite maintained despite prognathism
Distance between incisiors	<3 cm
Visibility of uvula	Not visible with mouth open and tongue extended
Shape of palate	Narrow or arched
Compliance of submandibular space	Stiff, indurated; presence of space-occupying lesion
Thyromental distance	<6 cm
Length of neck	Short
Thickness of neck	Thick
Cervical range of motion	Inability to touch chin to chest or to extend the neck

From Apfelbaum JL, Hagberg CA, Caplan RA, Blitt CD, Connis RT, Nickinovich DG, et al; American Society of Anesthesiologists Task Force on Management of the Difficult Airway. Practice guidelines for management of the difficult airway: an updated report by the American Society of Anesthesiologists Task Force on Management of the Difficult Airway. Anesthesiology. 2013 Feb;118(2):251-70; used with permission.

Assessment of Upper Airway Patency

The exchange of oxygen and carbon dioxide requires a patent upper airway to allow inhaled gasses to reach the alveoli. Assessment of the patency of the upper airway is important in the overall assessment of respiratory function, especially if the patient is neurologically compromised and cannot sustain airway patency spontaneously. Neurologic compromise may result from medications, metabolic conditions, ischemic intracranial events, or intracerebral hemorrhage. Nonneurologic causes include obstructive sleep apnea and masses of the upper airway, including the oropharynx, nasopharynx, and laryngopharynx. Trauma of the face and neck can also compromise the patency of the upper airway.

The physical examination is beneficial in determining patency of the upper airway. Observation and listening to breathing noises can help identify potential airway compromise, and characteritics of airway sounds and inspiratory and expiratory patterns may indicate a possible cause. Inspection of the visible portion of the upper airway is useful to determine whether patency may be compromised by any conditions, such as a large swollen tongue due to trauma or angioedema, prominent tonsils, or unilateral narrowing as seen in Ludwig angina.

Patency can be also assessed both qualitatively and quantitatively. Methods of qualitative assessment include watching for a matching chest rise on inspiration and noting the use of accessory muscles during normal breathing. Paradoxical breathing, where the chest moves in the opposite direction as the abdomen during respiratory effort, may be an early sign that alerts the clinician to the possibility

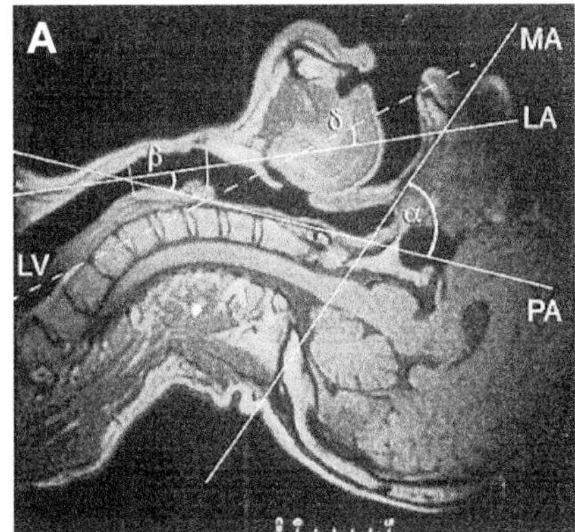

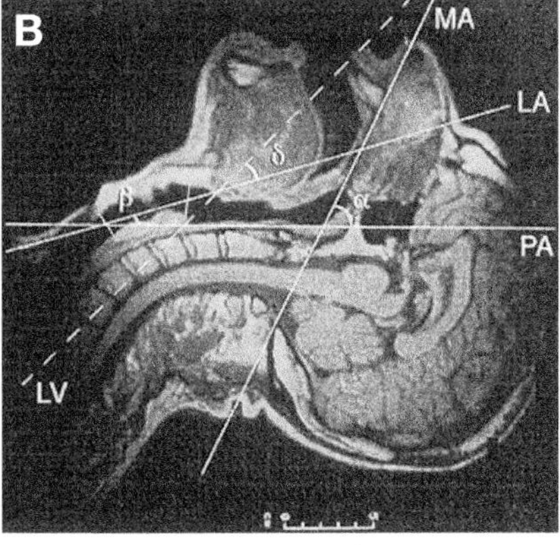

Figure 114.2. "Sniffing Position." A, Neck extension. B, Sniffing position. The measured angles (α, β, and δ) are not significantly different between the 2 positions. LA indicates laryngeal axis; LV, line of vision; MA, mouth axis; PA, pharyngeal axis. (From Adnet F, Borron SW, Dumas JL, Lapostolle F, Cupa M, Lapandry C. Study of the "sniffing position" by magnetic resonance imaging. Anesthesiology. 2001 Jan;94[1]:83-6; used with permission.)

of upper airway obstruction. Accessory muscle use may indicate increased effort of breathing and the potential for respiratory failure if not addressed. In addition, snoring, gurgling, or cessation of audible breath sounds may indicate impending or evolving upper airway obstruction. Stridor, an inspiratory crowing, can be particularly concerning because it indicates that compromise of patency may be evolving at the level of the glottis and surrounding extrathoracic structures.

A semiquantitative method for assessment of upper airway patency is *capnography*. Already the standard of care for general anesthesia, capnography is recognized as an invaluable tool for monitoring patients who may be having procedural sedation in the operating room, emergency department, ICU, and other nontraditional locations. In those settings, a closed system is usually not achieved, so it is not possible to fully capture all the exhaled gasses and thus get a true measurement of end-tidal carbon dioxide, but a capnogram shows an exhaled gas waveform over time and indicates ongoing ventilation.

Further investigation of the upper airway may include radiography. Ultrasonography is useful for evaluating the upper airway, specifically the glottis and adjacent structures.

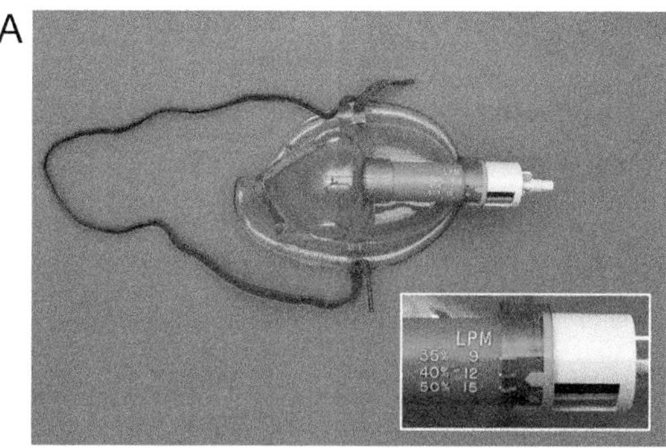

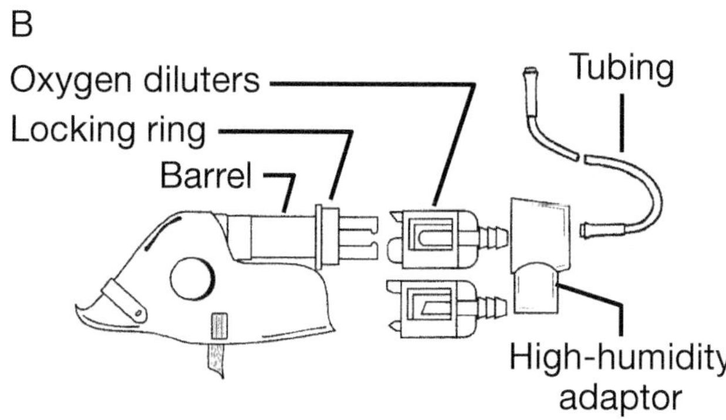

Figure 114.3. Venturi Mask. A, Entrainment valve is shown with the Venturi mask and in a close-up view (inset). LPM indicates liters per minute. B, Components of the Venturi mask.

Oxygen Delivery Devices

Invasive and noninvasive ventilation are reviewed elsewhere in this text, but various noninvasive oxygen delivery devices can be used to support the patient's oxygenation or ventilation passively. The simplest device is the standard nasal cannula. This device delivers a limited amount of supplemental oxygen (24%-44%) to the wearer. The amount of oxygen delivered is dependent on the patient's inspiratory flow: As inspiratory flow increases, room air entrainment increases, effectively diluting the delivered oxygen. Consequently use of this therapy should not be encouraged if a patient has severe hypoxemia. Flows greater than 4 L/min should be accompanied by humidification to avoid drying of the upper airway, which causes discomfort, a burning sensation, and sometimes bleeding.

Various masks are available. With simple face masks, delivery varies with inspiratory flow as described above. A more effective method incorporates a reservoir device, such as a nonrebreather mask, which provides a small reservoir to overcome the differential between the inspiratory flow of the patient and the oxygen flow. The nonrebreather mask can deliver 40% to 60% oxygen, although it is still subject to the patient's minute ventilation. Maximum efficiency is achieved if the mask is fitted tightly with 1-way valves, but this arrangement is not always well tolerated by patients.

Examples of high-flow devices include the Venturi mask (Figure 114.3) and the high-flow nasal cannula, a relatively new oxygen delivery device. Venturi masks can be regulated to deliver between 24% and 50% oxygen and are not dependent on humidification because of a high degree of ambient air entrainment. The amount of oxygen delivered is controlled by adjusting the entrainment valve.

The high-flow nasal cannula (Figure 114.4) can deliver high-flow oxygen therapy (HFOT) and still be well tolerated

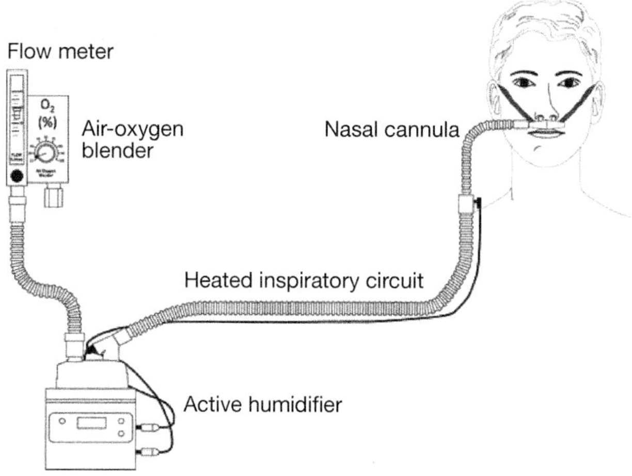

Figure 114.4. High-Flow Nasal Cannula Components. (From Nishimura M. High-flow nasal cannula oxygen therapy in adults. J Intensive Care. 2015 Mar 31;3[1]:15; used under Creative Commons Attribution License [http://creativecommons.org/licenses/by/4.0].)

because of efficient active humidification and heating. It is more effective than a Venturi mask in maintaining oxygenation for a specific fraction of inspired oxygen in recently extubated patients. Oxygen delivery with a high-flow nasal cannula has been shown to be as effective as noninvasive ventilation in preventing reintubation in the first 48 hours after extubation. A high-flow nasal cannula can also be used to augment oxygenation in the management of air embolism and pneumocephalus.

Summary

- The decision-making process requires an understanding of the ASA difficult airway algorithm.
- Oxygen supplementation can be achieved with various delivery devices to support patients who are in respiratory distress or who have been recently extubated.
- A high-flow nasal cannula is effective for supporting patients requiring HFOT and for preventing reintubation.
- Noninvasive ventilation is first-line therapy for patients who have chronic obstructive pulmonary disease exacerbation with acute respiratory acidosis, and it is recommended for patients who have respiratory failure after abdominal or thoracic surgery; after cardiothoracic surgery, HFOT is as efficient as noninvasive ventilation.

SUGGESTED READING

Adnet F, Borron SW, Dumas JL, Lapostolle F, Cupa M, Lapandry C. Study of the "sniffing position" by magnetic resonance imaging. Anesthesiology. 2001 Jan;94(1):83–6.

Apfelbaum JL, Caplan RA, Barker SJ, Connis RT, Cowles C, Ehrenwerth J, et al; American Society of Anesthesiologists Task Force on Operating Room Fires. Practice advisory for the prevention and management of operating room fires: an updated report by the American Society of Anesthesiologists Task Force on Operating Room Fires. Anesthesiology. 2013 Feb;118(2):271–90.

Apfelbaum JL, Hagberg CA, Caplan RA, Blitt CD, Connis RT, Nickinovich DG, et al; American Society of Anesthesiologists Task Force on Management of the Difficult Airway. Practice guidelines for management of the difficult airway: an updated report by the American Society of Anesthesiologists Task Force on Management of the Difficult Airway. Anesthesiology. 2013 Feb;118(2):251–70.

Benumof JL. Management of the difficult adult airway: with special emphasis on awake tracheal intubation. Anesthesiology. 1991 Dec;75(6):1087–110. Erratum in: Anesthesiology 1993 Jan;78(1):224.

Frat JP, Coudroy R, Thille AW. Non-invasive ventilation or high-flow oxygen therapy: when to choose one over the other? Respirology. 2018 Nov 8. [Epub ahead of print]

Hernandez G, Vaquero C, Colinas L, Cuena R, Gonzalez P, Canabal A, et al. Effect of postextubation high-flow nasal cannula vs noninvasive ventilation on reintubation and postextubation respiratory failure in high-risk patients: a randomized clinical trial. JAMA. 2016 Oct 18;316(15):1565–74. Errata in: JAMA. 2016 Nov 15;316(19):2047–8. JAMA. 2017 Feb 28;317(8):858.

Kallstrom TJ; American Association for Respiratory Care (AARC). AARC Clinical Practice Guideline: oxygen therapy for adults in the acute care facility: 2002 revision & update. Respir Care. 2002 Jun;47(6):717–20.

Krauss B, Hess DR. Capnography for procedural sedation and analgesia in the emergency department. Ann Emerg Med. 2007 Aug;50(2):172–81. Epub 2007 Jan 12.

Maggiore SM, Idone FA, Vaschetto R, Festa R, Cataldo A, Antonicelli F, et al. Nasal high-flow versus Venturi mask oxygen therapy after extubation: effects on oxygenation, comfort, and clinical outcome. Am J Respir Crit Care Med. 2014 Aug 1;190(3):282–8.

Nagler J, Krauss B. Capnography: a valuable tool for airway management. Emerg Med Clin North Am. 2008 Nov;26(4):881–97.

Naguib M, Brewer L, LaPierre C, Kopman AF, Johnson KB. The myth of rescue reversal in "can't intubate, can't ventilate" scenarios. Anesth Analg. 2016 Jul;123(1):82–92.

Rochwerg B, Granton D, Wang DX, Helviz Y, Einav S, Frat JP, et al. High flow nasal cannula compared with conventional oxygen therapy for acute hypoxemic respiratory failure: a systematic review and meta-analysis. Intensive Care Med. 2019 May;45(5):563–72. Epub 2019 Mar 19.

Shiga T, Wajima Z, Inoue T, Sakamoto A. Predicting difficult intubation in apparently normal patients: a meta-analysis of bedside screening test performance. Anesthesiology. 2005 Aug;103(2):429–37.

Werner SL, Jones RA, Emerman CL. Sonographic assessment of the epiglottis. Acad Emerg Med. 2004 Dec;11(12):1358–60.

Endotracheal Intubation Procedures

MATTHEW J. RITTER, MD

Goals

- Describe the approach to endotracheal intubation.
- Describe the different techniques for endotracheal intubation.
- Discuss the use of drugs to facilitate endotracheal intubation.

Introduction

Endotracheal intubation (ETI) is one of the most common procedures performed in the intensive care unit (ICU). It is also associated with a high incidence of complications.

Indications for ETI include acute hypoxemic or hypercapnic respiratory failure, loss of protective reflexes, and inability to manage secretions. Additionally, in the neurosciences ICU, intubation may be necessary for transient hyperventilation in patients with elevated intracranial pressure.

Approach to ETI

When the decision has been made to proceed with ETI, the use of a checklist (Figure 115.1) should be considered to ensure that all necessary equipment is present and properly functioning. In addition to obtaining medications to facilitate ETI, it is prudent to have vasoactive medications available at the bedside to treat any ensuing hypotension. Furthermore, the use of an intubation bundle can decrease the incidence of life-threatening complications, including severe hypoxemia and cardiovascular collapse.

Obtain assistance, if available, from a person experienced in airway management. Assess the patient's airway for predictors of difficult direct laryngoscopy. Although no single feature is guaranteed to predict easy or difficult direct laryngoscopy, the following criteria have traditionally been considered to be reliable predictors, especially when more than 1 is present: a Mallampati score of 3 or 4 (Figure 115.2), a short thyromental distance (<6 cm or <3 fingerbreadths), a limited interincisor distance (<3 cm or <2 fingerbreadths), a limited cervical spine range of motion, and an inability to perform an upper lip bite test. The MACOCHA score, developed and validated in a multicenter cohort trial, provides a clinical predictive score for intubation difficulty in the ICU and incorporates several risk factors: a Mallampati score of 3 or 4, reduced mobility of the cervical spine, limited mouth opening (<3 cm), obstructive sleep apnea, severe hypoxia or coma, and placement of the endotracheal tube by a person who is not an anesthesiologist.

Preoxygenation

Preoxygenation is often performed with a face mask, anesthesia bag, and high-flow oxygen or with a self-inflating bag and the attached oxygen reservoir. The use of bag-mask ventilation between induction and laryngoscopy provides higher oxygen saturation and a lower risk of severe hypoxemia. If the patient is already receiving noninvasive positive pressure support with continuous positive airway pressure (CPAP) or bilevel positive airway pressure (BiPAP), either method may be used instead. In fact, a study showed that, during intubation of patients with preexisting hypoxemia, the use of noninvasive ventilation with a positive end-expiratory pressure (PEEP) of 5 cm H_2O and pressure support adjusted to exhaled tidal volumes of 7 to 10 mL/kg decreased the incidence of severe hypoxemia after intubation from 42% to 7% when compared with oxygenation with 100% oxygen alone. Ideally, the head of the patient's bed is elevated during preoxygenation to prevent further reduction in functional residual capacity from upward pressure on the diaphragm and to promote venous drainage if the patient's intracranial pressure is increased. When it is not contraindicated, the sniffing position should be used (slight cervical flexion with atlantoaxial extension).

Preparation

- ☐ Discuss the need for intubation with the consultant physician and obtain informed consent
  - ☐ Confirm that no DNI orders exist
- ☐ Evaluate for difficult airway. If a difficult airway is identified or anticipated, notify Anesthesia airway backup before proceeding
  - ☐ If any intraoral appliance is present (ie, dentures), remove
- ☐ Identify and prepare *specific* backup plan for an *unexpected* difficult airway
- ☐ Verify that equipment includes (at a minimum)
  - ☐ Wall suction with Yankauer suction catheter in place
  - ☐ Resuscitation bag with 100% oxygen flowing
  - ☐ Appropriately sized anesthesia mask
  - ☐ Appropriately sized oropharyngeal or nasopharyngeal airway
  - ☐ Appropriately sized ETTs (≥2) with stylette and syringe
  - ☐ Functional intubation device (ie, laryngoscope, video laryngoscope)
  - ☐ ETT fastener (adhesive tape, twill tape, etc)
  - ☐ Capnometer
- ☐ Obtain adult intubation drug kit, draw up specific medications, and label syringes
  - ☐ Premedication ☐ Induction drug ☐ Paralytic drug
- ☐ Verify that personal protective equipment is in place
  - ☐ Eye protection, mask, and gloves (at a minimum)
- ☐ Ensure functional intravenous access
- ☐ Position patient appropriately (sniffing position unless contraindicated)
- ☐ Perform universal protocol (procedural pause)
  - ☐ Verify patient name, Mayo Clinic number, procedure, and code status
  - ☐ Verbally check medications ordered, doses, and availability
  - ☐ Ensure that a specific backup plan is articulated with the necessary airway equipment and personnel (ie, Anesthesia, Surgery) in place
  - ☐ Review individual roles
- ☐ Preoxygenate with supplemental oxygen sufficient to achieve Spo_2 appropriate for the situation

Intubation

- ☐ Consider premedication with midazolam (for amnestic effect) or fentanyl
- ☐ Administer induction drug
  - ☐ Etomidate ☐ Ketamine ☐ Propofol
- ☐ To minimize aspiration risk, consider applying cricoid pressure (Sellick maneuver) and maintain until ETT placement has been confirmed (this may increase the difficulty in visualizing the vocal cords)
- ☐ (Optional) Administer neuromuscular blockade and observe for onset of action
  - ☐ Succinylcholine ☐ Rocuronium
- ☐ Perform laryngoscopy and visualize the ETT passing between the vocal cords
- ☐ Confirm ETT placement with ≥2 of the following:
  - ☐ Capnometry
  - ☐ Bilateral breath sounds and absence of breath sounds over epigastrium
  - ☐ Flexible fiberoptic visualization of tracheal/bronchial anatomy

Post-Care

- ☐ Secure the ETT
- ☐ Initiate mechanical ventilation (mechanical ventilation orders placed in CPOE)
- ☐ Order long-acting analgesia and sedation
- ☐ Order a chest radiograph
- ☐ Anticipate and monitor for hemodynamic changes
- ☐ Fill out electronic procedural form

Figure 115.1. Mayo Clinic Intubation Checklist. CPOE indicates computerized physician order entry; DNI, do not intubate; ETT, endotracheal tube.

(Used with permission of Mayo Foundation for Medical Education and Research.)

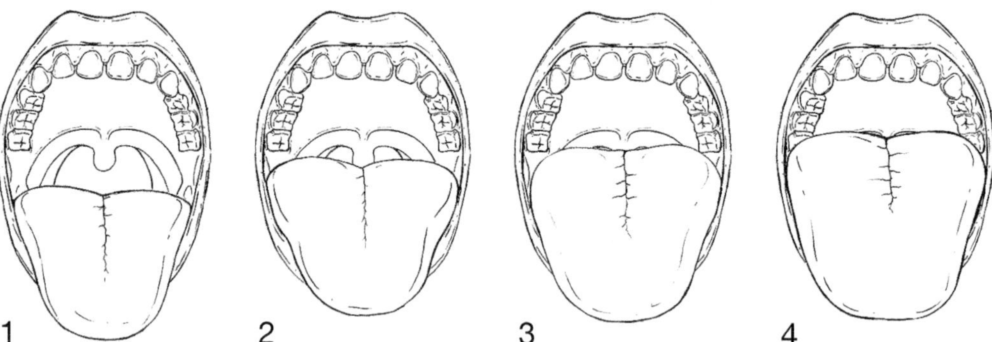

Figure 115.2. Mallampati Score. The 4 classes are characterized as follows: 1, the faucial/tonsillar pillars, uvula, and soft palate are all visible; 2, the faucial/tonsillar pillars, uvula, and soft palate are partially visible; 3, the base of the uvula, the soft palate, and the hard palate are visible; 4, only the hard palate is visible.

(From Kumar HV, Schroeder JW, Gang Z, Sheldon SH. Mallampati score and pediatric obstructive sleep apnea. J Clin Sleep Med. 2014 Sep 15;10[9]:985-90; used with permission.)

For a morbidly obese patient, elevating the upper portion of the patient's body or placing the patient in a ramp position may provide a better laryngoscopic view than the sniffing position alone.

Laryngoscopy

The decision on which technique to use to place the endotracheal tube is based on the history, examination, and urgency of intubation. Numerous techniques have been described (Box 115.1), but the most common are *direct laryngoscopy*, using a laryngoscope with a Macintosh (curved) blade or a Miller (straight) blade, and *indirect laryngoscopy*, using a video laryngoscope. When a Macintosh blade is used, the tip of the blade is placed in the vallecula between the epiglottis and the tongue base; upward force on the laryngoscope lifts the base of the tongue and the epiglottis, exposing the glottis (Figure 115.3). When a Miller blade is used, it is placed just posterior to the epiglottis; upward force on the laryngoscope lifts the epiglottis out of the way, exposing the glottis. The endotracheal tube should be advanced between the vocal cords until the cuff of the tube is 2 to 3 cm past the vocal cords. The choice of blade is mainly one of personal preference. Some find the Macintosh blade easier to use, while the Miller blade can be useful in a patient with a small mouth opening, an anterior larynx, or a long epiglottis that does not move out of the way with a Macintosh blade. With either blade, upward pressure should be applied, rather than rocking the blade back, to decrease the risk of dental trauma. If the patient requires cervical spine precautions, in-line stabilization must be maintained during direct laryngoscopy to prevent any unwanted movement.

Several studies have suggested that video laryngoscopy offers a higher success rate for ETI, a faster learning curve, and fewer complications. Video laryngoscopes have a wide viewing angle and do not require the sniffing position for ETI. Thus, if a patient has cervical spine precautions in-line stabilization is not necessary because the head position does not need to change. Use of a rigid endotracheal tube stylet greatly improves the ease of ETI when using video laryngoscopy. Novice users of video laryngoscopy often acquire an excellent view, yet encounter difficulty when attempting to pass the endotracheal tube through the glottis. This may be alleviated by slightly pulling the video laryngoscope out, thus allowing for more room for manipulation of the endotracheal tube. Sometimes, however, passing the endotracheal tube is difficult because the viewing angle provided by video

Box 115.1 • Methods for Translaryngeal Endotracheal Intubation

- Direct laryngoscopy
  - With Macintosh or Miller blade
  - With endotracheal tube introducer (intubating stylet, Eschmann stylet, or bougie)
- Indirect laryngoscopy
  - Video laryngoscopy
  - Fiberoptic intubation
    - Flexible fiberoptic bronchoscope
    - Rigid fiberoptic bronchoscope (optical stylets)
  - Nonfiberoptic optical laryngoscope
- Techniques that do not require visualization of the glottis
  - Intubating laryngeal mask airway
  - Lighted stylet intubation
  - Blind nasal intubation
  - Retrograde wire-assisted intubation

A

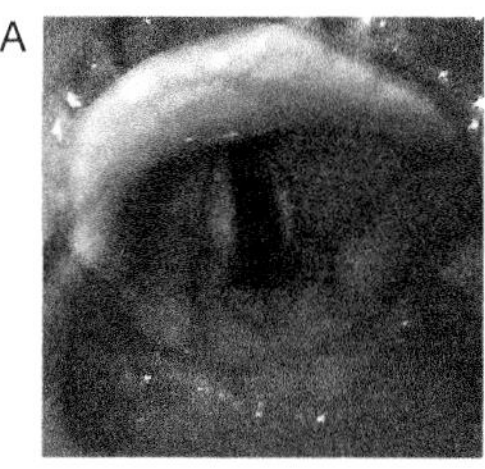

B

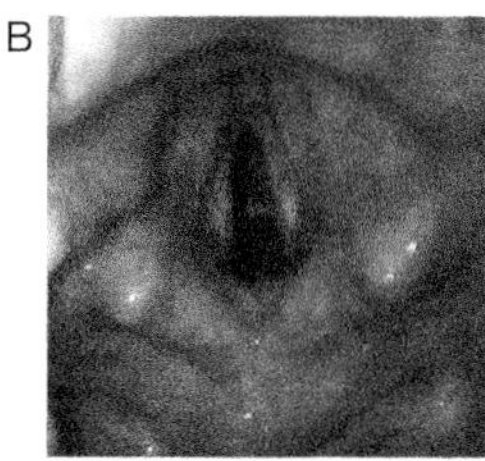

Figure 115.3. View of Glottis With Direct Laryngoscopy. A, When a Macintosh (curved) blade is used, the tip of the blade is in the vellecula, above (ie, anterior to) the epiglottis. B, When a Miller (straight) blade is used, the tip of the blade is posterior to the epiglottis, lifting it out of view.

laryngoscopy is anterior, while the endotracheal tube must pass posteriorly into the thorax after clearing the glottis.

Despite the improved success rates with video laryngoscopy in patients with normal or challenging airways, awake fiberoptic intubations are the gold standard for a patient with an airway that is known or predicted to be difficult. However, intubation with a flexible fiberoptic bronchoscope requires much more training and experience than intubation with either a direct laryngoscope or a video laryngoscope.

Decisions include whether the patient should be awake or sedated for intubation and whether spontaneous ventilation should be maintained or a paralytic should be administered to facilitate ETI. Debate continues as to whether patients in the ICU should be sedated and paralyzed for ETI. Maintenance of spontaneous ventilation may potentially prevent marked hypoxemia and provide a safety net if ETI is not successful or takes longer than expected. This approach is reasonable when ETI is being performed by someone who is relatively inexperienced or if experienced help is not readily available. Conversely, if the patient cannot be fully cooperative for the awake technique or if deeper sedation is warranted with or without paralysis (eg, to avoid increasing intracranial pressure), proceeding with a standard induction with muscle relaxation, when used as part of an intubation bundle, has been shown to be safe.

Pharmacologic Considerations

The choice of sedative hypnotic agent and muscle relaxant depends on the clinical scenario. Sedative and analgesic drugs are discussed in Chapter 135 ("Sedation and Analgesia"); however, a few points should be made about common agents used for sedation for ETI.

Propofol is frequently chosen for sedation for ETI. It has a rapid onset and can be continued for ongoing sedation after intubation. It results in a dose-dependent decrease in respiratory rate and can cause more hypotension than most sedatives. The hypotension is due to a decrease in systemic vascular resistance and venodilation rather than to a decrease in cardiac output as previously thought. Propofol markedly decreases cerebral blood flow and the cerebral metabolic rate.

Similarly, etomidate decreases cerebral blood flow and the cerebral metabolic rate. It provides more hemodynamic stability than propofol, but it has become unpopular because of concern over adrenal suppression and increased mortality when used in critically ill patients. Although a recent review did not identify an increase in mortality, an increased risk of adrenal dysfunction and a small increase in multiorgan system dysfunction were associated with its use.

Ketamine is stable from a cardiac standpoint. It produces bronchodilation and can help to maintain spontaneous breathing. Traditionally, ketamine was thought to increase intracranial pressure (and was therefore contraindicated in patients with elevated intracranial pressure), but data have shown mixed results.

Muscle relaxation often provides superior intubating conditions. Succinylcholine is the only depolarizing neuromuscular blocker. Rapid onset and short duration make it appealing for facilitating ETI for all urgent or emergent intubations. If succinylcholine is contraindicated or not desirable, rocuronium may be used for muscle relaxation for urgent intubation. The onset is slower than with succinylcholine, but it can still provide excellent intubating conditions within 60 seconds after a 1-mg/kg dose. In the past, use of nondepolarizing muscle relaxants was sometimes avoided because of the prolonged duration of action. With the recent approval of sugammadex, however, rocuronium (and possibly vecuronium) can be fully reversed within minutes of administration, making these muscle relaxants part of the ICU physician's armamentarium.

Confirmation of Endotracheal Tube Placement

Once intubation has been performed, tube placement in the trachea should be confirmed. Identification of carbon dioxide in exhaled gas, either qualitatively (with capnometry) or quantitatively (with capnography), is the current standard for verification of proper endotracheal tube placement. However, even end-tidal carbon dioxide is not a foolproof finding, because carbon dioxide may be absent or severely decreased in many patients, especially those with low cardiac output.

Several other techniques have been described, but they have drawbacks. Breath sounds may be absent with pneumothorax or difficult to appreciate if a patient has a large body habitus. Additionally, sounds resembling normal breath sounds can be heard with esophageal intubation, and the chest rise with esophageal intubation can be indistinguishable from that with endotracheal tube placement. Condensation in the endotracheal tube can occur in up to 85% of esophageal intubations. Furthermore, after esophageal intubation, several minutes may pass before oxygen saturation decreases, especially in patients with normal lung function (eg, those intubated for neurologic reasons).

Proper placement in the trachea rather than in a mainstem bronchus can be confirmed with bronchoscopy or chest radiography.

Summary

- Use of an intubation checklist and bundle can reduce the incidence of severe complications with ETI.
- Identification of predictors of difficult direct laryngoscopy can help with formulation of the most appropriate method of ETI.
- Indirect laryngoscopy with a video laryngoscope may be associated with a higher success rate and fewer complications than direct laryngoscopy.
- Maintenance of spontaneous respirations in patients with difficult airways is recommended whenever possible.

SUGGESTED READING

Andersen KH, Hald A. Assessing the position of the tracheal tube: the reliability of different methods. Anaesthesia. 1989 Dec;44(12):984–5.

Apfelbaum JL, Hagberg CA, Caplan RA, Blitt CD, Connis RT, Nickinovich DG, et al; American Society of Anesthesiologists Task Force on Management of the Difficult Airway. Practice guidelines for management of the difficult airway: an updated report by the American Society of Anesthesiologists Task Force on Management of the Difficult Airway. Anesthesiology. 2013 Feb;118(2):251–70.

Baillard C, Fosse JP, Sebbane M, Chanques G, Vincent F, Courouble P, et al. Noninvasive ventilation improves preoxygenation before intubation of hypoxic patients. Am J Respir Crit Care Med. 2006 Jul 15;174(2):171–7. Epub 2006 Apr 20.

Bruder EA, Ball IM, Ridi S, Pickett W, Hohl C. Single induction dose of etomidate versus other induction agents for endotracheal intubation in critically ill patients. Cochrane Database Syst Rev. 2015 Jan 8;1:CD010225.

Casey JD, Janz DR, Russell DW, Vonderhaar DJ, Joffe AM, Dischert KM, et al; PreVent Investigators and the Pragmatic Critical Care Research Group. Bag-mask ventilation during tracheal intubation of critically ill adults. N Engl J Med. 2019 Feb 28;380(9):811–21. Epub 2019 Feb 18.

Cavus E, Dorges V. Video laryngoscopes. In: Hagberg CA, editor. Benumof and Hagberg's airway management. 3rd ed. Philadelphia (PA): Elsevier/Saunders; c2013. p. 536–48.

Collins JS, Lemmens HJ, Brodsky JB, Brock-Utne JG, Levitan RM. Laryngoscopy and morbid obesity: a comparison of the "sniff" and "ramped" positions. Obes Surg. 2004 Oct;14(9):1171–5.

De Jong A, Jung B, Jaber S. Intubation in the ICU: we could improve our practice. Crit Care. 2014 Mar 18;18(2):209.

De Jong A, Molinari N, Terzi N, Mongardon N, Arnal JM, Guitton C, et al; AzuRea Network for the Frida-Rea Study Group. Early identification of patients at risk for difficult intubation in the intensive care unit: development and validation of the MACOCHA score in a multicenter cohort study. Am J Respir Crit Care Med. 2013 Apr 15;187(8):832–9.

de Wit F, van Vliet AL, de Wilde RB, Jansen JR, Vuyk J, Aarts LP, et al. The effect of propofol on haemodynamics: cardiac output, venous return, mean systemic filling pressure, and vascular resistances. Br J Anaesth. 2016 Jun;116(6):784–9.

Griesdale DE, Bosma TL, Kurth T, Isac G, Chittock DR. Complications of endotracheal intubation in the critically ill. Intensive Care Med. 2008 Oct;34(10):1835–42. Epub 2008 Jul 5.

Hoffman WE, Charbel FT, Ausman JI. Cerebral blood flow and metabolic response to etomidate and ischemia. Neurol Res. 1997 Feb;19(1):41–4.

Jaber S, Jung B, Corne P, Sebbane M, Muller L, Chanques G, et al. An intervention to decrease complications related to endotracheal intubation in the intensive care unit: a prospective, multiple-center study. Intensive Care Med. 2010 Feb;36(2):248–55. Epub 2009 Nov 17.

Kirkegaard-Nielsen H, Caldwell JE, Berry PD. Rapid tracheal intubation with rocuronium: a probability approach to determining dose. Anesthesiology. 1999 Jul;91(1):131–6.

Lapinsky SE. Endotracheal intubation in the ICU. Crit Care. 2015 Jun 17;19:258.

Levitan RM, Heitz JW, Sweeney M, Cooper RM. The complexities of tracheal intubation with direct laryngoscopy and alternative intubation devices. Ann Emerg Med. 2011 Mar;57(3):240–7. Epub 2010 Jul 31.

Mosier JM, Whitmore SP, Bloom JW, Snyder LS, Graham LA, Carr GE, et al. Video laryngoscopy improves intubation success and reduces esophageal intubations compared to direct laryngoscopy in the medical intensive care unit. Crit Care. 2013 Oct 14;17(5):R237.

Paolini JB, Donati F, Drolet P. Review article: video-laryngoscopy: another tool for difficult intubation or a new paradigm in airway management? Can J Anaesth. 2013 Feb;60(2):184–91. Epub 2012 Dec 12.

Park SO, Kim JW, Na JH, Lee KH, Lee KR, Hong DY, et al. Video laryngoscopy improves the first-attempt success in endotracheal intubation during cardiopulmonary resuscitation among novice physicians. Resuscitation. 2015 Apr;89:188–94. Epub 2014 Dec 22.

Pollard BJ, Junius F. Accidental intubation of the oesophagus. Anaesth Intensive Care. 1980 May;8(2):183–6.

Ramez Salem M, Baraka AS. Confirmation of endotracheal intubation. In: Hagberg CA, editor. Benumof and Hagberg's airway management. 3rd ed. Philadelphia (PA): Elsevier/Saunders; c2013. p. 657–82.

Seo SH, Lee JG, Yu SB, Kim DS, Ryu SJ, Kim KH. Predictors of difficult intubation defined by the intubation difficulty scale (IDS): predictive value of 7 airway assessment factors. Korean J Anesthesiol. 2012 Dec;63(6):491–7. Epub 2012 Dec 14.

Vandesteene A, Trempont V, Engelman E, Deloof T, Focroul M, Schoutens A, et al. Effect of propofol on cerebral blood flow and metabolism in man. Anaesthesia. 1988 Mar;43 Suppl:42–3.

Zeiler FA, Teitelbaum J, West M, Gillman LM. The ketamine effect on ICP in traumatic brain injury. Neurocrit Care. 2014 Aug;21(1):163–73.

Zeiler FA, Teitelbaum J, West M, Gillman LM. The ketamine effect on intracranial pressure in nontraumatic neurological illness. J Crit Care. 2014 Dec;29(6):1096–106. Epub 2014 Jun 4.

Noninvasive Positive Pressure Ventilation

KAREN W. HAMPTON, MS, RRT

Goals

- Understand noninvasive ventilation and the appropriate use of the technique.
- Describe how to initiate and manage noninvasive ventilation.
- Discuss common complications of noninvasive ventilation.

Introduction

Noninvasive positive pressure ventilation, also called noninvasive ventilation (NIV), is delivered through a noninvasive device, such as a full-face mask. Unlike the systems for invasive ventilation, which is delivered through an endotracheal or tracheostomy tube, the NIV delivery system is not a closed system, and so it leaks. The size of the leak affects the tidal volume delivered and the ability of the patient to trigger the machine into inspiration or cycle the machine into expiration. The acceptable leak for most systems is less than 35% of the peak inspiratory flow (leakage may be expressed as a percentage or as liters per minute).

Most NIV devices can be used with a specified respiratory rate. However, NIV is usually considered a backup for apnea, so a respiratory rate is typically not set with NIV unless the patient has a "do not intubate" directive and does not have an intact respiratory drive.

The indications for NIV and the goals for its use are based on many years of research and experience. The most commonly stated benefits for intensive care patients are the following:

- Decreased need for intubation
- Shortened intensive care unit (ICU) and hospital stays
- Decreased risk of nosocomial pneumonia
- Decreased mortality
- Improved patient comfort
- Decreased need for sedation
- Preservation of airway protective mechanisms

In addition to its use for short-term care, NIV is also beneficial for long-term care. For example, in patients with sleep-disordered breathing and neurologic disorders, NIV has been shown to increase functional capacity and prolong survival.

Patient Selection

When deciding whether a patient is a candidate for NIV, an important consideration is whether the patient's condition is easily reversible. If it is not, NIV may not be beneficial in preventing intubation. Airway protective mechanisms should also be assessed, and if patients cannot protect their airway, NIV should not be used. NIV is best for patients who are alert, able to protect their airway, and cooperative.

In an observational cohort study, NIV was not successful in 70.3% of patients with acute lung injury (which included all patients with shock). The conclusion of that study was that NIV should not be used, or should be used only with extreme caution, in patients with acute lung injury who have shock, metabolic acidosis, or profound hypoxemia.

In another study that compared NIV with mechanical ventilation in patients with acute respiratory failure, patients who first received NIV and then required intubation had high mortality (90%). That study was conducted before the standard Acute Respiratory Distress Syndrome Network (ARDSNet) lung protective strategies became standard practice. The reason for the increase in mortality is not fully understood.

Chronic Obstructive Pulmonary Disease Exacerbation

The most common use of NIV is for patients with exacerbation of chronic obstructive pulmonary disease (COPD). This use of NIV has been studied more often than any other use, and the studies have provided the strongest evidence for a decreased need for intubation in those patients. In addition, the use of NIV in patients with COPD has been shown to decrease ICU stay, complications, and mortality.

During an exacerbation of COPD, hyperinflation worsens and respiratory muscle activity increases, which increases the oxygen cost of breathing. Without intervention, patients are at risk for respiratory failure and death. The use of NIV in these patients is thought to decrease respiratory muscle activity and the respiratory rate. In addition, tidal volume and minute ventilation increase, allowing for better alveolar gas exchange.

Hypoxemic Respiratory Failure

The evidence for NIV use in patients with hypoxemic respiratory failure is inconsistent. Conditions causing hypoxemic respiratory failure are associated with impaired gas exchange (ratio of Pa_{O_2} to fraction of inspired oxygen [F_{IO_2}] <200) and increased respiratory rate (>30 breaths per minute). If NIV is initiated and the patient's gas exchange and overall condition improve, the patient has a decreased risk for complications associated with intubation.

Typically, NIV is difficult to manage if a patient has an increased respiratory rate. However, if the gas exchange improves, the respiratory rate may decrease after initiation of NIV; if improvement does not occur within a few hours, however, NIV probably will not be beneficial.

Neuromuscular Conditions

NIV has some value in patients with acute neuromuscular respiratory failure, such as in Guillain-Barré syndrome or myasthenic crisis, but appropriate patient selection is problematic. Generally, NIV is excellent for rescue therapy after weaning. It is useful if myasthenia gravis worsens before plasma exchange results in improvement. However, NIV may be dangerous for patients with worsening Guillain-Barré syndrome because plasma exchange rarely results in improvement quickly. The value of NIV in chronic forms, such as amyotrophic lateral sclerosis, is established.

Initiation of NIV

The NIV device most commonly used is a full-face mask, which must be properly sized to minimize leakage. Most masks have fitting guides to assist the clinician with choosing the correct size. Use of a mask that does not fit properly results in increased leakage and loss of volume. Although many clinicians tighten the mask to try to decrease the leakage, air pressure helps to seat the mask and minimize leaks without having to tighten the mask, so it is not uncommon for leakage to increase when a mask is too tight. Tightening the mask can also cause pressure-related skin issues and skin breakdown.

When therapy is initiated, the patient should be in an upright position. The initial pressure settings should be relatively low: Typically, the inspiratory positive airway pressure (IPAP) is started at 8 to 10 cm H_2O, and the expiratory positive airway pressure (EPAP) at 4 to 5 cm H_2O. Initial alarms should be silenced to minimize patient and family anxiety. Allowing the patient to hold the mask (if possible) during adjustment of the settings and fitting of the mask may also help to decrease anxiety and improve comfort.

Oxygen saturation should be monitored and F_{IO_2} adjusted to achieve the desired saturation. The IPAP and EPAP should be adjusted slowly to achieve the volume desired, but the clinician must remember that the difference between these 2 pressures is directly related to volume delivery and as IPAP and EPAP are increased, the potential for mask leaks increases. When the desired settings have been reached, the headgear for the mask may need to be adjusted. After the patient's condition has been stabilized, arterial blood gas (ABG) values may be needed to determine whether adequate ventilation is being delivered. If settings cannot be adjusted to reach the desired volume within 1 hour, NIV will probably be unsuccessful (Figure 116.1).

After Extubation

For patients at risk for respiratory failure after extubation, NIV application may be beneficial. In these patients, reintubation may be avoided if NIV is initiated soon after extubation. However, routine use of NIV after extubation is not recommended. Extubation failure, hospital stay, and mortality have not been significantly different between patients who were successfully extubated after a spontaneous breathing trial and patients who were routinely treated with NIV after extubation.

NIV Management

If a patient tolerates the initial phase of NIV, clinical improvement should be evident within the first 2 hours. The goal is to provide enough support to decrease the work of breathing and improve pH and Pa_{CO_2}. The oxygenation goal is for oxygen saturation to exceed 90%.

When IPAP and EPAP levels are being determined, the patient's clinical status must be observed. If the IPAP level is insufficient, the work of breathing and the respiratory rate may increase. The EPAP level may need to be adjusted to offset the intrinsic positive end-expiratory pressure. However, if EPAP is increased, the IPAP may also need to be increased to maintain the same pressure difference. The result of not doing so can be a decreased delivered tidal volume. The tidal volume should be 5 to 7 mL/kg of predicted body weight, and IPAP should not exceed 20 cm H_2O.

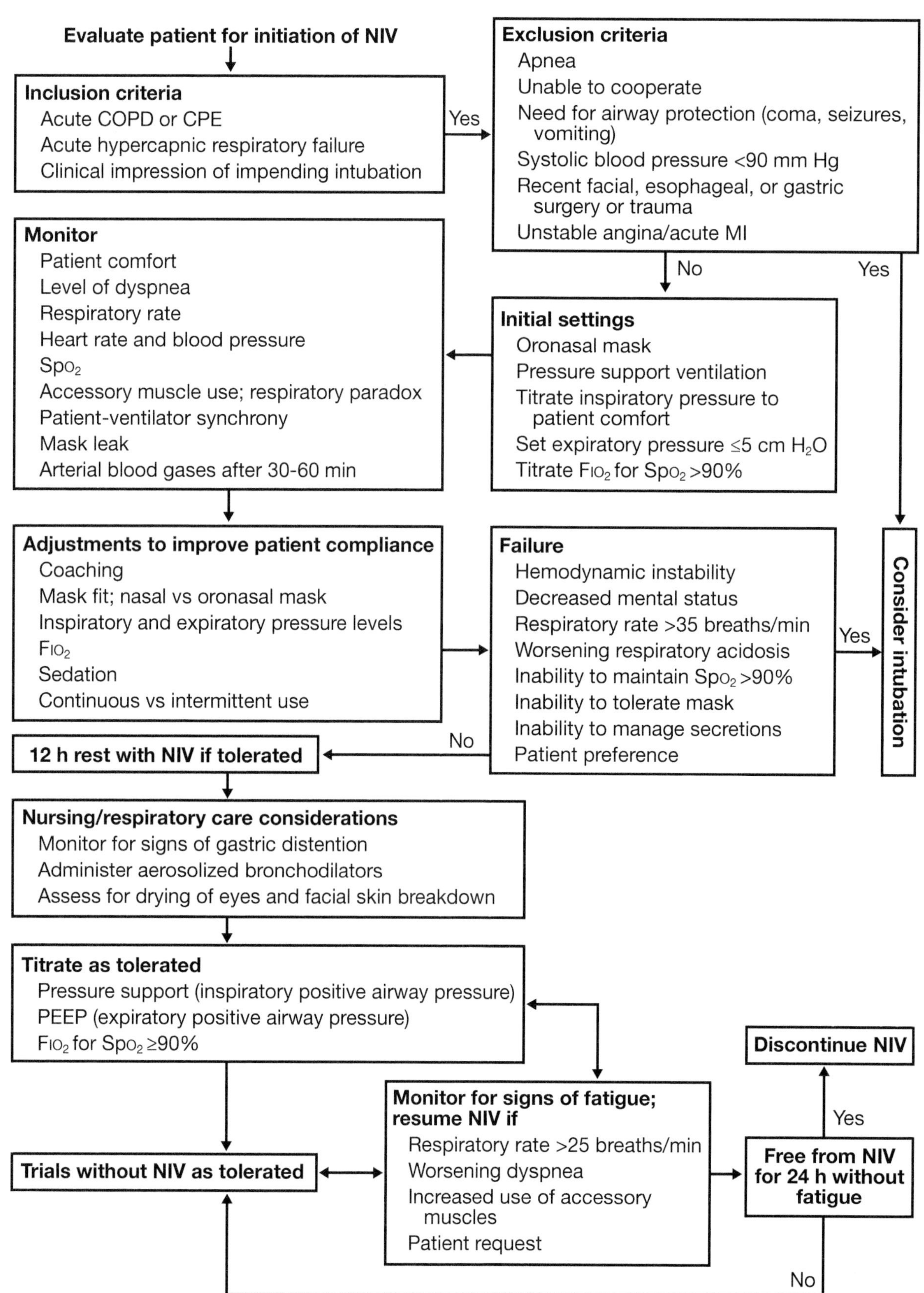

Figure 116.1. Initiation of Noninvasive Ventilation (NIV). COPD indicates chronic obstructive pulmonary disease; CPE, cardiogenic pulmonary edema; $F\text{IO}_2$, fraction of inspired oxygen; MI, myocardial infarction; PEEP, positive end-expiratory pressure; $\text{Sp}O_2$, oxygen saturation by pulse oximetry.

(From Hess DR. How to initiate a noninvasive ventilation program: bringing the evidence to the bedside. Respir Care. 2009 Feb;54[2]: 232–43; used with permission.)

If the patient's condition improves after 1 to 2 hours of support, the patient probably will not need to be intubated. ABG values should be used to verify ventilation, but the ABG values may not normalize for several hours after NIV is initiated. Decreased work of breathing is not a cause for alarm if the patient's clinical status is improving.

Complications

As with all positive pressure ventilation, NIV is associated with complications. The most common complication is mask discomfort. Higher flows and pressures can be uncomfortable for some patients initially. Mask leaks are often irritating to the eyes. A mask that has been tightened too much can cause pressure on the bridge of the nose or cheeks, causing skin breakdown. Use of a barrier under the mask may help decrease pressure-related complications.

Gastric insufflation is another common complication. An oral or nasogastric tube may be necessary. Patients with decreased protective airway mechanisms are at risk for aspiration and may not be candidates for NIV.

Humidification may not be needed for short-term use. If the patient is expected to require continuous NIV for several hours, humidification should be provided; otherwise, the higher flows required with NIV may cause irritation to the nasal mucosa and cause nasal congestion.

Summary

- NIV is a safe, useful tool in selected patients.
- Patients should be evaluated for proper mask fitting, airway protection, and reversible causes requiring NIV.
- One of the greatest barriers to successful use of NIV is lack of understanding.
- Initiation of NIV requires time to make the patient comfortable; without the patient's cooperation, therapy with NIV will probably be unsuccessful.

SUGGESTED READING

Antonelli M, Conti G, Rocco M, Bufi M, De Blasi RA, Vivino G, et al. A comparison of noninvasive positive-pressure ventilation and conventional mechanical ventilation in patients with acute respiratory failure. N Engl J Med. 1998 Aug 13;339(7):429–35.

Ergan B, Nasiłowski J, Winck JC. How should we monitor patients with acute respiratory failure treated with noninvasive ventilation? Eur Respir Rev. 2018 Apr 13;27(148). pii: 170101. Print 2018 Jun 30.

Gramlich T. Basic concepts of noninvasive positive pressure ventilation. In: Pilbeam SP, Cairo JM, editors. Mechanical ventilation: physiological and clinical applications. 4th ed. St. Louis (MO): Mosby Elsevier; c2006. p. 417–37.

Hess DR. How to initiate a noninvasive ventilation program: bringing the evidence to the bedside. Respir Care. 2009 Feb;54(2):232–43.

Hess DR. Noninvasive ventilation for acute respiratory failure. Respir Care. 2013 Jun;58(6):950–72.

Rana S, Jenad H, Gay PC, Buck CF, Hubmayr RD, Gajic O. Failure of non-invasive ventilation in patients with acute lung injury: observational cohort study. Crit Care. 2006;10(3):R79. Epub 2006 May 12.

Thille AW, Frat JP. Noninvasive ventilation as acute therapy. Curr Opin Crit Care. 2018 Dec;24(6):519–24.

Tracheostomy

SABA GHORAB, MD; DAVID G. LOTT, MD

Goals

- Discuss the indications for tracheostomy.
- Describe the techniques used to perform tracheostomy.
- Discuss the complications of tracheostomy.

Introduction

Tracheostomy is a procedure where a conduit is created between the skin and the trachea (Figure 117.1). One of the earliest recorded surgical procedures, tracheostomy dates to 100 BC. Sporadic use of tracheostomy for relief of upper airway obstruction, often with little success, has been reported for centuries. The first documented successful tracheostomy was performed in 1546 by an Italian physician, Antonio Musa Brasavola. In 1909, Chevalier Jackson described a reliable surgical tracheostomy (ST) technique that is still used today. The percutaneous approach gained popularity in 1985 when Ciaglia first used serial dilators with modification of the Seldinger guidewire technique for insertion. Advances in technology have led to the evolution of Ciaglia's original method, with emergence of bronchoscopically guided percutaneous dilatational tracheostomy (PDT) as a useful alternative to ST.

Tracheostomy is one of the most frequent procedures undertaken in critically ill patients. Each year, approximately 10% of critical care patients in the United States require a tracheostomy, most often for prolonged mechanical ventilation (Box 117.1). There are no contraindications to performing ST, but PDT is usually contraindicated for the following: emergent airway compromise; pediatric patients younger than 16 years; tracheomalacia; anatomical anomalies (abnormal or poorly palpable neck anatomy); morbid obesity; neck infection, burn, or trauma; cervical spine instability; uncorrectable bleeding diathesis; and clinically important ventilation requirements.

Benefits

Compared with conventional translaryngeal endotracheal intubation, tracheostomy offers many advantages, including improved patient comfort and reduced sedation requirements, thus enabling early mobilization, resumption of oral nutrition, return to speech, and administration of nursing care. Tracheostomy reduces airway resistance, allowing for less work of breathing and respiratory fatigue. Additionally, transtracheal pulmonary toilet reduces the risk of nosocomial pneumonia. These benefits of tracheostomy may expedite weaning from mechanical ventilation and decrease the hospital length of stay. Tracheostomy also minimizes the risk of laryngotracheal injury from prolonged translaryngeal intubation, including pressure ulcers, stenosis, malacia, and vocal fold dysfunction.

Techniques

The optimal technique is a topic of much debate. The traditional open tracheostomy is commonly performed in an operating room, whereas the percutaneous approach has been refined with widespread use of bedside bronchoscopically guided PDT in critical care units. Despite numerous studies comparing ST with PDT, consensus has not been reached on which method is superior. Nonetheless, when performed by experienced practitioners under controlled circumstances, both techniques are safe and have comparable complication profiles. The choice of approach should be made for each patient, taking into account patient factors, operator and institutional experience, and availability of resources.

Timing

Owing to substantial heterogeneity among studies, no consensus has been reached on when translaryngeal intubation should be replaced with tracheostomy. Compared with late tracheostomy (>10 days after intubation), early tracheostomy (≤10 days after intubation) has been shown to provide consistent morbidity benefits but not mortality benefits. For most critically ill patients, it is generally acceptable to wait 7 to 10 days to determine whether ongoing respiratory support will be needed. Patients with any of the following may benefit from early tracheostomy:

- Serious pulmonary disease (eg, chronic obstructive pulmonary disease, acute respiratory distress syndrome, or failed primary extubation).
- Respiratory failure after cardiovascular surgery.
- Disorders requiring neurocritical care (eg, basilar artery occlusion, cervical spinal cord injury, severe traumatic brain injury with prolonged coma, and axonal forms of Guillain-Barré syndrome).
- Polytrauma involving the head, neck, spine, or chest.
- Severe burns (>60% total surface body area) requiring multiple operations.
- Head or neck burns with associated inhalation injury.

Complications

Tracheostomy, regardless of the technique, is not risk-free. In critical care patients, even minor complications can be life-threatening and therefore require timely recognition and management. Tracheostomy complications are classified as *intraprocedural* (during or immediately after insertion), *early postprocedural* (≤1 week), or *late postprocedural* (>1 week) (Box 117.2).

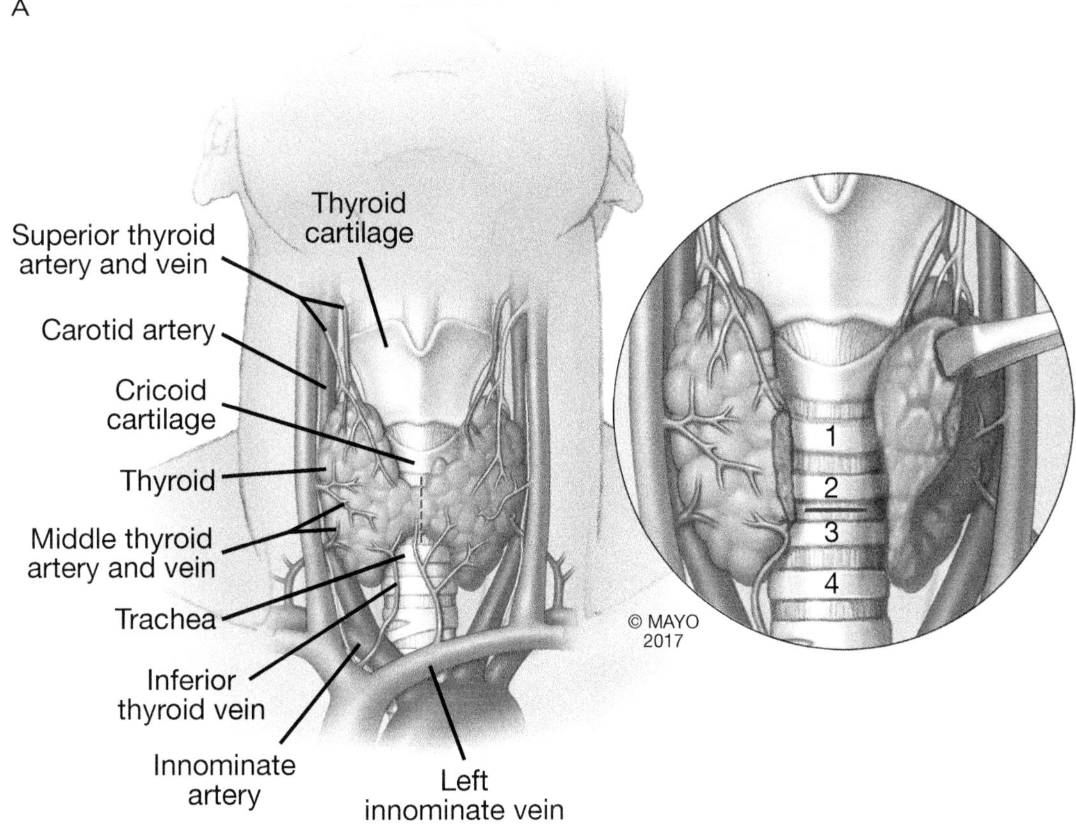

Figure 117.1. *Pertinent Cervical Anatomy During Tracheostomy Tube Placement. A, Anterior view. Surface anatomical landmarks include the thyroid notch (between the thyroid and cricoid cartilages), cricoid cartilage, and sternal notch. The thyroid gland isthmus may be divided (dashed line) to gain access to the trachea. The tracheal opening is typically made between the second and third tracheal rings (inset, solid line). The anterior jugular veins and a high-riding innominate artery are nearby vessels at risk for injury. B, Lateral view. The proper position of the tracheostomy tube is shown. Accidental penetration of the posterior tracheal wall may extend into the esophagus, which is situated directly posterior.*

(continued next page)

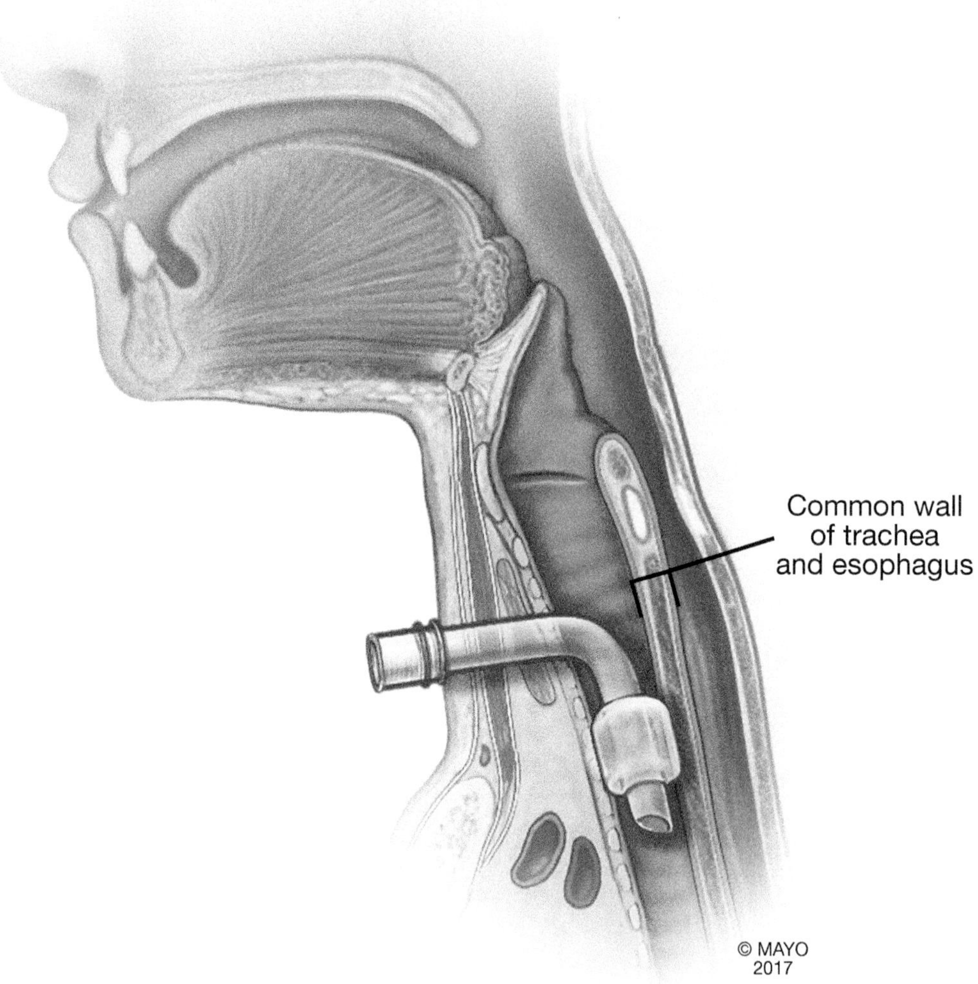

Figure 117.1. Continued

Hemorrhage

The most common postprocedural complication is hemorrhage, usually occurring within the first week and resulting from superficial vein injury. Minor hemorrhage is amenable to 1 or more local measures such as injection of lidocaine-epinephrine, cautery, or packing. Major hemorrhage is concerning for a tracheoarterial fistula and is often due to anterior tracheal wall erosion into the innominate artery. Tracheoinnominate fistula is the most lethal complication of tracheostomy. Even with urgent management, less than 20% of patients survive. It usually occurs within the first month with sentinel bleeding (in up to 50% patients) and progresses to massive hemoptysis causing imminent asphyxiation and exsanguination. If sentinel bleeding is suspected, immediate intraoperative evaluation must be undertaken. Management of massive hemorrhage includes 1 or both of the following: 1) tamponade with cuff overinflation or 2) translaryngeal intubation with direct digital compression of the innominate artery while expediting emergency surgical repair.

Loss of Airway

Loss of airway caused by tracheostomy tube obstruction or dislodgement warrants immediate translaryngeal intubation if attempts to restore tube patency are ineffective. Tube obstruction from mucus or blood clot can be relieved with suctioning or changing the inner cannula. Marked intraluminal blockage or angulation of the tube orifice against the tracheal wall may be mitigated by exchanging the tracheostomy tube. Tube replacement during the first week is particularly challenging because of the absence of stomal tract maturation. Successful tube reinsertion is

Box 117.1 • General Indications for Tracheostomy

- Mechanical ventilation for respiratory failure
  - Need for prolonged mechanical ventilation
  - Inability to wean patient from mechanical ventilation
- Pulmonary toilet
  - Copious respiratory secretions
  - Inability to mobilize or manage respiratory secretions because of inadequate or absent cough reflex
- Airway protection
  - Head and neck burns with associated inhalation injury
  - Polytrauma involving the head, neck, spine, or chest
  - Neurologic conditions (eg, stroke, traumatic brain injury, spinal cord injury, and neuromuscular disorders) causing loss of consciousness or altered mentation, bulbar dysfunction, or neuromuscular weakness
- Upper respiratory tract obstruction
  - Congenital anomaly (laryngeal hypoplasia or vascular ring)
  - Foreign body that cannot be dislodged
  - Inflammation and edema (from infection, anaphylaxis, trauma, or burns)
  - Laryngeal disorders (stenosis, tumor, or vocal fold immobility)
  - Severe obstructive sleep apnea not amendable to continuous positive airway pressure devices or sleep surgery
- Prophylaxis
  - In preparation for extensive head and neck procedures
  - Severe burns (>60% of total surface body area) requiring multiple operative procedures

Box 117.2 • Complications of Tracheostomy

- Intraprocedural (during or soon after insertion)
  - Airway fire
  - Multiple attempts
  - Paratracheal insertion
  - Posterior tracheal wall injury
- Early postprocedural (≤7 d; before complete stomal tract maturation)
  - Hemorrhage
  - Subcutaneous emphysema
  - Pneumothorax
  - Stomal infection
  - Loss of airway
    - Tube obstruction
    - Tube dislodgement
- Late postprocedural (>7 d)
  - Granulation tissue formation
  - Stenosis (subglottic, tracheal)
  - Tracheomalacia
  - Fistula
    - Tracheoesophageal
    - Tracheoinnominate
    - Tracheocutaneous
  - Scarring
  - Vocal fold dysfunction
  - Subjective phonetic changes
  - Subjective respiratory symptoms

dependent on appropriate tube selection and on adequate stomal tract visualization and stabilization. The following maneuvers may aid tube reinsertion: supine position, neck extension, clearance of secretions, gentle lateral traction of stay sutures, placement of retractors in the stoma, and use of the modified Seldinger technique with a suction catheter or flexible endoscope as a guide tube. Flexible endoscopy also offers adjunctive confirmation of correct tube placement or positioning. Inadvertent loss of the airway is minimized with routine cleaning, suturing the flange to the skin, using well-fitted tracheostomy ties or collars, and securing the tube during patient movement.

Tracheal Injury

Posterior tracheal wall injury is often due to poor control of the guidewire and guiding catheter during PDT; the risk is reduced with concomitant bronchoscopic guidance. Small tears heal spontaneously, whereas larger tears require emergent surgical intervention.

Late tracheal complications (eg, stenosis, tracheomalacia, and fistula) are precipitated by direct tube trauma or ischemia from high intracuff pressures and are worsened by persistent irritation from excess secretions, acid reflux, or infection. These factors elicit various degrees of tracheal inflammation, including mucosal ulceration, chondritis, and necrosis. Clinical manifestations of such complications include difficulty weaning the patient from the ventilator, a need for reintubation after decannulation, recurrent pulmonary aspiration or infection, and respiratory symptoms (eg, stridor, dyspnea, hemoptysis, cough, and sputum retention) months to years after decannulation. Diagnosis is made from the clinical history, physical examination findings, and the results of flexible bronchoscopy, pulmonary function testing, or computed tomography. Management includes placement of a longer tracheostomy tube, endoscopic dilation, endoscopic stenting, or definitive surgical repair.

Summary

- Benefits of tracheostomy over prolonged translaryngeal intubation include liberation from mechanical ventilation, improved patient comfort, early mobilization, resumption of oral nutrition and speech, and reduced risk of laryngotracheal injury.
- The most common indications for tracheostomy are to provide access for prolonged mechanical ventilation, to aid in weaning from mechanical ventilation, and to facilitate management of respiratory secretions.
- Bedside bronchoscopically guided PDT is a useful alternative to ST in select critical care patients.
- Before a tracheostomy is performed, it is generally acceptable to wait 7 to 10 days after intubation to determine whether ongoing respiratory support will be needed.

SUGGESTED READING

Appleby I. Tracheostomy. Anaesth Int Care Med. 2005;6(7):220–2.

Catalino MP, Lin FC, Davis N, Anderson K, Olm-Shipman C, Jordan JD. Early versus late tracheostomy after decompressive craniectomy for stroke. J Intensive Care. 2018 Jan 4;6:1.

Cheung NH, Napolitano LM. Tracheostomy: epidemiology, indications, timing, technique, and outcomes. Respir Care. 2014 Jun;59(6):895–915.

Cools-Lartigue J, Aboalsaud A, Gill H, Ferri L. Evolution of percutaneous dilatational tracheostomy: a review of current techniques and their pitfalls. World J Surg. 2013 Jul;37(7):1633–46.

Engels PT, Bagshaw SM, Meier M, Brindley PG. Tracheostomy: from insertion to decannulation. Can J Surg. 2009 Oct;52(5):427–33.

Fernandez-Bussy S, Mahajan B, Folch E, Caviedes I, Guerrero J, Majid A. Tracheostomy tube placement: early and late complications. J Bronchology Interv Pulmonol. 2015 Oct;22(4):357–64.

Hyzy RC. Overview of tracheostomy. In: Mathur PN, editor. UpToDate. Waltham (MA): UpToDate; c2016.

Johnson-Obaseki S, Veljkovic A, Javidnia H. Complication rates of open surgical versus percutaneous tracheostomy in critically ill patients. Laryngoscope. 2016 Nov;126(11):2459–67. Epub 2016 Apr 14.

Keeping A. Early versus late tracheostomy for critically ill patients: a clinical evidence synopsis of a recent Cochrane review. Can J Respir Ther. 2016 Winter;52(1):27–8.

Khammas AH, Dawood MR. Timing of tracheostomy in intensive care unit patients. Int Arch Otorhinolaryngol. 2018 Oct;22(4):437–42. Epub 2018 Aug 9.

Longworth A, Veitch D, Gudibande S, Whitehouse T, Snelson C, Veenith T. Tracheostomy in special groups of critically ill patients: who, when, and where? Indian J Crit Care Med. 2016 May;20(5):280–4.

Morris LL, Whitmer A, McIntosh E. Tracheostomy care and complications in the intensive care unit. Crit Care Nurse. 2013 Oct;33(5):18–30.

Silvester W, Goldsmith D, Uchino S, Bellomo R, Knight S, Seevanayagam S, et al. Percutaneous versus surgical tracheostomy: a randomized controlled study with long-term follow-up. Crit Care Med. 2006 Aug;34(8):2145–52.

Diagnostic and Interventional Bronchoscopy in the Intensive Care Unit

CESAR A. KELLER, MD

Goals

- Understand the diagnostic and therapeutic relevance of fiberoptic bronchoscopy for patients in the intensive care unit.
- Identify the most useful interventional aspects of fiberoptic bronchoscopy for critically ill patients.
- Know the safety issues related to fiberoptic bronchoscopy.

Introduction

In the 1960s, Shigeto Ikeda in Japan developed fiberoptic bronchoscopy (FOB), beginning a revolution in the diagnosis and treatment of diverse pulmonary conditions. FOB evolved with additional diagnostic and interventional tools. Forceps and probes were created for biopsies of endobronchial lesions and lung parenchyma. Needle sampling of mediastinal lesions was enhanced by creating endobronchial ultrasonography. Balloons were developed for dilatation of stenotic airways, and therapeutic modalities (eg, laser therapy, cryotherapy, argon plasma coagulation [APC], thermoplasty, and stent therapy) were developed to manage multiple airway conditions. Current explorations include the use of probe-based confocal endomicroscopy for optical biopsies that allow real-time visualization of alveoli, microvascular structures, and intra-alveolar cellularity.

FOB has become an essential bedside tool for diagnosis and management in critically ill patients. FOB is safe, even in patients with respiratory failure and, if done cautiously, in patients with increased intracranial pressure.

General Considerations

Indications and Contraindications

There are many indications for diagnostic or therapeutic bronchoscopic procedures in the intensive care unit (ICU) (Box 118.1). In critically ill patients, contrary to patients undergoing elective procedures, there are relative but not necessarily absolute contraindications for FOB. When a patient is acutely ill, the risk-benefit ratio must be considered; if the outcome depends on a diagnostic or therapeutic intervention, the procedure is performed with full disclosure of the risks involved. Standard diagnostic bronchoscopy, including bronchoalveolar lavage (BAL), is safe and well tolerated, even by patients with respiratory failure and patients requiring anticoagulation or hemodynamic support.

Complications

Procedure-related minor complications include sore throat, nasal or oral trauma, local bleeding, transient postprocedural fever, transient bronchospasm, hypoxemia, and hypotension. Worsening hypoxemia may require increased respiratory support or mechanical ventilation. Important complications include pneumothorax, bleeding, hypotension, arrhythmias, airway laceration or perforation, air embolism, pneumonia, and unintended stent migration. When bronchial biopsies are required, the risk of pneumothorax, bleeding, hypoxemia, hypotension, and arrhythmias increases. In most reviews, the overall incidence of complications is low (1%-7%). When transbronchial biopsies are performed in patients receiving mechanical ventilation, the incidence of pneumothorax increases to nearly 25% and the incidence of bleeding complications increases to about 10%. The risk of death related to interventional

Box 118.1 • Indications and Contraindications of Fiberoptic Bronchoscopy in the ICU

- Diagnostic indications and procedures
  - Clinical symptoms: cough, wheezing, sputum production, stridor, or hemoptysis
  - Ventilator-associated pneumonia or hospital-acquired pneumonia
  - Immunocompromised host with lung infiltrates
  - Undiagnosed lung infiltrates, lung masses, lung nodules, or mediastinal adenopathy
  - Persistent atelectasis or consolidation
  - Suspected airway trauma, surgical dehiscence, or bronchopleural fistula
  - Evaluation of complications related to artificial airways
  - Suspected infection or rejection in lung transplant patients
  - Procedures
    - Inspection, bronchial washings, bronchial brushings, tracheal or bronchial biopsies, transbronchial biopsies, and cryobiopsies (bronchial and transbronchial)
    - Transbronchial needle aspiration (by direct visualization or endobronchial ultrasound-guided biopsy[a])
- Therapeutic indications and procedures
  - Mucus impaction (excessive bronchial secretions)
    - Inspection and suctioning
  - Removal of aspirated foreign objects (eg, aspirated food)
    - Inspection, suctioning, use of forceps or snare devices, or APC
  - Difficult airway management
    - Bronchoscopic intubation
  - Bedside percutaneous dilatational tracheostomy
    - Bronchoscopic guidance
  - Active hemoptysis or blood clot removal
    - Suctioning, use of forceps, APC, or instillation of medications
  - Obstructive tracheal or bronchial lesions
    - Balloon bronchoplasty, APC, or cryotherapy
    - Stent therapy or endobronchial instillation of medications
    - Nd:YAG laser therapy,[a] brachytherapy,[a] or thermoplasty[a]
  - Bronchopleural fistula or persistent air leak
    - Endobronchial valve placement
- Contraindications (relative)
  - High F_{IO_2} or PEEP requirement (transbronchial biopsies)
  - Uncorrected coagulopathy or need for anticoagulation (biopsy procedures)
  - Severe pulmonary hypertension (PASP >50 mm Hg) (transbronchial biopsies)
  - Severe renal failure (transbronchial biopsies)
  - Cardiovascular decompensation or hemodynamic instability
  - Pacemaker and automatic implantable cardioverter-defibrillator (atrial premature contraction)

Abbreviations: APC, argon plasma coagulation; F_{IO_2}, fraction of inspired oxygen; ICU, intensive care unit; PASP, pulmonary artery systolic pressure; PEEP, positive end-expiratory pressure.

[a] Procedure is not typically done in the ICU.

bronchoscopy is low (0.01%). Interventional procedures are riskier in critically ill patients, but the benefit often justifies the risk.

Preparation

Before the procedure, all the information available on the patient should be reviewed. This information should include the history, physical examination findings, laboratory test results, findings from imaging studies, electrocardiographic results, and clinical data.

Bronchoscope selection reflects the intended use. The standard-diameter bronchoscope (external diameter, 4.9 mm; working and suction channel diameter, 2 mm) is used for most diagnostic procedures, including bronchial washings, BAL, bronchial brushings, and transbronchial biopsies. A large-diameter scope (external diameter, 6 mm; working channel diameter, 3 mm) allows passage of larger biopsy forceps, cryoprobes, balloon dilatation catheters, guidewires, and other probes. Small-diameter scopes (external diameters, 4.2 and 3.1 mm; working channel diameters, 2 and 1.2 mm, respectively) are useful with small-diameter endotracheal or tracheostomy tubes, or when inspection of distal airways is required (beyond fourth- or fifth-generation airways).

The equipment must be reviewed. For diagnostic procedures, the tools to collect specimens should be available. For interventional procedures, additional equipment (eg, balloon, pumps, stents, cryoprobes, and APC probes) should be readily available. If fluoroscopic guidance is required, the equipment should be operational and available. Equipment and supplies to manage possible adverse events should include cold saline, topical epinephrine, and thrombin to manage local bleeding; pneumothorax catheters and insertion kits to manage possible pneumothorax; endotracheal intubation and ventilation equipment to manage possible respiratory failure; and percutaneous tracheostomy equipment if the oral airway may be in jeopardy.

Cardiopulmonary monitoring should include heart rate, arterial blood pressure, oxygen saturation by pulse oximetry, and end-tidal carbon dioxide. Before the procedure, topical anesthesia should be administered as nebulized 4%

lidocaine; during the procedure, further topical instillations of 2% lidocaine or a similar agent should be available. Adequate intravenous access must be established to provide intravenous sedation and volume replacement therapy. Before the procedure is begun, team members participate in a time-out to confirm that the correct procedure is to be performed for the correct patient, who has given consent.

Sedation of spontaneously breathing patients is usually conscious sedation, in which benzodiazepines (eg, midazolam) are used in combination with opioids (fentanyl or morphine), and oxygen supplementation is administered through a nasal cannula or oxygen mask. These agents can be reversed if necessary with flumazenil (for benzodiazepines) or naloxone (for opioids). Alternatively, propofol can be used if a laryngeal mask airway is inserted for oxygenation and ventilation support. For patients receiving mechanical ventilation, an increased dose of the sedatives already being used is sufficient. For complex interventional procedures, paralyzing agents may be necessary.

Interventional procedures can be challenging in patients receiving mechanical ventilation through an endotracheal tube. FOB insertion increases airway resistance and peak pressures, it may cause auto-positive end-expiratory pressure, and it decreases effective minute ventilation. During the procedure, the operator should move the scope in and out frequently to allow adequate ventilation and oxygenation. In patients with small artificial airways, use of a small-diameter FOB may be helpful. In patients with severely reduced lung compliance, it is safer to perform manual ventilation with bag-valve-mask ventilation.

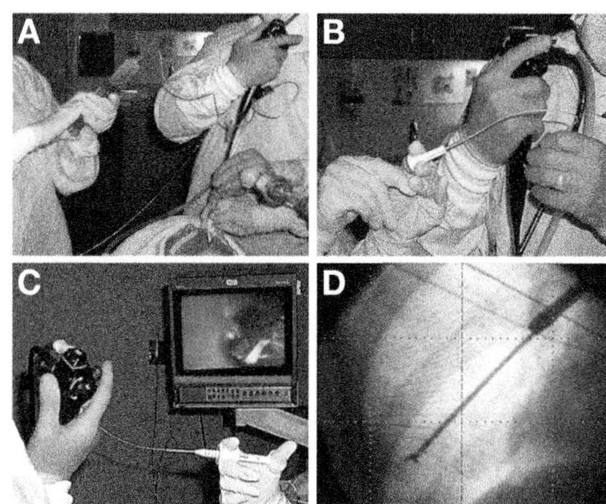

Figure 118.1. Diagnostic Bronchoscopy. A, During bronchoalveolar lavage, 60 to 100 mL of sterile saline solution is instilled through the working channel of a bronchoscope wedged into a distal bronchi, and then the fluid is gently aspirated. Alternatively, saline can be instilled into the distal bronchus and then aspirated into a mucus trap. B, Cytologic or protected brushings are done by advancing a brush enclosed in a catheter sheath. The brush is deployed in the area of interest to retrieve cells for cytology or bacterial sampling. C, For a bronchial biopsy, a forceps is advanced with bronchoscopic guidance into a target lesion, the forceps is opened and advanced into the lesion, and the forceps is closed to retrieve small pieces of tissue for histologic analysis. D, During transbronchial biopsies, the same forceps used for bronchial biopsies is used, advanced distally beyond the view of the bronchoscope, and blindly (or with fluoroscopic guidance) advanced into the alveolar space, where the forceps is opened and closed as the patient exhales. Several (4-10) small pieces of alveolated tissue are retrieved for histologic analysis and, if needed, for special staining and histochemistry studies.

Diagnostic Bronchoscopy

Airway Inspection

The FOB is advanced nasally or orally or through an artificial airway as indicated (Figure 118.1). Airways are inspected for various features, such as integrity, inflammation, infection or trauma, and presence of foreign objects, tumors, or nodules. If a patient has hemoptysis, all distal airways must be inspected to assess the origin of bleeding. After a transplant, anastomostic integrity and patency are evaluated.

Bronchial Washing

Bronchial washing samples are obtained by suctioning and retrieving excessive secretions present in proximal airways or by flushing sterile saline in proximal airways followed by suctioning secretions into a mucous trap. Culture results are interpreted in the context of possible contamination from proximal airways, and discriminating between active infections and colonization requires clinical decisions.

Bronchoalveolar Lavage

For BAL, the bronchoscope is advanced into a selected subsegment until it is wedged in the bronchus lumen. Sterile saline is instilled (40-100 mL) and gently aspirated until 20 to 30 mL is retrieved for analysis. BAL provides alveolar sampling for total and differential cell counts and for various microbiologic studies (eg, bacterial, viral, and fungal cultures and identification of *Legionella, Pneumocystis,* and other agents). Cytologic processing allows evaluation of neoplastic processes, and special stains allow evaluation of uncommon conditions (eg, pulmonary alveolar proteinosis, beryliosis, and diffuse alveolar hemorrhage).

Bronchial Brushing

Bronchial brushing is used to sample specific target areas for cytology. With the use of a specially designed sterile catheter fitted with a protective plug on the distal end that is ejected before deployment, bronchial brushing is also used to obtain samples for quantified cultures by avoiding contamination from the suction channel and proximal airways.

Endobronchial Biopsy

Endobronchial biopsy samples are obtained by advancing a forceps through the working channel and selecting lesions under direct visualization for retrieving tissue samples, which are subsequently preserved in formalin for histologic studies and special stains if indicated. Tissues can also be preserved in sterile saline for cultures, or they can be specially preserved for studies with electron microscopy.

Transbronchial Biopsy

Transbronchial biopsy samples can be obtained blindly for diagnosis of diffuse interstitial processes and acute rejection in lung transplant recipients. They may also be obtained with fluoroscopic guidance while the forceps is advanced to specific areas of interest. When the forceps is in position, it is opened and then closed to obtain alveolated tissue samples while the patient exhales. Typically, 4 to 10 biopsy samples are obtained. Other guidance maneuvers (eg, those involving ultrasonography, virtual bronchoscopic navigation, or electromagnetic technique guidance) are not typically done in ICU patients.

Cryobiopsy

Cryobiopsy samples are obtained through cryofixation with liquid nitrogen or carbon dioxide. Specially designed cryoprobes are advanced distally through the FOB under fluoroscopic guidance, the tip of the probe is frozen for 3 to 5 seconds, and the bronchoscope and probe are pulled out, detaching frozen alveolated tissue. Typically, the biopsy samples are 5 to 10 times larger than standard biopsy samples. Bleeding and pneumothorax are more common with this procedure, so cryobiopsy requires deep sedation, preventive intubation, and additional protective procedures, such as advancing a Fogarty catheter (which is inflated as soon as the cryoprobe is retrieved) into the bronchus to contain possible bleeding. Endobronchial cryobiopsies increase the diagnostic yield in patients with endobronchial tumors.

Transbronchial Needle Aspiration

In transbronchial needle aspiration, a catheter sheath containing a needle in the distal end is used to obtain cellular material for cytology and microbiology or a small core of tissue to sample mediastinal or peripheral nodules. The procedure is performed under direct visualization or endobronchial ultrasonography for central lesions or under navigational guidance for peripheral lesions. This technique is most commonly used for staging of non–small cell lung carcinoma and is not typically an ICU-related procedure.

Interventional Bronchoscopy

Fiberoptic Intubation

Patients who have difficult airways or who pose challenges for deep sedation can be intubated by sliding an endotracheal tube over the bronchoscope; the FOB is advanced between the vocal cords and is used as a guide for sliding the tube into the trachea. The technique offers several advantages: Deep sedation is avoided, intubation may be done with the patient in a sitting position to provide a ventilation advantage, and positioning of the endotracheal tube above the carina is immediately documented.

Percutaneous Dilatational Tracheostomy

When ICU patients are expected to need prolonged mechanical ventilation, they may benefit from bedside percutaneous dilatational tracheostomy (PDT) facilitated with bronchoscopic guidance. The FOB is advanced through the endotracheal tube for clearing secretions and for visualizing the entrance of the percutaneously inserted angiocatheter in the anterior trachea. A guidewire and dilators are advanced. Eventually the tracheostomy tube is deployed in the trachea. FOB helps clear blood and clots from the entrance point and is used to inspect and treat distal airways as needed for lacerations or bleeding. Bedside PDT, now the standard of care for patients requiring tracheostomy, is as safe as surgical tracheostomy.

Endobronchial Instillation of Medications and Abscess Drainage

FOB can be used to deliver medications directly or through custom-fitted catheters to specific areas of need. Instillation of cold saline, topical epinephrine, and thrombin are commonly used to manage bleeding that occurs from visible lesions or lacerations or after diagnostic procedures. Instillation of surfactant has been used to manage primary graft dysfunction in lung transplant recipients. In conjunction with APC, endobronchial instillation of medications has been used to successfully treat mucormycosis (with amphotericin B) and papillomatosis (with cidofovir). Fiberoptically guided placement of pigtail catheters may be used to drain abscess cavities refractory to antibiotic therapy.

Balloon Bronchoplasty

Balloon bronchoplasty involves advancing specially designed balloons through an FOB with a large working channel or through an FOB-placed guidewire to dilate tracheobronchial obstructive lesions secondary to various causes, including neoplasia, previous intubation, transplant surgery, infection, radiotherapy, and inhalation injury (Figure 118.2). These balloons can be dilated to diameters from 4 to 20 mm with specially designed pressure-measuring syringes that generate pressures from 3 to 9 atm. This therapy can be used alone or in combination with other therapies (eg, APC, cryotherapy, or stent therapy). Endobronchial insertion of a balloon catheter can be used as a temporizing maneuver to contain large localized bleeding or to selectively divert ventilation to the opposite lung in cases of air leak.

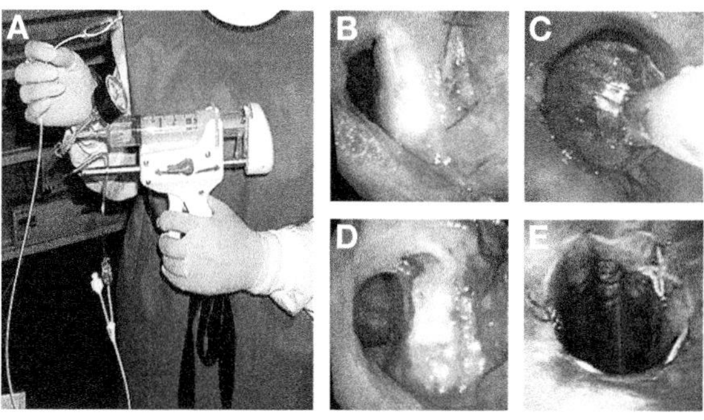

Figure 118.2. *Balloon Bronchoplasty. A, Balloon dilatation catheters are specially designed catheters that can be expanded with a calibrated syringe to 3 diameters (8, 9, and 10 mm and 10, 11, and 12 mm are the most commonly used) with different pressures (typically, 3-9 atm). Balloon length ranges from 2 to 4 cm. Two to 4 dilatations for about 30 seconds each are usually required at each diameter; the diameter is increased progressively until the desired final diameter is achieved. These catheters can be advanced under direct vision through the working channel of a large bronchoscope, or they can be advanced with fluoroscopic guidance through a guidewire previously inserted during fiberoptic bronchoscopy (FOB). B, This stenotic lesion, the persistent stenosis of a bronchial anastomosis, was visualized after lung transplant. C, This balloon was inflated to a diameter of 12 mm under direct FOB visualization to widen the stenotic lesion and improve airway patency. D, The stenotic lesion is shown after balloon dilatation (balloon bronchoplasty). E, A metallic self-expandable uncovered stent was deployed in the stenotic area after balloon dilatation. When a stent is deployed, balloon dilatation is usually performed within the stent to the maximum diameter of the stent. The blue thread at the proximal opening of the stent can be pulled with forceps, if necessary, to remove the stent or to move it to a more proximal position.*

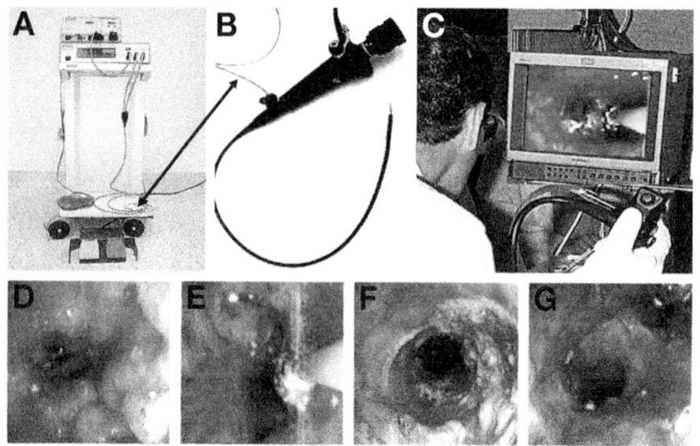

Figure 118.3. *Argon Plasma Coagulation (APC). A, An APC unit includes a grounding pad that may be placed on the lower abdomen or thigh, a pedal that allows the operator to deliver APC pulses, and a probe (arrow in panels A and B). Typical power settings are 20 to 40 W (the use of less power decreases the risk of complications such as ignition or air embolism) with an argon gas flow rate of 0.5 to 1 L/min (a lower flow rate is safer). B, The APC probe is advanced through the working channel of the fiberoptic bronchoscope, and the probe tip is advanced a few centimeters beyond the tip of the bronchoscope to ensure that the bronchoscope will not be burned. C, The probe tip is placed within 1 cm of the target lesion to achieve the therapeutic effect (thermal desiccation). APC is activated by pressing the foot switch that synchronizes the current with the transfer of an ionized plasma gas across the field to the target tissue (pulses are 1-5 seconds; shorter pulses are safer). With transient interruption of positive pressure ventilation and oxygenation during the APC pulses, airway ignition and air embolism are less likely to occur. D, This patient received a stent because of obstruction after severe fungal bronchitis. Excessive granulation tissue had formed after topical treatment with amphotericin and stent therapy. E, Granulation tissue was treated with APC. F, With APC therapy, the endobronchial obstruction progressively improved. G, APC therapy resulted in resolution of the endobronchial obstruction.*

Argon Plasma Coagulation

With APC, ionized argon gas conducts an electrical current through a probe that is easily advanced through the FOB working channel (Figure 118.3). The positively charged argon gas flows toward the negatively charged tissues, producing a noncontact diathermy. The generated heat vaporizes tissue water, resulting in coagulation, which helps to control bleeding, and desiccation, which destroys the target lesion obstructing the airway. Because desiccation occurs to a depth of only 2 to 3 mm, damage to underlying structures is prevented and the chances of perforation are minimized. Desiccated tissues can be removed with forceps or allowed to slough as the underlying mucosa heals. This therapy can be used for palliation of malignant obstructive lesions or for treatment of benign lesions and conditions, such as excessive granulation tissue, obstruction due to scarring, papillomatosis, carcinoids, and airway complications in lung transplant recipients. APC can produce endobronchial ignition in patients requiring a high fraction of inspired oxygen (F_{IO_2}), so the administration of APC and the use of interrupted ventilation and oxygenation must be closely coordinated during therapy to avoid luminal ignition. Patients with a pacemaker or automatic implantable cardioverter-defibrillator susceptible to electrical interference should not undergo APC without the approval of their cardiologist.

Cryotherapy

During cryotherapy, the tip of a cryoprobe touches cells, which are destroyed when ice crystals form in the cytosol, producing tissue death and necrosis. This technique allows relatively large pieces of tissue to be removed, restoring airway patency through an initial debulking in combination with a delayed effect that occurs days later when necrotic tissue sloughs. Cryotherapy poses no risk of accidental fire injury, even for patients who require a high FIO_2, and no cardiac risk for patients who require a pacemaker or defibrillation device.

Endobronchial Stenting

Self-expanding metallic stents (either uncovered or covered with translucent polyvinyl chloride) can be deployed with FOB and fluoroscopic guidance for palliative treatment of malignant lesions and for benign obstructive lesions from scarring or inflammation. Stent therapy is used commonly in lung transplant recipients to manage stenotic lesions and to manage postoperative fistulas or dehiscence (Figures 118.2 and 118.4). Stent placement requires follow-up bronchoscopy to clear secretions and manage complications such as granulation tissue. Current technology allows placement of removable stents in combination with other therapies to resolve the cause of obstruction.

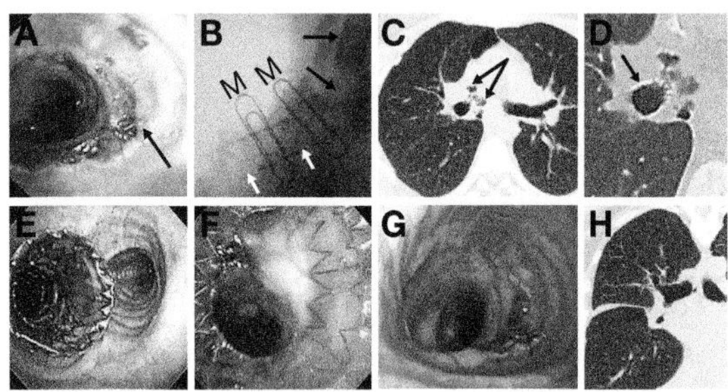

Figure 118.4. Stent Therapy for a Small Surgical Dehiscence. A, A 37-year-old woman with cystic fibrosis had dehiscence (arrow) on the right anastomosis within 2 weeks after bilateral lung transplant. B, A fluoroscopic image shows the tip of the previously inserted tracheostomy tube (upper black arrow) and the guidewire (lower black arrow) used to insert the stents (white arrows). Two paper clips (letter M*) were placed on the patient's chest as markers for deploying the stents. C, A computed tomographic scan shows evidence of dehiscence with the presence of free air (arrows) around the anastomosis. D, A computed tomographic scan shows stents in place (arrow) and free air in mediastinal structures. E, Two removable metallic self-expanding covered stents were placed to cover the dehiscent area. The proximal end of 1 stent is shown at the carina. A thread around the border of the stent can be pulled with a forceps to retrieve and remove the stent. F, The distal end of 1 stent is within the other stent, whose distal end opens just above the bifurcation between the right upper lobe bronchus and the right main bronchus. G, The right main anastomosis healed 1 month after transplant and after retrieval of the removable stents. H, A computed tomographic scan shows resolution of free air in the mediastinum and the intact anastomosis with the stents removed.*

Endobronchial Valve Placement

Critically ill, nonsurgical candidates who have large or persistent air leaks due to pneumothoraces and bronchopleural fistulas can be treated conservatively and effectively by temporarily inserting 1-way endobronchial valves originally designed to decrease lung volume in patients who have bullous emphysema (Figure 118.5).

Other Debulking Therapies

Debulking therapies such as Nd:YAG laser therapy, brachytherapy, and photodynamic therapy are not commonly used in the ICU. Brachytherapy and photodynamic therapy do not result in rapid debulking in critically ill patients, and laser therapy requires expensive and complex equipment not commonly available for bedside procedures.

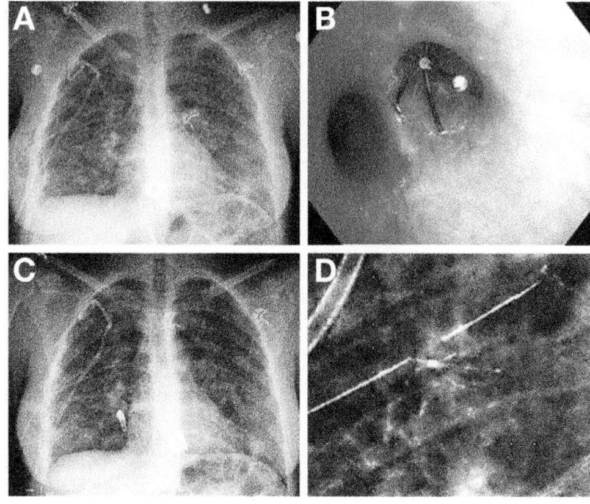

Figure 118.5. Endobronchial Valves. A, This radiograph is of a 16-year-old female patient with cystic fibrosis who had spontaneous pneumothorax with a persistent, large air leak for 21 days despite insertion of 2 chest tubes. B, Fiberoptic bronchoscopy was performed, and balloon occlusion of the posterior segment of the right upper lobe resulted in resolution of the air leak; therefore, a 7-mm endobronchial valve was deployed in that segment. C, A follow-up radiograph shows resolution of the pneumothorax. D, Enlargement shows the endobronchial valve in place. It was removed endoscopically 1 month after the bronchopleural fistula resolved.

Summary

- Bedside diagnostic and interventional bronchoscopy is immediately available to manage critical illness in patients requiring rapid diagnosis and resolution of acute airway complications.
- FOB and related interventional technologies are essential tools in the armamentarium of the critical care team.
- The critical care team should include expert users of FOB to make procedures safer for critically ill patients who may require a high level of respiratory, hemodynamic, neurologic, and metabolic support.
- Management of airway and pulmonary complications in critically ill patients usually requires the use of several complex interventional procedures.

SUGGESTED READING

Anders GT, Johnson JE, Bush BA, Matthews JI. Transbronchial biopsy without fluoroscopy: a seven-year perspective. Chest. 1988 Sep;94(3):557–60.

Baughman RP. Technical aspects of bronchoalveolar lavage: recommendations for a standard procedure. Semin Respir Crit Care Med. 2007 Oct;28(5):475–85.

Brodsky JB. Bronchoscopic procedures for central airway obstruction. J Cardiothorac Vasc Anesth. 2003 Oct;17(5):638–46.

Bulpa PA, Dive AM, Mertens L, Delos MA, Jamart J, Evrard PA, et al. Combined bronchoalveolar lavage and transbronchial lung biopsy: safety and yield in ventilated patients. Eur Respir J. 2003 Mar;21(3):489–94.

Colt HG, Crawford SW. In vitro study of the safety limits of bronchoscopic argon plasma coagulation in the presence of airway stents. Respirology. 2006 Sep;11(5):643–7.

Cracco C, Fartoukh M, Prodanovic H, Azoulay E, Chenivesse C, Lorut C, et al. Safety of performing fiberoptic bronchoscopy in critically ill hypoxemic patients with acute respiratory failure. Intensive Care Med. 2013 Jan;39(1):45–52. Epub 2012 Oct 16.

Crosta C, Spaggiari L, De Stefano A, Fiori G, Ravizza D, Pastorino U. Endoscopic argon plasma coagulation for palliative treatment of malignant airway obstructions: early results in 47 cases. Lung Cancer. 2001 Jul;33(1):75–80.

Erasmus DB, Keller CA, Alvarez FB. Large airway complications in 150 consecutive lung transplant recipients. J Bronchol. 2008 Jul;15(3):152–7.

Ergan B, Nava S. The use of bronchoscopy in critically ill patients: considerations and complications. Expert Rev Respir Med. 2018 Aug;12(8):651–63. Epub 2018 Jul 12.

Ferguson JS, Sprenger K, Van Natta T. Closure of a bronchopleural fistula using bronchoscopic placement of an endobronchial valve designed for the treatment of emphysema. Chest. 2006 Feb;129(2):479–81.

Folch E, Mehta AC. Airway interventions in the tracheobronchial tree. Semin Respir Crit Care Med. 2008 Aug;29(4):441–52.

Gottlieb J, Fuehner T, Dierich M, Wiesner O, Simon AR, Welte T. Are metallic stents really safe? A long-term analysis in lung transplant recipients. Eur Respir J. 2009 Dec;34(6):1417–22. Epub 2009 May 14.

Gruson D, Hilbert G, Valentino R, Vargas F, Chene G, Bebear C, et al. Utility of fiberoptic bronchoscopy in neutropenic patients admitted to the intensive care unit with pulmonary infiltrates. Crit Care Med. 2000 Jul;28(7):2224–30.

Haas AR, Vachani A, Sterman DH. Advances in diagnostic bronchoscopy. Am J Respir Crit Care Med. 2010 Sep 1;182(5):589–97. Epub 2010 Apr 8.

Heidegger T. Videos in clinical medicine: fiberoptic intubation. N Engl J Med. 2011 May 19;364(20):e42.

Herth F, Ernst A, Becker HD. Endoscopic drainage of lung abscesses: technique and outcome. Chest. 2005 Apr;127(4):1378–81.

Hetzel J, Eberhardt R, Herth FJ, Petermann C, Reichle G, Freitag L, et al. Cryobiopsy increases the diagnostic yield of endobronchial biopsy: a multicentre trial. Eur Respir J. 2012 Mar;39(3):685–90. Epub 2011 Aug 18.

Hinerman R, Alvarez F, Singh A, Keller C. Treatment of endobronchial mucormycosis with amphotericin B via flexible bronchoscopy. J Bronchol. 2002 Oct;9(4):294–7.

Hopkins PM, Aboyoun CL, Chhajed PN, Malouf MA, Plit ML, Rainer SP, et al. Prospective analysis of 1,235 transbronchial lung biopsies in lung transplant recipients. J Heart Lung Transplant. 2002 Oct;21(10):1062–7.

Jose RJ, Shaefi S, Navani N. Sedation for flexible bronchoscopy: current and emerging evidence. Eur Respir Rev. 2013 Jun 1;22(128):106–16.

Keller C, Frost A. Fiberoptic bronchoplasty: description of a simple adjunct technique for the management of bronchial stenosis following lung transplantation. Chest. 1992 Oct;102(4):995–8.

Keller CA, Hinerman R, Singh A, Alvarez F. The use of endoscopic argon plasma coagulation in airway complications after solid organ transplantation. Chest. 2001 Jun;119(6):1968–75.

Kermeen FD, McNeil KD, Fraser JF, McCarthy J, Ziegenfuss MD, Mullany D, et al. Resolution of severe ischemia-reperfusion injury post-lung transplantation after administration of endobronchial surfactant. J Heart Lung Transplant. 2007 Aug;26(8):850–6.

Kerwin AJ, Croce MA, Timmons SD, Maxwell RA, Malhotra AK, Fabian TC. Effects of fiberoptic bronchoscopy on intracranial pressure in patients with brain injury: a prospective clinical study. J Trauma. 2000 May;48(5):878–82.

Kornblith LZ, Burlew CC, Moore EE, Haenel JB, Kashuk JL, Biffl WL, et al. One thousand bedside percutaneous tracheostomies in the surgical intensive care unit: time to change the gold standard. J Am Coll Surg. 2011 Feb;212(2):163–70. Epub 2010 Dec 30.

Lawson RW, Peters JI, Shelledy DC. Effects of fiberoptic bronchoscopy during mechanical ventilation in a lung model. Chest. 2000 Sep;118(3):824–31.

Machuzak M, Santacruz JF, Gildea T, Murthy SC. Airway complications after lung transplantation. Thorac Surg Clin. 2015;25(1):55–75.

Madden BP, Datta S, Charokopos N. Experience with Ultraflex expandable metallic stents in the management of endobronchial pathology. Ann Thorac Surg. 2002 Mar;73(3):938–44.

Madden BP, Loke TK, Sheth AC. Do expandable metallic airway stents have a role in the management of patients with benign tracheobronchial disease? Ann Thorac Surg. 2006 Jul;82(1):274–8.

Matsuda M, Horai T, Nakamura S, Nishio H, Sakuma T, Ikegami H, et al. Bronchial brushing and bronchial biopsy: comparison of diagnostic accuracy and cell typing reliability in lung cancer. Thorax. 1986 Jun;41(6):475–8.

McArdle JR, Gildea TR, Mehta AC. Balloon bronchoplasty: its indications, benefits, and complications. J Bronchol. 2005 Apr;12(2):123–7.

Morice RC, Ece T, Ece F, Keus L. Endobronchial argon plasma coagulation for treatment of hemoptysis and neoplastic airway obstruction. Chest. 2001 Mar;119(3):781–7.

Panchabhai TS, Mehta AC. Historical perspectives of bronchoscopy: connecting the dots. Ann Am Thorac Soc. 2015 May;12(5):631–41.

Parekh PJ, Buerlein RC, Shams R, Herre J, Johnson DA. An update on the management of implanted cardiac devices during electrosurgical procedures. Gastrointest Endosc. 2013 Dec;78(6):836–41. Epub 2013 Oct 15.

Peikert T, Rana S, Edell ES. Safety, diagnostic yield, and therapeutic implications of flexible bronchoscopy in patients with febrile neutropenia and pulmonary infiltrates. Mayo Clin Proc. 2005 Nov;80(11):1414–20.

Poletti V, Casoni GL, Gurioli C, Ryu JH, Tomassetti S. Lung cryobiopsies: a paradigm shift in diagnostic bronchoscopy? Respirology. 2014 Jul;19(5):645–54. Epub 2014 May 26.

Prebil SE, Andrews J, Cribbs SK, Martin GS, Esper A. Safety of research bronchoscopy in critically ill patients. J Crit Care. 2014 Dec;29(6):961–4. Epub 2014 Jun 13.

Rea-Neto A, Youssef NC, Tuche F, Brunkhorst F, Ranieri VM, Reinhart K, et al. Diagnosis of ventilator-associated pneumonia: a systematic review of the literature. Crit Care. 2008;12(2):R56. Epub 2008 Apr 21.

Sakr L, Dutau H. Massive hemoptysis: an update on the role of bronchoscopy in diagnosis and management. Respiration. 2010;80(1):38–58. Epub 2010 Jan 8.

Thiberville L, Salaun M, Lachkar S, Dominique S, Moreno-Swirc S, Vever-Bizet C, et al. Confocal fluorescence endomicroscopy of the human airways. Proc Am Thorac Soc. 2009 Aug 15;6(5):444–9.

Travaline JM, McKenna RJ Jr, De Giacomo T, Venuta F, Hazelrigg SR, Boomer M, et al; Endobronchial Valve for Persistent Air Leak Group. Treatment of persistent pulmonary air leaks using endobronchial valves. Chest. 2009 Aug;136(2):355–60. Epub 2009 Apr 6. Erratum in: Chest. 2009 Sep;136(3):950.

Tukey MH, Wiener RS. Population-based estimates of transbronchial lung biopsy utilization and complications. Respir Med. 2012 Nov;106(11):1559–65. Epub 2012 Aug 28.

Vergnon JM, Huber RM, Moghissi K. Place of cryotherapy, brachytherapy and photodynamic therapy in therapeutic bronchoscopy of lung cancers. Eur Respir J. 2006 Jul;28(1):200–18.

Wahidi MM, Ernst A. Role of the interventional pulmonologist in the intensive care unit. J Intensive Care Med. 2005 May-Jun;20(3):141–6.

Wahidi MM, Herth FJ, Ernst A. State of the art: interventional pulmonology. Chest. 2007 Jan;131(1):261–74.

Waller EA, Aduen JF, Kramer DJ, Alvarez F, Heckman MG, Crook JE, et al. Safety of percutaneous dilatational tracheostomy with direct bronchoscopic guidance for solid organ allograft recipients. Mayo Clin Proc. 2007 Dec;82(12):1502–8.

Yasuo M, Tanabe T, Tsushima K, Nakamura M, Kanda S, Komatsu Y, et al. Endobronchial argon plasma coagulation for the management of post-intubation tracheal stenosis. Respirology. 2006 Sep;11(5):659–62.

Cardiovascular and Cardiopulmonary Monitoring and Access

Electrocardiographic Monitoring[a]

PRAGNESH P. PARIKH, MD; K. L. VENKATACHALAM, MD

Goals

- Explain the principles underlying electrocardiogram acquisition and display.
- Describe the approach to electrocardiographic evaluation.
- Differentiate between concerning and unconcerning electrocardiographic findings.

Introduction

Continuous electrocardiographic (ECG) monitoring is almost universal in patients in intensive care units, and 12-lead ECG is a frequently performed investigation. Both have the ability to detect many cardiac disturbances and the cardiac consequences of other conditions. Understanding the acquisition of the tracing, having a systematic approach to interpretation, and having the ability to differentiate concerning findings from nonconcerning ones and from artifacts are key skills for the intensivist.

Basic Cardiac Electrophysiology

Individual interconnected cardiac muscle cells are depolarized sequentially through organized electrical pathways starting at the sinoatrial node and progressing to the atrioventricular node and His-Purkinje system to the 2 ventricles. The electrical activity of the pacemaker cells in the sinoatrial node is modulated by sympathetic tone (increasing heart rate) and parasympathetic tone (decreasing heart rate) through multiple ion channels. The ECG is the composite representation of the depolarization of myocardial cells (muscle activity) and does not display the electrical activity of the conduction system itself. Even if ventricular depolarization (QRS) is noted on the ECG monitor, muscle contraction may not occur (as in pulseless electrical activity), and it is important to verify the presence of a pulse.

ECG Monitor

A block diagram of a typical ECG acquisition system in the intensive care unit and the derived ECG vectors are shown in Figure 119.1. The 3 limb connections—right arm (R_A), left arm (L_A), and left leg (L_L)—are connected to a switching network through protection circuitry to prevent damage to the electronics during defibrillation. Also entering this circuit are the 6 precordial connections (V_1 through V_6). Each of these 9 wires is incapable of producing meaningful signals by themselves and can do so only when analyzed with reference to another wire (the voltage difference between 2 wires is a "lead"). For the 3 limb connections, true bipolar leads are obtained by referencing each of them to 1 of the other 2 (R_A to L_A is lead I, R_A to L_L is lead II, and L_A to L_L is lead III). The vector sum of lead I and lead III equals that of lead II (Einthoven law). Three additional augmented leads—aVR, aVL, and aVF— provide intermediate vectors. The precordial and augmented leads need a reference electrode for the second wire and use the vector sum of the 3 limb wires to approximate a theoretical zero voltage point known as Wilson central terminal (WCT).

The 12 leads thus derived are sequentially switched rapidly to produce a snapshot of each lead, which is amplified, filtered, and digitized before being displayed. These signals are filtered from 0.05 to 100 Hz (diagnostic quality ECG) or from 0.5 to 40 Hz (monitor quality ECG). A notch filter is provided at 50/60 Hz to further reject line frequency interference. Pacemaker spikes are separated from the main

[a] Portions previously published in Venkatachalam KL, Herbrandson JE, Asirvatham SJ. Signals and signal processing for the electrophysiologist: part I: electrogram acquisition. Circ Arrhythm Electrophysiol. 2011 Dec;4(6):965-73; used with permission.

A

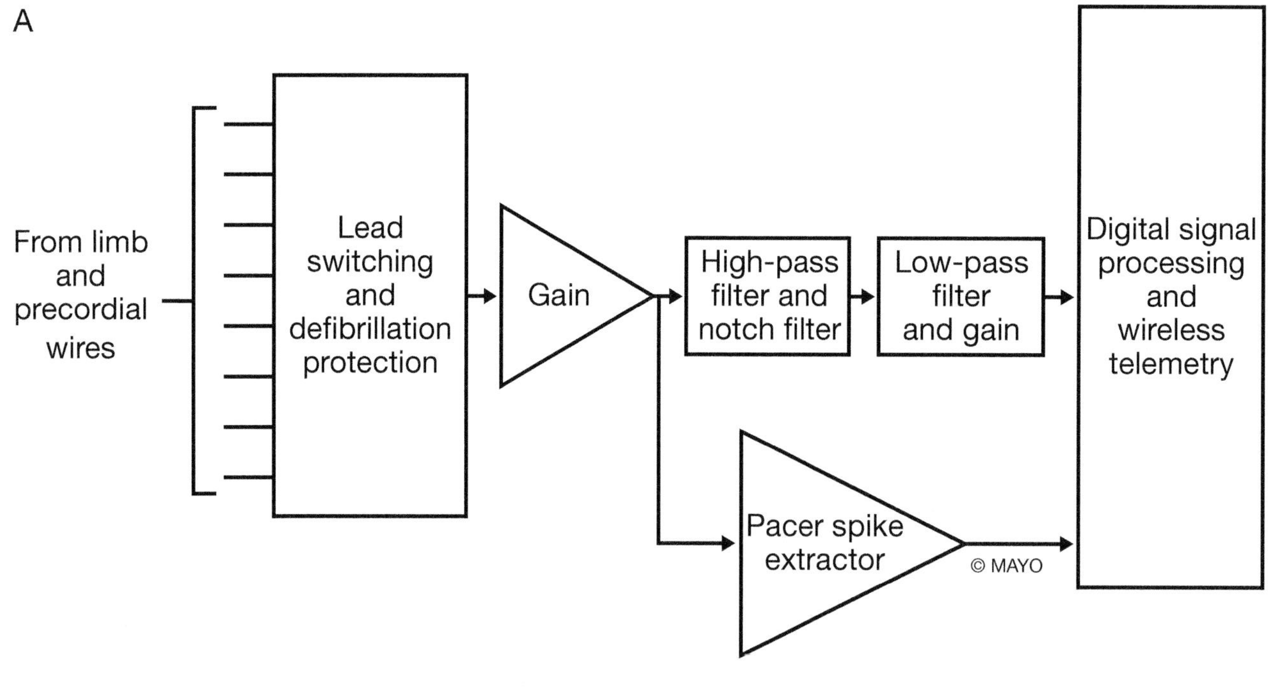

B

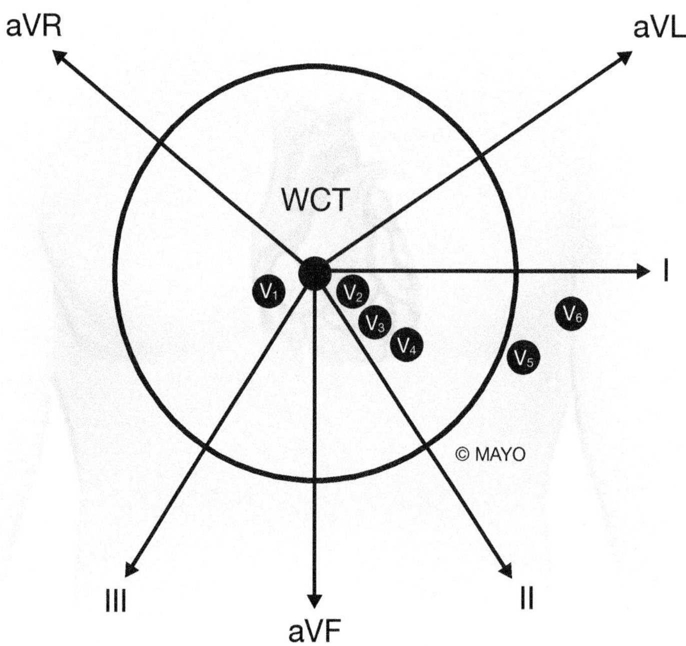

Figure 119.1. *Electrocardiographic (ECG) Monitoring. A, Block diagram of ECG machine. The limb and precordial signals are combined appropriately, amplified, and filtered before being processed and displayed. Special hardware and software processing are often used to separate and reinstall pacemaker spikes on the display. This additional processing is prone to interference, and identification of paced complexes independently, by morphologic features, is important. B, ECG 12-lead orientation, including Wilson central terminal (WCT). Often, monitoring systems used in the intensive care unit display only 3 leads at any given time. Selection of 3 orthogonal leads, such as leads I (lateral), II (inferior), and V (right anterior), is useful to obtain a snapshot of the entire cardiac activity. Lead II usually has the tallest QRS voltage.*

signal, and that timing information is sent to the system's microprocessor, which then reinserts an artificial pacemaker spike at the correct time onto the composite ECG signal. This step is done to prevent the amplifier circuitry from being overwhelmed by the pacemaker spikes, which have a substantially higher voltage than the QRS amplitude. The presence or absence of pacemaker spikes on the display is greatly influenced by the electrical noise in the intensive care unit and by the filtering being used and is not entirely reliable. Thus, recognizing a paced QRS morphologic pattern independently is very important.

For ambulatory or intensive care unit monitoring, multiple reduced electrode sets (3, 5, and 6 electrodes) of leads have been developed that use mathematical transformation to recreate all 12 leads.

Principles of ECG Evaluation

If the net vector (force and direction) of myocardial depolarization moves towards an ECG lead (pair of wires), it is inscribed as a positive deflection on the ECG. If it moves away from a lead, it is inscribed as a negative deflection. This powerful rule allows localization of ectopic beats, pacemaker leads, and accessory pathways (leads with negative deflection denote the origin of depolarization). The QRS amplitude on a particular lead is highest when the vector is parallel to that lead and is small or nonexistent when the vector is orthogonal (perpendicular) to that lead (Figure 119.2A). This allows determination of QRS axis. A lead with a large QRS should always be on display (usually lead II, because it is nearly parallel to the QRS vector). The amplitudes of QRS (depolarization) and T (repolarization)

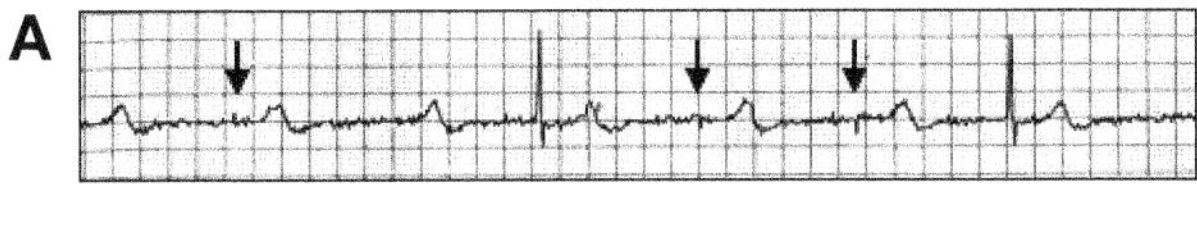

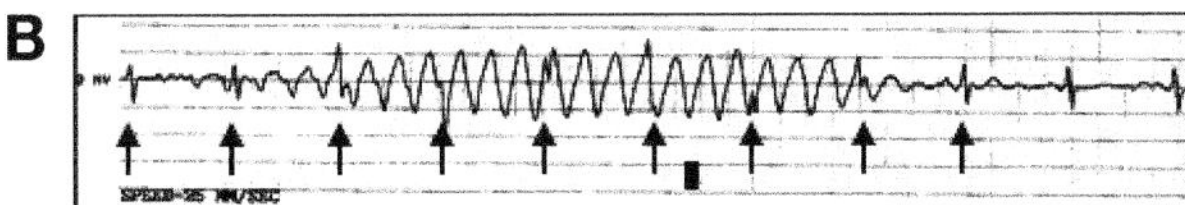

Figure 119.2. Mimicry on Electrocardiography. A, Orthogonal vectors mimicking ventricular asystole. QRS deflections are clearly seen, but the smaller deflections, which initially appear to be P waves with no associated QRS, are actually T waves. Looking closely, one can see small QRS deflections (arrows) before each T wave. They occur because the ECG monitor lead is perpendicular to the dominant QRS vector and the vector shifts with respiration. Switching to another lead will show the QRS and T. B, Noise mimicking ventricular tachycardia. The arrows show the presence of QRS deflections within the "ventricular tachycardia," confirming motion artifact.

Box 119.1 • High-Yield ECG Interpretation

When assessing a cardiac rhythm on ECG or monitor, independently evaluate the rhythm strip for atrial rhythm (P waves) and ventricular rhythm (QRS complexes) and their relationship to one another

Assess the ECG for life-threatening conditions (heart rate <50 bpm or >120 bpm and evidence for injury) initially, before doing a comprehensive evaluation. If QRS complexes are occurring between 3 and 6 large boxes apart on the ECG, the rate is unlikely to be a problem. ST depression in lead V_1 or ST elevation in any of the other leads could be due to injury

P waves from the sinus node area are biphasic (positive followed by negative) in lead V_1 and upright in leads I and II. Other P-wave morphologic patterns suggest ectopic atrial rhythm

Normal QRS complexes are upright in leads I and II and demonstrate gradual increase in positive amplitude (normal R-wave progression) from leads V_1 through V_6, with a transition from negative to positive by lead V_3 or V_4. Any variation from this pattern could be due to lead malposition, abnormal rotation of the heart, or weak forces in specific leads (eg, after a myocardial infarction)

Upright QRS in leads I and aVF suggests normal QRS axis. Left-axis deviation has a net negative QRS in lead II. Right-axis deviation has a net negative QRS in lead I. New right-axis deviation may suggest right heart strain due to pulmonary hypertension or pulmonary embolus

PR interval is a measure of conduction from the sinus node to the ventricles. Interval >200 ms (1 large box) represents first-degree AV block, which by itself is not clinically significant. However, marked PR prolongation (>300 ms) may be symptomatic. In this setting, use caution with AV nodal blocking agents. Second-degree AV block is characterized by periodic loss of AV conduction, which may or may not be clinically significant. Complete lack of communication between P waves and QRS (with more P waves than QRS waves) is third-degree AV block and is always clinically significant

The QRS duration is a measure of synchrony between the right and left ventricles. Conduction slowing may produce right bundle or left bundle branch block, typically asymptomatic. However, left bundle branch block obscures assessment of ST-segment changes during acute myocardial infarction. Right ventricular pacing may also produce a wide QRS complex, usually with a left bundle branch block configuration

QT interval is a measure of ventricular repolarization and varies with heart rate. The QT corrected for heart rate is referred to as QTc, and marked QTc prolongation predisposes to ventricular arrhythmias

Abbreviations: AV, atrioventricular; bpm, beats per minute; ECG, electrocardiographic.

Box 119.2 • Non–Life-Threatening ECG Findings

AV dissociation. If there are more QRS complexes than P waves, the AV node is not to blame. AV dissociation could be life-threatening in the setting of ventricular tachycardia. Having more P waves than QRS complexes could be an indication of complete heart block, except when the atrial rate is high enough that AV nodal block is expected, such as atrial flutter with 4:1 AV conduction

Flat line on monitor. No activity on the monitor strip (lack of even fine noise) suggests that the monitor amplifiers are resetting because of movement or intermittent lead connection. This finding could be mistaken for asystole

If a sustained wide-complex tachycardia is noted on monitor, a 12-lead ECG should be obtained as soon as possible to confirm that this is not supraventricular tachycardia with aberrant conduction

Occasional dropped pacemaker beats could be normal operation in which the pacemaker is checking pacemaker capture thresholds or trying to minimize ventricular pacing

Early repolarization may produce ST-segment elevation with no serious acute consequence

Abbreviations: AV, atrioventricular; ECG, electrocardiographic.

may also be different in different leads. Leads with a high QRS/T ratio should be displayed to minimize the risk of double-counting the QRS and T and calculating a heart rate

Box 119.3 • Concerning ECG Findings

All causes of ST-segment elevation (see Box 119.4)

All causes of wide-complex tachycardia (see Box 119.5)

T-wave peaking could be due to early injury or hyperkalemia

Bradycardia, AV block, and substantial pauses

QT prolongation (corrected QT >450 in men and >460 in women) due to medications, hypokalemia, hypocalcemia, hypomagnesemia, hypothermia, subarachnoid hemorrhage, or long QT syndromes. Ventricular pacing and bundle branch blocks also lengthen the QT interval. However, because this QT increase is due to the increase in QRS duration, it does not have the same risk of ventricular arrhythmias as an intrinsic QT prolongation

Pacemaker spikes falling on native P, QRS, or T waves could be a sign of pacemaker malfunction

Abbreviations: AV, atrioventricular; ECG, electrocardiographic.

Box 119.4 • Causes of ST-Segment Elevation on ECG Monitor in the ICU

Acute myocardial injury or infarction (often with cardiac biomarker elevation)

Myocarditis (often with cardiac biomarker elevation)

Stress (takotsubo) cardiomyopathy (often with cardiac biomarker elevation)

Subarachnoid hemorrhage

Electrolyte abnormalities

Acute pericarditis (diffuse ST elevation, PR elevation in aV_R, PR depression in inferior leads)

Ventricular pacing (pacemaker spikes may not always be visible, depending on cardiac monitor settings)

LV aneurysm (chronic ST elevation)

Bundle branch block or intraventricular conduction delay

Brugada syndrome (coved ST elevation in V_1)

Abbreviations: ECG, electrocardiographic; ICU, intensive care unit; LV, left ventricular.

that is twice the actual rate. Boxes 119.1 through 119.5 list the important, high-yield aspects of rhythm monitoring and interpretation in the intensive care unit.

Box 119.5 • Causes of Wide-Complex Tachycardia on ECG in the ICU

Ventricular tachycardia (especially if QRS duration is >140 ms with RBBB-like morphology or >160 ms with LBBB-like morphology)

Supraventricular tachycardia with aberrant conduction (the aberrancy will look like typical RBBB or typical LBBB)

Hyperkalemia (may become sinusoidal at very high serum potassium level)

Sinus tachycardia with ventricular pacing (the pacemaker spikes may not always be visible)

Antidromic tachycardia (supraventricular tachycardia using an accessory pathway antegrade and AV node retrograde), often cannot be distinguished from ventricular tachycardia

Pacemaker-mediated tachycardia (the pacemaker spikes may not always be visible)

Motion artifact and electrical interference (Figure 119.2B)

Abbreviations: AV, atrioventricular; ECG, electrocardiography; ICU, intensive care unit, LBBB, left bundle branch block; RBBB, right bundle branch block.

Summary

- View the ECG in groups (II, III, aVF are inferior; I, aVL, V_5, and V_6 are left lateral; V_1 and V_2 are septal; V_3 and V_4 are anterior). A negatively directed deflection in a particular lead group denotes the origin of that depolarization. Use this fact to localize ectopic beats and pacemaker leads.
- Rhythm strips showing "polymorphic ventricular tachycardia" are often normal sinus rhythm with motion artifact. Look for normal QRS deflections within the "ventricular tachycardia."
- "Asystole" may be artifact from electronic reset of the amplifier. The flat line noted in this instance is devoid of the usual low-level baseline noise of a normal rhythm strip and looks abnormally "clean." The accompanying arterial blood pressure tracing, if present, is normal.

SUGGESTED READING

Drew BJ, Califf RM, Funk M, Kaufman ES, Krucoff MW, Laks MM, et al; American Heart Association; Councils on Cardiovascular Nursing, Clinical Cardiology, and Cardiovascular Disease in the Young. Practice standards for electrocardiographic monitoring in hospital settings: an American Heart Association scientific statement from the Councils on Cardiovascular Nursing, Clinical Cardiology, and Cardiovascular Disease in the Young: endorsed by the International Society of Computerized Electrocardiology and the American Association of Critical-Care Nurses. Circulation. 2004 Oct 26;110(17):2721–46. Erratum in: Circulation. 2005 Jan 25;111(3):378.

Kligfield P, Gettes LS, Bailey JJ, Childers R, Deal BJ, Hancock EW, et al; American Heart Association Electrocardiography and Arrhythmias Committee, Council on Clinical Cardiology; American College of Cardiology Foundation; Heart Rhythm Society, Josephson M, Mason JW, Okin P, Surawicz B, Wellens H. Recommendations for the standardization and interpretation of the electrocardiogram: part I: the electrocardiogram and its technology: a scientific statement from the American Heart Association Electrocardiography and Arrhythmias Committee, Council on Clinical Cardiology; the American College of Cardiology Foundation; and the Heart Rhythm Society: endorsed by the International Society for Computerized Electrocardiology. Circulation. 2007 Mar 13;115(10):1306–24. Epub 2007 Feb 23.

Surawicz B, Knilans TK. Chou's electrocardiography in clinical practice: adult and pediatric. 6th ed. Philadelphia (PA): Saunders/Elsevier; c2008. 732 p.

Hemodynamic Monitoring

HANNELISA E. CALLISEN, PA-C; STACY L. LIBRICZ, PA-C, MS; AYAN SEN, MD

Goals

- To elucidate different methods of measuring perfusion pressure.
- To describe measures of oxygen delivery.
- To illustrate challenges and options with measurement of fluid responsiveness.
- To describe different methods of cardiac output assessment.

Introduction

In the critically ill patient, ensuring adequate oxygen delivery with sufficient perfusion pressure is vital. Basic physical examination remains the most invaluable and simplistic form of hemodynamic assessment, but technologic evolution has allowed for substantial advancement in monitoring techniques.

This chapter reviews the most common hemodynamic monitoring devices and techniques and focuses on the invasiveness, advantages, limitations, and technical aspects of each (Table 120.1).

Perfusion Pressure

Noninvasive: Oscillometry (Intermittent Cuff Method)

Noninvasive blood pressure monitoring by cuff uses the oscillometric method. Small-amplitude arterial wall oscillations are detected as a cuff is deflated. The initial increase in amplitude represents the systolic blood pressure, and the increase indicates the mean arterial pressure. Amplitude decreases until it ceases, which correlates with the diastolic blood pressure.

Noninvasive blood pressure monitoring requires either an automatic oscillometric device or auscultation. Automatic devices use different proprietary algorithms according to the manufacturer that result in computerized estimates of pressure. Auscultation relies on Korotkoff sounds made audible through the use of a stethoscope and sphygmomanometer. The appearance and subsequent muffling of these sounds represent the systolic and diastolic blood pressures. The mean arterial pressure must be mathematically estimated from the sum of diastolic blood pressure plus one-third the difference between diastolic and systolic pressures.

Limitations of this technique include overestimation and underestimation of blood pressure with mismatch of arm circumference to cuff size and less reliable readings with arrhythmias such as atrial fibrillation. The lack of continuous monitoring also increases the risk of delayed or missed recognition of hypotension or hypertension.

Invasive: Arterial Catheterization

Invasive blood pressure measurement with arterial catheterization has been regarded as the standard and is frequently used in the critical care setting. A catheter inserted in an artery (frequently radial, brachial, or femoral) is attached to a transduction system. This system includes stiff connection tubing filled with a column of saline that is pressurized to allow for a continuous flush into the bloodstream. Within this system is a transducer that converts mechanical energy to an electrical signal. A dome diaphragm within the transducer deforms according to pressure changes transmitted from arterial blood pulsation, which correlates to a proportional change in transducer

Table 120.1 • Hemodynamic Monitoring Devices and Techniques

Factor Monitored	Invasiveness	Technique	Devices or Technology
Cardiac output	Invasive	PATD	
		Bolus	PAC
		Continuous filament	PAC
		CPCA	
		TPTD	PiCCO
			PiCCOplus/PulseCO
			VolumeView/EV1000
		Lithium dilution	LiDCO
			LiDCOplus/PulseCO
		Other	Modelflow
		Non-CPCA	FloTrac-Vigileo
			LiDCOrapid
			PRAM/Mostcare
			ProAQT/Pulsioflex
	Semi-invasive	TEE Doppler	TEE
		Esophageal Doppler	CardioQ
	Noninvasive	Bioimpedance	
		Thoracic	BioZ
		Endotracheal	ECOM
		Electrical bioreactance	NICOM
		TTE Dopper	US, echo
		Capnography	$ETCO_2$ monitor
		Volume-clamp	Nexfin
			CNAP
			ClearSight
Fluid status and responsiveness	Invasive	Ventricular filling pressures	
		CVP	CVC (thoracic), PAC
		PAOP	PAC
		Global EDV	PiCCO/PiCCOplus
	Semi-invasive	SVV, SPV, PPV	Arterial line
			FloTrac-Vigileo
			LiDCO, LiDCOplus, LiDCOrapid
			PiCCO, PiCCOplus
			PRAM/Mostcare
			ProAQT/Pulsioflex
			VolumeView/EV1000
		End-expiratory occlusion test	Mechanical ventilator[a]
	Noninvasive	Passive leg raise	Blood pressure cuff[a]
		Cardiovascular US	US, echo
		Volume-clamp	Nexfin
			CNAP
			ClearSight
Perfusion pressure	Invasive	Arterial line	Arterial line
	Noninvasive	Oscillometry (interrmittent cuff)	Blood pressure cuff
		Volume-clamp	Nexfin
			CNAP
			ClearSight
Global oxygen delivery	Invasive	Central venous oxygen saturation	CVC (thoracic)
		Mixed venous oxygen saturation	PAC
	Semi-invasive	Biomarkers	Blood draw
	Noninvasive	Regional oximetry	INVOS
			NONIN
			FORE-SIGHT

Abbreviations: CPCA, calibrated pulse contour analysis; CVC, central venous catheter; CVP, central venous pressure; echo, echocardiography; EDV, end-diastolic volume; $ETCO_2$, end-tidal carbon dioxide (pressure); NICOM, noninvasive cardiac output monitor; PAC, pulmonary artery catheter; PAOP, pulmonary artery occlusion pressure; PATD, pulmonary artery thermodilution; PPV, pulse pressure variation; SPV, systolic pressure variation; SVV, stroke volume variation; TEE, transesophageal echocardiography; TPTD, transpulmonary thermodilution; TTE, transthoracic echocardiography; US, ultrasonography.

[a] May be used with more invasive hemodynamic monitoring.

current created by resistance changes across a Wheatstone bridge-type electrical circuit.

Calibration is required for this system to a "zero" value, defined as the isosbestic point, which is optimally equivalent to the hydrostatic pressure in the left atrium. Use of this technology necessitates leveling of the transducer to the height of the left atrium at all times.

The morphologic pattern of an arterial pulse waveform is created by atrioventricular valve closure, arterial wall compliance, and wave reflections and is further affected by heart rate, velocity of blood flow, vascular anatomy, and location of measurement. Pulse pressure increases the more distal to the aortic root.

Inherent risks with catheter insertion include bleeding, thrombosis, dislodgment, and infection. Accurate blood pressure reading requires that the invasive monitoring system is correctly damped with a frequency response that is greater than the natural frequency of the arterial pulse. Overdamping (or a decrease in frequency response) may be created by long tubing, microbubbles, thrombi, catheter kinks, and incompletely open stopcocks and results in an underestimation of blood pressure. Hyperresonance within the system can also occur and create underdamping or overestimation of blood pressure.

Oxygen Delivery

The premise of critical care hemodynamic assessment, and arguably most important, revolves around oxygen delivery (Do_2). In addition to adequate arterial oxygen content, Do_2 requires sufficient cardiac output (CO), which is determined by cardiac function and venous return.

Noninvasive: Regional Oximetry

Tissue and cerebral oximetry are 2 forms of regional oximetry most commonly used during certain operations, trauma resuscitation, and shock management. Near infrared spectroscopy is used to assess oxygen balance at a local level and may be indicative of oxygen or perfusion debt at different end-organs.

Semi-invasive: Biomarkers

Laboratory values that support adequate Do_2 include normal blood lactate level, base excess, and renal, hepatic, and cardiac biomarkers. Normal values, however, do not rule out inadequate Do_2, and abnormal values could be a result of other clinical situations. Lactate is frequently measured when there is a concern about insufficient Do_2 or blood pressure because it is produced during anaerobic metabolism, when oxygen is not available to cells for phosphorylation of adenosine triphosphate.

Invasive: Central and Mixed Venous Oxygen Saturations

Normal cellular respiration based on aerobic metabolism requires adequate Do_2, which increases or decreases according to metabolic rate or tissue oxygen demand. In normal physiology the Do_2 to oxygen consumption ($\dot{V}o_2$) ratio is 5:1; when the ratio is closer to 2:1, the oxygen extraction ratio is more than 50% and cellular respiration becomes supply-dependent.

The oxygen extraction ratio correlates with the difference between arterial and venous oxygen saturation. A venous sample is drawn either from near the right atrium by central venous catheter (CVC) to obtain a "central" venous oxygen saturation or from the distal port of a pulmonary artery catheter (PAC) to obtain a "mixed" venous saturation. It is mixed because it is an admixture of blood from the superior and inferior vena cava and the coronary sinus and can be obtained from intermittent blood sampling or continuous fiberoptic reflectance oximetry with a modified PAC. A normal oxygen extraction ratio is about 25% with a venous saturation of about 75% in nonhypoxic states.

The venous saturation is primarily influenced by hemoglobin, arterial oxygen saturation, CO, and $\dot{V}o_2$ and is therefore valuable for assessing and managing volume status, anemia, hypoxia, and cardiac function. Used as an indirect index of global tissue oxygenation, it does not indicate organ-specific malperfusion.

Fluid Status and Responsiveness

The goal of increasing venous return to augment stroke volume and improve CO will be effective only if the ventricles are fluid-responsive. Fluid responsiveness is represented by the ascending portion of the Frank-Starling curve (Figure 120.1). Because excessive fluid administration is correlated with worse outcomes, accurate assessment of preload and volume responsiveness is vital.

Noninvasive

Passive Leg Raise

The passive leg raise uses a patient's own pooled lower extremity venous blood as a temporary fluid challenge of about 300 mL. By passively elevating the legs to 45° from a semirecumbent position for 30 to 90 seconds, change in CO can be assessed as the venous reservoir in the lower half of the body partially empties, converts to stressed volume, and affects cardiac preload. Clinical studies have shown this assessment to be an accurate predictor of volume responsiveness, particularly if CO increased by at least 10%. Because it is exerted over a time with numerous cardiac and respiratory cycles, it is less sensitive to spontaneous breathing and cardiac arrhythmias.

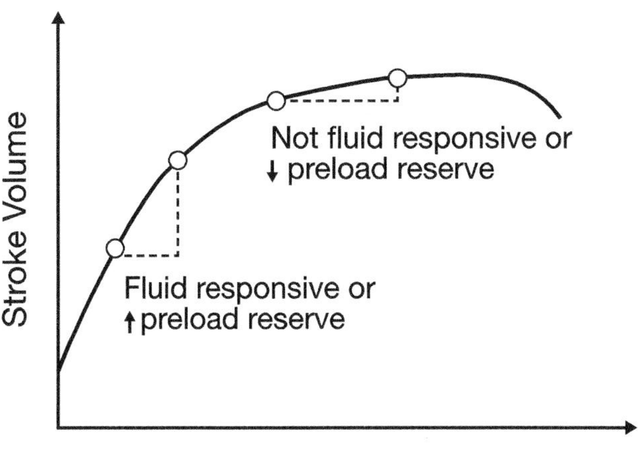

Figure 120.1. Cardiac Function Curve Based on the Frank-Starling Principle. A fluid challenge to ventricles functioning on the steep part of the curve (left side) results in a considerable increase in stroke volume, deeming them fluid-responsive with preload reserve. This increase is not seen in ventricles functioning on the horizontal part of the curve (top). EDV indicates end-diastolic volume.

Cardiovascular Sonography

Ultrasonography has been widely used for static noninvasive assessment of right atrial pressure or central venous pressure and for dynamic evaluation of inferior vena cava (IVC) diameter variation with respiration. Guidelines published by the American Society of Echocardiography in 2015 recommend that IVC diameter measurements should be obtained with the subcostal view with the IVC in its long axis at a point just caudal to its junction with the hepatic vein. Supine positioning is recommended, and there is no specification on measurement according to phase of respiration.

Although studies with variable findings have resulted in a difficult interpretation of the reliability and accuracy of this static measure, a review published by Ciozda et al (see Suggested Reading) concluded overall support for sonographic assessment of the IVC and found consistent positive correlation between IVC size and right atrial pressure and negative correlation between the IVC collapsibility index and right atrial pressure.

Inaccuracies in measurement may relate to patient positioning and operator skill. Right atrial pressure may also be highly dynamic and influenced by tricuspid valve regurgitation, positive end-expiratory pressure, and deep respiration.

Semi-invasive: Stroke Volume and Pulse Pressure Variation

The effect of positive pressure ventilation on heart-lung interaction is clear, and its effect on venous return and CO can be recognized through analysis of the morphologic pattern of the arterial waveform. In its simplest form, variations in pulse contour may be visualized on bedside arterial waveform tracings, often more pronounced in situations of intravascular volume depletion and increased chamber compliance.

Preload dependence can thereby be assessed by monitoring variation in stroke volume throughout the respiratory cycle, which, if present, correlates with the steep portion of the Frank-Starling curve (Figure 120.1). The use of pulse pressure as a surrogate for stroke volume has additionally led to the use of pulse pressure variation as a valid indicator of volume responsiveness in the right clinical context. Pulse pressure variation and stroke volume variation of more than 13% have been identified to predict a substantial response in cardiac index with a rapid volume challenge (Figure 120.2).

Some commercially available systems that calculate and use stroke volume variation include PiCCO (Pulsion Medical Systems), LiDCO (LiDCO, Ltd), and the FloTrac-Vigileo (Edwards Lifesciences) (discussed further in the Cardiac Output section below) (Figure 120.3).

Risks involved with this assessment are those that occur with arterial line cannulation. Limitations of use include less reliability in situations of spontaneous breathing, cardiac arrhythmias, low tidal volume or lung compliance, open chest, increased intra-abdominal pressure, very high respiratory rate, and right heart failure.

Invasive: Ventricular Filling Pressures

With use of a transducer system, additional vascular pressures can be monitored with the insertion of either a CVC or PAC in the internal jugular or subclavian vein. Despite their static nature and poor correlation to fluid responsiveness, ventricular filling pressures have long been used as surrogates for ventricular filling volumes in the assessment of preload.

The measurement of central venous pressure and pulmonary artery occlusion pressure are defined as the back pressures to systemic and pulmonary venous return, respectively. When used not as singular, static readings of intravascular volume but rather trended over time, they can provide valuable information about changes in fluid status and cardiac function.

Although misinterpretation is frequent, improper zeroing, leveling, and calibration of the transducer system may also lead to further inaccuracies.

Cardiac Output

Although a PAC is still considered the standard for CO monitoring, it is regarded as highly invasive and requires accurate data interpretation to be most beneficial. A drive for less invasive techniques has popularized several other methods, many of which are discussed below.

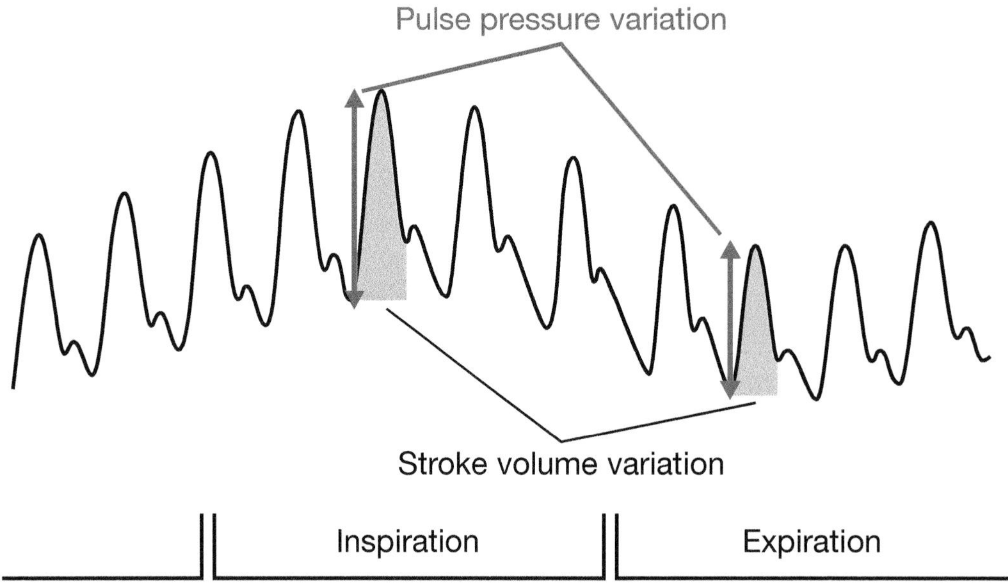

Figure 120.2. Stroke Volume Variation and Pulse Pressure Variation. These are noted during inspiration and expiration while patient receives positive pressure ventilation. Stroke volume is estimated from the systolic (shaded) portion of the arterial waveform.

		Parameter and equation		Normal range
Oxygen devlivery	DO_2	CO × CaO_2		
	CaO_2	Hb × 1.34 × SaO_2 + 0.003 × PaO_2		
	CO	HR × SV	*$\dot{V}O_2$ ÷ [(CaO_2 − CvO_2) × 10]*	4.0-8.0 L/min
	CI	CO ÷ BSA		2.5-4.0 L/min per m^3
	SV	EDV − ESV	*CO ÷ HR*	60-100 mL/beat
	RV preload	RVEDP / CVP/ RAP		2-6 mm Hg
	LV preload	LVEDP /PAOP / PCWP		8-15 mm Hg
	Contractility	EF: SV ÷ EDV		55%-75%
	RV afterload	PVR: 80 (MPAP − PAOP) ÷ CO		<250 dynes•s/cm^5
	LV afterload	SVR: 80 (MAP − CVP) ÷ CO		800-1,200 dynes•s/cm^5
Oxygen consumption	$\dot{V}O_2$	CO × (CaO_2 − CvO_2)		
	CvO_2	Hb × 1.34 × SvO_2 + 0.003 × PvO_2		
	OER	$\dot{V}O_2$ ÷ DO_2	*SaO_2 − SvO_2*	25%
Perfusion pressure	SBP			90-140 mm Hg
	DBP			60-90 mm Hg
	MAP	(SBP + 2 × DBP) ÷ 3	*(SVR × CO) + CVP*	70-105 mm Hg

Figure 120.3. Cardiac Hemodynamic Calculations and Normal Values. BSA indicates body surface area; Cao_2, arterial oxygen content; CI, cardiac index; CO, cardiac output; Cvo_2, venous oxygen content; CVP, central venous pressure; DBP, diastolic blood pressure; Do_2, oxygen delivery; EDV, end-diastolic volume; EF, ejection fraction; ESV, end-systolic volume; Hb, hemoglobin; HR, heart rate; LV, left ventricular; LVEDP, left ventricular end-diastolic pressure; MAP, mean arterial pressure; MPAP, mean pulmonary artery pressure; OER, oxygen extraction ratio; Pao_2, arterial partial pressure of oxygen; PAOP, pulmonary artery occlusion pressure; PCWP, pulmonary capillary wedge pressure; Pvo_2, venous partial pressure of oxygen; PVR, pulmonary vascular resistance; RAP, right atrial pressure; RV, right ventricular; RVEDP, right ventricular end-diastolic pressure; Sao_2, arterial oxygen saturation; SBP, systolic blood pressure; SV, stroke volume; Svo_2, mixed venous oxygen saturation; SVR, systemic vascular resistance; $\dot{V}o_2$, oxygen consumption. Equations in italics are additional inferred calculations.

Noninvasive

Volume-Clamp Method

A novel platform using an inflatable finger cuff and plethysmography is used to completely noninvasively monitor CO. The Nexfin device (BMEYE) uses this volume-clamp method to provide beat-by-beat stroke volume measurements by "re-creation" of a brachial artery pressure waveform and assessment of the pulsatile systolic area. This area divided by the aortic input impedance, derived from the Windkessel model, calculates the CO. This servo-controlled device alters cuff pressure to maintain a stable arterial diameter in the finger, which is measured with photoplethysmography. A benefit to this technology is the ability to additionally monitor stroke volume variation, arterial oxygen saturation, hemoglobin, and Do_2. Its use, however, may be limited to the surgical setting because its accuracy in critically ill or septic patients is concerning. Sensor dislocation and movement artifact further affect device signal and reliability.

Bioimpedance and Bioreactance

Electrical bioimpedance uses skin electrodes placed on the chest that conduct low-magnitude, high-frequency current. Variation in impedance or electrical amplitude induced by circulating blood flow in the chest is then detected with each cardiac cycle and generated into a waveform from which CO can be calculated. With bioreactance, an oscillating electrical current is delivered to the patient, and the changes in current frequency created by aortic blood flow are then measured and used to estimate CO. Although this method is easy to apply, its usefulness and clinical impact have been limited.

Transthoracic Echocardiography and Doppler

Echocardiography allows measurement of cardiac output with 2-dimensional transthoracic imaging or pulse-wave Doppler. Stroke volume and CO are calculated by measuring velocity time integral and left ventricular outflow tract diameter through the apical long-axis and parasternal long-axis views, respectively. This technique generally can provide reasonable measurements (discussed in more detail below). Although the use of echocardiography allows for the additional assessment of valvular function, volume status, and regional wall motion, it is limited by operator skill and provides only intermittent data.

Semi-invasive

Fick Method

Regarded as one of the most accurate methods of estimating CO, the Fick method is not confused by low-output states, valvular regurgitation, shunts, or arrhythmias. It is based on the Fick principle: the total uptake of (or release of) a substance by the peripheral tissues is equal to the product of the blood flow to the peripheral tissues and the arterial-venous concentration difference (gradient) of the substance. $\dot{V}o_2$ is the difference between inspired and expired O_2 and can be measured with an exhaled gas collection bag, although it is usually estimated. Conventionally, resting metabolic consumption of oxygen is 3.5 mL of O_2 per kilogram per minute, or 125 mL O_2 per square meter of body surface area per minute. The equation used is as follows:

$$CO = \frac{\dot{V}o_2}{Ca - Cv}$$

Where CA is oxygen concentration of arterial blood and Cv is oxygen concentration of mixed venous blood.

Noncalibrated Pulse Contour Analysis

Many less invasive CO monitoring systems use mathematical algorithms based on pulse contour analysis that calculate stroke volume with every beat. The available systems connect to invasive arterial lines and usually use special arterial sensors. Devices that use pulse contour analysis without other invasive calibration include the FloTrac-Vigileo (Edwards Lifesciences), LiDCOrapid (LiDCO, Ltd), PRAM-MostCare (Vytech), and ProAQT of the Pulsioflex device (Pulsion Medical Systems). Each uses a proprietary algorithm with unique characteristics to make hemodynamic assumptions.

The FloTrac-Vigileo device uses autocalibration once initial patient demographics are programmed into the system. It uses the mathematical Windkessel model based on the Ohm law, which relies on the concept that stroke volume is proportional to pulse pressure and inversely related to compliance. This strict relationship between compliance and pressure results in limited accuracy of this device when used in vasoplegic, hyperdynamic, or hemodynamically unstable states. In addition, all limitations of pressure monitoring with arterial lines apply and allow for factors such as damping, vessel tone, and catheter site to produce an inaccurate CO measurement.

Esophageal Doppler and Transesophageal Echocardiography

As with transthoracic echocardiography, transesophageal echocardiography is valuable for assessing global biventricular function, valvular disease, and preload. In critical care, it can be used to calculate stroke volume and CO with volumetric assessment (Simpson method) or Doppler technology. Use of Doppler allows for measuring of velocity time integral at the left ventricular outflow tract, which reflects the velocity of blood flow or the distance it travels over a time frame such as systole. When this is multiplied with the cross-sectional area of the left ventricular outflow tract, stroke volume can be calculated and then multiplied again with heart rate to estimate CO. Use of this tool requires access to equipment and adequate operator skill.

Specialized esophageal Doppler devices for continuous CO monitoring exist, such as the CardioQ (Deltex Medical). This technology uses velocity time integral to display "stroke distance" and nomogram data to get a cross-sectional area of the aorta. Because only about 70% of blood ejected from the left ventricle is observed in the descending aorta, accuracy of measurement has been questioned. Limitations to this device include inherent risk of injury to the esophagus and frequent need for repositioning to ensure a proper angle and adequate signal.

Invasive

Invasive CO monitoring usually involves the insertion of either a PAC or a CVC. PAC insertion requires knowledge of pressure waveform analysis and proper technique. Severe complications, although rare, include catheter malposition or tangling, pulmonary artery rupture, and pulmonary artery occlusion. A key advantage to PAC use is the additional information it provides about stroke volume, right atrial pressure, pulmonary artery pressures, pulmonary artery occlusion pressure, and mixed venous oxygen saturation.

Pulmonary Artery Thermodilution

Measurement of CO through a PAC uses thermodilution in either bolus or "continuous" form. Most commonly, a bolus of cold saline solution is used as the indicator and flushed into the right atrium. Its mixture or dilution in the right ventricle can be sampled over time in the pulmonary artery through a thermistor at the PAC tip. CO is calculated by the temperature-time curve that demonstrates an initial increase in indicator concentration and then a logarithmic decay, the slope of which is inversely related to blood flow. This method is based on the Stewart-Hamilton equation.

"Continuous" CO monitoring uses an adapted PAC that has a thermal filament or coil attached at the level of the right ventricle. This filament heats the blood according to a pseudorandom binary sequence and then the downstream temperature change is automatically measured by the thermistor at the tip. A classic thermodilution curve gets constructed and CO is calculated. The monitor displays a "continuous" CO by averaging readings over a certain time interval. Inaccuracies may occur with intracardiac shunts, central bloodstream temperature instability, rapid fluid resuscitation, and tricuspid valve regurgitation.

Calibrated Pulse Contour Analysis

Some devices use pulse contour analysis for CO assessment by calibrating it against another accepted method of CO monitoring such as thermodilution, indicator dilution, or sonography. These other techniques are discussed below.

Calibrated Pulse Contour Analysis and Transpulmonary Thermodilution

Similar to pulmonary artery thermodilution, transpulmonary thermodilution uses an injection of cold saline as the indicator and a temperature-time curve as the means to calculate CO. A 15-mL indicator solution is injected into the superior vena cava through a CVC, and the thermal changes are sensed at a thermistor-tipped arterial line, which is usually placed in the femoral artery because of its large diameter.

Combining data from transpulmonary thermodiluation with continuous PCA allows for the calculation of other hemodynamic parameters. The PiCCO and PiCCOplus/PulseCO devices estimate preload from global end-diastolic volume, left ventricular contractility with cardiac function index, and extravascular lung water. Although the PiCCO has demonstrated good accuracy, it requires recalibration with any marked changes in systemic vascular resistance or at least every 3 to 4 hours. It also remains relatively invasive and may be inaccurate in the setting of intracardiac shunts.

Lithium Dilution

Lithium dilution uses a small amount of lithium chloride as the indicator, which is then sensed on the arterial side by a lithium selective electrode. A lithium concentration curve is mapped out to calculate CO. The most commonly used devices are the LiDCO and LiDCOplus/PulseCO. Limitations are similar to those of transpulmonary thermodilution, and it is less reliable in unstable patients.

Summary

- Assessment and monitoring of hemodynamics is vital in neurocritically ill patients, who are often hemodynamically unstable.
- Perfusion pressure can be determined noninvasively with the blood pressure cuff method (oscillometry) or invasively with arterial catheterization.
- Oxygen delivery is largely assessed through regional or central venous oximetry and biomarkers such as lactate.
- The components of oxygen delivery, including cardiac output and preload, can be evaluated with several strategies, ranging from ultrasonography to pulse contour analysis to PAC.
- The method of invasiveness should be determined from the clinical situation and resources.
- Appropriate use and interpretation of any method is important, and users must be cognizant of the limitations of each.

SUGGESTED READING

Boyd JH, Forbes J, Nakada TA, Walley KR, Russell JA. Fluid resuscitation in septic shock: a positive fluid balance and elevated central venous pressure are associated with increased mortality. Crit Care Med. 2011 Feb;39(2):259–65.

Bur A, Herkner H, Vlcek M, Woisetschlager C, Derhaschnig U, Delle Karth G, et al. Factors influencing the accuracy of oscillometric blood pressure measurement in critically ill patients. Crit Care Med. 2003 Mar;31(3):793–9.

Cariou A, Monchi M, Dhainaut JF. Continuous cardiac output and mixed venous oxygen saturation monitoring. J Crit Care. 1998 Dec;13(4):198–213.

Ciozda W, Kedan I, Kehl DW, Zimmer R, Khandwalla R, Kimchi A. The efficacy of sonographic measurement of inferior vena cava diameter as an estimate of central venous pressure. Cardiovasc Ultrasound. 2016 Aug 20;14(1):33.

Davison DL, Patel K, Chawla LS. Hemodynamic monitoring in the critically ill: spanning the range of kidney function. Am J Kidney Dis. 2012 May;59(5):715–23. Epub 2012 Mar 3.

De Backer D, Bakker J, Cecconi M, Hajjar L, Liu DW, Lobo S, et al. Alternatives to the Swan-Ganz catheter. Intensive Care Med. 2018 Jun;44(6):730–41. Epub 2018 May 3.

De Backer D, Vincent JL. The pulmonary artery catheter: is it still alive? Curr Opin Crit Care. 2018 Jun;24(3):204–8.

Downs EA, Isbell JM. Impact of hemodynamic monitoring on clinical outcomes. Best Pract Res Clin Anaesthesiol. 2014 Dec;28(4):463–76. Epub 2014 Oct 7.

Esper SA, Pinsky MR. Arterial waveform analysis. Best Pract Res Clin Anaesthesiol. 2014 Dec;28(4):363–80. Epub 2014 Sep 6.

Fick A. [Uber die Messung des Blutquantums in den Herzventrikeln]. Seitung Physik Med Ges Wurzburg. 1870;2:290–1. German.

Geisen M, Rhodes A, Cecconi M. Less-invasive approaches to perioperative haemodynamic optimization. Curr Opin Crit Care. 2012 Aug;18(4):377–84.

Huang YC. Monitoring oxygen delivery in the critically ill. Chest. 2005 Nov;128(5 Suppl 2):554S–60S.

Hyttel-Sorensen S, Hessel TW, Greisen G. Peripheral tissue oximetry: comparing three commercial near-infrared spectroscopy oximeters on the forearm. J Clin Monit Comput. 2014 Apr;28(2):149–55. Epub 2013 Aug 30.

Jabot J, Teboul JL, Richard C, Monnet X. Passive leg raising for predicting fluid responsiveness: importance of the postural change. Intensive Care Med. 2009 Jan;35(1):85–90. Epub 2008 Sep 16.

Lang RM, Badano LP, Mor-Avi V, Afilalo J, Armstrong A, Ernande L, et al. Recommendations for cardiac chamber quantification by echocardiography in adults: an update from the American Society of Echocardiography and the European Association of Cardiovascular Imaging. J Am Soc Echocardiogr. 2015 Jan;28(1):1–39.e14.

Lazaridis C. Advanced hemodynamic monitoring: principles and practice in neurocritical care. Neurocrit Care. 2012 Feb;16(1):163–9.

Lesur O, Delile E, Asfar P, Radermacher P. Hemodynamic support in the early phase of septic shock: a review of challenges and unanswered questions. Ann Intensive Care. 2018 Oct 29;8(1):102.

Magder S. Invasive hemodynamic monitoring. Crit Care Clin. 2015 Jan;31(1):67–87.

Manoach S, Weingart SD, Charchaflieh J. The evolution and current use of invasive hemodynamic monitoring for predicting volume responsiveness during resuscitation, perioperative, and critical care. J Clin Anesth. 2012 May;24(3):242–50.

Marik PE, Cavallazzi R, Vasu T, Hirani A. Dynamic changes in arterial waveform derived variables and fluid responsiveness in mechanically ventilated patients: a systematic review of the literature. Crit Care Med. 2009 Sep;37(9):2642–7.

Michard F, Boussat S, Chemla D, Anguel N, Mercat A, Lecarpentier Y, et al. Relation between respiratory changes in arterial pulse pressure and fluid responsiveness in septic patients with acute circulatory failure. Am J Respir Crit Care Med. 2000 Jul;162(1):134–8.

Monnet X, Marik PE, Teboul JL. Prediction of fluid responsiveness: an update. Ann Intensive Care. 2016 Dec;6(1):111. Epub 2016 Nov 17.

Monnet X, Teboul JL. Assessment of volume responsiveness during mechanical ventilation: recent advances. Crit Care. 2013 Mar 19;17(2):217.

Monnet X, Teboul JL. Passive leg raising. Intensive Care Med. 2008 Apr;34(4):659–63. Epub 2008 Jan 23.

Muller JC, Kennard JW, Browne JS, Fecher AM, Hayward TZ. Hemodynamic monitoring in the intensive care unit. Nutr Clin Pract. 2012 Jun;27(3):340–51.

Naik BI, Durieux ME. Hemodynamic monitoring devices: putting it all together. Best Pract Res Clin Anaesthesiol. 2014 Dec;28(4):477–88. Epub 2014 Sep 26.

Nichols D, Nielsen ND. Oxygen delivery and consumption: a macrocirculatory perspective. Crit Care Clin. 2010 Apr;26(2):239–53.

Renner J, Scholz J, Bein B. Monitoring cardiac function: echocardiography, pulse contour analysis and beyond. Best Pract Res Clin Anaesthesiol. 2013 Jun;27(2):187–200.

Reuter DA, Huang C, Edrich T, Shernan SK, Eltzschig HK. Cardiac output monitoring using indicator-dilution techniques: basics, limits, and perspectives. Anesth Analg. 2010 Mar 1;110(3):799–811.

Saugel B, Cecconi M, Hajjar LA. Noninvasive cardiac output monitoring in cardiothoracic surgery patients: available methods and future directions. J Cardiothorac Vasc Anesth. 2018 Jun 27. [Epub ahead of print].

Saugel B, Dueck R, Wagner JY. Measurement of blood pressure. Best Pract Res Clin Anaesthesiol. 2014 Dec;28(4):309–22. Epub 2014 Sep 6.

Schloglhofer T, Gilly H, Schima H. Semi-invasive measurement of cardiac output based on pulse contour: a review and analysis. Can J Anaesth. 2014 May;61(5):452–79. Epub 2014 Mar 19.

Smulyan H, Safar ME. Blood pressure measurement: retrospective and prospective views. Am J Hypertens. 2011 Jun;24(6):628–34. Epub 2011 Feb 24.

Strumwasser A, Frankel H, Murthi S, Clark D, Kirton O; American Association for the Surgery of Trauma Committee on Critical Care. Hemodynamic monitoring of the injured patient: from central venous pressure to focused echocardiography. J Trauma Acute Care Surg. 2016 Mar;80(3):499–510.

Tanczos K, Molnar Z. The oxygen supply-demand balance: a monitoring challenge. Best Pract Res Clin Anaesthesiol. 2013 Jun;27(2):201–7.

van Montfrans GA. Oscillometric blood pressure measurement: progress and problems. Blood Press Monit. 2001 Dec;6(6):287–90.

Vincent JL, Rhodes A, Perel A, Martin GS, Della Rocca G, Vallet B, et al. Clinical review: update on hemodynamic monitoring: a consensus of 16. Crit Care. 2011 Aug 18;15(4):229.

Wesseling KH, Jansen JR, Settels JJ, Schreuder JJ. Computation of aortic flow from pressure in humans using a nonlinear, three-element model. J Appl Physiol (1985). 1993 May;74(5):2566–73.

Pulmonary Artery Catheterization

PHILIP E. LOWMAN, MD

Goals

- Outline the indications for and the technical aspects of pulmonary artery catheterization.
- Describe the physiologic data obtained from a pulmonary artery catheter.
- Discuss the limitations and complications of pulmonary artery catheterization.

Introduction

For years, the pulmonary artery catheter (PAC, better known as Swan-Ganz catheter) has been used largely to estimate and optimize hemodynamics according to the wedge pressure of the pulmonary artery. Its use dramatically declined after reports of complications and increased costs without benefit to patients. In the absence of reliable noninvasive devices, the catheter is used in severe cases and in cardiac surgery intensive care units.

Indications for Use of a PAC

In critically ill patients, hemodynamic derangements may cause or be the consequence of organ failure. Attempts to better define the nature of hemodynamic instability may aid in the diagnosis and management of complex and unstable conditions. The PAC has had a role in the care of patients with these conditions since its introduction in 1970 by Swan, Ganz, and colleagues. Although there is no indication for routine use of PACs in critically ill patients, frequently cited indications include the following:

1. Assessment and management of left and right ventricular dysfunction.
2. Assessment and management of complex cardiac conditions (eg, postoperative open heart surgery, tamponade, constrictive pericarditis, valvular disorders).
3. Diagnosis and management of pulmonary hypertension.
4. Monitoring response to therapy with, for example, inotropes, vasopressors, fluids, diuretics, positive end-expiratory pressure, and inhaled nitric oxide.
5. Obtaining core body temperature and mixed venous oxygen saturation.

Technical Aspects of Placing a PAC

Equipment

A PAC is a multilumen, polyvinyl chloride catheter, usually 110 cm in length with an external diameter of 5F to 8F (Figure 121.1). A balloon is incorporated within a centimeter of the distal tip. Catheter design may include a variable number of lumens used for pressure transduction of the pulmonary artery and right atrium, passage of electrical leads from a distally placed thermistor used for core temperature and thermodilution measurements, medication infusion and blood draws, passage of cardiac pacing electrodes, or balloon inflation. Some catheters incorporate a spiraled heating filament used when continuously measuring cardiac output.

An introducer sheath of appropriate caliber to accommodate the chosen PAC, usually 6F to 9F, should be present within a large vein (internal jugular, femoral, subclavian, basilic, brachial). A plastic sheath should be available to cover the PAC in order to maintain its sterility during placement and manipulation. An appropriate fluid-filled tubing system and transducer should be available, as should a monitor capable of displaying the gathered data, such as pressure waveforms and measurements, temperature, and cardiac output. Electrocardiographic and hemodynamic monitoring should be in place during catheter placement.

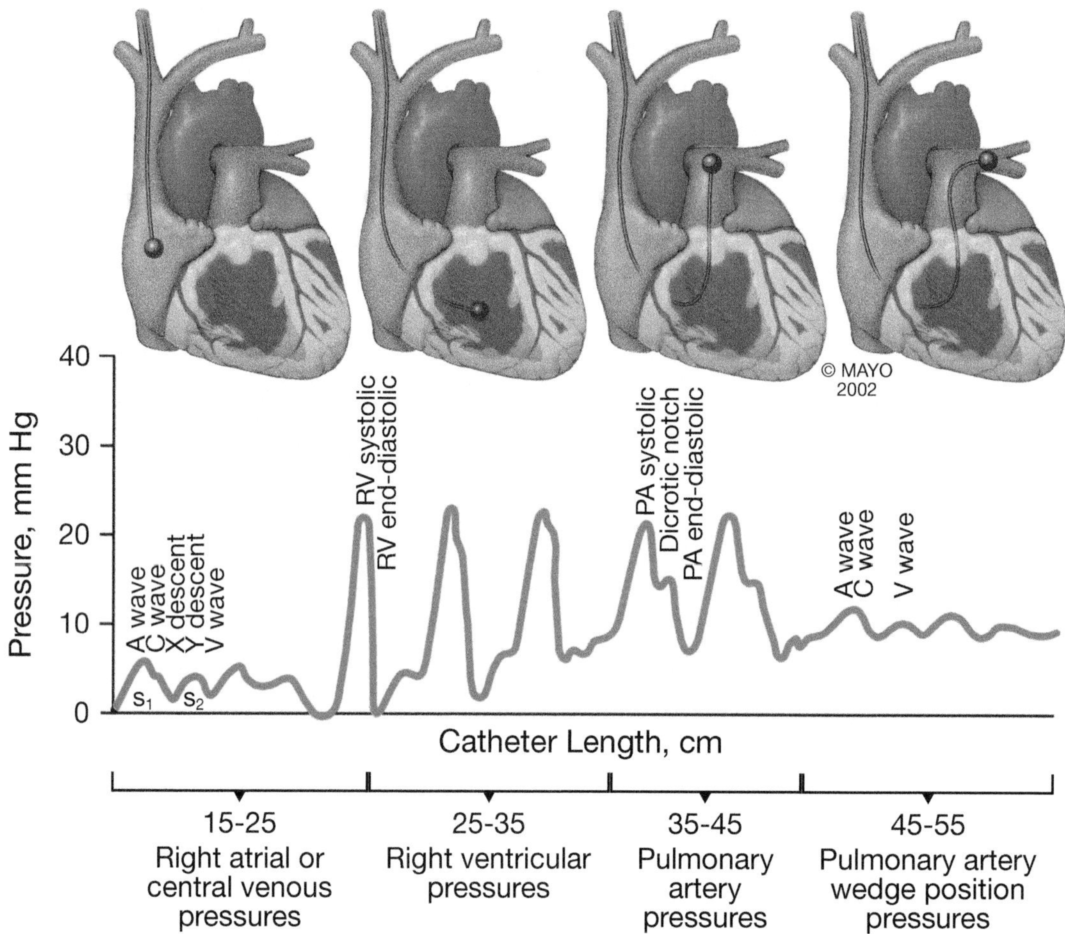

Figure 121.1. Advancement of Pulmonary Artery Balloon Flotation Catheter and Characteristic Tracings During Placement. PA indicates pulmonary artery; RV, right ventricular; S1, first heart sound; S2, second heart sound.

(From Wijdicks EFM. The practice of emergency and critical care neurology. 1st ed. Oxford [UK]: Oxford University Press; c2010. Chapter 22, monitoring devices; p. 261-78; used with permission of Mayo Foundation for Medical Education and Research.)

Insertion Technique

A sterile field should be established and an introducer sheath should be placed with the Seldinger technique into the patient's vein. The lumens of the PAC should be flushed with saline to ensure that no air can be embolized to the patient. Pressure transducers should be attached to the catheter, and the sterile sleeve should be passed over the PAC. The competency of the balloon should then be checked by inflating with a quantity of air described by the manufacturer, usually 1.0 to 1.5 mL. The catheter is then advanced into the introducer until a central venous or right atrial pressure waveform is seen (Figure 121.1). At this time, the balloon should be slowly inflated. The catheter is then "floated" in the direction of blood flow. As the pressure monitor at the tip of the PAC enters sequential chambers, the pressure waveform changes as shown in Figure 121.1. Movement from the right atrium into the right ventricle causes a systolic pressure step-up, and traversing the pulmonic valve from the right ventricle into the pulmonary artery causes an increase in diastolic pressure. The catheter should continue to be advanced with the balloon inflated until there is a loss of the pulmonary artery systolic upstroke and a decrease in pressure equal to or less than the pulmonary artery diastolic pressure. This final pressure represents the pulmonary artery occlusion pressure, or "wedge." The balloon should then be deflated and the catheter secured in sterile fashion. Radiographic confirmation of the catheter's final course and position should be obtained.

Measurements Obtained From the PAC

Direct Measurements

Direct measurements can be obtained of the pressures within the chambers through which the tip of the PAC

Table 121.1 • Values Obtained From a Pulmonary Artery Catheter

Value	Normal Range
Right atrial pressure	2-8 mm Hg
Right ventricle	
Systolic pressure	15-25 mm Hg
Diastolic pressure	2-8 mm Hg
Pulmonary artery	
Systolic pressure	15-25 mm Hg
Diastolic pressure	8-15 mm Hg
Mean	10-20 mm Hg
Occlusion (wedge) pressure	6-12 mm Hg
Cardiac output	4.0-8.0 L/min
Mixed venous saturation	60%-80%

passes. Cardiac output, temperature, and mixed venous oxyhemoglobin saturation can also be measured. Normal values obtained from a PAC are listed in Table 121.1. Typical abnormal profiles are shown in Table 121.2.

Indirect Measurements

After direct measurements are obtained from the PAC, other values can be derived from equations. These values include cardiac index, right ventricular stroke volume, pulmonary and systemic vascular resistances and resistance indices, ventricular stroke work indices, and oxygen delivery and consumption.

Table 121.2 • Interpretation of Pulmonary Artery Monitoring Profiles

Condition	PCWP	CO	SVR
Left ventricular failure	High	Low	High
Pulmonary edema			
Diastolic heart failure	High	Normal	Normal
Neurogenic	Normal	Normal or low	Normal
Sepsis			
Early	Low	High	Low
Late	Normal	Normal	High
Hypovolemia	Low	Low	High
Saddle pulmonary embolism	Normal	Low	High

Abbreviations: CO, cardiac output; PCWP, pulmonary capillary wedge pressure; SVR, systemic vascular resistance.

(From Wijdicks EFM. The practice of emergency and critical care neurology. 1st ed. Oxford [UK]: Oxford University Press; c2010. Chapter 22, Monitoring devices; p. 261-78; used with permission of Mayo Foundation for Medical Education and Research.)

Complications of PAC Use

Complications of PAC use are related to vascular access, monitoring, and interpretation. The complications related to vascular access that are not unique to PACs include pneumothorax, infection, vascular injury, and thromboembolic phenomena. Unique to PAC is the risk of knotting of the catheter within the cardiac chambers or around indwelling devices, balloon rupture, arrhythmias, and pulmonary arterial infarction or rupture.

Limitations of PAC Use

After its introduction, the PAC was widely used because of the belief that filling pressures would allow for optimization of left and right ventricular preload and management of volume status. It was used to develop commonly taught hemodynamic profiles for various shock states. Throughout the 1990s and early 2000s, increasing data emerged indicating that use of the PAC was not associated with improved outcomes. This understanding has led to a decline in its use and replacement with other methods of hemodynamic monitoring, such as pulse pressure analysis, echocardiographic and ultrasonographic evaluation, and electrical bioimpedence.

Summary

- Although the efficacy of PAC is debatable, it can provide some valuable information in a very select patient population, such as patients who have had cardiac surgery or transplant.
- The usefulness of PAC is subject to correct interpretation of measured and derived values and is highly operator-dependent.
- Trends, rather than absolute values obtained by the PAC, should be used to guide therapy.

SUGGESTED READING

Bossert T, Gummert JF, Bittner HB, Barten M, Walther T, Falk V, et al. Swan-Ganz catheter-induced severe complications in cardiac surgery: right ventricular perforation, knotting, and rupture of a pulmonary artery. J Card Surg. 2006 May-Jun;21(3):292–5.

Brennan JM, Blair JE, Hampole C, Goonewardena S, Vasaiwala S, Shah D, et al. Radial artery pulse pressure variation correlates with brachial artery peak velocity variation in ventilated subjects when measured by internal medicine residents using hand-carried ultrasound devices. Chest. 2007 May;131(5):1301–7.

Cohn JD, Engler PE, Timpawat C, Aguilar PS, Fillipone LA, Del Guercio LG, et al. Physiologic profiles in circulatory support and management of the critically ill. JACEP. 1977 Nov;6(11):479–85.

Connors AF Jr, Speroff T, Dawson NV, Thomas C, Harrell FE Jr, Wagner D, et al; SUPPORT Investigators. The effectiveness of right heart catheterization in the initial care of critically ill patients. JAMA. 1996 Sep 18;276(11):889–97.

De Backer D, Hajjar LA, Pinsky MR. Is there still a place for the Swan-Ganz catheter? We are not sure. Intensive Care Med. 2018 Jun;44(6):960–2. Epub 2018 May 23.

Demiselle J, Mercat A, Asfar P. Is there still a place for the Swan-Ganz catheter? Yes. Intensive Care Med. 2018 Jun;44(6):954–6. Epub 2018 May 23.

Kearney TJ, Shabot MM. Pulmonary artery rupture associated with the Swan-Ganz catheter. Chest. 1995 Nov;108(5):1349–52.

Summers RL, Shoemaker WC, Peacock WF, Ander DS, Coleman TG. Bench to bedside: electrophysiologic and clinical principles of noninvasive hemodynamic monitoring using impedance cardiography. Acad Emerg Med. 2003 Jun;10(6):669–80.

Swan HJ, Ganz W, Forrester J, Marcus H, Diamond G, Chonette D. Catheterization of the heart in man with use of a flow-directed balloon-tipped catheter. N Engl J Med. 1970 Aug 27;283(9):447–51.

Teboul JL, Cecconi M, Scheeren TWL. Is there still a place for the Swan-Ganz catheter? No. Intensive Care Med. 2018 Jun;44(6):957–9. Epub 2018 May 23.

Thakkar AB, Desai SP. Swan, Ganz, and their catheter: its evolution over the past half century. Ann Intern Med. 2018 Nov 6;169(9):636–42.

Thoracentesis and Chest Tubes

STACI E. BEAMER, MD

Goals

- Review the indications for thoracentesis and chest tube placement.
- Review the diagnostic work-up for and common causes of pleural effusions in patients receiving critical care.
- Discuss the procedure techniques for thoracentesis and chest tube placement.

Introduction

The pleural cavity is a negative-pressure airtight space that serves as the interface between the lung and the chest wall. Fluid is produced normally by the parietal pleura and absorbed by the visceral pleura as a result of difference in capillary pressure. The fluid is subsequently absorbed by the pleural lymphatics and ultimately into the thoracic duct. Disruption of the pleural space can result in a pneumothorax (air) or a pleural effusion (fluid). Pleural effusions can be caused by blood (hemothorax), infection (parapneumoic effusion or empyema), chyle (chylothorax), malignancy, inflammatory conditions, or imbalances in hydrostatic and oncotic pressures. Both types of pleural processes alter the negative pressure of the thorax. The resulting positive pressure causes partial or complete lung collapse and respiratory symptoms. Thoracentesis and chest tube placement are essential procedures for both diagnosis and treatment of pleural conditions.

Thoracentesis

A thoracentesis is a procedure in which a needle is guided into the affected pleural space with or without ultrasound guidance and a temporary drainage catheter is inserted. This procedure is used for both diagnostic and therapeutic purposes. The indication for a diagnostic thoracentesis is the presence of a clinically significant pleural effusion with no known cause. There are no contraindications for the procedure, but attention should be paid to a patient's anticoagulation status. A small sample is collected for fluid analysis to assist with determining cause and guiding further management. The amount of fluid available for analysis is important. Studies show increased rates of diagnosis of malignant pleural effusion with volumes of 50 to 60 mL, and thus obtaining this volume is recommended. A therapeutic thoracentesis is performed to drain large volumes of fluid in symptomatic patients. Historically, a maximum drainage amount of 1.5 L was removed to prevent re-expansion pulmonary edema. However, current literature indicates safe removal of large volumes of pleural fluid (>3 L) with no increased rate of re-expansion pulmonary edema. Removal of the entire pleural effusion is feasible and safe as long as the patient does not experience pain, chest discomfort, or pleural pressures less than −20 cm H_2O if pleural manometry is used.

Various commercial kits are available for thoracentesis. The procedure is performed in various positions depending on the mobility limitations of the patient. The pleural fluid can be identified by auscultation or percussion techniques. The use of ultrasound guidance can assist with localizing the fluid collection, determining fluid characteristics (increased viscosity, loculations), and improving visualization of adjacent structures such as the lung, heart, liver, and spleen. Once local anesthetic is provided, a small knife puncture is made in the skin to assist with needle access. The needle should be guided into the pleural space directly above a rib to avoid damage to the intercostal bundle (Figure 122.1). Aspiration is maintained until fluid appears in the syringe. The drainage catheter is carefully inserted over the needle and the appropriate apparatus connected to drain the fluid at a slow, steady rate. The catheter is removed during the expiratory phase to avoid air entry into the pleural space, and a dressing is placed.

Complications from thoracentesis include pneumothorax, hemothorax, intercostal nerve injury, re-expansion

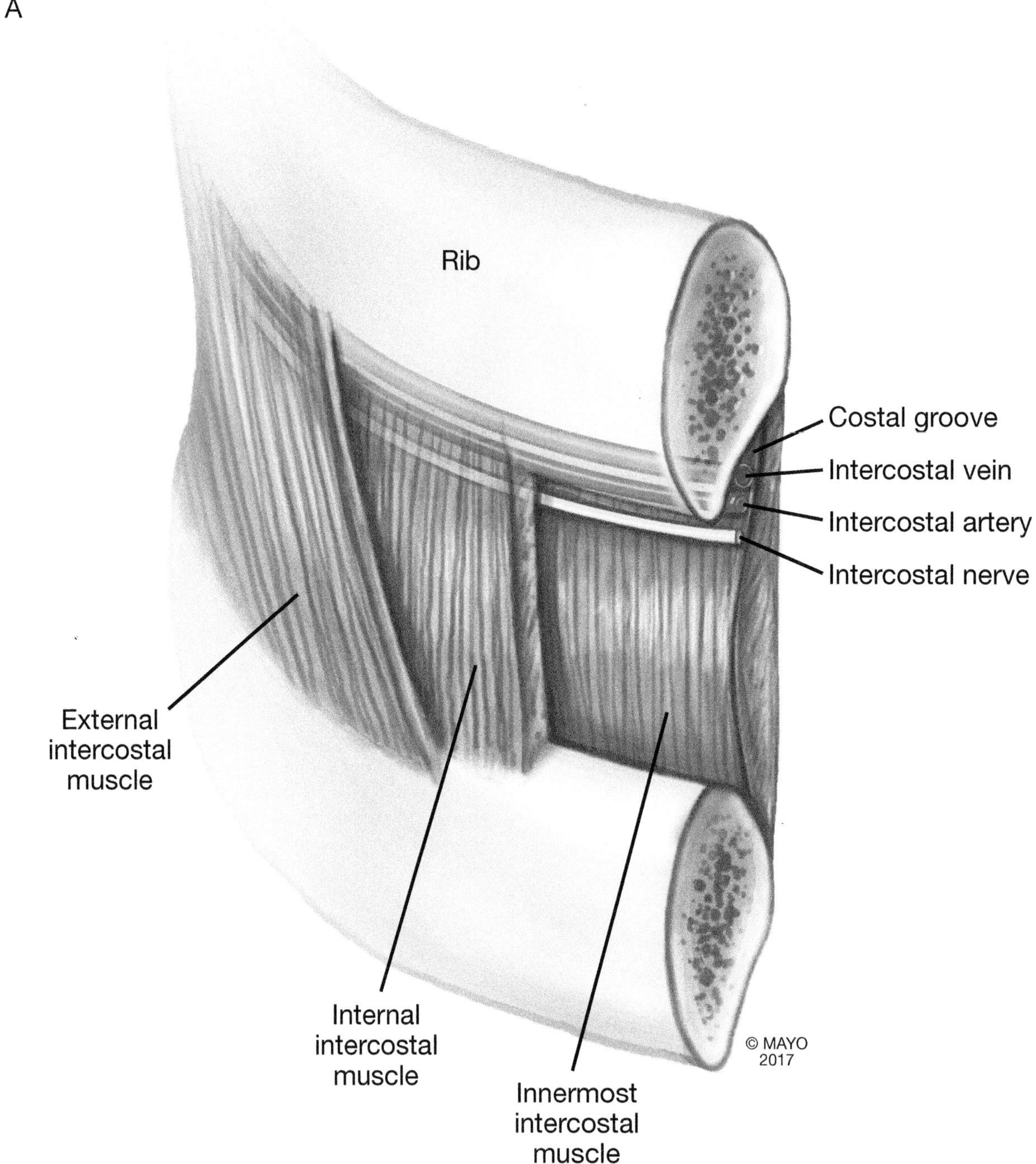

Figure 122.1. Anatomy Related to Thoracentesis (A and B) and Area of Needle Insertion (C). Blue triangle (C) indicates area of insertion of chest tube for management of pneumothorax.

pulmonary edema, and injury to nearby organs including the liver and spleen. The most common complication is pneumothorax with rates ranging from 4% to 20%. The use of ultrasound for thoracentesis is shown in studies to substantially reduce the risk of pneumothorax to 1% to 3%, increase therapeutic thoracentesis fluid yield, and reduce overall hospital costs due to the decreased complication rates. Thoracic ultrasound training and subsequent clinical application are strongly recommended for pleural drainage procedures.

The most common diagnostic tests performed on pleural fluid and the Light criteria are listed in Box 122.1. The Light

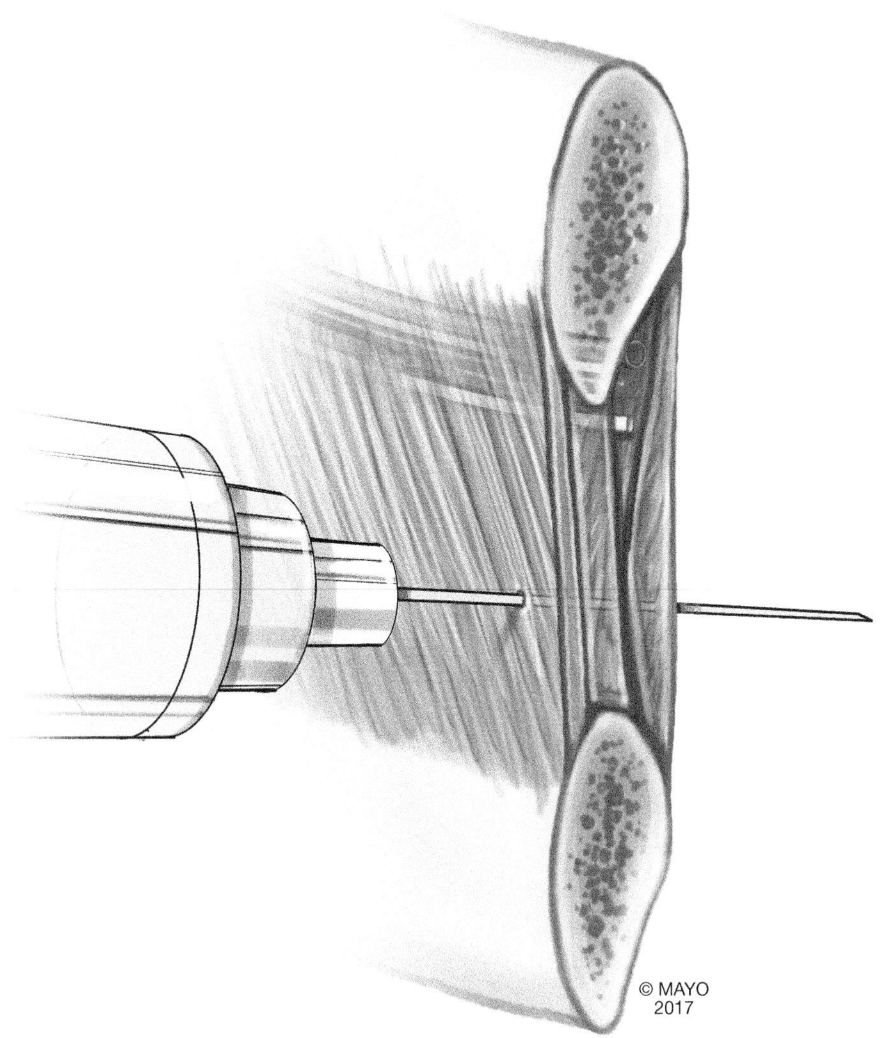

Figure 122.1. Continued (next page)

criteria are very sensitive for exudative effusions but have less specificity and thus can lead to misdiagnosis of some transudates as exudates. These tests are used as a guide to identify the cause of the pleural process and guide further management. Common causes of transudative and exudative effusions are listed in Box 122.2.

Chest Tubes

The indications for placement of tube thoracostomy are listed in Box 122.3. Chest tubes can be categorized by size (large bore >20F, small bore <20F) or by placement technique (Seldinger, trocar, blunt dissection). Benefits of large-bore chest tubes include decreased resistance to flow and decreased clogging, and disadvantages include patient discomfort, need for surgical expertise, and decreased efficacy in draining loculated collections. Large-bore tubes are appropriate for hemothorax, large pneumothorax, pneumothorax on ventilated patients, chest trauma, and empyema. Small-bore chest tubes include pigtail catheters and simple single-lumen catheters modified for pleural drainage. These tubes are placed using the Seldinger technique, often with ultrasound or computed tomography guidance. Small-bore tubes reduce patient discomfort and have lower rates of malposition, but disadvantages include lower flow rates and higher rates of clogging or kinking. Routine flushing of small-bore catheters and maintenance on wall suction can improve patency rates.

Chest tubes placed without image guidance for pneumothorax should be inserted into the triangle of safety (Figure 122.2, blue area) to avoid injuring important thoracic

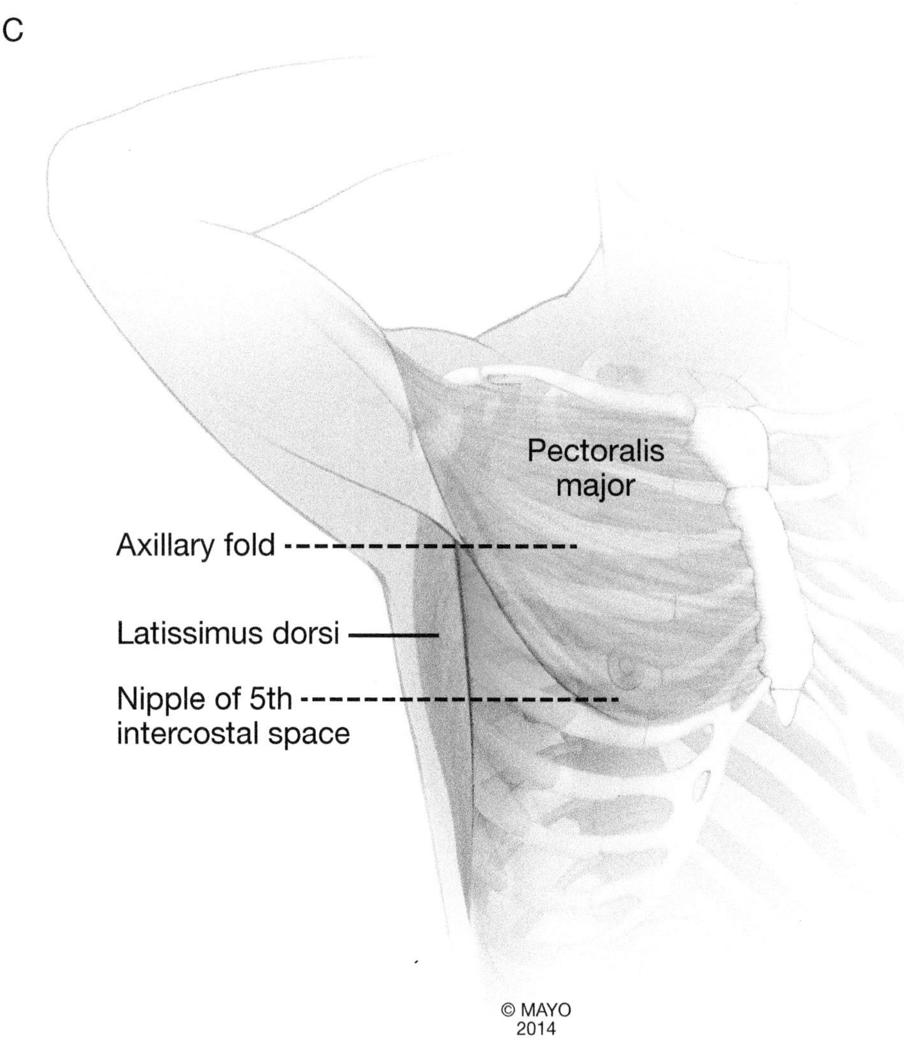

Figure 122.1. Continued

structures. The triangle is bordered anteriorly by the lateral border of the pectoralis major, posteriorly by the lateral border of the latissimus dorsi, and interiorly by the level of the fifth intercostal space. An example of large-bore silicone chest tube placement is illustrated in Figure 122.2.

After administration of topical anesthetic, a small incision is made along the selected interspace. The tissues are bluntly dissected to the level of the intercostal muscle and ribs. A clamp is used to penetrate the intercostal muscle directly above the rib to avoid damage to the neurovascular bundle. The thoracic entry site is spread large enough to allow passage of a finger to directly palpate the lung and assess for adhesions. This step reduces risks of intra-abdominal placement and lung injury due to adhesions. The tube is directed into place and secured.

Tubes for pneumothorax are guided anteriorly and apically because air will accumulate in this space. In contrast, tubes for effusions are guided posteriorly and basilar for more effective drainage. Chest tube placement for effusions can be dictated by the location of the fluid collection, particularly when small-bore tubes and ultrasound guidance are used.

Chest tubes are initially placed to suction to improve drainage of air or fluid unless a large-volume effusion or pneumothorax is present. In this circumstance, passive drainage on water seal is indicated to avoid re-expansion pulmonary edema. After the procedure, chest radiography is recommended to assess tube placement.

Complications of chest tubes include bleeding, damage to thoracic or abdominal organs, major vascular injury,

Box 122.1 • Pleural Fluid Diagnostic Tests and Light Criteria

Pleural fluid diagnostic tests
- Cell count
- Total protein
- LDH
- pH
- Amylase/lipase
- Glucose
- Gram stain, culture
- Triglycerides
- Adenosine deaminase
- Cytology

Light criteria
- Exudative effusion if 1 or more of the following criteria:
  - Pleural fluid protein/serum protein ratio >0.5
  - Pleural fluid LDH/serum LDH ratio >0.6
  - Pleural fluid LDH greater than two-thirds the upper limit of normal serum LDH

Abbreviation: LDH, lactate dehydrogenase.

Box 122.2 • Causes of Transudative and Exudative Effusions

Transudate
- Heart failure
- Hepatic hydrothorax
- Renal failure, nephrotic syndrome
- Peritoneal dialysis
- Atelectasis

Exudate
- Parapneumonic effusion, empyema, subphrenic abscess
- Malignancy
- Pulmonary embolism
- Pancreatitis
- Chylothorax
- Esophageal perforation
- Tuberculosis
- Viral infections
- Connective tissue diseases
- Acute respiratory distress syndrome

Box 122.3 • Indications for Chest Tube Insertion

Pneumothorax
- In all patients receiving mechanical ventilation
- Large pneumothorax
- Clinically unstable patient after needle decompression
- Pneumothorax caused by chest trauma
- Recurrent pneumothorax

Hemopneumothorax

Esophageal rupture with intrapleural leak

Malignant pleural effusion

Treatment with sclerosing agents or pleurodesis

Recurrent pleural effusion

Parapneumonic effusion or empyema

Chylothorax

Postoperative care

re-expansion pulmonary edema, and infection. It is important to assess the chest tube and drainage system frequently for air leaks and to assess the quantity and quality of pleural drainage. Chest tube removal is dictated by the resolution of air leaks or decreased daily pleural fluid drainage (<200-300 mL/24 h). Before chest tube removal, the pleural fluid should no longer be bloody, purulent, or chylous. Chest tube removal can result in aspiration of air into the pleural space with resulting pneumothorax. This complication is avoided by performing chest tube removal during the expiratory phase with the addition of a Valsalva maneuver if possible. Techniques for removing chest tubes also include removal at end-expiration when pleural pressures are similar to atmospheric pressure or at end-inspiration when the visceral and parietal pleura are closely approximated. Randomized control trials found no difference in rates of pneumothorax between the 2 techniques if a Valsalva maneuver was performed.

Summary

- A thoracentesis should be performed for clinically significant pleural effusions with unknown cause.
- Ultrasound guidance for thoracentesis and small-bore chest tube placement decreases procedure-associated complications.
- Large-bore chest tubes are recommended for hemothorax, empyema, trauma, and large pneumothorax or unstable pneumothorax.
- Chest tubes should be removed during the expiratory phase cycle with a Valsalva maneuver, if possible.

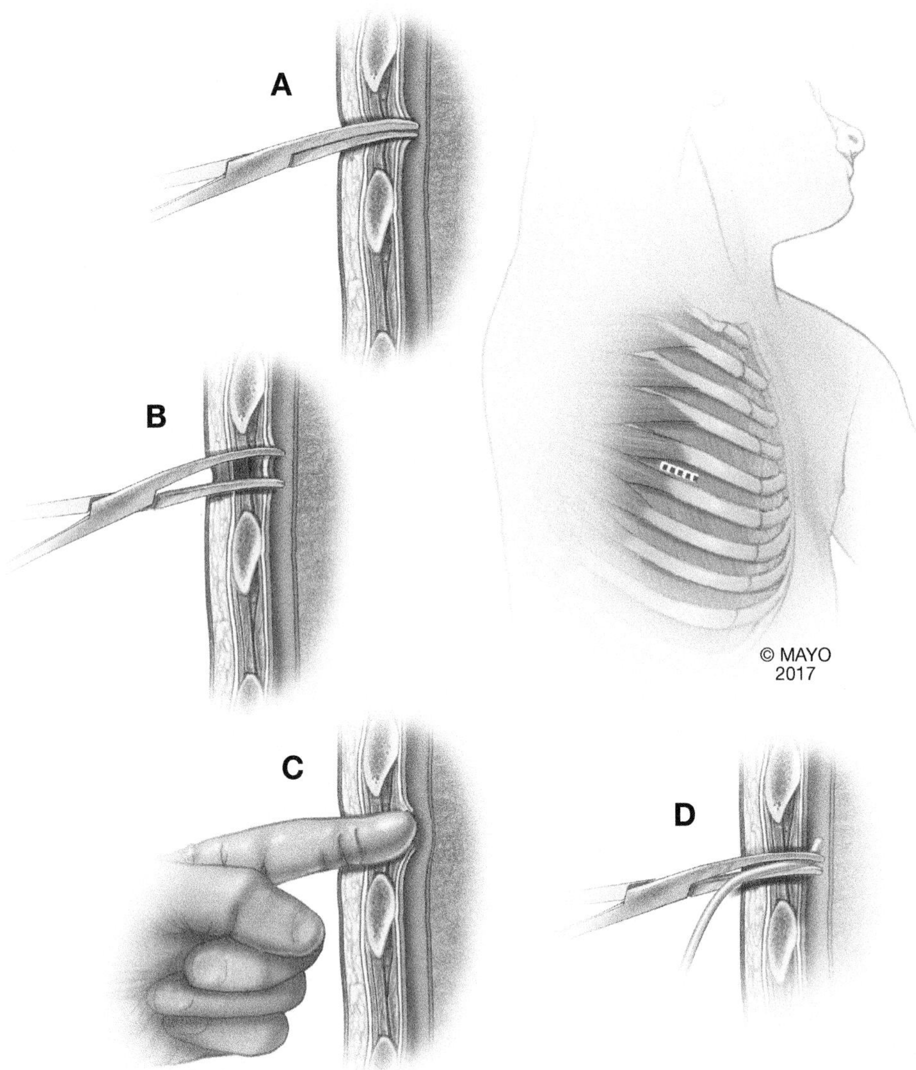

Figure 122.2. Placement of a Large-Bore Chest Tube. After administration of topical anesthetic, a small incision is made along the selected interspace (dashed line on chest wall). The tissues are bluntly dissected to the level of the intercostal muscle and ribs, and then a clamp is used to penetrate the intercostal muscle directly above the rib (A). The thoracic entry site is spread large enough to allow passage of a finger (B) to directly palpate the lung and assess for adhesions (C). The tube is directed into place (D) and then secured.

SUGGESTED READING

Cassivi SD, Deschamps C, Pastis NJ. Chest tube insertion and management. In: Spiro SG, Silvestri GA, Agusti A, editors. Clinical respiratory medicine. 4th ed. Philadelphia (PA): Elsevier Saunders; c2012. p. 862–8.

Cerfolio RJ, Bryant AS, Skylizard L, Minnich DJ. Optimal technique for the removal of chest tubes after pulmonary resection. J Thorac Cardiovasc Surg. 2013 Jun;145(6):1535–9. Epub 2013 Mar 15.

Cooke DT, David EA. Large-bore and small-bore chest tubes: types, function, and placement. Thorac Surg Clin. 2013 Feb;23(1):17–24.

Davies HE, Davies RJ, Davies CW; BTS Pleural Disease Guideline Group. Management of pleural infection in adults: British Thoracic Society Pleural Disease Guideline 2010. Thorax. 2010 Aug;65 Suppl 2: ii41–53.

Dev SP, Nascimiento B Jr, Simone C, Chien V. Videos in clinical medicine: chest-tube insertion. N Engl J Med. 2007 Oct 11;357(15):e15.

Feller-Kopman D, Berkowitz D, Boiselle P, Ernst A. Large-volume thoracentesis and the risk of reexpansion pulmonary edema. Ann Thorac Surg. 2007 Nov;84(5):1656–61.

Filosso PL, Guerrera F, Sandri A, Roffinella M, Solidoro P, Ruffini E, et al. Errors and complications in chest tube placement. Thorac Surg Clin. 2017 Feb;27(1):57–67.
Hashmi U, Nadeem M, Aleem A, Khan FUHH, Gull R, Ullah K, et al. Dysfunctional closed chest drainage: common causative factors and recommendations for prevention. Cureus. 2018 Mar 9;10(3):e2295.
Havelock T, Teoh R, Laws D, Gleeson F; BTS Pleural Disease Guideline Group. Pleural procedures and thoracic ultrasound: British Thoracic Society Pleural Disease Guideline 2010. Thorax. 2010 Aug;65 Suppl 2:ii61–76.
Jones CW, Rodriguez RD, Griffin RL, McGwin G, Jansen JO, Kerby JD, et al. Complications associated with placement of chest tubes: a trauma system perspective. J Surg Res. 2019 Jul;239:98–102. Epub 2019 Feb 27.
Lotano VE. Chest tube thoracostomy. In: Parrillo JE, Dellinger RP, editors. Critical care medicine: principles of diagnosis and management in the adult. 3rd ed. Philadelphia (PA): Mosby Elsevier; c2008. p. 271–80.
Macha DB, Thomas J, Nelson RC. Pigtail catheters used for percutaneous fluid drainage: comparison of performance characteristics. Radiology. 2006 Mar;238(3):1057–63.
Mahmood K, Wahidi MM. Straightening out chest tubes: what size, what type, and when. Clin Chest Med. 2013 Mar;34(1):63–71. Epub 2013 Jan 17.
Mercaldi CJ, Lanes SF. Ultrasound guidance decreases complications and improves the cost of care among patients undergoing thoracentesis and paracentesis. Chest. 2013 Feb 1;143(2):532–8.
Millar FR, Hillman T. Managing chest drains on medical wards. BMJ. 2018 Nov 21;363:k4639. Erratum in: BMJ. 2018 Dec 12;363:k5219.
Novoa NM, Jimenez MF, Varela G. When to remove a chest tube. Thorac Surg Clin. 2017 Feb;27(1):41–6.
Perazzo A, Gatto P, Barlascini C, Ferrari-Bravo M, Nicolini A. Can ultrasound guidance reduce the risk of pneumothorax following thoracentesis? J Bras Pneumol. 2014 Jan-Feb;40(1):6–12. English, Portuguese.
Shojaee S, Argento AC. Ultrasound-guided pleural access. Semin Respir Crit Care Med. 2014 Dec;35(6):693–705. Epub 2014 Dec 2.
Swiderek J, Morcos S, Donthireddy V, Surapaneni R, Jackson-Thompson V, Schultz L, et al. Prospective study to determine the volume of pleural fluid required to diagnose malignancy. Chest. 2010 Jan;137(1):68–73. Epub 2009 Sep 9.
Yarmus L, Feller-Kopman D. Pneumothorax in the critically ill patient. Chest. 2012 Apr;141(4):1098–105.

Central Line Placement

NICHOLAS D. WILL, MD; W. BRIAN BEAM, MD

Goals

- Discuss indications for placement of central venous catheters.
- Discuss approach to site selection and placement of central venous catheters.
- Discuss complications related to central venous catheters.

Introduction

Central venous catheter placement is one of the most commonly performed procedures in the intensive care unit. Common indications for central venous catheter placement include the need for vasoactive or caustic medication infusions, vascular access in patients with poor peripheral veins, long-term access for intravenous medications, infusion of parenteral nutrition, hemodynamic monitoring, transvenous cardiac pacing, and access for hemodialysis or plasmapheresis. There are no absolute contraindications to central venous catheter placement because it is a potentially lifesaving intervention, but careful planning and site selection are warranted in some cases, such as a patient with a known coagulopathy. Training is now feasible in institutions with simulation centers.

Catheter Types and Site Selection

The jugular, subclavian, and femoral veins are the most common sites of central line placement. The use of peripherally inserted central catheters is also becoming increasingly common. Lines can be tunneled or nontunneled. Because of the ease of bedside placement, nontunneled lines are most commonly placed in the intensive care unit. Tunneled lines require fluoroscopy for appropriate placement, which is usually done in the interventional radiology suite or operating room. Central lines are of various types, and the decision regarding the type of line to be placed should be based on the indication for the line. In general, because of their long length and relatively small diameter, lines such as standard triple-lumen catheters are a poor choice for patients who require high-volume fluid resuscitation because of their relatively slow flow rates, as predicted by the Poiseuille law.

The choice of access site depends on patient factors and clinician experience. Complications include infection, arterial puncture, pneumothorax, hematoma, venous air embolism, and thrombosis. Femoral access has been associated with the highest risk of infectious and thrombotic complications. Insertion sites that are contaminated or at risk for contamination such as sites in proximity to burns, skin breakdown, or a tracheostomy should be avoided. Subclavian lines have the lowest rate of infection and symptomatic deep vein thrombosis but have an increased risk of pneumothorax and should be avoided in a patient with limited pulmonary reserve or with coagulopathy because of the noncompressible nature of the vessels in this area. Internal jugular vein insertion has the highest rate of arterial puncture but is preferred because of the ease of insertion under ultrasound guidance and lower risk of infection compared with femoral lines (Figure 123.1).

Central venous catheter insertion should take place in an environment where sterility is able to be maintained. As part of a "bundle," hand washing, full-body sterile drape, sterile gloves, and masks have been shown to reduce catheter-associated bloodstream infections. In addition, skin preparation with a chlorhexidine solution is recommended. Antibiotics are generally not indicated, but they can be considered in high-risk immunocompromised patients. Although evidence is equivocal regarding overall benefit, silver sulfadiazine or chlorhexidine catheters can be considered in select patients, particularly if the catheter will remain in place for a prolonged time. For upper extremity

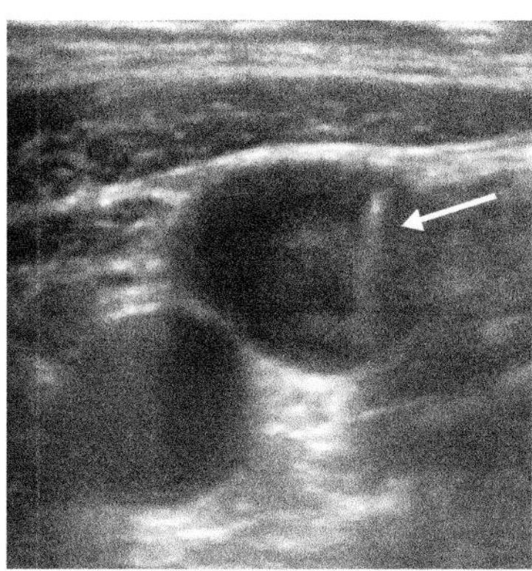

Figure 123.1. Ultrasound-Guided Image of Central Venous Catheter Placement. Right internal jugular vein is on right, and carotid artery is on left. Note that the guidewire is present in the internal jugular vein (arrow).

line placement, Trendelenburg positioning increases the cross-sectional area of the veins and may decrease the risk of venous air embolism by increasing venous pressures. Use of dynamic ultrasound guidance for line placement has been shown to decrease complications, access time, placement failure, and need for multiple attempts compared with the landmark technique. Venous cannulation should be verified before vessel dilation. This verification can be performed with ultrasound, manometry, pressure waveform analysis, or blood gas analysis. A chest radiograph should be obtained to verify line placement. If unintended arterial dilation and cannulation occur, a surgical consultation should be obtained before line removal.

Use of a chlorhexidine-impregnated dressing is recommended. The catheter site should be inspected daily, and the line should be promptly removed when no longer clinically indicated. If the catheter becomes infected and central access remains necessary, the catheter should be removed and a new catheter inserted at a new site.

Summary

- Common indications for central line insertion include medication infusions, monitoring, nutritional support, and the need for hemodialysis or plasmapheresis.
- Catheter type is determined by the clinical situation, and site selection should be individualized on the basis of patient factors and clinician experience.
- Complications include infection, arterial puncture, pneumothorax, hematoma, venous air embolism, and thrombosis.
- The risk of complications can be reduced by the use of sterile technique, careful site selection and patient positioning, ultrasound guidance, confirmation of venous cannulation, and prompt removal of unnecessary catheters.

SUGGESTED READING

Ablordeppey EA, Drewry AM, Beyer AB, Theodoro DL, Fowler SA, Fuller BM, et al. Diagnostic accuracy of central venous catheter confirmation by bedside ultrasound versus chest radiography in critically ill patients: a systematic review and meta-analysis. Crit Care Med. 2017 Apr;45(4):715–24.

Bauer PR, Daniels CE, Sampathkumar P. Complications of central venous catheterization. N Engl J Med. 2016 Apr 14;374(15):1491.

McGee DC, Gould MK. Preventing complications of central venous catheterization. N Engl J Med. 2003 Mar 20;348(12):1123–33.

Parienti JJ, Mongardon N, Megarbane B, Mira JP, Kalfon P, Gros A, et al; 3SITES Study Group. Intravascular complications of central venous catheterization by insertion site. N Engl J Med. 2015 Sep 24;373(13):1220–9.

Smith RN, Nolan JP. Central venous catheters. BMJ. 2013 Nov 11;347:f6570.

Soffler MI, Hayes MM, Smith CC. Central venous catheterization training: current perspectives on the role of simulation. Adv Med Educ Pract. 2018 May 25;9:395–403.

Taylor RW, Palagiri AV. Central venous catheterization. Crit Care Med. 2007 May;35(5):1390–6.

Interventional Radiology Procedures

RAHMI OKLU, MD, PhD

Goals

- Describe the general principles for interventional procedures in patients in the intensive care unit.
- Describe the more common interventional procedures performed.

Introduction

Most patients in an intensive care unit (ICU) are critically ill, hemodynamically unstable, and have multiple comorbidities. Interventional radiology (IR) procedures can offer therapeutic options for these patients and avoid the risks associated with invasive surgery and general anesthesia.

Preprocedural Concerns

Coagulation

Evidence regarding periprocedural coagulation management for patients undergoing image-guided procedures is limited. The Society of Interventional Radiology issued a consensus statement in 2012 offering periprocedural recommendations. Routine preprocedure laboratory testing should include prothrombin time, international normalized ratio, and platelet counts. For procedures with moderate or considerable risks of bleeding, the recommended limit is 1.5 for the international normalized ratio and concentration 50,000/mcL for the platelet count. Values beyond these recommended thresholds are relative, not absolute, contraindications. Some investigators advocate transfusing fresh frozen plasma to rapidly correct the international normalized ratio or platelet count in cases of thrombocytopenia. However, high-level evidence is lacking about transfusions before image-guided procedures. The decision to proceed with intervention despite suboptimal coagulation parameters depends on multiple factors, including operator experience, required urgency of intervention, patient comorbidities, and the planned procedure.

Nothing-by-Mouth Status

Conscious sedation is commonly used during IR procedures and typically consists of an intravenous analgesic and a benzodiazepine, usually fentanyl and midazolam. Because of the concern for aspiration after administration of these medications, there should be no intragastric contents, including secretions, before any procedure in which conscious sedation will be used. Patients in the ICU who can tolerate oral intake, should remain in nothing-by-mouth status for at least 8 hours unless the underlying condition necessitates urgent intervention. Some of the less invasive, usually superficial, procedures can be performed with local anesthetic or with current protocols for so-called conscious sedation.

Image-Guided Procedures

Preferably all interventions for critically ill patients are performed within the IR department. Because of the tenuous status of some patients in the ICU, select minor procedures can be performed at the bedside (eg, thoracenteses, paracenteses, and placement of nontunneled central lines) using portable ultrasound and radiographic units.

Drainage Procedures

Percutaneous drainage of abnormal fluid collections is indicated if the fluid is suspected to be infected (abscess), there is a need for fluid characterization, or the collection may be producing clinically relevant symptoms. The only absolute contraindication to percutaneous drainage is the absence of a safe track for the needle or drainage catheter to traverse. Complications of drainage procedures include septic shock, hemorrhage requiring blood transfusion, and transgression of nontarget structures.

Superficial collections are usually drained with a combination of ultrasound and fluoroscopic guidance, whereas deeper collections or collections adjacent to vital organs are often accessed under computed tomographic guidance. Catheter sizing is based on the fluid's viscosity. Drains are left in place until outputs diminish considerably (<10 mL/24 h over several days) or the patient's clinical status improves. Infusion of radiopaque contrast material into the catheter (a sinography) is also frequently performed before removing a drain. The sinogram defines the residual cavity and excludes the presence of any associated fistulous communication to the bowel, biliary tree, pancreas, or urinary tract.

Pleural Space Interventions

IR procedures involving the pleural space include thoracentesis, chest tube placement, and tunneled catheter insertion. Thoracentesis is the most common, accounting for approximately 178,000 procedures annually in the United States. Indications for draining pleural fluid include respiratory compromise; for small-bore chest tube placement, pneumothorax or empyema drainage; and for tunneled catheter insertion, recurrent symptomatic malignant effusions. Ultrasonography, catheter placement, and fluoroscopy are all used for pleural space interventions, depending on the indication and operator preference.

Paracentesis

Paracentesis is the drainage of ascites for therapeutic purposes in symptomatic patients or for diagnostic purposes in cases of suspected bacterial peritonitis. The procedure is low-risk, provides rapid relief, and is generally well tolerated. Ultrasonography is solely used with skin access sites at the most dependent areas of ascites accumulation (usually lateral lower quadrants or midline infraumbilical). Inferior epigastric arteries should be avoided and are usually located 4 to 8 cm lateral of midline.

Cholecystostomy

Decompression of an inflamed gallbladder by cholecystostomy is a temporizing procedure to stabilize a critically ill patient in whom definitive laparoscopic cholecystectomy is contraindicated. The gallbladder is drained under ultrasound guidance using transhepatic or direct transperitoneal access. The transhepatic approach offers a decreased risk of colonic perforation, catheter dislodgment, or intraperitoneal bile leakage. The catheter should remain in place for at least 3 weeks to allow the access tract to mature and not be removed until cystic duct patency is confirmed.

Percutaneous Nephrostomy

Nephrostomy tube placement is an excellent method to decompress the urinary collecting system in cases of urinary tract obstruction associated with leukocytosis, fever, and acute kidney injury. Ultrasound guidance is the preferred method of access in which proper catheter positioning is appreciated using fluoroscopy. Antibiotics are recommended before nephrostomy placement.

Central Venous Catheter Placement

Because of the multitude of indications, central venous access is almost universally required in the ICU setting and encompasses 4 subtypes of central venous catheters: peripherally inserted, temporary (nontunneled), permanent (tunneled), and implantable ports. Each of these catheters can be placed in the IR department with ultrasound and fluoroscopic guidance. Initial venous access is performed with ultrasound guidance, which offers multiple advantages compared with solely using anatomical skin surface landmarks for access. Benefits of using ultrasound include assessment of vessel patency, visualization of the needle tip within the tissues, and identifying variant anatomy. Fluoroscopy is used to confirm wire and catheter-tip positions intraprocedurally.

Gastrostomy Placement

Many patients in the ICU require nutritional support because of underlying neurologic disorders that place them at risk for aspiration (eg, residual stroke deficits, amyotrophic lateral sclerosis, multiple sclerosis) or the presence of head and neck cancer. Venting gastrostomy tubes can also decompress the stomach in cases of gastric or small bowel obstruction or altered gastric motility. Percutaneous gastrostomy placement with IR techniques has shown higher success rates and fewer tube-related complications than endoscopically placed gastrostomy tubes. The tube is placed with fluoroscopic guidance after gastric insufflation with air through a nasogastric tube. Insufflating air can displace the adjacent transverse colon and prevents traversing the posterior gastric wall. Ultrasound can also be used to demarcate the left hepatic lobe margin along the skin surface. Major complications (including hemorrhage, peritonitis, abscess formation, and bowel perforation) occur in 1.4% to 5.9% of cases.

Role of IR in the Management of Gastrointestinal Bleeding

Approximately 390,000 hospitalizations for gastrointestinal bleeding occur annually in the United States; associated mortality rates range from 3.0% to 8.8%. In cases of severe bleeding, administration of fluid or blood products and intervention are often required. If upper gastrointestinal (proximal to the ligament of Treitz) or colonic bleeding is suspected, endoscopy is the preferred initial therapeutic option. Tagged red blood cell scanning and computed tomographic angiography are useful adjuncts to help localize the site of bleeding. When bleeding is refractory to medical and endoscopic therapy, transcatheter embolization may be pursued. Adequate perception of bleeding under conventional angiography requires active bleeding rates of at least 0.5 to 1.0 mL/min, and the bleeding manifests as contrast extravasation into the bowel lumen. If possible, the chosen embolic agent should be deployed as close to the site of bleeding as possible to preserve collateral perfusion and thus avoid infarcting a segment of bowel.

Role of IR in the Management of Pulmonary Embolus

Percutaneous treatment of complete and partial occlusions of the proximal pulmonary arterial system is potentially lifesaving. Treatment ideally leads to rapid decrease in pulmonary artery pressure, right ventricular strain, and pulmonary vascular resistance; improved systemic perfusion; and facilitation of right ventricular recovery. Different percutaneous interventional techniques are used to facilitate clot removal and diminish thrombus burden (these are beyond the scope of this chapter). Approximate clinical success rates were 95% when percutaneous therapeutic interventions were used in combination with focal fibrinolytic therapy in patients with acute massive PE. Catheter thrombectomy is not recommended in patients with low-risk PE or acute submassive PE with minor right ventricular dysfunction, minor myocardial necrosis, and no clinical worsening.

Inferior Vena Cava Filter Placement

When there is active bleeding or anticoagulation is contraindicated in patients with acute PE (or central deep vein thrombosis), a prophylactic inferior vena cava (IVC) filter should be placed. If acute recurrent PE develops despite therapeutic anticoagulation, filter placement is also reasonable. A prospective randomized trial of 400 patients with deep vein thrombosis at high risk for PE found substantially reduced PE at 12 days and 8 years when an IVC filter was placed. This reduction was offset by an increased incidence of recurrent deep vein thrombosis 2 years after IVC filter placement. The filter is placed with ultrasound and fluoroscopic guidance. Some early complications include malpositioned devices, hematoma, air embolism, and arteriovenous fistula. Later complications include recurrent deep vein thrombosis (20.8%), IVC thrombosis (2%-10%), and IVC penetration (0.3%). Retrievable filters should be removed once the initial indication has resolved or contraindication to anticoagulation is no longer present.

Summary

- IR procedures can be helpful for placement of catheters (when multiple attempts have failed).
- IR procedures, when feasible, can avoid the risks associated with surgery and anesthesia in critically ill patients.
- Coagulation status nothing by mouth status should be evaluated before a procedure.

SUGGESTED READING

Bazarah SM, Al-Rawas M, Akbar H, Qari Y. Percutaneous gastrostomy and gastrojejunostomy: radiological and endoscopic approach. Ann Saudi Med. 2002 Jan-Mar;22(1–2):38–42.

Covarrubias DA, O'Connor OJ, McDermott S, Arellano RS. Radiologic percutaneous gastrostomy: review of potential complications and approach to managing the unexpected outcome. AJR Am J Roentgenol. 2013 Apr;200(4):921–31.

Daniels CE, Ryu JH. Improving the safety of thoracentesis. Curr Opin Pulm Med. 2011 Jul;17(4):232–6.

Decousus H, Leizorovicz A, Parent F, Page Y, Tardy B, Girard P, et al; Prevention du Risque d'Embolie Pulmonaire par Interruption Cave Study Group. A clinical trial of vena caval filters in the prevention of pulmonary embolism in patients with proximal deep-vein thrombosis. N Engl J Med. 1998 Feb 12;338(7):409–15.

Garcia-Blazquez V, Vicente-Bartulos A, Olavarria-Delgado A, Plana MN, van der Winden D, Zamora J; EBM-Connect Collaboration. Accuracy of CT angiography in the diagnosis of acute gastrointestinal bleeding: systematic review and meta-analysis. Eur Radiol. 2013 May;23(5):1181–90. Epub 2012 Nov 29.

Hann CL, Streiff MB. The role of vena caval filters in the management of venous thromboembolism. Blood Rev. 2005 Jul;19(4):179–202.

Jaff MR, McMurtry MS, Archer SL, Cushman M, Goldenberg N, Goldhaber SZ, et al; American Heart Association Council on Cardiopulmonary, Critical Care, Perioperative and Resuscitation; American Heart Association Council on Peripheral Vascular Disease; American Heart Association Council on Arteriosclerosis, Thrombosis and Vascular Biology. Management of massive and submassive pulmonary embolism, iliofemoral deep vein thrombosis, and chronic thromboembolic pulmonary hypertension: a scientific statement from the American Heart Association. Circulation. 2011 Apr 26;123(16):1788–830. Epub 2011 Mar 21. Errata in: Circulation. 2012 Aug 14;126(7):e104. Circulation. 2012 Mar 20;125(11):e495.

Jones PW, Moyers JP, Rogers JT, Rodriguez RM, Lee YC, Light RW. Ultrasound-guided thoracentesis: is it a safer method? Chest. 2003 Feb;123(2):418–23.

Kadir S, editor. Teaching atlas of interventional radiology: non-vascular interventional procedures. New York (NY): Thieme; c2006. 340 p.

Kucher N. Catheter embolectomy for acute pulmonary embolism. Chest. 2007 Aug;132(2):657–63.

Kuhle WG, Sheiman RG. Detection of active colonic hemorrhage with use of helical CT: findings in a swine model. Radiology. 2003 Sep;228(3):743–52.

McDermott S, Levis DA, Arellano RS. Chest drainage. Semin Intervent Radiol. 2012 Dec;29(4):247–55.

Mellouk Aid K, Tchala Vignon Zomahoun H, Soulaymani A, Lebascle K, Silvera S, Astagneau P, et al. MOrtality and infectious complications of therapeutic EndoVAscular

interventional radiology: a systematic and meta-analysis protocol. Syst Rev. 2017 Apr 24;6(1):89.
Mohan P, Manov J, Diaz-Bode A, Venkat S, Langston M, Naidu A, et al. Clinical predictors of arterial extravasation, rebleeding and mortality following angiographic interventions in gastrointestinal bleeding. J Gastrointestin Liver Dis. 2018 Sep;27(3):221–6.
Nicolaou S, Talsky A, Khashoggi K, Venu V. Ultrasound-guided interventional radiology in critical care. Crit Care Med. 2007 May;35(5 Suppl):S186–97.
Norfolk DR, Ancliffe PJ, Contreras M, Hunt BJ, Machin SJ, Murphy WG, et al. Consensus Conference on Platelet Transfusion, Royal College of Physicians of Edinburgh, 27–28 November 1997: synopsis of background papers. Br J Haematol. 1998 Jun;101(4):609–17.
Oakland K, Chadwick G, East JE, Guy R, Humphries A, Jairath V, et al. Diagnosis and management of acute lower gastrointestinal bleeding: guidelines from the British Society of Gastroenterology. Gut. 2019 May;68(5): 776–89. Epub 2019 Feb 12.
Patel IJ, Davidson JC, Nikolic B, Salazar GM, Schwartzberg MS, Walker TG, et al; Standards of Practice Committee, with Cardiovascular and Interventional Radiological Society of Europe (CIRSE) Endorsement. Consensus guidelines for periprocedural management of coagulation status and hemostasis risk in percutaneous image-guided interventions. J Vasc Interv Radiol. 2012 Jun;23(6):727–36. Epub 2012 Apr 17.
Pollak JS. Catheter-based therapies for pulmonary emboli. Clin Chest Med. 2018 Sep;39(3):651–8.
Reis SP, Zhao K, Ahmad N, Widemon RS, Root CW, Toomay SM, et al. Acute pulmonary embolism: endovascular therapy. Cardiovasc Diagn Ther. 2018 Jun;8(3):244–52.
Saber AA, Meslemani AM, Davis R, Pimentel R. Safety zones for anterior abdominal wall entry during laparoscopy: a CT scan mapping of epigastric vessels. Ann Surg. 2004 Feb;239(2):182–5.
Skaf E, Beemath A, Siddiqui T, Janjua M, Patel NR, Stein PD. Catheter-tip embolectomy in the management of acute massive pulmonary embolism. Am J Cardiol. 2007 Feb 1;99(3):415–20. Epub 2006 Dec 15.
Society of Cardiovascular and Interventional Radiology Standards of Practices Committee. Quality improvement guidelines for adult percutaneous abscess and fluid drainage. J Vasc Interv Radiol. 1995 Jan-Feb;6(1): 68–70.
Srygley FD, Gerardo CJ, Tran T, Fisher DA. Does this patient have a severe upper gastrointestinal bleed? JAMA. 2012 Mar 14;307(10):1072–9.
Stanworth SJ, Brunskill SJ, Hyde CJ, McClelland DB, Murphy MF. Is fresh frozen plasma clinically effective? A systematic review of randomized controlled trials. Br J Haematol. 2004 Jul;126(1):139–52.
Tan PL, Gibson M. Central venous catheters: the role of radiology. Clin Radiol. 2006 Jan;61(1):13–22.
Walker TG. Acute gastrointestinal hemorrhage. Tech Vasc Interv Radiol. 2009 Jun;12(2):80–91.
Wollman B, D'Agostino HB, Walus-Wigle JR, Easter DW, Beale A. Radiologic, endoscopic, and surgical gastrostomy: an institutional evaluation and meta-analysis of the literature. Radiology. 1995 Dec;197(3): 699–704.
Zurkiya O, Walker TG. Angiographic evaluation and management of nonvariceal gastrointestinal hemorrhage. AJR Am J Roentgenol. 2015 Oct;205(4):753–63.

Neuromonitoring and Procedures

Intracranial Pressure Monitoring and External Ventricular Drainage[a]

MAYA A. BABU, MD; JOHN L. D. ATKINSON, MD

Goals

- Recognize the indications for intracranial pressure monitoring and ventricular catheter placement.
- Review the basic intracranial pressure waveforms, the normal intracranial pressure values, and the factors that increase intracranial pressure.
- Review ventricular catheter insertion (the gold standard) for intracranial pressure measurement and the newer methods that use probes.

Introduction

The Monro-Kellie doctrine states that the cranial vault encloses a fixed space and that after trauma or injury, swelling of the brain parenchyma leads to increased pressure in the cerebrospinal fluid (CSF)-filled ventricles or in the vasculature because the sum of the volume of the blood, CSF, and parenchyma is fixed. Therefore, measurement of intracranial pressure (ICP) after an intracranial injury is clinically relevant. Several studies have shown that increased ICP has been associated with poor neurologic outcomes. Management of elevated ICP can improve neurologic outcomes and influence medical and surgical therapy, and accurate recording of ICP is helpful in assessing a patient's clinical status. Currently, the 2 most common forms of monitoring ICP involve 1) placement of a fiberoptic or strain gauge intraparenchymal monitor or 2) placement of a ventricular drain.

Indications for ICP Monitoring

According to the Brain Trauma Foundation *Guidelines for the Management of Severe Traumatic Brain Injury, Fourth Edition* (Carney et al, 2017; see Suggested Reading), "Management of severe TBI [traumatic brain injury] patients using information from ICP monitoring is recommended to reduce in-hospital and 2-week post-injury mortality" (a level IIB recommendation). Indications for monitoring, which were carried forward from the third edition, include the following:

1. "ICP should be monitored in all salvageable patients with a TBI (GCS [Glasgow Coma Scale] 3-8 after resuscitation) and an abnormal CT [computed tomographic] scan. An abnormal CT scan of the head is one that reveals hematomas, contusions, swelling, herniation, or compressed basal cisterns."
2. "ICP monitoring is indicated in patients with severe TBI with a normal CT scan if ≥2 of the following features are noted at admission: age >40 years, unilateral or bilateral motor posturing, or SBP [systolic blood pressure] <90 mm Hg."

Since this is not a level I evidence-based guideline, the practice of ICP monitoring is variable. Some neurotrauma specialists disagree as to which patient populations would benefit from invasive ICP monitoring and the extent to which monitoring should guide clinical practice. Most agree that elevated ICP has multifactorial causes, but monitoring is an intelligent approach to managing severe TBI, especially when mass lesions, loss of cisterns, and brain

[a] Portions previously published in Carney N, Totten AM, O'Reilly C, Ullman JS, Hawryluk GW, Bell MJ, et al. Guidelines for the management of severe traumatic brain injury, fourth edition. Neurosurgery. 2017 Jan 1;80(1):6-15; used with permission.

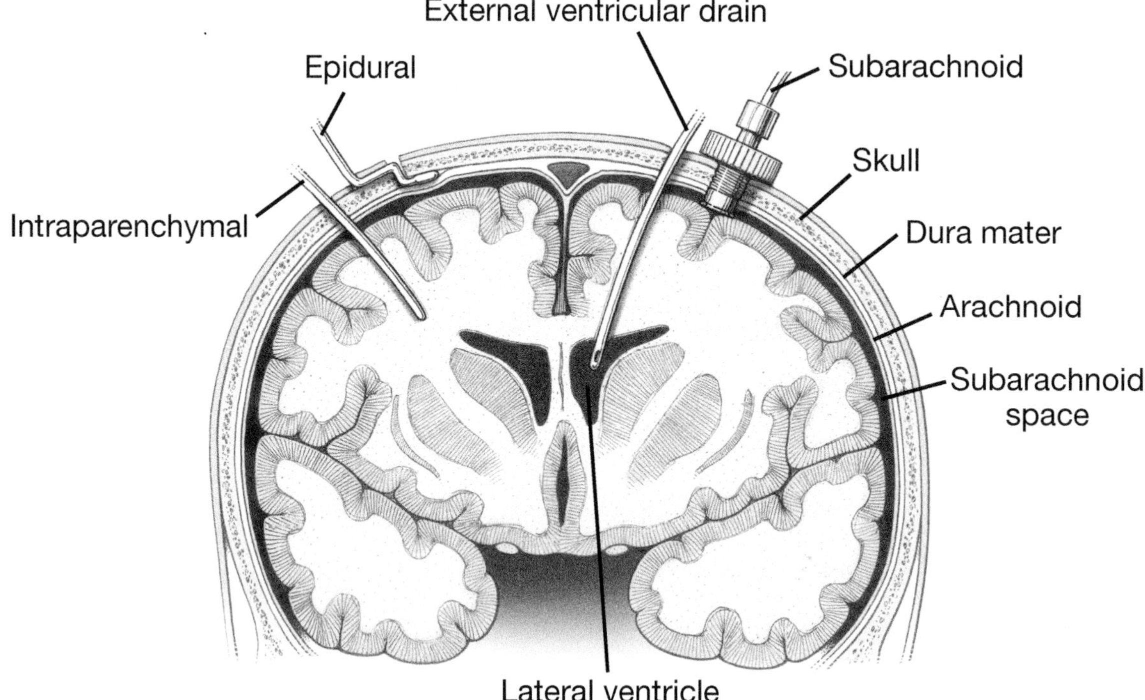

Figure 125.1. Intracranial Pressure Monitors. Monitoring sites are shown for an external ventricular drain and for intraparenchymal, epidural, and subarachnoid monitors.

(Modified from Freeman WD. Management of intracranial pressure. Continuum [Minneap Minn]. 2015 Oct;21[5 Neurocritical Care]:1299-323. Erratum in: Continuum [Minneap Minn]. 2015 Dec;21[6 Neuroinfectious Disease]:1550; used with permission of Mayo Foundation for Medical Education and Research.)

shifts are documented on CT. ICP monitoring is most beneficial as a warning system, so that if sudden or sustained elevations of ICP occur, follow-up CT scanning may correlate with increasing mass effect, and surgery may be necessary to maximize recovery.

External Ventricular Drainage

Several medical conditions can be managed with the use of an external ventricular drain (EVD) (Figure 125.1), including hydrocephalus secondary to subarachnoid hemorrhage, TBI, and intracranial hemorrhage with intraventricular extension.

The choroid plexus produces CSF, and the arachnoid granulations resorb CSF. The amount of CSF produced is 0.2 to 0.4 mL/min or 500 to 600 mL daily. Appropriate ranges for ICP vary with patient age and body position. For adults lying in the supine position, normal values are 5 to 15 mm Hg; for infants, 1 to 6 mm Hg.

Placement of an EVD has 3 purposes: 1) The EVD catheter can be connected to a drainage system that transduces the CSF flow waveform continuously and measures the ICP; elevated ICP can then be managed either with hyperosmolar or hypertonic solutions or with surgical intervention. 2) The EVD catheter can assist with CSF diversion; drainage of CSF temporarily creates more space for brain swelling and may help limit acute parenchymal damage. 3) The EVD catheter may be used to instill medications, such as tissue plasminogen activator (a thrombolytic agent) to treat a dense, obstructive intraventricular clot.

EVD Insertion

EVDs can be inserted at the bedside, as is often the situation in the intensive care unit, or in the sterile environment of the operating room. An intracranial access kit typically contains the supplies necessary for placing an EVD at the bedside. Placement of a bedside EVD is most often directed to the foramen of Monro, with a trajectory through the right frontal horn of the lateral ventricle. The most frequent entry site is the Kocher point, which is approximately 12 cm posterior to the nasion and 4 cm lateral to the midline, corresponding to the midpupillary line. This trajectory aligns with an approach through the right middle frontal gyrus, which is considered to be noneloquent cortex. A patient who requires an EVD is often obtunded, but if the patient is not intubated and is awake, sedative medications, (eg, midazolam or fentanyl) should be administered to help with pain control and agitation.

If the patient is in bed, the head of the bed should be elevated 45°.

The Kocher point should be marked and the hair in this region clipped, allowing ample room for subcutaneous tunneling of the EVD catheter. The region should be sterilized with cleansing agents that include iodine or isopropyl alcohol. Surgical drapes should be applied to create a sterile field and isolate the entry site. A procedural pause should be completed to verify the patient's medical record number and the procedure to be performed.

Lidocaine with epinephrine is typically infiltrated subcutaneously at the Kocher point to assist with pain control and hemostasis. A scalpel is used to make a stab incision at the Kocher point. A mastoid retractor is used to hold the skin edges apart. The bit of a manual drill is positioned perpendicular to the skull surface, and a hole is drilled through the outer and inner table of the skull. Care must be taken to avoid violating the dura.

When the dura is exposed, a Tuohy needle is used to create a shallow hole in the dura and pia and thereby help the EVD pass smoothly without obstruction by the dura or pia. In the coronal plane, the trajectory of the EVD is toward the medial canthus of the ipsilateral eye; in the antero-posterior plane, 1 cm anterior to the tragus. This trajectory can be verified with preprocedural CT of the head and may be modified if the ventricular caliber is diminished. The EVD and stylet should pass smoothly and any resistance should prompt questions about the trajectory and approach. Traversing the ventricular ependyma typically results in a haptic change, and a slight "pop" may be felt. CSF egress should be noted thereafter. The EVD should not be advanced more than about 7 cm. If no CSF egress is observed, the EVD should be removed and all landmarks and orientation rechecked for accuracy. If necessary, CT of the head may be repeated.

When CSF egress begins, the catheter should be tunneled under the skin and externalized several centimeters from the site of bone entry. The catheter should subsequently be secured to the skin with a silk suture or staples. The catheter can then be connected to the drainage apparatus, which in turn can be connected to monitors in the intensive care unit for continual monitoring of ICP. CT of the head is often performed to confirm placement of the distal tip of the EVD and to ensure that no hemorrhage occurred. The transducer should be at the level of the patient's external auditory meatus; otherwise, the readings may be influenced by patient positioning.

ICP Monitors

In addition to the EVD, several types of monitors for measuring ICP are commercially available (Figure 125.1). These intraparenchymal monitors measure transduced pressure, and some newer systems also measure the partial pressure of brain oxygen and parenchymal temperature.

Fiber optic pressure monitors measure ICP by measuring light emission through a fiber optic cable directed toward a displaceable mirror. Elevated ICP deforms the brain parenchyma and changes the orientation of the mirror, leading to differences in the intensity of light reflected, which can be converted into a measured ICP.

Strain gauge monitors measure ICP when the transducer wire is bent because of changes in ICP. The resistance of the wire changes, and from this change, ICP can be calculated.

Pneumatic sensors use a small balloon at the end of the catheter to measure pressure. They can also be used to assess intracranial compliance.

ICP Waveforms

The pressure wave of CSF flow has 3 parts: a percussion wave (P1), a tidal wave (P2), and a dicrotic wave (P3). The ICP waveform seems to blend 2 different frequencies, 1 mirroring the arterial pulse and the other, respirations. The component of the waveform caused by arterial pulsations in large intracranial vessels produces oscillation within the ventricular system. Thus, the CSF pressure wave tends to vary with systemic blood pressure. The dicrotic notch between P2 and P3 corresponds to the dicrotic notch of the arterial pulsation. ICP also varies with respiration and changes in central venous pressure, and intrathoracic pressure.

Summary

- ICP, the pressure within the intracranial vault, can increase if processes such as brain swelling or bleeding occur because the size of the intracranial vault in adults is fixed.
- ICP should be monitored in all patients who are expected to recover after a severe TBI, who are comatose (with a nonlocalizing motor response) after resuscitation, and who have abnormal CT findings.

SUGGESTED READING

Albeck MJ, Borgesen SE, Gjerris F, Schmidt JF, Sorensen PS. Intracranial pressure and cerebrospinal fluid outflow conductance in healthy subjects. J Neurosurg. 1991 Apr;74(4):597–600.

Bales JW, Bonow RH, Buckley RT, Barber J, Temkin N, Chesnut RM. Primary external ventricular drainage catheter versus intraparenchymal icp monitoring: outcome analysis. Neurocrit Care. 2019 Apr 29. [Epub ahead of print]

Becker DP, Miller JD, Ward JD, Greenberg RP, Young HF, Sakalas R. The outcome from severe head injury with early diagnosis and intensive management. J Neurosurg. 1977 Oct;47(4):491–502.

Bering EA Jr. Choroid plexus and arterial pulsation of cerebrospinal fluid: demonstration of the choroid plexuses as a cerebrospinal fluid pump. AMA Arch Neurol Psychiatry. 1955 Feb;73(2):165–72.

Brown PD, Davies SL, Speake T, Millar ID. Molecular mechanisms of cerebrospinal fluid production. Neuroscience. 2004;129(4):957–70.

Carney N, Totten AM, O'Reilly C, Ullman JS, Hawryluk GW, Bell MJ, et al. Guidelines for the management of severe traumatic brain injury, fourth edition. Neurosurgery. 2017 Jan 1;80(1):6–15.

Gopinath SP, Robertson CS, Contant CF, Narayan RK, Grossman RG. Clinical evaluation of a miniature strain-gauge transducer for monitoring intracranial pressure. Neurosurgery. 1995 Jun;36(6):1137–40.

Marshall LF, Smith RW, Shapiro HM. The outcome with aggressive treatment in severe head injuries. Part I: the significance of intracranial pressure monitoring. J Neurosurg. 1979 Jan;50(1):20–5.

Miller JD, Butterworth JF, Gudeman SK, Faulkner JE, Choi SC, Selhorst JB, et al. Further experience in the management of severe head injury. J Neurosurg. 1981 Mar;54(3):289–99.

Mokri B. The Monro-Kellie hypothesis: applications in CSF volume depletion. Neurology. 2001 Jun 26;56(12):1746–8.

Muralidharan R. External ventricular drains: management and complications. Surg Neurol Int. 2015 May 25;6(Suppl 6):S271–4.

Narayan RK, Kishore PR, Becker DP, Ward JD, Enas GG, Greenberg RP, et al. Intracranial pressure: to monitor or not to monitor? A review of our experience with severe head injury. J Neurosurg. 1982 May;56(5):650–9.

Piper I. Intracranial pressure and elastance. In: Reilly P, Bullock R, editors. Head injury: pathophysiology and management. Boca Raton (FL): CRC Press; c2005. p.93–112.

Raboel PH, Bartek J Jr, Andresen M, Bellander BM, Romner B. Intracranial pressure monitoring: invasive versus non-invasive methods: a review. Crit Care Res Pract. 2012;2012:950393. Epub 2012 Jun 8.

Reinstrup P, Unnerback M, Marklund N, Schalen W, Arrocha JC, Bloomfield EL, et al. Best zero level for external ICP transducer. Acta Neurochir (Wien). 2019 Apr;161(4):635–42. Epub 2019 Mar 8.

Schickner DJ, Young RF. Intracranial pressure monitoring: fiberoptic monitor compared with the ventricular catheter. Surg Neurol. 1992 Apr;37(4):251–4.

Lumbar Puncture

CHRISTINA C. SMITH, APRN

Goals

- Review the common indications for lumbar puncture.
- Review the procedure for performing lumbar puncture.
- Review basic cerebrospinal fluid data.
- Know how to distinguish between and manage bacterial (septic) and aseptic cerebrospinal fluid disorders.

Introduction

Lumbar puncture (LP) is used in the diagnosis of neurologic disorders such as central nervous system (CNS) infections, subarachnoid hemorrhage, CNS malignancies, and demyelinating diseases. Although LP is relatively safe, patients may have minor or major complications, including headache (10%-30% risk), bleeding (2%), severe radiculopathy (15%), and nerve damage (1%). Infection after a diagnostic lumbar puncture is exceedingly rare (the risk is increased with spinal anesthesia but infection is highly uncommon).

Contraindications

Contraindications to LP include increased intracranial pressure (ICP), coagulopathies, and infection at the puncture site (eg, skin infection or spinal abscess). Suspected bacteremia is not a contraindication to LP. Antimicrobial therapy should not be held for patients who may have acute bacterial meningitis if LP cannot be performed because of a contraindication or other reason. If increased ICP is suspected, computed tomography should be performed before LP to rule out a herniation syndrome.

Anticoagulation

If a patient has a coagulopathy, thrombocytopenia should be corrected so that the platelet count exceeds 80×10^9/L or the international normalized ratio does not exceed 1.4. Before elective LP in a patient receiving systemic anticoagulation, observational studies and expert opinion have suggested that intravenous unfractionated heparin should be stopped for at least 4 hours or until the activated partial thromboplastin time is normal; low-molecular-weight heparin should be stopped for 12 to 24 hours; and warfarin, for 5 to 7 days. Apixaban, edoxaban, and rivaroxaban should be held for 48 hours. Dabigatran should be held for 48 to 96 hours depending on the patient's renal function. Antiplatelet therapy with aspirin or nonsteroidal anti-inflammatory agents is generally not associated with an increased risk of bleeding after LP. If patients are receiving dual antiplatelet therapy, the risk-benefit ratio for withholding clopidogrel for 5 days but continuing aspirin should be considered.

Procedure

1. Obtain consent from the patient or legal representative.
2. Gather sterile supplies, LP kit, chlorhexadine wipes, and local anesthesia.
3. Position the patient in a left lateral fetal position with a pillow between the knees, in a prone position (typically used when fluoroscopic guidance is needed), or in a sitting position leaning over a chair (however, opening pressure [OP] cannot be measured in this position).
4. Locate the L3-4 and L4-5 intervertebral spaces by palpation.
5. Sterilize the skin (eg, with chlorhexadine swabs).
6. Don sterile equipment, including a face mask, and set up the collection tubes and manometer.
7. Use lidocaine to anesthetize the previously identified intervertebral spaces.
8. At L4-5, slowly advance a 20- or 22-gauge spinal needle and stylet, with the bevel cephalad, parallel to the bed

Table 126.1 • Typical CSF Findings for Leukocyte Count, Glucose Level, and Protein Level in Specific Conditions

CSF Finding	Condition
Many PMNs, low glucose, high protein	Bacterial meningitis Early viral or tuberculous meningitis Parameningeal infection Septic emboli Chemical meningitis Behçet disease Mollaret meningitis
Many lymphocytes, normal glucose, high protein	Viral meningitis or encephalitis Early fungal or tuberculous meningitis Active demyelinating disease Parasitic infection Partially treated bacterial meningitis Parameningeal infection Postinfectious encephalomyelitis
Many lymphocytes, low glucose, high protein	Tuberculous meningitis Fungal meningitis Partially treated meningitis Viral meningitis Leptomeningeal metastases

Abbreviations: CSF, cerebrospinal fluid; PMN, polymorphonuclear leukocyte.

but angled toward the umbilicus (ultrasonographic guidance may be used).

a. Remove the stylet as needed to check for flow of cerebrospinal fluid (CSF).
b. If the patient feels pain or tingling in a leg, the needle may be too lateral. Withdraw the needle and change the angle as necessary. If LP is unsuccessful at L4-5, anesthetize the L3-L4 (or L2-L3) intervertebral space and repeat the procedure. Do not attempt LP at a higher intervertebral level because of the risk of spinal cord puncture.

9. When CSF flow is seen, immediately attach a manometer to measure OP (normal OP is <200 mm H_2O). If the patient's legs are straightened, measurement will be more accurate.
   a. If OP is >400 mm H_2O, the risk of brain tissue shift is increased; the stylet should be replaced and mannitol administered to the patient. When the pressure is rechecked, if OP is <400 mm H_2O, the needle may be withdrawn. CSF should not be drained.
   b. If OP is normal, the manometer is removed and CSF is collected. For diagnostic purposes the required volume is typically 8-14 mL. For therapeutic purposes or for a high-volume collection, typically 30-40 mL is removed.
10. The stylet is reinserted, and the needle is removed. An adhesive bandage is applied at the site. The patient may lie down to help relieve a postprocedural headache.

If LP is difficult, imaging guidance can be used. Fluoroscopic guidance is used for patients who have undergone previous attempts that were unsuccessful and for patients who are obese or who have had previous surgery of the spine. Most fluoroscopically guided LPs are performed in the L2-L3 or L3-L4 intervertebral space with the patient in the prone position. Ultrasonographic guidance has been used to increase the success rate and decrease the risk of traumatic LP.

The most common complication of LP is postprocedural headache, which is typically positional (worse with standing). Another LP in the same region and injection of a small amount (20-30 mL) of the patient's venous blood is often immediately successful.

Interpretation of Results

Examination of the CSF often provides critical diagnostic information for infectious and noninfectious conditions (Tables 126.1 and 126.2). Examination should include at least a cell count and differential, glucose and protein levels, Gram stain, and culture. Knowledge of normal CSF values is critical for interpretation of the results. In adults, the normal CSF volume is 125 to 150 mL. Approximately 20% of the CSF volume is in the ventricles, and the remainder is in the subarachnoid space and spinal cord. The normal rate of CSF production is approximately 20 mL/h. CSF is typically acellular, but in adults it may normally contain up to 5 leukocytes/mcL and 5 erythrocytes/mcL. More than 3 polymorphonuclear leukocytes/mcL is abnormal in adults.

Summary

- LP is generally a safe procedure.
- LP cannot be performed in patients who have a mass or noncommunicating hydrocephalus, thrombocytopenia or other bleeding diathesis, lingering effects of anticoagulant therapy, or a possible spinal epidural abscess.
- Headache after LP can be successfully treated with a blood patch.

Table 126.2 • Diagnostic CSF Findings in Various Conditions

Condition	Opening Pressure, mm H_2O	Appearance	Cells/mcL	Protein, mg/dL	Glucose, mg/dL	Miscellaneous
Normal	60-200	Clear and colorless	0 PMNs 0 RBCs <5 monos	15-45	40-85	Lymphs 100 cells/mcL
Acute meningitis	Normal or increased	Turbid	>100 WBCs (mostly PMNs)	100-1,000	<40	Rapid antigen test: positive results
Viral meningoencephalitis	Normal	Normal	10-350 WBCs (mostly monos)	40-100	Normal	PMNs early
Guillain-Barré syndrome	Normal	Normal	Normal (≤100 monos)	50-1,000	Normal	Protein level is normal in early stages of disease
Tuberculous meningitis	Normal	Cloudy Clots on standing	50-500 lymphs and monos	60-700	<40	AFB culture and stain: positive results
Fungal meningitis	Normal or increased	Cloudy	30-300 monos (PMNs early)	100-700	<40	India ink preparation: positive results
Herpes simplex encephalitis	Normal or increased	Bloody	Increased monos and RBCs	High	Normal or low	PCR for antigen
Parameningeal infection	Increased	Normal	0-800 WBCs	High	Normal	Epidural abscess
Traumatic lumbar puncture	Normal	Bloody No xanthochromia	RBC:WBC ratio like in blood	Slightly increased	Normal	Less blood in subsequent tubes
Subarachnoid hemorrhage	Increased	Bloody Xanthochromia	RBC:WBC ratio 100:1	50-800	Normal	RBCs are present for about 2 wk
Multiple sclerosis	Normal	Normal	5-50 monos	Normal to 800	Normal	Oligoclonal IgG
Neurosyphilis	Normal	Normal	0-300 (various types)	High	Normal	Oligoclonal IgG antibodies to *Treponema*
Leptomeningeal metastasis	Normal	Typically normal	0-500 (various types)	Normal or increased	Normal	Cytologic evidence of tumor in 50% of patients
Pseudotumor cerebri	250-500	Normal	Normal	Normal	Normal	Perform high-volume lumbar puncture
Toxoplasmosis	Normal	Normal	Normal or elevated	Increased	Normal	CSF is often normal

Abbreviations: AFB, acid-fast bacilli; CSF, cerebrospinal fluid; Ig, immunoglobulin; lymph, lymphocyte; mono, monocyte; PCR, polymerase chain reaction; PMN, polymorphonuclear leukocyte; RBC, red blood cell; WBC, white blood cell.

SUGGESTED READING

Agrawal D. Lumbar puncture. N Engl J Med. 2007 Jan 25;356(4):424.

Costerus JM, Brouwer MC, van de Beek D. Technological advances and changing indications for lumbar puncture in neurological disorders. Lancet Neurol. 2018 Mar;17(3):268–78.

Greenberg MS, editor. Handbook of neurosurgery. 7th ed. Tampa (FL): Greenberg Graphics; New York (NY): Thieme Medical Publishers; c2010.

Layton KF, Kallmes DF, Horlocker TT. Recommendations for anticoagulated patients undergoing image-guided spinal procedures. AJNR Am J Neuroradiol. 2006 Mar;27(3):468–70.

Millington SJ, Silva Restrepo M, Koenig S. Better with ultrasound: lumbar puncture. Chest. 2018 Nov;154(5):1223–9. Epub 2018 Jul 20.

Quincke HI. Lumbar puncture. In: Church A, editor. Diseases of the nervous system. New York (NY): D. Appleton; c1910. p. 223.

Ruff RL, Dougherty JH Jr. Complications of lumbar puncture followed by anticoagulation. Stroke. 1981 Nov-Dec;12(6):879–81.

Shaikh F, Brzezinski J, Alexander S, Arzola C, Carvalho JC, Beyene J, et al. Ultrasound imaging for lumbar punctures and epidural catheterisations: systematic review and meta-analysis. BMJ. 2013 Mar 26;346: f1720.

Lumbar Drain

JAMIE J. VAN GOMPEL, MD

Goals

- Describe the indications, risks, and benefits of a lumbar drain.
- Describe the surgical procedure of lumbar drain placement.
- Describe the complications of lumbar drain placement.

Introduction

Lumbar drainage has a major role in neurosurgical and neurocritical care procedures. Lumbar drain insertion is a simple and, when done well, low-risk procedure. A lumbar drain is often necessary in the management of perioperative cerebrospinal fluid (CSF) leaks, the most common use, but it may be beneficial for patients with subarachnoid hemorrhage and communicating hydrocephalus and for patients undergoing surgery involving the aorta with possible damage to the spinal cord. CSF removal optimizes spinal cord blood flow. The rate of CSF leakage after endoscopic endonasal surgery has been reduced to 2% to 3%. The role of perioperative lumbar drainage in preventing this complication is controversial, with little evidence of its effect. However, insertion of lumbar drains in patients is not to be taken lightly. Serious complications can occur. This chapter describes lumbar drain insertion and some of the associated perils and pitfalls.

Technique

An important practical point is to know whether the patient will be conscious or sedated during the procedure. The risk of nerve root injury or epidural lumbar hematoma may be increased in a sedated patient. Most awake patients (other than pediatric patients) tolerate the procedure well with local infusion of lidocaine anesthetic (or other local anesthetic of choice), but the patient's level of associated pain and anxiety must be gauged. If a patient is anxious, conscious sedation may be useful for needle insertion, and performing the procedure in an operating room with an anesthesiologist's help may be beneficial.

Local anesthetic (approximately 3-5 mL) should be given at the point of entry. Time is allowed for infiltration, and then a long needle is used so the injection reaches the bone. Pain is sensed from bone, including the periosteum, so the space around the bone needs to be infiltrated without infiltrating beyond the bone. Awake patients experience pain when the dura is transgressed, and this should be anticipated by the person performing the procedure. In patients who are asleep, the procedure is relatively straightforward, and local anesthetic is not necessary.

The recommended position for placing lumbar drains is the left or right lateral decubitus position with the patient's knees tucked up as in a fetal position. A sitting position can be used if the patient's anatomy poses challenges, and fluoroscopy performed in an interventional radiology suite may be helpful if patients are older or have calcification of the posterior longitudinal ligament or dystrophic calcifications between the bones. Fluoroscopy is difficult with the patient in a lateral decubitus position, so it is often performed with the patient lying face down on the table. In this prone position, procedure time is important because of the patient's discomfort in the prone position while awake.

Two aspects of needle insertion are noteworthy. First, if the drain is being placed for long-term use, the distance in which the needle transgresses through soft tissue should be maximized. The soft tissue then acts like a gasket seal around the drain tubing to prevent CSF leaks around the drain itself. Furthermore, passing the tubing is difficult if it is perpendicular to the thecal sac; therefore, the entry point should be below the usual entry point. A common target is L3-4, but L2-3 is safe and often less deep in obese patients. For orientation, the L2 and L3 vertebrae can be palpated; typically, the iliac crest is palpated at the level of the

L4-5 interspace. The needle can be inserted here or at L3-4 or L2-3.

Second, although a common practice is to place 2 fingers on the spinous processes and insert the needle between them, a paramedian approach that is 10° to 15° from the midline (to the right or left, depending on the operator's handedness) is useful (Figure 127.1). This approach avoids the spinous processes, maximizes the shingled entrance in the laminar space, provides more tissue laxity for improving the seal around the catheter, and facilitates identification of the lamina and palpation with the needle. A good starting point is 1 cm inferior and 1 cm lateral to the lower aspect of the adjacent spinous process.

Typically, rather than starting with a Touhy needle, which is a large-bore needle with an angled open-bore tip and a catheter that is commonly threaded into the thecal space, a smaller 18- or 22-gauge needle is used first to find a trajectory in the approach. This smaller needle is often left in place while the trajectory is followed with the Touhy needle. The smaller needle also serves as an excellent marker for the depth into the thecal sac.

The Touhy needle is beveled with a large inner stylet, which should remain within the needle as the needle is advanced. Typically, the opening in the needle should be placed laterally until it is passed into the space and then turned superiorly to allow the catheter to pass cephalad within the thecal sac. With either the Touhy needle or a smaller lumbar puncture needle, the needle is passed through the skin and the lamina is felt; typically, the needle is stepped down by repositioning it and feeling the back side of the lamina, so that the needle can be slid under the lamina.

When the needle has entered the space, the posterior longitudinal ligament presents resistance, which often decreases as the needle enters the thecal space. When the large Touhy needle penetrates the space, it must frequently be advanced to the anterior aspect of the canal so that the entire needle tip is in the thecal sac. The inner stylet is then withdrawn, and CSF should flow. If CSF does not flow, or if the fluid is bloody, the needle should be redirected. A new trajectory usually requires a pronounced withdrawal of the needle through the soft tissue rather than simply making subtle movements, which do not change the needle

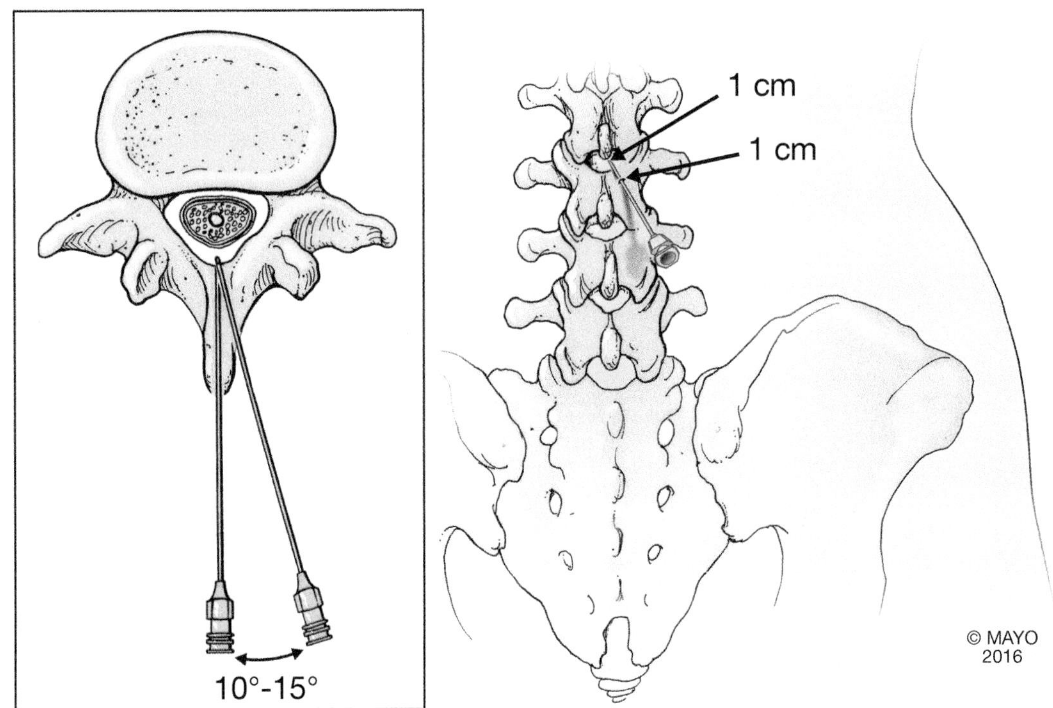

Figure 127.1. Paramedian Needle Insertion for Lumbar Puncture. The needle is introduced 10° to 15° off midline (inset shows vertebra in horizontal plane) and inserted at the disk space 1 cm inferior and 1 cm lateral to the lower aspect of the spinous process to improve the seal around the catheter.

(From Naveen N, Wong, CA. Spinal, epidural, and caudal anesthesia: anatomy, physiology, and technique. In: Chestnut's Obstetric Anesthesia: principles and practice. 5th ed. Philadelphia: Elsevier Saunders; 2015. p.229-60; used with permission of Mayo Foundation for Medical Education and Research.)

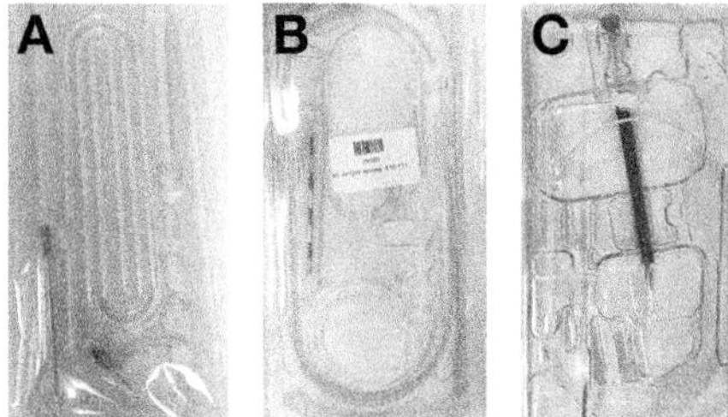

Figure 127.2. Lumbar Drains. A-C, Examples are shown from 3 manufacturers.

trajectory enough. When the needle has passed successfully into the thecal space and the CSF return is good, as much CSF should be left in the space as possible to aid in floating the soft catheter. In patients who have CSF hypotension syndrome caused by leaks elsewhere in the spine or skull base, it is sometimes difficult to achieve CSF return. Those patients should be placed in the reverse Trendelenburg position, or a small amount of fluid can be injected into the needle to confirm that the space has been entered. When the Touhy needle is within the space, it must be rotated so that the open-bore aspect is directed cephalad.

The catheter can be inserted with or without the inner stylet, which is a wire. If the inner stylet is used, it allows the distal tip of the catheter to pass more easily and it protects the catheter from the sharp edges of the Touhy needle if the catheter is in the epidural space during a retrieval attempt. Regardless, some people choose to pass the drainage tubing without the inner stylet and are successful.

Typically, black markings indicate the 10 to 20 cm of the distal catheter to be placed within the thecal sac. However the markings vary with the type of catheter; in the US market, 3 types are available (Figure 127.2). The catheter is held in place with 1 hand, while the introducing Touhy needle is pulled out slowly to avoid withdrawing too much of the catheter. The catheter is usually secured or held gently at the skin while the inner stylet is slowly withdrawn (pinching the catheter must be avoided because it hinders withdrawal). After the needle has been withdrawn and CSF return is confirmed, the catheter is secured. The catheter should pass easily. If the catheter is difficult to pass, it should not be forced. Instead, the needle may be repositioned; sometimes simply withdrawing it slightly is sufficient to allow the catheter to pass within the thecal space without difficulty.

When the inner stylet has been removed and good CSF return has been confirmed, the distal adapter is attached and it may be connected to a 10-mL syringe. A small tension-relief holder is then sutured to the skin. If a small aspect is left loose and close to the skin, a purse-string suture can be placed around the catheter to prevent CSF leakage around the catheter. All white or soft silicone portions of the catheter should be covered by a large transparent film dressing, which is typically wrapped twice around the patient, with the connection between the distal adapter to the intravenous (IV) tubing secured to the side so the patient does do not lie on it (Figure 127.3).

A good practice is to wrap transparent film dressing around the relatively strong IV tubing ("umbilicating" it) because if any white (silicone) portion of the catheter is left exposed, it may tear and cause complications. Even a small invisible tear in the catheter will allow CSF to leak onto the bed and cause substantial CSF hypotension within the head and permanent headaches while draining (Figure 127.4).

Drainage Management

Volume-driven drainage is typical. For example, CSF may be drained at 10 mL every 2 hours. A drainage rate of 20

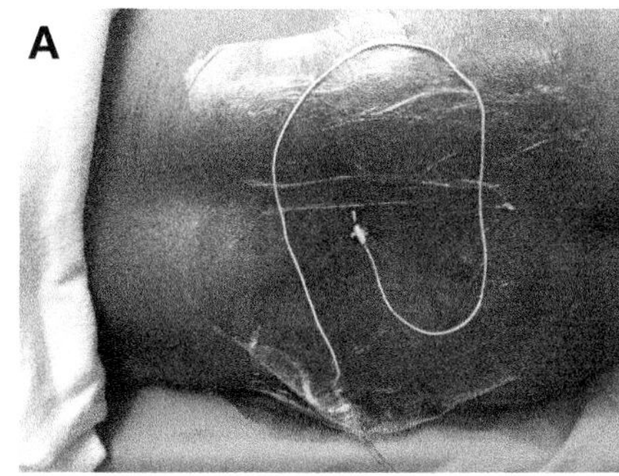

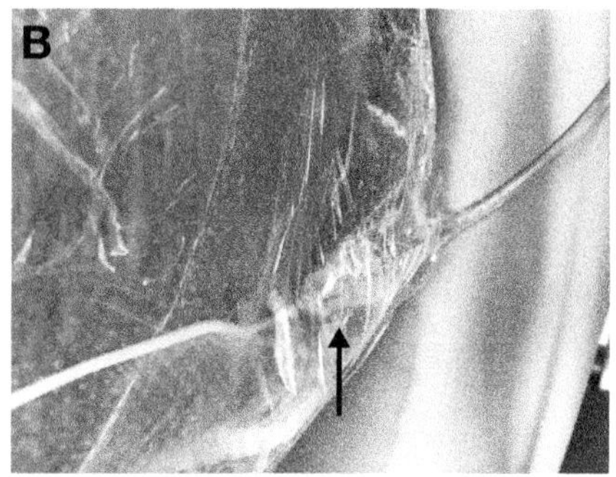

Figure 127.3. Well-Positioned Lumbar Drain. A, The soft silicone portion of the lumbar drain is completely covered with a large transparent film dressing with a loop designed for strain relief in case tension is accidentally applied to the catheter. A purse-string skin suture is placed around the entry point of the catheter. To prevent tearing, all the white (silicone) tubing must be protected under a dressing. B, The intravenous tubing is attached to the proximal catheter where the patient will not lie on it. The tubing is umbilicated (arrow) (ie, the dressing is wrapped around the tubing to prevent breakage of the proximal catheter), allowing patient movement and minimizing skin traction to improve patient comfort.

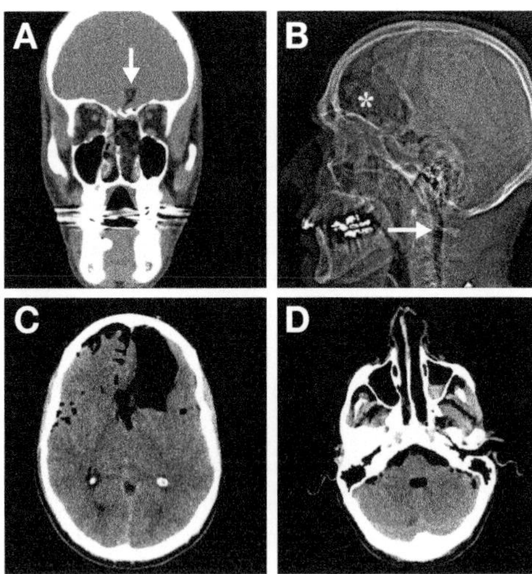

Figure 127.4. Pneumocephalus From Torn Catheter. A, Postoperative radiograph after a large encephalocele was resected and the skull base was reconstructed shows a small amount of fat (arrow) at the site with no pneumocephalus. Overnight a small invisible tear in the white silicone portion of the catheter allowed complete drainage of the intracranial cerebrospinal fluid and caused the patient to become comatose. B, Scout film for computed tomography (CT) shows a substantial frontal pneumocephalus (asterisk) and air down the spinal column (arrow). C and D, Axial CT images show tension pneumocephalus compression in the frontal lobes, in front of the brainstem, and in the fourth ventricle.

mL every 2 hours would be considered aggressive. Unlike an external ventricular drain (EVD) at the level of the external auditory meatus, a lumbar drain catheter carries CSF with a pressure of at least 10 cm H_2O because of resistance from the long, narrow tubing. If a patient has positional headaches, the drainage rate can be decreased. While the catheter is in place, patients may be given antibiotics such as cefepime and vancomycin for multidrug-resistant bacteria or cefazolin or vancomycin for skin flora.

Some drainage chambers limit the amount of drainage to a preset amount from 10 to 30 mL, which decreases the likelihood of an unmanaged open drain and substantial overdrainage. Similarly, pressure-driven drainage can use an EVD kit zeroed at the tragus, so that CSF can drain at 5 or 10 mm Hg when the kit is positioned above the tragus and be clamped if a maximum rate (eg, 5 or 10 mL/h) has been reached. This method may be easier for facilitating CSF drainage (like with an EVD).

Care After Lumbar Drain Removal

When the drain is removed, a single simple suture is typically placed with fast-absorbing chromic suture. Antibiotics can be discontinued when the drain is removed. The drain should be inspected for breakage. If it has broken, attempting to retrieve it is not recommended, but the patient should be advised that a retained object may be present. Patients may have positional headaches from a persistent fistula leaking CSF into the extrathecal space. These headaches are more common after lumbar drain placement than after simple lumbar puncture, but the rate is unknown. If the patient can tolerate these positional headaches, the headaches may be allowed to persist from 3 to 7 days. If they continue longer, a blood patch may help alleviate the symptoms. Infrequently, a patient needs another blood patch or a directed fibrin glue treatment. In extreme circumstances of persistent positional headaches, open surgical repair of the fistula may be necessary.

Summary

- All the white (soft silicone) portions of the catheter must be protected under a transparent film dressing.
- Patients must be monitored closely, especially for headaches and new neurologic symptoms, although they may not require an intensive care unit. Their symptoms should be monitored.
- After the drain is removed, 1 suture should be placed because patients may have CSF leakage from the incision.
- If excessive drainage occurs around the catheter, it should be removed or replaced because the leak, especially leaks anterior to the skull base or temporal bone, may indicate that a 1-way valve is allowing air into the intracranial space, and these patients can become comatose (Figure 127.4).
- Lumbar drains can be dangerous, and CSF leakage around the catheter predisposes patients to further infection; subtle leaks may be repaired with skin adhesive or fibrin sealant.

SUGGESTED READING

Caggiano C, Penn DL, Laws ER Jr. The role of the lumbar drain in endoscopic endonasal skull base surgery: a retrospective analysis of 811 cases. World Neurosurg. 2018 Sep;117:e575–9. Epub 2018 Jun 20.

Epstein NE. Cerebrospinal fluid drains reduce risk of spinal cord injury for thoracic/thoracoabdominal aneurysm surgery: a review. Surg Neurol Int. 2018 Feb 23;9:48.

Fedorow CA, Moon MC, Mutch WA, Grocott HP. Lumbar cerebrospinal fluid drainage for thoracoabdominal aortic surgery: rationale and practical considerations for management. Anesth Analg. 2010 Jul;111(1):46–58. Epub 2010 Jun 3.

Panni P, Donofrio CA, Barzaghi LR, Giudice L, Albano L, Righi C, et al. Safety and feasibility of lumbar drainage in the management of poor grade aneurysmal subarachnoid hemorrhage. J Clin Neurosci. 2019 Apr 22. pii:S0967-5868(18)31838-1. [Epub ahead of print]

Panni P, Fugate JE, Rabinstein AA, Lanzino G. Lumbar drainage and delayed cerebral ischemia in aneurysmal subarachnoid hemorrhage: a systematic review. J Neurosurg Sci. 2017 Dec;61(6):665–72. Epub 2015 Feb 4.

Ringel B, Carmel-Neiderman NN, Peri A, Ben Ner D, Safadi A, Abergel A, et al. Continuous lumbar drainage and the postoperative complication rate of open anterior skull base surgery. Laryngoscope. 2018 Sep 8. [Epub ahead of print].

Stokken J, Recinos PF, Woodard T, Sindwani R. The utility of lumbar drains in modern endoscopic skull base surgery. Curr Opin Otolaryngol Head Neck Surg. 2015 Feb;23(1):78–82.

Wolf S. Rationale for lumbar drains in aneurysmal subarachnoid hemorrhage. Curr Opin Crit Care. 2015 Apr;21(2):120–6.

Intraventricular Drug Administration

WILLIAM W. HORN JR, APRN; BENJAMIN L. BROWN, MD

Goals

- Know the indications for sterile intraventricular drug administration.
- Review the procedure of intraventricular drug administration.
- Review the risks, benefits, and complications of intraventricular drug administration.

Introduction

The blood-brain barrier prevents many medications from reaching brain tissue, and the intraventricular (IVT) route can be a useful alternative in appropriate situations. The administration of medications through extraventricular drains requires expertise. Permanently placed catheters such as Ommaya reservoirs can also be used for medication administration. These devices should be handled according to the manufacturer's recommendations to avoid damaging them. Many hospitals have practice protocols. Some guidelines on the procedure alone are provided below.

Indications

The most common indications for IVT delivery of medications are lysing a ventricular hematoma, treating cerebral vasospasm, treating ventriculitis, and administering intrathecal chemotherapy.

Preparation

When the IVT route is used appropriately, the risk of complications is 0% to 6%. The most recent computed tomographic (CT) scan of the patient's brain should be reviewed to determine the location of the catheter fenestrations. If the most recent CT scan is older than 48 to 72 hours, and if an IVT catheter was placed urgently, another CT scan should be performed to verify catheter tip placement. For long-term use of Ommaya reservoirs and catheters, repeating the CT scan may not be necessary unless the patient has undergone a surgical adjustment or the intracranial part of the catheter has been replaced. In optimal conditions, all the ventricular tip fenestrations are within the ventricle.

Inadequately or poorly placed ventricular catheters may prevent withdrawal of cerebrospinal fluid (CSF) or administration of medications and can result in hemorrhage along the catheter tract. Catheters that do not drain well can be assessed for external obstructions to the system. Sutures, staples, and other items used for fixation can kink the catheter and make CSF removal and medication administration difficult.

The use of isovolemic sterile technique is absolutely critical to avoid increasing the patient's intracranial pressure. With *isovolemic* technique, the volume to be injected intracranially should be the same as the volume of CSF withdrawn before the drug and flushing solution are injected. Most medications are reconstituted in less than 5 mL of sterile, preservative-free normal saline. Use of the proximal port of a drainage system requires 1 to 2 mL of flushing solution to fully clear the catheter and ensure that all the medication reaches the ventricular system. After the medication has been administered, the intracranial pressure and the patient's clinical status must be closely monitored.

Procedure

Necessary supplies include sterile attire (ie, hat, mask, gown, and gloves), preservative-free saline for flushing, two 3-way stopcocks, two 10-mL and one 5-mL syringes, sterile towels, and chlorhexidine swabs or an institution-specific disinfectant.

The injection port can be turned off to the drainage system while supplies are gathered and CSF is allowed to build up. The sterile towel pack is opened first, and the remaining sterile items are placed in the sterile field.

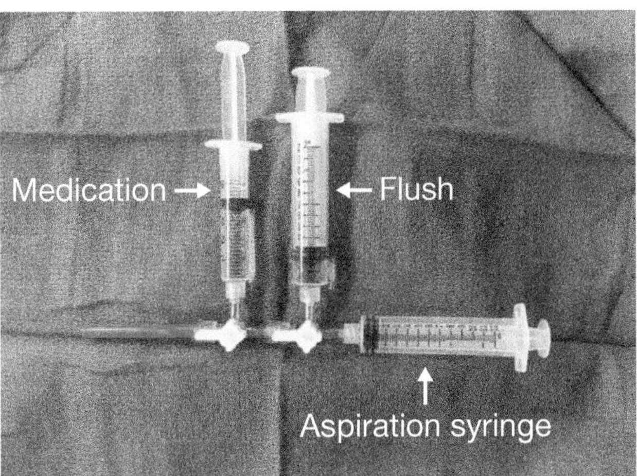

Figure 128.1. Apparatus for 2-Stopcock Method for Administration of Medication Into an Intraventricular Catheter.

The proceduralist, in sterile attire, assembles the injection apparatus. An assistant helps the proceduralist by drawing up the preservative-free saline flush and the medication to be administered (into a 5-mL sterile syringe if the volume permits). Use of different sizes of syringes helps to prevent confusion during administration. The 2 stopcocks should be connected to each other with an empty 10-mL syringe at the distal portion of the apparatus parallel to the medication syringe; the syringe containing the flushing solution should be placed on the other port of the distal stopcock (Figure 128.1). The medication to be administered should be placed at the closest port to the injection site.

After the administration apparatus has been assembled, a sterile field can be created with towels around the proximal injection port. After the sterile field has been created and the catheter port has been sterilized, the entire system can be connected to the drain port. The closest port to the brain should be used. After the ventricular system port is accessed, an amount of CSF equivalent to the total to be administered should be gently withdrawn. The stopcock is then opened to the medication syringe, and the medication is gently administered over several seconds. When the medication has been injected, the stopcock can be opened to the flushing syringe, and 2 mL of flushing solution can be gently injected to flush the medicine into the ventricle. The apparatus can then be removed. The system should remain closed for 1 hour for external ventricular catheters; the intracranial pressure is monitored, and the system is opened if the sustained pressure is greater than 20 mm Hg. If the patient has low pressure and the concern about the loss of medication is small, the drainage system can remain open at a pressure of 5 to 10 mm Hg higher than the original setting. Elevated pressures and the need to open the system require further attention. Patients with an Ommaya reservoir, which is an indwelling closed system, are monitored for headache and other clinical signs.

Complications

If any resistance to injection or aspiration is encountered during the process, the procedure should be stopped and the ventricular catheter assessed. Injury to healthy brain tissue must be avoided. A change in the patient's mental status or an increase in bloody drainage from the catheter should prompt an immediate neurologic reassessment and additional CT imaging. If fever develops in a patient while an extraventricular drain is in place, the patient should undergo a full diagnostic workup, including CSF sampling.

Summary

- Various medications can be administered through an external ventricular drain and an Ommaya reservoir.
- Sterile technique is critical in accessing an external ventricular drain or Ommaya system.
- With isovolemic drug administration, a specific volume of CSF is removed before a similar volume of drug is injected intracranially.

SUGGESTED READING

Calias P, Banks WA, Begley D, Scarpa M, Dickson P. Intrathecal delivery of protein therapeutics to the brain: a critical reassessment. Pharmacol Ther. 2014 Nov;144(2):114–22. Epub 2014 May 20.

Dabus G, Nogueira RG. Current options for the management of aneurysmal subarachnoid hemorrhage-induced cerebral vasospasm: a comprehensive review of the literature. Interv Neurol. 2013 Oct;2(1):30–51.

Dodson V, Majmundar N, El-Ghanem M, Amuluru K, Gupta G, Nuoman R, et al. Intracranial administration of nicardipine after aneurysmal subarachnoid hemorrhage: a review of the literature. World Neurosurg. 2019 Jan 29. pii:S1878-8750(19)30201-3. [Epub ahead of print]

Jones J, Schweder P, Drummond KJ, Kaye AH. Use of tissue plasminogen activator in the treatment of shunt blockage secondary to intraventricular haemorrhage. J Clin Neurosci. 2016 Dec;34:281–2. Epub 2016 Aug 10.

Transcranial Doppler Ultrasonography

MARK N. RUBIN, MD

Goals

- Review the physics of transcranial Doppler ultrasonography.
- Review the basic clinical applications of transcranial Doppler ultrasonography in intensive care unit and neuroscience intensive care unit emergencies.

Introduction

Transcranial Doppler (TCD) ultrasonography is a diagnostic technology for ascertaining numerous physiologic and pathologic phenomena by monitoring the direction and velocity of blood flow in intracranial vasculature. It is a noninvasive, point-of-care diagnostic tool that provides continuous and reproducible bedside data without the use of ionizing radiation. TCD ultrasonography involves holding an ultrasound probe over certain areas ("windows") around the skull best suited to provide adequate signals and information on blood velocity and direction of flow according to measured Doppler frequency shifts. The 2 types of probes are a 2-MHz "blind" probe for Doppler-only analysis and a multirange imaging probe for a transcranial color-coded duplex (TCCD) study.

From established patterns of normal and abnormal blood flow velocity and direction, these seemingly simple data are used in the intensive care unit (ICU) to noninvasively diagnose conditions such as the following: stenosis, occlusion, dissection, collateralization, hyperemia, cerebrovascular resistance, autoregulatory function, vasomotor reactivity, and microemboli. The most common indication for TCD or TCCD is vasospasm monitoring after aneurysmal subarachnoid hemorrhage (SAH). TCD correlates well with angiographic vasospasm in a middle cerebral artery (MCA). Additional common uses include diagnosis of cerebral circulatory arrest as a diagnostic adjunct to the clinical diagnosis of brain death, vascular changes from diffuse cerebral edema and dysautonomia after traumatic brain injury (TBI), and thrombosis localization in acute ischemic stroke (AIS). Other promising indications that require more investigation include monitoring for AIS thrombolysis, identifying vasomotor reactivity as a biologic marker of injury and recovery, and localizing epilepsy. (In this chapter, *TCD* refers to all TCD ultrasonography [eg, TCD and TCCD] unless otherwise specified.)

Pertinent Physics and Intracranial Hemodynamics

The *Doppler effect* is the shift in frequency emitted by a source moving in relation to an observer as perceived by the observer. The shift is to higher frequencies when the distance between the source and the observer decreases and to lower frequencies when the distance increases. In TCD, the source is a red blood cell reflecting an echo, and the observer is the ultrasound probe.

TCD instruments are generally calibrated to measure blood flow velocity when blood is moving either directly toward the ultrasound probe (0°) or directly away from it (180°). This principle is important because if insonation is at an angle other than 0° or 180°, only a fraction of the true velocity is measured.

Certain areas on and around the skull (*windows of insonation*) help the operator achieve insonation directly in line with blood flow and avoid signal attenuation from the skull and other tissue (Figure 129.1). The windows and the arteries that are examined at those windows are as follows:

- Transtemporal window: MCA, anterior cerebral artery (ACA), terminal portion of the internal carotid artery (ICA), and posterior cerebral artery (PCA).
- Transorbital (ophthalmic) window: ophthalmic artery and ICA at the siphon level.

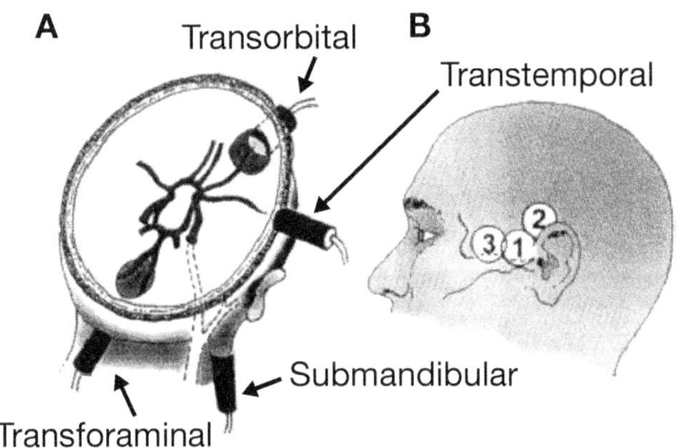

Figure 129.1. Transcranial Windows of Insonation. A, Probes are shown at 4 windows: transorbital, transtemporal, submandibular, and transforaminal. B, The transtemporal window has 3 aspects: middle (1), posterior (2), and anterior (3). (From Alexandrov AV, Rubiera M, Palazzo P, Neumyer MM. Intracranial cerebrovascular ultrasound examination techniques. In: Alexandrov AV, editor. Cerebrovascular ultrasound in stroke prevention and treatment. 2nd ed. West Sussex [UK]: Wiley-Blackwell; c2011. p. 13–25; used with permission.)

- Submandibular window: distal portion of the extracranial ICA.
- Transforaminal (occipital) window: basilar artery (BA) and vertebral artery (VA).

An understanding of intracranial hemodynamics, including relevant anatomy, physiology, and pathophysiology, is required in order to accurately obtain and interpret intracranial Doppler data. The typical vascular distributions and the myriad factors that can affect cerebral blood flow must be understood. The cerebral vasculature has mechanisms that compensate for changes in blood viscosity and cardiac output and keep cerebral blood flow (and cerebral blood flow velocity as measured with TCD) relatively constant; however, extreme rheologic changes or cardiac output changes will affect cerebral blood flow. For example, in larger arteries, plaque alters blood flow velocity. In smaller arteries, various precipitants (eg, arterial carbon dioxide, intracranial pressure [ICP], and mean arterial pressure [MAP]) alter the flow, and the upstream effects can be inferred from TCD.

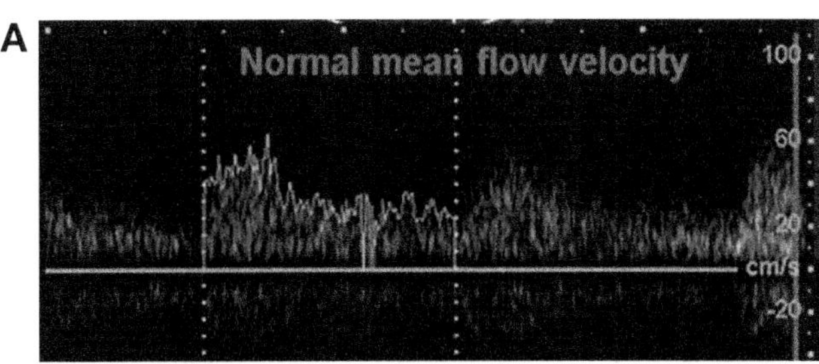

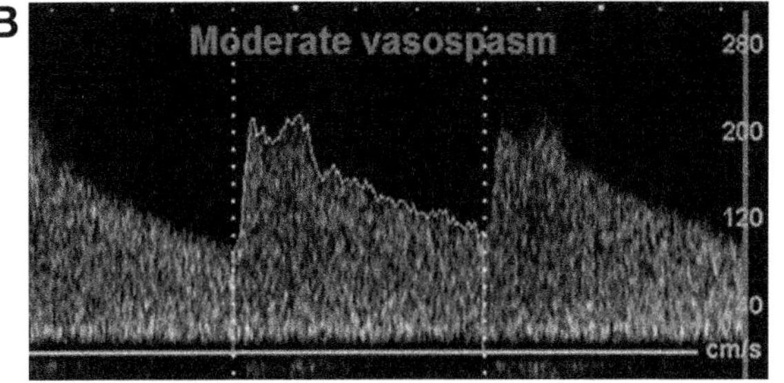

Figure 129.2. Transcranial Doppler Ultrasonograpy for Measurement of Blood Flow Velocity. A, Normal mean flow velocity. B, Moderate vasospasm.

Use of TCD in the ICU

Many normal physiologic and pathophysiologic states, including the common ones described below, can be inferred from TCD in a noninvasive manner at the bedside and can be of great value to the neurointensivist. The following conditions are not a comprehensive list, though, because any intracranial or systemic process that might affect cerebral blood flow may have a useful TCD biomarker.

Vasospasm After Aneurysmal SAH

TCD correlates well with angiographic vasospasm but not necessarily with symptomatic vasospasm (ie, clinical deficits). TCD is useful for measurement of blood flow velocity in all vessels in the circle of Willis, but especially for the MCA (Figure 129.2).

Trends in the baseline TCD mean flow velocity (MFV) over time in patients with SAH are recommended for screening for vasospasm. MFV is most sensitive and specific for angiographic vasospasm in the MCA, whereas it is less sensitive and specific for the first segments of the ACA and PCA.

The Lindegaard ratio (or the hemispheric ratio) is the ratio of the MCA flow velocity to the ipsilateral ICA flow velocity. The ratio is often used in conjunction with MCA MFV and accounts for hemodynamic augmentation from a hyperdynamic state (eg, from pressors or an endogenous hypersympathetic state). A Lindegaard ratio less than 3 suggests a hyperdynamic state with potential relative vasospasm as defined according to the MCA MFV (MCA MFV >120 cm/s indicates mild vasospasm; >150 cm/s, moderate; and >200 cm/s, severe). A Lindegaard ratio greater than 3 typically correlates with angiographic vasospasm seen on computed tomographic angiography (CTA) (>180 cm/s with perfusion impairment); a ratio greater than 6 indicates a high-grade angiographic spasm that may warrant an endovascular neurosurgery consultation.

Many confounders are related to the systemic illness associated with aneurysmal SAH: increased ICP, hemodynamic

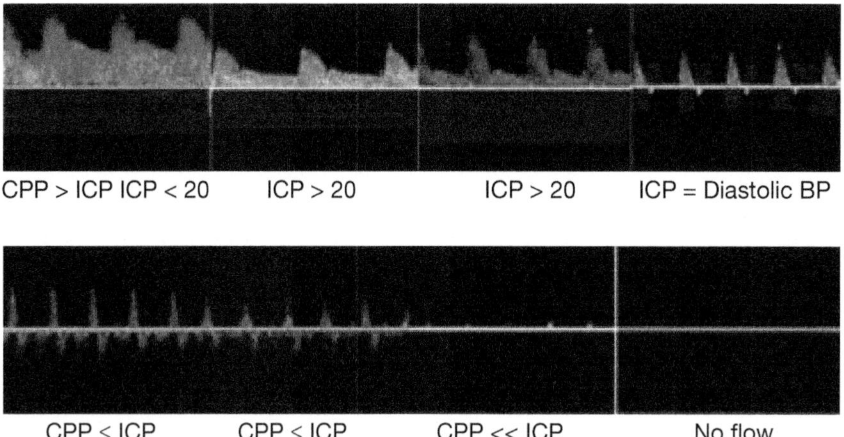

Figure 129.3. Cerebral Circulatory Arrest. Initially the cerebral perfusion pressure (CPP) exceeds the intracranial pressure (ICP). The ICP progressively increases, exceeding the diastolic blood pressure (BP) and the CPP, and then greatly exceeds the CPP such that no blood flow occurs. Units of measure for ICP are millimeters of mercury.

(From Tsivgoulis G, Neumyer MM, Alexandrov AV. Diagnostic criteria for cerebrovascular ultrasound. In: Alexandrov AV, editor. Cerebrovascular ultrasound in stroke prevention and treatment. 2nd ed. West Sussex [UK]: Wiley-Blackwell; c2011. p. 87–143; used with permission.)

instability, changes in Pa_{CO_2} or hematocrit, and collateralization. With established normative data, TCD can be used to compare extracranial and intracranial flow velocities to help localize an intracranial stenosis as distinguished from a hyperdynamic state that is increasing the blood flow velocity (Lindegaard ratio = MCA flow velocity/distal extracranial ICA flow velocity; Soustiel ratio = BA flow velocity/distal extracranial VA flow velocity). Velocity trends are checked in each vessel daily and correlated with symptoms or radiographic spasm as a noninvasive means of investigating the "spasm window." Velocities usually increase in the first 3 days after bleeding and decrease at 9 to 14 days.

Cerebral Circulatory Arrest

TCD can be used as ancillary testing to support a clinical suspicion for brain death, particularly with confounding factors (eg, an inability to perform an apnea test). Extremely elevated ICP forces arterial blood out. When ICP first exceeds diastolic flow, a characteristically peaked arterial waveform from systolic-only flow is present. Progressively increasing ICP eventually exceeds systolic pressure, resulting in a reverberating (oscillatory) column of blood and eventually no flow. Serial testing shows progression of the disease from normal to high resistance to oscillatory and, finally, to the absence of intracranial flow. If no flow is detected in the first TCD examination, the study is nondiagnostic because the absence of a signal may be from the absence of windows rather than from the absence of flow (Figure 129.3).

Traumatic Brain Injury

TBI is a major cause of progressive cerebral edema that leads to cerebral circulatory arrest and brain death. Along that spectrum of pathophysiologic changes, short of complete cerebral circulatory arrest, TCD can be used to monitor changes in patients with TBI. After the initial TBI, neurologic decline is often attributed to ischemia from low brain perfusion that results from a mismatch between demand and flow. TBI management hinges on optimizing real-time cerebral blood flow; however, the definition of *optimal* cerebral blood flow is controversial. Several methods have been used to estimate cerebral blood flow: Jugular venous oxygen, brain tissue oxygenation, and microdialysis are invasive surrogates of cerebral blood flow, and near-infrared spectroscopy is regional and has poor penetration into deeper areas of the brain.

The use of TCD to measure cerebral blood flow may be helpful for decisions related to management or prognosis. A *low-flow state* is defined as low overall MFV and peaked waveform of systolic-only flow with progression to cerebral circulatory arrest. Comatose patients with TBI and a low-flow state have a poor prognosis, and comatose patients without a low-flow state have a relatively good prognosis. Intracranial autoregulatory function is thought to be abnormal after TBI, and active research is investigating multimodal monitoring, including TCD, MAP, ICP, and other physiologic parameters that can help calculate a patient-specific optimal cerebral perfusion pressure.

Summary

- TCD is a noninvasive, bedside clinical procedure for detection of blood flow in the proximal cerebral intracranial arteries.
- In patients with SAH, TCD MFV trends are useful for screening for vasospasm; a high MCA MFV (>180 cm/s) and a high Lindegaard ratio (>3) correlate with

angiographic vasospasm, which occurs in up to two-thirds of patients (symptomatic vasospasm may occur with or without TCD evidence).

SUGGESTED READING

Aaslid R, Markwalder TM, Nornes H. Noninvasive transcranial Doppler ultrasound recording of flow velocity in basal cerebral arteries. J Neurosurg. 1982 Dec;57(6):769–74.

Alexandrov AV, Demchuk AM, Felberg RA, Christou I, Barber PA, Burgin WS, et al. High rate of complete recanalization and dramatic clinical recovery during tPA infusion when continuously monitored with 2-MHz transcranial Doppler monitoring. Stroke. 2000 Mar;31(3):610–4.

Alexandrov AV, Molina CA, Grotta JC, Garami Z, Ford SR, Alvarez-Sabin J, et al; CLOTBUST Investigators. Ultrasound-enhanced systemic thrombolysis for acute ischemic stroke. N Engl J Med. 2004 Nov 18;351(21):2170–8.

Alexandrov AV, Nguyen HT, Rubiera M, Alexandrov AW, Zhao L, Heliopoulos I, et al. Prevalence and risk factors associated with reversed Robin Hood syndrome in acute ischemic stroke. Stroke. 2009 Aug;40(8):2738–42. Epub 2009 May 21.

Blanco P, Abdo-Cuza A. Transcranial Doppler ultrasound in neurocritical care. J Ultrasound. 2018 Mar;21(1): 1–16. Epub 2018 Feb 10.

Bouzat P, Oddo M, Payen JF. Transcranial Doppler after traumatic brain injury: is there a role? Curr Opin Crit Care. 2014 Apr;20(2):153–60.

Chernyshev OY, Garami Z, Calleja S, Song J, Campbell MS, Noser EA, et al. Yield and accuracy of urgent combined carotid/transcranial ultrasound testing in acute cerebral ischemia. Stroke. 2005 Jan;36(1):32–7. Epub 2004 Nov 29.

Demchuk AM, Felburg RA, Alexandrov AV. Clinical recovery from acute ischemic stroke after early reperfusion of the brain with intravenous thrombolysis. N Engl J Med. 1999 Mar 18;340(11):894–5.

Lysakowski C, Walder B, Costanza MC, Tramer MR. Transcranial Doppler versus angiography in patients with vasospasm due to a ruptured cerebral aneurysm: a systematic review. Stroke. 2001 Oct;32(10):2292–8.

National Institute of Neurological Disorders and Stroke rt-PA Stroke Study Group. Tissue plasminogen activator for acute ischemic stroke. N Engl J Med. 1995 Dec 14;333(24):1581–7.

Robba C, Cardim D, Sekhon M, Budohoski K, Czosnyka M. Transcranial Doppler: a stethoscope for the brain-neurocritical care use. J Neurosci Res. 2018 Apr;96(4): 720–30. Epub 2017 Sep 7.

Robba C, Goffi A, Geeraerts T, Cardim D, Via G, Czosnyka M, et al. Brain ultrasonography: methodology, basic and advanced principles and clinical applications: a narrative review. Intensive Care Med. 2019 Apr 25. [Epub ahead of print]

Steiger HJ, Aaslid R, Stooss R, Seiler RW. Transcranial Doppler monitoring in head injury: relations between type of injury, flow velocities, vasoreactivity, and outcome. Neurosurgery. 1994 Jan;34(1):79–85.

Tsivgoulis G, Sharma VK, Lao AY, Malkoff MD, Alexandrov AV. Validation of transcranial Doppler with computed tomography angiography in acute cerebral ischemia. Stroke. 2007 Apr;38(4):1245–9. Epub 2007 Mar 1.

Ziegler D, Cravens G, Poche G, Gandhi R, Tellez M. Use of transcranial Doppler in patients with severe traumatic brain injuries. J Neurotrauma. 2017 Jan 1;34(1):121–7. Epub 2016 Jun 2.

Electroencephalography

AMY Z. CREPEAU, MD

Goals

- Provide an overview of electroencephalography in critically ill patients.
- Review indications for electroencephalography in critically ill patients.
- Review common electroencephalographic patterns in critically ill patients.

Introduction

Electroencephalography (EEG) in critically ill patients allows for monitoring of cerebral function when a clinical examination is limited because of altered mental status or coma. Continuous EEG (cEEG) has increasingly been used to monitor critically ill patients in the intensive care unit (ICU). Implementation of cEEG in the ICU presents a unique set of challenges, requiring special expertise and a multidisciplinary approach.

Status epilepticus is a recognized medical emergency. Convulsive status epilepticus is particularly dangerous, with a recognized mortality rate of up to 27%. The Department of Veterans Affairs Cooperative Study, a 1990s treatment trial for convulsive status epilepticus, described the concept of *subtle status epilepticus*, in which affected patients had an altered mental status with mild physical symptoms, such as finger or abdominal twitching, rather than generalized convulsions. Although the presentation was not as dramatic, those patients were less likely to regain consciousness within 12 hours, they had longer hospital stays, and they had a higher 30-day mortality. These data showed that "subtle" (or *nonconvulsive*) status epilepticus carries a danger of higher morbidity and mortality and that detection requires EEG monitoring.

Nonconvulsive Status Epilepticus

Nonconvulsive status epilepticus (NCSE) is a recognized cause of unexplained altered mental status (AMS). In a study of routine EEGs performed on hospitalized patients who had unexplained AMS, 8% of the EEGs showed NCSE. In another study of emergency department patients with AMS, 37% had electrographic evidence of NCSE. Although reported rates of NCSE on routine EEGs vary widely, those studies showed that EEG was necessary for diagnosis.

In critically ill patients, cEEG has been shown to increase the yield in detecting NCSE and nonconvulsive seizures. In a series of 570 patients undergoing cEEG in a neuroscience ICU, 10% of patients had NCSE sometime during monitoring, and 20% had nonconvulsive seizures. The yield of detecting seizures was 56% within the first hour of monitoring and increased to 93% with 24 to 48 hours of monitoring. NCSE can have many underlying causes. Although the highest incidence of NCSE is associated with acute neurologic injuries such as encephalitis, traumatic brain injury, and hypoxic-ischemic injury, NCSE or nonconvulsive seizures can also develop in patients who do not have a neurologic illness.

Detection of NCSE and nonconvulsive seizures is important because they have been shown to be associated with increased mortality and morbidity. In traumatic brain injury, seizures have been associated with increased length of stay and mortality. In patients with aneurysmal subarachnoid hemorrhage, NCSE or seizures are an independent risk factor for poor outcome. For patients with hypoxic-ischemic encephalopathy, nonconvulsive seizures and NCSE are considered malignant patterns that are strongly associated with poor outcomes.

Limited data suggest that nonconvulsive seizures can cause secondary neuronal injury in critically ill patients.

Seizures are an important risk factor for increased midline shift with intraparenchymal hemorrhage and are associated with prolonged increases in intracranial pressure in traumatic brain injury. Microdialysis data for cerebrospinal fluid have shown increased extracellular glutamate and lipid membrane breakdown, suggestive of associated neuronal injury.

NCSE and nonconvulsive seizures occur in critically ill patients with a wide range of underlying causes and are associated with increased morbidity and mortality. Detection requires cEEG, but implementation and interpretation of cEEG present numerous unique challenges.

Technical Considerations

The process of cEEG is labor intensive, requiring technicians for maintaining recordings, a reliable technologic infrastructure for transmitting EEG data, and experienced encephalographers for interpretating recordings. Not all institutions have EEG technicians available at all times for emergent EEG requests, leading to the use of less labor-intensive montages or electrodes to screen for NCSE or seizures.

Abbreviated electrode montages are appealing because neurologists or nurses can be trained to measure and apply fewer electrodes. Some studies have evaluated the use of abbreviated 4- or 6-channel hairline montages to screen for seizures. With a 4-channel subhairline montage, the sensitivity for detecting seizures was 68%; for detecting periodic patterns, 39%. The sensitivity was slightly higher with a 6-channel hairline montage (72% for detecting seizures and 54% for detecting periodic patterns). A limited montage with 7 electrodes showed similar results (70% sensitivity and 96% specificity) for detecting seizures. Disposable systems that are easier to set up are designed to be used by untrained staff, but those systems have not been shown to be reliable for long-term recordings.

Cup electrodes, which are applied with adhesive paste, allow for quality recordings with good impedances that remain stable over several days. Electrode montages can be modified to allow for skull defects or skin lesions, and electrodes that are compatible with magnetic resonance imaging and computed tomography are available. Cup electrodes must be applied by an experienced technician, though, and application is relatively time-consuming.

Needle electrodes can be applied more quickly and provide stable, reliable recordings. However, because they are placed under the skin, the risk of skin infection is a concern, and the electrodes can be applied only in comatose patients. The electrodes must be carefully maintained, and skin integrity must be checked regularly to prevent skin breakdown.

In the ICU, potential sources of artifact must be minimized. The patient must be grounded to prevent electrical injury and minimize artifact. Respirators, blood pressure cuffs, and dialysis machines can cause rhythmic or epileptiform-appearing artifacts, and chest compressions and suction can cause concerning patterns. Simultaneous video recording is crucial to distinguish between artifacts and cerebral patterns and to review clinical events.

The cost of cEEG can be a concern. The direct cost is multifactorial and depends on the equipment, personnel, and other considerations. However, studies examining the cost-benefit ratio of cEEG have been favorable. Among patients with traumatic brain injury, cEEG was associated with shorter admissions and improved outcomes, and it accounted for only 1% of total hospital costs. In a study of the Nationwide Inpatient Sample, use of cEEG in patients receiving mechanical ventilation was associated with lower inpatient mortality without a significant increase in total hospital charges. The use of cEEG is time and labor intensive, requiring many resources, but with appropriate planning and protocols, cEEG can be a valuable tool for monitoring cerebral function.

Common EEG Patterns in Critically Ill Patients

Interpretation of cEEG presents unique challenges, even for experienced electroencephalographers. The most common indication for cEEG is for the detection of NCSE. The Salzburg Consensus Criteria for Diagnosis of Non-Convulsive Status Epilepticus, published in 2013, outline electrographic criteria for NCSE, which was defined as 1) epileptiform discharges occurring at a frequency greater than 2.5 Hz or 2) epileptiform discharges of 2.5 Hz or less with EEG and clinical improvement with antiepileptic drugs, a subtle clinical correlate, or a typical evolution of the pattern. The criteria are slightly modified for patients with known epileptic encephalopathy (eg, Lennox-Gastaut syndrome) (Box 130.1) (Figure 130.1).

Critically ill patients commonly have rhythmic or periodic patterns that do not meet these criteria and are in the ictal-interictal continuum (IIC). These patterns have variable and arguable degrees of association with ictal activity and potential for neuronal injury. The 2012 version of the American Clinical Neurophysiology Society (ACNS) guidelines for critical care EEG terminology provides for a common language for describing these indeterminate patterns (Box 130.2). The terminology does not include *unequivocal electrographic seizures*, defined as clearly evolving discharges with a frequency of more than 4 Hz. The ACNS *main term 1* defines the location of the discharges as generalized, lateralized, bilateral independent, or multifocal. *Main term 2* describes the morphology as periodic discharges, rhythmic delta activity, or spike-and-wave or sharp-and-wave. Additional qualifiers are used to describe prevalence, duration, morphology, and response to stimulation. The use of

Box 130.1 • Salzburg Consensus Criteria for Diagnosis of Non-Convulsive Status Epilepticus

Patient without known epileptic encephalopathy

Epileptiform discharges >2.5 Hz

or

Epileptiform discharges ≤2.5 Hz or rhythmic delta activity >0.5 Hz *and* 1 of the following:

EEG and clinical improvement after IV antiepileptic drugs *or*

Subtle ictal phenomena that correlate with the pattern *or*

Typical spatiotemporal evolution

Or

Patient with known epileptic encephalopathy

Increase in features described above (compared with baseline) with associated clinical change

Improvement in clinical and EEG features with IV antiepileptic drugs

Abbreviations: EEG, electroencephalography; IV, intravenous.

From Beniczky S, Hirsch LJ, Kaplan PW, Pressler R, Bauer G, Aurlien H, et al. Unified EEG terminology and criteria for nonconvulsive status epilepticus. Epilepsia. 2013 Sep;54 Suppl 6:28-9; used with permission as modified from data in Kaplan PW. EEG criteria for nonconvulsive status epilepticus. Epilepsia. 2007;48 Suppl 8:39-41. Erratum in: Epilepsia. 2007 Dec;48(12):2383.

standardized terminology for these periodic patterns can assist with communication and future research endeavors.

Lateralized Periodic Discharges

Lateralized periodic discharges (LPDs), previously referred to as *periodic lateralized epileptiform discharges*, are waveforms with consistent morphology and duration, occurring at regular intervals, and limited to 1 hemisphere (Figure 130.2). LPDs are most commonly associated with underlying structural lesions such as strokes or tumors, and temporal LPDs are a hallmark finding in herpes simplex encephalitis. LPDs are associated with a risk of electrographic seizures, and when LPDs are accompanied by features such as underlying rhythmic slowing or superimposed fast activity, they carry an even higher risk. In general, LPDs are considered interictal when they occur at a frequency of less than 3 Hz and do not evolve. They do not consistently respond to antiepileptic treatment, and they occur in patients with no clinical signs of status epilepticus. However, when accompanied by clinical symptoms, LPDs represent the ictal end of the IIC. Time-locked, stereotyped sensory symptoms have been described and are associated with a central location. This suggests that symptoms are more likely to occur with LPDs when the location is next to eloquent cortex, such as the primary motor or sensory cortex.

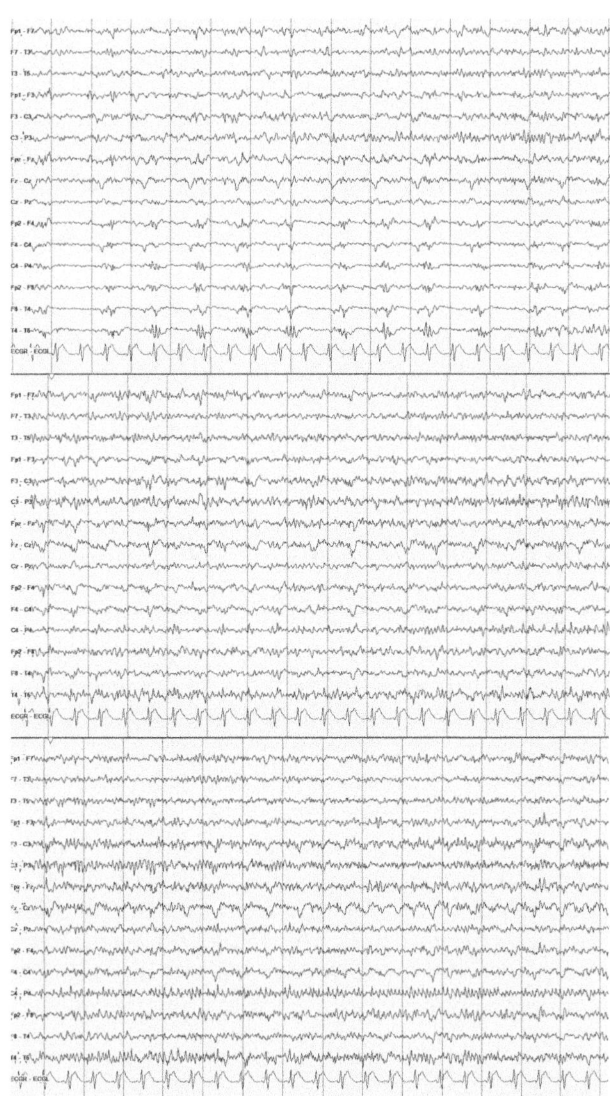

Figure 130.1. Evolving Electrographic Seizure. This pattern recurred continuously, representing nonconvulsive status epilepticus.

Lateralized Rhythmic Delta Activity

Lateralized rhythmic delta activity describes runs of sinusoidal or sharply contoured monomorphic delta activity. *Temporal intermittent rhythmic delta activity* is the former term that described this finding when located over the temporal head region. This finding, associated with remote or acute central nervous system lesions, carries the same risk of electrographic seizures as LPDs.

Generalized Periodic Discharges

Generalized periodic discharges (GPDs), previously known as *generalized periodic epileptiform discharges*, are a common finding on cEEG, with variable associations with NCSE or encephalopathy. In a large case-control study of GPDs in critically ill patients, the presence of

Box 130.2 • American Clinical Neurophysiology Society's Standardized Critical Care Electroencephalographic Terminology

Main term 1: location
- Generalized (G)
- Lateralized (L)
- Bilateral independent (BI)
- Multifocal (Mf)

Main term 2: morphology
- Periodic discharges (PDs)
- Rhythmic delta activity (RDA)
- Spike-and-wave or sharp-and-wave (SW)

Modified from Hirsch LJ, LaRoche SM, Gaspard N, Gerard E, Svoronos A, Herman ST, et al. American Clinical Neurophysiology Society's standardized critical care EEG terminology: 2012 version. J Clin Neurophysiol. 2013 Feb;30(1):1-27; used with permission.

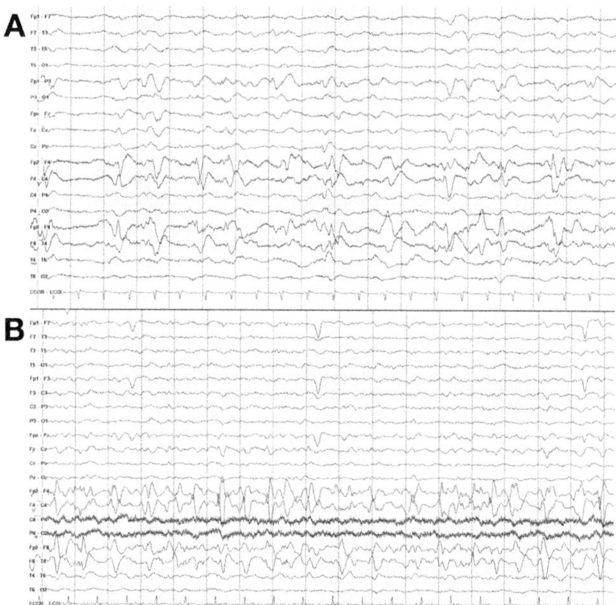

Figure 130.2. Lateralized Periodic Discharges (LPDs). A 62-year-old man was admitted with an aneurysmal subarachnoid hemorrhage and underwent a right frontocentral craniotomy. He remained comatose. A, Right frontal LPDs occurred at a frequency of up to 1 Hz. B, The frequency of the LPDs increased, and the patient's nurse observed periodic left facial and shoulder twitching. The changes in morphology, frequency, and clinical correlates suggest that the pattern changed from interictal to ictal.

GPDs was strongly associated with NCSE and nonconvulsive seizures. However, in certain circumstances, GPDs are not associated with seizures. The classic EEG finding in Creutzfeldt-Jakob disease is 1-Hz GPDs, yet the pattern does not respond to antiepileptic drugs and is not considered an ictal phenomenon. GPDs occur with baclofen toxicity and resolve with cessation of the medication. GPDs can result from many underlying causes, and the importance of the pattern is ultimately related to the cause.

Triphasic Waves

The pattern commonly known as *triphasic waves* is named *generalized periodic discharges with triphasic morphology*, according to the ACNS cEEG terminology (Figure 130.3). This pattern is associated with metabolic encephalopathy, although the relationship is not absolute, and interreader agreement is imperfect. The availability of clinical information yields high interreader agreement in differentiating triphasic waves from NCSE. However, in the absence of clinical information, agreement is only fair. A benzodiazepine challenge is not a reliable way to differentiate triphasic waves from NCSE because triphasic waves have been shown to have an EEG response to benzodiazepines. The presence of triphasic morphology with GPDs does not eliminate the risk of seizures. In a study of 20 cEEG samples with GPDs, patients with triphasic morphology were as likely to have seizures as those without. Although triphasic waves are associated with metabolic encephalopathy, cEEG is often warranted to monitor for the emergence of seizures.

Periodic Patterns

Periodic patterns are commonly seen when patients are critically ill. Determining the importance of the patterns requires consideration of the underlying cause, the patient's clinical state, and any additional data to guide interpretation and treatment decisions.

Additional Indications for cEEG Monitoring

Cardiac Arrest

If patients remain comatose after successful resuscitation from cardiac arrest, the 2010 American Heart Association guidelines recommend that EEG monitoring should be frequent or continuous to detect seizures and provide prognostic data.

Nonconvulsive seizures are common after cardiac arrest and occur in up to 40% of patients undergoing cEEG; status epilepticus occurs in up to 30% of this population. NCSE and seizures tend to occur within the first 12 hours after cardiac arrest, so for the purposes of seizure detection, the recommendation is to initiate cEEG as soon as the patient is clinically stable in the ICU. However, even with attempts at treatment, seizures and status epilepticus are strongly associated with poor outcomes.

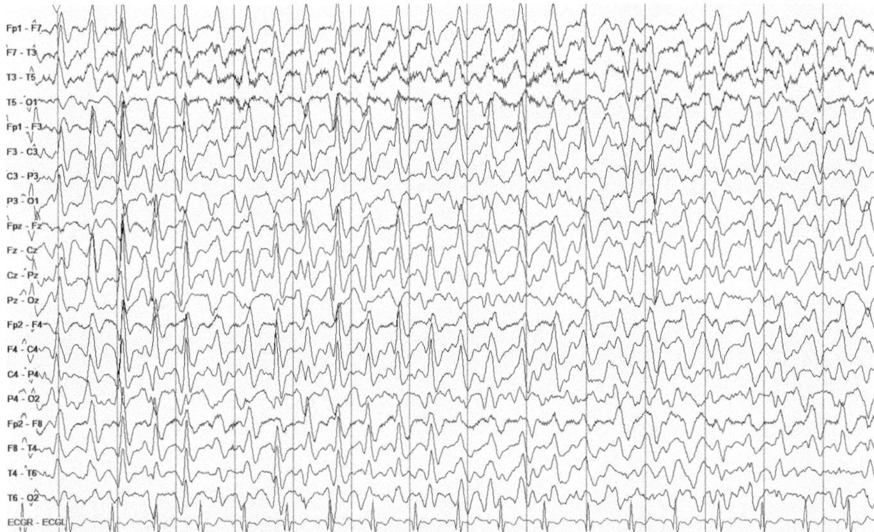

Figure 130.3. Generalized Periodic Discharges With Triphasic Morphology (Triphasic Waves).

The EEG background activity correlates with outcome. A continuous background within 12 hours of cardiac arrest is predictive of a good outcome, while an isoelectric (flat) background within 24 hours strongly correlates with a poor outcome. Lack of reactivity predicts a poor outcome, even during therapeutic hypothermia or targeted temperature management.

A *burst suppression pattern* or GPDs superimposed on a flat background have been associated with poor outcomes. Burst suppression from cerebral ischemia may be difficult to discern from burst suppression related to hypothermia or sedation. The distinction is crucial, though, because iatrogenic burst suppression does not correlate with outcome. Burst suppression with identical bursts, however, is a unique pattern that occurs only with cerebral ischemia and correlates strongly with poor outcome. When burst suppression is present, iatrogenic causes and the morphology of the bursts must be considered for an accurate prognosis (Box 130.3).

A prognosis after cardiac arrest must be based on many sources of data, including the physical examination, neuroimaging, and somatosensory evoked potentials. Concordance between EEG findings and these factors allows for the most informed conclusion.

Delayed Cerebral Ischemia

EEG shows reliable changes with alterations in cerebral blood flow, which have been well described from EEG monitoring for carotid endarterectomies. These changes can be monitored in real time with quantitative EEG algorithms for detection of delayed cerebral ischemia, such as with vasospasm after subarachnoid hemorrhage. Relative alpha variability measures the ratio of power in the bandwidths 6 to 14 Hz and 1 to 20 Hz. This algorithm was shown to be sensitive for detection of vasospasm before angiographic documentation. The alpha-delta ratio measures the ratio of alpha power (6-14 Hz) to delta power (1-4 Hz) for detection of delayed cerebral ischemia. A decrease of more than 10% from baseline over 6 consecutive hours was 100% sensitive and 76% specific for the detection of delayed cerebral ischemia.

Depth of Suppression

When barbiturates are administered for increased intracranial pressure, cEEG allows for monitoring of the depth of suppression. A trained ICU nurse can readily monitor suppression at the patient's bedside, and application of quantitative EEG algorithms aid in rapid review of suppression.

Box 130.3. • Prognostic Implications of EEG Findings After Cardiac Arrest

Poor prognosis (after accounting for sedatives and hypothermia)
- Status epilepticus
- Seizures
- Lack of reactivity
- Isoelectric (flat) background
- Generalized periodic discharges superimposed on a flat background
- Burst suppression with identical bursts

Good prognosis
- Continuous, reactive background

Abbreviation: EEG, electroencephalographic.

Summary

- NCSE and seizures are associated with increased morbidity and mortality; diagnosis requires EEG and cEEG to increase the yield of detection.
- The highest quality of cEEG recording that provides the greatest ability to detect seizures requires a full montage of electrodes, ideally with imaging-compatible cup electrodes.
- Periodic patterns of indeterminate importance are in the IIC and require consideration of the clinical state and the underlying cause.
- After cardiac arrest, cEEG provides important prognostic information for comatose patients.
- Other uses of cEEG include detecting delayed cerebral ischemia and monitoring the depth of suppression from barbiturates.

SUGGESTED READING

Alvarez V, Rossetti AO. Clinical use of EEG in the ICU: technical setting. J Clin Neurophysiol. 2015 Dec;32(6):481–5.

Amorim E, Rittenberger JC, Baldwin ME, Callaway CW, Popescu A; Post Cardiac Arrest Service. Malignant EEG patterns in cardiac arrest patients treated with targeted temperature management who survive to hospital discharge. Resuscitation. 2015 May;90:127–32. Epub 2015 Mar 14.

Beniczky S, Hirsch LJ, Kaplan PW, Pressler R, Bauer G, Aurlien H, et al. Unified EEG terminology and criteria for nonconvulsive status epilepticus. Epilepsia. 2013 Sep;54 Suppl 6:28–9.

Boulanger JM, Deacon C, Lecuyer D, Gosselin S, Reiher J. Triphasic waves versus nonconvulsive status epilepticus: EEG distinction. Can J Neurol Sci. 2006 May;33(2):175–80.

Butzkueven H, Evans AH, Pitman A, Leopold C, Jolley DJ, Kaye AH, et al. Onset seizures independently predict poor outcome after subarachnoid hemorrhage. Neurology. 2000 Nov 14;55(9):1315–20.

Chong DJ, Hirsch LJ. Which EEG patterns warrant treatment in the critically ill? Reviewing the evidence for treatment of periodic epileptiform discharges and related patterns. J Clin Neurophysiol. 2005 Apr;22(2):79–91.

Claassen J, Hirsch LJ, Kreiter KT, Du EY, Connolly ES, Emerson RG, et al. Quantitative continuous EEG for detecting delayed cerebral ischemia in patients with poor-grade subarachnoid hemorrhage. Clin Neurophysiol. 2004 Dec;115(12):2699–710.

Claassen J, Mayer SA, Kowalski RG, Emerson RG, Hirsch LJ. Detection of electrographic seizures with continuous EEG monitoring in critically ill patients. Neurology. 2004 May 25;62(10):1743–8.

Cloostermans MC, van Meulen FB, Eertman CJ, Hom HW, van Putten MJ. Continuous electroencephalography monitoring for early prediction of neurological outcome in postanoxic patients after cardiac arrest: a prospective cohort study. Crit Care Med. 2012 Oct;40(10):2867–75.

Crepeau AZ, Rabinstein AA, Fugate JE, Mandrekar J, Wijdicks EF, White RD, et al. Continuous EEG in therapeutic hypothermia after cardiac arrest: prognostic and clinical value. Neurology. 2013 Jan 22;80(4):339–44. Epub 2013 Jan 2.

Eertmans W, Genbrugge C, Haesen J, Drieskens C, Demeestere J, Vander Laenen M, et al. The prognostic value of simplified EEG in out-of-hospital cardiac arrest patients. Neurocrit Care. 2018 Aug 15. [Epub ahead of print]

Fakhoury T, Abou-Khalil B, Blumenkopf B. EEG changes in intrathecal baclofen overdose: a case report and review of the literature. Electroencephalogr Clin Neurophysiol. 1998 Nov;107(5):339–42.

Fatuzzo D, Beuchat I, Alvarez V, Novy J, Oddo M, Rossetti AO. Does continuous EEG influence prognosis in patients after cardiac arrest? Resuscitation. 2018 Nov;132:29–32. Epub 2018 Aug 25.

Foreman B, Claassen J, Abou Khaled K, Jirsch J, Alschuler DM, Wittman J, et al. Generalized periodic discharges in the critically ill: a case-control study of 200 patients. Neurology. 2012 Nov 6;79(19):1951–60. Epub 2012 Oct 3.

Foreman B, Mahulikar A, Tadi P, Claassen J, Szaflarski J, Halford JJ, et al; Critical Care EEG Monitoring Research Consortium (CCEMRC). Generalized periodic discharges and 'triphasic waves': a blinded evaluation of inter-rater agreement and clinical significance. Clin Neurophysiol. 2016 Feb;127(2):1073–80. Epub 2015 Aug 7.

Fountain NB, Waldman WA. Effects of benzodiazepines on triphasic waves: implications for nonconvulsive status epilepticus. J Clin Neurophysiol. 2001 Jul;18(4):345–52.

Gaspard N, Manganas L, Rampal N, Petroff OA, Hirsch LJ. Similarity of lateralized rhythmic delta activity to periodic lateralized epileptiform discharges in critically ill patients. JAMA Neurol. 2013 Oct;70(10):1288–95.

Hirsch LJ, LaRoche SM, Gaspard N, Gerard E, Svoronos A, Herman ST, et al. American Clinical Neurophysiology Society's standardized critical care EEG terminology: 2012 version. J Clin Neurophysiol. 2013 Feb;30(1):1–27.

Hofmeijer J, Tjepkema-Cloostermans MC, van Putten MJ. Burst-suppression with identical bursts: a distinct EEG pattern with poor outcome in postanoxic coma. Clin Neurophysiol. 2014 May;125(5):947–54. Epub 2013 Oct 26.

Knight WA, Hart KW, Adeoye OM, Bonomo JB, Keegan SP, Ficker DM, et al. The incidence of seizures in patients undergoing therapeutic hypothermia after resuscitation from cardiac arrest. Epilepsy Res. 2013 Oct;106(3):396–402. Epub 2013 Jul 29.

Lee H, Mizrahi MA, Hartings JA, Sharma S, Pahren L, Ngwenya LB, et al. Continuous electroencephalography after moderate to severe traumatic brain injury. Crit Care Med. 2019 Apr;47(4):574–82.

Little AS, Kerrigan JF, McDougall CG, Zabramski JM, Albuquerque FC, Nakaji P, et al. Nonconvulsive status epilepticus in patients suffering spontaneous subarachnoid hemorrhage. J Neurosurg. 2007 May;106(5):805–11.

Ney JP, van der Goes DN, Nuwer MR, Nelson L, Eccher MA. Continuous and routine EEG in intensive care: utilization and outcomes, United States 2005–2009. Neurology. 2013 Dec 3;81(23):2002–8. Epub 2013 Nov 1.

Peberdy MA, Callaway CW, Neumar RW, Geocadin RG, Zimmerman JL, Donnino M, et al; American Heart Association. Part 9: post-cardiac arrest care: 2010 American Heart Association guidelines for cardiopulmonary resuscitation and emergency cardiovascular care. Circulation. 2010 Nov 2;122(18 Suppl 3):S768–86. Errata in: Circulation. 2011 Feb 15;123(6):e237. Circulation. 2011 Oct 11;124(15):e403.

Privitera MD, Strawsburg RH. Electroencephalographic monitoring in the emergency department. Emerg Med Clin North Am. 1994 Nov;12(4):1089–100.

Reiher J, Rivest J, Grand'Maison F, Leduc CP. Periodic lateralized epileptiform discharges with transitional rhythmic discharges: association with seizures. Electroencephalogr Clin Neurophysiol. 1991 Jan;78(1):12–7.

Rittenberger JC, Popescu A, Brenner RP, Guyette FX, Callaway CW. Frequency and timing of nonconvulsive status epilepticus in comatose post-cardiac arrest subjects treated with hypothermia. Neurocrit Care. 2012 Feb;16(1):114–22.

Rossetti AO. Clinical neurophysiology for neurological prognostication of comatose patients after cardiac arrest. Clin Neurophysiol Pract. 2017 Mar 20;2:76–80.

Rossetti AO, Logroscino G, Liaudet L, Ruffieux C, Ribordy V, Schaller MD, et al. Status epilepticus: an independent outcome predictor after cerebral anoxia. Neurology. 2007 Jul 17;69(3):255–60.

Rossetti AO, Schindler K, Alvarez V, Sutter R, Novy J, Oddo M, et al. Does continuous video-EEG in patients with altered consciousness improve patient outcome? Current evidence and randomized controlled trial design. J Clin Neurophysiol. 2018 Sep;35(5):359–64.

Rossetti AO, Urbano LA, Delodder F, Kaplan PW, Oddo M. Prognostic value of continuous EEG monitoring during therapeutic hypothermia after cardiac arrest. Crit Care. 2010;14(5):R173. Epub 2010 Sep 29.

Rubin MN, Jeffery OJ, Fugate JE, Britton JW, Cascino GD, Worrell GA, et al. Efficacy of a reduced electroencephalography electrode array for detection of seizures. Neurohospitalist. 2014 Jan;4(1):6–8.

Sen-Gupta I, Schuele SU, Macken MP, Kwasny MJ, Gerard EE. "Ictal" lateralized periodic discharges. Epilepsy Behav. 2014 Jul;36:165–70. Epub 2014 Jun 13.

Sutter R. Are we prepared to detect subtle and nonconvulsive status epilepticus in critically ill patients? J Clin Neurophysiol. 2016 Feb;33(1):25–31.

Towne AR, Waterhouse EJ, Boggs JG, Garnett LK, Brown AJ, Smith JR Jr, et al. Prevalence of nonconvulsive status epilepticus in comatose patients. Neurology. 2000 Jan 25;54(2):340–5.

Treiman DM, Meyers PD, Walton NY, Collins JF, Colling C, Rowan AJ, et al; Veterans Affairs Status Epilepticus Cooperative Study Group. A comparison of four treatments for generalized convulsive status epilepticus. N Engl J Med. 1998 Sep 17;339(12):792–8.

Vespa P, Martin NA, Nenov V, Glenn T, Bergsneider M, Kelly D, et al. Delayed increase in extracellular glycerol with post-traumatic electrographic epileptic activity: support for the theory that seizures induce secondary injury. Acta Neurochir Suppl. 2002;81:355–7.

Vespa P, Prins M, Ronne-Engstrom E, Caron M, Shalmon E, Hovda DA, et al. Increase in extracellular glutamate caused by reduced cerebral perfusion pressure and seizures after human traumatic brain injury: a microdialysis study. J Neurosurg. 1998 Dec;89(6):971–82.

Vespa PM, Miller C, McArthur D, Eliseo M, Etchepare M, Hirt D, et al. Nonconvulsive electrographic seizures after traumatic brain injury result in a delayed, prolonged increase in intracranial pressure and metabolic crisis. Crit Care Med. 2007 Dec;35(12):2830–6.

Vespa PM, Nenov V, Nuwer MR. Continuous EEG monitoring in the intensive care unit: early findings and clinical efficacy. J Clin Neurophysiol. 1999 Jan;16(1):1–13.

Vespa PM, Nuwer MR, Juhasz C, Alexander M, Nenov V, Martin N, et al. Early detection of vasospasm after acute subarachnoid hemorrhage using continuous EEG ICU monitoring. Electroencephalogr Clin Neurophysiol. 1997 Dec;103(6):607–15.

Vespa PM, Nuwer MR, Nenov V, Ronne-Engstrom E, Hovda DA, Bergsneider M, et al. Increased incidence and impact of nonconvulsive and convulsive seizures after traumatic brain injury as detected by continuous electroencephalographic monitoring. J Neurosurg. 1999 Nov;91(5):750–60.

Vespa PM, O'Phelan K, Shah M, Mirabelli J, Starkman S, Kidwell C, et al. Acute seizures after intracerebral hemorrhage: a factor in progressive midline shift and outcome. Neurology. 2003 May 13;60(9):1441–6.

Young GB, Sharpe MD, Savard M, Al Thenayan E, Norton L, Davies-Schinkel C. Seizure detection with a commercially available bedside EEG monitor and the subhairline montage. Neurocrit Care. 2009 Dec;11(3):411–6.

Essentials of Multimodal Brain Monitoring

JENNIFER E. FUGATE, DO

Goals

- Describe the physiologic principles of multimodal monitoring.
- Describe the indications for multimodal monitoring.
- Review the physiologic inferences that can be made from multimodal monitoring but not from traditional single monitors.

Introduction

Intensive care unit (ICU) clinicians spend a substantial amount of time monitoring patients and their organ systems. Staples of systemic monitoring include continuous electrocardiography, pulse oximetry, serum laboratory values of liver and kidney function, urinary output, and ventilator parameters. Monitoring methods for the brain have lagged somewhat in technologic advances. For years, the only brain monitoring system was the neurologic examination, and it is still the foundation of all neuromonitoring. Neurointensivists must have a thorough knowledge of the anatomy and physiology of the central nervous system and be able to correctly interpret changes in the neurologic examination. Neuroimaging is essential to supplementing the clinical examination, and the technology has become increasingly sophisticated. Although computed tomography (CT) and magnetic resonance imaging (MRI) are crucial to defining appropriate diagnoses and treatment plans for patients with acute brain injury, they are not covered in this chapter.

Several devices are available for monitoring parameters of brain physiology, including intracranial pressure (ICP), cerebral blood flow (CBF), autoregulation, brain oxygenation, and brain metabolism (Figure 131.1). The most robust data for these monitoring devices come from patients with severe traumatic brain injury (TBI) and aneurysmal subarachnoid hemorrhage (aSAH). The rationale for monitoring different aspects of brain physiology (ie, multimodal monitoring) is to allow clinicians to track, prevent, and treat secondary brain injury; to facilitate care according to protocols for pathophysiologic processes; to detect deterioration in heavily sedated patients (in whom the neurologic examination is nearly useless); and to provide information that can be used as prognostic markers.

Intracranial Pressure

When a person is lying in a supine position, normal ICP is less than 15 mm Hg. An ICP exceeding 20 to 25 mm Hg has surpassed a generally accepted threshold and should be treated. Sustained intracranial hypertension is strongly associated with increased mortality, particularly in patients with TBI. Cerebral perfusion pressure (CPP), a concept rather than a directly measured value, is equal to mean arterial pressure (MAP) minus mean ICP. CPP is used as a surrogate for CBF; in theory, when ICP is high, CPP may become compromised and the brain may be at risk of injury due to global cerebral ischemia. General guidelines for when to use an ICP monitor are shown in Table 131.1.

The 2 reliable devices for measuring ICP are ventricular catheters (ie, external ventricular drains [EVDs]) and fiberoptic parenchymal monitors (Figure 131.2). Both are invasive, but the associated risks of infection and hemorrhage are minimal when the devices are placed and cared for by experienced operators. EVDs have the advantage that they can be used to treat increased ICP by diverting cerebrospinal fluid (CSF); EVDs are preferred for treatment of hydrocephalus. They produce a reliable measure of ICP, however, only when they are closed and not draining CSF. The benefit of parenchymal ICP monitoring is the relative ease of

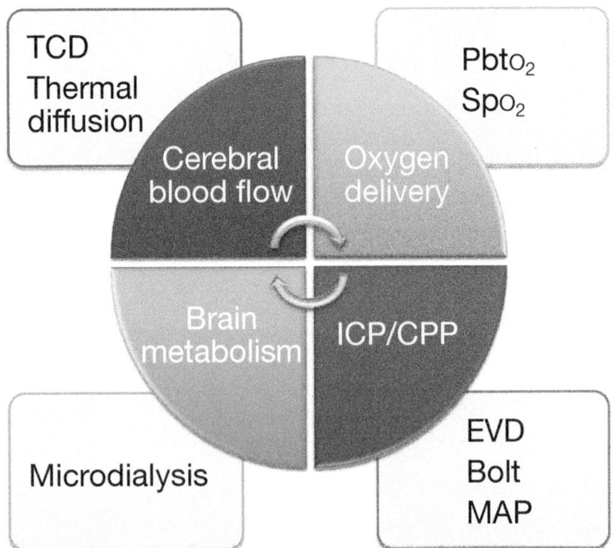

Figure 131.1. Overview of Multimodal Monitoring of Brain Physiology. CPP indicates cerebral perfusion pressure; EVD, external ventricular drain; ICP, intracranial pressure; MAP, mean arterial pressure; $Pbto_2$, partial pressure of oxygen in interstitial brain tissue; Spo_2, oxygen saturation by pulse oximetry; TCD, transcranial Doppler ultrasonography.

placement in addition to providing a continuous measure of ICP.

ICP measurements provide additional useful information because they are used to calculate secondary indexes of cerebral physiology. For example, the cerebrovascular *pressure reactivity index* (PRx), a moving correlation coefficient between mean ICP and slow fluctuations in MAP, reflects the ability of smooth muscle within cerebral arteriolar walls to react to changes in transmural pressure. Under normal circumstances, with increasing MAP, intact pressure reactivity will lead to vasoconstriction, a reduction in cerebral blood volume, and a reduction in ICP. Thus, as MAP increases, ICP decreases. PRx is calculated with a moving correlation coefficient between time-averaged values of ICP and MAP. A negative PRx reflects normal pressure reactivity of the blood vessels. A positive PRx signifies a nonreactive, passive arterial bed and dysfunctional cerebral autoregulation. Although PRx provides an indication of the status of cerebral autoregulation, it is not exact because other factors besides pressure reactivity contribute to autoregulation (eg, metabolic demand, $Paco_2$, and autonomic nervous system input).

ICP has been the focus of monitoring in neurocritical care units for decades, but interest has increased in the use of CPP-directed therapy. Brain Trauma Foundation guidelines recommend that for patients with severe TBI, the target CPP should be 50 to 70 mm Hg, but much research is being conducted to determine whether an individualized CPP may be superior. In theory, if autoregulation is impaired, a CPP that would otherwise be considered a goal may be too high and result in worsening brain edema,

Table 131.1 • Indications for Monitoring Intracranial Pressure

Acute Neurologic Disorder	Indications[a]
Traumatic brain injury	Coma and abnormal findings on CT of the head Coma and normal findings on CT of the head *and* 2 of the following 3: Age >40 y SBP <90 mm Hg Motor posturing (decorticate or decerebrate)
Subarachnoid hemorrhage	Hydrocephalus Diffuse brain edema and coma
Intracerebral hemorrhage	Hydrocephalus
Fulminant hepatic failure	Rapidly progressing grade 3 hepatic encephalopathy (incoherent speech and drowsy) Grade 4 hepatic encephalopathy (comatose, unresponsive to pain, and motor posturing) Diffuse brain edema
Acute bacterial meningitis	Diffuse brain edema
Other conditions with hydrocephalus (eg, cerebellar stroke, tumor)	Hydrocephalus

Abbreviations: CT, computed tomography; SBP, systolic blood pressure.
[a] *Coma* indicates Glasgow Coma Scale score less than 8.

higher ICP, and increased risk of hemorrhage. However, if autoregulation is intact, higher CPP levels may result in a compensatory vasoconstriction, reduced cerebral blood volume, and reduced ICP. Some research groups have proposed that an individualized "optimal CPP" may describe a target CPP at which autoregulation is optimal for each person. However, further large prospective studies are needed before this can be recommended for routine and widespread clinical use.

Brain Oxygenation

Adequate oxygenation is crucial to maintaining cell integrity. *Hypoxia* is defined as a reduction in tissue oxygenation to levels that are insufficient to maintain cellular metabolism and function. Inadequate oxygenation aggravates secondary brain injury, making detection and treatment of hypoxia (both brain and systemic) important in the care of critically ill patients. The introduction of monitoring the partial pressure of oxygen in interstitial brain tissue ($Pbto_2$) and the jugular bulb venous oxygen saturation ($Sjvo_2$) has allowed for continuous evaluation of the balance of oxygen delivery and use within the white matter of the brain. Brain Trauma Foundation guidelines recommend placement of brain oxygenation monitors when

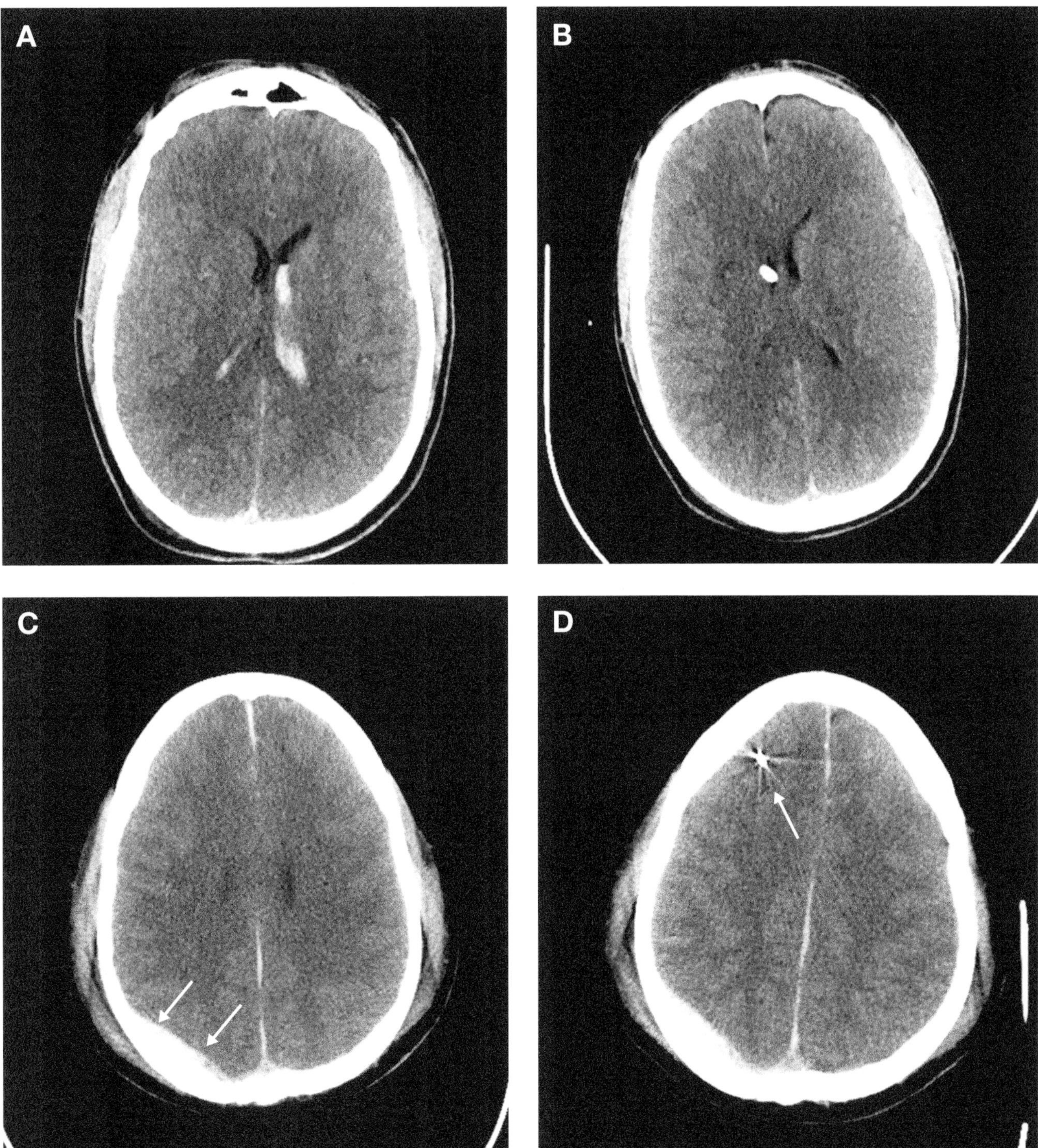

Figure 131.2. Intracranial Pressure Monitors. Axial noncontrast computed tomographic scans of the head show placement of intracranial pressure monitors. A and B, A patient with intraventricular hemorrhage (A) underwent placement of a right frontal external ventricular drain; the tip of the catheter is visualized in the right lateral ventricle (B). C and D, A patient with traumatic brain injury and right posterior subdural hematoma (C; arrows) underwent placement of a right frontal intraparenchymal fiberoptic intracranial pressure monitor (D; arrow).

hyperventilatory strategies are used after TBI. More recent guidelines from various international ICU societies recommend monitor placement in any patient thought to be at risk for cerebral ischemia.

Monitoring $Pbto_2$ requires an invasive probe that is placed through a bolt or through a craniotomy site. The probe provides a continuous measure of the partial pressure of oxygen within the adjacent white matter. Normal values for $Pbto_2$ have been documented as 20 to 35 mm Hg, and recent guidelines suggest a treatment threshold of 20 mm Hg. Low levels of $Pbto_2$ (<10 mm Hg) have been associated with morbidity, death, and extracellular evidence of metabolic crises. With the use of $Pbto_2$ as a target in CPP-driven therapies and in a few preliminary small studies, outcomes have improved with this approach, but $Pbto_2$ is not specific for failure of adequate perfusion. A product of both CBF and blood oxygen tension, $Pbto_2$ provides information to assess for adequate oxygen delivery and to identify hypoxia not related to perfusion. Clinical data are still emerging. Retrospective studies have had mixed results, but more reliable information is awaited from an ongoing phase 3 trial, Brain Oxygenation Optimization in Severe TBI—Phase 3 (BOOST-3), which is comparing therapy directed by $Pbto_2$ with therapy not directed by $Pbto_2$ to determine whether $Pbto_2$-directed therapy results in improved clinical outcomes.

In contrast to $Pbto_2$, which provides regional information (within a diameter of about 5 mm of the probe), $Sjvo_2$ provides a global measure of cerebral oxygen use. The monitoring of $Sjvo_2$ requires central catheter placement, usually in the dominant internal jugular vein, and positioning superiorly in the jugular bulb. Normal values range between 55% and 75%. $Sjvo_2$ levels less than 55% imply increased oxygen extraction and brain tissue possibly at risk for ischemia. These low values have been associated with poor outcomes, especially in patients with values that do not improve with treatment aimed at improving CBF. $Sjvo_2$ levels greater than 75% may signify hyperemia, decreased metabolic demand, or cell death. The accuracy and safety of $Sjvo_2$ monitoring is limited in comparison to $Pbto_2$ monitoring, and it shares the similar limitation of providing nonspecific data. Enthusiasm for $Sjvo_2$ monitoring has been limited because of the technical difficulties involved with placing and maintaining the device. $Sjvo_2$ monitoring can be susceptible to positioning artifacts and complications associated with catheter insertion (eg, carotid puncture, infection, accidental misplacement, and jugular thrombosis).

Cerebral Microdialysis

Cerebral microdialysis allows the measurement of concentrations of interstitial markers of brain metabolism with a perfusion pump and a small 2-lumen probe inserted into the brain parenchyma. Microdialysis is recommended for patients who are at risk for (or already have) cerebral ischemia, hypoxia, energy failure, or glucose deprivation. Microdialysis should be used only in combination with other monitoring tools. A standard cerebral microdialysis membrane (with a 20-kDa molecular weight cutoff) can be used to recover glucose, pyruvate, lactate, glycerol, and glutamate. The rationale for collecting these substances is that they are useful for identifying a transition from aerobic to anaerobic metabolism, which may signify energy failure. These markers are not specific for ischemia alone but reflect overall energy metabolism in the brain. The most sensitive marker for ischemia is an increased lactate to pyruvate ratio (LPR). In observational studies, an LPR greater than 40 and persistently low brain glucose levels have been associated with unfavorable clinical outcomes. Microdialysis has also been used to monitor extracellular concentrations of neurotransmitters, such as glutamate and γ-aminobutyric acid, and markers of cellular damage, such as glycerol.

Microdialysis is used mostly as a research tool; it is performed as a routine part of clinical management in only a few centers in the world. One limitation of microdialysis is that data are delayed because fluid travels relatively slowly through the catheter and the collection occurs over approximately 60 minutes. This can be a labor- and resource-intensive process, further limiting its widespread applicability.

Cerebral Blood Flow

Thresholds of CBF that define ischemia have been derived from experimental models, and there is much interest in developing methods to monitor CBF in patients. Radiographic methods used to estimate CBF (eg, CT perfusion, MRI perfusion studies, arterial spin labeling, and positron emission tomography) are beyond the scope of this chapter, but they have shown that cellular injury can occur in the absence of traditionally defined thresholds for ischemia. CBF data should be interpreted in the clinical context and in combination with data from other monitoring devices.

Blood flow can be monitored continuously in a small region of the brain with invasive thermal diffusion flowmetry (TDF) or, less commonly, laser Doppler flowmetry. TDF uses an intraparenchymal probe with a thermistor and a temperature sensor. The distal thermistor is heated by 2°C, and the thermal gradient between the thermistor and the proximal temperature sensor is measured, providing a quantified regional CBF measurement in milliliters per 100 grams per minute. Mean values of 18 to 25 mL/100 g/min are considered normal; however, trends rather than absolute values may be better for detecting early neurologic deterioration or for assessing a response to therapy. The process

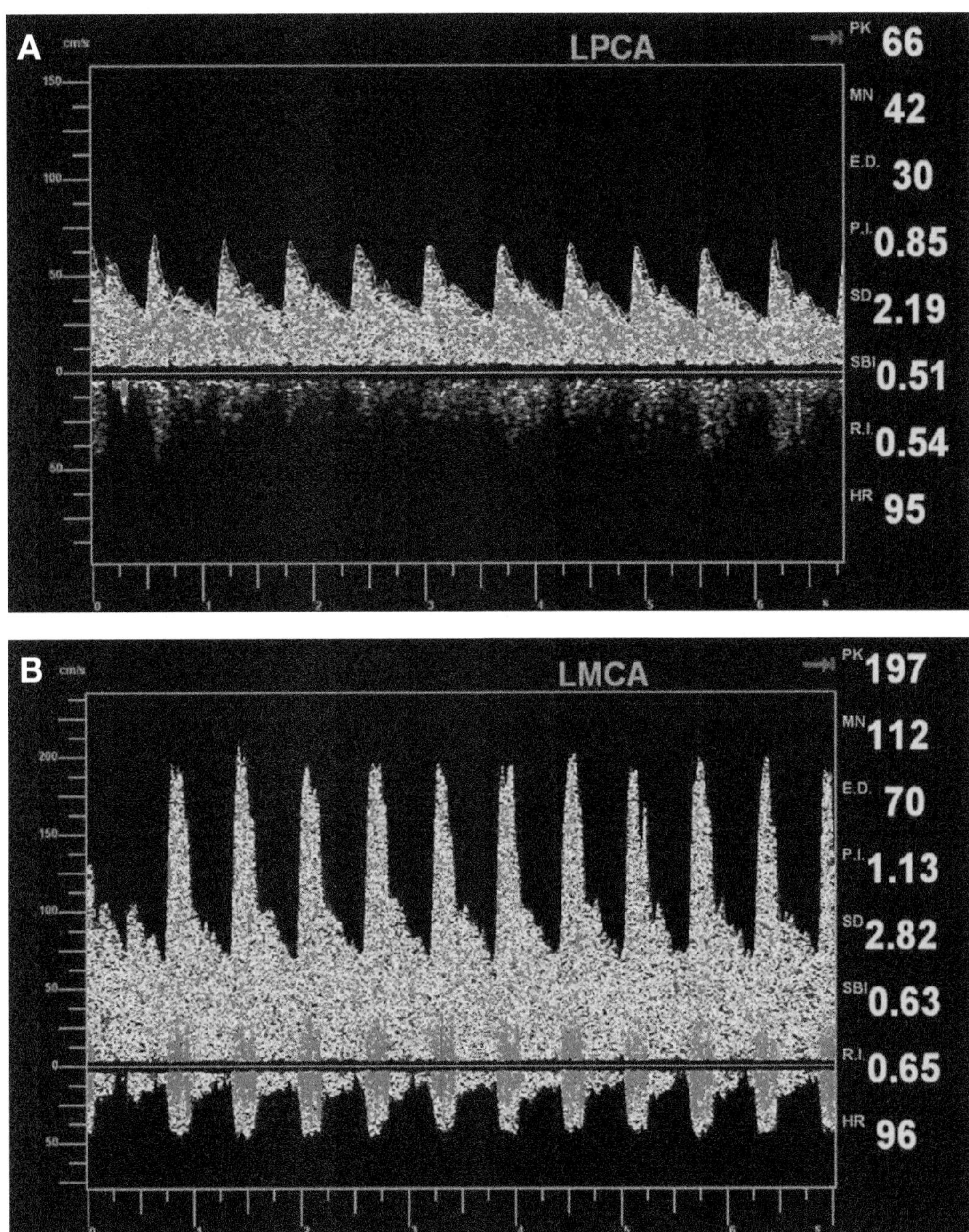

Figure 131.3. Transcranial Doppler Ultrasonography. A, Spectral waveforms (reflecting arterial pulse waveforms) were obtained with transcranial Doppler ultrasonography of the left posterior cerebral artery (LPCA) (mean flow velocity, 42 cm/s). B, Spectral waveform of the left middle cerebral artery (LMCA) shows mean flow velocity of 112 cm/s.

has several limitations: 1) Reliability is decreased when patients have an elevated systemic temperature; 2) limited data correlate with clinical outcomes; 3) only a small region of the brain is monitored; and 4) the optimal placement site is uncertain.

Blood flow to larger regions of the brain can be estimated with transcranial Doppler ultrasonography (TCD). TCD provides information on flow velocity and direction of flow in a segment of blood vessel being investigated. Most centers use TCD as an intermittent study, but a head frame can be used for continuous monitoring. Generally when a head frame is used, the patient must be heavily sedated because small movements decrease the accuracy of the probe. Within the segment of artery studied, TCD provides beat-to-beat information from peak systole through end diastole and creates the spectral waveform (Figure 131.3).

Table 131.2 • Brain Monitoring Modalities

Method	Variable Measured	Anatomical Resolution	Temporal Resolution	Advantages	Disadvantages
Fiberoptic catheter	ICP	Global	Continuous	Reliable Quantitative Allows calculation of secondary indexes	Invasive
EVD	ICP	Global	Intermittent or continuous	Reliable Quantitative Therapeutic Allows calculation of secondary indexes	Invasive
$Pbto_2$	Brain tissue oxygenation	Regional	Continuous	Sensitive Quantitative	Invasive Measures small region of brain
$Sjvo_2$	Cerebral hemispheric oxygenation	Global	Continuous	Quantitative	Invasive Susceptible to artifacts Thrombosis
Microdialysis	Brain metabolism	Regional	Intermittent	Sensitive Quantitative	Invasive Labor intensive
Thermal diffusion flowmetry	Cortical CBF	Regional	Continuous	Robust information	Qualitative Measures small region of brain Not well standardized
TCD	CBF	Regional	Continuous	Noninvasive	Operator dependent Difficult to keep probes in place

Abbreviations: CBF, cerebral blood flow; EVD, external ventricular drain; ICP, intracranial pressure; $Pbto_2$, partial pressure of oxygen in interstitial brain tissue; $Sjvo_2$, jugular bulb venous oxygenation saturation; TCD, transcranial Doppler ultrasonography.

In the ICU, TCD has been used primarily to monitor for vasospasm in aSAH and to identify hypoperfusion or hyperperfusion in patients with TBI. When monitoring for vasospasm, traditionally the mean blood flow velocity has been used to identify thresholds that correlate with the presence of angiographic vasospasm, and this is best studied in the proximal middle cerebral artery (MCA). A mean flow velocity less than 120 cm/s in the MCA is strongly suggestive of the absence of vasospasm. Values greater than 160 cm/s in the MCA are correlated with the presence of vasospasm, and values greater than 200 cm/s suggest the presence of severe vasospasm. The inclusion of the Lindegaard ratio (the ratio of the flow velocity in the MCA to the flow velocity in the extracranial internal carotid artery) or the relative rate of change of velocities improves accuracy. A Lindegaard ratio greater than 3 is consistent with the presence of intracranial vasospasm, and a ratio greater than 6 suggests severe vasospasm. As in any method of ultrasonography, the accuracy of TCD results is largely dependent on operator variability, which is a major limitation of this monitoring device. In addition, about 10% of patients have suboptimal bone windows for insonation.

Current Status

Devices are becoming more widely available to monitor various pathophysiologic parameters of the acutely injured brain (Table 131.2). These neurophysiologic data should always be integrated with the clinical examination and neuroimaging findings and should never be interpreted in isolation. The tremendous amount of data that can be generated with these monitors highlights the need for further development in bioinformatics, data acquisition, and data display techniques. Patient outcomes cannot be expected to be improved with the use of monitors alone but rather by the actions and changes in management that are provoked by data provided by the monitors. Much of the data for multimodal monitoring are from single-center observational studies, and prospective, multicenter, randomized trials are still needed.

Summary

- A main goal of multimodal monitoring is to detect and limit secondary brain injury, an important cause of morbidity and death among patients with acute brain injury.
- Measurement of ICP, the cornerstone of monitoring, is most accurate with an intraparenchymal fiberoptic catheter or, if hydrocephalus is present, with an EVD.
- CPP should be between 50 and 70 mm Hg in most patients; individualized CPP values that reflect the patient's autoregulation status are the subject of ongoing research.
- Brain oxygen delivery and use can be measured regionally with an intraparenchymal catheter or globally with a probe that measures $SjvO_2$.
- Cerebral microdialysis can assist in identifying neuroglycopenia and cellular metabolic crises.

SUGGESTED READING

Bohman LE, Pisapia JM, Sanborn MR, Frangos S, Lin E, Kumar M, et al. Response of brain oxygen to therapy correlates with long-term outcome after subarachnoid hemorrhage. Neurocrit Care. 2013 Dec;19(3):320–8.

Bratton SL, Chestnut RM, Ghajar J, McConnell Hammond FF, Harris OA, Hartl R, et al; Brain Trauma Foundation; American Association of Neurological Surgeons; Congress of Neurological Surgeons; Joint Section on Neurotrauma and Critical Care, AANS/CNS. Guidelines for the management of severe traumatic brain injury. II. Hyperosmolar therapy. J Neurotrauma. 2007;24 Suppl 1:S14–20. Erratum in: J Neurotrauma. 2008 Mar;25(3):276–8.

Chesnut RM, Temkin N, Carney N, Dikmen S, Rondina C, Videtta W, et al; Global Neurotrauma Research Group. A trial of intracranial-pressure monitoring in traumatic brain injury. N Engl J Med. 2012 Dec 27;367(26):2471–81. Epub 2012 Dec 12. Erratum in: N Engl J Med. 2013 Dec 19;369(25):2465.

Dawes AJ, Sacks GD, Cryer HG, Gruen JP, Preston C, Gorospe D, et al; Los Angeles County Trauma Consortium. Intracranial pressure monitoring and inpatient mortality in severe traumatic brain injury: a propensity score-matched analysis. J Trauma Acute Care Surg. 2015 Mar;78(3):492–501.

Helbok R, Olson DM, Le Roux PD, Vespa P; Participants in the International Multidisciplinary Consensus Conference on Multimodality Monitoring. Intracranial pressure and cerebral perfusion pressure monitoring in non-TBI patients: special considerations. Neurocrit Care. 2014 Dec;21 Suppl 2:S85–94.

Hiler M, Czosnyka M, Hutchinson P, Balestreri M, Smielewski P, Matta B, et al. Predictive value of initial computerized tomography scan, intracranial pressure, and state of autoregulation in patients with traumatic brain injury. J Neurosurg. 2006 May;104(5):731–7.

Korbakis G, Vespa PM. Multimodal neurologic monitoring. Handb Clin Neurol. 2017;140:91–105.

Lara LR, Puttgen HA. Multimodality monitoring in the neurocritical care unit. Continuum (Minneap Minn). 2018 Dec;24(6):1776–88.

Le Roux P, Menon DK, Citerio G, Vespa P, Bader MK, Brophy GM, et al. Consensus summary statement of the International Multidisciplinary Consensus Conference on Multimodality Monitoring in Neurocritical Care: a statement for healthcare professionals from the Neurocritical Care Society and the European Society of Intensive Care Medicine. Neurocrit Care. 2014 Dec;21 Suppl 2:S1–26.

Marcoux J, McArthur DA, Miller C, Glenn TC, Villablanca P, Martin NA, et al. Persistent metabolic crisis as measured by elevated cerebral microdialysis lactate-pyruvate ratio predicts chronic frontal lobe brain atrophy after traumatic brain injury. Crit Care Med. 2008 Oct;36(10):2871–7.

Sorrentino E, Diedler J, Kasprowicz M, Budohoski KP, Haubrich C, Smielewski P, et al. Critical thresholds for cerebrovascular reactivity after traumatic brain injury. Neurocrit Care. 2012 Apr;16(2):258–66.

Stocker RA. Intensive care in traumatic brain injury including multi-modal monitoring and neuroprotection. Med Sci (Basel). 2019 Feb 26;7(3). pii: E37.

Timofeev I, Carpenter KL, Nortje J, Al-Rawi PG, O'Connell MT, Czosnyka M, et al. Cerebral extracellular chemistry and outcome following traumatic brain injury: a microdialysis study of 223 patients. Brain. 2011 Feb;134(Pt 2):484–94. Epub 2011 Jan 18.

Vajkoczy P, Horn P, Thome C, Munch E, Schmiedek P. Regional cerebral blood flow monitoring in the diagnosis of delayed ischemia following aneurysmal subarachnoid hemorrhage. J Neurosurg. 2003 Jun;98(6):1227–34.

Vik A, Nag T, Fredriksli OA, Skandsen T, Moen KG, Schirmer-Mikalsen K, et al. Relationship of "dose" of intracranial hypertension to outcome in severe traumatic brain injury. J Neurosurg. 2008 Oct;109(4):678–84.

Essentials of Cranial Neuroimaging

E. PAUL LINDELL, MD

Goals

- Review the basic neuroimaging aspects of cranial computed tomography and magnetic resonance imaging and the advantages and disadvantages of each method.
- Describe the computed tomographic appearance of ischemic stroke, including its changing features over time, and the intracranial hemorrhage patterns on noncontrast cranial computed tomography.
- Recognize the neuroimaging appearance of other conditions, such as brain tumors.

Introduction

Critically ill patients may have a wide array of neuroimaging abnormalities, including ischemic stroke, intracranial hemorrhage (ICH), and anoxic or hypoxic brain injury. Recognition of common and life-threatening patterns is essential to proper treatment. Critically ill patients are in an unstable condition, so moving them to a computed tomographic (CT) or magnetic resonance imaging (MRI) suite presents logistic and safety challenges that involve nursing care, transport of the ventilator and other intravenous tubing, and vasopressor medications. Portable head CT scanners are available, but they are not widely prevalent in most intensive care units (ICUs). Although MRI is now more widely available, it is difficult to use with ICU patients, and MRI is contraindicated until a metallic safety questionnaire has excluded unsecured metal from gunshot wounds, items inside the head (eg, brain aneurysm clips), and pacemakers. CT has a faster acquisition time than MRI and is more commonly used to obtain emergent neuroimaging data, such as massive stroke or intracranial structural information.

Computed Tomography

CT is the most easily available cross-sectional imaging modality for the evaluation of ICU patients. It offers excellent imaging with short acquisition times for the brain, skull, spine, and spinal cord. It is available at most hospitals, and in most locations the turnaround time for interpretations is minimal. For most neurologic and neurosurgical emergencies, noncontrast CT of the head provides an abundance of useful information.

CT uses x-rays to make radiographic sections (tomograms) through tissue, which are reconstructed with a computer in 2-dimensional or 3-dimensional projection. CT density is measured in Hounsfield units (HU). The Hounsfield unit scale is a linear transformation of the attenuation coefficient of the x-ray beam. For water, the CT density is 0 HU; for air, -1,000 HU (Table 132.1).

Most CT studies include several sets of images, each with a different purpose and strength. The images can be reconstructed at various thicknesses and, if acquired helically, in any plane, including curved. Some images have had mathematical filters applied to enhance fine detail, as in dedicated bone images. Typical CT of the head includes detailed images of the brain and bone. The typical thickness of a section is 5 mm, although thinner sections are occasionally desired. The signal to noise ratio on thinner images is lower, which renders them less clear. This is an advantage for examining bone but a disadvantage for examining the brain.

CT images are viewed on a workstation with changeable parameters called the window width and the window level (or window center). *Window width* refers to the displayed densities on the image, which include the Hounsfield units of the tissue density of interest and excludes the remainder (eg, bone window, lung window, or brain window). For example, to distinguish between gray and white matter to

Table 132.1 • CT Appearance of Common Substances

Substance	HU	Appearance
Air	−1,000	Black
Fat	−100	Dark
Water	0	Dark
Muscle	40	Gray
Brain	30-50	Gray
Contrast material	130	Bright white
Bone	≥400-3,000	Very bright white

Abbreviations: CT, computed tomographic; HU, Hounsfield units.

evaluate for a stroke, a brain window should be centered at a width of 80 HU and a level of 20 to 45 HU. Thus, a typical brain window, expressed as window width/window level, is 80/40; a subdural window for extra-axial hemorrhage, such as subdural bleeding, is 200/50; for soft tissue evaluations, 350/50 is optimal; and for bone and fracture evaluation, 4,000/400 is typical.

For CT of the head, reconstruction is typically in a para-axial plane parallel to the canthomeatal line. Structures of the face, skull base, temporal bone, and neck (after trauma or bony injury) can sometimes be evaluated with basic CT of the head, but further evaluation may require dedicated CT of the face or orbits with fine (1-mm) sections, CT of the cervical spine, or CT of the neck soft tissue.

Comparative CT studies are quite useful. A previous CT study, if it exists, can provide critical chronologic information about current imaging findings to help determine whether a condition is acute, subacute, or chronic. Comparison of symmetry between the 2 sides of the brain is helpful in CT analysis to determine the side with a pathologic or disease process (Figure 132.1). The first step is to compare each section for differences in the gyri and sulci between the hemispheres. Next, the cisterns are compared (eg, the suprasellar, prepontine, quadrigeminal plate, ambient, cerebellopontine angle, and perimedullary cisterns) (Figure 132.1B and C). A similar evaluation of the ventricular system should be performed. Evaluation of the parenchyma for a uniform junction between gray matter and white matter and positive identification of the basal ganglia are critical for identifying common patterns of ischemia or anoxia (Figure 132.2). The density difference at the gray matter–white matter junction is largely due to blood pool differences between the cortex and the white matter; the differential is lost in ischemia due to reduced or absent blood flow. CT evaluation includes examination of all features and a search for abnormal densities.

Hydrocephalus

Obstructive hydrocephalus is suspected when 1 or more ventricles are asymmetrically larger than the others along the course of cerebrospinal fluid (CSF) flow. Obstructing masses or a mass effect typically occurs at the level of the ventricular conduits, such as the cerebral aqueduct. Communicating hydrocephalus occurs when all the ventricles are similarly enlarged. This typically results from slow egress of CSF through the arachnoid granulations. Accompanying progressive global sulcal effacement may be a more sensitive clue than ventricular size measurements.

Intracranial Hemorrhage

Blood from acute hemorrhage is usually brighter or denser than white matter but could be isodense compared with gray matter depending on the time frame. The density of gray matter is mostly due to the blood volume in the cortex. Extravasated blood from a hyperacute hemorrhage (seconds to minutes), such as an isodense subdural hematoma, can be difficult to identify apart from sulcal asymmetry or a subtle mass effect but is obvious when large enough (Figure 132.3). As the hemorrhage becomes acute (minutes to hours), the blood clots and changes density from a colloidal suspension to a solid with hypodense plasma (Figure 132.3B), and the dense bright material is essentially packed red blood cells.

An intraparenchymal hematoma (IPH) matures similarly over time and creates a hypodense rim that is perihematomal edema from plasma exudation from the central venous blood. After about 1 week, an IPH begins to be resorbed as liquid and slowly becomes less dense over days to weeks. Chronic hematomas (often subdural) appear as a black or dark density like CSF. An important clue is when an IPH or subdural hematoma has an unusual fluid-fluid level, which can be due to anticoagulation or to a severe bleeding disorder, coagulopathy, or clotting disorder.

Ischemia

The most subtle and earliest sign of ischemia on noncontrast CT of the head is the loss of the gray matter–white matter differentiation (Figure 132.1B) and local effacement of sulci and a mass effect in a distribution at and distal to the occlusion. Clinical neuroanatomical localization on neurologic examination of the brain area responsible for the observed deficits is helpful to guide evaluation of the CT scan for detection of early brain ischemia. Common patterns of involvement include the *insular ribbon sign*, which occurs with loss of the gray matter–white matter differentiation of the insular cortex and frequently with loss of delineation of the adjacent basal ganglia with an occlusion of the M1 segment of the middle cerebral artery (MCA) (Figure 132.1B, right panel, shows less CSF space in the

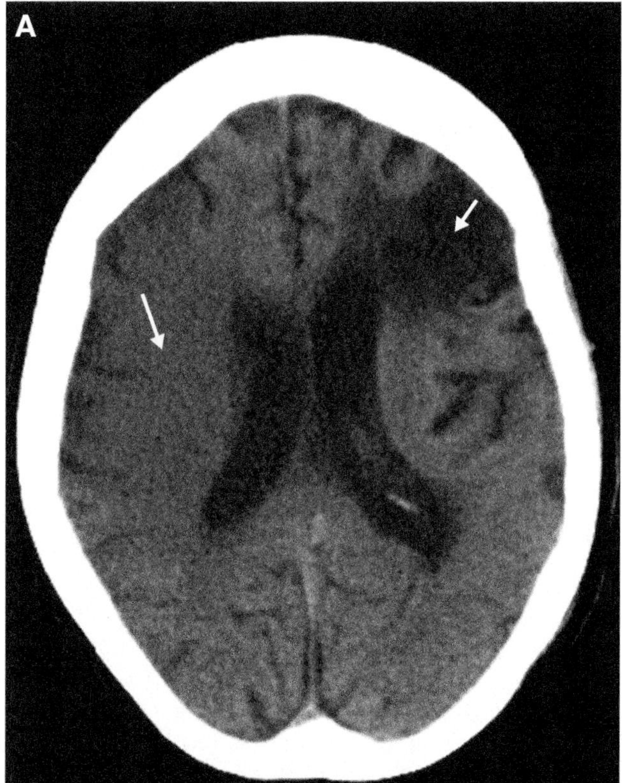

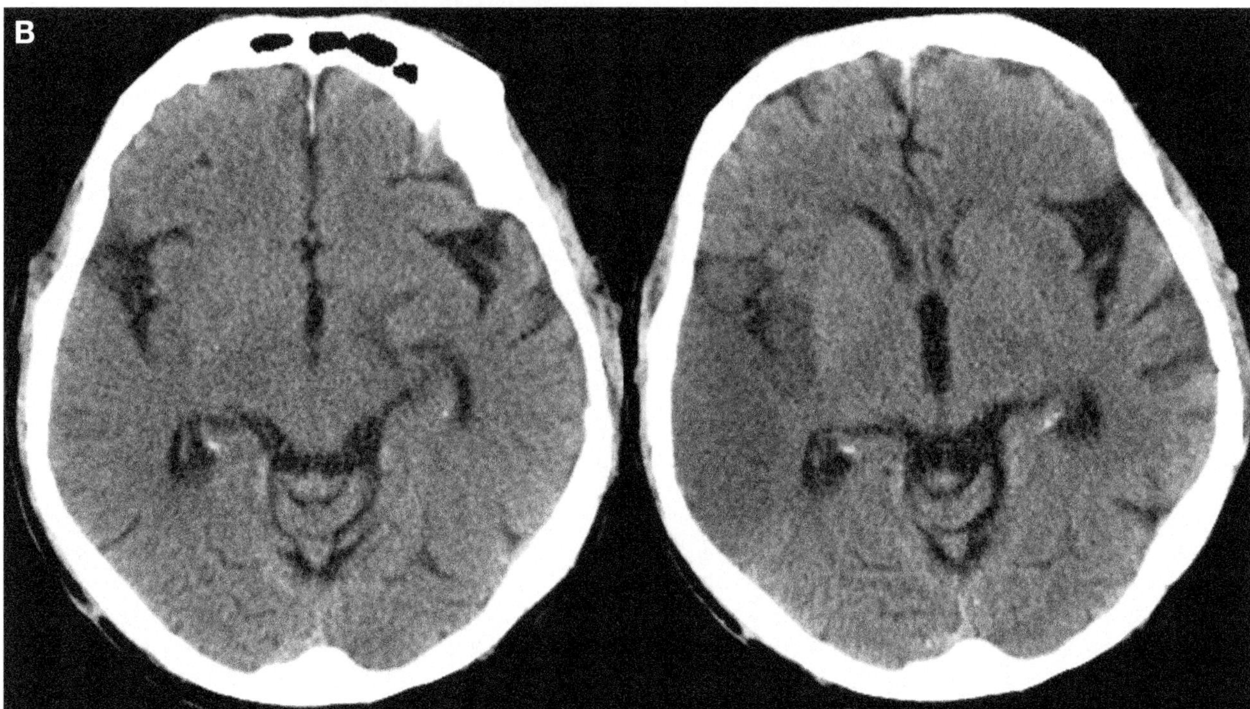

Figure 132.1. *Computed Tomographic Examples of Acute, Chronic, and Evolving Ischemic and Hemorrhagic Brain Infarcts. A, Acute and chronic infarcts. An acute infarct (left arrow) of the right middle cerebral artery (MCA) distribution is characterized by local effacement of sulci, loss of gray matter–white matter distinction, and low density from early infarction and edema. A chronic infarct (right arrow) appears black with a density close to that of water. The affected area, the anterior left MCA distribution, has regional volume loss from encephalomalacia, which appears as chronic involutional changes, typically seen in a chronic infarct. B, Infarct evolution. Left, At 2 hours, the acute right MCA infarct has a subtle loss of the gray matter–white matter junction. Right, At 24 hours, the acute right MCA infarct has regional sulcal effacement, darker density, and early edema. C, Infarct evolution with asymmetry. Upper left, Left MCA infarct on day 1 shows loss of gray matter–white matter distinction. Upper right, Left MCA infarct on day 5 shows edema and early mass effect on the frontal horn of the left lateral ventricle and loss of the left sylvian fissure. Lower left, Left MCA infarct on day 8 shows progressive edema and mass effect with midline shift. Lower right, Left MCA infarct on day 13 shows hemorrhagic transformation and midline shift.*

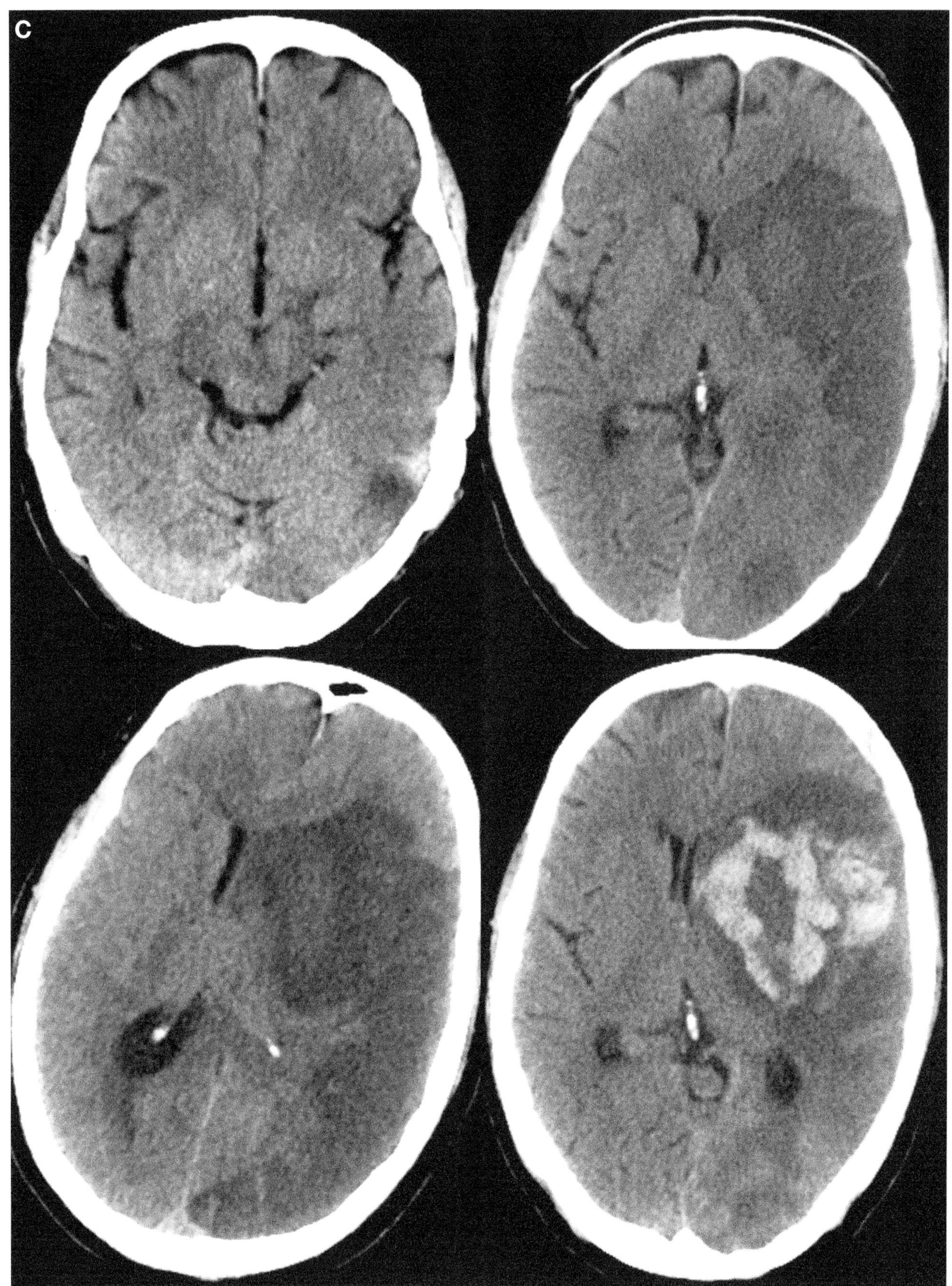

Figure 132.1. Continued

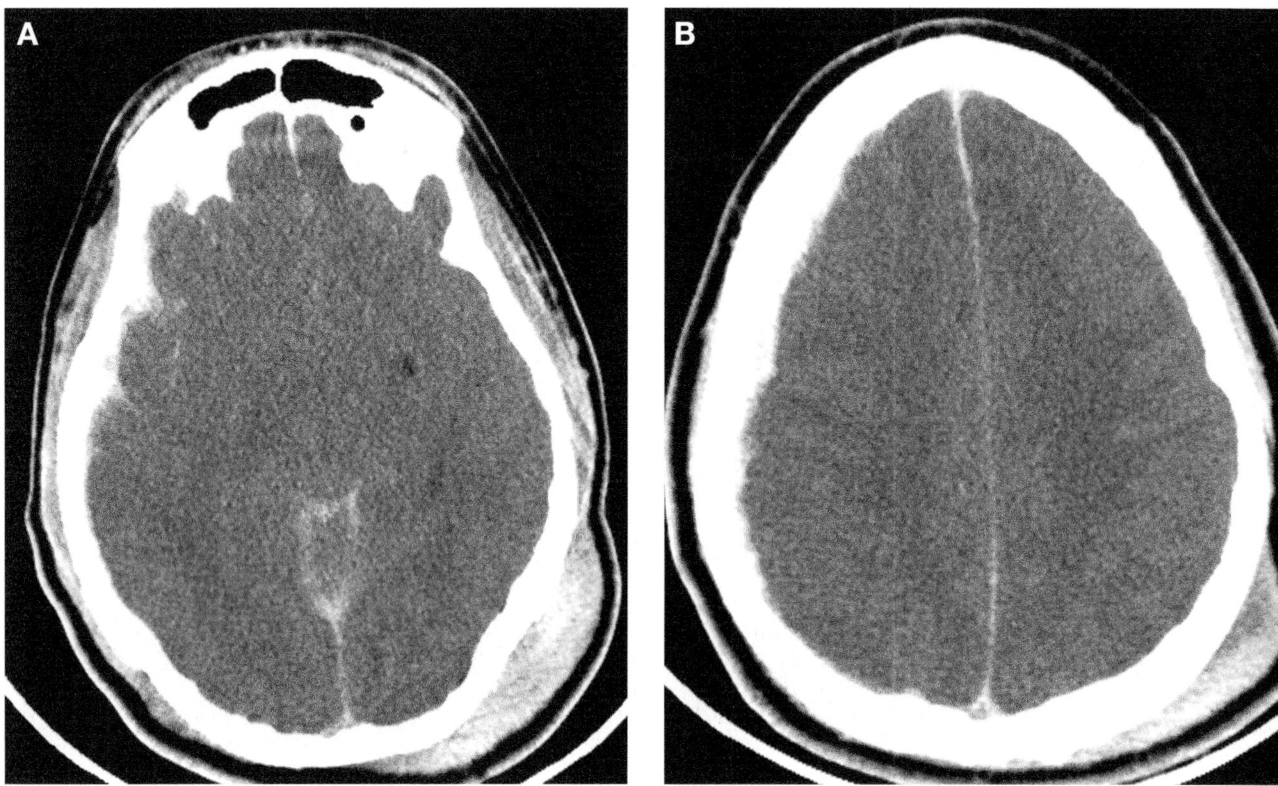

Figure 132.2. Brain Edema in Anoxic-Ischemic Encephalopathy. Because of its resemblance to subarachnoid hemorrhage (SAH), global anoxia is called pseudo-SAH. A and B, On computed tomography, global anoxia is characterized by loss of the gray matter–white matter junction.

insula compared with the contralateral side). Occasionally a thrombus is visualized in a vessel as the *hyperdense artery sign*, but it can be difficult to separate from arterial mural calcification, so it is often apparent retrospectively.

Use of Contrast Agents

Noncontrast CT can be used to answer most neurologic questions in the neurocritical care setting. For ICU patients, iodinated contrast material is most useful with CT angiography (CTA). CTA is a powerful technique that, like noncontrast CT, is nearly universally available. The resolution of CTA is less than that of formal digital subtraction cerebral angiography, but it is comparable to magnetic resonance angiography. The cervical vessels, the circle of Willis, and the M1 and larger M2 segments of the MCA can be visualized well. If clinically indicated, the dural venous sinuses and the larger cortical veins can be visualized well with CT venography. Dynamic lesions, such as dural arteriovenous fistulas and arteriovenous malformations, can be detected with CTA but are usually better evaluated with MRI or cerebral angiography.

Iodinated contrast material has been reported to cause renal dysfunction in patients with compromised renal function, although recent research suggests that this may be less of a problem than previously thought. Patients with an estimated glomerular filtration rate (eGFR) greater than 30 mL/min/1.73 m^2 are generally considered good candidates for administration of iodinated contrast material. Discussion with the radiologist is recommended for patients who have an eGFR less than 30 mL/min/1.73 m^2 or a potential dye allergy. Use of iodinated contrast material is unnecessary for CT of the head for the typical ICU patient.

Although MRI can be useful to evaluate for metastatic disease and less useful to evaluate for infection, such as meningitis, MRI is considerably superior to CT in both of these clinical situations. A potentially strong indication for use of an iodinated contrast agent is for extracranial head and neck infections unless MRI can be performed in a safe and timely manner.

Perfusion Imaging

Perfusion imaging can be performed with either CT or MRI. With CT perfusion imaging of the brain, a bolus of contrast material is injected while either continuous or short-interval scans are obtained. Numerous mathematical models are available to analyze the data. The analysis is roughly based on the central volume theory of flow being equal to the volume per unit time. The commonly

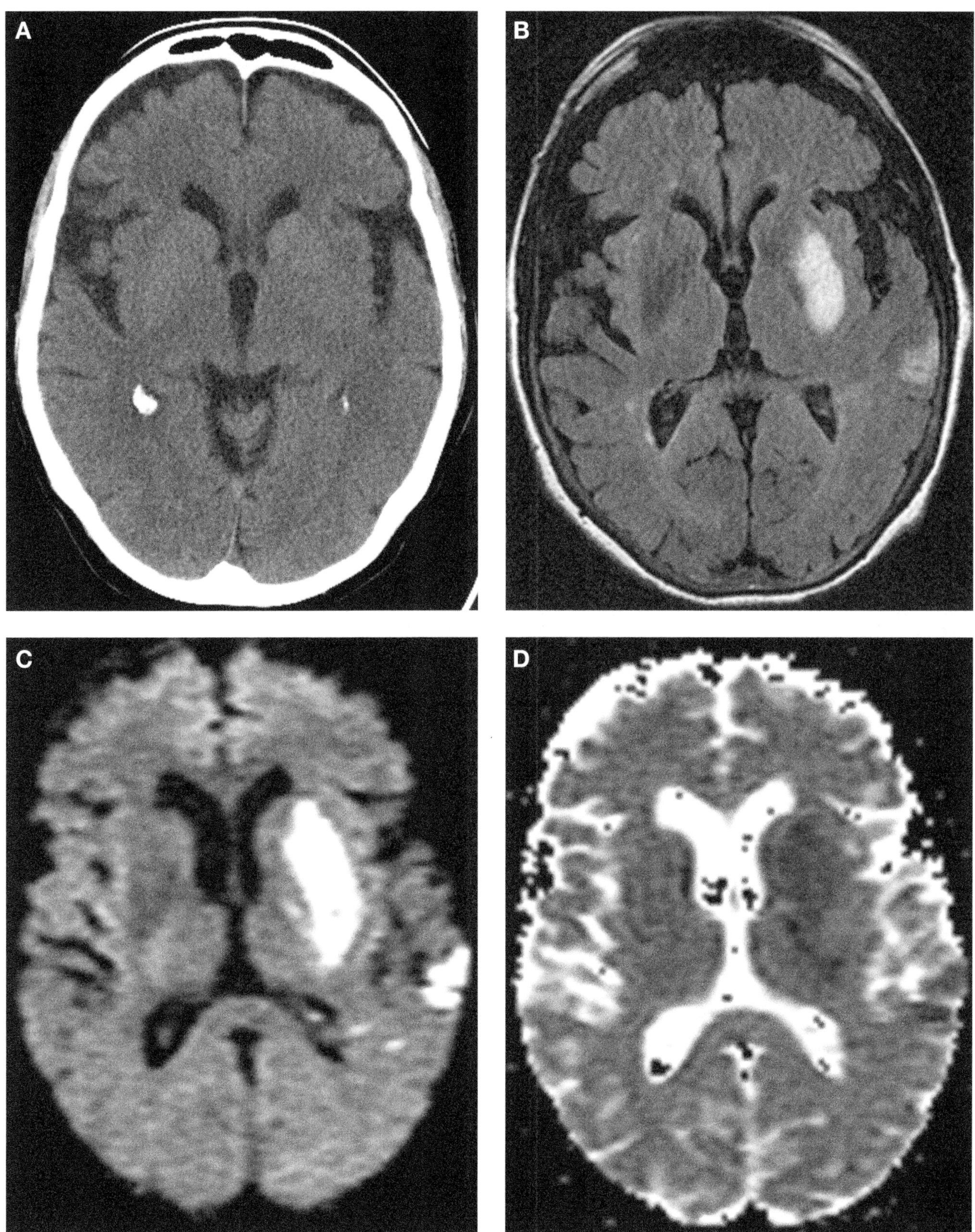

Figure 132.3. *Cerebral Infarction on Computed Tomography (CT) and Magnetic Resonance Imaging (MRI). A, CT shows left basal ganglial loss of the gray matter–white matter junction. B, Fluid-attenuated inversion recovery (FLAIR) MRI shows high signal intensity. C and D, Diffusion-weighted MRI (C) and the apparent diffusion coefficient (ADC) map (D) show a signal pattern of restricted diffusion of water. The dark signal on the ADC map is restricted compared with the internal reference of ventricular cerebrospinal fluid, which is nonrestricted.*

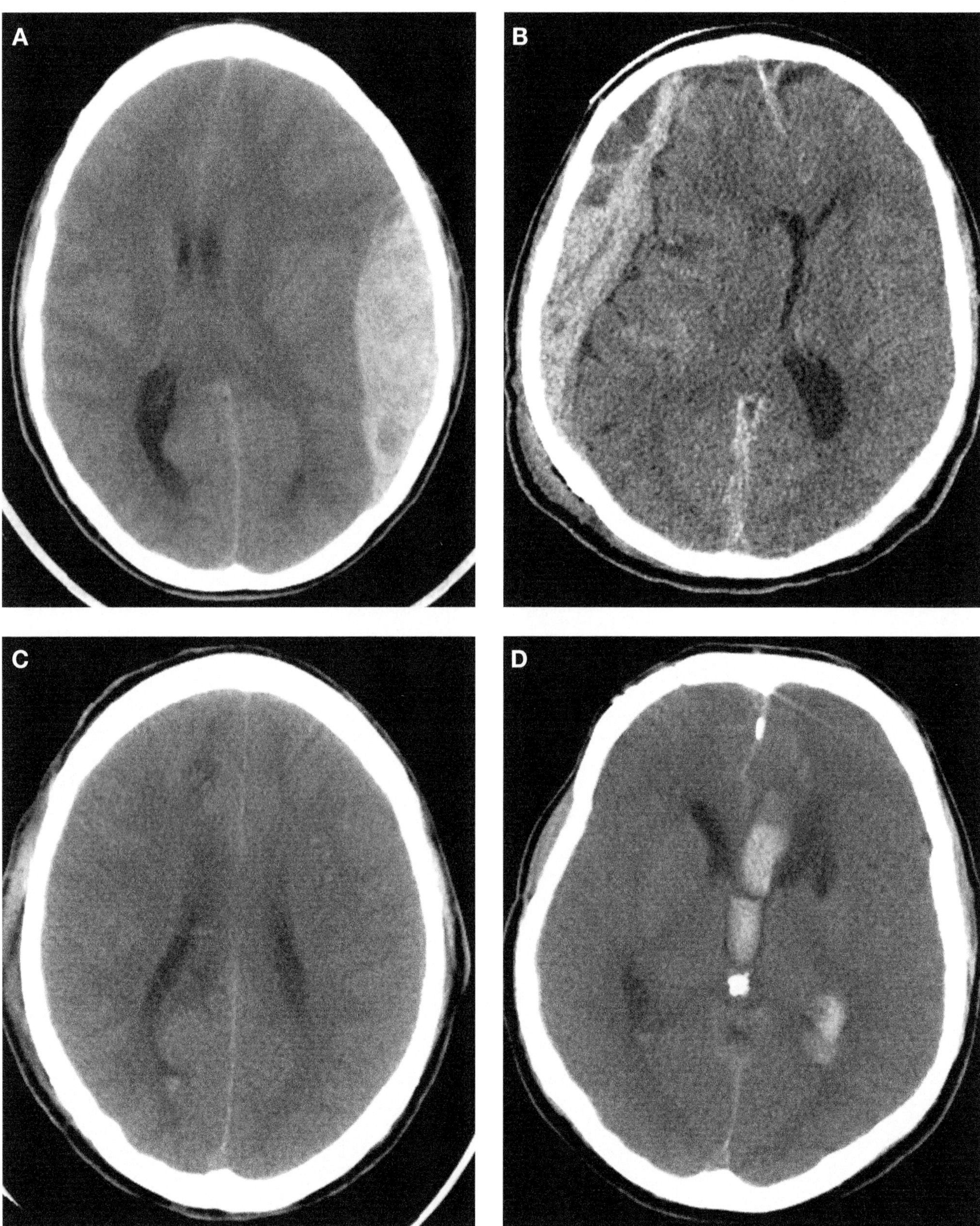

Figure 132.4. *Intracranial Hemorrhage on Computed Tomography. A, Epidural hematoma. The spread of blood is limited by the coronal suture anteriorly. B, Subdural hematoma. Blood crosses the coronal suture and extends along the falx cerebri, following the extent of the subdural space. Small amounts of posttraumatic subarachnoid hemorrhage are apparent in multiple sulci. C, Diffuse axonal injury. Multiple hemorrhages are apparent at the gray matter–white matter junction and within the corpus callosum. A small amount of posttraumatic intraventricular blood is present. D, Intraventricular blood with hydrocephalus. Clot retraction suggests an acute to subacute duration.*

calculated parameters include cerebral blood flow (CBF), cerebral blood volume (CBV), and mean transit time. The analysis of perfusion scans requires the recognition that the maps and values are only snapshots of a dynamic process. The hallmark of brain ischemia is a mismatch of CBF and CBV. The more preserved the CBV is, the greater is the contribution from collateral flow to the affected portion of the brain. The resolution of the perfusion scans is relatively low, and small lacunar infarcts are often not readily apparent.

Magnetic Resonance Imaging

MRI uses a strong, static magnetic field to align tissue protons in 1 plane and then radiofrequency energy and field gradients to image the body. CT uses ionizing radiation, but MRI does not. The large magnetic field used in MRI results in safety issues that include the projectile effect and induced currents in implanted devices such as pacemakers. Explicit listing of all implanted devices is recommended as part of a patient's admission history and physical examination. Most patients also carry a wallet card or similar information about the safety of their implanted device and MRI compatibility to help with screening safety.

MRI examinations consist of several sequences, each of which takes several minutes to acquire and process. Each sequence provides different information about the normal and pathologic tissues imaged. The information from each sequence must be synthesized with the others to allow for a cohesive description. If CT examinations are like a solo musician, MRI examinations are like a complete symphony orchestra, and listening to only the string section would provide an incomplete perception of the piece. MRI images are manipulated with a similar window and level adjustment to make different sequences; however, MRI has no scaled reference, such as Hounsfield units in CT. Each MRI sequence uses different tissue physics to detect abnormalities or highlight different tissues. For example, T1- and T2-weighted MRI sequences have quite different appearances, with T2-weighted sequences showing CSF spaces as very bright. Diffusion-weighted imaging is used to detect poor intracellular water diffusion; thus, infarcted (dead) brain tissue appears white, but "T2 shine through" must also be compared on these sequences.

While CT uses iodinated contrast material to alter the density and enhance the image contrast of tissues, MRI uses gadolinium-based contrast material, which changes the magnetic relaxivity of perfused tissues. The renal function considerations are similar for gadolinium-enhanced MRI. Patients with an eGFR greater than 30 mL/min/1.73 m^2 are considered good candidates for gadolinium administration. Those with eGFR less than 30 mL/min/1.73 m^2 are not considered good candidates because the risk of nephrogenic systemic fibrosis is higher. If a patient has an eGFR less than 30 mL/min/1.73 m^2, a potential allergy, or an implanted device, a discussion with the radiologist is recommended.

Epidural Hematoma

Epidural hematomas expand the potential epidural space by dissecting the endosteum from the calvaria (Figure 132.4). The endosteum is the outer layer of the 2 apposed layers of dura mater. Because the endosteum is tightly applied to the bone, high pressure is required for blood to accumulate. Typically this involves laceration of an epidural artery, such as the middle meningeal artery, or a larger dural sinus such as the transverse sinus. The vascular laceration is nearly always accompanied by a fracture. An epidural hematoma is classically described as lenticular shaped, but a more reliable characteristic for identification is the limitation of the hematoma by the calvarial suture lines. The endosteum is essentially fixed at the sutures, and this limits the extent of the hematoma extension.

Subdural Hematoma

Subdural hematomas (Figure 132.4) lie in the subdural space, which may be better termed the *epiarachnoid space*. This potential space is between the arachnoid membrane and the inner of the 2 apposed layers of dura mater. The transmitted forces during trauma are thought to lacerate vessels that transit this space. Blood accumulating in the space separates the inner layer of dura from the arachnoid. With no limitation to extension at the sutures, subdural hematomas cross suture lines. In addition, the space extends along the tentorium cerebelli and falx cerebri, which are common locations for subdural hematoma extension.

Parenchymal Hematoma

Parenchymal hematomas are centered in the brain parenchyma. During the first 3 to 5 days, the associated vasogenic edema increases and causes a progressively greater mass effect, even if the hematoma size is stable. Unlike epidural and subdural hemorrhages, parenchymal hematomas require additional imaging to exclude treatable underlying causes, such as arteriovenous malformations and underlying tumor. Parenchymal hematomas mature from the periphery to a central location. After trauma, cortical contusions appear over the course of a few days. They are particularly common in the inferior frontal lobes and the anterior temporal lobes.

Subarachnoid Hemorrhage

Subarachnoid hemorrhage occurs in the subarachnoid space between the pia mater, which courses over all gyri and into all sulci, and the arachnoid membrane. It appears as a higher density than cortex on CT and fills the affected sulci. Subarachnoid hemorrhage is a common finding after trauma and frequently occurs in a peripheral location. When it occurs more centrally, particularly in the suprasellar cistern and in the absence of obvious trauma, aneurysmal rupture must be considered. Barring additional hemorrhage, subarachnoid hemorrhage tends to clear and wash out along the path of CSF flow from central to peripheral and from inferior to superior over the convexities.

Summary

- Noncontrast serial cranial CT is most commonly done in the ICU setting.
- MRI poses challenges, such as requiring longer acquisition times, and may not be an alternative for patients who are hemodynamically unstable or who have metallic equipment that cannot be used near MRI scanners.
- Basic stroke and brain injury patterns (eg, subarachnoid hemorrhage, subdural hematoma, and epidural hematoma) can be easily recognized by intensivists and neurointensivists.
- The clinical history and the ICU neurologic examination must be used to help guide which type of neuroimaging test is best and safest for each patient.
- A radiologist should be consulted for specific and challenging clinical neuroimaging questions (eg, distinguishing posterior reversible encephalopathy syndrome, anoxic injury, and Creutzfeldt-Jakob disease from infarct or encephalitis).

SUGGESTED READING

American College of Radiology. Appropriateness criteria [Internet]. c2018 [cited 2018 Oct 9]. Available from: https://acsearch.acr.org/list.

Atlas SW, editor. Magnetic resonance imaging of the brain and spine. 4th ed. Philadelphia (PA): Wolters Kluwer Health/Lippincott Williams & Wilkins; c2009. 1,890 p.

Brinjikji W, Demchuk AM, Murad MH, Rabinstein AA, McDonald RJ, McDonald JS, et al. Neurons over nephrons: systematic review and meta-analysis of contrast-induced nephropathy in patients with acute stroke. Stroke. 2017 Jul;48(7):1862–8. Epub 2017 Jun 5.

Mamoulakis C, Tsarouhas K, Fragkiadoulaki I, Heretis I, Wilks MF, Spandidos DA, et al. Contrast-induced nephropathy: basic concepts, pathophysiological implications and prevention strategies. Pharmacol Ther. 2017 Dec;180:99–112. Epub 2017 Jun 19.

Masaryk T, Kolonick R, Painter T, Weinreb DB. The economic and clinical benefits of portable head/neck CT imaging in the intensive care unit. Radiol Manage. 2008 Mar-Apr;30(2):50–4.

Nadgir R, Yousem DM. Neuroradiology: the requisites. 4th ed. Philadelphia (PA): Elsevier; c2017. 630 p.

Radiopaedia. Cases: system: central nervous system [Internet]. c2005-2018 [cited 2018 Oct 9]. Available from: https://radiopaedia.org/encyclopaedia/cases/central-nervous-system?page=1.

Questions and Answers

Abbreviations Used

ADC	apparent diffusion coefficient
APC	argon plasma coagulation
BAL	bronchoalveolar lavage
cEEG,	continuous electroencephalography
$CHADS_2$-VASc	congestive heart failure, hypertension, age 75 years or older, diabetes mellitus, previous stroke or transient ischemic attack or thromboembolism, vascular disease, age 65 to 74 years, sex category (eg, female)
CO	cardiac output
COPD	chronic obstructive pulmonary disease
CSF	cerebrospinal fluid
CT	computed tomography
CVP	central venous pressure
Do_2	oxygen delivery
DWI	diffusion-weighted imaging
ED	emergency department
EEG	electroencephalography
Fio_2	fraction of inspired oxygen
FOB	fiberoptic bronchoscopy
GPD	generalized periodic discharge
HFNC	high-flow nasal cannula
ICA	internal carotid artery
ICP	intracranial pressure
ICU	intensive care unit
IR	interventional radiology
LP	lumbar puncture
LPD	lateral periodic discharge
MCA	middle cerebral artery
MFV	mean flow velocity
MRI	magnetic resonance imaging
NCSE	nonconvulsive status epilepticus
NIV	noninvasive ventilation
OER	oxygen extraction ratio
OSA	obstructive sleep apnea
PAC	pulmonary artery catheter
PAOP	pulmonary artery occlusion pressure
$Pbto_2$	partial pressure of oxygen in interstitial brain tissue
PDT	percutaneous dilatational tracheostomy
PEEP	positive end-expiratory pressure
PET	positron emission tomography
PLED	periodic lateralized epileptiform discharge
PRx	pressure reactivity index
SAH	subarachnoid hemorrhage
Sao_2	arterial oxygen saturation
SV	stroke volume
Svo_2	mixed venous oxygen saturation
SVV	stroke volume variation
TBI	traumatic brain injury
TCD	transcranial Doppler
$\dot{V}o_2$	oxygen consumption

Questions

Multiple Choice (choose the best answer)

Airway Procedures and Modes of Ventilation

VI.1. Which of the following is most useful for predicting difficulty with intubation?

a. Mallampati score alone
b. Sternomental distance in combination with Mallampati score
c. Thyromental distance in combination with Mallampati score
d. Mouth opening in combination with thyromental distance

VI.2. How does the HFNC compare with the Venturi mask and NIV for oxygen delivery?

a. The HFNC is inferior to the Venturi mask in maintaining oxygenation for a specific Fio_2.
b. The HFNC is inferior to NIV in preventing reintubation within 48 hours.
c. The HFNC is superior to the Venturi mask and to NIV in preventing reintubation within 48 hours.
d. The HFNC is noninferior to NIV in preventing reintubation within 48 hours.

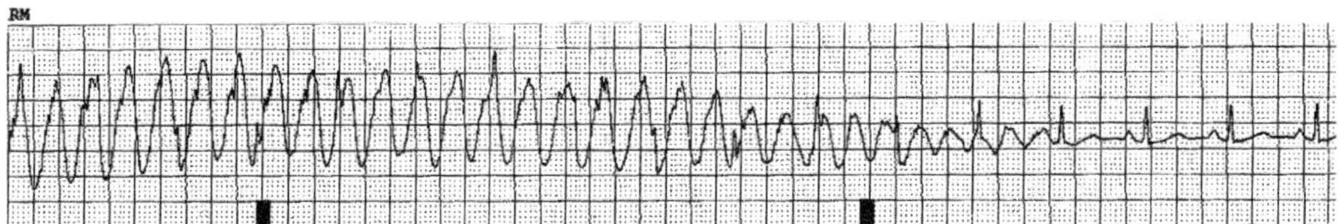

Figure VI.Q9.

VI.3. Which of the following is most reliable for confirming proper endotracheal tube placement?
a. Bilateral breath sounds
b. Symmetric chest rise with inspiration
c. Condensation in the endotracheal tube with exhalation
d. End-tidal carbon dioxide detection

VI.4. A patient with which of the following would *not* likely be a candidate for NIV?
a. Nocturnal NIV for OSA
b. Stable COPD
c. Exacerbation of COPD
d. Absent cough reflex

VI.5. Which of the following is *not* a criterion for discontinuing NIV and transitioning to invasive ventilation?
a. Worsening pH and $Paco_2$
b. Decreased level of consciousness
c. Decreased work of breathing
d. Inability to tolerate mask

VI.6. Which of the following is *false* about tracheostomy management?
a. PDT should generally be performed in patients 16 years or older.
b. Loss of tracheostomy airway in a patient in stable condition should be managed with immediate translaryngeal intubation.
c. The late postprocedural tracheostomy complication rate is affected by the duration of the preceding translaryngeal intubation.
d. Massive hemorrhage from a tracheoinnominate fistula may be preceded by sentinel bleeding.

VI.7. A 68-year-old man who is receiving immunosuppressive therapy for a previous kidney transplant is admitted to the ICU with fever for the past 48 hours, dyspnea, and progressive hypoxemia requiring intubation and mechanical ventilation (Fio_2 of 1.0 and PEEP of 8 cm H_2O to achieve an Sao_2 of 94%). He is hemodynamically stable after receiving intravenous fluid support, but he has abnormal renal function (serum creatinine, 3.5 mg/dL; serum urea nitrogen, 75 mg/dL). He receives subcutaneous heparin twice daily for deep vein thrombosis prophylaxis. His hemoglobin on admission is 6.9 g/dL. A bedside echocardiogram shows normal right and left ventricular contractility with normal ejection fraction. Chest radiography shows diffuse bilateral alveolar infiltrates without cardiomegaly, and his endotracheal tube appears to be in a good position. These infiltrates were not present at a routine visit with his nephrologist 2 weeks before. You discuss with the ICU team the best approach for diagnosing his condition. What would be the best diagnostic pulmonary procedure?
a. FOB to obtain bronchial washing samples
b. FOB to obtain bronchial brushing and bronchial biopsy samples
c. FOB to obtain BAL samples
d. FOB with bedside fluoroscopic guidance to obtain transbronchial biopsy samples

VI.8. A 70-year-old man who received a left lung transplant for COPD 5 years ago is admitted to the ICU with progressive respiratory distress, wheezing, and hypoxemia. He undergoes fiberoptic intubation and receives ventilator support (Fio_2 of 1.0). On bronchoscopic inspection of the proximal airways at intubation, a mass was partially occluding the right main bronchus and extending to the carina; the mass, with an unknown origin, was not present at the patient's latest recheck 6 months ago. He has a history of coronary artery disease and sick sinus syndrome; a dual-chamber pacemaker is in place. In addition to immediate medical management, which initial interventional procedure would be best to manage his condition?
a. Fiberoptic placement of a brachytherapy catheter
b. APC
c. Cryotherapy
d. Placement of endobronchial valves in the native emphysematous lung

Cardiovascular and Cardiopulmonary Monitoring and Access

VI.9. After laparoscopic cholecystectomy, a 66-year-old woman has an ischemic cardiomyopathy with an ejection fraction of 45%. The monitor shows several episodes, one of which is shown (Figure VI.Q9).
What is the next best step in the management of this rhythm disturbance?
a. Increased β-blockade
b. Urgent coronary angiography
c. Implantation of a cardioverter-defibrillator
d. Observation

VI.10. A 77-year-old man with hypertension, diet-controlled diabetes mellitus, and peripheral vascular disease has had left hip surgery. The only medications he is receiving are metoprolol and aspirin. A rhythm strip from his hospitalization is shown (Figure VI.Q10). On the basis of this strip, for what is he at greatest risk?
a. Myocardial infarction
b. Cerebrovascular accident
c. Sudden cardiac death
d. Hypotension

VI.11. The morphologic pattern or shape of an arterial line waveform is *not* affected by which of the following variables?
a. Location of arterial line cannulation
b. Heart rate
c. Transducer height
d. Velocity of blood flow

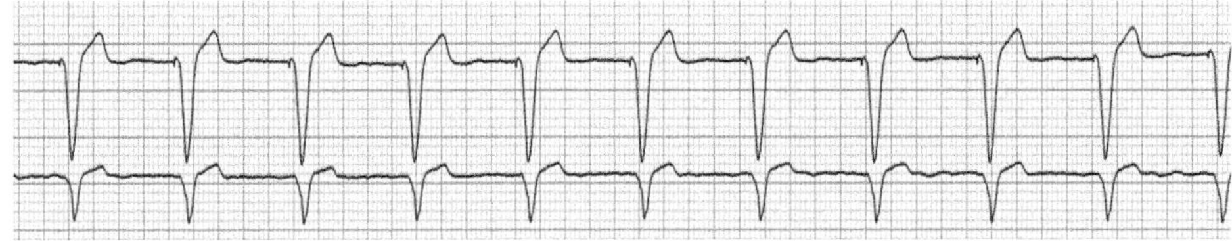

Figure VI.Q10.

VI.12. On the basis of the difference between a patient's arterial and central venous oxygen saturation, the OER is 55%. Which of the following clinical situations is *least* likely to cause this ratio?
a. Considerable anemia
b. Hypovolemia
c. Seizure
d. Fluid overload

VI.13. A hypotensive patient with ventricular function represented by the steep or ascending portion of the Frank-Starling curve would likely have which of the following responses?
a. Be responsive to a fluid bolus
b. Have a low SVV (<13%)
c. Have an increased PAOP
d. Benefit from the initiation of a vasopressor

VI.14. CO monitoring devices that also predict fluid response by analyzing arterial waveforms for pulse pressure variation or SVV (eg, FloTrac-Vigileo, PiCCO, LiDCO) require which of the following factors to be most reliable?
a. Spontaneous breathing
b. High respiratory rate
c. Low tidal volumes
d. Normal sinus rhythm

VI.15. PAOP is measured as a surrogate of which of the following?
a. Right ventricular afterload
b. Left ventricular preload
c. Right ventricular preload
d. Systemic vascular resistance

VI.16. A 74-year-old man presents for evaluation of dyspnea at rest. His past medical history is significant for stage 3 chronic kidney disease, hypertension, and diet-controlled diabetes mellitus. An echocardiogram is notable for preserved left ventricular systolic function, grade 1 diastolic dysfunction, biatrial enlargement, and right ventricular systolic pressure of 68 mm Hg (normal, 15-25 mm Hg). A PAC is placed and the findings are shown (Table VI.Q16).

Table VI.Q16. • PAC Results

Chamber	Pressure, mm Hg
Right atrium	14
Right ventricle	66/15
Pulmonary artery	65/37, mean 46
Pulmonary artery occlusion	Mean 36

Which of the following is the most appropriate next step in therapy?
a. Initiation of oral sildenafil therapy
b. Trial of inhaled nitric oxide
c. Referral for pulmonary thromboendarterectomy
d. Intravenous furosemide

VI.17. A 71-year-old woman referred for evaluation of worsening dyspnea on exertion is to undergo right heart catheterization. Her previously diagnosed mild pulmonary arterial hypertension (mean pulmonary artery pressure 34 mm Hg) was treated with sildenafil and warfarin by her local pulmonologist. A PAC is placed under fluoroscopic guidance into the right pulmonary artery, and the pulmonary artery pressure is 62/28 mm Hg (mean 39 mm Hg). Several attempts at obtaining occlusion pressure are met with overwedging, and the catheter must be repositioned several times. Suddenly, the patient coughs up approximately 100 mL of bright red blood, and Sao_2 decreases to 83% despite 50% Fio_2 administered with a Venturi mask. Which of the following interventions is the least appropriate next step in management?
a. Selective bronchial intubation of the left mainstem bronchus
b. Placement of a bronchial blocker in the right mainstem bronchus
c. Arranging for emergency interventional radiologic evaluation
d. Positioning the patient left-side down to minimize blood flow to the hemorrhaging lung

VI.18. Small-bore chest tubes are *not* indicated in which of the following types of pleural processes?
a. Parapneumonic effusion
b. Pneumothorax in a spontaneously ventilated patient
c. Traumatic hemothorax
d. Hepatic hydrothorax

VI.19. Which of the following is *false* regarding bedside procedures using ultrasound guidance?
a. Ultrasound is operator-dependent.
b. Ultrasound use increases yield of pleural drainage.
c. Ultrasound results in increased risk of solid-organ injury.
d. Ultrasound decreases the risk of post-procedure pneumothorax.

VI.20. A 24-year-old man is involved in a motor vehicle accident. He was unrestrained and was ejected from the car. On admission, 18- and 14-gauge peripheral intravenous lines were placed. The trauma survey and subsequent imaging found a grade 3 splenic laceration and a distal closed radius fracture. The surgical team plans nonoperative management of the splenic laceration, and the patient is admitted to the ICU for further management. He is afebrile, heart rate is 105 beats per minute, blood pressure is 110/70 mm Hg, hemoglobin level is 10.2 g/dL, platelet count is 130×10^9/L, and white blood cell count is 9.5×10^9/L. You are called to the bedside a few hours after the admission and the patient's heart rate is 130 beats per minute, blood pressure is 80/40 mm Hg, and temperature is 37.2°C. On physical examination, breath sounds are bilateral and equal, the patient feels slightly cool peripherally with capillary refill of 3 seconds, the abdomen is diffusely tender and more distended than on admission, and the patient opens his eyes but will not respond to questions. What is the best next step in the management of this patient?
a. Place a right internal jugular triple-lumen catheter to allow for monitoring of the CVP to assist in fluid management decisions.
b. Place a right internal jugular triple-lumen catheter and start an infusion of norepinephrine to support the blood pressure.
c. Place a right 9F single-lumen introducer and initiate massive transfusion protocol.
d. Give a bolus of 1 L lactated Ringer solution and check the hemoglobin level.

VI.21. A 65-year-old woman presents to the ED with 4 days of progressive shortness of breath, fever, and productive cough. Initial vital signs include the following: heart rate is 110 beats per minute; blood pressure, 85/44 mm Hg; respiratory rate, 24 breaths per minute; temperature, 38.5°C; and oxygen saturation, 92% while breathing 3 L supplemental oxygen by nasal cannula. Chest radiography shows an infiltrate of the left lower lobe. Blood specimens are obtained for culture, and the patient is given appropriate empiric antibiotics. Despite receiving 3 L of lactated Ringer solution in the ED, her blood pressure is 80/40 mm Hg on arrival to the ICU. You prepare to place a central line for infusion of norepinephrine. Regarding site selection and technique for central line placement, which of the following is true?
a. Femoral vein cannulation has been associated with the lowest incidence of catheter-related infections.
b. Although common, the use of ultrasound for central line placement has not been shown to change the incidence of complications compared with the landmark technique.

c. If a subclavian line is going to be placed, an initial attempt on the right side would be associated with the lowest risk of serious respiratory complications.
d. The subclavian site is associated with the lowest risk of thrombotic complications.

VI.22. A patient is in the surgical ICU for development of sepsis after an anastomotic leak after bowel surgery. The patient is intubated, receiving mechanical ventilation, and sedated. Pressors are being administered. CT shows an abdominal fluid collection that is concerning for an abscess. Which of the following is correct regarding this situation?
a. The patient is too unstable to undergo transport for an IR procedure.
b. Before IR drain placement, the international normalized ratio should be checked.
c. Because the patient has a postsurgical complication, open drainage with laparotomy is the preferred management.
d. The fluid collection must be visible on ultrasonography for an interventional procedure to be performed safely.

VI.23. After a brainstem stroke, a patient has had many aspiration events associated with incoordinated swallowing. A feeding gastrostomy tube is now to be placed with an IR procedure. Most recently, she has been fed by nasogastric tube. Which of the following is appropriate?
a. Planned tracheal intubation to prevent aspiration during the procedure
b. Holding nasogastric feeding and oral intake for 8 hours before the procedure
c. Preprocedural evaluation by anesthesiology for general anesthesia
d. Removal of the nasogastric tube at least 12 hours before the procedure

Neuromonitoring and Procedures

VI.24. Which statement is consistent with the Monro-Kellie doctrine?
a. The skull is a closed vault.
b. The sum of the volume of the intracranial contents (including the blood, CSF, and brain tissue) is dynamic.
c. The CSF and blood compartment are more than 50% of the intracranial volume.
d. The pressure gradient across the brain parenchyma varies with respirations.

VI.25. According to the fourth edition of the Brain Trauma Foundation guidelines, ICP should be monitored if patients have which of the following conditions?
a. Coma
b. Blood on the tentorium
c. Brainstem hemorrhage
d. Blood in the dependent parts of the lateral ventricles

VI.26. What is the approximate amount of CSF produced daily?
a. 500 mL
b. 1,000 mL
c. 2,000 mL
d. 3,000 mL

VI.27. What is the normal range for ICP values in healthy infants?
a. 0.1 to 1.5 mm Hg
b. 1 to 6 mm Hg
c. 6 to 10 mm Hg
d. 11 to 15 mm Hg

VI.28. For how many days before LP should warfarin therapy be stopped?
a. 1
b. 2
c. 3
d. 5

VI.29. How should one proceed with a patient with fever, coma, and suspected meningitis?
a. Wait to begin antibiotic therapy until after you have received CSF results.
b. Perform an LP before CT, submit the CSF samples for testing, and then start antibiotic therapy.
c. Obtain blood cultures, start empirical antibiotic therapy, perform CT, and then perform an LP as soon as possible.
d. Perform MRI with a contrast agent to document meningeal enhancement.

VI.30. A patient presents to the ED with fever, headache, seizure, and coma. EEG shows left PLEDs. Noncontrast CT of the head does not show any serious abnormalities. Which of the following is the best course of action?
a. First treat the seizures aggressively, and then perform LP.
b. Start empirical therapy with antibiotics and acyclovir because of concern about herpes simplex encephalitis, and then perform LP.
c. Perform MRI because of concern about a temporal lobe abscess, and then perform LP.
d. Start empirical therapy with corticosteroids for paraneoplastic encephalitis, and then perform LP.

VI.31. What is the estimated risk of infection with prolonged use of a lumbar drain?
a. 1% or less
b. 2% to 3%
c. 4% to 6%
d. More than 10%

VI.32. What is the effect of lumbar drainage in patients with SAH?
a. Improves long-term functional outcomes
b. Worsens long-term functional outcomes
c. Decreases mortality associated with SAH
d. Decreases the prevalence of delayed ischemic neurologic deficits

VI.33. While administering a medication into an external ventricular drain, you encounter resistance to administration. Which of the following is the most likely cause?
a. Elevated ICP
b. Migration of the catheter from the optimal position
c. Evolving meningitis
d. Debris at the tip of the catheter or a kink in the tubing

VI.34. In addition to sterile technique, which of the following is the fundamental basic principle of intraventricular administration of medication?
a. Administration according to institutional protocol
b. Hypervolemic administration
c. Isovolemic administration
d. Hypovolemic administration

VI.35. Which of the following is incorrect about TCD ultrasonography?
a. Can be used in a patient with a bone flap off
b. Involves a minimal amount of ionizing radiation
c. Provides highly reproducible results
d. Provides real-time physiologic data

VI.36. TCD ultrasonography in a patient with aneurysmal SAH in your ICU originally showed an MCA MFV of less than 120 cm/s daily until day 10; now the left MCA MFV is 250 cm/s. The ipsilateral ICA MFV is 40 cm/s. The patient has also become aphasic and weaker on the right side. Which of the following is the clinical concern?
a. The patient does not have vasospasm but does have a hyperdynamic cardiac state according to the Lindegaard ratio (left MCA/left ICA) and should receive triple-*H* therapy (induced hypertension, induced hypervolemia, and hemodilution).
b. The patient does not have vasospasm and should undergo EEG for subclinical seizure.

c. The patient could be hypoxemic according to the TCD values and should undergo immediate arterial blood gas testing and possibly a blood transfusion.
d. This patient likely has severe, symptomatic left MCA vasospasm (Lindegaard ratio = 6.25), which correlates well with angiographic vasospasm of the MCA after aneurysmal SAH.

VI.37. A 35-year-old man presents with a rather sudden progressive decline in consciousness and weakness. He takes many drugs according to his wife, but she does not know which ones. On examination, he is comatose with normal pupils and cranial nerve reflexes but a remarkable flaccid weakness. His past medical history is remarkable for low back pain, with a recent exacerbation due to heavy lifting. His EEG shows GPDs. What is the most likely cause of his presentation?
a. Herpes simplex encephalitis
b. Baclofen toxicity
c. Creutzfeldt-Jakob disease
d. Opioid toxicity

VI.38. A 62-year-old woman with a left parasagittal meningioma is admitted after a witnessed generalized tonic-clonic seizure. She is postictal in the ED. Her EEG shows diffuse slowing and left central LPDs at a frequency of 1 Hz. What feature would lead you to consider this an ictal pattern rather than an interictal pattern?
a. Subtle right shoulder twitches about once per second
b. An EEG 3 months ago showing left central LPDs at a frequency of 0.5 Hz
c. Decreased frequency of discharges after intravenous administration of fosphenytoin
d. Known history of focal epilepsy

VI.39. A 73-year-old man is successfully resuscitated after cardiac arrest, but he remains comatose. He is admitted to the ICU, where targeted temperature management and cEEG are begun according to the ICU protocol. At 12 hours after cardiac arrest, while he is receiving midazolam, which EEG feature would be most favorable?
a. Burst suppression
b. Continuous, reactive background
c. Markedly suppressed background
d. Alpha coma

VI.40. Which of the following is most strongly associated with sustained intracranial hypertension (ICP>30 mm Hg) in a patient with TBI?
a. Pinpoint pupils
b. Progression to brain death
c. Tachycardia
d. Seizures

VI.41. Which of the following PRx values would be expected in a patient with intact cerebrovascular autoregulation?
a. 1.3
b. 1.0
c. 0.7
d. −0.3

VI.42. Which of the following is recommended by guidelines as a treatment threshold while monitoring for brain hypoxia with $Pbto_2$?
a. 10 mm Hg
b. 15 mm Hg
c. 20 mm Hg
d. 25 mm Hg

VI.43. When cerebral microdialysis is used to evaluate brain metabolism, which of the following is the most sensitive marker of brain ischemia?
a. Increased lactate level
b. Decreased oxygen level
c. Decreased lactate to pyruvate ratio
d. Increased lactate to pyruvate ratio

VI.44. If a patient with an aneurysmal SAH undergoes TCD ultrasonography of the MCA, which of the following would be consistent with angiographic vasospasm?
a. Peak systolic velocity of 165 cm/s
b. End-diastolic velocity of 90 cm/s
c. Lindegaard ratio of 2.5
d. Lindegaard ratio of 5

VI.45. After undergoing surgery for an intramedullary tumor, a female patient had labile blood pressures and a generalized tonic-clonic seizure. On examination, she seems to have marked visual disturbances and does not recognize her surroundings; otherwise, the neurologic examination findings are unremarkable. A CT image is shown (Figure VI.Q45).

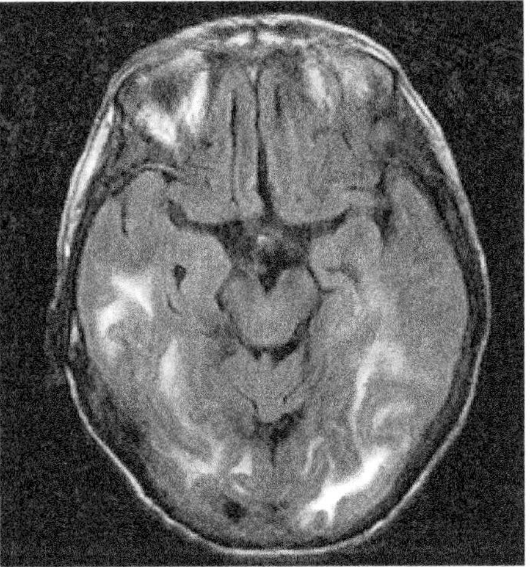

Figure VI.Q45.

What is your diagnosis and next management step?
a. The diagnosis is bilateral occipital infarctions, cause unknown; order urgent CT angiography.
b. The diagnosis is posterior reversible encephalopathy syndrome; control the patient's hypertension.
c. The diagnosis is most likely an infectious process; examine the CSF and consider use of broad-spectrum antibiotics.
d. The diagnosis is most likely anoxic-ischemic injury; no further therapeutic options are available.

VI.46. If DWI MRI shows a bright area and a black ADC map over the entire left MCA territory, which of the following would be the most likely physiologic explanation?
a. Normal brain tissue
b. Dense brain tumor, such as meningioma
c. Chronic left MCA infarct
d. Acute left MCA infarct

Answers

Airway Procedures and Modes of Ventilation

VI.1. Answer c.

In a meta-analysis that compared sternomental distance, thyromental distance, Mallampati score, and mouth opening, the best predictor of difficult intubation was an unfavorable Mallampati score in combination with an unfavorable thyromental distance.

Shiga T, Wajima Z, Inoue T, Sakamoto A. Predicting difficult intubation in apparently normal patients: a meta-analysis of bedside screening test performance. Anesthesiology. 2005 Aug;103(2):429–37.

VI.2. Answer d.

A Venturi mask can deliver a maximum of 50% oxygen, and HFNC maintains better oxygenation for a specific FIO_2. It is noninferior to NIV in preventing reintubation in the first 48 hours after extubation.

Hernandez G, Vaquero C, Colinas L, Cuena R, Gonzalez P, Canabal A, et al. Effect of postextubation high-flow nasal cannula vs noninvasive ventilation on reintubation and postextubation respiratory failure in high-risk patients: a randomized clinical trial. JAMA. 2016 Oct 18;316(15):1565–74. Errata in: JAMA. 2016 Nov 15;316(19):2047–8. JAMA. 2017 Feb 28;317(8):858.
Maggiore SM, Idone FA, Vaschetto R, Festa R, Cataldo A, Antonicelli F, et al. Nasal high-flow versus Venturi mask oxygen therapy after extubation: effects on oxygenation, comfort, and clinical outcome. Am J Respir Crit Care Med. 2014 Aug 1;190(3):282–8.

VI.3. Answer d.

Breath sounds may be absent with pneumothorax or difficult to appreciate with a large body habitus. Additionally, sounds resembling normal breath sounds can be heard with esophageal intubation, and the chest rise with esophageal intubation can be indistinguishable from that with endotracheal tube placement. Condensation in the endotracheal tube can occur in up to 85% of esophageal intubations. Identification of carbon dioxide in exhaled gas, either with capnometry or capnography, is the current standard for verification of proper endotracheal tube placement. These methods are not foolproof, however, because carbon dioxide may be absent or severely decreased in many patients, especially those with low CO.

Andersen KH, Hald A. Assessing the position of the tracheal tube: the reliability of different methods. Anaesthesia. 1989 Dec;44(12):984–5.
Pollard BJ, Junius F. Accidental intubation of the oesophagus. Anaesth Intensive Care. 1980 May;8(2):183–6.
Ramez Salem M, Baraka AS. Confirmation of endotracheal intubation. In: Hagberg CA, editor. Benumof and Hagberg's airway management. 3rd ed. Philadelphia (PA): Elsevier/Saunders; c2013. p. 657–82.

VI.4. Answer d.

Airway protection is imperative when considering a patient for NIV. Lack of airway protection puts the patient at risk for aspiration. Patient selection for NIV should include patients most likely to benefit, such as those with COPD or acute pulmonary edema. Patients who do not have an intact respiratory drive because of respiratory or cardiac arrest should not be considered candidates for NIV. Patients who cannot protect the airway should be considered for tracheal intubation instead.

Gramlich T. Basic concepts of noninvasive positive pressure ventilation. In: Pilbeam SP, Cairo JM, editors. Mechanical ventilation: physiological and clinical applications. 4th ed. St. Louis (MO): Mosby Elsevier; c2006. p. 417–37.
Hess DR. How to initiate a noninvasive ventilation program: bringing the evidence to the bedside. Respir Care. 2009 Feb;54(2):232–43.

VI.5. Answer c.

NIV should be terminated in favor of invasive ventilation if the patient's condition does not improve during the initial phase of NIV initiation. Arterial blood gas results should show improvements in pH and $PaCO_2$, and the clinical status should be improving. Recognizing NIV failure is important because avoiding delay in transitioning to invasive ventilation when needed could prevent emergent intubation and decrease harm to the patient.

Gramlich T. Basic concepts of noninvasive positive pressure ventilation. In: Pilbeam SP, Cairo JM, editors. Mechanical ventilation: physiological and clinical applications. 4th ed. St. Louis (MO): Mosby Elsevier; c2006. p. 417–37.
Hess DR. Noninvasive ventilation for acute respiratory failure. Respir Care. 2013 Jun;58(6):950–72.

VI.6. Answer b.

Loss of tracheostomy airway in a patient in stable condition can be managed first with attempts to alleviate any obstruction or to reposition the tracheostomy tube. If the initial efforts to achieve tube patency fail, translaryngeal intubation may be undertaken. If the patient's condition is unstable, translaryngeal intubation should be performed immediately. PDT is generally contraindicated in the pediatric population, whereas the traditional surgical approach may be used in all patient populations. The postprocedural tracheostomy complication rate is affected by the duration of the preceding translaryngeal intubation. Tracheal stenosis is the most common late complication, with almost all patients having some degree of narrowing. In approximately 10% of patients, clinically important stenosis develops 6 to 8 weeks after decannulation, indicative of a reduction in luminal diameter by more than 50%. Before massive life-threatening hemorrhage, sentinel bleeding may occur in up to 50% of patients with a tracheoinnominate fistula.

Engels PT, Bagshaw SM, Meier M, Brindley PG. Tracheostomy: from insertion to decannulation. Can J Surg. 2009 Oct;52(5):427–33.
Fernandez-Bussy S, Mahajan B, Folch E, Caviedes I, Guerrero J, Majid A. Tracheostomy tube placement: early and late complications. J Bronchology Interv Pulmonol. 2015 Oct;22(4):357–64.

VI.7. Answer c.

The patient appears to have an alveolar process, and results from bronchial washings may be related to upper airway contamination in an intubated patient in the ICU. Bronchial brushings and bronchial biopsies are better suited for patients thought to have malignant processes in the proximal airways. The yield of transbronchial biopsy is not better than BAL in the clinical circumstances described for this patient, and the risk of pneumothorax or bleeding is high for this patient who requires a high FIO_2 and PEEP and may have a coagulopathy from renal disease. Although transbronchial biopsies could be planned, they should be done only if the initial BAL samples did not provide the diagnosis. FOB and BAL can be done with a reasonable margin of safety in critically ill patients who require mechanical ventilation. A good BAL sample can be processed to rule out common or opportunistic infections, alveolar hemorrhage syndrome, and underlying neoplasia in patients with acute diffuse alveolar infiltrates.

Bulpa PA, Dive AM, Mertens L, Delos MA, Jamart J, Evrard PA, et al. Combined bronchoalveolar lavage and transbronchial lung biopsy: safety and yield in ventilated patients. Eur Respir J. 2003 Mar;21(3):489–94.

Cracco C, Fartoukh M, Prodanovic H, Azoulay E, Chenivesse C, Lorut C, et al. Safety of performing fiberoptic bronchoscopy in critically ill hypoxemic patients with acute respiratory failure. Intensive Care Med. 2013 Jan;39(1):45–52. Epub 2012 Oct 16.

VI.8. Answer c.

Cryotherapy could be used with a dual purpose: Large cryobiopsy samples could be obtained to debulk the mass and to establish a diagnosis. Cryotherapy poses no risk of ignition or electrical interference with this patient's pacemaker. Although brachytherapy can be used in the management of endobronchial neoplasia refractory to standard therapy, a diagnosis has not been established for this patient, and the effect of brachytherapy is delayed, but this patient needs immediate relief. APC could provide rapid relief from the obstruction, but this patient would be at high risk for complications such as endobronchial ignition because he requires 100% oxygen and because APC could produce electrical interference with his pacemaker. Although APC could be used if delivery of the high F_{IO_2} were interrupted and if the pacemaker pacing were interrupted (with the cardiologist's approval), these issues make APC a less useful option. Although fiberoptic placement of endobronchial valves in study trials has reduced lung volume in patients with emphysema, the only indication for these valves in the ICU is persistent air leak in patients with pneumothorax or bronchopleural fistula refractory to standard care.

Folch E, Mehta AC. Airway interventions in the tracheobronchial tree. Semin Respir Crit Care Med. 2008 Aug;29(4):441–52.

Cardiovascular and Cardiopulmonary Monitoring and Access

VI.9. Answer d.

The rhythm strip shows what appears to be polymorphic ventricular tachycardia. However, marching back the sinus QRS complexes from the end of the rhythm strip shows narrow complex depolarizations (from sinus rhythm) hidden within the "polymorphic ventricular tachycardia." This finding is motion artifact and does not need any intervention.

Knight BP, Pelosi F, Michaud GF, Strickberger SA, Morady F. Clinical consequences of electrocardiographic artifact mimicking ventricular tachycardia. N Engl J Med. 1999 Oct 21;341(17):1270–4.

Krasnow AZ, Bloomfield DK. Artifacts in portable electrocardiographic monitoring. Am Heart J. 1976 Mar;91(3):349–57.

VI.10. Answer b.

The strip shows atrial fibrillation with ventricular pacing. It is important to not overlook atrial arrhythmias when evaluating pacemaker rhythm strips. The $CHADS_2$-VASc score is 5, and thus he is at high risk for stroke. Aspirin is not sufficient, and he needs to be treated with oral anticoagulation.

January CT, Wann LS, Alpert JS, Calkins H, Cigarroa JE, Cleveland JC Jr, et al; American College of Cardiology/American Heart Association Task Force on Practice Guidelines. 2014 AHA/ACC/HRS guideline for the management of patients with atrial fibrillation: a report of the American College of Cardiology/American Heart Association Task Force on Practice Guidelines and the Heart Rhythm Society. J Am Coll Cardiol. 2014 Dec 2;64(21):e1–76. Epub 2014 Mar 28. Erratum in: J Am Coll Cardiol. 2014 Dec 2;64(21):2305–7.

Lip GY, Nieuwlaat R, Pisters R, Lane DA, Crijns HJ. Refining clinical risk stratification for predicting stroke and thromboembolism in atrial fibrillation using a novel risk factor-based approach: the euro heart survey on atrial fibrillation. Chest. 2010 Feb;137(2):263–72. Epub 2009 Sep 17.

VI.11. Answer c.

The morphologic pattern of the arterial line waveform is dependent on physiologic parameters such as atrioventricular valve closure, arterial compliance or stiffness, wave reflections, and properties related to the monitoring device itself. Because each component of the waveform, including diastolic pressure, peak pressure, ejection time, valve closure, rate of pressure increase during systole, and mean arterial pressure are all dependent on cardiovascular physiologic features, the location of arterial cannulation, the heart rate, and the velocity of blood flow all affect the waveform morphologic pattern. Complications of the monitoring device itself may also lead to inaccurate waveform display by means of overdamping or underdamping. This is usually created by long tubing, microbubbles, thrombi, or stopcock malposition resulting in an inaccurate frequency response by the transducer. Once calibrated or zeroed, the transducer height must remain level with the right atrium. If the transducer is not level, the pressure readings will be underestimates or overestimates, but the waveform morphologic pattern should not be affected.

Esper SA, Pinsky MR. Arterial waveform analysis. Best Pract Res Clin Anaesthesiol. 2014 Dec;28(4):363–80. Epub 2014 Sep 6.

Saugel B, Dueck R, Wagner JY. Measurement of blood pressure. Best Pract Res Clin Anaesthesiol. 2014 Dec;28(4):309–22. Epub 2014 Sep 6.

VI.12. Answer d.

The OER is increased with hypovolema, seizures, fever, and pain. Shock usually occurs when there is an imbalance of oxygen supply and oxygen demand resulting in an excessive oxygen debt. To prevent or correct this issue, one must either aim to improve Do_2 or target the cause of excessive $\dot{V}o_2$. The central or mixed venous oxygen saturation, primarily influenced by hemoglobin, Sao_2, CO, and $\dot{V}o_2$, is a good indicator of total body oxygenation. The difference between Sao_2 and Svo_2 provides the OER, which identifies an increase in $\dot{V}o_2$ due to either a pathologic increase in metabolism or a deficiency in Do_2. Anemia and hypovolemia result in reduced Do_2, which may increase $\dot{V}o_2$ at the tissue level and result in a higher OER.

Huang YC. Monitoring oxygen delivery in the critically ill. Chest. 2005 Nov;128(5 Suppl 2):554S-60S.

Nichols D, Nielsen ND. Oxygen delivery and consumption: a macrocirculatory perspective. Crit Care Clin. 2010 Apr;26(2):239–53.

VI.13. Answer a.

The ascending steep portion of the Frank-Starling curve identifies physiology in which a ventricle increases its force of contraction and ultimately stroke volume in response to an increase in preload. With a higher left ventricular preload, as seen on the flat portion of the curve, there is less of a contractile response to fluid and thereby no substantial improvement in SV. A hypotensive patient with ventricles functioning on the steep end would be described as fluid-responsive and would likely have an increased SVV with low filling pressures (CVP, PAOP). An increase in preload from a fluid bolus may improve SV and CO, whereas initiation of use of a vasopressor would potentially increase afterload and have a detrimental effect on CO.

Marik PE, Cavallazzi R, Vasu T, Hirani A. Dynamic changes in arterial waveform derived variables and fluid responsiveness in mechanically ventilated patients: a systematic review of the literature. Crit Care Med. 2009 Sep;37(9):2642–7.

Monnet X, Marik PE, Teboul JL. Prediction of fluid responsiveness: an update. Ann Intensive Care. 2016 Dec;6(1):111. Epub 2016 Nov 17.

VI.14. Answer d.

Devices that use arterial waveform analysis estimate pulse pressure variation and SVV in the respiratory cycle according to predictable heart-lung interactions. Cardiac and respiratory variables that alter pulse pressure regardless of preload may result in an inaccurate prediction of fluid response with these devices. For this reason they are best used with patients receiving controlled mechanical ventilation void of any breathing efforts, because any initiation by the patient would lead to irregular changes in intrathoracic pressure. Small tidal volumes may not induce considerable change in intrathoracic pressure and subsequently venous return, even in fluid-responsive patients, and thus readings are false-negative. A high respiratory rate may result in inaccurate readings, because the number of cardiac cycles per respiratory cycle are too few to demonstrate SVV. Normal sinus rhythm is necessary because arrhythmias may induce their own beat-to-beat variation in pulse pressure and SV.

Lazaridis C. Advanced hemodynamic monitoring: principles and practice in neurocritical care. Neurocrit Care. 2012 Feb;16(1):163–9.

Monnet X, Teboul JL. Assessment of volume responsiveness during mechanical ventilation: recent advances. Crit Care. 2013 Mar 19;17(2):217.

VI.15. Answer b.

Despite their static nature and poor correlation with fluid responsiveness, ventricular filling pressures are often measured as surrogates for ventricular filling volumes. The PAOP is assumed to be the back-pressure on pulmonary venous return induced by left ventricular preload.

Busse L, Davison DL, Junker C, Chawla LS. Hemodynamic monitoring in the critical care environment. Adv Chronic Kidney Dis. 2013 Jan;20(1):21–9.

Kumar A, Anel R, Bunnell E, Habet K, Zanotti S, Marshall S, et al. Pulmonary artery occlusion pressure and central venous pressure fail to predict ventricular filling volume, cardiac performance, or the response to volume infusion in normal subjects. Crit Care Med. 2004 Mar;32(3):691–9.

VI.16. Answer d.

This man presents with signs of group 2 pulmonary hypertension due to left heart disease. Signs of this include his echocardiographic findings of left atrial enlargement and grade 1 diastolic dysfunction. His risk factors include kidney disease (which predisposes to volume overload) and untreated hypertension leading to left ventricular hypertrophy. Initiation of diuresis to decrease his PAOP may improve his pulmonary artery pressure. Initiating use of pulmonary vasodilators is inappropriate and potentially dangerous in the setting of pulmonary venous hypertension (choices *a* and *b* are incorrect). There is no evidence of chronic thromboembolic pulmonary hypertension (choice *c* is incorrect).

Lam CS, Donal E, Kraigher-Krainer E, Vasan RS. Epidemiology and clinical course of heart failure with preserved ejection fraction. Eur J Heart Fail. 2011 Jan;13(1):18–28. Epub 2010 Aug 3.

Vachiery JL, Adir Y, Barbera JA, Champion H, Coghlan JG, Cottin V, et al. Pulmonary hypertension due to left heart diseases. J Am Coll Cardiol. 2013 Dec 24;62(25 Suppl):D100–8.

VI.17. Answer d.

In this patient, pulmonary artery rupture has developed as a result of catheterization with serial balloon inflation. Risk factors for pulmonary artery rupture include female sex, advanced age, preexisting pulmonary hypertension, and use of anticoagulant. The treatment of choice to control the hemorrhage is emergency angiography-directed embolization (choice *c* is incorrect). If this is unsuccessful, emergency lobectomy may be required. Adjunctive treatment involves prevention of asphyxiation. This includes protection of nonbleeding lung and isolation of the bleeding (choices *a* and *b* are incorrect). The patient should be positioned with the bleeding side in the dependent position to prevent spillage of blood to the contralateral lung (choice *d* is correct).

Hannan AT, Brown M, Bigman O. Pulmonary artery catheter-induced hemorrhage. Chest. 1984 Jan;85(1):128–31.

Karak P, Dimick R, Hamrick KM, Schwartzberg M, Saddekni S. Immediate transcatheter embolization of Swan-Ganz catheter-induced pulmonary artery pseudoaneurysm. Chest. 1997 May;111(5):1450–2.

VI.18. Answer c.

Small-bore chest tubes can adequately drain many types of pleural effusions or a pneumothorax. The benefits to patients include less discomfort and better positioning with image guidance. However, because of the size of the tube, there is higher resistance to flow and higher rates of clogging. A hemothorax has higher viscosity and is better drained with a large-bore chest tube.

Cooke DT, David EA. Large-bore and small-bore chest tubes: types, function, and placement. Thorac Surg Clin. 2013 Feb;23(1):17–24.

Dev SP, Nascimiento B Jr, Simone C, Chien V. Videos in clinical medicine: chest-tube insertion. N Engl J Med. 2007 Oct 11;357(15):e15.

VI.19. Answer c.

Ultrasound guidance is shown to reduce procedural complications, including pneumothorax and solid-organ injury. Appropriate training with ultrasound is essential because it is operator-dependent. Tube location is enhanced with bedside ultrasound and thus can improve pleural fluid drainage.

Mercaldi CJ, Lanes SF. Ultrasound guidance decreases complications and improves the cost of care among patients undergoing thoracentesis and paracentesis. Chest. 2013 Feb 1;143(2):532–8.

Shojaee S, Argento AC. Ultrasound-guided pleural access. Semin Respir Crit Care Med. 2014 Dec;35(6):693–705. Epub 2014 Dec 2.

VI.20. Answer d.

This patient had a recent traumatic injury and a known splenic laceration. He is now hypotensive and showing signs of decreased global perfusion. Initial steps should include treating and looking for causes of the hypotension. He most likely has bleeding related to his known splenic laceration, and thus giving fluid resuscitation and checking the hemoglobin level is the most appropriate next step. Although a 9F introducer would be a reasonable choice for volume resuscitation, given that the patient already has 2 large-bore peripheral intravenous lines, placing a central line would likely only delay resuscitation and definitive treatment. In general, small-bore central lines are poor choices for volume resuscitation because of the high resistance of the catheter (Poiseuille law). CVP has been shown to be unreliable as a predictor of blood volume. In this case, hypovolemia can more readily be diagnosed on the basis of the history and examination. Use of vasoactive medications when the patient is hypovolemic will likely only worsen tissue perfusion, although sometimes they are necessary as a temporizing measure while volume status is optimized.

Marik PE, Baram M, Vahid B. Does central venous pressure predict fluid responsiveness? A systematic review of the literature and the tale of seven mares. Chest. 2008 Jul;134(1):172–8.

Reddick AD, Ronald J, Morrison WG. Intravenous fluid resuscitation: was Poiseuille right? Emerg Med J. 2011 Mar;28(3):201–2. Epub 2010 Jun 26.

VI.21. Answer d.

This patient has signs of septic shock, and placement of a central venous catheter for vasopressor infusion is appropriate. The subclavian site is associated with a lower risk of both catheter-associated bloodstream infections and symptomatic deep vein thromboses. These benefits are tempered by an increased risk of mechanical complications, mainly pneumothorax. Thus, the risks and benefits of each line site need to be individualized to the patient presentation and clinician experience. Theoretically, a pneumothorax can be rapidly diagnosed and treated with placement of a chest tube; alternatively, diagnosis and treatment of a catheter-associated bloodstream infection or deep vein thrombosis can be challenging to treat effectively. Nevertheless, a pneumothorax could be life-threatening in this patient who is presenting with signs of progressive hypoxemic respiratory failure. In general, if the risk of pneumothorax is present, then insertion on the side of the diseased lung would be favored (argument against choice *c*). Choice *b* is incorrect because the use of dynamic ultrasound guidance for line placement has been shown to decrease complications, access time, placement failure, and need for multiple attempts compared with the landmark technique.

Parienti JJ, Mongardon N, Megarbane B, Mira JP, Kalfon P, Gros A, et al; 3SITES Study Group. Intravascular complications of central venous catheterization by insertion site. N Engl J Med. 2015 Sep 24;373(13):1220–9.

Shekelle PG, Wachter RM, Pronovost PJ, Schoelles K, McDonald KM, Dy SM, et al. Making health care safer II: an updated critical analysis of the evidence for patient safety practices. Comparative Effectiveness Review No. 211. (Prepared by the Southern California-RAND Evidence-based Practice Center under Contract No. 290–2007-10062-I). AHRQ Publication No. 13-E001-EF. Rockville (MD): Agency for Healthcare Research and Quality. March 2013. Available from: https://archive.ahrq.gov/research/findings/evidence-based-reports/ptsafetyII-full.pdf.

VI.22. Answer b.

The international normalized ratio should be lower than 1.5 before undertaking the IR procedure. An interventional approach to this patient is feasible providing a safe track from skin to the collection can be identified. An IR procedure avoids the risks of surgery and general anesthesia in this critically ill patient if there is no immediate indication for surgical intervention. Ultrasonographic visualization is not necessary; a computed tomography–guided procedure can be performed. Although patient stability during transfer should always be considered, critical illness is not a contraindication to transfer for IR procedures when appropriate support can be given. In this case, the risks of the alternatives, transfer to the operating room for surgery or no intervention, should be considered.

Patel IJ, Davidson JC, Nikolic B, Salazar GM, Schwartzberg MS, Walker TG, et al; Standards of Practice Committee, with Cardiovascular and Interventional Radiological Society of Europe (CIRSE) Endorsement. Consensus guidelines for periprocedural management of coagulation status and hemostasis risk in percutaneous image-guided interventions. J Vasc Interv Radiol. 2012 Jun;23(6):727–36. Epub 2012 Apr 17.

Society of Cardiovascular and Interventional Radiology Standards of Practices Committee. Quality improvement guidelines for adult percutaneous abscess and fluid drainage. J Vasc Interv Radiol. 1995 Jan-Feb;6(1):68–70.

VI.23. Answer b.

Before an IR procedure, nothing should be given by mouth for 8 hours to decrease the risk of aspiration associated with sedation. This recommendation includes nasogastric feeding. Endotracheal intubation is not necessary for interventional gastrostomy. IR procedures typically do not require use of general anesthesia; a combination of sedation and local anesthesia is sufficient for most patients. There is no reason to remove the nasogastric tube before gastrostomy because the stomach is distended with air through the nasogastric tube during the procedure.

Bazarah SM, Al-Rawas M, Akbar H, Qari Y. Percutaneous gastrostomy and gastrojejunostomy: radiological and endoscopic approach. Ann Saudi Med. 2002 Jan-Mar;22(1–2):38–42.

Neuromonitoring and Procedures

VI.24. Answer a.

The Monro-Kellie doctrine states that the size of the cranial vault is fixed, and the brain parenchyma, blood, blood vessels, and ventricular system occupy a fixed space. If a compartment enlarges (eg, from a brain contusion or hematoma), the remaining structures are compressed and may cause brain tissue shift through the tentorium or foramen magnum, resulting in signs of brainstem dysfunction.

Wilson MH. Monro-Kellie 2.0: the dynamic vascular and venous pathophysiological components of intracranial pressure. J Cereb Blood Flow Metab. 2016 Aug;36(8):1338–50. Epub 2016 May 12.

VI.25. Answer a.

The guidelines suggest that any patient who is comatose should undergo monitoring because elevated ICP may be the treatable culprit. CT evidence of blood on the tentorium or in the lateral ventricles is an indicator of trauma but not an indicator of severity.

Carney N, Totten AM, O'Reilly C, Ullman JS, Hawryluk GW, Bell MJ, et al. Guidelines for the management of severe traumatic brain injury, fourth edition. Neurosurgery. 2017 Jan 1;80(1):6–15.

VI.26. Answer a.

The choroid plexus normally produces 500 to 600 mL of CSF daily.

Sakka L, Coll G, Chazal J. Anatomy and physiology of cerebrospinal fluid. Eur Ann Otorhinolaryngol Head Neck Dis. 2011 Dec;128(6):309–16. Epub 2011 Nov 18.

VI.27. Answer b.

The normal range for ICP in infants is 1 to 6 mm Hg.

Dunn LT. Raised intracranial pressure. J Neurol Neurosurg Psychiatry. 2002 Sep;73(Suppl 1):i23–7.

VI.28. Answer d.

Warfarin therapy should be stopped for 5 days because warfarin has a relatively long half-life. If warfarin therapy cannot be stopped for 5 days before LP, prothrombin complex concentrate should be administered.

Laible M, Beynon C, Sander P, Purrucker J, Muller OJ, Mohlenbruch M, et al. Treatment with prothrombin complex concentrate to enable emergency lumbar puncture in patients receiving vitamin K antagonists. Ann Emerg Med. 2016 Sep;68(3):340–4. Epub 2016 Apr 14.

VI.29. Answer c.

First obtain urgent blood cultures, and then start antibiotic therapy immediately in patients with suspected bacterial meningitis. LP should be performed only if CT of the brain does not show any abnormalities. MRI has no role in an acute setting but can strongly suggest inflammation when there is gadolinium enhancement.

Costerus JM, Brouwer MC, Bijlsma MW, van de Beek D. Community-acquired bacterial meningitis. Curr Opin Infect Dis. 2017 Feb;30(1):135–41.

VI.30. Answer b.

This patient most likely has acute herpes simplex encephalitis. Starting empirical therapy with acyclovir and antibiotics would be reasonable before performing LP. The CT results are sufficient to exclude a supratentorial cause of mass effect before LP. Although MRI would delay care, it may show a temporal DWI pattern with herpes simplex encephalitis, but MRI could be performed after antiviral therapy is started. Corticosteroids are not recommended for immediate empirical therapy because paraneoplastic encephalitis typically progresses more slowly than more common life-threatening disorders, such as herpes simplex encephalitis and bacterial encephalitis, which should be excluded first.

Kennedy PG, Steiner I. Recent issues in herpes simplex encephalitis. J Neurovirol. 2013 Aug;19(4):346–50. Epub 2013 Jun 18.

VI.31. Answer a.

Although large, high-quality studies have not accurately assessed this risk, the rate of infection is probably 1% or less if the patients receive appropriate antibiotics to suppress the skin flora. However, some studies have reported a risk of suspected infections as high as 6%. CSF leakage around the catheter is probably a risk for infection and complications, and any leakage should be evaluated immediately.

Citerio G, Signorini L, Bronco A, Vargiolu A, Rota M, Latronico N; Infezioni LIquorali Catetere Correlate Study Investigators. External ventricular and lumbar drain device infections in ICU patients: a prospective multicenter Italian study. Crit Care Med. 2015 Aug;43(8):1630–7.

Stokken J, Recinos PF, Woodard T, Sindwani R. The utility of lumbar drains in modern endoscopic skull base surgery. Curr Opin Otolaryngol Head Neck Surg. 2015 Feb;23(1):78–82.

VI.32. Answer d.

In the only randomized trial that compared lumbar drainage with no lumbar drainage in addition to standard care for patients with SAH, lumbar drainage of CSF after aneurysmal SAH decreased the prevalence of delayed ischemic neurologic deficits and improved early clinical outcomes but did not improve 6-month outcomes. Mortality was not affected.

Al-Tamimi YZ, Bhargava D, Feltbower RG, Hall G, Goddard AJ, Quinn AC, et al. Lumbar drainage of cerebrospinal fluid after aneurysmal subarachnoid hemorrhage: a prospective, randomized, controlled trial (LUMAS). Stroke. 2012 Mar;43(3):677–82. Epub 2012 Jan 26.

VI.33. Answer b.

The most likely cause of resistance to administration of medication into an external ventricular drain is obstruction or migration of the catheter.

Hanley DF, Lane K, McBee N, Ziai W, Tuhrim S, Lees KR, et al; CLEAR III Investigators. Thrombolytic removal of intraventricular haemorrhage in treatment of severe stroke: results of the randomised, multicentre, multiregion, placebo-controlled CLEAR III trial. Lancet. 2017 Feb 11;389(10069):603–11. Epub 2017 Jan 10.

Stuart D, Christian R, Uschmann H, Palokas M. Effectiveness of intrathecal nicardipine on cerebral vasospasm in non-traumatic subarachnoid hemorrhage: a systematic review. JBI Database System Rev Implement Rep. 2018 Oct;16(10):2013–26.

VI.34. Answer c.

For intraventricular administration of medication, isovolemic administration is the standard recommendation.

Abdelmalik PA, Ziai WC. Spontaneous intraventricular hemorrhage: when should intraventricular tPA be considered? Semin Respir Crit Care Med. 2017 Dec;38(6):745–59. Epub 2017 Dec 20.

Jones J, Schweder P, Drummond KJ, Kaye AH. Use of tissue plasminogen activator in the treatment of shunt blockage secondary to intraventricular haemorrhage. J Clin Neurosci. 2016 Dec;34:281–2. Epub 2016 Aug 10.

Ko SB, Choi HA, Helbok R, Kurtz P, Schmidt JM, Badjatia N, et al. Acute effects of intraventricular nicardipine on cerebral hemodynamics: a preliminary finding. Clin Neurol Neurosurg. 2016 May;144:48–52. Epub 2016 Mar 2.

Lu N, Jackson D, Luke S, Festic E, Hanel RA, Freeman WD. Intraventricular nicardipine for aneurysmal subarachnoid hemorrhage related vasospasm: assessment of 90 days outcome. Neurocrit Care. 2012 Jun;16(3):368–75.

VI.35. Answer b.

The use of TCD ultrasonography does not require any ionizing radiation.

VI.36. Answer d.

The TCD values are sensitive and specific for angiographically proven vasospsasm of the MCA. The patient is symptomatic (left hemisphere MCA deficits of aphasia and hemiparesis) and should be treated emergently because the left MCA could become infarcted. Treatment may include medical and endovascular approaches, including short-term induced hypertension and relatively modest hypervolemia (positive fluid balance of ≥500 mL). Hemodilution was originally described as part of the so-called triple-*H* therapy but is now considered more theoretical. Hemodilution, which yields diminishing returns on the oxygen delivery equation and hemoglobin delivery, was originally proposed to reduce blood viscosity in "dehydrated" patients with SAH and a high hematocrit. The Neurocritical Care Society guidelines describe management of acute SAH vasospasm, but this patient has classic symptomatic TCD findings for acute symptomatic (delayed arterial) vasospasm.

AAN statement of TCD sensitivity and specificity. Available from: https://www.aan.com/Guidelines/Home/GetGuidelineContent/147.

Diringer MN, Bleck TP, Claude Hemphill J 3rd, Menon D, Shutter L, Vespa P, et al; Neurocritical Care Society. Critical care management of patients following aneurysmal subarachnoid hemorrhage: recommendations from the Neurocritical Care Society's Multidisciplinary Consensus Conference. Neurocrit Care. 2011 Sep;15(2):211–40.

VI.37. Answer b.

GPDs are a known EEG finding in baclofen toxicity, which would fit with the patient's recent exacerbation of back pain and clinical presentation. Herpes simplex encephalitis is associated with temporal lateralized periodic discharges on EEG. Although GPDs can be seen with Creutzfeldt-Jakob disease, the clinical presentation does not fit.

Fakhoury T, Abou-Khalil B, Blumenkopf B. EEG changes in intrathecal baclofen overdose: a case report and review of the literature. Electroencephalogr Clin Neurophysiol. 1998 Nov;107(5):339–42.

Foreman B, Claassen J, Abou Khaled K, Jirsch J, Alschuler DM, Wittman J, et al. Generalized periodic discharges in the critically ill: a case-control study of 200 patients. Neurology. 2012 Nov 6;79(19):1951–60. Epub 2012 Oct 3.

VI.38. Answer a.

The timing and neuroanatomy of the right shoulder twitches correlate with an ictal pattern. This would be considered a subtle ictal phenomenon, meeting the criteria for ictal LPDs or NCSE.

Although this patient has focal epilepsy, this is not the same as epileptic encephalopathy (such as in Lennox-Gastaut syndrome), and an increase in features compared with baseline cannot be used to diagnose NCSE. The response to antiepileptic drugs must be both electrographic and clinical. Her known history of epilepsy is not relevant for distinguishing between ictal and interictal patterns.

Beniczky S, Hirsch LJ, Kaplan PW, Pressler R, Bauer G, Aurlien H, et al. Unified EEG terminology and criteria for nonconvulsive status epilepticus. Epilepsia. 2013 Sep;54 Suppl 6:28–9.

Sen-Gupta I, Schuele SU, Macken MP, Kwasny MJ, Gerard EE. "Ictal" lateralized periodic discharges. Epilepsy Behav. 2014 Jul;36:165–70. Epub 2014 Jun 13.

VI.39. Answer b.

After cardiac arrest, a continuous, reactive background is associated with the potential for a good neurologic outcome. Burst suppression may be iatrogenic or, if the bursts are identical, correlated with a poor outcome. A persistently low amplitude on EEG is strongly correlated with a poor outcome. Alpha coma consists of monomorphic, nonreactive alpha activity, and while the background is continuous, the lack of variability and reactivity typically suggests a poor outcome.

Berkhoff M, Donati F, Bassetti C. Postanoxic alpha (theta) coma: a reappraisal of its prognostic significance. Clin Neurophysiol. 2000 Feb;111(2):297–304.

Cloostermans MC, van Meulen FB, Eertman CJ, Hom HW, van Putten MJ. Continuous electroencephalography monitoring for early prediction of neurological outcome in postanoxic patients after cardiac arrest: a prospective cohort study. Crit Care Med. 2012 Oct;40(10):2867–75.

VI.40. Answer b.

Sustained, high intracranial hypertension in patients with TBI is most strongly associated with brain tissue shift and progressive loss of brainstem reflexes and eventually loss of vasoregulation and respiration. A typical Cushing reflex can occur with bradycardia, hypertension, and fixed, dilated pupils.

Chambers IR, Treadwell L, Mendelow AD. Determination of threshold levels of cerebral perfusion pressure and intracranial pressure in severe head injury by using receiver-operating characteristic curves: an observational study in 291 patients. J Neurosurg. 2001 Mar;94(3):412–6.

Marmarou A, Saad A, Aygok G, Rigsbee M. Contribution of raised ICP and hypotension to CPP reduction in severe brain injury: correlation to outcome. Acta Neurochir Suppl. 2005;95:277–80.

VI.41. Answer d.

The PRx is an indicator of cerebral autoregulation. A moving correlation coefficient between ICP and slow fluctuations of mean arterial pressure, PRx ranges from −1 to 1. A negative value reflects intact autoregulation, and a positive value reflects impaired autoregulation.

Czosnyka M, Smielewski P, Kirkpatrick P, Laing RJ, Menon D, Pickard JD. Continuous assessment of the cerebral vasomotor reactivity in head injury. Neurosurgery. 1997 Jul;41(1):11–7.

Sorrentino E, Diedler J, Kasprowicz M, Budohoski KP, Haubrich C, Smielewski P, et al. Critical thresholds for cerebrovascular reactivity after traumatic brain injury. Neurocrit Care. 2012 Apr;16(2):258–66.

VI.42. Answer c.

Normal values for $Pbto_2$ have been documented as 20 to 35 mm Hg. Low levels (<10 mm Hg) have been associated with metabolic crises, morbidity, and death. Recent international guidelines from many ICU societies recommend a treatment threshold of 20 mm Hg.

Le Roux P, Menon DK, Citerio G, Vespa P, Bader MK, Brophy GM, et al. Consensus summary statement of the International Multidisciplinary Consensus Conference on Multimodality Monitoring in Neurocritical Care: a statement for healthcare professionals from the Neurocritical Care Society and the European Society of Intensive Care Medicine. Neurocrit Care. 2014 Dec;21 Suppl 2:S1–26.

Roh D, Park S. Brain multimodality monitoring: updated perspectives. Curr Neurol Neurosci Rep. 2016 Jun;16(6):56.

VI.43. Answer d.

The chemical markers obtained from microdialysis are not specific for brain ischemia but reflect overall energy metabolism in the brain. The most sensitive marker for brain ischemia is an increased ratio of lactate to pyruvate. Oxygenation is not measured by cerebral microdialysis.

Carpenter KL, Young AM, Hutchinson PJ. Advanced monitoring in traumatic brain injury: microdialysis. Curr Opin Crit Care. 2017 Apr;23(2):103–9.

Tisdall MM, Smith M. Cerebral microdialysis: research technique or clinical tool. Br J Anaesth. 2006 Jul;97(1):18–25. Epub 2006 May 12.

VI.44. Answer d.

A MFV less than 120 cm/s in the MCA is strongly suggestive of the absence of vasospasm. MFV values greater than 160 cm/s in the MCA are correlated with the presence of vasospasm, and values greater than 200 cm/s suggest the presence of severe vasospasm. A Lindegaard ratio (the ratio of the flow velocity in the MCA to the flow velocity in the extracranial ICA) greater than 3 is consistent with the presence of intracranial vasospasm. Peak systolic and end-diastolic values are not well validated for the presence of angiographic vasospasm.

Le Roux P, Menon DK, Citerio G, Vespa P, Bader MK, Brophy GM, et al. Consensus summary statement of the International Multidisciplinary Consensus Conference on Multimodality Monitoring in Neurocritical Care: a statement for healthcare professionals from the Neurocritical Care Society and the European Society of Intensive Care Medicine. Neurocrit Care. 2014 Dec;21 Suppl 2:S1–26.

Miller C, Armonda R; Participants in the International Multidisciplinary Consensus Conference on Multimodality Monitoring. Monitoring of cerebral blood flow and ischemia in the critically ill. Neurocrit Care. 2014 Dec;21 Suppl 2: S121–8.

VI.45. Answer b.

The image is characteristic of posterior reversible encephalopathy syndrome. MRI may show abnormalities in other areas, such as the thalami.

Hinchey J, Chaves C, Appignani B, Breen J, Pao L, Wang A, et al. A reversible posterior leukoencephalopathy syndrome. N Engl J Med. 1996 Feb 22;334(8):494–500.

VI.46. Answer d.

A bright or white area on DWI MRI suggests acute injury, and when ADC is black in the same distribution, this is most commonly an acute infarct pattern. The brightness may remain for a few weeks, and "T2 shine through" can occur on DWI from various causes (eg, edema and tumors). ADC is helpful because when DWI shows white and ADC shows black for the same brain territory, the pattern usually indicates an infarct. When ADC is not black, and DWI is gray or white, edema or tumor may be present rather than infarction.

Atlas SW, editor. Magnetic resonance imaging of the brain and spine. 4th ed. Philadelphia: Lippincott Williams & Wilkins; c2009. 1,890 p.

Section VII

Pharmacotherapeutics

133 Anticonvulsant Drugs

ANTENEH M. FEYISSA, MD; JEFFREY W. BRITTON, MD

Goals

- Review antiseizure drugs commonly used in intensive care units.
- Review selection and dosing of antiseizure drugs.
- Review common adverse effects and drug interactions of antiseizure drugs.

Introduction

Seizures are a common occurrence in intensive care units (ICUs) in which patients with acute brain injury are treated. The increased use of continuous electroencephalographic (EEG) monitoring has led to an increase in seizure detection in this setting. For example, in 1 study, 34% of patients in an ICU had nonconvulsive seizures shown on continuous EEG, and 76% of these were in nonconvulsive status epilepticus. Independent variables predicting seizure detection in this setting are age, cardiopulmonary arrest, and use of continuous EEG.

Seizures that complicate the status of critically ill patients should not be considered benign. Although there is controversy as to the degree to which brief seizures independently affect outcome, most intensivists will treat seizures detected in the ICU. During repetitive seizures or status epilepticus, intracranial pressure increases in parallel with cerebral blood flow, brain temperature, and lactate:pyruvate ratio and contributes to immediate metabolic stress and may lead to injurious effects due to deficits in brain tissue oxygen tension. This chapter reviews the main options for antiseizure drugs (ASDs), focusing on adverse effect profile, dosing, and clinically relevant drug interactions. These recommendations apply to patients with single seizures. Status epilepticus is discussed in Chapter 98.

Clinical Presentation and Diagnosis of Seizures

Seizure manifestationsrange from clinical focal or generalized convulsions to subclinical seizures. Although seizures may occur as single events in the ICU, affected patients are at considerable risk of repetitive seizures, and this risk prompts a lower threshold for initiation of ASD therapy. In addition, status epilepticus may develop, and it requires emergency treatment. Because subclinical seizures may contribute to persistent alteration of responsiveness and present without obvious clinical manifestations, one has to be aware of this possibility and evaluate patients who have altered consciousness with EEG. In fact, with use of continuous EEG monitoring, 20% of patients with acute brain injury may have nonconvulsive status epilepticus, and 8% of comatose patients in a general ICU may have nonconvulsive seizures. Causes of seizures in the ICU include the primary neurologic abnormality and consequences of critical illness or iatrogenic factors. Common causes of seizures in the ICU include stroke and head trauma, medications with epileptogenic potential, alcohol withdrawal, and electrolyte derangements (Boxes 133.1 and 133.2).

Management of Seizures

Seizure management follows rules similar to those in other hospital settings. Because seizures in the ICU are frequently resistant to treatment, familiarity of the medical and nursing staff with the detection, diagnosis, and treatment of seizures is essential (Box 133.3).

ASDs are commonly used in the ICU, and selection depends largely on the type of seizure being treated and the potential adverse effects relative to a patient's clinical

Box 133.1 • Common Causes of Seizures in the Intensive Care Unit: Neurologic Abnormalities

- Cerebrovascular
  - Ischemic stroke
  - Hemorrhagic stroke
  - Subarachnoid hemorrhage
  - Subdural and cerebral hemorrhage
  - Arteriovenous malformation
  - Cerebral sinus thrombosis
  - Hyperperfusion syndrome
- Brain tumor
  - Primary
  - Metastatic
- Infection of the central nervous system
  - Abscess, empyema
  - Meningitis
  - Encephalitis
- Antibody mediated (noninfectious encephalitis)
  - Autoimmune
  - Paraneoplastic
- Inflammatory disease
  - Vasculitis
  - Acute demyelinating encephalomyelitis
- Traumatic brain injury
  - Depressed skull fracture
  - Cerebral contusion
  - Subdural, epidural hemorrhage
- ASD noncompliance
- Inherited metabolic disturbance

Abbreviation: ASD, antiseizure drug.

Box 133.2 • Common Causes of Seizures in the Intensive Care Unit: Complications of Critical Illness

- Hypoxia
- Toxicities
  - Antibiotics (cefepime and other β-lactams)
  - Antidepressants (eg, bupropion)
  - Antipsychotics (eg, clozapine)
  - Bronchodilators
  - Local anesthetics
  - General anesthetics
  - Opioids
  - Immunosuppressives
  - Cocaine, amphetamines (eg, theophylline)
  - Phencyclidine
- Drug withdrawals
  - Barbiturates
  - Benzodiazepines
  - Opioids
  - Alcohol
- Systemic infection
  - Sepsis
  - Fever
- Metabolic abnormalities
  - Acidosis
  - Hyponatremia
  - Hypocalcemia
  - Hypophosphatemia
  - Hypoglycemia
  - Renal, hepatic dysfunction

situation (Table 133.1). There may be serious overprescription and drugs often can be discontinued after dismissal from the ICU. As a means to reduce adverse effects, rational ASD selection practices should be used to avoid medications with redundant mechanisms of action. For example, concomitant use of sodium channel blocking ASDs such as lacosamide, lamotrigine, carbamazepine, and phenytoin may result in diplopia, ataxia, and vertigo at higher rates than when any agent is administrated alone. Alternatively, combinations of ASDs with different primary mechanisms of action may be beneficial in some cases (rational polypharmacy). Data on the value of rational polypharmacy are limited. One combination of ASD therapies for which some data suggest benefit is that of valproic acid and lamotrigine. In addition, some data suggest a possible favorable pharmacodynamic interaction between levetiracetam and lacosamide.

Typically, intravenous formulations are preferred in the ICU, and oral formulations are suggested for patients who can swallow. Some ASDs have complex pharmacokinetics that require therapeutic monitoring. Measuring serum concentrations of old- and new-generation ASDs is useful 1) for diagnosis of toxicity, 2) for guiding dosage adjustment in situations associated with increased pharmacokinetic variability (eg, elderly patients, renal and hepatic comorbidities, drug formulation changes), 3) when a potentially important pharmacokinetic change is anticipated (eg, addition or elimination of an interacting drug), and 4) for guiding dose adjustments for ASDs with dose-dependent pharmacokinetics, particularly enzyme-inducing ASDs. ASD levels must always be interpreted in the context of a patient's clinical response. Table 133.1 lists mechanisms of action, common adverse effects, and serum reference ranges of some of the commonly used ASDs. For drugs that have high protein

Box 133.3 • Suggestions for Treating Seizures in the ICU

Brief single seizure (<60 s) (isolated seizures)

Observe, ensure adequate O_2 saturation and vital signs, eliminate cause

Initiate antiseizure therapy if recurrence risk is high[a]

- Phenytoin 15-20 mg/kg IV or fosphenytoin 15-20 mg/kg PE IV or IM loading; oral loading 15 mg/kg in increments of 300 mg q3h, maintenance dose 300-400 mg/day
- IV or PO valproic acid, 20-30 mg/kg load, maintenance 500-1,000 mg twice daily
- IV levetiracetam 1,500-3,000 mg load, maintenance 500-1,500 mg twice daily
- Lacosamide 200-400 mg load, maintenance 100-200 mg twice daily
- Oral carbamazepine 400-800 mg/day or oral oxcarbazepine 1,200-2,400 mg/day

Seizure precautions: padding bed rails, increased observation

Prolonged seizure (<5 min) or >1 seizure (impending status epilepticus)

Observe, ensure adequate O_2 saturation and vital signs, eliminate and treat underlying cause

Immediately administer IV benzodiazepine-lorazepam 1-4 mg, diazepam 10-20 mg, midazolam 2-10 mg with *concurrent* loading dose phenytoin or fosphenytoin PE or 15-20 mg/kg or other ASDs

Consider emergency EEG to exclude nonconvulsive seizures

Seizure precautions: padding bed rails, increased observation

Abbreviations: ASD, antiseizure drug; EEG, electroencephalography; ICU, intensive care unit; IM, intramuscular; IV, intravenous; PE, phenytoin sodium equivalents; PO, oral.

[a] Such as new cortical lesion, hyperammonemia, or hyponatremia.

binding (Table 133.2), particularly phenytoin and valproic acid, serum free levels should be followed.

Considerations for Choosing ASDs

Underlying Medical Conditions

Patients requiring ICU care often have underlying comorbidities that may predispose to seizures or affect medication management. For example, in patients with porphyria, enzyme-inducing ASDs may increase heme synthesis and precipitate hepatic failure and so should be avoided. Several ASDs are associated with hepatotoxicity, including phenobarbital, phenytoin, carbamazepine, and felbamate, and some are associated with hyperammonemia, such as valproic acid and topiramate. Generally, valproic acid should not be used in patients with considerable hepatic dysfunction. Because of complexities of metabolism, protein-binding, renal elimination, and other pharmacokinetic parameters, the dosing of ASDs in patients with substantial renal impairment also deserves careful attention. For example, decreased renal excretion can lead to toxicity with use of renally eliminated ASDs, and failure to account for clearance may result in breakthrough seizures in patients receiving hemodialysis. Patients receiving dialysis may require reduced maintenance doses and a supplemental dose for certain medications after dialysis. The metabolism of ASDs commonly used in ICU practice is summarized in Table 133.2. Table 133.2 also lists drugs requiring hepatic and renal dosing.

Interactions Between ASDs

Although monotherapy is wanted in the management of epilepsy, combinations of ASDs are used frequently in patients with refractory seizures. These increase the possibility of drug-drug interactions. Drug-drug interactions are relevant for patients with epilepsy for various reasons: 1) many ASDs have a narrow therapeutic index, and even relatively modest alterations in their pharmacokinetics can result in loss of response or toxic effects (especially phenytoin); and 2) many traditional ASDs (carbamazepine, valproic acid, and phenytoin) have inducing effects on the cytochrome P450 system, affecting dosing for other ASDs metabolized by the same system. Most clinically important ASD interactions result from induction or inhibition of drug-metabolizing enzymes. Consideration of other mechanisms is also important, including pharmacodynamic interactions, which may influence toleration of therapy. These may be prevented by avoiding polytherapy when possible and by selecting comedications that are less likely to interact. If the use of potentially interacting drugs cannot be avoided, the risk of adverse clinical consequences may be mitigated by dose adjustments guided by careful monitoring of clinical response and measurement of serum drug concentrations. The common drug interactions of ASDs are summarized in Table 133.2.

Interactions Between ASDs and Other Drugs

ASDs may also interact with non-ASDs used in the ICU. Most clinically important interactions of ASDs result from induction or inhibition of drug metabolism. Carbamazepine, phenytoin, phenobarbital, and primidone are strong enzyme inducers and can reduce the efficacy of coadministered medications metabolized by these same

Table 133.1 • Mechanism of Action, Dosage, and Adverse Effects of Commonly Used ASDs in the ICU

Drug	Mechanism of Action	Starting/Loading Dose	Maintenance Dose	Reference Range, mg/dL	Common Adverse Effects
Lorazepam	GABAergic	0.1 mg/kg IV[a]	NA	NA	Sedation, respiratory depression, arrhythmia, and hypotension
Diazepam	GABAergic	10 mg IM or 20 mg rectal	NA	NA	Sedation, respiratory depression, arrhythmia, and hypotension
Midazolam	GABAergic	10 mg IM; 5-30 mg IV[a]	NA	NA	Sedation, respiratory depression, arrhythmia, and hypotension
Fosphenytoin	Sodium channel inhibitors	20 mg/kg PE IV/IM[a]	NA	NA	Cardiorespiratory depression, arrhythmia, hypotension, nonallergic pruritus
Phenytoin	Sodium channel inhibitors	20 mg/kg IV[a]	300-400 mg daily	10-20	Nystagmus, ataxia, diplopia, dysarthria, gum hypertrophy; IV administration may lead to purple glove syndrome
Levetiracetam	Synaptic vesicle protein (SV2A) binding	60 mg/kg IV; maximum 4,500 mg/dose[a]	1,000-1,500 mg twice daily	12-46	Irritability, sleepiness, hostility, depression, psychosis
Valproic acid	Multiple mechanisms	40 mg/kg IV; maximum 3,000 mg/dose[a]	10-30 mg/kg twice daily	50-100	Nausea, tremor, hepato-pancreato-toxicity, thrombocytopenia
Lacosamide	Sodium channel modulation	200 mg IV, 100 mg 12 hours later[a]	100-200 mg twice daily	10-20	Nausea, visual blurring, diplopia, PR interval prolongation
Phenobarbital	GABAergic	15 mg/kg IV[a]	50-100 mg twice daily	10-40	Sedation, dysarthria, ataxia, and nystagmus
Carbamazepine	Sodium channel blocker	100-200 mg twice daily	200-400 mg twice daily	4-12	Nausea, dizziness, ataxia, diplopia, rash, hyponatremia
Oxcarbazepine	Sodium channel blocker	150-300 mg twice daily	300-600 mg twice daily	3-35	Dizziness, diplopia, rash, hyponatremia (>CBZ), leukopenia
Eslicarbazepine	Sodium channel blocker	400 mg once daily	800-1,600 mg once daily	3-35	Similar to those of oxcarbazepine but less frequent
Topiramate	Multiple mechanisms	25 mg twice daily	100-200 mg twice daily	5-20	Paresthesia, metabolic acidosis, impaired language fluency and cognition, renal calculi
Zonisamide	T-type calcium inhibitor	100 mg once daily	100-200 mg twice daily	10-40	Dizziness, somnolence, fever from reduced sweating pancreatitis, renal calculi
Gabapentin	Calcium channel modulation	100-300 mg 3 times daily	600-1,200 mg 3 times daily	2-20	Somnolence, dizziness, weight gain

Table 133.1 • Continued

Drug	Mechanism of Action	Starting/Loading Dose	Maintenance Dose	Reference Range, mg/dL	Common Adverse Effects
Lamotrigine	Sodium channel blocker (possibly calcium channel blocker)	25 mg	100-200 mg twice daily	2.5-15	Hypersensitivity reaction, Stevens-Johnson syndrome, dizziness, insomnia
Clobazam	GABAergic	5 mg twice daily	10-20 mg twice daily	0.03-0.3	Salivation, sedation, aggressive behavior, irritability
Rufinamide	Sodium channel modulator	200-400 mg twice daily	800-1,600 mg twice daily	30-40	QT shortening, rash, nausea, sleepiness, dizziness
Felbamate	GABA potentiation and glutamate/NMDA inhibition	400 mg twice daily	400-900 mg 3 times daily	30-60	Hepatic toxicity, aplastic anemia, insomnia, weight loss
Ethosuximide	T-type calcium inhibitor	250 mg once daily	250-750 mg twice daily	40-100	Nausea, abdominal discomfort, drowsiness, dizziness
Perampanel	AMPA receptor antagonist	2 mg once daily	8-10 mg once daily	NA	Dizziness, somnolence, irritability, falls, ataxia, hostility, homicidal ideation and threats, psychosis, delirium

Abbreviations: AMPA, α-amino-3-hydroxy-5-methyl-4-isoxazole propionic acid; ASD, antiseizure drug; CBZ, carbamazepine; GABA, γ-aminobutyric acid; ICU, intensive care unit; IM, intramuscular; IV, intravenous; NA, not applicable; NMDA, *N*-methyl-D-aspartate; PE, phenytoin sodium equivalents.
[a] Loading dose for acute seizure according to the Guideline Committee of the American Epilepsy Society. Epilepsy Curr. 2016 Jan-Feb;16(1):48-61.

Table 133.2 • Metabolism and Drug Interaction of ASDs Commonly Used in the ICU

Drug	Metabolism	Protein Binding[a]	Adjustment in Liver/Renal Impairment	Half-life[b]	Dialyzability	Expected Changes in Plasma Levels When Other ASDs Are Added
Lorazepam	Glucuronide conjugation	High	No/No	Intermediate	No	↓ by PHT, CBZ, PB, PRM
Diazepam	*N*-demethylation by CYP3A4 and 2C19	High	No/No	Very short	No	↓ by PHT, CBZ, PB, PRM
Midazolam	Hydroxylation by CYP3A4	High	No/No	Very short	No	↓ by PHT, CBZ, PB, PRM
Fosphenytoin	Oxidation; CYP450 inducer (CYP2C9/19)	High	Yes/No	Intermediate	5%	NA
Phenytoin	Oxidation; CYP450 inducer (CYP2C9/19)	High	Yes/No	Intermediate	5%	↑ by FBM, OXC VPA: free level ↑, total level ↓
Levetiracetam	Hydrolytic metabolism, no effects on CYP	Low	No/Yes	Short	50% (SD)	No interactions

(*continued*)

Table 133.2 • Continued

Drug	Metabolism	Protein Binding[a]	Adjustment in Liver/Renal Impairment	Half-life[b]	Dialyzability	Expected Changes in Plasma Levels When Other ASDs Are Added
Valproic acid	Oxidation and glucuronide conjugation; CYP inhibitor	High	Yes/No	Intermediate	<20%	Free level ↑ by PHT, total ↑ by FBM
Lacosamide	Demethylation (CYP3A4/ CYP2C19)	Low	No/Yes	Intermediate	50% (SD)	None clinically relevant
Phenobarbital	Oxidation, CYP inducer (CYP2C9/ 19)	Low	Yes/No	Long	<10%	↑ by FBM, VPA
Carbamazepine	Oxidation (CYP3A4), carbamazepine-10,11-epoxide, CYP inducer	Intermediate	Yes/No	Intermediate	<5%	Active metabolite ↑ by FBM, VPA ↓ by PHT, PB, PRM
Oxcarbazepine	Glucuronide conjugation to monohydroxy derivative, CYP inhibitor	Low	No/Yes	Short	No	None clinically relevant
Eslicarbazepine	Glucuronide conjugation	Low	No/Yes	Intermediate	No	None clinically relevant
Topiramate	Variably metabolized, weak CYP inducer	Low	No/Yes	Intermediate	50% (SD)	↓ by CBZ, PHT, PB, PRM
Zonisamide	Oxidation (CYP3A4), reduction, and *N*-acetylation (>50%): no effect on CYP	Low	No/Yes	Long	50%	↓ by CBZ, PHT, PB, PRM
Gabapentin	Excreted unchanged	Low	No/Yes	Short	>50% (SD)	No interactions
Lamotrigine	Glucuronide conjugation; no effect on CYP	Intermediate	Yes/No	Intermediate	20%	↓ by CBZ, PHT, PB, PRM ↑ by VPA
Clobazam	Oxidation (CYP3A4 and CYP2C19) to desmethyl-clobazam	High	Yes/No	Long	No	↓ by PHT, CBZ, PB, PRM
Rufinamide	Hydrolytic metabolism, modest CYP inducer	Intermediate	Yes/No	Short	<30%	↓ by PHT, PB, CBZ, PRM ↑ by VPA
Felbamate	Oxidation (CYP3A4)	Low	Yes/Yes	Long	No SD	↓ by CBZ, PHT
Ethosuxamide	Oxidation (CYP3A4); no effect on CYP	Low	No/No	Long	50% (SD)	↓ by CBZ, PHT, PB, PRM
Perampanel	Oxidation (CYP3A4)	High	Yes/Yes	Long	Unknown	↓ by CBZ, OXC, PHT

Abbreviations: ASD, antiseizure drug; CBZ, carbamazepine; CYP, cytochrome P450; FBM, felbamate; ICU, intensive care unit; NA, not applicable; OXC, oxcarbazepine; PB, phenobarbital; PHT, phenytoin; PRM, primidone; SD, supplementary dose is required after hemodialysis; VPA, valproic acid.

[a] Low, less than 50%; intermediate, 50% to 85%; high, more than 85%.

[b] Short, less than 10 hours; intermediate, 10-30 hours; long, more than 30 hours.

Table 133.3 • List of Non-ASDs That Interact With ASD Metabolism[a]

Non-ASDs	ASDs						
	Carbamazepine	Phenytoin	Phenobarbital	Valproic Acid	Lamatrigine	Perampanel	Topiramate
Drugs that increase ASD serum concentration or active metabolite	Fluoxetine, trazodone, fluvoxamine, propoxyphene, clarithromycin, erythromycin, fluconazole, ketoconazole, metronidazole, ritonavir, diltiazem, verapamil, omeprazole, cimetidine, risperidone, quetiapine	Fluoxetine, trazodone, imipramine, chloramphenicol, fluconazole, isoniazid, amiodarone, diltiazem, tacrolimus	Chloramphenicol, propoxyphene	Sertraline, erythromycin, isoniazid, cimetidine	Sertraline	Ketoconazole	Hydrochlorothiazide, lithium
Drugs in which serum concentration is potentially decreased by coadminstration of ASD	Oral contraceptives Antidepressants (eg, amitriptyline, mirtazapine, citalopram) Antimicrobials (eg, albendazole, indinavir, metronidazole) Antineoplastics (eg, methotrexate, cyclophosphamide, tamoxifen) Antipsychotics (eg, clozapine, haloperidol, quetiapine) Cardiovascular agents (eg, amiodarone, digoxin, warfarin) Immunosuppressants (eg, cyclosporine, sirolimus, methylprednisolone, dexamethasone) Others (eg, fentanyl, methadone, vecuronium)	Same as carbamazepine	Same as carbamazepine	Rifampin	None	None	Ethinyl estradiol, pioglitazone

Abbreviation: ASD, antiseizure drug.

[a] This table is not complete, and online references and pharmacy services should be consulted to determine potential drug-drug interactions in an individual patient.

systems. For example, carbamazepine may result in considerable reduction in rivaroxaban concentration, leading to reduction in anticoagulant effect. When enzyme-inducing ASDs are coadministered with immunosuppressant medications such as corticosteroids, interactions may lead to a reduction in anti-inflammatory effect. Furthermore, enzyme-inducing ASDs may alter warfarin metabolism. There can initially be an increase in anticoagulant action of warfarin when phenytoin is co-administered related to protein-binding interactions and competition for hepatic enzyme degradation sites, but then a decrease in anticoagulant activity may occur due to subsequent increase in warfarin metabolism. Therefore, closely following the international normalized ratio status is important in patients receiving warfarin and enzyme-inducing ASDs. The interactions of ASDs with commonly used antidepressants, antipsychotic drugs, oral anticoagulants, and antimicrobials are listed in Table 133.3.

Summary

- When combination therapy is needed, ASD combinations with the potential for synergistic efficacy and limited toxicity should be carefully selected.
- Combining more than 1 sodium channel blocking ASD such as lacosamide, lamotrigine, carbamazepine, or oxcarbazepine may result in additive adverse effects.
- Patients requiring ICU care often have underlying chronic or acute comorbid medical conditions that may affect seizure management. For example, patients receiving dialysis may require reduced maintenance doses and a supplemental dose after dialysis (such as levetiracetam).
- Enzyme-inducing ASDs, including carbamazepine, phenytoin, and phenobarbital, may reduce the efficacy of coadministered medications, including immunosuppressants, anticoagulants, and antimicrobials.

SUGGESTED READING

Brodie MJ, Sills GJ. Combining antiepileptic drugs: rational polytherapy? Seizure. 2011 Jun;20(5):369–75. Epub 2011 Feb 8.

Claassen J, Mayer SA, Kowalski RG, Emerson RG, Hirsch LJ. Detection of electrographic seizures with continuous EEG monitoring in critically ill patients. Neurology. 2004 May 25;62(10):1743–8.

Carnovale C, Pozzi M, Mazhar F, Mosini G, Gentili M, Peeters GGAM, et al. Interactions between antiepileptic and antibiotic drugs: a systematic review and meta-analysis with dosing implications. Clin Pharmacokinet. 2018 Nov 7. [Epub ahead of print]

French JA, Gazzola DM. Antiepileptic drug treatment: new drugs and new strategies. Continuum (Minneap Minn). 2013 Jun;19(3 Epilepsy):643–55.

Jordan KG. Continuous EEG and evoked potential monitoring in the neuroscience intensive care unit. J Clin Neurophysiol. 1993 Oct;10(4):445–75.

Mora Rodriguez KA, Benbadis SR. Managing antiepileptic medication in dialysis patients. Curr Treat Options Neurol. 2018 Sep 27;20(11):45.

Patsalos PN, Berry DJ, Bourgeois BF, Cloyd JC, Glauser TA, Johannessen SI, et al. Antiepileptic drugs: best practice guidelines for therapeutic drug monitoring: a position paper by the subcommission on therapeutic drug monitoring, ILAE Commission on Therapeutic Strategies. Epilepsia. 2008 Jul;49(7):1239–76.

Perucca E. Clinically relevant drug interactions with antiepileptic drugs. Br J Clin Pharmacol. 2006 Mar;61(3):246–55.

Ruiz-Gimenez J, Sanchez-Alvarez JC, Canadillas-Hidalgo F, Serrano-Castro PJ; Andalusian Epilepsy Society. Antiepileptic treatment in patients with epilepsy and other comorbidities. Seizure. 2010 Sep;19(7):375–82. Epub 2010 Jun 15.

Shandra A, Shandra P, Kaschenko O, Matagne A, Stohr T. Synergism of lacosamide with established antiepileptic drugs in the 6-Hz seizure model in mice. Epilepsia. 2013 Jul;54(7):1167–75. Epub 2013 Jun 10.

Titoff V, Moury HN, Titoff IB, Kelly KM. Seizures, antiepileptic drugs, and CKD. Am J Kidney Dis. 2019 Jan;73(1):90–101. Epub 2018 May 18.

Vorderwulbecke BJ, Lichtner G, von Dincklage F, Holtkamp M. Acute antiepileptic drug use in intensive care units. J Neurol. 2018 Dec;265(12):2841–50. Epub 2018 Sep 26.

134 Effects of Targeted Temperature Management on Drugs

LAUREN K. NG TUCKER, MD

Goals

- Outline the effects of common drugs used during targeted temperature management.
- Review the physiologic effects of hypothermia on drug metabolism and clearance.

Introduction

Targeted temperature management (TTM), also known as hypothermia therapy, has increased in popularity in the past several years and has proven benefits only in the setting of cardiac arrest. It has been unsuccessful or not sufficiently proven for use in traumatic brain injury, bacterial meningitis, cerebral hemorrhage, and ischemic stroke. TTM has been shown to decrease intracranial pressure and is used in the management of refractory intracranial pressure despite recent evidence suggesting harm.

Physiologic Mechanisms and Effects

TTM is believed to work through various physiologic mechanisms to produce its neuroprotective effects. These mechanisms are outlined below in Box 134.1. In addition, known physiologic effects of hypothermia are outlined in Table 134.1.

Although TTM has become commonplace in the intensive care unit setting, little is known regarding the pharmacologic effects on the body. Research in this field has mainly centered on the cytochrome P450 system. Given the known effect of decreased cytochrome P450 and hepatic metabolism in TTM, it is not surprising that many of the drugs have decreased clearance. Table 134.2 summarizes various animal and human studies on the effects of hypothermia on pharmacokinetics and pharmacodynamics. Renal and hepatic disease, obesity, advanced age, and hypothermia all have effects on medications. The most important effect of TTM on hepatic function is a decrease in the metabolic clearance of many drugs, including midazolam, fentanyl, phenobarbital, phenytoin, and neuromuscular junction blockers. Pharmacokinetics in induced hypothermia are substantially changed, often approaching a 10% decrease per 1°C decrease, a factor often underappreciated by clinicians.

Box 134.1 • Physiologic Mechanisms of TTM

- Decreases cerebral metabolism 6%-10% for every 1°C reduction in temperature
- Decreases metabolic rate and O_2 and CO_2 consumption decrease to 50%-65% of normal at a core temperature of 32°C
- Decreases insulin secretion and moderately increases insulin resistance
- Interrupts apoptotic pathway
- Blocks neuroexcitatory cascade by disrupting calcium homeostasis
- Suppresses ischemia-induced inflammatory reactions and release of proinflammatory cytokines
- Prevents and mitigates reperfusion-related DNA injury, lipid peroxidation, and leukotriene production and decreases nitric oxide production
- Impairs neutrophil and macrophage function
- Reduces free radical production

Table 134.1 • Physiologic Effects of Hypothermia

Organ System	Physiologic Effects of Hypothermia
Body metabolism	Decreased metabolic rate by 8% per 1°C decrease in temperature Decreased oxygen consumption Decreased carbon dioxide production Decreased rate of drug metabolism Increased fat metabolism
Cardiovascular	Decreased heart rate and cardiac output Increased contractility Increased plasma norepinephrine levels Increased activation of sympathetic nervous system Increased venous return Peripheral vasoconstriction Arrhythmias
Endocrine	Decreased insulin secretion and sensitivity
Gastrointestinal	Decreased motility, mild ileus Impaired active drug transport
Hematologic	Platelet dysfunction and mild decrease in platelet count
Hepatic	Decreased metabolic rate Decreased isoform-specific cytochrome P450 metabolism
Immunologic	Depressed immune function Increased infection rates
Renal	Cold diuresis Decreased active tubular secretion Decreased antidiuretic hormone Decreased antidiuretic hormone receptors No effect on passive filtration Hypokalemia, hypophosphatemia, hypomagnesemia, and hypocalcemia

Table 134.2 • Pharmacokinetic and Pharmacodynamic Effects of Hypothermia on Medications

Drug	Metabolism	Vd	CL	EC_{50}
Atropine	Hepatic		↓ 37%-77%	
Chlorzoxazone	CYP2E1	↑ 27%	↓ 54%	
Diazepam	CYP2C19, CYP3A4		↓ 29%-72%	
Dobutamine				↓ 24%-67%
Doxorubicin	Hepatic		↓ 29%	
Epinephrine				↓ 28%-88%
Fentanyl	CYP3A4		↓ 31%-52% conversion rate of 3A4	
Gentamicin	Renal	↓ 32%	↓ 51%	
Isoprenaline	Hepatic			↓ 71%-78%
Midazolam	CYP3A4	↑ 83%	↓ 11% per °C	
Morphine	UGT, CYP2C, CYP3A4	↓ 33%	↓ 70%	↑ 366%
Neostigmine	Hepatic	Unaltered	Unaltered	EC_{95} ↓ 13% DOA unaltered
Oxazepam	Hepatic		↓ 42%-48%	
Pancuronium		↓ 40%	↓ 2%-61%	Variable data
Pentobarbital	Hepatic	↓ 20%	↓ 50%-75%	

Table 134.2 • Continued

Drug	Metabolism	Vd	CL	EC_{50}
Phenazone	Hepatic	↓ 20%	↓ 45%	
Phenobarbital	CYP2C9, UGT	↑ 25%		
Phenytoin	CYP2C9, CYP2C19	Unaltered	↓ 67%	
Procaine	Plasma cholinesterase		↓ 64%-91%	
Propofol	Hepatic		↓ 25%	Unaltered
Propranolol	Hepatic			
Quinidine	Hepatic		↓ Metabolism 50%	
Rocuronium	CYP2D6, renal		↓ 51%	
Sulfanilamide			↓ 69%-71%	
Theophylline	CYP1A2, CYP2E1, CYP3A3	↓ 11%		
Tubocurarine		↓ 18%	↓ 44%-61%	↑ 30%-47%
Vecuronium	CYP450s		↓ 11.3% per °C	↓ 5% DOA prolonged

Abbreviations: CL, clearance; CYP, cytochrome P450; DOA, duration of action; EC_{50}, concentration of drug that gives half-maximal response; EC_{95}, effective concentration at 95% of maximal effect; UGT, uridine diphosphate glucuronosyltransferase; Vd, volume of distribution.

Summary

- TTM (which often leads to some degree of hypothermia) delays clearance of drugs through several mechanisms.
- In hypothermia, most sedatives and intravenous opioids have a marked decrease in clearance, which may cause failure to fully awaken.
- The physiologic effects of deep hypothermia (33°C) affect multiple organs and can be profound.

SUGGESTED READING

Anderson KB, Poloyac SM. Therapeutic hypothermia: implications on drug therapy. In: Sadaka F, editor. Therapeutic hypothermia in brain injury. London (United Kingdom): InTech; c2013. p. 131–48.

Andrews PJ, Sinclair HL, Rodriguez A, Harris BA, Battison CG, Rhodes JK, et al; Eurotherm3235 Trial Collaborators. Hypothermia for intracranial hypertension after traumatic brain injury. N Engl J Med. 2015 Dec 17;373(25):2403–12. Epub 2015 Oct 7.

Bernard SA, Gray TW, Buist MD, Jones BM, Silvester W, Gutteridge G, et al. Treatment of comatose survivors of out-of-hospital cardiac arrest with induced hypothermia. N Engl J Med. 2002 Feb 21;346(8):557–63.

Chen J, Liu L, Zhang H, Geng X, Jiao L, Li G, et al. Endovascular hypothermia in acute ischemic stroke: pilot study of selective intra-arterial cold saline infusion. Stroke. 2016 Jul;47(7):1933–5. Epub 2016 May 19.

Clifton GL, Miller ER, Choi SC, Levin HS, McCauley S, Smith KR Jr, et al. Lack of effect of induction of hypothermia after acute brain injury. N Engl J Med. 2001 Feb 22;344(8):556–63.

Fukuoka N, Aibiki M, Tsukamoto T, Seki K, Morita S. Biphasic concentration change during continuous midazolam administration in brain-injured patients undergoing therapeutic moderate hypothermia. Resuscitation. 2004 Feb;60(2):225–30.

Hostler D, Zhou J, Tortorici MA, Bies RR, Rittenberger JC, Empey PE, et al. Mild hypothermia alters midazolam pharmacokinetics in normal healthy volunteers. Drug Metab Dispos. 2010 May;38(5):781–8. Epub 2010 Feb 17.

Hypothermia After Cardiac Arrest Study Group. Mild therapeutic hypothermia to improve the neurologic outcome after cardiac arrest. N Engl J Med. 2002 Feb 21;346(8):549–56. Erratum in: N Engl J Med 2002 May 30;346(22):1756.

Karcioglu O, Topacoglu H, Dikme O, Dikme O. A systematic review of safety and adverse effects in the practice of therapeutic hypothermia. Am J Emerg Med. 2018 Oct;36(10):1886–94. Epub 2018 Jul 11.

Kaufmann J, Wellnhofer E, Stockmann H, Graf K, Fleck E, Schroeder T, et al. Clopidogrel pharmacokinetics and pharmacodynamics in out-of-hospital cardiac arrest patients with acute coronary syndrome undergoing target temperature management. Resuscitation. 2016 May;102:63–9. Epub 2016 Feb 23.

Krieger DW, De Georgia MA, Abou-Chebl A, Andrefsky JC, Sila CA, Katzan IL, et al. Cooling for acute ischemic brain damage (cool aid): an open pilot study of induced hypothermia in acute ischemic stroke. Stroke. 2001 Aug;32(8):1847–54.

Miyata K, Ohnishi H, Maekawa K, Mikami T, Akiyama Y, Iihoshi S, et al. Therapeutic temperature modulation in severe or moderate traumatic brain injury: a propensity score analysis of data from the Nationwide Japan Neurotrauma Data Bank. J Neurosurg. 2016 Feb;124(2):527–37. Epub 2015 Sep 18.

Polderman KH. Mechanisms of action, physiological effects, and complications of hypothermia. Crit Care Med. 2009 Jul;37(7 Suppl):S186–202.

Schreckinger M, Marion DW. Contemporary management of traumatic intracranial hypertension: is there a role for therapeutic hypothermia? Neurocrit Care. 2009 Dec;11(3):427–36.

Tortorici MA, Kochanek PM, Poloyac SM. Effects of hypothermia on drug disposition, metabolism, and response: a focus of hypothermia-mediated alterations on the cytochrome P450 enzyme system. Crit Care Med. 2007 Sep;35(9):2196–204.

van den Broek MP, Groenendaal F, Egberts AC, Rademaker CM. Effects of hypothermia on pharmacokinetics and pharmacodynamics: a systematic review of preclinical and clinical studies. Clin Pharmacokinet. 2010 May;49(5):277–94.

van der Worp HB, Macleod MR, Bath PM, Demotes J, Durand-Zaleski I, Gebhardt B, et al; EuroHYP-1 investigators. EuroHYP-1: European multicenter, randomized, phase III clinical trial of therapeutic hypothermia plus best medical treatment vs. best medical treatment alone for acute ischemic stroke. Int J Stroke. 2014 Jul;9(5):642–5. Epub 2014 May 15.

Zhou J, Poloyac SM. The effect of therapeutic hypothermia on drug metabolism and response: cellular mechanisms to organ function. Expert Opin Drug Metab Toxicol. 2011 Jul;7(7):803–16. Epub 2011 Apr 8.

135 Sedation and Analgesia

JUAN G. RIPOLL SANZ, MD; JOSE L. DIAZ-GOMEZ, MD

Goals

- Provide an overview of commonly used sedative and analgesic drugs.
- Provide criteria for sedation depth.
- Provide criteria for anxiolysis.
- Provide criteria for pain management.

Introduction

Although sedatives and analgesics differ in pharmacologic properties, both produce sedation. Opioids are the most commonly used and most effective analgesics. However, the 2 have clear distinctions. Sedatives should be considered the primary choice for sedation in intensive care units (ICUs), and opioids are preferred for pain management after major surgery, periprocedural use to avoid pain in conscious patients, patients with polytrauma (particularly major fractures), or patients who are known to chronically use these agents and in whom quick withdrawal may have major consequences for management.

Patients receiving neurocritical care often have pain, discomfort, anxiety, and agitation at the same time. Interventions such as mobilization of traumatized patients, dressing changes, endotracheal suctioning, and intravascular invasive procedures are common in the ICU.

Sedatives and analgesics are among the most commonly administered drugs in the ICU. They provide anxiolysis, diminish stress response, facilitate nursing care, and improve patient tolerance to mechanical ventilation. Nevertheless, they increase the in-hospital length of stay, prolong mechanical ventilation, and may increase health care costs.

Contemporary critical care management of any critically ill patient emphasizes the need to reduce paralysis and continuous deep sedation to improve patient outcomes and diminish length of stay in mechanically ventilated patients in the ICU. This substantial change has required a pharmacologic reappraisal of the medications used, dosing intervals, routes of administration, adverse effects of medications, and sedation scales for appropriate titration. Neurocritically ill patients, especially, may be the more challenging population in the ICU for sedation management because of the overlapping of discomfort and pain and, most importantly, masking of neurologic deterioration, which can be adequately assessed only clinically.

Need for Analgesia and Sedation

Before sedation in the ICU, all possible treatable causes of acute confusional state, sympathetic hyperactivity, and agitation must be excluded (Box 135.1). The term *sedation* is mistakenly used to replace analgesia, anxiolysis, or antipsychosis.

Pain

Pain is prevalent among patients admitted to the ICU. Short-term effects of untreated pain include higher-energy expenditure and immunomodulation. Conversely, long-term complications include an increased risk of posttraumatic stress disorder. Most patients in the ICU who have had a neurosurgical procedure have moderate to severe pain during the first 24 to 48 hours, especially during the first 12 hours. The deleterious effects of pain after a neurologic injury may increase intracranial pressure. Current evidence shows that pain resulting from intracranial procedures and brain injury is intense rather than minimal and it affects a patient's recovery.

Monitoring of Pain

The standard technique to assess the level of pain in patients with intact linguistic, cognitive, and social function is self-reporting. Patients' rating of their own pain is associated with better management and has the advantage

Box 135.1 • Common Conditions Affecting Cognition and Behavior in an Intensive Care Unit

Respiratory
- Hypoxemia
- Hypercarbia

Metabolic Disturbances
- Hyponatremia
- Hypernatremia
- Hypercalcemia
- Hyperamylasemia
- Hyperammonemia

Cardiovascular
- Ischemia
- Hypotension

Concomitant Medications
- Psychoactive medications
- Antipsychotics
- Antidepressants
- Anticonvulsants
- Peptic ulcer prophylactics
- Promotility agents
- Corticosteroids
- Antibiotics
- Antiretrovirals

Miscellaneous
- Infections

of rapidly matching the nociceptive perception with the analgesic intervention. Scales such as the numerical rating scale (1-10) or visual analog scale (1-100) have been successfully used for patients who are neurocritically ill. When self-reporting is impossible to obtain, physicians should consider behavioral pain scales exclusively developed for critically ill patients.

Behavioral pain scales, including the critical care observation tool, behavioral pain scale, and the nonverbal pain scale, are reasonably accurate methods for assessing pain in neurocritically ill patients who cannot self-report their level of pain. Although widely used, such scales are of limited value in the context of diseases limiting movement or paralysis induced by medications.

Physiologic measurements such as high blood pressure and tachycardia are inaccurate and correlate poorly with more intuitive measures of pain. Indeed, vital signs lack specificity because they are highly influenced by the administration of drugs (eg, opioids, sedatives, pressors) or additional ICU stressors. In a study of sedated patients who had had painful cardiac surgical procedures and were unable to communicate and had minimal or absent behavioral responses, alternative physiologic indicators of pain, such as pupil size, were more sensitive than traditional behavioral indicators.

Pain Management

Pain is a risk factor for development of agitation when inappropriately managed. Thus, clinicians should ensure that adequate analgesia is attained before administering any sedative agent. Among neurologically ill patients, analgesia needs to be thoroughly titrated to reduce pain or discomfort to less than 3 on a 0 to 10 ordinal scale to ensure patient responsiveness while controlling overt discomfort.

Among the most commonly used medications for analgesia are the nonsteroidal anti-inflammatory drugs, acetaminophen, ketamine, α_2-agonists, opioids, corticosteroids, and local anesthetics (Table 135.1). Routes of analgesia are diverse and include oral, intermittent and continuous intravenous, topical, epidural and spinal, local cutaneous, and intra-articular.

Anxiolysis

Anxiety is considered a psychologic state that manifests as apprehension, nervous tension, or, in its most severe state, profound agitation. Physiologically, it presents with changes in heart rate, blood pressure, and respiratory rate or as an overall sympathetic activation (also known as flight-or-fight response). The ICU environment has numerous psychologic stressors to neurocritically ill patients. Treatment options for anxiety include sedative or hypnotic agents such as barbiturates or propofol and benzodiazepines. Pharmacologic agents that provide simultaneous analgesia and anxiolysis, including ketamine, low-dose narcotics and α_2-agonists are also commonly used (Table 135.1).

Monitoring Sedation

Although sedative drugs have suitable therapeutic indices, they might result in an inappropriate level of sedation when administered without monitoring tools. Oversedation and undersedation have deleterious effects in patients receiving critical care, as evidenced by increased morbidity and mortality.

Among the most popularly used scales are the Richmond agitation-sedation scale, adaptation to the intensive care environment scale, and the Riker sedation agitation scale. The use of sedation scales in the ICU has been shown to decrease the number of days on mechanical ventilation, reduce health care costs, minimize the amount of drug administered, and improve communication among health care providers.

Table 135.1 • Common Sedative Agents Used

Class	Drug	Mechanism of Action	Analgesia	Sedation	Starting Dose	Adverse Effects
Remifentanil	Opioids	Mu-receptor agonist	High	Low	0.5-1 mcg/kg IV bolus	Arterial hypotension Respiratory depression and apnea Hyperalgesia after discontinuation
Fentanyl	Opioids	Mu-receptor agonist	High	Low	25-50 mcg IV every 5-10 min	Arterial hypotension Respiratory depression and apnea Ileus Prolonged sedation if continuous infusion is administered
Morphine sulfate	Opioids	Mu-receptor agonist	High	Low	5-20 mg IM every 4 h *or* 2-10 mg IV every 4 h	Arterial hypotension Histamine release Respiratory depression Dysphoria
Ketamine	Phencyclidine derivative	NMDA-receptor blockade	High	Low	0.2 mg/kg	Arterial hypertension Tachycardia Hypersalivation Hallucinations
Haloperidol	Butyrophenone Typical antipsychotic	Block dopamine, acetylcholine, serotonin, histamine, and adrenergic receptors	None	Low	0.5-5 mg IV	Arterial hypotension Extrapyramidal symptoms Acute dystonia Neuroleptic malignant syndrome Decreased seizure threshold
Quetiapine	Atypical antipsychotic	Block dopamine, acetylcholine, serotonin, histamine, and adrenergic receptors	None	Moderate	25-50 mg PO twice daily	Prolonged sedation with initial higher doses Anticholinergic effects Hyperglycemia with prolonged administration
Risperidone	Atypical antipsychotic	Block dopamine, acetylcholine, serotonin, histamine, and adrenergic receptors	None	Moderate	0.5 mg PO	Anticholinergic effects
Olanzapine	Atypical antipsychotic	Block dopamine, acetylcholine, serotonin, histamine, and adrenergic receptors	None	Moderate	2.5-5 mg PO daily	Anticholinergic effects
Dexmedetomidine	α_2-Agonist	α_2-Receptor agonist	Moderate	Moderate	1 mcg/kg IV bolus over 10 min	Arterial hypotension Bradycardia after achieving steady state Transient hypertension during initial priming bolus

(*continued*)

Table 135.1 • Continued

Class	Drug	Mechanism of Action	Analgesia	Sedation	Starting Dose	Adverse Effects
Propofol	Hypnotic	Predominantly GABA-receptor agonist. Some effects on cannabinoid and glutamate receptors	None	High	1.0-2.5 mg/kg IV (anesthesia induction) 5 mcg/kg per min IV (sedation)	Arterial hypotension Bradycardia Apnea PRIS: Features of PRIS Metabolic acidosis Cardiogenic shock Rhabdomyolysis (increased CK, hypertriglyceridemia, acute renal failure) Risk factors for PRIS: High doses (>80 mcg/kg per min) for more than 48 h, low BMI, younger age, and concomitant vasopressors use
Midazolam	Benzodiazepines	$GABA_A$-receptor agonist	None	High	0.5-1 mg IV every 5-30 min	Prolonged arousal time if continuous infusion More relevant effect in the setting of kidney failure because an active metabolite may accumulate
Lorazepam	Benzodiazepines	$GABA_A$-receptor agonist	None	High	0.25 mg-1 mg IV every 5-30 min	Propylene glycol toxicity may occur with high-dose infusion (arterial hypotension, bradycardia, lactic acidosis, hyperosmolality, and seizures)
Diazepam	Benzodiazepines	$GABA_A$-receptor agonist	Low	High	2 mg IV every 30-60 min	

Abbreviations: BMI, body mass index; CK, creatine kinase; GABA, γ-aminobutyric acid; IM, intramuscularly; IV, intravenously; NMDA, *N*-methyl-D-aspartate; PO, orally; PRIS, propofol-related infusion syndrome.

Choice of Sedative Agent

Despite multiple clinical trials comparing sedative regimens in the ICU, no drug is superior to all others. The evidence for use in neurocritical care is even more inconclusive because of the lack of studies addressing the choice of sedative. The ideal sedative for use in the neuroICU has a rapid onset, has a short half-life, reduces the intracranial pressure while maintaining adequate cerebral blood flow, diminishes brain metabolic demands, and preserves a clear neurologic examination. Nevertheless, no such agent exists. The most common sedative agents used in the neuroICU are listed in Table 135.1.

Summary

- Pain management and sedation should be considered 2 different approaches.
- Sedation scales are available to control depth of sedation.
- Clinical assessment of pain is required and can be graded.
- Some patients (eg, those with severe trauma) need substantial doses of opioids.

SUGGESTED READING

Arbour C, Gelinas C. Behavioral and physiologic indicators of pain in nonverbal patients with a traumatic brain injury: an integrative review. Pain Manag Nurs. 2014 Jun;15(2):506–18. Epub 2012 Jun 23.

Beretta L, De Vitis A, Grandi E. Sedation in neurocritical patients: is it useful? Minerva Anestesiol. 2011 Aug;77(8):828–34.

Blaise GA, Nugent M, McMichan JC, Durant PA. Side effects of nalbuphine while reversing opioid-induced respiratory depression: report of four cases. Can J Anaesth. 1990 Oct;37(7):794–7.

Brook AD, Ahrens TS, Schaiff R, Prentice D, Sherman G, Shannon W, et al. Effect of a nursing-implemented sedation protocol on the duration of mechanical ventilation. Crit Care Med. 1999 Dec;27(12):2609–15.

Carrasco G. Instruments for monitoring intensive care unit sedation. Crit Care. 2000;4(4):217–25. Epub 2000 Jul 13.

Chiu AW, Contreras S, Mehta S, Korman J, Perreault MM, Williamson DR, et al. Iatrogenic opioid withdrawal in critically ill patients: a review of assessment tools and management. Ann Pharmacother. 2017 Dec;51(12):1099–1111. Epub 2017 Aug 9.

Coleman RM, Tousignant-Laflamme Y, Ouellet P, Parenteau-Goudreault E, Cogan J, Bourgault P. The use of the bispectral index in the detection of pain in mechanically ventilated adults in the intensive care unit: a review of the literature. Pain Res Manag. 2015 Jan-Feb;20(1):e33–7. Epub 2014 Jul 22.

Gelinas C, Arbour C. Behavioral and physiologic indicators during a nociceptive procedure in conscious and unconscious mechanically ventilated adults: similar or different? J Crit Care. 2009 Dec;24(4):628.e7–17. Epub 2009 Mar 27.

Gelinas C, Fillion L, Puntillo KA, Viens C, Fortier M. Validation of the critical-care pain observation tool in adult patients. Am J Crit Care. 2006 Jul;15(4):420–7.

Gelinas C, Klein K, Naidech AM, Skrobik Y. Pain, sedation, and delirium management in the neurocritically ill: lessons learned from recent research. Semin Respir Crit Care Med. 2013 Apr;34(2):236–43. Epub 2013 May 28.

Gelinas C, Tousignant-Laflamme Y, Tanguay A, Bourgault P. Exploring the validity of the bispectral index, the Critical-Care Pain Observation Tool and vital signs for the detection of pain in sedated and mechanically ventilated critically ill adults: a pilot study. Intensive Crit Care Nurs. 2011 Feb;27(1):46–52. Epub 2010 Dec 18.

Gottschalk A, Yaster M. The perioperative management of pain from intracranial surgery. Neurocrit Care. 2009;10(3):387–402. Epub 2008 Oct 1.

Hogarth DK, Hall J. Management of sedation in mechanically ventilated patients. Curr Opin Crit Care. 2004 Feb;10(1):40–6.

Jacobi J, Fraser GL, Coursin DB, Riker RR, Fontaine D, Wittbrodt ET, et al; Task Force of the American College of Critical Care Medicine (ACCM) of the Society of Critical Care Medicine (SCCM), American Society of Health-System Pharmacists (ASHP), American College of Chest Physicians. Clinical practice guidelines for the sustained use of sedatives and analgesics in the critically ill adult. Crit Care Med. 2002 Jan;30(1):119–41. Erratum in: Crit Care Med 2002 Mar;30(3):726.

Jeitziner MM, Schwendimann R, Hamers JP, Rohrer O, Hantikainen V, Jakob SM. Assessment of pain in sedated and mechanically ventilated patients: an observational study. Acta Anaesthesiol Scand. 2012 May;56(5):645–54. Epub 2012 Mar 7.

Kress JP, Pohlman AS, O'Connor MF, Hall JB. Daily interruption of sedative infusions in critically ill patients undergoing mechanical ventilation. N Engl J Med. 2000 May 18;342(20):1471–7.

Leslie K, Troedel S, Irwin K, Pearce F, Ugoni A, Gillies R, et al. Quality of recovery from anesthesia in neurosurgical patients. Anesthesiology. 2003 Nov;99(5):1158–65.

Li D, Miaskowski C, Burkhardt D, Puntillo K. Evaluations of physiologic reactivity and reflexive behaviors during noxious procedures in sedated critically ill patients. J Crit Care. 2009 Sep;24(3):472.e9–13. Epub 2009 Jan 17.

Makii JM, Mirski MA, Lewin JJ 3rd. Sedation and analgesia in critically ill neurologic patients. J Pharm Pract. 2010 Oct;23(5):455–69. Epub 2010 Aug 4.

Mei W, Seeling M, Franck M, Radtke F, Brantner B, Wernecke KD, et al. Independent risk factors for postoperative pain in need of intervention early after awakening from general anaesthesia. Eur J Pain. 2010 Feb;14(2):149.e1–7. Epub 2009 May 6.

Mirrakhimov AE, Voore P, Halytskyy O, Khan M, Ali AM. Propofol infusion syndrome in adults: a clinical update. Crit Care Res Pract. 2015;2015:260385. Epub 2015 Apr 12.

Mirski MA, Hemstreet MK. Critical care sedation for neuroscience patients. J Neurol Sci. 2007 Oct 15;261(1–2):16–34. Epub 2007 Jul 13.

Mirski MA, Lewin JJ. Sedation and pain management in acute neurological disease. Semin Neurol. 2008 Nov;28(5):611–30. Epub 2008 Dec 29.

Mirski MA, Muffelman B, Ulatowski JA, Hanley DF. Sedation for the critically ill neurologic patient. Crit Care Med. 1995 Dec;23(12):2038–53.

Mondello E, Siliotti R, Gravino E, Coluzzi F, David T, Sinardi AU. Sedation monitoring in ICU. Minerva Anestesiol. 2005 Sep;71(9):487–96.

Myhren H, Ekeberg O, Toien K, Karlsson S, Stokland O. Posttraumatic stress, anxiety and depression symptoms in patients during the first year post intensive care unit discharge. Crit Care. 2010;14(1):R14. Epub 2010 Feb 8.

Odhner M, Wegman D, Freeland N, Steinmetz A, Ingersoll GL. Assessing pain control in nonverbal critically ill adults. Dimens Crit Care Nurs. 2003 Nov-Dec;22(6):260–7.

Opdenakker O, Vanstraelen A, De Sloovere V, Meyfroidt G. Sedatives in neurocritical care: an update on pharmacological agents and modes of sedation. Curr Opin Crit Care. 2019 Apr;25(2):97–104.

Ostermann ME, Keenan SP, Seiferling RA, Sibbald WJ. Sedation in the intensive care unit: a systematic review. JAMA. 2000 Mar 15;283(11):1451–9.

Page GG, Blakely WP, Ben-Eliyahu S. Evidence that postoperative pain is a mediator of the tumor-promoting effects of surgery in rats. Pain. 2001 Feb 1;90(1–2):191–9.

Payen JF, Bru O, Bosson JL, Lagrasta A, Novel E, Deschaux I, et al. Assessing pain in critically ill sedated patients by using a behavioral pain scale. Crit Care Med. 2001 Dec;29(12):2258–63.

Roberts DJ, Haroon B, Hall RI. Sedation for critically ill or injured adults in the intensive care unit: a shifting paradigm. Drugs. 2012 Oct 1;72(14):1881–916.

Smithburger PL, Patel MK. Pharmacologic considerations surrounding sedation, delirium, and sleep in critically ill adults: a narrative review. J Pharm Pract. 2019 Apr 7:897190019840120. [Epub ahead of print]

Stein-Parbury J, McKinley S. Patients' experiences of being in an intensive care unit: a select literature review. Am J Crit Care. 2000 Jan;9(1):20–7.

Tsaousi GG, Pourzitaki C, Aloisio S, Bilotta F. Dexmedetomidine as a sedative and analgesic adjuvant in spine surgery: a systematic review and meta-analysis of randomized controlled trials. Eur J Clin Pharmacol. 2018 Nov;74(11):1377–89. Epub 2018 Jul 14.

Tung A, Rosenthal M. Patients requiring sedation. Crit Care Clin. 1995 Oct;11(4):791–802.

Vincent JL, Shehabi Y, Walsh TS, Pandharipande PP, Ball JA, Spronk P, et al. Comfort and patient-centred care without excessive sedation: the eCASH concept. Intensive Care Med. 2016 Jun;42(6):962–71. Epub 2016 Apr 13.

136 Inotropes, Vasopressors, and Antihypertensive Agents

JUAN N. PULIDO, MD

Goals

- Explain pharmacologic manipulation of hemodynamics.
- Discuss various vasoactive agents, including inotropes, vasopressors, and vasodilators.
- Explain that inotropes augment cardiac contractility and vasopressors increase vascular tone.
- Explain that intravenous antihypertensive agents include vasodilators, sympatholytics, and diuretics.

Introduction

Pharmacologic manipulation of the cardiovascular system is considered one of the cornerstones of day-to-day management of critically ill patients. For formulation of an adequate hemodynamic plan, it is crucial 1) to have a thorough understanding of cardiovascular physiology and its intricate relationship with the autonomic nervous system and 2) to identify a clear hemodynamic goal, such as maintenance of oxygen delivery and perfusion in shock, permissive hypertension in acute stroke, or blood pressure control in hypertensive emergencies.

Hemodynamic pharmacologic support comes second to understanding the physiologic need at hand. Cardiac output (CO) and systemic vascular resistance (SVR) are the main determinants of mean arterial pressure (MAP). CO is determined by heart rate and rhythm and stroke volume. Stroke volume can be manipulated by changes in preload, contractility, and afterload (Figure 136.1). Consequently, pharmacologic manipulation of hemodynamics can be targeted to any of these variables: cardiac contractility (inotrope), afterload or SVR (vasopressor or vasodilator), preload (fluid challenge or diuretic), and heart rate and rhythm (chronotrope, pacing, maintenance of atrioventricular synchrony). All drugs or agents that have an effect on myocardial contractility or vascular tone, regardless of the mechanism of action, belong to the broad family of vasoactive agents. Some have more or less effect on vasculature tone and are further classified depending on their role in cardiac contractility and vascular resistance (inotropes vs vasopressors or negative inotropes vs vasodilators). This chapter focuses on inotropes, vasopressors, and antihypertensive agents.

Formulation of a Hemodynamic Plan

Before any vasoactive drug is prescribed, a rapid, organized approach should be followed, as outlined in Box 136.1.

Inotropes

Inotropy refers to the force and velocity of cardiac contraction, and lusitropy is the rate of myocardial relaxation. Both processes are highly energy-consuming, which is one of the major limitations of inotropic support. All drugs that augment cardiac contractility are denominated inotropes. All inotropes ultimately increase the availability of cardiac myocite sarcoplasmic calcium by various mechanisms. Most commonly, this process is initiated by increasing intracellular cyclic adenosine monophosphate, either by increased protein G-mediated production (adrenergic agents, glucagon) or decreased degradation (phosphodiestarase inhibitors). Other mechanisms include inhibition of the sodium-potassium adenosine triphosphatase pump (digoxin), increasing calcium availability (calcium salts), or calcium-troponin sensitization (levosimendan). Inotropes conceptually differ from vasopressors,

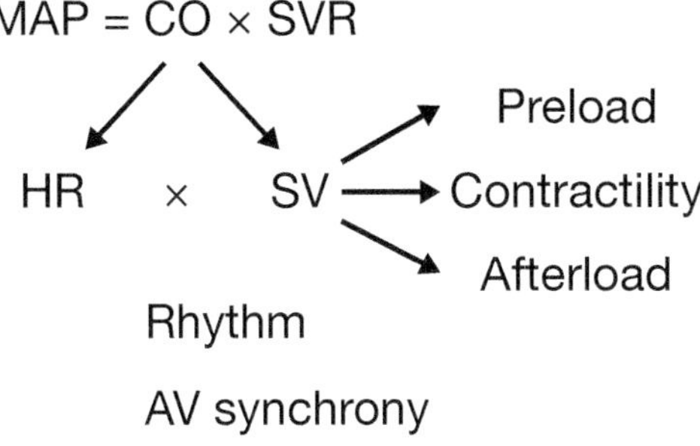

Figure 136.1. Hemodynamic Determinants of Mean Arterial Pressure (MAP). AV indicates atrioventricular; CO, cardiac output; HR, heart rate; SV, stroke volume; SVR, systemic vascular resistance.

Box 136.1 • Hemodynamic Plan

1. Have a clear physiologic and hemodynamic goal in mind.
   - Is CO the main problem or main target?
     - Contractility
       - Inotropes (inodilators vs inoconstrictors) vs negative inotropes
     - Preload
       - Fluid challenge or passive leg raise vs diuretics
     - Heart rate and rhythm
       - Maintenance of atrioventricular synchrony, pacing, chronotropes
   - Is SVR the main problem or main target?
     - Vasopressors
     - Vasodilators
2. Understand the mechanism of action and potential synergism.
   - Adrenergic (agonists or antagonists)
   - Nonadrenergic
3. Understand the adverse effects of the different agents.
   - Unwarranted cardiovascular effects:
     - Arrhythmias
     - Increase in oxygen consumption
     - Cardiac or tissue ischemia
   - Noncardiovascular effects
   - Effects in other organs
     - Cerebral vasodilation and intracranial pressure concerns
     - Coronary vasodilation or coronary steal phenomena
     - Inhibition of hypoxic pulmonary vasoconstriction
     - Renal, hepatic
   - Toxicity

which primarily cause vasoconstriction with subsequent increase in SVR and MAP.

Despite clear-cut definitions, there is overlap between these 2 major vasoactive classes. A particular agent can behave as an inotrope or vasopressor depending on the dose used and individual pleiotropic effect. For example, norepinephrine is primarily a vasopressor but also has inotropic properties because of concomitant, albeit less prominent, activation of β_1 receptors. Epinephrine and dopamine are predominantly inotropes but also exert vasopressor effects as a result of concomitant direct α_1 stimulation and, therefore, are considered part of both vasoactive classes.

Inotropes are functionally classified depending on concomitant stimulation (inoconstrictors) or inhibition (inodilators) of vascular smooth muscle tone. However, the more common classification is based on initial pharmacologic target, with 2 basic classes: adrenergic (sympathomimetic) and nonadrenergic agents (Table 136.1 and Figure 136.2).

The therapeutic effect of inotropic agents, as well as the adverse effects, largely depends on the relative proportion of sympathetic receptors stimulated (β_1, β_2, α_1) or, in the case of the nonadrenergic agents, on the specific pharmacodynamic targets in and outside the cardiac muscle. With application of the basic principles of formulating a pharmacologic plan for hemodynamic support, specific drugs can be used to achieve the desired physiologic effects. The concept of synergy emerges with use of 2 types of inotropes with different mechanism of action and receptor activation, theoretically potentiating the effect (adrenergic agent + phosphodiesterase inhibitor).

The major indication for inotropic support is cardiogenic shock. Despite the emphasis of a physiologic-based pharmacologic plan, important data favor specific inotropes over others. Norepinephrine is superior to dopamine for the treatment of shock regardless of the type of shock and the physiologic rationale. It is also essential to recognize that all inotropic agents increase myocardial oxygen consumption. Therefore, although this therapy is sometimes necessary to maintain perfusion and oxygen delivery during acute illness, it can be detrimental, and early mechanical circulatory support should be considered in select cases, depending on the cause, recoverability, and bridging options.

The adverse effect profile and the time of offset are other aspects that have to be considered when initiating vasoactive support. In addition to increased myocardial oxygen consumption and tachycardia, all inotropic agents, with the exception of digoxin, are arrhythmogenic. Digoxin is an unusual inotrope because it blocks atrioventricular conduction and causes bradycardia and arterial vasoconstriction with preferential use in patients with uncontrolled tachyarrhythmias and known low cardiac function. The vast majority of inotropes have a short half-life (2-5 minutes), with the notable exception of milrinone (1-2 hours) and levosimendan (1-80 hours because of its active metabolite), factors that are important considerations when weaning is attempted.

Table 136.1 • Inotropes

Drug (Class)	Action	HR	Con	Preload	SVR	BP	CO	Indication	Dose/Comments	Adverse Effects
Dobutamine (adrenergic, ID)	$\beta_1 > \beta_2$	↑↑	↑↑	No effect	↓	Var	↑	↓CO ↑SVR, MAP RV failure Bradycardia	250 mg/250 mL = 1 mg/mL 2-20 mcg/kg per min	Arrhythmias ↑MVO_2 Myocardial ischemia Hypotension
Dopamine (adrenergic, IC)	α_1, β_{1-2}, D_1 Indirect NE release	↑	↑	↑	No effect	↑	↑	↓CO ↓SVR, MAP	400 mg/250 mL = 1,600 mcg/mL 2-20 mcg/kg per min Variable individual dose response No benefit of low-dose "renal dose"	Arrhythmias ↑MVO_2 Myocardial ischemia HTN
Epinephrine (adrenergic, IC)	β_1, β_2, α_1, α_2	↑↑	↑↑	↑	No effect	↑↑	↑	Cardiac arrest Anaphylaxis Cardiogenic shock	4 mg/250 mL = 16 mcg/mL 2-10 mcg/IV bolus 0.01-0.2 mcg/kg per min 1-20 mcg per min	Arrhythmias ↑MVO_2 Hyperglycemia, ischemia Hyperlactatemia HTN
Isoproterenol (adrenergic, ID)	Strong β_1, β_2	↑↑	↑↑	No effect	↓	Var	↑	RV failure Bradycardia after heart transplant	0.01-0.1 mcg/kg per min 1-10 mcg/min	Arrhythmias ↑MVO_2 Myocardial ischemia, hypotension
Norepinephrine (adrenergic, IC)	α_1, α_2, β_1 Intense α_{1-2} constriction	Var	↑	↑	↑↑	↑	No effect	↓SVR +/- ↓CO Shock (distributive, cardiogenic)	4 mg/250 mL = 16 mcg/mL 0.01-0.3 mcg/kg per min 2-30 mcg per min	Tissue ischemia Arrhythmias HTN
Milrinone (nonadrenergic, ID)	PDE inhibitor	No effect	↑↑	↓	↓	Var	↑	↓CO w/↑SVR RV failure Pulm HTN	25-75 mcg/kg load 0.125-0.75 mcg/kg per min Long offset of action Fewer arrhythmias	Hypotension
Digoxin (nonadrenergic, IC)	(-) Na-K ATPase ↑ Ca+	↓	↑	No effect	↑	↑	No effect	Tachycardia ↓CO	0.5 mg IV Digitalization 1 mg first 24 h Use with caution in CKD and electrolyte abnormalities	Bradycardia Toxicity
Glucagon (nonadrenergic, IC)	Nonadrenergic ↑ cAMP	↑	↑↑	No effect	No effect	↑	↑	β-B or CCB toxicity Refractory hypoglycemia	1-5 mg IV 25-75 mcg per min	Hyperglycemia Tachycardia Nausea, vomiting
Calcium salts (nonadrenergic, IC)	↑ Ca+	No effect	↑	No effect	↑	↑	↑	HypoCa HyperK HypoMg CCB hypotension	10% = 100 mg/mL 200-1,000 mg IV CaCl only central admin	Phlebitis
Levosimendan (nonadrenergic, ID)	Ca sensitizer Binds to TnC (+) K_{ATP} channels vasodilation	No effect	↑↑	↓	↓	Var	↑	↓CO w/↑SVR RV failure Pulm HTN ↓ Arrhythmia	6-24 mcg/kg IV bolus 0.05-0.4 mcg/kg per min Up to 24 h Active metabolite 80 h Very long offset of action	Hypotension Hypokalemia

Abbreviations: ATPase, adenosine triphosphatase; β-B, beta-blocker; BP, blood pressure; Ca, calcium; CaCl, calcium chroride; cAMP, cyclic adenosine monophosphate; CCB, calcium channel blocker; CKD, chronic kidney disease; CO, cardiac output; Con, contractility; HR, heart rate; HTN, hypertension; HyperK, hyperkalemia; HypoCa, hypocalcemia; HypoMg, hypomagnesemia; IC, inoconstrictor; ID, inodilator; IV, intravenous; K_{ATP}, adenosine triphosphate–sensitive potassium channel; MAP, mean arterial pressure; MVO_2, myocardial oxygen consumption; Na-K, sodium-potassium; NE, norepinephrine; PDE, phosphodiesterase; Pulm, pulmonary; RV, right ventricle; SVR, systemic vascular resistance; TnC, cardiac troponin C; Var, variable.

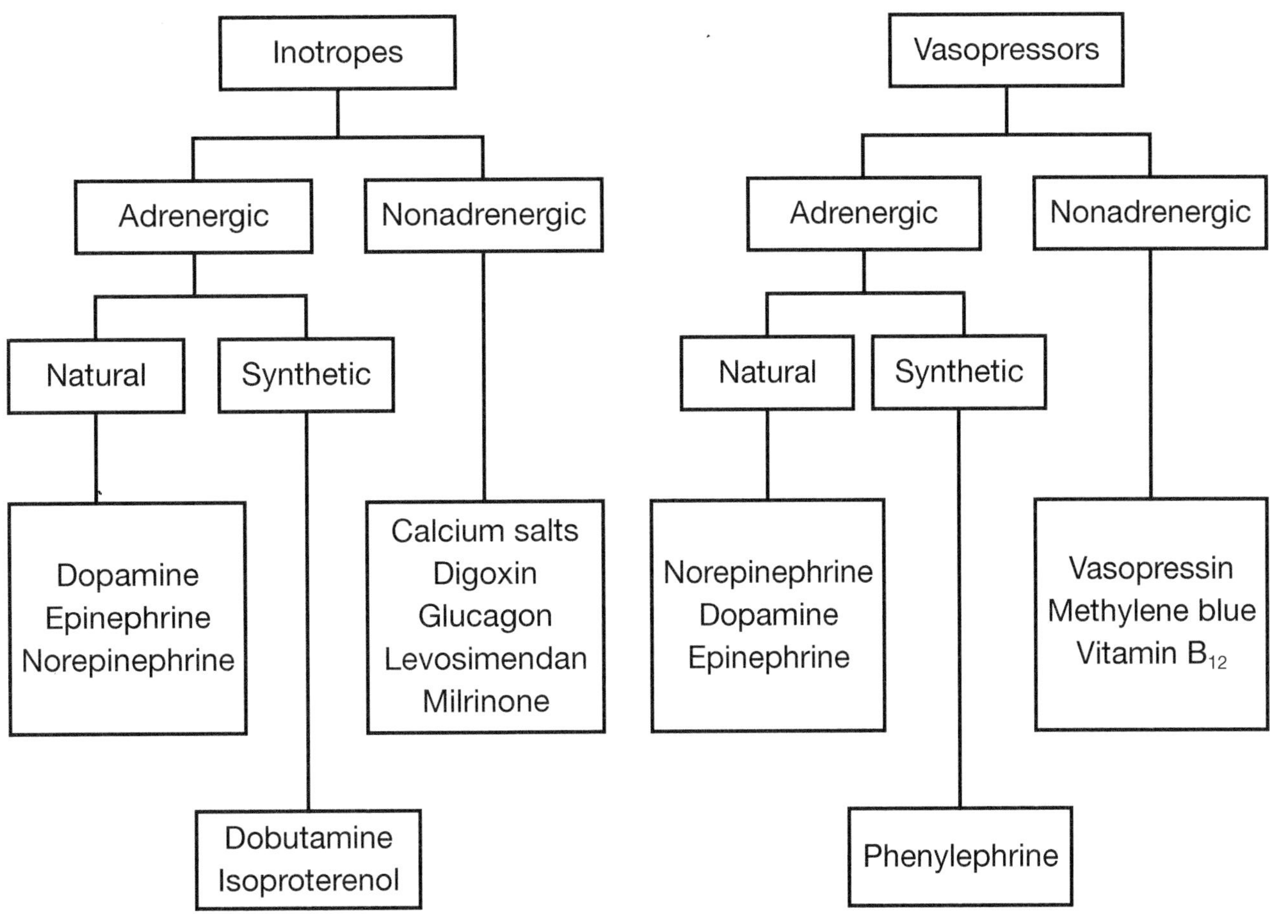

Figure 136.2. Classification of Inotropes and Vasopressors.

Table 136.1 lists the different inotropic agents and their hemodynamic effects, dosages, uses, and adverse effects.

Vasopressors

Vasopressors are drugs that produce vascular smooth muscle contraction with resultant increased SVR and MAP. These agents cause vasoconstriction by 2 major pathways:

1. Calcium-calmodulin–mediated phosphorylation of myosin through second messenger systems (phospholipase C, diacylglycerol, and inositol triphosphate) activated by G-protein–α_1-coupled adrenergic receptor or V_1 receptors.
2. Inhibition of cyclic guanosine monophosphate-nitric oxide–induced vasodilatation

The effect of cellular membrane potential on vascular smooth muscle tone is particularly important because hyperpolarization reduces the ability of the cell to constrict. During vasoconstriction, the adenosine triphosphate–sensitive potassium channel remains closed, maintaining potassium inside the cell and allowing the entrance of calcium for subsequent contraction. However, during shock, particularly with the presence of lactic acid, reduced local adenosine triphosphate stores, and high hydrogen ion concentrations, the membrane becomes hyperpolarized and the channel remains open with subsequent vasodilatation despite attempts of second messenger-mediated vasoconstriction. This phenomenon explains the relative lack of efficacy and tachyphylaxis of vasopressors in shock with acidosis.

Other pathways such as the nitric oxide-cyclic guanosine monophosphate pathway can be inhibited with methylene blue or with high-dose vitamin B_{12} (hydroxocobalamine) with resultant synergy when the response to standard vasopressors is poor. These agents are usually reserved for refractory vasoplegia.

In cases of refractory shock, the role of cortisol in the vascular and cardiac myocite response to catecholamines has to be considered. Also, depending on the situation (sepsis, vasoplegia), stress-dose steroid administration and buffer therapy should be considered to reduce the vascular

Table 136.2 • Vasopressors

Drug (Class)	Action	HR	Con	Preload	SVR	BP	CO	Indication	Dose/Comments	Adverse Effects
Norepinephrine (adrenergic, IC)	α_1, α_2, β_1 Intense α_{1-2} constriction	Var	↑	↑↑	↑↑	↑	No effect	↓SVR Shock Distributive, cardiogenic	4 mg/250 mL = 16 mcg/mL 0.01-0.3 mcg/kg per min 2-30 mcg/min	Tissue ischemia, arrhythmias, HTN
Phenylephrine (adrenergic, PVC)	α_1	No effect	No effect	↑	↑↑	↑	No effect	↓SVR TET spell HOCM	10 mg/250 mL= 40 mcg/mL 50-100 mcg IV 10-80 mcg/min Tachyphylaxis	Bradycardia HTN
Dopamine (adrenergic, IC)	α_1, β_{1-2}, D_1 1-3 mcg/kg per mg = D_1 3-10 = β_{1-2}>D >10 = α>β	No effect	↑	↑	-/↑	↑	↑	Low CO Low SVR	400 mg/250 mL = 1,600 mcg/mL 2-20 mcg/kg per min Variable individual dose response No benefit of low-dose "renal dose"	Arrhythmias, ↑MVO_2 Myocardial ischemia, HTN
Epinephrine (adrenergic, IC)	β_1, β_2, α_1, α_2 1-3 mcg/mg = β 3-10 = β & α >10 = α & β	↑↑	↑↑	↑	-/↓ 1-3 -/↓ 3-10 ↑↑ 10-20	↑	↑	Cardiac arrest Anaphylaxis Cardiogenic shock	4 mg/250 mL = 16 mcg/mL 2-10 mcg/IV bolus 0.01-0.2 mcg/kg per min 1-20 mcg per min	Arrhythmias, ↑MVO_2 Hyperglycemia, ischemia, hyperlactatemia, HTN
Vasopressin (nonadrenergic, PVC)	V_1 receptors No α-β activity ADH	-/↓	No effect	No effect	↑↑	↑	Var	↓SVR Shock 2nd line Pulm HTN	0.01-0.04 U/min Maximum 0.1 unit/min in severe vasoplegia Shock and pulm HTN No effect in pulm vasculature	Tissue ischemia, water intoxication
Methylene blue (nonadrenergic, PVC)	(-) cGMP (-) NO synthase	-/↓	No effect	No effect	↑↑	↑	Var	↓SVR Refractory shock 3rd line	1.5-2 mg/kg 15-30 min 0.25-1 mg/kg per h Avoid if SSRI, MAOI, TCA	Serotonin syndrome
Hydroxocobalamine (nonadrenergic, PVC)	(-) cGMP (-) NO synthase	-/↓	No effect	No effect	↑↑	↑	Var	↓SVR Refractory shock 3rd line	5 g/200 mL = 25 mg/mL Infuse total dose 15-120 min	None

Abbreviations: ADH, antidiuretic hormone; BP, blood pressure; cGMP, cyclic guanosine monophosphate; CO, cardiac output; Con, contractility; HOCM, hypertrophic obstructive cardiomyopathy with dynamic outflow tract obstruction; HR, heart rate; HTN, hypertension; IC, inoconstrictor; IV, intravenous; MAOI, monoamine oxidase inhibitor; MVO_2, myocardial oxygen consumption; NO, nitric oxide; Pulm, pulmonary; PVC, pure vasoconstrictor; SSRI, selective serotonin reuptake inhibitor; SVR, systemic vascular resistance; TCA, tricyclic antidepressant; TET, tetralogy of Fallot; Var, variable.

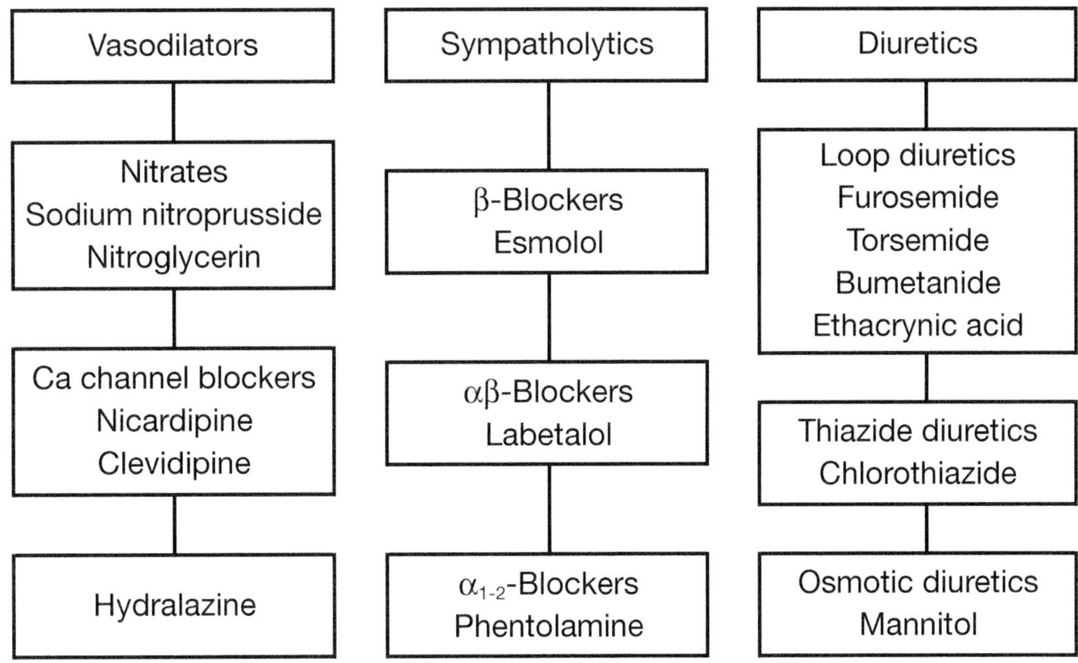

Figure 136.3. Classification of Intravenous Antihypertensive Agents.

smooth muscle membrane hyperpolarization in case of severe acidosis.

As described above, certain vasopressors also have inotropic properties (inoconstrictors), but, in addition there are pure vasoconstrictor agents without any effect in cardiac contractility. The vasopressors are also classified on the basis of initial pharmacologic target, with 2 basic classes: adrenergic (sympathomimetic) and nonadrenergic (Table 136.2 and Figure 136.2). The appropriate use of these agents follows the same principles of formulating a hemodynamic support plan described above, including the concept of synergy. Table 136.2 lists the different vasopressors and their hemodynamic effects, dosages, uses, and adverse effects.

Intravenous Antihypertensive Agents

The category of antihypertensive drugs is broad and complex. The intravenous antihypertensive agents more commonly used for critical care are discussed here. As discussed above, MAP is closely regulated by CO and SVR. Intravenous drugs that reduce contractility (negative inotropes), reduce preload (diuretics or venodilators), or relax vascular tone (vasodilators) are used to mitigate or control blood pressure to the desired target.

Blood pressure goals vary considerably among many disease states, and these goals change from time to time as new evidence emerges. Not uncommonly, vasodilator therapy is changed to vasopressor therapy when blood pressure has to be tightly regulated. Use of intravenous hypertensive agents requires a clear understanding of the physiologic goals and the same basic principles described above for formulating an adequate pharmacologic hemodynamic plan. The agent of choice should be selected on the basis of the rapidity of blood pressure control required (aortic dissection, hypertensive emergencies), underlying cardiovascular function, drug effects in other organ systems, and drug toxicity.

Moreover, unique pathophysiologic principles related to specific disease states should be considered when formulating an antihypertensive hemodynamic plan:

1. Reduction of shear stress and contractility before reduction in SVR in blood pressure control for aortic dissection.
2. Preferential arterial vs venous dilatation (increased venous capacitance) in acute conditions such hypertensive emergency with acute pulmonary edema, when modification of afterload vs preload is of differential importance.
3. Specific organ blood flow considerations, such as coronary and cerebral vasodilation as a desired or unwarranted effect and pulmonary vasodilatation causing pulmonary shunt and hypoxemia.

In general, the mechanism of action of antihypertensive agents is opposite that of the inotrope or vasopressor

Table 136.3 • Antihypertensive Agents

Drug (Class)	Action	Onset (Min)	Duration	HR	SVR	CO	Indication	Dose/Comments	Adverse Effects
Vasodilators									
Sodium nitroprusside (nitrate)	NO (+) cGMP	<2	1-2 min	↑	↓	↑	HTN emergency Need for rapid titration arterial > venous	0.3-3 mcg/kg per min Caution: coronary steal, ↑ ICP, ↑ CBF, AS, HOCM, AKI	Cyanide, thiocyanate toxicity Methemoglobinemia Hypotension
Nitroglycerin (nitrate)	(+) cGMP Requires glutathione	<2	1-2 min	No effect	↓	↑	Potent venodilator, venous > arterial Coronary vasodilator Angina APE	5-200 mcg/min Tolerance Caution: patients on PDE inhibitor	Headache Methemoglobinemia Profound hypotension if PDE inhibitor
Nicardipine (Ca channel blocker)	CCB DHP	5-15	30-120 min	-/↑	↓	↑	HTN emergency Coronary vasospasm arterial > venous	2.5-15 mg/h Caution: AS, HOCM	Hypotension AKI
Clevidipine (Ca channel blocker)	CCB DHP	2	90 s	↑	↓	↑	HTN emergency Need for rapid titration arterial > venous	1-32 mg/h Caution: AS, HOCM Soy or egg allergy	Tachycardia AKI
Hydralazine (vasodilator)	(+) cGMP	5-20	2-8 h	↑	↓	↑	HTN No need for strict titration	2.5 – 20 mg IV every 4-6 h Unpredictable effect, duration	Headache Drug-induced SLE
Sympatholytics									
Esmolol (β-blocker)	(-) β_1	1-2	10-30 min	↓	↓	↓	Tachycardia HTN Aortic dissection	0.5 mg/kg IV 50-300 mcg/kg per min Large volume	Angioedema Bronchospasm AV block
Labetalol (αβ-blocker)	(-) α_1, $\beta_{1\text{-}2}$	2-5	2-4 h	↓	↓	-/↓	HTN Aortic dissection Preeclampsia	10-80 mg IV every 10 min 2 mg/min	Bronchospasm CHF
Phentolamine (α-blocker)	(-) $\alpha_{1\text{-}2}$	2	10-15 min	↑	↓	↑	IV extravasation Pheochromocytoma	2.5-5 mg IV	Angina Tachycardia Nausea

Diuretics									
Furosemide	Loop	2-10	1-2 h	-/↑	-	↓	Diuresis	0.1-1 mg/kg IV 0.1-0.4 mg/kg per h	Azotemia ↓ K, Mg, H Ototoxicity
Torsemide	Loop	2-10	3-4 h	-/↑	-	↓	Diuresis	10-20 mg IV	As above
Bumetanide	Loop	2-10	1 h	-/↑	-	↓	Diuresis	0.5-1 mg q 2-3 h 0.5-2 mg/h	As above
Ethacrynic acid	Loop	2-10	1 h	-/↑	-	↓	Diuresis	0.5-1 mg IV	As above
Chlorothiazide	Distal	15	1-2 h	-/↑	-	↓	Diuresis	250-1,000 mg IV every 12-24 h	Azotemia ↓ K, Mg, H Pancreatitis
Mannitol	Osmotic	30-60	6-8 h	-/↑	-	Var	Decrease ICP Diuresis	0.25-1 g/kg IV ↓ ICP	Pulm edema Seizures

Abbreviations: AKI, acute kidney injury; APE, acute pulmonary edema; AS, aortic stenosis; AV, atrioventricular; Ca, calcium; CBF, cerebral blood flow; CCB, calcium channel blocker; cGMP, cyclic guanine monophosphate; CHF, congestive heart failure; CO, cardiac output; Cor, coronary; DHP, dihydropyridine; H, hydrogen; HOCM, hypertrophic obstructive cardiomyopathy; HR, heart rate; HTN, hypertension; ICP, intracranial pressure; IV, intravenous; K, potassium; M, magnesium; NO, nitric oxide; PDE, phosphodiesterase; pulm, pulmonary; SLE, systemic lupus erythematosus; SVR, systemic vascular resistance; Var, variable.

counterparts, with the exception of diuretics. Broadly, these medications are classified in 3 main groups depending on mechanism of action: vasodilators, sympatholytics (adrenergic antagoists), and diuretics (Figure 136.3 and Table 136.3). The appropriate use of these agents generally has to follow clinical context considering the hemodynamic goal, disease state, rapidity of effect needed, mechanism of action, and adverse effects. Table 136.3 lists the different intravenous antihypertensive agents and their onset of action, hemodynamic effects, dosing, uses, and adverse effects.

Summary

- An understanding of each patient's CO and vascular physiology is needed with clear goals in mind up front for optimal selection of inotrope, vasopressor, and antihypertensives.
- Proper selection of an agent is based on a patient's physiology and comorbidities.
- Norepinephrine increases shock control in sepsis.

SUGGESTED READING

Abe K. Vasodilators during cerebral aneurysm surgery. Can J Anaesth. 1993 Aug;40(8):775–90.

Basir MB, Schreiber TL, Grines CL, Dixon SR, Moses JW, Maini BS, et al. Effect of early initiation of mechanical circulatory support on survival in cardiogenic shock. Am J Cardiol. 2017 Mar 15;119(6):845–51. Epub 2016 Dec 18.

Bellomo R, Chapman M, Finfer S, Hickling K, Myburgh J; Australian and New Zealand Intensive Care Society (ANZICS) Clinical Trials Group. Low-dose dopamine in patients with early renal dysfunction: a placebo-controlled randomised trial. Lancet. 2000 Dec 23–30;356(9248):2139–43.

Brater DC. Diuretic therapy. N Engl J Med. 1998 Aug 6;339(6):387–95.

Colley PS, Cheney FW Jr, Hlastala MP. Ventilation-perfusion and gas exchange effects of sodium nitroprusside in dogs with normal and edematous lungs. Anesthesiology. 1979 Jun;50(6):489–95.

De Backer D, Biston P, Devriendt J, Madl C, Chochrad D, Aldecoa C, et al; SOAP II Investigators. Comparison of dopamine and norepinephrine in the treatment of shock. N Engl J Med. 2010 Mar 4;362(9):779–89.

den Ouden DT, Meinders AE. Vasopressin: physiology and clinical use in patients with vasodilatory shock: a review. Neth J Med. 2005 Jan;63(1):4–13.

Gamper G, Havel C, Arrich J, Losert H, Pace NL, Mullner M, et al. Vasopressors for hypotensive shock. Cochrane Database Syst Rev. 2016 Feb 15;2:CD003709.

Gheorghiade M, St Clair J, St Clair C, Beller GA. Hemodynamic effects of intravenous digoxin in patients with severe heart failure initially treated with diuretics and vasodilators. J Am Coll Cardiol. 1987 Apr;9(4):849–57.

Hollenberg SM. Vasoactive drugs in circulatory shock. Am J Respir Crit Care Med. 2011 Apr 1;183(7):847–55. Epub 2010 Nov 19.

Hosseinian L, Weiner M, Levin MA, Fischer GW. Methylene blue: magic bullet for vasoplegia? Anesth Analg. 2016 Jan;122(1):194–201.

Jentzer JC, Coons JC, Link CB, Schmidhofer M. Pharmacotherapy update on the use of vasopressors and inotropes in the intensive care unit. J Cardiovasc Pharmacol Ther. 2015 May;20(3):249–60. Epub 2014 Nov 28.

Landry DW, Oliver JA. The pathogenesis of vasodilatory shock. N Engl J Med. 2001 Aug 23;345(8):588–95.

Overgaard CB, Dzavik V. Inotropes and vasopressors: review of physiology and clinical use in cardiovascular disease. Circulation. 2008 Sep 2;118(10):1047–56.

Permpikul C, Tongyoo S, Viarasilpa T, Trainarongsakul T, Chakorn T, Udompanturak S. Early use of Norepinephrine in Septic Shock Resuscitation (CENSER): a randomized trial. Am J Respir Crit Care Med. 2019 May 1;199(9):1097–1105.

Roderique JD, VanDyck K, Holman B, Tang D, Chui B, Spiess BD. The use of high-dose hydroxocobalamin for vasoplegic syndrome. Ann Thorac Surg. 2014 May;97(5):1785–6.

Rotando A, Picard L, Delibert S, Chase K, Jones CMC, Acquisto NM. Push dose pressors: experience in critically ill patients outside of the operating room. Am J Emerg Med. 2019 Mar;37(3):494–8. Epub 2018 Dec 3.

Stevenson LW. Clinical use of inotropic therapy for heart failure: looking backward or forward? Part I: inotropic infusions during hospitalization. Circulation. 2003 Jul 22;108(3):367–72.

Varon J, Marik PE. Clinical review: the management of hypertensive crises. Crit Care. 2003 Oct;7(5):374–84. Epub 2003 Jul 16.

Vasu TS, Cavallazzi R, Hirani A, Kaplan G, Leiby B, Marik PE. Norepinephrine or dopamine for septic shock: systematic review of randomized clinical trials. J Intensive Care Med. 2012 May-Jun;27(3):172–8. Epub 2011 Mar 24.

Xing F, Hu X, Jiang J, Ma Y, Tang A. A meta-analysis of low-dose dopamine in heart failure. Int J Cardiol. 2016 Nov 1;222:1003–11. Epub 2016 Aug 5.

Antibiotics, Antivirals, and Antifungals

DAVID A. SOTELLO AVILES, MD; WALTER C. HELLINGER, MD

Goals

- Describe rational use of antimicrobials.
- Review the pharmacologic characteristics and clinical applications of the antibacterial, antifungal, and antiviral agents.
- Provide a working knowledge of antimicrobial drug dosing, adjustment of dosing for renal or hepatic insufficiency, drug-drug interactions, and antimicrobial allergies or intolerances.

Introduction

Antimicrobial therapy, particularly antibiotics, are often used in critically ill patients, but the indications are often questionable at best. Antimicrobial therapy should not be initiated before a susceptible pathogen is strongly suspected or confirmed or before appropriate diagnostic specimens, including those for cultures, are collected. Important principles are 1) the limited and adjunctive role of antibiotics in the management of many infections that require source control (eg, removal of infected devices, drainage of abscesses) and 2) mitigation of predisposing anatomical or physiologic conditions (eg, recurrent respiratory aspiration, obstruction of the urine collection system). Selecting antimicrobial agents is based on clinical and microbiologic findings. Physicians need to distinguish between empiric prescribing, when infection syndromes and pathogens are suspected, and therapeutic prescribing, when infection syndromes are confirmed and pathogens identified. Knowledge of antimicrobial drug dosing, adjustment of dosing for renal or hepatic insufficiency, drug-drug interactions, and antimicrobial intolerances is required.

For easy reference this chapter summarizes clinical applications of the antibacterial, antifungal, and antiviral agents.

Antibiotics

The spectrums of frequently used antibiotics are shown in Table 137.1. These β-lactams inhibit the synthesis of the bacterial peptidoglycan cell wall by attachment to, and inactivation of, bacterial penicillin-binding proteins, the peptidases that extend and cross-link cell wall peptides. This class of antibiotics encompasses several families, including penicillins, cephalosporins, carbapenems and monobactams, which share a common core structure, the β-lactam ring, but differ in their spectrums of activity, pharmacology, and therapeutic applications.

Penicillins

Penicillin is active against many gram-positive cocci, gram-positive bacilli, anaerobes, and spirochetes. Resistance to penicillin and derivatives is mediated through 1) production of a β-lactamase, which hydrolyzes the β-lactam ring; 2) alterations in the outer cell membranes of gram-negative bacteria that prevent penicillin from reaching peptidases at the peptidoglycan cell wall; or 3) alteration in conformation of peptidases that prevents penicillin and other β-lactam antibiotic binding and thereby results in intrinsic β-lactam antibiotic resistance, as occurs in methicillin-resistant staphylococci and penicillin-resistant pneumococci.

Aminopenicillins (eg, ampicillin, amoxicillin), by virtue of having greater lipid solubility than penicillin, are able to cross the outer cell membrane of gram-negative pathogens and are thereby active against many non–β-lactamase-producing strains of common gram-negative pathogens, such as *Escherichia coli, Proteus*, and *Salmonella*. The aminopenicillins, unlike the antistaphylococcal penicillins described above, share penicillin's excellent activity against streptococci, including enterococci.

Table 137.1 • Spectrum of Antibiotics Used in the Intensive Care Unit

Group	Gram-Positive	Gram-Negative	*Pseudomonas aeruginosa*	Anaerobes	MSSA	MRSA	*Listeria* spp	GN ESBL	GN Carbapenemase Producers	Other Coverage
Antistaphylococcal penicillins	+++	+	–		+++		–	–	–	
Aminopenicillins	++	++	–	+	–	–	+++	–	–	Enterococci (not VRE)
Carboxypenicillins, ureidopenicillins	+++	+++	+++	+	–	–	++	–	–	
Ureidopenicillin + β-lactamase inhibitor	+++	+++	+++	+++	++	–	++	+	–	
Cephalosporins										
1st-Generation	+++	+	–	+	+++	–	–	–	–	
2nd-Generation	+++	++	–	+	++	–	–	–	–	
3rd-Generation	++	+++	–	+	++	–	–	–	–	*Borrelia* spp, *Neisseria gonorrhoeae*
4th-Generation	++	+++	+++	+	++	–	–	–	–	
Ceftaroline	+++	+++	–	+	+++	+++	–	–	–	
Carbapenems	+++	+++	+++	+++	+++	–	++	+++	–	Enterococci (not including ertapenem)
Vancomycin	+++	–	–	–	++	+++	–	–	–	Enterococci *Clostridium difficile* (oral)
Daptomycin	+++	–	–	–	+++	+++	–	–	–	Enterococci
Linezolid	+++	–	–	–	+++	+++	+	–	–	
Quinolones	++	+++	++	–	+	–	++	±	±	*Chlamydia* spp, *Mycoplasma* spp, *Legionella* spp, *Salmonella* spp, *Brucella* spp
Macrolides	++	+	–	–	++	–	–	–	–	*Chlamydia* spp, *Mycoplasma* spp, *Legionella* spp, *Rickettsiae* spp, *Corynebacterium diphtheriae*, *Bordetella pertussis*

Tetracyclines	+++	++	–	–	++	++	–	±	±	*Mycoplasma* spp, *Chlamydia* spp, *Coxiella burnetii, Rickettsia* spp, *Anaplasma, Borrelia* spp
Tigecycline (glycylcycline)	+++	+++	–	–	++	+++	–	++	++	Same as tetracyclines
Clindamycin	+++	–	–	++	++	++	–	–	–	
Metronidazole	–	–	–	+++	–	–	–	–	–	*C difficile*, many protozoal microorganisms
Trimethoprim-sulfamethoxazole	++	++	–	–	++	++	++	+	+	*Pneumocystis jiroveci, Nocardia* spp, *Stenotrophomonas* spp, *Burkholderia* spp, *Toxoplasma*
Aminoglycosides	+	+++	++	–	–	+	++	+	+	Synergy for *Enterococcus, Streptococcus, Staphylococcus aureus*

Abbreviations: ESBL, extended-spectrum β-lactamases; GN, gram-negative; MRSA, methicillin-resistant *Staphylococcus aureus*; MSSA, methicillin-susceptible *S aureus*; spp, species; VRE, vancomycin-resistant enterococci; plus and minus symbols indicate degree of effectiveness.

The extended-spectrum penicillins (carboxypenicillins and ureidopenicillins), like the aminopenicillins, retain the base spectrum of activity of penicillin and extend it to provide activity against gram-negative bacteria that are not susceptible to the aminopenicillins. They are active against *Pseudomonas aeruginosa*.

Penicillins are minimally metabolized and are cleared primarily by the renal system, and quickly. The serum half-life of penicillins is less than 60 minutes; optimally, they are administered every 4 to 6 hours. The antistaphylococcal penicillins, the aminopenicillins, and the ureidopenicillins are excreted in the bile; the biliary excretion of the antistaphylococcal penicillins is such that they can be administered without dose adjustment to patients with renal failure receiving dialysis who have unimpaired hepatic function. With the exception of the antistaphylococcal penicillins, dose reduction is generally required in the setting of renal dysfunction.

One of the more common adverse effects of the penicillins is hypersensitivity reactions, including rash, anaphylactic shock, and interstitial nephritis. Hepatobiliary toxicity (hepatocellular enzyme increase) may occur during administration of antistaphylococcal penicillins. The penicillins have poor central nervous system (CNS) penetration, which is improved in the setting of meningeal inflammation.

Cephalosporins

Cephalosporins are grouped by the generations in which they were released, chronologically. The different generations do differ in their spectrum of activity and pharmacology. The first- and second-generation cephalosporins are more active against gram-positive bacteria, and the third- and fourth-generation cephalosporins are more active against gram-negative bacteria. Some third-generation (eg, ceftazidime) and the fourth-generation cephalosporins (eg, cefepime) are active against *P aeruginosa*. Neither the cephalosporins nor the penicillins are active against *Legionella, Mycoplasma, Chlamydia*, or *Rickettsia* species. With the single exception of ceftaroline (see below), the cephalosporins are not active against enterococci. The mechanisms of bacterial resistance, excretion, and adverse reactions are similar to those of the penicillins. The serum half-lives of the third- and fourth-generation agents, particularly ceftriaxone, are, in general, longer than those of the first- and second-generation agents. All agents are principally eliminated by renal excretion and must be adjusted for renal insufficiency, except for ceftriaxone, which is so efficiently excreted in the bile that it can be given, like the antistaphylococcal penicillins, without dose adjustment to patients in renal failure receiving dialysis who have unimpaired hepatic function. All of the third-generation cephalosporins, except cefoperazone, and the only fourth-generation agent, cefepime, can penetrate the blood-brain barrier and achieve CNS concentrations suitable for treatment of susceptible pathogens.

Recently released fifth-generation cephalosporins are, unlike all other β-lactam antibiotics, active against methicillin-resistant staphylococci and penicillin-resistant pneumococci. Agents in this class include ceftaroline and ceftobiprole (not available in the United States). Neither is active against *P aeruginosa*.

Carbapenems

This family of β-lactam antibiotics includes agents with the broadest spectrum of activity of all antimicrobials approved for systemic administration to humans. Imipenem, the first carbapenem to be released, is active against streptococci, enterococci, methicillin-susceptible *S aureus*, most anaerobes, and most gram-negative pathogens (including *Pseudomonas*). Subsequently released meropenem and doripenem have spectrums of activity and pharmacologic features similar to those of imipenem, without imipenem's epileptogenicity and infusion-related emesis. Imipenem, meropenem, and doripenem must be administered every 6 to 8 hours to patients who have normal renal function. The most recently released ertapenem can be administered once every 24 hours because of its longer serum half-life. Ertapenem, however, lacks activity against enterococci, *Pseudomonas*, and *Acinetobacter*. Because of their very broad spectrum of activity, these agents can be used to treat a wide variety of infections, including polymicrobial infections, and meropenem is safe and effective for a wide range of bacterial CNS infections. Given their exceptional activity against common nosocomial aerobic gram-negative bacterial pathogens, however, many institutions have elected to discourage frequent use of these agents when other less broadly active agents can be used together or in combination so as to prevent the appearance and spread of carbapenem resistance.

Monobactams

Aztreonam is the single member of this family. Its spectrum of activity is limited to aerobic gram-negative pathogens, including *P aeruginosa*. Aztreonam has the unusual property of infrequently producing cross-reactive hypersensitivity in patients who are allergic to penicillins or cephalosporins, the exception being ceftazidime, from which aztreonam was created by removal of its 6-member dihydrothiazine ring.

β-Lactam–β-Lactamase Inhibitor Combinations

β-Lactamase inhibitors are relatively small compounds that serve as suicide inhibitors of β-lactamases produced by staphylococci, anaerobes, and aerobic gram-negative bacilli. When combined with β-lactam antibiotics, these inhibitors extend the spectrum of the coadministered agents to second-line antistaphylococcal activity, first-line antianaerobic activity, and broader aerobic gram-negative activity. Examples of these agents include clavulanate, sulbactam, and tazobactam, which have been combined with aminopenicillins (amoxicillin-clavulanate, ampicillin-sulbactam), ureidopenicillins (ticarcillin-clavulanate, piperacillin-tazobactam), and cephalosporins (ceftazidime-tazobactam). The spectrum of activity and pharmacologic features of the β-lactam antibiotics remain unchanged when administered with a β-lactamase inhibitor.

Two recently released β-lactam–β-lactamase inhibitor combinations, ceftazidime-avibactam and ceftolozane-tazobactam, provide reliable activity against an array of extended-spectrum β-lactamases, which are responsible for conferring broad resistance of common gram-negative bacterial pathogens (eg, *E coli, Klebsiella pneumoniae*) to most penicillins and cephalosporins. Ceftazidime-avibactam is also active against many carbapenem-resistant Enterobacteriaceae organisms, although not metallo-β-lactamse (eg, New Delhi metallo-β-lactamase 1)–producing strains.

Quinolones

The quinolone antibiotics block bacterial DNA gyrase and topoisomerase IV, which are responsible for bacterial DNA synthesis and postreplication DNA modification. Most are fluorinated derivatives of nalidixic acid, which was released in the 1960s. The first fluoroquinolone antibiotics to be released (eg, norfloxacin, ciprofloxacin, ofloxacin) were active against *S aureus* and aerobic gram-negative bacilli and cocci, including, with respect to ciprofloxacin, *P aeruginosa*. A subsequent generation of fluoroquinolones (eg, levofloxacin, moxifloxacin, gemifloxacin), also known as respiratory quinolones, have reliable activity against penicillin-resistant *Streptococcus pneumoniae*. Levofloxacin is distinguished in this later generation by activity against many aerobic gram-negative bacteria, including *Pseudomonas*. The fluoroquinolones are active in vivo against a wide array of intracellular pathogens, including *Mycoplasma, Chlamydia, Legionella, Salmonella*, and *Brucella*. They are also active against *Mycobacterium tuberculosis* and *Bacillus anthracis*.

Quinolones are efficiently absorbed from the gastrointestinal tract, more than 95% for many compounds, a trait that facilitates administration and reduces the cost of therapy. They achieve excellent penetration of the genitourinary tract, lungs, prostate, bones, and joints. They can be used to treat respiratory, gastrointestinal, genitourinary, and musculoskeletal infections. Most may be administered once or twice daily and require dose adjustment for renal impairment. Toxicities include tendinopathy (more common in older patients), impairment of bone development in immature animals (an effect that has restricted their use in the pediatric population), neuropathy, and prolongation of the QT interval. Bacterial resistance to fluoroquinolones, especially in health care–associated infection, has increased because of their widespread use. As for all other antibiotics, susceptibility to these agents must be examined in pathogens for which they are prescribed.

Glycopeptides

These antibiotics, of which vancomycin is the best known, are frequently used in the treatment of infections of patients in the intensive care unit (ICU). Most importantly, they are active against methicillin-resistant staphylococci, both coagulase-positive (ie, *S aureus*) and coagulase-negative. In addition, they are active against *Bacillus, Corynebacterium, Actinomyces, Clostridium*, and many *Enterococcus* species. They are not active against gram-negative bacteria or mycobacteria. Because of their negligible absorption after oral administration, their use is restricted to parenteral administration, with the exception of intraluminal therapy of *Clostridium difficile* infection. Their bactericidal mechanism of action is through inhibition of the cell wall synthesis by binding to the D-alanyl–D-alanine terminus of peptide cell wall precursors. Resistance is most common among *Enterococcus* species (especially *Enterococcus faecium*) and is rare, fortunately, in *S aureus*.

Vancomycin is inferior to antistaphylococcal penicillins for treatment of methicillin susceptible *S aureus*. Vancomycin can pass the blood-brain barrier to a limited degree, achieving therapeutic concentrations in the cerebrospinal fluid, most reliably so in the setting of meningeal inflammation. It is excreted without metabolism renally. A not-infrequent toxicity is infusion-related red-man syndrome that follows histamine release from direct, nonallergic vancomycin-mediated mast cell destabilization; it can usually be mitigated or avoided by slowing the rate of infusion. Nephrotoxicity was a common complication of originally released vancomycin formulations in the 1960s. Although less common now, nephrotoxicity still occurs, and its risk of occurrence is reduced by monitoring of serum levels to avoid excessive increases. Ototoxicity has also been reported with supratherapeutic levels.

Rational Use of Less Commonly Prescribed Antibiotics

Daptomycin is a lipopeptide that disrupts the bacterial cell membrane function in a calcium-dependent mechanism; this effect, in turn, results in depolarization, loss of membrane potential, and cell death. Its spectrum of activity is very similar to that of vancomycin. Muscular toxicity is the most common adverse effect. It is inactivated by pulmonary surfactant and, therefore, cannot be used for treatment of pneumonia. Bacterial resistance may develop during treatment, particularly in settings of high inocula or foreign body–associated infection. Therefore, appropriate dosing, sometimes in combination with other agents, and appropriate source control of infection (ie, débridement of devitalized tissues, removal of infected foreign bodies) are indicated.

Linezolid is an oxazolidinone that has excellent coverage against gram-positive organisms, including *Staphylococci* and *Enterococci* species. It inhibits protein synthesis by binding to the 50S ribosomal subunit. It achieves excellent absorption after oral administration and is commonly used for treatment of infections caused by *S aureus* (including methicillin-resistant *S aureus*), *E faecium* (vancomycin-resistant), and other streptococcal infections. Major adverse effects include myelosuppression, usually developing after 14 or more days of administration, and interaction with commonly used drugs such as selective serotonin reuptake inhibitors may lead to a serotonin syndrome.

The macrolides are useful for treatment of gram-positive infections such as *Streptococci* species and for treatment of *Moraxella catarrhalis*, nontuberculous mycobacteria, and intracellular organisms including *Chlamydia, Mycoplasma, Legionella,* and *Rickettsiae* species. They are agents of choice when treating *Corynebacterium diphtheriae* and *Bordetella pertussis*.

Tetracyclines are active against intra-cellular pathogens including *Mycoplasma, Chlamydia, Legionella, Coxiella burnetti, Rickettsia* species, and *Anaplasma phagocytophilum*, and spirochetes, including *Borrelia* species (eg, *Borrelia burgdorferi*, the agent of Lyme disease), *Treponema pallidum*, and *Listeria*. Members including doxycycline and minocycline have near 100% oral bioavailability and readily cross the blood-brain barrier, reaching therapeutic cerebrospinal fluid concentrations. Dosage adjustment is generally not required for renal dysfunction, but caution is advised during administration in the setting of hepatic dysfunction. Common important adverse effects include gastrointestinal upset, esophageal ulceration, and photosensitizing rash.

Tigecycline is a glycylcycline derivative of minocycline that has broad antimicrobial activity including methicillin-resistant *S aureus, Acinetobacter baumannii*, and some multiply drug-resistant aerobic gram-negative pathogens, excluding *P aeruginosa*. The therapeutic niche of tigecycline remains to be determined.

Clindamycin is active against many gram-positive pathogens, including *Streptococcus* species and *S aureus*, and has broad activity against anaerobic pathogens, including *Bacteroides fragilis*. Its administration may be more strongly associated with a risk of *C difficile* colitis than many other antibiotics.

Metronidazole is a nitroimidazole active against many anaerobic protozoal and bacterial microorganisms. It has excellent oral bioavailability and tissue distribution, including the CNS. It is commonly used for CNS infections when anaerobic coverage is required and for treatment of mild to moderate *C difficile* infections.

Trimethoprim-sulfamethoxazole is active against many strains of methicillin-resistant *S aureus, Streptococcus* species, and other aerobic gram-positive and gram-negative pathogens, including multiply drug-resistant pathogens such as *Burkholderia* species and *Stenotrophomonas*. It is also first-line agent in the treatment of *Pneumocystis jirovec i, Toxoplasma gondii*, and many *Nocardia* species.

Aminoglycosides exert their antimicrobial effect by inhibiting bacterial protein synthesis. They are active against aerobic gram-negative bacteria and some mycobacteria. In combination with agents that interfere with bacterial cell wall synthesis or repair, they can synergistically inhibit some bacterial pathogens including strains of *Enterococcus* species, *Streptococcus* species, *S aureus*, and *Pseudomonas*. They are not used as monotherapy when equally active agents in less toxic classes of antibiotics are available. They are not absorbed after oral administration. Their distribution after parenteral administration is primarily the extracellular fluid space, except the CNS, because they do not efficiently cross the blood-brain barrier. Their most important toxicities are nephrotoxicity, ototoxicity, and vestibular toxicity, which can be prevented or mitigated by appropriate dosing, by laboratory monitoring of renal function and serum drug concentrations, and by clinical monitoring of hearing, tinnitus, and vertigo. These toxicities are reversed after immediate discontinuation of aminoglycoside administration.

Antifungals

The antifungals most frequently used in the ICU are the polyenes, which include amphotericin B and its lipid formulations, the azoles, and the echinocandins. The antifungals most commonly used in the ICU are summarized in Table 137.2.

Amphotericin B (deoxycolate) disrupts the structure and function of the fungal cell membrane by binding to membrane sterols. It is one of the most potent antifungals available, but it has considerable adverse effects, including infusion-related pyrogenic reactions and nephrotoxicity. New lipid formulations of amphotericin B deoxycholate, including liposomal, lipid complex, and colloidal dispersion (not available in the United States) agents, provide broad and potent antifungal activity at lower risk of pyrogenic reactions and nephrotoxicity.

The azole antifungals impair the fungal synthesis of ergosterol, which is required for cell membrane synthesis. The azole antifungals as a group have a broad range of antifungal activity, including *Candida* species, the geographically restricted dimorphic fungi, molds such as *Aspergillus* species, *Fusarium*, and the agents of mucormycosis and phaeohyphomycosis. However, the spectrum of activity of individual agents is generally limited to only some of these pathogens. The predominant toxicities of the azole antifungal agents are generally hepatic. Because they are metabolized through the P450 system, they can affect (generally increase) the serum levels of similarly metabolized coadministered compounds (eg, warfarin and the calcineurin inhibitors such as tacrolimus).

Echinocandins (caspofungin, micafungin, anidulafungin) block cell wall biosynthesis through inhibition of the 1,3-β-D-glucan synthase complex. They are broadly active against *Candida* species for which they are often the agent of choice while speciation and antifungal susceptibility test results are awaited. However, they are not reliably active against *Candida parapsilosis*. They have some fungistatic activity against *Aspergillus*. They are not active against cryptococci.

Antivirals

For the management of infections caused by herpes simplex virus (HSV type 1, HSV type 2) or varicella-zoster virus (VZV), acyclovir, a nucleoside analog that acts by inhibiting DNA synthesis, is generally used. Intravenous administration is required for treatment of neuroinvasive or disseminated infections because the absorption of acyclovir after oral administration is insufficient to provide reliable serum, tissue, and CNS concentrations. The valine ester of acyclovir, valacyclovir, is much better absorbed after oral administration and can sometimes be used to treat stable or improving disseminated or neuroinvasive infection. Higher doses of acyclovir and valacyclovir are required for treatment of VZV infections than for HSV infections because of the lower susceptibility of VZV to these agents relative to that of HSV. Acyclovir and valacyclovir are usually well tolerated; nephrotoxicity may occasionally complicate intravenous administration of high-dose acyclovir. Dose adjustment for renal dysfunction is required, and adequate hydration is recommended.

For the management of infections due to cytomegalovirus, intravenously administered ganciclovir or oral administration of its better absorbed valine ester, valganciclovir, are generally used. These agents are active against HSV-1, HSV-2, and VZV and have mechanisms of action that are similar to that of acyclovir. The most common adverse effect of ganciclovir or valganciclovir is myelosuppression, which can limit their use. Resistance to ganciclovir by cytomegalovirus has been reported and, in that setting, the more (renally) toxic agents, foscarnet or cidofovir, can be considered.

The most frequently used antivirals for influenza are the neuraminidase inhibitors: oseltamivir or zanamivir. They inhibit neuraminidases of influenza A and B. These compounds are generally well tolerated. Oseltamivir has been associated with gastrointestinal upset, and zanamivir,

Table 137.2 • Spectrum of Antifungals Most Commonly Used in the Intensive Care Unit

Agent	*Candida* spp	*Aspergillus* spp	Other Molds	Mucorales	*Cryptococcus* spp	*Histoplasma*	*Blastomyces*	*Coccidioides*
Fluconazole	++	–	–	–	+++	+	+	+++
Itraconazole	++	+	+	–	++	+++	+++	+++
Voriconazole	++	+++	+	–	++	+	+	+
Posaconazole	++	+++	++	+	++	+	+	+
Isavuconazole	++	+++	+	++	+	Unknown	Unknown	Unknown
Amphotericin B	+++	++	+++	+++	+++	+++	+++	+++
Echinocandins	+++	+	+	–	–	–	–	–

Abbreviations: plus and minus symbols indicate degree of effectiveness.

which is administered as an inhaled powder, has been associated with airway hyperreactivity. Ribavirin can be considered for the management of respiratory syncytial virus pneumonia.

For patients who are receiving treatment for infection due to HIV on ICU admission, their antiretroviral therapy should be continued as long as there are no contraindications to its administration, there are no likely interactions with other administered medications, and reliable absorption of all agents is anticipated. For patients in whom HIV is newly diagnosed, early initiation of antiretroviral therapy is recommended, although in critically ill patients consideration needs to be given to the possibility of unidentified opportunistic coinfection and to the development of immune reconstitution syndrome. Drug dosing adjustments for renal or hepatic impairment are commonly required for antiretroviral agents. An antiretroviral regimen should, in general, be initiated in the context of a plan for continued outpatient administration to prevent gaps in therapy that could increase the risk for the development of antiretroviral-resistant HIV infection.

Summary

- Appropriate selection and de-escalation of antimicrobials are crucially important in the ICU.
- Antifungals are highly toxic but can be part of empirical therapy in immunocompromised patients.
- Antivirals are used only if there is evidence of neuroinvasive disease of a disseminatated infection.

SUGGESTED READING

Acosta EP, Flexner C. Antiviral agents (nonretroviral). In: Brunton LL, editor. Goodman & Gilman's the pharmacological basis of therapeutics. 12th ed. New York (NY): McGraw-Hill Medical; c2011. p. 1593–1622.

Aguilar-Zapata D, Petraitiene R, Petraitis V. Echinocandins: the expanding antifungal armamentarium. Clin Infect Dis. 2015 Dec 1;61 Suppl 6:S604–11.

Baddour LM, Wilson WR, Bayer AS, Fowler VG Jr, Tleyjeh IM, Rybak MJ, et al; American Heart Association Committee on Rheumatic Fever, Endocarditis, and Kawasaki Disease of the Council on Cardiovascular Disease in the Young, Council on Clinical Cardiology, Council on Cardiovascular Surgery and Anesthesia, and Stroke Council. Infective endocarditis in adults: diagnosis, antimicrobial therapy, and management of complications: a scientific statement for healthcare professionals from the American Heart Association. Circulation. 2015 Oct 13;132(15):1435–86. Epub 2015 Sep 15. Errata in: Circulation. 2015 Oct 27;132(17):e215. Circulation. 2016 Aug 23;134(8):e113.

Bennett JE. Antifungal agents. In: Brunton LL, editor. Goodman & Gilman's the pharmacological basis of therapeutics. 12th ed. New York (NY): McGraw-Hill Medical; c2011. p. 1571–92.

Campion M, Scully G. Antibiotic use in the intensive care unit: optimization and de-escalation. J Intensive Care Med. 2018 Dec;33(12):647–55. Epub 2018 Mar 13.

Guilhaumou R, Benaboud S, Bennis Y, Dahyot-Fizelier C, Dailly E, Gandia P, et al. Optimization of the treatment with beta-lactam antibiotics in critically ill patients-guidelines from the French Society of Pharmacology and Therapeutics (Societe Francaise de Pharmacologie et Therapeutique-SFPT) and the French Society of Anaesthesia and Intensive Care Medicine (Societe Francaise d'Anesthesie et Reanimation-SFAR). Crit Care. 2019 Mar 29;23(1):104.

Heavner MS, Claeys KC, Masich AM, Gonzales JP. Pharmacokinetic and pharmacodynamic considerations of antibiotics of last resort in treating gram-negative infections in adult critically ill patients. Curr Infect Dis Rep. 2018 Apr 5;20(5):10.

Hooper DC, Strahilevitz J. Quinolones. In: Bennett JE, Dolin R, Blaser MJ, editors. Mandell, Douglas, and Bennett's principles and practice of infectious diseases. 8th ed. Philadelphia (PA): Elsevier/Saunders; c2015. p. 419–39.e8.

INSIGHT START Study Group, Lundgren JD, Babiker AG, Gordin F, Emery S, Grund B, Sharma S, et al. Initiation of antiretroviral therapy in early asymptomatic HIV infection. N Engl J Med. 2015 Aug 27;373(9):795–807. Epub 2015 Jul 20.

Leggett JE. Aminoglycosides. In: Bennett JE, Dolin R, Blaser MJ, editors. Mandell, Douglas, and Bennett's principles and practice of infectious diseases. 8th ed. Philadelphia (PA): Elsevier/Saunders; c2015. p. 310–21.e7.

MacDougall C, Chambers HF. Protein synthesis inhibitors and miscellaneous antibacterial agents. In: Brunton LL, editor. Goodman & Gilman's the pharmacological basis of therapeutics. 12th ed. New York (NY): McGraw-Hill Medical; c2011. p. 1521–47.

Marcelin JR, Wilson JW, Razonable RR; Mayo Clinic Hematology/Oncology and Transplant Infectious Diseases Services. Oral ribavirin therapy for respiratory syncytial virus infections in moderately to severely immunocompromised patients. Transpl Infect Dis. 2014 Apr;16(2):242–50. Epub 2014 Mar 13.

Marston HD, Dixon DM, Knisely JM, Palmore TN, Fauci AS. Antimicrobial resistance. JAMA. 2016 Sep 20;316(11):1193–1204.

Moffa M, Brook I. Tetracyclines, glycylcyclines, and chloramphenicol. In: Bennett JE, Dolin R, Blaser MJ, editors. Mandell, Douglas, and Bennett's principles and practice of infectious diseases. 8th ed. Philadelphia (PA): Elsevier/Saunders; c2015. p. 322–38.e6.

Murray BE, Arias CA, Nannini EC. Glycopeptides (vancomycin and teicoplanin), streptogramins (quinupristin-dalfopristin), lipopeptides (daptomycin), and lipoglycopeptides (telavancin). In: Bennett JE, Dolin R, Blaser MJ, editors. Mandell, Douglas, and Bennett's principles and practice of infectious diseases. 8th ed. Philadelphia (PA): Elsevier/Saunders; c2015. p. 377–400.e4.

Nagel JL, Aronoff DM. Metronidazole. In: Bennett JE, Dolin R, Blaser MJ, editors. Mandell, Douglas, and Bennett's principles and practice of infectious diseases. 8th ed. Philadelphia (PA): Elsevier/Saunders; c2015. p. 350–7.e2.

Ostrosky-Zeichner L, Rex JH. Antifungal and antiviral therapy. In: Parrillo JE, Dellinger RP, editors. Critical care medicine: principles of diagnosis and management in the adult. 4th ed. Philadelphia (PA): Elsevier/Saunders; c2014. p. 886–900.e7.

Pappas PG, Kauffman CA, Andes DR, Clancy CJ, Marr KA, Ostrosky-Zeichner L, et al. Clinical practice guideline for the management of candidiasis: 2016 update by the Infectious Diseases Society of America. Clin Infect Dis. 2016 Feb 15;62(4):e1–50. Epub 2015 Dec 16.

Petri WA Jr. Penicillins, cephalosporins, and other β-lactam antibiotics. In: Brunton LL, editor. Goodman & Gilman's the pharmacological basis of therapeutics. 12th ed. New York (NY): McGraw-Hill Medical; c2011. p. 1477–1503.

Petri WA Jr. Sulfonamides, trimethoprim-sulfamethoxazole, quinolones, and agents for urinary tract infections. In: Brunton LL, editor. Goodman & Gilman's the pharmacological basis of therapeutics. 12th ed. New York (NY): McGraw-Hill Medical; c2011. p. 1463–76.

Sivapalasingam S, Steigbigel NH. Macrolides, clindamycin, and ketolides. In: Bennett JE, Dolin R, Blaser MJ, editors. Mandell, Douglas, and Bennett's principles and practice of infectious diseases. 8th ed. Philadelphia (PA): Elsevier/Saunders; c2015. p. 358–76.e6.

Tan DH, Walmsley SL. Management of persons infected with human immunodeficiency virus requiring admission to the intensive care unit. Crit Care Clin. 2013 Jul;29(3):603–20. Epub 2013 May 8.

The Sandford guide to antimicrobial therapy. Tigecycline. Mobile device application [cited 2016 May 10]. Available from: https://www.sanfordguide.com/products/digital-subscriptions/sanford-guide-to-antimicrobial-therapy-mobile/.

Zinner SH, Mayer KH. Sulfonamides and trimethoprim. In: Bennett JE, Dolin R, Blaser MJ, editors. Mandell, Douglas, and Bennett's principles and practice of infectious diseases. 8th ed. Philadelphia (PA): Elsevier/Saunders; c2015. p. 410–8.e2.

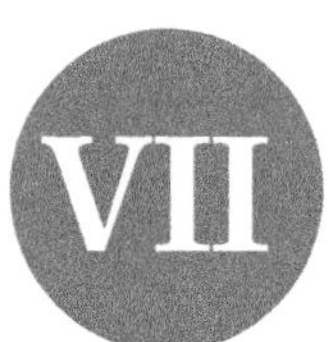

Questions and Answers

Abbreviations Used

ASD antiseizure drug
CBZ carbamazepine
CNS central nervous system
CRRT chronic renal replacement therapy
CVP central venous pressure
CYP cytochrome P450
FDA US Food and Drug Administration
ICU intensive care unit
INR international normalized ratio
MAP mean arterial pressure
MRSA methicillin-resistant *Staphylococcus aureus*
MSSA methicillin-susceptible *Staphylococcus aureus*
$\dot{V}/\dot{Q}$ ventilation-perfusion

Questions

Multiple Choice (choose the best answer)

VII.1. A 66-year-old woman with temporal lobe epilepsy who is receiving phenytoin was admitted with status epilepticus because she missed a few doses of phenytoin. While she was hospitalized, atrial fibrillation was diagnosed and, at the time of discharge, warfarin 5 mg daily was prescribed. Which of the following statements regarding the potential drug-drug interactions is *not* accurate?

a. Initially, the patient may have a supratherapeutic INR.
b. If she continues to receive the same dose of warfarin, the INR might be subtherapeutic in a few weeks.
c. Phenytoin can displace warfarin from protein-binding sites and cause a subtherapeutic INR.
d. Hemorrhagic complications may result from inhibition of warfarin metabolism by phenytoin.

VII.2. A 75-year-old man with focal seizures who is receiving CBZ 400 mg twice daily is admitted to the ICU with subarachnoid hemorrhage. In the ICU, the patient was found to have antiphospholipid syndrome, and his hematologist is planning to initiate rivaroxaban therapy. What is the best course of action?

a. Preemptively increase the dose of CBZ to 600 mg twice daily.
b. Start a lower dose of rivaroxaban than usual.
c. Transition to another ASD and discontinue CBZ therapy before initiating rivaroxaban therapy.
d. Reassure the patient, because there is no clinically relevant drug interaction between the 2 drugs.

VII.3. A 35-year-old man with primary generalized epilepsy receiving a maintenance dose of lamotrigine 250 mg twice daily was admitted to the ICU with acute repetitive seizures. The seizures were aborted with midazolam infusion, and, at the time of discharge, the consulting neurologist recommends adding valproic acid therapy as an adjunct to lamotrigine. Which action should be considered before starting valproic acid therapy?

a. The dose of lamotrigine needs to be doubled in lieu of adding valproic acid.
b. Start therapy with valproic acid 500 mg twice daily to prevent breakthrough seizures.
c. Reduce the dose of lamotrigine by half to avoid potential toxicity.
d. There is no need for dose adjustment for either ASD.

VII.4. A 51-year-old woman with a history of systemic lupus erythematosus and seizure disorder had a prolonged ICU course that included sepsis, respiratory failure requiring prolonged mechanical ventilation, and acute renal failure. At home, she was maintained on levetiracetam 500 mg twice daily and is also receiving CRRT. Approximately 6 hours after a hemodialysis session, the patient became confused, and emergency electroencephalography showed subclinical seizures. These seizures might have been avoided if which of the following had occurred?

a. The patient had received a supplemental dose of levetiracetam immediately after CRRT.
b. The patient had received a supplemental dose of levetiracetam during CRRT.
c. The patient had received a supplemental dose of levetiracetam just before CRRT.
d. Therapy was changed to phenytoin just before CRRT.

VII.5. A 45-year-old man presented with ventricular fibrillation cardiac arrest with return of spontaneous circulation after cardiopulmonary resuscitation. He remains unresponsive, and targeted temperature management is initiated. Which of the following medications has not been shown to be affected by hypothermia?

a. Propranolol
b. Levetiracetam
c. Epinephrine
d. Vecuronium

VII.6. A 52-year-old woman presents with a poor-grade subarachnoid hemorrhage with obstructive hydrocephalus and refractory intracranial pressure despite first- and second-line therapy. The ICU team decides to initiate a hypothermia protocol for intracranial pressure control. What effect will hypothermia have on midazolam?
a. Midazolam concentrations decrease 5-fold with temperatures less than 35°C.
b. Midazolam volume of distribution decreases 43%.
c. Midazolam clearance decreases 11% for each degree Celsius reduction in core temperature.
d. Midazolam elimination remains unchanged.

VII.7. A 50-year-old woman who was admitted to the ICU with flail chest, acute respiratory failure, and traumatic brain injury after a motor vehicle accident has severe psychomotor agitation. She has been receiving a continuous infusion of propofol (50 mcg/kg per minute). Her bedside nurse is very concerned because the intracranial pressure on ventriculostomy monitoring is persistently more than 20 mm Hg during the past 15 minutes. What should be the immediate intervention?
a. Administer a bolus of propofol and increase continuous infusion if the Richmond agitation-sedation scale is score +3.
b. Evaluate pain and causes of respiratory derangement and administer a fentanyl bolus if pain is suspected.
c. Perform a comprehensive neurologic examination and do not modify the sedation regimen for further neurologic assessment.
d. Induce a barbiturate coma and immediately obtain a computed tomogram of the head.

VII.8. A 27-year-old man is admitted to the ICU with a diagnosis of severe acute respiratory distress syndrome due to influenza infection. The patient has required higher doses of sedatives (propofol and fentanyl) because of ventilator dyssynchrony during pressure-controlled ventilation mode during the past few days. The patient requires increasing doses of vasopressors and fluid boluses for suspected worsening kidney dysfunction and superimposed pneumonia. However, all culture results are negative, and the white blood cell count and procalcitonin levels are normal. What is the most appropriate next step?
a. Obtain a computed tomogram of the chest to better characterize superimposed bacterial pneumonia.
b. Switch the mechanical ventilator mode to airway pressure release ventilation and decrease sedation.
c. Continue aggressive fluid resuscitation and vasopressor support for septic shock.
d. Order immediate testing for triglyceride and creatine kinase levels, and perform point-of-care echocardiography.

VII.9. A 58-year-old man is in septic shock caused by severe community-acquired pneumonia. Appropriate antibiotic therapy was started in the emergency department. After 5 L of crystalloid boluses, the patient is febrile, tachycardic with a heart rate of 128 beats per minute, hypotensive with an MAP of 48 mm Hg, and a CVP of 7 mm Hg, and acidotic with a pH of 7.23. What is the *best* next course of action?
a. Continue fluid resuscitation and add norepinephrine, titrating to an MAP of more than 60 mm Hg.
b. Stop fluid resuscitation and start dobutamine therapy.
c. Transfuse 2 U of red blood cells and start vasopressin therapy, titrating to an MAP of more than 60 mm Hg.
d. Start dopamine therapy at 30 mcg/kg per minute.

VII.10. The patient described in the previous question now has cold extremities, he is receiving norepinephrine at 0.2 mcg/kg per minute (20 mcg/min), CVP is 14 mm Hg (positive end-expiratory pressure is 5 cm H_2O), MAP is 60 mm Hg, mild metabolic acidosis remains, central venous oxygen saturation is 51%, and hemoglobin level is 11 g/dL. Which of the following choices is *least* appropriate?
a. Start therapy with dobutamine.
b. Transfuse 2 U of red blood cells.
c. Start therapy with vasopressin.
d. Start therapy with milrinone.

VII.11. Which of the following statements is *true*?
a. The cardiac and vascular myocyte share the same mechanism of adrenergic receptor activity.
b. It is optimal to combine catecholamines to achieve a desirable effect.
c. Levosimendan is an example of the new-generation vasoconstrictors.
d. Combinations of a β-agonist with phosphodiesterase inhibitors are synergistic.

VII.12. If infusion of the following agents is stopped, for which one will the effect *not* be immediately seen?
a. Norepinephrine
b. Epinephrine
c. Nitroprusside
d. Milrinone

VII.13. Which of the following antihypertensive agents can cause hypoxemia in patients with respiratory failure and $\dot{V}/\dot{Q}$ mismatch?
a. Labetalol
b. Esmolol
c. Sodium nitroprusside
d. Furosemide

VII.14. A patient admitted to the ICU had development of fever, and blood culture results are positive for *Enterococcus faecalis*. Which of the following antibiotics is *never* effective against *E faecalis*?
a. Daptomycin
b. Linezolid
c. Ampicillin-sulbactam
d. Ceftriaxone

VII.15. A patient is admitted for a craniotomy related to an epidural abscess. Intraoperative culture results are positive against MSSA. The patient has no allergies to any medication. Which of the following antibiotics is the preferred choice?
a. Nafcillin
b. Ceftriaxone
c. Daptomycin
d. Vancomycin

VII.16. Which of the following agents is best used for treatment of multidrug-resistant *Pseudomonas aeruginosa*?
a. Levofloxacin
b. Cefepime
c. Aztreonam
d. Ceftolozane-tazobactam

VII.17. A patient was admitted to the ICU for new-onset seizures that, after extensive workup, were found to be due to a *Candida albicans* (pansusceptible) brain abscess. Which of the following is *not* an adequate option in the management of this infection?
a. Fluconazole
b. Caspofungin
c. Voriconazole
d. Amphotericin B

VII.18. A 24-year-old man with a past medical history of systemic lupus erythematosus has been receiving high-dose prednisone for the past few weeks for lupus nephritis. He was admitted to the neurocritical care unit after new-onset seizures. Brain magnetic resonance imaging showed a frontal abscess. Blood cultures were positive for *P aeruginosa*, resistant to all β-lactam antibiotics except carbapenems. The microorganism was also resistant to ciprofloxacin and aminoglycosides. What is the antibiotic of choice?
a. Imipenem-cilastin
b. Meropenem
c. Ertapenem
d. Cefepime

Answers

VII.1. Answer d.

When phenytoin and warfarin are coadministered, there can initially be an increase in the anticoagulant action of warfarin due to protein displacement, but then a decrease in anticoagulant activity may occur due to an increase in warfarin metabolism.

Perucca E. Clinically relevant drug interactions with antiepileptic drugs. Br J Clin Pharmacol. 2006 Mar;61(3):246–55.

Zaccara G, Perucca E. Interactions between antiepileptic drugs, and between antiepileptic drugs and other drugs. Epileptic Disord. 2014 Dec;16(4):409–31.

VII.2. Answer c.

Choice *d* is incorrect because CYP3A4 inducers may lead to increased rivaroxaban clearance. Similarly, given increased rivaroxaban clearance associated with CBZ, choice *b* is incorrect because reducing the dose would exacerbate the issue of adequacy of anticoagulant effect, and choice *a* is incorrect because increasing the CBZ dose would increase the potential for increased rivaroxaban clearance. Strong CYP3A4 inducers such as carbamazepine can result in considerable reduction in rivaroxaban concentration. Because monitoring the degree of anticoagulation effect is difficult in patients receiving direct factor Xa inhibitors such as rivaroxaban, it is probably best to consider transition to an ASD with less potential for drug-drug interaction. If patients are already receiving CBZ, then replacing it before initiating rivaroxaban should be considered, if feasible.

Perucca E. Clinically relevant drug interactions with antiepileptic drugs. Br J Clin Pharmacol. 2006 Mar;61(3):246–55.

Zaccara G, Perucca E. Interactions between antiepileptic drugs, and between antiepileptic drugs and other drugs. Epileptic Disord. 2014 Dec;16(4):409–31.

VII.3. Answer c.

Valproic acid can inhibit metabolism of lamotrigine and could result in toxicity of the latter. Therefore, the dose of lamotrigine should be reduced by a minimum of 50% when initiating valproic acid in patients who are already receiving the maximum tolerated dose of lamotrigine. A 50% reduction would still supersede the FDA-approved lamotrigine dose for use in combination with valproate, which is set at 150 mg daily. It would be prudent to consider initiating valproic acid therapy at a low dose and increase by 250 to 500 mg daily per week to the target.

Perucca E. Clinically relevant drug interactions with antiepileptic drugs. Br J Clin Pharmacol. 2006 Mar;61(3):246–55.

Zaccara G, Perucca E. Interactions between antiepileptic drugs, and between antiepileptic drugs and other drugs. Epileptic Disord. 2014 Dec;16(4):409–31.

VII.4. Answer a.

Drug properties that affect CRRT drug elimination include volume of distribution, protein binding, renal and nonrenal clearance, and, to a lesser degree, molecular weight and charge of the molecule. Levetiracetam has properties that support its removal during CRRT, including a small volume of distribution at 0.7 L/kg, low protein binding at less than 10%, high renal clearance at more than 90 mL/min per 1.73 m^2, and small molecular weight at 170 Da. Patients receiving CRRT require a reduced maintenance dose of levetiracetam based on baseline creatinine clearance and a supplemental dose after dialysis. Other ASDs that require a supplemental dose after CRRT include lacosamide, topiramate, and gabapentin.

Bansal AD, Hill CE, Berns JS. Use of antiepileptic drugs in patients with chronic kidney disease and end stage renal disease. Semin Dial. 2015 Jul-Aug;28(4):404–12. Epub 2015 May 1.

VII.5. Answer b.

Most of the data regarding the effects of hypothermia are focused on hepatic elimination and decreased activity of the CYP450 system. Potential mechanisms behind hypothermia's effects on the CYP450 system include decreased affinity of the CYP450 for specific substrates, decreased rate of redox reactions performed by CYP450, and changes in reductase activity. Propranolol, epinephrine, and vecuronium are all primarily hepatically eliminated, and either human or animal studies have shown changes in pharmacokinetics and pharmacodynamics in the setting of hypothermia. The effects on renal elimination are unknown, and there are no studies on the effects of hypothermia on levetiracetam (therefore, choice *b* is correct).

Anderson KB, Poloyac SM. Therapeutic hypothermia: implications on drug therapy. In: Sadaka F, editor. Therapeutic hypothermia in brain injury. London (UK): InTech; c2013. p. 131–48.

VII.6. Answer c.

Midazolam is metabolized by CYP3A4 and CYP3A5, which are impaired in hypothermia. A study showed a decrease in midazolam elimination constant, 5-fold increase in midazolam concentrations at temperatures less than 35°C, and increased volume of distribution by 83%. Midazolam pharmacokinetics in hypothermia in normal healthy volunteers showed decreased clearance by 11% for each degree Celsius reduction in core temperature (thus, choice *c* is correct).

Anderson KB, Poloyac SM. Therapeutic hypothermia: implications on drug therapy. In: Sadaka F, editor. Therapeutic hypothermia in brain injury. London (UK): InTech; c2013. p. 131–48.

VII.7. Answer b.

A higher dose of propofol can mask pain and avoid proper recognition of underlying complications in mechanically ventilated patients in the ICU (ventilator dyssynchrony, hypercapnia, hypoxemia). Sustained intracranial hypertension will have detrimental effects on the mental status, and its immediate treatment should be guided by its cause. Barbiturate coma is an effective intervention for intracranial hypertension. Pain is a very common condition in traumatized patients in the ICU. This patient was not receiving analgesics after severe chest and brain trauma. Thus, an initial measure should be rapid assessment of pain and appropriate treatment with opioids such as fentanyl given its short duration of action. In addition, the underlying respiratory status must be evaluated more carefully because potentially life-threatening complications such as pneumothorax with associated hypercapnia and hypoxemia can be missed when symptoms are treated rather than investigated through proper evaluation of increased intracranial pressure in neurocritically ill patients. In general, both immediate treatment of possible cause (pain, discomfort, or anxiety) and a methodic approach to the identification of increased intracranial pressure are recommended.

Gelinas C, Tousignant-Laflamme Y, Tanguay A, Bourgault P. Exploring the validity of the bispectral index, the Critical-Care Pain Observation Tool and vital signs for the detection of pain in sedated and mechanically ventilated critically ill adults: a pilot study. Intensive Crit Care Nurs. 2011 Feb;27(1):46–52. Epub 2010 Dec 18.

Gottschalk A, Yaster M. The perioperative management of pain from intracranial surgery. Neurocrit Care. 2009;10(3):387–402. Epub 2008 Oct 1.

Mirski MA, Hemstreet MK. Critical care sedation for neuroscience patients. J Neurol Sci. 2007 Oct 15;261(1–2):16–34. Epub 2007 Jul 13.

VII.8. Answer d.

Although the patient is at risk for bacterial pneumonia after influenza infection, computed tomography of the chest would not easily differentiate viral from bacterial infection. The airway pressure release ventilation mode has the advantage of reducing the use of sedatives. However, it will not lead to treatment of the specific cause of cardiovascular and renal deterioration in this patient. Further diagnostic workup must be initiated. Continuation of initial measures for presumptive septic shock will not lead to proper recognition of a life-threatening complication of sedative administration in the ICU. A propofol-related infusion syndrome has been described primarily in young patients receiving high-dosage infusions. The syndrome is due to impairment of mitochondrial β-oxidation of fatty acids, disruption of the electron transport chain, and blockage of β-adrenoreceptors and cardiac calcium channels. A propofol-related infusion syndrome is suspected in patients receiving more than 80 mcg/kg per minute for more than 48 hours who have development of persistent metabolic acidosis with hyperlactatemia, hyperkalemia, refractory hypotension, rhabdomyolysis, and ventricular dysfunction. A recent comprehensive review of this syndrome in adult patients cited the following risk factors for this life-threatening complication: high dosage and prolonged continuous infusion, high acuity, concomitant use of corticosteroids and catecholamines, and low carbohydrate intake.

Mirrakhimov AE, Voore P, Halytskyy O, Khan M, Ali AM. Propofol infusion syndrome in adults: a clinical update. Crit Care Res Pract. 2015;2015:260385. Epub 2015 Apr 12.

VII.9. Answer a.

A patient in persistent shock with a low MAP and low CVP who is acidotic despite fluid resuscitation requires continuation of fluid administration and initiation of vasopressor therapy because both systemic vascular resistance and cardiac output need to be optimized. Norepinephrine is the inoconstrictor of choice in septic shock. Dobutamine can be detrimental because of the predominant hypotension. There is no indication for blood transfusion. Dopamine is inferior to norepinephrine in the treatment of septic shock, and the dosage provided is wrong. Stress-dose corticosteroids can be used if the patient requires multiple vasopressors and should not be used as a last resort.

De Backer D, Biston P, Devriendt J, Madl C, Chochrad D, Aldecoa C, et al; SOAP II Investigators. Comparison of dopamine and norepinephrine in the treatment of shock. N Engl J Med. 2010 Mar 4;362(9):779–89.

Overgaard CB, Dzavik V. Inotropes and vasopressors: review of physiology and clinical use in cardiovascular disease. Circulation. 2008 Sep 2;118(10):1047–56.

VII.10. Answer b.

The hemodynamic profile has changed from distributive to cardiogenic shock, and the patient would benefit from an inotrope, such as dobutamine or milrinone. There is no indication for blood transfusion, and it would be harmful. Vasopressin could be considered because the norepinephrine required to maintain borderline MAP is at a high dose. However, it would not increase cardiac output and oxygen delivery. Vasopressin should be considered if there is evidence of persistent vasodilatation at high doses of norepinephrine and high central venous oxygen saturation. It is not the best option, but it is also not the worst.

Overgaard CB, Dzavik V. Inotropes and vasopressors: review of physiology and clinical use in cardiovascular disease. Circulation. 2008 Sep 2;118(10):1047–56.

VII.11. Answer d.

Whenever 2 drugs with different mechanisms of action are used, the result can be synergistic. An example of synergy is the use of epinephrine and milrinone for cardiogenic shock or of norepinephrine and vasopressin for vasodilatory shock. Cardiac and vascular smooth muscle cells have different second-messenger systems and receptor mechanisms that respond to adrenergic activity. Levosimendan is a new-generation inodilator that sensitizes calcium-troponin complex in the cardiac myocite and stimulates the adenosine triphosphate–sensitive potassium channel, causing potent vasodilatation in the vascular smooth muscle.

Bers DM. Cardiac excitation-contraction coupling. Nature. 2002 Jan 10;415(6868):198–205.

Landry DW, Oliver JA. The pathogenesis of vasodilatory shock. N Engl J Med. 2001 Aug 23;345(8):588–95.

Overgaard CB, Dzavik V. Inotropes and vasopressors: review of physiology and clinical use in cardiovascular disease. Circulation. 2008 Sep 2;118(10):1047–56.

VII.12. Answer d.

Most vasoactive agents that can be used as continuous infusions have a rapid onset of action and a short offset of action. Important exceptions are milrinone and levosimendan, for which the effect is not offset for hours. This difference has to be considered when weaning inotropic support.

Gamper G, Havel C, Arrich J, Losert H, Pace NL, Mullner M, et al. Vasopressors for hypotensive shock. Cochrane Database Syst Rev. 2016 Feb 15;2:CD003709.

Overgaard CB, Dzavik V. Inotropes and vasopressors: review of physiology and clinical use in cardiovascular disease. Circulation. 2008 Sep 2;118(10):1047–56.

Stevenson LW. Clinical use of inotropic therapy for heart failure: looking backward or forward? Part I: inotropic infusions during hospitalization. Circulation. 2003 Jul 22;108(3): 367–72.

VII.13. Answer c.

Intravenous vasodilators, such as sodium nitroprusside, can inhibit hypoxic pulmonary vasoconstriction and cause hypoxemia from $\dot{V}/\dot{Q}$ mismatch or shunting, among other important adverse effects such as intense cerebral vasodilatation resulting in increased cerebral blood flow and intracranial pressure.

Abe K. Vasodilators during cerebral aneurysm surgery. Can J Anaesth. 1993 Aug;40(8):775–90.

Colley PS, Cheney FW Jr, Hlastala MP. Ventilation-perfusion and gas exchange effects of sodium nitroprusside in dogs with normal and edematous lungs. Anesthesiology. 1979 Jun;50(6):489–95.

VII.14. Answer d.

Cephalosporins (all generations) are not effective against *Enterococcus* species as monotherapy, with the exception of the fifth-generation ceftaroline, which has some activity.

The Sandford guide to antimicrobial therapy. Antibacterial agents. Mobile device application [cited 2016 Oct 27]. Available from: https://www.sanfordguide.com/products/digital-subscriptions/sanford-guide-to-antimicrobial-therapy-mobile/.

The Sandford guide to antimicrobial therapy. Tigecycline. Mobile device application [cited 2016 Oct 27]. Available from: https://www.sanfordguide.com/products/digital-subscriptions/sanford-guide-to-antimicrobial-therapy-mobile/.

VII.15. Answer a.

All the options are active against MSSA, but the treatment of choice for this microorganism is the antistaphylococcal penicillins (eg, nafcillin, oxacillin). Ceftriaxone can be effective against MSSA, but it is inferior to nafcillin. Vancomycin is effective against MSSA and MRSA, but it is also inferior to antistaphylococcal penicillins. Daptomycin is effective against MSSA and MRSA, but its cost makes it prohibitive.

Baddour LM, Wilson WR, Bayer AS, Fowler VG Jr, Tleyjeh IM, Rybak MJ, et al; American Heart Association Committee on Rheumatic Fever, Endocarditis, and Kawasaki Disease of the Council on Cardiovascular Disease in the Young, Council on Clinical Cardiology, Council on Cardiovascular Surgery and Anesthesia, and Stroke Council. Infective endocarditis in adults: diagnosis, antimicrobial therapy, and management of complications: a scientific statement for healthcare professionals from the American Heart Association. Circulation. 2015 Oct 13;132(15):1435–86. Epub 2015 Sep 15. Errata in: Circulation. 2015 Oct 27;132(17):e215. Circulation. 2016 Aug 23;134(8):e113.

Murray BE, Arias CA, Nannini EC. Glycopeptides (vancomycin and teicoplanin), streptogramins (quinupristin-dalfopristin), lipopeptides (daptomycin), and lipoglycopeptides (telavancin). In: Bennett JE, Dolin R, Blaser MJ, editors. Mandell, Douglas, and Bennett's principles and practice of infectious diseases. 8th ed. Philadelphia (PA): Elsevier/Saunders; c2015. p. 377–400.e4.

Petri WA Jr. Penicillins, cephalosporins, and other β-lactam antibiotics. In: Brunton LL, editor. Goodman & Gilman's the pharmacological basis of therapeutics. 12th ed. New York (NY): McGraw-Hill Medical; c2011. p. 1477–1503.

VII.16. Answer d.

Psuedomonas aeruginosa can be a multidrug-resistant microorganism and develop resistance to one or many of the known agents against *P aeruginosa*. Ceftolozane-tazobactam is a newly developed agent that may be used for treatment of multidrug-resistant *P aeruginosa*.

Viale P, Giannella M, Tedeschi S, Lewis R. Treatment of MDR-Gram negative infections in the 21st century: a never ending threat for clinicians. Curr Opin Pharmacol. 2015 Oct;24:30–7. Epub 2015 Jul 24.

VII.17. Answer b.

All the options are effective for the treatment of infections due to *Candida* species. The microorganism involved in this case is susceptible to all antifungal agents. For CNS infections, drugs with adequate tissue penetration must be considered. Echinocandins (eg, caspofungin) are well distributed throughout the body, with the exception of the CNS, eye, and urine.

Pappas PG, Kauffman CA, Andes DR, Clancy CJ, Marr KA, Ostrosky-Zeichner L, et al. Clinical practice guideline for the management of candidiasis: 2016 update by the Infectious Diseases Society of America. Clin Infect Dis. 2016 Feb 15;62(4):e1–50. Epub 2015 Dec 16.

VII.18. Answer b.

This patient's brain abscess is possibly related to recent immunosuppression from corticosteroid use. Blood culture results indicate a multidrug-resistant *P aeruginosa* (making it the likely cause of the brain abscess). The microorganism carries an extended-spectrum β-lactamase, which precludes use of all β-lactam antibiotics with the exclusion of the carbapenems, which have excellent CNS penetration. Because the patient was admitted for recent new-onset seizures, imipenem is not an appropriate choice because of its epileptogenic potential. Ertapenem lacks coverage for *P aeruginosa*.

Doi Y, Chambers HF. Penicillins and β-lactamase inhibitors. In: Bennett JE, Dolin R, Blaser MJ, editors. Mandell, Douglas, and Bennett's principles and practice of infectious diseases. 8th ed. Philadelphia (PA): Elsevier/Saunders; c2015. p. 263–77.e3.

Petri WA Jr. Penicillins, cephalosporins, and other β-lactam antibiotics. In: Brunton LL, editor. Goodman & Gilman's the pharmacological basis of therapeutics. 12th ed. New York (NY): McGraw-Hill Medical; c2011. p. 1477–1503.

Section VIII

Ethics in the Neurointensive Care Unit

138 Palliative and End-of-Life Care in the Intensive Care Unit

MAISHA T. ROBINSON, MD

Goals

- Describe the principles and role of palliative care in the intensive care unit.
- Discuss the process of withdrawal of life-sustaining interventions.
- Explain the models of palliative care delivery in the intensive care unit.

Introduction

Palliative medicine is the specialty that focuses on improving the quality of life for patients and families when the patients have serious or advanced medical conditions. The approach to care is patient centered and goal oriented. It can be performed at any stage of illness with or without a palliative medicine consultative service. All clinicians, including intensive care unit (ICU) physicians, who care for patients with serious or advanced illnesses should be able to provide adequate palliative care.

Critically ill patients are admitted to the ICU for aggressive management of their underlying conditions. Given that goal, integration of palliative care into the patients' management plans may seem counterintuitive. However, a growing body of literature suggests that the provision of high-quality care to critically ill patients with neurologic conditions should include a palliative approach. This involves the recognition, assessment, and treatment of suffering in all forms.

Palliative care among patients with neurologic disease often involves establishing goals of care, managing symptoms, providing support to caregivers, and making complex decisions. Providing social support for families and addressing goals of care were the most common needs in a single-center study in a neuroscience ICU in which 62% of patients had at least 1 palliative need identified on a palliative care screen.

Palliative care checklists and trigger criteria have been suggested as tools to identify ICU patients who may benefit from palliative care. Screening protocols have included patient characteristics and medical conditions that portend a poor prognosis, such as the presence of at least 2 medical comorbidities in a patient who is at least 80 years old, the presence of metastatic cancer, a history of cardiac arrest, and intracerebral hemorrhage that requires mechanical ventilation. When palliative care has been provided proactively, the length of stay in the ICU was shortened. Additionally, the frequency of family meetings increased, and they occurred earlier during ICU admission.

End-of-Life Care in the ICU

Patients in the neuroscience ICU have catastrophic conditions characterized by an acute or rapidly progressive process that affects mobility, independence, communication, and quality of life. Mortality and morbidity in the ICU are high, and only a minority of patients with traumatic and anoxic brain injuries, ischemic strokes, and intracerebral hemorrhages achieve functional independence at 1 year. Some patients and families decide to withhold or withdraw life-sustaining interventions when the expected outcome does not align with the previously expressed wishes of the patient. This decision may be influenced by the severity of illness, the patient's age, the presence or absence of a surgical intervention, the patient's race and ethnicity, the burden of treatment, and a patient's known wishes.

Terminal extubation involves compassionately weaning a patient from a ventilator or removing respiratory support if no appreciable benefit to continuing these interventions occurs or if the overall prognosis is not acceptable to the patient, as documented in an advance directive or as indicated by the health care surrogate. With the endotracheal tube in place, the fraction of inspired oxygen, positive end-expiratory pressure, respiratory rate, and tidal volume are reduced. Preemptive treatment is recommended for expected symptoms with the appropriate titration of medications after extubation to maintain comfort. Common symptoms after extubation include labored breathing and terminal secretions, often referred to as the *death rattle*. Pharmacologic management of distress symptoms for both the patient and the family includes the use of opioids, sedatives, and anticholinergics. Patients are treated for distress if they might still be aware of symptoms but not if they are deeply comatose from a catastrophic disorder.

Local hospice agencies may provide additional support for family members and bereavement counseling. Palliative care includes but is not synonymous with both end-of-life care and hospice care. Hospice care is specialized care for terminally ill people who are expected to live 6 months or less if the disease follows its normal trajectory.

Models of Palliative Care in the ICU

Models for incorporating palliative care into the ICU are integrative or consultative. *Integrative models* rely on the ICU team to provide primary palliative care after receiving education and training in the principles of palliative care. ICU clinicians should be able to provide generalist-level palliative care, which includes eliciting code status, initiating basic discussions about prognosis and goals of care, and managing common symptoms.

Consultative models involve the assessment and management of medical conditions by palliative medicine interdisciplinary teams, which may include physicians, nurses, chaplains, and social workers. In this model, the palliative care team provides specialist-level care for advanced or complex palliative needs and addresses the 8 domains of palliative care.

The ideal model is a combination of these models, known as a *mixed model*, which is common in other consultative services. The advantage of this model in the ICU, where prognostic uncertainty is common and where health care surrogates are often unsure of the patients' wishes, is that patients and surrogate decision-makers benefit from the expertise of both teams as they make complex decisions about treatments and estimate the patient's future quality of life.

Principles of Palliative Care

The provision of high-quality palliative care is based on 8 domains of care:

- Structures and processes of care
- Physical aspects of care
- Psychological and psychiatric aspects of care
- Social aspects of care
- Spiritual, religious, and existential aspects of care
- Cultural aspects of care
- Care of the imminently dying patient
- Ethical and legal aspects of care

Box 138.1 • Principles of Palliative Care

Understand the diagnosis and prognosis.

- Ensure that patients and family members understand the disease process and the expected prognosis.
- Use prognostic scales to estimate life expectancy.

Bridge communication and knowledge gaps.

- Relay additional clinical or prognostic information to the patient and family to help guide care decisions.
- Provide the care teams with salient background details related to the patient's and family's preferences for care.
- Organize care team meetings.
- Arrange family meetings.

Establish goals of care.

- Understand what is important to the patient given the patient's current condition.
- Know the available treatment options and the intentions for these treatments, therapies, and procedures.
- Identify the surrogate decision maker (if it is not the patient), and review advance care planning documentation.
- Align the patient's preferences with appropriate treatments.

Alleviate suffering.

- Assess physical symptoms.
- Inquire about mood and coping strategies.
- Determine the role of religion or spirituality in the patient's life.
- Provide suggestions and treatments based on symptoms.

Manage end-of-life care.

- Recognize impending death.
- Provide anticipatory guidance to the patient and family.
- Engage hospice care as appropriate.
- Anticipate and alleviate symptom burden.

Provide support.

- Assess caregiver burden.
- Offer bereavement support.

Incorporating components of these domains of care into the management plans for ICU patients provides a holistic approach to care that aims to reduce suffering among patients and family members despite the patient's critical illness. Essential principles of palliative care include ensuring that patient and family members understand the disease process and the expected prognosis; developing reasonable goals of care according to what is important to the patient and the available treatment options; addressing suffering of all forms (physical, spiritual and existential, and psychological); bridging communication and knowledge gaps; and providing emotional support to patients and their families (Box 138.1). Appropriate end-of-life care management involves the recognition of impending death, symptom management, and family or caregiver bereavement support.

Benefits of Palliative Care

Palliative care benefits patients by improving symptom control, and palliative care benefits families by potentially decreasing the risk of prolonged grief and posttraumatic stress disorder. Palliative care may reduce ICU length of stay, and it reduces health care use by patients who are unlikely to benefit from invasive procedures and recurrent hospitalizations.

Summary

- The delivery of high-quality care in the ICU may involve the incorporation of palliative care.
- Common palliative needs in the ICU are to provide caregiver support and to clarify the goals of care.
- Multiple factors affect the withdrawal of life-sustaining care, and terminal extubation should involve anticipating and alleviating suffering.
- Palliative care delivery models include integrative, consultative, and mixed models.

SUGGESTED READING

Ahluwalia SC, Chen C, Raaen L, Motala A, Walling AM, Chamberlin M, et al. A systematic review in support of the national consensus project clinical practice guidelines for quality palliative care, fourth edition. J Pain Symptom Manage. 2018 Dec;56(6):831–70. Epub 2018 Oct 31.

Aslakson RA, Curtis JR, Nelson JE. The changing role of palliative care in the ICU. Crit Care Med. 2014 Nov;42(11):2418–28.

Billings JA. Humane terminal extubation reconsidered: the role for preemptive analgesia and sedation. Crit Care Med. 2012 Feb;40(2):625–30.

Boersma I, Miyasaki J, Kutner J, Kluger B. Palliative care and neurology: time for a paradigm shift. Neurology. 2014 Aug 5;83(6):561–7. Epub 2014 Jul 2.

Borasio GD. The role of palliative care in patients with neurological diseases. Nat Rev Neurol. 2013 May;9(5):292–5. Epub 2013 Apr 2.

Braus N, Campbell TC, Kwekkeboom KL, Ferguson S, Harvey C, Krupp AE, et al. Prospective study of a proactive palliative care rounding intervention in a medical ICU. Intensive Care Med. 2016 Jan;42(1):54–62. Epub 2015 Nov 10.

Brizzi K, Creutzfeldt CJ. Neuropalliative care: a practical guide for the neurologist. Semin Neurol. 2018 Oct;38(5):569–75. Epub 2018 Oct 15.

Campbell ML, Guzman JA. A proactive approach to improve end-of-life care in a medical intensive care unit for patients with terminal dementia. Crit Care Med. 2004 Sep;32(9):1839–43.

Campbell ML, Guzman JA. Impact of a proactive approach to improve end-of-life care in a medical ICU. Chest. 2003 Jan;123(1):266–71.

Casarett D, Johnson M, Smith D, Richardson D. The optimal delivery of palliative care: a national comparison of the outcomes of consultation teams vs inpatient units. Arch Intern Med. 2011 Apr 11;171(7):649–55.

Center to Advance Palliative Care (CAPC). About palliative care: definition of palliative care [Internet]. New York (NY): CAPC [cited 2016 Dec 30]. Available from: https://www.capc.org/about/palliative-care/.

Centers for Medicare & Medicaid Services. Medicare hospice benefits [Internet]. Baltimore (MD): US Department of Health & Human Services. c2017 [cited 2016 Nov 22]. Available from: https://www.medicare.gov/pubs/pdf/02154-Medicare-Hospice-Benefits.pdf.

Cook D, Rocker G. Dying with dignity in the intensive care unit. N Engl J Med. 2014 Jun 26;370(26):2506–14.

Creutzfeldt CJ, Engelberg RA, Healey L, Cheever CS, Becker KJ, Holloway RG, et al. Palliative care needs in the neuro-ICU. Crit Care Med. 2015 Aug;43(8):1677–84.

Creutzfeldt CJ, Kluger BM, Holloway RG, editors. Neuropalliative care: a guide to improving the lives of patients and families affected by neurologic disease. Cham (Switzerland): Springer International Publishing; 2019. 312 p.

Diringer MN, Edwards DF, Aiyagari V, Hollingsworth H. Factors associated with withdrawal of mechanical ventilation in a neurology/neurosurgery intensive care unit. Crit Care Med. 2001 Sep;29(9):1792–7.

Frontera JA, Curtis JR, Nelson JE, Campbell M, Gabriel M, Mosenthal AC, et al; Improving Palliative Care in the ICU Project Advisory Board. Integrating palliative care into the care of neurocritically ill patients: a report from the Improving Palliative Care in the ICU Project Advisory Board and the Center to Advance Palliative Care. Crit Care Med. 2015 Sep;43(9):1964–77.

Higginson IJ, Finlay I, Goodwin DM, Cook AM, Hood K, Edwards AG, et al. Do hospital-based palliative teams improve care for patients or families at the end of life? J Pain Symptom Manage. 2002 Feb;23(2):96–106.

Holloway RG, Arnold RM, Creutzfeldt CJ, Lewis EF, Lutz BJ, McCann RM, et al; American Heart Association Stroke Council, Council on Cardiovascular and Stroke Nursing, and Council on Clinical Cardiology. Palliative and end-of-life care in stroke: a statement for healthcare professionals from the American Heart Association/American Stroke Association. Stroke. 2014 Jun;45(6):1887–916. Epub 2014 Mar 27.

Holloway RG, Benesch CG, Burgin WS, Zentner JB. Prognosis and decision making in severe stroke. JAMA. 2005 Aug 10;294(6):725–33.

Institute of Medicine of the National Academies. Dying in America: improving quality and honoring individual preferences near the end of life [Internet]. Washington (DC): Institute of Medicine of the National Academies. c2014 [cited 2016 Dec 30]. Available from: http://nationalacademies.org/hmd/~/media/Files/Report%20Files/2014/EOL/Key%20Findings%20and%20Recommendations.pdf.

Kluger BM, Bernat JL. Palliative care and inpatient neurology: Where to next? Neurology. 2019 Apr 23;92(17): 784–5. Epub 2019 Mar 27.

Kompanje EJ, van der Hoven B, Bakker J. Anticipation of distress after discontinuation of mechanical ventilation in the ICU at the end of life. Intensive Care Med. 2008 Sep;34(9):1593–9. Epub 2008 May 31.

Mayer SA, Kossoff SB. Withdrawal of life support in the neurological intensive care unit. Neurology. 1999 May 12;52(8):1602–9.

Morrison RS, Penrod JD, Cassel JB, Caust-Ellenbogen M, Litke A, Spragens L, et al; Palliative Care Leadership Centers' Outcomes Group. Cost savings associated with US hospital palliative care consultation programs. Arch Intern Med. 2008 Sep 8;168(16):1783–90.

National Consensus Project for Quality Palliative Care. Clinical practice guidelines for quality palliative care. 3rd ed [Internet]. Pittsburgh (PA): National Consensus Project for Quality Palliative Care. c2013 [cited 2017 Jun 4]. Available from: https://www.hpna.org/multimedia/NCP_Clinical_Practice_Guidelines_3rd_Edition.pdf.

Nelson JE, Bassett R, Boss RD, Brasel KJ, Campbell ML, Cortez TB, et al; Improve Palliative Care in the Intensive Care Unit Project. Models for structuring a clinical initiative to enhance palliative care in the intensive care unit: a report from the IPAL-ICU Project (Improving Palliative Care in the ICU). Crit Care Med. 2010 Sep;38(9):1765–72.

Norton SA, Hogan LA, Holloway RG, Temkin-Greener H, Buckley MJ, Quill TE. Proactive palliative care in the medical intensive care unit: effects on length of stay for selected high-risk patients. Crit Care Med. 2007 Jun;35(6):1530–5.

Quill TE, Abernethy AP. Generalist plus specialist palliative care: creating a more sustainable model. N Engl J Med. 2013 Mar 28;368(13):1173–5. Epub 2013 Mar 6.

Taylor BL, O'Riordan DL, Pantilat SZ, Creutzfeldt CJ. Inpatients with neurologic disease referred for palliative care consultation. Neurology. 2019 Apr 23;92(17):e1975–e1981. Epub 2019 Mar 27.

World Health Organization (WHO). WHO definition of palliative care [Internet]. Geneva (UN): World Health Organization. [cited 2016 Nov 30]. Available from: http://www.who.int/cancer/palliative/definition/en/.

139 Communicating With Families

CORY INGRAM, MD

Goals

- Discuss professionalism and effective communication.
- Discuss the techniques of communicating with families.
- Discuss mutual decision making.

Introduction

Professionalism guides how intensivists provide care, and communicating effectively is a core principle of professionalism. Communicating with families is common in intensive care units because patients may be in extremis or unable to understand their critical illness.

Medical professionalism dates back to the Hippocratic oath, an early description of expected physician behavior. The current Charter on Medical Professionalism outlines 3 fundamental principles: 1) primacy of patient welfare, 2) patient autonomy, and 3) social justice. The charter also identifies 10 professional responsibilities for clinicians: 1) commitment to professional competence, 2) honesty with patients, 3) patient confidentiality, 4) maintaining appropriate relations with patients, 5) improving quality of care, 6) improving access to care, 7) just distribution of finite resources, 8) scientific knowledge, 9) maintaining trust by managing conflicts of interest, and 10) professional responsibilities.

Interpersonal and communication skills are core competency areas at all levels of medical training and practice. The Accreditation Council for Graduate Medical Education included interpersonal and communication skills as a general competence, and the American Board of Medical Specialties endorsed the same competencies for practicing physicians. Nonetheless, a physician must rely on experience to recommend certain options to patients' families, guide them toward understanding, and proceed with the best professional choice.

Principles of Communicating With Families

Clinicians learn communication skills from informal observation of peers or mentors and from trial and error. Poor communication is common between clinicians and families, and it is a major reason for dissatisfaction with medical care. Miscommunication erodes trust, confuses families, and, in more extreme situations, results in anger or an increased medicolegal risk.

Good communication with family members (and significant others) is increasingly considered in quality metrics and research protocols. Families value receiving honest, understandable, and timely information; being given support and reassurance; and understanding the prognosis while maintaining hope. Special challenges arise when the medical situation and outcomes are not what anyone wants to hear or discuss.

Training clinicians in communicating with families increases family satisfaction. Family decision makers feel more confident in their decisions when communication is clear and understood; they feel less confident when communication is ambiguous or ridden with platitudes or medical jargon. Additionally, communicating with families improves clinical outcomes for patients. The mnemonic *VALUE* is a reminder of a communication strategy (Table 139.1):

- Value what surrogates communicate
- Acknowledge their emotions
- Listen carefully
- Understand who the patient is as a person
- Elicit questions

The VALUE trial randomly assigned 126 surrogate decision makers to receive either the VALUE communication intervention or routine care. The participants in the

Table 139.1 • Communication Techniques

Technique	Components
VALUE	Value what surrogates communicate Acknowledge emotion Listen carefully Understand who the patient is as a person Elicit questions
Ask-Tell-Ask	Question Share Question again
Hope and Worry	I hope this too, and I worry that we may not achieve that
Hoping for a miracle	Seek understanding Share the professional obligation Find common ground
NURSE	Name the emotion Understand the emotion Respect the emotion Support the caregiver Explore the emotion

intervention group had less depression, anxiety, and post-traumatic stress symptoms.

Talking With Families

Setting Up the Conversation

All family members should be invited to conversations unless a patient previously requested that someone should not participate. All pertinent health care teams should also be invited. Nurses, chaplains, and social workers can reinforce and support the family through various aspects of their respective disciplines. Evidence indicates that families value such an approach and communication outcomes are better.

Preparing Before the Meeting

When several health care providers communicate with the family, they should all have a similar view and understanding of the clinical situation to help prevent confusing or conflicting information arising during the conversations. The providers must identify who will lead the conversation with the family.

Introducing Participants and Setting the Agenda

Most conversations with a family start with introductions of the medical staff and family members, which should include their name, their relationship to the patient, and their role in making decisions. After introductions, the goals of the conversation should be clearly defined and understood by all participants. Adequate time must be allowed for all to speak, and the health care providers should not dominate the conversation.

Avoiding the Patient's Anonymity

An important goal is to better understand who the patient is as a person. Helping family members focus on personal aspects of their loved one may be a welcome departure from the serious medical topics to come. Simply providing a few minutes to talk about the personal context of the situation and the patient often lessens the tension in the room.

Understanding the Illness

Often conversations with families resemble a medical encyclopedic summary of the history of the illness. A more helpful approach is to listen and hear about the patient's illness in the patient's and family's own words as they provide their understanding of the situation.

Sharing Clinical Information

Ask-Tell-Ask is a helpful communication technique that can be used to learn how much information families want to know (Table 139.1). If families want to know details about the prognosis, drawings, brochures, pictures, and other resources can help increase their understanding. The facilitator and other health care providers may choose to offer questions that the family may benefit from having answered. If a family wants to know a prognosis, it should be provided with a range (days to weeks, weeks to months, or years). Clinicians are often reluctant to talk about prognosis for fear of dashing a family's hope, but families are often more optimistic than the clinical teams. Discussions of prognosis often involve talking about the best, worst, and common clinical outcome scenarios for the patient's condition.

Understanding Goals of Care

If a patient has an irreversible illness and is in a critical situation, the next step should be identified. The best care possible is the care that would best match the preferences and priorities of the patient and family. A care plan recommendation may be appropriate. Identification of how and when the outcomes will be evaluated is often referred to as a time-limited trial.

Dealing With Conflict

A family conference may expose a family's unrealistic expectations for the clinical situation. One framework used when people may be hoping for a miracle is to seek to understand, share the professional obligation, and find common ground (Table 139.1).

Responding to Emotion

Caring for a loved one is an emotional experience, and emotional responses can include anger, grief, guilt, fear, anxiety, sadness, and isolation. The use of empathetic statements increases a family's satisfaction with communication. The *NURSE* mnemonic offers a practical framework for clinicians responding to a caregiver's emotion (Table 139.1): naming, understanding, and respecting the emotion; supporting the caregiver; and exploring the emotion. Emotion is a bridge that connects the family and the medical team, leads to better clinician-patient relationships, and improves the patient's and family's experience.

Summary

- Communicating with families about medical care for their loved ones is foundational to medical professionalism, and good communication makes the experience more enjoyable for the families and the clinicians.
- Family conversations should be arranged to ensure participation of the appropriate medical colleagues and family members. A facilitator should lead the conversation and follow a set structure.
- Conversations should focus on the personal and medical aspects, and the family should speak at least as much as the facilitator. Questions to the family should be asked in plain language, and the family's understanding should be evaluated regularly.

SUGGESTED READING

ABIM Foundation. American Board of Internal Medicine; ACP-ASIM Foundation; American College of Physicians-American Society of Internal Medicine; European Federation of Internal Medicine. Medical professionalism in the new millennium: a physician charter. Ann Intern Med. 2002 Feb 5;136(3):243–6.

Accreditation Council for Graduate Medical Education (ACGME). Common program requirements. c2017 [cited 2017 May 2]. Available from: https://www.acgme.org/Portals/0/PFAssets/ProgramRequirements/CPRs_2017-07-01.pdf.

Anderson WG, Cimino JW, Ernecoff NC, Ungar A, Shotsberger KJ, Pollice LA, et al. A multicenter study of key stakeholders' perspectives on communicating with surrogates about prognosis in intensive care units. Ann Am Thorac Soc. 2015 Feb;12(2):142–52.

Back AL, Arnold RM, Quill TE. Hope for the best, and prepare for the worst. Ann Intern Med. 2003 Mar 4;138(5):439–43.

Barrier PA, Li JT, Jensen NM. Two words to improve physician-patient communication: what else? Mayo Clin Proc. 2003 Feb;78(2):211–4.

Beck CS. The needs of the patient come first. Mayo Clin Proc. 2000 Mar;75(3):224.

Byock I. The best care possible: a physician's quest to transform care through the end of life. New York (NY): Avery; c2012. 320 p.

Byock I, Ingram C. Palliative care in advanced dementia. In: Quinn JF, editor. Dementia. 1st ed. Chichester (West Sussex): John Wiley & Sons; c2013. p. 188.

Clarke EB, Curtis JR, Luce JM, Levy M, Danis M, Nelson J, et al; Robert Wood Johnson Foundation Critical Care End-Of-Life Peer Workgroup Members. Quality indicators for end-of-life care in the intensive care unit. Crit Care Med. 2003 Sep;31(9):2255–62.

Curtis JR. Communicating about end-of-life care with patients and families in the intensive care unit. Crit Care Clin. 2004 Jul;20(3):363–80.

DeAngelis CD. Medical professionalism. JAMA. 2015 May 12;313(18):1837–8.

DeLisser HM. A practical approach to the family that expects a miracle. Chest. 2009 Jun;135(6):1643–7.

Garrouste-Orgeas M, Max A, Lerin T, Gregoire C, Ruckly S, Kloeckner M, et al. Impact of proactive nurse participation in ICU family conferences: a mixed-method study. Crit Care Med. 2016 Jun;44(6):1116–28.

Halpern SD, Becker D, Curtis JR, Fowler R, Hyzy R, Kaplan LJ, et al; Choosing Wisely Taskforce; American Thoracic Society; American Association of Critical-Care Nurses; Society of Critical Care Medicine. An official American Thoracic Society/American Association of Critical-Care Nurses/American College of Chest Physicians/Society of Critical Care Medicine policy statement: the Choosing Wisely Top 5 list in Critical Care Medicine. Am J Respir Crit Care Med. 2014 Oct 1;190(7):818–26.

Hiltunen EF, Puopolo AL, Marks GK, Marsden C, Kennard MJ, Follen MA, et al. The nurse's role in end-of-life treatment discussions: preliminary report from the SUPPORT Project. J Cardiovasc Nurs. 1995 Apr;9(3):68–77.

Hwang DY, Yagoda D, Perrey HM, Tehan TM, Guanci M, Ananian L, et al. Consistency of communication among intensive care unit staff as perceived by family members of patients surviving to discharge. J Crit Care. 2014 Feb;29(1):134–8.

Ingram C. A paradigm shift: healing, quality of life, and a professional choice. J Pain Symptom Manage. 2014 Jan;47(1):198–201.

Lautrette A, Darmon M, Megarbane B, Joly LM, Chevret S, Adrie C, et al. A communication strategy and brochure for relatives of patients dying in the ICU. N Engl J Med. 2007 Feb 1;356(5):469–78. Erratum in: N Engl J Med. 2007 Jul 12;357(2):203.

Leske JS. Overview of family needs after critical illness: from assessment to intervention. AACN Clin Issues Crit Care Nurs. 1991 May;2(2):220–9.

Levy MM. End-of-life care in the intensive care unit: can we do better? Crit Care Med. 2001 Feb;29(2 Suppl):N56–61.

Lilly CM, Sonna LA, Haley KJ, Massaro AF. Intensive communication: four-year follow-up from a clinical practice study. Crit Care Med. 2003 May;31(5 Suppl):S394–9.

Majesko A, Hong SY, Weissfeld L, White DB. Identifying family members who may struggle in the role of surrogate decision maker. Crit Care Med. 2012 Aug;40(8):2281–6.

Mayo WJ. The necessity of cooperation in medicine. Mayo Clin Proc. 2000 Jun;75(6):553–6.

McAdam JL, Dracup KA, White DB, Fontaine DK, Puntillo KA. Symptom experiences of family members of intensive care unit patients at high risk for dying. Crit Care Med. 2010 Apr;38(4):1078–85.

McCannon JB, O'Donnell WJ, Thompson BT, El-Jawahri A, Chang Y, Anamian L, et al. Augmenting communication and decision making in the intensive care unit with a cardiopulmonary resuscitation video decision support tool: a temporal intervention study. J Palliat Med. 2012 Dec;15(12):1382–7. Epub 2012 Oct 25.

Mularski RA, Curtis JR, Billings JA, Burt R, Byock I, Fuhrman C, et al. Proposed quality measures for palliative care in the critically ill: a consensus from the Robert Wood Johnson Foundation Critical Care Workgroup. Crit Care Med. 2006 Nov;34(11 Suppl):S404–11.

Nelson JE, Mulkerin CM, Adams LL, Pronovost PJ. Improving comfort and communication in the ICU: a practical new tool for palliative care performance measurement and feedback. Qual Saf Health Care. 2006 Aug;15(4):264–71.

Nelson JE, Puntillo KA, Pronovost PJ, Walker AS, McAdam JL, Ilaoa D, et al. In their own words: patients and families define high-quality palliative care in the intensive care unit. Crit Care Med. 2010 Mar;38(3):808–18.

October TW, Dizon ZB, Roter DL. Is it my turn to speak? An analysis of the dialogue in the family-physician intensive care unit conference. Patient Educ Couns. 2018 Apr;101(4):647–52. Epub 2017 Oct 28.

Peigne V, Chaize M, Falissard B, Kentish-Barnes N, Rusinova K, Megarbane B, et al. Important questions asked by family members of intensive care unit patients. Crit Care Med. 2011 Jun;39(6):1365–71.

Phillips RS, Wenger NS, Teno J, Oye RK, Youngner S, Califf R, et al; SUPPORT Investigators. Choices of seriously ill patients about cardiopulmonary resuscitation: correlates and outcomes: study to understand prognoses and preferences for outcomes and risks of treatments. Am J Med. 1996 Feb;100(2):128–37.

Pochard F, Azoulay E, Chevret S, Lemaire F, Hubert P, Canoui P, et al; French FAMIREA Group. Symptoms of anxiety and depression in family members of intensive care unit patients: ethical hypothesis regarding decision-making capacity. Crit Care Med. 2001 Oct;29(10):1893–7.

Pollak KI, Alexander SC, Tulsky JA, Lyna P, Coffman CJ, Dolor RJ, et al. Physician empathy and listening: associations with patient satisfaction and autonomy. J Am Board Fam Med. 2011 Nov-Dec;24(6):665–72.

Powazki R, Walsh D, Hauser K, Davis MP. Communication in palliative medicine: a clinical review of family conferences. J Palliat Med. 2014 Oct;17(10):1167–77. Epub 2014 Jul 3.

Rubenfeld GD, Curtis JR; End-of-Life Care in the ICU Working Group. End-of-life care in the intensive care unit: a research agenda. Crit Care Med. 2001 Oct;29(10):2001–6.

Selph RB, Shiang J, Engelberg R, Curtis JR, White DB. Empathy and life support decisions in intensive care units. J Gen Intern Med. 2008 Sep;23(9):1311–7.

Shaw DJ, Davidson JE, Smilde RI, Sondoozi T, Agan D. Multidisciplinary team training to enhance family communication in the ICU. Crit Care Med. 2014 Feb;42(2):265–71.

Smith RC. The patient's story: integrated patient-doctor interviewing. Boston (MA): Little, Brown; c1996. 242 p.

Wenrich MD, Curtis JR, Shannon SE, Carline JD, Ambrozy DM, Ramsey PG. Communicating with dying patients within the spectrum of medical care from terminal diagnosis to death. Arch Intern Med. 2001 Mar 26;161(6):868–74.

White DB, Ernecoff N, Buddadhumaruk P, Hong S, Weissfeld L, Curtis JR, et al. Prevalence of and factors related to discordance about prognosis between physicians and surrogate decision makers of critically ill patients. JAMA. 2016 May 17;315(19):2086–94.

Wittenberg E, Kravits K, Goldsmith J, Ferrell B, Fujinami R. Validation of a model of family caregiver communication types and related caregiver outcomes. Palliat Support Care. 2017 Feb;15(1):3–11. Epub 2016 Apr 1.

Wysham NG, Mularski RA, Schmidt DM, Nord SC, Louis DL, Shuster E, et al. Long-term persistence of quality improvements for an intensive care unit communication initiative using the VALUE strategy. J Crit Care. 2014 Jun;29(3):450–4. Epub 2013 Dec 21.

140 Brain Death

EELCO F. M. WIJDICKS, MD, PhD

Goals

- Describe clinical examination in brain death.
- Describe confounders and pitfalls in the diagnosis of brain death.
- Describe the preconditions and technique for the apnea test.

Introduction

The fundamental neurologic principle that all brainstem function must have irreversibly ceased—in the overwhelming proportion of patients, but not exclusively, from massive damage to both cerebral hemispheres—must be understood before brain death testing proceeds. *Brain death* is a nonfunctioning, destroyed ("dead") brain in a patient with the absence of breathing and circulation if support is not provided. This is different from prolonged coma, and where the brainstem and thus the vital functions of breathing and maintaining blood pressure are partly or fully intact.

The American Academy of Neurology issued a new guideline in 2010, and this guideline is the standard for neurology practice. It stipulates that the clinical diagnosis of brain death is determined only after a comprehensive clinical examination that includes at least 25 assessments (Box 140.1). These assessments involve several categories, including exclusion of confounding factors, a set of neurologic tests as part of of the neurologic examination, and the performance of a carbon dioxide challenge to document the absence of breathing.

Clinical Criteria

The diagnosis of brain death is based on neurologic common sense (Box 140.1). First, of course, brain death determination should never proceed if computed tomography (CT) shows an abnormality that would not produce a loss of all brain function or that may actually be reversible (eg, cerebellar hematoma requiring decompression or hydrocephalus requiring a ventriculostomy). Second, it is critically important to exclude all possible lingering effects of sedation or the use of illegal drugs or alcohol or drugs or agents that block neuromuscular traffic. If a drug has been recently administered, a reasonable guideline is to calculate 5 times the drug's elimination half-life in hours and allow that time to pass before clinical examination is performed (if kidney and liver function are normal). Targeted temperature management after cardiopulmonary resuscitation may have substantially slowed the metabolism of medications such as lorazepam and fentanyl used during an intervention. Moreover, organ function and thus drug clearance may be abnormal after prolonged resuscitation, causing shock liver or acute tubular necrosis of the kidney. An alcohol level below the legal alcohol limit for driving (blood alcohol content 0.08%) is acceptable for proceeding with the determination of brain death.

Furthermore, absence of severe electrolyte, acid-base, or endocrine disturbances (defined by marked acidosis or any substantial deviation from the normal values) should be documented. Cutoff values are not known. The patient should be normothermic or mildly hypothermic (≥36°C), and systolic blood pressure should be at least 100 mm Hg.

Clinical Examination

The clinical requirements are shown in Box 140.1. Standard noxious stimuli include compression of the supraorbital nerves, forceful nail bed pressure, and temporomandibular joint compression. The challenge is to recognize "spinal responses." They may occur with neck flexion and nail bed compression but are absent with supraorbital nerve compression. Usually triple flexion responses are seen. After the neurologic examination of the brainstem

Box 140.1 • Checklist of 25 Assessments for Declaration of Brain Death

Prerequisites (all must be checked)

1. □ Coma—irreversible and cause known
2. □ Neuroimaging explains coma
3. □ Sedative drug effect absent (if indicated, order a toxicology screen)
4. □ No residual effect of paralytic drug (if indicated, use peripheral nerve stimulator)
5. □ Absence of severe acid-base, electrolyte, or endocrine abnormality
6. □ Normal or near-normal temperature (core temperature ≥36°C)
7. □ Systolic blood pressure ≥100 mm Hg
8. □ No spontaneous respirations

Examination (all must be checked)

9. □ Pupils nonreactive to bright light (typically midposition at 5-7 mm)
10. □ Corneal reflexes absent (use both saline jet and tissue touch)
11. □ Eyes immobile, oculocephalic reflexes absent (tested only if cervical spine integrity is ensured)
12. □ Oculovestibular reflexes absent (50 mL of ice water in each ear sequentially)
13. □ No facial movement to noxious stimuli at supraorbital nerve or temporomandibular joint compression (absent snout and routing reflexes in neonates)
14. □ Gag reflex absent (gloved index finger to posterior pharynx)
15. □ Cough reflex absent to tracheal suctioning (≥2 passes)
16. □ No motor response to noxious stimuli in all 4 limbs (triple flexion response is most common spinal-mediated reflex)

Apnea testing (all must be checked)

17. □ Patient hemodynamically stable (systolic blood pressure ≥100 mm Hg)
18. □ Ventilator adjusted to normocapnia ($Paco_2$ 35-45 mm Hg)
19. □ Patient preoxygenated with 100% oxygen for 10 min (Pao_2 ≥200 mm Hg)
20. □ Patient maintains oxygenation with a PEEP of 5 cm H_2O (if not, consider recruitment maneuver)
21. □ Disconnect ventilator
22. □ Provide oxygen with an insufflation catheter to the level of the carina at 6 L/min or attach T-piece with CPAP valve (at 10-20 cm H_2O) and resuscitation bag
23. □ Spontaneous respirations absent
24. □ Arterial blood gas sample drawn at 8-10 min; patient reconnected to ventilator
25. □ $Paco_2$ ≥60 mm Hg, or increase of 20 mm Hg from normal baseline value

or

Apnea test aborted and confirmatory ancillary test performed (EEG or cerebral blood flow study)

Additional examinations

- Newborn (gestational age ≥37 wk) to age 30 d: 2 examinations, 2 separate physicians, 24 h apart
- Age 30 d to 18 y: 2 examinations, 2 separate physicians, 12 h apart
- Age ≥18 y: 1 examination (a second examination is needed in Alabama, California, Florida, Iowa, Kentucky, and Louisiana)

Documentation

- Time of death (use time of final blood gas result or time of completion of ancillary test)

Abbreviations: CPAP, continuous positive airway pressure; EEG, electroencephalography; PEEP, positive end-expiratory pressure.

From Wijdicks EF, Varelas PN, Gronseth GS, Greer DM; American Academy of Neurology. Evidence-based guideline update: determining brain death in adults: report of the Quality Standards Subcommittee of the American Academy of Neurology. Neurology. 2010 Jun 8;74(23):1911-8; used with permission.

is completed, using typical neurologic examination skills, an apnea test can begin (Box 140.1). The apnea test should be performed by the same examiner and not by another specialist. Dividing the examination into separate portions performed by different examiners will lead to errors, delay, and incomplete or inaccurate testing.

Ancillary Tests

None of the ancillary tests should replace a clinical assessment. Catheter angiography is subject to variability because the extent of skull base and intracranial arterial opacification can vary with the catheter tip position in relation to the carotid bifurcation and vertebral artery origins. CT angiography uses a venous injection, and the timing of the contrast bolus to the brain, especially if the intracranial pressure is elevated, may be delayed and result in false-positive results. It is, however, widely accepted that a cerebral flow study that unambiguously shows the absence of intracranial flow could replace an apnea test if it cannot be safely performed. Under no circumstance should an ancillary test replace a neurologic examination confounded by the effects of a lingering drug or unknown illegal drug ingestion.

Common Pitfalls

Some common mistakes are shown in Box 140.2. Most pitfalls relate to premature assessment of the patient or misjudgment of triggering of the ventilator because of ventilator autocycling. When in doubt, a fully executed apnea test allows discrimination between a patient's respiratory drive

Box 140.2 • Common Misjudgments in Determinations of Brain Death

Incomplete testing
Failure to recognize ventilator autocycling
Examination of a patient who has confounders (eg, recently administered medication or use of drugs or alcohol)
Use of a cerebral blood flow study as a diagnostic test
Misinterpretation of ancillary tests
Misinterpretation of spinal reflexes
Premature discussion with patient's family about brain death and organ donation

and an artifactual mechanical drive. Misinterpretation of ancillary test results often occurs when artifacts are thought to be signs of cerebral blood flow or electrical activity.

Ethical Issues

A diagnosis of brain death in the United States leads to organ transplant in about 70% of cases. The organ donation agency will become involved after the diagnosis is made, but the agency may have been called earlier when the patient met specific criteria. Ethical tensions may occur between the attending intensivist and the organ donation representative if there is uncertainty about whether a neurologic injury is unsurvivable, defined as 1) no medical intervention is planned or medical intervention was unsuccessful, 2) no neurosurgical options exist for the patient, and 3) uncertainty exists about a confounder. If all 3 criteria are met, the organ donation agency may contact the intensivist to allow for more effective communication if the patient has 1) a loss of pupillary and corneal reflexes or gag reflexes or 2) a FOUR (Full Outline of Unresponsiveness) score of 2 or less.

Ethical controversies have occurred when families have intervened with neurologic testing. They may object to a full examination, knowing that it could lead to a declaration of death, or refuse to let the physician perform an apnea test. Brain death determination is a medical decision of death based on a neurologic examination, which, in itself, does not require informed consent. The negligible incidence of harm associated with apnea testing, once the prerequisites are fulfilled, does not justify an additional informed consent requirement. When families deny brain death as a neurologic criterion for death, support is continued until the legal issues have been resolved.

A rare ethical issue is brain death and organ donation if a pregnant woman has a viable baby. Providing support until delivery is rarely successful, but support should be provided if several more weeks would allow delivery of a potentially healthy baby.

Summary

- Brain death examination requires a detailed clinical assessment.
- Pitfalls are common, and each needs to be anticipated.
- Ancillary tests are not needed unless the apnea test cannot be performed.

SUGGESTED READING

Lewis A, Bernat JL, Blosser S, Bonnie RJ, Epstein LG, Hutchins J, et al. An interdisciplinary response to contemporary concerns about brain death determination. Neurology. 2018 Feb 27;90(9):423–6. Epub 2018 Jan 31.

Nakagawa TA, Ashwal S, Mathur M, Mysore MR, Bruce D, Conway EE Jr, et al; Society of Critical Care Medicine; Section on Critical Care and Section on Neurology of the American Academy of Pediatrics; Child Neurology Society. Guidelines for the determination of brain death in infants and children: an update of the 1987 Task Force recommendations. Crit Care Med. 2011 Sep;39(9):2139–55.

Wijdicks EF. The case against confirmatory tests for determining brain death in adults. Neurology. 2010 Jul 6;75(1):77–83.

Wijdicks EFM. Critical synopsis and key questions in brain death determination. Intensive Care Med. 2019 Mar;45(3):306–309. Epub 2019 Feb 6.

Wijdicks EF. Brain death. 3rd ed. New York (NY): Oxford University Press; c2017. 284 p.

Wijdicks EF, Rabinstein AA, Manno EM, Atkinson JD. Pronouncing brain death: contemporary practice and safety of the apnea test. Neurology. 2008 Oct 14;71(16):1240–4.

Wijdicks EF, Varelas PN, Gronseth GS, Greer DM; American Academy of Neurology. Evidence-based guideline update: determining brain death in adults: report of the Quality Standards Subcommittee of the American Academy of Neurology. Neurology. 2010 Jun 8;74(23):1911–8.

Minimally Conscious State and Persistent Vegetative State

DAVID T. JONES, MD

Goals

- Describe the clinical characteristics of disorders of consciousness.
- Describe the clinical trajectory of each disorder of consciousness.
- Describe magnetic resonance imaging findings in disorders of consciousness.

Introduction

Advances in critical care medicine have allowed for more patients to survive catastrophic brain injuries. However, the degree of recovery from serious neurologic injury is highly variable.

Coma

An acute, severe neurologic insult can cause a state of pathologic unconsciousness referred to as a coma. A comatose state is characterized by a patent having a lack of awareness of the environment, an absence of sleep-wake cycles, and an inability to be awakened. Common causes of brain injuries leading to a comatose state include cardiac arrest, a severe vascular event, a profound metabolic disturbance (eg, hypoglycemia), carbon monoxide or other poisoning, intoxications, or overdoses. The duration of a comatose state is rarely longer than days to weeks. With successful life-sustaining measures and avoidance of progression to brain death, the comatose patient recovers consciousness or remains in an intermediate state of consciousness between some degree of awareness and interaction with the external environment and complete lack of awareness and interaction (Table 141.1).

Prolonged States of Unconsciousness

The transition from a comatose state to an intermediate state of consciousness is marked by the return of sleep-wake cycles and spontaneous eye opening or wakefulness. If this clinical transition in conscious state is not accompanied by visual tracking or other signs of nonreflexive environmental interaction (eg, intermittent wakefulness without evidence of awareness), the state of consciousness is referred to as the *persistent vegetative state* (PVS). Given that this state may not be permanent, and the potential for an erroneous negative connotation of the word *vegetative* (because of its similarity to *vegetable*), some have suggested that the term *unresponsive wakefulness syndrome* replace *PVS*.

If a patient has awareness at any time, this state is referred to as a *minimally conscious state* (MCS). Evidence of awareness is identified from a detailed clinical examination focused on eliciting nonreflexive patient interactions with the environment (Box 141.1 and Figure 141.1). When distinguishing PVS from MCS, the clinician must consider the possibility that a patient has some level of awareness but cannot show evidence of it on clinical evaluation because of the lack of control of voluntary muscles, as in so-called locked-in syndrome (LIS).

In the classical form of LIS, a lesion in the ventral pons causes a complete loss of voluntary muscle control except for vertical eye movements and blinking. Therefore, a detailed assessment of the patient's eye movements should be performed to distinguish MCS from LIS. The patient's own image reflected in a mirror held by the examiner and moved across the visual field provides a strong stimulus to test for interaction with environmental stimuli. Rarely, total LIS has occurred without voluntary control of eye movements.

Table 141.1 • States of Impaired Consciousness

State	Wakefulness	Awareness	Interaction
Coma	–	–	–
PVS/UWS	+	–	–
MCS	+	+ or –	+ or –
LIS	+	+	Eyes only

Abbreviations: LIS, locked-in syndrome; MCS, minimally conscious state; PVS, persistent vegetative state; UWS, unresponsive wakefulness syndrome; –, absent; +, present.

Some investigators have advocated supplementing traditional bedside clinical evaluations of awareness with task-based functional neuroimaging or task-based quantitative electrophysiology. This approach would provide evidence of a patient's awareness with the use of only volitional changes in brain activity, and consequently the assessment would be independent from a physician's assessment of a patient's volitional control of muscle movements. However, these techniques have many technical confounding factors, and published studies of their clinical application are limited and lack detailed accounts of long-term clinical outcome. Currently, clinical indications do not exist for the use of imaging or electrophysiologic technologies to supplement detailed bedside clinical evaluation of a patient's level of consciousness.

Default Mode Network

From a basic science perspective, advanced neuroimaging investigations of clinical states of impaired consciousness have begun to shed light on the brain networks associated with consciousness. The *default mode network* has been shown to have decreasing levels of functional connectivity with a progression from full consciousness to MCS, PVS, coma, and absence in brain death (Figure 141.2). Assessment of the integrity of the default mode network may be important in the assessment of states of impaired consciousness in the future, but now its use is only investigational. Future studies may be used to complement existing ancillary clinical tools for prognostication, such as somatosensory evoked potentials.

Box 141.1. • Physical Examination Findings Consistent With Minimally Conscious State

Auditory: Reproducible or consistent movement to command

Visual: Fixation, pursuit, tracking own image in mirror, reaching for object, or object recognition

Motor: Localization to noxious stimuli, object manipulation, or automatic behavioral motor response

Verbal: Intelligible verbalization

Prognosis

Long-term outcome data are sparse for MCS, but consensus does exist for patients in a PVS. If a nontraumatic mechanism of injury leads to a PVS that lasts longer than 3 months, the PVS is considered chronic, but if the patient had a traumatic brain injury, the general consensus is that only if a PVS lasts longer than 1 year should the condition be considered chronic.

The few studies that have addressed long-term outcome from the MCS have focused mainly on traumatic injuries and have shown variable levels of recovery. One study followed 18 patients who were in an MCS from a traumatic brain injury for 2 to 5 years and found that 9 patients were independent in some self-care activities. The reports of variable levels of recovery from the MCS after traumatic brain injury have led to many ongoing research efforts to supplement the bedside clinical evaluation with functional neuroimaging and quantitative electrophysiology, but these efforts have not yielded long-term outcome data. However, early results have been publicized to the lay public, so clinicians must stay current on these developments so that they can adequately counsel the family members of patients in states of impaired consciousness. The most important prognostic factors for long-term outcome in states of impaired consciousness are the mechanism of brain injury and the age of the patient: Patients who are younger and have traumatic brain injury have better long-term outcomes than older patients and patients who have nontraumatic brain injury.

According to the recent American Academy of Neurology practice guideline, the term *permanent vegetative state* should not be used. This recommendation reflects the frequency of recovery after 3 months among patients with nontraumatic vegetative state and the frequency of recovery after 12 months among patients with traumatic vegetative state.

Summary

- Patients in coma usually recover, and prolonged unconsciousness is rare.
- PVS is less common than MCS.
- The prognosis for a patient in a state of impaired consciousness depends on the mechanism of brain injury and the age of the patient.

JFK Coma Recovery Scale–Revised Record Form								
Patient: Date:								
Auditory Function Scale								
4–Consistent movement to comand[a]								
3–Reproducible movement to command[a]								
2–Localization to sound								
1–Auditory startle								
0–None								
Visual Function Scale								
5–Object recognition[a]								
4–Object localization: reaching[a]								
3–Visual pursuit[a]								
2–Fixation[a]								
1–Visual startle								
0–None								
Motor Function Scale								
6–Functional object use[b]								
5–Automatic motor response[a]								
4–Object manipulation[a]								
3–Localization to noxious stimulation[a]								
2–Flexion withdrawal								
1–Abnormal posturing								
0–None/flaccid								
Oromotor/Verbal Function Scale								
3–Intelligible verbalization[a]								
2–Vocalization/oral movement								
1–Oral reflexive movement								
0–None								
Communication Scale								
3–Oriented[b]								
2–Functional: accurate[b]								
1–Nonfunctional: intentional[a]								
0–None								
Arousal Scale								
3–Attention[a]								
2–Eye opening without stimulation								
1–Eye opening with stimulation								
0–Unarousable								
Total Score								

Figure 141.1. *Record Form for the JFK Coma Recovery Scale—Revised. Superscript* a *indicates minimally conscious state (MCS); superscript* b, *emergence from MCS.*

(From Giacino JT, Kalmar K, Whyte J. The JFK coma recovery scale-revised: measurement characteristics and diagnostic utility. Arch Phys Med Rehabil. 2004 Dec;85[12]:2020-9; used with permission.)

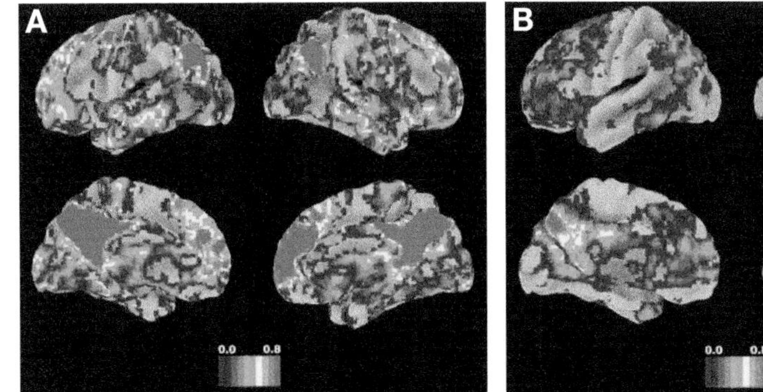

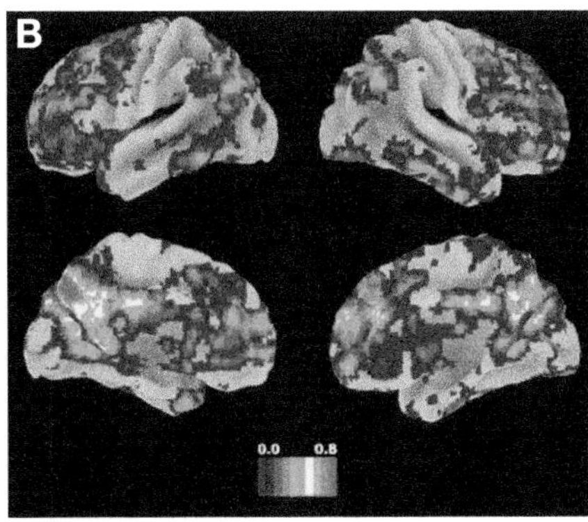

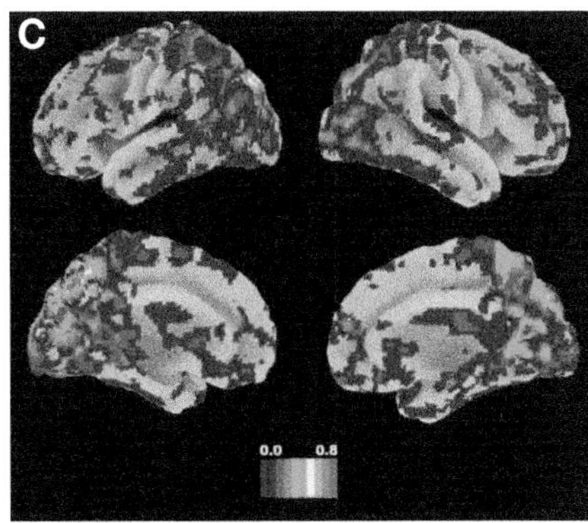

Figure 141.2. Default Mode Network (DMN) in Various States of Consciousness. The functional connectivity within the DMN is displayed on surface renderings for a state of normal wakefulness (A), a minimally conscious state (MCS) (B), and a persistent vegetative state (PVS) (C). The color bars encode the strength of connectivity, with red being the strongest and purple the weakest. Connectivity within the DMN is strong in the fully conscious state and impaired in the MCS; systems-level organization of the brain's DMN is almost completely absent in the PVS.

(From Jones DT. Cortical circuitry, networks, and function. In: Flemming KD, Jones LK Jr, editors. Mayo Clinic neurology board review: basic sciences and psychiatry for initial certification. Vol. 1. Oxford [UK]: Oxford University Press; c2015. p. 185-92. [Mayo Clinic Scientific Press series]; used with permission of Mayo Foundation for Medical Education and Research.)

SUGGESTED READING

Giacino JT, Katz DI, Schiff ND, Whyte J, Ashman EJ, Ashwal S, et al. Practice guideline update recommendations summary: disorders of consciousness: report of the Guideline Development, Dissemination, and Implementation Subcommittee of the American Academy of Neurology; the American Congress of Rehabilitation Medicine; and the National Institute on Disability, Independent Living, and Rehabilitation Research. Neurology. 2018 Sep 4;91(10):450–60. Epub 2018 Aug 8.

Span-Sluyter CAMFH, Lavrijsen JCM, van Leeuwen E, Koopmans RTCM. Moral dilemmas and conflicts concerning patients in a vegetative state/unresponsive wakefulness syndrome: shared or non-shared decision making? A qualitative study of the professional perspective in two moral case deliberations. BMC Med Ethics. 2018 Feb 22;19(1):10.

Wade DT. How often is the diagnosis of the permanent vegetative state incorrect? A review of the evidence. Eur J Neurol. 2018 Apr;25(4):619–25. Epub 2018 Feb 16.

Wijdicks EF. Being comatose: why definition matters. Lancet Neurol. 2012 Aug;11(8):657–8.

Wijdicks EFM. Who improves from coma, how do they improve, and then what? Nat Rev Neurol. 2018 Dec;14(12):694–6.

Wijdicks EFM. The comatose patient. 2nd ed. Oxford (UK): Oxford University Press; c2014. 784 p.

Ethical Concerns and Care Before Organ Donation

DIANE C. MCLAUGHLIN, APRN; LAUREN K. NG TUCKER, MD

Goals

- Describe the ethical considerations associated with different types of organ donation protocols.
- Describe consent for organ donation.
- Describe the initial critical care support of the potential donor.

Introduction

Organ donation usually proceeds smoothly and compassionately without raising any ethical concerns, and the involved family members are usually very satisfied. When concerns do arise, they typically involve 3 issues: consent for organ donation, critical care of the potential organ donor with brain death, and donation after cardiac death.

Consent for Organ Donation

Consent for organ donation typically occurs in 1 of 2 ways: 1) *first-person consent*, when the donor's driver's license shows the organ donor designation or when the donor has enrolled in an organ donor registry, or 2) *informed consent* of the patient's family. Conflict can occur when a patient's family opposes organ donation, but the patient has given first-person consent. Despite the recommendations from many organizations to respect first-person consent, those situations must be considered individually. The organ procurement organizations must collaborate with hospital ethics committees and the family to come up with a solution. If a patient's wishes related to organ donation are unknown, the surrogate's decision should be respected in the same way as in other end-of-life decisions.

Critical Care of Potential Donors After Brain Death

Despite the legal determination of brain death, the Centers for Medicare and Medicaid Services requires patients to be maintained on full life support until they can be evaluated as potential organ donors. This is done to preserve their organs for possible donation until consent can be obtained or declined or the patient is determined to be ineligible for donation. If the patient does not become an organ donor, life support can be discontinued according to institutional policies.

Hemodynamic instability is common after brain death. A catecholamine surge that occurs immediately before brain death leads to hypertension, arrhythmias, cardiac stunning, and neurogenic pulmonary edema. Immediately after brain death, sympathetic tone is lost and hypotension develops. Later, hypertension may occur as a result of sympathetic overdrive generated by the spinal cord. Pituitary hormonal secretion stops after brain death, and the patient enters a hypopituitary state characterized by low serum levels of cortisol, thyroid analogues, insulin, and antidiuretic hormone, resulting in diabetes insipidus and intravascular volume depletion.

Successful care of potential donors requires prompt management of volume status and hypotension, with hormonal supplementation for deficiencies (Box 142.1). Hemodynamic management of hypotension requires both judicious administration of fluids to achieve euvolemia and supportive therapy with inotropes or vasopressors. Whereas norepinephrine is the drug of choice in many intensive care units, its use in potential donors is typically avoided because doses larger than 0.05 mcg/kg/min are associated with graft dysfunction in heart transplant recipients. Instead, epinephrine is the drug of choice. Hormone supplementation with corticosteroids and levothyroxine often

Box 142.1 • Initial Supportive Care of Potential Donors After Brain Death

Target mean arterial pressure >65 mm Hg
Phenylephrine (50-200 mcg/min) if systolic blood pressure <100 mm Hg
Thyroxine infusion (10-50 mcg/h) if blood pressure is still unstable
Vasopressin (0.2-0.3 units/h) if urine output >300 mL/h
Methylprednisolone (15 mg/kg)
Target normoglycemia (140-180 mg/dL)

improves hemodynamic stability and may decrease vasopressor requirements. Vasopressin is useful for maintaining blood pressure and even more so for managing diabetes insipidus.

Maintenance of potential organ donors with full life support can cause ethical conflict for health care providers. According to the Uniform Anatomical Gift Act, hospitals cannot legally remove life-sustaining treatment until the organ procurement organization has evaluated the patient's potential as an organ donor. The term *maintenance* is not explicitly defined, however, so the meaning is subject to broad interpretation. This can cause concern because the team must continue to treat a patient who has already been declared brain dead. The team must also continue treatment without expressing the purpose of the treatment to family.

Donation After Cardiac Death

Donation after cardiac death may be the biggest source of ethical conflict for health care providers. After cardiac death, potential donors are not brain dead, but usually they have had a severe neurologic insult and require mechanical ventilation. For organ donation, life-sustaining measures are withdrawn and the patient dies a natural death after being transferred to the operating room. After the patient has been extubated, and after respiratory and circulatory activities have ceased, a 5-minute waiting period is observed to ensure that the patient does not undergo autoresuscitation (with resumption of circulation) before organs are recovered. However, the duration of cardiac cessation necessary to declare death is controversial, and recommendations from different organizations and countries range from 2 to 10 minutes. With rare exceptions, eligible donors undergo circulatory arrest within 60 minutes after respiratory support is discontinued. If patients continue to breathe after extubation, they become ineligible for donation and standard palliative care is begun.

The main ethical conflicts involving potential donors after cardiac death are the irreversibility of circulatory cessation and the timing of the declaration of death as mentioned above. According to the Uniform Determination of Death Act of 1981, *circulatory death* is defined as the irreversible loss of circulatory and respiratory function after a period of unresponsiveness, the presence of apnea, and the absence of circulation. The debate lies with the interpretation of *irreversible*. Many experts hold that circulation will not return after several minutes despite attempts with cardiac resuscitation. Another ethical conflict is that certain actions are taken to evaluate or optimize organs for donation that do not benefit the patient. Several organizations (including the American Thoracic Society, the International Society for Heart and Lung Transplantation, the Society of Critical Care Medicine, the Association of Organ Procurement Organizations, and the United Network for Organ Sharing) released a statement that said that these acts can be justified by supporting the donor's interest in becoming an organ donor after death.

Summary

- After the brain death of a donor, the maintenance of adequate blood pressure requires the incremental use of vasopressors.
- Ventricular tachycardia and ventricular fibrillation are the most common terminal arrhythmias and are treated with amiodarone.
- Donation after cardiac death should be considered for each patient younger than 60 years who is transitioning to comfort care.

SUGGESTED READING

Aulisio MP, Devita M, Luebke D. Taking values seriously: ethical challenges in organ donation and transplantation for critical care professionals. Crit Care Med. 2007 Feb;35(2 Suppl):S95–101.

Citerio G, Cypel M, Dobb GJ, Dominguez-Gil B, Frontera JA, Greer DM, et al. Organ donation in adults: a critical care perspective. Intensive Care Med. 2016 Mar;42(3):305–15. Epub 2016 Jan 11.

Frontera JA, Kalb T. How I manage the adult potential organ donor: donation after neurological death (part 1). Neurocrit Care. 2010 Feb;12(1):103–10.

Gries CJ, White DB, Truog RD, Dubois J, Cosio CC, Dhanani S, et al; American Thoracic Society Health Policy Committee. An official American Thoracic Society/International Society for Heart and Lung Transplantation/Society of Critical Care Medicine/Association of Organ and Procurement Organizations/United Network of Organ Sharing Statement: ethical and policy considerations in organ donation after circulatory determination of death. Am J Respir Crit Care Med. 2013 Jul 1;188(1):103–9.

Kotloff RM, Blosser S, Fulda GJ, Malinoski D, Ahya VN, Angel L, et al; Society of Critical Care Medicine/American College of Chest Physicians/Association of Organ Procurement Organizations Donor Management Task Force. Management of the Potential Organ Donor in the ICU: Society of Critical Care Medicine/American College of Chest Physicians/Association of Organ

Procurement Organizations Consensus Statement. Crit Care Med. 2015 Jun;43(6):1291–325.
Manno EM. Nonheart-beating donation in the neurologically devastated patient. Neurocrit Care. 2005;3(2):111–4.
Meyfroidt G, Gunst J, Martin-Loeches I, Smith M, Robba C, Taccone FS, et al. Management of the brain-dead donor in the ICU: general and specific therapy to improve transplantable organ quality. Intensive Care Med. 2019 Mar;45(3):343–53. Epub 2019 Feb 11.
Morrissey PE, Monaco AP. Donation after circulatory death: current practices, ongoing challenges, and potential improvements. Transplantation. 2014 Feb 15;97(3):258–64.
Park J, Yang NR, Lee YJ, Hong KS. A single-center experience with an intensivist-led brain-dead donor management program. Ann Transplant. 2018 Dec 4;23:828–35.
Sade RM. Consequences of the dead donor rule. Ann Thorac Surg. 2014 Apr;97(4):1131–2.
Smith M, Dominguez-Gil B, Greer DM, Manara AR, Souter MJ. Organ donation after circulatory death: current status and future potential. Intensive Care Med. 2019 Mar;45(3):310–21. Epub 2019 Feb 6.
Tullius SG, Rabb H. Improving the supply and quality of deceased-donor organs for transplantation. N Engl J Med. 2018 May 17;378(20):1920–9.
Venkat A, Baker EF, Schears RM. Ethical controversies surrounding the management of potential organ donors in the emergency department. J Emerg Med. 2014 Aug;47(2):232–6. Epub 2014 May 29.

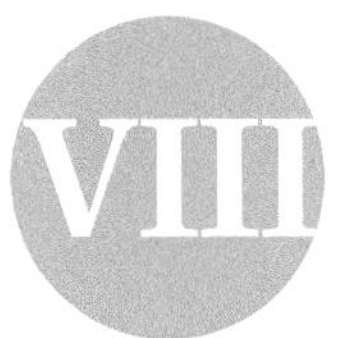

Questions and Answers

Abbreviations Used

CMS Centers for Medicare & Medicaid Services
DNR do-not-resuscitate
ICU intensive care unit
OPO organ procurement organization

Questions

Multiple Choice (choose the best answer)

VIII.1. A critically ill, 85-year-old widower with a history of end-stage renal disease and diabetes mellitus is admitted to the neuroscience ICU with a pontine hemorrhage. He was intubated upon arrival. His son is his health care surrogate, and he is unsure whether the patient has an advance directive. Which of the following is the most appropriate next step in this patient's care?
a. Continue aggressive care until the advance directive status can be clarified.
b. Request a palliative care consultation to discuss end-of-life issues.
c. Establish goals of care with the patient's son.
d. Arrange a family meeting if the patient's condition does not improve.

VIII.2. Which of the following most accurately describes the process of terminally weaning a patient from the ventilator?
a. The fraction of inspired oxygen should be reduced to 21%, but positive end-expiratory pressure should not be reduced before the endotracheal tube is removed.
b. Patients should be premedicated only if they are already receiving opioids before extubation.
c. Changes in breathing patterns are uncommon after extubation.
d. Medications should be titrated according to signs and symptoms after extubation to ensure patient comfort.

VIII.3. What is the best care possible for a patient?
a. The care that helps the patient live the longest
b. The care that provides the best quality of life for the patient
c. The care that allows the patient to be at home the most
d. The care that best matches the preferences and priorities of the patient and family

VIII.4. What is the most common error in brain death determination?
a. Failure to do an apnea test
b. Failure to do an ancillary test
c. Failure to do a toxicology screen
d. Failure to do a second examination

VIII.5. What is the most common error in apnea testing?
a. Failure to preoxygenate with 100% oxygen
b. Failure to use arterial blood gas testing
c. Failure to achieve a normal $Paco_2$
d. Failure to place the oxygen catheter at the carina

VIII.6. After how many months would a traumatic persistent vegetative state first be considered permanent?
a. 3
b. 6
c. 12
d. Not fully known

VIII.7. During bedside clinical evaluation, a patient has spontaneous eye opening, reflexive responses to painful stimuli, and visual tracking of the patient's own reflection in a mirror but is not responsive in any other way. Which of the following describes the patient's clinical state?
a. Minimally conscious state
b. Delirium
c. Persistent vegetative state
d. Stupor

VIII.8. A man has been declared brain dead after a gunshot wound to the head. What should the attending physician do?
a. Call the local OPO to ensure that the patient has been referred and to determine his eligibility to donate.
b. Determine whether the patient may be a viable candidate for organ donation, and discuss donation with the family.
c. Remove ventilator support because the patient is legally dead.
d. Continue all treatment until the patient undergoes cardiac death.

VIII.9. You are asked to be the declaring physician for a donation after cardiac death. Life-supporting measures are discontinued, and circulatory arrest occurs soon. After 5 minutes, the patient remains pulseless. What should you do?
a. Confirm death and allow the recovery team to proceed.
b. Attempt resuscitation, and if a pulse does not return, allow the recovery team to proceed.

c. Refuse to pronounce the patient dead until confirmatory testing can be conducted.
d. Confirm with the family members that they would like organ donation to proceed.

VIII.10. You are caring for a patient with a subarachnoid hemorrhage who was admitted to the ICU earlier today with unresponsive coma but intact respiratory drive and pupillary response. You are called in the middle of the night because the patient has become hemodynamically unstable and hypotensive. Upon examination, you find that the patient no longer has brainstem reflexes and has most likely progressed to brain death. The patient's family is coming from out of town but has been informed that this progression would probably occur. Which should you do next?
a. Perform brain death testing.
b. Write a DNR order, but do not escalate care since this patient is clearly brain dead.
c. Pronounce the patient dead, and discontinue mechanical ventilation.
d. Order vasopressors to attempt to improve the patient's hemodynamic stability.

VIII.11. For the past week, you have cared for a 17-year-old male patient who survived a motorcycle crash. He remains in an unresponsive coma with a questionable pupillary response and occasional initiation of respirations. His parents have decided to compassionately wean him from life support. When you are preparing to write the order to extubate the patient, the bedside nurse tells you that the parents commented on how proud the patient was when he received his driver's license and registered to be an organ donor. What should you do?
a. Continue with the current plan to discontinue life support and withdraw care.
b. Make a referral to an OPO for a possible donation after cardiac death.
c. Explain to the patient's parents that because he is not brain dead, he is not a candidate for organ donation.
d. Talk to the patient's parents and suggest that they wait a few more days to see whether the patient progresses to brain death.

Answers

VIII.1. Answer c.

Clinicians in the ICU should be able to provide generalist-level palliative care, which includes establishing goals of care and discussing preferences for life-prolonging measures with the health care surrogate. If specialist-level palliative care is needed, a formal palliative care consultation may be requested.

Institute of Medicine of the National Academies. Dying in America: improving quality and honoring individual preferences near the end of life [Internet]. Washington (DC): Institute of Medicine of the National Academies. c2014 [cited 2016 Dec 30]. Available from: http://nationalacademies.org/hmd/~/media/Files/Report%20Files/2014/EOL/Key%20Findings%20and%20Recommendations.pdf.

Quill TE, Abernethy AP. Generalist plus specialist palliative care: creating a more sustainable model. N Engl J Med. 2013 Mar 28;368(13):1173–5. Epub 2013 Mar 6.

VIII.2. Answer d.

Medications should be titrated according to signs and symptoms after extubation to ensure patient comfort. The process of compassionately weaning a patient from a ventilator involves decreasing all ventilator parameters before the endotracheal tube is removed. The patient should be premedicated with opioids, sedatives, and anticholinergic medications, and these medications should be titrated according to the patient's signs and symptoms after extubation. Audible secretions and labored, agonal breathing are common after extubation.

Billings JA. Humane terminal extubation reconsidered: the role for preemptive analgesia and sedation. Crit Care Med. 2012 Feb;40(2):625–30.

Kompanje EJ, van der Hoven B, Bakker J. Anticipation of distress after discontinuation of mechanical ventilation in the ICU at the end of life. Intensive Care Med. 2008 Sep;34(9):1593–9. Epub 2008 May 31.

Mayer SA, Kossoff SB. Withdrawal of life support in the neurological intensive care unit. Neurology. 1999 May 12;52(8):1602–9.

VIII.3. Answer d.

The patient and family should make decisions according to their preferences and priorities.

Peigne V, Chaize M, Falissard B, Kentish-Barnes N, Rusinova K, Megarbane B, et al. Important questions asked by family members of intensive care unit patients. Crit Care Med. 2011 Jun;39(6):1365–71.

VIII.4. Answer c.

Failure to recognize possible drug or alcohol intoxication is the most common mistake. A good history and toxicology screening are required.

Wijdicks EF, Varelas PN, Gronseth GS, Greer DM; American Academy of Neurology. Evidence-based guideline update: determining brain death in adults: report of the Quality Standards Subcommittee of the American Academy of Neurology. Neurology. 2010 Jun 8;74(23):1911–8.

VIII.5. Answer a.

Failure to preoxygenate and obtain arterial hyperoxygenation is common when the investigator assumes that the tracheal catheter is sufficient. If the Pao_2 is not more than 200 mm Hg, the test may lead to early hypoxemia and failure to complete an apnea test.

Wijdicks EF, Varelas PN, Gronseth GS, Greer DM; American Academy of Neurology. Evidence-based guideline update: determining brain death in adults: report of the Quality Standards Subcommittee of the American Academy of Neurology. Neurology. 2010 Jun 8;74(23):1911–8.

VIII.6. Answer d.

Recovery from a persistent vegetative state to a minimally conscious state is possible after traumatic brain injury, and firm time cutoffs have been questioned recently. Because recovery is possible, use of the term *permanent* is discouraged.

Estraneo A, Moretta P, Loreto V, Lanzillo B, Santoro L, Trojano L. Late recovery after traumatic, anoxic, or hemorrhagic long-lasting vegetative state. Neurology. 2010 Jul 20;75(3):239–45. Epub 2010 Jun 16.

VIII.7. Answer a.

Minimally conscious state is distinguished from persistent vegetative state by the presence of behaviors associated with conscious awareness. These behaviors occur inconstantly but are reproducible or sustained long enough that they are distinguishable from reflexive behavior. Only 1 behavior (eg, tracking the patient's own image in the mirror) is required to meet this criterion.

Giacino JT, Ashwal S, Childs N, Cranford R, Jennett B, Katz DI, et al. The minimally conscious state: definition and diagnostic criteria. Neurology. 2002 Feb 12;58(3):349–53.

VIII.8. Answer a.

The CMS Hospital Conditions of Participation legislation requires hospitals that receive federal reimbursement to notify the local OPO of all imminent deaths in a timely manner, which is defined in a contract between the OPO and the hospital. Furthermore, it is the responsibility of the OPO and not the hospital medical personnel to determine medical suitability, and only a trained, designated requestor or OPO representative may approach the family of a potential donor about consent for organ donation.

Park J, Yang NR, Lee YJ, Hong KS. A single-center experience with an intensivist-led brain-dead donor management program. Ann Transplant. 2018 Dec 4;23:828–35.

Tullius SG, Rabb H. Improving the supply and quality of deceased-donor organs for transplantation. N Engl J Med. 2018 May 17;378(20):1920–9.

VIII.9. Answer a.

Resuscitation should not be attempted because a DNR order is in effect when life support is discontinued, regardless of the organ donor status. Additional confirmatory testing beyond standard care is unnecessary. When consent is obtained, the consent stands unless it is explicitly revoked by the legal next of kin.

Park J, Yang NR, Lee YJ, Hong KS. A single-center experience with an intensivist-led brain-dead donor management program. Ann Transplant. 2018 Dec 4;23:828–35.

Tullius SG, Rabb H. Improving the supply and quality of deceased-donor organs for transplantation. N Engl J Med. 2018 May 17;378(20):1920–9.

VIII.10. Answer d.

With the patient's unstable condition, brain death testing could be challenging. A DNR status needs to be directed by the patient or legal next of kin. Pronouncing the patient dead would be incorrect because the CMS Hospital Conditions of Participation legislation requires that families of potential donors be offered the option of organ donation if deemed appropriate by the OPO. An attempt to improve the patient's hemodynamic stability would be the best way to preserve the option of organ donation.

Park J, Yang NR, Lee YJ, Hong KS. A single-center experience with an intensivist-led brain-dead donor management program. Ann Transplant. 2018 Dec 4;23:828–35.

Tullius SG, Rabb H. Improving the supply and quality of deceased-donor organs for transplantation. N Engl J Med. 2018 May 17;378(20):1920–9.

VIII.11. Answer b.

The hospital is required to notify the local OPO of the imminent death in a timely manner. Therefore, continuing with the current plan would be incorrect, and telling the parents that the patient is not a candidate for organ donation would be incorrect because only the OPO can determine a patient's eligibility to donate organs. Suggesting that the parents wait a few more days would also be incorrect because only a trained designated requestor or OPO representative can approach families for organ donation.

Department of Health and Human Services (US). Medicare and medicaid programs; hospital conditions of participation; identification of potential organ, tissue, and eye donors and transplant hospitals' provision of transplant-related data. Final rules. Fed Regist. 1998 Jun 22;63(119):33856–75.

Index

Note: Page numbers followed by *f*, *t*, or *b* denote figures, tables, or boxes, respectively.

For the benefit of digital users, indexed terms that span two pages (e.g., 52–53) may, on occasion, appear on only one of those pages.

A

B

C

D

E

F

G

H

I

M

N

Q

R

S

T

U

W

X

Y

Z